# The COMPLETE SOLUTION for Modern Dental Assisting



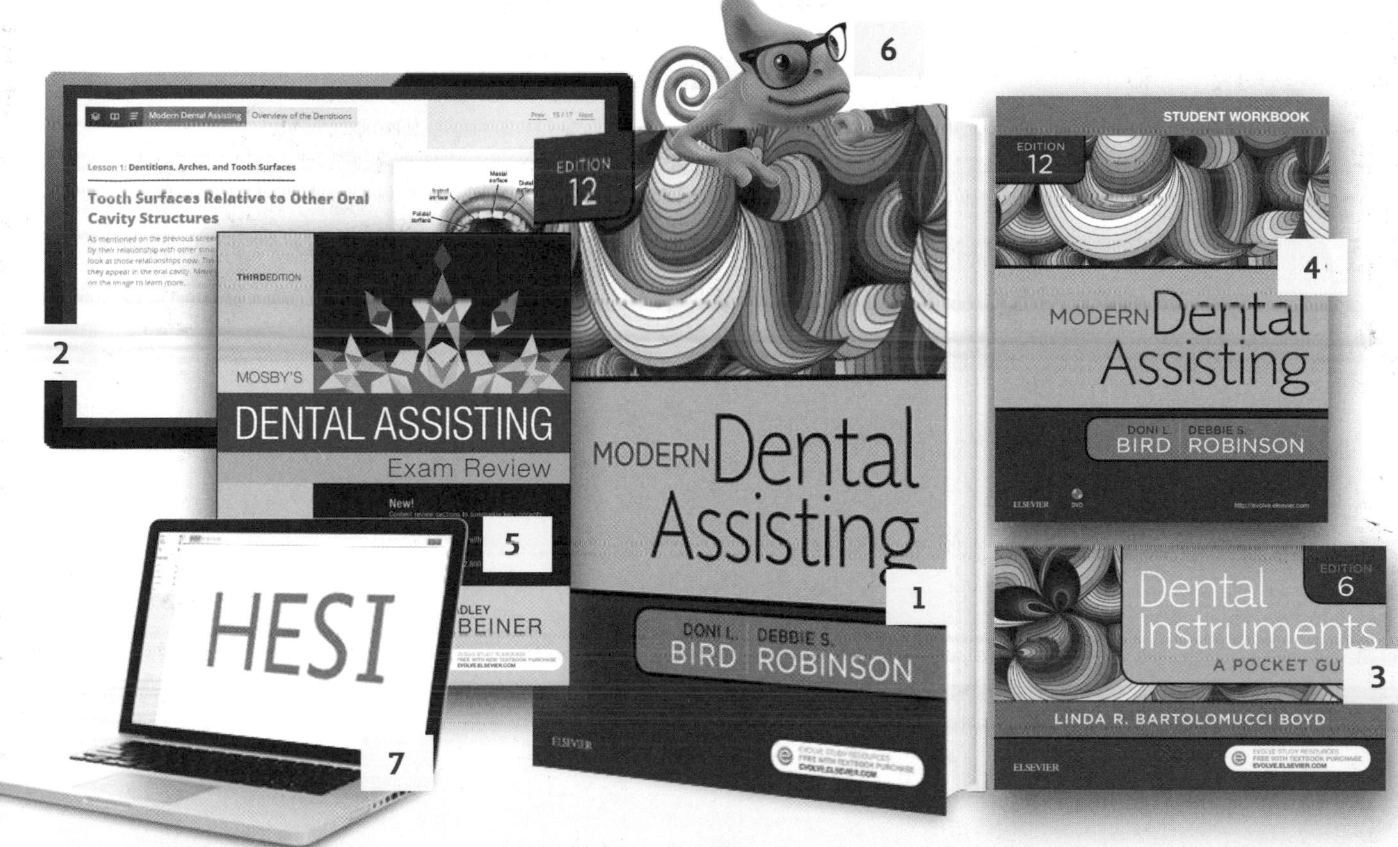


1. **Modern Dental Assisting, 12th Edition**
   ISBN: 978-0-323-43030-2

2. **Dental Assisting Online for Modern Dental Assisting, 12th Edition**
   ISBN: 978-0-323-47399-6

3. **Dental Instruments: A Pocket Guide, 6th Edition**
   ISBN: 978-0-323-47405-4

4. **Student Workbook for Modern Dental Assisting, 12th Edition**
   ISBN: 978-0-323-43031-9

5. **Mosby's Dental Assisting Exam Review, 3rd Edition**
   ISBN: 978-0-323-39630-1

6. **Elsevier Adaptive Quizzing for Modern Dental Assisting, 12th Edition**
   ISBN: 978-0-323-49633-9

7. **HESI Review & Testing for Dental Assisting**
   **Instructors:** Contact your Elsevier Education Solutions Consultant for details.
   **Students:** Ask your instructor about adding HESI to help you prepare for the board exam.

**Visit evolve.elsevier.com to get all the resources you need to become a successful dental assistant!**

17-NHPtc-0022 TM/CH 1/17

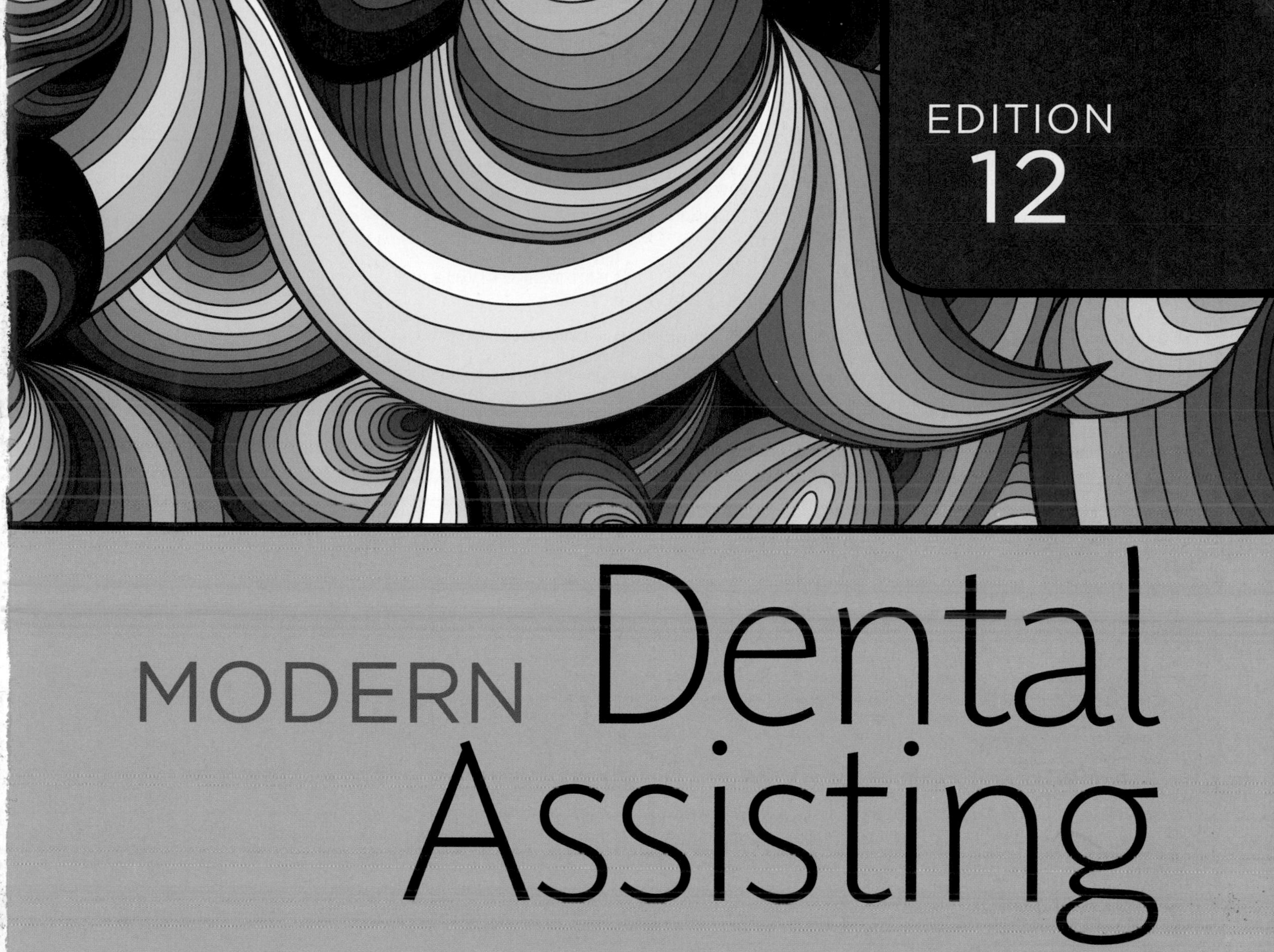


# MODERN Dental Assisting

**DONI L. BIRD, CDA, RDA, RDH, MA**

Dental Education Consultant
DB Bird Management
Instructor, Continuing Education
Former Director, Allied Dental Education Program
Santa Rosa Junior College
Santa Rosa, California

**DEBBIE S. ROBINSON, CDA, MS**

Research Associate and Project Manager
Gillings School of Global Public Health
Former Director, Dental Assisting and Dental Assisting Specialty Program
University of North Carolina
Chapel Hill, North Carolina

ELSEVIER

ELSEVIER

3251 Riverport Lane
St. Louis, Missouri 63043

MODERN DENTAL ASSISTING, TWELFTH EDITION ISBN: 978-0-323-43030-2



**Library of Congress Cataloging-in-Publication Data-**
Names: Bird, Doni, author. | Robinson, Debbie (Debbie S.), author.
Title: Modern dental assisting / Doni L. Bird, Debbie S. Robinson.
Description: 12th edition. | St. Louis, Missouri : Elsevier, [2018] |
Includes bibliographical references and index.
Identifiers: LCCN 2017001893 | ISBN 9780323430302 (hardcover : alk. paper)
Subjects: | MESH: Dental Assistants | Dental Care
Classification: LCC RK60.5 | NLM WU 90 | DDC 617.6/0233--dc23 LC record available at https://lccn.loc.gov/2017001893

*Senior Content Strategist:* Kristin Wilhelm
*Content Development Manager:* Luke Held
*Content Development Specialist:* Kelly Skelton
*Publishing Services Manager:* Jeff Patterson
*Senior Project Manager:* Tracey Schriefer
*Design Direction:* Brian Salisbury



Printed in Canada.

Last digit is the print number: 9 8 7 6 5 4 3 2 1

# REVIEWERS*

**Teresa A. Bailey, CDA, EFDA, MS**
Dental Assisting Program Chair
Ivy Tech Community College
Anderson, Indiana

**Patricia A. Capps, CDA, RDH, EFDA, BSDH, MS**
Clinical Associate Professor
Indiana University School of Dentistry
Indianapolis, Indiana

**Charmaine M. Chappell, BS, MBA, CDA**
Dental Assisting Program Coordinator
Centura College
North Chesterfield, Virginia

**Lisa Childers, BA, CDA, RDA**
Program Director/Instructor
Arkansas Northeastern College
Blytheville, Arkansas

**Jamie Collins, RDH, CDA**
Dental Assisting Instructor
College of Western Idaho
Nampa, Idaho

**Sharron J. Cook, CDA, BS**
Dental Assisting Program Director
Columbus Technical College
Columbus, Georgia

**Nicole Gard Day, BSDH, RDH**
Professional Item Writer
Riverton, Wyoming
*Revised Mock Dental Assisting Board Examination (Evolve)*

**Margaret Dennett, CDA, MCE**
Instructor
Vancouver Community College
Vancouver, British Columbia

**Liz Eccles, CDA, PID, Prostho**
Instructor, Dental Assistant Program
Vancouver Island University
Nanaimo, British Columbia

**Helen Fairchild, RDA, MHRM**
Dean, Dental Programs
Carrington College
Sacramento, California

**Robin McKay Ganshorn, Cert. (Bus.), RDA, FCP, BBA, MAED**
Instructor, Dental Assisting Program
School of Health Sciences
Saskatchewan Polytechnic—Regina Campus
Regina, Saskatchewan, Canada
*Reviewed Canadian Content Corner (Evolve)*

**Aimee M. Gaspari, ED, CDA, EFDA**
Dental Assisting Instructor
YTI Career Institute
Lancaster, Pennsylvania
*Revised Chapter Practice Quizzes (Evolve)*

**Kathy Gibson, MS Ed, CDA**
Associate Professor
Coordinator for Dental Assisting
John A. Logan College
Carterville, Illinois
*Reviewed Video Review Questions and Answers (Evolve)*

**Lola Giusti, DDS, MA**
Associate Professor
Department of Dental Practice
Arthur A. Dugoni School of Dentistry
University of the Pacific
San Francisco, California

**Heidi Gottfried-Arvold, CDA, MS**
Program Director, Dental Assistant Program
Gateway Technical College
Kenosha, Wisconsin

**DeBorah LaVeaux-Jackson, RDA, N2O, CERAC**
Dental Program Director
Brightwood College–Dallas
Dallas, Texas

**Laura E. Magana, Cirujano Dentista U.A.S.L.P.**
Dental Assistant Program Director
Brightwood College
Corpus Christi, Texas

**Alicia Melendez, RDA, CDA, AAS, BS**
Dean of Curriculum—Dental Assistant
Zenith Education Group
Minneapolis, Minnesota

---

* Individuals in this listing reviewed either one or more of the following Modern Dental Assisting products: textbook or Evolve content.

**Glenda L. Miller, CDA, EFDA, BS**
Professor, Dental Assisting
Florida State College at Jacksonville
Jacksonville, Florida

**Rina A. Nowka, RDH, MA**
Clinical Dental Hygiene Instructor
Bergen Community College
Paramus, New Jersey,
Dental Radiology Curriculum Developer and Instructor
New Jersey Health Professionals Development Institute
River Edge, New Jersey

**Donna Passino, CDA, EFDA**
Adjunct Dental Instructor
Penn Foster
Scranton, Pennsylvania

**Pamela Pemberton**
Texas State Technical College Waco
Waco, Texas

**Beatrice Pena, CDA, RDA, AAS**
Clinic Manager, Quality Assurance
The University of Texas Health Science Center San Antonio
San Antonio, Texas

**Dawn Roberts**
WorWic Community College
Delmar, Maryland

**Raeleen Roberts, D.A., EFDA**
Dental Assisting Coordinator
Eastern Idaho Falls Technical College
Idaho Falls, Idaho

**Joseph W. Robertson, DDS, BS**
Faculty
Department of Nursing and Health Professions
Oakland Community College
Bloomfield Hills, Michigan
*Revised Test Bank (Evolve)*

**Denise Romero, CDA, COA, RDA, OA, MA**
Pasadena City College
Pasadena, California

**Cheryl Russell-Julien, CDA, PDA, CDA II, DHE**
Director
Hands On Practical Solutions
Ottawa, Ontario

**Dana Scott, CDA, RDA, CDPMA**
Dental Assisting Program Director
Amarillo College
Amarillo, Texas

**Judy Shannon, RDH, CDA, MEd**
Director of Dental Assisting
Massasoit Community College
Canton, Massachussetts

**Roxanne Terranova, CDA, RDA, MSM**
Dental Assisting Coordinator
Camden County College
Blackwood, New Jersey

**Laura J. Webb, RDH, MS, CDA, MAADH**
Allied Dental Education Program Consultant & Continuing Education Provider
LJW Education Services
Fallon, Nevada

# ACKNOWLEDGMENTS

Thank you to our publishing family at Elsevier: Kristin Wilhelm, Senior Content Strategist; Kelly Skelton, Content Development Specialist; Jeff Patterson, Publishing Services Manager; Tracey Schriefer, Senior Project Manager; Traci Cahill, Marketing Manager; and Brian Salisbury, Designer. In addition, a huge thank you to the sales associates nationwide who really do the legwork to get "MDA" to the instructors and dental assisting programs. We truly appreciate everyone's support, advice, contributions, and collaboration in creating such a comprehensive learning package.

We sincerely appreciate and thank the reviewers who took the time to review our work carefully and to provide constructive suggestions and recommendations.

Finally, a special thank you to our family, friends, and colleagues for their ongoing patience, adjustments to their schedules, and support that go hand in hand with working in the publishing world.

**Doni and Debbie**

# ABOUT THE AUTHORS

**DONI L. BIRD** served for many years as the director of the Allied Dental Education Programs at Santa Rosa Junior College (SRJC) in Santa Rosa, California, before her retirement in 2012. She continues to teach continuing education courses at SRJC. Before becoming a dental assisting educator, she practiced as a dental assistant in private practice and at Mount Zion Hospital and Medical Center in San Francisco. Doni holds a Bachelor's Degree in Education and Master's Degree in Education from San Francisco State University and a degree in dental hygiene from the University of New Mexico in Albuquerque. She has served as a member and Chairman of the Board of Directors of the Organization for Safety, Asepsis and Prevention (OSAP). She is a member of the American Dental Assistants Association (ADAA) and has served as president of the Northern California Dental Assistants Association and as chairman of the Dental Assisting National Board (DANB). She has served on the Board of Directors of the California Association of Dental Assisting Teachers (CADAT) and serves as a consultant in dental assisting education to the Commission on Dental Accreditation (CODA) of the American Dental Association (ADA). She has served as a member and president of the California Dental Hygiene Educators Association and a member of the Foundation Board of the California Dental Association. Doni has written many articles and presented numerous continuing education programs at major state and national meetings.

**DEBBIE S. ROBINSON** is currently a Research Associate Professor at the University of North Carolina, where she is involved in clinical research within the Gilling's School of Global Public Health. Her educational background includes an associate degree in Dental Assisting from Broward Community College, a Bachelor's degree in Health Administration from Florida Atlantic University, and a Master's of Science degree in Dental Auxiliary Teachers Education from the University of North Carolina. Her clinical experience includes practicing as a clinical chairside assistant for 7 years in a pediatric dental office, as well as in the dental research center and the special patient care clinic at the University of North Carolina (UNC) Dental School. With more than 20 years of teaching, Debbie has held teaching positions in the community college setting in Florida and North Carolina. She has served as Clinical Assistant Professor and Director of the Dental Assisting Program and Dental Assisting Specialty Program at UNC School of Dentistry. She has presented continuing education for practicing dental assistants at local, state, and international meetings. She has served as a member of the Dental Assisting National Board (DANB) test construction committee for two terms and has authored and co-authored journal articles for *The Dental Assistant.* Additional endeavors include consulting with community colleges and proprietary schools on the development of new curriculums for dental assisting programs across the country.

Congratulations on your choice of a career in dental assisting!

When Hazel O. Torres and Ann Ehrlich published the first edition of *Modern Dental Assisting* in 1976, their goal was to provide dental assisting students and educators with the most comprehensive textbook ever for dental assisting education. It provided the background, principles, and techniques necessary to become an educationally qualified and competent dental assistant.

Since then, some amazing changes have taken place in the profession of dental assisting. It is now recognized that oral health and general health are interwoven and that people cannot be healthy without oral health. Advances in scientific research, the prevention of oral diseases, emerging technology, and regulatory changes have significantly influenced the evolving roles and responsibilities of today's dental assistant.

In the 12th Edition of *Modern Dental Assisting*, we uphold the same core educational values and goals instilled in us by Hazel Torres and Ann Ehrlich. However, the knowledge and skills necessary to reach competency in each of the many new techniques and procedures have been greatly expanded.

Chapters are revised to reflect changes resulting from evidence-based research, the increasing use of digital imaging, advancement of dental materials, and advances in technology that have allowed new functions to be delegated to dental assistants in some states and provinces. Every effort is made to create a balance to retain foundational knowledge while incorporating the most current principles and procedures to remain on the cutting edge of dental assisting practice today.

Our team of authors and editors has listened to dental assisting educators and students throughout the United States and Canada and has responded to their requests. Our reviewers, who represent a diverse community of dental assisting educators throughout North America, have helped us to ensure inclusion of the most current knowledge.

## Who Will Benefit from This Book?

Whether you are a new student to dental assisting or expanding your role in this profession, *Modern Dental Assisting* will provide you with the tools and resources to move forward.

## Organization

The book is divided into 11 parts—from historical and scientific information to the general and specialized practice of dentistry. Each part opener provides an introduction and lists the related chapters that are found within that section.

The ease of reading each comprehensive chapter and the additional materials provides students with the maximum opportunity to learn. The driving force in the development of this package was to create a competent dental assistant. With that goal in mind, this package meets and exceeds accreditation standards and certification requirements.

## The Learning Package

The 12th Edition of *Modern Dental Assisting* is designed as a comprehensive learning package.

**The Student Package Includes the following:**

- Textbook
- Evolve Resources
- Student Workbook (sold separately)
- *Dental Assisting Online* (sold separately)

**The Faculty Package Includes All Student Resources, Plus the following:**

- Evolve Resources instructor-only assets
- TEACH Instructor Resources
- Accreditation Mapping Guides

The entire package has been designed with the student and educator in mind.

## New to This Edition

### Textbook

- **NEW content** addresses public health and access to care, Ebola, Zika virus, teledentistry, and the oral–systemic health connection.
- **NEW illustrations** focus on dental anatomy, tooth morphology, and more.
- **NEW, full-color photos** show the latest technology, instruments, and procedures.

### Evolve Resources

#### *For Instructors*

- **Test Bank:** 2500-question test bank includes many questions that focus on the application of chapter objectives in realistic clinical situations. Questions include answers, rationales, page number references, cognitive level, and CDA exam blueprint category. The test bank helps students prepare for the Dental Assisting National Board (DANB) examination.

#### *For Students*

- **Animations** from the new Elsevier Collection feature foundational A&P information with cutting-edge graphics.

## Student Workbook

- **Additional labeling exercises** for anatomy and tooth morphology help students master the foundational content that is essential to successful dental assisting practice.
- **Externship Guide** provides resources to document assigned externship sites, including a record of clinical activities and time sheets.

## Dental Assisting Online

- **New art** corresponding with the textbook, focusing on dental anatomy, tooth morphology, and instruments, and equipment.
- **Module exams with cognitive leveling** for questions based on Bloom's Taxonomy.
- **Updated glossary** with additional terms from the textbook.

## Support

If you have questions or need assistance with ordering or adopting the *Modern Dental Assisting* learning package, contact Educator Support at 1-800-222-9570 or via e-mail at sales.inquiry@elsevier.com.

If you have questions or need assistance with the electronic components of the *Modern Dental Assisting* learning package, you can contact Technical Support at 1-800-692-9010 (Option 2) or via e-mail at technical.support@elsevier.com or through the Support section of the main Evolve Web site at http://evolve.elsevier.com.

**Doni L. Bird**
**Debbie S. Robinson**

# THE LEARNING PACKAGE

*Modern Dental Assisting* is the ideal learning package for preparing students to become dental assistants. It provides a solid foundation for the basic and advanced clinical skills students must master to achieve competence, and its student-friendly style clarifies even the most complex concepts and procedures to help prepare for Dental Assisting National Board (DANB) certification.

## Textbook

- Comprehensive coverage that spans the entire dental assisting curriculum
- Cutting-edge content and approachable writing style
- Expert authorship
- Top-notch art program
- Step-by-step procedures for basic and expanded functions with icons
- *Recall* questions throughout chapters that summarize key issues and facts
- *CDC* boxes highlighting specific recommendations of the Centers for Disease Control and Prevention
- *Legal and Ethical Implications* features
- *Patient Education* features with tips and strategies
- *Eye to the Future* features that introduce cutting-edge and evolving research and practice
- *Critical Thinking* questions and mini-scenarios that encourage content application
- Key terms, definitions, and phonetic pronunciations presented at the beginning of each chapter and highlighted in boldface color within the text discussion
- A back-of-book Glossary with chapter cross-references
- Learning and Performance Outcomes at the beginning of each chapter
- Electronic Resources also at the beginning of each chapter to highlight ancillary content applicable to that chapter

## Evolve Resources

Elsevier has created a Web site dedicated solely to support this learning package: http://evolve.elsevier.com/Bird/modern. The Web site includes a *Student site* and an *Instructor site.*

### Student Site

- Audio Glossary
- Canadian Content to supplement topics that differ between Canada and the United States, such as nutrition and privacy regulations
- Mock dental assisting board examination
- Practice quizzes for each chapter
- Tray setup questions and identification exercises
- Video clips of dental assisting procedures
- Video scripts in English and Spanish
- Video review questions and answers

#### *Plus* The Interactive Dental Office Online!

The interactive portion of this learning package offers exercises for the immediate application of knowledge to help the student develop and retain critical thinking and problem-solving skills. The *Interactive Dental Office* is built around 25 in-depth patient case studies with questions, charting and tooth-numbering exercises, and radiographic mounting exercises to help students assimilate content from various chapters and apply it in a realistic, patient-centered setting. A content mapping guide indicates the corresponding chapter to each activity for every patient.

### Faculty Site

- Access to all the student resources
- Competency skill sheets for all procedures in the book
- Image collection
- Mapping guides for ADA accreditation, for the Dental Board of California, and for syllabus conversion
- Test Bank with more than 2500 questions, answers, rationales for correct and incorrect choices, page-number references for remediation, cognitive level, CDA exam blueprint category, and chapter objectives to which the question maps; available in ExamView
- TEACH Instructor Resources (explained in more detail in the next section)
    - TEACH Lesson Plans
    - TEACH PowerPoints
    - TEACH Student Handouts
    - TEACH Answer Key

#### *TEACH Instructor Resources*

TEACH for *Modern Dental Assisting* stands for *Total Education and Curriculum Help* and is an all-in-one resource designed to save educators time and take the guesswork out of classroom planning and preparation. TEACH includes detailed Lesson Plans, providing a chapter teaching focus; chapter pretest and background questions to help gauge students' baseline knowledge; lesson preparation checklist; materials and supply list; key terms covered in each lesson; homework assignments; lecture outline; and related class discussions, activities, and critical thinking questions all designed to fit into 50-minute classroom increments to ease the work involved in classroom preparation. Online activities are also provided to further enhance the learning experience outside the classroom. These Lesson Plans are centered around the mapping of textbook, ancillary, and Evolve content to specific chapter learning and performance outcomes. In addition, the lecture outlines reflect the detailed chapter lecture slides that come as part of TEACH. These PowerPoint slides provide teaching notes and talking points for educators as a ready-to-use classroom resource. A PDF file of the PowerPoint slides from each chapter is also provided. It contains the slides without the instructor talking points, so it can be distributed directly to students. Finally, an answer key is provided for the textbook *Recall* questions and the *Student Workbook* questions and exercises.

Note: If you are unable to access TEACH on the Web site, contact your Elsevier Education Solutions Consultant.

## Student Workbook

The Student Workbook is an optional supplement to the learning process (sold separately). The content of the workbook matches the book chapter by chapter to help students master and apply key concepts and procedures to a clinical situation through short-answer and multiple-choice questions, as well as fill-in-the-blank statements. Case study scenarios and associated questions encourage application of key concepts. Clinical competency forms are located within appropriate chapters of the Student Workbook, allowing students to evaluate both their strengths and weaknesses in performing procedures. A Dentrix software DVD is included, along with practice exercises in relevant chapters, so that students can become familiar with working in dental office systems. As a bonus, flashcards are located in the back of the workbook as a study tool, focusing on terms, instruments, and procedures.

New to this edition is the Externship Guide. An externship is an integral part of a dental assistant's education, and the guide includes resources for students to stay organized. These include time sheets, record of clinical activities, and student journal prompts.

## *Dental Assisting Online for Modern Dental Assisting*

This first-of-its-kind online course (sold separately) contains 42 modules, each of which correlates to a specific chapter in the textbook. Modules take the most challenging content within the corresponding chapters and presents it in an interactive and engaging way to help promote true content mastery. Brief summary content screens are interspersed with interactive exercises, videos, animations, and quizzes to provide a range of audio and visual learning opportunities that reach far beyond the traditional model of classroom instruction and encourage students to immerse themselves in the learning process and develop a more comprehensive understanding of the material presented in the textbook. A turnkey design makes incorporating the course into your program easy and seamless.

# HOW TO USE
# *Modern Dental Assisting*

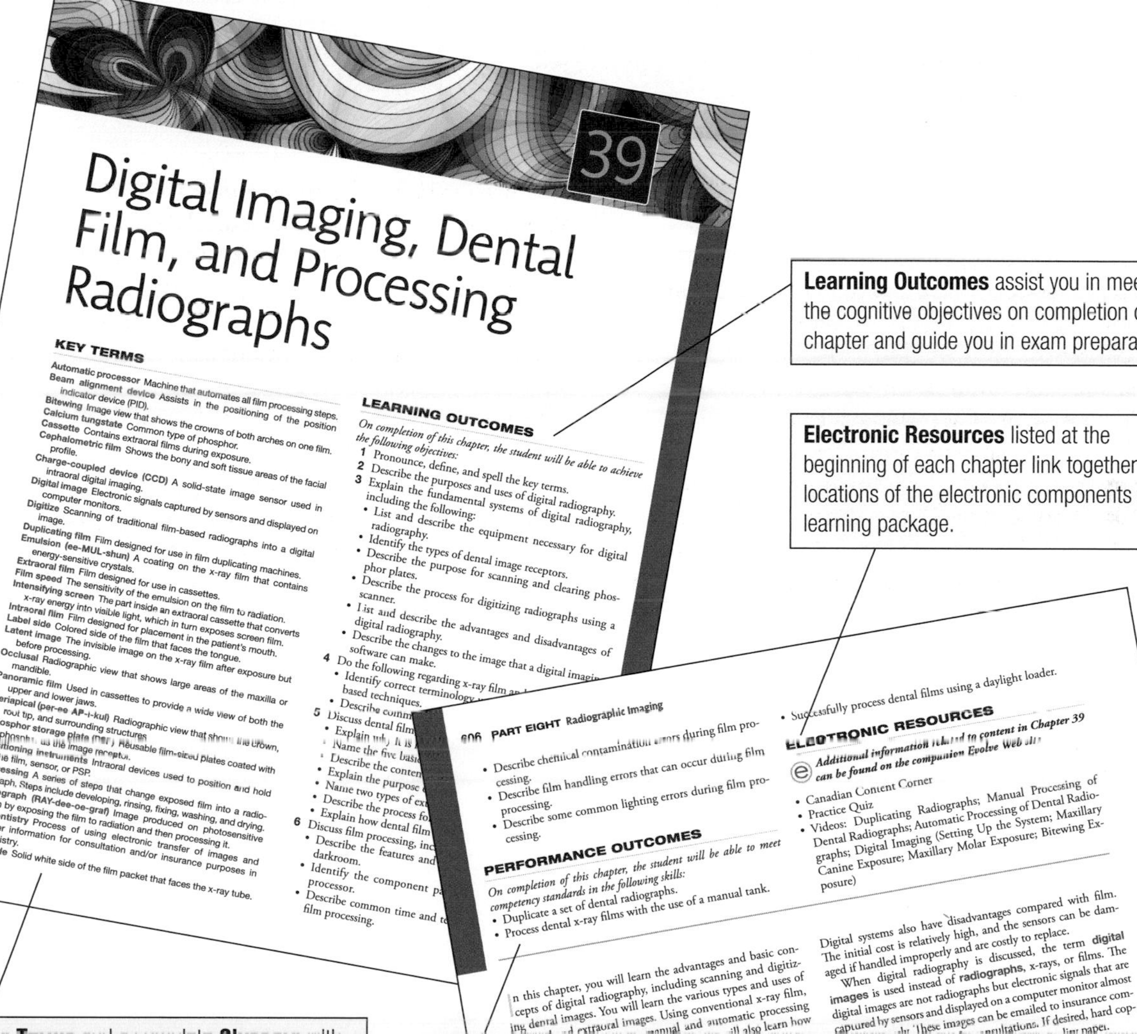

39

# Digital Imaging, Dental Film, and Processing Radiographs

**KEY TERMS**

**Automatic processor** Machine that automates all film processing steps.
**Beam alignment device** Assists in the positioning of the position indicator device (PID).
**Bitewing** Image view that shows the crowns of both arches on one film.
**Calcium tungstate** Common type of phosphor.
**Cassette** Contains extraoral films during exposure.
**Cephalometric film** Shows the bony and soft tissue areas of the facial profile.
**Charge-coupled device (CCD)** A solid-state image sensor used in intraoral digital imaging.
**Digital image** Electronic signals captured by sensors and displayed on computer monitors.
**Digitize** Scanning of traditional film-based radiographs into a digital image.
**Duplicating film** Film designed for use in film duplicating machines.
**Emulsion (ee-MUL-shun)** A coating on the x-ray film that contains energy-sensitive crystals.
**Extraoral film** Film designed for use in cassettes.
**Film speed** The sensitivity of the emulsion on the film to radiation.
**Intensifying screen** The part inside an extraoral cassette that converts x-ray energy into visible light, which in turn exposes screen film.
**Intraoral film** Film designed for placement in the patient's mouth.
**Label side** Colored side of the film that faces the tongue.
**Latent image** The invisible image on the x-ray film after exposure but before processing.
**Occlusal** Radiographic view that shows large areas of the maxilla or mandible.
**Panoramic film** Used in cassettes to provide a wide view of both the upper and lower jaws.
**Periapical (per-ee-AP-i-kul)** Radiographic view that shows the crown, root tip, and surrounding structures.
**Phosphor storage plate (PSP)** Reusable film-sized plates coated with phosphors, as the image receptor.
**Positioning instruments** Intraoral devices used to position and hold the film, sensor, or PSP.
**Processing** A series of steps that change exposed film into a radiograph. Steps include developing, rinsing, fixing, washing, and drying.
**Radiograph (RAY-dee-oe-graf)** Image produced on photosensitive film by exposing the film to radiation and then processing it.
**Teledentistry** Process of using electronic transfer of images and other information for consultation and/or insurance purposes in dentistry.
**Tube side** Solid white side of the film packet that faces the x-ray tube.

**LEARNING OUTCOMES**

*On completion of this chapter, the student will be able to achieve the following objectives:*

1 Pronounce, define, and spell the key terms.
2 Describe the purposes and uses of digital radiography.
3 Explain the fundamental systems of digital radiography, including the following:
- List and describe the equipment necessary for digital radiography.
- Identify the types of dental image receptors.
- Describe the purpose for scanning and clearing phosphor plates.
- Describe the process for digitizing radiographs using a scanner.
- List and describe the advantages and disadvantages of digital radiography.
- Describe the changes to the image that a digital imaging software can make.

4 Do the following regarding x-ray film and ...
- Identify correct terminology ...
based techniques.
- Describe comm...

5 Discuss dental film...
- Explain why it is ...
- Name the five basic...
- Describe the conten...
- Explain the purpose ...
- Name two types of ex...
- Describe the process fo...
- Explain how dental film...

6 Discuss film processing, inc...
- Describe the features and ... darkroom.
- Identify the component p... processor.
- Describe common time and te... film processing.

606 PART EIGHT Radiographic Imaging

- Describe chemical contamination errors during film processing.
- Describe film handling errors that can occur during film processing.
- Describe some common lighting errors during film processing.

- Successfully process dental films using a daylight loader.

**PERFORMANCE OUTCOMES**

*On completion of this chapter, the student will be able to meet competency standards in the following skills:*
- Duplicate a set of dental radiographs.
- Process dental x-ray films with the use of a manual tank.

**ELECTRONIC RESOURCES**

*Additional information related to content in Chapter 39 can be found on the companion Evolve Web site.*
- Canadian Content Corner
- Practice Quiz
- Videos: Duplicating Radiographs; Manual Processing of Dental Radiographs; Automatic Processing of Dental Radiographs; Digital Imaging (Setting Up the System; Maxillary Canine Exposure; Maxillary Molar Exposure; Bitewing Exposure)

In this chapter, you will learn the advantages and basic concepts of digital radiography, including scanning and digitizing dental images. You will learn the various types and uses of intraoral and extraoral images. Using conventional x-ray film, you will learn how to use manual and automatic processing techniques and how to duplicate films. You will also learn how to recognize common errors in film processing and how to prevent them from occurring.

## Digital Radiography

Digital radiography has revolutionized dentistry (Fig. 39.1). Digital imaging eliminates chemical processing and hazardous wastes from chemicals and lead foil. Images can be electronically transferred to other healthcare providers without loss of the original image quality. A significant advantage is that it requires less radiation than film, thus reducing radiation to the patient. Finally, digital imaging allows enhancements, measurements, and corrections that are not available with film (Fig. 39.2).

Digital systems also have disadvantages compared with film. The initial cost is relatively high, and the sensors can be damaged if handled improperly and are costly to replace.

When digital radiography is discussed, the term **digital images** is used instead of **radiographs**, x-rays, or films. The digital images are not radiographs but electronic signals that are captured by sensors and displayed on a computer monitor almost instantly. These images can be emailed to insurance companies and other dentists for consultations. If desired, hard copies of these images can be printed on high-quality paper.

Although digital imaging systems are high tech, a conventional x-ray machine is still needed to expose the image, and the position of the image receptor (sensor or phosphor storage plate [PSP]) in the mouth is identical to positioning with film. In addition, strict infection control measures must be used because the sensors and PSPs are reused time and again. U.S. Food and Drug Administration (FDA)–cleared disposable, fluid-impervious barriers must be used on digital image sensors and phosphor plates. Digital image receptors are *not* able to tolerate heat sterilization.

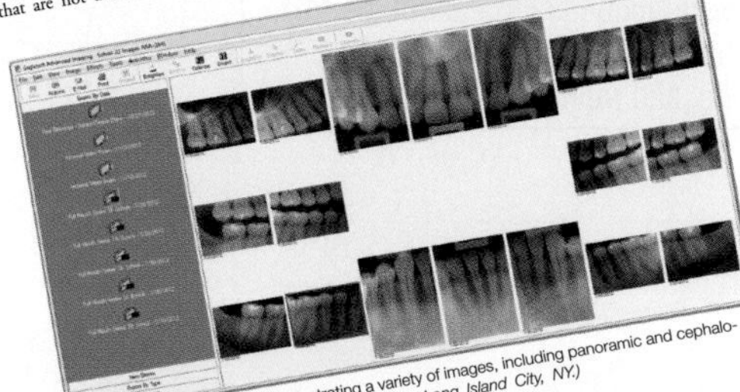

**FIG. 39.1** Computer monitor illustrating a variety of images, including panoramic and cephalometric images. (*Courtesy Sirona Dental, Inc., Long Island City, NY.*)

**Learning Outcomes** assist you in meeting the cognitive objectives on completion of the chapter and guide you in exam preparation.

**Electronic Resources** listed at the beginning of each chapter link together the locations of the electronic components of the learning package.

**Key Terms** and a complete **Glossary** with definitions and pronunciations reinforce new terminology. In the pronunciations, the main accented syllable is bolded. If there is a secondary accented syllable, it is italicized.

**Performance Outcomes** help you to master the clinical skills necessary to become a competent dental assistant.

**Patient Education** offers tips and strategies to help you interact and share information with patients.

**Legal and Ethical Implications** help you focus on the legal and ethical behaviors you will need to know to protect yourself, your patients, and the practice for which you work.

**Eye to the Future** introduces you to cutting-edge research, future trends, and topics relating to the chapter content.

**Critical Thinking** questions and scenarios at the end of each chapter reinforce your ability to solve problems and make appropriate decisions.

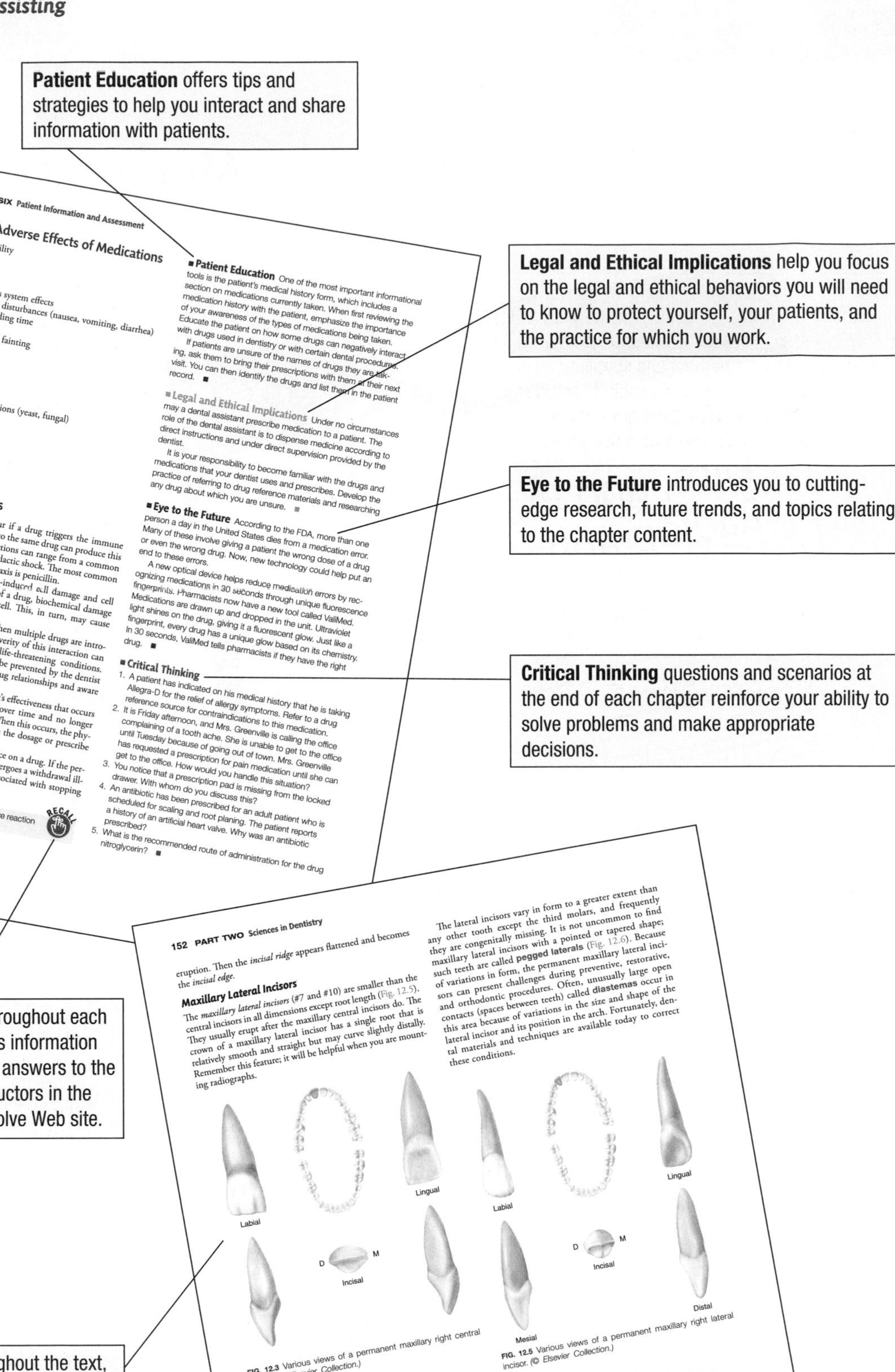

**Recall Questions** are interspersed throughout each chapter to help you retain the previous information before going on to the next topic. The answers to the Recall questions are available to instructors in the TEACH resources, available on the Evolve Web site.

**Outstanding artwork** abounds throughout the text, with a mixture of high-quality color illustrations, clinical photographs, and radiographs.

**Expanded Function procedures** include a list of prerequisite skills required of dental assistants.

**Step-by-step procedures** in the textbook include illustrations, the equipment and supplies you will need, icons, and the rationale behind certain steps. At the end of many procedures are samples of how you would enter the procedure in the patient's chart.

**Procedural icons** are located with each procedure to remind you at a glance of those important precautions that are required during the performance of a procedure.

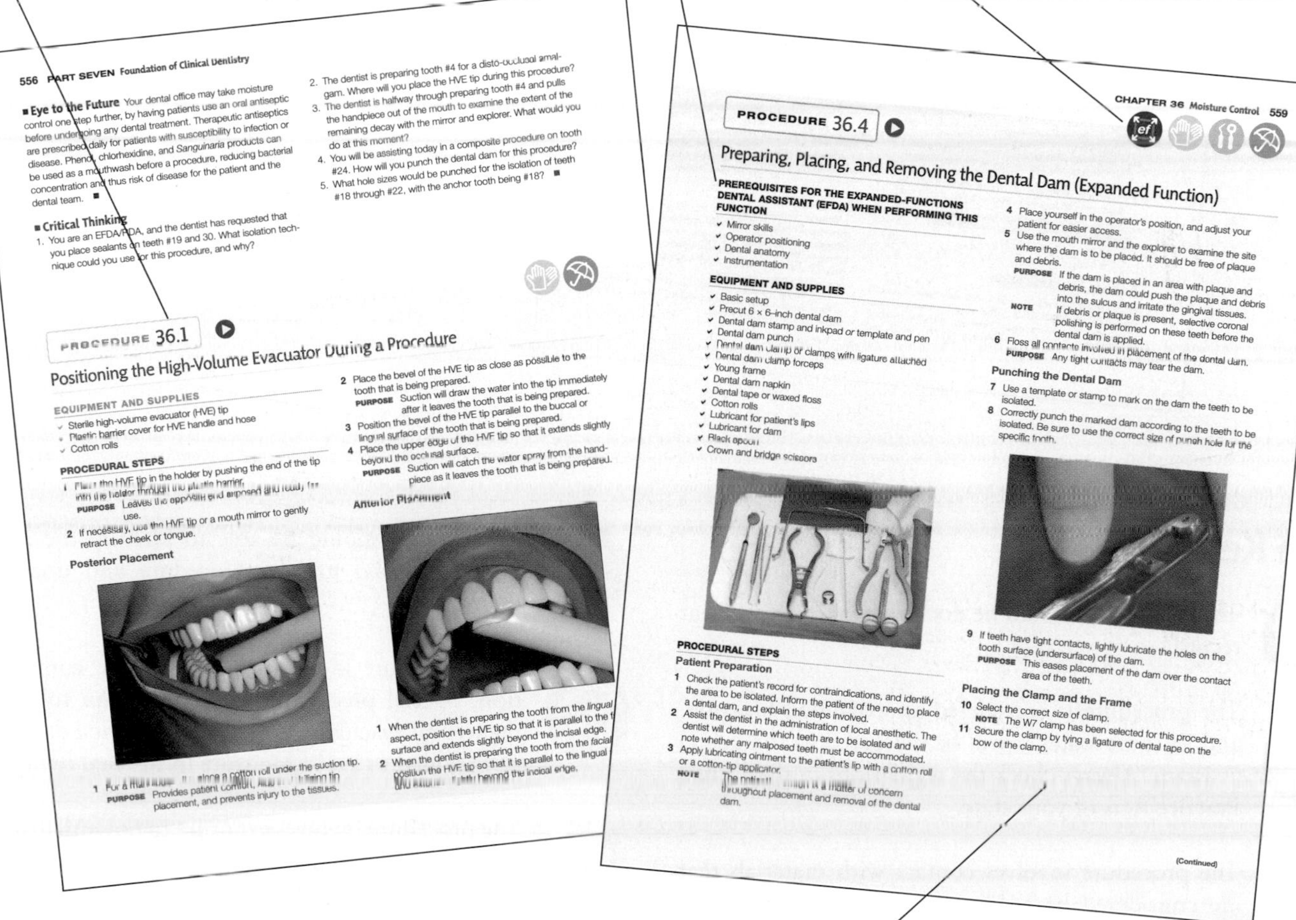

**Expanded Function procedures** feature a different color background to further differentiate them from the more foundational procedures.

**Transfer surfaces** are not directly touched but often are touched by contaminated instruments. Transfer surfaces include instrument trays and handpiece holders.

**Splash, spatter, and droplet surfaces** do not actually contact members of the dental team or contaminated instruments or supplies. Countertops are a major example.

Touch and transfer surfaces should be barrier protected or cleaned and disinfected between patients. Splash, spatter, and droplet surfaces should be cleaned at least once daily (Table 20.1).

CDC

### CDC Recommendations for Environmental Infection Control

**General Recommendations**

- Follow the manufacturers' instructions for correct use of cleaning and EPA-registered hospital disinfecting products. (Categories IB, IC)
- Do not use liquid chemical sterilants/high-level disinfectants for disinfection of environmental surfaces (clinical contact or housekeeping). (Categories IB, IC)
- Use PPE, as appropriate, when cleaning and disinfecting environmental surfaces. (Category IC)

**Clinical Contact Surfaces**

- Use surface barriers to protect clinical contact surfaces, particularly those that are difficult to clean, and change barriers between patients. (Category II)
- Clean and disinfect clinical contact surfaces that are not barrier protected by using an EPA-registered hospital disinfectant with low-level (i.e., HIV and HBV label claims) to intermediate-level (i.e., tuberculocidal claim) activity after each patient. Use an intermediate-level disinfectant if visibly soiled with blood. (Category IB)

**Housekeeping Surfaces**

- Clean housekeeping surfaces (e.g., floors, walls, sinks) with a detergent and water or an EPA-registered hospital disinfectant/detergent on a routine basis, depending on the nature of the surface and the type and degree of contamination, and as appropriate according to location within the facility, and when visibly soiled. (Category IB)
- Clean mops and cloths after use and allow to dry before reuse, or use single-use disposable mop heads or cloths. (Category II)
- Prepare fresh cleaning or EPA-registered disinfecting solutions daily and as instructed by the manufacturer. (Category II)
- Clean walls, blinds, and window curtains in patient care areas when they are visibly dusty or soiled. (Category II)

*EPA*, Environmental Protection Agency; *HBV*, hepatitis B virus; *HIV*, human immunodeficiency virus; *PPE*, personal protective equipment.

## Surface Contamination

Two methods that may be used to deal with surface contamination are (1) to prevent the surface from becoming contaminated with the use of a **surface barrier**, and (2) to preclean and disinfect the surface between patients (Fig. 20.2). Each

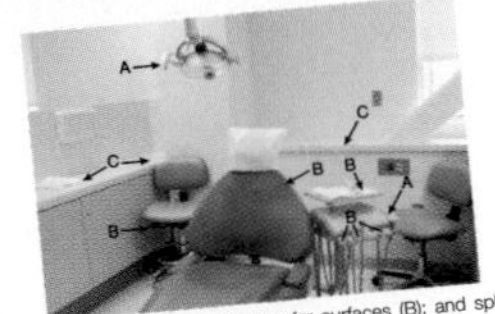


**FIG. 20.1** Touch surfaces (A); transfer surfaces (B); and splash, spatter, and droplet surfaces (C).

has advantages and disadvantages, and most dental offices use a combination of surface disinfection and surface barriers.

Smooth, hard surfaces such as countertops, trays, handles, supply containers, and bottles can be quickly and easily cleaned. Surfaces with crevices, knobs, or other difficult-to-clean features, such as light handles, air-water syringe handles, and electrical switches (which can short-circuit), are better protected with surface barriers.

It is the responsibility of the dental assistant to make certain that equipment and treatment room surfaces are properly managed to prevent patient-to-patient disease transmission.

### Surface Barriers

Placing barriers on surfaces and equipment can prevent contamination of clinical contact areas, but barriers are especially important for those areas that are difficult to clean (Fig. 20.3).

All surface barriers should be resistant to fluids. Fluid-resistant barriers prevent microorganisms in saliva, blood, and other liquids from soaking through the barrier material to contact the surface underneath (Fig. 20.4). Some plastic bags are specially designed to fit the shapes of dental chairs, air-water syringes, hoses, pens, and light handles (Fig. 20.5). Other types of barrier materials include clear plastic wrap, bags, tubing, plastic tape, and plastic-backed paper, and sticky tape is frequently used as a plastic barrier to protect smooth surfaces, such as touch pads on equipment or electrical switches on chairs and x-ray equipment. Aluminum foil can also be used because it is easily formed around any shape. See Procedure 20.1: Placing and Removing Surface Barriers.

Between patients, while you are still gloved, you should remove and discard contaminated barriers. If, when removing contaminated barriers, you are careful not to touch the surface below, you do not have to clean and disinfect the surface. However, if you do inadvertently touch a surface, you will have to clean and disinfect that surface.

Even though surfaces have been covered with barriers, the surfaces should still be cleaned and disinfected at the beginning and at the end of each workday.

**CDC feature boxes** highlight the latest guidelines developed by the Centers for Disease Control and Prevention for safe dental practice.

## Icon Key

The procedure should be documented in the patient record.

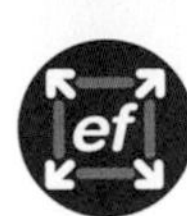


The procedure is considered an expanded function, and in some states it will be delegated to the dental assistant. Always check the regulations in the Dental Practice Acts of your state.

The procedure involves contact with materials that are considered hazardous. Special handling or disposal techniques are required.

The student should be able to identify the instruments required for the procedure and document their use.

The procedure is sensitive to moisture contamination. Special precautions such as cotton roll placement, oral evacuation, and use of a dental dam must be included to avoid moisture in the oral cavity.

The procedure involves exposure to potentially infectious materials and requires the use of appropriate personal protective equipment, such as a mask, eyewear, and gloves.

The procedure is supplemented by a video on the Evolve site.

*In memory of our colleagues Margaret M. (Peggy) Walsh, RDH, MS, EdD, and Michelle Leonardi Darby, BSDH, MS, co-authors of* Dental Hygiene: Theory and Practice, *and to Donna Phinney, CDA, BA, MEd, co-author of* Comprehensive Dental Assisting. *Their contributions to dental assisting and dental hygiene education will always be remembered.*

CONTENTS

## PART 4
## Infection Prevention in Dentistry



## PART 5
## Occupational Health and Safety



## PART 6
## Patient Information and Assessment

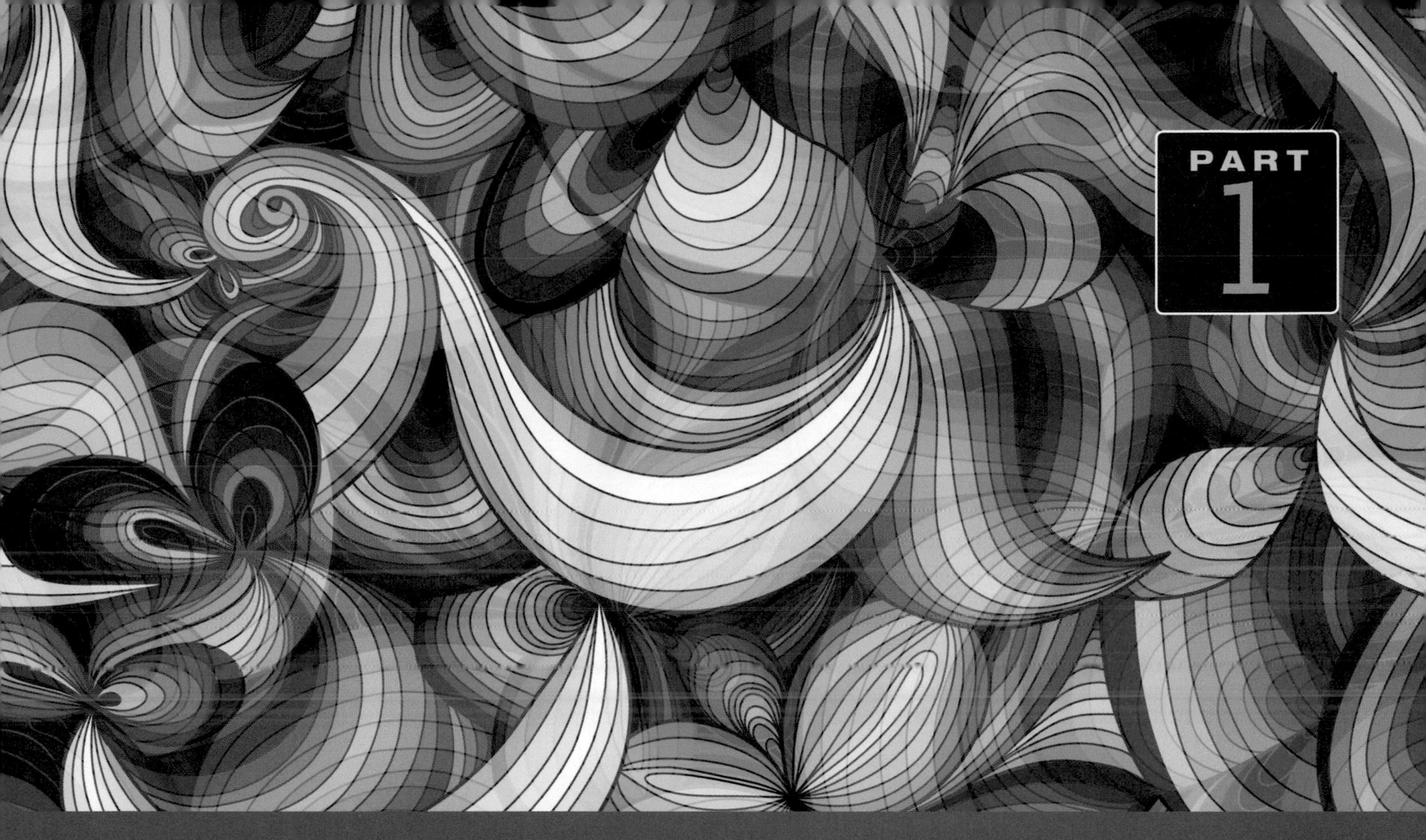


# The Dental Assisting Profession

Dental assistants are important members of the dental healthcare team. A career as a dental assistant can be exciting, challenging, and very rewarding. The educated dental assistant can look forward to job satisfaction, variety, and financial reward. It is a career that offers opportunities for recent high school graduates, as well as for individuals who may be older and wish to return to school and change careers.

*Professionalism* is difficult to define. It is an attitude that is apparent in everything a person says and does, at and away from the office. Professionalism distinguishes people who "have a job" from those who "pursue a career." By always behaving in a professional manner, the dental assistant earns respect and recognition as a dental healthcare professional.

The chapters in this section are designed to provide an overview of the dental profession. It begins with a look at the history of dentistry through the ages, introduces the other members of the dental healthcare team, and explains the legal and ethical responsibilities expected of a dental professional.

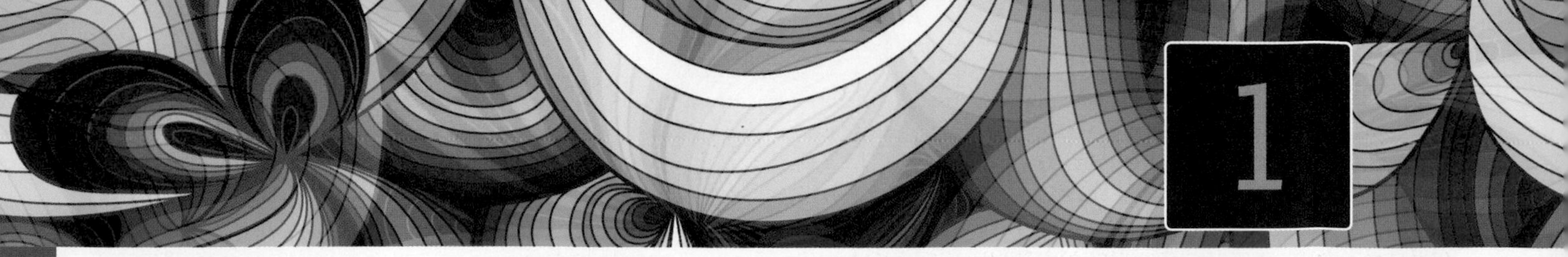


# History of Dentistry

## KEY TERMS

**Commission on Dental Accreditation of the American Dental Association** Commission that accredits dental, dental assisting, dental hygiene, and dental laboratory educational programs.

**Dental treatise (TREE-tis)** Formal article or book based on dental evidence and facts.

**Forensic (fuh-REN-zik) dentistry** Area of dentistry that establishes the identity of an individual on the basis of dental evidence such as dental records, impressions, bite marks, and so forth.

**Periodontal (per-ee-oe-DON-tul) disease** Infections and other conditions of the structures that support the teeth (gums and bone).

**Preceptorship (PREE-sep-tor-ship)** Study under the guidance of a dentist or other professional.

**Saint Apollonia** Recognized as the Patroness of Dentistry.

**Silver amalgam (uh-MAL-gum) paste** A mixture of mercury, silver, and tin.

**Teledentistry** The process of using electronic transfer of images and other information for consultation and/or insurance purposes in dentistry.

## LEARNING OUTCOMES

*On completion of this chapter, the student will be able to achieve the following objectives:*

1. Pronounce, define, and spell the key terms.
2. Compare and contrast the early contributions in dentistry of ancient cultures in Egypt, Greece, China, and Rome, including the following:
   - The role of Hippocrates in history.
   - The basic premise of the Hippocratic Oath.
   - The culture that first developed a silver amalgam paste for filling teeth.
   - Important Romans who contributed to oral hygiene and dentistry.
3. Identify the important contributions of the Renaissance period in dental history, including Leonardo da Vinci's contribution to dentistry.
4. Identify the important contributions of early America in dental history, including the individual credited with beginning the science of forensic dentistry.
5. List the important contributions in dental education and professional development, including the following:
   - The contributions of Horace H. Hayden and Chapin A. Harris.
   - Two major contributions of G. V. Black.
   - The scientist who discovered x-rays.
   - The physician who first used nitrous oxide for tooth extractions.
6. Identify key women in dental history, including the following:
   - The woman dentist who discovered oral hairy leukoplakia.
   - The first woman to graduate from a college of dentistry.
   - The first woman to practice dentistry in the United States.
7. Identify key African Americans in dental history, including the following:
   - The first African American woman to receive a dental degree in the United States.
   - The first African American to receive the DMD degree from Harvard University.
8. Identify key American Indians in dental history, including the following:
   - The first American Indian to receive a dental degree in the United States.
   - The first American Indian woman to receive a dental degree in the United States.
9. Identify key historical contributors in the field of dental assisting and dental hygiene, including the following:
   - The first dentist to employ a dental assistant.
   - The contributions of Ann Ehrlich and Hazel Torres to dental assisting education.
   - The first person to become a dental hygienist.
   - The contribution of Dr. Alfred C. Fones to the dental profession.
10. Explain the process of dental accreditation and its importance.
11. Discuss the purpose and activities of the National Museum of Dentistry.

## ELECTRONIC RESOURCES

***Additional information related to content in Chapter 1 can be found on the companion Evolve Web site.***

- Practice Quiz
- Canadian Content Corner

Dentistry has a long and fascinating history. From the earliest times, humans have suffered from dental pain and have sought a variety of means to alleviate it. As they developed tools, humans also cleaned and cared for their teeth and oral cavity. Early toothbrushes ranged from wooden sticks with frayed ends for scraping the tongue to ivory-handled brushes with animal-hair bristles for cleaning the teeth.

It is easy to believe that the ideas and techniques used in dentistry today are new or have been recently discovered or invented. Actually, many of the remarkable techniques in modern dentistry can be traced to the earliest times in every culture. People may think of "cosmetic dentistry" as a relatively new field, but skulls of ninth-century BC Mayans have numerous inlays of decorative jade and turquoise on the front teeth. Skulls of the Incas discovered in Ecuador have gold pounded into prepared holes in the teeth, similar to modern gold inlay restorations. As early as the sixth century BC, the Etruscans were able to make false teeth using gold and cattle teeth (Fig. 1.1). More than 2200 years ago, a cleft palate was repaired on a child in China. Muhammad introduced basic oral hygiene into the ritual of Islam in the seventh century AD. He recognized the value of Siwak, a tree twig containing natural minerals, as an oral hygiene device.

As B. W. Weinberger noted in *Dentistry: An Illustrated History* (Ring, 1995), a profession that is ignorant of its past experiences has lost a valuable asset because "it has missed its best guide to the future." Table 1.1 lists major highlights in the history of dentistry.

# Early Times

## The Egyptians

As long as 4600 years ago in Egypt, physicians began to specialize in healing certain parts of the body. A physician named **Hesi-Re** was the earliest dentist whose name is known. He practiced about 3000 BC and was called "Chief of the Toothers and the Physicians." Three teeth fastened together with gold wire, apparently an early fixed bridge, were found with the remains of an Egyptian who lived about 3100 BC.

A radiograph of the skull of Thuya, mother-in-law of Pharaoh Amenhotep III, showed bone loss in her jaws, an indication of **periodontal disease**. Some dental problems have been attributed to the Egyptian diet, which was primarily vegetarian. Grain was ground with stone pestles, which mixed sand and grit into the food, resulting in severe wear of the *occlusal* (biting) tooth surfaces and exposure of the pulp.

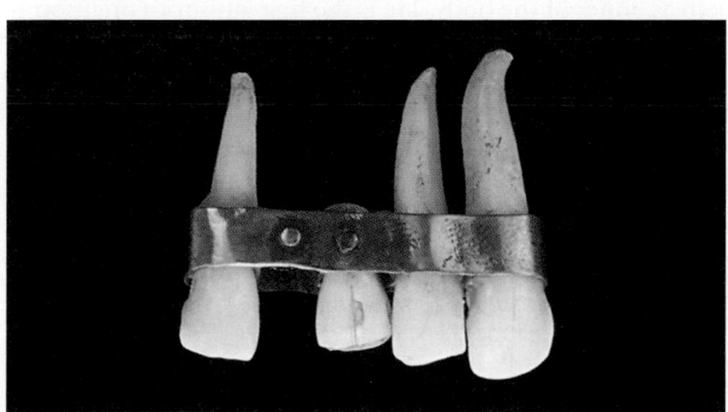

FIG. 1.1 Ancient Etruscan gold-banded bridge with built-in calf's tooth. *(Courtesy Musée de l'Ecole Dentaire de Paris.)*

1 Who was Hesi-Re?
2 How long has dental disease existed?

## The Greeks

During the fifth century BC in Greece, the practice of medicine and dentistry was based on the worship practices of the priesthood. Priests would give patients a sleeping potion and perform healing rituals. During this period, **Hippocrates** (460–377 BC) began to outline a rational approach to treating patients. He suggested that four main fluids in the body—blood, black bile, yellow bile, and phlegm—along with heat, cold, dry air, and wet air, must remain in balance, or disease would occur. His approach to treatment of patients earned him the title "Father of Medicine."

Hippocrates stressed the importance of keeping the teeth in good condition. His writings described the teeth, their formation, and their eruption, as well as diseases of the teeth and methods of treatment. He also developed a dentifrice and mouthwash. The famous Hippocratic Oath, a solemn obligation to refrain from wrongdoing and to treat patients with confidentiality and to the best of one's ability, still serves as the basis of the code of ethics for medical and dental professions.

**Aristotle** (384–322 BC), the great philosopher, referred to teeth in many of his writings. However, he mistakenly stated that the gingiva was responsible for tooth formation, and that men had 32 teeth and women had only 30. Many of his erroneous ideas were not corrected until the Renaissance.

**Diocles of Carystus,** an Athenian physician of Aristotle's time, recommended rubbing the gums and teeth with bare fingers and "finely pulverized mint" to remove adherent food particles. Other materials used to clean the teeth included pumice, talc, emery, ground alabaster, coral powder, and iron rust.

## The Chinese

By 2000 BC, the Chinese were practicing dentistry. They used arsenic to treat decayed teeth. This probably relieved the toothache. About the second century AD, the Chinese developed a **silver amalgam paste** for fillings, more than a thousand years before dentists in the West used a similar substance. In the eleventh century, **T'ing To-t'ung** and **Yu Shu** described the entire process of chewing and swallowing. Their description of the process was accurate, but they were incorrect about what happened to the food when it reached the stomach. They believed that digestion was a result of vapors arising from the spleen.

## The Romans

When the medical profession in Rome was just beginning, dentistry was already being practiced. Several Roman physicians wrote extensively about dental treatment, although many people still believed that a "toothworm" was responsible for toothaches. In addition to extracting teeth, the Romans were

**TABLE 1.1** Highlights in the History of Dentistry

| Date | Group/Individual | Event |
|---|---|---|
| 3000–2151 BC | Egyptians | Hesi-Re is earliest dentist known by name. |
| 2700 BC | Chinese | Chinese Canon of Medicine refers to dentistry. |
| 900–300 BC | Mayans | Teeth receive attention for religious reasons or self-adornment. |
| 460–322 BC | Greeks | Hippocrates and Aristotle write about tooth decay. |
| 166–201 AD | Romans | Restore decayed teeth with gold crowns. |
| 570–950 | Muslims | Use Siwak as a primitive toothbrush. |
| 1510–1590 | Ambroise Paré | Writes extensively about dentistry, including extractions. |
| 1678–1761 | Pierre Fauchard | Becomes "Father of Modern Dentistry." |
| 1728–1793 | John Hunter | Performs first scientific study of teeth. |
| 1826 | M. Taveau | Introduces amalgam as "silver paste." |
| 1844 | Horace Wells | Uses nitrous oxide for relief of dental pain. |
| 1859 | | American Dental Association is founded. |
| 1885 | C. Edmund Kells | Employs first dental assistant. |
| 1895 | G. V. Black | Becomes "Grand Old Man of Dentistry" and perfects amalgam. |
| 1895 | W. C. Roentgen | Discovers x-rays. |
| 1908 | Frederick McKay | Discovers that fluoride is connected with prevention of dental caries. |
| 1913 | Alfred C. Fones | Establishes first dental hygiene school in Bridgeport, Connecticut. |
| 1923 | | American Dental Hygiene Association is founded. |
| 1924 | | American Dental Assistants Association is founded. |
| 1948 | | Dental Assisting National Board is founded. |
| 1970 | Congress | Creates Occupational Safety and Health Administration. |
| 1978 | *Journal of the American Dental Association* | Publishes a report on infection control for dental offices. |
| 1980 | | First cases of what later became known as acquired immunodeficiency syndrome (AIDS) are reported. |
| 1982 | | First hepatitis B vaccine becomes commercially available. |
| 1983 | | Human immunodeficiency virus (HIV) is identified as the cause of AIDS. |
| 2000 | | *Oral Health in America: A Report of the Surgeon General* is released. |
| 2003 | Centers for Disease Control and Prevention | Releases *Guidelines for Infection Control in Dental Health-Care Settings—2003.* |

skilled in restoring decayed teeth with gold crowns and replacing missing teeth by means of fixed bridgework.

The Romans had a high regard for oral hygiene and developed tooth-cleaning powders made from eggshells, bones, and oyster shells mixed with honey. Dinner guests of upper-class Romans picked their teeth between courses with elaborately decorated toothpicks of metal, often gold, and were invited to take their gold toothpicks home as gifts.

**Saint Apollonia** was one of a group of virgin martyrs who suffered in Alexandria during a local uprising against the Christians before the persecution of Decius. According to legend, her torture included having all of her teeth violently pulled out or shattered. For this reason, she is popularly regarded as the patroness of dentistry and those suffering from toothache or other dental problems (Fig. 1.2).

**Cornelius Celsus** (25 BC–50 AD) wrote *De Medicina,* a digest of medical and surgical science from the earliest times to the period of Augustus Caesar. This book contains the earliest record of orthodontic treatment.

**Claudius Galen** (130–200 AD) is considered to be the greatest physician after Hippocrates. In his writings, Galen listed the teeth as bones of the body. He is the first author to mention the nerves in the teeth: "The teeth are furnished with nerves both because as naked bones they have need of sensitivity so that the animal may avoid being injured or destroyed by mechanical or physical agencies, and because the teeth, together with the tongue and other parts of the mouth, are designed for the perception of various flavors" (Guerini, 1909).

RECALL

3 Who is the "Father of Medicine"?
4 What is the Hippocratic Oath?
5 Who is the Patroness of Dentistry?
6 Were Western dentists the first to use silver amalgam as fillings?

RECALL

13 Who founded the first dental school in America?
14 Who earned the title of "Grand Old Man of Dentistry"?
15 Who was the first dentist to use nitrous oxide?
16 Who was the first woman in the United States to graduate from a dental school?
17 Who was the first person to discover oral "hairy" leukoplakia?

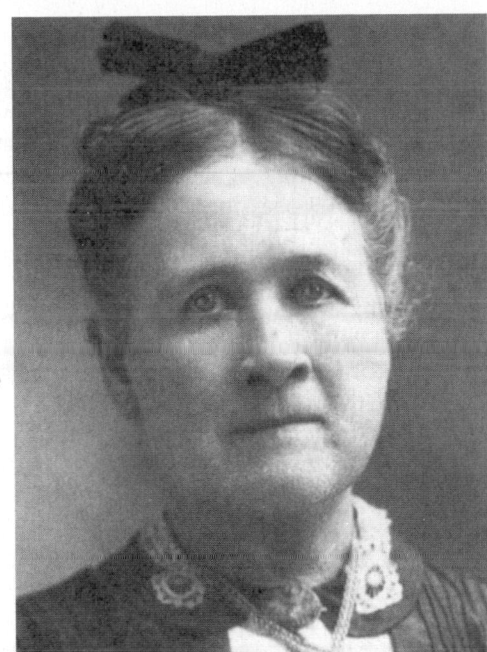

**FIG. 1.9** Lucy B. Hobbs-Taylor, the first female graduate of dental school. *(Courtesy Kansas State Historical Society, Topeka, KS.)*

## African Americans in Dental History

African Americans were not accepted for training at any dental schools until 1867, when Harvard University initiated its first dental class and accepted **Robert Tanner Freeman** as its first African American student (Fig. 1.11). **George Franklin Grant** graduated from Harvard in 1870 and later was appointed to the school's dental faculty.

**Ida Gray-Rollins** (1867–1953) was the first African American woman in the country to earn a formal DDS degree and the first African American woman to practice dentistry in Chicago. She graduated from the University of Michigan School of Dentistry and practiced dentistry in Chicago until she retired in 1928. In 1929 she married William Rollins and used the name Dr. Ida Gray-Rollins for the rest of her life (see Table 1.2).

African Americans have been appointed deans and faculty members at a number of American dental schools (Table 1.3).

## American Indians in Dental History

**Dr. George Blue Spruce, Jr.,** is the first American Indian dentist in the United States. He graduated Dental School from Creighton University in 1956, where he was the only American Indian on campus (Fig. 1.12). He began treating patients on American Indian reservations and later in his career became an Assistant Surgeon General in the United States Public Health Service. He is currently the Assistant Dean for American Indian Affairs at the Arizona School of Dentistry and Oral Health.

*Never be afraid to go after your dream. You, too, can meet and beat the challenges that come your way. Sometimes simply discovering and sharing your dreams can be a big step forward.*

DR. GEORGE BLUE SPRUCE, JR.

**TABLE 1.2** Highlights of Women in Dentistry

| Date | Group/Individual | Event |
|---|---|---|
| 1859 | Emeline Robert Jones | First woman to establish a regular dental practice in the United States. |
| 1866 | Lucy B. Hobbs-Taylor | First woman to graduate from a recognized dental college in the United States; received credit for time as a preceptor in her husband's practice. |
| 1869 | Henriette Hirschfeld | First woman to complete the full dental curriculum in a U.S. dental school. |
| 1870 | Nellie E. Pooler Chapman | First woman to practice dentistry in California. |
| 1873 | Emilie Foeking | First female graduate of the Baltimore College of Dental Surgery. Wrote a thesis titled *Is Woman Adapted to the Dental Profession?* |
| 1876 | Jennie D. Spurrier | First female dentist in Illinois. Her first patient needed an extraction, for which she was paid 50 cents. She had the coin engraved with the date and "My first." |
| 1885 | Malvina Cueria | First female dental assistant. |
| 1890 | Ida Gray-Rollins | First African American female dental graduate from a U.S. dental college. |
| 1892 | Mary Stillwell-Kuedsel | Founded the Women's Dental Association of the United States with 12 charter members. |
| 1906 | Irene Newman | First dental hygienist. |
| 1927 | M. Evangeline Jordan | Author of the first textbook on pediatric dentistry. |
| 1951 | Helen E. Myers | U.S. Army's first female dentist. |
| 1984 | Deborah Greenspan | Discovered and published first paper on oral "hairy" leukoplakia. |
| 1991 | Geraldine T. Morrow | First female president of the American Dental Association. |



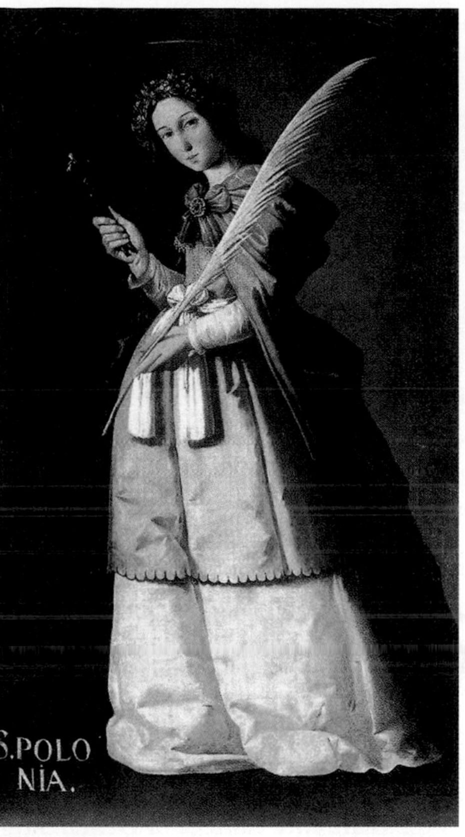


**FIG. 1.2** Saint Apollonia is an oil-on-canvas painted by Spanish artist Francisco de Zurbaran in 1636. It is currently held and exhibited at the Louvre in Paris. *(By Francisco de Zurbarán, via Wikimedia Commons.)*

## The Renaissance

One of the most important achievements of the Renaissance was the separation of science from theology and superstition. During the fifteenth and sixteenth centuries, new interest arose in the study of anatomy and the human body. Artists became more aware of human anatomy and used it to enhance their artwork. **Leonardo da Vinci** (1452–1519) sketched every internal and external structure of the body. He also studied the skull in great detail and was the first anatomist to describe the differences between molars and premolars.

**Ambroise Paré** (pah-RAY) (1510–1590) began his career in Paris in about 1525 as an apprentice to a barber surgeon. His extensive writings describe dental extraction methods and reimplantation of teeth. He described a toothache as "the most atrocious pain that can torment a man without being followed by death" (Ring, 1985). At that time, the practice was to treat soldiers with gunshots by washing the wound with boiling oil, which caused extreme pain. After one battle, the supply of oil was depleted, and Paré had to treat a soldier's wounds with a mixture of egg whites, oil of roses, and turpentine. After using this soothing mixture, Paré vowed that he would "never so cruelly burn poor wounded men." He is also credited with being the first to use artificial eyes, hands, and legs. Paré is known as the "Father of Modern Surgery."

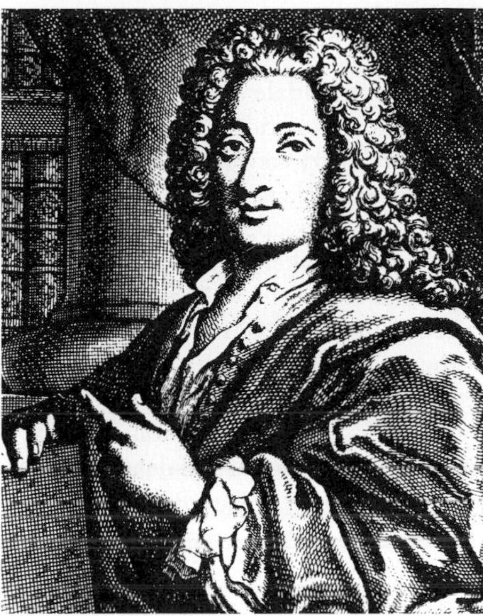

**FIG. 1.3** Pierre Fauchard, the "Father of Modern Dentistry." *(From Fauchard P: Le Chirurgien dentiste ou traité des dents, Paris, 1746, Pierre-Jean Mariette.)*

**Pierre Fauchard** (fo-SHAR) (1678–1761), a physician who earned great fame and respect in his lifetime, willingly shared his knowledge at a time when physicians typically guarded their knowledge and skills (Fig. 1.3). Fauchard developed dentistry as an independent profession and originated the title of "surgeon dentist," a term the French still use today. In the United States, the degree conferred on dentists is Doctor of Dental Surgery (DDS).

Fauchard dispelled the theory that tooth decay was caused by a toothworm. He was ahead of his time in understanding periodontal disease and recognized that scaling the teeth could prevent gum disease. In his book, *Le Chirurgien Dentiste,* Fauchard covered the entire field of dentistry and described his method of removing caries from a tooth and filling the cavity with lead or tin. He suggested using either human teeth or teeth carved from hippopotamus or elephant ivory to make denture teeth. Although advanced in his thinking, Fauchard firmly believed that to ensure good health, people should rinse their mouth every morning with several spoonfuls of their own fresh urine.

**Chapin A. Harris,** the great American dentist, said of Fauchard: "Considering the circumstances under which he lived, Fauchard deserves to be remembered as a noble pioneer and sure founder of dental science. That his practice was crude was due to his times, that it was scientific and comparatively superior and successful was due to himself" (Ring, 1985). Fauchard is known as the "Father of Modern Dentistry."

7 Which artist first distinguished molars from premolars?
8 Who is the "Father of Modern Surgery"?
9 Who is the "Father of Modern Dentistry"?

## Early America

In 1766 **Robert Woofendale** was one of the first dentists to travel throughout the American colonies. His advertisement in *The New York Mercury* stated that he "performs all operations upon the teeth, sockets, gums and palate, likewise fixes artificial teeth, so as to escape discernment" (Ring, 1985). A short time later, **John Baker** arrived from Cork County, Ireland, where he studied dentistry. Although he was a physician, Baker practiced dentistry in Boston, New York, Philadelphia, and many other colonial cities. He was one of George Washington's dentists (Fig. 1.4).

**Paul Revere** (1735–1818), the famous colonial patriot, was a silversmith by trade, but he studied dentistry as an apprentice under Dr. Baker in Boston. When Baker moved to New York in 1768, Revere took over his practice. However, Revere was primarily interested in using his skills as a silversmith to make artificial teeth and surgical instruments. After 6 years of part-time work, he gave up his dental practice.

Paul Revere is credited with beginning the science of **forensic dentistry** and performed the first identification of a corpse recorded in dental history. Dr. Joseph Warren was killed at the Battle of Bunker Hill in 1775 and was buried by the British in a mass grave. A year later, the bodies were exhumed but were unrecognizable. Revere studied the skulls and identified Warren's body on the basis of a two-unit bridge he had made.

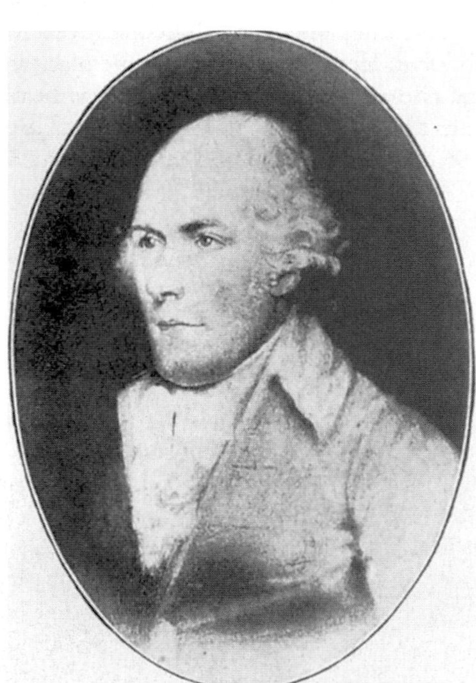

FIG. 1.4 John Greenwood, dentist to George Washington, was the second son of Isaac Greenwood, who is regarded as the first native-born American dentist. John Greenwood served in the colonial army at age 14 during the Revolutionary War and later became a dentist. *(From Kock CRD: History of dental surgery, vol 3, Fort Wayne, Indiana, 1910, National Art Publishing.)*

RECALL

10 Who was John Baker's famous patient?
11 Which famous colonial patriot first used forensic evidence?
12 Who was Robert Woofendale?

## Educational and Professional Development in the United States

In the early days, no colleges for dentistry existed in the United States. Dentists learned their profession through a **preceptorship** while studying and learning under the direction of a skilled professional. During 1839 and 1840 **Horace H. Hayden** and **Chapin A. Harris** set the foundation for the profession of dentistry.

Horace H. Hayden (1769–1844) was inspired by his own dentist, John Greenwood, and became a reputable dentist. He lectured to medical students on the topic of dentistry and wrote for professional journals. Chapin A. Harris (1806–1860), a preceptorial student of Hayden, was instrumental in establishing the first nationwide association of dentists in the United States. His book, *The Dental Art: A Practical Treatise on Dental Surgery,* was reissued over 74 years in 13 editions; no other **dental treatise** can match this record. Together, in 1840 Hayden and Harris established the first dental college in the world, the **Baltimore College of Dental Surgery,** which is now the University of Maryland, School of Dentistry.

**Dr. Green Vardiman Black** (1836–1915), known worldwide as **G. V. Black,** earned the title of the "Grand Old Man of Dentistry" through his unmatched contributions to the profession (Figs. 1.5 and 1.6). Dr. Black believed that dentistry should stand as a profession independent from and equal to that of medicine. He invented numerous machines for testing metal alloys and dental instruments. He taught in dental schools, became a dean, and wrote more than 500 articles and several books. Two of his major contributions to dentistry were (1) the principle of *extension for prevention,* in which the margins of a filling were extended to within reach of a toothbrush for cleaning the tooth, and (2) standardized rules of cavity preparation and filling.

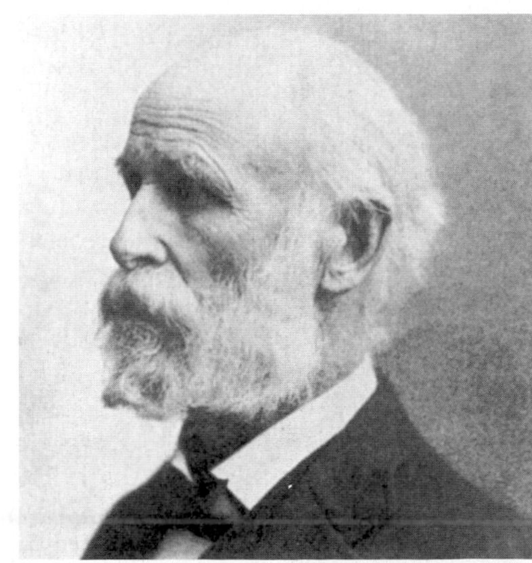

FIG. 1.5 G. V. Black, the "Grand Old Man of Dentistry." *(From Kock CRD: History of dental surgery, vol 1, Chicago, 1909, National Art Publishing.)*

A man of vision, Black told his dental students at Northwestern University, "The day is surely coming, and perhaps within the lifetime of you young men before me, when we will be engaged in practicing preventive, rather than reparative, dentistry" (Ring, 1985).

**Wilhelm Conrad Roentgen** (RENT-ken) (1845–1923) was a Bavarian physicist who discovered x-rays in 1895 (Fig. 1.7). His discovery revolutionized diagnostic capabilities and forever changed the practice of medicine and dentistry (see Chapter 38).

**Horace Wells** (1815–1848) is the dentist credited with the discovery of inhalation anesthesia in 1844, one of the most important medical discoveries of all time. Before this innovation, the only remedies for pain were brute force, alcohol (brandy, rum, whiskey), and opium. Oral drugs could not be properly dosed, and patients were generally undermedicated or overmedicated. If an operation lasted longer than 20 minutes, it was possible for the patient to die of exhaustion or shock. Realizing the potential for pain-free dental surgery with the use of nitrous oxide, Wells said, "Let it be as free as the air we breathe" (Ring, 1985) (see Chapter 37).

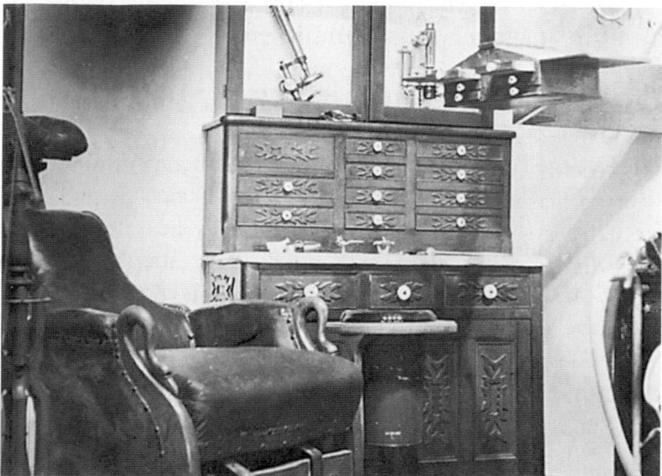

FIG. 1.6 Black's dental treatment room, as reconstructed in a Smithsonian exhibit.

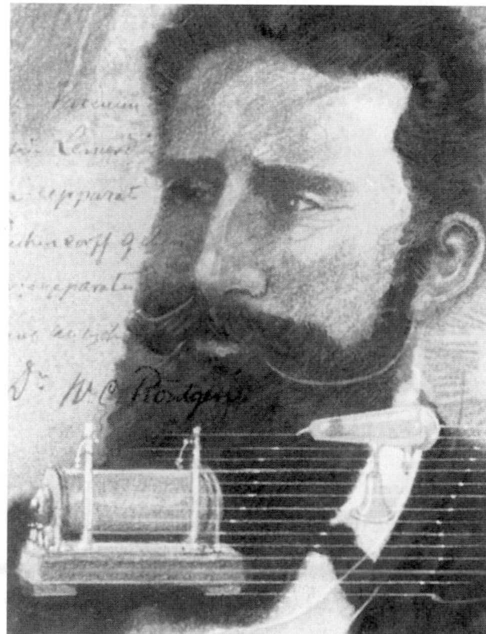

FIG. 1.7 W. C. Roentgen discovered the early potential of an x-ray beam in 1895. *(Courtesy Carestream Health, Rochester, NY.)*

## Women in Dental History

In the eighteenth and early nineteenth centuries, dental schools throughout the world did not accept women. Yet women such as Nellie E. Pooler Chapman and Lucy B. Hobbs-Taylor broke those barriers and led the way for other women to follow as dental professionals (Figs. 1.8 and 1.9).

Today, women represent almost 50 percent of students in some dental schools, and are active in dental associations, specialty organizations, public health, and the military (Table 1.2).

**Dr. Deborah Greenspan** is recognized worldwide for her research into the dental issues related to the human immunodeficiency virus (HIV) and acquired immunodeficiency syndrome (AIDS). She discovered oral "hairy" leukoplakia (see Chapter 17) and opened a new arena of research into both HIV/AIDS and Epstein-Barr virus. Her work has influenced oral healthcare worldwide. She is a professor and Chair of the Oral Facial Sciences Department at the University of California San Francisco School of Dentistry.

**Dr. Faith Sai So Leong** was 13 years old and spoke no English when she immigrated to the United States in 1894. When she was 24 years old, she became the first woman to graduate from the College of Physicians and Surgeons (now the University of the Pacific Arthur A. Dugoni School of Dentistry) in 1904. She practiced dentistry in San Francisco (Fig. 1.10).

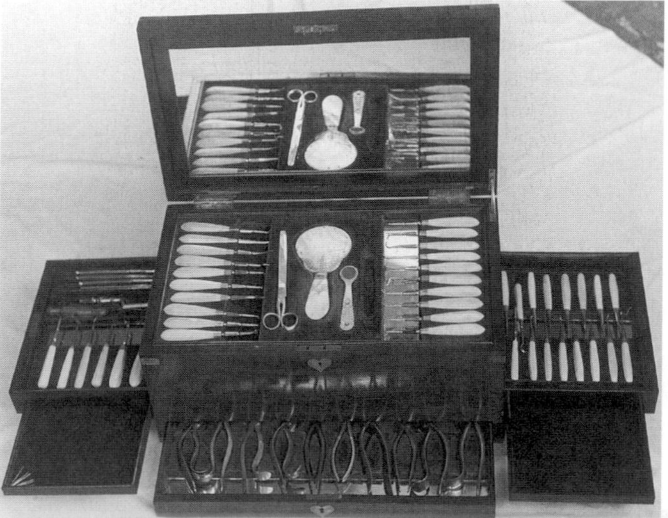

FIG. 1.8 Dental instrument kit belonging to Nellie E. Pooler Chapman. She practiced dentistry in Nevada City, California. She died in 1906. *(Courtesy School of Dentistry, University of California San Francisco.)*

**Jessica A. Rickert** became the first recognized American Indian female dentist in 1975. She attended the University of Michigan, School of Dentistry, and she was the only American Indian in a class of approximately 150 students. During this time there were very few female dentists or female dental students. She received the 2005 Access Recognition Award from the American Dental Association (ADA) for leadership in helping people in need gain access to dental care. In particular, she was nominated for her work in educating American Indians on dental care and encouraging them to pursue careers in the dental field. In 2009 she was honored for her work by being inducted into the Michigan Women's Hall of Fame (Fig. 1.13).

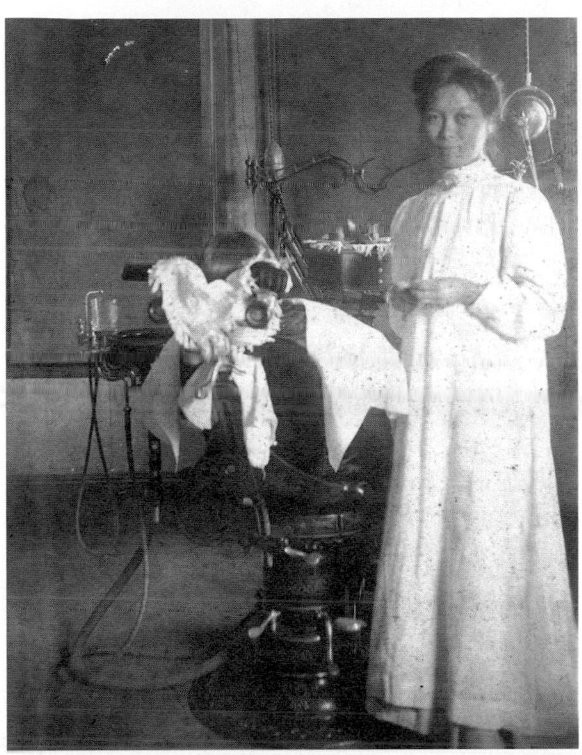

**FIG. 1.10** Dr. Faith Sai So Leong, the first female graduate at College of Physicians and Surgeons (now the University of Pacific Arthur A. Dugoni School of Dentistry).

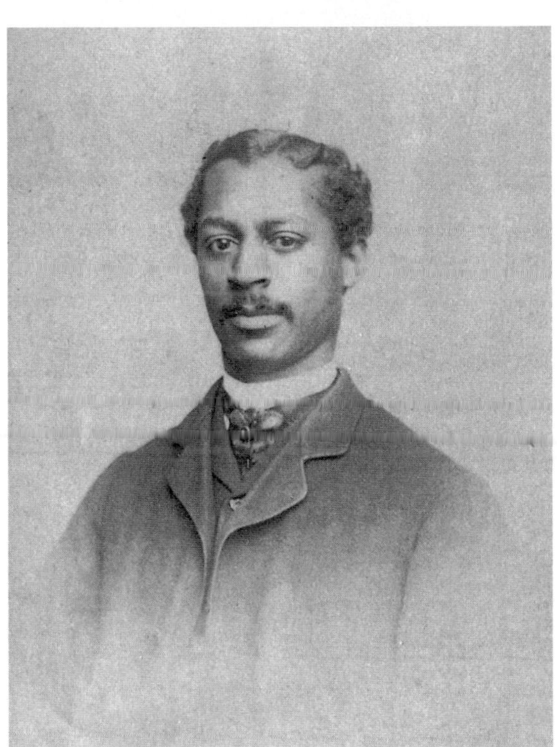

**FIG. 1.11** Robert Tanner Freeman, the first African American graduate of Harvard School of Dental Medicine. *(Courtesy Harvard Medical Library in the Francis A. Countway Library of Medicine, Boston, MA.)*

**TABLE 1.3** Highlights of African Americans in Dentistry

| | | |
|---|---|---|
| 1765 | Peter Hawkins | Native-born, an itinerant preacher in Richmond, Virginia, did extractions for parishioners. |
| 1851 | John S. Rock | Awarded a silver medal for making artificial teeth. Examples of his work were exhibited by the Benjamin Franklin Institute. |
| 1869 | Robert Tanner Freeman | First African American dentist to receive the DMD degree from Harvard University. |
| 1963 | Andrew Z. Kellar | Published "The Epidemiology of Lip, Oral and Pharyngeal Cancers" in *American Journal of Public Health.* |
| 1967 | Van E. Collins | First African American dentist in regular military service to be promoted to the rank of colonel. |
| 1973 | Konneta Putman | Installed as the president of the American Dental Hygienists Association. |
| 1975 | Jeanne C. Sinkford | First African American female dean of a U.S. dental school. |
| 1989 | Raymond J. Fonseca | Appointed dental dean at the University of Pennsylvania. |
| 1994 | Juliann Bluitt | The first woman dentist elected president of the American College of Dentists. |
| 1994 | Caswell A. Evans | The first African American dentist elected president of the American Public Health Association. |
| | Eugenia Mobley | The first African American woman dentist to earn a degree in public health and the second female dean of a U.S. dental school. |
| | Clifton O. Dummett | Distinguished professor emeritus of the University of Southern California School of Dentistry and author and historian for the National Dental Association. |

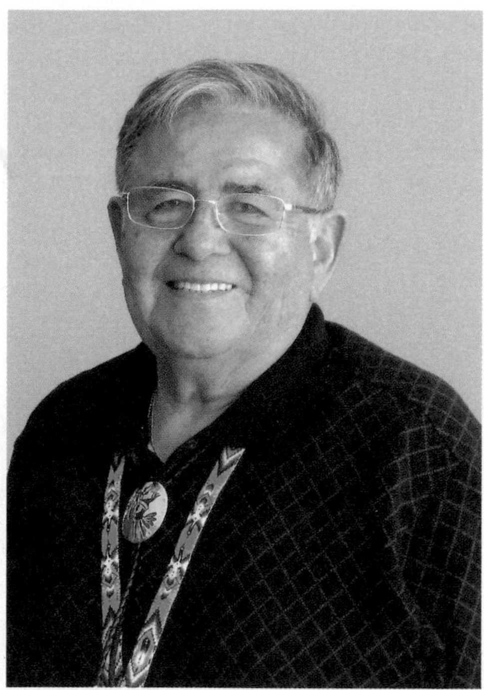

**FIG. 1.12** Dr. George Blue Spruce, Jr. *(Courtesy Dr. George Blue Spruce, Jr.)*

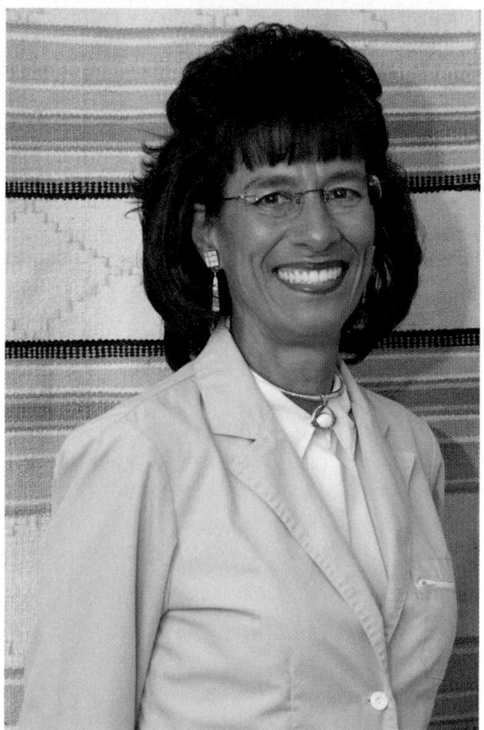

**FIG. 1.13** Dr. Jessica Rickert. *(Courtesy Dr. Jessica Rickert/ William A. Strait Photography.)*

## History of Dental Assisting

**C. Edmund Kells** (1856–1928), a New Orleans dentist, is usually credited with employing the first dental assistant (Fig. 1.14). In 1885 the first "lady assistant" was really a "lady in attendance," who made it respectable for a woman patient to visit a dental office unaccompanied. The assistant helped with office duties, and by 1900 Kells was working with both a chairside dental assistant and a secretarial assistant. Soon other dentists saw the value of dental assistants and began to train dental assistants in their own offices.

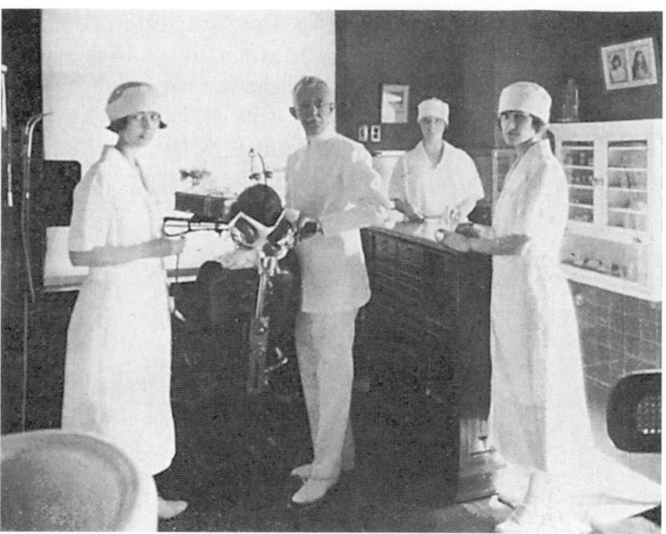

**FIG. 1.14** C. Edmund Kells and his "working unit," about 1900. Assistant on the left is keeping cold air on the cavity, while assistant on the right mixes materials, and "secretary" records details. *(From Kells CE: The dentist's own book, St Louis, 1925, Mosby.)*

In 1930 a curriculum committee was formed to draft courses of training to be used as educational guides. In 1948 the Certifying Board of the American Dental Assistants Association was established (now the Dental Assisting National Board [DANB]). By 1950 one- and two-year programs were available for dental assisting education.

**Hazel O. Torres** and **Ann Ehrlich** forever set the standard for dental assisting textbooks in 1976, when their coauthored *Modern Dental Assisting* became the first major textbook written by dental assistants for dental assistants. Now in its eleventh edition, *Modern Dental Assisting* is the premier international learning system for dental assisting education.

Hazel Torres (Fig. 1.15) described herself as a sponge for knowledge. She began her career as an on-the-job trained dental assistant, continued her education, and later developed and taught in two dental assisting programs at community colleges in California. Among her many contributions to the profession of dental assisting, she was the first dental assistant to serve as a member of the California Board of Dental Examiners and served as a commissioner on the Commission of Dental Accreditation of the American Dental Association. She served as president of the American Dental Assistants Association (ADAA) and was awarded the Lifetime Achievement Award.

Ann Ehrlich (Fig. 1.16) began her career as a "wet-fingered" dental assistant in New Jersey. She had a passion for dental assisting and later completed her master's degree and became an educator and taught dental assisting full time at the University of North Carolina. As a member of the ADAA, for years she assumed an important role in the authoring and publication of the *Journal of the American Dental Assistants Association.* She also served as a consultant to the Dental Assisting National Board.

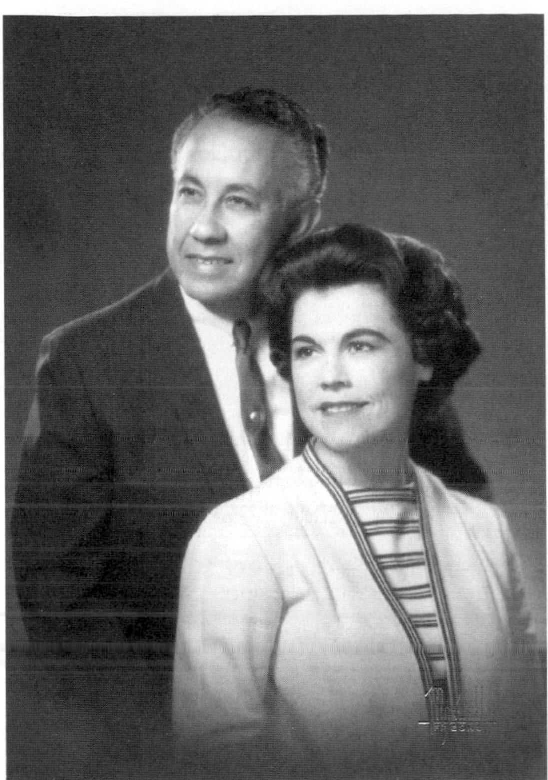

**FIG. 1.15** Hazel O. Torres, CDA, RDAEF, MA, founding coauthor of the *Modern Dental Assisting* textbook, shown here with her husband, Carl.

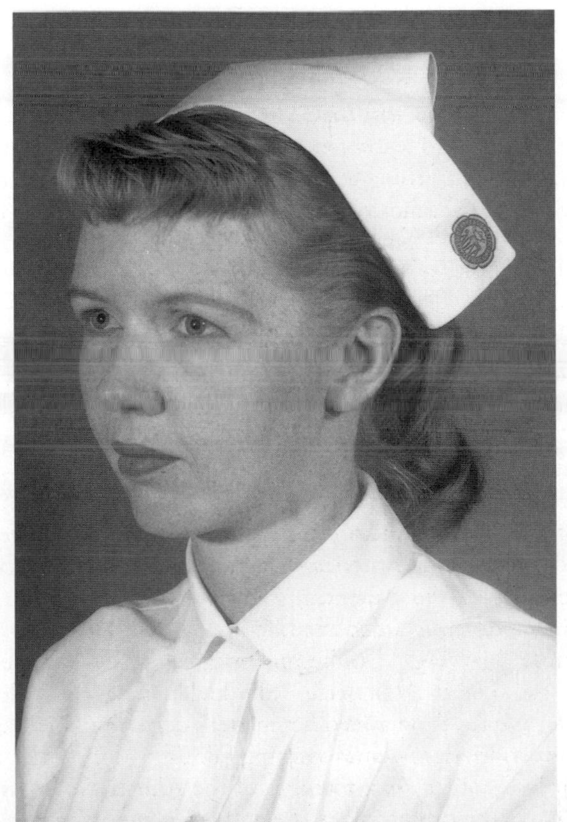

**FIG. 1.16** Ann Ehrlich, CDA, MA, founding coauthor of the *Modern Dental Assisting* textbook.

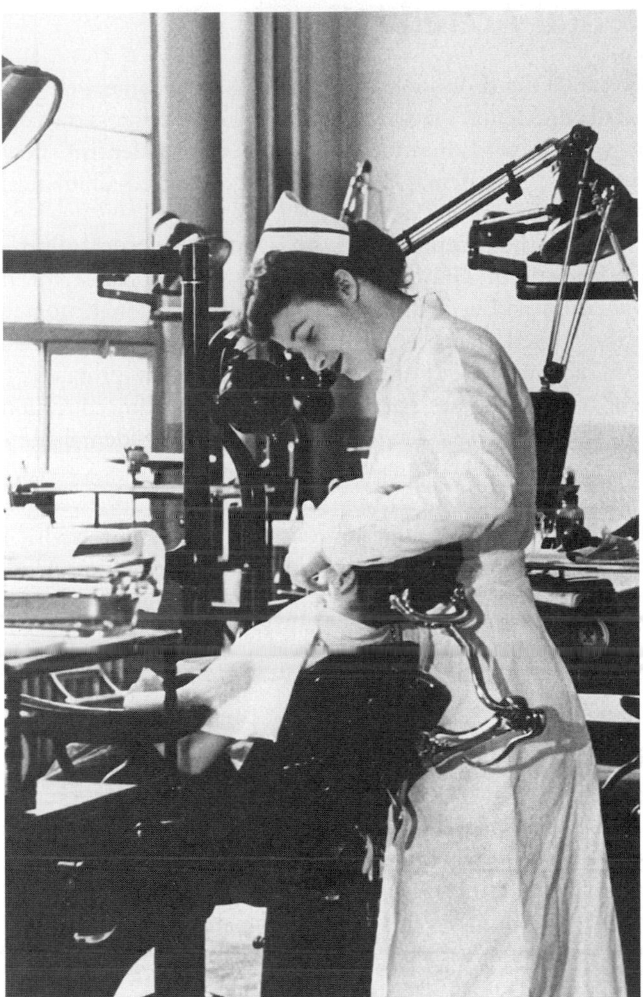

**FIG. 1.17** Dental hygienist during the 1960s working in a standing position. *(Courtesy Fr. Edward J. Dowling, S. J. Marine Historical Collection, University of Detroit, Mercy, Detroit, MI.)*

RECALL

**18** Who was the first African American to graduate from the dental school at Harvard University?

**19** Who was the first African American female dentist in the United States?

**20** Who was the first American Indian dentist in the United States?

## History of Dental Hygiene

The first person to become a dental hygienist was **Irene Newman,** a dental assistant in Bridgeport, Connecticut, in the early 1900s. At that time **Alfred C. Fones,** a dentist, believed that women could be trained to provide preventive services and thus give the dentist time to perform more complex procedures. Dr. Fones trained Irene Newman in dental hygiene and then developed a school for dental hygienists in 1913 (Fig. 1.17). The school exists today in Connecticut as the University of Bridgeport, Fones School of Dental Hygiene.

## Dental Accreditation

By 1900, the profession of dentistry had become well established, and dental schools were being founded across the country (Fig. 1.18). Educational requirements for dentists, dental hygienists, and dental assistants have increased dramatically over the years.

Today, the **Commission on Dental Accreditation of the American Dental Association** is responsible for the evaluation and accreditation of dental educational programs in the United States. These include graduate dental programs, postgraduate specialty programs, and residency programs for dentists. The Commission also sets standards for educational programs in dental assisting, dental hygiene, and dental laboratory technology.

To maintain accreditation status, schools are reviewed every seven years through comprehensive self-study and a visit by members of an accreditation team. The accreditation process provides assurance to students and to the public that the program continues to meet the high standards set forth by the dental profession (Fig. 1.19).

## National Museum of Dentistry

The **Dr. Samuel D. Harris National Museum of Dentistry** is an affiliate of the Smithsonian Institution and is the largest and most comprehensive museum of dentistry in the world. In 2003 it was declared the nation's official dental museum by a joint resolution of the U.S. Congress. The museum is located on the grounds of the Baltimore College of Dental Surgery in Baltimore, Maryland, the world's first dental college. The museum's name honors Dr. Samuel D. Harris, a retired pediatric dentist who in 1992 was instrumental in founding the museum (Fig. 1.20).

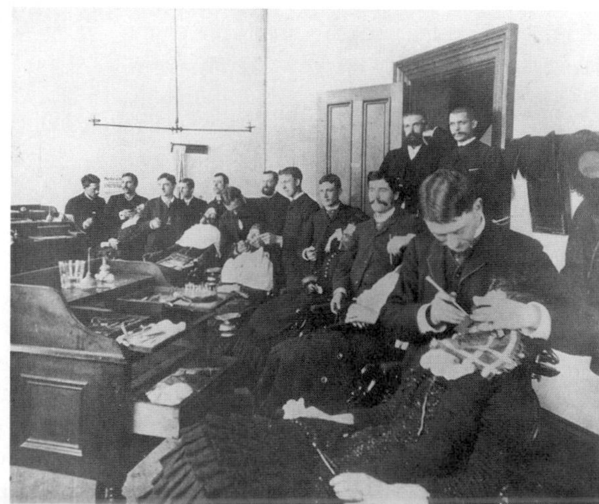

**FIG. 1.18** Dental students at the University of California San Francisco, School of Dentistry, treat patients in the dental clinic in the early 1900s. *(Courtesy School of Dentistry, University of California San Francisco.)*

The museum provides many interactive exhibits, historic artifacts, and engaging educational programs. Visitors learn about the heritage and future of dentistry, achievements of dental professionals, and the importance of oral health in a healthy life. To obtain more information, visit the Web site at www.dental.umaryland.edu/museum/index.html.

RECALL

**21** Who was the first dentist to use a dental assistant?
**22** Who founded dental hygiene education in America?
**23** Where is the Dr. Samuel D. Harris National Museum of Dentistry located?

■ **Legal and Ethical Implications** The public views the profession of dentistry with respect and trust. As important members of the oral healthcare profession, dental assistants should remember the trials and errors, struggles, and contributions made over the years to advance the dental profession.

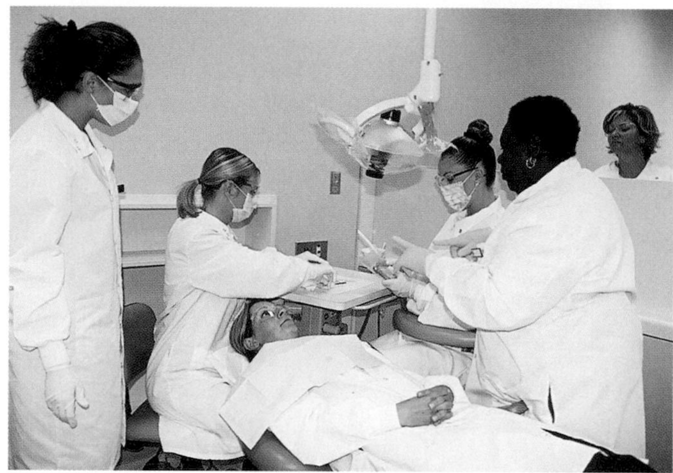

**FIG. 1.19** Modern dental-assisting students practicing chairside skills with their instructor in an accredited dental-assisting program.

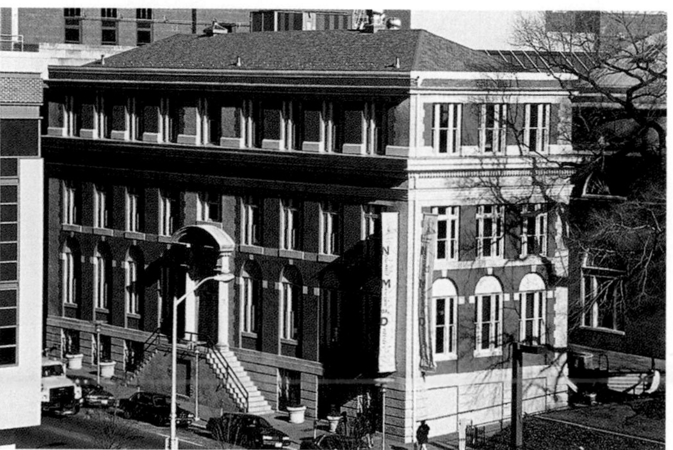

**FIG. 1.20** Dr. Samuel D. Harris National Museum of Dentistry. *(Courtesy National Museum of Dentistry, Baltimore, MD.)*

Remember: to learn, we must stand on the shoulders of those who went before us. ■

## ■ Eye to the Future

**Teledentistry** uses information technology and telecommunications to provide oral healthcare to patients in remote or underserved areas by collaborating with dentists and specialists in other areas. It is also used in providing oral health education and public awareness.

Teledentistry can also be used by general dentists to consult with specialists in other states or other areas of the world. It can also improve services to underserved populations such as in rural or less developed areas.

Dentists, dental hygienists, and dental assistants are equipped with portable imaging equipment and electronic patient record systems, which they use to gather radiographs, photographs, medical histories, and dental charts that are uploaded to a secure Web site where they are reviewed by a dentist or specialist in another location. Teledentistry is especially useful in providing oral healthcare in underserved areas such as geographically remote areas, nursing homes, schools, and facilities for the disabled.

The expanding use of teledentistry makes this an exciting time to be entering the dental healthcare profession. ■

## ■ Critical Thinking

1. What would you say to a 50-year-old patient who was reluctant to come to the dentist because of his negative experiences in the dental office as a child?
2. What would you tell the mother of a child who believes dental decay began when soft drinks and candy were discovered?
3. Who can serve as historic role models for young women today who face any type of discrimination in their career choices?
4. What would you say to someone who does not understand why you are studying the history of dentistry?
5. Do you think that the Hippocratic Oath is important today? Why? ■

2

# The Professional Dental Assistant

## KEY TERMS

**American Dental Assistants Association (ADAA)** Professional organization that represents the profession of dental assisting on a national level.

**Certified dental assistant (CDA)** The nationally recognized credential of the dental assistant who has passed the DANB certification examination and keeps current in practice through continuing education.

**Dental Assisting National Board (DANB)** National agency responsible for administering the certification examination and issuing the credential of certified dental assistant.

**HIPAA** The Health Insurance Portability and Accountability Act of 1996 specifies federal regulations that ensure privacy regarding a patient's healthcare information.

**Professional** Person who meets the standards of a profession.

## LEARNING OUTCOMES

*On completion of this chapter, the student will be able to achieve the following objectives:*

1 Pronounce, define, and spell the key terms.

2 Describe and demonstrate the characteristics of a professional dental assistant, including the following:
- Explain why confidentiality is very important in a dental office.
- Identify the purpose of the Health Insurance Portability and Accountability Act of 1996 (HIPAA).

3 Identify the educational requirements and career opportunities for the educationally qualified dental assistant.

4 Explain the role and purpose of the American Dental Assistants Association (ADAA) and the Dental Assisting National Board (DANB), including benefits of membership and certification.

## ELECTRONIC RESOURCES

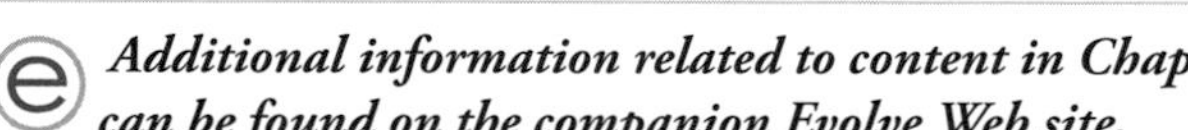
***Additional information related to content in Chapter 2 can be found on the companion Evolve Web site.***

- Practice Quiz
- Canadian Content Corner

A highly skilled dental assistant is a vital member of the dental healthcare team. Reducing patient anxiety, making decisions, simplifying treatment procedures, maintaining appropriate infection control measures, and improving the quality of patient care are all part of a dental assistant's day (Fig. 2.1).

You chose an exciting and challenging career when you decided to become a professional dental assistant. A career in dental assisting offers variety, job satisfaction, opportunity for service, and financial reward. It is a career that requires dedication, personal responsibility, integrity, and a commitment to continuing education.

## Characteristics of a Professional Dental Assistant

Becoming a dental assistant involves more than acquiring the knowledge and developing the skills necessary to perform a variety of duties. Becoming a dental assistant is about becoming a **professional**.

*Professionalism* is an attitude that is apparent in everything you do and say, in and out of the dental office. Professionalism is what distinguishes people who "have a job" from those who "pursue a career." The public's expectations of healthcare workers are higher than expectations of individuals in other occupations. The dental assistant must demonstrate patience and compassion when communicating with patients and other team members. When you demonstrate your professionalism, you receive respect and acknowledgment from your colleagues and patients as a valued member of the dental healthcare team.

### Professional Appearance

A dental assistant's professional appearance promotes the patient's confidence in the entire office and improves his or her dental experience. The essential aspects of a professional

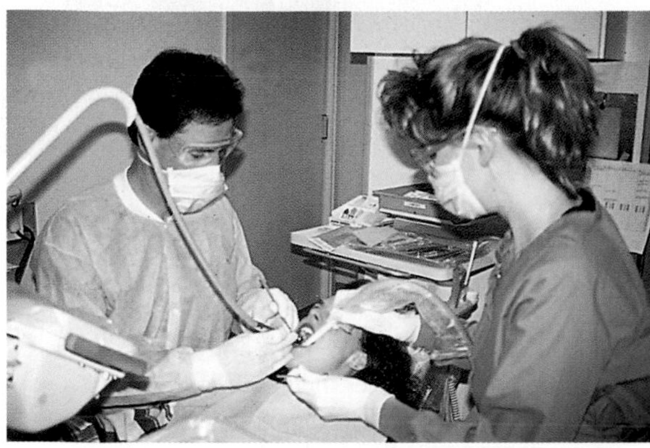

FIG. 2.1 The dental assistant is an important member of the dental healthcare team.

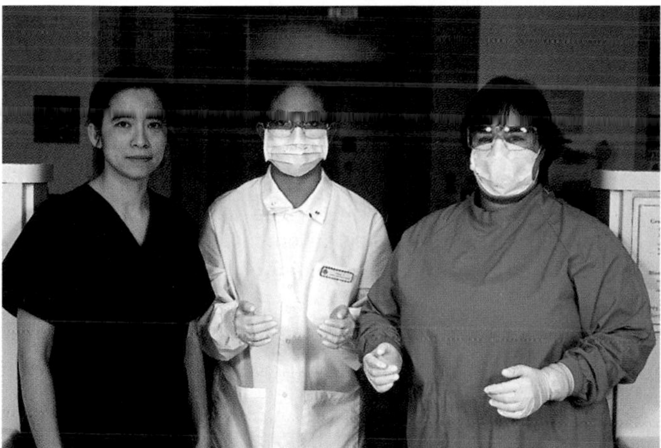

FIG. 2.2 The professional dental assistant's attire may vary depending on the duties performed. *Left,* Scrubs are acceptable at times. *Center,* Full personal protective wear is indicated for chairside procedures. *Right,* Surgical gowns may be indicated for surgery or hospital dentistry.

appearance include (1) good health, (2) good grooming, and (3) appropriate dress.

To stay in *good health,* you must get an adequate amount of rest, eat well-balanced meals, and exercise enough to keep fit. Dental assisting is a physically demanding profession.

*Good grooming* requires paying attention to the details of your personal appearance. Personal cleanliness involves taking a daily bath or shower, using a deodorant, and practicing good oral hygiene. Do not use perfume or cologne. You are working in very close personal proximity to coworkers and patients, who may be allergic to or irritated by some scents. Avoid the use of tobacco products because the odor lingers on your hair and clothing and is offensive to many patients and dental team members.

*Appropriate dress* involves wearing clothing appropriate for the type of position in which the dental assistant is working (see Chapter 3). Regardless of the type of professional wear, it must be clean, wrinkle free, and worn over appropriate undergarments (Fig. 2.2). In any dental position, excessive makeup and jewelry are not considered appropriate for a professional appearance. Infection control requirements must also be considered when one is selecting clinical wear (see Chapter 19).

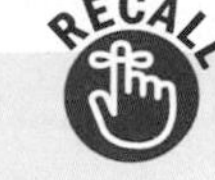


1 How can a dental assistant demonstrate "professionalism"?
2 Name the three essential aspects of a professional appearance.

## Knowledge and Skills

Depending on the type of dental practice, the duties of a dental assistant will vary. Ideally, dental assistants should have both front desk and chairside (clinical) skills. This is very convenient when a team member is absent from the office. Generally, dental assistants choose to stay in the position they prefer. Regardless of the type of dental practice, the day of a dental assistant is never boring or "routine."

### Guidelines for a Professional Appearance

- Uniform or scrubs should be clean, pressed, and in good repair*
- Shoes and laces should be clean and in good condition*
- Hair should be styled so that it stays out of your face*
- Jewelry should be avoided*
- Fingernails should be clean and short*
- Artificial fingernails should not be worn; they can harbor bacteria*
- Perfumes and body scents should not be worn
- Tobacco products should not be used
- Makeup should be subtle and natural
- Avoid visible tattoos, body piercings, bright fingernail polish, and extreme hairdos
- Bathe each day and use deodorant
- Maintain good oral hygiene

*Special implications for infection control and prevention of disease transmission.

## Teamwork

Teamwork is extremely important in a dental office. The letters in the word *team* mean that "***T***ogether, ***E***veryone ***A***ccomplishes ***M***ore." Dental assistants should offer to do an absent colleague's work and should be willing to help coworkers when other tasks are completed. When several assistants work in an office, each should be able and willing to substitute for the others in an emergency.

## Attitude

Patients, coworkers, and employers appreciate the dental assistant who has a good attitude. It is important for the dental assistant to show a willingness to get along by avoiding gossiping or criticizing others. It is important to show appreciation for what others have done and to be willing to pitch in and help. The dental office can be a stressful place for patients and staff, so it is important to maintain a positive attitude.

## Dedication

Professional dental assistants are dedicated to their dental practice, their patients, and the profession of dental assisting. Dedication is possible only if the assistant truly cares for people, is empathetic to their needs, and maintains a positive attitude.

## Responsibility and Initiative

The dental assistant can demonstrate work responsibility by (1) arriving on time, (2) staying for the full shift, (3) being a cooperative team member, and (4) not asking to leave early. Assistants should understand what is expected of them regularly and, if time permits, should volunteer to help others who may be overworked.

You can show a willingness to learn additional skills by asking questions and observing others. Show initiative by finding tasks to perform without being asked. Show responsibility by calling the office when you are ill or unavoidably late. Do *not* discuss your personal problems in the dental office with your patients or with other staff members.

**3** How can you demonstrate that you are a responsible person?

## Confidentiality

*Everything* that is said or done in the dental office must remain confidential. Dental assistants have access to a vast amount of personal and financial information about their patients. Such information must be held in strict confidence and must not be discussed with others. Breaches of confidentiality can result in lawsuits against all parties involved.

You cannot reveal the identity of a patient or any information from his or her records without the patient's written consent. *Never* discuss patients with anyone outside the dental office.

**HIPAA** (Health Insurance Portability and Accountability Act of 1996) is a set of federal privacy laws. These laws apply to all types of healthcare providers regarding methods that must be used to ensure that patient privacy is protected while health information is shared among healthcare providers. You will learn the details of these laws in Chapter 63.

## Personal Qualities

Many people do not enjoy a visit to the dentist and they are often stressed or intimidated by being in the dental office. The dental assistant must (1) demonstrate sensitivity to the patient's needs, (2) show empathy, (3) say "the right thing at the right time," and (4) *be sincere.*

Never discuss aspects of your personal life with your patients. By learning to be a good listener, you will develop sensitivity to the opinions and concerns of others. It is nearly impossible to build *rapport* (good relations) with patients in your office if they do not trust you.

# Educational Requirements

## Types of Programs

Dental assistants can receive their formal education through various types of programs. These include academic programs at community colleges, vocational schools, career colleges, technical institutes, universities, and dental schools. Most academic programs require 8 to 11 months to complete. Some schools offer accelerated programs, part-time programs, or training via distance education. Graduates of these programs usually receive certificates.

# Career Opportunities

## Employment Settings

Today, many dentists employ two or more dental assistants. Employment opportunities for dental assistants are excellent. The types of practice settings available to dental assistants include the following:

- Solo practice (practices with only one dentist)
- Group practice (practices with two or more dentists)
- Specialty practices (such as orthodontics, oral surgery, endodontics, periodontics, and pediatric dentistry)
- Office managers
- Financial coordinators
- Scheduling coordinators
- Public health dentistry (settings such as schools and clinics)
- Hospital dental clinics
- Dental school clinics

## Other Career Opportunities

In addition to assisting in the delivery of dental care, other excellent career opportunities are available for dental assistants. These opportunities include the following:

- Insurance company workers, processing dental insurance claims
- Teachers, teaching dental assisting in vocational schools, technical institutes, community colleges, dental schools, and universities (some may require associate or baccalaureate college degrees)
- Dental product sales representatives

## Salaries

The salary of a dental assistant depends primarily on the skills and abilities of the individual and the responsibility associated with the specific position. Earning potential can also be influenced by the geographic location of the place of employment.

Generally, dental assistants earn salaries equal to those of other healthcare professionals with similar training and experience, such as medical assistants, physical therapy assistants, occupational therapy assistants, veterinary technicians, and pharmacy technicians.

# Professional Organizations

## American Dental Assistants Association

The **American Dental Assistants Association (ADAA)** is the organization that represents the profession of dental assisting. The ADAA was formed in 1924 by **Juliette A. Southard** (Fig. 2.3). Her vision was of "an educated, efficient dental assistant with her own place in the profession of dentistry."

The ADAA is a national nonprofit corporation based in Bloomingdale, Illinois. Membership is *tripartite,* which means that when you join the ADAA, you become a member of (1) the state component, (2) the local component, and (3) the national organization (Fig. 2.4). By becoming a member of the ADAA, dental assistants can be proactive and take leadership positions within organized dentistry and the healthcare profession.

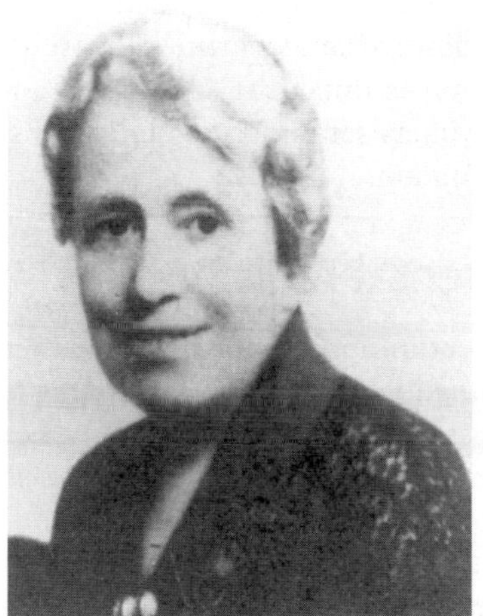

FIG. 2.3 Juliette A. Southard, founder of the American Dental Assistants Association (ADAA). *(Courtesy ADAA, Chicago, IL.)*

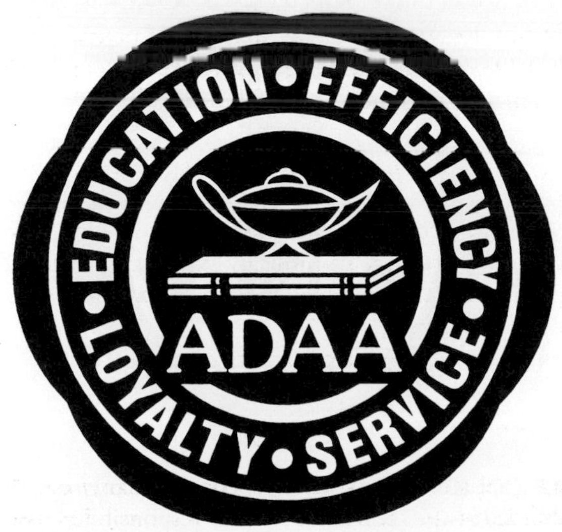


FIG. 2.4 The seal of the American Dental Assistants Association (ADAA). *(Courtesy ADAA, Chicago, IL.)*

### Benefits of Membership

By joining the ADAA, you can grow personally and professionally and keep abreast of legislative issues and current information. ADAA members have the opportunity to attend local, state, and national meetings, where they can participate in workshops, earn continuing education credit, hear prominent speakers, and establish lifelong friendships with other dental assistants.

Other benefits of membership include a subscription to *The Dental Assistant,* the journal of the ADAA; professional liability, accidental death and dismemberment, and medical insurance options; awards and scholarship opportunities; credit card options; and other discounts. Student membership is available for those enrolled in formal training programs.

Participating in ADAA activities enhances "people skills" and teaches leadership. You can influence the future of your profession and show that you are serious about your career.

### Many Roles of Dental Assistants

**Chairside Dental Assistant**

Works directly with the dentist in the treatment area. Primary responsibilities in this role include, but are not limited to, the following:

- Seating and preparing for patients
- Charting
- Instituting infection control procedures
- Mixing and passing dental materials
- Assisting the dentist during procedures
- Ensuring patient comfort
- Exposing and processing radiographs
- Pouring and trimming models, as well as performing other laboratory procedures
- Providing patient education
- Providing postoperative instructions to patients
- Overseeing inventory control and ordering dental supplies
- Ensuring compliance with regulations of the Occupational Safety and Health Administration (OSHA)

**Expanded-Functions Dental Assistant**

Delegation of the following functions varies among states, depending on the individual state's or province's Dental Practice Act:

- Placing dental sealants
- Taking impressions
- Fabricating temporary crowns and bridges
- Placing retraction cord
- Applying fluoride
- Applying topical anesthetic
- Placing and removing dental dams
- Placing and removing matrices and wedges
- Applying liners, varnishes, and bases
- Placing, carving, and finishing amalgam or composite restorations

*Continued*

- Removing sutures
- Placing and removing periodontal dressings
- Performing additional functions as specified in the Dental Practice Act of the state in which the dental assistant is employed

It is important to be aware of the laws of the state, province, or territory in which you practice.

**Administrative Assistant**

Also known as the *secretarial assistant, business assistant,* or *receptionist.* The administrative assistant is responsible for the efficient operation of the business office and performs the following duties:

- Greeting patients and answering the phone
- Scheduling patient visits
- Managing patient records
- Managing accounts receivable and accounts payable
- Managing the recall system
- Maintaining privacy of patient information
- Overseeing and monitoring practice marketing activities

## Check Your Personal Qualities as a Dental Assistant

- How do I interact with patients?
- Am I friendly? Do I have a pleasant attitude?
- Do I listen more than I talk?
- Am I courteous?
- Am I considerate, respectful, and kind?
- Do I control my temper?
- Do I try to see the other person's point of view?
- Am I responsible?
- Am I dependable?
- Am I attentive to details?
- Am I calm in an emergency?
- Am I responsible for my own actions?
- Do I tend to blame others or find fault with others?
- Do I offer to help others without being asked?
- Do I avoid office gossip?

## Mission Statement of the American Dental Assistants Association (ADAA)

To advance the careers of dental assistants and to promote the dental-assisting profession in matters of education, legislation, credentialing, and professional activities that enhance the delivery of quality dental healthcare to the public.

## Where to Obtain More Information: ADAA

American Dental Assistants Association
140 North Bloomingdale Road
Bloomingdale, IL 60108-1017
Phone: 630-994-4247
Toll Free: 877-874-3785
Fax: 630-351-8490
www.dentalassistant.org

4 What is the purpose of the ADAA?
5 What are some benefits of being a member of the ADAA?

## Dental Assisting National Board

The **Dental Assisting National Board (DANB)** is the nationally recognized agency responsible for testing dental assistants and issuing the credential of **Certified Dental Assistant™ (CDA®)**. The American Dental Association recognizes DANB as the national certifying board for dental assistants. Certification is voluntary and is not mandatory in all states, although some states require a dental assistant to be a CDA certificant to legally perform specific "expanded functions" within the state.

By earning DANB certification, dental assistants demonstrate their commitment to excellence. In addition, a CDA certificant in the dental office promotes the image of professionalism.

For dental assistants or dental hygienists to be permitted to teach in a Commission on Dental Accreditation (CODA)-accredited dental assisting program, they must be currently certified by DANB. Unless the dental assisting program administrator/director is a dentist, he or she must also hold CDA certification to direct the educational program.

DANB also offers state-specific dental assisting expanded-function examinations.

## Certified Dental Assistant

To earn CDA certification, an assistant must take and pass a national examination that is developed and administered by DANB. Successful completion of the DANB examination and annual certification renewal entitles the assistant to use the CDA credential, wear the official certification pin (Fig. 2.5), and display the CDA certificate.

DANB offers five national certifications: **Certified Dental Assistant™ (CDA®), Certified Orthodontic Assistant (COA®), National Entry Level Dental Assistant (NELDA®),**

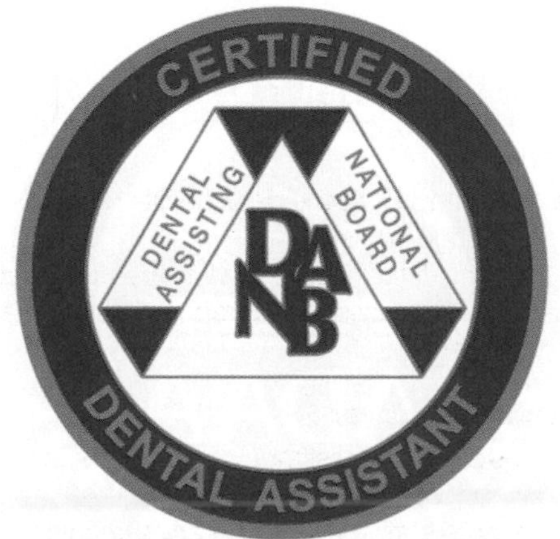


**FIG. 2.5** Official DANB CDA Pin Design. *(Courtesy DANB, Chicago, IL.)*

**Certified Restorative Functions Dental Assistant (CRFDA®)** and **Certified Preventive Functions Dental Assistant (CPFDA®).** DANB offers the option to take any of its certification examinations and the component exams comprising the certification exam by computer at secure, proctored test sites around the United States.

**CERTIFIED DENTAL ASSISTANT (CDA) EXAMINATION.** The CDA examination contains three separate component exams: General Chairside Assisting (GC), Radiation Health and Safety (RHS®), and Infection Control (ICE®).

**CERTIFIED ORTHODONTIC ASSISTANT (COA) EXAMINATION.** The COA examination contains two separate component exams: Orthodontic Assisting (OA) and Infection Control (ICE).

**NATIONAL ENTRY LEVEL DENTAL ASSISTANT (NELDA) EXAMINATION.** The NELDA examination consists of three component exams: Radiation Health and Safety (RHS), Infection Control (ICE), and Anatomy, Morphology and Physiology (AMP).

**CERTIFIED RESTORATIVE FUNCTIONS DENTAL ASSISTANT (CRFDA) EXAMINATION.** The CRFDA examination consists of six component exams: Anatomy, Morphology and Physiology (AMP), Impressions (IM), Temporaries (TPM), Isolation (IS), Sealants (SE), and Restorative Functions (RF).

**CERTIFIED PREVENTIVE FUNCTIONS DENTAL ASSISTANT (CPFDA).** The CPFDA examination consists of four component exams: Coronal Polish (CP), Sealants (SE), Topical Anesthetic (TA), and Topical Fluoride (TF).

### Where to Obtain More Information: DANB

Dental Assisting National Board
444 N. Michigan Avenue, Suite 900
Chicago, IL 60611
Phone: 800-FOR-DANB or 312-642-3368
Fax: 312-642-8507
www.danb.org

### Benefits of DANB Certification

**For the Patient**

- Provides assurance that the dental assistant has the necessary knowledge and skills
- Strengthens a patient's confidence in the dental team
- Enhances the dental assistant's reputation regarding delivery of quality services

**For the Dentist-Employer**

- Provides a level of professionalism that is beneficial to the practice
- CDA certificants stay in the field nearly three times as long as noncertified dental assistants
- Some states allow CDA certificants to perform expanded duties

**For the Dental Assistant**

- Certification provides a sense of personal achievement
- Promotes the dental assistant's professional pride
- Demonstrates a commitment to excellence and lifelong learning
- Provides greater earning power and job satisfaction. DANB certificants earn nearly $2 more per hour than dental assistants who are not certified
- Provides career advancement because DANB is recognized or required by 39 states, the District of Columbia, the U.S. Air Force and the Department of Veterans Affairs

*CDA®, COA®, NELDA®, CFRDA®, and CPFDA® are registered certification marks of the Dental Assisting National Board, Inc. (DANB). ICE®, and RHS® are registered service marks of DANB. The pin design is a registered trademark of DANB. This publication is not affiliated with or endorsed or reviewed by DANB.*

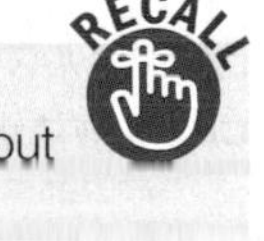


6 Which credentials are issued by the DANB?
7 Where can you obtain additional information about the DANB examinations?

## ■ Eye to the Future

Increased demand for dental care and a shortage of dental professionals have created many opportunities for qualified dental assistants. The current demand for educationally qualified dental assistants is at an all-time high. Employment opportunities are abundant and extremely varied. The future is promising and challenging for the educationally qualified dental assistant.

Visit the ADAA Web page and the DANB Web page to enhance your knowledge and pride in your chosen profession. ■

## ■ Critical Thinking

1. Imagine yourself as a nervous dental patient entering the dental office to have your wisdom teeth extracted. The dental assistant who greets you has long red artificial fingernails, dangling earrings, a tattoo on her arm, and long hair hanging over her shoulders. What is your first impression of the office and the dentist?
2. Dr. Wong is interviewing two dental assistants for a chairside position in his new office. Both are recent graduates of a local dental-assisting program. Both seem capable, but only one is a CDA and a member of the ADAA. Who do you think Dr. Wong would prefer to hire? Why?
3. While you and a friend are having lunch at a local restaurant, you remember an embarrassing but funny event that happened to a patient in your dental office. You want to share this story, but do you? Why or why not?
4. Do you have a preference for administrative or clinical duties? Why?
5. Sylvia, a dental assistant in your office, is always the first one out the door at 5:00 PM. You always stay and finish up, but you are becoming very tired of Sylvia's irresponsible behavior. How do you handle this situation? ■

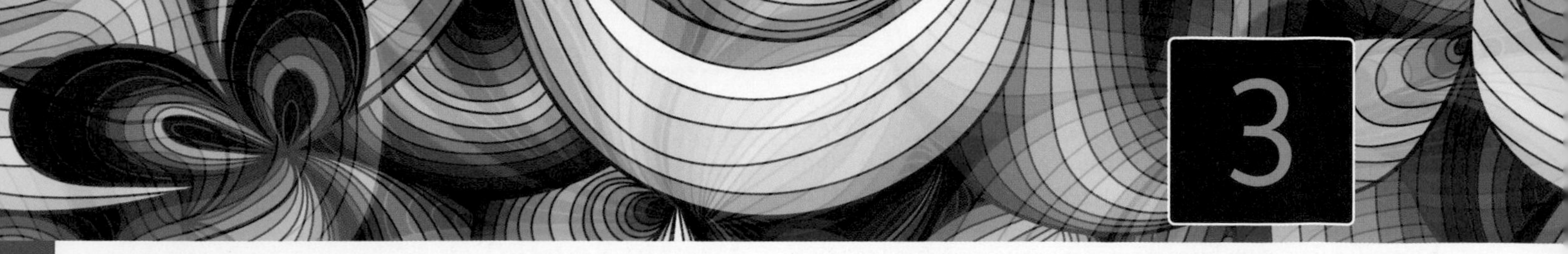

3

# The Dental Healthcare Team

## KEY TERMS

**Certified dental technician (CDT)** A dental laboratory technician who has passed a written national examination and who performs dental laboratory services such as fabricating crowns, bridges, and dentures, as specified by the dentist's written prescription.
**Dental assistant** Oral healthcare professional trained to provide supportive procedures for the dentist and for patients.
**Dental equipment technician** Specialist who installs and maintains dental equipment.
**Dental hygienist (hy-JEN-ist)** Licensed oral healthcare professional who provides preventive, therapeutic, and educational services.
**Dental laboratory technician** Professional who performs dental laboratory services such as fabricating crowns, bridges, and dentures, as specified by the dentist's written prescription. Most frequently trained on the job as an apprentice.
**Dental public health** Specialty that promotes oral health through organized community efforts.
**Dental spa** Dental practices that offer many services not normally associated with dental carefacials, paraffin wax hand treatment, reflexology, micro-dermabrasion, massage therapy, and many other pampering, therapeutic, and rejuvenation offerings.
**Dental supply person** Representative of a dental supply company who provides dental supplies, product information, services, and repairs.
**Dentist** Oral healthcare provider licensed to practice dentistry.
**Detail person** Representative of a specific company who provides information concerning the company's product.
**Endodontics (en-do-DON-tiks)** Dental specialty that diagnoses and treats diseases of the pulp.
**Oral and maxillofacial radiology (ray-dee-OL-o-jee)** Dental specialty that deals with the diagnosis of disease through various forms of imaging, including x-ray films (radiographs).
**Oral and maxillofacial (mak-sil-oe-FAY-shul) surgery** Dental surgical specialty that diagnoses and treats conditions of the mouth, face, upper jaw (maxilla), and associated areas.
**Oral pathology (puh-THOL-uh-jee)** Dental specialty that diagnoses and treats diseases of the oral structures.
**Orthodontics (or-thoe-DON-tiks)** Specialty within dentistry that focuses on preventing, intercepting, and correcting skeletal and dental problems.
**Pediatric (pee-dee-AT-rik) dentistry** Dental specialty concerned with neonatal through adolescent patients, as well as patients with special needs in these age groups.
**Periodontics (per-ee-oe-DON-tiks)** Dental specialty involved with the diagnosis and treatment of diseases of the supporting tissues.
**Prosthodontics (pros-thoe-DON-tiks)** Dental specialty that provides restoration and replacement of natural teeth.

## LEARNING OUTCOMES

*On completion of this chapter, the student will be able to achieve the following objectives:*

1. Pronounce, define, and spell the key terms.
2. List the members of the dental healthcare team and explain their roles, including the following:
   - Identify the minimal educational requirements for each member of the dental healthcare team.
   - Name and describe the nine dental specialties recognized by the American Dental Association (ADA).
   - Describe the various job opportunities and responsibilities that are available to a qualified dental assistant.

## ELECTRONIC RESOURCES

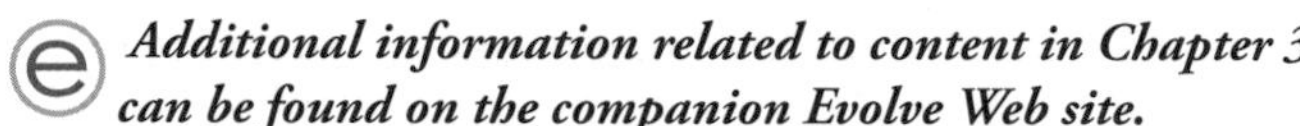

***Additional information related to content in Chapter 3 can be found on the companion Evolve Web site.***

- Practice Quiz
- Canadian Content Corner

The goal of the dental healthcare team is to provide quality oral healthcare for patients in the practice. The **dentist** is the individual who is legally responsible for the care of patients and the supervision of all other members of the team. Because of this, the dentist is often referred to as the leader of the team.

The dental healthcare team consists of the following:

- Dentist (general dentist or specialist)
- Dental assistant (clinical, expanded-functions, business)
- Dental hygienist
- Dental laboratory technician

## Dentist

Dentists trained in the United States must graduate from a dental university approved by the Commission on Dental

Accreditation of the American Dental Association (ADA). Most dentists have attained an undergraduate degree before they are admitted to a dental university. Dental education programs usually last 4 academic years. On graduation, the dentist must successfully pass the written National Board Dental Examination (NBDE) and a state-specific clinical examination to obtain a license to practice dentistry in a particular state.

Training in the dental university includes dental sciences and intensive clinical practice on patients in the university's clinic. When dentists graduate from a dental university, they are awarded the *Doctor of Dental Surgery* (DDS) or the *Doctor of Medical Dentistry* (DMD), depending on which dental school they attended. Before going into practice, all dentists must pass a *written* national board examination. Dentists are then required to take a *clinical* board examination in the state or region in which they choose to practice.

Dentists have a variety of practice options available to them. Some will choose to practice alone, some may choose to have a practice partner, and others may enter a large group practice. Other options for dentists include the military, public health, community clinics, research, teaching, or returning to school for specialty training.

Although a general dentist is trained and is legally permitted to perform all dental functions, many dentists prefer to refer more difficult cases to specialists who have advanced training in certain areas. Most dentists are members of their professional organization, the *American Dental Association (ADA).*

## Dental Specialist

The ADA recognizes nine dental specialties. Depending on the type of specialty, additional education required to become a specialist takes from 2 to 6 years to complete. Most dentists who are specialists belong to a professional organization created for their specialty, in addition to maintaining membership in the ADA.

1 Name the members of the dental healthcare team.
2 Name the nine dental specialties.

## Registered Dental Hygienist

Generally, a *registered dental hygienist (RDH)* removes deposits on the teeth, exposes radiographs, places topical fluoride and dental sealants, and provides patients with home care instructions (Fig. 3.1). Duties delegated to the **dental hygienist** vary from state to state. In many states, dental hygienists are allowed to administer local anesthesia. It is important for

### Roles and Responsibilities of Dental Healthcare Team Members

**Dentist or Dental Specialist**

- Is legally responsible for the care of the patient
- Assesses the patient's oral health needs as related to physical and emotional well-being
- Uses up-to-date diagnostic skills
- Uses current techniques and skills in all aspects of patient care
- Provides legally required supervision for dental auxiliaries

**Clinical Dental Assistant (Chairside Assistant, Circulating Assistant)**

- Seats and prepares patients
- Maintains and prepares treatment rooms and instruments
- Assists dentist at chairside during patient treatment
- Prepares and delivers dental materials
- Provides postoperative patient instructions
- Oversees infection control program
- Performs radiographic procedures
- Performs basic laboratory procedures (e.g., pouring impressions to create diagnostic casts)
- Provides assurance and support for the patient
- Ensures that patient privacy measures are followed

**Expanded-Functions Dental Assistant (EFDA)**

- Performs only those intraoral (inside mouth) procedures that are legal in the state in which the EFDA practices
- Check with your state board of dentistry for a current listing of dental assistant duties

**Dental Hygienist**

- Assesses the periodontal status of patients, including measurement of the depth of periodontal pockets and assessment of conditions of the oral tissues
- Performs dental prophylaxis (e.g., removal of plaque from crowns and root surfaces)
- Performs scaling and root-planing procedures
- Exposes, processes, and evaluates the quality of radiographs
- Performs additional procedures, such as administration of local anesthetic and administration of nitrous oxide if allowed by the state

**Business Assistant (Administrative Assistant, Secretarial Assistant, Receptionist)**

- Greets patients and answers the phone
- Makes and confirms appointments
- Manages patient records, payroll, insurance billing, and financial arrangements
- Ensures that patient privacy measures are in place and followed
- Oversees patient relations

**Dental Laboratory Technician**

- Performs laboratory work only under the licensed dentist's prescription
- Constructs and repairs prosthetic devices (e.g., full and partial dentures)
- Constructs restorations (e.g., crowns, bridges, inlays, veneers)

## Dental Specialties Recognized by the American Dental Association

Dental public health involves development of policies at county, state, and national levels for programs to control and prevent disease. Examples include dental public health professionals involved with community fluoridation issues, community oral health education, and Head Start programs. Dental public health also includes dental screenings within a community to assess the needs of the community. In dental public health, the community, rather than the individual, is the patient. For additional information, contact the American Association of Public Health Dentistry (www.aaphd.org).

Endodontics involves the cause, diagnosis, prevention, and treatment of diseases and injuries to the pulp and associated structures. The common term for much of the treatment is *root canal.* The specialist is an *endodontist* (see Chapter 54). For additional information, contact the American Association of Endodontics (www.aae.org).

Oral and maxillofacial radiology became the first new dental specialty in 36 years when it was granted recognition by the American Dental Association (ADA) in 1999. The *dental radiologist* uses new and sophisticated imaging techniques to locate tumors and infectious diseases of the jaws, head, and neck, and assists in the diagnosis of patients with trauma and temporomandibular disorders (see Chapter 42). For additional information, contact the American Academy of Oral and Maxillofacial Radiology (www.aaomr.org).

Oral and maxillofacial surgery involves the diagnosis and surgical treatment of diseases, injuries, and defects of the oral and maxillofacial regions. It consists of much more than tooth extractions. The specialist is an *oral and maxillofacial surgeon* (see Chapter 56). For additional information, contact the American Association of Oral and Maxillofacial Surgeons (www.aaoms.org).

Oral pathology involves examination of the nature of diseases that affect the oral cavity and adjacent structures. A major function is to perform biopsies and work closely with oral surgeons to provide a diagnosis. The specialist is an *oral pathologist* (see Chapter 17). For additional information, contact the American Academy of Oral and Maxillofacial Pathology (www.aaomp@b-online.com).

Orthodontics involves the diagnosis, treatment, and prevention of malocclusions of the teeth and associated structures. This specialty entails much more than fitting of braces. The specialist is an *orthodontist* (see Chapter 60). For additional information, contact the American Association of Orthodontists (www.aaortho.org).

Pediatric dentistry involves the oral healthcare of children from birth to adolescence. The *pediatric dentist* often treats children with emotional and behavioral problems (see Chapter 57). For additional information, contact the American Academy of Pediatric Dentistry (www.aapd.org).

Periodontics involves the diagnosis and treatment of diseases of the oral tissues that support and surround the teeth. The specialist is a *periodontist* (see Chapter 55). For additional information, contact the American Academy of Periodontology (www.perio.org).

Prosthodontics involves the restoration and replacement of natural teeth with artificial constructs such as crowns, bridges, and dentures. The specialist is a *prosthodontist* (see Chapters 50, 52, and 53). For additional information, contact the American College of Prosthodontists (www.prosthodontists.org).

dental hygienists to have a thorough understanding of the laws of the state, province, or territory in which they practice. Employment opportunities for dental hygienists are found in private and specialty dental offices, health clinics, school systems, research facilities, public health departments, and educational programs, as well as in the marketing and sales of dental products.

The minimal education required for a registered dental hygienist is 2 academic years of college study and an associate's degree in an ADA-accredited dental hygiene program. Dental hygiene is also offered in bachelor's and master's degree programs.

The RDH must pass both written national or regional board examinations and clinical state board examinations to be licensed by the state in which he or she plans to practice. In most states, the RDH is required to work under the supervision of a licensed dentist.

Dental hygienists may be members of their professional organization, the *American Dental Hygienists Association (ADHA).* For additional information on dental hygiene, visit the Web site at http://www.adha.org.

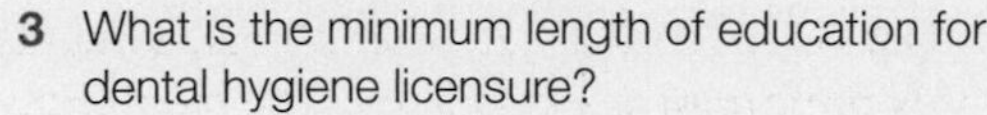

**3** What is the minimum length of education for dental hygiene licensure?

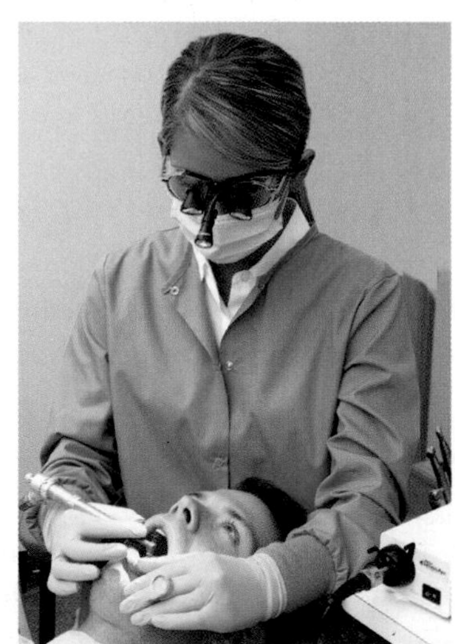

**FIG. 3.1** Dental hygienist performing an oral prophylaxis. *(From Darby M, Walsh M: Dental hygiene: theory and practice, ed 4, St Louis, 2015, Elsevier.)*

## Dental Assistant

An educationally qualified **dental assistant** is able to assume many activities that do not require the professional skill and judgment of the dentist. However, responsibilities assigned to

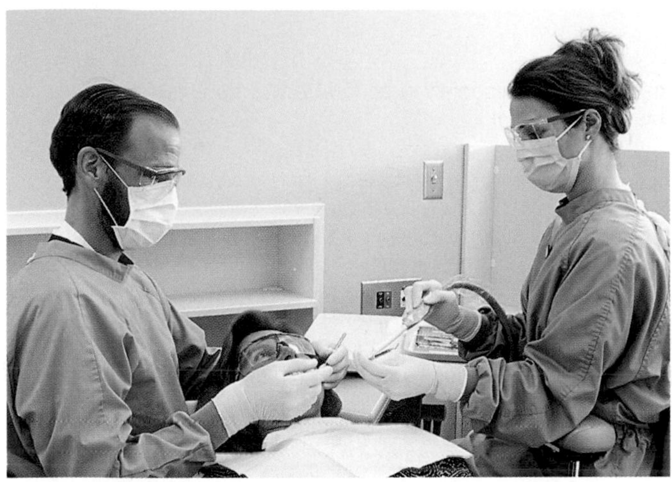

FIG. 3.2 Dentist and chairside dental assistant working together.

a dental assistant are limited by the regulations of the Dental Practice Act of the state in which the practice is located (see Chapter 5).

Although not all states require formal education for dental assistants, minimal standards for schools accredited by the Commission on Dental Accreditation require a program of approximately 1 academic year in length, conducted in a post–high school educational institution. The curriculum must include didactic, laboratory, and clinical content. Dental assistants may also receive training at vocational schools or proprietary schools accredited through the state's Board of Dentistry.

As modern dentistry changes and procedures and techniques become more complex, the role of the dental assistant will continue to evolve. Many important and varied roles are available within dentistry for dental assistants. Each dental practice is unique and has specific needs, and the educationally qualified dental assistant is quick to adapt to new situations as the need arises.

## Clinical Dental Assistant

The clinical dental assistant is directly involved in patient care. The role of the clinical dental assistant is usually defined as *chairside* or *circulating assistant.*

### Chairside Assistant

The chairside assistant works primarily with the dentist who uses four-handed dentistry techniques. The term *four-handed dentistry* describes the seated dentist and chairside assistant working as an efficient team (Fig. 3.2). The chairside assistant mixes dental materials, exchanges instruments, and provides oral evacuation during dental procedures. An equally important role of the chairside dental assistant is to make the patient feel comfortable and relaxed.

### Circulating Assistant

The circulating assistant serves as an extra pair of hands where needed throughout the clinical areas of the practice. This is referred to as *six-handed dentistry* (Fig. 3.3).

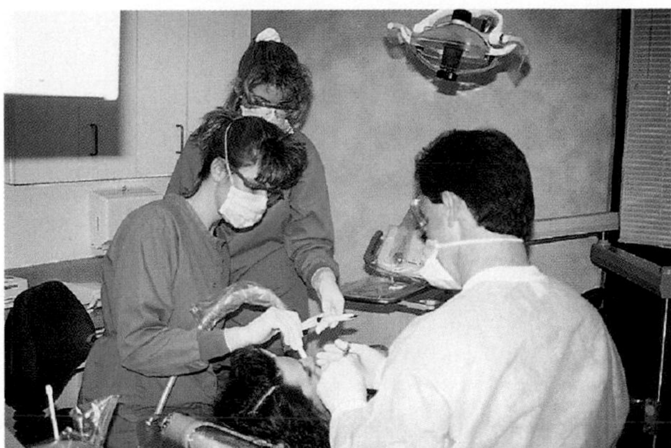

FIG. 3.3 Chairside dental assistant supported by a circulating dental assistant.

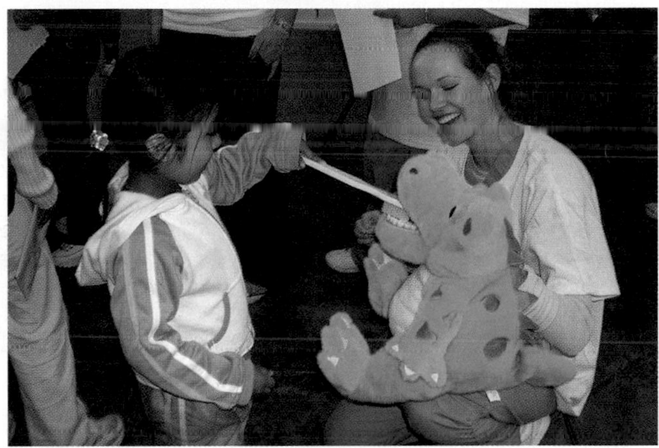

FIG. 3.4 Dental assistants find volunteering at community dental health events very rewarding.

In many practices, the circulating assistant is responsible for seating and dismissing patients, as well as for preparing and caring for instruments and treatment rooms.

### Community Work

Many dental assistants find it personally rewarding to volunteer for participation in activities such as the national Give Kids a Smile Day, community health fairs, preschool visitations, and other oral health education events (Fig. 3.4).

### Mobile Dental Facilities

Some communities and nonprofit agencies own vans that are fully equipped with dental operatories, sterilization equipment, and x-ray machines. The vans are operated and staffed by dentists and dental assistants, and they travel to underserved areas and provide much-needed dental services (Fig. 3.5).

## Sterilization Assistant

In many offices, the responsibility for sterilization procedures is delegated to a specific individual. In other offices, all dental assistants share this important responsibility. The sterilization

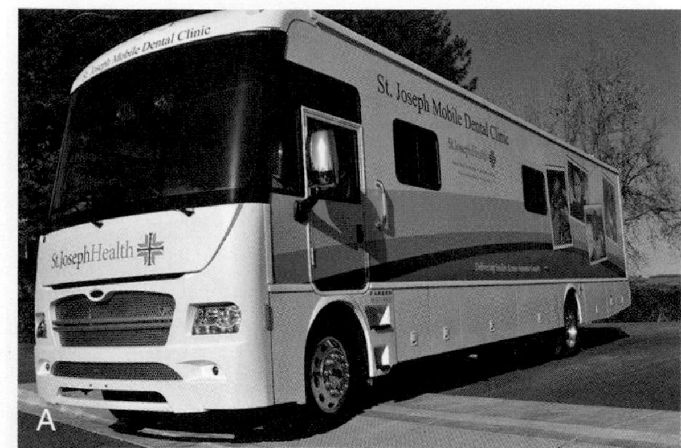


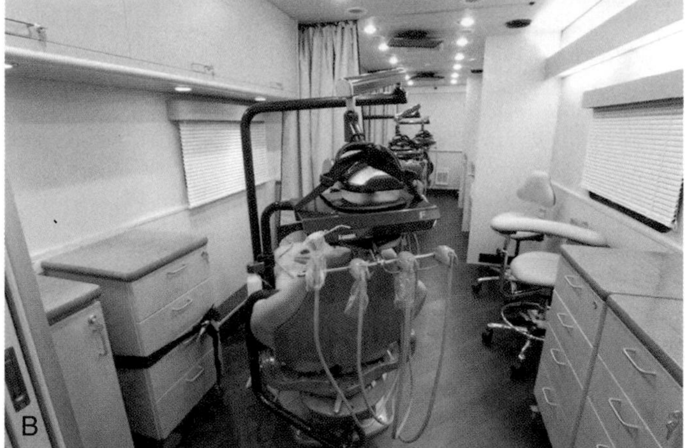

FIG. 3.5 A, Mobile dental van. B, Treatment area inside the dental van. *(Courtesy St. Joseph Health, Sonoma County, CA.)*

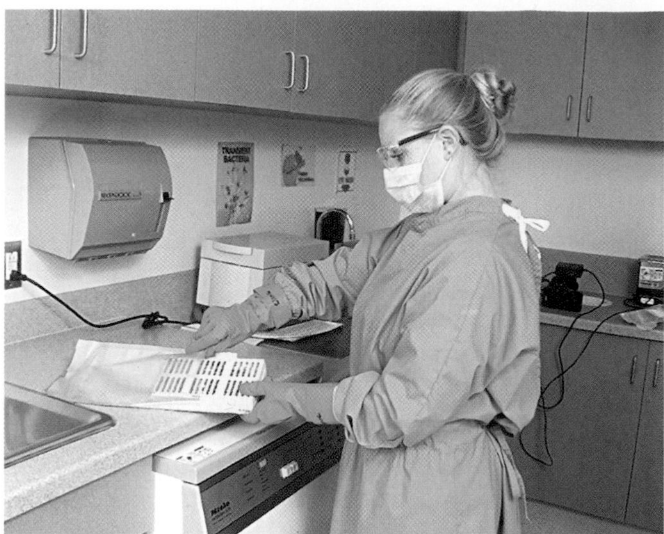

FIG. 3.6 A sterilization assistant is an important member of the team.

assistant efficiently and safely processes all instruments and manages biohazard waste. Other responsibilities include weekly monitoring of sterilizers and maintenance of sterilization monitoring reports (Fig. 3.6). The sterilization assistant is also responsible for selecting infection control products and for performing quality assurance procedures (see Chapters 20 and 21).

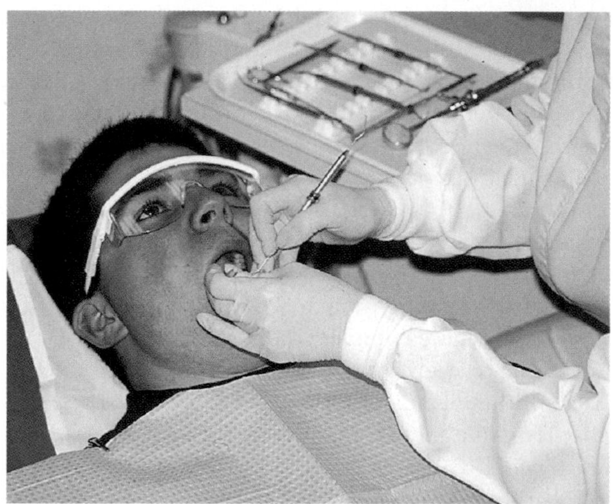

FIG. 3.7 Expanded-functions dental assistant (EFDA) removing excess cement. *(Courtesy Pamela Landry, RDA.)*

## Expanded-Functions Dental Assistant

An expanded-functions dental assistant (EFDA) has received additional training and is legally permitted to provide certain intraoral patient care procedures beyond the duties traditionally performed by a dental assistant (Fig. 3.7). Duties delegated to the EFDA vary according to the Dental Practice Act in each state, province, or territory. It is important that a dental assistant perform only those functions allowed by law (see Chapter 5).

## Business Assistant

Business assistants, also known as *administrative assistants, secretarial assistants,* and *receptionists,* are primarily responsible for the smooth and efficient operation of the business office (Fig. 3.8). Two or more assistants may work in the business area of a dental office. The duties of a business assistant include scheduling appointments, communicating on the phone, coordinating financial arrangements with patients, and handling dental insurance claims. It is not uncommon for a chairside dental assistant to move into a business office position. It is very helpful when the individual at the desk has an excellent understanding of how the clinical practice functions.

## Dental Laboratory Technician

The **dental laboratory technician** usually does not work in the dental office with the other team members, although some dental offices have "in-house" laboratories. Many dental technicians choose to be employed in private laboratories, and others choose to own and operate their own laboratory (Fig. 3.9). In either case, the dental laboratory technician may legally

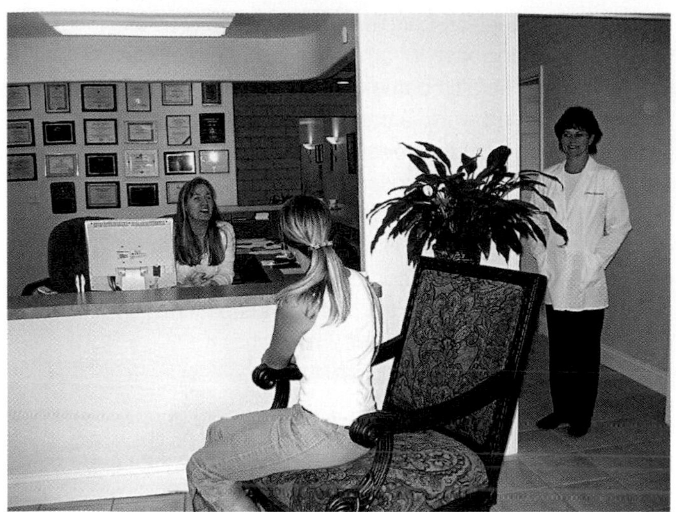

**FIG. 3.8** A patient is greeted by the business assistant before meeting the dental hygienist. *(Courtesy Dr. Peter Pang, Sonoma, CA.)*

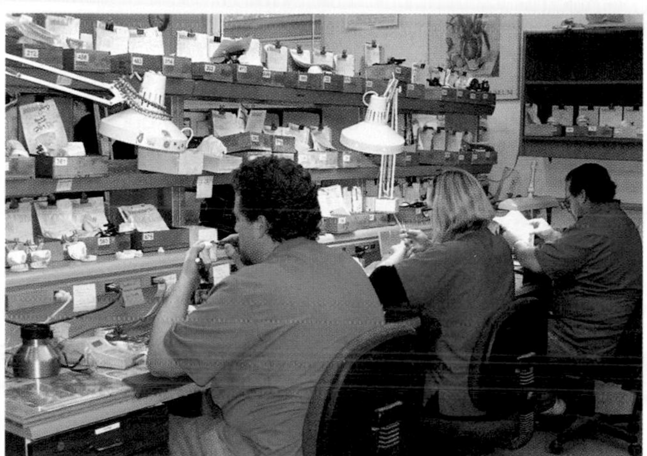

**FIG. 3.9** Dental laboratory technicians working in a large commercial dental laboratory. *(Courtesy Dental Masters Laboratory, Santa Rosa, CA.)*

perform only those tasks specified by the *written prescription* of the dentist (Fig. 3.10). Dental technicians make crowns, bridges, and dentures from impressions taken by the dentist and sent to the dental laboratory. The dental assistant often communicates with the dental laboratory technician regarding the length of time needed to return a case, or to relay special instructions from the dentist about a case. It is important to have a good working relationship with the dental laboratory.

In most states, dental laboratory technicians are not required to have formal education. They can receive their training through apprenticeships, commercial schools, or ADA-accredited programs. Many have received their training in ADA-accredited programs that are 2 years in length. Dental laboratory technicians have extensive knowledge of dental anatomy and materials and exhibit excellent manual dexterity.

To become a **certified dental technician (CDT)**, the dental laboratory technician must pass a written examination. Dental technicians may be members of their professional organization, the *American Dental Laboratory Technician Association (ADLTA).*

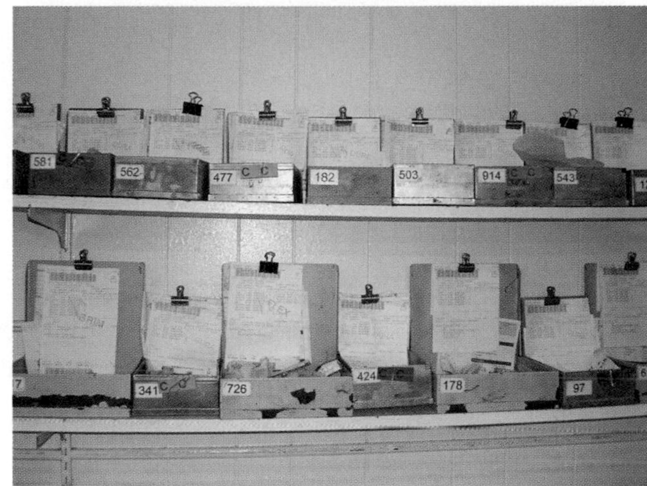

**FIG. 3.10** Laboratory cases are stored in work pans. The dentist's written laboratory prescription is posted on each work pan.

RECALL

4 What is the minimum length of education for an ADA-accredited dental assisting program?
5 What is the minimum length of education for an ADA-accredited dental laboratory technician program?
6 What is required before a dental laboratory technician can perform a task?

## Supporting Services

Often, people in supporting service positions are former dental assistants, dental hygienists, or dental laboratory technicians. Although not official members of the dental healthcare team, individuals in this group are important and provide necessary services and support to the dental office. The **dental supply person** is a representative from a dental supply company who routinely calls on dental offices. This person provides services such as taking orders for supplies, providing new product information, and helping to arrange for service and repairs. The dental supply person visits the dental office frequently.

The **detail person** is a representative of a *specific company*, often a drug or dental product manufacturer, who visits the dental office to provide the dentist with information concerning the specific company's product.

The **dental equipment technician** is a specialist who installs and maintains dental equipment. This service may be provided under a maintenance contract or on an as-needed basis. Sometimes, the dental supply person and the equipment technician work for the same company, and one phone call is all that is necessary.

**■ Legal and Ethical Implications** On occasion, you will be asked to perform tasks that are beyond your level of training, or are illegal in your state. Always remember that many opportunities in the field of dentistry are available for those who are educationally qualified without having to sacrifice ethical standards.

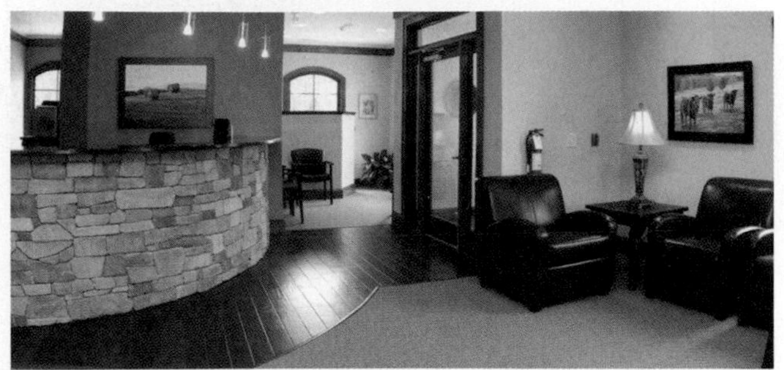

**FIG. 3.11** Entrance to the treatment areas of a modern dental spa–type office. *(Courtesy Patterson Dental, St Paul, MN.)*

All truly successful dental health professionals have a passion for their profession and pride in the quality of care they deliver. You can demonstrate pride in your profession by becoming a member of your professional organization, the American Dental Assistants Association (ADAA). A frequently quoted saying in dentistry is, *"Patients don't care how much you know, until they know how much you care."* ■

**■ Eye to the Future** Because many people fear going to the dentist, a new trend in dentistry, called **dental spas**, is spreading across the country (Fig. 3.11). Dental spas are most prevalent in cosmetic dental practices. To ease the patient's anxiety and avoid the sterile feel and smell of traditional dental offices, dental spas offer a soothing and peaceful atmosphere. Scented aromatherapy candles are often located throughout the office. A wide variety of amenities are offered in dental spas, including warm paraffin baths for the hands, massage blankets, assorted teas, and warm aromatherapy neck pillows. Each room often has its own cable television and a large selection of videos. At the end of the dental procedure, patients are offered a warm lemon-scented towel and a cool, refreshing bottle of water. Spa dentistry puts patients at ease during dental treatment. Many of the techniques used in spa dentistry may be implemented in any type of dental practice to minimize the patient's anxiety and enhance the dental environment. ■

## ■ Critical Thinking

1. How do you think you will fit into the dental profession?
2. Do you have a preference for a business office position or a chairside position? Why?
3. Do you think you might want to work for a specialist? If so, which one and why?
4. Did you learn anything in this chapter that surprised you? If so, what?
5. Where would you like to see yourself in 10 years?
6. Are any dental spas located in your area?

Dentistry is an excellent profession with many opportunities for the person who is willing to participate as a member of the dental healthcare team, accepts responsibilities, and meets high standards. ■

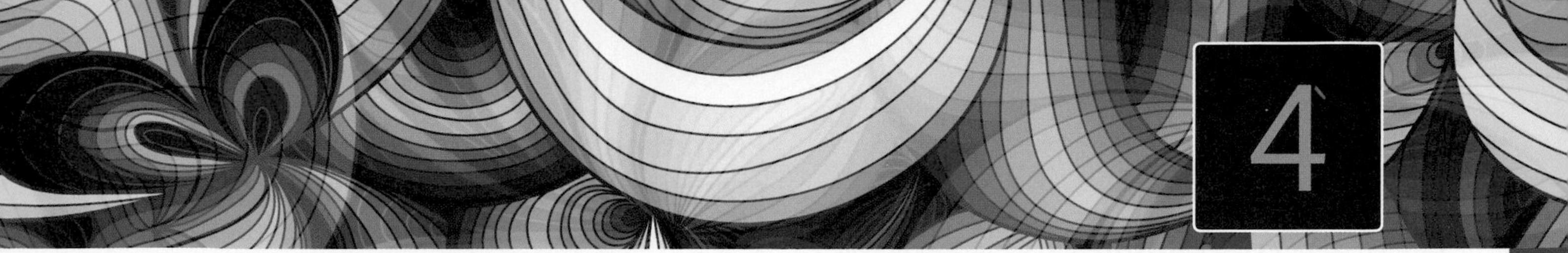


# Dental Ethics

## KEY TERMS

**Autonomy (aw-TON-uh-mee)** Self-determination.
**Beneficence** Of benefit to the patient.
**Code of ethics** Voluntary standards of behavior established by a profession.
**Confidentiality** Never revealing any personal information about the patient.
**Ethics** Moral standards of conduct; rules or principles that govern proper conduct.
**HIPAA** The Health Insurance Portability and Accountability Act of 1996; specifies federal regulations that ensure privacy regarding a patient's healthcare information.
**Justice** Fair treatment of the patient.
**Laws** Minimum standards of behavior established by statutes for a population or profession.
**Nonmaleficence** Of no harm to the patient.
**Veracity** Truthfulness; not lying to the patient.

## LEARNING OUTCOMES

*On completion of this chapter, the student will be able to achieve the following objectives:*

1 Pronounce, define, and spell the key terms.
2 Explain ethics, including sources for ethics, the basic principles of ethics, and why continuing education is an important ethical obligation for dental assistants.
3 Discuss the American Dental Assistants Association Code of Ethics.
4 Do the following regarding the application of ethical principles:
- Define an ethical dilemma.
- Give examples for each principle of ethics.
- Give examples of personal ethics and unethical behaviors.
- Develop case studies that involve ethical dilemmas.
- Describe the steps involved in ethical decision making.

## ELECTRONIC RESOURCES

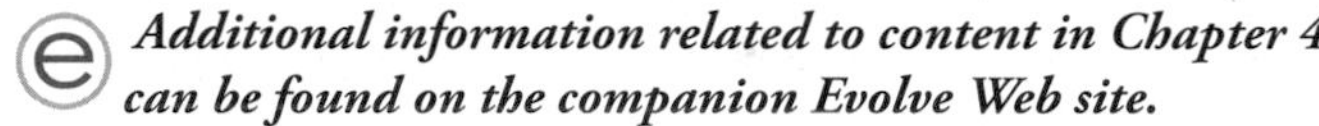
***Additional information related to content in Chapter 4 can be found on the companion Evolve Web site.***

- Practice Quiz
- Canadian Content Corner

Dental assistants are oral healthcare professionals. As members of a profession, they must practice in accordance with both ethical and legal standards that the public expects from healthcare providers. The connection between law and ethics is very close. Chapter 5 discusses the legal aspects of dental practice.

**Ethics** refers to moral conduct (right and wrong behavior, "good" and "evil"). Ethics includes values, high standards of conduct, and personal obligations reflected in our interactions with other professionals and patients. Ethics involves very few absolutes and many gray areas. Ethical issues are subject to individual interpretation regarding the right or wrong of particular situations. Dental healthcare professionals should practice ethical behavior as they provide dental care to their patients.

As a general rule, *ethical standards* are always of a higher order than minimum legal standards established by law. A behavior can be unethical and still be legal, but it cannot be illegal and still be ethical. The study of ethics seeks to answer two basic questions:

1. *What* should I do?
2. *Why* should I do it?

Ethics refers to what you *should* do, not what you *must* do. The law deals with what you *must* do (see Chapter 5).

1 What is the difference between ethics and law?

## Sources for Ethics

Ethical decisions are present in every part of our lives. Ethics is involved in the way we treat other humans, animals, and the environment. You have been learning personal ethics throughout your life in a variety of ways from the following sources:

- Basic instinct (tells you "right" from "wrong")
- Parents ("How would you feel if someone did that to you?")
- Teachers ("Study hard; don't cheat.")
- Religion ("Do unto others as you would have them do unto you.")
- Observation of other people's behavior

## Basic Principles of Ethics

Actions and decisions of healthcare providers are guided by ethical principles. The following six basic principles of ethics have been developed over time. These principles guide healthcare providers by helping to identify, clarify, and justify moral (ethical) choices (Table 4.1).

### Regard for Self-Determination (Autonomy)

Self-determination includes the right to privacy, freedom of choice, and acceptance of responsibility for one's actions. **Autonomy** refers to a person's freedom to think, judge, and act independently without undue influence. People are free to do what they like, as long as they do not break the law or cause harm to others. For example, patients have the right to participate in decisions related to dental care, and they have the right to refuse recommended treatment.

### To "Do No Harm" (Nonmaleficence)

The principle of **nonmaleficence** comes from Hippocrates' dictate to "do no harm." It is the most basic element in morality. It relates to all levels of interpersonal and professional behavior. For example, if an action may cause harm (physical or mental) to another, it cannot be considered moral. An example of this principle in practice is the patient who wants the dentist to provide a treatment that the dentist believes is not in the best interest of the patient. The dentist is bound by the ethical principle to "do no harm."

**TABLE 4.1** Basic Ethical Principles

| Principle | Description |
|---|---|
| Autonomy | Self-determination, right to freedom of choice, self-responsibility |
| Nonmaleficence | To do no harm |
| Beneficence | To do good or provide a benefit |
| Justice | Fairness |
| Veracity | To tell the truth |
| Confidentiality | Never revealing any personal information about the patient |

### Promotion of Well-Being (Beneficence)

The principle of **beneficence** is based on the idea that actions are ethical as long as they will benefit a person or a community. Sometimes, *not causing* harm is not enough, and one wants to help others. Volunteering in dental health education programs is an example of this type of behavior.

### Regard for Justice

**Justice** involves treating people fairly and giving people what they deserve and are entitled to receive. This concept is demonstrated in the philosophy that all patients should receive the same quality of dental care, regardless of their socioeconomic status, ethnicity, level of education, or ability to pay.

### Veracity

The principle of **veracity** involves telling the truth. It is in the patient's best interest to know the truth about his or her condition. Incomplete information, such as omission of information about a less expensive option for treatment, can threaten the trust between the patient and the dentist. Another example is telling a child that a dental treatment will not hurt, when in fact it may.

### Confidentiality

**Confidentiality** is a very important issue in the healthcare profession. Patients have a right to privacy concerning their healthcare and treatment choices (Fig. 4.1). Healthcare professionals must be very careful to avoid revealing any personal information about the patient. Respecting a patient's privacy is a legal and ethical obligation. It is unethical to reveal any personal information about a patient. However, conflicts do arise surrounding the principle of confidentiality. Legal requirements mandate that the healthcare provider report cases of suspected child abuse or elder abuse to protect individuals from harm. Issues may arise when dealing

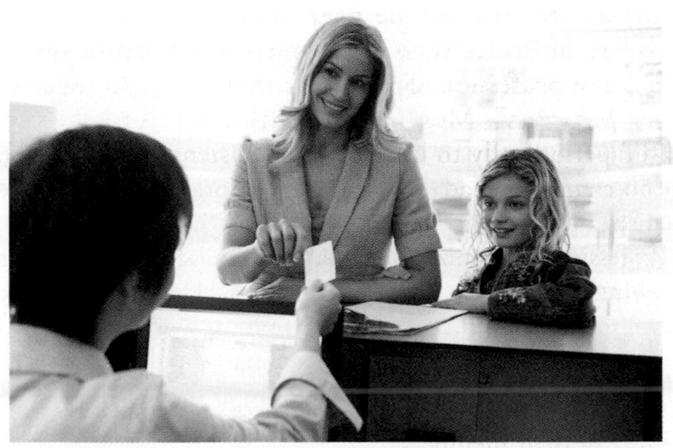

**FIG. 4.1** Patients have the right to expect confidentiality regarding their conversations in the dental office. *(Copyright © FangXiaNuo/E+/Getty Images.)*

with adolescents, who may or may not be adults according to the legal system. Sometimes, the patient's right to confidentiality has to be balanced against the rights of other individuals. In any situation, the healthcare provider must explain to the patient that professional and legal responsibilities are clear regarding disclosure, and that every attempt will be made to help the patient as much as possible.

## Privacy

In addition to moral and ethical principles regarding patient confidentiality, **HIPAA** (Health Insurance Portability and Accountability Act of 1996) has put forth very definite legal requirements related to confidentiality of patients' health information (see Chapters 5 and 63).

## Continuing Education

It is the ethical obligation of dental assistants to maintain and update their knowledge and skills. Continuing education (CE) is an important and stimulating part of the dental assistant's life. Because continuing education is so important, the Dental Assisting National Board (DANB) requires evidence of continuing education for the Certified Dental Assistant (CDA) to remain certified, and many states that license or register dental assistants require continuing education as part of the license renewal process. The type and amount of CE vary from state to state. CE courses are readily available at professional association meetings and through approved home study courses; an increasing number of CE courses are becoming available online.

2 What are the six basic principles of ethics?

# Professional Code of Ethics

All professions (e.g., dental, medical, legal), similar to the American Dental Assistants Association (ADAA), have a written **code of ethics**. These are *voluntary* standards that are set by members of the profession. They are not **laws**. The code of ethics serves as a method of self-regulation within the profession. Remember that the code states the "ideal behavior." Most professional codes of ethics are revised periodically to keep them consistent with the times, but no change is made involving the moral intent or overall idealism.

Professional organizations establish a code of ethics for the following reasons:

- To demonstrate the standard of care that the public can expect from their members
- To enhance the ethical consciousness and ethical responsibility of their members
- To guide members in making informed ethical decisions
- To establish a standard for professional judgment and conduct

## American Dental Assistants Association (ADAA): Principles of Ethics (2011)

**Foreword**

The Principles of Professional Ethics lists legal and ethical guidelines expected by patients, employers, and employees and, in many areas, required by regulatory boards.

- Cause no harm.
- Uphold all federal, state, and local laws and regulations.
- Be truthful and honest in verbal, financial, and treatment endeavors.
- Recognize and report signs of abuse to proper authorities.
- Assist in informed decision making of treatment options while respecting the rights of patients to determine the final course of treatment to be rendered.
- Do not discriminate against others.
- Support, promote, and participate in access to care efforts through education, professional activities, and programs.
- Deliver optimum care using professional knowledge, judgment, and skill within the law.
- Be compassionate, respectful, kind, and fair to employers, coworkers, and patients.
- Refrain from denigrating by word, print, or in electronic communication your employer, workplace, or colleagues at all times.
- Create and maintain a safe work environment.
- Assist in conflict management when necessary to maintain harmony within the workplace.
- Strive for self-improvement through continuing education.
- Strive for a healthy lifestyle, which may prevent physical or mental impairment caused by any type of illness.
- Refrain from any substance abuse.
- Never misrepresent professional credentials or education.

Adapted from ADAA House of Delegates, 2011; reviewed 2013.

## American Dental Assistants Association (ADAA): Code of Member Conduct (2011)

**Foreword**

As an organization charged with representing a part of the profession involved in the practice of dentistry, the American Dental Assistants Association has delineated a Code of Conduct for members, officers, and trustees. They are general goals to which each member should aspire and are not intended to be enforceable as rules of conduct for dental assistants.

**Code of Conduct as a Member of the ADAA**

As a member of the American Dental Assistants Association, I pledge to:

- Abide by the Bylaws of the Association;
- Maintain loyalty to the Association;
- Pursue the objectives of the Association;
- Hold in confidence the information entrusted to me by the Association;
- Serve all members of the Association in an impartial manner;
- Maintain respect for the members and the employees of the Association;

Continued

- Exercise and insist on sound business principles in the conduct of the affairs of the Association;
- Use legal and ethical means to influence legislation or regulation affecting members of the Association;
- Issue no false or misleading statements to fellow members or to the public;
- Refrain from disseminating malicious information concerning the Association or any member or employee of the American Dental Assistants Association;
- Maintain high standards of personal conduct and integrity;
- Cooperate in a reasonable and proper manner with staff and members;
- Accept no personal compensation from fellow members, except as approved by the Association;
- Ensure public confidence in the integrity and service of the Association;
- Promote and maintain the highest standards of performance in service to the Association.

From ADAA House of Delegates, 2011; reviewed 2013.

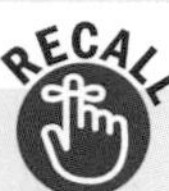


**3** What establishes a guide to professional behavior?

# Applying Ethical Principles

We face ethical issues every day in our personal and professional lives. The following are examples in which ethical principles must be applied:

- A woman chooses not to have dental radiographs taken because she is afraid of radiation exposure. She has the right to accept or refuse radiographs. She also has the right to be fully informed about her oral healthcare, and her dentist would likely explain the risks of conditions that remain undetected through lack of dental radiographs. The dentist is facing an ethical dilemma that involves the principle of autonomy.
- Several dental assistants in your office enjoy gossiping about the receptionist. By refusing to participate in office gossip, you are applying the principle of nonmaleficence (doing no harm).
- A student in your dental-assisting class is struggling with her studies. You could ignore the student because you have too much to do, or you could apply the principle of beneficence (well-being) by offering to help her study.
- You find a wallet that contains a large amount of cash and identification cards of the owner. By returning the wallet and the cash, you are applying the principle of justice.
- When you tell a patient that he or she may feel some discomfort after the local anesthetic wears off, you are applying the principle of veracity.
- You are tempted to tell your friends that a very popular celebrity, who came to have her teeth whitened, was a patient in your dental practice but you do not. You are demonstrating the principle of confidentiality.

# Ethical Dilemmas

An everyday problem that can be solved by applying an ethical principle is different from an *ethical dilemma.* An ethical dilemma occurs when one or more ethical principles are in conflict, for example, when the principle of avoiding harm is in conflict with the principle of autonomy in a specific situation.

## *Case Example*

A patient who has had a recent heart attack wishes to have some veneers placed on her front teeth immediately because she is going on a cruise in 3 weeks. The dentist wants to wait a while for her medical condition to stabilize before beginning the cosmetic procedure. The patient is very insistent about her wishes. The dentist now has an ethical dilemma to solve.

In the case study just described, the conflict is between the patient's ethical right to *self-determination (autonomy)* and the dentist's ethical obligation to "do no harm."

An ethical dilemma is different from a situation in which a dentist knowingly charges an insurance company for a procedure that was not performed. This clearly involves unethical and illegal behavior.

Another example of principles in conflict occurs when the dentist believes that a treatment is in the best interest of the patient, and the patient chooses another option (autonomy versus "do no harm"). The dentist may choose to perform the procedure that the patient prefers *only* if that procedure is within the standards of patient care. It would be unethical under the principle of "do no harm" for the dentist to perform a procedure that is below the standard of care just because the patient wants it. For example, a patient may want to have all of his healthy teeth extracted so he does not have to brush and floss (autonomy). In this case, it would be unethical for a dentist to comply with the patient's wishes.

## *Steps for Solving Ethical Dilemmas*

Many ethical dilemmas do not have quick or easy solutions. When an ethical dilemma is particularly complex, the following steps can be used as a "road map." It sometimes helps to write down the alternatives when evaluating all the options.

1. *Identify the alternatives.* Answer these questions: What alternatives do I have? What are the likely outcomes of each alternative?
2. *Determine the professional implications.* With each alternative, determine what "should" and "should not" be done professionally. You must carefully consider all specific professional obligations relevant to the situation.
3. *Rank the alternatives.* Then select the best alternative. If you think two alternatives are equal, you must choose one or the other. This step allows you to know that you have done your best, given the circumstances.
4. *Choose a course of action.* When you follow these steps and make a judgment and a decision about what should and should not be done ethically and professionally, you will be more comfortable with your decision.

**■ Legal and Ethical Implications** You may be faced with a situation in which your dentist-employer's conduct violates ethical standards. Before you make any judgments, be absolutely certain of all information and circumstances. If violations of ethical conduct have occurred, you must answer the following questions:

- Do you want to remain at your job under these circumstances?
- Should you discuss the situation with your employer?
- Should you seek other employment?
- If you remain, will it affect you in the future in your dealings with other employers?
- What options do you have?

These decisions are difficult, especially if you like your employer and enjoy your job. A dental assistant is not *legally* obligated to report questionable actions of the dentist or to attempt to alter the circumstances. However, as an *ethical* dental assistant, you have to live with the decisions you make. You will not want to participate in substandard care or unlawful practices that may be harmful to patients. ■

**■ Eye to the Future** You may be faced with ethical dilemmas daily when you are working in a dental practice. Many professional ethical judgments are straightforward. When you are faced with more complex issues, however, remember the steps for solving ethical dilemmas. Remember also that the correct alternative is not always the easiest choice, but it is always the best choice. ■

## ■ Critical Thinking

1. Susan, the office manager in your dental office, enjoys sharing personal information about the dentist and his wife with members of the staff. You are uncomfortable with her behavior but you know she is responsible for your evaluation, so you are reluctant to speak to her. What can you do?
2. You have just begun working for Dr. Wong as a dental assistant. You know that confidential papers, case histories, and the appointment book should be kept from curious eyes to protect patients, as well as the dentist and office staff. The receptionist does not always follow these practices, however, and insists that this involves no ethical issues with any of the patients. Is there anything you can do to protect your patients' privacy?
3. The president of the local dental assistant society asks you to volunteer for upcoming dental screenings at an urban school on Saturday. You had planned to spend some time with friends you have not seen in a while. You know volunteers are difficult to find and this is a worthwhile project, but it has been weeks since you and your friends got together. What will you do? Why? ■

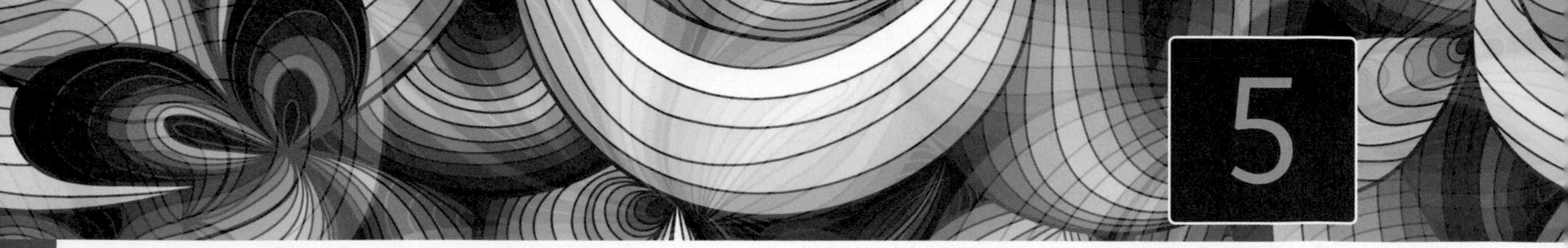

5

# Dentistry and the Law

## KEY TERMS

**Abandonment** Withdrawing a patient from treatment without giving reasonable notice or providing a competent replacement.
**Administrative law** Category of law that involves regulations established by government agencies.
**Board of dentistry** State agency that adopts rules and regulations and implements the specific state's Dental Practice Act.
**Child abuse** Any act that endangers or impairs a child's physical or emotional health or development.
**Civil law** Category of law that deals with relations of individuals, corporations, or other organizations.
**Contract law** Category of law that involves an agreement for services in exchange for a payment (contract).
**Criminal law** Category of law that involves violations against the state or government.
**Dental auxiliary (awg-ZIL-yuh-ree)** Dental assistants, dental hygienists, and dental laboratory technicians.
**Direct supervision** Level of supervision in which the dentist is physically present when the dental auxiliary performs delegated functions.
**Due care** Just, proper, and sufficient care, or the absence of negligence.
**Elder abuse** Includes physical or sexual abuse, financial exploitation, emotional confinement, passive neglect, or willful deprivation of an elderly person.
**Expanded functions** Specific intraoral functions delegated to an auxiliary that require increased skill and training.
**Expressed contract** A contract that is established through verbal or written words.
**Felony** A major crime, such as fraud or drug abuse. Conviction can result in imprisonment of 1 year or longer.
**General supervision** Level of supervision in which the dental auxiliary performs delegated functions according to the instructions of the dentist, who is not necessarily physically present.
**HIPAA** The Health Insurance Portability and Accountability Act of 1996; specifies federal regulations ensuring privacy regarding a patient's healthcare information.
**Implied consent** Type of consent in which the patient's action indicates consent for treatment.
**Implied contract** Contract that is established by actions, not words.
**Informed consent** Permission granted by a patient after he or she is informed about the details of a procedure.
**Infraction** Minor offense that usually results in only a fine.
**Licensure** License to practice in a specific state.
**Malpractice** Professional negligence.
**Mandated reporters** Designated professionals who are required by law to report known or suspected child abuse.
**Misdemeanor** Offense that may result in imprisonment of 6 months to 1 year.
**Patient of record** Individual who has been examined and diagnosed by the dentist and has had treatment planned.
**Reciprocity (re-si-PROS-i-tee)** System that allows individuals in one state to obtain a license in another state without retesting.
***Res gestae*** Latin for "things done." Statements made by a person present at the time of an alleged negligent act that are admissible as evidence in a court of law.
***Res ipsa loquitur*** Latin phrase for "the thing speaks for itself."
***Respondeat superior*** Latin for "Let the master answer." Legal doctrine that holds an employer liable for acts of the employee.
**Spousal abuse** Domestic violence intentionally inflicted by a family member or members.
**Standard of care** Level of knowledge, skill, and care comparable with that of other dentists who are treating similar patients under similar conditions.
**State Dental Practice Act** Document of law that specifies legal requirements for practicing dentistry in a particular state.
**Statutory law** Law enacted by legislation through U.S. Congress, state legislature, or local legislative bodies.
**Tort law** Involving an act that brings harm to a person or damage to property.
**Written consent** Consent that involves a written explanation of diagnostic findings, prescribed treatment, and reasonable expectations about treatment results.

## LEARNING OUTCOMES

*On completion of this chapter, the student will be able to achieve the following objectives:*

1. Pronounce, define, and spell the key terms.
2. Explain the types of statutory law, including the difference between criminal law and civil law.
3. Explain the purpose of the state Dental Practice Act and the role of the Board of Dentistry, including the following:
   - State the purpose for licensing dental health professionals.
   - Give an example of *respondeat superior.*
   - Explain the difference between general supervision and direct supervision.
   - Explain the legal ramifications of the unlicensed practice of dentistry.
4. Explain the dynamics of the dentist-patient relationship, including the concept of standard of care, the circumstances required for patient abandonment, and the dentist's obligation of due care.
5. Explain malpractice in dentistry, including the following:
   - List the "four D's" required for a successful malpractice lawsuit.
   - Explain the difference between an act of omission and an act of commission.
   - Define the doctrine of *res ipsa loquitur.*

6 Describe strategies of risk management in dentistry, including the following:
- Describe ways to avoid malpractice suits.
- Give an example of *res gestae.*
- Describe the difference between written and implied consent.
- Explain when it is necessary to obtain an informed refusal.
- Describe the exceptions to disclosure.
- Describe the procedure for obtaining consent for minor patients.
- Describe the procedure for documenting informed consent and the content of informed consent forms.
- Provide requirements for conditions for patient referral and ramifications of failure to refer.
- Explain the principle of contributory negligence.

7 Discuss the protocol of working with patient records, including the guidelines for charting entries in clinical records.

8 Explain the role of dental professionals in reporting abuse and neglect of patients, including the following:
- Discuss the indications of spousal, child, and elder abuse and neglect.
- Describe signs of dental neglect.
- Explain the purpose of HIPAA.

## ELECTRONIC RESOURCES

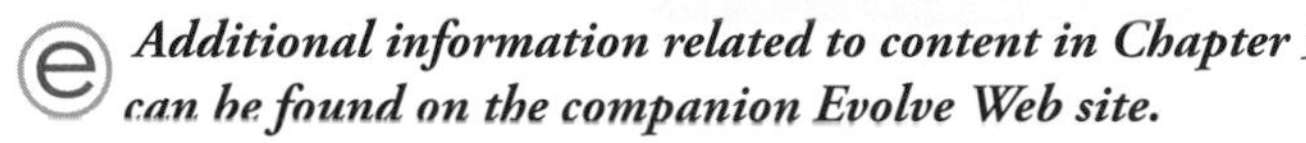
***Additional information related to content in Chapter 5 can be found on the companion Evolve Web site.***

- Practice Quiz
- Canadian Content Corner

Every state government has the responsibility to protect the health, welfare, and safety of its citizens. To do this, regulations are written and legislation is passed. When the U.S. Congress, a state legislature, or a local legislative body passes legislation, it becomes **statutory law**. As a dental assistant, you must understand the law to protect yourself, the dentist, and the patient.

## Statutory Law

Statutory law consists of two types: criminal law and civil law. **Criminal law** involves crimes against society. In criminal law, a governmental agency such as law enforcement or the board of dentistry initiates legal action. **Civil law** involves crimes against an individual, with another individual initiating legal action (i.e., lawsuit) (Fig. 5.1).

### Criminal Law

Criminal law seeks to punish the offender, but civil law seeks to compensate the victim. For example, a dental assistant who performs a procedure that is not legal is in violation of criminal law. Insurance fraud is another criminal act that may be committed in a dental office.

Criminal offenses are classified as follows:

- **Felony**: Major crime, such as insurance fraud or drug abuse in the dental setting. Conviction may result in imprisonment for 1 year or longer.
- **Misdemeanor**: A lesser offense that may result in a variety of penalties, including fines, loss or suspension of the license to practice dentistry, mandatory continuing education, counseling, or community service. An example of a misdemeanor is a dentist who violates a regulation of the Dental Practice Act by failing to follow infection control regulations.
- **Infraction**: Minor offense (e.g., traffic violation) that usually results in only a fine. For example, if a dentist does not pay his or her license renewal fee on time, a penalty fee is added to the original renewal fee.

### Civil Law

Civil law is concerned with relations of individuals, corporations, or other organizations. Classifications of civil law that affect the practice of dentistry are as follows:

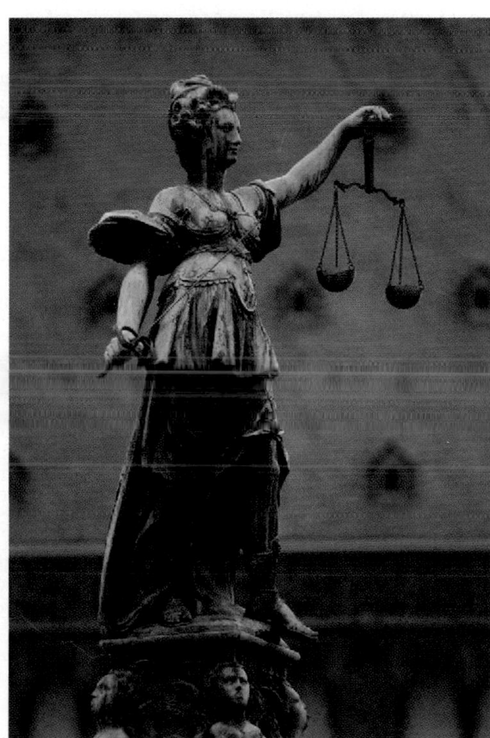

FIG. 5.1 "Lady Justice." Justitia was the Roman goddess of justice and is the figure depicted in statues across the world, often holding both scales and a sword. Her scales imply the weighting of justice, and the blindfold represents the impartiality of justice. *(From Proctor DB et al: Kinn's the medical assistant, ed 13, St Louis, Elsevier, 2017.)*

- **Contract law** refers to a binding agreement between two or more people. This could involve employment contracts or contracts for patient treatment.
- **Tort law** involves acts (intentional or unintentional) that bring harm to a person or damages to property. An example would be a malpractice suit in which a patient alleges that a dentist caused harm or damage to him or her.
- **Administrative law** involves regulations established by government agencies, for example, violations of the Occupational Safety and Health Administration (OSHA) regulations. Regulations of the Dental Practice Act are also examples of administrative law.

### Contract Law

For a contract or agreement to be *binding,* it must be established between two competent people. This eliminates mentally incompetent persons, those under the influence of alcohol or drugs, and minors. The agreement must also include an exchange of a service for payment. When the dentist accepts the patient and the patient arrives for care, the dentist has the legal obligation under contract law to provide dental care. A contract can be either *expressed* or *implied,* as follows:

- **Expressed contracts** are established through the written word or by a verbal agreement. Expressed contracts are commonly used when the required treatment is extensive or will take a long time to complete (e.g., orthodontics, full mouth reconstruction).
- **Implied contracts** are established by *actions,* not by words. Most dental contracts are implied contracts. For example, if a patient comes to the dentist with a toothache and allows the dentist to examine him or her, it is implied that the patient wants treatment.

### Tort Law

A tort is a civil wrong. A tort can be *intentional* or *unintentional.* For example, a breach of confidentiality is an intentional tort. If a dental assistant mounts radiographic films on the wrong side and the dentist notices and corrects the error, no harm is done to the patient and no tort would occur. However, a tort would occur if the dentist extracted a tooth on the wrong side of the mouth as a result of not noticing the error.

In addition, a tort can be an act of *omission* (i.e., not doing something that should have been done) or an act of *commission* (i.e., doing something that should not have been done). For example, failing to recognize periodontal disease or not taking radiographs would be an act of *omission.* Taking out the wrong tooth or causing nerve injury during an extraction would be an act of *commission.*

RECALL

1. What are the two types of statutory law?
2. What is the difference between an act of omission and an act of commission?
3. What is the difference between an expressed contract and an implied contract?

## State Dental Practice Act

To protect the public from incompetent dental healthcare providers, each state has established a **state Dental Practice Act.** The Dental Practice Act specifies the legal requirements for the practice of dentistry within each state. It may be a single law or a compilation of laws that regulate the practice of dentistry. Regulations regarding dental assistants vary greatly from state to state. It is important to have a clear understanding of the law in *your* state as it relates to dental assisting and the practice of dentistry. Each state's Dental Practice Act is now accessible on the Internet. You will find links to each state's Dental Practice Act at www.ada.org.

### Contents of a Typical Dental Practice Act

- Requirements for licensure
- Requirements for license renewal
- Grounds for suspension or revocation of a license
- Requirements for continuing dental education
- Duties to be delegated to dental assistants and dental hygienists
- Infection control regulations
- Requirements for the use of radiation and qualifications for healthcare professionals who expose dental radiographs

## Board of Dentistry

An administrative board, usually called the **board of dentistry**, interprets and implements state regulations. The governor of the state usually appoints the members of the state board of dentistry, also referred to as the *dental board* in some states. In addition to licensed dentists, some states have dental hygienists, dental assistants, and consumers as members of the board.

The board adopts rules and regulations that define, interpret, and implement the intent of the Dental Practice Act. The board is also responsible for enforcement of regulations for the practice of dentistry within the state.

**Licensure** (having a license to practice in a specific state) is one method of supervising individuals who practice in the state. The purpose of licensure is to protect the public from unqualified or incompetent practitioners. Requirements for licensure vary from state to state, but dentists and dental hygienists *must* be licensed by the state in which they practice.

An increasing number of states are requiring either licensing or registration for dental assistants in their states. It is essential to understand the requirements for practice in your state. In every state, any person who practices dentistry without a license is guilty of an illegal act.

Some states have a reciprocity agreement with another state or a plan for licensure by credential. **Reciprocity** is an agreement between two or more states that allows a dentist or dental hygienist who is licensed in one state to receive, *usually without further examination or requirements,* a license to practice in any of the other states in the reciprocity agreement. Reciprocity agreements are usually made between states with adjoining borders and similar testing requirements. States without reciprocity agreements require dentists and dental hygienists licensed in another state to take their state board examination.

**Licensure by credential** allows an individual who is currently licensed in one state to become licensed in another state *if* certain requirements are met. Examples of such requirements could include never having had a license suspended or revoked, or having been in practice for a specified amount of time, or having been a faculty member in a dental school, or having completed a specific number of continuing education units. The requirements for licensure by credential vary according to the state.

The state board of dentistry has the authority not only to *issue* a license but also to *revoke, suspend,* or *deny renewal* of a license. Most states will take action if the licensed person has a felony conviction or a misdemeanor involving drug addiction, moral corruptness, or incompetence, or a mental/physical disability that may cause harm to patients.

4 What is the purpose of licensure?
5 What authority does a state board of dentistry have?
6 What is meant by reciprocity and licensure by credential?

## Expanded Functions and Supervision

**Expanded functions** are specific intraoral tasks delegated to qualified dental auxiliaries who have advanced skill and training. When these functions are included in the Dental Practice Act, the dentist may delegate them to the dental assistant. Some states require additional education, certification, or registration to perform these functions.

As with all functions performed by the dental assistant, expanded functions are included in the doctrine of ***respondeat superior*** ("let the master answer"). This means that the employer is responsible for any harm caused by the actions of the employee while the employee is carrying out the business of the employer. In a dental practice, this means that the patient may sue the dentist for an error committed by the dental assistant.

However, the employee is also responsible for his or her own actions, and the injured patient may also file suit against the dental assistant. The dentist's liability insurance cannot be counted on to provide complete coverage for the dental assistant. Many dental assistants who provide direct patient care choose to carry their own liability insurance.

In states that allow the dentist to delegate expanded functions to a **dental auxiliary** (dental assistant or dental hygienist), the rules in the state Dental Practice Act are usually specific regarding the types of auxiliary supervision that the dentist must provide. The following terms are used often in dental practice acts:

- A **patient of record** is an individual who has been examined and diagnosed by a licensed dentist and has had his or her treatment planned by the dentist.
- **Direct supervision** generally means that the dentist has delegated a specific procedure to be performed for a patient of record by a legally qualified dental auxiliary (who meets the requirements of the state board of dentistry). The dentist must examine the patient before delegating the procedure and again when the procedure is complete. *The dentist must be physically present in the office at the time the procedures are performed.*
- **General supervision** (indirect supervision) generally means that the dentist has authorized and delegated specific procedures that may be performed by a legally qualified dental auxiliary for a patient of record. Exposing radiographs and recementing a temporary crown that has become dislodged are examples of functions that are often delegated under general supervision.

7 What does *respondeat superior* mean?
8 What is the difference between direct supervision and general supervision?

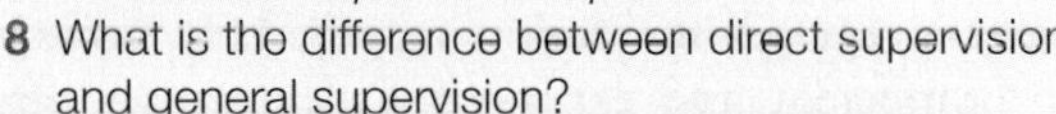

## Unlicensed Practice of Dentistry

As a dental assistant, you may legally perform *only* those functions that have been delegated to you under the Dental Practice Act of the state in which you practice. Performing procedures that are not legal is the same as practicing dentistry without a license, which is a *criminal act.* Ignorance of the Dental Practice Act is no excuse for illegally practicing dentistry. *If the dentist asks you to perform an expanded function that is not legal in your state and you choose to do so, you are committing a criminal act.*

### Expanded Functions Delegated to Qualified Dental Assistants*

- Inspecting oral cavity with mouth mirror
- Applying topical anesthetics
- Polishing coronal surfaces of teeth
- Assisting with administration of nitrous oxide
- Applying topical anticarcinogenic agents
- Fitting trial endodontic file points
- Determining root length and endodontic file length
- Making impressions for intraoral appliances
- Making impressions for study casts
- Removing sutures
- Performing preliminary oral examinations
- Placing and removing matrices and wedges
- Placing and removing temporary or sedative restorations
- Placing and removing temporary crowns and bridges
- Preparing teeth for etching
- Placing and removing rubber dams
- Placing and removing periodontal dressings
- Placing, condensing, and carving amalgam restorations
- Placing and finishing composite resin restorations
- Applying cavity liners and bases
- Applying pit-and-fissure sealants
- Placing and removing orthodontic arch wires, brackets, and bands

*Check with your state's board of dentistry for information pertaining to your state. Locate your state's Dental Practice Act on the Internet at http://www.ada.org.

# Dentist-Patient Relationship

## Duty of Care/Standard of Care

The concept of *duty of care* (also known as the **standard of care**) is commonly misunderstood among dental professionals. Many assume that it is a law or regulation and that it provides specific steps that a dentist must follow. It is, in fact, not a black-and-white rule at all. Instead, it is a legal *concept* that provides general boundaries within which a dentist must perform in a given situation.

The standard of care that a dentist must meet is simply the customary practice of reputable dentists who have similar training and experience, who practice in similar disciplines, or who practice in the same area or a similar locality (e.g., urban, remote rural). When a dentist fails to meet the standard of care and the patient is injured, the dentist may be held liable for malpractice. Competent and experienced dentists are often called as witnesses to testify in court (Fig. 5.2).

The duty of care owed by a dentist to a patient includes (1) being licensed; (2) using reasonable skill, care, and judgment; and (3) using standard drugs, materials, and techniques. The dentist may refuse to treat a patient; however, this action must *not* be based on the patient's race, color, or creed.

In addition, the Americans with Disabilities Act protects patients with infectious diseases such as human immunodeficiency virus (HIV) infection. For example, a patient with HIV cannot be refused treatment simply because of the presence of the disease. The only exception would be the patient with HIV who has a special condition (e.g., severe periodontal disease) that requires the care of a specialist, if the dentist would refer any patient with the same condition to a specialist, regardless of HIV status. In other words, a patient cannot be refused treatment *only* on the basis of HIV status.

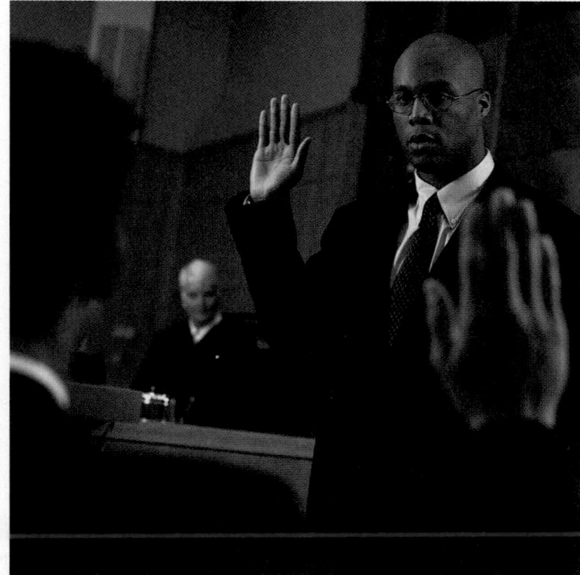

**FIG. 5.2** Witnesses must be credible and tell the truth on the stand in court to avoid charges of perjury. *(From Proctor DB et al: Kinn's the medical assistant, ed 13, St Louis, Elsevier, 2017.)*

### Dentist's Duty of Care to the Patient

- Be properly licensed
- Use reasonable skill, care, and judgment
- Use standard drugs, materials, and techniques
- Use "standard precautions" in treatment of all patients
- Maintain confidentiality of all information
- Obtain and update patients' medical-dental health history
- Make appropriate referrals, and request consultation when indicated
- Maintain a strong level of knowledge and competence in keeping with advances in the dental profession
- Do not exceed the scope of practice or allow assistants under general supervision to perform unlawful acts
- Complete patients' care in a timely manner
- Do not use experimental procedures
- Obtain informed consent from the patient or guardian before beginning an examination or treatment
- Arrange for patients' care during a temporary absence
- Give adequate instructions to patients
- Achieve reasonable treatment results

## Abandonment

**Abandonment** refers to discontinuation of care after treatment has begun, but before it has been completed. The dentist may be liable for abandonment if the dentist ends the dentist-patient relationship without giving the patient reasonable notice. Even if a patient refuses to follow instructions and fails to keep appointments, the dentist may not legally refuse to give the patient another appointment. The dentist may not dismiss or refuse to treat a patient of record without giving the patient written notification of termination. After notification, care must continue for a reasonable length of time, usually 30 days, to allow the patient time to find another dentist. It could even be considered abandonment if a dentist left the area for a weekend without making arrangements with another dentist to be available for emergencies, or without leaving a number that the patient can call for care.

## Patient Responsibilities

The patient also has legal duties to the dentist. The patient is legally required to pay a reasonable and agreed-on fee for services. The patient also is expected to cooperate and follow instructions regarding treatment and home care.

## Due Care

**Due care** is a legal term that means proper and sufficient care or the absence of negligence. The dentist has a legal obligation to provide due care in treating patients. This obligation applies to all treatment procedures.

When a drug is administered and prescribed, due care implies that the dentist is familiar with the drug and its properties. The dentist must also have adequate information regarding the patient's health to know whether the drug is suitable for the patient, or whether the patient's health record contraindicates its use. Therefore a complete, up-to-date health history is essential.

## Malpractice

Although patients may bring a lawsuit against the dentist, this does not mean that they will win. The following four conditions, sometimes called the "four D's," must *all* be present for a malpractice lawsuit to be successful:

1. *Duty.* A dentist-patient relationship must exist to establish the duty.
2. *Derelict* (lacking a sense of duty, negligent). Negligence occurred because the standard of care was not met.
3. *Direct cause.* The negligent act was the direct cause of the injury.
4. *Damages.* Pain and suffering, loss of income, and medical bills are included in damages.

If a dentist injects local anesthetic on the wrong side of a patient's mouth, for example, probably no grounds exist for a malpractice suit because no "damages" occurred to the patient. Although negligence ("derelict") may have occurred, all four conditions were not present.

### Acts of Omission and Commission

**Malpractice** is *professional negligence,* or failure to provide due care, or the lack of due care. In dentistry, the two types of malpractice are acts of omission and acts of commission.

An act of omission is failure to perform an act that a "reasonable and prudent professional" *would* perform. An example would be a dentist who fails to diagnose periodontal disease because the dentist did not take radiographs or perform a periodontal probing.

An act of commission is performance of an act that a "reasonable and prudent professional" *would not* perform. An example would be a dentist who administers 15 cartridges of a local anesthetic to a small child, resulting in a life-threatening overdose.

### Doctrine of *Res Ipsa Loquitur*

Sometimes an expert witness is not necessary in a malpractice suit. Under the doctrine of **res ipsa loquitur** ("the act speaks for itself"), the evidence is clear. An example is the dentist who extracted the wrong tooth or broke an instrument during a root canal and left the instrument in the tooth.

RECALL

9 What is meant by abandonment?
10 Can a dentist refuse to treat a patient only because he or she has HIV infection?
11 What are the "four D's" necessary for a successful malpractice suit?
12 What does *res ipsa loquitur* mean?
13 What are the best defenses against a malpractice suit?

## Risk Management

In this age of increasing *litigiousness* (proneness to engage in lawsuits), the dental team must constantly be aware of the need to avoid malpractice risks in the dental practice. Risk management refers to the procedures and practices that are used to avoid lawsuits. Major areas of risk management include (1) excellent communication with patients, (2) maintaining accurate and complete records, (3) receiving informed consent, and (4) doing everything possible to maintain the highest standards of clinical excellence.

Legal authorities note that legal problems with patients are best avoided by maintaining a climate of *good rapport* and *open communication* with all patients. When patients become angry or frustrated and believe they are not being heard, they are more likely to file a lawsuit.

### Avoiding Malpractice Lawsuits

Prevention and good communication between provider and patient are the best defenses against malpractice. Patients are less likely to initiate a lawsuit when they have a clear understanding of the following:

- Planned treatment
- Reasonable treatment results
- Potential treatment complications
- Their own financial obligations

The dental assistant can play an important role in prevention of malpractice litigation by being aware of signs of patient dissatisfaction and alerting the dentist when signs are noted (Fig. 5.3).

### "Silence Is Golden"

The dental assistant must never make critical remarks about dental treatment rendered by an employer or another dentist.

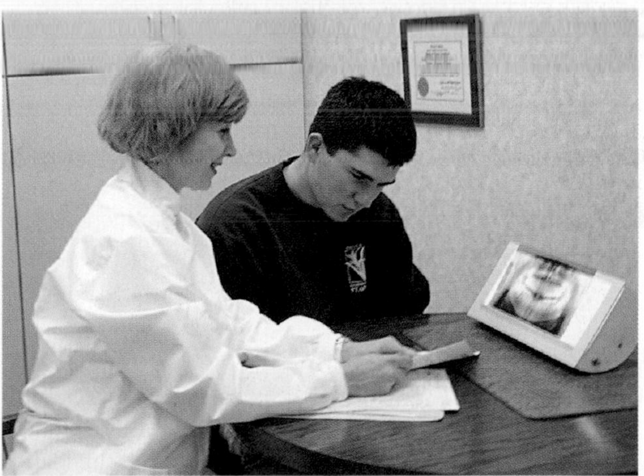

**FIG. 5.3** An important role of the dental assistant is to facilitate good communication with the patient. *(Courtesy Pamela Landry, RDA.)*

The dental assistant should never discuss other patients and should avoid discussing the dentist's professional liability insurance.

Under the concept of **res gestae** ("things done"), statements made spontaneously by anyone (including the dental assistant) at the time of an alleged negligent act are admissible as evidence and may be damaging to the dentist and dental assistant in a court of law. Comments such as "whoops" or "uh-oh" may unnecessarily frighten the patient and should be avoided.

**14** What is meant by *res gestae*?

## Guidelines for Informed Consent

The concept of **informed consent** is based on the idea that it is the patient who must pay the bill and endure the pain and suffering that may result from treatment. Therefore the patient has the right to know all important facts about the proposed treatment.

### Informed Patient Consent

Informed consent to dental treatment is based on information provided by the dentist. This means that the dentist must give the patient enough information about his or her condition and all available treatment options. The patient and dentist should then discuss these options, and the patient must choose the most suitable treatment alternative.

When a patient enters a dentist's office, the patient gives **implied consent**, at least for the dental examination. Provided the patient is capable, implied consent is given when the patient agrees to treatment, or at least does not object to treatment. In a court of law, implied consent is a less reliable form of consent in a malpractice suit. **Written consent** is the preferred means of obtaining and documenting the patient's consent to and understanding of the procedure.

#### Guidelines for Informed Consent

The patient should be informed about the following:

- Nature of the proposed treatment, including the cost and expected time for healing
- Benefits of the proposed treatment, as well as the consequences of *not* having the treatment
- Common, severe risks associated with the proposed treatment
- Reasonable alternatives to the proposed treatment, including risks and benefits of each alternative

### Informed Refusal

If a patient refuses proposed treatment, the dentist must inform the patient about the likely consequences and must obtain the patient's informed refusal. However, obtaining the patient's informed refusal does not release the dentist from the responsibility of providing the standard of care. A patient may not consent to substandard care, and the dentist may not legally or ethically agree to provide such care. For example, if a patient refuses radiographs, the dentist may refer the patient to another provider because the dentist believes radiographs are a necessary standard of care. Another dentist, however, may be willing to treat the patient without radiograph films and may request that the patient sign a written and dated informed refusal for radiographs. This statement is then filed with the patient's record.

## Exceptions to Disclosure

The dentist does not have a duty to disclose information about proposed treatment in the following situations:

- The patient asks not to be advised.
- The procedure is simple and straightforward, and life-threatening risks (e.g., death from a filling) are remote.
- Treatment risk is minor, and treatment rarely results in serious adverse effects (e.g., discomfort while biting down as radiograph films are taken).
- Information would be so upsetting that the patient would be unable to weigh risks and benefits rationally; this is known as the *therapeutic exception*.

## Informed Consent for Minors

The parent, custodial parent, or legal guardian must give consent for minor children. When parents live separately, the child's personal information form should indicate which parent is the custodial parent. When separated parents share custody, the child's record should contain letters from both parents providing consent and authorization to treat. Asking in advance for a parent's or a custodial parent's "blanket" consent for emergency treatment avoids confusion and delays should the child require emergency care when a parent or guardian is not present.

## Documenting Informed Consent

Most states do not require a specific means for documenting discussions on informed consent. At minimum, the patient's record should indicate that the patient received information about risks, benefits, and treatment alternatives and consented to or refused the proposed treatment.

When treatment is extensive, invasive, or risky, a written informed consent document is recommended. The patient, the dentist, and a witness should sign the written consent form. The patient should receive a copy of the form, and the original should be kept in the patient's chart.

#### Clinical Situations that Require Written Informed Consent

- New drugs are used
- Experimentation or clinical testing is involved
- Patient's identifiable photograph is used
- General anesthesia is administered
- Minors are treated in a public program
- Treatment takes longer than 1 year to complete

## Content of Informed Consent Forms

Informed consent is a *process,* not just a form. It involves face-to-face discussion between the dentist and the patient. Enough time should be made available to answer all of the patient's questions and concerns.

Many types of commercial informed consent forms are available from professional organizations and insurance companies. Dentists often choose to develop their own forms. In any case, informed consent forms should contain the following:

- Nature of the proposed treatment
- Benefits and treatment alternatives
- Risks and potential consequences associated with not performing treatment
- Other information as necessary for a particular case

This form should be signed by the patient, the dentist, and a witness. The patient should be given a copy of the form, and the original should be kept in the patient's chart.

The signed informed consent form and documented discussion do not absolutely protect the dentist against the patient who alleges that he or she was not fully informed about a procedure. However, thorough documentation greatly increases the dentist's chance of defense against such allegations.

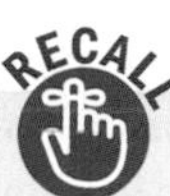


**15** What is the difference between implied consent and written consent?

## Patient Referral

Dentists usually refer a patient who has an unusual case or a condition beyond their scope of expertise. The dentist must inform the patient that the needed treatment cannot be performed properly in the dentist's office and that the services of a specialist are required. The dentist should assist the patient in finding an appropriate specialist.

### *Failure to Refer*

Many malpractice claims involve failure of the general dentist to refer the patient to a specialist when the patient's oral condition requires special attention.

Failure to recognize periodontal disease and refer the patient to a periodontist is a very common cause for this type of malpractice suit. Periodontal disease is a silent disease; patients rarely experience pain and often are not even aware that a problem exists. Therefore it is important that the general dentist establish a patient's baseline oral condition and record changes in periodontal health over time. It is also important to make an entry in the chart each time that the patient has been informed of the condition and the need for treatment and/or referral.

When a patient is referred to a specialist, the referral should be thoroughly documented in the patient's chart. Documentation should include a description of the problem, reasons for referral, the name and specialty of the referral dentist, and whether or not the patient has agreed to the referral.

## Guarantees

Outcomes of dental care cannot be completely predicted. Neither the dentist nor the staff should make a promise or a claim about the outcome of care because this could be interpreted as a "guarantee." It is unethical to make guarantees; in some states, it is illegal.

## Contributory Negligence

The patient's record should include notation of any broken appointments or last-minute cancellations. These actions may be interpreted as "contributory negligence" on the part of the patient. Contributory negligence occurs when a patient's action (or lack of action) negatively affects the treatment outcome. Documentation of broken and cancelled appointments helps protect the practice from legal recourse should a patient claim negligence against the dentist.

For example, a dentist and a dental hygienist explain the need for improved home care to a patient and document these instructions on the patient's chart. At each visit, however, the patient's home care remains unimproved despite continued warnings. The patient's periodontal condition continues to decline. The patient's lack of home care constitutes contributory negligence that led to the development of periodontal disease.

**16** Why should broken appointments be noted on the patient's chart?

# Patient Records

Records regarding patient care are referred to as the *dental chart* or *patient record.* These records are important legal documents that must be protected and handled with care (see Chapter 26). All examination records, diagnoses, radiographs, consent forms, updated medical histories, copies of medical and laboratory prescriptions, and correspondence to or about a patient are filed together in the patient's folder. Financial information is *not* included in the patient chart (Fig. 5.1).

Patient records are acceptable in court and clearly show the dates and details of services rendered for each patient. Nothing should be left to memory. Incomplete or unclear records are damaging evidence in a malpractice case. Every entry in a chart should be made as if the chart will be seen in a court of law. Patient records must never be altered. If an error is made on the patient's chart, it must be corrected properly (see Chapter 26). The dental assistant should never use white correction fluid to attempt to cover up the original entry.

## Ownership of Dental Records and Radiographs

The dentist technically "owns" all patient records and radiographs. According to some state laws, however, patients have

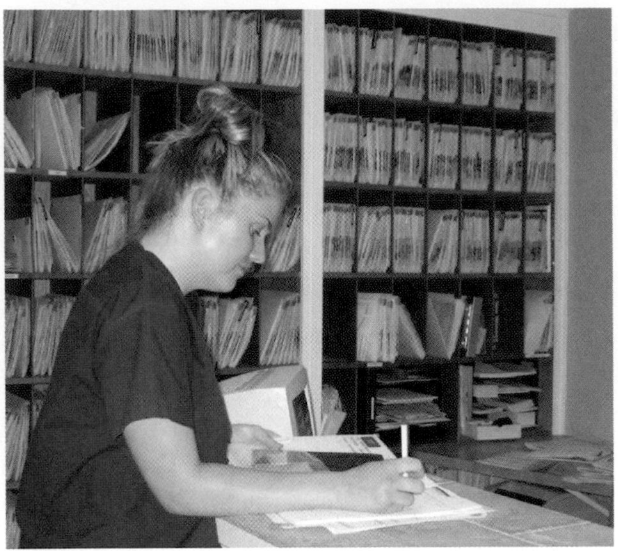

**FIG. 5.4** Patient records must be handled with care.

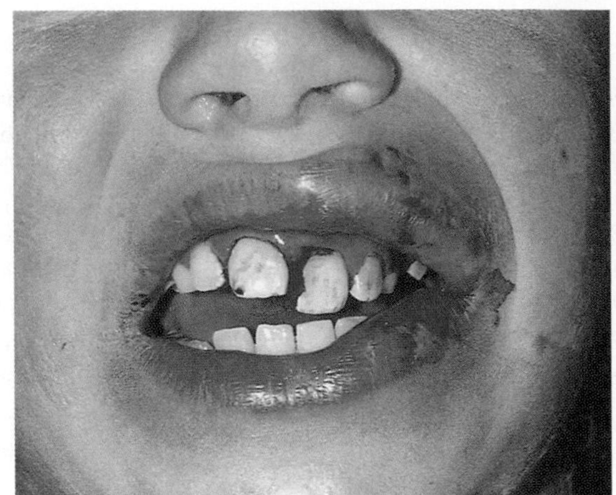

**FIG. 5.5** This boy was a victim of child abuse.

the right to *access* (review) and *retrieve* (remove) their records and radiographs.

Original records and radiographs cannot be taken from the practice without the dentist's permission. In most situations, duplicate radiographs and a photocopy of the record will satisfy patient needs. If the patient disagrees with practice policies on this, the dental assistant should not attempt to make a decision but should refer the matter to the dentist immediately.

### Guidelines for Charting Entries in Clinical Records

- Keep a separate chart for each patient. Do not use a "group" chart for an entire family.
- Business and financial information is not part of the clinical record. Do not include these records in the chart.
- It is better to chart too much information than too little.
- Make the chart entry during the examination or patient visit. The longer the time between the procedure and the charting entry, the greater the chance for error.
- Write legibly, and record the entry accurately in ink. Date and initial the entry.
- The chart entry should be sufficiently complete to indicate that nothing was neglected; this includes the reason for the visit, details of the treatment provided, and a record of all instructions to the patient, prescriptions, and referrals.
- Never change the chart after a problem arises. If a charting error occurs, correct it properly (see Chapter 26).

## Reporting Abuse and Neglect

Dentists, dental hygienists, and dental assistants may be the first to recognize signs of abuse and may be instrumental in enhancing the victim's chances of obtaining assistance. Abuse can occur inside or outside of the home, for example, in day care centers or nursing homes. Because many injuries occur around the mouth, neck, face, and head, members of the dental health team are in an excellent position to recognize the signs of abuse and to report cases of suspected abuse to authorities. Many states identify dental professionals as **mandated reporters**. In these states, dental professionals must report suspected abuse if they observe signs of abuse, or if they have reasonable suspicion of abuse. The report may be made to a social work agency, a county welfare or probation department, or a police or sheriff's department. Basic types of abuse are **child abuse**, **spousal abuse**, **elder abuse**, and dental neglect.

### Child Abuse

Cases of child abuse and neglect are increasingly reported throughout the United States. Approximately 75 percent of child abuse injuries involve the head, neck, or mouth area (Fig. 5.5). A child is defined as any patient who is 18 years of age or younger.

The primary intent of reporting abuse is *to protect the child.* It is equally important that help be provided for the parents. Parents may be unable to ask for help directly, and child abuse may be a means of revealing family problems. A report of abuse may lead to changes in the home that can reduce the risk of abuse.

*Child abuse* is legally defined as any act of omission or commission that endangers or impairs a child's physical or emotional health and development. These acts include (1) physical abuse and corporal punishment resulting in injury, (2) emotional abuse, (3) emotional deprivation, (4) physical neglect or inadequate supervision, and (5) sexual abuse or exploitation.

Warning signs of child abuse include repeated injury (multiple bruises), unusual sites of accidental injury such as the neck or cheeks, neglected appearance of the patient, strict and overly critical parents, and extremely isolated families. It is very important that unusual or frequent injuries be documented so that patterns, if present, can be identified.

## Domestic Violence

*Domestic violence* is the term used to describe battering, abuse, or control over an intimate individual within the same household. It happens to women more often than to men. Even though some states require that spousal abuse must be reported, adherence to this mandate can be difficult because the victim may deny the incident or may say that the report was filed without her permission. Spousal abuse should be reported with the consent of the abused spouse. This abuse usually starts with controlling behavior on the part of the abusive spouse that becomes more frequent and more aggressive. The dental professional must be sensitive and supportive and must document evidence that may suggest abuse.

## Elder Abuse

Elder abuse occurs when a relative (i.e., child, spouse, or other family member) or a healthcare provider abuses an elderly patient. An elder is defined as a person 65 years of age or older. Elder abuse can be physical, sexual, or emotional; it can consist of passive neglect, willful deprivation, and, most commonly, financial exploitation. As with child and spousal abuse, dental professionals should look for signs of physical abuse and for behavior that suggests abuse, such as being withdrawn. Other indications include poor personal hygiene, lack of appropriate dress, and the presence of unusual injuries. One of the problems with identifying elder abuse is that the elderly person may not wish to report the actions of a son or daughter. Another concern of the elderly victim may be the thought of the consequences of reporting abuse, and worry about who will then take care of them. Reports may be made to local social agencies that help the elderly.

As the elderly population grows and begins to rely on primary care providers, it is becoming more important for dental professionals to be aware of and to document all signs of potential elder abuse.

## Dental Neglect

Dental neglect is the willful failure of a person or guardian to seek and obtain appropriate treatment for caries and oral infection. Dental neglect consists of the following:

- Untreated rampant caries, easily detected by a layperson
- Chronic pain
- Delay or retardation in a child's growth or development
- Child's difficulty with or inability to perform daily activities such as playing or going to school

### Indicators of Child Abuse and Neglect

**Behavioral Indicators**

- Child is wary of adult contacts.
- Child is apprehensive when other children cry.
- Child is afraid to go home.
- Child is frightened of parents.
- Child exhibits overly compliant, passive, and undemanding behaviors to avoid confrontation with abuser.
- Child lags in development of motor skills, toilet training, socialization, or language. (Developmental lags may also result from physical abuse, medical neglect, or nutritional deficiency.)

**Dental Neglect or Abuse**

- Untreated rampant caries that is easily detectable by a layperson
- Untreated pain, infection, bleeding, or trauma affecting the orofacial region
- Injuries or tears to the labial frenum, indicating forced feedings

**Other Indicators**

- Child displays cigarette burns or bite marks.
- Child displays cuts, bleeding, or finger marks on ears, or "cauliflower ear."
- Child displays bald or sparse spots on scalp, indicating malnutrition or hair pulling.
- Child is dirty, is unkempt, or has poor oral hygiene.
- Child is dressed inappropriately for weather to conceal bruises or injuries (e.g., long sleeves on a hot day).
- Child shows evidence of poor supervision, such as repeated falls down stairs, repeated ingestion of harmful substances, or being left alone in a car or on the street.
- Mentally or physically disabled children are especially vulnerable and are often targets for abuse because of the difficulties caregivers face in meeting the needs of these children.

## Immunity

In states that legally mandate the reporting of child, spousal, or elder abuse, immunity is granted from criminal and civil liability for reporting as required. This means that the dental professional cannot be sued for reporting suspicions in an attempt to protect a potential victim.

## HIPAA

In 1996 Congress enacted the Health Insurance Portability and Accountability Act (**HIPAA**). The purpose of HIPAA is to provide consumers with greater access to healthcare insurance, to protect the privacy of protected health information, and to promote greater standardization and to enhance efficiency in the healthcare industry. Dentists and all dental health professionals must follow the HIPAA regulations (see Chapter 63).

### Purpose of HIPAA

- To ensure portability of health benefits for employees who change jobs and whose eligibility for benefits may have changed because of a change in health status
- To provide tax credits for employers to encourage employee medical savings accounts
- To reduce fraud and abuse (principally in Medicare and Medicaid)
- To encourage administrative simplification in healthcare, while maintaining patient confidentiality

## HIPAA: Summary of the Health Insurance Portability and Accountability Act of 1996

The Health Insurance Portability and Accountability Act of 1996 (HIPAA) was signed into law by President Bill Clinton on August 21, 1996. Conclusive regulations were issued on August 17, 2000, to take effect by October 16, 2002. HIPAA requires that transactions of all patient healthcare information be formatted in a standardized electronic style. In addition to protecting the privacy and security of patient information, HIPAA includes legislation on the formation of medical savings accounts, the authorization of a fraud and abuse control program, the easy transport of health insurance coverage, and the simplification of administrative terms and conditions.

HIPAA encompasses privacy requirements that can be broken down into three types: privacy standards, patients' rights, and administrative requirements.

### Privacy Standards

A central concern of HIPAA is the careful use and disclosure of protected health information (PHI), which generally is electronically controlled health information that is able to be distinguished individually. PHI also refers to verbal communication, although the HIPAA Privacy Rule is not intended to hinder necessary verbal communication. The U.S. Department of Health and Human Services (USDHHS) does not require restructuring, such as soundproofing, architectural changes, and so forth, but some caution is necessary when health information is exchanged through conversation.

An Acknowledgment of Receipt of Notice of Privacy Practices, which allows patient information to be used or divulged for treatment, payment, or healthcare operations (TPO), should be procured from each patient. A detailed and time-sensitive authorization can also be issued, which allows the dentist to release information in special circumstances other than TPO. A *written consent* is also an option. Dentists can disclose PHI *without* acknowledgment, consent, or authorization in very special situations, for example, perceived child abuse, public health supervision, fraud investigation, or law enforcement with valid permission (e.g., a warrant). When divulging PHI, a dentist must try to disclose only the *minimum necessary* information to help safeguard the patient's information as much as possible.

It is important that dental professionals adhere to HIPAA standards because healthcare providers (as well as healthcare clearinghouses and healthcare plans) who convey *electronically* formatted health information via an outside billing service or merchant are considered *covered entities.* Covered entities may be dealt serious civil and criminal penalties for violation of HIPAA legislation. Failure to comply with HIPAA privacy requirements may result in civil penalties of up to $100 per offense with an annual maximum of $25,000 for repeated failure to comply with the same requirement. Criminal penalties resulting from the illegal mishandling of private health information can range from $50,000 and/or 1 year in prison to $250,000 and/or 10 years in prison.

### Patients' Rights

HIPAA allows patients, authorized representatives, and parents of minors, as well as minors, to become more aware of the health information privacy to which they are entitled. These rights include, but are not limited to, the right to view and copy their health information, the right to dispute alleged breaches of policies and regulations, and the right to request alternative forms of communicating with their dentist. If any health information is released for any reason other than TPO, the patient is entitled to an account of the transaction. Therefore it is important for dentists to keep accurate records of such information and to provide them when necessary.

The HIPAA Privacy Rule ensures that the parents of a minor have access to their child's health information. This privilege may be overruled, for example, in cases where child abuse is suspected, or the parent consents to a term of confidentiality between the dentist and the minor. Parents' rights to access their child's PHI also may be restricted in situations where a legal entity, such as a court, intervenes and the law does not require a parent's consent. For a full list of patients' rights provided by HIPAA, be sure to acquire a copy of the law and to read it well.

### Administrative Requirements

Complying with HIPAA legislation may seem like a chore, but it does not need to be so. It is recommended that you become appropriately familiar with the law, organize the requirements into simpler tasks, begin compliance early, and document your progress in compliance. An important first step is to evaluate the information and practices currently in place in your office.

Dentists will need to write a *privacy policy* for their office, a document for their patients that details the office's practices concerning PHI. The *HIPAA Privacy Kit* of the American Dental Association (ADA) includes forms that you (the dentist) can use to customize your privacy policy. It is useful to try to understand the role of healthcare information for your patients and the ways in which they deal with this information while they are visiting your office. Train your staff; make sure they are familiar with the terms of HIPAA and your office's privacy policy and related forms. HIPAA requires that you designate a *privacy officer,* a person in your office who will be responsible for applying the new policies in your office, fielding complaints, and making choices involving the minimum necessary requirements. Another person in the role of *contact person* will process complaints.

A *Notice of Privacy Practices*—a document that details the patient's rights and the dental office's obligations concerning PHI—also must be drawn up. Further, any role of a third party with access to PHI must be clearly documented. This third party is known as a *business associate* (BA) and is defined as any entity who, on behalf of the dentist, takes part in any activity that involves exposure of PHI. The *HIPAA Privacy Kit* provides a copy of the USDHHS "Business Associate Contract Terms," which presents a concrete format for detailing BA interactions.

The original HIPAA privacy compliance date, including all staff training, was April 14, 2003, although many covered entities that submitted a request and a compliance plan by October 15, 2002, were granted 1-year extensions. Contact your local branch of the ADA for details. It is recommended that dentists prepare their offices ahead of time for all deadlines pertaining to preparation of privacy policies and forms and business associate contracts, as well as employee training sessions.

For a comprehensive discussion of all of these terms and requirements, a complete list of HIPAA policies and procedures, and a full collection of HIPAA privacy forms, contact the American Dental Association for a *HIPAA Privacy Kit.* The relevant ADA Web site is www.ada.org/goto/hipaa. Other Web sites that may provide useful information about HIPAA are the following:

- USDHHS Office of Civil Rights: www.hhs.gov/ocr/hipaa
- Work Group on Electronic Data Interchange: www.wedi.org/SNIP
- Phoenix Health: www.hipaadvisory.com
- USDHHS Office of the Assistant Secretary for Planning and Evaluation: http://aspe.os.dhhs.gov/admnsimp/

Data from HIPAA Privacy Kit and American Dental Association (www.ada.org).

**17** What is the primary purpose of reporting suspected cases of child abuse?
**18** What are mandated reporters?

**■ Legal and Ethical Implications** The practice of dentistry is subject to a variety of laws and regulations that are meant to protect the public. Dental assisting is a highly skilled profession that requires education and competence in a variety of procedures.

As a dental assistant, you should have a general understanding of how laws affect the practice of dentistry and how you can minimize the risk of malpractice liability. Legally and ethically, you must be aware of the laws that govern the practice of dentistry in your state, and you must always practice within the law. ■

**■ Eye to the Future** The number of lawsuits in dentistry increases each year. Remember, you may become involved in a malpractice suit or may be called to testify even if you are no longer employed by the practice. ■

## ■ Critical Thinking

Mrs. Jensen has been a patient in your office for longer than 10 years. At best, she has been difficult and demanding. She has failed to keep some appointments and often arrives late for appointments. When Mrs. Jensen phoned the office to make an appointment, the receptionist told her that Dr. Klein would no longer be able to treat her. Mrs. Jensen became very angry and threatened to call her attorney.

1. Does Mrs. Jensen have a basis for legal action? If so, on what grounds?
2. Even though the receptionist told Mrs. Jensen that she could not be seen again in the dental office, is Dr. Klein still liable? Why or why not?
3. What would have been a better way to dismiss Mrs. Jensen from the practice of dentistry, and how can you minimize the risk of malpractice liability? ■

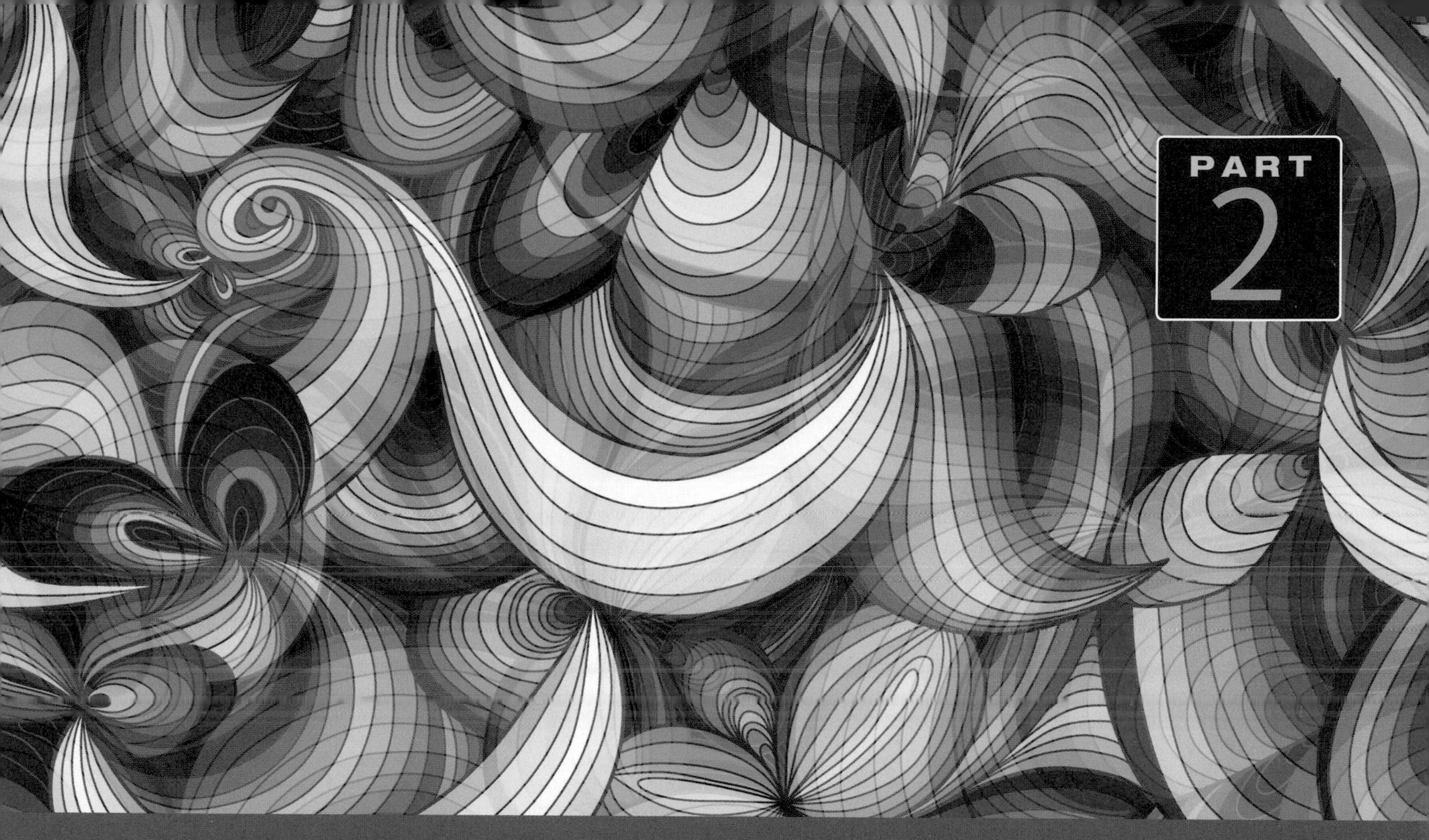

PART 2

# Sciences in Dentistry

The sciences are the foundation for your career as a dental assistant. The human body is wonderful, complex, and fascinating. As you study the information in this section, think about your own body. It will make this information even more relevant to you.

The chapters in this section provide an overview of basic human anatomy and physiology, and provide a look into the future of regenerative medicine through stem cell research. You will be able to identify the structures of the oral cavity in detail and will learn how the teeth begin to develop before birth. You will use your knowledge of dentition every day in your career as a dental assistant.

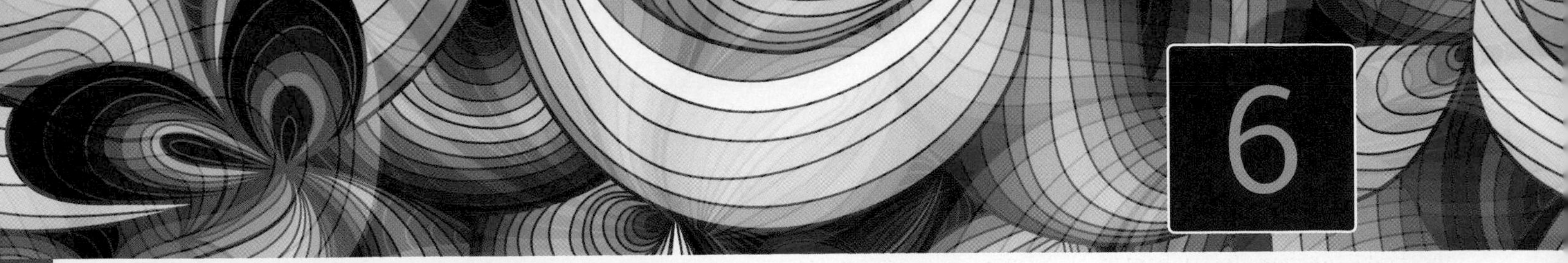

6

# General Anatomy

## KEY TERMS

**Abdominal cavity** Contains the stomach, liver, gallbladder, spleen, and most of the intestines.
**Abdominopelvic cavity** Part of the ventral cavity that contains the abdominal and pelvic cavities.
**Anatomical (anatomic) position (an-uh-TOM-i-kul, an-uh-TOM-ik)** The body standing erect with face forward, feet together, arms hanging at the sides, and palms forward.
**Anatomy (uh-NAT-uh-mee)** Study of the shape and structure of the human body.
**Anterior** Toward the front.
**Appendicular (ap-en-DIK-yoo-ler)** Pertaining to the body region that consists of the arms and legs.
**Axial (AK-see-ul)** Referring to the body region that comprises the head, neck, and trunk.
**Connective tissue** The major support material of the body.
**Cranial (KRAY-nee-ul) cavity** Space that houses the brain.
**Cytoplasm (SI-toe-plaz-em)** Gel-like fluid inside the cell.
**Differentiation** Term for the specialization function of cells.
**Distal** Farther away from the trunk of the body; opposite of proximal.
**Dorsal cavity** Cavity located in the back of the body.
**Epithelial (ep-i-THEE-lee-ul) tissue** Type of tissue that forms the covering of all body surfaces.
**Frontal plane** Vertical plane that divides the body into anterior (front) and posterior (back) portions.
**Horizontal plane** Plane that divides the body into superior (upper) and inferior (lower) portions.
**Medial** Toward or nearer to the midline of the body.
**Midsagittal plane** Imaginary line that divides the patient's face into equal right and left sides.
**Muscle tissue** Tissue with the ability to lengthen or shorten to provide movement to body parts.
**National Institute of Dental and Craniofacial Research (NIDCR)** The federal government's lead agency for scientific research on oral, dental, and craniofacial disease.
**Nerve tissue** Responsible for coordinating and controlling body activities.
**Nucleus (NOO-klee-us)** "Control center" of the cell.
**Organelle (or-guh-NEL)** Specialized part of a cell that performs a specific function.
**Parietal (puh-RYE-e-tul)** Pertaining to the walls of a body cavity.
**Pelvic cavity** Contains portions of the large and small intestines, the rectum, the urinary bladder, and the reproductive organs.
**Physiology (fiz-ee-OL-uh-jee)** Study of the functions of the human body.
**Planes** Three imaginary lines used to divide the body into sections.
**Posterior** Toward the back.
**Proximal** Closer to the trunk of the body; opposite of distal.
**Regenerative medicine** Process of creating living, functional tissues to repair or replace tissue or organ function through the use of stem cells.
**Sagittal (SADJ-ih-tal) plane** Any vertical plane parallel to the midline that divides the body into unequal left and right portions.
**Spinal cavity** Space in the body that contains the spinal cord.
**Stem cell** Immature, unspecialized cells capable of replication and differentiation into other types of cells or tissues.
**Superior** Above another portion, or closer to the head.
**Thoracic cavity** Contains the heart, lungs, esophagus, and trachea.
**Ventral cavity** Cavity located at the front of the body.
**Visceral (VIS-er-ul)** Pertaining to internal organs or the covering of those organs.

## LEARNING OUTCOMES

*On completion of this chapter, the student will be able to achieve the following objectives:*

1. Pronounce, define, and spell the key terms.
2. Identify the planes and associated body directions used to divide the body into sections.
3. Identify and describe the four levels of organization in the human body, including the following:
   - Describe the components of a cell, including the different types of stem cells.
   - Identify and describe the four types of tissue in the human body.
   - Explain the difference between an organ and a body system.
4. Identify the two major body cavities and their components, as well as name and locate the two reference regions of the body.

## ELECTRONIC RESOURCES

***Additional information related to content in Chapter 6 can be found on the companion Evolve Web site.***

- Animations: Directions of the Body
- Practice Quiz

You may ask yourself, Why is it important for the dental assistant to have a basic understanding of the structure and anatomy of the human body? Think about this: Yes, you could learn to drive a car without any knowledge of motors, radiators, tires, fuel, batteries, oil pressure, and so on. However, when you have a basic understanding of the parts and operating systems of your car and how they function, you are better equipped to deal with routine maintenance and unexpected malfunctions. Because of your knowledge, you are in fact a better and safer motorist on the road.

**Anatomy** is the scientific study of the *shape* and *structure* of the human body. **Physiology** is the scientific study of how the body *functions* (see Chapter 7). Studies of anatomy and physiology are closely related because one continuously influences the other. Remember that *function affects structure, and structure affects function.*

To communicate effectively as a health professional, you must begin by learning some basic terms that relate to the anatomy of the body. This chapter discusses terms used to describe regions of the body and directional terms used in describing the body. You are learning a new vocabulary that will continue to grow as you progress through the book. The basic anatomical reference systems are (1) planes and body directions, (2) structural units, and (3) body cavities.

## Planes and Body Directions

The word *anatomy* comes from the Greek words *ana* and *tome-*, which means to "cut up." In the study of anatomy, the human body is described as if it were dissected. Terms used to describe *directions* in relation to the whole body are easier to understand if you think of them as *pairs of opposite directions,* such as up and down, left and right, or front and back (Table 6.1).

When the human body is described, it is assumed that the body is in "anatomical position." **Anatomical (or anatomic) position** refers to the body standing erect with face forward, feet together, and arms hanging at the sides (Fig. 6.1).

To help visualize the relationships of internal body parts, imaginary lines called **planes** are used to divide the body into sections.

The **midsagittal plane**, also known as the *median plane* or *midline plane,* is the vertical plane that divides the body into equal left and right halves.

The **sagittal plane** is any vertical plane parallel to the midline that divides the body, from top to bottom, into unequal left and right portions.

The **horizontal plane**, also known as the *transverse plane,* divides the body into *superior* (upper) and *inferior* (lower) portions.

The **frontal plane**, also known as the *coronal plane,* is any vertical plane at right angles to the midsagittal plane that divides the body into **anterior** (front) and **posterior** (back) portions.

1 What is the difference between anatomy and physiology?
2 What imaginary lines are used to divide the body into sections?

## Structural Units

The human body is incredibly complex. However, the study of anatomy is not difficult when it is broken down into small units.

The study of the human body begins with the smallest units and builds systematically to larger and larger units, finally resulting in the complete body. The human body has four organizational levels. From the simplest to the most complex, these consist of (1) cells, (2) tissues, (3) organs, and (4) body systems (Fig. 6.2).

### Cells

Cells are the basic units of structure of the human body. Every human life begins as a single cell, a fertilized egg. This single cell divides into 2 cells, then 4, 8, 16, and so on, until the adult human body is complete and has an estimated 75 trillion cells. Each tiny cell has the following unique capabilities: (1) to react to stimuli and transform nutrients into energy, (2) to grow, and (3) to reproduce (Fig. 6.3).

Cells have different shapes. Some cells are shaped like columns, and others are shaped like cubes or spheres. For example, red blood cells resemble shallow saucers, nerve cells look like threads, and cheek cells resemble flat paving stones. The life span of cells varies depending on the type. For example, cells in the lining of the intestines die after 1½ days, red blood cells die after 120 days, and nerve cells can live for 100 years.

**TABLE 6.1** Directional Terms for the Human Body

| Term | Definition | Example |
|---|---|---|
| **Superior** | Above another part, or closer to head | Nose is superior to mouth. |
| Inferior | Below another part, or closer to feet | Heart is inferior to neck. |
| **Proximal** | Closer to a point of attachment, or closer to trunk of body | Elbow is proximal to wrist. |
| **Distal** | Farther from a point of attachment, or farther from trunk of body | Fingers are distal to wrist. |
| Lateral | The side, or away from the midline | Ears are lateral to eyes. |
| **Medial** | Toward, or nearer the midline | Nose is medial to ears. |
| Dorsal | On the back | Spine is on dorsal side of body. |
| Ventral | On the front | Face is on ventral side of body. |
| Anterior | Toward the front | Heart is anterior to spine. |
| Posterior | Toward the back | Ear is posterior to nose. |

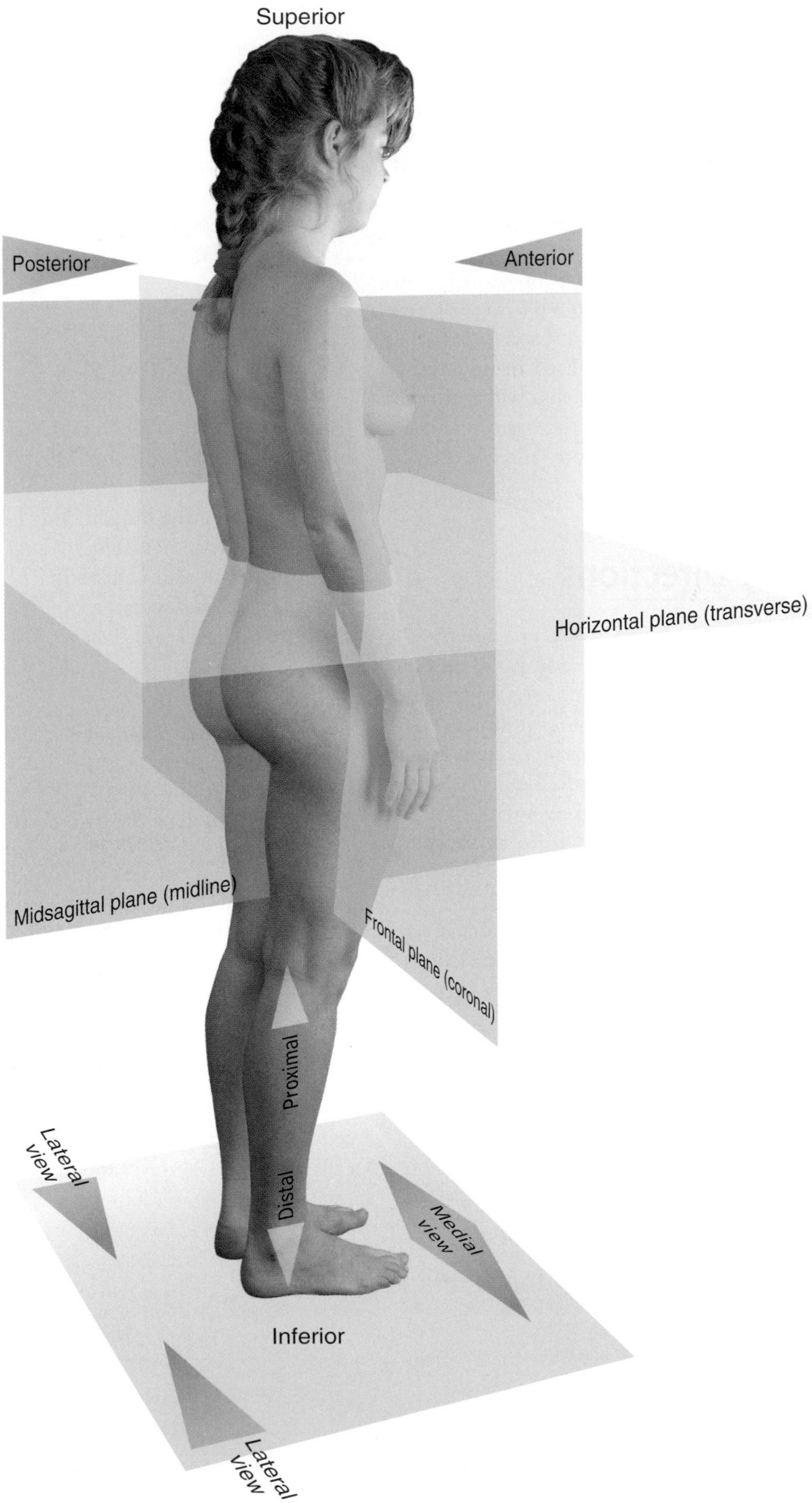

**FIG. 6.1** Body in anatomical (anatomic) position. *(Modified from Abrahams PH, Marks SC Jr, Hutchins RT: McMinn's color atlas of human anatomy, St Louis, Mosby, 2003.)*

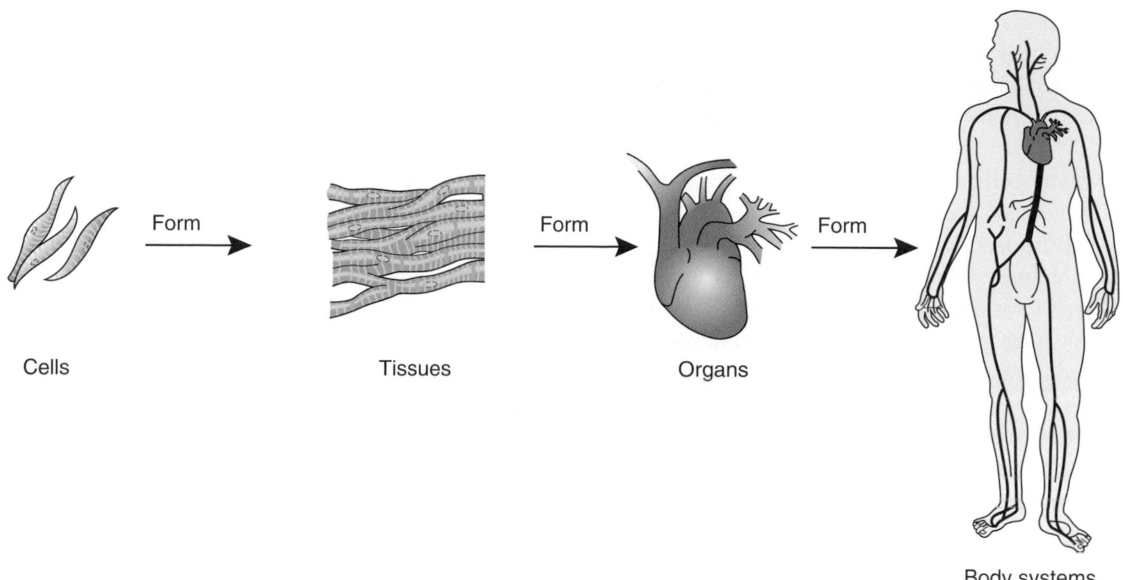


**FIG. 6.2** Organizational levels of the body. The human body develops from the simplest to the most complex forms.

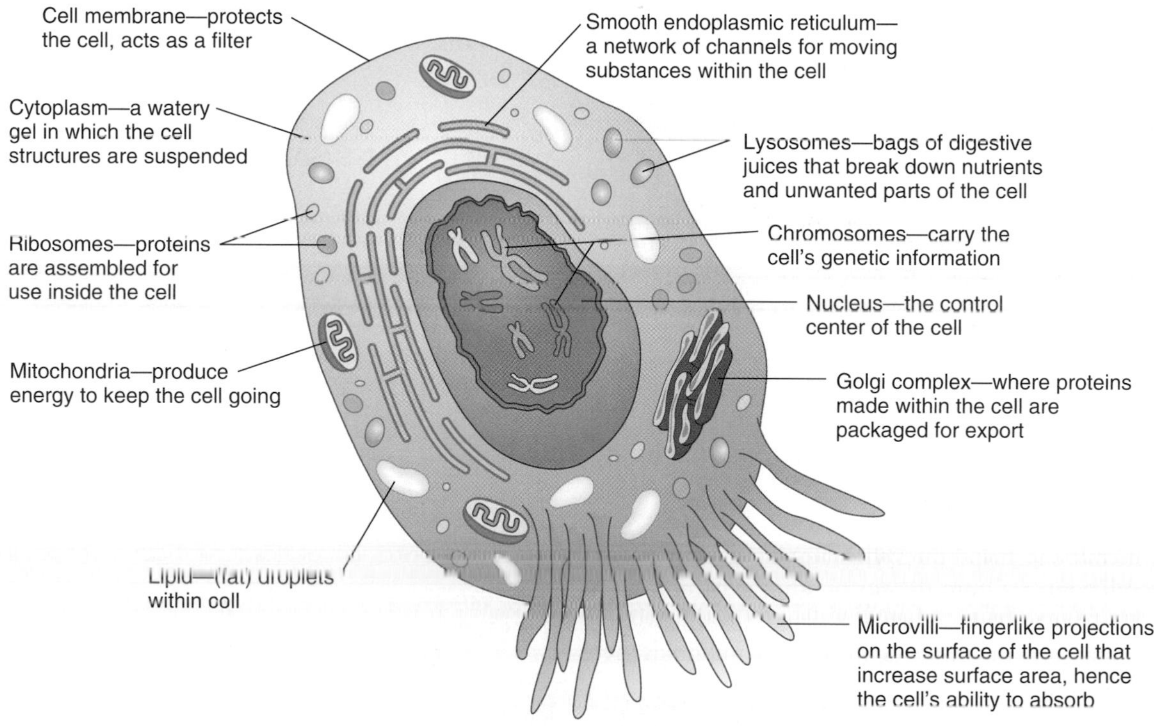


**FIG. 6.3** Basic human cell.

Different types of cells have different functions; brain cells, for example, have a different function than blood cells. The term for this specialized function of cells is **differentiation**. The human body contains many types of cells, each with a specific purpose.

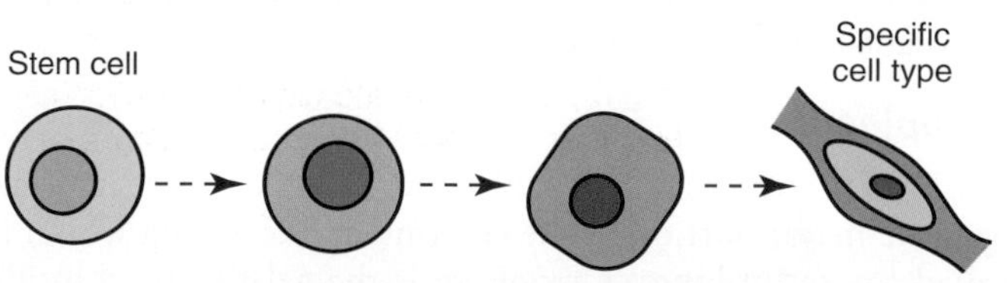


**FIG. 6.4** The evolution of a stem cell.

## *Stem Cells*

**Stem cells** are immature, *unspecialized* cells in the body. Stem cells can be induced to become other types of cells in the body (Fig. 6.4). Stem cells divide and grow rapidly and differentiate into other tissue types, such as muscle, nerve, and components of the blood. Stem cells can be found in different organs and tissues in the human body at all stages of life. Stem cells are identified by two primary sources: *embryonic stem cells* and *adult stem cells.*

**Embryonic stem cells** come from embryos that develop from eggs that have been fertilized in a test tube and then are used for research purposes. They are not derived from eggs fertilized in a woman's body. The embryos are usually 4 or 5 days old and are referred to as blastocysts (see Chapter 8). Currently no treatments or human trials using embryonic stem cells have been approved in the United States. Many countries have placed legal restrictions on producing human embryonic stem cells for research development and testing.

**Adult stem cells** can actually be found in the tissues of both adults and children. The term *adult stem cell* is used to make a distinction from the embryonic stem cell. Adult stem cells can be found in bone marrow and are easy to obtain. Stem cells from bone marrow have been used in bone marrow transplant procedures for many years. Adult stem cells are also found in blood, skin, dental pulp, retina, skeletal muscle, and the brain.

### Stem Cells in Medicine

Through the use of stem cells, a new field of medicine called regenerative medicine offers hope to those who suffer from Parkinson's disease, diabetes, and autoimmune, liver, and cardiovascular disease; and for those requiring regeneration following brain or spinal cord injury. The U.S. Food and Drug Administration has approved some new therapies, and others are currently in review. Scientists are working to develop new technologies and procedures for future approval.

### *Cell Membrane*

Each cell has a thin membrane that surrounds it. This membrane serves two purposes:

- The cell membrane helps the cell maintain its form and separates cell contents from the surrounding environment. Imagine the cell membrane as being similar to the thin white membrane that lines the inside of an eggshell and holds the rest of the egg in place.
- The cell membrane has special physical and chemical properties that allow it to recognize and interact with other cells. Basically, it "decides" what may enter or leave the cell. For example, nutrients are allowed to pass through, and waste products are allowed to leave. This maintains the healthy balance that helps the cell to survive.

### *Cytoplasm*

The overall structure of a cell is very similar to that of an egg; the major portion of the cell (much like an egg white) is called the **cytoplasm**. Cytoplasm is the gel-like fluid inside the cell. It consists primarily of water. About two thirds of the body's water is found in the cytoplasm of cells. When viewed with an ordinary light, cytoplasm appears homogeneous and empty. However, when viewed through an electron microscope, the cytoplasm is seen to be highly organized with numerous small structures called **organelles** suspended within it. Each organelle, or "little organ," has a definite structure and a specific role in the function of a cell. Organelles manufacture, modify, store, and transport proteins and dispose of cellular wastes.

### *Nucleus*

The "control center" of the cell, called the **nucleus**, can be compared to an egg yolk. The nucleus directs the metabolic activities of the cell. All cells have at least one nucleus at some time during their existence. Some cells (e.g., red blood cells) lose their nucleus as they mature. Other cells (e.g., skeletal muscle cells) have more than one nucleus.

The nucleus of every cell contains a complete set of the body's chromosomes, which include *DNA* (deoxyribonucleic acid) and *RNA* (ribonucleic acid), two chemicals that carry all genetic information.

Human life begins as the result of cell division. For this reason, all the cells in your body (except for egg or sperm cells) contain the same information as the fertilized egg from which you began.

### Visualizing the Semipermeable Function of the Cell

Visualize a teabag in a cup of water. The teabag paper acts as a semipermeable membrane that holds the tea leaves in the bag. It does, however, permit water to enter the bag. The smallest particles mix with the water, which carries them back through the porous teabag into the cup of water. We know that this occurs because color and flavor changes in the water are evident.

3 What is the portion of the cell that carries genetic information?

## Tissues

Tissues are formed when many millions of the same type of cell join together to perform a specific function for the body. Four main tissue types have been identified in the human body: (1) epithelial, (2) connective, (3) muscle, and (4) nerve tissue (Table 6.2).

**Epithelial tissue** forms a covering for the external and internal body surfaces (e.g., the skin on the outside of the body, the lining of the oral cavity and intestines). The purposes of epithelial cells are to (1) provide protection, (2) produce secretions, and (3) regulate the passage of materials across them. Some epithelial cells are *specialized,* meaning that they have special functions associated with skin color, hair, nails, mucus production, and sweat regulation.

**TABLE 6.2** Types of Tissues and Functions in the Body

| Tissue Type | Function | Appearance |
|---|---|---|
| **Epithelial Tissue Covering and Lining** | • Skin protects the body from exposure to disease-causing organisms.<br>• Epithelium lines internal organs and body cavities (e.g., nose, mouth, lungs, stomach). | 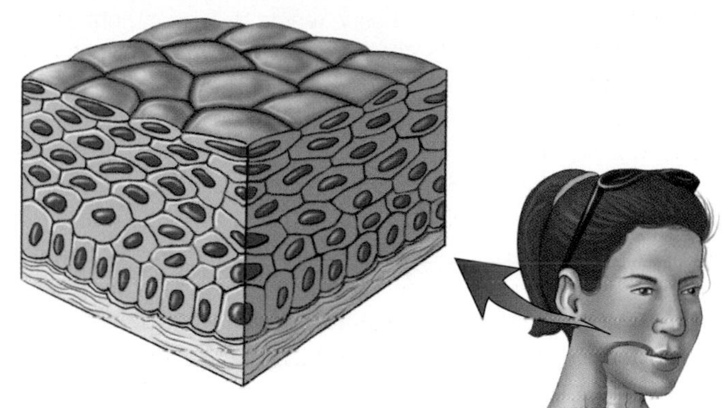 |
| **Epithelial Tissue Glandular or Secretory** | • Epithelial tissues secrete substances such as digestive juices, hormones, milk, perspiration, and mucus. | |

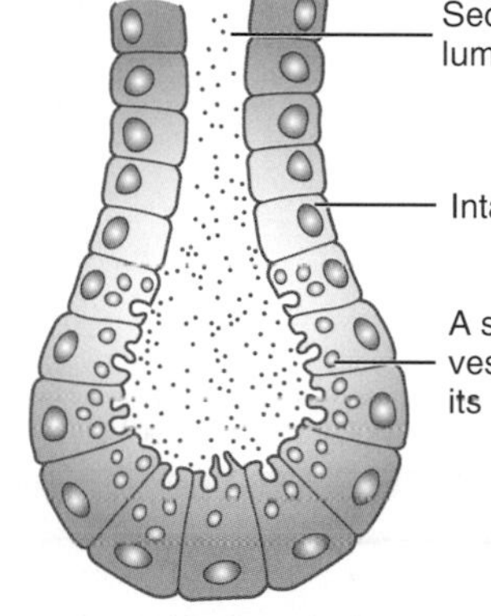

Merocrine gland

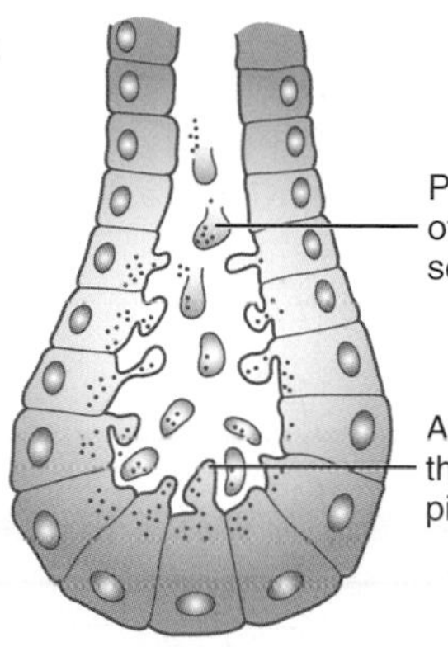

Apocrine gland

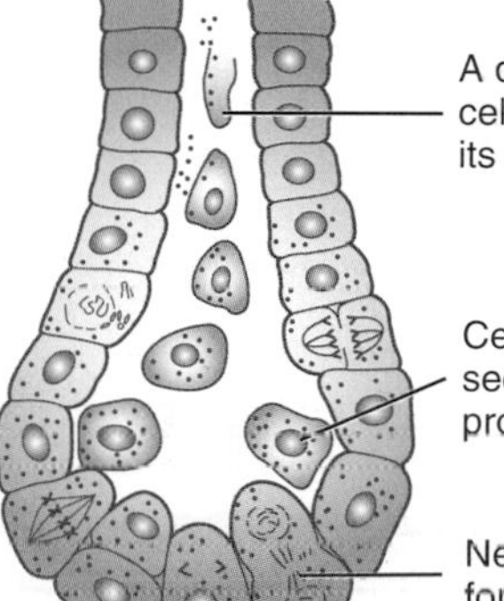

Holocrine gland

| Tissue Type | Function | Appearance |
|---|---|---|
| **Muscle Tissue Striated** | • Also called *skeletal* and *voluntary,* these muscles are attached to bones, tendons, or other muscles.<br>• Striated (striped) muscles are responsible for voluntary movement. |  |
| **Muscle Tissue Smooth** | • Also known as **visceral**, *nonstriated,* and *involuntary,* these muscles provide involuntary movement (e.g., digestion).<br>• Smooth muscles are found in visceral (internal) organs, as well as in hollow body cavities. | 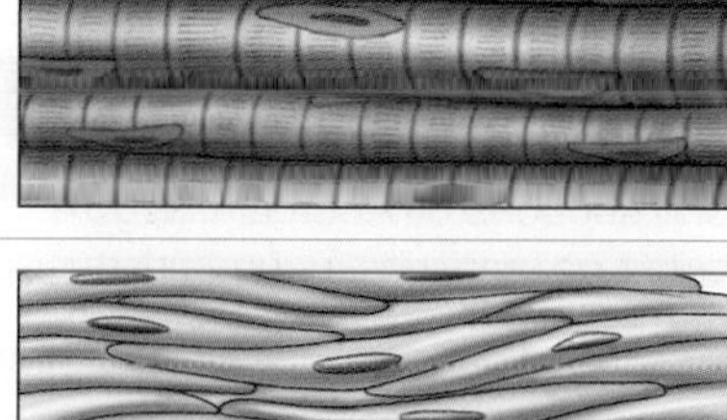 |
| **Muscle Tissue Cardiac** | • Tissue makes up the walls of the heart.<br>• Muscles help pump blood out of the heart.<br>• Even though muscle has striations, movement is involuntary. | 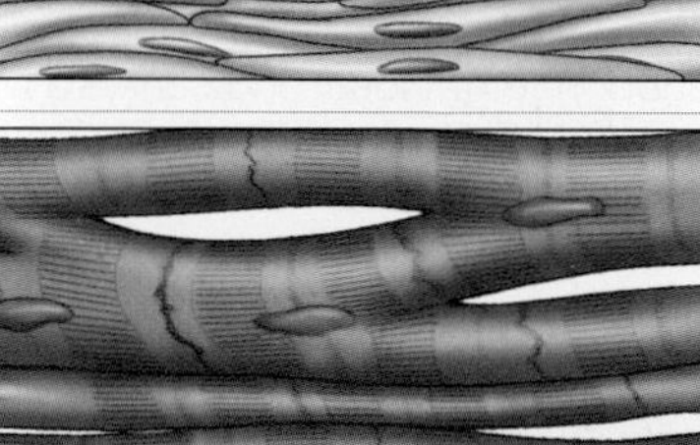 |

*Continued*

**TABLE 6.2** Types of Tissues and Functions in the Body—cont'd

| Tissue Type | Function | Appearance |
|---|---|---|
| **Nerve Tissue Neuronal** | • Tissue reacts to environmental stimuli.<br>• Nerves carry messages (impulses) to and from the brain.<br>• Tissues are found in the brain, spinal cord, and sense organs. | **Nervous Tissue**<br>Dendrites<br>Cell body<br>Axon |
| **Connective Tissue Adipose (fat)** | • Tissues store fat.<br>• Tissues provide energy source when needed.<br>• Fat cushions, supports, and insulates the body. | |
| **Connective Tissue Supportive** | • *Osseous tissue* (bone) protects and supports other organs (e.g., spinal column, ribs around heart and lungs). | |
| | • *Cartilage* provides firm flexible support (e.g., nose) and serves as a shock absorber at the joints. | 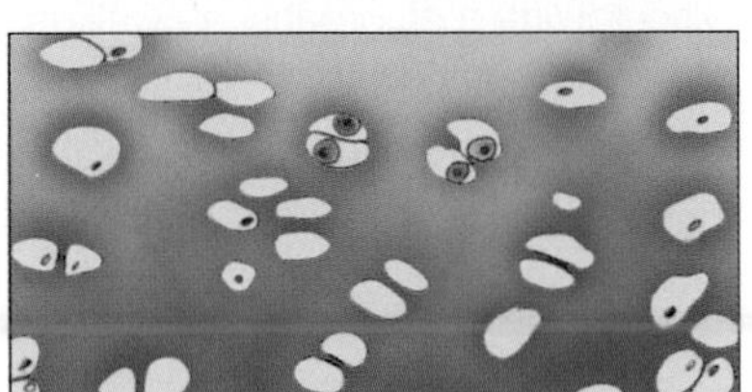 |

**TABLE 6.2** Types of Tissues and Functions in the Body—cont'd

| Tissue Type | Function | Appearance |
|---|---|---|
| **Connective Tissue Dense Fibrous** | • Ligaments are strong, flexible bands that hold bones together at the joints.<br>• *Tendons* are white glossy bands that attach skeletal muscles to the bones. | |
| **Connective Tissue Vascular** | • Blood transports nutrients and oxygen to body cells and carries away waste products.<br>• Lymph transports tissue, fluid, proteins, fat, and other materials from the tissues to the capillaries. | Red blood cells<br>White blood cells<br>Platelets<br>Plasma |

Images of epithelial tissue (glandular or secretory) and connective tissue (vascular) from Applegate EJ: *The anatomy and physiology learning system*, ed 4, St Louis, Saunders, 2011. All other images from Herlihy B: *The human body in health and illness*, ed 5, St Louis, 2014, Saunders.

**Connective tissue** is the major support material of the body. It provides support for the body and connects its organs and tissues. Fat, tendons, ligaments, bone, cartilage, blood, and lymph are all types of connective tissue. Specific types of connective tissue can store fat, destroy bacteria, produce blood cells, and develop antibodies against infection and disease.

**Muscle tissue** has the ability to lengthen and shorten and thus move body parts. Skeletal muscles are either *voluntary* or *involuntary*. For example, when you decide to move your arms or legs, the muscle movement is voluntary. However, the beating of your heart, the churning of your stomach, and changes in the pupils of your eyes are controlled by involuntary muscle movements.

**Nerve tissue** is found in the brain, spinal cord, and nerves. It is responsible for coordinating and controlling many body activities. It stimulates muscle contraction and plays a major role in emotions, memory, and reasoning. Nerve tissue also has the unique ability to react to environmental changes, such as heat, cold, light, or pressure. Nerve tissue carries messages from all areas of the body to the brain and from the brain to all areas of the body. To perform these functions, cells in nerve tissue must communicate with one another by way of electrical nerve impulses.

**4** What are the four types of tissue in the human body?

## Organs

Organs are formed when several types of tissue group together to perform a single function. For example, the stomach is an organ that contains each of the four tissue types (nerve, connective, muscle, and epithelial) and performs the digestive functions of the body. The heart and lungs are other organs that contain all four major tissue types.

## Body Systems

A body system is composed of a group of organs that work together to perform a major function to keep the body healthy and functional. For example, the digestive system is responsible for ingestion of food, digestion, and absorption of nutrition. Organs of the digestive system include the esophagus, stomach, and small and large intestines. Each organ has its specific job to do, and when each of the digestive organs performs its function as required, proper digestion, absorption, and elimination of food occur. The body comprises 10 major body systems (see Chapter 7).

**5** What are the four organizational levels of the human body, from simplest to most complex?

## Body Cavities

Organs of the body are located in areas called *body cavities*. Two main body cavities have been identified (Fig. 6.5).

- The cavity located at the back of the body is known as the **dorsal cavity**. The cavity located at the front of the body is called the **ventral cavity**. Each of the two major body cavities is further divided into smaller cavities. **Parietal** refers to the walls of a body cavity. The dorsal cavity is divided into the **cranial**

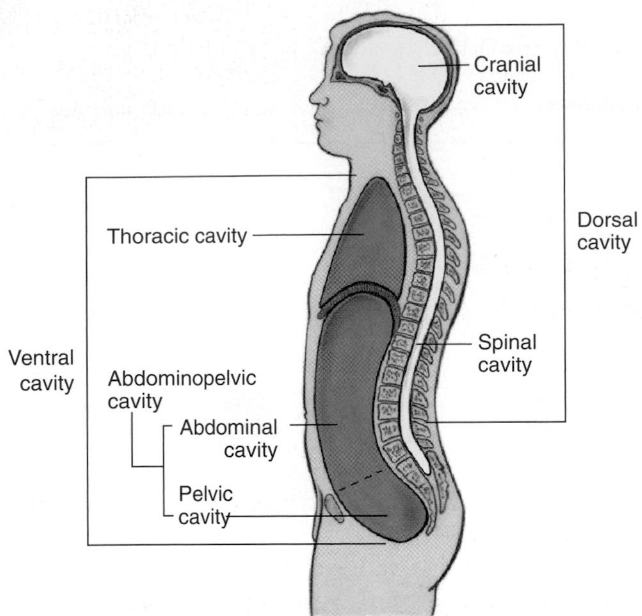


**FIG. 6.5** Spaces within the body that house specific organs are referred to as body cavities. *(From Applegate EJ: The anatomy and physiology learning system, ed 4, St Louis, Saunders, 2011.)*

**cavity**, which contains the brain, and the **spinal cavity**, which contains the spinal cord. The cranial and spinal cavities join with each other to form a continuous space.

- The ventral cavity is much larger than the dorsal cavity and is subdivided into the **thoracic cavity** and the **abdominopelvic** (abdominal and pelvic) **cavity**. The thoracic cavity contains the heart, lungs, esophagus, and trachea. The **abdominal cavity** houses the stomach, liver, gallbladder, spleen, and most of the intestines. The **pelvic cavity** contains portions of the small and large intestines, the rectum, the urinary bladder, and internal reproductive organs.

## Body Regions

For reference, the body is divided into two major regions. The **axial** division consists of the head, neck, and trunk, and the **appendicular** region comprises the arms and legs.

**6** What are the two major body cavities?
**7** Which components make up the axial and appendicular regions of the human body?

**■ Legal and Ethical Implications** A wise person once said, *"Patients don't care how much you know, until they know how much you care."* Never forget that your patients are more than cells, organs, and body systems. They are the most important people in the dental office. Treat patients as you would want to be treated in the healthcare environment. ■

**■ Eye to the Future** As the federal government's lead agency for scientific research on oral, dental, and craniofacial disease, the **National Institute of Dental and Craniofacial Research (NIDCR)** is truly the Eye to the Future. Using the latest molecular and genetic tools, NIDCR scientists conduct research on the full spectrum of topics related to oral, dental, and craniofacial health and disease. NIDCR shares its research findings with the public, health professionals, and policy makers. It also produces and distributes health education materials for consumers, as well as for dentists, physicians, and other healthcare professionals. The NIDCR Web page is easy to read and contains the most current scientific information and NIDCR research findings and clinical trials. The NIDCR also supports training and career development programs for everyone from high school students to independent scientists. As a dental-assisting student, you will find a visit to the NIDCR Web site fascinating: www.nidcr.nih.gov/Research/. ■

**■ Critical Thinking**

1. Why is it important for the dental assistant to study general anatomy?
2. How would you explain the process of cells developing into organs?
3. What benefits can you imagine for future use of stem cell therapies? ■

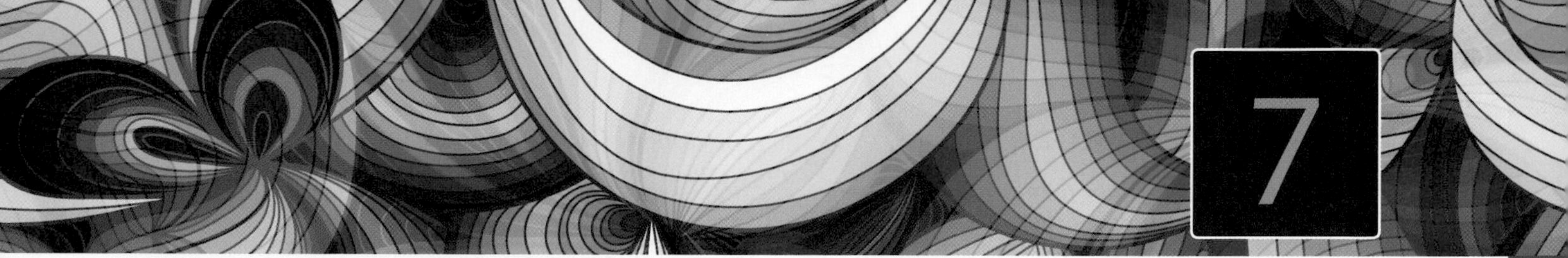

7

# General Physiology

## KEY TERMS

**Apocrine sweat glands** Large sweat glands that are found under the arms, around the nipples, and in the genital region.
**Appendicular (ap-en-DIK-yoo-lur) skeleton** Portion of the skeleton that consists of the upper extremities and shoulder girdle plus the lower extremities and pelvic girdle.
**Arteries** Large blood vessels that carry blood away from the heart.
**Articulation (ahr-tik-yoo-LAY-shun)** Another term for joint.
**Axial (AK-see-ul) skeleton** Portion of the skeleton that consists of the skull, spinal column, ribs, and sternum.
**Bone marrow** Gelatinous material that produces white blood cells, red blood cells, or platelets.
**Cancellous (KAN-sil-us) bone** Lightweight bone found in the interior of bones; also known as spongy bone.
**Capillaries** A system of microscopic vessels that connects the arterial and venous systems.
**Cartilage** Tough, connective, nonvascular elastic tissue.
**Central nervous system (CNS)** The brain and spinal cord.
**Compact bone** Outer layer of bones, where needed for strength; also known as cortical bone.
**Gomphosis** A type of fibrous joint such as a tooth into the alveolus.
**Integumentary (in-teg-yoo-MEN-tuh-ree) system** The skin system.
**Involuntary muscles** Muscles that function automatically without conscious control.
**Joints** Structural areas where two or more bones come together.
**Muscle insertion** Location where the muscle ends; the portion away from the body's midline.
**Muscle origin** Location where the muscle begins; the portion toward the body's midline.
**Neurons** Direct nerve impulses.
**Osteoblasts (OS-tee-oh-blasts)** Cells that form bone.
**Pericardium (per-i-KAHR-dee-um)** Double-walled sac that encloses the heart.
**Periosteum (per-ee-OS-tee-um)** Specialized connective tissue that covers all bones of the body.
**Peripheral nervous system (PNS)** Cranial nerves and spinal nerves.
**Peristalsis (per-i-STAHL-sis)** Rhythmic action that moves food through the digestive tract.
**Plasma** A straw-colored fluid that transports nutrients, hormones, and waste products.
**Red blood cells** Cells that contain the blood protein hemoglobin, which plays an essential role in oxygen transport; also known as erythrocytes.
**Sebaceous glands** Oil glands that keep the hair and skin soft and are associated with sex hormones.
**Sharpey's fibers** Tissues that anchor the periosteum to the bone.
**Sudoriferous (soo-doe-RIF-ur-us) glands** Sweat glands that are widely distributed over the body and provide heat regulation.
**Veins** Blood vessels that carry blood to the heart.
**White blood cells** Cells that have the primary function of fighting disease in the body; also known as leukocytes.

## LEARNING OUTCOMES

*On completion of this chapter, the student will be able to achieve the following objectives:*

1 Pronounce, define, and spell the key terms.
2 Explain why understanding physiology is important to the dental assistant.
3 Locate the skeletal system; explain its purpose, components, and functions; and describe the signs and symptoms of its common disorders.
4 Locate the muscular system; explain its purpose, components, and functions; and describe the signs and symptoms of its common disorders.
5 Locate the cardiovascular system; explain its purpose, components, and functions; and describe the signs and symptoms of its common disorders.
6 Locate the nervous system; explain its purpose, components, and functions; and describe the signs and symptoms of its common disorders.
7 Locate the respiratory system; explain its purpose, components, and functions; and describe the signs and symptoms of its common disorders.
8 Locate the digestive system; explain its purpose, components, and functions; and describe the signs and symptoms of its common disorders.
9 Locate the endocrine system; explain its purpose, components, and functions; and describe the signs and symptoms of its common disorders.
10 Locate the urinary system; explain its purpose, components, and functions; and describe the signs and symptoms of its common disorders.
11 Locate the integumentary system; explain its purpose, components, and functions; and describe the signs and symptoms of its common disorders.
12 Locate the reproductive system; explain its purpose, components, and functions; and describe the signs and symptoms of its common disorders.
13 Give examples of conditions that require interaction among body systems.

## ELECTRONIC RESOURCES

*Additional information related to content in Chapter 7 can be found on the companion Evolve Web site.*

- Animations: Overview of the following body systems: Cardiovascular, Digestive, Endocrine, Integumentary, Lymphatic, Musculoskeletal, Nervous, Reproductive, Respiratory, Urinary, Vascular
- Practice Quiz

# Physiology and Dental Assisting

You may be wondering why you are studying physiology in a dental assisting program. The answer is that a foundation in physiology will help you become a more valuable member of the dental healthcare team. As you continue your dental assisting education, you will recognize the importance of physiology in your personal life and in your career.

The human body is the most incredible creation, with its senses and strengths, an ingenious defense system, and mental capabilities. The human body is a masterpiece more amazing than science fiction.

### Physiology and the Dental Assistant

- Medical conditions on the patient's health history
- Effects of commonly used medications
- Recognizing medically compromised patients
- Interpretation of radiographic dental images
- Infection control and prevention of disease transmission
- Performing lifesaving procedures (e.g., cardiopulmonary resuscitation [CPR])
- Recognize potential medical emergencies in the dental office
- Understanding various disease processes
- Maintain a healthy body through ergonomics
- Proper nutrition and dental health
- Exposure to harmful chemicals
- Communicate using proper terminology
- Recommendations from the American Heart Association

The study of the human body is as old as human history, because people have always had a fascination about how the body is put together, how it works, why it becomes diseased, and why it wears out.

Physiology is the study of how living organisms *function.* It continues beyond the study of anatomy into how the body works, what it can do, and why (see Chapter 6).

# Body Systems

The human body has ten systems: (1) skeletal, (2) muscular, (3) cardiovascular (including lymphatic and immune systems), (4) nervous, (5) respiratory, (6) digestive, (7) endocrine, (8) urinary, (9) integumentary (skin), and (10) reproductive. Each system has specific organs within it, and each body system performs specific functions. When all ten systems are functioning well, the person is healthy (Table 7.1). This chapter summarizes each of these body systems, their components and functions, and the disorders that affect them.

**TABLE 7.1** Major Body Systems

| Body System | Components | Major Functions |
|---|---|---|
| Skeletal system | 206 bones | Protection, support, and shape; hematopoietic; storage of certain minerals |
| Muscular system | Striated, smooth, and cardiac muscle | Holding body erect, locomotion, movement of body fluids, production of body heat, communication |
| Cardiovascular system | Heart, arteries, veins, blood | Respiratory, nutritive, excretory |
| Lymphatic and immune systems | White blood cells; lymph fluid, vessels, and nodes; spleen and tonsils | Defense against disease, conservation of plasma proteins and fluid, lipid absorption |
| Nervous system | Central and peripheral nervous systems, special sense organs | Reception of stimuli, transmission of messages, coordinating mechanism |
| Respiratory system | Nose, paranasal sinuses, pharynx, epiglottis, larynx, trachea, bronchi, and lungs | Transport of oxygen to cells, excretion of carbon dioxide and some water wastes |
| Digestive system | Mouth, pharynx, esophagus, stomach, intestines, and accessory organs | Digestion of food, absorption of nutrients, elimination of solid wastes |
| Urinary system | Kidneys, ureters, bladder, and urethra | Formation and elimination of urine, maintenance of homeostasis |
| Integumentary system | Skin, hair, nails, and sweat and sebaceous glands | Protection of body, regulation of body temperature |
| Endocrine system | Adrenals, gonads, pancreas, parathyroids, pineal, pituitary, thymus, and thyroid | Integration of bodily functions, control of growth, maintenance of homeostasis |
| Reproductive system | *Male:* testes, penis<br>*Female:* ovaries, fallopian tubes, uterus, vagina | Production of new life<br>Production of new life |

## Skeletal System

The skull, spine, and rib cage form the **axial skeleton** and account for 80 of the 206 bones in the human body. The shoulders, arms, hands, hips, legs, and feet form the **appendicular skeleton**. The skull consists of 28 bones and is discussed in detail in Chapter 9 (Fig. 7.1).

The axial skeleton (80 bones) consists of the skull, spinal column, ribs, and sternum. Its function is to protect the major organs of the nervous, respiratory, and circulatory systems.

The appendicular skeleton (126 bones) consists of the upper extremities and shoulder area plus the lower extremities and pelvic area. It protects the organs of digestion and reproduction.

Many disorders can affect the skeletal system (Table 7.2).

## Bone

The bones of the human body weigh only approximately 20 pounds. The bones of the body allow us to stand and walk, and they protect internal organs. The skull protects the brain, and the rib cage shields the heart and lungs. Bone is a living connective tissue that is capable of repairing itself when injured. It consists of an organic component (the cells and matrix) and an inorganic component (minerals). The minerals, primarily *calcium* and *phosphate,* give rigidity to bone. These minerals stored in bones also act as reservoirs to maintain essential blood mineral concentrations when the body's supply is inadequate. The three layers of bone are (1) periosteum, (2) compact bone, and (3) cancellous bone and marrow (Fig. 7.2).

The **periosteum** (Latin for "surrounding the bone") is the first layer of bone. It is a thin layer of whitish connective tissue and contains nerves and blood vessels. It supplies the cells from which the hard bone below the periosteum is built up. It is necessary for bone growth and repair, for nutrition, and for carrying away waste. It is the periosteum that is responsible for the life of the bone, and it is capable of repair. The inner layer is loose connective tissue that contains **osteoblasts**, or cells associated with bone formation. The periosteum is anchored to bone by

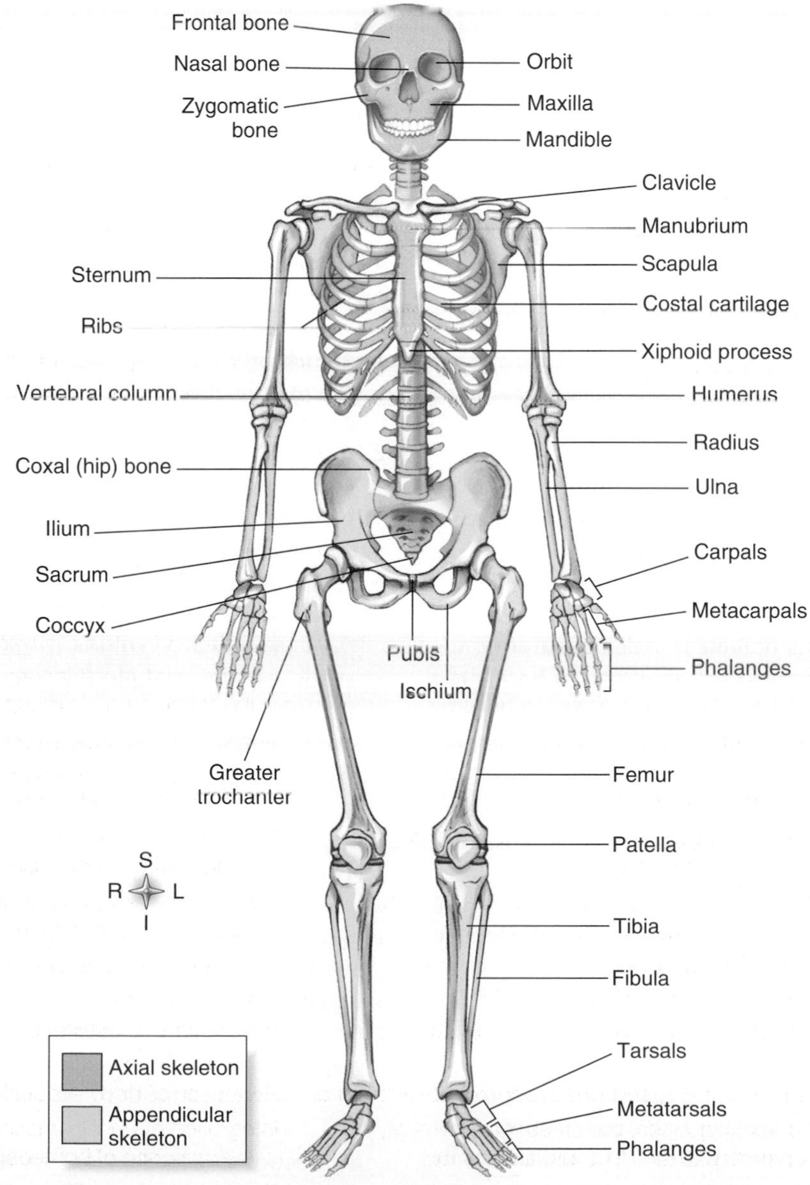


**FIG. 7.1** The skeletal system. *(From Patton KT, Thibodeau GA: Anatomy and physiology, ed 8, St Louis, Mosby, 2013.)*

**TABLE 7.2 Disorders of the Skeletal System**

| Disorder | Description | Signs and Symptoms |
|---|---|---|
| Arthritis | Inflammation of a joint. More than 100 forms are known, and all have different causes. | Swelling and pain, usually with structural changes; mobility impairment and difficulty in performing daily tasks |
| Fracture | Broken bones caused by stress on the bone. Fractures can occur in any bone in the body and are classified by type. | Severe pain, swelling, and disfigurement, depending on the type of fracture |
| Gout | Inflammatory joint reaction caused by accumulation of uric acid crystals. The area that is usually affected is the big toe. | The joint usually becomes red, warm, shiny, swollen, and very sensitive to the touch |
| Osteomyelitis | Infection of the bone that is caused by bacteria, fungi, or contaminated foreign material such as an artificial joint. | Sudden onset of fever, limited movement, and severe pain in the body part involved |
| Osteoporosis | Age-related disease in which bone is demineralized, resulting in loss of bone density and fracture. | Frequent fractures, especially of the vertebrae, wrist, or hip; back pain and decreased height |
| Sprain | Injury to a joint. The joint is usually stretched beyond its normal range of movement. | Pain, swelling, bruising, abnormal movement, and joint weakness (depending on severity) |

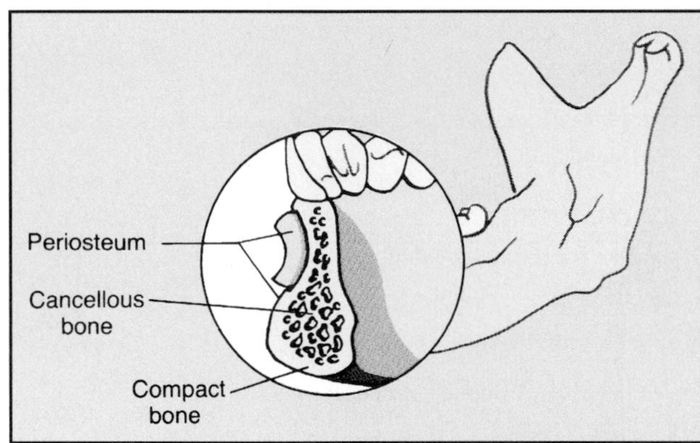


**FIG. 7.2** The structure of bone.

**Sharpey's fibers**, which penetrate the underlying bone matrix. Beneath the periosteum is dense, rigid compact bone.

**Compact bone** is hard, dense, and very strong (Fig. 7.3,*B*; see also Fig. 7.2). It forms the outer layer of bone, where it is needed for strength. This layer of bone is so dense that surgeons must use a saw or a bone bur instead of a knife to cut through it.

**Cancellous bone** is found inside the bone. It is lighter in weight and is not as strong as compact bone. *Trabeculae* (plural of *trabecula*) are bony spicules in cancellous bone that form a honeycomb pattern of spaces that are filled with *bone marrow.* On a radiograph, trabeculae appear as a weblike structure (see Fig. 7.3,*A*).

**Bone marrow** is a gelatinous material that produces white blood cells (which fight infection), red blood cells (which carry oxygen), or platelets (which help to stop bleeding).

## Cartilage

**Cartilage** is strong but is more elastic than bone. It is found where bones join together. Cartilage is a tough, nonvascular (not associated with blood) connective tissue. In addition to its presence in the ends of bones, cartilage forms the nose and ears.

RECALL

1 What are the two divisions of the skeleton?
2 What is the connective tissue that covers all bones?
3 What are the two types of bone, and what are their features?
4 Where is cartilage found?

## Joints

**Joints**, or **articulations**, are the areas where two bones come together (Fig. 7.4). The three basic types of joints are as follows:

1. *Fibrous joints,* such as sutures of the skull, do not move. A *suture* is the jagged line at which bones articulate and form a joint that does not move.
2. *Cartilaginous joints* are made of connective tissue and cartilage. They move only very slightly. An example is the joints between the bones of the vertebrae.
3. *Synovial joints* are movable joints that account for most of the joints in the body. Some synovial joints are lined with a fibrous sac called a *bursa.* The bursa is filled with *synovial fluid* and acts as a cushion to ease movement. Examples of synovial joints include the knee and elbow (hinge type); the hips and shoulders (ball-and-socket type); gliding joints (wrists); pivot joints (base of the skull); saddle joints (the thumb); and **gomphoses** (attachments of teeth to sockets).

Ball-and-socket joints allow for movements such as flexion, extension, and limited rotation. Hinge joints allow movement in only one direction, similar to the hinge on a door. Gliding joints allow the bones to slide. The pivot joint at the base of the skull allows the head to rotate. The saddle joint allows movements such as touching the thumb to the fingers. Gomphoses are specialized joints that allow only very slight movement, such as attaching a tooth to the socket.

5 Articulation is another term for what structure?

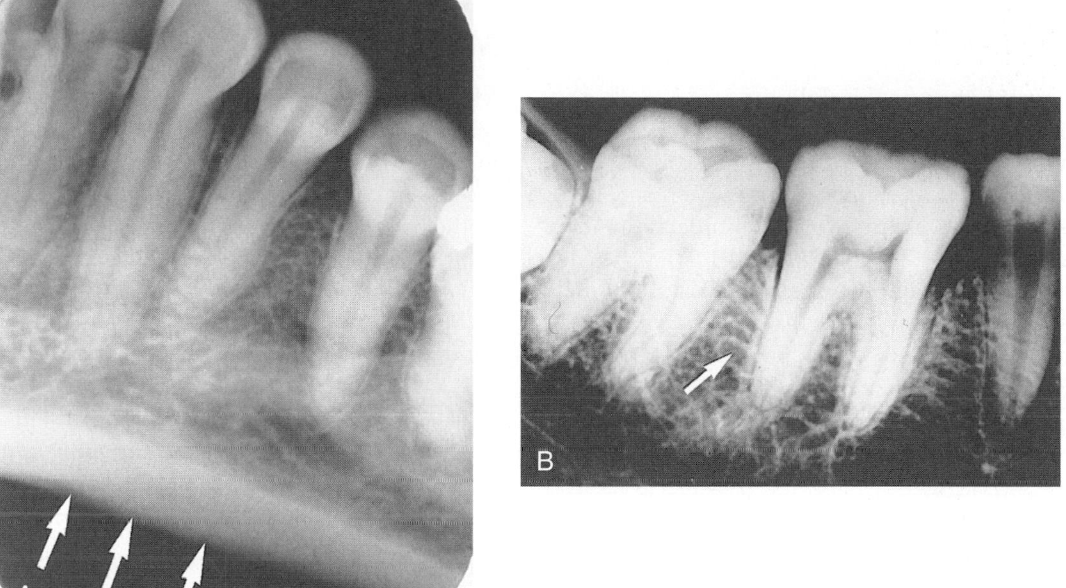


**FIG. 7.3** A, Cortical bone *(arrows)* appears hard and dense. B, Cancellous bone forms trabeculae *(arrow)*. *(From Haring JI, Lind LJ: Radiographic interpretation for the dental hygienist, Philadelphia, Saunders, 1993.)*

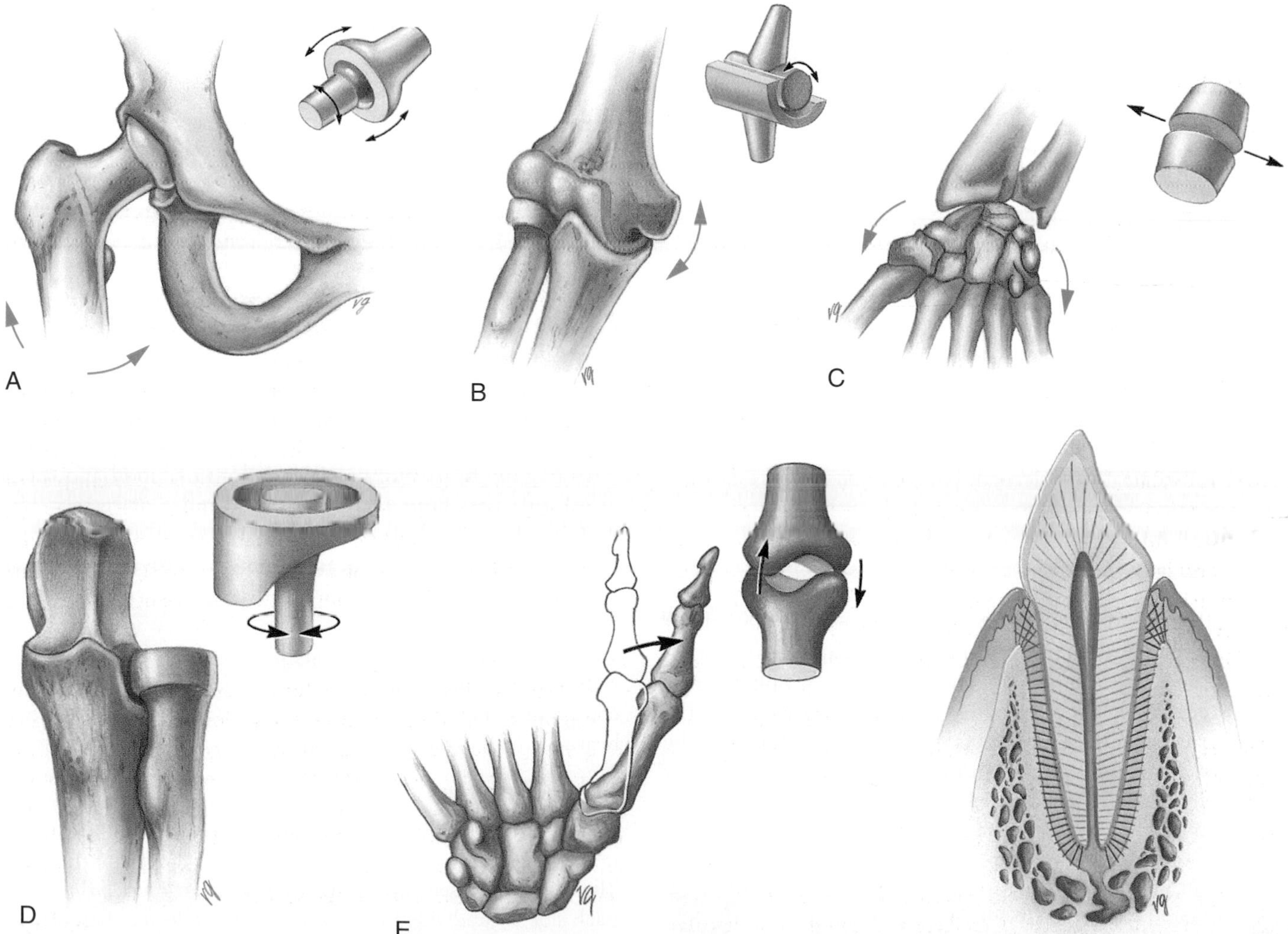

**FIG. 7.4** Types of joints. A, Ball-and-socket. B, Hinge. C, Gliding. D, Pivot. E, Saddle. F, Gomphosis. *(From Gerdin J: Health careers today, ed 6, St Louis, Elsevier, 2017.)*

## Muscular System

The muscular system gives us the ability to stand, walk, run, jump, move our eyes, smile, and frown (Figs. 7.5 and 7.6). For muscles to make the body move, they must work together. Each muscle consists of muscle tissue, connective tissue, nerve tissue, and vascular (blood) tissue. Many disorders can affect the muscular system (Table 7.3).

The muscular system is composed of more than 600 individual muscles. However, only three *types of muscles* have been identified: *striated, smooth,* and *cardiac.*

### Striated Muscle

Striated muscles are so named because dark and light bands within the muscle fibers create a striped, or striated, appearance. Striated muscles are also known as skeletal, or voluntary, muscles. These muscles attach to the bones of the skeleton and make voluntary bodily motion possible. *Voluntary muscles* are so named because we have conscious (voluntary) control over these muscles. For example, you decide when to move your arms or legs.

### Smooth Muscle

Smooth muscle fibers move the internal organs, such as the digestive tract, blood vessels, and secretory ducts leading from the glands. In contrast to the marked contraction and relaxation of striated muscles, smooth muscles produce relatively slow contraction.

Smooth muscles are also known as unstriated, involuntary, or visceral muscles. *Unstriated muscles* do not have the dark and light bands that produce the striped appearance seen in striated muscles. **Involuntary muscles** are so named because they are under the control of the autonomic nervous system and are not controlled voluntarily. For example, you do not decide when to begin digesting your lunch. *Visceral muscles* are so named because they are found in all the visceral (internal) organs except the heart. They are also found in hollow structures, such as the digestive and urinary tracts.

### Cardiac Muscle

Cardiac muscle is striated in appearance but resembles smooth muscle in its action. Cardiac muscle forms most of the walls of the heart, and contraction of this muscle results in the heartbeat. Over a lifetime, the human heart beats 4 billion times and pumps 600,000 tons of blood. Physiologists think the reason cardiac muscle is so durable is that it combines the power of striated voluntary muscles with the steady reliability of smooth, involuntary ones. Moreover, the cardiac fibers connect with each other and create a mutually supportive network of communications.

RECALL

6 What are the three types of muscle tissue?

7 What distinguishes the appearance of each muscle type?

### Muscle Function

Muscles are the only bodily tissues that have the ability to contract and relax. *Contraction* is the tightening of a muscle, during which it becomes shorter and thicker. *Relaxation* occurs when a muscle returns to its original form or shape. Muscles of the body are arranged in opposing pairs, so that when one muscle contracts, the other muscle relaxes. These opposing actions make motion possible.

**Muscle origin** is the place where the muscle begins (originates). This refers to the more fixed attachment, or the portion of the muscle that is toward the midline of the body.

**Muscle insertion** is the place where the muscle ends (inserts). This refers to the more movable attachment, or the portion of the muscle that is away from the midline of the body.

8 What are four disorders of the muscular system?

## Cardiovascular System

The cardiovascular system consists of the (1) circulatory system, (2) heart, and (3) lymphatic system. These systems provide life-sustaining functions for the survival of bodily cells and tissues. Disorders of the heart and lymphatic system have specific signs and symptoms (Tables 7.4 and 7.5).

### Circulatory System

The two primary functions of the circulatory system are as follows:

1. Transports (a) oxygen and nutrients *to* the body cells, (b) carbon dioxide and waste products *from* the body cells, and (c) hormones and antibodies throughout the body
2. Regulates body temperature and maintains chemical stability

### Heart

Each day the heart pumps 4000 gallons of blood at a speed of 40 miles per hour through 70,000 miles of vessels (Fig. 7.7). The heart is a hollow muscle that consists of four chambers. Heart size varies from individual to individual, but the heart is about the size of a closed fist. The heart is protected by the thoracic cavity and is located between the lungs and above the diaphragm. The heart is enclosed within a double-walled membranous sac known as the **pericardium**. Pericardial fluid between layers prevents friction when the heart beats.

#### *Heart Chambers*

The heart functions as a double pump; the right side pumps blood to the lungs, and the left side sends blood to the rest of the body. The coronary vessels supply blood to the heart muscle (Fig. 7.8). Each side is subdivided into an upper and a lower chamber, for a total of four chambers. The upper chambers, the *atria,* receive blood. The lower chambers, the *ventricles,* pump blood.

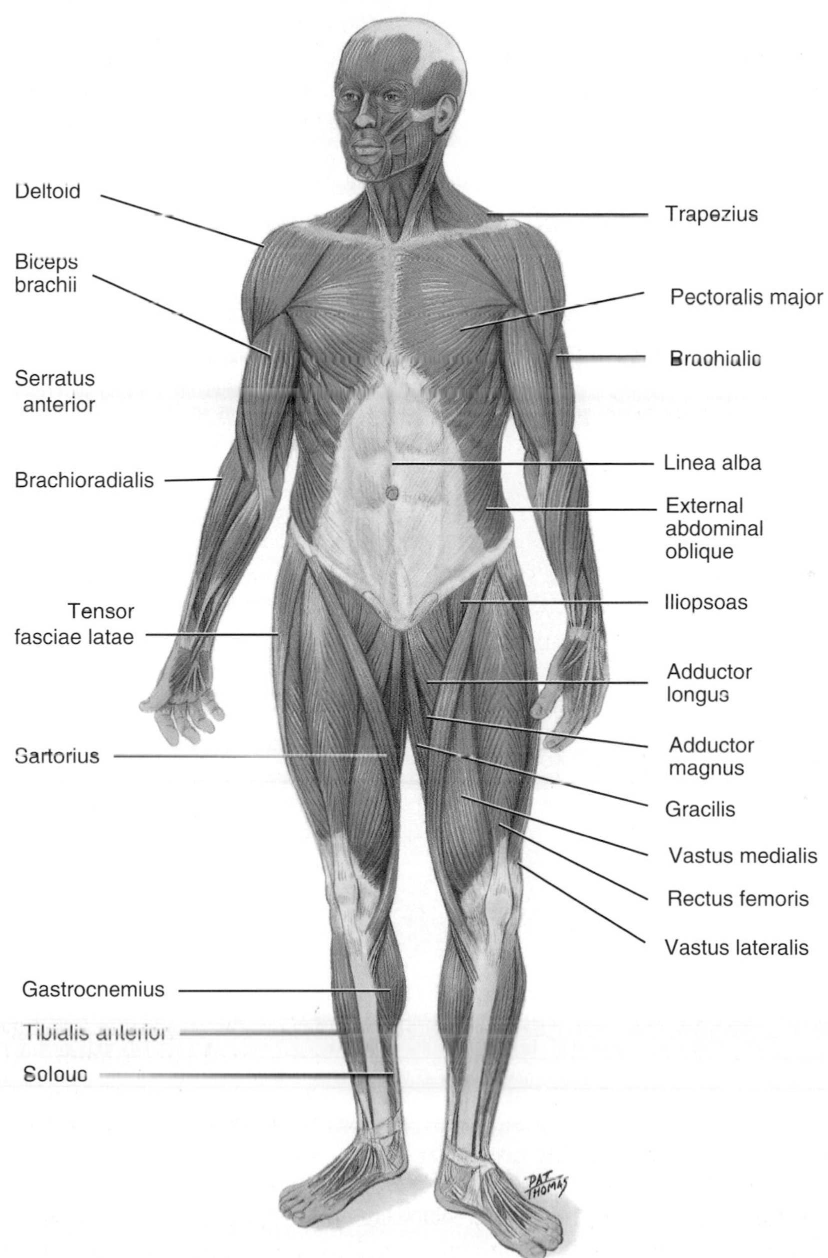


**FIG. 7.5** Muscles of the body, anterior view. *(From Applegate EJ: The anatomy and physiology learning system, ed 4, St Louis, 2011, Saunders.)*

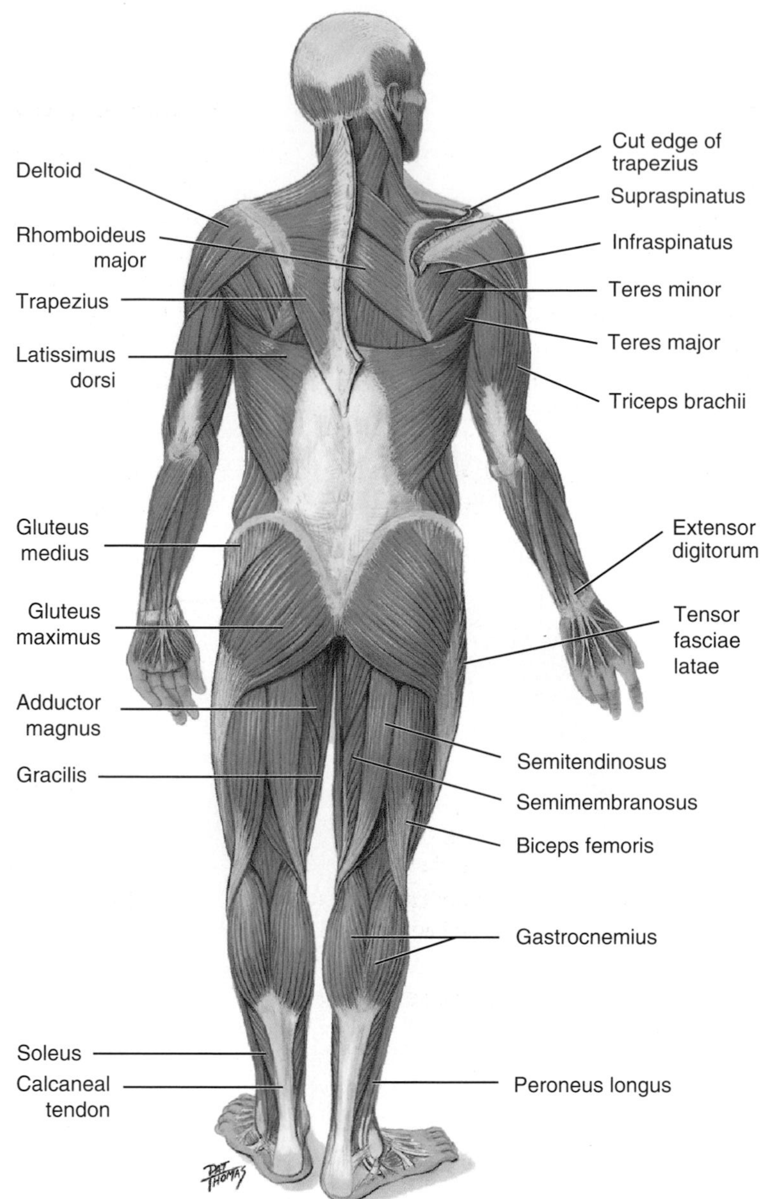


**FIG. 7.6** Muscles of the body, posterior view. *(From Applegate EJ: The anatomy and physiology learning system, ed 4, St Louis, 2011, Saunders.)*

**TABLE 7.3** Disorders of the Muscular System

| Disorder | Description | Signs and Symptoms |
|---|---|---|
| Contusions | Soft tissue trauma | Swelling, tenderness, and localized hemorrhage and bruising can restrict range of motion without producing loss of joint stability. |
| Strain | Injury of a muscle that has been stretched beyond its capacity | Small blood vessels around the area rupture, causing swelling in the area. The area becomes tender, and painful muscle spasms may occur. |
| Progressive muscular dystrophy | Includes nine types, all with unknown causes | Progressive muscle atrophy with organ involvement and weakness. |
| Sprain | Injury to a joint that has been stretched beyond its normal range of motion, resulting in a tear | Depending on the severity of damage, it may include pain in the affected area, swelling, bruising, abnormal motion, and joint weakness. |

## TABLE 7.4 Disorders of the Heart

| Disorder | Description | Signs and Symptoms |
|---|---|---|
| Cardiomyopathy | Heart muscle disease; cause is unknown; usually leads to heart failure | Fatigue, weakness, heart failure, chest pain, and shortness of breath |
| Coronary artery disease | Caused by a buildup of cholesterol plaques in coronary arteries, which reduce blood flow to the heart | Chest pain, shortness of breath; pain may radiate to neck, jaw, arm, or back; ashen or gray color and anxiety are also common |
| Endocarditis | Inflammation of the endocardial layer of the heart; can be caused by bacteria, virus, tuberculosis, or cancer | High fever, heart murmur, blood clots, joint pain, fatigue, shortness of breath, and chest pain |
| Heart failure | The heart can no longer pump an adequate supply of blood; can be caused by disease, congenital problems, hypertension, lung disease, or valve problems | Breathlessness, weakness, fatigue, dizziness, confusion, hypotension, or death |
| Pericarditis | Inflammation of the pericardial layer of the heart; can be caused by bacteria, virus, tuberculosis, or cancer | High fever, heart murmur, blood clots, enlarged spleen, fatigue, joint pain, weight loss, or shortness of breath |

## TABLE 7.5 Disorders of the Lymphatic System

| Disorder | Description | Signs and Symptoms |
|---|---|---|
| Lymphangitis | Inflammation of peripheral lymphatic vessels, usually caused by infection | Red streaks that extend up the arm or leg, with enlarged, tender lymph nodes |
| Lymphadenopathy | Swelling or enlargement of one or more lymph nodes; can result from infection, inflamma-tion, or neoplasm | Painful swelling of lymph nodes |
| Lymphedema | Swelling of soft tissues caused by increased lymph | Painful swelling of limbs |

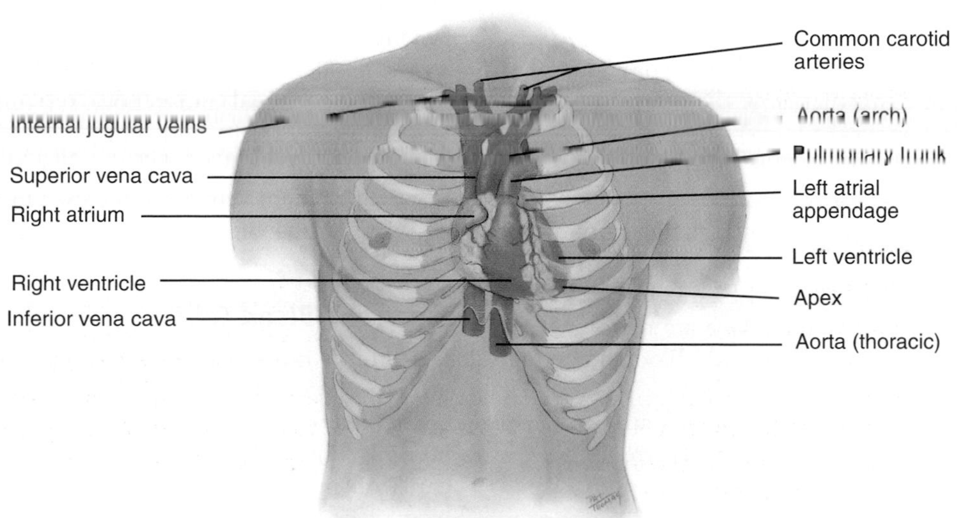


**FIG. 7.7** The heart and great vessels.

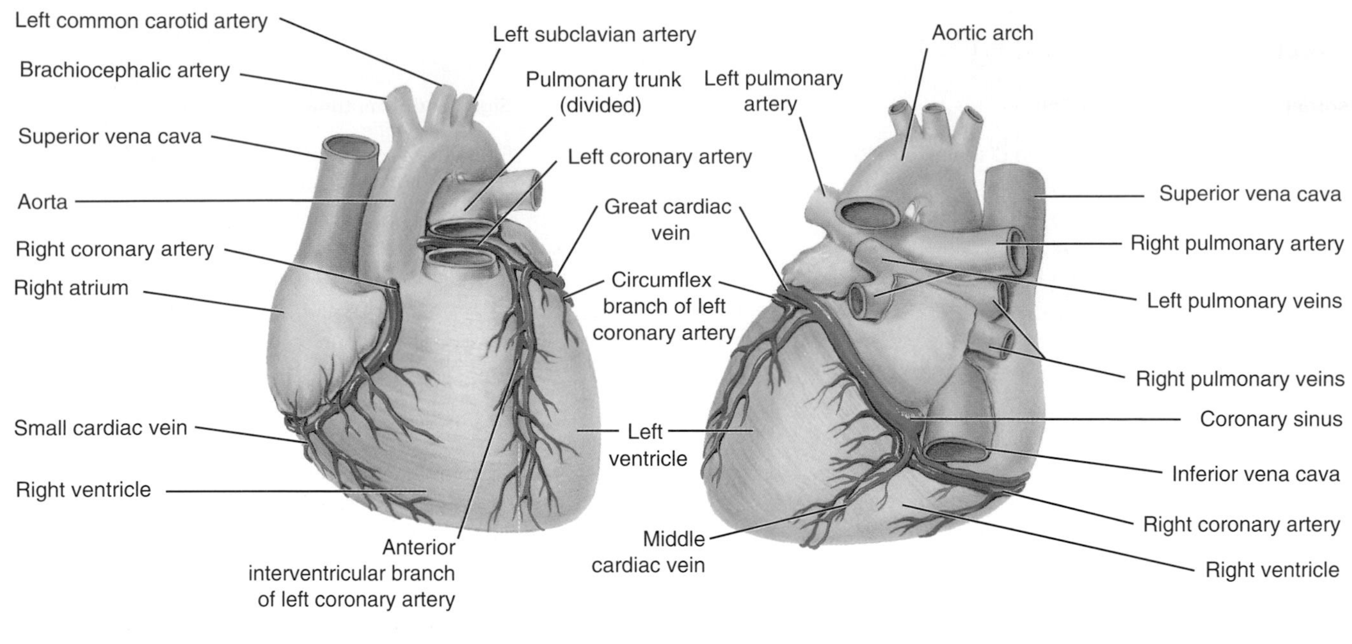


**FIG. 7.8** Coronary vessels. *(From Applegate EJ: The anatomy and physiology learning system, ed 4, St Louis, 2011, Saunders.)*

## Heart Valves

One-way valves prevent the backflow of blood and separate the chambers of the heart by opening and closing with each heartbeat. The *tricuspid valve* (with three "cusps," or triangular segments) is found between the right atrium and the right ventricle. The *mitral valve* has two cusps and lies between the left atrium and the left ventricle. Two *semilunar valves* have three crescent-shaped flaps. The *pulmonary semilunar valve* allows blood to flow from the right ventricle into the pulmonary artery. Blood flows from the left ventricle into the aorta through the *aortic semilunar valve.*

## Blood Flow through the Heart

The *right atrium* receives blood from the superior and inferior venae cavae, the largest veins that enter the heart. This blood comes from all tissues (except the lungs), contains waste materials, and is oxygen poor. Blood flows from the right atrium into the right ventricle.

The *right ventricle* receives blood from the right atrium and pumps it into the pulmonary artery, which carries it to the lungs.

The *left atrium* receives oxygenated blood from the lungs through the four pulmonary veins. (These are the only veins in the body that contain oxygen-rich blood.) Blood flows from here into the left ventricle.

The *left ventricle* receives blood from the left atrium. Blood then goes into the aorta, the largest of the arteries, and is pumped to all parts of the body, except the lungs.

RECALL

**9** What are the two primary functions of the circulatory system?

**10** What are the upper and lower chambers of the heart?

## Blood Vessels

Three major types of blood vessels are found in the body: (1) arteries, (2) veins, and (3) capillaries.

The **arteries** are the large blood vessels that carry blood away from the heart to all regions of the body (Fig. 7.9). The walls of the arteries are composed of three layers. This structure makes arteries both muscular and elastic, so they can expand and contract with the pumping beat of the heart.

The **veins** form a low-pressure collecting system that returns waste-filled blood to the heart. Veins have thinner walls compared to arteries, and they are less elastic. Veins have valves that allow blood to flow toward the heart but prevent it from flowing away from the heart.

The **capillaries** form a system of microscopic vessels that connect the arterial and venous systems. Blood flows rapidly along the arteries and veins; however, this flow is much slower through the expanded area provided by the capillaries. Slower flow allows time for the exchange of oxygen, nutrients, and waste materials between tissue fluids and surrounding cells.

## Blood and Blood Cells

Hematology is the study of blood. The body contains approximately 4 to 5 L of blood, which accounts for about 8 percent of the body's weight. Blood separates into solid and liquid portions when spun in a centrifuge (Fig. 7.10). The solid parts, called *formed elements,* are the red blood cells, white blood cells, and plasma. One drop of blood contains 5 million red blood cells, 7500 white blood cells, and 300,000 platelets.

**Plasma** is a straw-colored fluid that transports nutrients, hormones, and waste products. Plasma is 91 percent water.

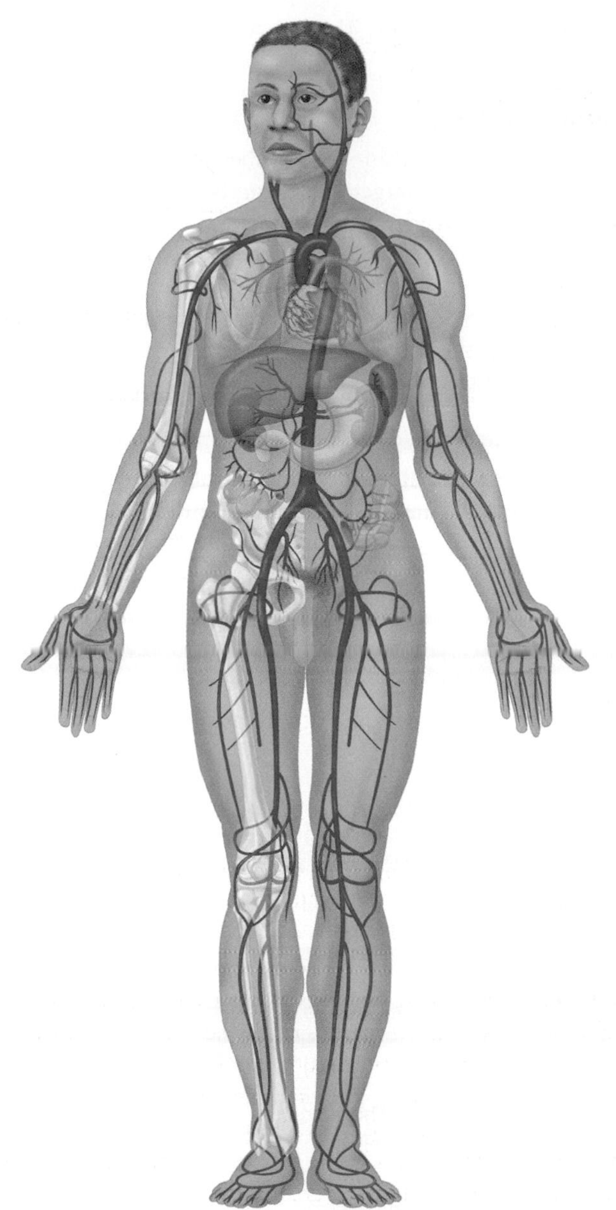

FIG. 7.9 Arteries carry blood from the heart to the body. *(From Patton KT, Thibodeau GA: Anatomy and physiology, ed 8, St Louis, Mosby, 2013.)*

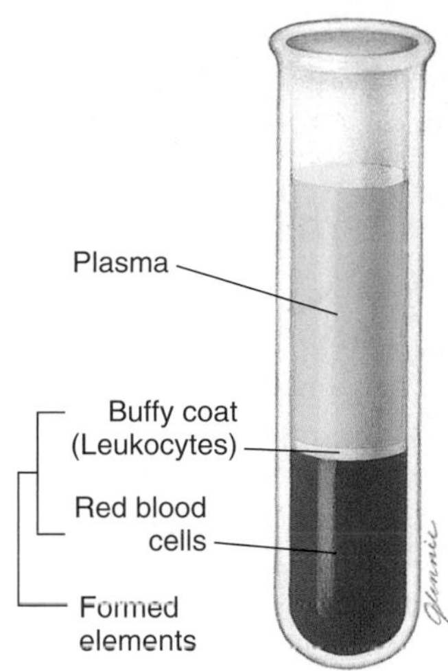


FIG. 7.10 Hematocrit. *(From Gerdin J: Health careers today, ed 6, St Louis, Elsevier, 2017.)*

The remaining 9 percent consists mainly of plasma proteins, including albumin and globulin.

**Red blood cells**, also known as *erythrocytes,* contain the blood protein *hemoglobin,* which plays an essential role in oxygen transport. Erythrocytes are produced by the red bone marrow. When erythrocytes are no longer useful, they are destroyed by macrophages in the spleen, liver, and bone marrow.

**White blood cells**, also known as *leukocytes,* have the primary function of fighting disease in the body. The five major groups of leukocytes are as follows:

1. *Basophils* have imprecisely understood functions.
2. *Eosinophils* increase in number in allergic conditions.
3. *Lymphocytes* are important in the immune process for protecting the body.
4. *Monocytes* act as *macrophages* and dispose of dead and dying cells and other debris.
5. *Neutrophils* fight disease by engulfing germs.

Thrombocytes, also known as *platelets,* are the smallest formed elements of the blood. They are manufactured in the bone marrow and play an important role in the clotting of blood. Thrombocytes usually are produced in red bone marrow and live for about 5 to 9 days.

RECALL

**11** What are the names and functions of the three main types of blood vessels?

## Blood Typing and Rh Factor

The safe administration of blood from donor to recipient requires typing and cross-matching. *Blood typing* is based on the antigens and antibodies found in the blood. The most important classifications are A, AB, B, and O. Patients who receive blood that is incompatible with their own may experience a serious and possibly fatal reaction.

The *Rh factor,* named for its discovery through research with rhesus monkeys, is an additional antigen that is present on the surfaces of the red blood cells of some individuals. In addition to matching these blood types, the Rh factor must be matched according to whether it is positive or negative. A person whose blood contains the factor is *Rh positive.* A person whose blood does *not* contain the factor is *Rh negative.* Anti-Rh antibodies are not naturally found in plasma as they are in blood types, but they do develop if the patient is exposed to the Rh factor. For example, an Rh-negative mother who gives birth to an Rh-positive baby will not have a blood reaction with the first pregnancy, but after blood is mixed during delivery, the mother will develop anti-Rh antibodies in her serum. A subsequent Rh-positive fetus may develop erythroblastosis fetalis if maternal anti-Rh antibodies react with fetal Rh antigen. This condition can cause the death of the fetus. Immediately after delivery of

Rh-positive babies, Rh-negative mothers are given an injection of anti-Rh gamma globulin to prevent the development of anti-Rh antibodies.

## Lymphatic System

The structures of the lymphatic system include lymph vessels, lymph nodes, lymph fluid, and lymphoid organs (Fig. 7.11). Drainage vessels absorb excess protein from tissues and return it to the bloodstream. Lymphoid organs contribute to the immune system to assist with destruction of harmful microorganisms (see Chapter 19 for a discussion of immunity and how it relates to disease transmission). Fluid leaves circulatory capillaries to bathe tissues and cells to keep them moist. This same clear, light-yellow fluid, called *lymph,* is reabsorbed by the lymphatic system and is returned to the blood through the veins. This one-way flowing system moves fluid toward the heart.

### Lymph Vessels

*Lymph capillaries* are thin-walled tubes that carry lymph from tissue spaces to the larger *lymphatic vessels.* Similar to veins, lymphatic vessels have valves that prevent the backflow of fluid. Lymph fluid always flows toward the thoracic cavity, where it empties into veins in the upper thoracic region. Specialized lymph vessels, called *lacteals,* are located in the small intestine. Lacteals aid in the absorption of fats from the small intestine into the bloodstream.

### Lymph Nodes

Lymph nodes are small round or oval structures that are located in lymph vessels. They fight disease by producing antibodies;

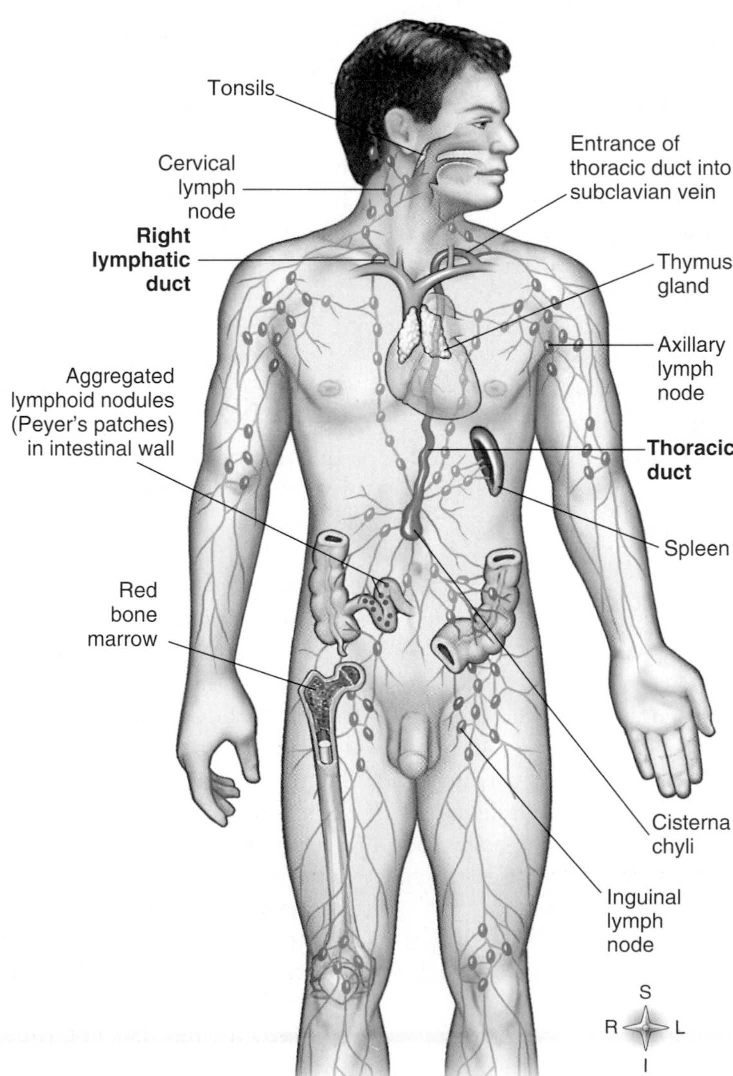


**FIG. 7.11** Lymphatic system. *(From Patton KT, Thibodeau GA: Anatomy and physiology, ed 8, St Louis, Mosby, 2013.)*

this is part of the immune reaction. In acute infection, the lymph nodes become swollen and tender as a result of the collection of lymphocytes gathered to destroy invading substances (see Table 7.5).

Major lymph node sites of the body include *cervical nodes* (in the neck), *axillary nodes* (under the arms), and *inguinal nodes* (in the lower abdomen).

### Lymph Fluid

Lymph, also known as *tissue fluid,* is a clear and colorless fluid. Lymph flows in the spaces between cells and tissues, so that it can carry substances from these tissues back into the bloodstream.

### Lymphoid Organs

**TONSILS.** The tonsils are masses of lymphatic tissue that are located in the upper portions of the nose and throat, where they form a protective ring of lymphatic tissue (Fig. 7.12).

The *nasopharyngeal tonsils,* also known as *adenoids,* are found in the nasopharynx. The *palatine tonsils* are located in the oropharynx between the anterior and posterior pillars of fauces (throat) and are visible through the mouth. The *lingual tonsils* are located on the back of the tongue.

All these tonsils are removed during a tonsillectomy. Tonsils place lymphocytes into the lymph to destroy invading microorganisms; they may become infected during this process.

**SPLEEN.** The spleen is the largest of the lymphoid organs. It is about the size of a clenched fist and is located in the upper left quadrant of the abdomen, just below the diaphragm and behind the stomach. The spleen produces lymphocytes and monocytes, which are important components of the immune system. It also filters microorganisms and other debris not destroyed by the lymphatic system. Other splenic functions include storing red blood cells, maintaining an appropriate balance between cells and plasma in the blood, and removing and destroying nonviable (worn out) red blood cells.

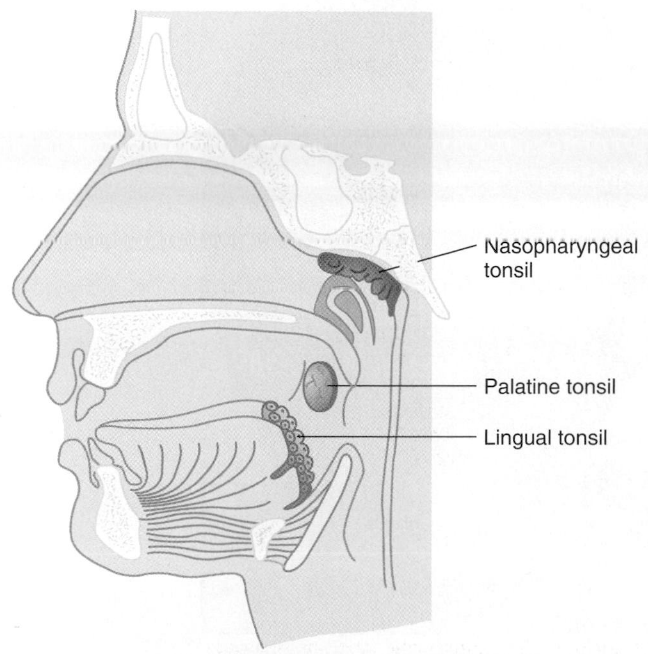


**FIG. 7.12** The tonsils.

**12** What is the primary function of the lymphatic system?
**13** What structures make up the lymphatic system?

## Nervous System

The nervous system is the communication system of the body. Instructions and directions are sent out by this system to various organs in the body. The nervous system can be compared to computer communications, with the brain and spinal cord serving as the main computer and the nerves as cables that carry messages to and from this center. Many disorders can affect the nervous system (Table 7.6 and Fig. 7.13).

The nervous system is composed of the central and peripheral nervous systems. The **central nervous system (CNS)** consists of the brain and the spinal cord (Fig. 7.14). The **peripheral nervous system (PNS)** consists of the cranial nerves and the spinal nerves. The PNS also includes the autonomic nervous system, which is divided into the *sympathetic* and *parasympathetic* nervous systems.

**14** What two systems make up the nervous system?
**15** What are the two divisions of the autonomic nervous system?

### Neurons

The basic function of the **neurons** is to direct communication or nerve impulses. Neurons have the properties of *excitability,* which is the ability to respond to a stimulus, and *conductivity,* which refers to transmission of an impulse.

Three types of neurons may be described, according to their functions, as follows:

1. *Sensory neurons* emerge from the skin or sense organs and carry impulses toward the brain and spinal cord.
2. *Motor neurons* carry impulses away from the brain and spinal cord and toward the muscles and glands.
3. *Associative neurons* carry impulses from one neuron to another.

A *synapse* is the space between two neurons or between a neuron and a receptor organ. A *neurotransmitter* is a chemical substance that allows the impulse to jump across the synapse from one neuron to another.

Some nerves have a white protective covering called the *myelin sheath.* Nerves covered with myelin are referred to as *white matter.* Nerves that do not have the protective myelin sheath are gray and make up the *gray matter* of the brain and spinal cord.

**16** What are the three types of neurons, as categorized according to function?

## TABLE 7.6 Disorders of the Nervous System

| Disorder | Description | Signs and Symptoms |
|---|---|---|
| Head injury | Can be caused by blunt trauma to the head or a break in the skull | Symptoms vary, depending on the area of the brain involved in the injury, but can include bleeding, swelling, or increased intracranial pressure. |
| Brain tumors | Can be benign (noncancerous) or malignant (cancerous) | Depends on the location of the tumor, which exerts pressure on surrounding tissue. |
| Migraine headache | Vasodilation and increased blood flow to the head | Throbbing sensation, severe head pain, nausea, vomiting, and blurred vision. |
| Cerebrovascular accident | Interruption in blood flow to the brain; can be caused by a hemorrhage or a blood clot and is commonly called a *stroke* | Numbness, altered mental status, vertigo, loss of muscle coordination, and others. |
| Epilepsy | Seizures | *Grand mal:* rigid and jerking motions.<br>*Petit mal:* stare, amnesia for event. |
| Multiple sclerosis (MS) | A progressive neurologic condition with demyelination and scarring of sites along the central nervous system | Visual problems and sensory, motor, and emotional problems can occur. |
| Alzheimer's disease | Chronic, progressive degenerative disease with no cure | Loss of recent memory for events, persons, and places. Over time, confusion and disorientation increase, leading to physical deterioration and death. |
| Bell's palsy | Paralysis of the facial (seventh cranial) nerve that causes distortion on the affected side of the face | The person may not be able to open an eye or close the mouth. The condition may be unilateral or bilateral. |
| Trigeminal neuralgia | A neurologic condition of the trigeminal facial nerve | Also known as tic *douloureux.* Severe pain caused by inflammation of the trigeminal (fifth cranial) nerve. This pain, which has been described as excruciating, stabbing, and searing, may last for a few seconds; however, the initial incident is usually followed by other episodes, often of increasing severity. Depending on which of the three nerve branches is affected, pain could occur around the eyes and over the forehead; in the upper lip, nose, and cheek; or in the tongue and lower lip. |
| Parkinson's disease | A slowly progressive, degenerative neurologic disorder | Resting tremors of hands, rigidity of movement, shuffling gait, masklike face, and stooped appearance. |

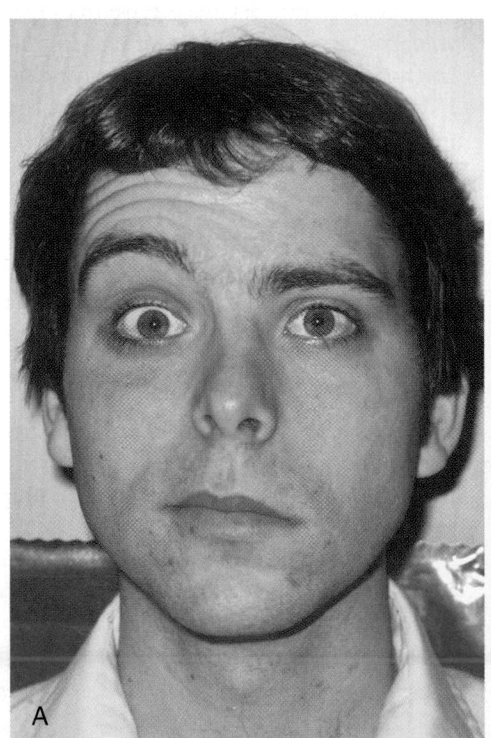


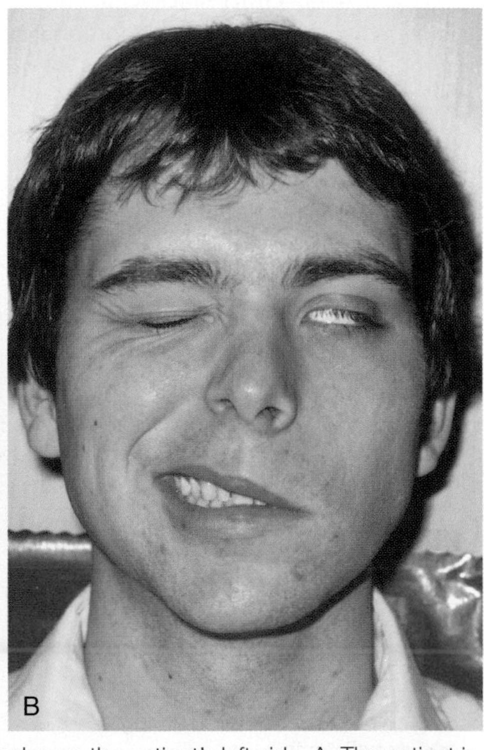


**FIG. 7.13** Bell's palsy. Paralysis of the facial muscles on the patient's left side. A, The patient is trying to raise his eyebrows. B, The patient is attempting to close his eyes and smile. *(Courtesy Dr. Bruce B. Brehm.)*

## Central Nervous System

The brain is enclosed in the cranium for protection, whereas the vertebrae protect the spinal cord.

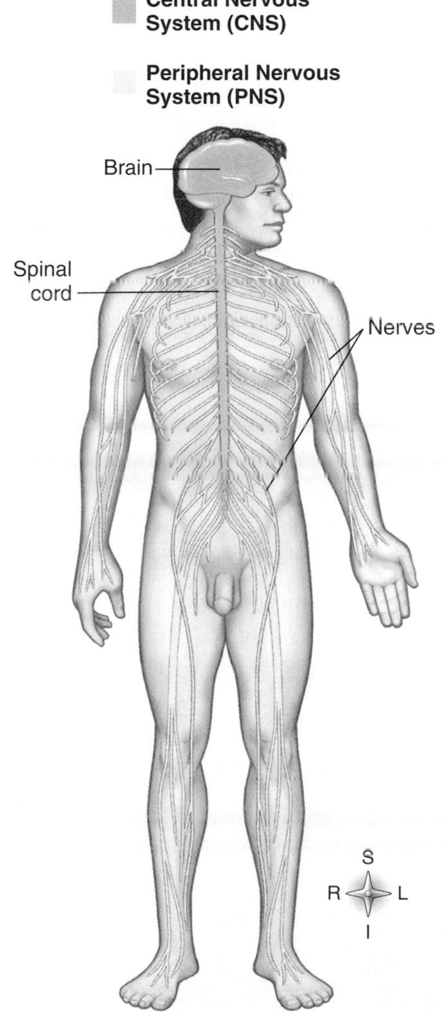


**FIG. 7.14** The central nervous system. *(From Patton KT, Thibodeau GA: Anatomy and physiology, ed 8, St Louis, Mosby, 2013.)*

### Brain

The brain is the primary center for regulating and coordinating body activities; each part of the brain controls a different aspect of bodily functions. The largest part of the brain is the *cerebrum,* which is divided into the right and left cerebral hemispheres. The brain is organized so that the left side of the brain controls the right side of the body and the right side of the brain controls the left side of the body.

### Spinal Cord

The spinal cord carries all the nerves that affect the limbs and the lower part of the body. The spine is the pathway for impulses that pass to and from the brain. *Cerebrospinal fluid* flows throughout the brain and around the spinal cord. Its primary function is to cushion these organs from shock and injury.

## Peripheral Nervous System

The PNS consists of the nerves that branch out from the brain and the spinal cord. The PNS has two divisions. The *autonomic nervous system* (ANS) controls unconscious activities, such as breathing, heart rate, body temperature, blood pressure, and pupil size. The *somatic nervous system* (SNS) controls conscious activities.

## Respiratory System

The term *respiration* means "breathing" or "to breathe." The respiratory system delivers *oxygen* to the millions of cells in the body and transports the waste product *carbon dioxide* out of the body. The respiratory system comprises the nose, paranasal sinuses, pharynx, epiglottis, larynx, trachea, alveoli, and lungs. Disorders of the respiratory system have specific signs and symptoms (Table 7.7).

**TABLE 7.7** Disorders of the Respiratory System

| Disorder | Description | Signs and Symptoms |
|---|---|---|
| Tonsillitis | Inflammation of the tonsils; adenoids also may be involved | Severely dry, scratchy, and sore throat; may include fever, chills, headache, muscle aches, and general body aching |
| Sinusitis | Acute inflammation of a sinus | Fever, chills, nasal obstruction, pain, and tenderness over the affected sinus |
| Pneumonia | Acute inflammation of the lungs; can be viral, bacterial, or nonbacterial | Fever, chills, productive cough, and general malaise |
| Pharyngitis (sore throat) | Inflammation of the throat caused by virus, bacteria, or irritants | Sore red throat, chills, high temperature, headache, and difficulty in swallowing |
| Tuberculosis | Infectious disease caused by infected droplets that contain tubercle bacteria | Early symptoms include low-grade fever, chills, night sweats, weakness, and fatigue; later, coughing of sputum that contains blood and chest pain |
| Lung cancer | Suspected causes include smoking and air pollutants | Cough, pain, shortness of breath, weight loss, and general malaise |

## Structures

### Nose

Air enters the body through the nostrils *(nares)* of the nose and passes through the *nasal cavity* (Fig. 7.15). The nose is divided by a wall of cartilage called the *nasal septum.*

The nose and the respiratory system are lined with mucous membrane, which is a specialized form of epithelial tissue. Incoming air is filtered by the *cilia,* which are thin hairs that are attached to the mucous membrane just inside the nostrils.

*Mucus* secreted by the mucous membranes helps moisten and warm the air as it enters the nose. (Notice the difference in spelling between *mucous,* the word used to describe the membrane, and *mucus,* the secretion of the membrane.)

### Pharynx

After passing through the nasal cavity, air reaches the pharynx, which is commonly known as the *throat.* The three divisions of the pharynx are the nasopharynx, oropharynx, and laryngopharynx.

The *nasopharynx* is located behind the nose and above the soft palate. The *eustachian tube,* the narrow tube that leads from the middle ear, opens into the nasopharynx.

The *oropharynx* extends from the soft palate above to the level of the epiglottis below. This is the part of the throat that

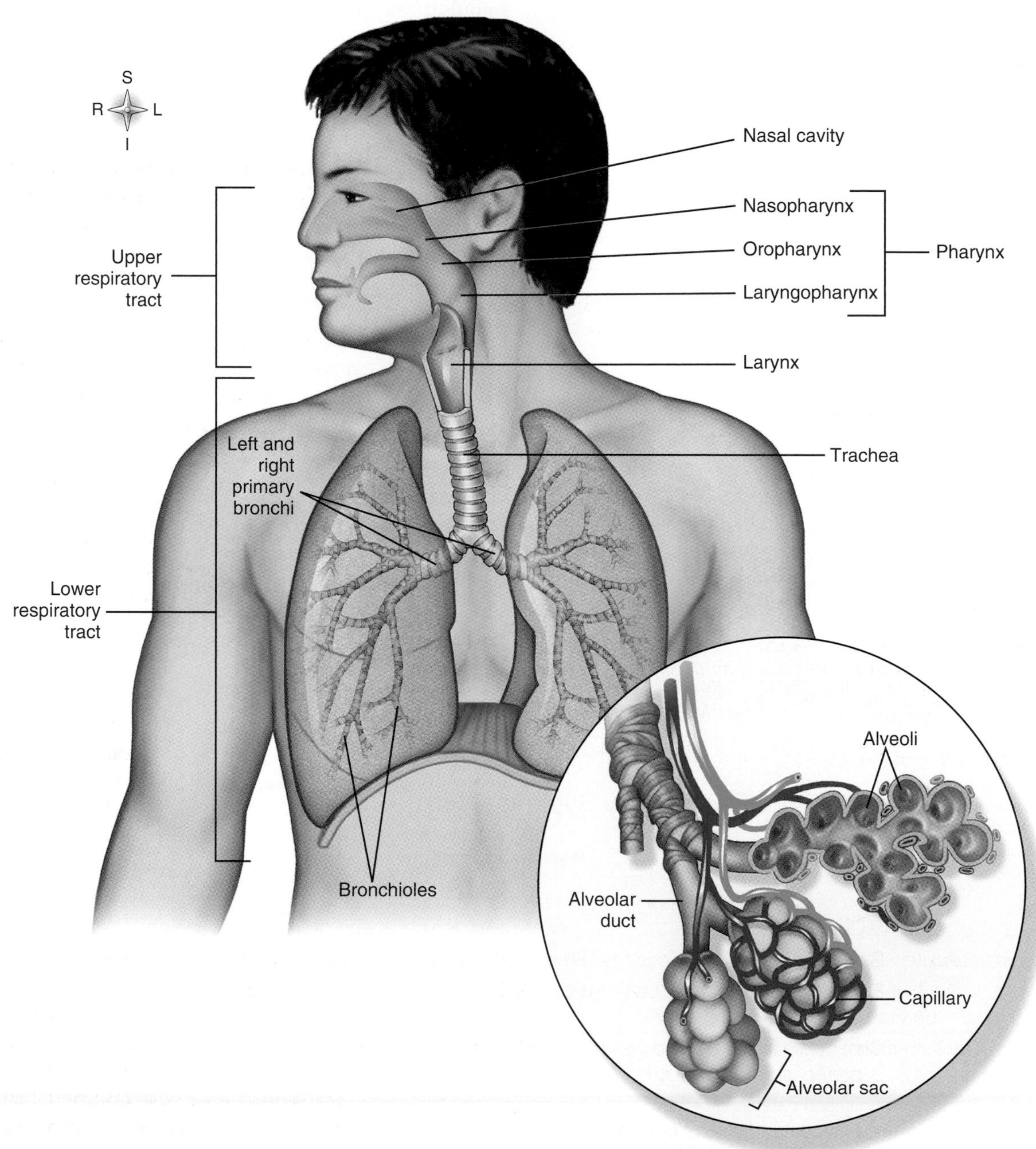


**FIG. 7.15** Structure of the respiratory system. *(From Patton KT, Thibodeau GA: Anatomy and physiology, ed 8, St Louis, Mosby, 2013.)*

is visible when one is looking into the mouth. This opening leads to both the stomach and the lungs. If a patient aspirates an object during treatment, such as a sharp tooth fragment, it could go to the lung or the digestive system. (As used here, *aspirate* means to inhale or swallow accidentally.)

The *laryngopharynx* extends from the level of the epiglottis above to the larynx below. The nasopharynx contains the adenoids; the oropharynx contains the palatine tonsils.

### Epiglottis

The oropharynx and the laryngopharynx serve as a common passageway for food from the mouth and air from the nose. During swallowing, the epiglottis acts as a lid and covers the larynx so that food does *not* enter the lungs.

### Larynx

The larynx, also known as the *voice box,* contains the vocal bands, which make speech possible. The larynx is protected and is held open by a series of cartilaginous structures. The largest cartilage forms the prominent projection in front of the neck, which is commonly known as the "Adam's apple."

### Trachea

Air passes from the larynx to the trachea. The trachea extends from the neck into the chest, directly in front of the esophagus. It is protected and held open by a series of C-shaped cartilaginous rings.

### Lungs

The trachea divides into two branches called *bronchi.* Each bronchus leads to a lung, where it divides and subdivides into increasingly smaller branches; *bronchioles* are the smallest of these branches. *Alveoli* are tiny grapelike clusters found at the end of each bronchiole. The walls of the alveoli are very thin and are surrounded by a network of capillaries. During respiration, exchange of gases between the lungs and the blood takes place in the alveoli. Oxygen from the air passes through the thin walls of the alveoli into the bloodstream, and carbon dioxide passes from the blood into the alveoli to be expelled into the air.

**17** What is the function of the respiratory system?

## Digestive System

The digestive system works similarly to an assembly line, but in reverse. It takes in whole foods and breaks them down into their chemical components. Food that has been eaten is broken down by digestive juices into small absorbable nutrients that generate energy and provide the body with the nutrients, water, and electrolytes necessary for life. The digestive system functions under involuntary control. We decide what and when we eat, but once we swallow our food, our digestive system takes over without our conscious thought. Disorders of the digestive system are variable and range from common (e.g., gastroesophageal reflux) to life-threatening events (e.g., peritonitis) (Table 7.8).

### Digestive Process

The digestive system provides nutrition for the body through the following five basic actions:

1. *Ingestion.* Food is taken into the mouth.
2. *Digestion.* The digestive process begins in the mouth with *mastication* (chewing), which consists of mixing the food with saliva and swallowing it. A digestive enzyme called *salivary amylase* begins the process of breaking down carbohydrates into simpler forms that the body can use. After the food is swallowed, the churning action of the stomach mixes it with gastric juice. The digestion of carbohydrates continues in the stomach, and the digestion of protein begins.
3. *Movement.* After swallowing, **peristalsis** occurs; this consists of rhythmic, wavelike contractions that move food through the digestive tract.
4. *Absorption.* Nutritional elements in the gastrointestinal tract pass through its lining and into the bloodstream. Absorption of nutrients occurs mostly in the small intestines.
5. *Elimination.* In the large intestine, excess water is absorbed, and solid by-products of digestion are eliminated from the body in feces.

### Structures

The major structures of the digestive system are the mouth, pharynx, esophagus, stomach, small intestine, large intestine, liver, gallbladder, and pancreas (Fig. 7.16).

**TABLE 7.8** Disorders of the Digestive System

| Disorder | Description | Signs and Symptoms |
|---|---|---|
| Gastroesophageal reflux | Backward flow of gastric juices into the esophagus | Heartburn, difficulty swallowing |
| Peptic ulcer | Erosion of the gastric mucosa that exposes it to gastric juice and pepsin | Feeling of pressure, burning, heaviness, or hunger; change in appetite and weight loss |
| Ulcerative colitis and Crohn's disease | Chronic inflammatory process of bowel that results in poor absorption of nutrients | Abdominal pain, cramping, or diarrhea with weight loss; may have anemia, fatigue; possibly bloody stools, pain, and cramping |
| Hemorrhoids | Varicose or dilated veins in the anal canal | Itching and pain and burning with defecation |
| Peritonitis | Inflammation of the lining of the abdominal cavity; a life-threatening condition | Fever, acute pain, cramping, signs of shock, tenderness, and rigid or distended abdomen |

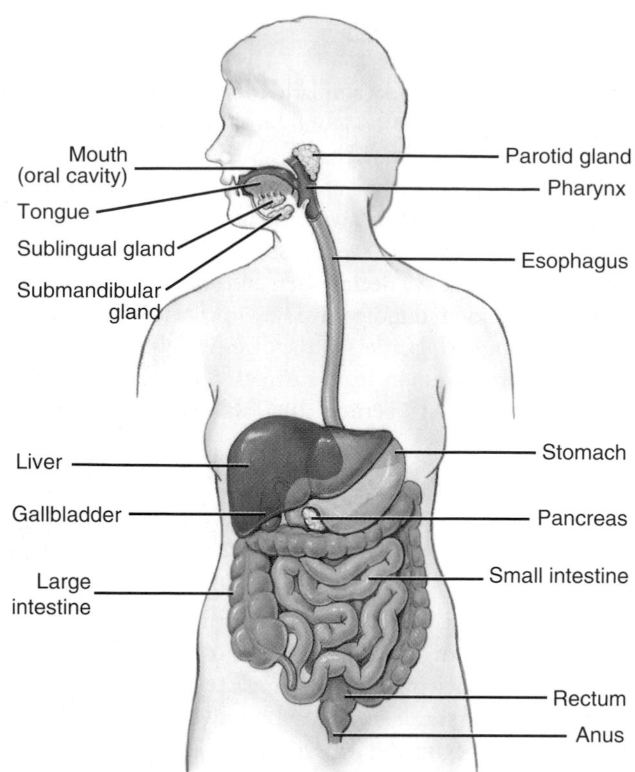


**FIG. 7.16** Major structures of the digestive system. *(From Applegate EJ: The anatomy and physiology learning system, ed 4, St Louis, Saunders, 2011.)*

### Mouth

Many structures are associated with the *mouth,* which is known as the oral region of the head. Each of these structures is discussed in detail in Chapter 10.

### Pharynx

The *pharynx* is a fibromuscular tube that connects the nasal and oral cavities to the larynx and esophagus. It serves as a passageway for food and air.

### Esophagus

The *esophagus* is a tubelike structure approximately 10 inches in length that transports food from the pharynx to the stomach.

### Stomach

The *stomach* is a saclike organ that lies in the abdominal cavity just under the diaphragm. Glands within the stomach produce the gastric juices that aid in digestion and the mucus that forms the protective coating of the stomach lining.

### Small Intestine

The *small intestine* extends from the stomach to the first part of the large intestine. It consists of three parts: duodenum, jejunum, and ileum.

### Large Intestine

The *large intestine* extends from the end of the small intestine to the anus. It is divided into four parts: cecum, colon, sigmoid colon, and rectum and anus.

### Liver, Gallbladder, and Pancreas

The *liver* is located in the right upper quadrant of the abdomen. It removes excess *glucose* (sugar) from the bloodstream and stores it as *glycogen* (starch). When the blood sugar level is low, the liver converts glycogen back into glucose and releases it for use by the body.

The liver destroys old erythrocytes, removes poisons from the blood, and manufactures some blood proteins. It also manufactures *bile,* a digestive juice.

The *gallbladder* is a pear-shaped sac that is located under the liver. It stores and concentrates bile for later use. When needed, bile is emptied into the duodenum of the small intestine.

The *pancreas* produces pancreatic juices, which contain digestive enzymes. These juices are emptied into the duodenum of the small intestine.

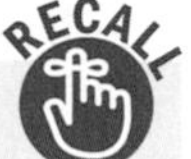


18 What is the role of the digestive system?
19 What are the five actions of the digestive system?

## Endocrine System

The endocrine system uses chemical messengers called *hormones* that move through the bloodstream and can reach every cell in the body.

Hormones help maintain a constant environment inside the body, adjusting the amount of salt and water in the tissues, sugar in the blood, and salt in sweat to suit the particular conditions that exist. Hormones produce long-term changes, such as a child's growth and sexual maturation, and rhythmic ones, such as the menstrual cycle. They trigger swift, dramatic responses in the body whenever illness or injury strikes, or whenever the brain perceives danger. Hormones have a lot to do with emotions such as fear, anger, joy, and despair.

Hormones are secreted directly into the bloodstream (not through a duct). The endocrine glands include the *thyroid* and *parathyroid, ovaries, testes, pituitary, pancreas,* and *adrenal medulla.* The major endocrine glands are scattered throughout the body but are considered to function as one system (Fig. 7.17).

System components are interrelated, and secretion from one gland can affect glands elsewhere. Many disorders can affect the endocrine system (Table 7.9).

20 What is the primary function of the endocrine system?

## Urinary System

The urinary system is also known as the *excretory system* (Fig. 7.18). Its principal function is to maintain fluid volume and the composition of body fluids. To accomplish this, gallons of fluid are filtered out of the bloodstream and through tubules of the kidneys. Waste products leave the body in the form of urine, and needed substances are returned to the blood. Disorders of the urinary system range from incontinence to renal failure (Table 7.10).

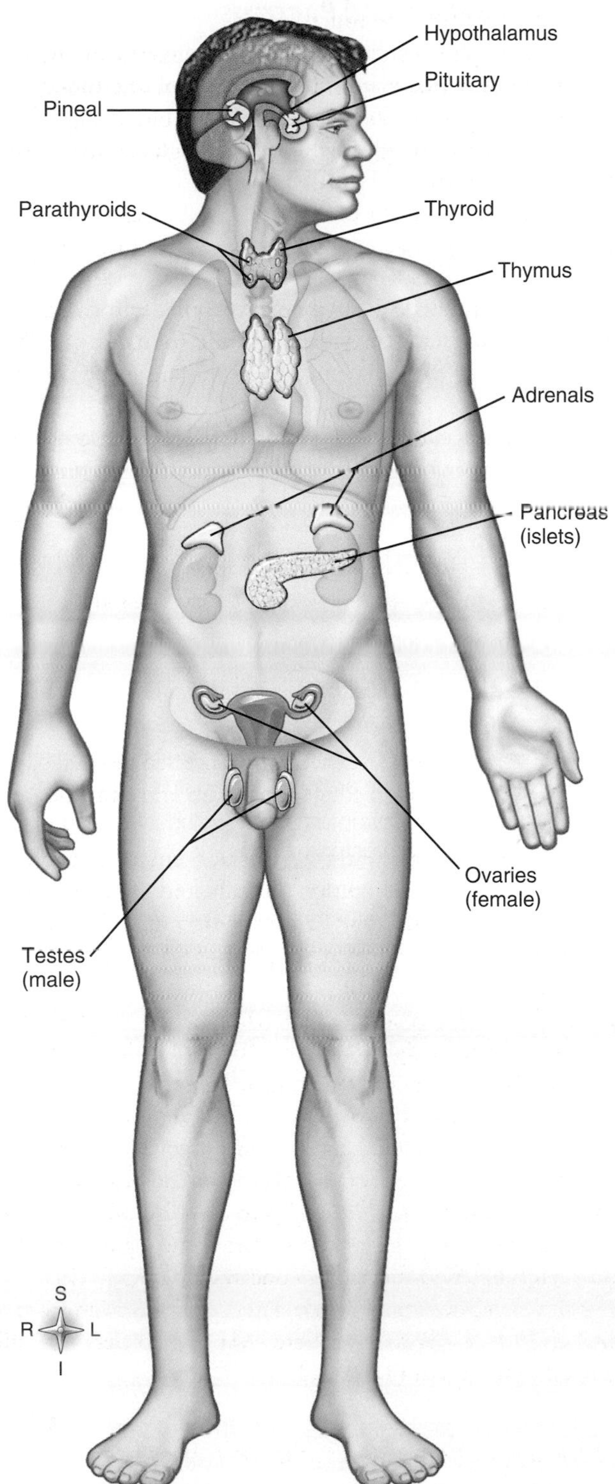


FIG. 7.17 Endocrine glands. *(From Patton KT, Thibodeau GA: Anatomy and physiology, ed 8, St Louis, Mosby, 2013.)*

The urinary system consists of (1) the *kidneys,* where urine is formed to carry away waste materials from the blood; (2) the *ureters,* which transport urine from the kidneys; (3) the *bladder,* where urine is stored until it can be eliminated; and (4) the *urethra,* through which the bladder is emptied to the outside through the process of urination. The kidneys require a large blood supply and are connected close to the body's main artery, the aorta. More than 2 pints of blood pass through the kidneys every minute.

**TABLE 7.9 Disorders of the Endocrine System**

| Disorder | Description | Signs and Symptoms |
|---|---|---|
| Hypothyroidism | Decreased level of activity of the thyroid gland | Decreased level of metabolism, sensitivity to cold, weight gain, or thick hair |
| Hyperthyroidism | Excessive level of activity of the thyroid gland | Nervousness, agitation, irritability, inability to concentrate, heat intolerance, or weight loss with increased appetite |
| Diabetes mellitus | Impaired glucose uptake by the cells | *Type 1 diabetes:* insulin dependence, weight loss, fatigue, and frequent urination<br>*Type 2 diabetes:* no insulin dependence; symptoms less severe than type 1, and may include blurred vision |

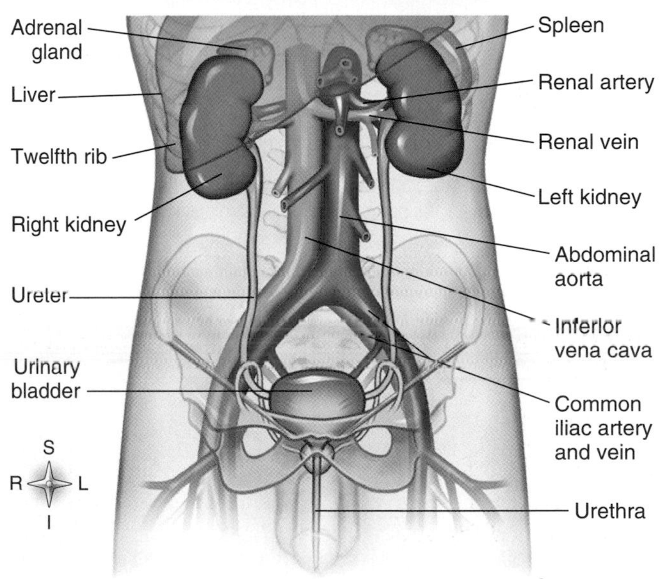


FIG. 7.18 The urinary system. *(From Patton KT, Thibodeau GA: Anatomy and physiology, ed 8, St Louis, Mosby, 2013.)*

**21** What is the primary function of the urinary system? RECALL

## Integumentary System

The skin is the body's first line of defense against disease. The **integumentary system**, or *skin system,* has many important functions, as follows:

- Helps to regulate body temperature
- Provides a barrier that prevents bacteria from entering the body
- Excretes liquids and salts

**TABLE 7.10 Disorders of the Urinary System**

| Disorder | Description | Signs and Symptoms |
|---|---|---|
| Renal failure | Loss of kidney function | Rapid retention of fluid and metabolic wastes |
| Urinary incontinence | Inability to control urination; bladder pressure increases | Incontinence during coughing, sneezing, or laughing; can be a symptom of urinary tract infection and other diseases, including Parkinson's disease and multiple sclerosis |
| Cystitis | Inflammation of the bladder | Painful urination, urgency, low back pain, and fever |

- Provides sensitivity to touch
- Uses ultraviolet rays from the sun to convert chemicals into the vitamin D necessary for absorption of calcium

Disorders of the integumentary system range from abscess to carcinoma (Table 7.11 and Fig. 7.19).

## Skin Structures

The skin is composed of different layers, including epidermis, dermis, and subcutaneous fat.

### Epidermis

The *epidermis* is the outer layer of the skin. It has no blood supply of its own. Cells of the epidermis receive their

**TABLE 7.11 Disorders of the Integumentary System**

| Disorder | Description | Signs and Symptoms |
|---|---|---|
| Abscess | Usually the result of a wound that allows bacteria to invade the dermis | Red, tender nodule that enlarges and becomes more painful as it grows |
| Acne | One of the most common skin diseases; inflammation of the sebaceous glands causes pimples or blackheads | Face and the upper body are the most common sites; inflamed lesions are papules, pustules, and cysts |
| Eczema | Nonspecific dermatitis; may be acute or chronic | Severe itching; symptoms may include weeping vesicles and crusted patches |
| Basal cell carcinoma | Most common of all human cancers; primary cause is exposure to sun radiation | A pearly, nodular border; the tumor enlarges, developing a central crater that continually repeats the cycle of eroding, crusting, bleeding, and healing |

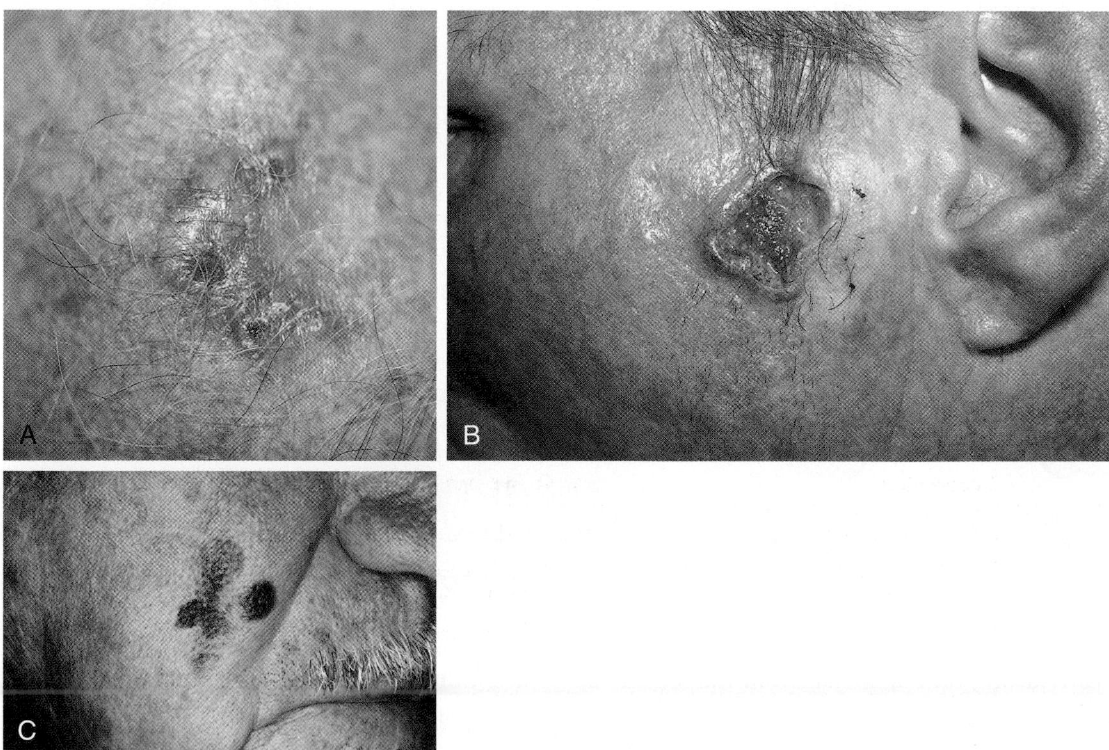


**FIG. 7.19** The three most common forms of skin cancer. A, Squamous cell. B, Basal cell. C, Malignant melanoma. *(From James WD, Berger TG, Elston DM: Andrews' diseases of the skin: clinical dermatology, ed 11, St Louis, Saunders, 2012.)*

nutrients from vessels in the underlying tissue. As new cells are pushed to the surface, older cells die and are *sloughed* (cast) off.

### Dermis

The *dermis* is a thick connective tissue layer that gives bulk to the skin. The dermal layer contains many free nerve endings and receptors, which allow for detection of touch, temperature, and pain. With age, connective tissue becomes less elasticized, and wrinkles develop.

### Subcutaneous Fat

*Subcutaneous fat* is a layer of loose connective tissue that anchors the skin to underlying organs. It insulates the body against heat loss and cushions underlying organs. The distribution of subcutaneous fat is responsible for the differences in body contours between men and women.

## Skin Appendages

The skin has a number of appendages, including hair, nails, and glands.

### Hair

*Hair* is found on almost all skin surfaces. It is enclosed in a follicle and consists of a root and a shaft. The bulk of the shaft consists of dead material and protein. Hair color and skin color are determined by the melanin produced in the epidermis.

### Nails

As with hair, *nails* primarily consist of nonliving matter. Nails contain a root and a body. The body is the visible portion, and the root is covered by skin called the *cuticle.* The extensive blood supply in the underlying dermis gives nails their pink color.

### Glands

The three types of glands in the skin are sebaceous, sudoriferous, and apocrine sweat glands.

**Sebaceous glands** are found in all areas of the body except the palms of the hands and the soles of the feet. They are oil glands that keep the hair and skin soft. They are also associated with sex hormones and become active during puberty. Sebaceous activity decreases with age, which is why hair and skin become dry as aging occurs.

**Sudoriferous glands** are distributed all over the body and provide heat regulation by secreting sweat. Sweat is also produced in response to stress.

**Apocrine sweat glands**, the largest glands, are found under the arms, around the nipples, and in the genital region. Bacterial action causes secretions to break down, producing body odor.

**22** What are the functions of the skin?
**23** What are the appendages to the skin?

## Reproductive System

### Female

The female reproductive system consists of external and internal genitalia. External genitalia include the *mons pubis, labia majora,* and *labia minora,* along with the *vulva* and the *clitoris.* Internal genitalia consist of the *ovaries, fallopian tubes, uterus,* and *vagina.* Fertility, the normal functioning of the reproductive system, begins at puberty (the onset of menstruation) and ceases at menopause. Many disorders can affect the female reproductive system (Table 7.12).

### Male

The male reproductive system produces and transports sperm. This system consists of *testes, excretory ducts,* and *accessory organs.* Accessory organs include the *prostate* and *seminal vesicles.* In the male, several organs serve as parts of both the urinary tract and the reproductive system. A disorder may interfere with the function of either system or of both systems (Table 7.13).

**TABLE 7.12** Disorders of the Female Reproductive System

| Disorder | Description | Signs and Symptoms |
|---|---|---|
| Vaginitis | Inflammation of the vagina | Vaginal discharge, itching, and pain, especially on urination |
| Ovarian tumors | Enlargements of normal ovarian structures | Feeling of pelvic pressure, urinary frequency, constipation, and backache |
| Toxic shock syndrome | Infection related to menstruation and tampon use | Flulike symptoms for the first 24 hours; onset of high fever, headache, sore throat, vomiting, generalized rash, and hypotension |
| Pelvic inflammatory disease (PID) | Inflammation of several reproductive organs | Foul-smelling vaginal discharge and abdominal pain; general symptoms of an infection |
| Breast cancer | Uncontrolled growth of cancer cells within the breast; these cells spread to other areas of the body | Abnormal mass of tissue in the breast; dimpling, nipple retraction, or enlargement of the breast may be noted |

**TABLE 7.13 Disorders of the Male Reproductive System**

| Disorder | Description | Signs and Symptoms |
|---|---|---|
| Testicular cancer | Rare, usually occurs in men younger than 40; most common type of cancer in men between 20 and 35 years of age | Begins as a painless lump in the testicle; may spread through lymphatic system to lymph nodes in abdomen, chest, neck, or lungs |
| Orchitis | Infection or inflammation of one or both testes | Pain in the involved testes; high temperature with red, swollen, and tender testes |
| Epididymitis | Inflammation or infection of the epididymis | Pain and tenderness in the groin area and scrotum; high fever and symptoms of urinary tract infection may be present |
| Prostate cancer | Cause is unknown; third leading cause of cancer death in men; more common in men older than 40 years | Urinary frequency, difficulty in urinating, and urinary retention |

## Interaction among the Ten Body Systems

Body systems do not operate independently; they exert important effects on each other. For example, when you exercise hard, your muscular system needs extra oxygen, so your respiratory system works harder than usual to supply it. The ovaries and testes clearly belong to the reproductive system. However, because one of their functions is to produce hormones, they are also components of the endocrine system. The muscular system clearly depends on the skeletal system. A healthy respiratory system is of no value if the circulatory system fails. When something happens in one system, the event usually affects other systems. For example, if your nervous system reacts to upsetting information while you are eating, your digestive system may not function as well as usual.

**■ Legal and Ethical Implications** Oral health is a necessary component for overall general health. New research is pointing to associations between chronic oral infection and heart and lung disease, stroke, low birth weight, and premature birth. An association has been recognized between periodontal disease and diabetes. An individual cannot be healthy without oral health. Oral health and general health are not separate entities. Risk factors that affect general health, such as tobacco use and poor nutrition, also affect oral health.

In this country today, inequities and disparities may prevent people from achieving optimal oral health. Barriers to oral health include lack of access to care, whether because of limited income or lack of insurance, transportation difficulties, and lack of flexibility to take time off from work to see a dentist. Individuals with disabilities and those with complex health problems may face additional barriers to care. Many challenges remain for eliminating social, political, and economic barriers to oral health and general well-being. ■

**■ Eye to the Future** As a dental assistant, you need a strong foundation in anatomy and physiology. This information can help you both personally and professionally. For example, it is important for you to understand how the muscular system works, so you can protect the muscles in your neck and back from fatigue and strain while assisting during long procedures. Also, you will see patients with muscular problems, who will need your understanding and assistance.

You will be better prepared to assist during a medical emergency in the dental office when you understand the circulatory and respiratory systems. Prescription medications may adversely affect a patient's dental treatment. You should be alert for signs and symptoms of various systemic disorders in yourself and in your family members, as well as in your patients. ■

### ■ Critical Thinking

1. The respiratory system is exposed to the atmosphere and is susceptible to airborne infection, contaminants, and irritants. What can you do to protect your respiratory system?
2. If a patient with severe arthritis in her hands came into your dental office, what dental treatment–related difficulties might she experience?
3. When 80-year-old Mrs. McBride comes into the office, the receptionist comments on how nice her hair looks. Mrs. McBride thanks the receptionist and then mentions that her hair used to be much softer and had more shine when she was younger. Do you think Mrs. McBride's hair has actually changed? Why or why not?
4. Mr. Cardono has been a patient in your office for several years. While you update his health history, Mr. Cardono states that his immunity must be down because he recently has had several severe sore throats and colds. Which body system is responsible for the decline in his immunity? ■

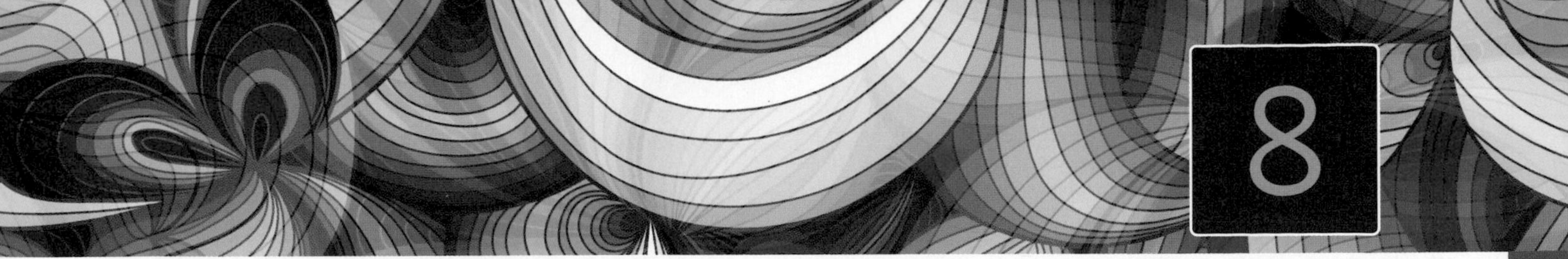

8

# Oral Embryology and Histology

## KEY TERMS

**Alveolar crest** Highest point of the alveolar ridge.

**Alveolar socket** Cavity within the alveolar process that surrounds the root of a tooth.

**Ameloblasts (uh-MEL-oe-blasts)** Cells that form enamel.

**Anatomical crown** Portion of the tooth that is covered with enamel.

**Apex** Tapered end of each root tip.

**Apical foramen** Natural opening in the root.

**Cementoblasts (se-MEN-toe-blasts)** Cells that form cementum.

**Cementoclasts (se-MEN-toe-klasts)** Cells that resorb cementum.

**Cementum** Specialized, calcified connective tissue that covers the anatomic root of a tooth.

**Clinical crown** That portion of the tooth that is visible in the oral cavity.

**Conception** Union of the male sperm and the female ovum.

**Coronal pulp** Part that lies within the crown portion of the tooth.

**Cortical plate** Dense outer covering of spongy bone that makes up the central part of the alveolar process.

**Dental lamina** Thickened band of oral epithelium that follows the curve of each developing arch.

**Dental papilla** Gingivae between the teeth.

**Dental sac** Connective tissue that envelops the developing tooth.

**Dentin** Hard portion of the root that surrounds the pulp and is covered by enamel on the crown and by cementum on the root.

**Dentinal fiber** Fibers found in dentinal tubules.

**Dentinal tubules** Microscopic canals found in dentin.

**Deposition** The process by which the body adds new bone.

**Embryo** An organism in the earliest stages of development.

**Embryology (em-bree-OL-uh-jee)** The study of prenatal development.

**Embryonic (em-bree-ON-ik) period** Stage of human development that occurs from the beginning of the second week to the end of the eighth week.

**Enamel lamellae** Thin, leaflike structures that extend from the enamel surface toward the detinoenamel junction and consist of organic material with little mineral content.

**Enamel organ** Part of a developing tooth destined to produce enamel.

**Enamel spindles** The ends of odontoblasts (dentin-forming cells) that extend across the detinoenamel junction a short distance into the enamel.

**Enamel tufts** The hypocalcified or uncalcified ends of groups of enamel prisms that start at the detinoenamel junction and may extend to the inner third of the enamel.

**Exfoliation (eks-foe-lee-AY-shun)** The normal process of shedding the primary teeth.

**Fetal period** Stage of human development that starts at the beginning of the ninth week and ends at birth.

**Fibroblast** Type of cell in connective tissue responsible for the formation of the intercellular substance of pulp.

**Gestation (jes-TAY-shun)** Stage of human development that starts at fertilization and ends at birth.

**Histology (his-TOL-uh-jee)** The study of the structure and function of body tissues on a microscopic level.

**Hunter-Schreger bands** Alternating light and dark bands in the enamel that are produced when enamel prisms intertwine or change direction.

**Hydroxyapatite** Mineral compound that is the principal inorganic component of bone and teeth.

**Hyoid arch** The second branchial arch, which forms the styloid process, stapes of the ear, stylohyoid ligament, and part of the hyoid bone.

**Lamina dura** Thin, compact bone that lines the alveolar socket; also known as the cribriform plate.

**Lining mucosa** Mucous membrane that covers the inside of the cheeks, vestibule, lips, soft palate, and underside of the tongue and acts as a cushion for underlying structures.

**Mandibular (man-DIB-yoo-lur) arch** The lower jaw.

**Masticatory (MAS-ti-kuh-tor-ee) mucosa** Oral mucosa that covers the hard palate, dorsum of the tongue, and gingiva.

**Meiosis (mye-OE-sis)** Reproductive cell production that ensures the correct number of chromosomes.

**Modeling** Bone changes that involve deposition and resorption of bone and occur along articulations as they increase in size and shape to keep up with the growth of surrounding tissues; also known as displacement.

**Odontoblasts (o-DON-to-blasts)** Cells that form dentin.

**Odontogenesis (o-don-to-JEN-eh-sis)** Formation of new teeth.

**Osteoblasts (OS-tee-oe-blasts)** Cells that form bone.

**Osteoclasts (OS-tee-oe-klasts)** Cells that resorb bone.

**Periodontium (per-ee-oe-DON-shee-um)** Structures that surround, support, and are attached to the teeth.

**Preimplantation period** Stage of development that occurs during the first week after fertilization.

**Prenatal (pree-NAY-tul) development** Stage of human development that starts at pregnancy and ends at birth.

**Primary cementum** Cementum that covers the root of the tooth and is formed outward from the cementodentinal junction for the full length of the root.

**Primary dentin** Dentin that forms before eruption and that makes up the bulk of the tooth.

**Primary palate** The shelf that separates the oral and nasal cavities.

**Prism** A calcified column or rod.

**Pulp chamber** The space occupied by pulp.

**Radicular pulp** The other portion of pulp known as root pulp.

**Remodeling** Growth and change in shape of existing bone that involves deposition and resorption of bone.

**Resorption (ree-SORP-shun)** The body's processes of eliminating existing bone or hard tissue structure.

**Secondary cementum** Cementum that is formed on the apical half of the root; also known as cellular cementum.

**Secondary dentin** Dentin that forms after eruption and continues at a very slow rate throughout the life of the tooth.

**Secondary palate** The final palate formed during embryonic development.

**Specialized mucosa** Mucous membrane on the tongue in the form of lingual papillae, which are structures associated with sensations of taste.

**Stomodeum** The primitive mouth.

**Stratified squamous (SKWA-mus) epithelium** Layers of flat, formed epithelium.

**Striae of Retzius** Incremental rings that represent variations in deposition of the enamel matrix during tooth formation.

**Succedaneous (suk-se-DAY-ne-us) teeth** Permanent teeth that replace primary teeth.

**Tertiary dentin** Dentin that forms in response to irritation and appears as a localized deposit on the wall of the pulp chamber; also known as reparative dentin.

**Tooth buds** Enlargements produced by the formation of dental lamina.

**Zygote** Fertilized egg.

## LEARNING OUTCOMES

*On completion of this chapter, the student will be able to achieve the following objectives:*

1. Pronounce, define, and spell the key terms.
2. Define embryology and discuss this important phase of development, including the following:
   - Describe the three periods of prenatal development.
   - Discuss prenatal influences on dental development.
   - Describe the stages of development of the hard and soft palates.
   - Describe the stages in the development of a tooth.
   - Name the genetic and environmental factors that can affect dental development.
   - Describe the functions of osteoclasts and osteoblasts.
3. Describe the life cycle of a tooth.
4. Define histology and discuss its importance, including the following:
   - Explain the difference between clinical and anatomical crowns.
   - Name and describe the tissues of the teeth.
   - Name and describe the three types of dentin.
   - Describe the structure and location of dental pulp.
   - Name and describe the components of the periodontium, including the functions of periodontal ligaments.
   - Describe the various types of oral mucosa and give an example of each.

## ELECTRONIC RESOURCES

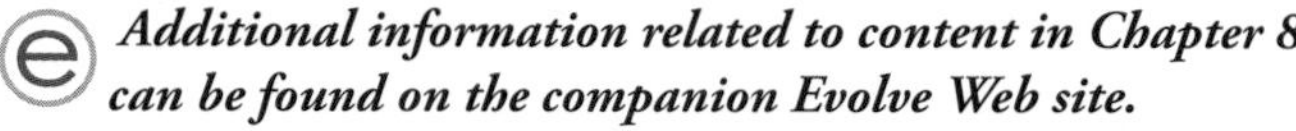


- Practice Quiz

**Embryology** is the study of **prenatal development** throughout the stages before birth. The first part of this chapter discusses development with emphasis on the formation of the teeth and structures of the oral cavity. Learning about the development of the oral structures provides the foundation for later understanding of developmental problems that may occur in these structures.

**Histology** is the study of the structure and function of tissues on a *microscopic level.* The second part of this chapter covers the histology of the teeth, their supporting structures, and the oral mucosa, which surrounds the teeth and lines the mouth. By understanding the histology of oral tissues, the dental assistant can better understand the disease processes that occur in the oral cavity.

# Oral Embryology

*Pregnancy* begins with **conception**, which is also known as *fertilization.* **Gestation**, the period from fertilization to birth, has an average duration of 9 months from conception to birth, or 40 weeks from the last menstrual period (LMP). The due date is usually figured out with a convenient rule of thumb; count back 3 months from the day the LMP began, then add a year and a week. The date you come up with is just a guide; the baby may arrive anywhere from 2 weeks earlier to 2 weeks later. The sex of the baby is established at conception and will be apparent in a few weeks. This little 1-inch being weighs only about .04 ounce (1 gram) and could fit comfortably on a tablespoon.

A physician usually describes prenatal development in weeks on the basis of the date of the LMP. In embryology, *developmental age* is based on the date of conception, which is assumed to have occurred 2 weeks after the LMP. Developmental ages noted in this chapter are based on the date of conception.

## Prenatal Development

Prenatal development consists of three distinct periods: (1) preimplantation, (2) embryonic, and (3) fetal (Fig. 8.1).

The **preimplantation period** takes place during the first week. At the beginning of the week, an ovum (egg) is penetrated by and united with a sperm during fertilization (Fig. 8.2). This penetration of the egg by a sperm cell has an immediate effect on the surface of the egg: The outer coating of the egg changes, so that no other sperm cell can enter. The union of the egg and the sperm subsequently forms a fertilized egg, or **zygote**. In the zygote, 23 chromosomes in the sperm unite with 23 chromosomes in the egg, providing a new life with a full complement of 46 chromosomes. These chromosomes will determine its inherited characteristics and will direct its growth and development. The process of joining the parents' chromosomes is called **meiosis**. Meiosis ensures that the future **embryo** will have the correct number of chromosomes.

The **embryonic period** extends from the beginning of the second week to the end of the eighth week, and the new individual is known as an embryo. This period is the *most critical time* because during these weeks, development begins in

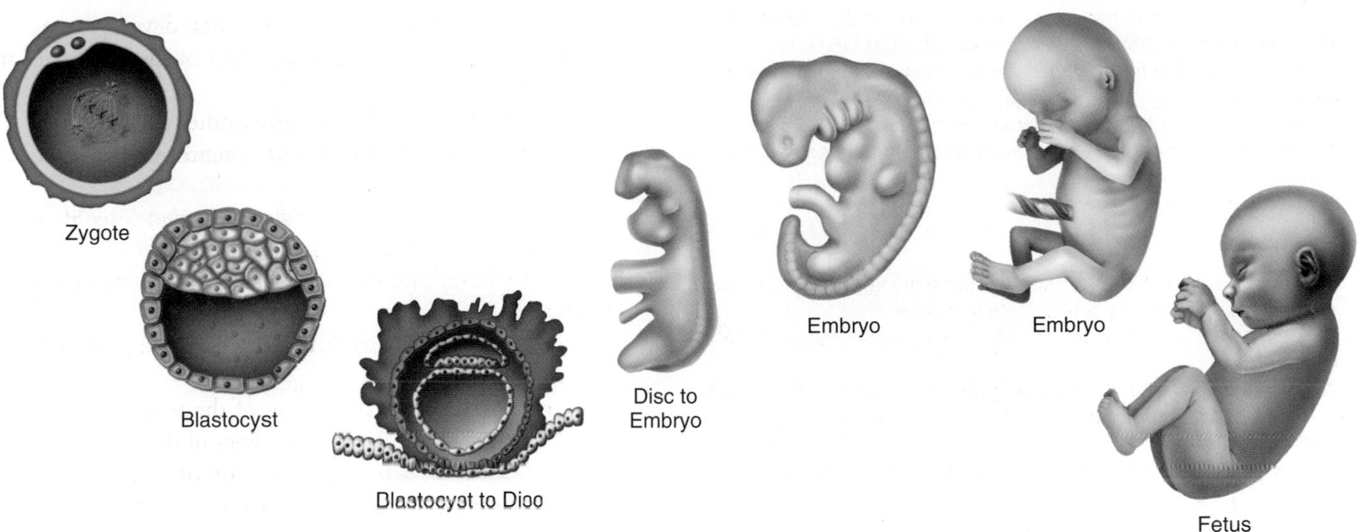


FIG. 8.1 Periods and structures in prenatal development. Note that the size of the structures is neither accurate nor comparative. *(© Elsevier Collection.)*

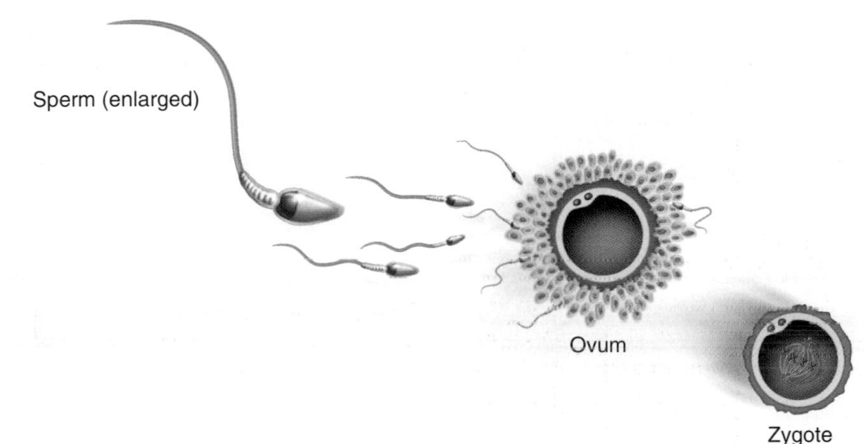


FIG. 8.2 Sperm fertilizes the ovum and unites with it to form the zygote after the process of meiosis and during the first week of prenatal development. Chromosomes from the ovum and sperm join to form a zygote—a new individual. *(© Elsevier Collection.)*

all major structures of the body. The cells begin to *proliferate* (increase in number), *differentiate* (change into tissues and organs), and *integrate* (form systems). Many of these key developments occur before the mother even knows that she is pregnant. At about the end of the eighth week of pregnancy, a baby graduates from embryo to fetus. This name change signifies a change in the baby's level of development. While an embryo, the baby looks very much like a tadpole, but as a fetus, it has a distinctly human appearance.

The **fetal period** continues from the ninth week and lasts until birth. During the fetal phase, body systems continue to develop and mature. The fetus has distinguishable ears, arms, hands, legs, and feet, as well as the fingerprints and footprints that will set it apart from other human beings. Because all organ systems are formed during the embryonic period, the fetus is less vulnerable than the embryo to malformations caused by radiation, viruses, and drugs (Table 8.1). The fetal stage is a period of growth and maturation (Fig. 8.3).

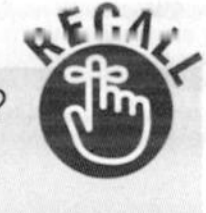


1 What are the three periods of prenatal development?
2 Which period of prenatal development is the most critical, and why?

## Embryonic Development of the Face and Oral Cavity

The face and its related tissues begin to form during the fourth week of prenatal development within the embryonic period. During this time, the rapidly growing brain of the embryo bulges over the oropharyngeal membrane, beating heart, and stomodeum (Fig. 8.4).

### *Primary Embryonic Layers*

During the third week of development, the cells of the embryo form the three primary embryonic layers: *ectoderm, mesoderm,* and *endoderm.* The cells within each layer multiply and

**TABLE 8.1** Developmental Disturbances

| Developmental Period | Developmental Disturbance | Examples of Disturbances |
|---|---|---|
| Preimplantation period | Child with Down syndrome 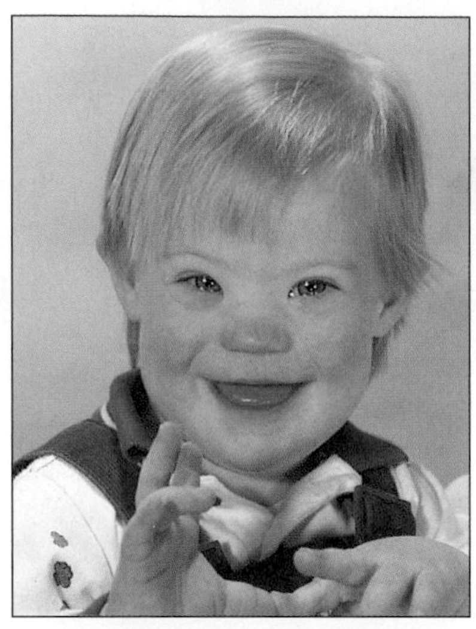 | If any disturbances occur in meiosis during fertilization, major congenital malformations result. Down syndrome is caused by an extra chromosome. A child with this syndrome has a flat, broad face with wide-set eyes, a flat-bridged nose, oblique eyelid fissures, and other defects. An affected child can have various levels of intellectual disability. Children with Down syndrome have increased levels of periodontal (gum) disease and abnormally shaped teeth.<br>Implantation may occur outside the uterus; this is called ectopic (ek-TOP-ik) pregnancy. Most such pregnancies occur within the fallopian tube. Tubal pregnancies usually rupture, causing loss of the embryo and threatening the life of the pregnant woman. |
| Embryonic period | Child with fetal alcohol syndrome 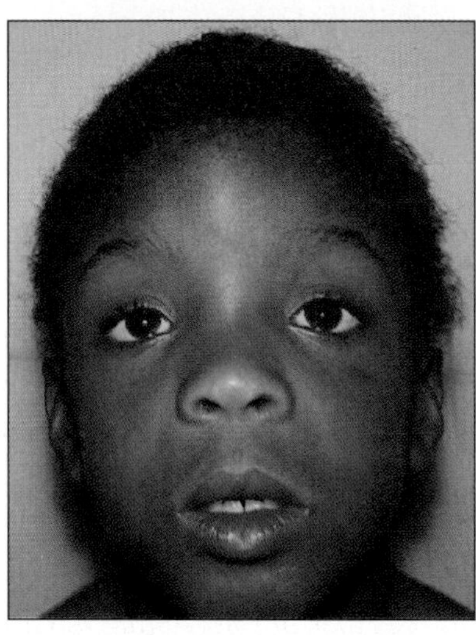 | Developmental disturbances during this period may cause major congenital malformations.<br>Caused by the rubella (roo-BELL-ah) virus, German measles in the mother can result in cardiac defects and deafness in the child.<br>Exposure to high levels of radiation may result in cell death and retardation of mental development and physical growth.<br>Fetal alcohol syndrome can occur when a pregnant woman ingests alcohol. |
| Fetal period | Endogenous developmental stain: tetracycline 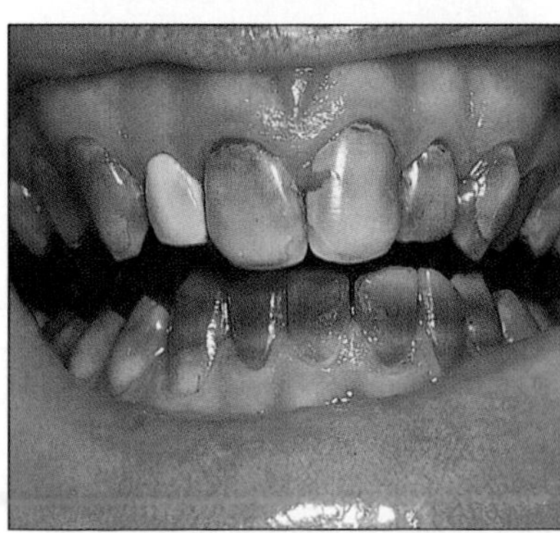 | In amniocentesis (am-nee-o-sen-TEE-sis), a common prenatal diagnostic procedure, amniotic fluid is sampled during the fourteenth to sixteenth weeks to determine whether a birth defect is present in the fetus.<br>When a pregnant woman takes the systemic antibiotic tetracycline (tet-rah-SI-kleen) during the fetal period, permanent staining of the child's primary teeth may result. |

Preimplantation and embryonic periods from Zitelli BJ, McIntire SC, Nowalk AJ: *Zitelli and Davis' atlas of pediatric physical diagnosis,* ed 6, St Louis, Saunders, 2013. Fetal period courtesy Dr. George Taybos, Jackson, MS.

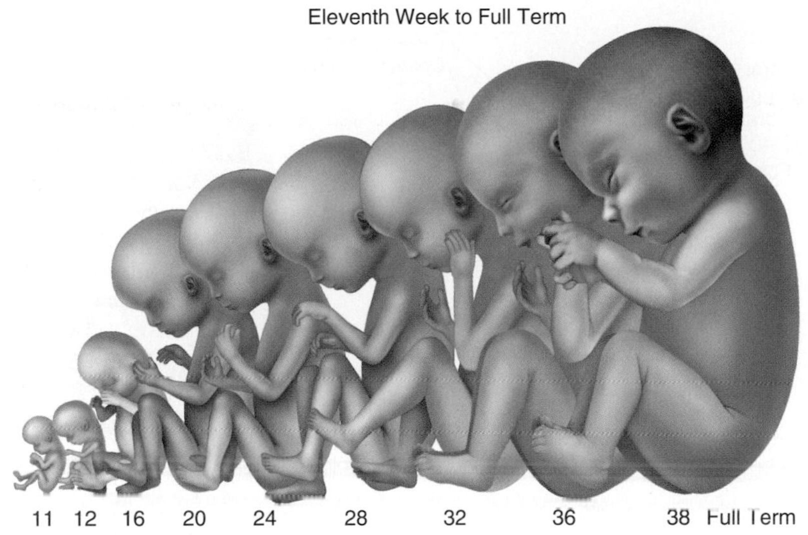


**FIG. 8.3** A fetus at various weeks of development. *(© Elsevier Collection.)*

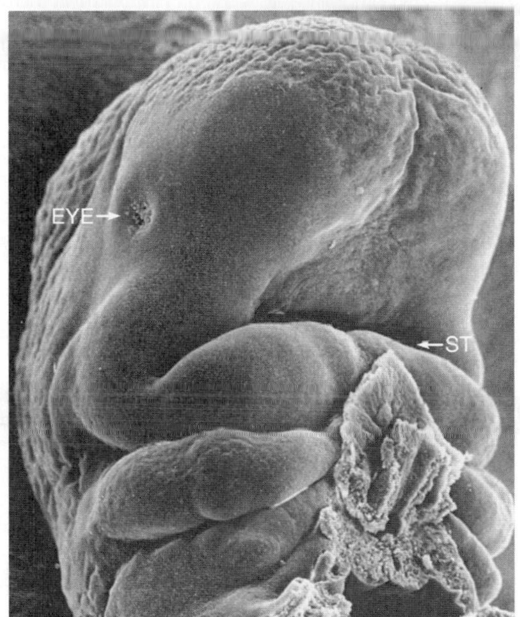


**FIG. 8.4** Scanning electron micrograph of the head and neck of an embryo at 4 weeks shows development of the brain, face, and heart. Note the stomodeum *(ST)*, or "primitive mouth," and the developing eye.

differentiate into specialized cells needed to form the organs and tissues of the body.

## Structures Formed by Specialized Cells of Primary Embryonic Layers

**Ectoderm (Outer Layer)**

- Skin, brain, spinal cord
- Hair, nails
- Enamel of teeth
- Lining of oral cavity

**Mesoderm (Middle Layer)**

- Bones, muscles
- Circulatory system
- Kidneys, ducts
- Reproductive system
- Lining of abdominal cavity
- Dentin, pulp, and cementum of teeth

**Endoderm (Inner Layer)**

- Lining of digestive system
- Lining of lungs
- Parts of urogenital system

**3** What are the three primary embryonic layers?

## Early Development of the Mouth

During the fourth week, the **stomodeum** (primitive mouth) and the primitive pharynx merge, and the stomodeum extends into part of the mouth. By the beginning of the fifth week, the embryo is approximately 5 mm. The heart is prominent and bulging (Fig. 8.5).

The site of the face is indicated from above by the region just in front of the bulging forebrain (future forehead) and from below by the first pair of branchial arches (future jaws).

## Branchial Arches

By the end of the fourth week, six pairs of branchial arches have formed. The first two of these arches give rise to the structures of the head and neck (see Chapter 9).

The *first branchial arch,* also known as the **mandibular arch**, forms the bones, muscles, and nerves of the face. The first arch also forms the lower lip, the muscles of mastication, and the anterior portion of the alveolar process of the mandible.

The *second branchial arch,* also known as the **hyoid arch**, forms the styloid process, stapes of the ear, stylohyoid ligament, and part of the hyoid bone. The second arch also forms the side and front of the neck, as well as some muscles of facial expression.

The *third branchial arch* forms the body of the hyoid and the posterior tongue. The *fourth, fifth,* and *sixth branchial arches*

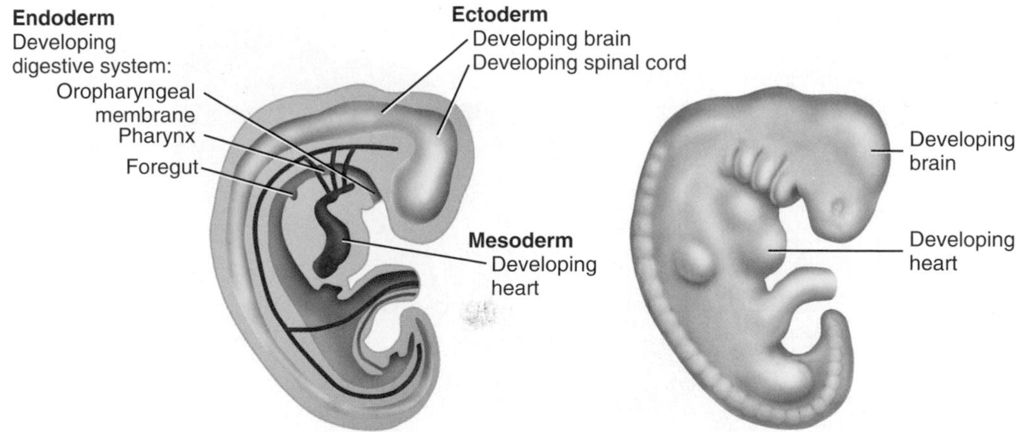


FIG. 8.5 A human embryo during the fifth week of development. *(© Elsevier Collection.)*

form the structures of the lower throat, including the thyroid cartilage, and the muscles and nerves of the pharynx and larynx.

RECALL

4 Which branchial arch forms the bones, muscles, nerves of the face, and lower lip?

5 Which branchial arch forms the side and front of the neck?

## *Hard and Soft Palates*

Formation of the palate takes several weeks to occur. It is formed from two separate embryonic structures: the **primary palate** and the **secondary palate**. This process begins in the fifth week of prenatal development. The hard and soft palates are formed by the union of the primary and secondary palates. This fusion makes a Y-shaped pattern in the roof of the mouth. This pattern is visible in the bony hard palate of an infant; however, the bones continue to fuse, and these lines are no longer visible in the adult hard palate.

Fusion usually begins from the anterior during the ninth week. The palate is then completed during the twelfth week within the fetal period. Thus the palate is formed in three consecutive stages: (1) formation of the primary palate, (2) formation of the secondary palate, and (3) fusion of the palate (Fig. 8.6). Any disruption in this process may result in a cleft lip or cleft palate (Fig. 8.7) (see Chapter 10).

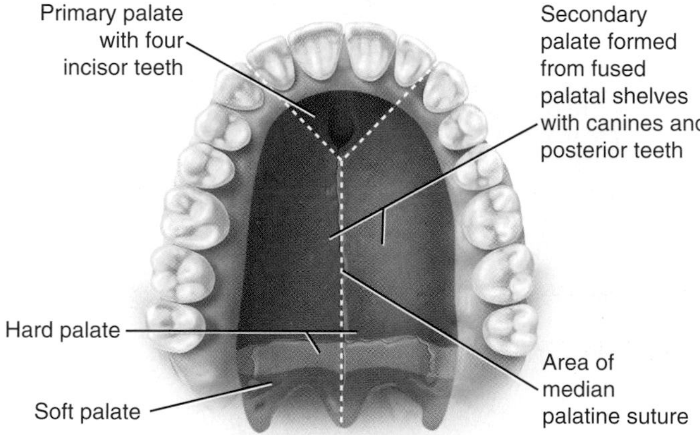


FIG. 8.6 Adult palate and developmental divisions. *(© Elsevier Collection.)*

RECALL

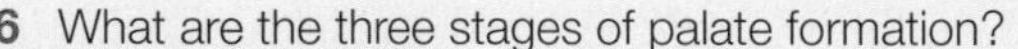

6 What are the three stages of palate formation?

## *Facial Development*

The development of the human face occurs primarily between the fifth and eighth weeks. The face develops from the frontonasal process, which covers the forebrain, and the first branchial arch. Forward growth of the structures of the mouth produces striking age-related changes in the silhouette of the developing head, as follows:

- In the embryo at 1 month, the overhanging forehead is the dominant feature.
- During the second month, rapid growth of the nose and upper jaw occurs, and the lower jaw appears to lag behind.
- In the third month, the fetus definitely resembles a human, although the head is still disproportionately large.
- At 4 months, the face looks human, the hard and soft palates are differentiated, and formation has begun on all primary dentition (arrangement and number of teeth).
- During the last trimester, fat is laid down in the cheeks; these "sucking pads" give a healthy full-term fetus the characteristic round contour of the face.

7 When does development of the human face occur?

## *Tooth Development*

When the embryo is 5 to 6 weeks old, the first signs of tooth development are found in the anterior mandibular region (Table 8.2). Shortly after the mandibular anteriors develop, the anterior maxillary teeth begin to develop, and the process of tooth development progresses toward the posterior in both jaws.

By the seventeenth week, all primary teeth are developed and the development of permanent teeth has begun.

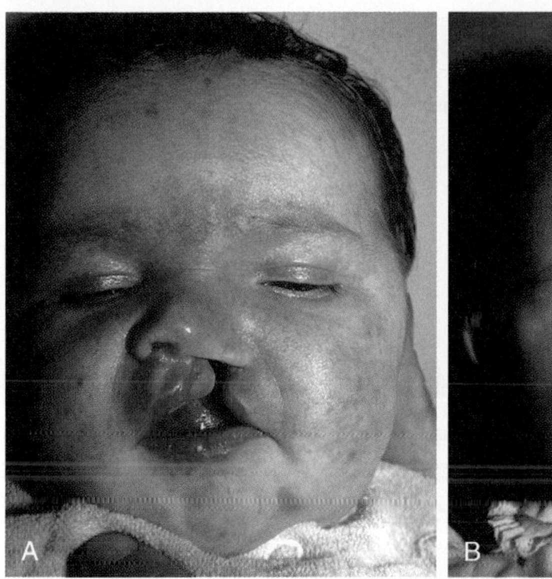


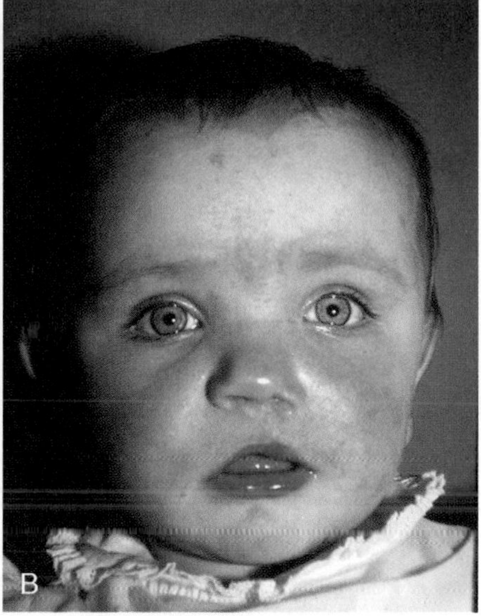


**FIG. 8.7** A, An infant with a left unilateral complete cleft lip and palate. B, The infant after corrective surgeries are performed. *(From Kaban L, Troulis M: Pediatric oral and maxillofacial surgery, St Louis, 2004, Saunders.)*

**TABLE 8.2** Stages of Tooth Development

| Stage/Time Span* | Microscopic Appearance | Main Processes Involved | Description |
|---|---|---|---|
| Initiation stage/sixth to seventh week | 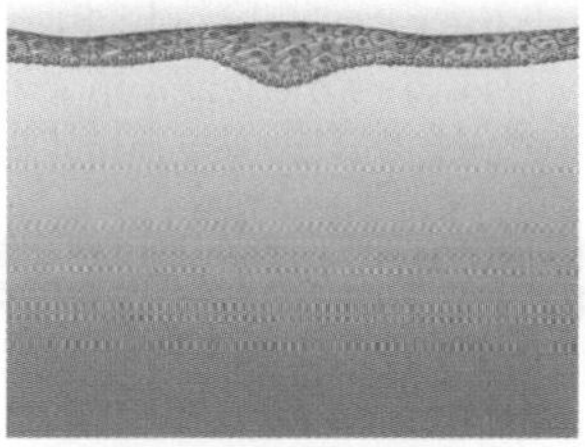 | Induction | Ectoderm lining stomodeum gives rise to oral epithelium and then to dental lamina, adjacent to deeper mesenchyme and neural crest cells and separated by a basement membrane. |
| Bud stage/eighth week | 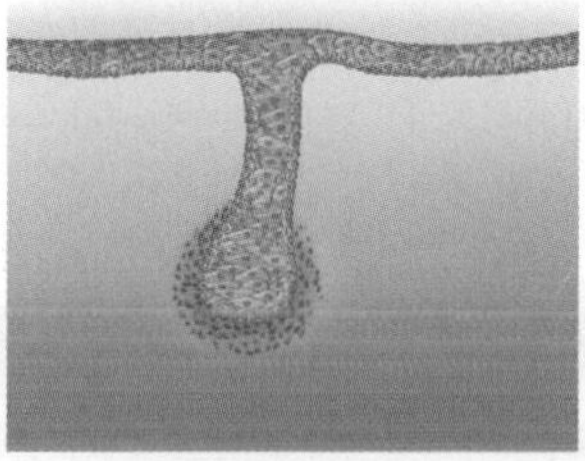 | Proliferation | Growth of dental lamina into bud that penetrates growing mesenchyme. |
| Cap stage/ninth to tenth week | 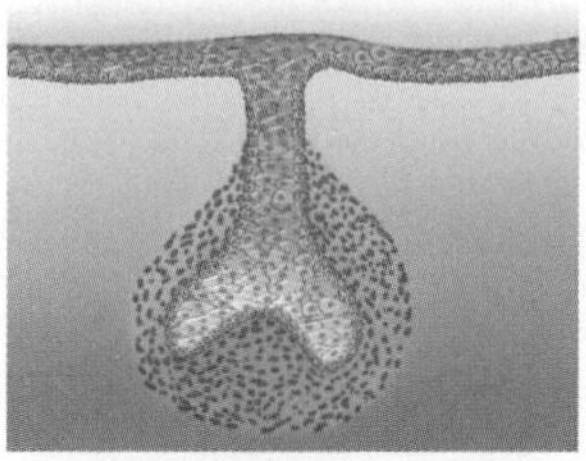 | Proliferation, differentiation, morphogenesis | Enamel organ forms into cap, surrounding mass of dental papilla from the mesenchyme and surrounded by mass of dental sac also from the mesenchyme; formation of the tooth germ. |
| Bell stage/eleventh to twelfth week | 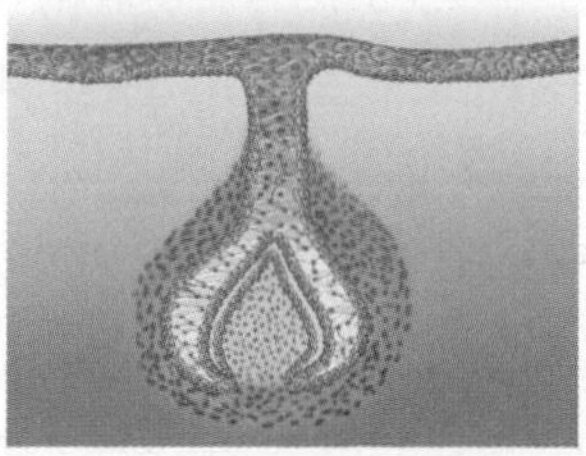 | Proliferation, differentiation, morphogenesis | Differentiation of enamel organ into bell with four cell types and dental papilla into two cell types. |

*Continued*

**TABLE 8.2 Stages of Tooth Development—cont'd**

| Stage/Time Span* | Microscopic Appearance | Main Processes Involved | Description |
|---|---|---|---|
| Apposition stage/varies per tooth | 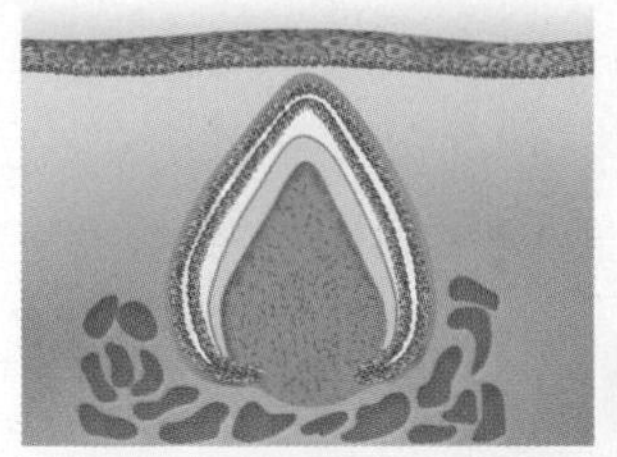 | Induction, proliferation | Dental tissues secreted as matrix in successive layers. |
| Maturation stage/varies per tooth | 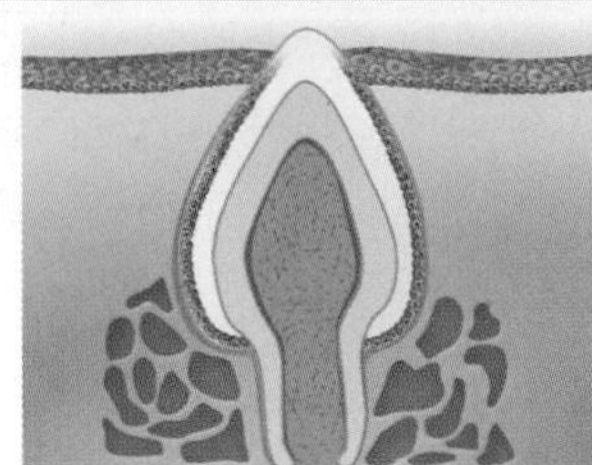 | Maturation | Dental tissues fully mineralize to their mature levels. |

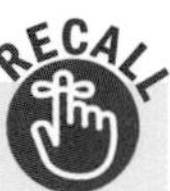

*Note that these are approximate prenatal time spans for development of the primary dentition.

Data from Fehrenbach MJ, Popowics T: *Illustrated dental embryology, histology, and anatomy,* ed 4, St Louis, 2016, Saunders. Images © Elsevier Collection.

RECALL

8 How old is the embryo when the first signs of tooth development are found?

## Developmental Disturbances

Disturbances at any stage of dental development may cause a wide variety of *anomalies* (abnormalities). Developmental disturbances can be caused by genetic and environmental factors (Table 8.3; also see Table 8.1). See Chapter 17 for pictures of these conditions.

### Genetic Factors

In prenatal tooth development, the genetic factor that is most often a matter of concern is tooth and jaw size. A child may inherit large teeth from one parent and a small jaw from the other, or small teeth and a large jaw. A large discrepancy in the size relationship of teeth and jaws may cause malocclusion (poor tooth position or contact) as the child develops. Less common genetic factors appear in the dentition as anomalies.

### Environmental Factors

Adverse environmental influences called *teratogens* include infections, drugs, and exposure to radiation. Drugs taken during pregnancy may cause birth defects. Such drugs include prescribed medication, over-the-counter remedies such as aspirin and cold tablets, and abused drugs, including alcohol. Antibiotics, particularly tetracycline, taken during pregnancy may result in a yellow-gray-brown stain on the primary teeth. Women of childbearing age should avoid teratogens from the time of their first missed menstrual period.

The mother's dental health is also of concern. Toxins from a dental infection may be dangerous to both mother and child (e.g., toxins from periodontal disease in the mother are linked to low birth weight in the infant). Fever in the mother during pregnancy will leave marks on the developing teeth of the fetus.

Good nutrition *before* pregnancy helps carry mother and child through the first weeks, which are critical for the developing child. This is also the time when morning sickness affects many expectant mothers, and some women find it difficult to eat.

### Known Teratogens Involved in Congenital Malformations

- *Drugs:* ethanol, tetracycline, phenytoin (Dilantin), lithium, methotrexate, aminopterin, diethylstilbestrol, warfarin, thalidomide, isotretinoin (retinoic acid), androgens, progesterone
- *Chemicals:* methylmercury, polychlorinated biphenyls
- *Infection:* rubella, herpes simplex, human immunodeficiency virus (HIV), syphilis
- *Radiation:* high levels of ionizing type*

*Diagnostic levels of radiation should be avoided but have not been directly linked to congenital malformations.

Modified from Fehrenbach MJ, Popowics T: Illustrated dental embryology, histology, and anatomy, ed 4, St Louis, 2016, Saunders.

9 What are the two major categories of factors that can adversely influence dental development?

## Facial Development After Birth

The shape of the face changes considerably from newborn to adult (Fig. 8.8). After the immediate postnatal period, most facial growth takes place in predictable *growth spurts,* which occur during youth and early adolescence. Facial bones grow and are reshaped to achieve normal growth and development.

TABLE 8.3 Dental Developmental Disturbances

| Disturbance | Stage | Description | Etiologic Factors | Clinical Ramifications |
|---|---|---|---|---|
| Anodontia | Initiation stage | Absence of single or multiple teeth | Hereditary, endocrine dysfunction, systemic disease, excessive radiation exposure | May cause disruption of occlusion and esthetic problems. May need partial or full dentures, bridges, or implants to replace teeth. |
| Supernumerary teeth | Initiation stage | Development of one or more extra teeth | Hereditary | Occurs commonly between the maxillary centrals, distal to third molars, and the premolar region. May cause crowding, failure of normal eruption, and disruption of occlusion. |
| Macrodontia/microdontia | Bud stage | Abnormally large or small tooth | Developmental or hereditary | Commonly involves permanent maxillary lateral incisor and third molar |
| Dens in dente | Cap stage | Enamel organ invaginates into the dental papilla | Hereditary | Commonly affects the permanent maxillary lateral incisor. Tooth may have deep lingual pit and endodontic therapy may be required. |
| Germination | Cap stage | Tooth germ tries to divide | Hereditary | Large single-rooted tooth with one pulp cavity that exhibits "twinning" in crown area. Normal number of teeth in dentition. May cause problems in appearance and spacing. |
| Fusion | Cap stage | Union of two adjacent tooth germs | Pressure on area | Large tooth with two pulp cavities. Extra tooth in dentition. May cause problems in appearance and spacing. |
| Tubercle | Cap stage | Extra cusp caused by effects on enamel organ | Trauma, pressure, or metabolic disease | Common or permanent molars or cingulum of anterior teeth. |
| Enamel pearl | Apposition and maturation stages | Sphere of enamel on root | Displacement of ameloblasts to root surface | May be confused with calculus deposit on root. |
| Enamel dysplasia | Apposition and maturation stages | Faulty development of enamel from interference involving ameloblasts | Local or systemic or hereditary | Pitting and intrinsic color changes in enamel. |
| Dentinal dysplasia | Apposition and maturation stages | Faulty development of dentin from interference with odontoblasts | Local or systemic or hereditary | Intrinsic color changes and changes in thickness of dentin possible. Problems in function or esthetics |
| Concrescence | Apposition and maturation stages | Union of root structure of two or more teeth by cementum | Traumatic injury or crowding of teeth | Common with permanent maxillary molars. |

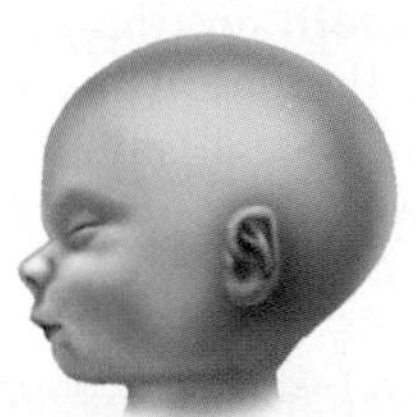

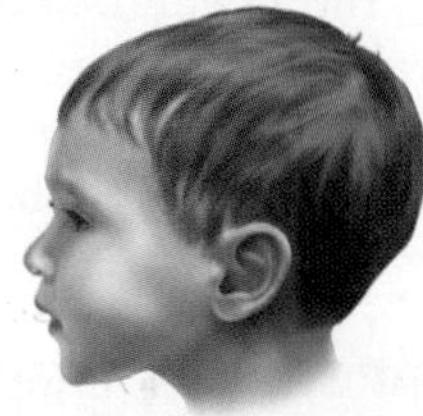

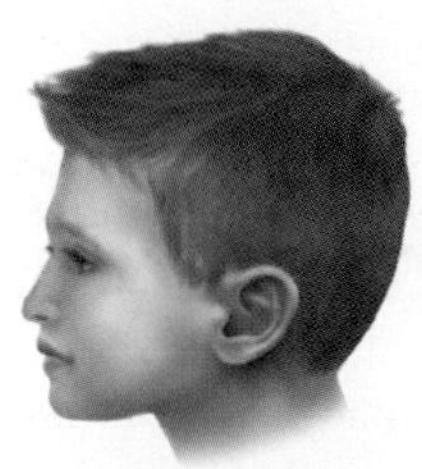

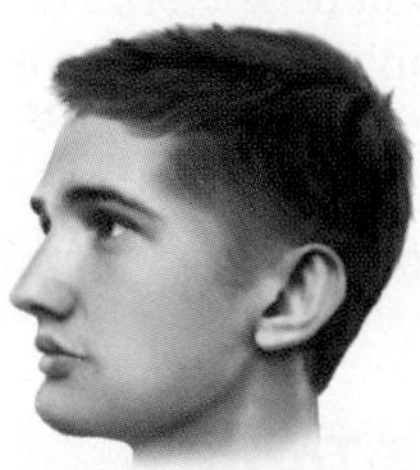


**FIG. 8.8** Changes in facial contours from birth to adulthood. *(© Elsevier Collection.)*

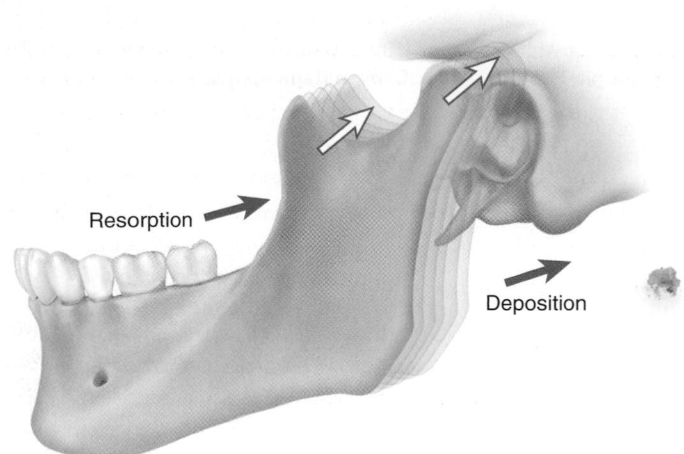


**FIG. 8.9** The mandible grows by displacement, resorption, and deposition. Note how space is created to accommodate the third molar. *(© Elsevier Collection.)*

This process involves the **deposition** of new bone in some areas and the **resorption** of existing bone from other areas.

Deposition is the process of "laying down" or adding new bone. **Osteoblasts** are the cells that are responsible for new bone formation. Examples of new bone formation include healing of a fractured bone and creation of new bone to fill the socket left after tooth extraction.

Resorption occurs when the body removes bone. **Osteoclasts** are the cells responsible for this process, in which bone cells are resorbed (taken away) by the body. The roots of primary teeth resorb before the tooth is lost. Resorption also occurs with loss of bone from the alveolar ridge during periodontal disease.

**Modeling**, also known as *displacement,* describes bone changes that occur along the articulations (joints) of bones as they increase in size and shape to keep up with the growth of surrounding tissues.

**Remodeling** describes growth and changes in the shape of existing bone. Modeling and remodeling involve both deposition and resorption of bone (Fig. 8.9).

### Tooth Movement

Remodeling occurs in response to forces placed on the tooth within its socket. To understand this concept, imagine yourself standing in a swimming pool. As you step forward, the water moves from in front of you and fills in the space in back of you. Similarly, when force is applied to a tooth and the tooth moves, the bone in front will be *resorbed* and will be *deposited* in back of the tooth to fill in the space (Fig. 8.10).

**10** What is the process of adding bone?
**11** What is the process of bone loss or removal?

## Life Cycle of a Tooth

The process of tooth formation, called **odontogenesis**, is divided into three primary periods: growth, calcification, and eruption (see Table 8.2).

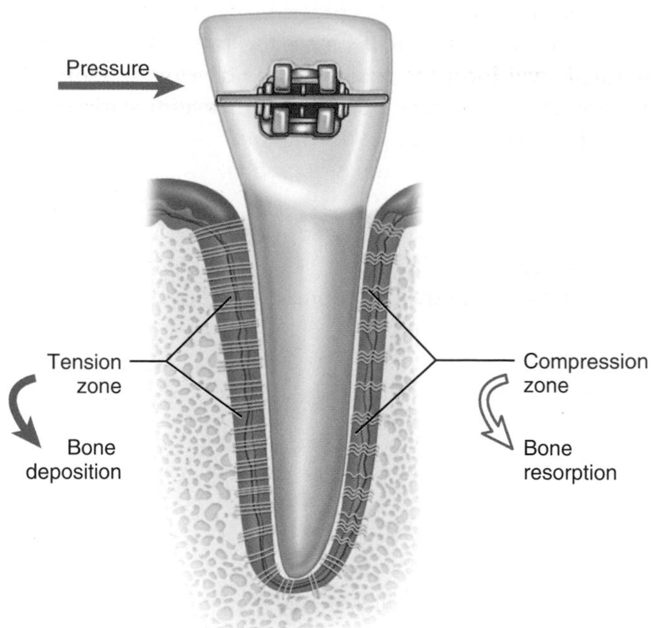


**FIG. 8.10** Process of orthodontic tooth movement. *(© Elsevier Collection.)*

### Growth Periods

The growth periods are divided into three stages: bud, cap, and bell.

**BUD STAGE.** The bud stage, also known as *initiation,* is the beginning of development for each tooth. This stage follows a definite pattern, and it takes place at a different time for each type of tooth.

Initiation starts with the formation of the **dental lamina**, which is a thickened band of oral epithelium that follows the curve of each developing dental arch. Almost as soon as the dental lamina is formed, it produces ten enlargements in each arch. These are the **tooth buds** for the *primary teeth.*

The *permanent teeth* develop similarly. The dental lamina continues to grow in a posterior direction to produce tooth buds for the three permanent molars, which will develop distal to the primary teeth on each quadrant. The tooth bud for the first permanent molar forms at about the seventeenth week of fetal life; the tooth buds for the second molars form about 6 months after birth; and buds for the third molars form at about 5 years.

The **succedaneous teeth** are the *permanent* teeth that replace the primary teeth. These teeth develop from tooth buds in the deep portion of the dental lamina on the lingual side of the primary teeth. These teeth begin to form as early as 24 weeks.

**CAP STAGE.** During the cap stage, also known as *proliferation,* the cells of the tooth grow and increase in number. This growth causes regular changes in size and proportion of the developing tooth, and the solid-looking tooth bud changes into a hollow, caplike shape.

The primary embryonic ectoderm layer, which has differentiated into *oral epithelium,* becomes the **enamel organ**, which eventually will form the enamel of the developing tooth. The primary embryonic mesoderm layer, now differentiated into connective tissue known as *mesenchyme,* becomes the **dental papilla**, which will form the pulp and **dentin** of the tooth. As the enamel organ and dental papilla of the tooth develop, the mesenchyme surrounding them condenses to form a capsule-like structure, called the **dental sac**. This sac will give rise to the **cementum** and the periodontal ligament.

**BELL STAGE.** During the bell stage, the cells differentiate and become specialized in a process called *histodifferentiation,* as follows:

- Epithelial cells become **ameloblasts**, which are the enamel-forming cells.
- Peripheral cells of the dental papilla become **odontoblasts**, which are the dentin-forming cells.
- Inner cells of the dental sac differentiate into **cementoblasts**, which are cementum-forming cells.
- As the tooth continues to develop, the dental organ continues to change. It assumes a shape described as resembling a bell. As these developments take place, the dental lamina, which thus far has connected the dental organ to the oral epithelium, breaks apart.

The basic shape and relative size of each tooth are established during the process of *morphodifferentiation.* The *dentinoenamel junction* (DEJ) and the *cementodentinal junction* are formed and act as a blueprint for the developing tooth.

In accordance with this pattern, the ameloblasts deposit enamel and the odontoblasts deposit dentin to give the completed tooth its characteristic shape and size. This process starts at the top of the tooth and moves downward toward the future root. Development of the root, or roots, begins after enamel and dentin formation has reached the future *cementoenamel junction* (CEJ).

As part of this process, the inner cells of the dental sac differentiate into cementoblasts, which produce cementum to cover the developing root.

12 What are the three primary periods in tooth formation?
13 What are the three stages in the growth period?

## Calcification

Calcification is the process by which the structural outline formed during the growth stage is hardened by the deposit of calcium and other mineral salts. Enamel is built layer by layer by the ameloblasts, which work outward from the DEJ, starting at the top of the crown of each tooth and spreading downward over its sides.

**PITS AND FISSURES.** If the tooth has several cusps, a cap of enamel forms over each cusp. As growth continues, the cusps eventually *coalesce* (fuse together) to form a solid enamel covering for the occlusal surface of the tooth.

Pits and fissures may be formed during this process. A *fissure* is a fault along a developmental groove on the occlusal surface that is caused by incomplete or imperfect joining of the lobes during tooth formation. A *pit* results when two developmental grooves cross each other, forming a deep area that is too small for the bristle of a toothbrush to clean. The enamel may be particularly thin; these areas are often inaccessible for cleaning and thus are sites where decay frequently begins (see Chapter 59).

## Eruption of Primary Teeth

Once it has passed through the previous stages, a tooth must be able to achieve its normal position. *Eruption* is movement of the tooth into its functional position in the oral cavity.

Eruption of the primary dentition takes place in chronologic order, as does the permanent dentition later (Fig. 8.11). This process involves active eruption, which is the actual vertical movement of the tooth. We know *how* tooth eruption occurs, but *why* it occurs is still uncertain. No one can specify the exact forces that "push" teeth through the soft tissues.

Active eruption of a primary tooth involves many stages in the movement of the tooth (Fig. 8.12). The period of tissue disintegration causes an inflammatory response known as "teething," which may be accompanied by tenderness and swelling of local tissues.

## Shedding of Primary Teeth

Shedding, or **exfoliation**, is the normal process by which primary teeth are lost as succedaneous (permanent) teeth develop. When it is time for a primary tooth to be lost, osteoclasts cause resorption of the root, beginning at the **apex** and continuing in the direction of the crown. Eventually, the crown of the tooth is lost because of lack of support.

The process of shedding is intermittent because at the same time that osteoblasts replace resorbed bone, odontoblasts and cementoblasts are replacing resorbed portions of the root. Thus a primary tooth may tighten after it has been loose. Finally, the primary tooth will be lost (Fig. 8.13).

## Eruption of Permanent Teeth

The process of eruption for a succedaneous tooth is the same as for a primary tooth. The permanent tooth erupts into the oral cavity in a position lingual to the roots of the shedding (or shed) primary anterior tooth or between the roots of the shedding primary posterior tooth (Fig. 8.14).

When a permanent tooth starts to erupt before the primary tooth is fully shed, problems in spacing can arise. Thus it is important for children with retained primary teeth to seek dental consultation early.

RECALL

14 When a tooth has several cusps, what structures are formed when the cusps join together?
15 What is the name of the process by which teeth move into the oral cavity?

## Oral Histology

Oral histology is the study of the *structure and function* of the teeth and oral tissues. This section discusses anatomic parts and histology of the teeth, the supporting structures, and the oral mucosa, which surrounds the teeth and lines the mouth.

Each tooth consists of a crown and one or more roots. The size and shape of the crown and the size and number of roots vary according to the type of tooth (see Chapter 11).

### Crown

In the crown, dentin is covered by enamel, and in each root, dentin is covered by cementum. The inner portion of the dentin of both the crown and the root also covers the pulp cavity of the tooth close to the CEJ. The CEJ is the external line at the neck or cervix of the tooth where the enamel of the crown and the cementum of the root usually meet (Fig. 8.15).

Portions of the crown are usually defined in more specific ways. The **anatomical crown** is the portion of the tooth

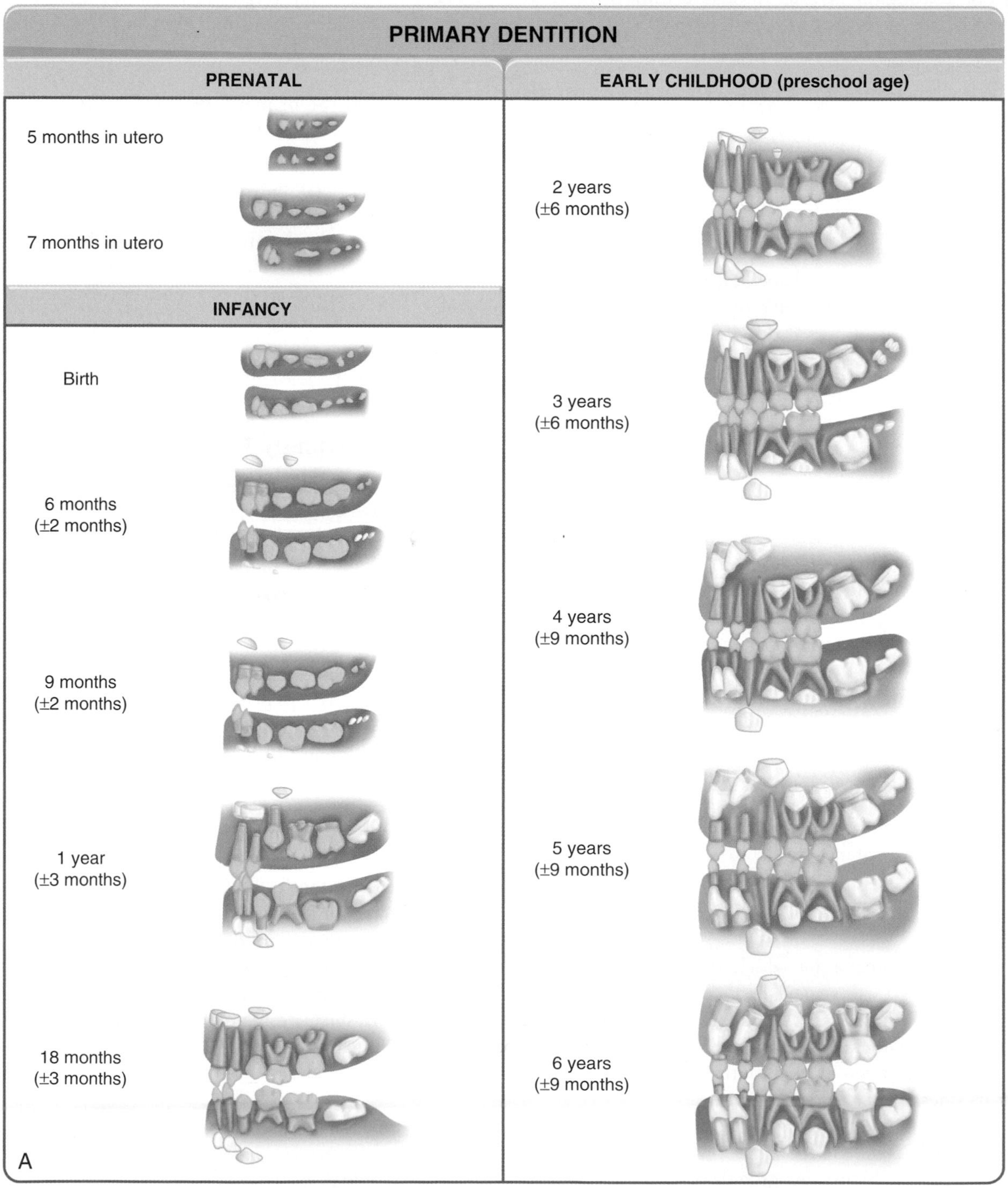

**FIG. 8.11** A, Chronologic order of eruption of the primary dentition.

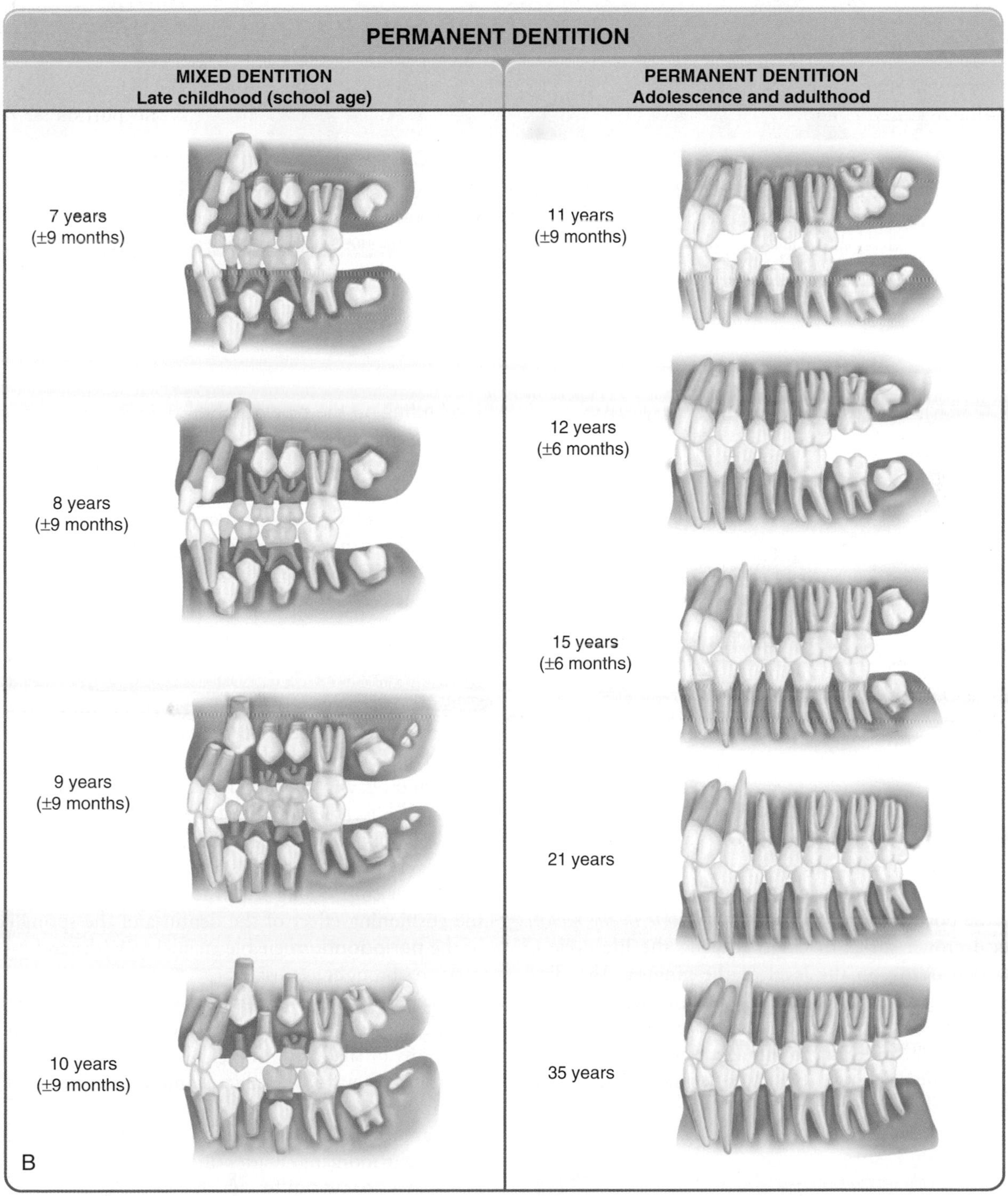


**FIG. 8.11, cont'd** B, Permanent dentition. *(© Elsevier Collection.)*

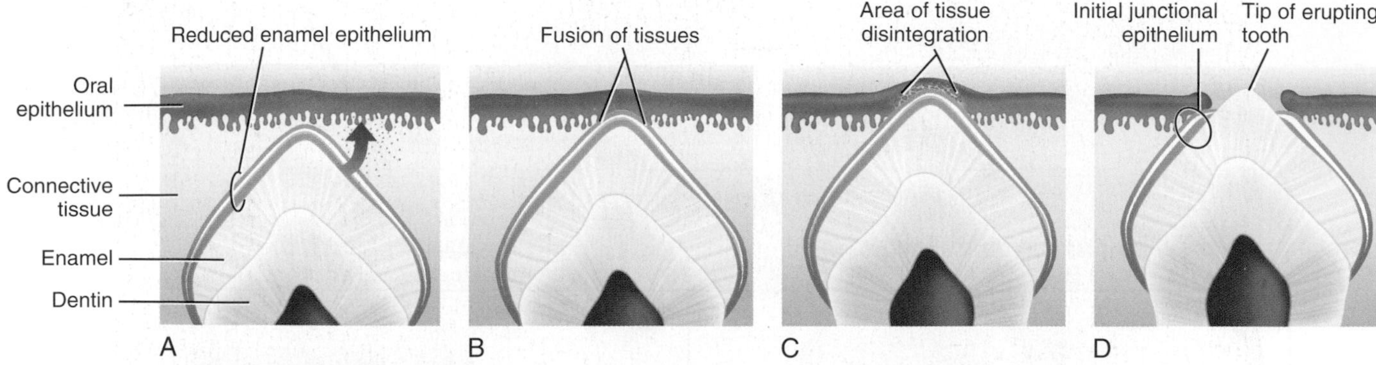


**FIG. 8.12** Stages in the process of tooth eruption. A, Oral cavity before the eruption process begins. Reduced enamel epithelium covers the newly formed enamel. B, Fusion of the reduced enamel epithelium with the oral epithelium. C, Disintegration of central fused tissue, leaving a tunnel for tooth movement. D, Coronal fused tissues peel back from the crown during eruption, leaving the initial junctional epithelium near the cementoenamel junction. *(© Elsevier Collection.)*

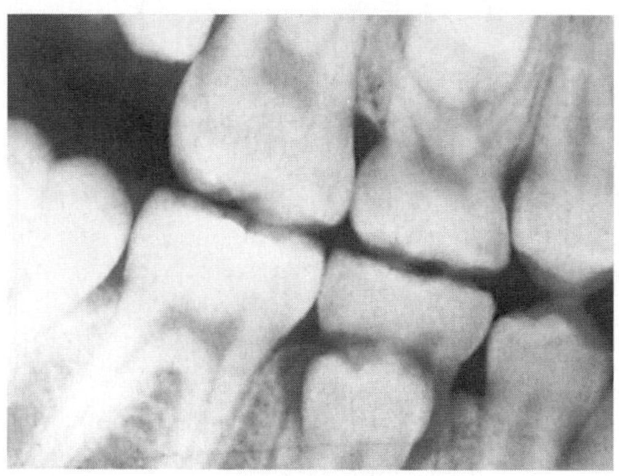

**FIG. 8.13** Radiograph shows normal resorption of the roots of a mandibular primary molar before it is shed.

that is *covered with enamel* (Fig. 8.16). The size of the anatomical crown remains constant throughout the life of the tooth, regardless of the position of the gingiva. The **clinical crown** is the portion of the tooth that is *visible in the mouth.* The clinical crown varies in length during the life cycle of the tooth depending on the level of the gingiva. The clinical crown is shorter as the tooth erupts into position, and it becomes longer as surrounding tissues recede. The phrase "long in the tooth," referring to old age, refers to the process by which the clinical crown becomes longer as the gingiva recedes around the tooth.

RECALL

**16** What is the difference between the anatomical crown and the clinical crown?

**17** Where is the CEJ?

## Root

The root of the tooth is that portion that is normally embedded in the alveolar process and is covered with cementum. Depending on the type of tooth, the root may have one, two, or three branches. *Bifurcation* means division into two roots. *Trifurcation* means division into three roots.

The tapered end of each root tip is known as the apex. Any structure or object that is situated at the apex is said to be *apical.* Anything that surrounds the apex is *periapical* (*peri-* means around, and *apical* refers to the apex).

## Enamel

Enamel, which makes up the anatomical crown of the tooth, is the hardest material in the body. This hardness is important because enamel forms the protective covering for the softer underlying dentin. It also provides a strong surface for crushing, grinding, and chewing food.

Enamel is able to withstand crushing stresses to about 100,000 pounds per square inch. Although enamel is strong, it is also very brittle, and this brittleness may cause the enamel to fracture or chip. Along with the strength of enamel, however, the cushioning effect of the dentin and the springlike action of the **periodontium** enable enamel to withstand most of the pressures brought against it.

Enamel is *translucent* (allows some light to pass through it) and ranges in color from yellow to grayish white. These variations in shade are caused by differences in the thickness and translucency of the enamel and in the color of the dentin beneath it.

Enamel, which is formed by ameloblasts, consists of 96 to 99 percent inorganic matter and only 1 to 4 percent organic matrix. **Hydroxyapatite**, which consists primarily of calcium, is the most abundant mineral component. Hydroxyapatite is the material that is lost in the process of dental decay (see Chapter 13).

Enamel is similar to bone in its hardness and mineral content. Different from bone, however, mature enamel does not contain cells that are capable of remodeling and repair. Nevertheless, some remineralization is possible (see Chapter 15).

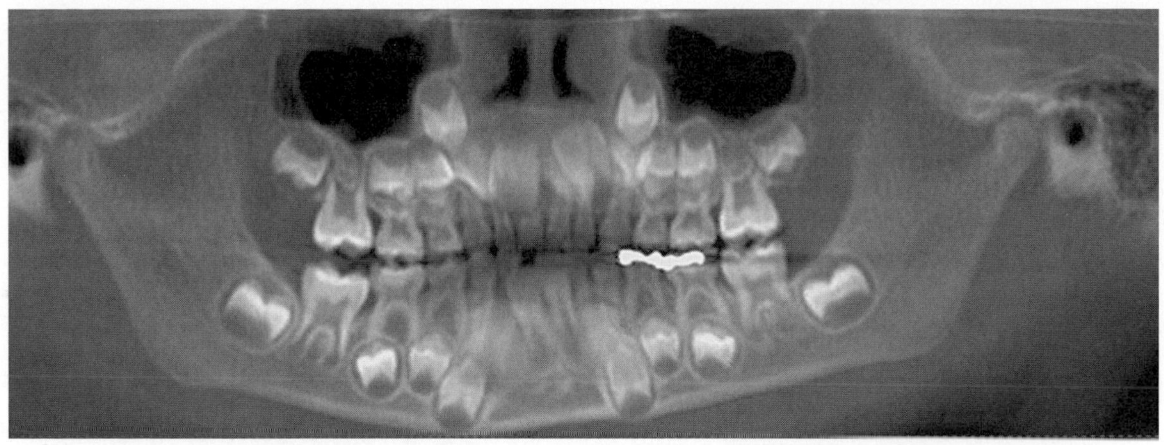

**FIG. 8.14** Panoramic image revealing mixed dentition of a 6-year-old child. *(Courtesy Carolina OMF Imaging, W. Bruce Howerton Jr, DDS, MS, Raleigh, NC.)*

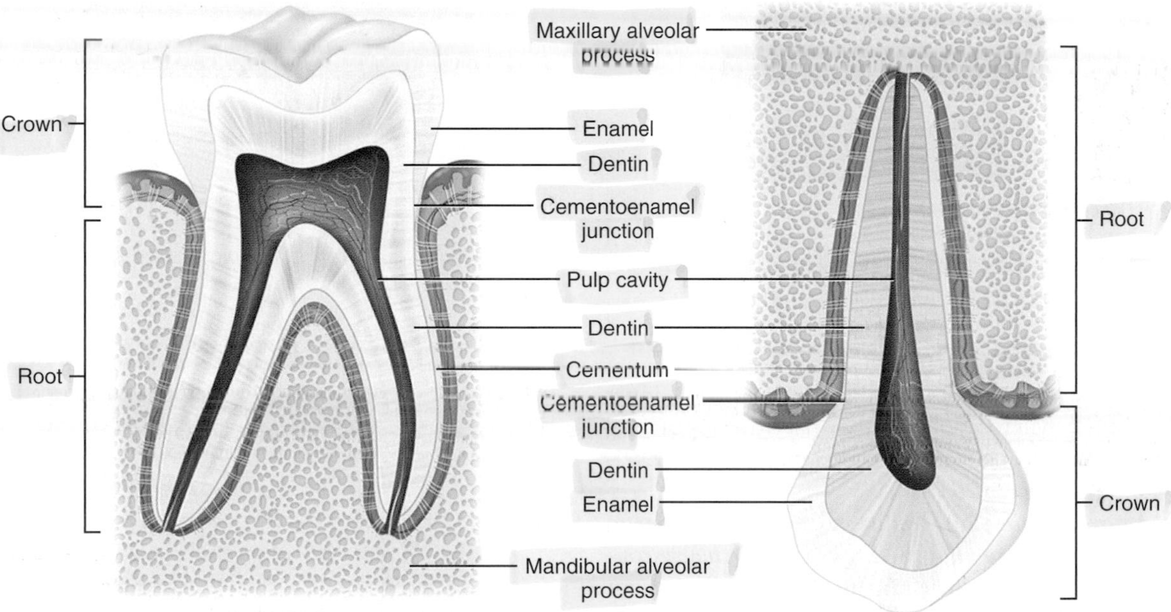


**FIG. 8.15** Anterior (top or front) tooth and posterior (bottom or back) tooth show the dental tissues. *(© Elsevier Collection.)*

Enamel is composed of millions of calcified enamel **prisms**, which are also known as *enamel rods.* These extend from the surface of the tooth to the DEJ. Enamel prisms tend to be grouped into rows and organized around the circumference of the long axis of the tooth. Prisms within each row follow a course that is generally perpendicular to the surface of the tooth. This organization into rows is clinically important because enamel tends to fracture along the interfacial planes of adjacent groups of prisms.

The diameter of a prism is approximately 5 to 8 microns, depending on its location (1 micron is equal to one millionth of a meter). In cross section, the prisms appear to be keyhole-shaped structures that consist of a head and a tail (Fig. 8.17). If a handful of straws were held together, the ends would resemble the structure of enamel rods.

Each prism appears to be encased in a *prism sheath,* and an *interprismatic substance,* also known as an *interrod substance,* holds the sheathed prisms together. Of all these hard structures, the prisms are hardest, and the interprismatic substance is weakest. These differences make it possible to "acid-etch" teeth for the direct bonding of restorative materials (see Chapter 43).

**Hunter-Schreger bands**, which microscopically appear as alternating light and dark bands in the enamel, are caused by enamel prisms that intertwine or change direction.

The **striae of Retzius**, also known as the *strips of Retzius,* are incremental rings, similar to growth rings of a tree that represent variations in the deposition of enamel matrix during formation of the tooth. Enamel produced prenatally contains only a few of these incremental lines; however, the shock of birth is registered as a ring known as the *neonatal* line.

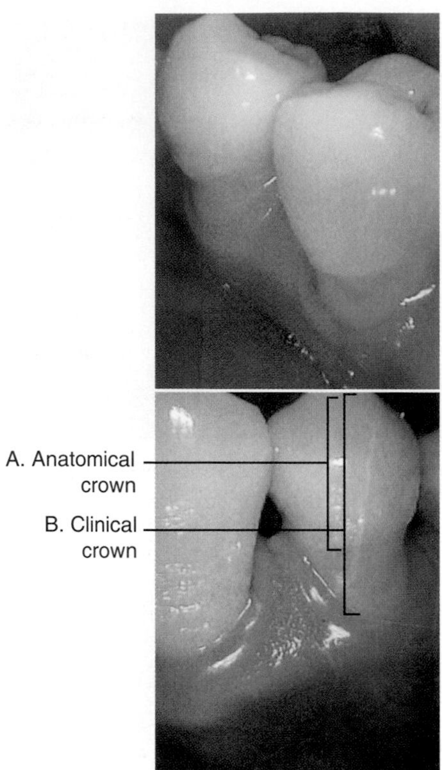


**FIG. 8.16** A, The anatomical crown is the portion of the tooth that is covered with enamel and remains the same. B, The clinical crown is the portion of the tooth that is visible in the mouth and may vary because of changes in the position of the gingiva.

**Enamel tufts** start at the DEJ and may extend to the inner third of the enamel. Microscopically, they have the appearance of tufts of grass. Enamel tufts are the hypocalcified or uncalcified ends of groups of enamel prisms.

**Enamel lamellae** are thin, leaflike structures that extend from the enamel surface toward the DEJ. These lamellae consist of organic material with little mineral content. (The singular form is *lamella.*)

**Enamel spindles** are the ends of odontoblasts (dentin-forming cells) that extend across the DEJ a short distance into the enamel.

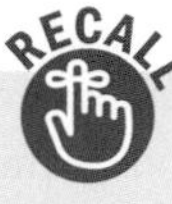


**18** What is the hardest substance in the human body?
**19** What is the most abundant mineral component of enamel?

## Dentin

Dentin, which makes up the main portion of the tooth structure, extends almost the entire length of the tooth. It is covered by enamel on the crown and by cementum on the root.

In the primary teeth, dentin is very light yellow. In the permanent teeth, it is light yellow and somewhat transparent. The color may darken with age.

Dentin is a mineralized tissue that is harder than bone and cementum but not as hard as enamel. Although hard, dentin has elastic properties that are important in the support of enamel, which is brittle.

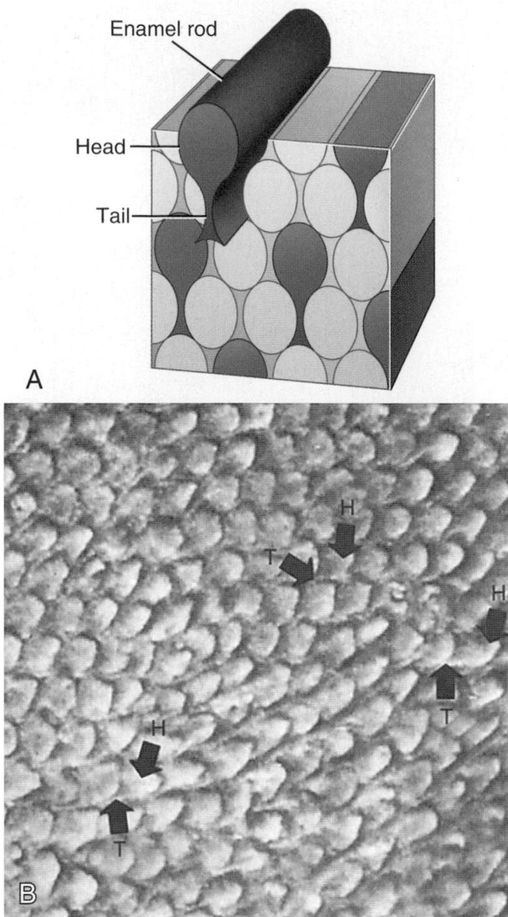


**FIG. 8.17** Enamel rod, the basic unit of enamel. A, Relationship of the rod to enamel. B, Scanning electron micrograph of enamel shows head *(H)* and tail *(T)*. *(A, © Elsevier Collection. B, From Fehrenbach MJ, Popowics T: Illustrated dental embryology, histology, and anatomy, ed 4, St Louis, 2016, Saunders.)*

Dentin is composed of 70 percent inorganic material and 30 percent organic matter and water. The rapid penetration and spreading of the caries in dentin are caused in part by its high content of organic substances.

Dentin is formed by the odontoblasts, beginning at growth centers along the DEJ and proceeding inward toward what will become the **pulp chamber** of the tooth. The internal surface of the dentin forms the walls of the pulp cavity. Odontoblasts line these walls, and from there, they continue to form and repair the dentin.

Dentin is penetrated through its entire thickness by microscopic canals called **dentinal tubules** (Fig. 8.18). Each dentinal tubule contains a **dentinal fiber**. These fibers, which terminate in a branching network at the junction with the enamel or cementum, transmit pain stimuli and make dentin an excellent thermal conductor.

Because of the presence of dentinal fibers within the dentin, it is considered to be a living tissue. During operative procedures, dentin must be protected from dehydration and thermal shock.

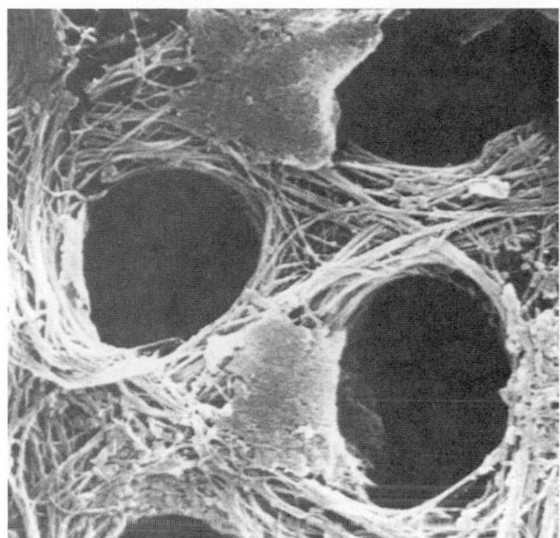

**FIG. 8.18** Scanning electron micrograph of dentinal tubules.

When 1 mm of dentin is exposed, about 30,000 dentinal fibers are exposed, and thus 30,000 living cells may be damaged.

Because it is capable of continued growth and repair, dentin is available in three major types:

1. **Primary dentin**, which is formed before eruption, forms the bulk of the tooth.
2. **Secondary dentin** begins formation after eruption; this continues at a very slow rate throughout the life of the tooth and results in gradual narrowing of the pulp chamber with age.
3. **Tertiary dentin**, also known as *reparative dentin*, is formed in response to irritation and appears as a localized deposit on the wall of the pulp chamber. This may occur in response to *attrition* (wearing away of tooth through normal use), erosion, dental caries, dental treatment, or other irritants.

RECALL

20 How does dentin transmit sensations of pain?
21 What are the three types of dentin?

## Cementum

Cementum is bonelike, rigid connective tissue that covers the root of the tooth. It overlies the dentin and joins the enamel at the CEJ. A primary function of cementum is to anchor the tooth to the bony socket with attachment fibers within the periodontium.

Cementum is light yellow and is easily distinguishable from enamel by its lack of luster and its darker hue. It is somewhat lighter in color than dentin.

Cementum, which is formed by cementoblasts, is not quite as hard as dentin or bone. In contrast to bone, cementum does not resorb and form again. This difference is important because it makes orthodontic treatment possible. However, cementum is capable of some repair through the deposition of new layers.

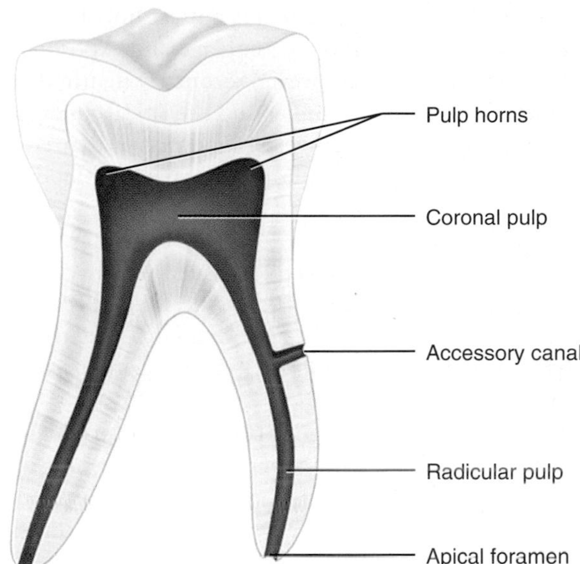


**FIG. 8.19** The dental pulp. *(© Elsevier Collection.)*

As the root develops, **primary cementum**, also known as *acellular cementum*, is formed outward from the cementodentinal junction for the full length of the root. After the tooth has reached functional occlusion, **secondary cementum**, also known as *cellular cementum*, continues to form on the apical half of the root.

As a result, the cervical half of the root is covered by a thin layer of primary cementum, and the apical half of the root has a covering of thickened cementum. This continued growth in the apical area helps maintain the total length of the tooth by compensating for enamel lost by attrition.

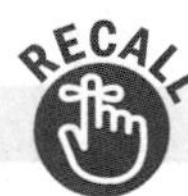

22 What are the two types of cementum?

## Pulp

The inner aspect of the dentin forms the boundaries of the pulp chamber (Fig. 8.19). As with the dentin surrounding it, the contours of the pulp chamber follow the contours of the exterior surface of the tooth.

At the time of eruption, the pulp chamber is large; however, as the result of continuous deposition of dentin, it becomes smaller with age.

The portion of the pulp that lies within the crown portion of the tooth is called the **coronal pulp**. This structure includes the *pulp horns,* which are extensions of the pulp that project toward the cusp tips and incisal edges.

The other portion of the pulp, which is more apically located, is referred to as the **radicular pulp**, or the *root pulp.* During development of the root, the continued deposition of dentin causes this area to become longer and narrower.

The radicular portion of the pulp in each root is continuous with the tissues of the periapical area via an **apical foramen**.

In young teeth, the apical foramen is not yet fully formed, and this opening is wide. With increasing age and exposure of the tooth to functional stress, however, secondary dentin decreases the diameter of the pulp chamber and the apical foramen.

Pulp is made up of blood vessels and nerves that enter the pulp chamber through the apical foramen. The blood supply is derived from branches of the dental arteries and from the periodontal ligament.

Pulp also contains connective tissue, which consists of cells, intercellular substance, and tissue fluid. **Fibroblasts**, one type of cell that is present in connective tissue, are responsible for the formation of the intercellular substance of the pulp.

The tissue fluid interchange between the pulp and the dentin serves the important function of keeping tissue supplied with moisture and nutrients. The rich blood supply also has an important defense function in response to bacterial invasion of the tooth.

The nerve supply of the pulp receives and transmits pain stimuli. When the stimulus is weak, the response of the pulpal system is weak, and the interaction goes unnoticed. When the stimulus is great, the reaction is stronger, and pain quickly calls attention to the threatened condition of the tooth.

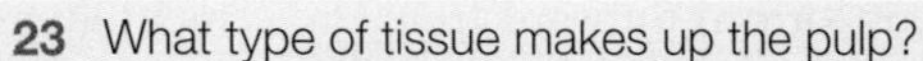
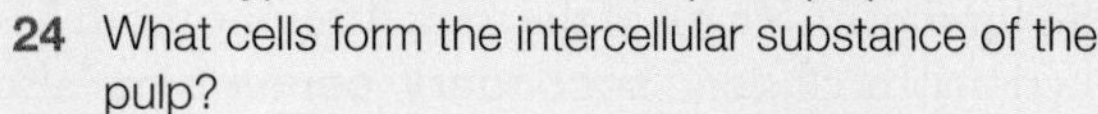

**23** What type of tissue makes up the pulp?
**24** What cells form the intercellular substance of the pulp?

## Periodontium

The periodontium, which supports the teeth within the alveolar bone, consists of *cementum, alveolar bone,* and the *periodontal ligaments.* These tissues also protect and nourish the teeth. The periodontium is divided into two major units: the attachment apparatus and the gingival unit.

### *Attachment Apparatus*

The attachment apparatus consists of the cementum (see earlier discussion), the alveolar process, and the periodontal ligaments (Fig. 8.20). These tissues work together to support, maintain, and retain the tooth in its functional position within the jaw.

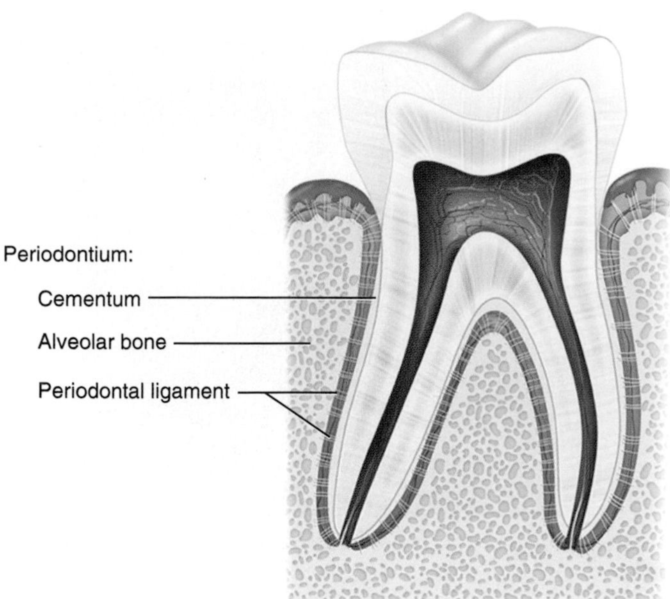


**FIG. 8.20** Periodontium of the tooth with its components identified. *(© Elsevier Collection.)*

**ALVEOLAR PROCESS.** Alveolar processes are extensions of bone from the body of the mandible and the maxilla, which support the teeth in their functional positions within the jaws (Fig. 8.21). Osteoblasts are responsible for the formation of this bone, and osteoclasts are responsible for resorption and remodeling of the bone.

The alveolar process develops in response to the growth of developing teeth. After teeth have been lost, bone from the alveolar process is resorbed, and the ridge decreases in size and changes in shape.

The **cortical plate** is the dense outer covering of the spongy bone that makes up the central part of the alveolar process. The cortical plate provides strength and protection and is the place where skeletal muscles attach. The cortical plate of the mandible is denser than that of the maxilla and has fewer openings for the passage of nerves and vessels. This structural difference affects the technique of injection for local anesthetic and extractions.

The **alveolar crest** is the highest point of the alveolar ridge. At this location, alveolar bone fuses with cortical plates on the facial and lingual sides of the crest of the alveolar process. In a healthy mouth, the distance between the CEJ and the alveolar crest is fairly constant (Fig. 8.22). Early periodontal disease results in flattening of the alveolar crest.

The **alveolar socket** is the cavity within the alveolar process that surrounds the root of a tooth. The tooth does not actually contact the bone at this point. Instead, it is suspended in place within the socket by the periodontal ligaments. The bony projection that separates one socket from another is called the *interdental septum.* The bone that separates the roots of a multirooted tooth is called the *interradicular septum.*

The **lamina dura**, also known as the *cribriform plate,* consists of thin, compact bone that lines the alveolar socket. The lamina dura is pierced by many small openings, which allow blood vessels and nerve fibers within the bone to communicate freely with those in the periodontal ligament. On a dental radiograph, the lamina dura appears as a thin white line around the root of the tooth (see Chapter 41).

**25** What are the functions of osteoblasts and osteoclasts?

**PERIODONTAL LIGAMENT.** The periodontal ligament is dense connective tissue organized into fiber groups that connects the cementum covering the root of the tooth with the alveolar bone of the socket wall. At one end, the fibers are embedded in cementum; at the other end, they are embedded

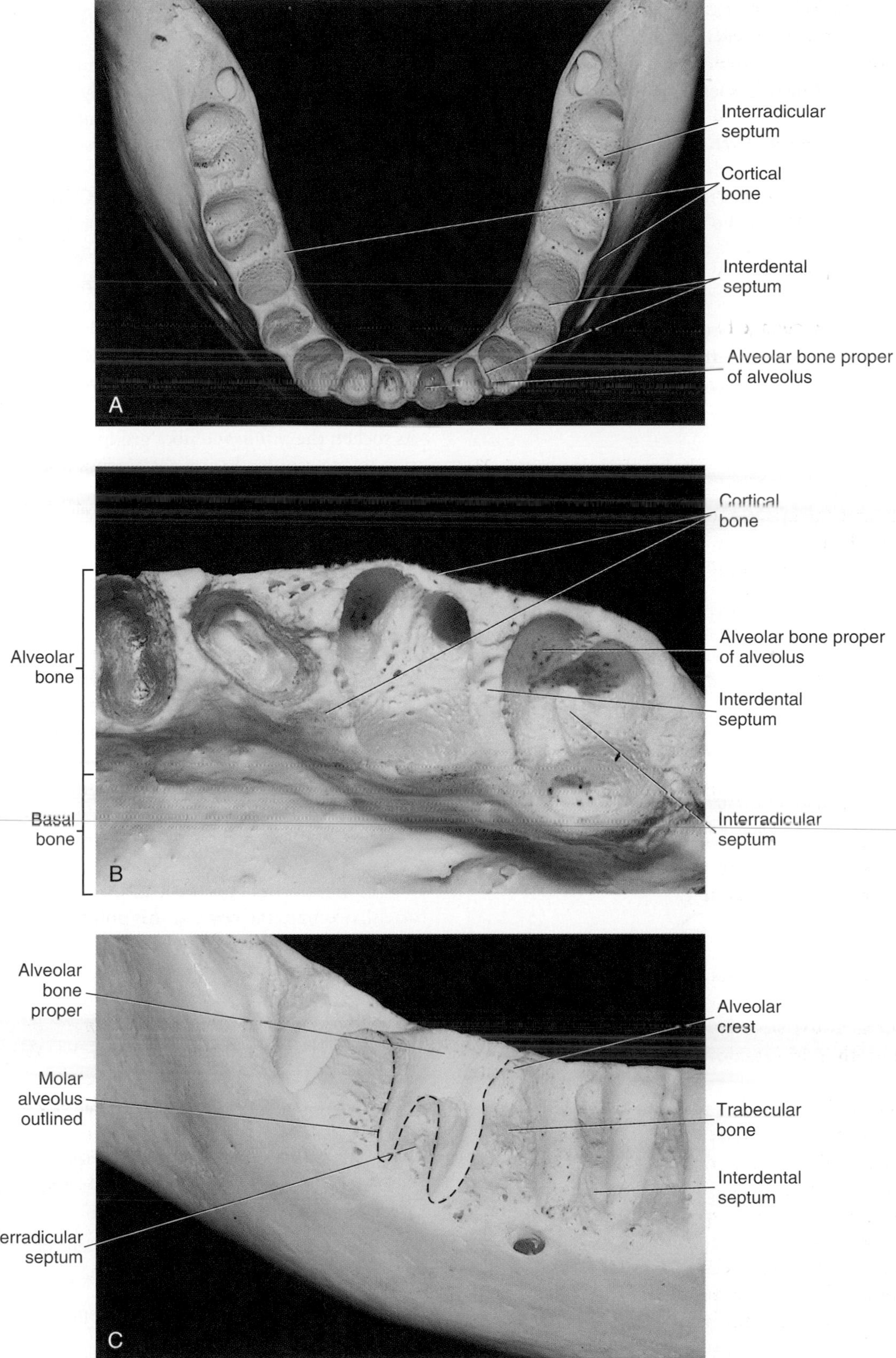


**FIG. 8.21** Anatomy of the alveolar bone. A, Mandibular arch of a skull with the teeth removed. B, Portion of the maxilla of a skull with the teeth removed. C, Cross section of the mandible with the teeth removed. *(From Fehrenbach MJ, Popowics T: Illustrated dental embryology, histology, and anatomy, ed 4, St Louis, 2016, Saunders.)*

in bone. These embedded portions become mineralized and are known as *Sharpey's fibers.*

The periodontal ligament ranges in width from 0.1 to 0.38 mm; the thinnest portion is noted around the middle third of the root. With age, the width of these ligaments tends to narrow.

**SUPPORTIVE AND PROTECTIVE FUNCTIONS.** Fiber groups are designed to support the tooth in its socket and to hold it firmly in normal relationship to surrounding soft and hard tissues. This arrangement allows the tooth to withstand the pressures and forces of mastication.

**SENSORY FUNCTION.** The nerve supply for the ligament comes from the nerves just before they enter the apical foramen. Also, nerve fibers in the surrounding alveolar bone provide the tooth with the protective "sense of touch." Note how it feels when you bite into food.

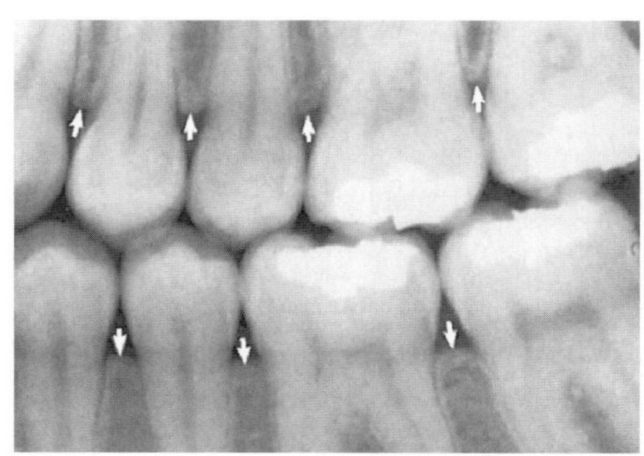

**FIG. 8.22** The alveolar crest as it appears on a radiograph. *(From Haring JI, Lind LJ: Radiographic interpretation for the dental hygienist, Philadelphia, 1993, Saunders.)*

Nerve fibers also act as the sensory receptors needed for proper positioning of the jaws during normal function.

**NUTRITIVE FUNCTION.** The ligaments receive their nutrition from the blood vessels that also supply the tooth and its alveolar bone. Blood vessels enter the dental pulp through the apical foramen and from the vessels that supply surrounding alveolar bone.

**FORMATIVE AND RESORPTIVE FUNCTIONS.** The fibroblasts of the periodontal ligament permit the continuous and rapid remodeling that is required for these fiber groups. Cementoblasts and **cementoclasts** (cementum-resorbing cells) are also involved in these remodeling functions, as are osteoblasts and osteoclasts.

**PERIODONTAL LIGAMENT FIBER GROUPS.** The periodontal ligament consists of three different types of fiber groups (Fig. 8.23). The *periodontal* fiber groups support the tooth in its socket; the *transseptal* fiber groups support the tooth in relation to adjacent teeth; and the *gingival* fiber groups support the gingiva that surrounds the tooth.

**PERIODONTAL FIBER GROUPS.** *Alveolar crest fibers* run from the crest of the alveolar bone to the cementum in the region of the CEJ. Their primary function is to retain the tooth in the socket and to oppose lateral forces.

*Horizontal fibers* course at right angles to the long axis of the tooth, from the cementum to the bone. Their primary function is to restrain lateral tooth movement.

*Oblique fibers* run in an upward direction, from cementum to bone. These fiber bundles, which are the most numerous fibers, constitute the main attachment of the tooth. Their primary function is to resist forces placed on the long axis of the tooth.

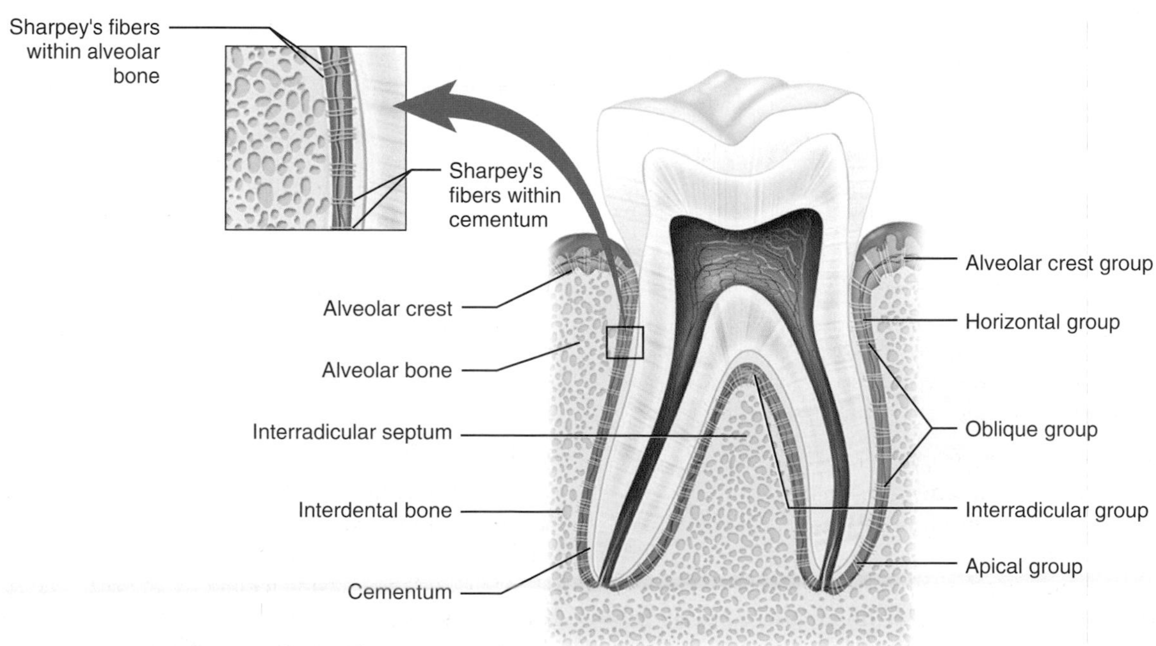


**FIG. 8.23** Periodontal fiber groups. *(© Elsevier Collection.)*

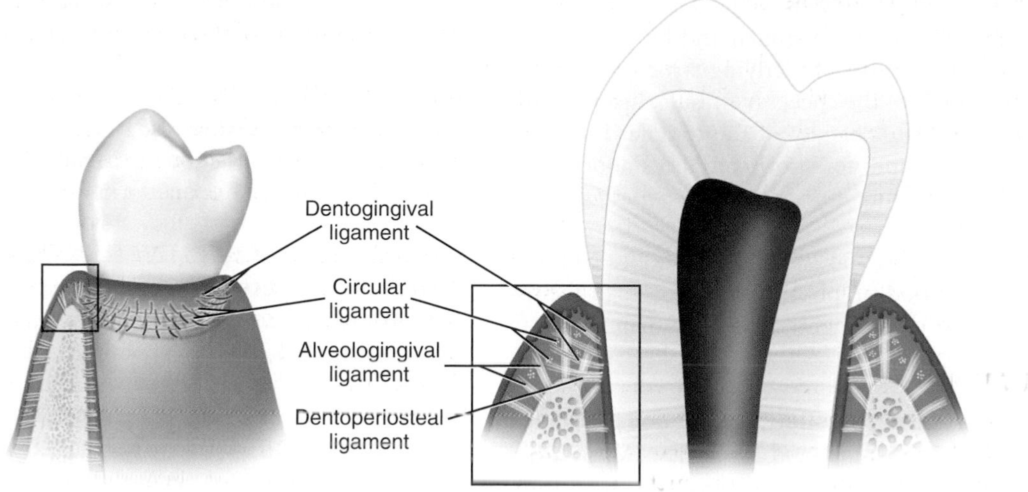


**FIG. 8.24** Some of the fiber subgroups of the gingival fiber group: circular, dentogingival, alveologingival, and dentoperiosteal ligaments. *(© Elsevier Collection.)*

*Apical fibers* radiate outward from the apical cementum and insert into the surrounding bone. Their primary functions are to (1) prevent the tooth from tipping; (2) resist luxation (twisting); and (3) protect blood, lymph, and nerve supplies.

*Interradicular fibers* are found only in multirooted teeth. They course from the cementum of the root and insert into the interradicular septum. Their primary function is to enhance resistance to tipping and twisting.

**TRANSSEPTAL FIBER GROUPS.** *Transseptal fibers,* also known as *interdental fibers,* are located interproximally above the crest of the alveolar bone between the teeth. These fibers originate in the cervical cementum of one tooth and insert into the cervical cementum of an adjacent tooth. Their primary function is to support the interproximal gingiva and to aid in securing the position of the adjacent tooth.

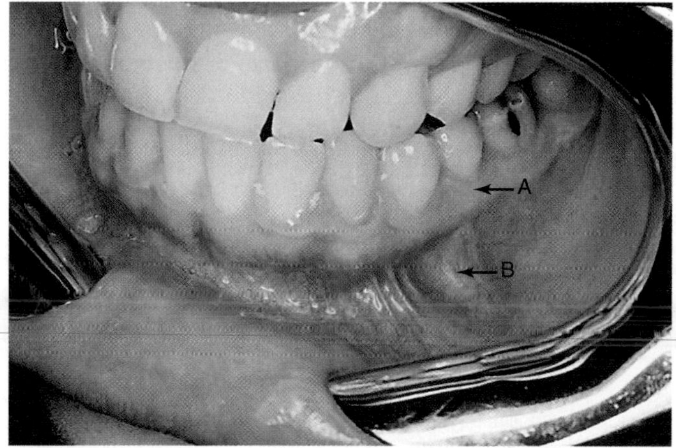


**FIG. 8.25** A, A dense masticatory type of mucosa makes up the gingiva. B, The delicate lining type of mucosa covers the vestibule.

**GINGIVAL FIBER GROUPS.** *Gingival fibers* are regarded as part of the periodontal ligaments, even though they do *not* support the tooth in relation to the jaws. They function to support marginal gingival tissues to maintain their relation to the tooth (Fig. 8.24). This function is similar to a sphincter-like "pulling of purse strings."

The gingival fibers are located in the *lamina propria* (connective tissues of the gingiva) and do *not* insert into the alveolar bone. Gingival fibers are divided into the following four groups:

1. *Dentogingival fibers* extend from the cervical cementum outward and upward into the lamina propria.
2. *Alveologingival fibers* extend upward from the alveolar crest into the lamina propria.
3. *Circular fibers* form a band around the neck of the tooth and are interlaced by other groups of fibers in the unattached gingiva.
4. *Dentoperiosteal fibers* extend facially and lingually from the cementum, pass over the crest of the alveolar bone, and insert into the periosteum of the alveolar process. Their primary function is to support the tooth and the gingiva.

**26** What are the functions of the periodontal ligaments?

**27** To which structures are the periodontal ligaments attached?

## Gingival Unit

*Oral mucosa* almost continuously lines the oral cavity. Oral mucosa is composed of **stratified squamous epithelium** that overlies connective tissue. The oral mucosa includes ducts of salivary glands in various regions of the oral cavity. Although oral mucosa is present throughout the mouth, different types of mucosal tissues are present in different regions of the mouth. The three main types of oral mucosa found in the oral cavity are lining, masticatory, and specialized mucosa (Fig. 8.25).

**LINING MUCOSA.** **Lining mucosa** is noted for its softer texture, moist surface, and ability to stretch and be compressed, thereby acting as a cushion for underlying structures. Lining mucosa covers the inside of the cheeks, vestibule, lips, soft palate, and ventral surface (underside) of the tongue. Run your tongue over these areas, and note how soft and smooth these tissues are. Beneath the lining mucosa is the *submucosa,* which contains blood vessels and nerves.

Because lining mucosa is not attached to bone, it moves freely. The abundant blood supply and the thinness of the tissue give the lining mucosa a brighter red color than is seen in the masticatory mucosa.

**MASTICATORY MUCOSA.** **Masticatory mucosa** is noted for its rubbery surface texture and resiliency. Masticatory mucosa includes the attached gingiva, hard palate, and dorsum (upper surface) of the tongue (see Chapter 10).

Masticatory mucosa is light pink and is *keratinized,* which means that it has a tough, protective outer layer. Lining mucosa lacks this protective layer.

Submucosa is present beneath the masticatory mucosa. The masticatory mucosa is firmly affixed to the bone and does not move. Run your tongue across the roof of your mouth and compare the texture of the mucosa on your palate with that on the inside of your cheeks. This tissue is a dense covering that is designed to withstand the vigorous activity of chewing and swallowing food.

**SPECIALIZED MUCOSA.** On the top surface, or *dorsal* surface, of the tongue, both masticatory mucosa and **specialized mucosa** are present in the form of lingual papillae. These *papillae* are associated with sensations of taste (see Chapter 10).

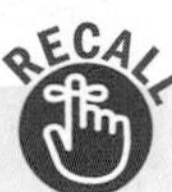


**28** List the three types of oral mucosa, and provide an example of each.

## ■ Legal and Ethical Implications

The most critical time of development occurs during the embryonic period, because this is when the major organs are forming. Frequently, a woman is not yet aware that she is pregnant. Therefore a woman should always be concerned about good nutrition and a healthy lifestyle, in case she might be pregnant.

As a healthcare professional, do you think that you have an ethical responsibility to provide pregnant patients with information about dental development? ■

## ■ Eye to the Future

Medical technology has made it possible to detect fetal abnormalities at an early stage in a child's development. This has opened a new frontier of medicine: treating sick babies before they are born. Infants with various disorders have been saved from severe illness, retardation, and even death. Until recently, the only point of access to the fetus has been through the placenta. A new technique can correct some deficiencies with an injection into the amniotic fluid that allows the fetus to swallow the medication. Guided by computers and ultrasound images and using sensitive instruments, physicians can now give blood transfusions to babies while they are still in the uterus. In other cases, physicians can drain excess fluid from the baby's brain and can successfully perform fetal surgery. ■

## ■ Critical Thinking

1. A 9-year-old child arrives at your office for an emergency appointment. He was in a bicycle accident and chipped his two front teeth. The child's mother asks you if you think the chip in the teeth will eventually repair itself. How would you explain the situation to her?
2. Leanne Morris is a patient in your office. As you begin to update her health history, Leanne is very excited and tells you that she is pregnant. She asks you questions regarding the development of her baby's teeth. What information would the dentist want to provide?
3. Karen Kelleher made an appointment for her young son Willy because his primary tooth was loose, and she thought the dentist might need to remove it. When they arrived for the appointment, the tooth was no longer loose. Mrs. Kelleher was embarrassed and insisted that it had been loose earlier in the week. What would you say to her? ■

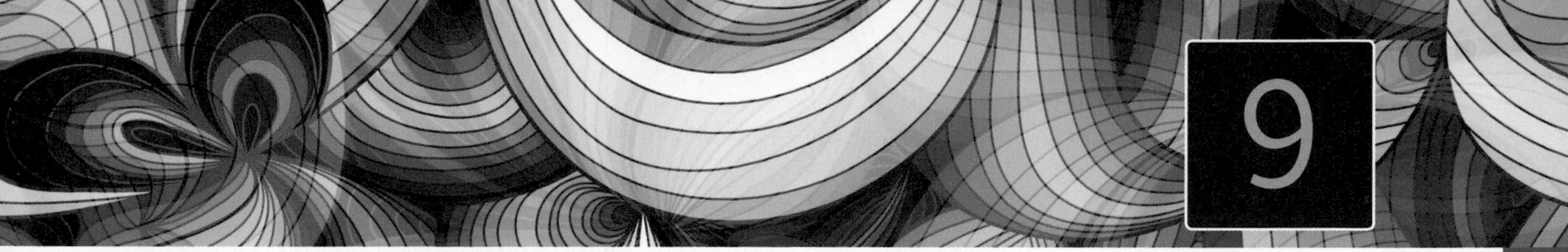

9

# Head and Neck Anatomy

## KEY TERMS

**Alveolar process** Portion of the maxillary bones that forms the support for teeth of the maxillary arch.

**Articular (ahr-TIK-yoo-luer) disc** Cushion of dense, specialized connective tissue that divides the articular space into upper and lower compartments; also known as the *meniscus.*

**Articular eminence** Raised portion of the temporal bone just anterior to the glenoid fossa.

**Articular space** Space between the capsular ligament and between the surfaces of the glenoid fossa and the condyle.

**Buccal (BUK-ul)** Region of the head that refers to structures closest to the inner cheek.

**Circumvallate lingual papillae (sir-kum-VAL-ayt LING-gwul puh-PIL-ee)** Large tissue projections on the tongue.

**Condyloid process** The posterior process of each ramus; articulates with a fossa in the temporal bones to form the temporomandibular joint; also known as the *mandibular condyle.*

**Coronal suture** Line of articulation between the frontal bone and parietal bones.

**Cranium (KRAY-nee-um)** Eight bones that cover and protect the brain.

**External auditory meatus** Bony passage of the outer ear.

**Foramen** A small round opening in a bone through which blood vessels, nerves, and ligaments pass; plural, *foramina.*

**Foramen magnum** Large opening in the occipital bone that connects the vertical canal and the cranial cavity.

**Fossa (FOS-ah, FAW-suh)** Hollow, grooved, or depressed area in a bone.

**Frontal** Region of the head pertaining to the forehead.

**Frontal process** Process of the zygomatic bone that extends upward to articulate with the frontal bone at the outer edge of the orbit.

**Glenoid fossa** Area of the temporal bone where condyles of the mandible articulate with the skull.

**Greater palatine (PA-luh-tine) nerve** Nerve that serves the posterior hard palate and the posterior lingual gingiva.

**Hamulus** A hook-shaped process.

**Infraorbital (in-fruh-OR-bi-tul)** Region of the head below the orbital region.

**Lacrimal (LAK-ri-mul) bones** Paired facial bones that help form the medial wall of the orbit.

**Lambdoid suture** Line of junction between the occipital and parietal bones.

**Lateral pterygoid plate** Point of origin for internal and external pterygoid muscles.

**Lymphadenopathy (lim-fad-uh-NOP-uh-thee)** Disease or swelling of the lymph nodes.

**Masseter (muh-SEE-tur)** The strongest and most obvious muscle of mastication.

**Mastoid process** Projection on the temporal bone located behind the ear.

**Maxillary tuberosity** Large, rounded area on the outer surface of the maxillary bones in the area of the posterior teeth.

**Meatus** The external opening of a canal.

**Medial pterygoid plate** Plate that ends in the hook-shaped hamulus.

**Mental** Region of the head pertaining to or located near the chin.

**Mental protuberance** Part of the mandible that forms the chin.

**Nasal** Region of the head that pertains to or is located near the nose.

**Nasal conchae** Projecting structures found in each lateral wall of the nasal cavity and extending inward from the maxilla; singular, *concha.*

**Occipital (ok-SIP-i-tul)** Region of the head overlying the occipital bone and covered by the scalp.

**Oral** Region of the head pertaining to or located near the mouth.

**Orbital** Region of the head pertaining to or located around the eye.

**Ossicles** The bones of the middle ear.

**Parietal (puh-RYE-e-tul)** Pertaining to the walls of a body cavity.

**Parotid (puh-ROT-id) duct** Duct associated with the parotid salivary gland, which opens into the oral cavity at the parotid papilla.

**Process** A prominence or projection on a bone.

**Pterygoid process** Process of the sphenoid bone, consisting of two plates.

**Sagittal suture** Suture that is located at the midline of the skull, where the two parietal bones are joined.

**Sphenoid sinuses** Sinuses that are located in the sphenoid bone.

**Sternocleidomastoid (stur-noe-klye-doe-MAS-toid)** Major cervical muscle.

**Styloid process** Process that extends from the undersurface of the temporal bone.

**Symphysis menti (SIM-fi-sis MEN-tee)** The separation of the mandible at the chin that occurs at birth.

**Temporal** Region of the head superior to the zygomatic arch.

**Temporal process** Process that articulates with the zygomatic process of the temporal bone to form the zygomatic arch, which creates the prominence of the cheek.

**Temporomandibular (tem-puh-roe-man-DIB-yoo-lur) joint (TMJ)** Joint on each side of head that allows movement of the mandible.

**Trapezius (truh-PEE-zee-us)** Major cervical muscle.

**Trigeminal nerve** The nerve that is the primary source of innervation for the oral cavity.

**Zygomatic** Region of the head pertaining to or located near the zygomatic bone (cheekbone).

**Zygomatic arch** The arch formed when the temporal process of the zygomatic bone articulates with the zygomatic process of the temporal bone.

**Zygomatic process** The process of the maxillary bones that extends upward to articulate with the zygomatic bone.

## LEARNING OUTCOMES

*On completion of this chapter, the student will be able to achieve the following objectives:*

1. Pronounce, define, and spell the key terms.
2. Identify the regions of the head.

3 Locate and identify the bones of the skull, including the following:
- Name and locate the bones of the cranium, the face, and the hyoid bone.
- Discuss the postnatal development of the skull.
- Differentiate between the male and female skull.

4 Discuss the temporomandibular joints, including the following:
- Identify the components of the temporomandibular joint.
- Describe the action and movement of the temporomandibular joint.
- Describe the symptoms of temporomandibular joint disorders.

5 Locate and identify the muscles of the head and neck.

6 Identify the locations of minor and major salivary glands and associated ducts, and name the three large paired salivary glands.

7 Identify and trace the routes of the blood vessels of the head and neck.

8 Identify and locate the nerves of the head and neck, including the following:
- Name the twelve cranial nerves.
- Name the maxillary and mandibular divisions of the trigeminal nerve.

9 Discuss the importance of lymph nodes, including the following:
- Explain the structure and function of lymph nodes.
- Identify the locations of the lymph nodes of the head and neck.
- Identify the locations of major lymph node sites of the body.

10 Identify the paranasal sinuses and explain their function.

## ELECTRONIC RESOURCES

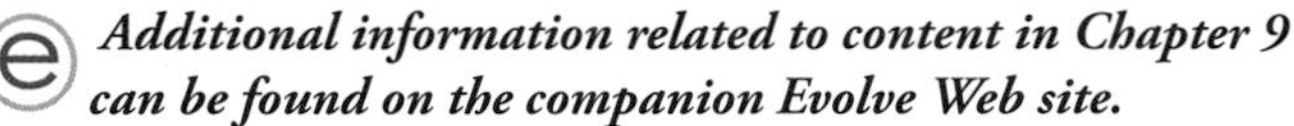


***Additional information related to content in Chapter 9 can be found on the companion Evolve Web site.***

- Practice Quiz

In this chapter, you will learn the anatomical basis for the clinical practice of dental assisting. You will learn the names and locations of bones of the skull and face, facial nerves, lymph nodes, and salivary glands. You will identify muscles of the head and neck, including the facial muscles, which create facial expressions and help to open and close the mouth and swallow food.

You will find that knowledge of anatomical landmarks is a necessity as you begin to mount radiographs.

## Regions of the Head

The head can be divided into eleven regions: **frontal**, **parietal**, **occipital**, **temporal**, **orbital**, **nasal**, **infraorbital**, **zygomatic**, **buccal**, **oral**, and **mental**. As you continue this chapter, you will encounter references to these regions of the head (Fig. 9.1).

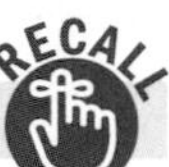


1 What are the eleven regions of the head?

## Bones of the Skull

The human skull is divided into two sections: the cranium and the face. The **cranium** is composed of eight bones that cover and protect the brain; the face consists of fourteen bones (Table 9.1). Specific anatomical terms are used to describe landmarks on these bones (Table 9.2).

## Bones of the Cranium

The cranial bones are the single frontal, occipital, sphenoid, and ethmoid bones and the paired parietal and temporal bones.

### *Parietal Bones*

The two parietal bones form most of the roof and upper sides of the cranium. The two parietal bones are joined at the **sagittal suture** at the midline of the skull. The line of articulation between the frontal bone and the parietal bones is called the **coronal suture** (Fig. 9.2). In a newborn, the anterior *fontanelle* is the soft spot where the sutures between the frontal and parietal bones have not yet closed. This spot disappears as the child grows and the sutures close.

### *Frontal Bone*

The frontal bone forms the forehead, part of the floor of the cranium, and most of the roof of the orbits. (The *orbit* is the bony cavity that protects the eye.) The frontal bone contains the two *frontal sinuses,* with one located above each eye (Fig. 9.3).

### *Occipital Bone*

The occipital bone forms the back and base of the cranium (Fig. 9.4). It joins the parietal bones at the **lambdoid suture**. The spinal cord passes through the **foramen magnum** of the occipital bone.

### *Temporal Bones*

Paired temporal bones form the sides and base of the cranium (see Fig. 9.2). Each temporal bone encloses an ear and contains the **external auditory meatus**, which is the bony passage of the outer ear.

The **mastoid process** is a projection on the temporal bone located just behind the ear. The mastoid process is composed of air spaces that communicate with the middle ear cavity.

The lower portion of each temporal bone bears the **glenoid fossa** for articulation with the mandible. The **styloid process** extends from the undersurface of the temporal bone.

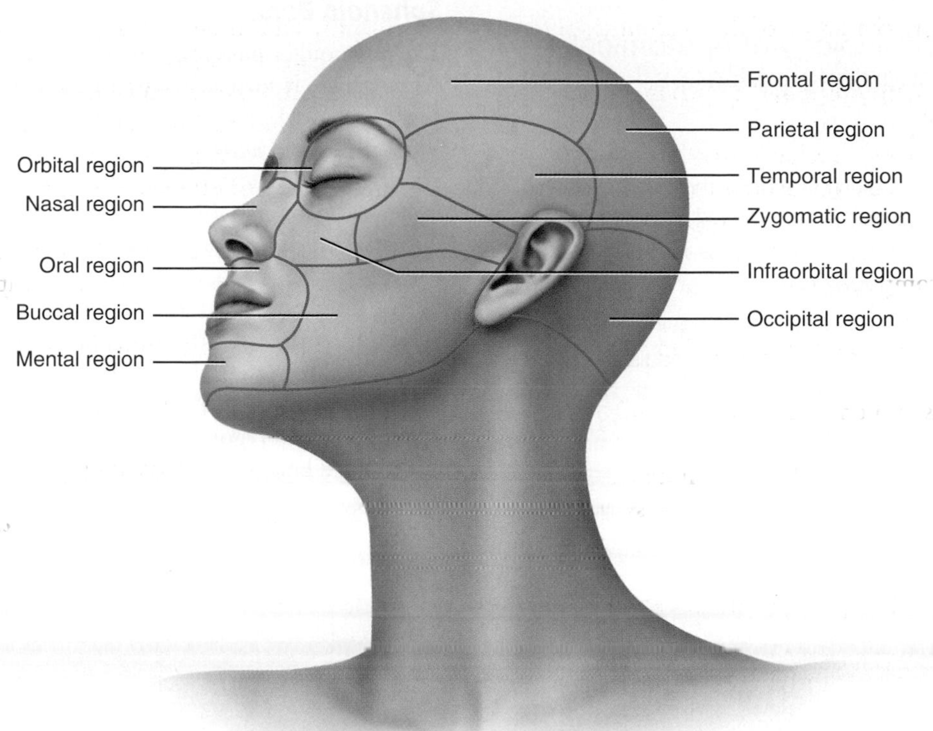


**FIG. 9.1** Regions of the head: frontal, parietal, occipital, temporal, orbital, nasal, infraorbital, zygomatic, buccal, oral, and mental. *(© Elsevier Collection.)*

**TABLE 9.1** Bones of the Skull

| Bone | Number | Location |
|---|---|---|
| **Eight Bones of the Cranium** | | |
| Frontal | 1 | Forms the forehead, most of the orbital roof, and the anterior cranial floor |
| Parietal | 2 | Form most of the roof and upper sides of the cranium |
| Occipital | 1 | Forms the back and base of the cranium |
| Temporal | 2 | Form the sides and base of the cranium |
| Sphenoid | 1 | Forms part of the anterior base of the skull and part of the walls of the orbit |
| Ethmoid | 1 | Forms part of the orbit and the floor of the cranium |
| **Fourteen Bones of the Face** | | |
| Zygomatic | 2 | Form the prominence of the cheeks and part of the orbit |
| Maxillary | 2 | Form the upper jaw |
| Palatine | 2 | Form the posterior part of the hard palate and the floor of the nose |
| Nasal | 2 | Form the bridge of the nose |
| Lacrimal | 2 | Form part of the orbit at the inner angle of the eye |
| Vomer | 1 | Forms the base for the nasal septum |
| Inferior conchae | 2 | Form part of the interior of the nose |
| Mandible | 1 | Forms the lower jaw |
| **Six Auditory Ossicles** | | |
| Malleus, incus, stapes | 6 | Bones of the middle ear |

**TABLE 9.2** Terminology of Anatomical Landmarks of Bones

| Term | Definition |
|---|---|
| Foramen | A natural opening in a bone through which blood vessels, nerves, and ligaments pass |
| Fossa | A hollow, grooved, or depressed area in a bone |
| Meatus | The external opening of a canal |
| **Process** | A prominence or projection on a bone |
| Suture | The jagged line where bones articulate and form a joint that does not move |
| Symphysis | The site where bones come together to form a cartilaginous joint |
| Tubercle | A small, rough projection on a bone |
| Tuberosity | A large, rounded process on a bone |

### Sphenoid Bone

The sphenoid bone is made up of a body and paired greater and lesser wings. It forms the anterior part of the base of the skull (see Fig. 9.2).

Each *greater wing* articulates with the temporal bone on either side and anteriorly with the frontal and zygomatic bones to form part of the orbit. Each *lesser wing* articulates with the ethmoid and frontal bones and also forms part of the orbit.

The **sphenoid sinuses** are located in the sphenoid bone just posterior to the eye. The **pterygoid process**, which extends downward from the sphenoid bone, consists of two plates. The **lateral pterygoid plate** is the point of origin for the internal and external pterygoid muscles. The **medial pterygoid plate** ends in the hook-shaped **hamulus** (Fig. 9.5), which is visible on some dental radiographs.

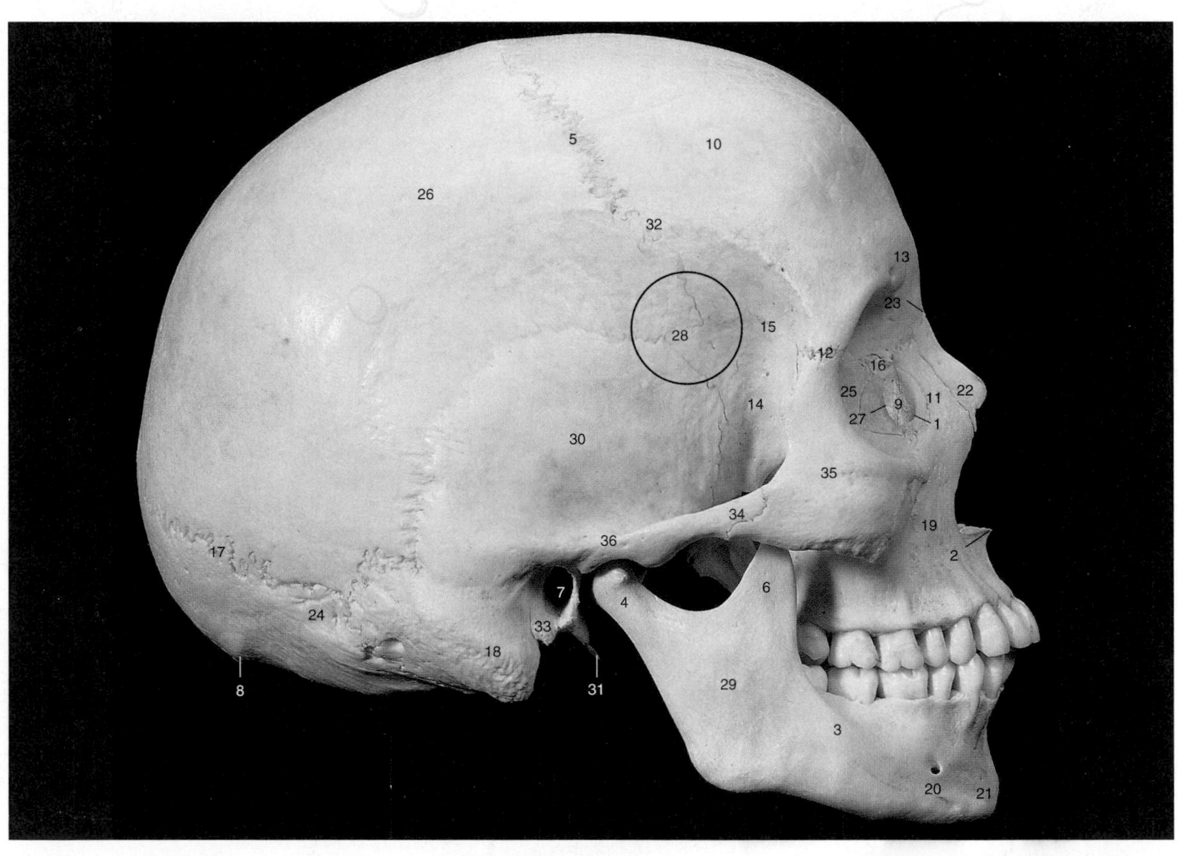


*1,* Anterior lacrimal crest
*2,* Anterior nasal spine
*3,* Body of mandible
*4,* Condyle of mandible
*5,* Coronal suture
*6,* Coronoid process of mandible
*7,* External acoustic meatus of temporal bone
*8,* External occipital protuberance (inion)
*9,* Fossa for lacrimal sac
*10,* Frontal bone
*11,* Frontal process of maxilla
*12,* Frontozygomatic suture
*13,* Glabella
*14,* Greater wing of sphenoid bone
*15,* Inferior temporal line
*16,* Lacrimal bone
*17,* Lambdoid suture
*18,* Mastoid process of temporal bone
*19,* Maxilla
*20,* Mental foramen
*21,* Mental protuberance
*22,* Nasal bone
*23,* Nasion
*24,* Occipital bone
*25,* Orbital part of ethmoid bone
*26,* Parietal bone
*27,* Posterior lacrimal crest
*28,* Pterion (encircled)
*29,* Ramus of mandible
*30,* Squamous part of temporal bone
*31,* Styloid process of temporal bone
*32,* Superior temporal line
*33,* Tympanic part of temporal bone
*34,* Zygomatic arch
*35,* Zygomatic bone
*36,* Zygomatic process of temporal bone

**FIG. 9.2** Lateral view of the skull. *(From Abrahams PH, Spratt JD, Loukas M, et al: McMinn and Abrahams' color atlas of human anatomy, ed 7, St Louis, 2014, Mosby.)*

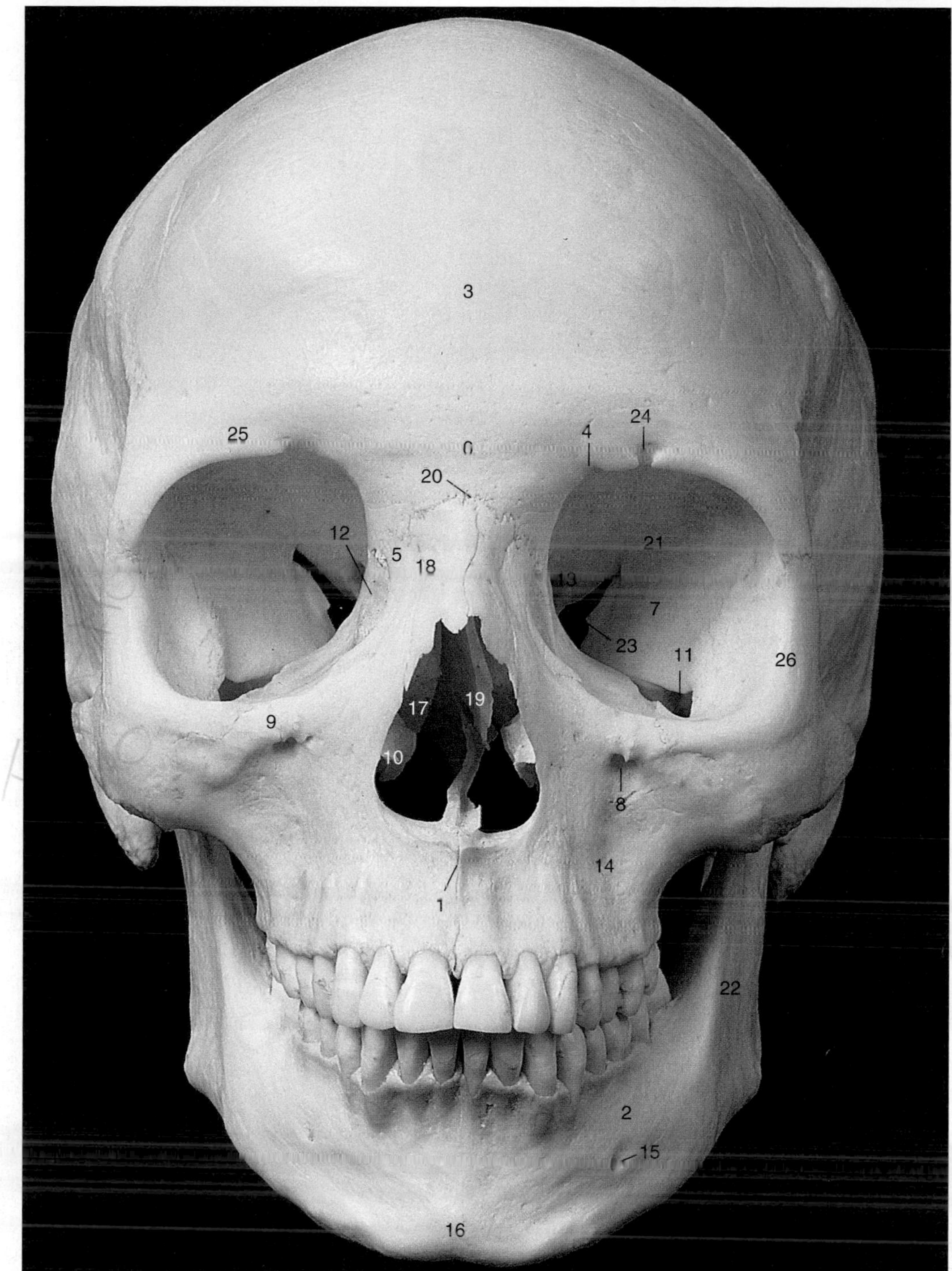


*1,* Anterior nasal spine
*2,* Body of mandible
*3,* Frontal bone
*4,* Frontal notch
*5,* Frontal process of maxilla
*6,* Glabella
*7,* Greater wing of sphenoid bone
*8,* Infraorbital foramen
*9,* Infraorbital margin
*10,* Inferior nasal concha
*11,* Inferior orbital fissure
*12,* Lacrimal bone
*13,* Lesser wing of sphenoid bone
*14,* Maxilla
*15,* Mental foramen
*16,* Mental protuberance
*17,* Middle nasal concha
*18,* Nasal bone
*19,* Nasal septum
*20,* Nasion
*21,* Orbit (orbital cavity)
*22,* Ramus of mandible
*23,* Superior orbital fissure
*24,* Supraorbital foramen
*25,* Supraorbital margin
*26,* Zygomatic bone

**FIG. 9.3** Frontal view of the skull. *(From Abrahams PH, Spratt JD, Loukas M, et al: McMinn and Abrahams' color atlas of human anatomy, ed 7, St Louis, 2014, Mosby.)*

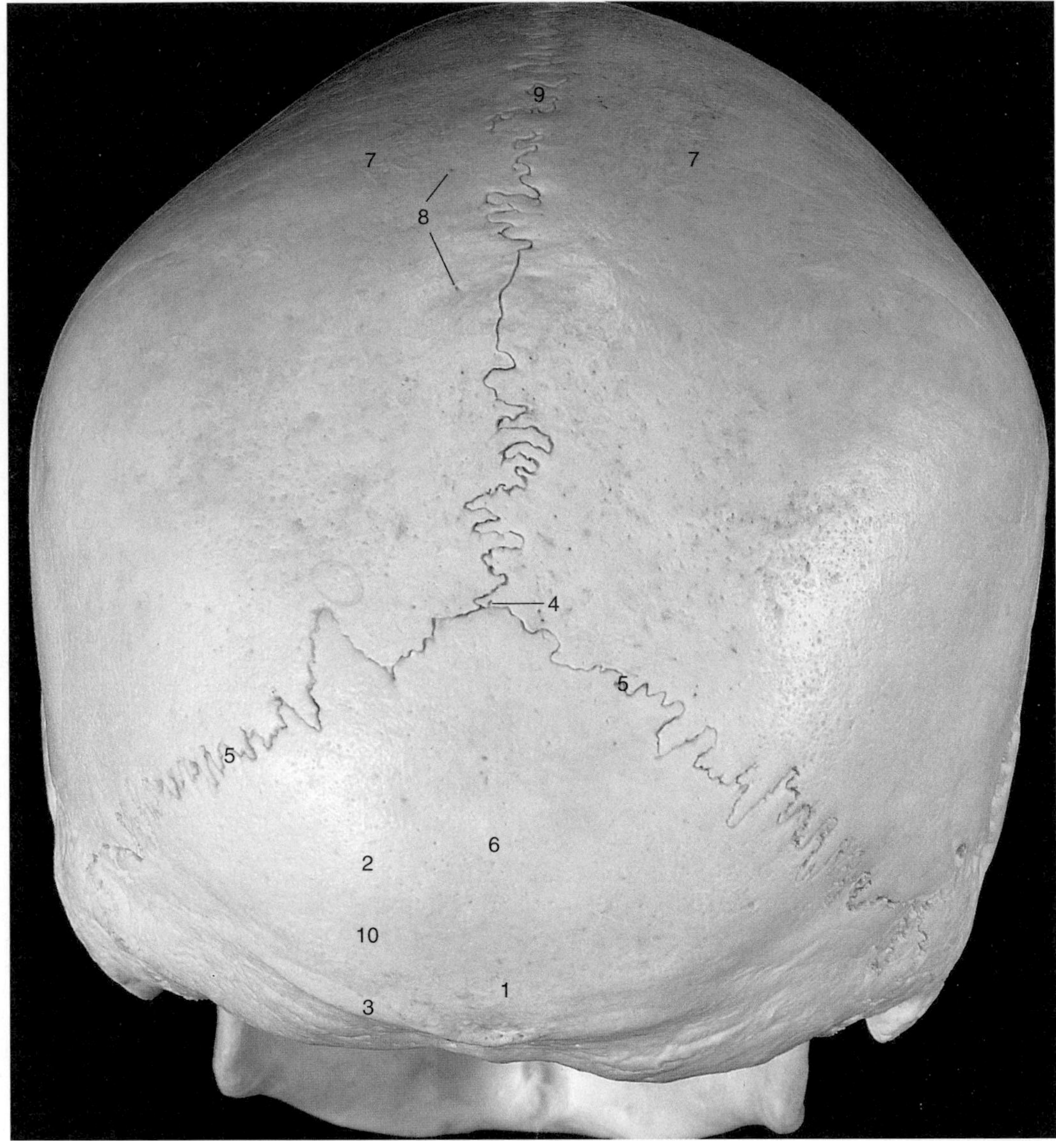


*1*, External occipital protuberance (inion)
*2*, Highest nuchal line
*3*, Inferior nuchal line
*4*, Lambda
*5*, Lambdoid suture
*6*, Occipital bone
*7*, Parietal bone
*8*, Parietal foramen
*9*, Sagittal suture
*10*, Superior nuchal line

**FIG. 9.4** Posterior view of the skull. *(From Abrahams PH, Spratt JD, Loukas M, et al: McMinn and Abrahams' color atlas of human anatomy, ed 7, St Louis, 2014, Mosby.)*

### *Ethmoid Bone*

The ethmoid bone forms part of the floor of the cranium, the orbit, and the nasal cavity. This complex bone contains honeycomb-like spaces and the *ethmoid sinuses.* The *medial concha* and *superior concha,* which are scroll-like structures, extend from the ethmoid bone.

### *Auditory Ossicles*

The six auditory **ossicles** are the bones of the middle ear. Each ear contains one *malleus, incus,* and *stapes.*

RECALL

**2** What bone forms the forehead?
**3** What bone forms the back and base of the cranium?

## Bones of the Face

From an anterior view of the skull, the bones one sees are the lacrimal bone, nasal bone, vomer, nasal conchae, zygomatic bone, maxilla, and mandible (Fig. 9.6).

### *Zygomatic Bones*

The two zygomatic bones, also known as the *malar bones,* form the prominence of the cheek and the lateral wall and floor of the orbit. The **frontal process** of the zygomatic bone extends upward to articulate with the frontal bone at the outer edge of the orbit (see Fig. 9.3).

The zygomatic bones rest on the maxillary bones, and each articulates with the right or left zygomatic process.

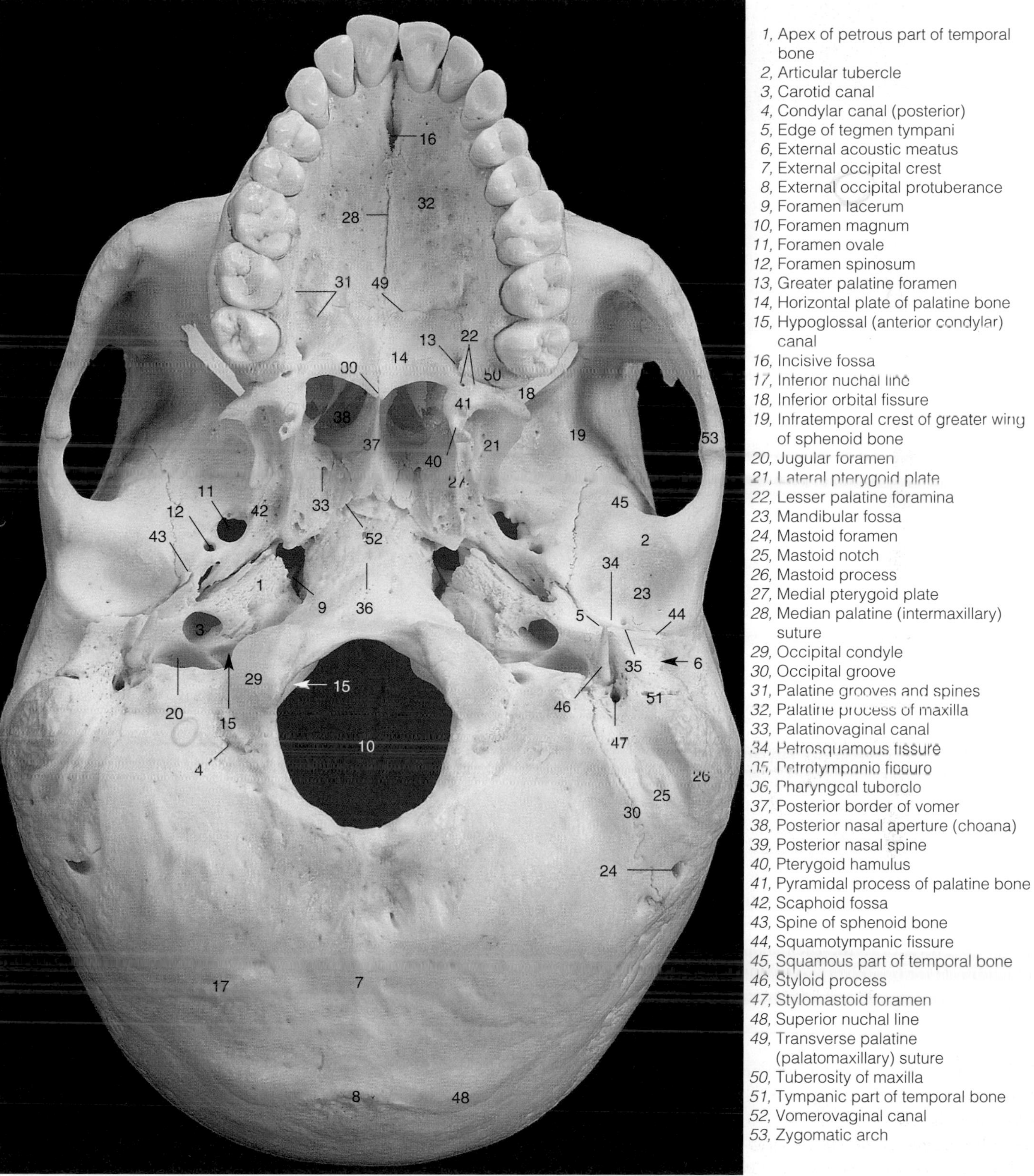

*1,* Apex of petrous part of temporal bone
*2,* Articular tubercle
*3,* Carotid canal
*4,* Condylar canal (posterior)
*5,* Edge of tegmen tympani
*6,* External acoustic meatus
*7,* External occipital crest
*8,* External occipital protuberance
*9,* Foramen lacerum
*10,* Foramen magnum
*11,* Foramen ovale
*12,* Foramen spinosum
*13,* Greater palatine foramen
*14,* Horizontal plate of palatine bone
*15,* Hypoglossal (anterior condylar) canal
*16,* Incisive fossa
*17,* Inferior nuchal line
*18,* Inferior orbital fissure
*19,* Infratemporal crest of greater wing of sphenoid bone
*20,* Jugular foramen
*21,* Lateral pterygoid plate
*22,* Lesser palatine foramina
*23,* Mandibular fossa
*24,* Mastoid foramen
*25,* Mastoid notch
*26,* Mastoid process
*27,* Medial pterygoid plate
*28,* Median palatine (intermaxillary) suture
*29,* Occipital condyle
*30,* Occipital groove
*31,* Palatine grooves and spines
*32,* Palatine process of maxilla
*33,* Palatinovaginal canal
*34,* Petrosquamous fissure
*35,* Petrotympanic fissure
*36,* Pharyngeal tubercle
*37,* Posterior border of vomer
*38,* Posterior nasal aperture (choana)
*39,* Posterior nasal spine
*40,* Pterygoid hamulus
*41,* Pyramidal process of palatine bone
*42,* Scaphoid fossa
*43,* Spine of sphenoid bone
*44,* Squamotympanic fissure
*45,* Squamous part of temporal bone
*46,* Styloid process
*47,* Stylomastoid foramen
*48,* Superior nuchal line
*49,* Transverse palatine (palatomaxillary) suture
*50,* Tuberosity of maxilla
*51,* Tympanic part of temporal bone
*52,* Vomerovaginal canal
*53,* Zygomatic arch

**FIG. 9.5** View of external base of the skull. *(From Abrahams PH, Spratt JD, Loukas M, et al: McMinn and Abrahams' color atlas of human anatomy, ed 7, St Louis, 2014, Mosby.)*

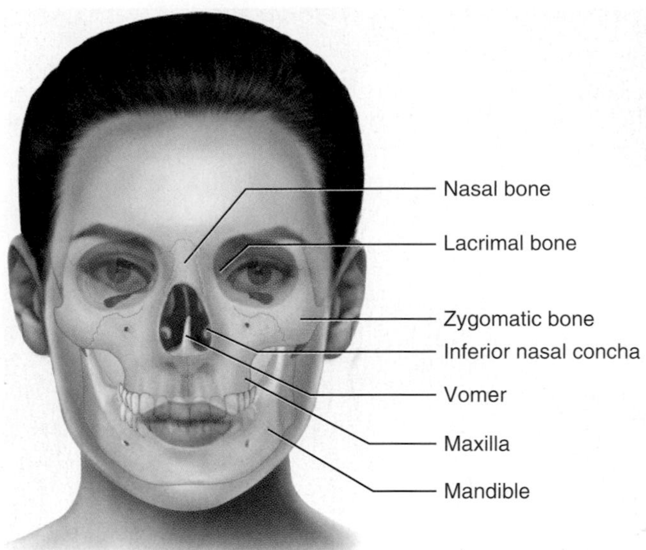


**FIG. 9.6** Anterior view of the facial bones and overlying facial tissue. *(© Elsevier Collection.)*

The **temporal process** of the zygomatic bone articulates with the zygomatic process of the temporal bone to form the **zygomatic arch**, which creates the prominence of the cheek. The zygomatic bones are useful in identifying maxillary radiographs.

### Maxillary Bones

The two maxillary bones, also known as the *maxillae* (singular, *maxilla*), form the upper jaw and part of the hard palate. The maxillary bones are joined together at the midline by the *maxillary suture.* The **zygomatic process** of the maxillary bones extends upward to articulate with the zygomatic bone.

The maxillary bones contain the *maxillary sinuses.* The **alveolar process** of the maxillary bones forms the support for the teeth of the maxillary arch. The **maxillary tuberosity** is a larger, rounded area on the outer surface of the maxillary bones in the area of the posterior teeth. The maxillary tuberosity is also a useful landmark for mounting maxillary radiographs.

### Palatine Bones

The two palatine bones are not strictly considered facial bones but are discussed here for ease of learning. Each palatine bone consists of two plates: the horizontal and vertical plates (Fig. 9.7).

The *horizontal plates* of the palatine bones form the posterior part of the hard palate of the mouth and the floor of the nose. The *vertical plates* form part of the lateral walls of the nasal cavity. Anteriorly, they articulate (join) with the maxillary bone.

### Nasal Bones

The two nasal bones form the bridge of the nose. Superiorly, they articulate with the frontal bone and make up a small portion of the nasal septum (see Fig. 9.3).

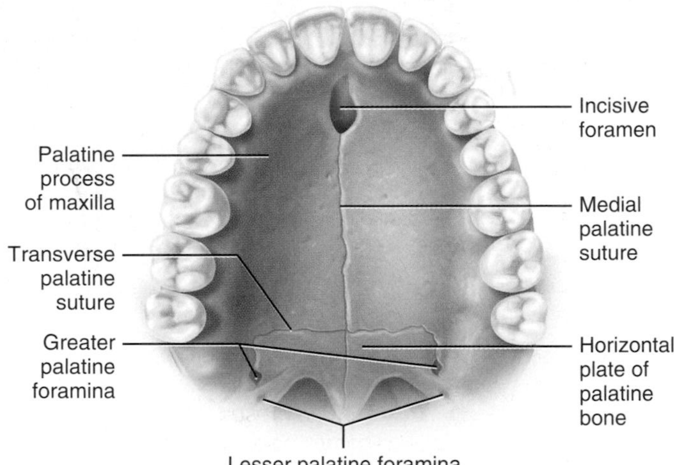


**FIG. 9.7** Bones and landmarks of the hard palate. *(© Elsevier Collection.)*

### Lacrimal Bones

The two **lacrimal bones** make up part of the orbit at the inner angle of the eye. These small, thin bones lie directly behind the frontal processes of the maxillary bones (see Fig. 9.3).

### Vomer

The vomer is a single, flat bone that forms the base for the nasal septum (see Fig. 9.6).

### Nasal Conchae

Each lateral wall of the nasal cavity consists of three projecting structures that extend inward from the maxilla, called the nasal conchae (singular, *concha*). Each concha extends scroll-like into the nasal cavity. The superior, middle, and inferior **nasal conchae** are formed from the ethmoid bone (see Fig. 9.6).

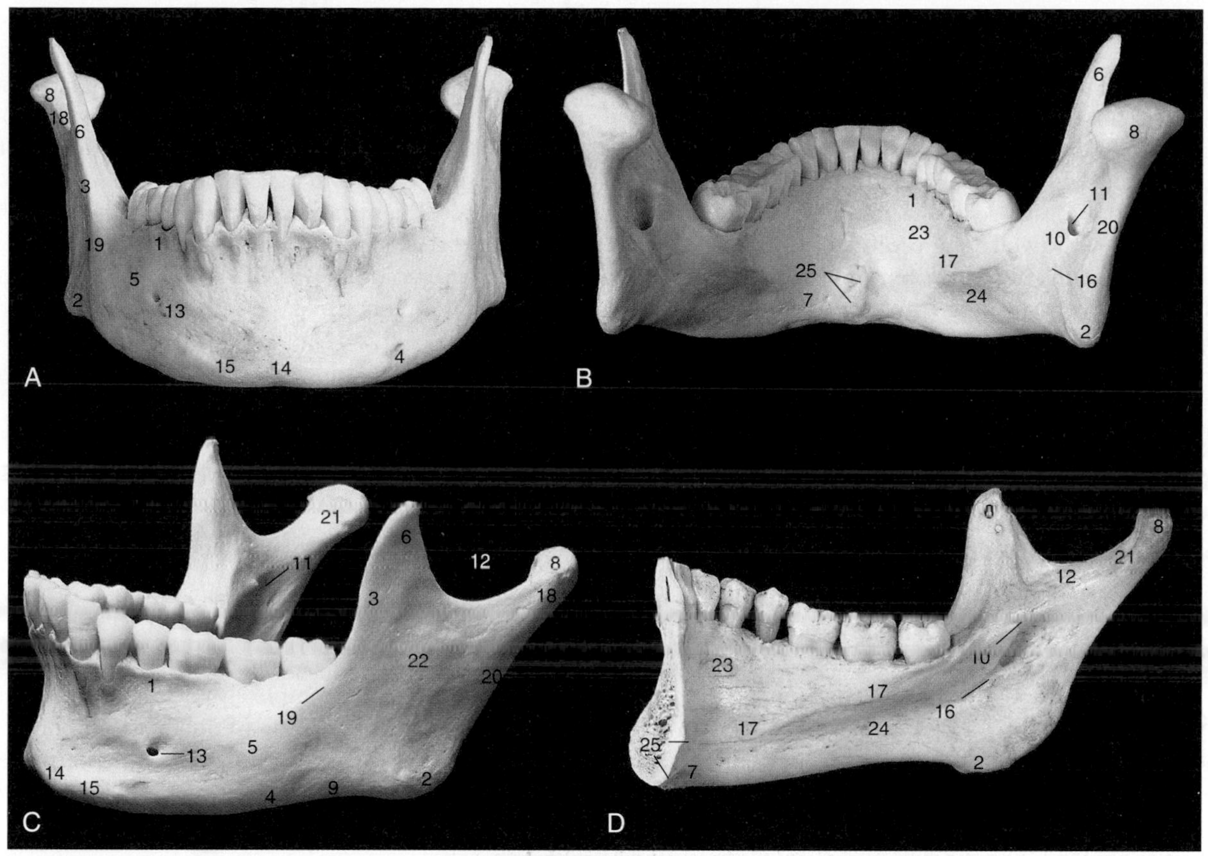


*1*, Alveolar part
*2*, Angle
*3*, Anterior border of ramus
*4*, Base
*5*, Body
*6*, Coronoid process
*7*, Digastric fossa
*8*, Head
*9*, Inferior border of ramus
*10*, Lingula
*11*, Mandibular foramen
*12*, Mandibular notch
*13*, Mental foramen
*14*, Mental protuberance
*15*, Mental tubercle
*16*, Mylohyoid groove
*17*, Mylohyoid line
*18*, Neck
*19*, Oblique line
*20*, Posterior border of ramus
*21*, Pterygoid fovea
*22*, Ramus
*23*, Sublingual fossa
*24*, Submandibular fossa
*25*, Superior and inferior mental spines (genial tubercles)

**FIG. 9.8** The mandible. A, From the front. B, From behind and above. C, From the left and front. D, Internal view from the left. *(From Malamed S: Handbook of local anesthesia, ed 6, St Louis, 2013, Mosby. Data from Abrahams PH, Spratt JD, Loukas M, et al: McMinn and Abrahams' color atlas of human anatomy, ed 7, St Louis, 2014, Mosby.)*

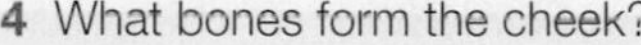
**4** What bones form the cheek?

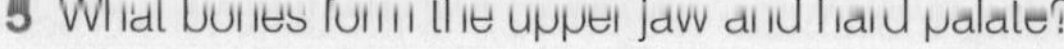
**5** What bones form the upper jaw and hard palate?

## Mandible

The mandible forms the lower jaw and is the movable bone of the skull. The alveolar process of the mandible supports the teeth of the mandibular arch (Fig. 9.8).

The U-shaped mandible, which is the strongest and longest bone of the face, develops prenatally as two parts; in early childhood, however, it ossifies (hardens) into a single bone. This symphysis is located at the midline and forms the **mental protuberance**, commonly known as the *chin.*

A mental **foramen** is located on the facial surface on the left and right between the apices of the first and second mandibular premolars. Other structures include the following:

- *Genial tubercles*—small, rounded and raised areas on the inner (medial) surface of the mandible near the symphysis
- *Mylohyoid ridge*—on the lingual surface of the body of the mandible
- *Angle of the mandible*—area where the mandible meets the ramus
- *Mandibular notch*—on the border of the mandible just anterior to the angle of the mandible
- *Ramus*—the upright portion at each end of the mandible
- *Coronoid process*—the anterior portion of each ramus
- *Condyloid process*—the posterior process of each ramus; articulates with a **fossa** in the temporal bones to form the temporomandibular joint; also known as the *mandibular condyle*
- *Sigmoid notch*—structure separating the coronoid and condyloid processes
- *Mandibular foramen*—on the lingual surface of each ramus
- *Oblique ridge*—on the facial surface of the mandible near the base of the ramus
- *Retromolar area*—portion of the mandible directly posterior to the last molar on each side

## Hyoid Bone

The hyoid bone is unique because it does not articulate with any other bone. Instead, the hyoid is suspended between the mandible and the larynx, where it functions as a primary support for the tongue and other muscles.

The hyoid bone is shaped like a horseshoe and consists of a central body with two lateral projections. Externally, its position is noted in the neck between the mandible and the larynx. The hyoid is suspended from the styloid process of the temporal bone by two *stylohyoid ligaments.*

6 What is the only movable bone in the skull?
7 Where is the mental foramen located?

## Postnatal Development

At birth, the cranial vault is large, and the cranial base and face are small. The face lacks vertical dimension because the teeth have not yet erupted (Figs. 9.9 and 9.10).

### *Fusion of Bones*

Several bones of the skull have not fused as single bones at the time of birth. For example, the frontal bone is separated by an interfrontal suture, and various components of the temporal, occipital, sphenoid, and ethmoid will fuse during infancy and early childhood.

### *Development of the Facial Bones*

**MANDIBLE.** At birth, the mandible is present in two halves separated by the **symphysis menti**. During the first year of life, the symphysis menti fuses; later, the condylar process lengthens. The chin (mental protuberance) reaches full development after puberty. Males have more pronounced development of the chin than do females.

**MAXILLA.** At birth, the maxilla is entirely filled with developing tooth buds (see Chapter 11). Vertical growth of the upper face is caused largely by dentoalveolar development and formation of the maxillary sinuses.

## Differences between Male and Female Skulls

Generally speaking, female skulls tend to be smaller and lighter and to have thinner walls. The female forehead usually retains a rounded anterior contour, and the teeth are smaller, with rounded incisal edges. Male skulls are larger and heavier and have more rugged muscle markings and prominences. Male teeth are larger and are squared incisally, and the forehead is flatter as a result of developing frontal sinuses, which are larger in men.

8 What is the difference between the teeth of males and females?

## Temporomandibular Joints

The **temporomandibular joint (TMJ)** is a joint on each side of the head that allows movement of the mandible for speech and *mastication* (chewing). The TMJ receives its name from the two bones that enter into its formation: the *temporal bone* and the *mandible.* The mandible is attached to the cranium by the ligaments of the TMJ. The mandible is held in position by the muscles of mastication (Fig. 9.11). The TMJ is made up of the following three bony parts:

1. The glenoid fossa, which is lined with fibrous connective tissue, is an oval depression in the temporal bone just anterior to the external auditory **meatus**.
2. The **articular eminence** is a raised portion of the temporal bone just anterior to the glenoid fossa.
3. The **condyloid process** of the mandible lies in the glenoid fossa.

## Capsular Ligament

A fibrous joint capsule completely encloses the TMJ. This capsule wraps around the margin of the temporal bone's articular eminence and articular fossa superiorly. Inferiorly, the capsule wraps around the circumference of the mandibular condyle, including the condylar neck.

## Articular Space

The **articular space** is the area between the capsular ligament and the surfaces of the glenoid fossa and condyle.

The **articular disc**, also known as the *meniscus,* is a cushion of dense, specialized connective tissue that divides the articular space into upper and lower compartments. These compartments are filled with *synovial fluid,* which helps lubricate the joint and fills the synovial cavities.

## Jaw Movement

The TMJ performs two basic types of movement: (1) a hinge action and (2) a gliding movement (Fig. 9.12). With these two types of movement, the jaws can open and close and shift from side to side.

### *Hinge Action*

The hinge action is the first phase in mouth opening; only the lower compartment of the joint is used. During hinge action, the condylar head rotates around a point on the undersurface of the articular disc, and the body of the mandible drops almost passively downward and backward.

The jaw is opened through combined actions of the external pterygoid, digastric, mylohyoid, and geniohyoid muscles. The jaw is closed by the actions of the temporal, masseter, and internal pterygoid muscles.

### *Gliding Movement*

Gliding movement allows the lower jaw to move forward or backward. It involves both the lower and upper compartments

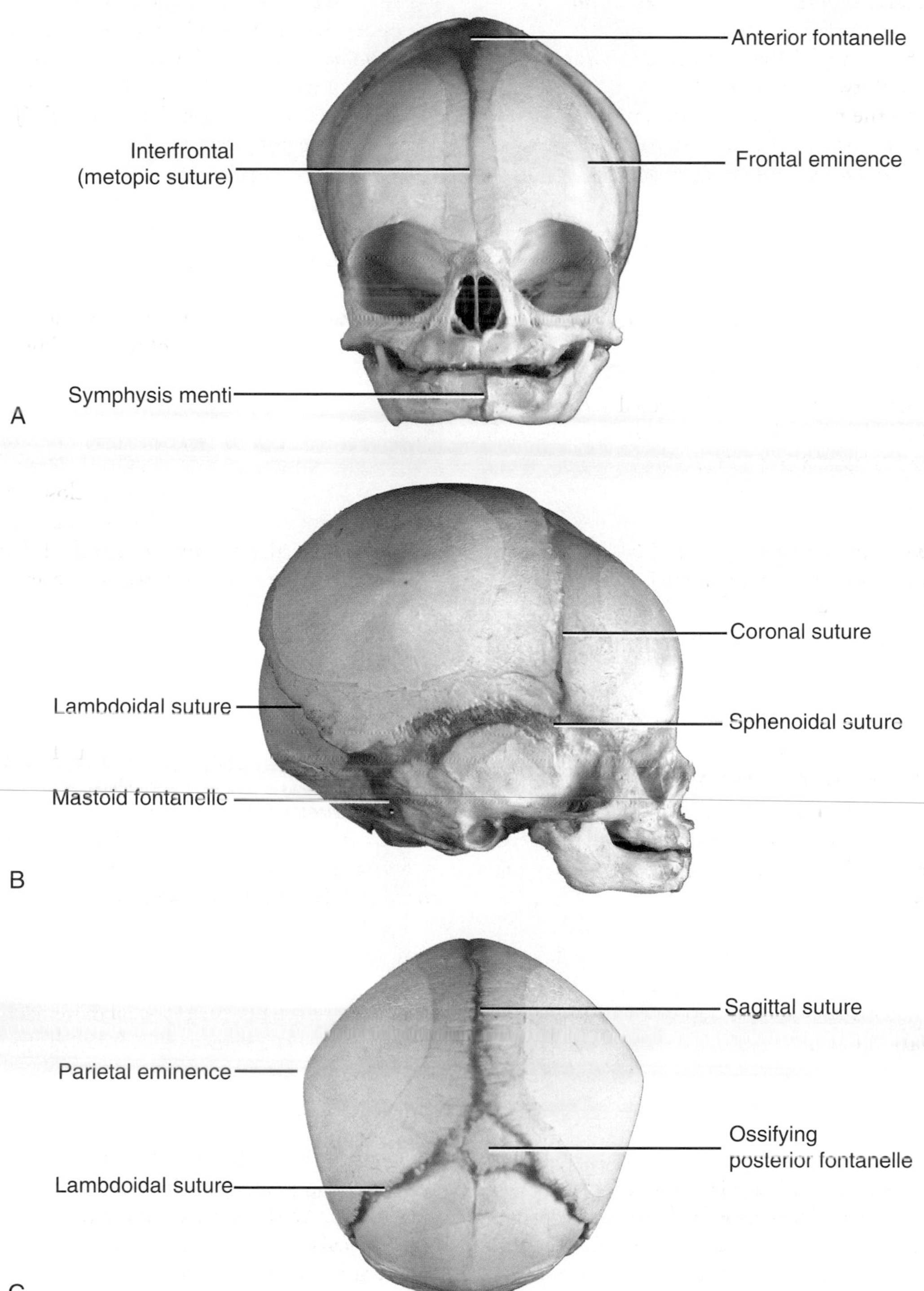


**FIG. 9.9** The fetal skull. A, Anterior view. B, Lateral view. C, Posterior view. *(From Liebgott B: The anatomical basis of dentistry, ed 3, St Louis, 2010, Mosby.)*

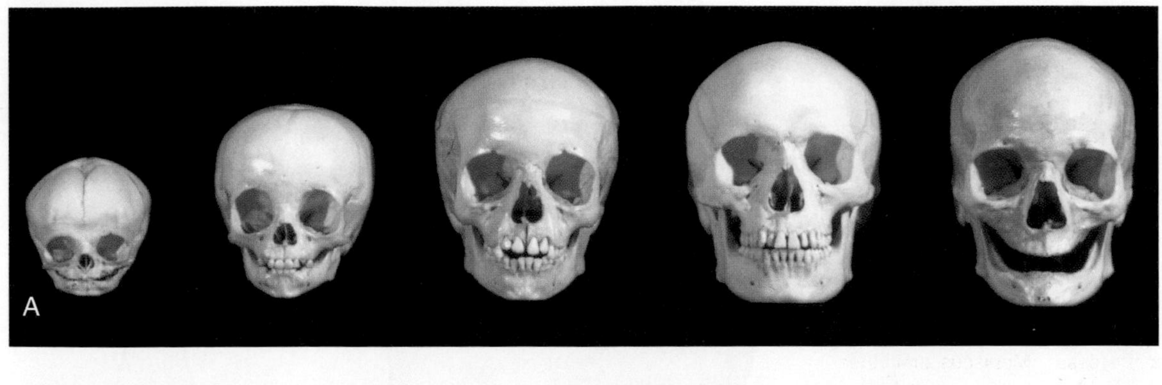


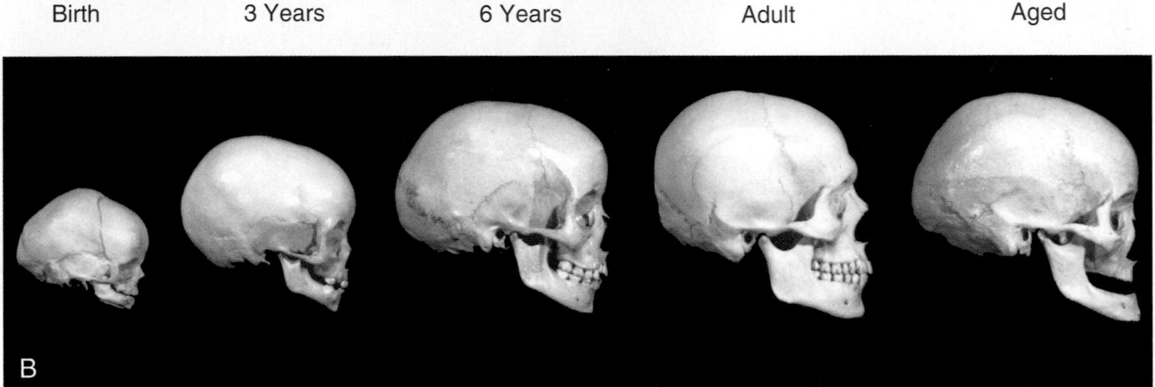


**FIG. 9.10** Stages of postnatal development of the human skull. A, Anterior view. B, Lateral view. *(From Liebgott B: The anatomical basis of dentistry, ed 3, St Louis, 2010, Mosby.)*

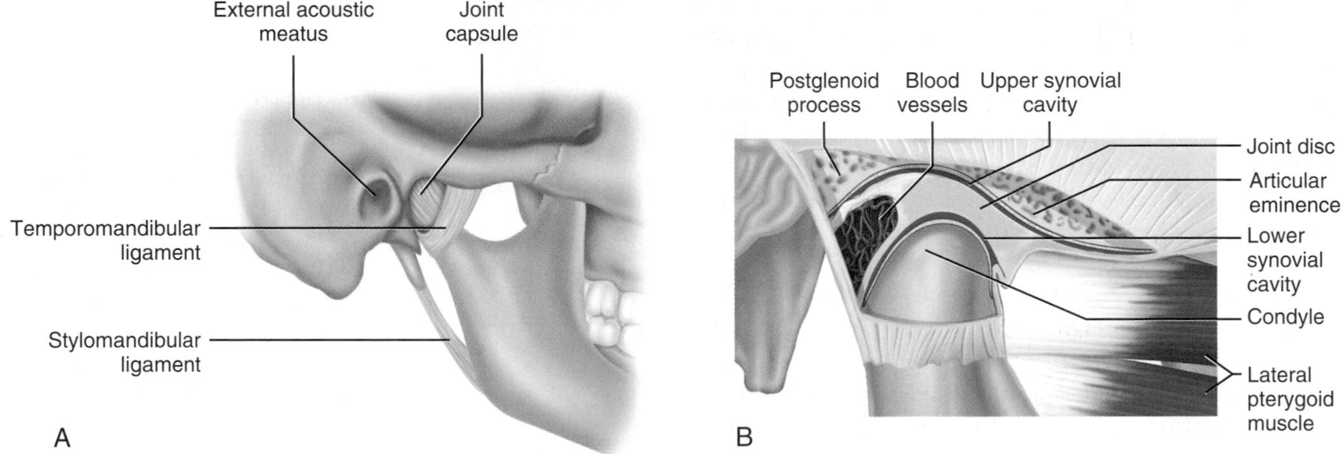


**FIG. 9.11** Lateral view of the joint capsule of the temporomandibular joint and its lateral temporomandibular ligament. Note in Fig. B that the capsule has been removed to show the upper and lower synovial cavities and their relationship to the articular disc. *(© Elsevier Collection.)*

of the joint. The condyle and articular disc "glide" forward and downward along the articular eminence (projection). This movement occurs only during protrusion and lateral movements of the mandible and in combination with the hinge action during wider opening of the mouth.

Protrusion is the forward movement of the mandible. This happens when the internal and external pterygoid muscles on both sides contract together. The reversal of this movement is the backward movement of the mandible, called *retrusion*.

Lateral movement (sideways movement) of the mandible occurs when the internal and external pterygoid muscles on the same side of the face contract together.

Side-to-side *grinding movements* result from alternating contractions of the internal and external pterygoid muscles, first on one side and then on the other.

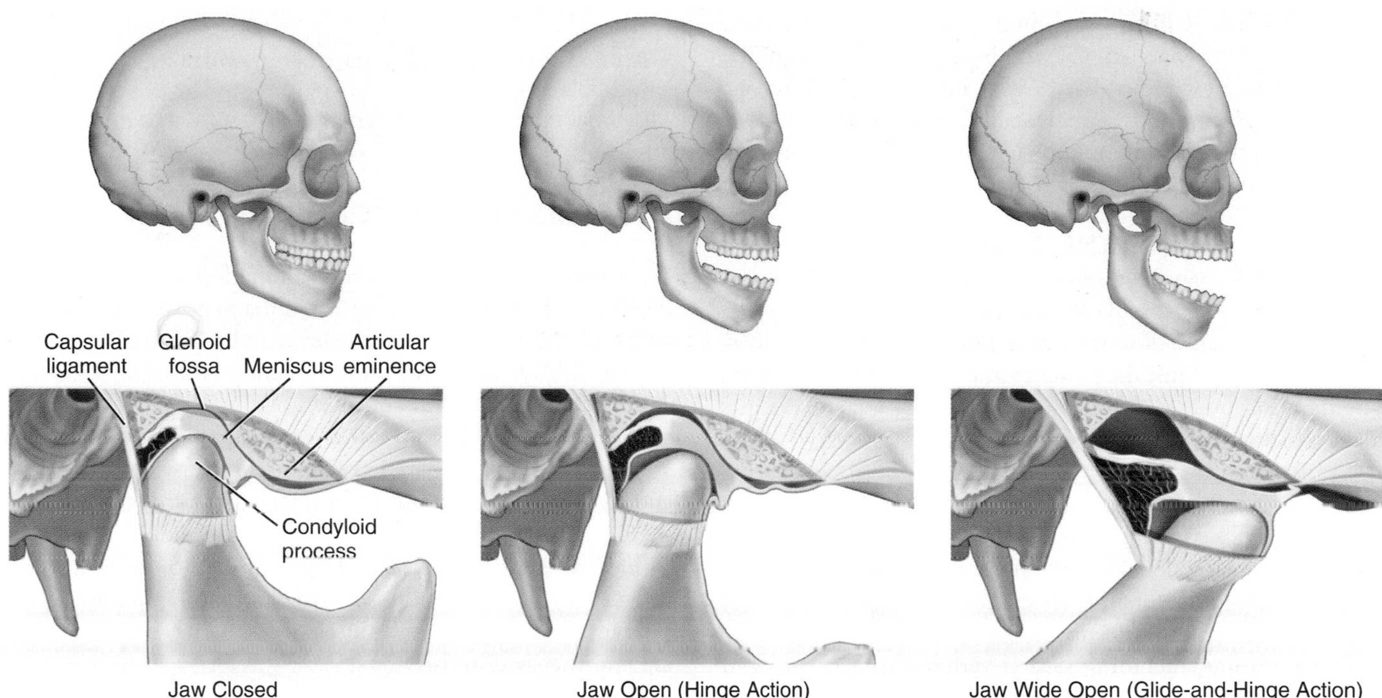


**FIG. 9.12** Hinge and gliding actions of the temporomandibular joint. *(© Elsevier Collection.)*

## Temporomandibular Disorders

A patient may experience a disease process associated with one or both of the TMJs, or a *temporomandibular disorder (TMD).* TMD is a complex disorder that involves many factors, such as stress, clenching, and bruxism. *Clenching* is holding the teeth tightly together for prolonged periods. *Bruxism* is habitual grinding of the teeth, especially at night. TMD can also be caused by trauma to the jaw, systemic diseases such as osteoarthritis, or wear as a result of aging (Table 9.3).

Diagnosis and treatment of TMD can be difficult (Fig. 9.13). Frequently, the diagnosis of TMD requires a multidisciplinary approach. For a complete analysis of the patient's condition, some cases require involvement of dentists, physicians, psychiatrists, psychologists, neurologists, neurosurgeons, and others.

### *Symptoms*

One reason TMD is difficult to diagnose is that the symptoms are so varied. Pain, joint sounds, and limitations in movement occur most often.

**PAIN.** Patients with TMD may report a wide range of pain types, including headache; pain in and around the ear (when no infection is present); pain on chewing; and pain in the face, head, and neck. *Spasms* ("cramps") of the muscles of mastication can become part of a cycle that results in tissue damage, increased pain, muscle tenderness, and more spasms.

**TABLE 9.3** Categories of Temporomandibular Disorders (TMDs)

| Category | Description |
|---|---|
| Acute masticatory muscle complaints | These are characterized by muscle inflammation, muscle spasms, and protective muscle splinting. |
| Articular disc derangement | The disc, which allows smooth movement of the joint, may be displaced or damaged. This may cause clicking sounds, limited ability to open the mouth, and other symptoms associated with TMDs. |
| Extrinsic trauma | These injuries from external causes may involve dislocation of the joint, fracture of the bones, and internal derangement of the joint. |
| Joint diseases | Degenerative and inflammatory forms of arthritis may severely damage the joint. |
| Chronic mandibular hypomobility | *Hypomobility* means a limited ability to move. In the mandible, this may be influenced by damage to the joint (the bony portions or the articular capsule), contracture (shortening) of muscles of mastication, or damage to the articular disc. |

**JOINT SOUNDS.** Clicking, popping, or crepitus may be heard when the mouth is opened. *Crepitus* is the cracking sound that may be heard in a joint. The dentist may use a stethoscope to listen for these sounds. Patients also report hearing *cracking* or *grinding* sounds. It is unknown whether joint sounds are related to problems with the jaws.

**LIMITATIONS IN MOVEMENT.** Limitations in movement lead to difficulty and pain on chewing, yawning, or widely opening the mouth. *Trismus,* spasm of the muscles of mastication, is the most common cause of restricted mandibular movement. Trismus may severely limit the patient's ability to open the mouth. Patients' descriptions of this condition include a jaw that "gets stuck," "locks," or "goes out."

### Causes

TMDs are often considered to be related to stress. Frequently, oral habits such as clenching the teeth or bruxism are important contributing factors. Other causes of TMDs include (1) accidents involving injuries to the jaw, head, or neck; (2) diseases of the joint, including several varieties of arthritis; and (3) *malocclusion,* in which the teeth come together in a manner that produces abnormal strain on the joint and surrounding tissues.

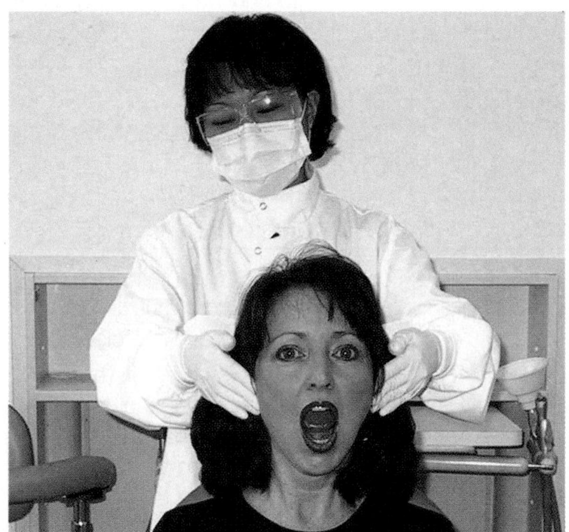

**FIG. 9.13** Palpation of the patient during movements of both temporomandibular joints.

9 What are the two basic types of movement by the TMJ?
10 What symptoms might a patient with a TMD have?

## Muscles of the Head and Neck

To perform a thorough patient examination, it is necessary to determine the location and action of many muscles of the head and neck. Malfunction of muscles may be involved in malocclusion, TMD, and even spread of dental infection.

Muscles must *expand* and *contract* to make movement possible. Each muscle has a point of origin that is fixed (nonmovable) and a point of insertion (movable). Muscles of the head and neck are divided into seven main groups: (1) muscles of the neck, (2) muscles of facial expression, (3) muscles of mastication, (4) muscles of the floor of the mouth, (5) muscles of the tongue, (6) muscles of the soft palate, and (7) muscles of the pharynx. Other groups of muscles of the ears, eyes, and nose are not discussed in this book.

## Major Muscles of the Neck

The two muscles of the neck discussed in this text are superficial and are easily palpated on the neck. These cervical muscles are the **sternocleidomastoid** and **trapezius**. These muscles can become painful when dental assistants use improper posture while assisting (Table 9.4 and Fig. 9.14).

## Major Muscles of Facial Expression

The muscles of facial expression are paired muscles (left and right) that originate from the bone and insert on skin tissue. These muscles cause wrinkles at right angles to the action line of the muscle. The seventh cranial (facial) nerve innervates all the muscles of facial expression (Table 9.5).

## Major Muscles of Mastication

The muscles of mastication are four pairs of muscles attached to the mandible that include the *temporalis,* **masseter**, *internal (medial) pterygoid,* and *external (lateral) pterygoid* (Fig. 9.15).

**TABLE 9.4** Major Muscles of the Neck

| Muscle | Origin | Insertion | Function |
|---|---|---|---|
| Sternocleidomastoid | Clavicle (collarbone) and lateral surfaces of sternum | Posterior and inferior to external acoustic meatus | Divides neck region into anterior and posterior cervical triangles; serves as landmark of neck during extraoral examination |
| Trapezius | External surface of occipital bone | Lateral third of clavicle and parts of scapula | Lifts clavicle and scapula (shoulder blade), as when shoulders are shrugged |

These muscles work with the TMJ to make all movements of the mandible possible. The mandibular division of the fifth cranial (trigeminal) nerve innervates all muscles of mastication (Table 9.6).

## Muscles of the Floor of the Mouth

The muscles of the floor of the mouth are the *digastric, mylohyoid, stylohyoid,* and *geniohyoid* (Fig. 9.16). These muscles are located between the mandible and the hyoid bone (Table 9.7). Different nerve branches innervate the muscles on the floor of the mouth.

## Muscles of the Tongue

The tongue has two groups of muscles: *intrinsic* (within the tongue) and *extrinsic*. Intrinsic muscles are responsible for shaping the tongue during speaking, chewing, and swallowing. Extrinsic muscles (Table 9.8) assist in the movement and functioning of the tongue and include the *genioglossus, hyoglossus, styloglossus,* and *palatoglossus* (Fig. 9.17). All muscles of the tongue, except the palatoglossus, are innervated by the hypoglossal nerve. The palatoglossus muscle is discussed with the palate. Muscles of the tongue and the floor of the mouth attach to the hyoid bone.

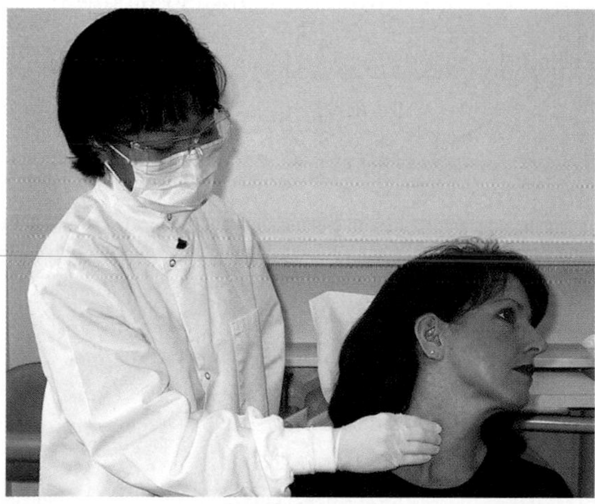

**FIG. 9.14** Palpation of the sternocleidomastoid muscle by having the patient turn the head to the opposite side.

## Muscles of the Soft Palate

The soft palate has two major muscles called the *palatoglossus* and *palatopharyngeus* (Table 9.9). The *pharyngeal plexus* innervates both of these muscles.

RECALL

**11** Which cranial nerve innervates all muscles of mastication?

**12** What is the name of the horseshoe-shaped bone at which the muscles of the tongue and the floor of the mouth attach?

# Salivary Glands

The salivary glands produce *saliva,* which lubricates and cleanses the oral cavity and aids in digestion of food through an enzymatic process. Saliva also helps maintain the integrity of tooth surfaces through a process of *remineralization.* In addition, saliva is involved in the formation of dental plaque, and it supplies minerals for supragingival calculus formation. These processes are discussed in detail in Chapters 13 and 14.

The salivary glands produce two types of saliva. *Serous* saliva is watery, mainly protein fluid. *Mucous* saliva is very thick, mainly carbohydrate fluid. Salivary glands are classified by their size as major or minor (Fig. 9.18).

## Minor Salivary Glands

The minor salivary glands are smaller and more numerous than the major salivary glands. The minor glands are scattered in the tissues of the buccal, labial, and lingual mucosa; the soft palate; the lateral portions of the hard palate; and the floor of the mouth. *Von Ebner's salivary gland* is associated with the **circumvallate lingual papillae** on the tongue.

## Major Salivary Glands

The three large paired salivary glands are the *parotid, submandibular,* and *sublingual* glands.

**TABLE 9.5** Major Muscles of Facial Expression

| Muscle | Origin | Insertion | Function |
|---|---|---|---|
| Orbicularis oris | From muscle fibers around mouth; no skeletal attachment | Into itself and surrounding skin | Closes and puckers lips; aids in chewing and speaking by pressing lips against teeth |
| Buccinator | Posterior portion of alveolar processes of maxillary bone and mandible | Fibers of orbicularis oris, at angle of mouth | Compresses cheeks against teeth and retracts angle of mouth |
| Mentalis | Incisive fossa of mandible | Skin of chin | Raises and wrinkles skin of chin and pushes up lower lip |
| Zygomatic major | Zygomatic bone | Into fibers of orbicularis oris | Draws angles of mouth upward and backward, as in laughing |

The *parotid salivary gland* is the largest of the major salivary glands, but it provides only 25 percent of the total volume of saliva. It is located in an area just below and in front of the ear. Saliva passes from the parotid gland into the mouth through the **parotid duct**, also known as *Stensen's duct.*

The *submandibular salivary gland,* about the size of a walnut, is the second largest salivary gland. This gland provides 60 to 65 percent of the total volume of saliva. It lies beneath the mandible in the *submandibular fossa,* posterior to the sublingual salivary gland. The gland releases saliva into the oral cavity through the *submandibular duct,* also known as *Wharton's duct,* which ends in the sublingual caruncles. Ducts visible in the oral cavity are shown in Chapter 10.

The *sublingual salivary gland* is the smallest of the three major salivary glands. It provides only 10 percent of the total salivary volume. This gland releases saliva into the oral cavity through the *sublingual duct,* also known as *Bartholin's duct.* Other smaller ducts of the sublingual gland open along the sublingual fold. A stone, or *sialolith,* may block the salivary glands in the duct opening, preventing saliva from flowing into the mouth. Salivary stones may be removed surgically (Fig. 9.19).

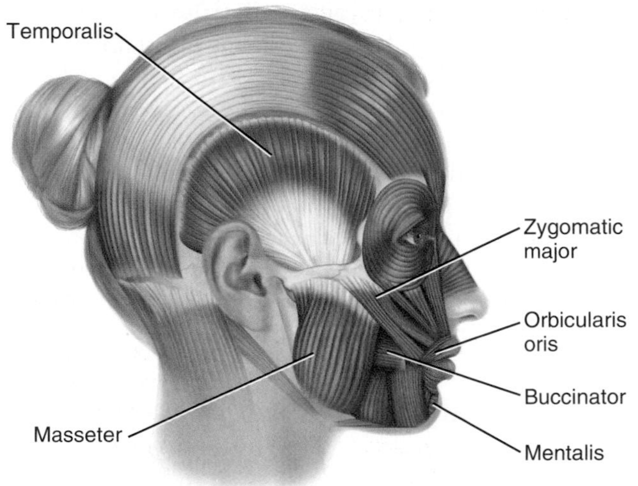


**FIG. 9.15** Major muscles of mastication include the temporalis and masseter muscles shown here. *(© Elsevier Collection.)*

**13** Which of the major salivary glands is the largest?
**14** What is another name for the parotid duct?

# Blood Supply to the Head and Neck

It is important to be able to locate the larger blood vessels of the head and neck, because these vessels may become compromised as the result of disease or during a dental procedure such as injection of a local anesthetic. Blood vessels may also spread infection in the head and neck area.

## Major Arteries of the Face and Oral Cavity

The *aorta* ascends from the left ventricle of the heart. The *common carotid artery* arises from the aorta and subdivides into the internal and external carotid arteries. The *internal carotid artery* supplies blood to the brain and eyes. The *external carotid artery* provides the major blood supply to the face and mouth (Table 9.10 and Fig. 9.20).

### External Carotid Artery

The branches of the external carotid artery are named according to the areas they supply. These branches supply the tongue, face, ears, and wall of the cranium.

**TABLE 9.6** Major Muscles of Mastication

| Muscle | Origin | Insertion | Function |
|---|---|---|---|
| Temporal | Temporal fossa of temporal bone | Coronoid process and anterior border of mandibular ramus | Raises mandible and closes jaws |
| Masseter | **Superficial part:** lower border of zygomatic arch<br>**Deep part:** posterior and medial side of zygomatic arch | **Superficial part:** angle and lower lateral side of mandibular ramus<br>**Deep part:** upper lateral ramus and mandibular coronoid process | Raises mandible and closes jaws |
| Internal (medial) pterygoid | Medial surface of lateral pterygoid plate of sphenoid bone, palatine bone, and tuberosity of maxillary bone | Into inner (medial) surface of ramus and angle of mandible | **Closes jaw:** acting with lateral pterygoid on same side, pulls mandible to one side; medial and lateral pterygoids on both sides act together to bring lower jaw forward* |
| External (lateral) pterygoid | Originates from two heads; upper head originates from greater wing of sphenoid bone | Into neck of condyle of mandible and into articular disc and capsular ligament of TMJ | Depresses mandible to open jaw* |

*When both pterygoid muscles contract together, the main action is to bring the lower jaw forward, thus causing protrusion of the mandible. If only one lateral pterygoid muscle is contracted, the lower jaw shifts to the opposite side, causing lateral deviation of the mandible.

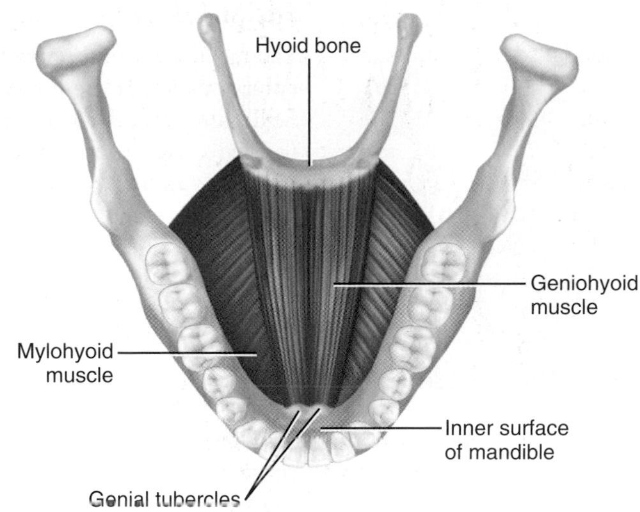


**FIG. 9.16** View from above the floor of the oral cavity showing the origin and insertion of the geniohyoid muscle. *(© Elsevier Collection.)*

## TABLE 9.7 Muscles of the Floor of the Mouth

| Muscle | Origin | Insertion | Function | Innervation |
|---|---|---|---|---|
| Mylohyoid | Left and right portions are joined at the midline; each portion originates on mylohyoid line of mandible | Body of hyoid bone | Forms floor of mouth; elevates (raises) tongue and depresses (lowers) jaw | **Posterior belly:** facial nerve **Anterior belly:** mandibular branch of trigeminal nerve |
| Digastric | **Anterior belly:** lower border of mandible **Posterior belly:** mastoid process of temporal bone | Body and great horn of hyoid bone | Each digastric muscle demarcates superior portion of anterior cervical triangle, forming (with the mandible) a submandibular triangle on each side of neck | **Anterior belly:** facial nerve **Posterior belly:** facial nerve (seventh cranial nerve) |
| Stylohyoid | Styloid process of temporal bone | Body of hyoid bone | Assists in swallowing by raising hyoid bone | Facial nerve |
| Geniohyoid | Medial (inner) surface of mandible, near symphysis | Body of hyoid bone | Draws tongue and hyoid bone forward | Hypoglossal nerve |

## TABLE 9.8 Extrinsic Muscles of the Tongue

| Muscle | Origin | Insertion | Function |
|---|---|---|---|
| Genioglossus | Medial (inner) surface of mandible, near symphysis | Hyoid bone and inferior (lower) surface of tongue | Depresses and protrudes tongue |
| Hyoglossus | Body of hyoid bone | Side of tongue | Retracts and pulls down side of tongue |
| Styloglossus | Styloid process of temporal bone | Side and undersurface of tongue | Retracts tongue |

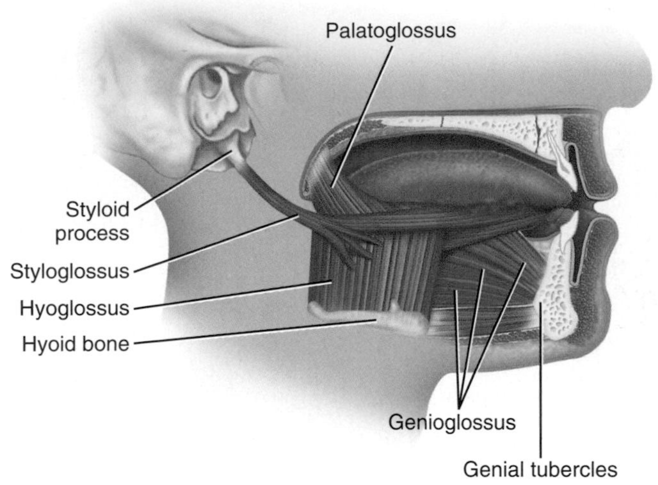

FIG. 9.17 Extrinsic muscles of the tongue. (© *Elsevier Collection.)*

### *Facial Artery*

The facial artery is another branch of the external carotid. It enters the face at the inferior border of the mandible and can be detected by gentle palpation of the mandibular notch. The facial artery passes forward and upward across the cheek toward the angle of the mouth. Then it continues upward alongside the nose and ends at the medial *canthus* (inner corner) of the eye. The facial artery has six branches that supply the pharyngeal muscles, soft palate, tonsils, posterior tongue, submandibular gland, muscles of the face, nasal septum, nose, and eyelids.

### *Lingual Artery*

The lingual artery is also a branch of the external carotid. It consists of several branches to the entire tongue, floor of the mouth, lingual gingiva, and a portion of the soft palate and tonsils.

**TABLE 9.9** Major Muscles of the Soft Palate

| Muscle | Origin | Insertion | Function |
|---|---|---|---|
| Palatoglossus | Anterior arch on each side of throat; arises from soft palate | Along posterior side of tongue | Elevates base of tongue, arching tongue against soft palate; depresses soft palate toward tongue |
| Palatopharyngeal | Posterior border of thyroid cartilage and connective tissue of pharynx | Thyroid cartilage and wall of pharynx | Forms posterior pillar of fauces; serves to narrow fauces and helps shut off nasopharynx* |

*The nasopharynx is the portion of the pharynx that is superior to the level of the soft palate.

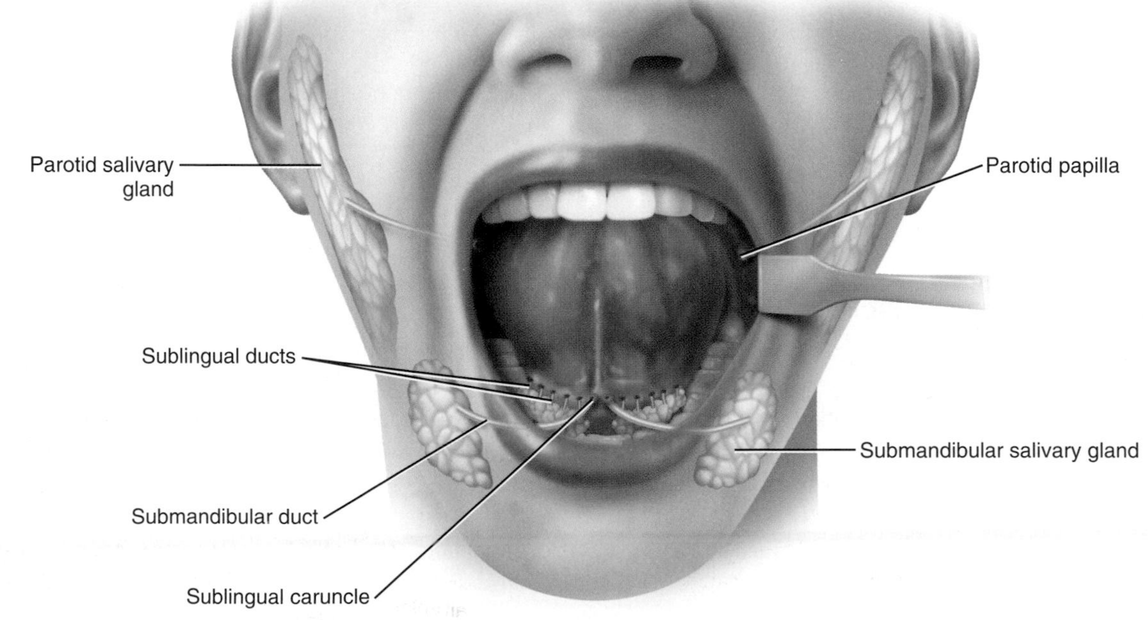

**FIG. 9.18** The salivary glands. (© *Elsevier Collection.)*

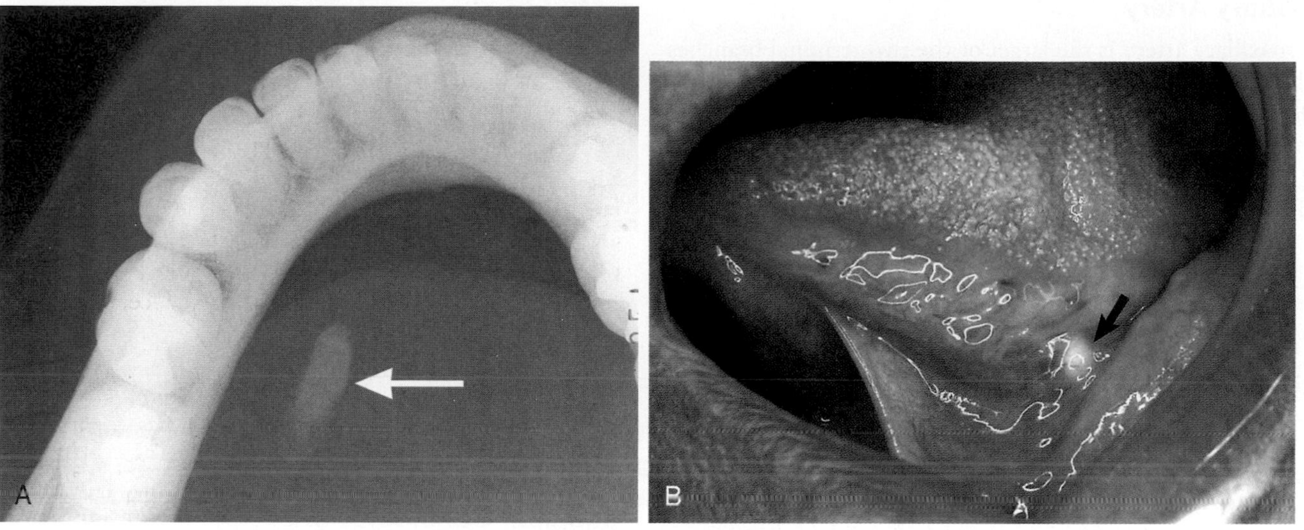


**FIG. 9.19** Sialoliths. A, Occlusal radiograph showing a sialolith *(arrow)* in Wharton's duct. B, Sialolith *(arrow)* in a minor salivary gland on the floor of the mouth. *(From Ibsen O, Phelan J: Oral pathology for the dental hygienist, ed 6, St Louis, 2014, Saunders; A, courtesy Dr. Barry Wolinsky.)*

**TABLE 9.10** Major Arteries to the Face and Oral Cavity

| Structure | Blood Supply |
|---|---|
| Muscles of facial expression | Branches and small arteries from maxillary, facial, and ophthalmic arteries |
| Maxillary bones | Anterior, middle, and posterior alveolar arteries |
| Maxillary teeth | Anterior, middle, and posterior alveolar arteries |
| Mandible | Inferior alveolar arteries |
| Mandibular teeth | Inferior alveolar arteries |
| Tongue | Lingual artery |
| Muscles of mastication | Facial arteries |

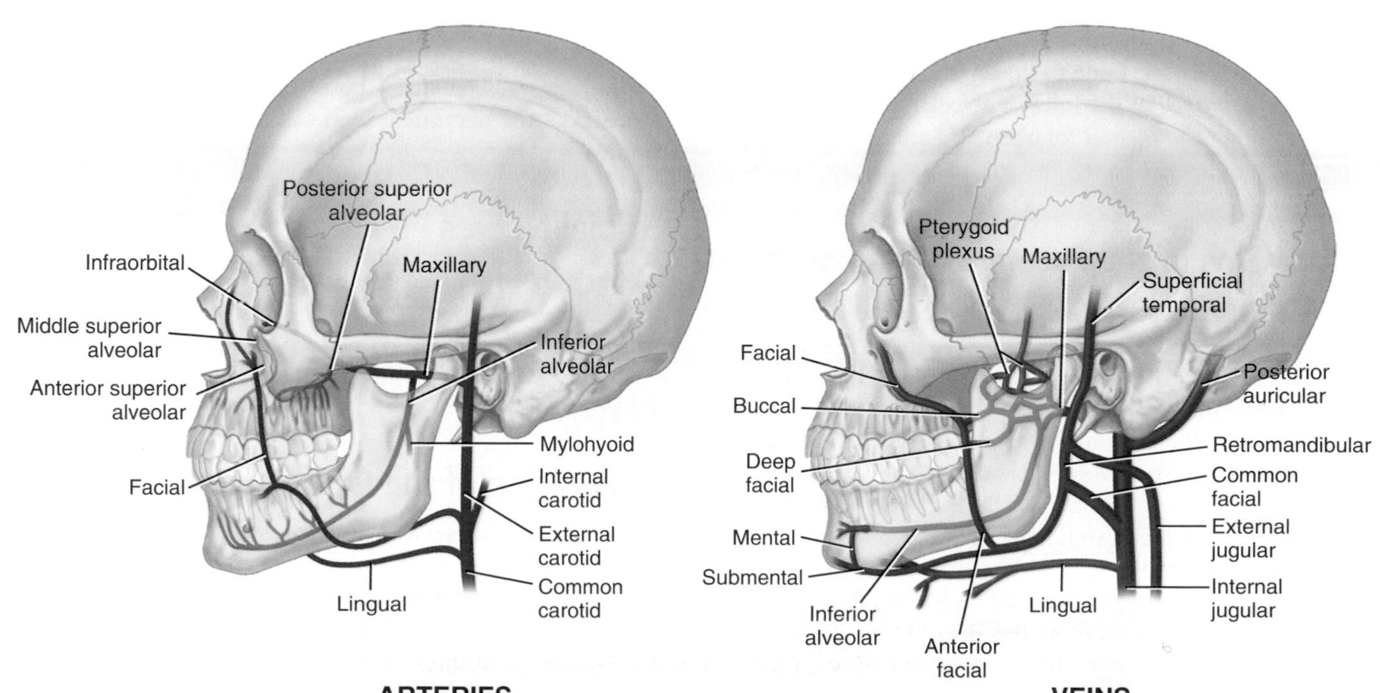


**FIG. 9.20** Major arteries and veins of the face and oral cavity. *(© Elsevier Collection.)*

### Maxillary Artery

The maxillary artery is the larger of the two terminal branches of the external carotid. It arises behind the angle of the mandible and supplies the deep structures of the face. The maxillary artery divides into three sections: *inferior alveolar, pterygoid,* and *pterygopalatine.*

The *pterygoid artery* supplies blood to the temporal muscle, masseter muscle, pterygoid muscles, and buccinator muscles. The pterygoid artery divides into the following five branches:

1. *Anterior* and *middle superior alveolar arteries,* with distribution to the maxillary incisors and cuspid teeth and to the maxillary sinuses
2. *Posterior superior alveolar artery,* with distribution to the maxillary molars and premolars and gingivae
3. *Infraorbital artery,* with distribution to the face
4. *Greater palatine artery,* with distribution to the hard palate and lingual gingiva
5. *Anterior superior alveolar artery,* with distribution to the anterior teeth

The **inferior alveolar artery** also comes from the maxillary artery. It enters the mandibular canal, along with the inferior alveolar nerve. It branches into the following five arteries:

1. The *lingual artery* has distribution along the surface of the tongue.
2. The *inferior alveolar artery* descends close to the medial surface of the mandibular ramus to the mandibular foramen; it then continues along the mandibular canal. Opposite the first premolar, it divides into the incisive and mental branches.
3. The *mylohyoid artery* branches from the inferior alveolar artery before entering the mandibular canal. It supplies the mylohyoid muscle.
4. The *incisive branch* of the inferior alveolar artery continues anteriorly within the bone to supply the anterior teeth.
5. The *mental branch* of the inferior alveolar artery passes outward through the mental foramen and anteriorly to supply the chin and lower lip.

## Major Veins of the Face and Oral Cavity

The *maxillary vein* receives branches that correspond to those of the maxillary artery. These branches form the *pterygoid plexus.* The trunk of the maxillary vein passes backward behind the neck of the mandible.

The union of the temporal and maxillary veins forms the *retromandibular vein.* It descends within the parotid gland and divides into two branches. The *anterior branch* passes inward to join the facial vein. The *posterior branch* is joined by the posterior auricular vein and becomes the external jugular vein.

The *external jugular vein* empties into the *subclavian vein.* The *facial vein* begins near the side of the nose. It passes downward and crosses over the body of the mandible with the facial artery. It then passes outward and backward to unite with the anterior division of the retromandibular vein to form the *common facial vein,* which enters the internal jugular vein.

The *deep facial vein* courses from the pterygoid plexus to the facial vein. The *lingual veins* begin on the dorsum (top), sides, and undersurface of the tongue. They pass backward, following the course of the lingual artery and its branches, and terminate in the internal jugular vein.

The *internal jugular vein,* which corresponds to the common carotid artery, empties into the *superior vena cava,* which returns blood from the upper portion of the body to the right atrium of the heart.

### Clinical Considerations: Facial Paralysis

The removal of an impacted third molar could be complicated by the relationship of the location of the nerves in the area to the tooth. For example, if the dentist damaged the nerve while attempting to remove the tooth, paralysis of the tongue or lip could result. Depending on the extent of injury that occurs to the nerve, paralysis could be temporary or permanent.

RECALL

**15** What five arteries branch from the inferior alveolar artery?
**16** What artery supplies the maxillary molars and premolars and the gingivae?

## Nerves of the Head and Neck

A thorough understanding of the nerves of the head and neck is important for the use of local anesthesia during dental treatment, and because the nerves are related to certain conditions of the face, such as facial paralysis (Fig. 9.21). Also, some disorders of the nervous system can affect the head and neck region.

### Cranial Nerves

Twelve pairs of *cranial nerves* are connected to the brain. These nerves serve both sensory and motor functions. The cranial nerves are generally named for the area or function that they serve and are identified with Roman numerals I to XII (Fig. 9.22).

### Innervation of the Oral Cavity

The **trigeminal nerve** is the primary source of innervation for the oral cavity (Figs. 9.23 and 9.24).

The trigeminal nerve subdivides into three main divisions: *ophthalmic, maxillary,* and *mandibular.* The ophthalmic nerve is not discussed in this chapter.

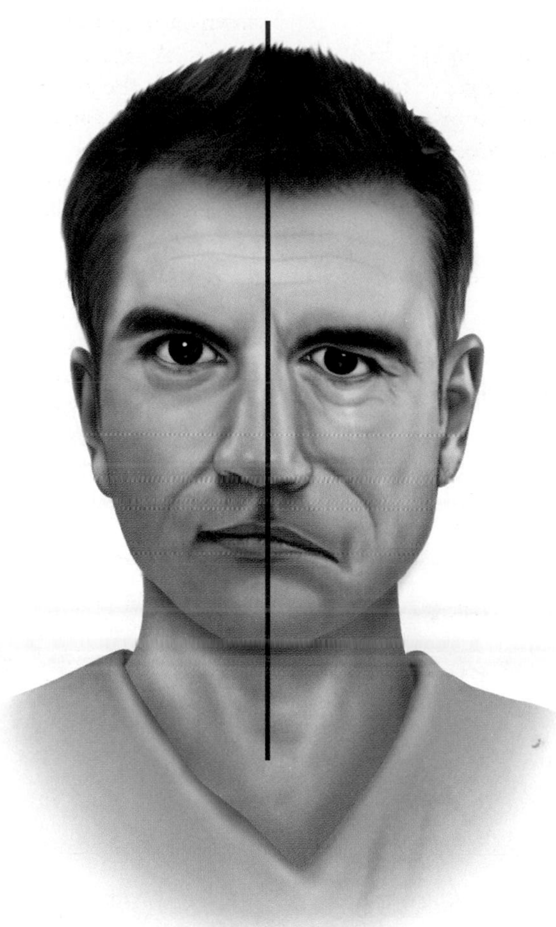

**FIG. 9.21** Facial paralysis resulting from damage to lower motor neurons of the facial nerve (cranial nerve VII). *(© Elsevier Collection.)*

## Maxillary Division of Trigeminal Nerve

The maxillary division of the trigeminal nerve supplies the maxillary teeth, periosteum, mucous membranes, maxillary sinuses, and soft palate. The maxillary division subdivides to provide the following innervation:

- The *nasopalatine nerve,* which passes through the incisive foramen, supplies the mucoperiosteum palatal to the maxillary anterior teeth. (*Mucoperiosteum* is periosteum that has a mucous membrane surface.)
- The **greater palatine nerve**, which passes through the posterior palatine foramen and forward over the palate, supplies the mucoperiosteum, intermingling with the nasopalatine nerve.
- The *anterior superior alveolar nerve* supplies the maxillary central, lateral, and cuspid teeth, along with their periodontal membranes and gingivae. This nerve also supplies the maxillary sinus.
- The *middle superior alveolar nerve* supplies the maxillary first and second premolars, the mesiobuccal root of the maxillary first molar, and the maxillary sinus.
- The *posterior superior alveolar nerve* supplies the other roots of the maxillary first molar and the maxillary second and third molars. It also branches forward to serve the lateral wall of the maxillary sinus.

## Mandibular Division of the Trigeminal Nerve

The mandibular division of the trigeminal nerve subdivides to provide the following innervation:

- The *buccal nerve* (long buccal) supplies branches to the buccal mucous membrane and to the mucoperiosteum of the mandibular molars.
- The *lingual nerve* supplies the anterior two thirds of the tongue and branches to supply the lingual mucous membrane and mucoperiosteum.
- The *inferior alveolar nerve* subdivides into the following:
  - The *mylohyoid nerve* supplies the mylohyoid muscles and the anterior belly of the digastric muscle.
  - *Small dental nerves* supply the molar and premolar teeth, alveolar process, and periosteum.

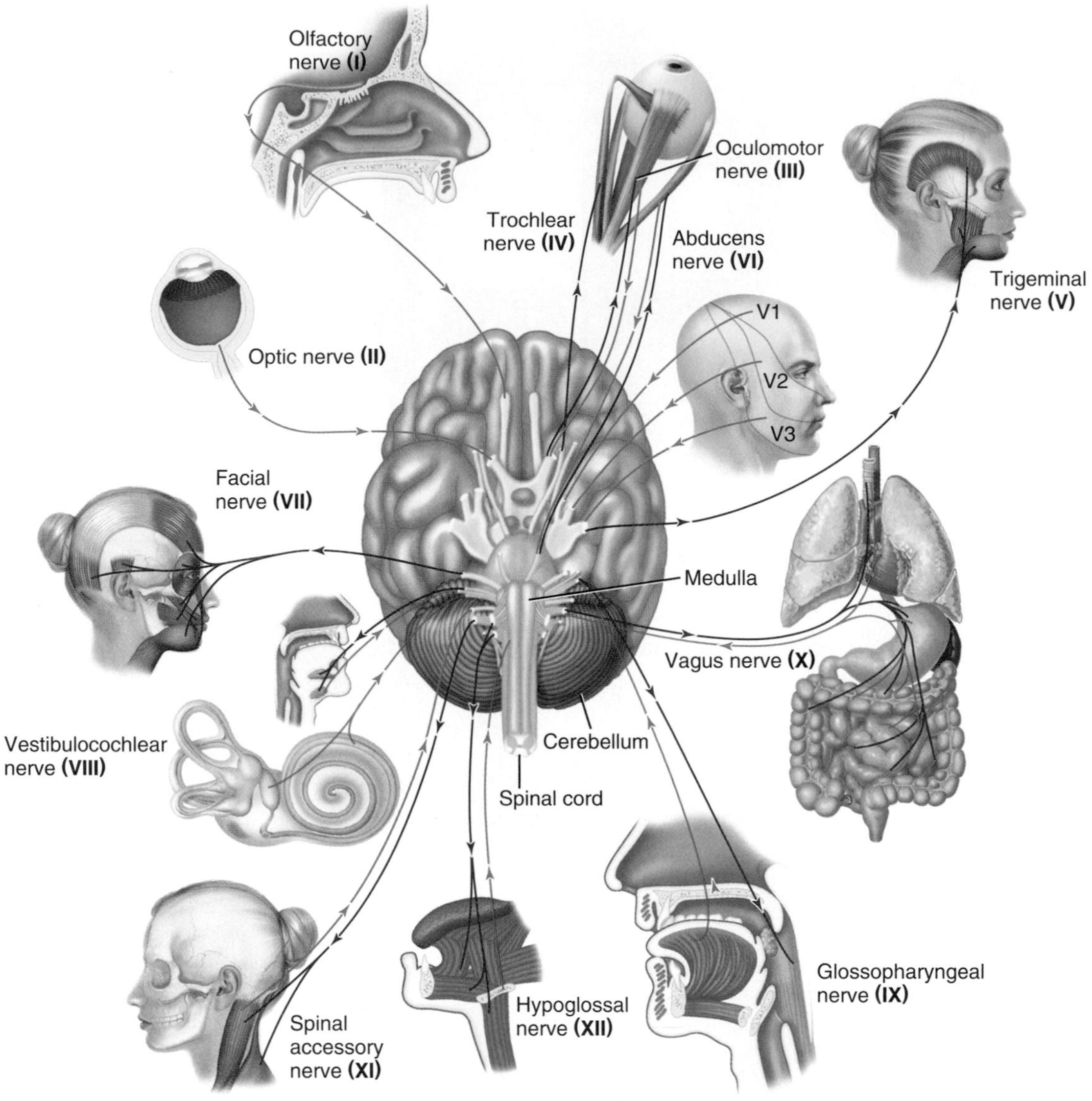


| NERVE | TYPE | FUNCTION |
|---|---|---|
| (I) Olfactory | Sensory | Sense of smell |
| (II) Optic | Sensory | Sense of sight |
| (III) Oculomotor | Motor | Movement of eye muscles |
| (IV) Trochlear | Motor | Movement of eye muscles |
| (V) Trigeminal | Motor | Movement of muscles of mastication and other cranial muscles |
| | Sensory | General sensations for face, head, skin, teeth, oral cavity, and tongue |
| (VI) Abducens | Motor | Movement of eye muscles |
| (VII) Facial | Motor | Facial expression, functions of glands and muscles |
| | Sensory | Sense of taste on tongue |
| (VIII) Vestibulocochlear | Sensory | Senses of sound and balance |
| (IX) Glossopharyngeal | Motor | Functioning of parotid gland |
| | Sensory | General sensation of skin around ear |
| (X) Vagus | Motor | Moves muscles in soft palate, pharynx, and larynx |
| | Sensory | General sensation on skin around ear and sense of taste |
| (XI) Accessory | Motor | Movement of muscles of the neck, soft palate, and pharynx |
| (XII) Hypoglossal | Motor | Movement of muscles of the tongue |

**FIG. 9.22** The twelve cranial nerves. *(© Elsevier Collection.)*

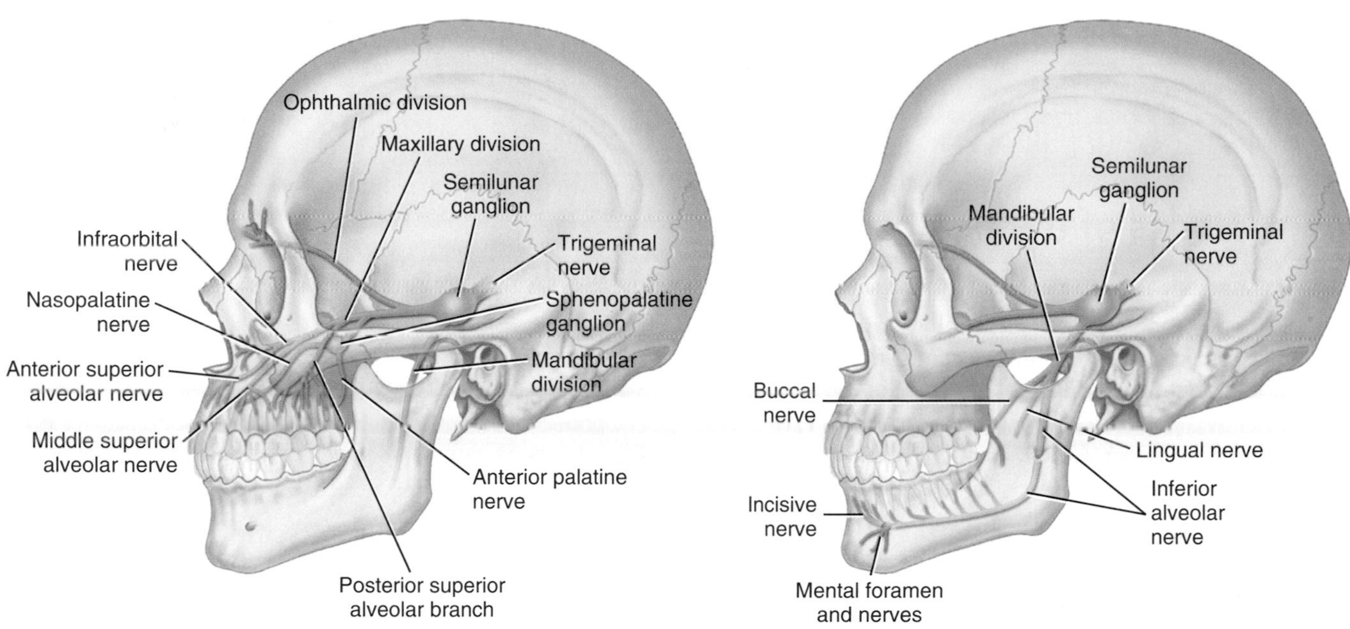


**FIG. 9.23** Maxillary and mandibular innervation. *(© Elsevier Collection.)*

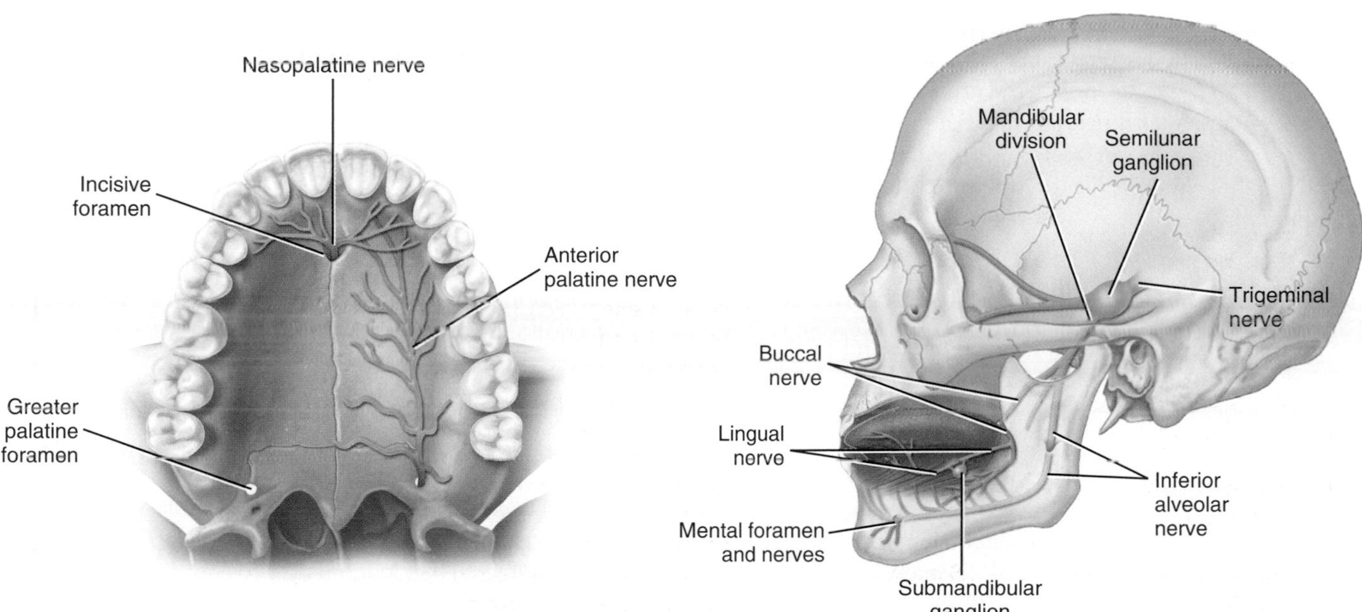


**FIG. 9.24** Palatal, lingual, and buccal innervation. *(© Elsevier Collection.)*

- The *mental nerve* moves outward and anteriorly through the mental foramen and supplies the chin and mucous membrane of the lower lip.
- The *incisive nerve* continues anteriorly within the bone and gives off small branches to supply the incisor teeth.

**17** How many pairs of cranial nerves are connected to the brain?
**18** Which division of the trigeminal nerve subdivides into the buccal, lingual, and inferior alveolar nerves?

# Lymph Nodes of the Head and Neck

A dental professional must examine and palpate the lymph nodes of the head and neck very carefully during an extraoral examination. Enlarged lymph nodes could indicate infection or cancer. Lymph nodes for the oral cavity drain intraoral structures such as the teeth, as well as the eyes, ears, nasal cavity, and deeper areas of the throat. Often, a patient needs a referral to a physician when lymph nodes are palpable because of a disease process in these other regions.

## Structure and Function

*Lymph nodes* are small round or oval structures that are located in lymph vessels. They fight disease by producing antibodies; this is part of the immune reaction. In acute infection, lymph nodes become swollen and tender as a result of the collection of lymphocytes gathered to destroy invading substances.

Major lymph nodes of the body include *cervical nodes* (in the neck), *axillary nodes* (under the arms), and *inguinal nodes* (in the lower abdomen). Lymph nodes of the head are classified as *superficial* (near the surface) or *deep.* All nodes of the head drain the right or the left tissues in the area, depending on their location.

## Superficial Lymph Nodes of the Head

Five groups of superficial lymph nodes are found in the head: occipital, retroauricular, anterior auricular, superficial parotid, and facial nodes (Fig. 9.25, *A*).

## Deep Cervical Lymph Nodes

Deep cervical lymph nodes are located along the length of the internal jugular vein on each side of the neck, deep to the sternocleidomastoid muscle (Fig. 9.25, *B*).

## Lymphadenopathy

When a patient has an infection or cancer in a region, the lymph nodes in that region will respond by increasing in size and becoming very firm. This change in size and consistency is called **lymphadenopathy.** It results from an increase in the size of individual lymphocytes (lymphocyte cells are the body's main defense) and in overall cell count in the lymphoid tissue. With increased size and number of lymphocytes, the body is better able to fight the disease process.

The dentist will make an appropriate referral to a physician when any enlarged lymph nodes are found during an examination (see Fig. 9.13).

### Clinical Considerations: Toothache and Sinus Pain

A patient who is suffering from a toothache on the maxillary arch may actually have an infected sinus. The roots of the maxillary teeth lie in close proximity to the sinus floor. Because the teeth and the maxillary sinus share a common nerve supply, sinusitis (inflammation of the sinus) may cause a generalized aching of the maxillary teeth.

RECALL

**19** During what type of dental examination are lymph nodes palpated?
**20** What is the term for enlarged or palpable lymph nodes?

# Paranasal Sinuses

The paranasal sinuses are air-containing spaces within the skull that communicate with the nasal cavity (Fig. 9.26). (A *sinus* is an air-filled cavity within a bone.) Functions of the sinuses include (1) producing mucus; (2) making the bones of the skull lighter; and (3) providing resonance, which helps produce sound.

The sinuses are named for the bones in which they are located, as follows:

- *Maxillary sinuses*—the largest of the paranasal sinuses
- *Frontal sinuses*—located within the forehead just above the left and right eyes
- *Ethmoid sinuses*—irregularly shaped air cells separated from the orbital cavity by a very thin layer of bone
- *Sphenoid sinuses*—located close to the optic nerves, where an infection may damage vision

■ **Eye to the Future** Saliva has long been recognized for its protective and lubricating properties. Today, saliva is recognized as the strongest link between oral and systemic health. Changes in salivary flow and function are extremely sensitive to subtle changes in general health.

Recent research has found a new role for saliva as an effective laboratory tool. Saliva is now used in inexpensive, noninvasive, and easy-to-use diagnostic aids for oral and systemic diseases. For example, human immunodeficiency virus (HIV) antibodies in saliva have led to the development of test kits. These test kits provide the sensitivity of a blood test, without the discomfort of a needle stick. In laboratory tests, saliva is also reliable for diagnosing viral hepatitis A, B, and C. Saliva has been used as a diagnostic aid for Alzheimer's disease, cystic fibrosis, diabetes, and diseases of the adrenal

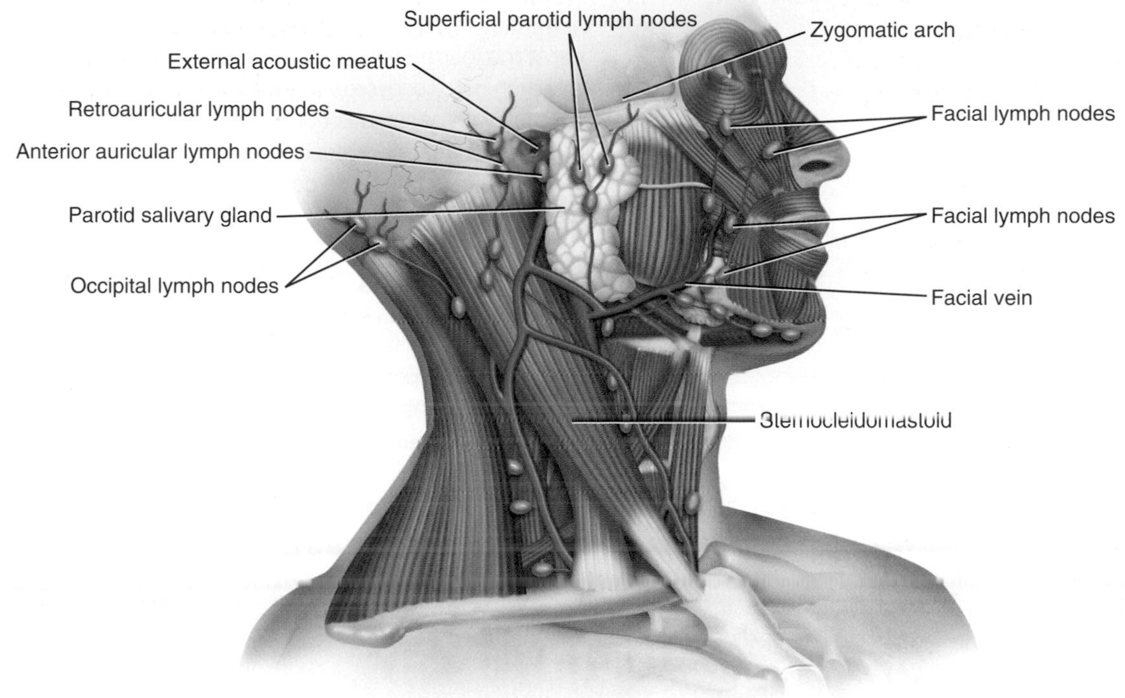


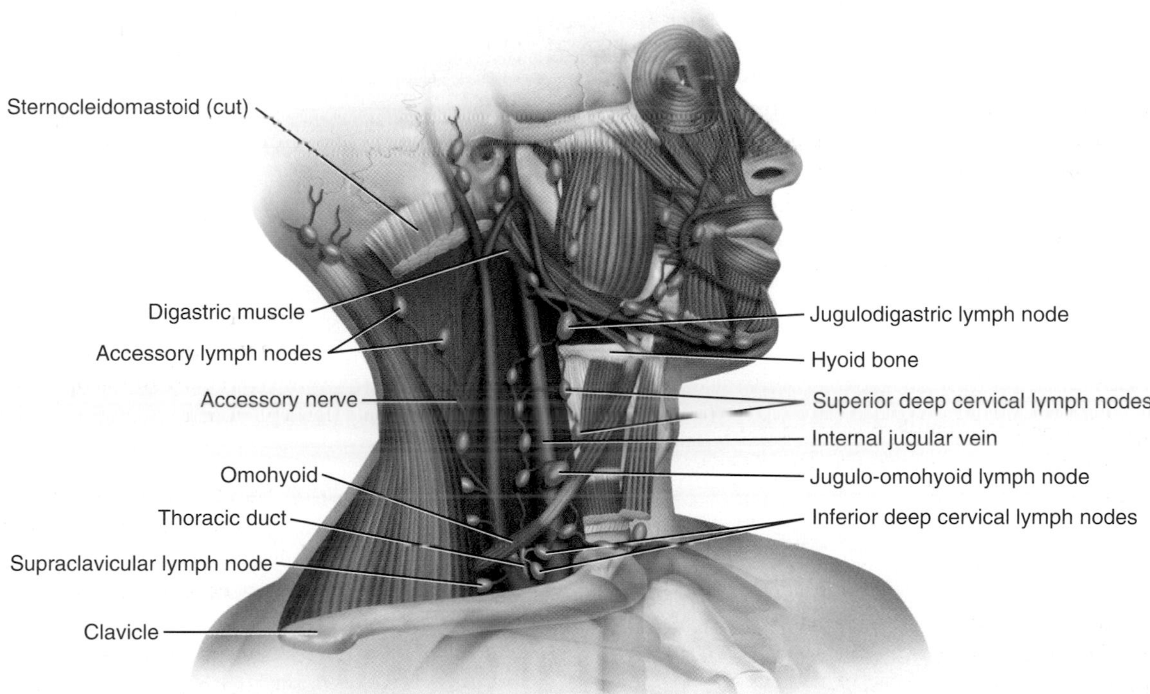


**FIG. 9.25** A, Superficial lymph nodes of the head and associated structures. B, Deep cervical lymph nodes and associated structures. *(© Elsevier Collection.)*

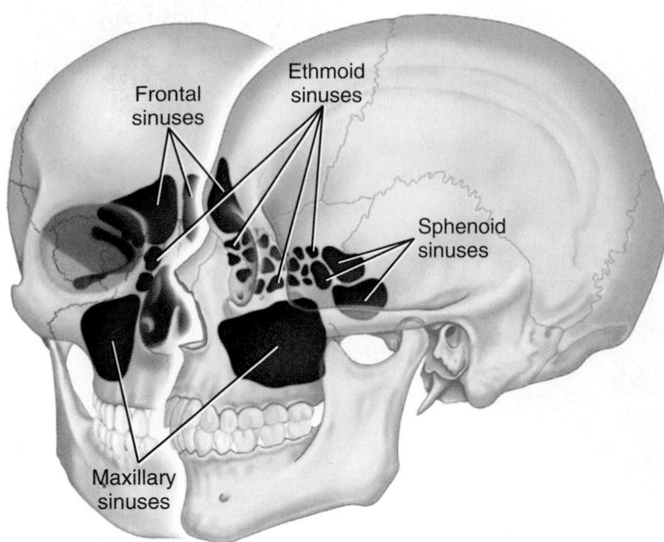


**FIG. 9.26** The paranasal sinuses. *(© Elsevier Collection.)*

cortex. Saliva is also proving to be an effective tool for monitoring levels of hormones, medications, and illicit drugs.

According to the American Cancer Society, pancreatic cancer is the fourth-leading cause of cancer deaths. Very recent research has discovered markers in saliva that can differentiate patients with pancreatic cancer from patients without pancreatic cancer. Imagine a deadly cancer that has had no early-stage detection methods can now be diagnosed in its early stages in saliva. ■

## ■ Critical Thinking

1. While reading the newspaper, you notice an advertisement for an automobile with an "occipital headrest" on the passenger side. What type of headrest do you think this could be? Why?
2. If your dental-assisting program has one or more skulls that you can look at, compare the size of the skulls and the shape of the teeth. See if you can determine whether it is the skull of a male or a female. ■

10

# Landmarks of the Face and Oral Cavity

## KEY TERMS

**Ala (AY-lah)** Winglike tip of the outer side of each nostril; plural, *alae*.

**Angle of the mandible** The lower posterior of the ramus.

**Angular cheilosis** Inflammation at the corners of the mouth that may be caused by nutritional deficiency of the B-complex vitamins, but most commonly is a fungal condition.

**Anterior faucial pillar** Anterior arch of the soft palate.

**Anterior naris (NAY-ris)** The nostril; plural, *nares.*

**Buccal vestibule** Area between the cheeks and the teeth or alveolar ridge.

**Canthus (KAN-thus)** Fold of tissue at the corner of the eyelids.

**Filiform papillae** Threadlike elevations that cover most of the tongue.

**Fordyce's (FOR-dise-ez) spots** Normal variations that may appear on the buccal mucosa.

**Frenum (FRE-num)** Band of tissue that passes from the facial oral mucosa at the midline of the arch to the midline of the inner surface of the lip; also called *frenulum;* plural, *frenula.*

**Fungiform papillae** Knoblike projections on the tongue.

**Gingiva (JIN-ji-vuh)** Masticatory mucosa that covers the alveolar processes of the jaws and surrounds the necks of the teeth; plural, *gingivae.*

**Glabella (glah-BEL-uh)** Smooth surface of the frontal bone; also, the anatomical part directly above the root of the nose.

**Incisive papilla** Pear-shaped pad of tissue that covers the incisive foramen.

**Isthmus of fauces** The opening between the two arches of the soft palate.

**Labia** The gateway to the oral cavity; commonly known as "lips."

**Labial (LAY-bee-ul) commissure** The angle at the corner of the mouth where the upper and lower lips join.

**Labial frenum** Band of tissue that passes from the facial oral mucosa at the midline of the arch to the midline of the inner surface of the lip; also called *frenulum;* plural, *frenula.*

**Linea alba** Normal variation noted on the buccal mucosa.

**Lingual frenum** The thin fold of mucous membrane that extends from the floor of the mouth to the underside of the tongue.

**Mental protuberance** Part of the mandible that forms the chin.

**Mucobuccal fold** Base of the vestibule where the buccal mucosa meets the alveolar mucosa.

**Mucogingival junction** Distinct line of color change in the tissue where the alveolar membrane meets with attached gingivae.

**Nasion (NAY-ze-on)** Midpoint between the eyes just below the eyebrows.

**Nasolabial sulcus** The groove extending upward between the labial commissure and the nasal ala.

**Oral cavity proper** The space on the tongue side within the upper and lower dental arches.

**Parotid papilla** Small elevation of tissue located on the inner surface of the cheek.

**Philtrum (FIL-trum)** Rectangular area from under the nose to the midline of the upper lip.

**Posterior faucial pillar** Posterior arch of the soft palate.

**Root** Facial landmark commonly called the "bridge" of the nose.

**Septum (SEP-tum)** 1. Dental dam material located between the holes of the punched dam. 2. Tissue that divides the nasal cavity into two nasal fossae.

**Tragus (TRAY-gus)** Cartilaginous projection anterior to the external opening of the ear.

**Uvula** Pear-shaped projection at the end of the soft palate.

**Vallate papillae** The largest papillae on the tongue, arranged in the form of a V.

**Vermilion (vur-MIL-yun) border** Darker-colored border around the lips.

**Vestibule** Space between the teeth and the inner mucosal lining of the lips and cheeks.

**Zygomatic arch** The arch formed when the temporal process of the zygomatic bone articulates with the zygomatic process of the temporal bone.

## LEARNING OUTCOMES

*On completion of this chapter, the student will be able to achieve the following objectives:*

1. Pronounce, define, and spell the key terms.
2. Name and identify the landmarks of the face.
3. Name and identify the landmarks of the oral cavity, including the following:
   - Describe the structures found in the vestibular region of the oral cavity.
   - Describe the characteristics of normal gingival tissue.
4. Name and identify the landmarks of the oral cavity proper, including the following:
   - Locate and identify the structures of the tongue.
   - Locate and describe the functions of the taste buds.

## ELECTRONIC RESOURCES

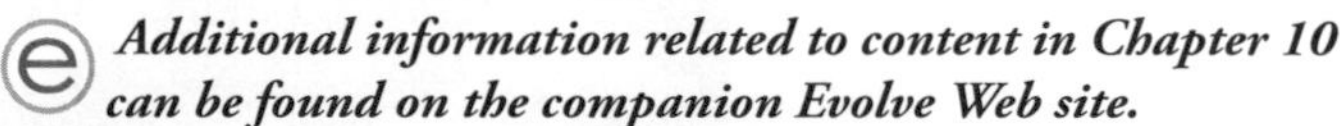
***Additional information related to content in Chapter 10 can be found on the companion Evolve Web site.***

- Practice Quiz

The dental assistant must be thoroughly knowledgeable about the landmarks of the face and oral cavity. In addition to serving as useful reference points for dental radiography and other procedures, facial features provide essential landmarks for many deeper structures. Any deviation from normal in surface features may be clinically significant.

You may wish to examine your own face and mouth or those of a partner. An operatory with a dental chair and a light is an ideal setting. However, use of a flashlight and a tongue depressor in the laboratory setting is adequate for intraoral inspection.

## Landmarks of the Face

The *face* is defined as the part of the head that is visible in a frontal view and is anterior to the ears and all that lies between the hairline and the chin.

### Regions of the Face

The facial region can be subdivided into nine areas (Fig. 10.1):

1. *Forehead,* extending from the eyebrows to the hairline
2. *Temples,* or temporal area posterior to the eyes
3. *Orbital* area, containing the eye and covered by the eyelids
4. *External nose*
5. *Zygomatic (malar) area,* the prominence of the cheek
6. *Mouth and lips*
7. *Cheeks*
8. *Chin*
9. *External ear*

### Features of the Face

The dental assistant should be able to identify the following thirteen important facial features (Fig. 10.2):

1. The outer **canthus** of the eye is the fold of tissue at the outer corner of the eyelids.
2. The inner canthus of the eye is the fold of tissue at the inner corner of the eyelids.
3. The **ala** of the nose is the winglike tip on the outer side of each nostril.
4. The **philtrum** is the rectangular area between the two ridges running from under the nose to the midline of the upper lip.
5. The **tragus** of the ear is the cartilaginous projection anterior to the external opening of the ear.
6. The **nasion** is the midpoint between the eyes just below the eyebrows. On the skull, this is the point where the two nasal bones and the frontal bone join.
7. The **glabella** is the smooth surface of the frontal bone; also, the anatomical area directly above the root of the nose.
8. The **root** is commonly called the "bridge" of the nose.
9. The **septum** is the tissue that divides the nasal cavity into two nasal fossae.
10. The **anterior naris** is the nostril.
11. The **mental protuberance** of the mandible forms the chin.
12. The **angle of the mandible** is the lower posterior of the ramus.
13. The **zygomatic arch** creates the prominence of the cheek.

1 What are the nine regions of the face?

### Skin

The skin of the face is thin to medium in relative thickness. It is soft and movable over a layer of loose connective tissue. The skin around the external ear and the ala of the nose is fixed to underlying cartilage. Facial skin contains many sweat and

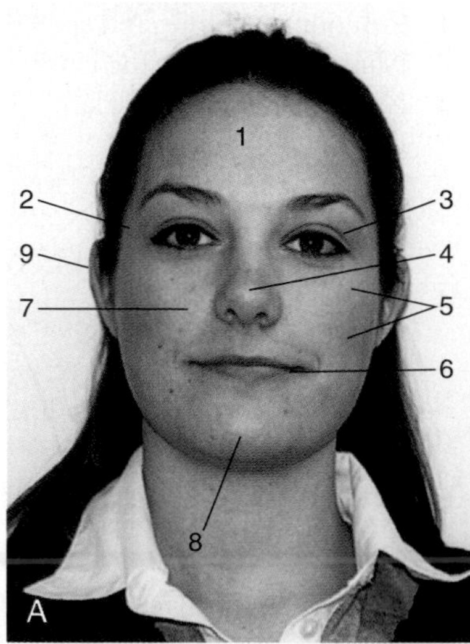


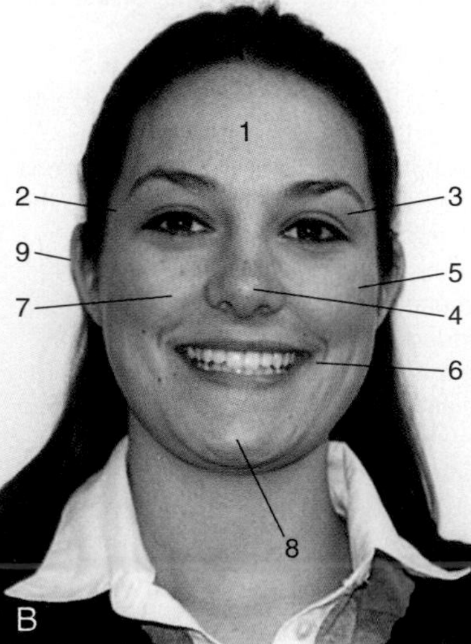


**FIG. 10.1** Regions of the face. A, At rest. B, Smiling. See the Regions of the Face section for which regions correspond to each number.

sebaceous glands. The connective tissue below the skin contains variable amounts of fat that smooth out the contours of the face, particularly between the muscles of facial expression (see Chapter 9). Located within the connective tissue are sensory and motor nerves of facial expression.

## Lips

The lips, also known as **labia**, provide the gateway to the oral cavity. They are formed externally by the skin and internally by mucous membrane (Fig. 10.3). The lips are outlined by the **vermilion border**, which is darker in color than the surrounding skin. Grasp your upper or lower lip between your thumb and forefinger to feel the pulsations of the labial branches of the facial artery.

The **labial commissure** is the angle at the corner of the mouth where the upper and lower lips join. The upper and lower lips are continuous at the angles of the mouth and blend with the cheeks.

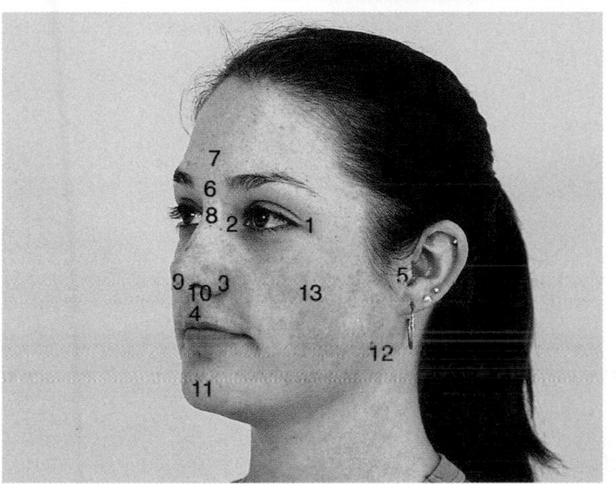


**FIG. 10.2** Features of the face. See the Features of the Face section for which regions correspond to each number.

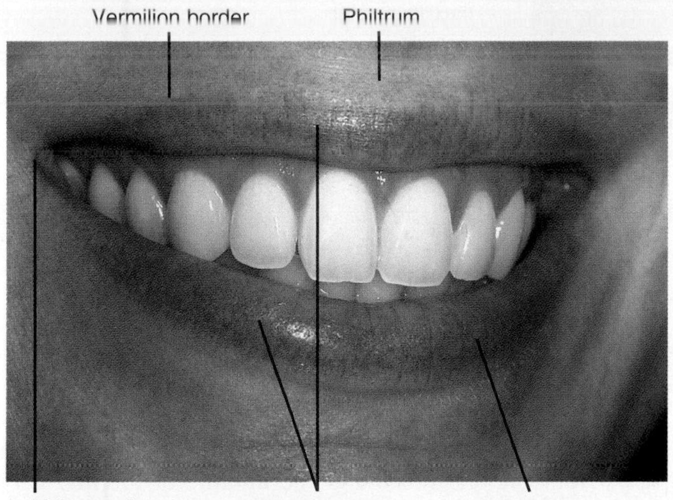


**FIG. 10.3** Frontal view of the lips.

The **nasolabial sulcus** is the groove that extends upward between each labial commissure and nasal ala.

### Clinical Considerations: Lips

The dentist will examine the lips before examining the oral cavity because the lips may have a variety of lesions or diseases.

Normally, a distinct border is seen between the lips and the surrounding skin of the face; this is called the *vermilion border.* During a clinical examination, the dentist will look for any disappearance of the vermilion border of the lips. When this occurs, it could simply be caused by scar tissue from past injuries, or it may be the result of changes caused by exposure to the sun. However, changes in the vermilion border may also be associated with oral cancer. A biopsy is the only way to determine whether cells are cancerous.

An inflammation or cracking at the corners of the mouth could be a condition called angular cheilosis, which is associated with vitamin B deficiency. Herpes labialis, or cold sores, may be present on the lips and can be very painful.

2 What is the area of color change around the border of the lips?

## The Oral Cavity

The entire oral cavity is lined with *mucous membrane* tissue. This type of tissue is moist and is adapted to meet the needs of the area it covers.

The oral cavity consists of the following two areas:

- The **vestibule** is the space between the teeth and the inner mucosal lining of the lips and cheeks.
- The **oral cavity proper** is the space on the tongue side within the upper and lower dental arches.

### The Vestibule

The intraoral vestibule begins on the inside of the lips and then extends from the lips onto the alveolar process of both arches. The vestibules are lined with mucosal tissue (Fig. 10.4). The vestibular mucosa is thin, red, and loosely bound to underlying alveolar bone. The base of each vestibule, where the buccal mucosa meets the alveolar mucosa, is called the **mucobuccal fold** (Fig. 10.5).

A distinct line of color change can be seen in the tissue where the alveolar membrane meets with attached gingivae. This line is called the **mucogingival junction** (Fig. 10.6). The attached gingiva is a lighter color and has a stippled surface.

The inside surfaces of the cheeks form the side walls of the oral cavity. The **buccal vestibule** is the area between the cheeks and the teeth or alveolar ridge. (*Buccal* means pertaining to the cheek.) A small elevation of tissue called the **parotid papilla** is located on the inner surface of the cheek on the buccal mucosa, just opposite the second maxillary molar. The parotid papilla protects the opening of the

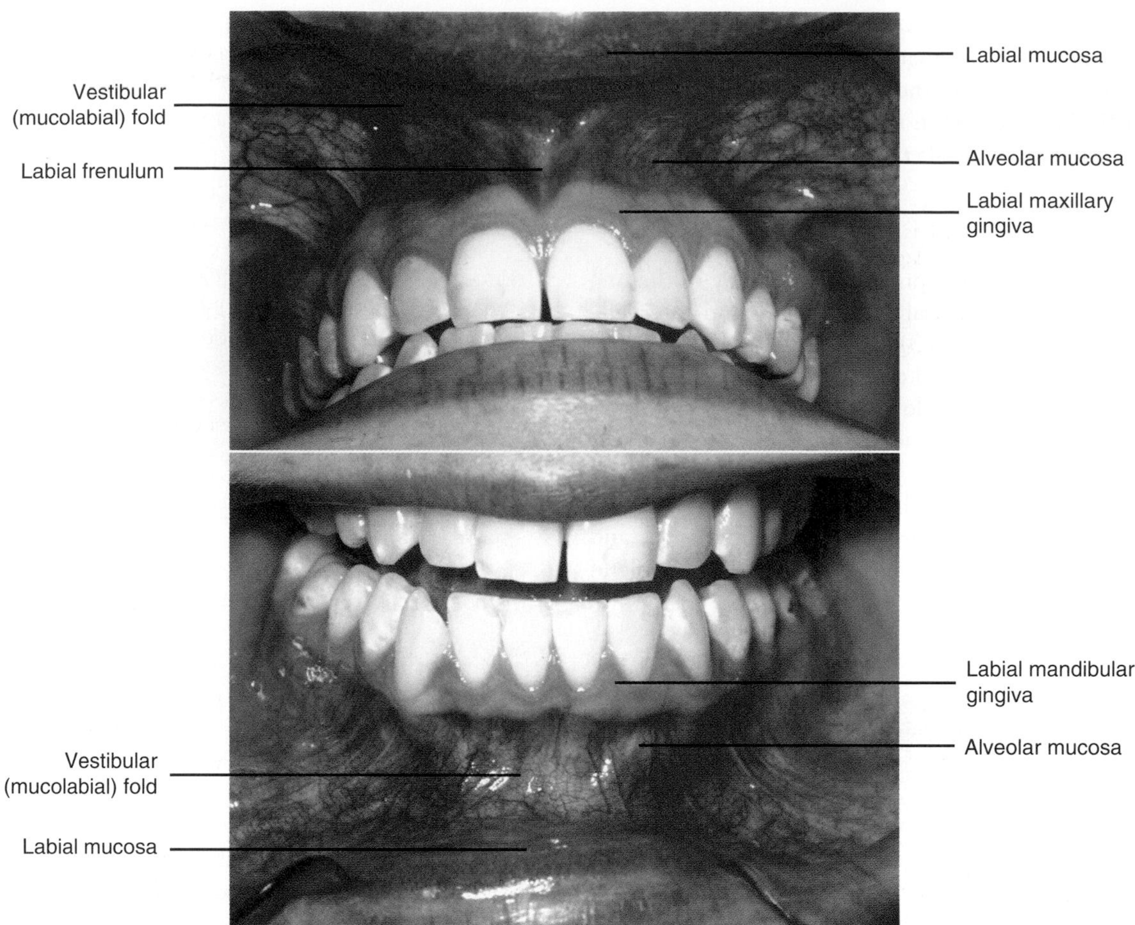


**FIG. 10.4** Vestibule and vestibular tissue of the oral cavity. *(From Liebgott B: The anatomical basis of dentistry, ed 3, St Louis, 2010, Mosby.)*

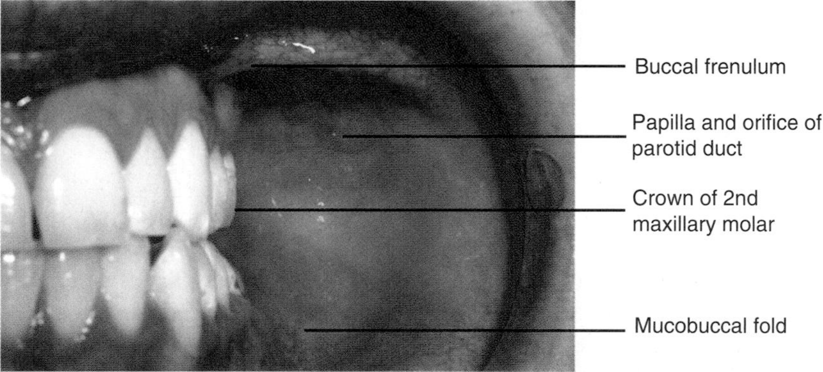


**FIG. 10.5** Buccal vestibule and buccal mucosa of the cheek. The opening of the parotid duct is seen opposite the second maxillary molar. *(From Liebgott B: The anatomical basis of dentistry, ed 3, St Louis, 2010, Mosby.)*

parotid duct (Stensen's duct) of the parotid salivary gland (see Fig. 10.5).

**Fordyce's spots** (or *granules*) are normal, small, yellowish elevations that may appear on the buccal mucosa. Another normal variation noted on the buccal mucosa is the **linea alba**. This white ridge of raised tissue extends horizontally at the level where the maxillary and mandibular teeth come together (Fig. 10.7).

## Labial and Other Frenula

A **frenum**, or *frenulum* (plural, *frenula*), is a narrow band of tissue that connects two structures. The *maxillary* **labial frenum** passes from the oral mucosa at the midline of the maxillary arch to the midline of the inner surface of the upper lip. The *mandibular labial frenum* passes from the oral mucosa at the

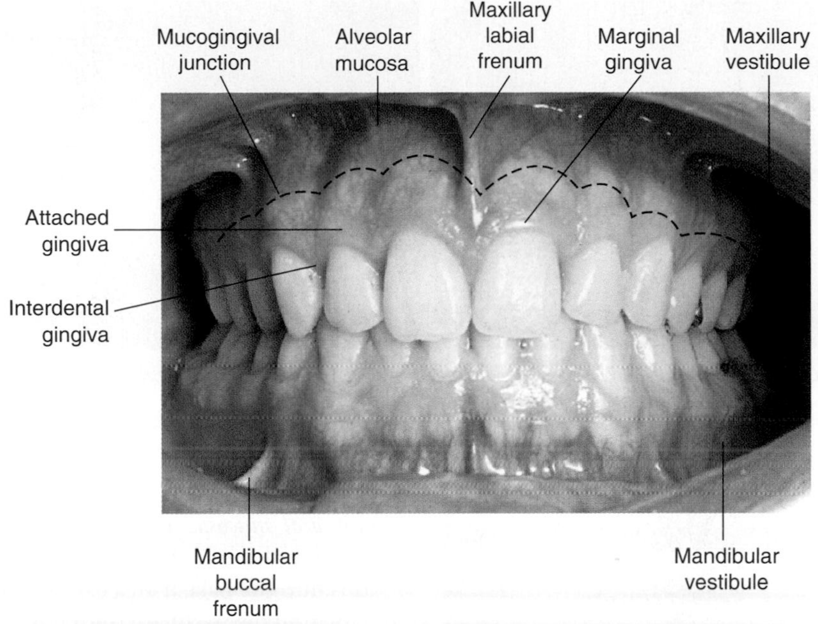


**FIG. 10.6** View of gingivae and associated anatomical landmarks.

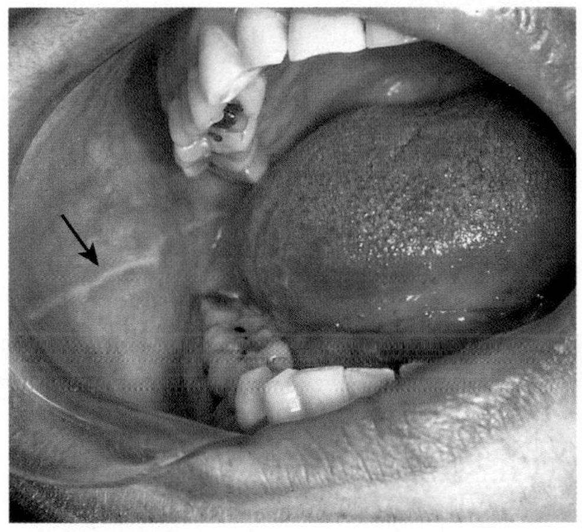

**FIG. 10.7** Linea alba *(arrow). (From Ibsen O, Phelan J: Oral pathology for the dental hygienist, ed 6, St Louis, 2014, Saunders.)*

midline of the mandibular arch to the midline of the inner surface of the lower lip.

In the area of the first maxillary permanent molar, the *buccal frenum* passes from the oral mucosa of the outer surface of the maxillary arch to the inner surface of the cheek. The **lingual frenum** passes from the floor of the mouth to the midline of the ventral border of the tongue (see Fig. 10.5).

RECALL

3 What types of tissue cover the oral cavity?
4 What are the two regions of the oral cavity?
5 What is the name of the structure that passes from the oral mucosa to the facial midline of the mandibular arch?

## Gingiva

The **gingiva** (plural, *gingivae*), commonly referred to as the "gums," is masticatory mucosa that covers the alveolar processes of the jaws and surrounds the necks of the teeth (see Fig. 10.6). Normal gingival tissue has the following characteristics:

- Gingiva surrounds the tooth like a collar and is self-cleansing.
- Gingiva is firm and resistant and can be tightly adapted to the tooth and bone.
- Surfaces of the attached gingiva and interdental papillae are stippled and resemble the rind of an orange.
- The color of the gingival surface varies according to the individual's pigmentation (Fig. 10.8).

### Unattached Gingiva

Unattached gingiva, also known as *marginal gingiva* or *free gingiva,* is the border of the gingiva that surrounds the teeth in a collar-like fashion (Fig. 10.9).

The unattached gingiva, which is usually light pink or coral, is not bound to the underlying tissue of the tooth. It consists of the tissues from the top of the gingival margin to the base of the gingival sulcus. The unattached gingiva is usually about 1 mm wide, and it forms the soft wall of the gingival sulcus. (The *sulcus* is the space between the tooth and the gum where popcorn husks become lodged.) The unattached gingiva is the first tissue to respond to inflammation.

### Interdental Gingiva

The interdental gingiva, also known as *interdental papilla* (plural, *papillae*), is the extension of the free gingiva that fills the interproximal embrasure between two adjacent teeth.

### Gingival Groove

The gingival groove, also known as the *free gingival groove,* is a shallow groove that runs parallel to the margin of the unattached gingiva and marks the beginning of the attached gingiva.

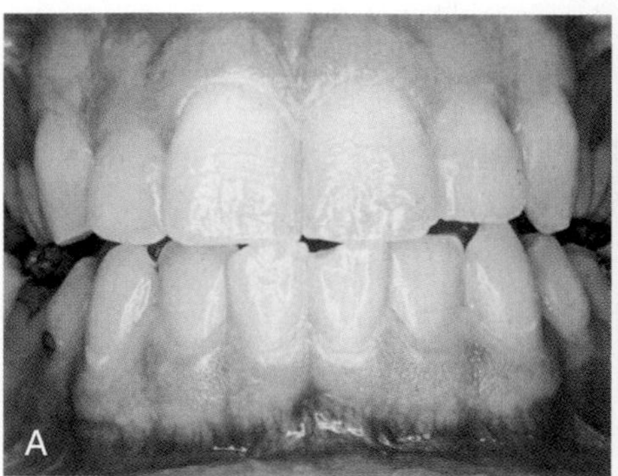


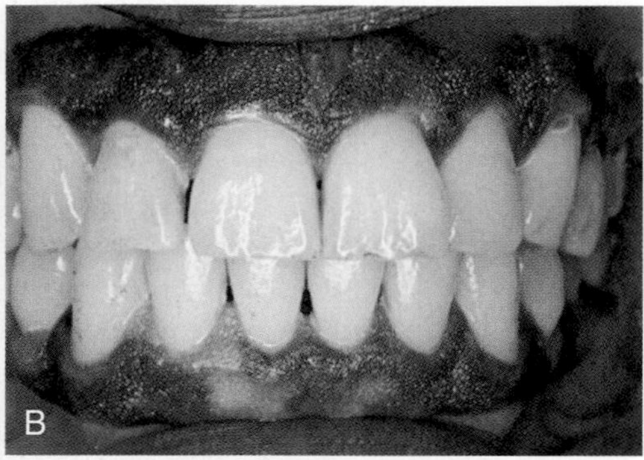


**FIG. 10.8** A, Clinically normal gingivae in light-skinned individual. B, Clinically normal pigmented gingivae in a dark-skinned individual. *(From Glickman I, Smulow JB: Periodontal disease: clinical, radiographic, and histopathologic features, Philadelphia, 1974, Saunders.)*

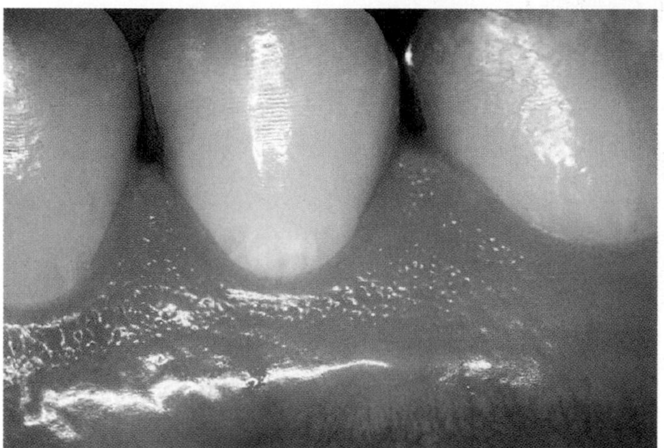

**FIG. 10.9** Close-up view of gingivae and associated anatomical landmarks.

### *Attached Gingiva*

The attached gingiva extends from the base of the sulcus to the mucogingival junction. It is a stippled, dense tissue that is self-protecting, firmly bound, and resilient.

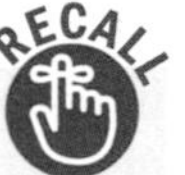


6 What is the anatomical term for the gums?
7 What is another term for unattached gingiva?
8 What is another term for interdental gingiva?

# The Oral Cavity Proper

Hold your teeth together, and with your tongue, feel the areas of the oral cavity proper. The oral cavity proper is the area inside of the dental arches. In back of your last molar is a space that links the vestibule with the oral cavity proper.

## Hard Palate

With your tongue, feel your hard palate, or the roof of your mouth. The hard palate separates the nasal cavity above from the oral cavity below (Fig. 10.10, *A*). The nasal surfaces are covered with *respiratory mucosa,* and the oral surfaces are covered with *oral mucosa.* The mucosa of the hard palate is tightly bound to the underlying bone, which is why submucosal injections into the palatal area can be extremely painful.

Behind the maxillary central incisors is the **incisive papilla**, a pear-shaped pad of tissue that covers the incisive foramen. This is the site of injection for anesthesia of the nasopalatine nerve. Extending laterally from the incisive papilla are irregular ridges or folds of masticatory mucosa, called palatal *rugae.* Running posteriorly from the incisive papilla is the midline palatal *raphe.* Numerous minor palatal glands open onto the palatal mucosa as small pits.

## Soft Palate

Move your tongue to the back of your hard palate, and feel where the soft palate begins. The soft palate is the movable posterior third of the palate (Fig. 10.10, *B*). It has no bony support and hangs into the pharynx behind it. The soft palate ends with a pear-shaped hanging projection of tissue, called the **uvula** (see Fig. 10.10, *B*).

The soft palate is supported posteriorly by two arches, the *fauces.* The *anterior arch* runs from the soft palate down to the lateral aspects of the tongue as the **anterior faucial pillar**. The *posterior arch* is the free posterior border of the soft palate and is called the **posterior faucial pillar** (see Fig. 10.10, *B*). The opening between the two arches, called the **isthmus of fauces**, contains the palatine tonsil.

RECALL

9 What is the pear-shaped pad of tissue behind the maxillary incisors?
10 What is the hanging projection of tissue at the border of the soft palate?

## Tongue

The tongue is composed mainly of muscles. It is covered on top with a thick layer of mucous membrane and thousands of tiny projections called *papillae.* Inside the papillae are the sensory organs and nerves for both taste and touch. On a healthy tongue, the papillae are usually pinkish-white and velvety smooth.

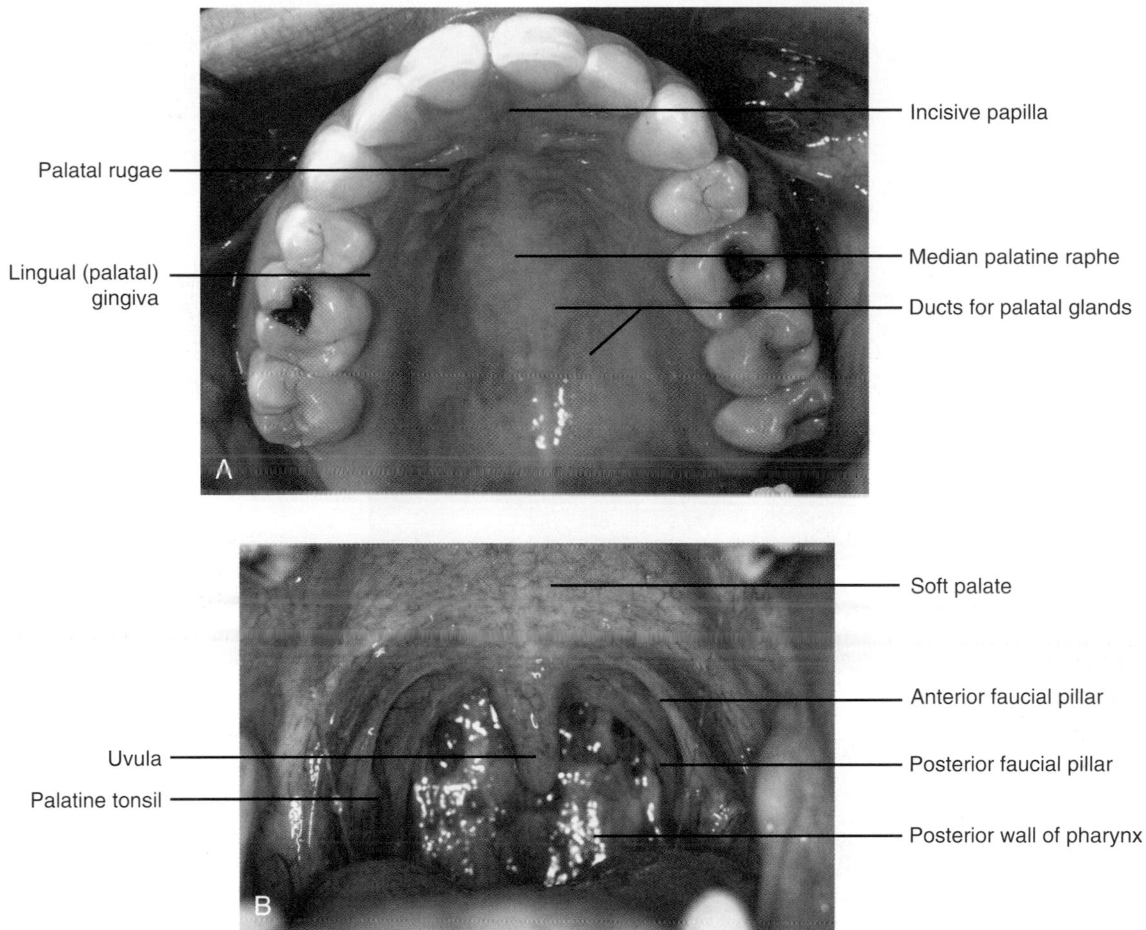


**FIG. 10.10** A, Surface features of the hard palate. B, Surface features of the soft palate. *(From Liebgott B: The anatomical basis of dentistry, ed 3, St Louis, 2010, Mosby.)*

The tongue is one of the body's most versatile organs and is responsible for a number of functions: (1) speaking, (2) positioning food while eating, (3) tasting and tactile sensations, (4) swallowing, and (5) cleansing the oral cavity. After eating, note how your tongue moves from crevice to crevice, seeking out and removing bits of retained food in your mouth.

The anterior two thirds of the tongue, called the *body*, is found in the oral cavity. The *root* of the tongue is the posterior part that turns vertically downward to the pharynx. The *dorsum* comprises the superior (upper) and posterior roughened aspects of the tongue. It is covered with small papillae of various shapes and colors (Fig. 10.11).

The *sublingual surface* of the tongue is covered with thin, smooth, transparent mucosa through which many underlying vessels can be seen (Fig. 10.12). Two small papillae are seen on either side of the lingual frenulum (frenum) just behind the central incisors. Through these papillae into the mouth are the openings of the submandibular ducts. The saliva enters the oral cavity through these ducts. Salivary glands are discussed in detail in Chapter 9.

On either side of the lingual surface are two smaller *fimbriated folds.* The lingual frenum is the thin fold of mucous membrane that extends from the floor of the mouth to the underside of the tongue.

## Clinical Considerations: Gag Reflex

When working in a patient's mouth, the dental assistant must be very careful not to accidentally trigger the gag reflex. Touching the membranes of the soft palate, the fauces, and the posterior portion of the tongue can trigger the gag reflex and may cause gagging or vomiting.

## Clinical Considerations: Lingual Frenula

Mobility of the tongue can be severely limited when the lingual frenum is unusually short. When this occurs, speech can be difficult for the patient, and performing dental procedures such as radiographs and taking impressions can be difficult for the operator. The condition is commonly called "tongue tied," and it can be easily corrected through a surgical procedure called a *lingual frenectomy,* during which the lingual frenulum is cut.

RECALL

**11** What is the term for the upper surface of the tongue?
**12** What is the thin fold of mucous membrane that extends from the floor of the mouth to the underside of the tongue?

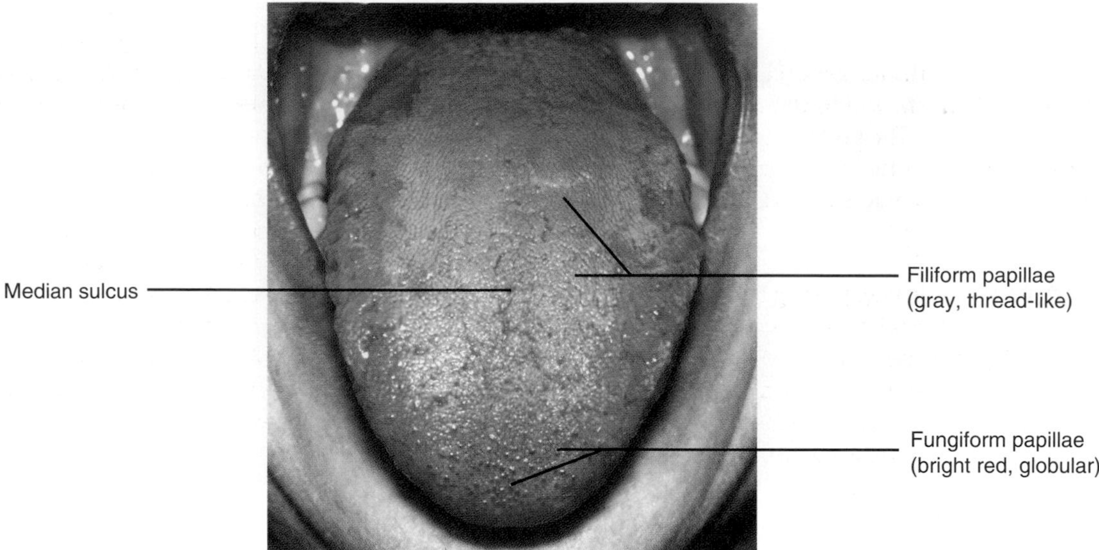


**FIG. 10.11** Dorsum of the tongue. *(From Liebgott B: The anatomical basis of dentistry, ed 3, St Louis, 2010, Mosby.)*

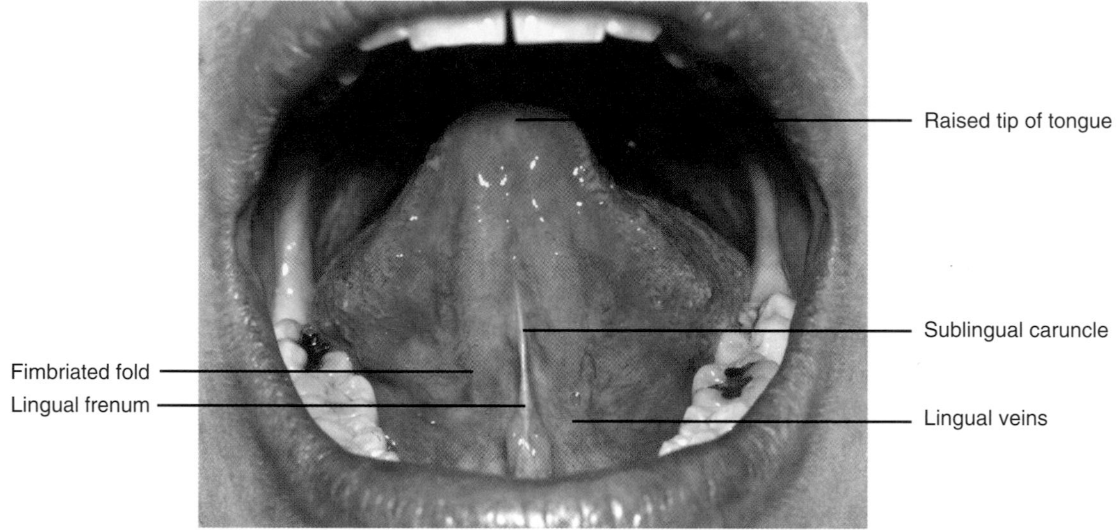


**FIG. 10.12** Sublingual aspect of the tongue. *(From Liebgott B: The anatomical basis of dentistry, ed 3, St Louis, 2010, Mosby.)*

## Taste Buds

The taste buds are the organs that allow us to enjoy the flavors of food and that give us warning when foods are too hot. They are located on the dorsum (top side) of the tongue. Saliva is necessary to stimulate the taste buds to detect flavors. If your mouth were dry, you would not be able to taste anything.

The taste buds are located on the **fungiform papillae** and in the trough of the large **vallate papillae**, which form a V on the posterior portion of the tongue. The sense of *touch* is provided by numerous **filiform papillae** that cover the entire surface of the tongue. These filiform papillae contain no taste receptors.

Although thousands of flavors are known, it is believed that only four primary tastes combine to create all flavors. These primary tastes are salty, sweet, sour, and bitter.

You may note that some substances taste sweet when they enter the mouth but taste bitter by the time they reach the back. Saccharin is an example of one such substance. Of the four primary tastes, the one that is most easily distinguished is bitter. It is thought that this unmistakable taste would serve as a protective mechanism. Many deadly toxins taste bitter, and a person spits them out before they can do harm.

## Teeth

Humans have two sets of teeth during a lifetime. These teeth sit in bony sockets called *alveoli,* within the alveolar process of the maxilla and the mandible. The portion of the tooth that is visible in the oral cavity, called the *crown,* is surrounded by a cuff of gingival tissue. Dental anatomy is discussed in detail in Chapters 11 and 12.

■ **Eye to the Future** You can help prevent the early signs of aging by protecting your lips and the skin on your face from drying and chapping. Drying of the skin can be caused by soaps and detergents, dry indoor air, and exposure to sun or windy weather. Even the face masks you wear in the dental office can cause irritation to your face. You should gently pat, not vigorously rub, your skin dry after washing. Use emollient creams or lotions liberally and regularly to soften and moisturize your skin. ■

### ■ Critical Thinking

1. The dentist asked you to take an alginate impression of the maxillary and mandibular arches on Mr. Wong, but you are having a difficult time moving the patient's tongue out of the way to seat the impression tray. Mr. Wong tells you that he is "tongue tied." What does this mean?
2. Sixteen-year-old Letecia Williams is in your office complaining of a painful bump on her palate in back of her upper front teeth. She explains that she ate very hot pizza and burned the roof of her mouth. What is the normal oral landmark that may have been burned by the pizza?
3. Thirteen-year-old Ronnie is curious about the sensation of taste. He asks you to explain how the tongue can taste sweet and sour. How would you answer? ■

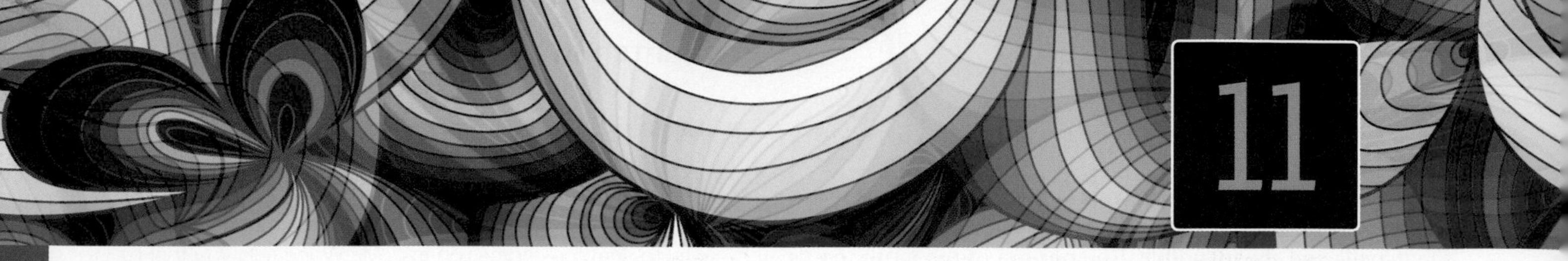

11

# Overview of the Dentitions

## KEY TERMS

**Angle's classification** System developed by Dr. Edward H. Angle to describe and classify occlusion and malocclusion.
**Anterior** Toward the front.
**Apical third** Division of the root nearest the tip of the root.
**Buccal surface** Tooth surface closest to the inner cheek.
**Buccolingual division** Lengthwise division of the crown in a labial or buccolingual direction, consisting of the *facial* or *buccal/labial* third, *middle* third, and *lingual* third.
**Centric occlusion** Maximum contact between the occluding surfaces of the maxillary and mandibular teeth.
**Cervical third** Division of the root nearest the neck of the tooth.
**Concave** Curved inward.
**Contact area** Area of the mesial or distal surface of a tooth that touches the adjacent tooth in the same arch.
**Convex** Curved outward.
**Curve of Spee** Curvature formed by the maxillary and mandibular arches in occlusion.
**Curve of Wilson** Cross-arch curvature of the occlusal plane.
**Deciduous (duh-SID-yoo-us)** Pertaining to first dentition of 20 teeth; often called "baby teeth" or primary teeth.
**Dentition (den-TI-shun)** Natural teeth in the dental arch.
**Distal surface** Surface of tooth distant from the midline.
**Distoclusion (DIS-toe-kloo-shun)** A class II malocclusion in which the mesiobuccal cusp of the maxillary first molar occludes (by more than the width of a premolar) mesial to the mesiobuccal groove of the mandibular first molar.
**Embrasure (em-BRAY-zhur)** Triangular space in a gingival direction between the proximal surfaces of two adjoining teeth in contact.
**Facial surface** Tooth surface closest to the face. Facial surfaces closest to the lips are called *labial surfaces*, and facial surfaces closest to the inner cheek are called *buccal surfaces*; therefore the term *facial* can be substituted for *labial* and *buccal*, and vice versa.
**Functional occlusion** Contact of the teeth during biting and chewing movements.
**Incisal surface** Chewing surface of anterior teeth.
**Interproximal (in-tur-PROK-si-mul) space** The area between adjacent tooth surfaces.
**Labial surface** Facial surface closest to the lips.
**Labioversion** The inclination of the teeth to extend facially beyond the normal overlap of the incisal edge of the maxillary incisors over the mandibular incisors.
**Line angle** Junction of two walls in a cavity preparation.
**Lingual surface** Surface of mandibular and maxillary teeth closest to the tongue; also called *palatal surface*.
**Linguoversion** Position in which the maxillary incisors are behind the mandibular incisors.
**Malocclusion (MAL-o-kloo-zhun)** Occlusion that is deviated from a class I normal occlusion.
**Mandibular (man-DIB-you-ler) arch** The lower jaw.
**Masticatory (MAS-ti-kuh-tor-ee) surface** The chewing surface of the teeth.
**Maxillary (MAK-si-lar-ee) arch** The upper jaw.
**Mesial surface** Surface of the tooth toward the midline.
**Mesioclusion (MEE-zee-oe-kloo-zhun)** Term used for class III malocclusion.
**Mesiodistal division** Lengthwise division of the crown in a mesiodistal (front-to-back) direction, consisting of the *mesial* third, *middle* third, and *distal* third.
**Middle third** Division of the root in the middle.
**Mixed dentition** A mixture of permanent teeth and primary teeth that occurs until all primary teeth have been lost, usually between ages 6 and 12.
**Nasmyth's membrane** Residue from epithelial tissue on the crowns of newly erupted teeth that may become extrinsically stained.
**Neutroclusion** An ideal mesiodistal relationship between the jaws and the dental arches.
**Occlusal surface** Chewing surface of posterior teeth.
**Occlusion (oe-KLOO-zhun)** The natural contact of the maxillary and mandibular teeth in all positions.
**Occlusocervical division** Crosswise division of the crown that is parallel to the occlusal or incisal surface, consisting of the *occlusal* third, *middle* third, and *cervical* third.
**Palatal surface** Lingual surface of maxillary teeth.
**Permanent dentition** The set of 32 secondary teeth.
**Point angle** Angle formed by the junction of three surfaces.
**Posterior** Toward the back.
**Primary dentition** The first set of 20 primary teeth.
**Proximal surfaces** The surfaces next to each other when teeth are adjacent in the arch.
**Quadrant** One quarter of the dentition.
**Sextant** One sixth of the dentition.
**Succedaneous (suk-se-DAY-nee-us) teeth** Permanent teeth that replace primary teeth.

## LEARNING OUTCOMES

*On completion of this chapter, the student will be able to achieve the following objectives:*

1. Pronounce, define, and spell the key terms.
2. Name the three dentition periods and explain the differences between them.
3. Name the two dental arches and explain two ways that the arches can be divided.
4. Describe the types and functions of teeth.
5. Name and identify tooth surfaces.
6. Describe the anatomical features of the teeth.
7. Explain the concepts of angles and division of teeth.
8. Discuss occlusion and malocclusion of teeth, including the following:

- Explain the terms occlusion, centric occlusion, and malocclusion.
- Explain Angle's classification of malocclusion.

9 Explain the three factors of stabilization of the arches.
10 Name and describe the three primary systems of tooth numbering, and identify teeth using each system.

## ELECTRONIC RESOURCES

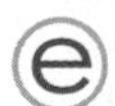

***Additional information related to content in Chapter 11 can be found on the companion Evolve Web site.***

- Practice Quiz
- Canadian Content Corner

In this chapter, you will learn the names and locations of various types of teeth in the human dentition. You will also learn their functions and how they relate to each other in the same dental arch and to teeth in the opposing arch. In preparation for learning dental charting, you will learn the common systems of tooth numbering, as well as the patterns of tooth eruption.

# Dentition Periods

During a lifetime, people have two sets of teeth: the primary dentition and the permanent dentition. **Dentition** describes the natural teeth in the dental arch. Although only two sets of teeth develop, *three dentition periods* have been identified. These periods are *primary, mixed,* and *permanent.*

The first set of 20 primary teeth is called the **primary dentition**, commonly referred to as the "baby teeth." You may also hear the term **deciduous** dentition. This is an older dental term that is less frequently used to describe the primary dentition.

The **permanent dentition** refers to the 32 secondary teeth, or "adult teeth." The permanent teeth that replace the primary teeth are called **succedaneous teeth**, meaning that these teeth "succeed" (come after) deciduous teeth. Because 20 primary teeth are present, 20 succedaneous teeth have also been noted. Molars are *not* succedaneous teeth because premolars replace the primary molars.

The **mixed dentition** period takes place between about 6 and 12 years of age. Until a child is about 6 years old, the primary dentition is in place. At about that age, the first permanent teeth begin to emerge into the mouth, and there is a mixture of permanent teeth and primary teeth until about age 12, when all primary teeth have been lost (Table 11.1).

## Primary Dentition

Only primary teeth are present in the mouth during the primary dentition period. This period occurs between approximately 6 months and 6 years of age (Table 11.2). The primary dentition period begins with the eruption of the primary mandibular central incisors and ends when the first permanent mandibular molar erupts (Fig. 11.1).

## Mixed Dentition

### Clinical Considerations: Nasmyth's Membrane

During the early eruption of all teeth of both dentitions, a thin residue of epithelium tissue called the Nasmyth's membrane may form over the crown of the teeth. This residue may become stained from food debris. It is removed by a gentle coronal polish (see Chapter 58).

While in the mixed dentition period, children lose their primary teeth, and permanent teeth begin to erupt. During this period, children have both primary and permanent teeth in their mouth (Fig. 11.2). The mixed dentition period begins with the eruption of the first permanent tooth and ends with the shedding of the last primary tooth.

The mixed dentition period is often a difficult time for children because color differences between the primary and permanent teeth become apparent (primary teeth are whiter than permanent teeth), and they may notice the difference in crown

**TABLE 11.1 Dentition Periods and Clinical Considerations**

| Dentition Period | Approximate Time Span | Teeth Marking Start of Period | Dentition Present | Growth of Jawbones |
|---|---|---|---|---|
| Primary dentition period | 6 months to 6 years | Eruption of primary mandibular central incisor | Primary | Beginning |
| Mixed dentition | 6 years to 12 years | Eruption of permanent mandibular first molar | Primary and permanent | Fastest and most noticeable |
| Permanent dentition period | After 12 years | Shedding of primary maxillary second molar | Usually permanent | Slowest and least noticeable |

Adapted from Fehrenbach MJ, Popowics T: *Illustrated dental embryology, histology, and anatomy,* ed 4, St Louis, 2016, Saunders; and Nelson SJ, Ash MM: *Wheeler's dental anatomy, physiology, and occlusion,* ed 9, St Louis, 2010, Saunders.

**TABLE 11.2 Primary Dentition in Order of Eruption**

| Dentition | Date of Eruption | Date of Exfoliation |
|---|---|---|
| **Maxillary Teeth** | | |
| Central incisor | 6–10 months | 6–7 years |
| Lateral incisor | 9–12 months | 7–8 years |
| First molar | 12–18 months | 9–11 years |
| Canine | 16–22 months | 10–12 years |
| Second molar | 24–32 months | 10–12 years |
| **Mandibular Teeth** | | |
| Central incisor | 6–10 months | 6–7 years |
| Lateral incisor | 7–10 months | 7–8 years |
| First molar | 12–18 months | 9–11 years |
| Canine | 16–22 months | 9–12 years |
| Second molar | 20–32 months | 10–12 years |

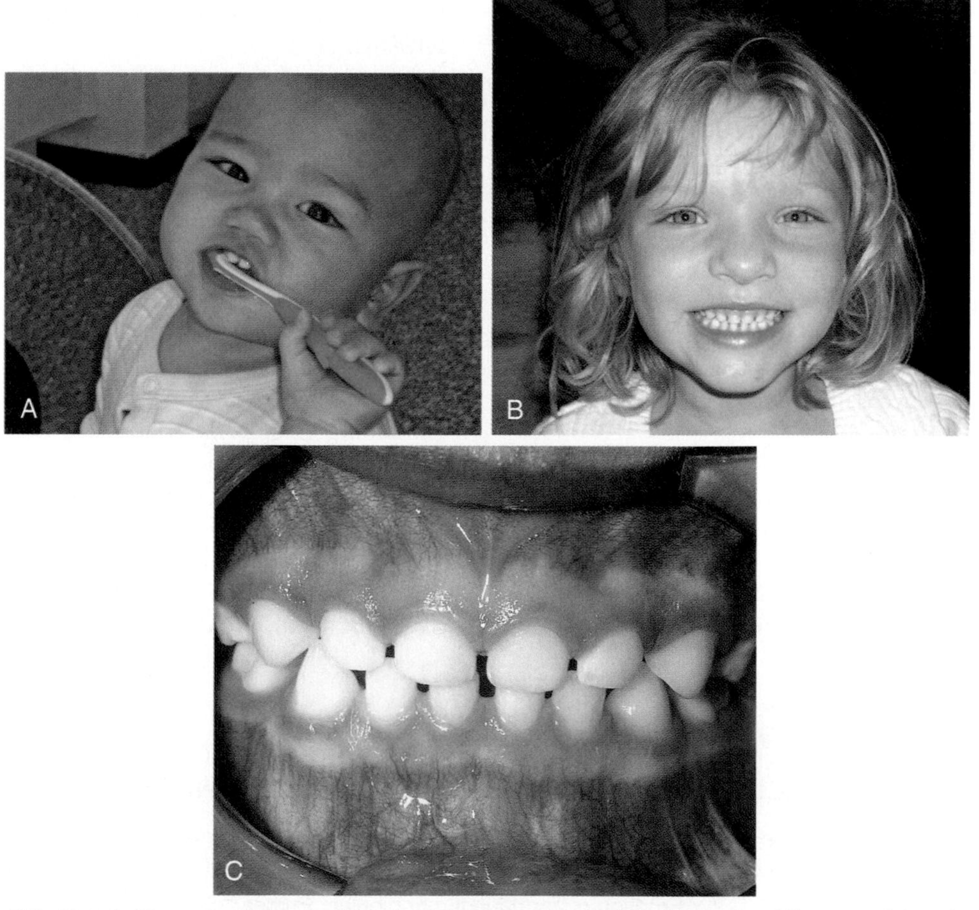

**FIG. 11.1** A, Example of the dentition in a 9-month-old child. B, Example of the complete primary dentition. C, Labial view of the primary dentition. Note the attrition of the masticatory surfaces of the dentition. Primate spaces of the primary dentition are indicated by the arrows. *(C, From Fehrenbach MJ, Popowics T: Illustrated dental embryology, histology, and anatomy, ed 4, St Louis, 2016, Saunders.)*

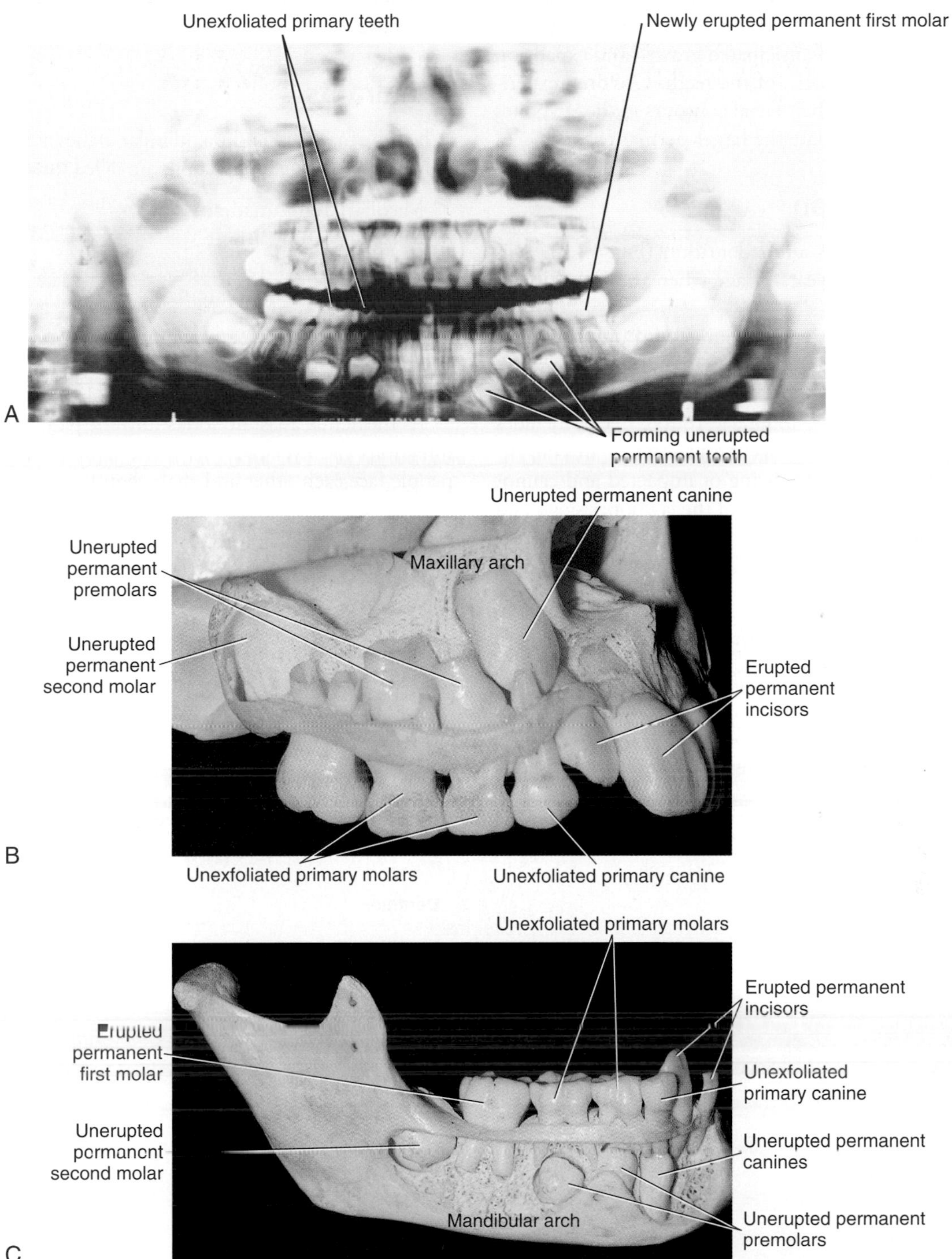


**FIG. 11.2** Examples of mixed dentition with primary teeth being shed and the permanent dentition erupting. A, Radiograph of mixed dentition. Note the permanent teeth still forming within the jaw bones of each arch. B and C, Maxilla and mandible of a skull, with a section of facial compact bone removed. *(From Fehrenbach MJ, Popowics T: Illustrated dental embryology, histology, and anatomy, ed 4, St Louis, 2016, Saunders.)*

size between larger permanent teeth and smaller primary teeth. Some children may notice crowding of the teeth as they shift positions during eruption.

Decisions regarding dental treatment are often based on the dentition period. For example, orthodontic treatment may be started or delayed because of anticipated growth and expansion of the jawbones and movement of the teeth. Children experience noticeable changes in their facial contours as the jawbones begin to grow to accommodate the larger permanent teeth.

## Permanent Dentition

The permanent dentition is adult dentition (Fig. 11.3). This period begins at about 12 years of age when the last primary tooth is shed (Table 11.3).

After eruption of the permanent canines and premolars and eruption of second permanent molars, the permanent dentition is complete at about age 14 to 15, except for the third molars, which are not completed until about age 18 to 25. This includes eruption of all permanent teeth, except for teeth that are congenitally (from the time of birth) missing or impacted and cannot erupt (usually, third molars). Growth of the jawbones slows and eventually stops. Minimal growth of the jaw occurs overall during the permanent dentition period because puberty has passed.

# Dental Arches

In the human mouth, there are two dental arches: the maxillary and the mandibular. The layperson may refer to the maxillary arch as the upper jaw and the mandibular arch as the lower jaw.

The **maxillary arch** *(upper arch),* which is actually part of the skull, is not capable of movement. The teeth in the upper arch are set in the *maxilla,* the maxillary bone.

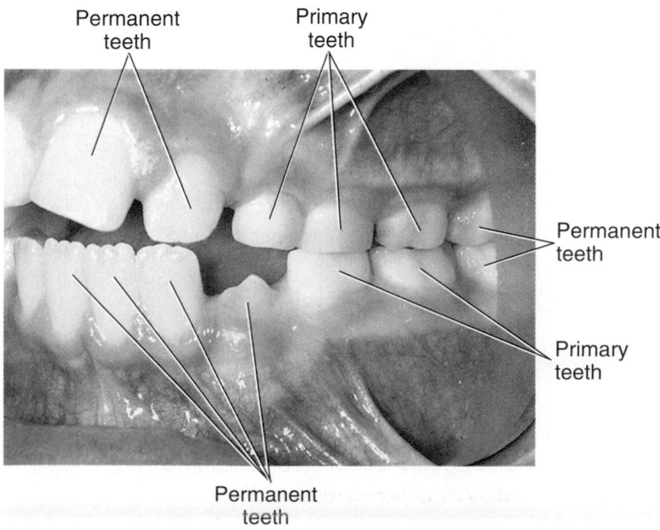


**FIG. 11.3** An example of the oral cavity during the mixed dentition period. The primary and permanent teeth are identified. *(From Fehrenbach MJ, Popowics T: Illustrated dental embryology, histology, and anatomy, ed 4, St Louis, 2016, Saunders.)*

The **mandibular arch** *(lower arch)* is movable through the action of the temporomandibular joint, and it applies force against the immovable maxillary arch (see Chapter 9).

When the teeth of both arches are in contact, the teeth are in **occlusion**.

## Quadrants

When the maxillary and mandibular arches are each divided into halves, the resulting four sections are called **quadrants**, as follows:

- Maxillary right quadrant
- Maxillary left quadrant
- Mandibular left quadrant
- Mandibular right quadrant

Each quadrant of permanent dentition contains *eight* permanent teeth (4 × 8 = 32), and a quadrant of primary dentition contains *five* teeth (4 × 5 = 20) (Fig. 11.4).

As the dental assistant looks into the patient's oral cavity, the directions are reversed. This is the same concept as when two people face each other and shake hands.

## Sextants

Each arch can also be divided into sextants rather than quadrants. A **sextant** is one sixth of the dentition. There are three sextants in each arch. The dental arch is divided as follows (Fig. 11.5):

- Maxillary right posterior sextant
- Maxillary anterior sextant

**TABLE 11.3** Permanent Dentition in Order of Eruption

| Dentition | Eruption Date |
|---|---|
| **Maxillary Teeth** | |
| First molar | 6–7 years |
| Central incisor | 7–8 years |
| Lateral incisor | 8–9 years |
| First premolar | 10–11 years |
| Second premolar | 10–12 years |
| Canine | 11–12 years |
| Second molar | 12–13 years |
| Third molar | 17–21 years |
| **Mandibular Teeth** | |
| First molar | 6–7 years |
| Central incisor | 6–7 years |
| Lateral incisor | 7–8 years |
| Cuspid | 9–10 years |
| First premolar | 10–11 years |
| Second premolar | 12–13 years |
| Second molar | 11–13 years |
| Third molar | 17–21 years |

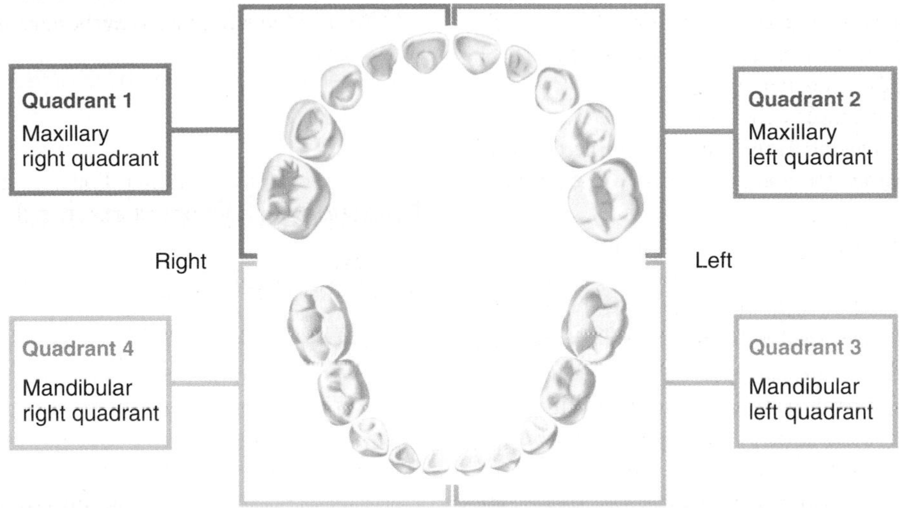


A **Primary Dentition**

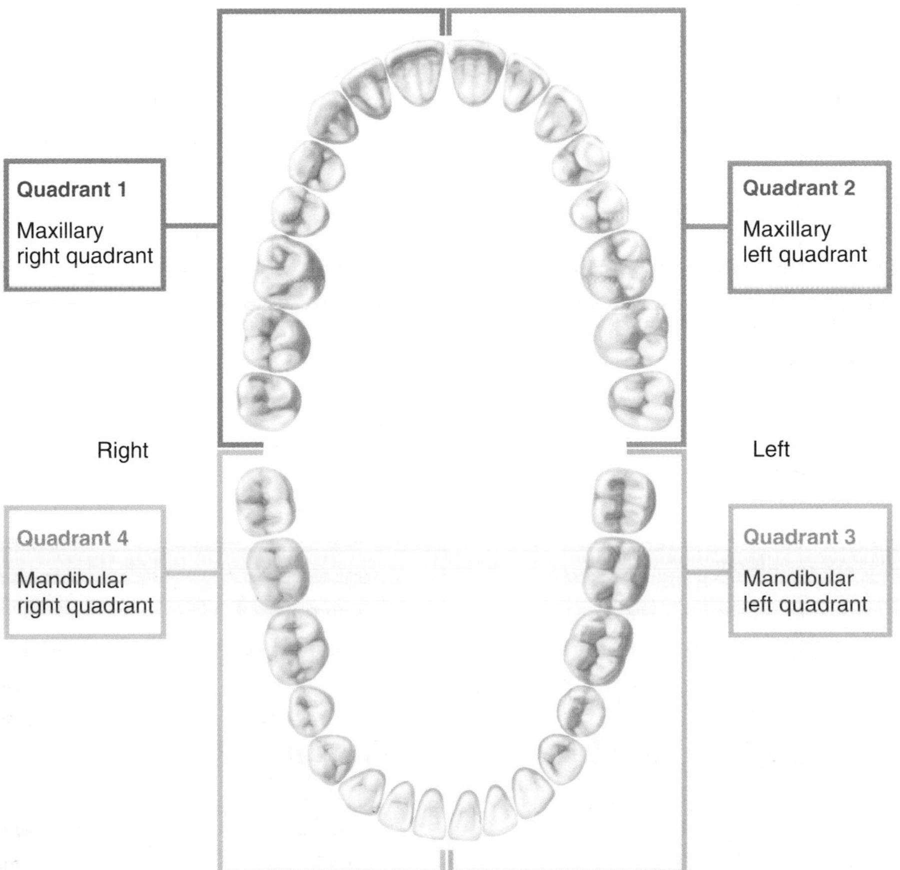


B **Permanent Dentition**

**FIG. 11.4** A, Primary dentition separated into quadrants. B, Permanent dentition separated into quadrants. *(© Elsevier Collection.)*

- Maxillary left posterior sextant
- Mandibular right posterior sextant
- Mandibular anterior sextant
- Mandibular left posterior sextant

## Anterior and Posterior Teeth

To assist in describing their locations and functions, teeth are classified as being **anterior** (toward the front) or **posterior** (toward the back).

The anterior teeth are the incisors and canines. These are the teeth that are usually visible when people smile. The anterior teeth are aligned in a gentle curve. The posterior teeth are the premolars and molars. These teeth are aligned with little or no curvature and appear to be in an almost straight line. Remembering how these teeth are aligned in the dental arch will be important when you begin exposing radiographs.

RECALL

1 What are the two sets of teeth that people have in their lifetime?
2 How many teeth are in each dentition?
3 What is the term for the four sections of the divided dental arches?
4 What are the terms for the front teeth and for the back teeth?

## Types and Functions of Teeth

Humans are omnivorous, which means they eat both meat and plants. To accommodate this variety in diet, human teeth are designed for cutting, tearing, and grinding different types of food.

The permanent dentition is divided into four types of teeth: *incisors, canines, premolars,* and *molars.* The primary dentition consists of incisors, canines, and molars. There are no premolars in the primary dentition (Fig. 11.6).

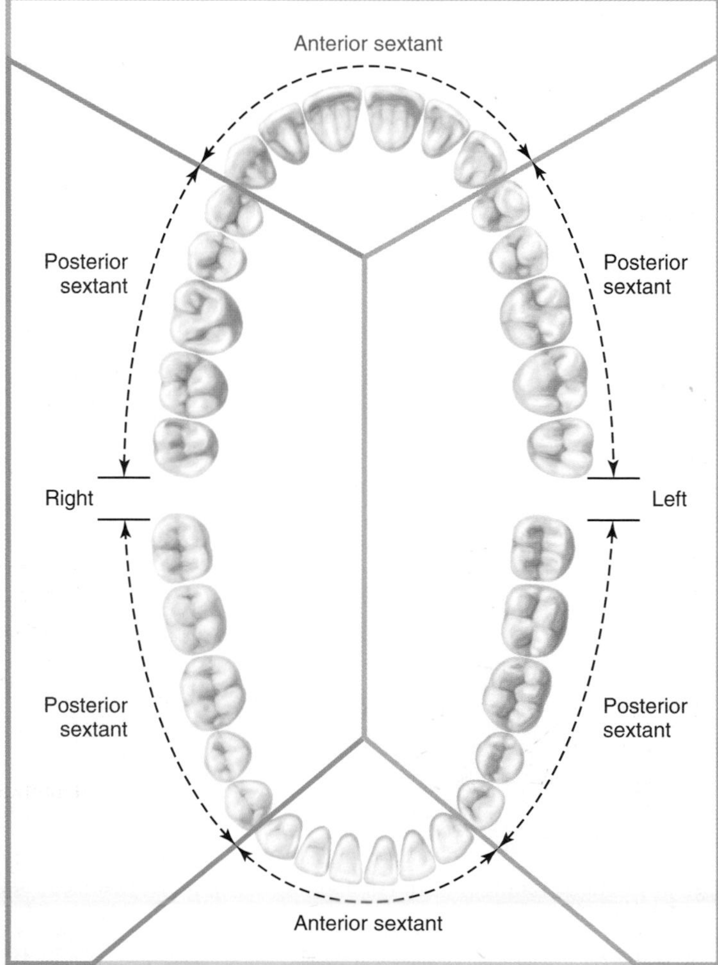


**FIG. 11.5** Permanent dentition separated into sextants. *(© Elsevier Collection.)*

## Incisors

Incisors are single-rooted teeth with a relatively sharp, thin edge. Located at the front of the mouth, they are designed to cut food without the application of heavy force (an incisor is something that makes an incision, or cut). The tongue side, or lingual surface, is shaped like a shovel to aid in guiding food into the mouth.

## Canines

The canines, also known as cuspids, are located at the "corner" of the arch. They are designed for cutting and tearing foods, which requires the application of force. These teeth in dogs are designed for tearing food or protecting themselves.

The canines are the longest teeth in the human dentition. They are also some of the best-anchored and most stable teeth because they have the longest roots. Canines are usually the last teeth to be lost. Because of its sturdy crown, long root, and location in the arch, the canine is referred to as the "cornerstone" of the dental arch.

## Premolars

There are four maxillary and four mandibular premolars. The premolars are a cross between canines and molars. You may hear the older term *bicuspids* used occasionally. This term is inaccurate because it refers to *two* ("bi") cusps, and some premolars have three cusps. Therefore the newer term *premolar* is preferred. The pointed buccal cusps hold the food while the lingual cusps grind it. Premolars are not as long as canines, and they have a broader surface for chewing food. (There are no premolars in the primary dentition.)

## Molars

Molars are much larger than premolars, usually having four or more cusps. The function of the 12 molars is to chew or grind up food. There are four or five cusps on the occlusal (biting) surface of each molar, depending on its location.

Maxillary and mandibular molars differ greatly from each other in shape, size, and number of cusps and roots. The unique characteristics of each tooth are discussed in Chapter 12.

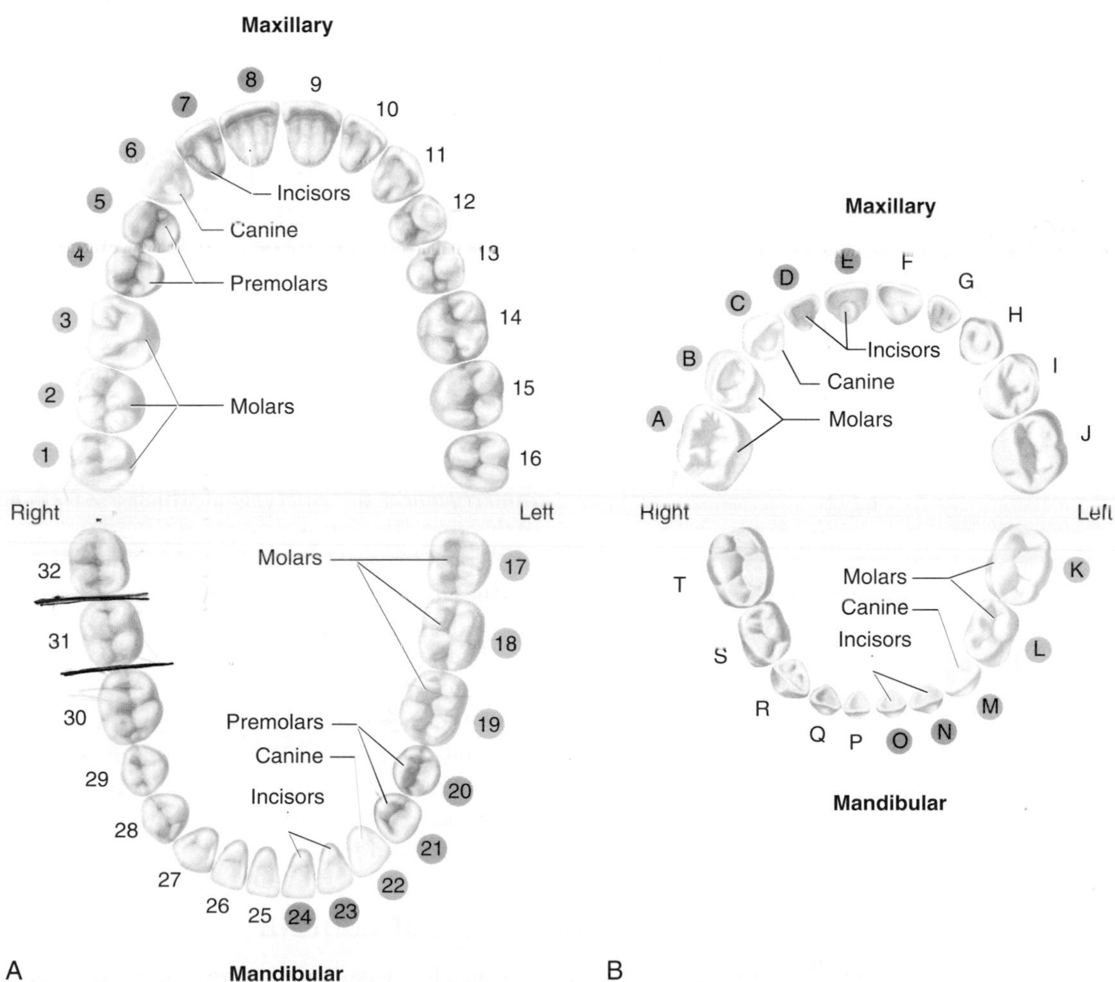


**FIG. 11.6** A, Occlusal view of the permanent dentition. Types of teeth are identified through the Universal/National System. B, Occlusal view of the primary dentition. *(© Elsevier Collection.)*

5 What are the four types of teeth?
6 Which tooth is referred to as the "cornerstone" of the dental arch?

## Tooth Surfaces

Imagine each tooth as being similar to a box with sides. Each tooth has five surfaces: (1) facial, (2) lingual, (3) masticatory (occlusal), (4) mesial, and (5) distal. Some surfaces of the tooth are identified by their relationship to other orofacial structures (Fig. 11.7).

The **facial surface** is the surface closest to the face. The facial surfaces closest to the lips are also called **labial surfaces**. Facial surfaces closest to the inner cheek are also referred to as **buccal surfaces**. Therefore the term *facial* can be substituted for *labial* and *buccal,* and vice versa.

The **lingual surface** is the surface of mandibular and maxillary teeth that is closest to the tongue. The lingual surface of maxillary teeth may also be referred to as the **palatal surface** because that surface is near the palate.

The **masticatory surface** is the chewing surface. On anterior teeth, it is the **incisal surface** (or *incisal edge*), and it is the **occlusal surface** on posterior teeth.

The **mesial surface** is the surface of the tooth *toward* the midline. The **distal surface** is the surface of the tooth *distant from* the midline.

When teeth are adjacent (next) to each other in the arch, the surfaces adjacent to each other are called **proximal surfaces**. For example, the distal surface of the first molar and the mesial surface of the second molar are proximal surfaces. The area between adjacent tooth surfaces is called the **interproximal space**.

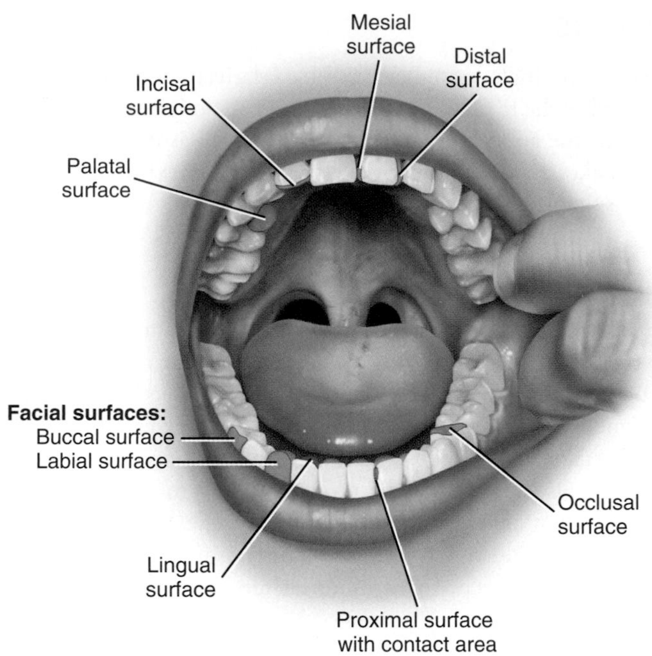


**FIG. 11.7** Surfaces of the teeth and their relationships to other oral cavity structures, to the midline, and to other teeth. *(© Elsevier Collection.)*

## Anatomic Features of Teeth

All teeth have contours, contacts, and embrasures. These anatomic features of the teeth help to maintain their position in the arch and to protect the tissues during mastication.

### Contours

All teeth have a curved surface except when the tooth is fractured or worn. Some surfaces are **convex**; others are **concave**. Although the general contours vary, the general principle that the *crown of the tooth narrows toward the cervical line* is true for all types of teeth.

#### Facial and Lingual Contours

Curvatures found on the facial and lingual surfaces provide natural passageways for food. This action protects the gingiva from the impact of foods during mastication. The normal contour of a tooth provides the gingiva with adequate stimulation for health, while protecting it from damage that may be caused by food (Fig. 11.8, *A*).

When a tooth is restored, it is important to return it to a normal contour. With *inadequate contour,* the gingiva may be traumatized when food pushes against it (Fig. 11.8, *B*). With *overcontouring,* the gingiva will lack adequate stimulation and will be difficult to clean (Fig. 11.8, *C*).

#### Mesial and Distal Contours

The contours of the mesial and distal surfaces provide normal contact and *embrasure* form. These contours tend to be self-cleansing and further contribute to self-preservation of the tooth.

### Contacts

The **contact area** is the area of the mesial or distal surface of a tooth that touches the adjacent tooth in the same arch. The *contact point* is the *exact spot* at which the teeth actually touch each other. The terms *contact* and *contact area* are frequently used interchangeably to refer to the contact point.

The crown of each tooth in the dental arches should be in contact with its adjacent tooth or teeth. A proper contact relationship between adjacent teeth serves the following three purposes:

1. Prevents food from being trapped between the teeth.
2. Stabilizes the dental arches by holding the teeth in either arch in positive contact with each other.
3. Protects the interproximal gingival tissue from trauma during mastication.

### Height of Contour

The height of contour is the "bulge," or widest point, on a specific surface of the crown. Contact areas on the mesial and distal surfaces are usually considered the height of contour on

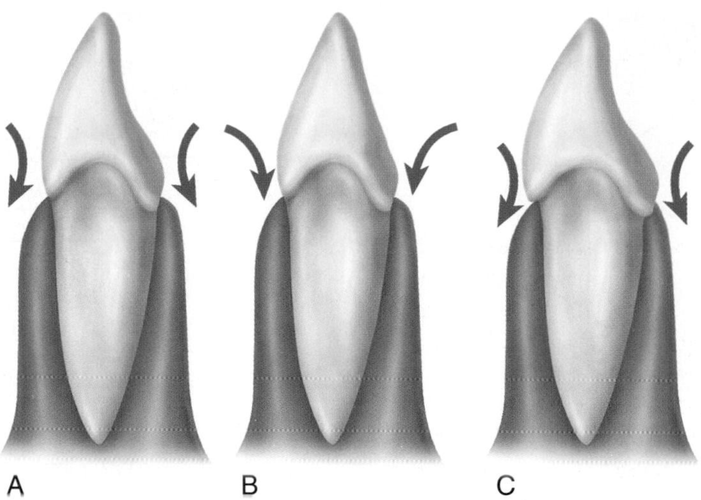


**FIG. 11.8** Tooth contours. A, Normal contour. B, Inadequate contour. C, Overcontouring. *(© Elsevier Collection.)*

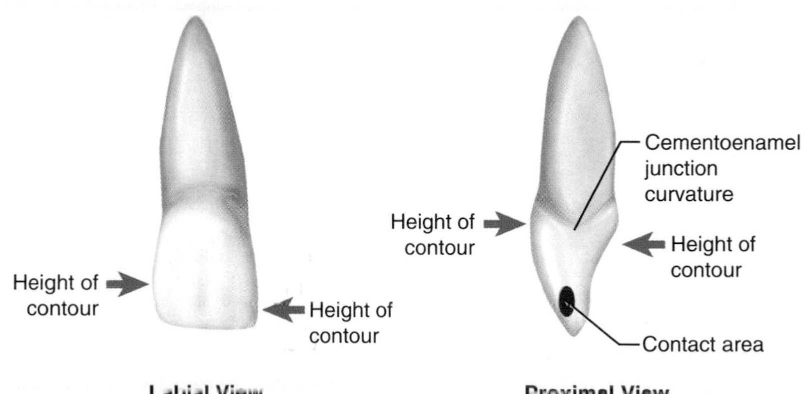


**FIG. 11.9** Example of a permanent anterior tooth with the contact area and the height of contour identified. *(© Elsevier Collection.)*

the proximal surfaces. Facial and lingual surfaces also have a height of contour (Fig. 11.9).

## Embrasures

An **embrasure** is a triangular space near the gingiva between the proximal surfaces of two adjoining teeth. Embrasures are continuous with the interproximal spaces between teeth. All tooth contours, including contact areas and embrasures, are important in the function and health of the oral tissues (Fig. 11.10).

### Clinical Considerations: Anatomical Features of the Teeth

Temporary crowns, bridges, and restorations must have proper contour, contacts, and embrasures to ensure the health of the oral tissues and the comfort of the patient. The dental assistant must have a thorough understanding of the anatomical features of the teeth to fabricate and place temporary restorations.

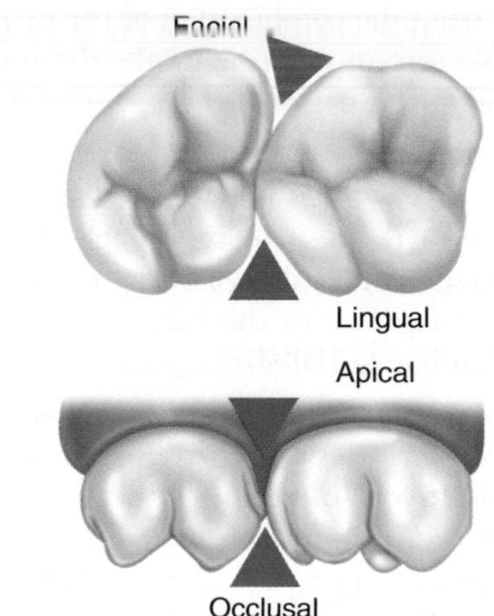


**FIG. 11.10** Embrasures may diverge facially, lingually, occlusally, or apically. *(© Elsevier Collection.)*

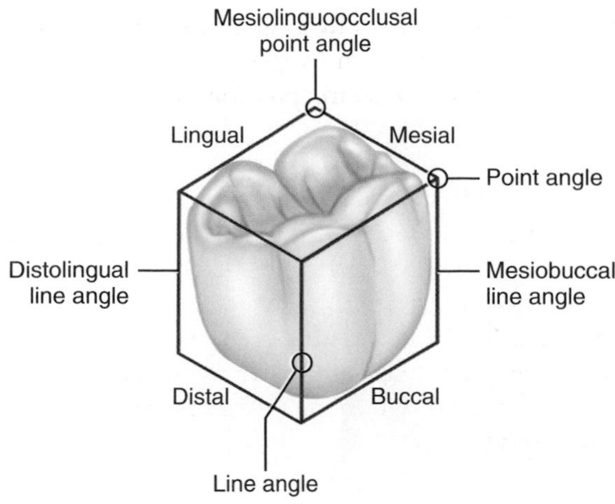


**FIG. 11.11** Line and point angles. *(© Elsevier Collection.)*

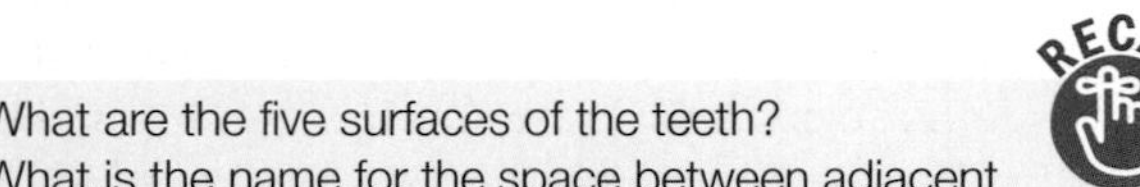

7 What are the five surfaces of the teeth?
8 What is the name for the space between adjacent teeth?
9 What is the name of the area where adjacent teeth physically touch?
10 What is the name of the triangular space toward the gingiva between adjacent teeth?

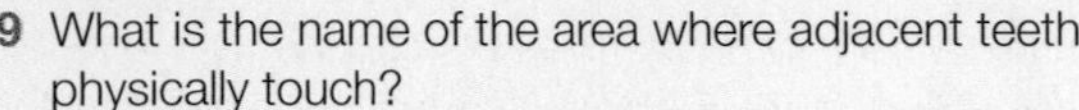

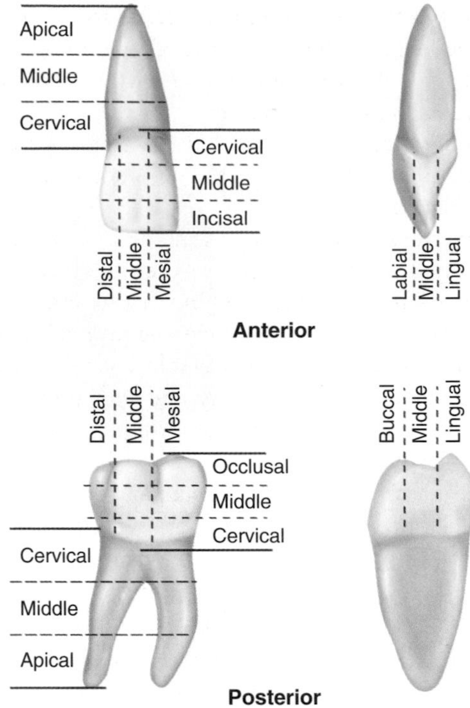


**FIG. 11.12** An anterior tooth and a posterior tooth, with designations for crown and root thirds. *(© Elsevier Collection.)*

# Angles and Divisions of Teeth

For better description of the teeth, the crowns and roots of the teeth have been divided into thirds, and junctions of the crown surfaces are described as **line angles** and **point angles**. Actually, there are no angles or points on the teeth. Line and point angles are used only as descriptive terms to indicate specific locations.

## Line and Point Angles

A line angle is formed by the junction of two surfaces and derives its name from the combination of the two surfaces that join. For example, on an anterior tooth, the junction of the mesial and labial surfaces is called the *mesiolabial line angle* (Fig. 11.11).

A point angle is that angle formed by the junction of *three* surfaces at one point. These angles also get their name from the combination of names of the surfaces that form them. For example, the junction of the mesial, buccal, and occlusal surface of a molar is called the *mesiobucco-occlusal point angle.*

When these words are combined, the last two letters of the first word are dropped and the letter *o* is substituted.

## Divisions into Thirds

To help identify a specific area of the tooth, each surface is divided into imaginary thirds (Fig. 11.12). These thirds are named according to the areas they approximate.

The *root* of the tooth is divided crosswise into thirds: the **apical third** (nearest the tip of the root), **middle third**, and **cervical third** (nearest the neck of the tooth).

The *crown* of the tooth is divided into thirds in three divisions:

- **Occlusocervical division**: The crosswise division parallel to the occlusal or incisal surface. The occlusocervical division consists of the *occlusal* third, *middle* third, and *cervical* third.
- **Mesiodistal division**: The lengthwise division in a mesial-distal (front-to-back) direction. The mesiodistal division consists of the *mesial* third, *middle* third, and *distal* third.
- **Buccolingual division**: The lengthwise division in a labial or buccal-lingual direction. The buccolingual division consists of the *facial* or *buccal/labial* third, *middle* third, and *lingual* third.

11 What is the term for the junction of two tooth surfaces?
12 What is the name for the third of the tooth nearest the end of the root?

# Occlusion and Malocclusion

*Occlusion* is defined as the relationship between the maxillary and mandibular teeth when the upper and lower jaws are in a fully closed position. Occlusion also refers to the relationship between the teeth in the same arch. Occlusion-related problems could affect the teeth, joints, and muscles of the head and neck and cause periodontal trauma.

Occlusion develops in a child as the primary teeth erupt. Habits such as thumb sucking or improper swallowing habits can affect the occlusion.

Proper occlusion of erupting permanent teeth depends on the occlusion of the primary teeth as they are shed. Correction of improper occlusion is discussed in Chapter 60.

**Centric occlusion** occurs when the jaws are closed in a position that produces maximal stable contact between the occluding surfaces of the maxillary and mandibular teeth. In this position, the condyles are in the most posterior, unstrained position in the glenoid fossa.

Centric occlusion serves as the standard for a normal occlusion. In normal occlusion, the lingual cusps of the posterior maxillary teeth fit into the central fossae of the occlusal surfaces of the posterior mandibular teeth. This positioning allows effective grinding of food. Centric occlusion widely distributes occlusal forces and affords the greatest comfort and stability (Fig. 11.13).

**Functional occlusion**, also known as *physiologic occlusion,* is the term used to describe contact of the teeth during biting and chewing movements.

**Malocclusion** refers to abnormal or malpositioned relationships of the maxillary teeth to the mandibular teeth when they are in centric occlusion. Treatment of malocclusion is discussed in Chapter 60.

RECALL

13 What is the name for the position of the teeth when they are in chewing movements?
14 What is the term for teeth that are in poor occlusion?

## Angle's Classification

**Angle's classification** system was developed by Dr. Edward H. Angle to describe and classify occlusion and malocclusion.

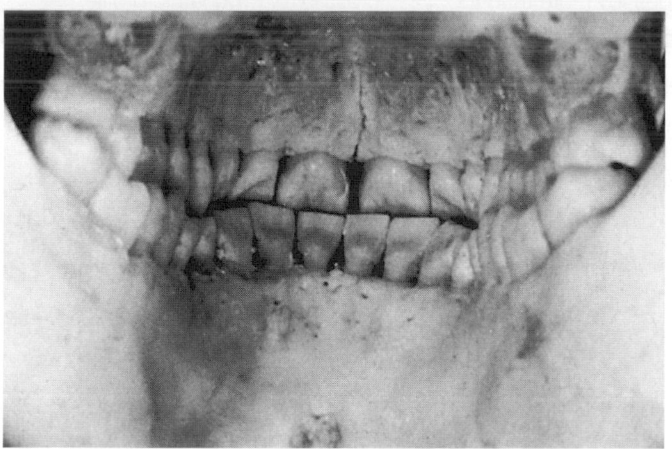

**FIG. 11.13** Skull showing lingual view of the teeth in centric occlusion. *(From Nelson SJ, Ash MM: Wheeler's dental anatomy, physiology, and occlusion, ed 9, St Louis, 2010, Saunders.)*

The basis of this system is that the *permanent maxillary first molar* is the key to occlusion. Angle's system assumes that the patient is occluding in a centric position (Table 11.4).

### *Class I*

In class I, or **neutroclusion**, an ideal mesiodistal relationship exists between the jaws and the dental arches. The mesiobuccal cusp of the permanent maxillary first molar occludes with the mesiobuccal groove of the mandibular first molar.

Class I may include the situation in which the anterior or individual teeth are malaligned in their position in the arch. However, the relationship of the permanent first molars determines the classification.

### *Class II*

In class II, or **distoclusion**, the mesiobuccal cusp of the maxillary first molar occludes (by more than the width of a premolar) mesial to the mesiobuccal groove of the mandibular first molar. The mandibular dental arch is in a *distal* relationship to the maxillary arch. This frequently gives the appearance of protrusion of the maxillary anterior teeth over the mandibular anterior teeth.

The major group of class II malocclusion has two subgroups—*division 1* and *division 2*—that are based on the position of the anterior teeth, the shape of the palate, and the resulting profile.

**DIVISION 1.** The lips are usually flat and parted, with the lower lip tucked behind the upper incisors. The upper lip appears short and drawn up over the protruding anterior teeth of the maxillary arch.

Also in class II, division 1, the maxillary incisors are in labioversion. **Labioversion** is the inclination of the teeth to extend facially beyond the normal overlap of the incisal edge of the maxillary incisors over the mandibular incisors.

**DIVISION 2.** Class II, division 2, includes class II malocclusions in which the maxillary incisors are *not* in labioversion. The maxillary central incisors are nearly normal anteroposteriorly, and they may be slightly in linguoversion. The maxillary lateral incisors may be tipped labially and mesially.

**Linguoversion** refers to the position of the maxillary incisors behind the mandibular incisors. Normally, the maxillary incisors slightly overlap the front of the mandibular incisors.

### *Class III*

In a class III malocclusion, or **mesioclusion**, the body of the mandible must be in an abnormal *mesial* relationship to the maxilla. This frequently gives the appearance of protrusion of the mandible.

The mesiobuccal cusp of the maxillary first molar occludes in the interdental space between the distal cusp of the mandibular first permanent molar and the mesial cusp of the mandibular second permanent molar.

15 What is the technical term for class III malocclusion?
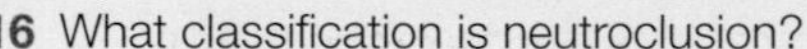
16 What classification is neutroclusion?

## TABLE 11.4 Angle's Classifications of Malocclusion

| Class | Model | Arch Relationships | Descriptions |
|---|---|---|---|
| **Class I** | 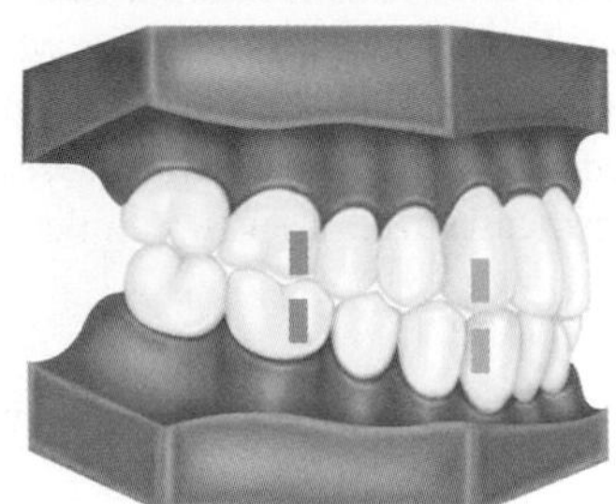 | **Molar:** MB cusp of the maxillary first molar occludes with the MB groove of the mandibular first molar.<br>**Canines:** Maxillary occludes with the distal half of the mandibular canine and the mesial half of the mandibular first premolar. | Dental malalignment(s), such as crowding or spacing, present (see text). Mesognathic profile. |
| **Class II** | 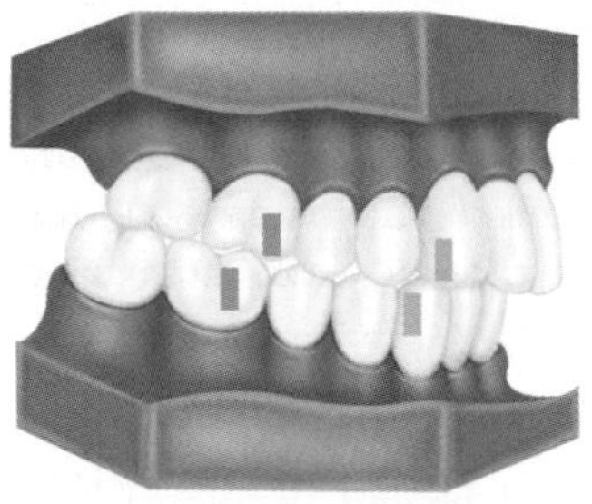 | **Molar:** MB cusp of the maxillary first molar occludes (by more than the width of a premolar) mesial to the MB groove of the mandibular first molar.<br>**Canines**: Distal surface of the mandibular canine is distal to the mesial surface of the maxillary canine by at least the width of a premolar. | **Division 1:** Maxillary anteriors protrude facially from the mandibular anteriors, with deep overbite. Retrognathic profile. |
| | | | **Division 2:** Maxillary central incisors are upright or retruded, and lateral incisors are tipped labially or overlap the central incisors with deep overbite. Mesognathic profile. |
| **Class III** | 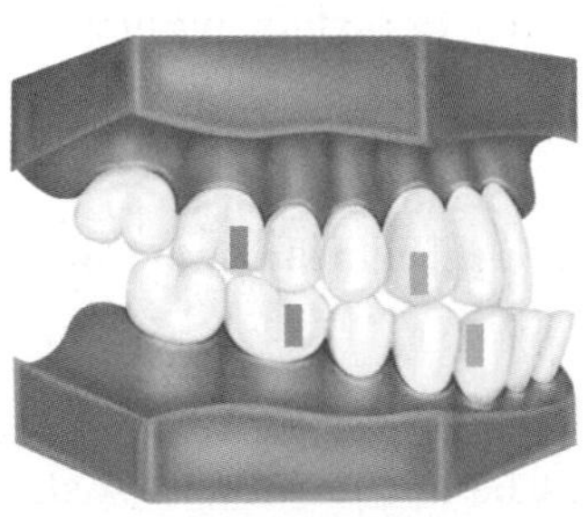 | **Molar:** MB cusp of the maxillary first molar occludes (by more than the width of a premolar) distal to the MB groove of the mandibular first molar.<br>**Canines:** Distal surface of the mandibular mesial to the mesial surface of the maxillary by at least the width of a premolar. | Mandibular incisors in complete cross-bite. Prognathic profile. |

Data from Fehrenbach MJ, Popowics T: *Illustrated dental embryology, histology, and anatomy,* ed 4, St Louis, 2016, Saunders. Images © Elsevier Collection.

*MB,* Mesiobuccal.

*Note:* This system deals with the classification of the permanent dentition.

## Stabilization of the Arches

In a healthy mouth with properly maintained dentition, the dental arches remain stable and efficient. However, malocclusion or the loss of one or more teeth may greatly reduce the functioning and stability of the dentition (Fig. 11.14).

### Closure

The anterior teeth are not designed to fully support the occlusal forces on the entire dental arch; therefore as the jaws close, the stronger posterior teeth come together first. After they have assumed most of the load, the more delicate anterior teeth come together.

### Curve of Spee

The occlusal surfaces of the posterior teeth do not form a flat plane. Those of the mandibular arch form a slightly curved plane, which appears concave (curved inward, like the inside of a bowl). The maxillary arch forms a curved plane that appears convex (curved outward, like the outside of a bowl). The curvature formed by the maxillary and mandibular arches in occlusion is known as the **curve of Spee** (Fig. 11.15, *A*). On a radiograph, the occlusal line of the teeth appears to be smiling.

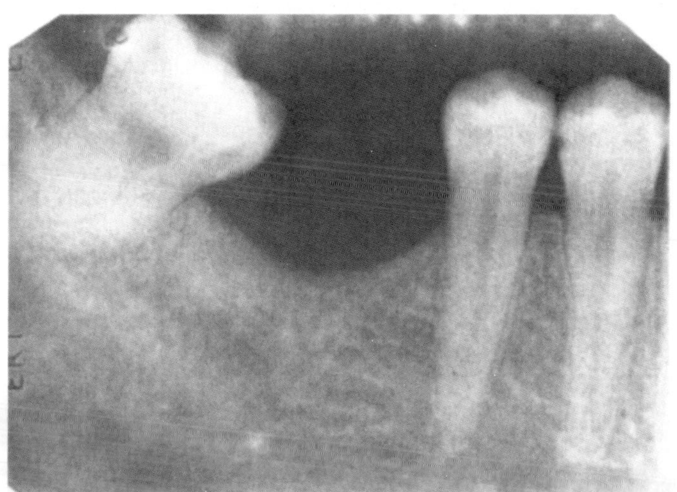

FIG. 11.14 Radiograph shows the mesial drift of the mandibular second molar after the first molar has been lost.

### Curve of Wilson

The **curve of Wilson** is the cross-arch curvature of the posterior occlusal plane. The downward curvature of the arc is defined by a line drawn across the occlusal surface of the left mandibular first molar, extending across the arch and through the occlusal surface of the right mandibular first molar (Fig. 11.15, *B*).

**17** What is the name for the curve of the occlusal plane?

## Tooth-Numbering Systems

Numbering systems are used as a simplified means of identifying the teeth for charting and descriptive purpose. Three basic numbering systems are used, and the dental assistant must be familiar with each system.

### Universal/National System

The system most often used in the United States is the Universal/National System, which was approved by the American Dental Association (ADA) in 1968. In the Universal/National System, the permanent teeth are numbered from 1 to 32. Numbering begins with the upper-right third molar (tooth #1), works around to the upper-left third molar (tooth #16), drops to the lower-left third molar (tooth #17), and works around to the lower-right third molar (tooth #32) (see Fig. 11.6, *A*).

The primary teeth are lettered with capital letters from *A* to *T*. Lettering begins with the upper-right second primary molar (tooth A), works around to the upper-left second primary molar (tooth J), drops to the lower-left second primary molar

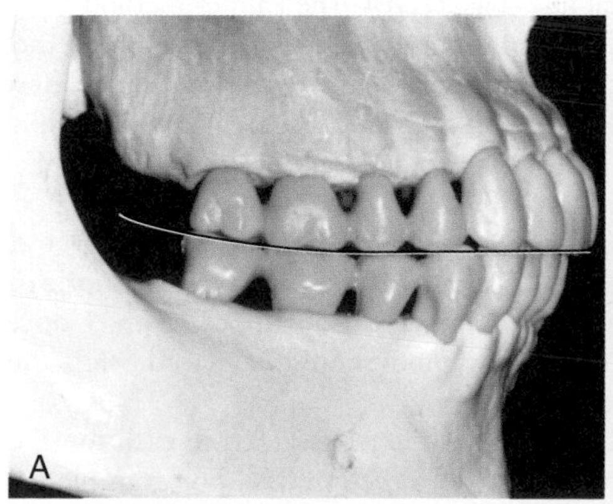


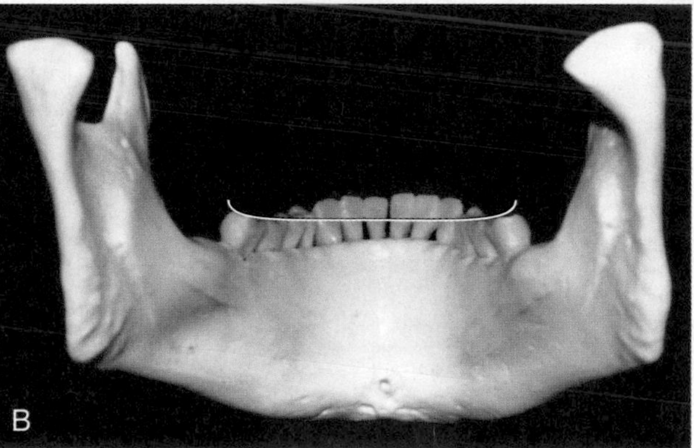


FIG. 11.15 Curves noted in the dental arch. A, Curve of Spee. B, Curve of Wilson. *(From Fehrenbach MJ, Popowics T: Illustrated dental embryology, histology, and anatomy, ed 4, St Louis, 2016, Saunders.)*

(tooth K), and works around to the lower-right second primary molar (tooth T) (see Fig. 11.6, *B*).

## International Standards Organization System

To meet the need for a numbering system that could be used internationally, as well as by electronic data transfer, the World Health Organization accepted the International Standards Organization (ISO) System for teeth. In 1996 the ADA accepted the ISO system, in addition to the Universal/National System. The ISO System is based on the Fédération Dentaire Internationale (FDI) System and is used in most countries.

**The Palmer Notation System for Permanent Teeth**

| Maxillary Right | | Maxillary Left |
|---|---|---|
| | 8 7 6 5 4 3 2 1 \| 1 2 3 4 5 6 7 8 | |
| | 8 7 6 5 4 3 2 1 \| 1 2 3 4 5 6 7 8 | |
| Mandibular Right | | Mandibular Left |

| Tooth Numbers | |
|---|---|
| Central incisors | #1 |
| Lateral incisors | #2 |
| Canines | #3 |
| 1st premolar | #4 |
| 2nd premolar | #5 |
| 1st molar | #6 |
| 2nd molar | #7 |
| 3rd molar | #8 |

Examples of Charting

1| Maxillary right central incisor
2| Mandibular right lateral incisor
|4 Maxillary left first premolar
|8 Mandibular left third molar

**The Palmer Notation System for Primary Teeth**

| Maxillary Right | | Maxillary Left |
|---|---|---|
| | E D C B A \| A B C D E | |
| | E D C B A \| A B C D E | |
| Mandibular Right | | Mandibular Left |

Examples of Charting

A| Maxillary right central incisor
B| Mandibular right lateral incisor
|C Maxillary left canine
|D Mandibular left first primary molar

| Tooth Letters | |
|---|---|
| Central incisors | A |
| Lateral incisors | B |
| Canines | C |
| 1st primary molar | D |
| 2nd primary molar | E |

**FIG. 11.16** Palmer Notation System.

The ISO/FDI system uses a two-digit tooth-recording system. The first digit indicates the quadrant, and the second digit indicates the tooth within the quadrant, with numbering from the midline toward the posterior. Permanent teeth are numbered as follows:

- The maxillary right quadrant is digit 1 and contains teeth #11 to #18
- The maxillary left quadrant is digit 2 and contains teeth #21 to #28
- The mandibular left quadrant is digit 3 and contains teeth #31 to #38
- The mandibular right quadrant is digit 4 and contains teeth #41 to #48

Primary teeth are numbered as follows:

- The maxillary right quadrant is digit 5 and contains teeth #51 to #55
- The maxillary left quadrant is digit 6 and contains teeth #61 to #65
- The mandibular left quadrant is digit 7 and contains teeth #71 to #75
- The mandibular right quadrant is digit 8 and contains teeth #81 to #85

The digits should be pronounced separately. For example, the permanent canines are teeth #1-3 ("number one-three"), #2-3 ("number two-three"), #3-3 ("number three-three"), and #4-3 ("number four-three").

To prevent miscommunication internationally, the ISO/FDI System also has designated areas in the oral cavity. A two-digit number designates these, and at least one of the two digits is zero (0). In this system, for example, 00 ("zero-zero") designates the whole oral cavity, and 01 ("zero-one") indicates the maxillary area only.

## Palmer Notation System

In the Palmer Notation System, each of the four quadrants is given its own tooth bracket made up of a vertical line and a horizontal line (Fig. 11.16). The Palmer method is a shorthand diagram of the teeth presented as if one is viewing the patient's teeth from the outside. The teeth in the right quadrant would have the vertical midline bracket to the right of the tooth numbers or letters, just as when one is looking at the patient. The midline is to the right of the teeth in the right quadrant.

For example, if the tooth is a maxillary tooth, the number or letter should be written above the horizontal line of the bracket, thus indicating an upper tooth. Conversely, a mandibular tooth symbol should be placed below the line, indicating a lower tooth.

The number or letter assigned to each tooth depends on its position relative to the midline. For example, central incisors, the teeth closest to the midline, have the lowest number, 1, for permanent teeth and the letter A for primary teeth. All central incisors, maxillary and mandibular, are given the number 1. All lateral incisors are given the number 2, all canines are given the number 3, premolars are numbers 4 and 5, molars are 6 and 7, and third molars are number 8.

## Example of Palmer Notation System

| | |
|---|---|
| Maxillary right lateral incisor | 2 |
| Maxillary left first premolar | 4 |
| Mandibular right third molar | 8 |
| Mandibular central incisor | 1 |

**■ Legal and Ethical Implications** Extreme care must be taken when tooth numbers are entered on records or when verbal instructions regarding a specific tooth are carried out. Errors have resulted in extraction of the wrong tooth.

Remember that all dental records are legal documents. Learn the charting systems, and make your charting entries accurately. You may have to explain them in a court of law. ■

**■ Eye to the Future** Primary teeth hold a substantial supply of stem cells in their dental pulp. Scientists at the National Institute of Dental and Craniofacial Research found that stem cells stay alive in the tooth for a brief period after the tooth is outside of the child's mouth. This creates the possibility of collecting these cells for research.

Stem cells may help repair damage to major organs, encourage bone regeneration, and cause specialized dentin formation. This research was published in the online version of *Proceedings of the National Academy of Sciences*. ■

## ■ Critical Thinking

1. While you are taking radiographs of 6-year-old Melissa's teeth, her mother expresses concern that Melissa's erupting permanent teeth look yellow compared to her nice white baby teeth. What could you say to Melissa's mother about her child's teeth?
2. You and another dental assistant are planning to speak to a group of young mothers about dental health and the importance of primary teeth. What information would you include in your presentation about primary teeth?
3. Dr. Ortega asks you to take a radiograph of tooth letters K and T. Which teeth are these?
4. Dr. Lane has just extracted the maxillary left third molar and the mandibular left third molar. What Universal tooth numbers would you enter on the insurance form? ■

12

# Tooth Morphology

## KEY TERMS

**Bicanineate** A two-cusp type of mandibular second premolar.
**Bifurcated** Divided into two.
**Bifurcation** Area in which two roots divide.
**Canine eminence (EM-i-nens)** External vertical bony ridge on the labial surface of the canines.
**Central groove** Most prominent developmental groove on the posterior teeth.
**Cingulum (SING-gyoo-lum)** Raised, rounded area on the cervical third of the lingual surface.
**Cusp** Major elevation on the masticatory surfaces of canines and posterior teeth.
**Cusp of Carabelli** The fifth supplemental cusp found lingual to the mesiolingual cusp.
**Diastema (dye-uh-STEE-muh)** A space between two teeth.
**Fossa (FOS-ah, FAW-seh)** Wide, shallow depression on the lingual surfaces of anterior teeth.
**Furcation (fur-KAY-shun)** Area between two or more root branches.
**Imbrication (im-bri-KAY-shun) lines** Slight ridges that run mesiodistally in the cervical third of the teeth.
**Incisal edge** Ridge on permanent incisors that appears flattened on labial, lingual, or incisal view after tooth eruption.
**Inclined cuspal planes** Sloping areas between the cusp ridges.
**Mamelon (MAM-uh-lon)** Rounded enamel extension on the incisal ridges of incisors.
**Marginal groove** A developmental groove that crosses a marginal ridge and serves as a spillway, allowing food to escape during mastication.
**Marginal ridge** Rounded, raised border on the mesial and distal portions of the lingual surfaces of anterior teeth and the occlusal table of posterior teeth.
**Molars** Teeth located in the posterior aspect of the upper and lower jaws.
**Morphology (mor-FOL-uh-jee)** Study of form and shape, as of the teeth.
**Nonsuccedaneous (non-suk-se-DAY-nee-us)** Pertaining to a permanent tooth that does not replace a primary tooth.
**Pegged laterals** Incisors with a pointed or tapered shape.
**Succedaneous (suk-se-DAY-nee-us)** Permanent teeth that replace primary teeth.
**Triangular groove** A developmental groove that separates a marginal ridge from the triangular ridge of a cusp.
**Tricanineate** A three-cusp type of mandibular second premolar.
**Trifurcated** Divided into three.
**Trifurcation** Area in which three roots divide.

## LEARNING OUTCOMES

*On completion of this chapter, the student will be able to achieve the following objectives:*

1. Pronounce, define, and spell the key terms.
2. Discuss the anterior permanent dentition, including the following:
   - Identify the location of each anterior permanent tooth.
   - Use the correct terminology when discussing features of the anterior permanent dentition.
   - Describe the general and specific features of each tooth in the anterior permanent dentition.
   - Discuss clinical considerations of each tooth in the anterior permanent dentition.
3. Discuss the posterior permanent dentition, including the following:
   - Identify the location of each posterior permanent tooth.
   - Use the correct terminology when discussing features of the posterior permanent dentition.
   - Describe the general and specific features of each tooth in the posterior permanent dentition.
   - Discuss clinical considerations of each tooth in the posterior permanent dentition.
4. Discuss the primary dentition, including the following:
   - Compare and contrast the features of the primary and permanent dentitions.
   - Describe the general and specific features of the primary dentition.
   - Discuss clinical considerations of the primary dentition.

## ELECTRONIC RESOURCES

e ***Additional information related to content in Chapter 12 can be found on the companion Evolve Web site.***

- Practice Quiz

As a dental assistant, you will find that a thorough understanding of tooth **morphology** (the shape of teeth) is especially useful in the following clinical situations:

- Mounting dental radiographs (see Chapter 41)
- Assisting in charting a mouth with missing teeth and teeth that have "drifted"
- Selecting temporary crowns from a box with a variety of shapes
- Forming matrix bands before application (see Chapter 48)
- Selecting rubber dam clamps (see Chapter 36)
- Fabricating temporary crowns and bridges (see Chapter 51)

As you study tooth morphology, remember that there is always a certain amount of normal variation among individual teeth, just as there is variation among individual people. Every tooth may not meet all the criteria for identification. When you understand the characteristics of each tooth, however, you will be able to differentiate among teeth, as well as between the left teeth and the right teeth in any particular group.

# Anterior Permanent Dentition

The permanent anterior teeth include two *central incisors,* two *lateral incisors,* and two *canines.* The central incisors are closest to the midline, the lateral incisors are the second teeth from the midline, and the canines are the third teeth from the midline. All anterior teeth are **succedaneous**, which means they replace primary teeth of the same type.

The anterior teeth play an important role in a person's appearance (Fig. 12.1). The size, shape, color, and position of the anterior teeth directly relate to how a person looks. Many people are extremely self-conscious about the appearance of their front (anterior) teeth. The anterior teeth also play an important role in speech and are necessary for formation of *s* and *t* sounds.

All anterior teeth have a **cingulum**, a rounded, raised area on the cervical third of the lingual surface. The lingual surface has rounded, raised borders on the mesial and distal surfaces called **marginal ridges**. Some anterior teeth have a **fossa**, a wide, shallow depression on the lingual surfaces (Fig. 12.2).

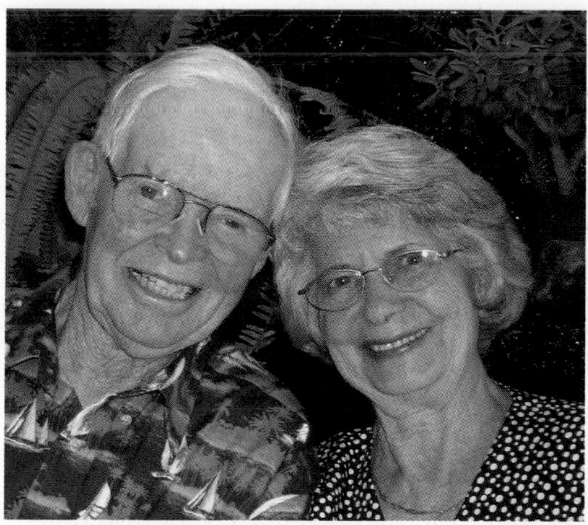

**FIG. 12.1** Attractive teeth are important for a nice smile at any age.

Rub your tongue up and down on the lingual side of your front teeth. The bump or raised area you feel near the gingiva is the cingulum, and the deeper area is the fossa.

## Permanent Incisors

There are eight permanent incisors—four maxillary and four mandibular. The maxillary group comprises two central incisors and two lateral incisors, as does the mandibular group. These teeth complement each other in form and function. The central incisors erupt about a year or so before the lateral incisors do.

### Maxillary Central Incisors

The *maxillary central incisors* (#8 and #9) have unique anatomic features (Fig. 12.3). They are larger than mandibular central incisors in all dimensions, especially in width (mesiodistally). The labial surfaces are more rounded from the incisal aspect. The root of the maxillary central is shorter than the roots of other permanent maxillary teeth. The marginal ridges, lingual fossa, and cingulum are more prominent on the maxillary central incisor than on the mandibular central incisor.

When an incisor is newly erupted, the incisal portion is rounded; this is called the *incisal ridge.* The term *edge* implies an angle formed by the merging of two flat surfaces. Therefore an **incisal edge** does not exist on an incisor until occlusal wear has created a flattened surface on the incisal portion. The incisal edge is also known as the *incisal surface* or *incisal plane.* The incisal edges of maxillary incisors have a lingual inclination (slant). The incisal edges of mandibular incisors have a labial inclination. The incisal planes of mandibular and maxillary incisors are parallel to each other and work together to create a cutting action, similar to that produced by the blades of a pair of scissors.

When newly erupted, the central and lateral incisors have three **mamelons**, or rounded enamel extensions, on the incisal ridge, or edge (Fig. 12.4). These mamelons usually undergo attrition (wearing away of a tooth surface) shortly after

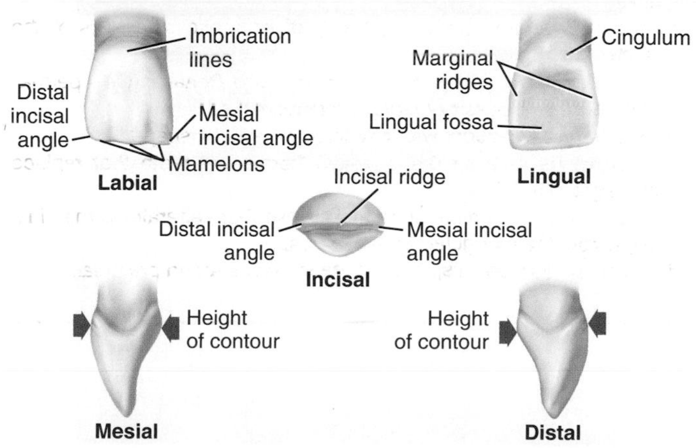


**FIG. 12.2** Various views of a newly erupted permanent maxillary incisor show its features. *(© Elsevier Collection.)*

eruption. Then the *incisal ridge* appears flattened and becomes the *incisal edge.*

### Maxillary Lateral Incisors

The *maxillary lateral incisors* (#7 and #10) are smaller than the central incisors in all dimensions except root length (Fig. 12.5). They usually erupt after the maxillary central incisors do. The crown of a maxillary lateral incisor has a single root that is relatively smooth and straight but may curve slightly distally. Remember this feature; it will be helpful when you are mounting radiographs.

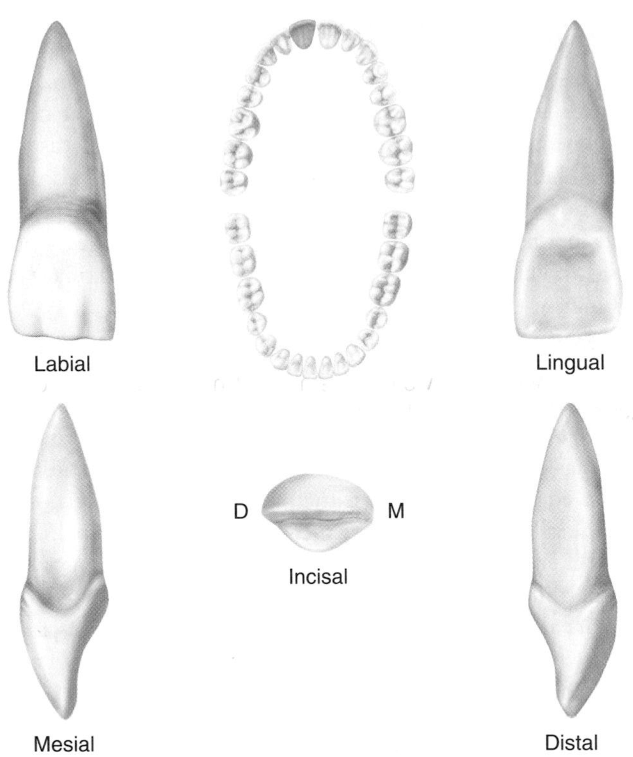


**FIG. 12.3** Various views of a permanent maxillary right central incisor. *(© Elsevier Collection.)*

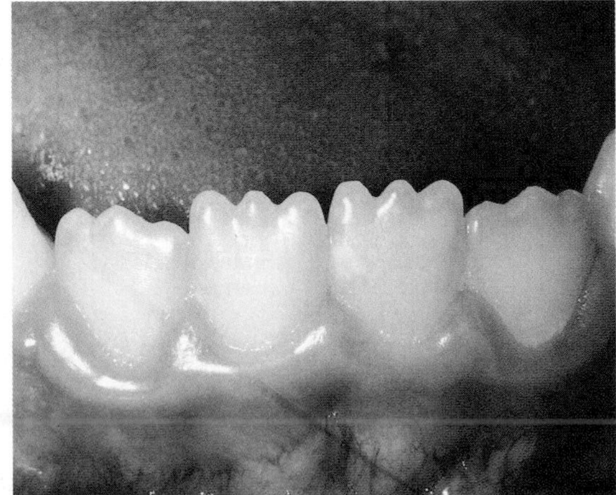

**FIG. 12.4** Mamelons are the rounded portions of the incisal edge of the incisors.

The lateral incisors vary in form to a greater extent than any other tooth except the third molars, and frequently they are congenitally missing. It is not uncommon to find maxillary lateral incisors with a pointed or tapered shape; such teeth are called **pegged laterals** (Fig. 12.6). Because of variations in form, the permanent maxillary lateral incisors can present challenges during preventive, restorative, and orthodontic procedures. Often, unusually large open contacts (spaces between teeth) called **diastemas** occur in this area because of variations in the size and shape of the lateral incisor and its position in the arch. Fortunately, dental materials and techniques are available today to correct these conditions.

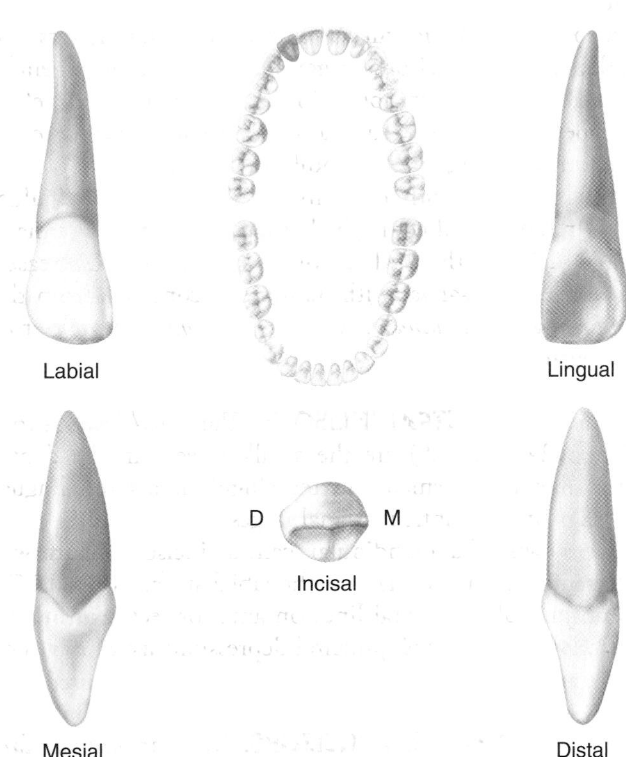


**FIG. 12.5** Various views of a permanent maxillary right lateral incisor. *(© Elsevier Collection.)*

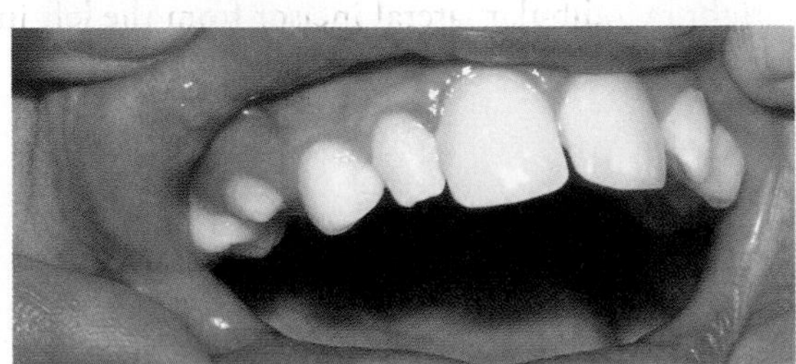

**FIG. 12.6** Pegged maxillary lateral incisor. Note the conical shape. The maxillary third molars differ from the other teeth considerably in terms of size, contour, and relative position. *(From Ibsen OC, Phelan JA: Oral pathology for the dental hygienist, ed 6, St Louis, 2014, Saunders.)*

RECALL

1 How many anterior teeth are included in the permanent dentition?
2 What is the term for the permanent teeth that replace primary teeth?
3 What is the term for the rounded, raised area on the cervical third of the lingual surface of anterior teeth?
4 What effect do newly erupted central and lateral incisors have on the incisal ridge?

## Mandibular Incisors

The permanent *mandibular incisors* are the smallest teeth of the permanent dentition and the most symmetric. The central and lateral incisors of the mandibular arch closely resemble each other.

In contrast to the maxillary central and lateral incisors, the mandibular lateral incisor is larger than the mandibular central incisor. The lower, mandibular incisors generally erupt before the upper, maxillary incisors do. It is rare for developmental disturbances to occur with mandibular incisors.

Supragingival tooth deposits such as plaque, calculus, and stain tend to collect in the lingual concavity of the mandibular incisors. The buildup of these deposits is increased by the release of saliva, with its mineral contents, from the *sublingual* and *submandibular salivary glands* in the floor of the mouth.

**MANDIBULAR CENTRAL INCISORS.** The *mandibular central incisors* (#24 and #25) are the smallest teeth in the dental arches. They have a small centered cingulum, a subtle lingual fossa, and equally subtle marginal ridges.

The crown of a mandibular central incisor is narrower on the lingual surface than on the labial surface (Fig. 12.7). Developmental horizontal lines on anterior teeth, or **imbrication lines**, and developmental depressions usually are not obvious.

**MANDIBULAR LATERAL INCISORS.** The *mandibular lateral incisors* (#23 and #26) are slightly larger than the mandibular central incisors but otherwise are similar. The lateral teeth usually erupt after the mandibular central incisors do. The mesial side of the crown is often longer than the distal side, causing the incisal ridge, which is straight, to slope downward in a distal direction. This helps in differentiating the right mandibular lateral incisor from the left incisor (Fig. 12.8).

### Clinical Considerations: Incisors

The maxillary and mandibular incisors function together to perform a scissors-like action. The anterior teeth are the most noticeable teeth in a person's smile. Knowing the location of the grooves and ridges and understanding their characteristics is important for the dental assistant who is constructing temporary crowns or bridges, or who is finishing and polishing existing restorations.

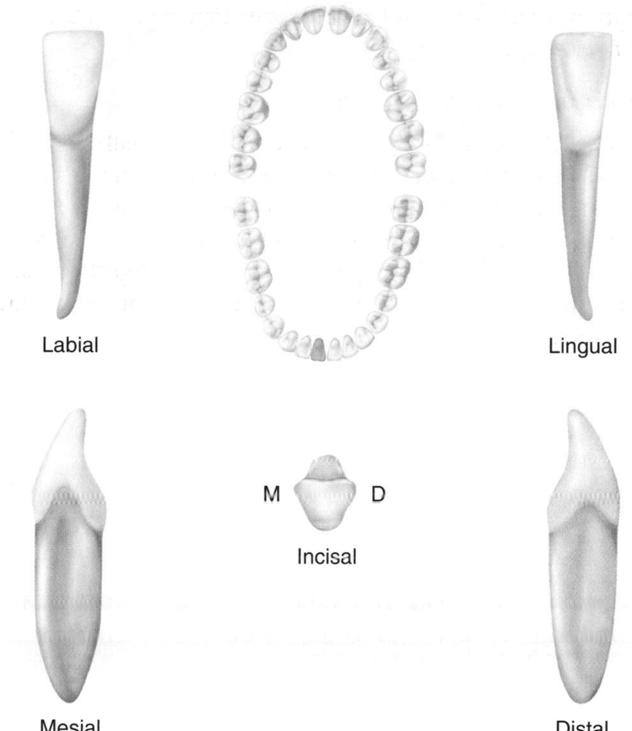


**FIG. 12.7** Various views of a permanent mandibular right central incisor. *(© Elsevier Collection.)*

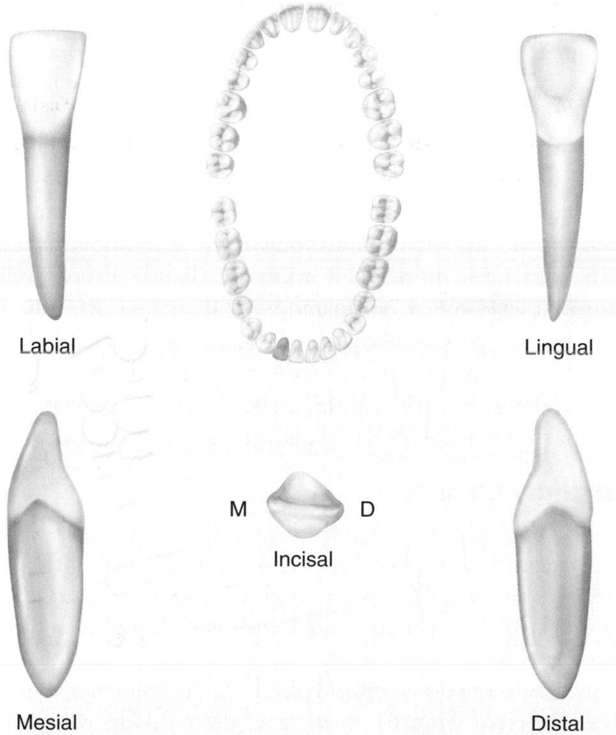


**FIG. 12.8** Various views of a permanent mandibular right lateral incisor. *(© Elsevier Collection.)*

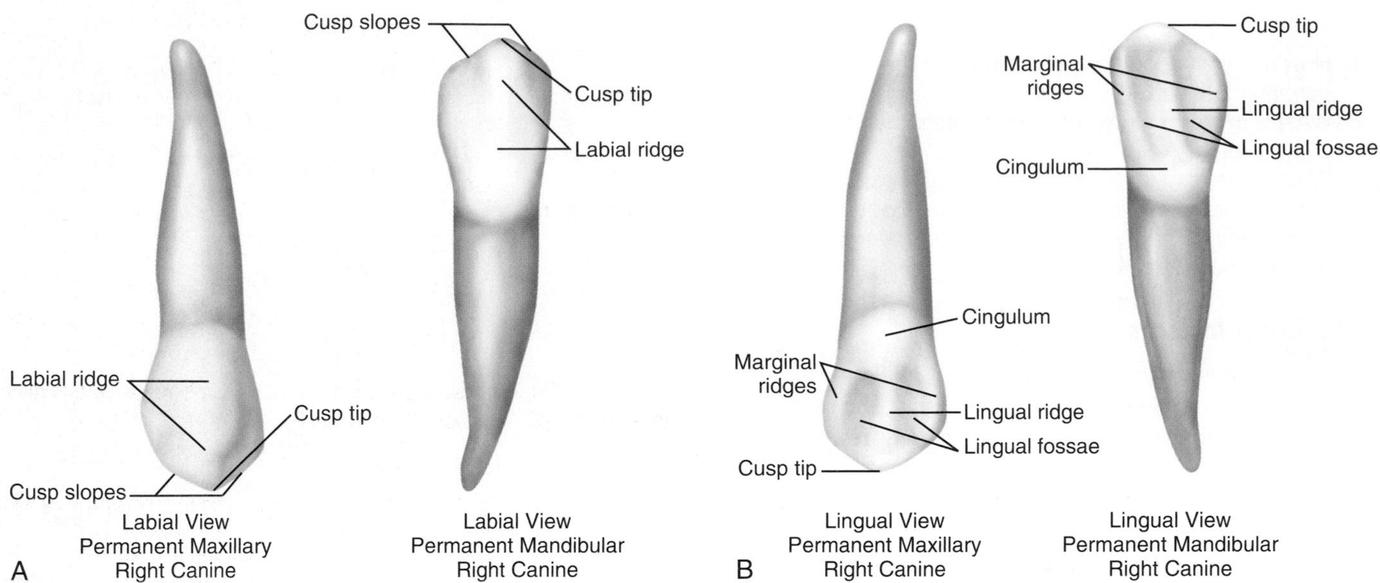


**FIG. 12.9** Views of permanent mandibular and maxillary canines. A, Labial view. B, Lingual view. *(© Elsevier Collection.)*

## Permanent Canines

The permanent canines are the four anterior teeth that are located at the corner of each quadrant for each dental arch (Fig. 12.9, *A*). They are commonly referred to as the "cornerstone" of the dental arches. These teeth are the most stable in the mouth. Their name is derived from the Latin word for *dog* ("canus") because canines resemble dogs' teeth. The permanent canines are the longest teeth in the dentition. The canine has a particularly long, thick root. The root is usually the same length as or twice the length of the crown. The crown of the canine is shaped in a manner that promotes cleanliness. Because of their self-cleansing shape and sturdy anchorage in the jaws, the canines are usually the last teeth to be lost.

Another important characteristic of the canines is the cosmetic value of the **canine eminence**. This is the bony ridge over the labial portion of the roots of the canines that forms facial contours. Patients commonly call the canines their "eyeteeth" and often notice the normally slightly deeper yellow color of their canines compared with their incisors. You may hear the term *cuspid* used instead of *canine.* This is an older term that was used because these were the only teeth in the permanent dentition that had one cusp. A **cusp** is a major elevation on the masticatory surface of a canine or posterior tooth.

### Maxillary Canines

The *maxillary canines* (#6 and #11) usually erupt after the mandibular canines, the maxillary incisors, and possibly the maxillary premolars do. The maxillary canines have a larger and more developed cusp compared with the mandibular canines (Fig. 12.9, *B*, and Fig. 12.10).

Similar to the other anterior teeth, each canine has an incisal edge. Different from the incisors is the cusp tip, which is in line with the long axis of the root. The cusp tip is sharper on a maxillary canine. Because of the cusp tip, the incisal edge of the canine is divided into two cusp slopes, or ridges, rather than being nearly straight across, as is an incisor. The mesial cusp slope is usually shorter than the distal cusp slope in maxillary and mandibular canines when they first erupt. The length of these cusp slopes and the cusp tip can change with attrition.

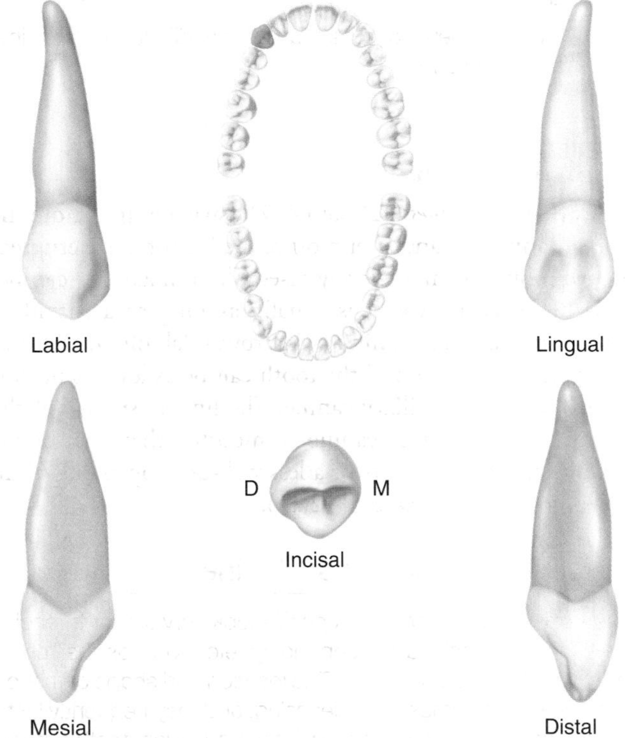


**FIG. 12.10** Various views of a permanent maxillary right canine. *(© Elsevier Collection.)*

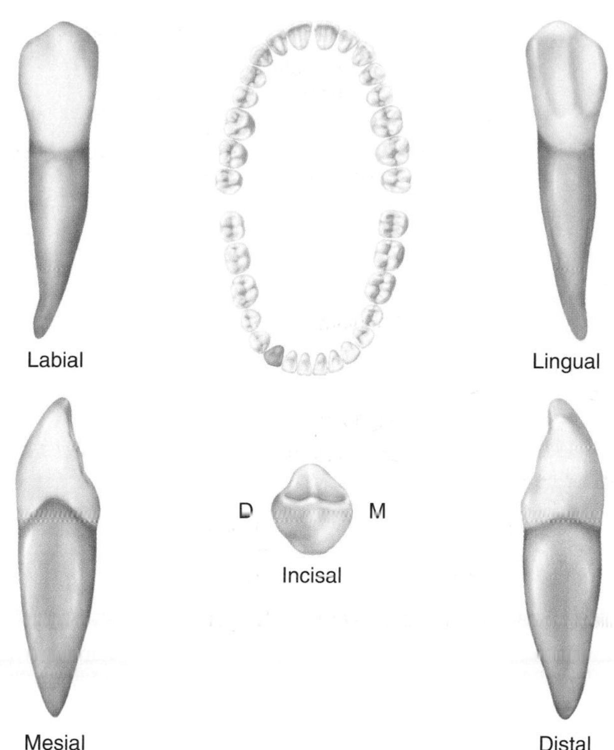


FIG. 12.11 Various views of a permanent mandibular right canine. *(© Elsevier Collection.)*

### *Mandibular Canines*

The *mandibular canines* (#22 and #27) usually erupt before the maxillary canines do and after most of the incisors have erupted.

A mandibular canine closely resembles a maxillary canine. Although the entire tooth is usually as long as a maxillary canine, a mandibular canine is narrower labiolingually and mesiodistally. The crown of the tooth can be as long as or longer than that of a maxillary canine. The lingual surface of the crown of the mandibular canine is smoother than that of the maxillary canine; it consists of a less well-developed cingulum and two marginal ridges (Fig. 12.11).

### Clinical Considerations: Canines

The maxillary and mandibular canines look very similar to each other. The four canines are commonly referred to as the "cornerstone" of the dental arches. The location and shape of these teeth make them almost self-cleansing, and they frequently last throughout a person's life, or they may be the last teeth a person loses. The canines are also very important in establishing a natural facial contour.

RECALL

5 Which teeth are the longest ones in the permanent dentition?
6 Which teeth are the smallest ones in the permanent dentition?
7 What is the name for developmental horizontal lines on the anterior teeth?

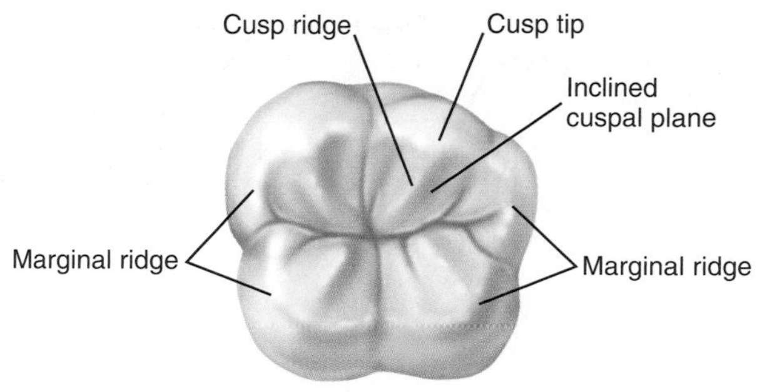


FIG. 12.12 Occlusal surface on a permanent posterior tooth and its features. *(© Elsevier Collection.)*

## Posterior Permanent Dentition

The permanent posterior teeth include the *premolars* and the **molars**. The crown of each posterior tooth consists of an occlusal surface and marginal ridges on the mesial and distal surfaces (Fig. 12.12).

The occlusal surfaces include two or more cusps. Imagine each cusp as a mountain with sloping areas, or cusp ridges, that extend from the top of the mountain; between the ridges are sloping areas called **inclined cuspal planes**. Each cusp usually has four inclined cuspal planes. Some inclined planes are important in occlusion of the teeth.

The marginal ridges border the occlusal surface and create an inner occlusal table. Each shallow, wide depression on the occlusal table is a fossa. One type of fossa on the posterior teeth, the *central fossa,* is located where the cusp ridges converge at a central point, where the grooves meet. Another type of fossa is the *triangular fossa,* which has a triangular shape at the convergence of the cusp ridges and is associated with termination of the triangular grooves.

Sometimes located in the deepest portions of the fossa are occlusal *developmental pits.* Each pit is a sharp pinpoint depression where two or more grooves meet.

*Developmental grooves* are also found on the occlusal table (Fig. 12.13). The developmental grooves on each different posterior tooth type are located in the same place and mark the junction among the developmental lobes. The grooves are sharp, deep, V-shaped linear depressions. The most prominent developmental groove on the posterior teeth is the **central groove**, which generally travels mesiodistally and divides the occlusal table in half.

Other developmental grooves include **marginal grooves**, which cross marginal ridges and serve as a spillway, allowing food to escape during mastication. **Triangular grooves** separate a marginal ridge from the triangular ridge of a cusp.

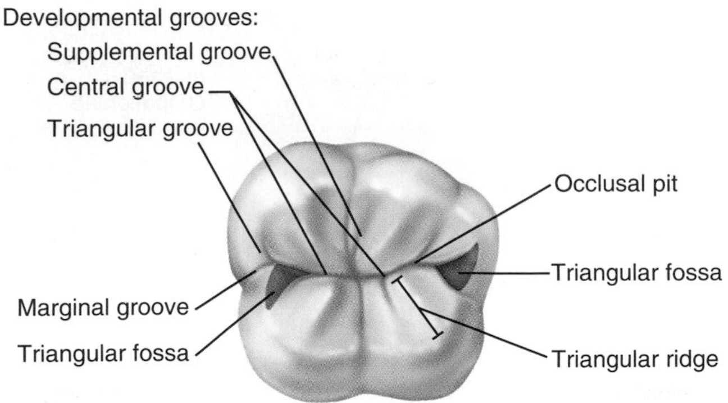


**FIG. 12.13** Other features of the occlusal table on a permanent posterior tooth, including the central groove. *(© Elsevier Collection.)*

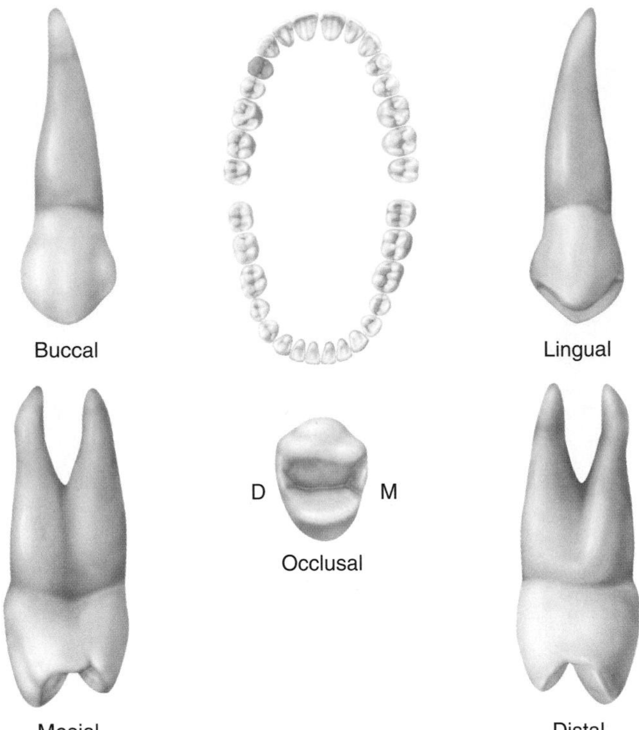


**FIG. 12.14** Various views of a permanent maxillary first premolar. *(© Elsevier Collection.)*

## Clinical Considerations: Posterior Teeth

The permanent posterior teeth are responsible for the major portion of chewing. The pits and grooves on these teeth make them highly susceptible to tooth decay. The occlusal surfaces should be carefully checked at each recall for signs of decay. Dental sealants are often placed on posterior teeth soon after they erupt. Dental sealants are discussed in Chapter 59.

# Permanent Premolars

Each quadrant of the arch has a *first premolar* and a *second premolar.* The first premolar is distal to the canine. The second premolar is behind the first premolar. These teeth occlude with opposing teeth when the jaws are brought together. Premolars are efficient as grinding teeth, and they function similarly to molars. The permanent premolars are succedaneous and replace the primary first and second molars. The crowns of the premolars are shorter than the crowns of the anterior teeth. The buccal surface of the premolars is rounded, and a prominent vertical buccal ridge is noted in the center of the crown. Two buccal depressions are present on each side of the buccal ridge. Premolars are *always* anterior to molars.

## Clinical Considerations: Premolars

The maxillary and mandibular premolars work with the molars in the chewing of food. The first premolars help the canines in shearing or cutting bits of food. The premolars also support the corners of the mouth and cheeks. When people lose all of their molars, they usually can still chew if they have their premolars. Unfortunately, the fact that a person is missing one or more maxillary premolars is very noticeable when he or she smiles.

Modified from Fehrenbach MJ, Popowics T: Illustrated dental embryology, histology, and anatomy, ed 4, St Louis, 2016, Saunders.

### *Maxillary First Premolars*

Each maxillary first premolar has two cusps (buccal and lingual) and two roots (facial and lingual) (Fig. 12.14). A maxillary first premolar (#5 and #12) is larger than a maxillary second premolar (#4 and #13). Both maxillary premolars erupt earlier than do mandibular premolars.

The buccal cusp is long and sharp to assist the canine with tearing. The facial cusp of the maxillary first premolar is much more prominent in size than the lingual cusp. It is longer and wider across and is similar to the canine from the facial side. The central groove extends between the mesial and distal grooves. The mesial marginal ridges border the mesial groove, and the distal marginal ridge borders the distal groove.

The maxillary first premolar has a **bifurcated** root. This means that the root is divided into two roots—one buccal and one lingual. A **furcation** is the area between two or more root branches. Some first premolars have roots that are joined together, or *fused.* These roots are shorter and resemble the roots of the molars.

### *Maxillary Second Premolars*

Each maxillary second premolar (#4 and #13) has two cusps (buccal and lingual) and one root. The maxillary second premolar (Fig. 12.15) differs from the first premolar in the following ways:

- The cusps, one buccal and one lingual, are more equal in length on the second premolar.
- The lingual cusp is larger than and almost the same height as the buccal cusp on the maxillary second premolar.

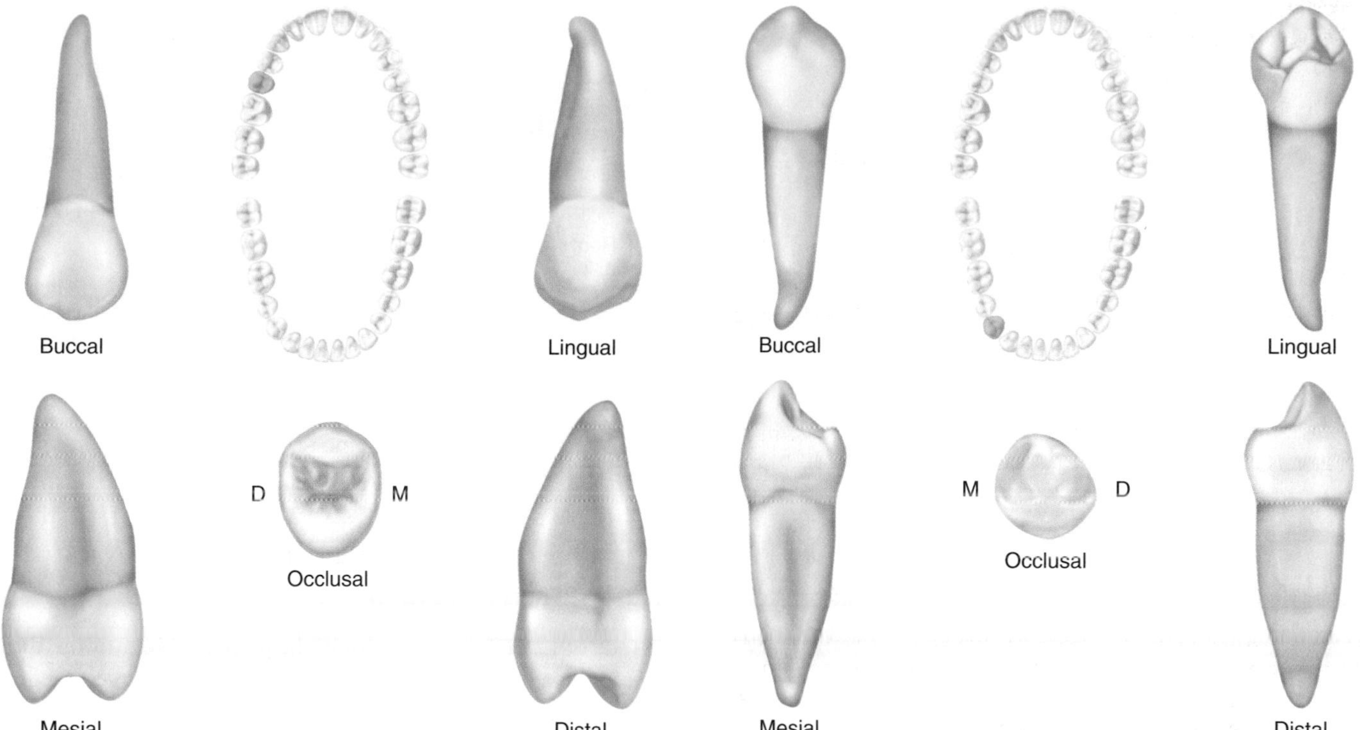


**FIG. 12.15** Various views of a permanent maxillary right second premolar. *(© Elsevier Collection.)*

**FIG. 12.16** Various views of a permanent mandibular right first premolar. *(© Elsevier Collection.)*

- The mesiobuccal cusp slope is shorter than the distobuccal cusp slope on the second premolar.
- The cusps of the secondary premolar are not as sharp as those of the maxillary first premolar.
- The second premolar has only one root and therefore only one root canal.
- The second premolar has a very slight depression on the mesial root.
- The second premolar is wider buccolingually than mesiodistally.

## Mandibular First Premolars

The mandibular first premolars (#21 and #28) have a long and well-formed buccal cusp and a nonfunctioning lingual cusp. The lingual cusp may be small.

Mandibular first premolars are smaller and shorter than mandibular second premolars (Fig. 12.16). The mandibular premolars do not resemble each other as much as the maxillary premolars do. Generally, both mandibular premolars erupt into the oral cavity later than do the maxillary premolars.

The permanent premolars have equal buccolingual and mesiodistal widths when viewed from the occlusal, making the outline almost round. In addition, both types of premolars have a similar buccal outline of both the crown and the root.

The mesial and distal contact areas of mandibular premolars are positioned at nearly the same level. The crowns incline lingually, bringing the cusps into proper occlusion with the teeth on the opposing arch.

## Mandibular Second Premolars

The permanent mandibular second premolars (#20 and #29) erupt distal to the mandibular first premolars. Thus they are the succedaneous replacements for the primary mandibular second molars (Fig. 12.17).

Two forms of the mandibular second premolar have been identified: the *three-cusp type,* or **tricanineate** form, and the *two-cusp type,* or **bicanineate** form. The more common three-cusp type consists of one large buccal cusp and two smaller lingual cusps. Less often, they are made up of a larger buccal cusp and a single smaller lingual cusp. The three-cusp type appears more angular from the occlusal view, and the two-cusp type appears more rounded.

In tricanineate premolars, the groove pattern is typically Y-shaped. In the two-cusp type, the groove pattern may be U-shaped (also called C-shaped) or H-grooved, depending on whether the central developmental groove is straight mesiodistally or curved buccally at its ends (Fig. 12.18).

Both types of mandibular second premolars have a greater number of supplemental grooves than do the mandibular first premolars. The single root of the mandibular second premolar is larger and longer than that of the first mandibular premolar but shorter than that of the maxillary premolars.

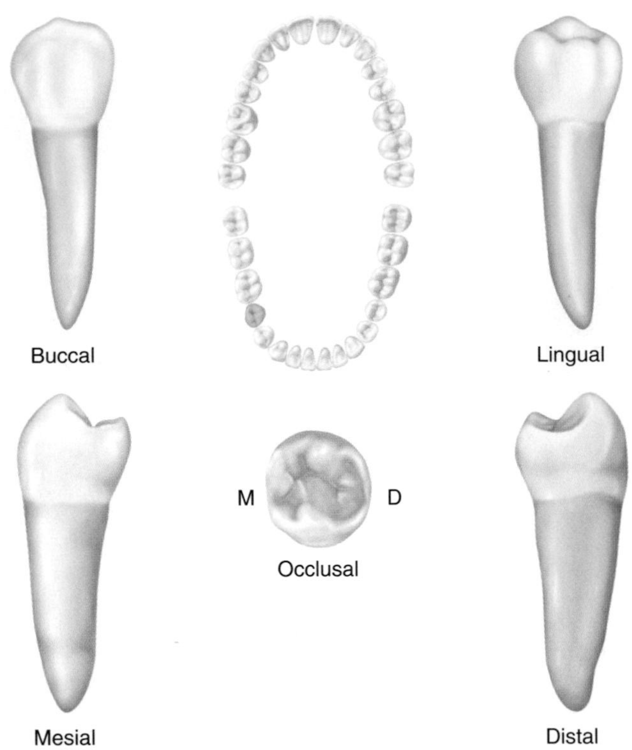


**FIG. 12.17** Various views of a permanent mandibular second premolar. *(© Elsevier Collection.)*

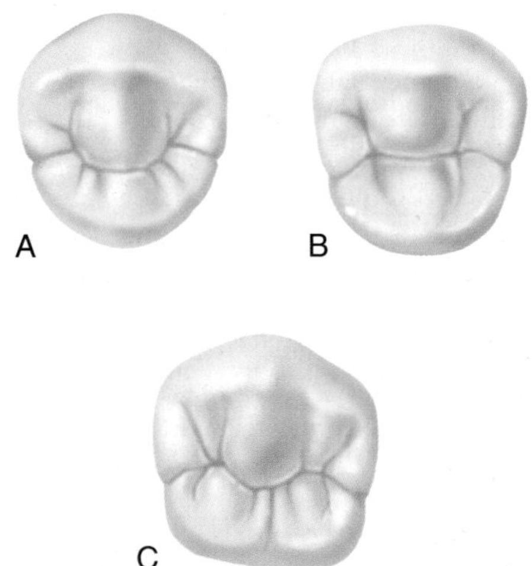


**FIG. 12.18** Occlusal views of a permanent mandibular second premolar. A, U-type. B, H-type. C, Y-type. *(© Elsevier Collection.)*

RECALL

8 What feature borders the occlusal table of a posterior tooth?
9 What are the pinpoint depressions where two or more grooves meet?
10 What are the two forms of mandibular second premolars?

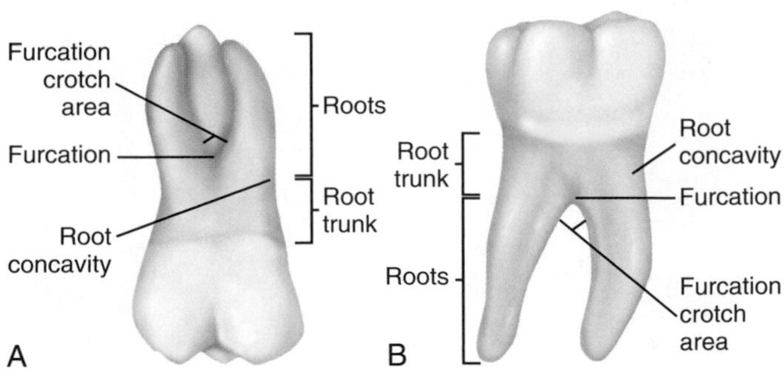


**FIG. 12.19** A, Maxillary first molar. B, Mandibular first molar. *(© Elsevier Collection.)*

## Permanent Molars

A total of 12 molars are present in the permanent dentition, three in each quadrant. The permanent molars are the largest teeth in the dentition. The name *molar* comes from the Latin word for "grinding"—one of the functions of the molar teeth. Three types of molars are present: the first molar, the second molar, and the third molar. The first and second molars are called the 6-year and 12-year molars, respectively, because of the approximate age of individuals at eruption. The molar crowns consist of four or five short, blunt cusps, and each molar has two or three roots that help to support the larger crown (Fig. 12.19).

### Maxillary Molars

The *maxillary molars* assist the mandibular molars in performing the major portion of the work of mastication. These are usually the first permanent teeth to erupt into the maxillary arch. Because of their size and their "anchorage" in the jaws, the molars are the largest and strongest maxillary teeth. Each maxillary molar usually includes four major cusps, with two cusps on the buccal portion of the occlusal table and two on the lingual portion.

Each maxillary molar has three well-separated and well-developed roots. A tooth with three roots is said to be **trifurcated**, which means divided into thirds. A **trifurcation** is the area at which three roots divide. Because maxillary molars are trifurcated, these three divisions are usually located on the mesial, buccal, and distal surfaces. They provide the tooth with maximum anchorage against occlusal forces. All maxillary molars are wider buccolingually than mesiodistally.

#### Clinical Considerations: Maxillary Molars

The roots of the maxillary molars are positioned in close proximity to the walls and floor of the sinus. On rare occasions, the maxillary sinus may be accidentally perforated by an instrument during surgical removal of a maxillary molar.

*Continued*

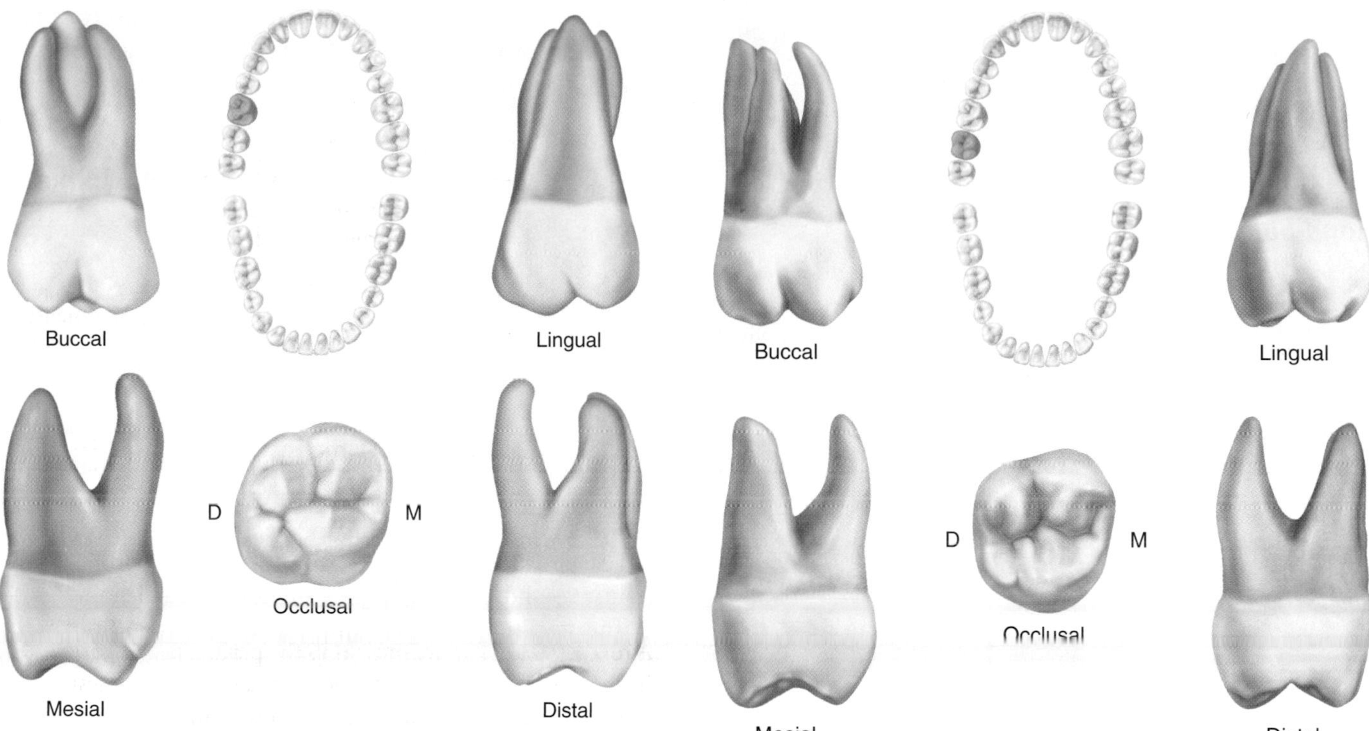


**FIG. 12.20** Various views of a permanent maxillary right first molar. *(© Elsevier Collection.)*

**FIG. 12.21** Various views of a permanent maxillary right second molar. *(© Elsevier Collection.)*

Because the maxillary molar roots are close to the sinus, some patients confuse the pain caused by a sinus infection with pain related to their maxillary teeth, and vice versa. Diagnostic tests are necessary to determine the cause.

If the maxillary first molar is lost to caries or periodontal disease, the second molar can tip and drift into the open space, causing difficulty in chewing and furthering periodontal disease.

Third molars often present oral hygiene problems for patients because this area is difficult to reach with a toothbrush.

Modified from Fehrenbach MJ, Popowics T: Illustrated dental embryology, histology, and anatomy, ed 4, St Louis, 2016, Saunders.

**MAXILLARY FIRST MOLARS.** The maxillary first molars (#3 and #14) are the first permanent teeth to erupt into the maxillary arch (Fig. 12.20). They erupt distal to the primary maxillary second molars and thus are **nonsuccedaneous**, meaning they do *not* replace the primary teeth.

The maxillary first molar, the largest tooth in the maxillary arch, also has the largest crown in the permanent dentition. This molar is composed of five developmental lobes: two buccal and three lingual. Four of the cusps (mesiolingual, distolingual, mesiobuccal, and distobuccal) are well-developed, functioning cusps, and the fifth supplemental cusp is of little practical use. The fifth cusp is called the **cusp of Carabelli**. When present, this cusp is located lingual to the mesiolingual cusp. However, it often is so poorly developed that it is scarcely distinguishable.

**MAXILLARY SECOND MOLARS.** The maxillary second molars (#2 and #15) supplement the first molars in function (Fig. 12.21). These molars erupt distal to the permanent maxillary first molars and are nonsuccedaneous.

The crown is somewhat shorter than that of the first molar, and the maxillary second molar usually has four cusps (mesiobuccal, distobuccal, mesiolingual, and distolingual). No fifth cusp is present. Three roots (mesiobuccal, distobuccal, and lingual) are observed. The roots of the secondary molars are smaller than the roots of the first molars. The lingual root is the largest and longest.

The buccal groove is located farther distally on the buccal surface of the second than the first maxillary molar. The mesiobuccal cusp of the second maxillary molar is longer and has a less sharp cusp tip than the distobuccal cusp.

**MAXILLARY THIRD MOLARS.** The maxillary third molars (#1 and #16) often appear as a developmental anomaly. The maxillary third molar differs considerably in size, contour, and relative position from the other teeth. Maxillary third molars are more likely than other teeth in the arch to be out of position. They are seldom as well developed as the maxillary second molar, to which they bear some resemblance.

The third molar supplements the second molar in function. Its fundamental design is similar, but the crown is smaller, and the roots usually are shorter. The roots of this tooth tend to fuse, and the result is a single, tapered root (Figs. 12.22 and 12.23). People sometimes refer to this tooth as the "wisdom" tooth because it is the last to erupt, usually at about age 17 years.

RECALL

11 What is the term for a tooth with three roots?
12 What is the term for a tooth that does not replace a primary tooth?
13 What is the name of the fifth cusp on a maxillary first molar?
14 Which teeth are referred to as the "wisdom" teeth?

## Mandibular Molars

The *mandibular molars* erupt 6 months to 1 year before the corresponding permanent maxillary molars erupt. The crown of a mandibular molar includes four or five major cusps, of which two lingual cusps are always of about the same width. All mandibular molars are wider mesiodistally than buccolingually.

Each mandibular molar has *two* well-developed roots: one mesial and one distal. As was mentioned earlier, a tooth with two roots is bifurcated, which means divided into two. Each root has its own root canal. A **bifurcation** is the area at which the two roots divide.

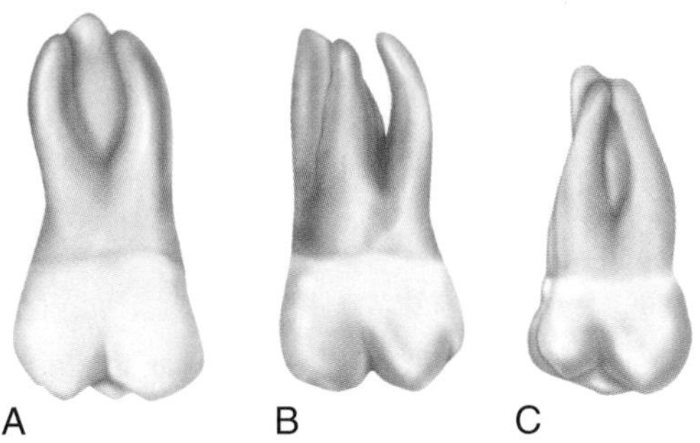


**FIG. 12.22** Buccal views of permanent maxillary right molars. A, First molar. B, Second molar. C, Third molar. Notice how the roots tend to be located closer together when the molars are farther distally. Third molar roots are often fused. *(© Elsevier Collection.)*

### Clinical Considerations: Mandibular Molars

The mandibular molars can make positioning of the oral evacuator difficult because of the lingual inclination of the crowns. In addition, patients often have problems with their oral hygiene because of the lingual inclination of the molar teeth; they may miss cleaning the lingual gingiva with the toothbrush.

**MANDIBULAR FIRST MOLARS.** The permanent mandibular first molars (#19 and #30) erupt between 6 and 7 years of age. These teeth are usually the first permanent teeth to erupt in the oral cavity (Fig. 12.24). They erupt distal to the primary mandibular second molars and thus are nonsuccedaneous.

The two roots, mesial and distal, of a mandibular first molar are larger and more divergent than those of a second molar, leaving the roots widely separated buccally. Usually, both roots are the same in length. However, if one is longer, it is the mesial root, which is also wider and stronger than the distal root. The pulp cavity of a mandibular first molar may have three root canals: distal, mesiobuccal, and mesiolingual.

The mesiobuccal cusp is the largest, widest, and highest cusp on the buccal portion. The distobuccal cusp is slightly smaller,

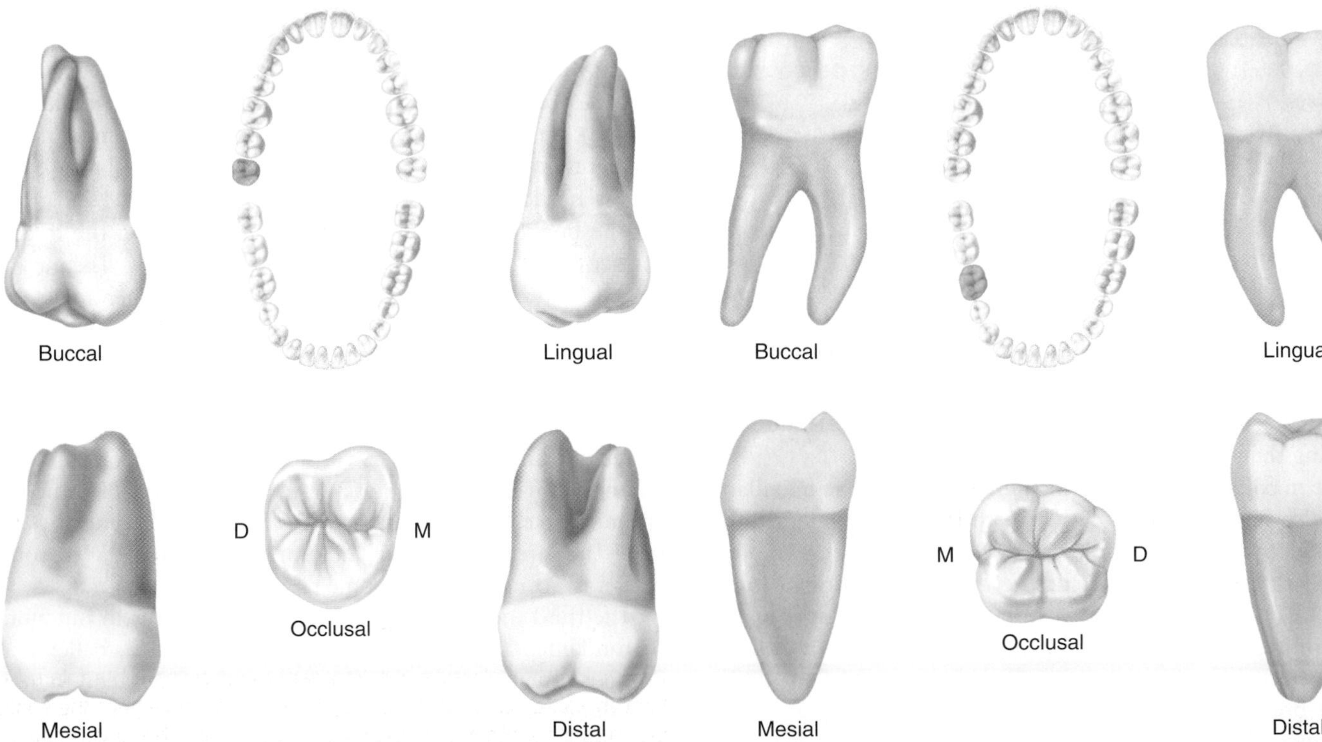


**FIG. 12.23** Various views of permanent maxillary right third molars. *(© Elsevier Collection.)*

**FIG. 12.24** Various views of a permanent mandibular right first molar. *(© Elsevier Collection.)*

shorter, and sharper than the mesiobuccal cusp. The distal cusp is the lowest cusp and is slightly sharper than the other two.

**MANDIBULAR SECOND MOLARS.** The mandibular second molars (#18 and #31) erupt between 11 and 12 years of age (Fig. 12.25). These teeth erupt distal to the permanent first molars and thus are nonsuccedaneous.

The crown of the mandibular second molar is slightly smaller than that of the first molar in all directions. The crown has four well-developed cusps (mesiolingual, distolingual, mesiobuccal, and distobuccal) and two roots (mesial and distal).

The two roots of the mandibular second molar are smaller, shorter, less divergent, and closer together than those of the first molar. These roots are not as broad buccolingually as those of the first molar and are not as widely separated.

The mesiolingual cusp and the distolingual cusp are the same in size and shape as the buccal cusps.

**MANDIBULAR THIRD MOLARS.** The mandibular third molars (#17 and #32) are similar to the maxillary third molars in that they vary greatly in shape and have no standard form. There is no typical mandibular third molar. This molar is usually smaller in all dimensions than the second molar. The third molar usually consists of four developmental lobes.

The crown of a mandibular third molar tapers distally when viewed from the mesial aspect. The occlusal outline of the crown is more oval than rectangular, although the crown frequently resembles that of a second molar. The two mesial cusps are larger than the two distal cusps. The occlusal surface appears wrinkled (Fig. 12.26).

A mandibular third molar usually has two roots that are fused, irregularly curved, and shorter than those of a mandibular second molar. Third molars are frequently impacted. Third molars often present with anomalies in form and position. A common anomaly is that the multiple roots are fused to form a single root (Fig. 12.27).

**15** How many roots do mandibular molars have?

## Primary Dentition

A total of 20 primary teeth are included in the primary dentition: 10 in the maxillary arch and 10 in the mandibular

**FIG. 12.25** Various views of a permanent mandibular right second molar. *(© Elsevier Collection.)*

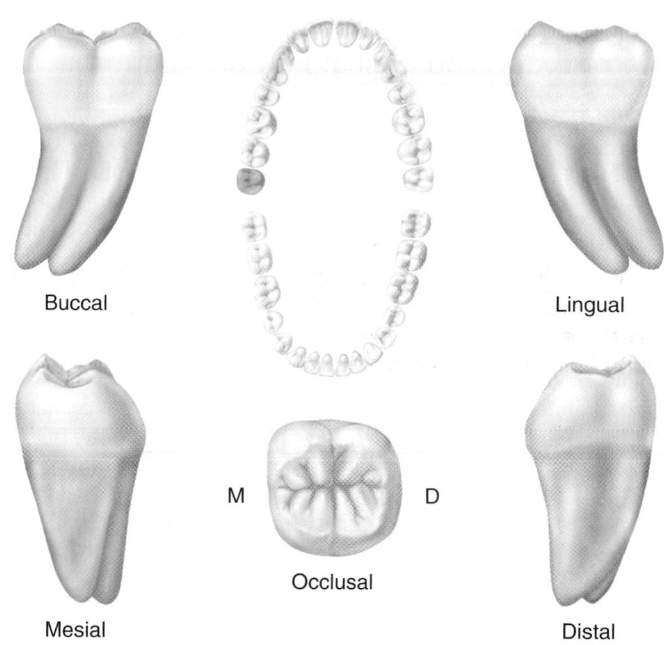


**FIG. 12.26** Various views of the permanent mandibular right third molar. *(© Elsevier Collection.)*

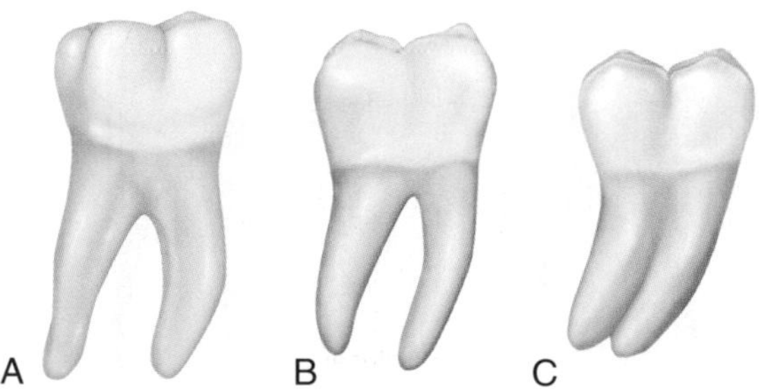


**FIG. 12.27** Buccal views of permanent mandibular right molars. A, First molar. B, Second molar. C, Third molar. Note that the roots are closer together and become shorter from the first molar to the third molar. Third molar roots are often fused. *(© Elsevier Collection.)*

arch. These teeth include incisors, canines, and molars. The primary teeth are numbered in the Universal/National Teeth-Numbering System with the use of capital letters A through T.

The primary teeth are smaller overall and have whiter enamel than the permanent teeth. This is so because of the increased opacity of the enamel that covers the underlying dentin. The crown of any primary tooth is short in relation to its total length. The crowns are narrower at the *cementoenamel junction* (CEJ). The roots of primary teeth are also narrower and longer than the crown.

The pulp chambers and the pulp horns in the primary teeth are relatively large in proportion to those of the permanent teeth. A thick layer of dentin is present between the pulp chambers and the enamel, especially in the primary mandibular second molar. However, the enamel layer is relatively thin (Fig. 12.28).

### Clinical Considerations: Primary Teeth

Some parents think that "baby teeth" are only temporary and are not really important because these teeth will be replaced by permanent ones. However, when primary teeth are lost prematurely, serious problems with tooth alignment, spacing, and occlusion can result later on. The primary teeth play an important role in "saving" space for the permanent teeth.

In addition to facilitating chewing, enhancing appearance, and assisting with speech for about 5 to 11 years, primary teeth support the cheeks and lips, resulting in a normal facial appearance. Because enamel and dentin are thinner in primary teeth, decay can travel quickly through the enamel to the pulp, possibly causing loss of the tooth.

Early dental health education and dental care are essential for keeping the primary dentition healthy. Primary teeth are essential for clear speech.

Modified from Fehrenbach MJ, Popowics T: Illustrated dental embryology, histology, and anatomy, ed 4, St Louis, 2016, Saunders.

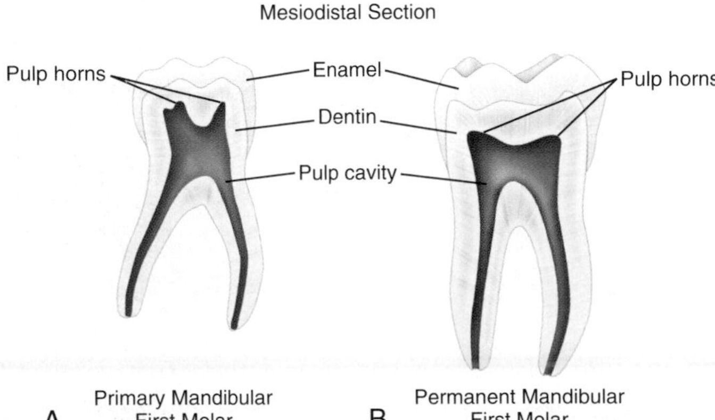


**FIG. 12.28** Illustration showing the differences between (A) primary and (B) permanent teeth. *(© Elsevier Collection.)*

## Primary Incisors

The crowns and roots of deciduous incisors are smaller than those of their permanent successors. The roots are twice as long as the crowns and taper toward the apex.

### *Maxillary Central Incisors*

The crown of the primary maxillary central incisor (E and F) is wider mesiodistally than incisocervically—the opposite of its permanent successor. It is the only tooth of either dentition with this crown dimension.

The primary maxillary incisors have no mamelons. These teeth rarely have developmental depressions or imbrication lines. The cingulum and marginal ridges are more prominent than on the permanent successor, and the lingual fossa is deeper (Fig. 12.29).

### *Maxillary Lateral Incisors*

The crown of the primary maxillary lateral incisor (D and G) is similar to that of the central incisor but is much smaller in all dimensions (Fig. 12.30).

The incisal angles on the lateral incisor are also more rounded than on the central incisor. The lateral root is longer in proportion to its crown, and its apex is sharper.

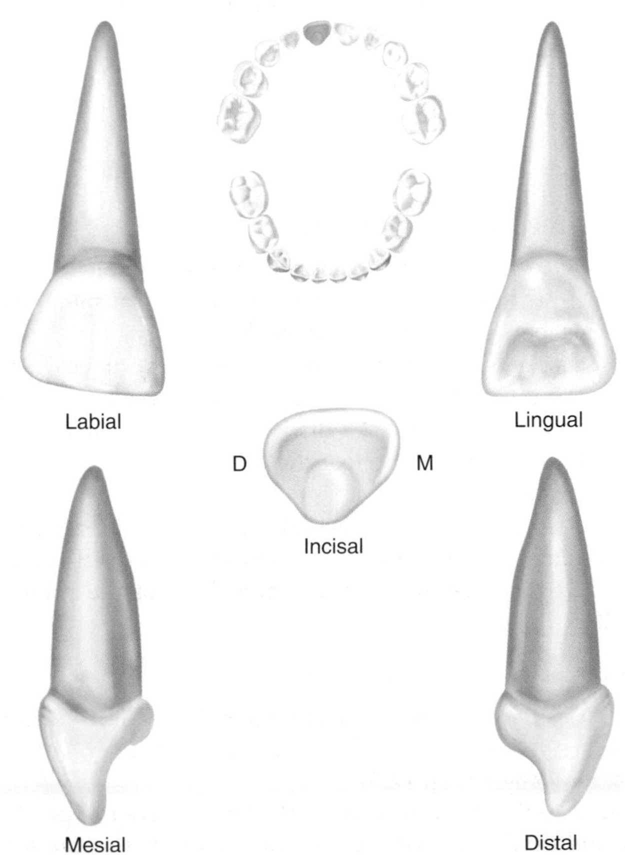


**FIG. 12.29** Various views of a primary maxillary right central incisor. *(© Elsevier Collection.)*

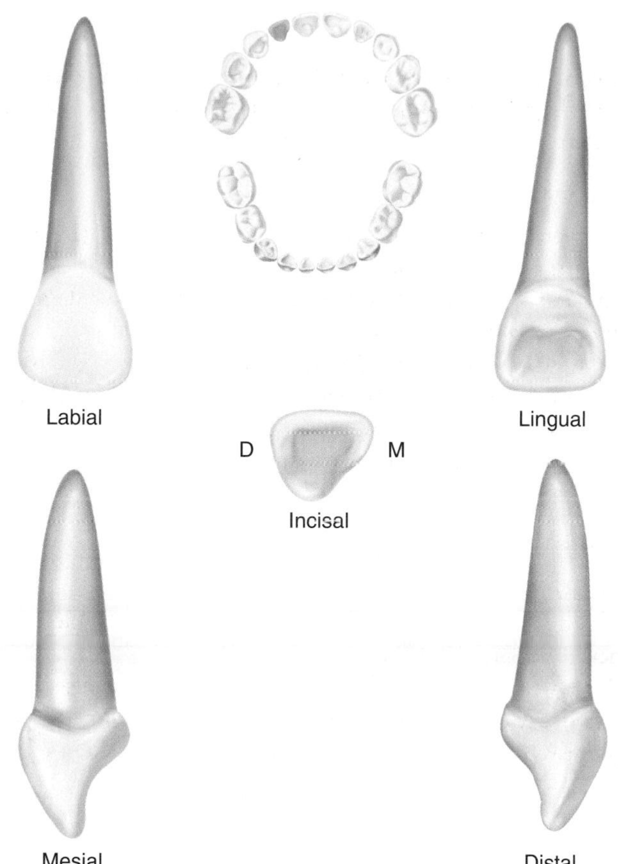


FIG. 12.30 Various views of a primary maxillary lateral incisor. (© Elsevier Collection.)

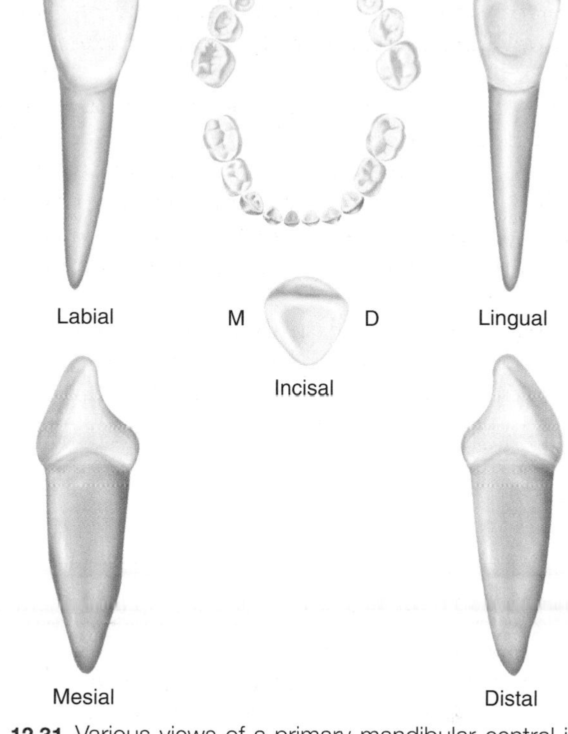


FIG. 12.31 Various views of a primary mandibular central incisor. (© Elsevier Collection.)

## Mandibular Central Incisors

The crown of the primary mandibular incisor (O and P) resembles that of the primary mandibular lateral incisor more than its permanent central successor does (Fig. 12.31).

The mandibular central incisor is extremely symmetric. It is also not as constricted at the cementoenamel junction as is the primary maxillary incisor. Its mesial and distal outlines from the labial aspect also show that the crown tapers evenly from the contact areas.

The lingual surface of the mandibular central incisor appears smooth and tapers toward the prominent cingulum. The marginal ridges are less pronounced than those of the primary maxillary incisor.

## Mandibular Lateral Incisors

The crown of the primary lateral incisor (Q and N) is similar in form to that of the central incisor in the same arch, but it is wider and longer (Fig. 12.32).

The incisal edge of the mandibular lateral incisor slopes distally, and the distoincisal angle is more rounded. The root may have a distal curvature in its apical third and usually has a distal longitudinal groove.

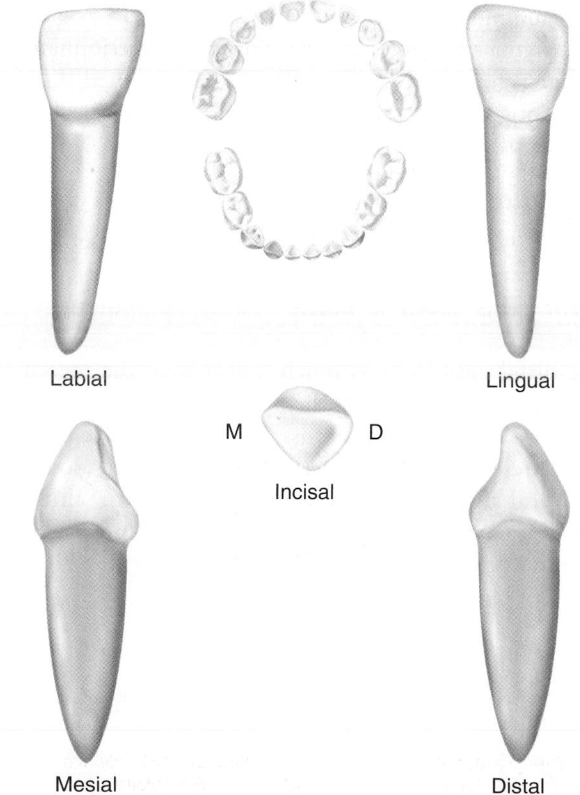


FIG. 12.32 Various views of a primary mandibular lateral incisor. (© Elsevier Collection.)

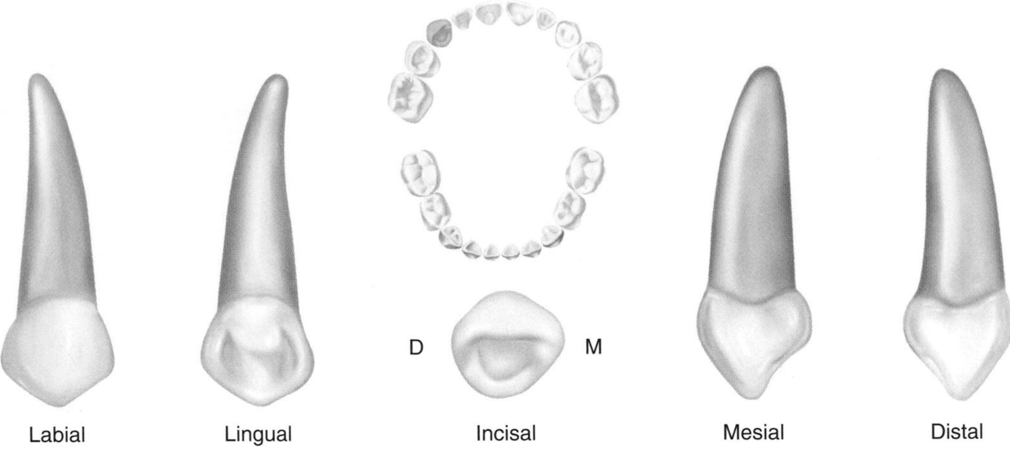

**FIG. 12.33** Various views of a primary maxillary canine. *(© Elsevier Collection.)*

## Primary Canines

There are four primary canines, two in each dental arch. These primary canines differ from the outline of their permanent successors in the following ways.

### *Maxillary Canines*

When first erupted, the crown of the primary maxillary canine (C and H) has a relatively longer and sharper cusp than its permanent successor (Fig. 12.33). The mesial and distal outlines of the primary maxillary canine are rounder.

On the lingual surface, the cingulum is well developed, as are the lingual ridge and marginal ridges. The mesiolingual and distolingual fossae are shallow. The root is inclined distally, is twice as long as the crown, and is more slender than the root of its successor.

### *Mandibular Canines*

The primary mandibular canine (M and R) resembles the primary maxillary canine, although some dimensions are different. This tooth is much smaller labiolingually (Fig. 12.34).

The distal cusp slope is much longer than the mesial cusp slope. The lingual surface of the primary mandibular canine is marked by a shallow lingual fossa. The incisal edge is straight and is centered over the crown labiolingually. The root is long, narrow, and almost twice the length of the crown, although it is shorter and more tapered than the root of a primary maxillary canine.

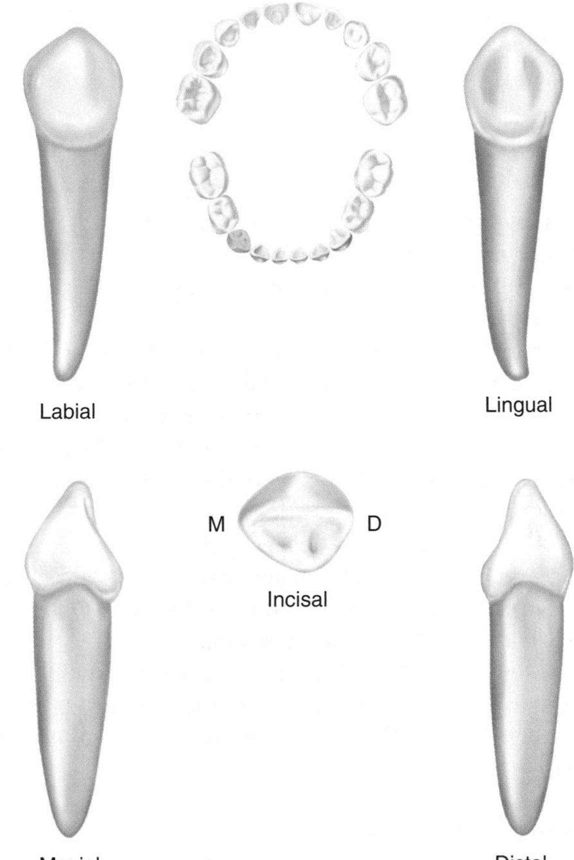

**FIG. 12.34** Various views of a primary mandibular canine. *(© Elsevier Collection.)*

RECALL

16 How thick is the enamel covering on a primary tooth?
17 What method of identification is used in the Universal/National Tooth-Numbering System for the primary dentition?
18 Do primary anterior incisors have mamelons?

## Primary Molars

The primary dentition consists of a total of eight primary molars. Each quadrant includes a first primary molar and a second primary molar. Each molar crown is wider than it is tall. The permanent premolars replace the primary molars when they are exfoliated.

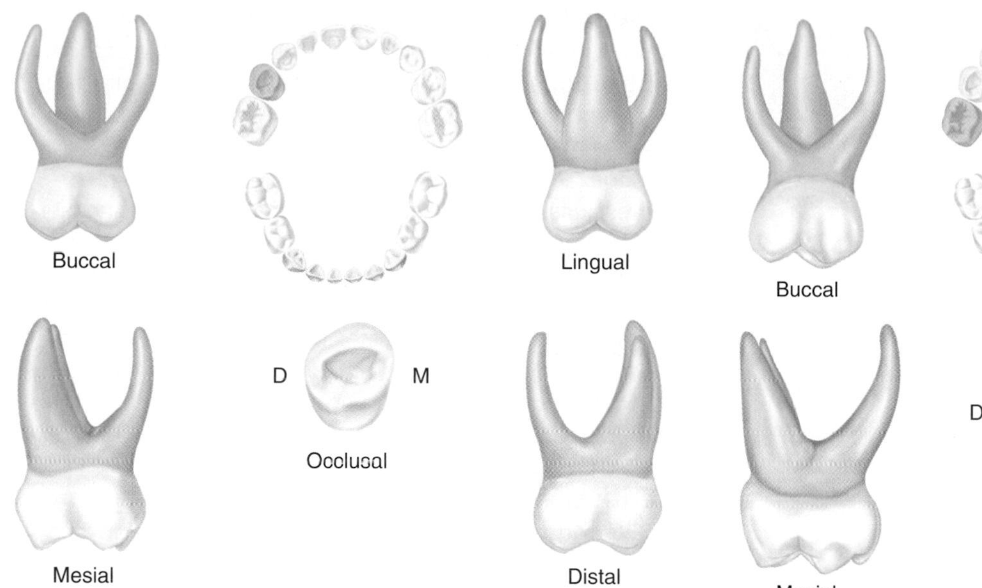


FIG. 12.35 Various views of a primary maxillary first molar. (© Elsevier Collection.)

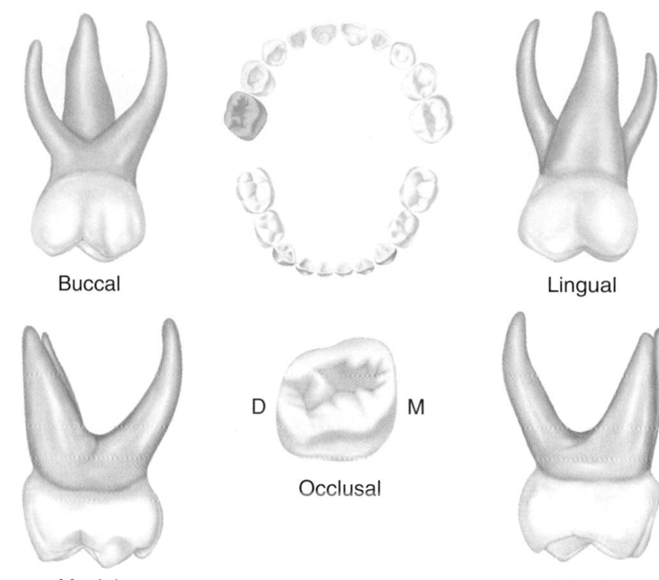


FIG. 12.36 Various views of a primary maxillary second molar. (© Elsevier Collection.)

## Maxillary First Molars

The crown of the primary maxillary first molar (B and I) does not resemble any other crown of either dentition (Fig. 12.35). The height of contour on the buccal surface is at the cervical one third of the tooth, and on the lingual side it is at the middle one third.

The occlusal table may have four cusps (mesiobuccal, mesiolingual, distobuccal, and distolingual); the two mesial cusps are the largest cusps, and the two distal cusps are very small. The primary maxillary first molar frequently has only three cusps because the distolingual cusp may be absent. The occlusal table also has a prominent transverse ridge.

This tooth also has an H-shaped groove pattern and three fossae: central, mesial triangular, and distal triangular. The central groove connects the central pit with the mesial pit and the distal pit at each end of the occlusal table.

The primary maxillary first molar has three roots, which are thinner and have greater flare than those of the permanent maxillary first molar. The lingual root is the longest and most divergent.

## Maxillary Second Molars

The primary maxillary second molar (A and J) is larger than the primary maxillary first molar (Fig. 12.36). This tooth most closely resembles the permanent maxillary first molar in form but is smaller in all dimensions. The second molar usually has a cusp of Carabelli, the minor fifth cusp.

## Mandibular First Molars

The crown of the primary mandibular first molar (L and S) is different from that of any other tooth of either dentition (Fig. 12.37). The tooth has a prominent buccal cervical ridge, also on the mesial half of the buccal surface, similar to other primary molars. The height of contour on the buccal surface is seen at the cervical one third of the tooth; on the lingual side, it is noted at the middle one third. The mesiolingual line angle of the crown is rounder than other line angles.

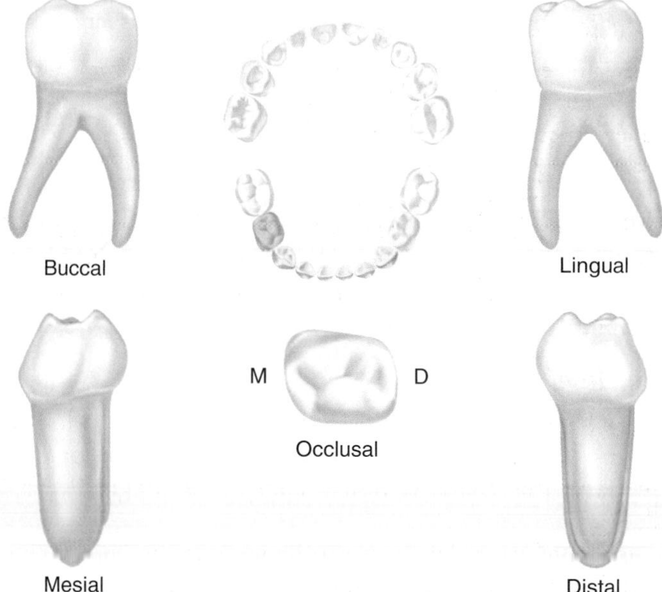


FIG. 12.37 Various views of a primary mandibular first molar. (© Elsevier Collection.)

The primary mandibular first molar has four cusps; the mesial cusps are larger. The mesiolingual cusp is long, pointed, and angled into the occlusal table. A transverse ridge passes between the mesiobuccal and mesiolingual cusps. The tooth has two roots, which are positioned similarly to those of other primary and permanent mandibular molars.

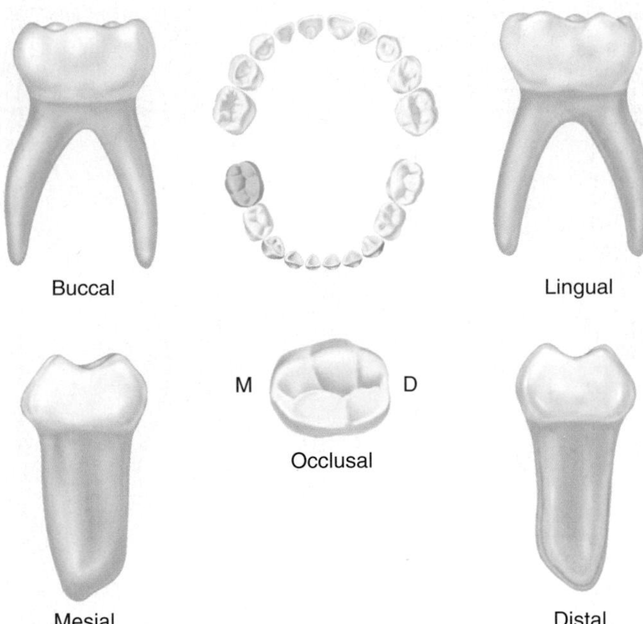


**FIG. 12.38** Various views of a primary mandibular second molar. *(© Elsevier Collection.)*

## Mandibular Second Molars

The primary mandibular second molar (K and T) is larger than the primary mandibular first molar (Fig. 12.38). Because it has five cusps, the second molar most closely resembles in form the permanent mandibular first molar that erupts distal to it. The three buccal cusps are nearly equal in size, however, and the primary mandibular second molar has an overall oval occlusal shape.

RECALL

**19** Which primary molar has an H-shaped groove pattern on the occlusal surface?
**20** Which primary mandibular molar is the largest?

## ■ Eye to the Future

As a practicing dental assistant, you will be surprised at how often your knowledge of tooth morphology and the other dental sciences will directly relate to patient care and your understanding of dental treatment plans.

For example, while exposing radiographs or making impressions, you may note that the anatomy of the lingual surfaces of the patient's maxillary anterior teeth has an unusually smooth, glassy appearance. You may see few if any stains or lines on the teeth and may observe a slight loss of occlusal anatomy on the posterior teeth. These oral manifestations are commonly associated with bulimia. Erosion is caused by acidic gastric fluids produced by chronic vomiting and movement of the tongue. ■

## ■ Critical Thinking

1. Eight-year-old Lucinda Alvarez is at your dental office for a 6-month checkup. While you are waiting for Dr. Miller to come to the treatment room, Lucinda asks you why the edges on your front teeth are flat and hers have "ruffled edges." What would you tell her?
2. Sharon Jackson brings her 10-year-old son into your office for an emergency visit because she is certain that one of his permanent molars "fell out." When Mrs. Jackson shows you the tooth, you immediately recognize it as a primary molar that was exfoliated naturally. How would you explain to her the differences between a primary molar and a permanent molar?
3. Michael Hughes is a 14-year-old who is very interested in his teeth. He wants to know how many teeth he will have as an adult, and how many different types of teeth there are. What will you tell him?
4. A young mother brings her 4-year-old son into your dental office with a toothache. The mother is shocked and embarrassed when the dentist tells her that the decay has gone into the pulp chamber. Another dentist saw the child just over a year ago. How do you think this happened? ■

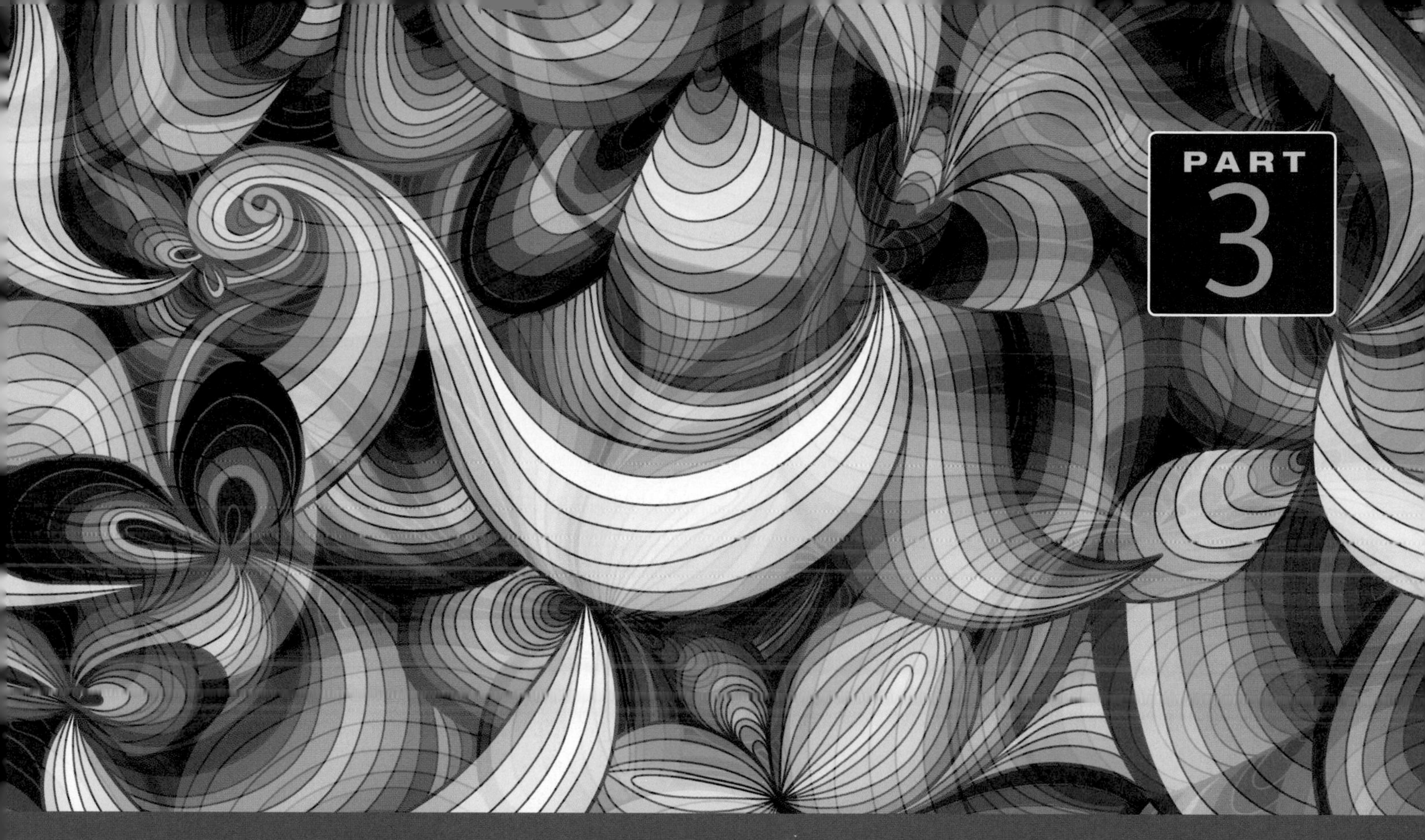


# Oral Health and Prevention of Dental Disease

*"The mouth is the gateway to the rest of the body, a mirror of our overall well-being."*

**Harold C. Slavkin, DDS**

Former Director, National Institute of Dental and Craniofacial Research
Former Dean, University of Southern California, School of Dentistry

The U.S. Surgeon General's report *Oral Health in America* (http://www.nidcr.nih.gov/DataStatistics/SurgeonGeneral/sgr/welcome.htm) has alerted Americans to the full meaning of oral health and its importance to general health and well-being. A major theme of this report is that "oral health means much more than healthy teeth." It means being free of chronic oral-facial pain, oral and pharyngeal (throat) cancers, oral soft tissue lesions, birth defects such as cleft lip and palate, and scores of other diseases and disorders. *You cannot be healthy without oral health. Oral health* and *general health* should not be interpreted as separate entities. Oral health is a critical component of health.

Every day in the United States, millions of people, including children, working families, and the elderly, live in constant pain as a result of oral disease or injury to the mouth. The chapters in this section discuss the two most important infectious dental diseases—*dental caries* and *periodontal disease*—and describe measures that are effective in improving oral health and preventing oral disease. Also discussed in this section is the role of nutrition in general health and how it relates to oral health in particular.

13

# Dental Caries

## KEY TERMS

**CAMBRA** Caries management by risk assessment.
**Caries (KAR-eez)** The infectious disease process of tooth decay.
**Caries Risk Test (CRT)** Test for cariogenic bacteria.
**Cariology (KAR-ee-all-o-gee)** The science and study of dental caries.
**Carious (KAR-ee-us) lesion** White spots, brown spots, and decay on tooth surfaces.
**Cavitation (ka-vi-TAY-shun)** Formation of a cavity or hole.
**Demineralization (dee-min-ur-ul-i-ZAY-shun)** Loss of minerals from the tooth.
**Early childhood caries (ECC)** Decay in any primary teeth.
**Evidence based** Information based on documented evidence from critically reviewed research.
**Fermentable (fur-MEN-tuh-bul) carbohydrates** Simple carbohydrates, such as sucrose, fructose, lactose, and glucose.
**Fluoride (FLOOR-ide)** Mineral to make teeth more resistant to decay.
**Incipient (in-SIP-ee-ent) caries** Tooth decay that is beginning to form or become apparent.
**Lactobacilli (lak-toe-buh-SIL-eye)** Bacteria that produce lactic acid from carbohydrates associated with causing dental caries.
**Mutans streptococci (strep-toe-KOK-sye)** Type of bacteria primarily responsible for dental caries.
**Oral biofilm** Also called plaque, a highly organized complex of microorganisms that adheres to surfaces where moisture and nutrients are available.
**Pellicle (PEL-i-kul)** Thin film coating of salivary materials deposited on tooth surfaces.
**Plaque (plak)** Soft deposit on teeth that consists of organized complex of bacteria and bacterial by-products.
**Rampant (RAM-punt) caries** Decay that develops rapidly and is widespread throughout the mouth.
**Remineralization** Replacement of minerals in the tooth.
**Root caries** Decay on the root surface of teeth that have gingival recession.
**Saliva flow rate test** Determines flow rate of saliva in milliliters per minute.
**Xerostomia (zeer-oe-STOE-mee-uh)** Dryness of the mouth caused by reduction of saliva.
**Xylitol (ZY-li-toll)** Ingredient in chewing gum that has an antibacterial effect against decay-causing bacteria.

## LEARNING OUTCOMES

*On completion of this chapter, the student will be able to achieve the following objectives:*

1. Pronounce, define, and spell the key terms.
2. Classify dental caries as an infectious disease, and name the two types of bacteria that cause dental caries.
3. Explain the caries process, including the following:
   - List the factors that cause dental caries.
   - Describe how dental caries is transmitted.
   - Name the four areas of a tooth where dental caries can occur.
   - Explain the development of dental caries.
   - Explain why secondary (recurrent) caries are difficult to diagnose.
   - Identify the risk factors for root caries.
4. Discuss early childhood caries (ECC), including the following:
   - Name the most common chronic disease in children.
   - Explain the risk factors for early childhood caries.
   - Explain how ECC is transmitted.
   - Explain the consequences of early childhood caries.
5. Explain the importance of saliva related to tooth decay.
6. Describe the advantages and disadvantages of each method of detecting dental caries.
7. Explain the goal of CAMBRA.
8. List the methods of caries intervention.
9. Describe the current caries risk assessment tests.

## PERFORMANCE OUTCOMES

*On completion of this chapter, the student will be able to meet competency standards in the following skills:*

- Perform a caries detection procedure using an electronic caries detection device.
- Perform a caries risk test and compare the density of bacterial colonies versus evaluation pictures.

## ELECTRONIC RESOURCES

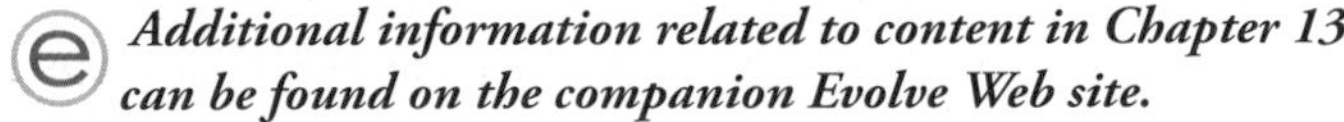
***Additional information related to content in Chapter 13 can be found on the companion Evolve Web site.***

- Practice Quiz

Dental **caries** (tooth decay) is an infectious and communicable disease. It is a worldwide health concern, affecting humans of all ages. *Dental caries is the single most common chronic disease in children.* In fact, five times more children in the United States have untreated dental disease than have childhood asthma. This results in more than 50 million missed school hours every year. Caries is not just a child's disease. Because of recession of the gingival tissues, many older adults experience root caries. This chapter discusses **cariology**, which includes the causes of caries, the process by which caries occurs, and the science and practice of caries management and prevention.

Caries has plagued humankind since the beginning of recorded history. Since the late nineteenth century, dentists have been fighting tooth decay by drilling out the decayed tooth structure and filling the tooth with a restorative material. Although this treatment eliminates decay that is already present, it does nothing to lower levels of bacteria in the mouth that may cause additional caries. Today, the emphasis in fighting caries is shifting from the traditional approach of restoring (filling) teeth to newer strategies of managing caries by determining the risk for caries in an individual and then implementing appropriate methods of preventing future caries. Advances in science and new technologies have placed the emphasis on *prevention* and *early intervention.*

## Bacterial Infection

Caries is a *transmissible* bacterial infection. The two specific groups of bacteria in the mouth that are responsible for caries are the **mutans streptococci** (MS) *(Streptococcus mutans)* and the **lactobacilli** (LB).

MS, which are considered to be *major pathogenic* (disease-producing) bacteria, are found in relatively large numbers in dental plaque. The presence of LB in a patient's mouth indicates that the patient has a high sugar intake. MS and LB, separately or together, are the primary causative agents of caries.

It is important to note that the oral cavity of a newborn does not contain MS. However, these bacteria are transmitted through contact with saliva (most frequently the mother's saliva) to the infant. Mothers are the most common source of disease-causing MS because of the close and frequent contact that takes place between mother and child during the first few years. For example, a mother kisses her baby and may also taste food on a spoon before giving it to her baby. Science has proved that when mothers have high counts of MS in their mouths, their infants have high counts of the same bacteria in their mouths. Children also may be infected by a caregiver or even by siblings.

Remember, caries is an infectious disease. When the number of caries-causing bacteria in the mouth increases, the risk for developing caries also increases.

1 What two types of bacteria primarily cause dental caries?

2 Which of the above two types of bacteria is most responsible for dental caries?

## Oral Biofilm

**Oral biofilm** (also known as **plaque**, **dental plaque biofilm, microbial biofilm**) is a colorless, soft, sticky coating made up of communities of microorganisms that adheres to tooth surfaces, dental appliances, restorations of the teeth, the oral mucosa, the tongue, and alveolar bone.

Dental caries and gingival and periodontal infections are caused by microorganisms in dental plaque (Fig. 13.1). The relationship of oral biofilm and periodontal disease is discussed in Chapter 55. If toothbrushing and flossing are not thorough, the oral biofilm remains attached to the oral surfaces. Even self-cleansing movements of the tongue, or rinsing and spraying of the mouth with water or even mouthwash, will not dislodge the biofilm.

If you were to look at biofilm under a microscope, you would see colonies of bacteria embedded in an adhesive substance called the **pellicle**. Formation of plaque on a tooth concentrates millions of microorganisms on that tooth. A milligram of wet plaque may contain as many as 200 to 500 million microorganisms. A similar amount of saliva flowing through the oral cavity contains less than 1 percent of this number of organisms, so it is clear that bacteria in plaque that is attached to the tooth are a major part of the problem.

## Enamel Structure

To gain an understanding of how bacterial infection leads to the caries process, it is important to review the structure of enamel. Enamel is the most highly mineralized tissue in the body, and it is stronger than bone. Refer to Chapter 8 for an in-depth discussion of the structure of enamel.

Enamel consists of microscopic crystals of hydroxyapatite arranged in structural layers or rods, also known as *prisms.* These crystals are surrounded by water, and primary teeth are made up of slightly more water than are permanent teeth. The water in enamel allows acids to flow into the tooth and minerals to flow out of the tooth. Carbonated apatite, a mineral in enamel, makes it easier for the tooth structure to dissolve.

RECALL

3 What is the soft, sticky bacterial mass that adheres to the teeth?

4 What is the mineral in the enamel that makes the tooth structure easier to dissolve?

## The Caries Process

Caries is a disease caused by multiple factors (Fig. 13.2). For caries to develop, the following three factors must be present at the same time:

1. A susceptible tooth.
2. A diet rich in **fermentable carbohydrates**.
3. Specific bacteria. (Regardless of other factors, caries cannot occur without the presence of bacteria.)

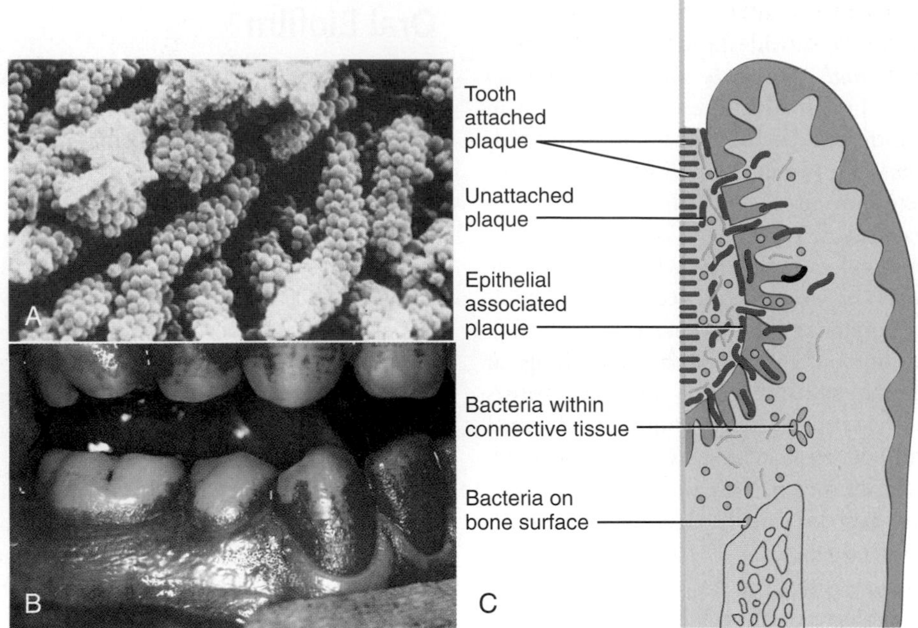


**FIG. 13.1** Oral biofilm. A, Long-standing supragingival plaque near the gingival margin demonstrates "corncob" arrangement. A central gram-negative filamentous core supports the outer coccal cells, which are firmly attached. B, Disclosed supragingival plaque covering one third to two thirds of the clinical crown. C, Diagram depicting the plaque bacteria associated with tooth surface and periodontal tissues. *(From Newman MG, Takei HH, Klokkevold PR, et al: Carranza's clinical periodontology, ed 12, St Louis, 2015, Saunders.)*

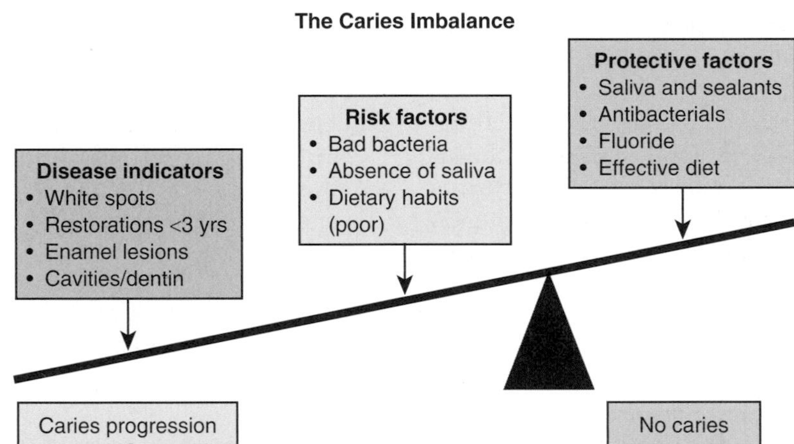


**FIG. 13.2** Factors involved in the formation of carious defects. *(Courtesy Dr. John D. B. Featherstone, School of Dentistry, University of California San Francisco.)*

Bacteria in dental plaque feed on fermentable carbohydrates found in a regular diet, such as sugars (including fruit sugars) and cooked starch (e.g., bread, potatoes, rice, pasta). Just as human wastes are a by-product of eating, these bacteria produce acids as a by-product of their metabolism. Within about 5 minutes after eating or drinking, bacteria begin to produce acids as a by-product of their digesting your food. These acids can penetrate into the hard substance of the tooth and dissolve some of the minerals (calcium and phosphate). If acid attacks are infrequent and of short duration, saliva can help repair the damage by neutralizing the acids and supplying minerals and **fluoride** to replace those lost from the tooth. When fermentable carbohydrates are eaten frequently, more acid is produced and the risk for decay increases. If this process continues, caries develops.

**Carious lesions** can occur in four general areas of the tooth:

1. *Pit-and-fissure caries* occurs primarily on occlusal surfaces, on buccal and lingual grooves of posterior teeth, and on lingual pits of the maxillary incisors.
2. *Smooth surface caries* occurs on enamel surfaces, including mesial, distal, facial, and lingual surfaces.

3. *Root surface caries* occurs on any surface of the exposed root.
4. *Secondary caries,* or *recurrent caries,* occurs on the tooth that surrounds a restoration.

5 What are the three factors necessary for the formation of dental caries?

## Stages of Caries Development

It can take months or even years for a carious lesion to develop. Carious lesions occur when more minerals are lost (demineralization) from the enamel than are deposited (remineralization). **Demineralization** occurs when calcium and phosphate dissolve from hydroxyapatite crystals in the enamel. In **remineralization**, calcium and phosphate are redeposited in previously demineralized areas. The processes of demineralization and remineralization may occur without loss of tooth structure.

Dental caries is not simply a continual, cumulative loss of minerals from the tooth. Rather, caries is a dynamic, ongoing process that is characterized by *alternating periods* of demineralization and remineralization (Fig. 13.3).

Carious lesions develop in two distinct stages:

1. The first stage, **incipient caries** or *incipient lesions,* occurs when caries begins to demineralize the enamel (Fig. 13.4, *A*).
2. The second stage, the *overt lesion,* or *frank lesion,* is characterized by **cavitation**—the development of a cavity or a hole (Fig. 13.4, *B*).

At times, onset of the incipient lesion is followed rapidly by the development of cavitation, with multiple lesions throughout the mouth. This condition is known as **rampant caries** (Figs. 13.5 and 13.6; also see Fig. 13.4, *C*). Usually, rampant caries occurs after excessive and frequent intake of sucrose or after **xerostomia** (dry mouth).

### How to Control Tooth Decay

- **Diet:** Limit quantities of sugary and starchy foods, snacks, drinks, and candy (three snacks per day).
- **Fluorides:** Fluorides help make the tooth resistant to being dissolved by acids (see Chapter 15).
- **Remove plaque:** Perform thorough brushing and flossing to remove plaque from all tooth surfaces.
- **Saliva:** Saliva neutralizes acids and provides minerals and proteins that protect the tooth. After you have had a snack, chew some sugar-free gum to increase the flow of saliva and neutralize acids. Choose gums that contain xylitol or gums that contain baking soda (see Chapter 15).
- **Antibacterial mouth rinses:** The dentist can prescribe these rinses for patients who are at high risk for caries, to reduce the numbers of bacteria that cause tooth decay.
- **Dental sealants:** Sealants are an excellent preventive measure that can be used for children and young adults who are at risk for decay (see Chapter 59).

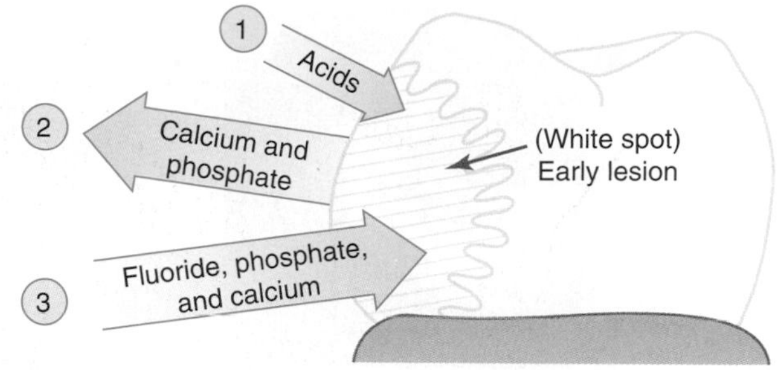


1. The tooth is attacked by acids in plaque and saliva.
2. Calcium and phosphate dissolve from the enamel in the process of demineralization.
3. Fluoride, phosphate, and calcium re-enter the enamel in a process called remineralization.

**FIG. 13.3** Demineralization and remineralization of the tooth.

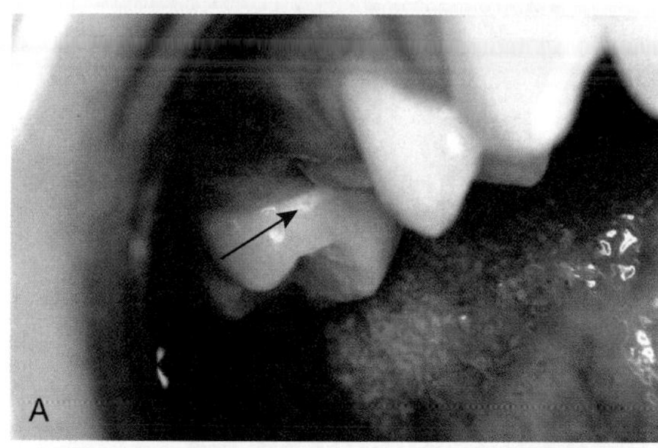


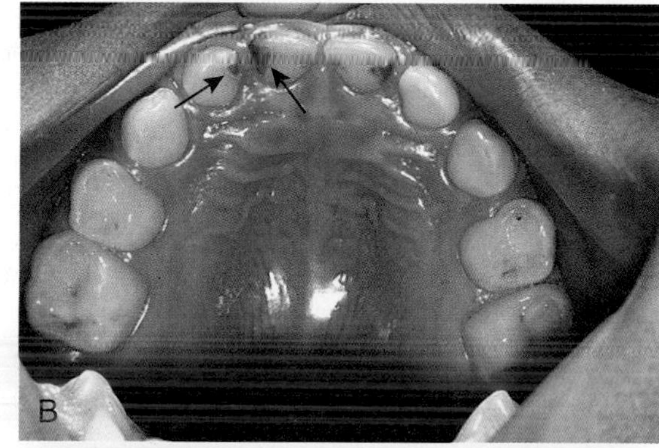


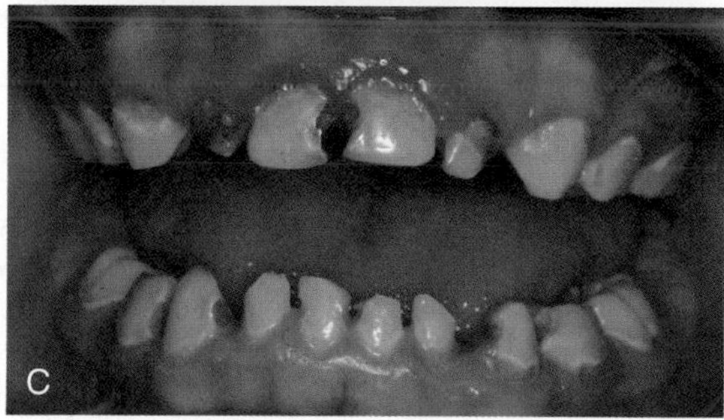


**FIG. 13.4** A, Early carious lesion, or white spot of demineralization. B, Overt carious lesion. C, Rampant caries. *(A, Courtesy Dr. John D. B. Featherstone, School of Dentistry, University of California San Francisco. B and C, Courtesy Dr. Frank Hodges, Santa Rosa, CA.)*

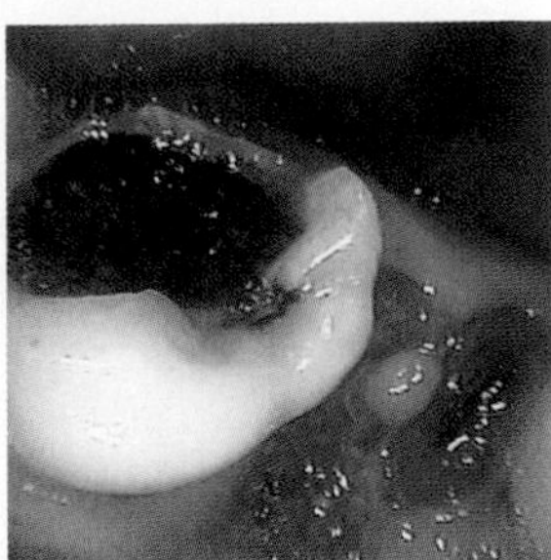

FIG. 13.5 Severely decayed molar on a child.

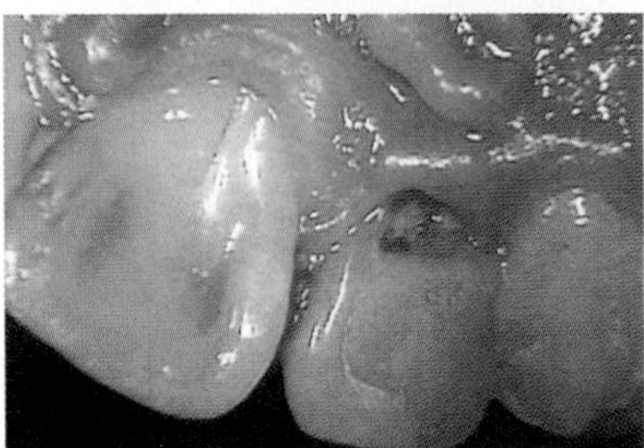

FIG. 13.6 Decay on the lingual surface of a maxillary lateral incisor.

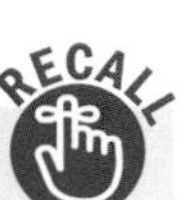


6 What is the term for the dissolution of calcium and phosphate from the tooth?
7 What is the term for rapid and extensive formation of caries?

## Secondary (Recurrent) Caries

Secondary, or recurrent, caries starts to form in tiny spaces between the tooth and the margins of a restoration. Bacteria are able to thrive in these areas. This type of caries is difficult to diagnose because it cannot be seen easily, and it cannot be detected with an explorer. Radiographs are required to detect this type of caries.

When dental restorations must be replaced, the reason is usually recurrent caries under the existing restoration. New restorative materials that bond to the tooth structure may help prevent recurrent decay by eliminating the tiny space between the tooth and the filling material, where microleakage can occur. Restorative materials that slowly release fluoride also can help to prevent secondary caries (Fig. 13.7).

## Root Caries

Tooth decay can occur at any age. However, as patients age they may become at risk for **root caries**. Root caries occurs on the root of teeth that have gingival recession that exposes root surfaces. The cementum covering root surfaces is more susceptible to caries than enamel because it has less mineral content and is more soluble, and therefore is more susceptible to root caries.

People are living longer and are keeping their teeth longer, and older people often take many medications that may cause xerostomia (reduced salivary flow). Patients who have undergone radiation treatment for head or neck cancer are also at a greater risk for root caries because their normal salivary flow is reduced. Whatever the reason, reduced flow of saliva is a risk factor for the development of all types of caries.

Root caries have a different clinical appearance. Similar to coronal caries, root caries undergo periods of demineralization and remineralization (Fig. 13.8).

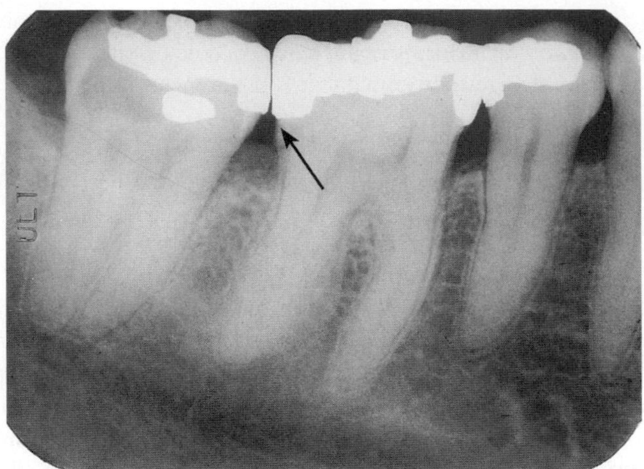

FIG. 13.7 Radiograph shows recurrent decay *(arrows)* under an amalgam restoration.

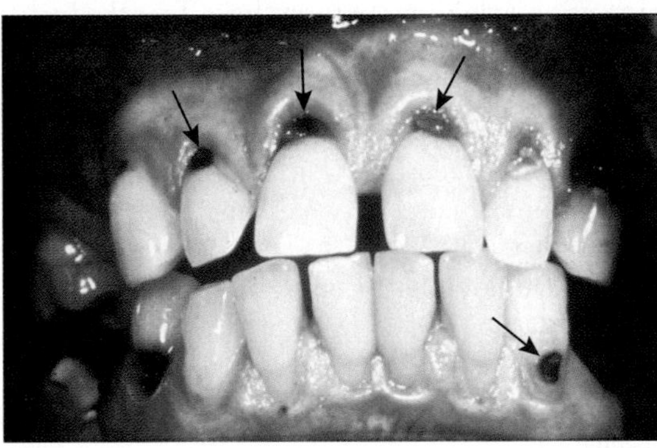

FIG. 13.8 Root surface caries. *(Courtesy Dr. John D. B. Featherstone, School of Dentistry, University of California San Francisco.)*

### Prevention of Root Caries

- Thorough plaque removal with brushing and flossing
- Nutritional counseling
- Patient education
- In-office and/or prescription fluoride products (containing 5000 ppm)
- Remineralization products that contain calcium phosphate
- For patients with xerostomia, stimulate saliva with use of sugarless chewing gum or sugarless candies, or apply saliva substitutes, such as gels, sprays, or liquids

No one method will be ideal for all patients, so recommendations should be based on the individual patient's needs and caries risk assessment.

RECALL

8 What is the term for caries that occurs under or adjacent to existing dental restorations?
9 Why are exposed root surfaces more susceptible to caries than enamel?

## Early Childhood Caries

**Early childhood caries (ECC)** is an infectious disease that can happen in any family. Many children live with the constant pain of decayed teeth and swollen gums (Fig. 13.9). In some states, ECC affects one third of preschool children.

Tooth decay is the single most prevalent disease of childhood. Untreated tooth decay in children results in pain and infection. Children who suffer from ECC often miss school or are unable to concentrate when they are in school. ECC can also affect a child's ability to sleep and overall health and well-being. Many children with severe ECC must be hospitalized for treatment, and this can be very expensive (Fig. 13.10). ECC can be prevented by providing appropriate education for parents and oral healthcare for the child.

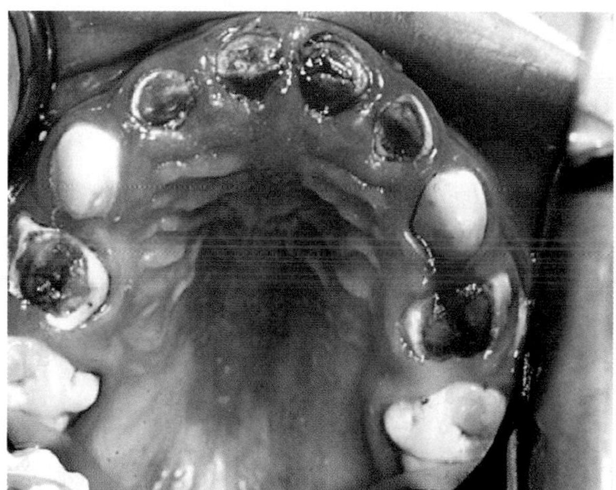

**FIG. 13.9** Rampant early childhood caries. *(Courtesy Dr. Frank Hodges, Santa Rosa, CA.)*

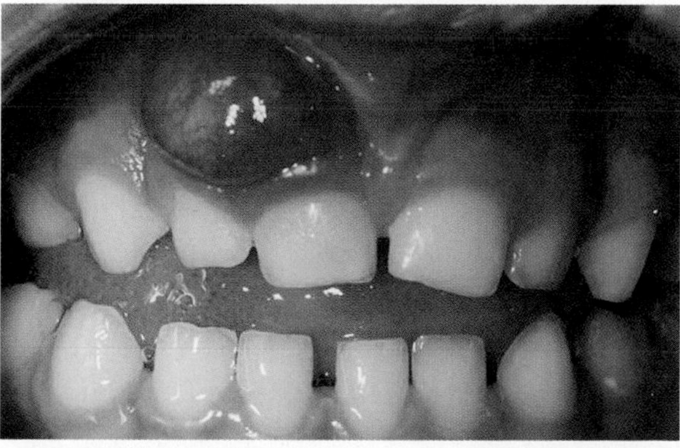

**FIG. 13.10** Child suffering from an abscess. *(Courtesy Dr. Frank Hodges, Santa Rosa, CA.)*

### Risk Factors

ECC is common among families of lower socioeconomic status. The rate of untreated dental disease among low-income children ages 2 to 5 years is almost 5 times higher than that seen in high-income families. ECC is more common among particular ethnic groups (Fig. 13.11), in those families who have limited access to dental care, and in areas where water fluoridation is lacking. ECC is also more common among children with special needs.

#### Risk Factors for Early Childhood Caries

- Low-income families
- Particular ethnic groups
- Limited access to care
- Lack of water fluoridation

See Chapter 15 for additional information about water fluoridation.

### How Children Get Early Childhood Caries

ECC is a transmissible disease. Bacteria present in the parent's or caregiver's mouth are passed to the child. It is important for parents to keep their own teeth healthy to keep their children's teeth healthy. Parents should substitute healthful foods and snacks for those that are sugary, starchy, or sticky. If a baby sleeps with a bottle, the chances of decay are increased (Fig. 13.12). *Baby bottle tooth decay* is another term for ECC. Refer to Chapter 15 for additional information on prevention of ECC.

## The Importance of Saliva

Saliva is like a miracle fluid that provides *physical, chemical,* and *antibacterial* protective measures for the teeth.

The **physical protection** is dependent on the water content in the saliva and the amount or flow of saliva. If enough saliva is present, it provides a cleansing effect. The fluid dilutes and removes acid components from the dental plaque. If the saliva is thick, it is less effective than a thin or more watery saliva in clearing carbohydrates.

The **chemical protection** provided by saliva is especially important because saliva contains calcium, phosphate, and fluoride. Saliva keeps calcium in the mouth, ready to be used during remineralization. Saliva also includes buffers, bicarbonate, phosphate, and small proteins that neutralize acids after fermentable carbohydrates are ingested.

The **antibacterial protection** provided by saliva depends on substances found within the saliva, such as immunoglobulins, that work against bacteria. However, if the bacterial count in the mouth becomes very high, these substances may not be able to provide enough antibacterial protection.

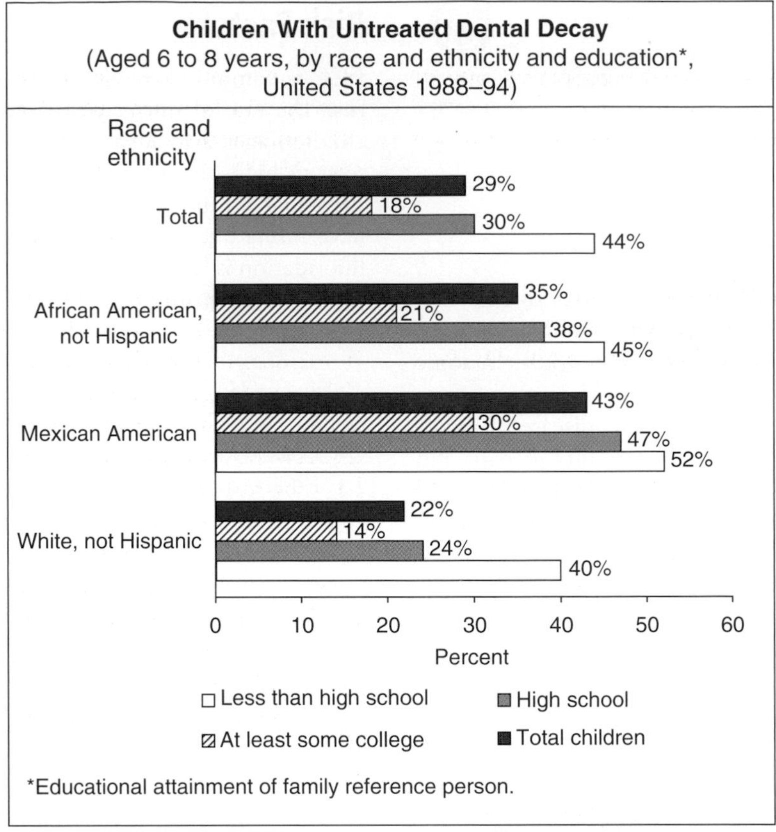


**FIG. 13.11** Children with untreated dental decay. *(From National Center for Health Statistics: National Health and Nutrition Examination Survey, 1988–1994. Hyattsville, MD: Centers for Disease Control and Prevention, unpublished data. In U.S. Department of Health and Human Services: Healthy People 2010: Objectives for improving health, Rockville, MD, 1999, USDHHS. Available at* http://www.healthypeople.gov/document/HTML/Volume2/21Oral.htm.*)*

A good flow of saliva is necessary to control caries. If salivary function is reduced for any reason, such as illness, medication, or radiation therapy, the teeth are at increased risk for decay.

## Saliva's Beneficial Actions

- Provides calcium and phosphate for remineralization
- Carries topical fluoride around the mouth for remineralization
- Neutralizes organic acids produced in plaque biofilm
- Discourages the growth of bacteria, inhibiting infection
- Recycles ingested fluoride into the mouth
- Protects hard and soft tissues from drying
- Facilitates chewing and swallowing
- Speeds oral clearance of food

From Eakle SW, Featherstone JDB: Caries risk instruction [course handout], San Francisco, 2002, University of California School of Dentistry.

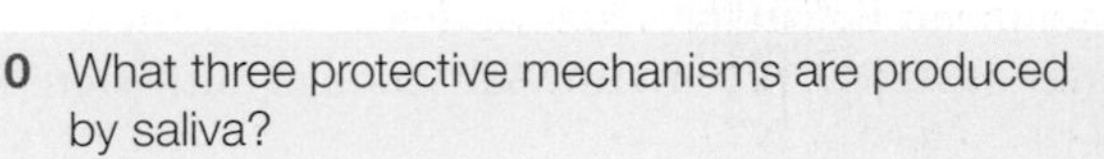


**10** What three protective mechanisms are produced by saliva?

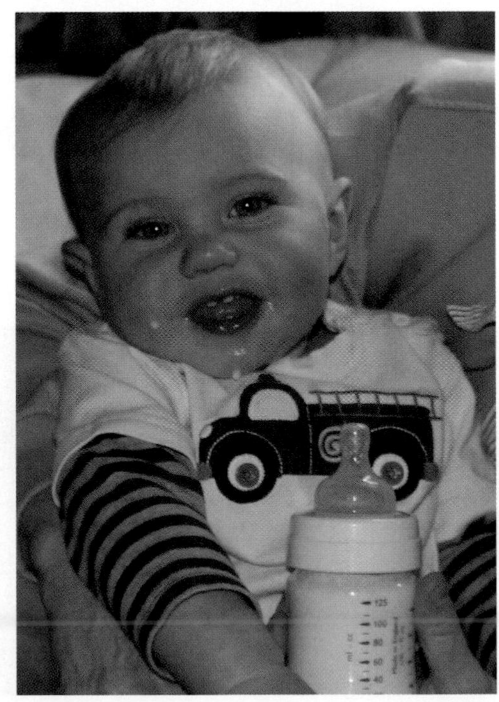

**FIG. 13.12** Milk or formula will remain on babies' teeth if they are put to sleep with a bottle.

## Caries Diagnosis

Accurately diagnosing early dental caries is a challenge for the dentist. The following methods are used to detect dental caries, and each has specific limitations. (Detection of dental caries is also discussed in Chapter 28.)

### Dental Explorer

When a sharp explorer tip is pressed into an area of suspected caries, it will "stick" when it is being removed. New research shows that this technique has limitations on the occlusal surface.

### Radiographs

Although useful for detection of interproximal caries, early caries on occlusal surfaces is not visible on radiographs. In addition, the extent of caries can be misdiagnosed easily because the caries is often two times deeper and more widespread than it appears on radiographs.

### Visual Appearance

The appearance of darkly stained grooves in the teeth may indicate caries, although dark grooves may simply reveal a stain caused by coffee or tea. Gray shadowing underneath enamel can also indicate decay.

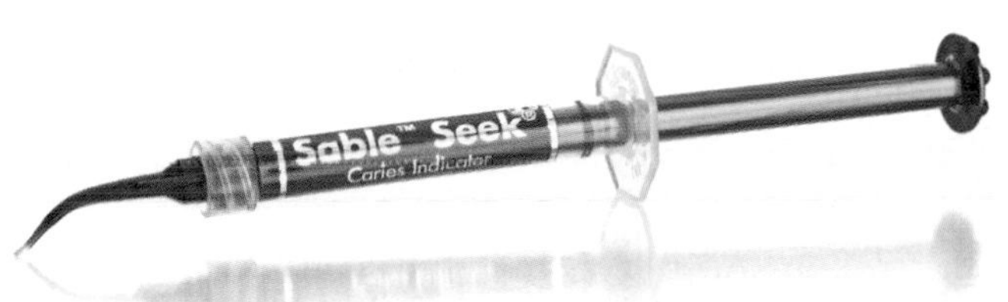


**FIG. 13.13** Special types of dyes, when applied to a preparation, can indicate with color any areas of decay and thus aid in earlier caries detection. *(Courtesy Ultradent, South Jordan, UT.)*

### Indicator Dyes

Special dyes are available for use during operative procedures; these products, when applied to the inside of a preparation, can indicate through a color change whether decay remains (Fig. 13.13).

### Caries Detection Devices

With new technology, several types of devices have been developed that can provide a higher level of discrimination in the diagnosis of dental caries. Some devices detect bacterial by-products and quantify sound signals to aid in caries detection; some detect differences in tooth structure and display the information on a screen (Fig. 13.14). Others have software that can be used to analyze density changes on digital radiographs and to outline potential lesions. Some systems are useful for detecting caries on both occlusal and interproximal surfaces of posterior teeth. However, none can be used independently to determine appropriate treatment. It is important to note that the dentist ultimately makes a diagnosis of caries, and no single instrument or technique in itself has been found to be 100% effective in all cases.

### Laser Caries Detector

The laser caries detector is one type of recently developed device that is used to diagnose caries and reveal bacterial activity underneath the enamel surface (Fig. 13.15). The laser caries detector does not detect interproximal caries, subgingival caries, or secondary caries under crowns, inlays, or restorations. However, caries detectors may be used to aid in monitoring progression or arrestment of caries by comparing a patient's readings from visit to visit.

When the laser beam passes through a change in the density of the tooth, it gives off a fluorescent light of different wavelengths. A clean, healthy tooth exhibits little or

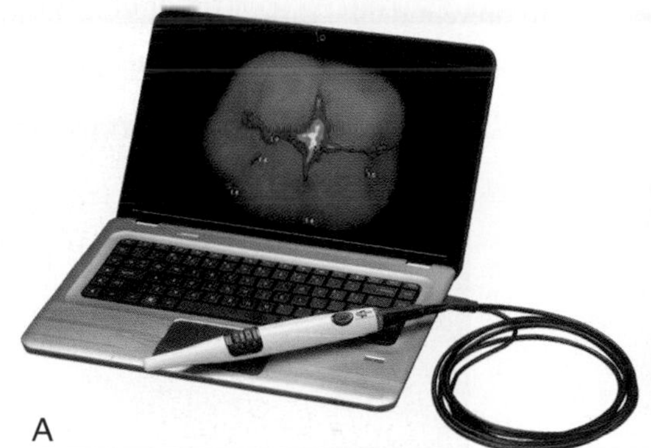


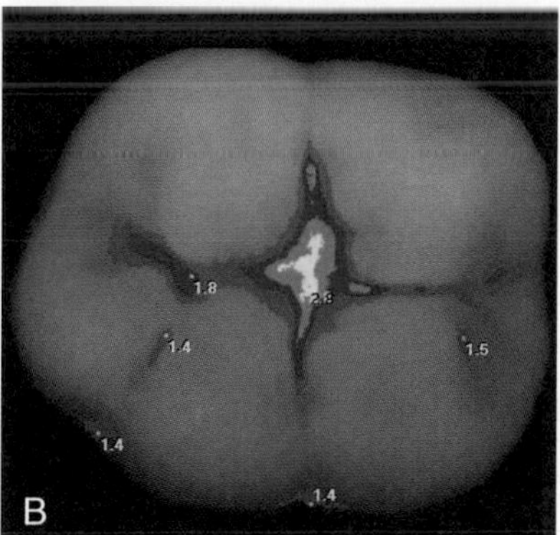


**FIG. 13.14** Spectra Fluorescence Caries Detection Aid System. A, Lightweight handpiece with high resolution, auto-exposure CCD sensor connects to a computer. B, Doppler radar-like images provide both color and numerical indicators; in active mode carious regions appear red, healthy enamel appears green. *(Courtesy Air Techniques, Inc., Melville, NY.)*

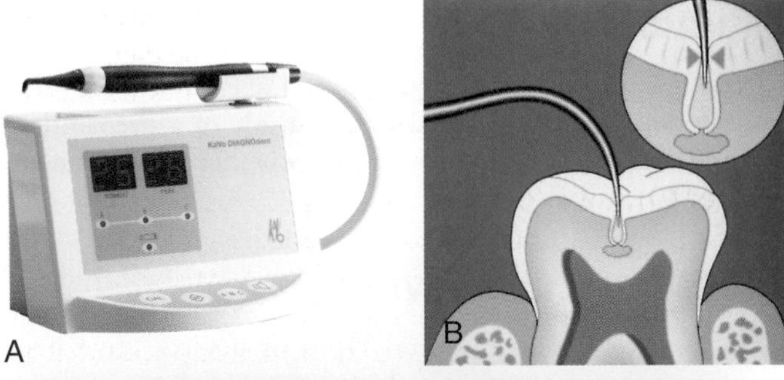


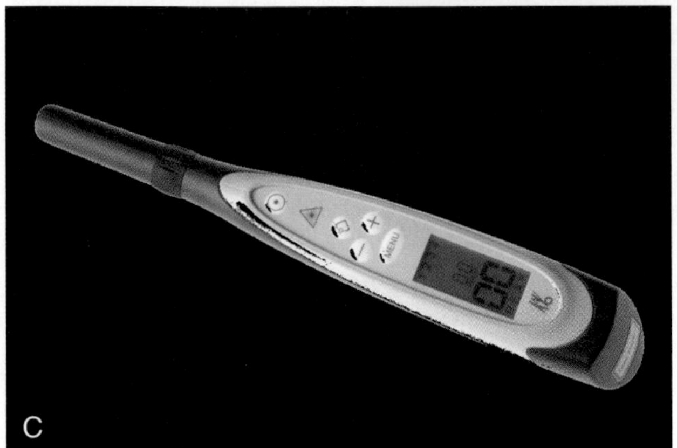


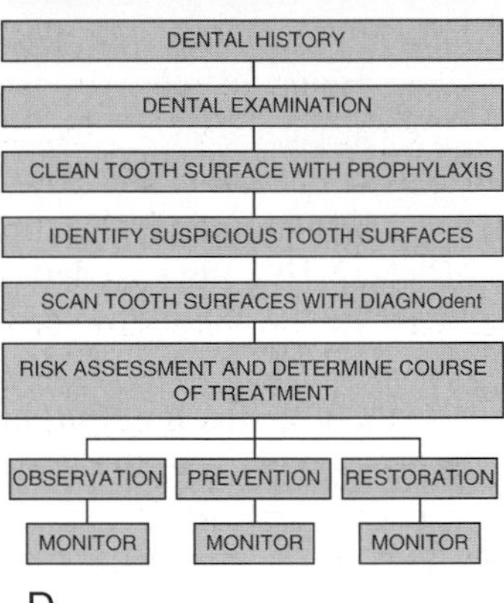


**FIG. 13.15** A and B, The DIAGNOdent directs a laser beam into the occlusal surface. C, The DIAGNOdent pen is an even newer device that provides the same early caries detection in a more portable handheld device. D, The dental treatment sequence. *(Courtesy KaVo Kerr, Orange, CA.)*

no fluorescence, resulting in very low readings (Figs. 13.16 and 13.17). The laser wavelength is translated into a number from 0 to 99 that appears on the face of the unit. See Procedure 13.1: Performing Caries Detection Using the KaVo DIAGNOdent Caries Detection Device (Expanded Function).

However, carious tooth structure shows higher degrees of fluorescence. As the amount of decay increases, readings reveal higher degrees of fluorescence. False-positives may arise because of fluorescence caused by plaque or calculus in the fissures, or as the result of discoloration or food debris lodged in or on the surface of the tooth. Therefore one should not rely totally on the readings; the laser caries detector is not a stand-alone diagnostic tool.

Use of this laser has its limitations. For example, the laser cannot be used to diagnose interproximal caries because access to those surfaces is limited. It cannot detect caries located under dental sealants or under an amalgam restoration, although it can detect decay around the occlusal margins of a restoration.

### Calibration of the Tip

Because of slight natural variations in the fluorescence of healthy tooth structure, it is recommended to establish a *zero baseline* specific to each patient.

## CAMBRA

Caries management by risk assessment (**CAMBRA**) is an **evidence-based** strategy for preventive and reparative care for early dental caries that can be used in any dental office.

The goal of CAMBRA is to assess the risk of caries in an individual. A dental health professional first assesses an individual's risk factors and protective factors, and then determines the level of risk for caries (low, moderate, high, or extreme). Based on the determined level of risk, the dental professional develops an individualized preventive plan for each patient. Then, depending on the patient's level of risk, the dental health professional provides specific products and recommendations to prevent dental caries.

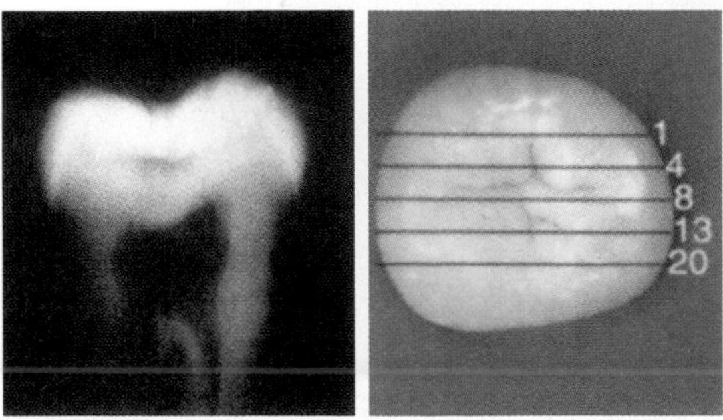


**FIG. 13.16** Visual and radiographic appearance of seemingly intact molar. *(Courtesy KaVo Kerr, Orange, CA.)*

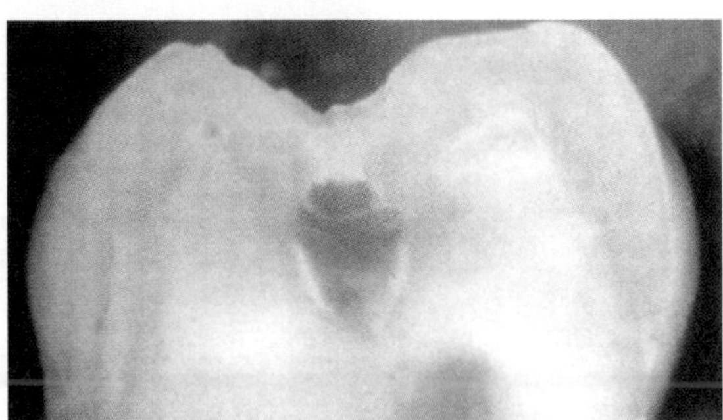

**FIG. 13.17** Cross section of molar shows decay. *(Courtesy KaVo Kerr, Orange, CA.)*

### CAMBRA Techniques

- Risk assessment
- Fluoride application
- Dietary counseling
- Application of dental sealants
- Fluoridated drinking water, toothpastes, and rinses
- Xylitol gum
- Calcium phosphate products
- Professionally applied fluoride foams and varnishes

See Chapter 15 for additional information.

## Methods of Caries Intervention

Even though the dentist restores (fills) the carious tooth, the risk for further decay to that tooth remains. This is so because restoring teeth has no effect on bacteria that continue to live in the mouth. Dental caries occurs when more disease-causing agents (e.g., bacteria, fermentable carbohydrates) than protective agents (e.g., saliva, fluoride) are present in the mouth. The caries process can be interrupted or prevented in the following ways (Fig. 13.18):

- *Fluoride.* Various forms of fluoride are available to strengthen teeth against solubility and acid.
- *Antibacterial rinses.* For patients at high risk for caries, products such as chlorhexidine mouth rinses reduce the numbers of cariogenic bacteria in the mouth. Patients rinse once daily for 1 minute at bedtime. This should be repeated for 1 week every month.
- *Decreased fermentable carbohydrates.* Our diet today includes fast foods, frequent snacking, and regular intake of foods that have a high sugar content. All of these factors put teeth at risk for caries. It is important to reduce the quantity and frequency of fermentable carbohydrates in the diet.
- *Increased salivary flow.* Saliva can tilt the caries balance by neutralizing acids that cause demineralization; it can also aid in remineralization of tooth surfaces. Chewing sugarless gum with sweeteners such as aspartame or sorbitol, as well as newer types with the noncariogenic sweetener **xylitol**, increases the flow of saliva and thereby reduces the acid challenge to the teeth. Chewing one stick three times a day, preferably after meals, helps to neutralize any acids that are present and promotes remineralization.

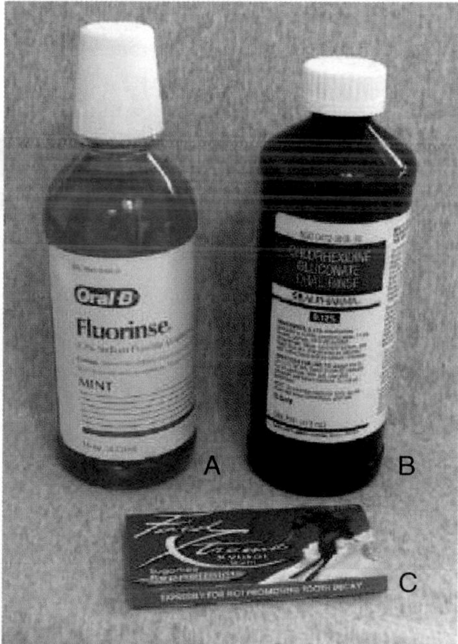


**FIG. 13.18** Preventive measures against caries. A, Fluoride rinse. B, Chlorhexidine rinse. C, Xylitol gum.

These methods of caries intervention are discussed in greater detail in Chapter 15.

## Caries Risk Assessment Tests

*Caries risk assessment* tests are used to identify the factors that contribute to an increased risk for dental caries. There are commercial **Caries Risk Tests (CRT)** available that are used to detect the numbers of MS and LB bacteria present in the saliva. High bacterial counts indicate a high caries risk, and low counts indicate a low risk for caries.

One example of a caries risk test is the **saliva flow rate test**. This type of test measures the amount of saliva in the mouth in milliliters per minute. The patient chews a paraffin pellet for 3 to 5 minutes and then spits all generated saliva into a paper cup. Using a pipette, measure the amount of saliva (in milliliters = ml) and divide that amount by the time, to determine the ml/minute of stimulated salivary flow. Flow rates of 1 ml/minute and above are considered normal. A level of 0.7 ml/minute is low, and a level of 0.5 ml/minute or less is dry, indicating a high risk for caries. Determining the reason for a low flow rate is an important step in patient treatment. Procedure 13.2: Performing Caries Risk Assessment (Expanded Function) describes the steps involved in bacterial caries risk assessment.

The **CariScreen Caries Susceptibility Test** is a simple 1-minute chair-side bacterial test for assessing caries risk. The patent-pending CariScreen uses ATP (adenosine triphosphate) driven bioluminescence to identify the oral bacterial load and has been proven to correlate with risk for decay (Fig. 13.19).

By determining the patient's risk for developing dental caries, and by beginning appropriate preventive treatment, the healthcare worker can help prevent dental caries from occurring. Patients with high numbers of bacteria in the mouth are likely to develop carious lesions if preventive measures are not provided (Fig. 13.20).

### Dental Assistant's Role in Caries Risk Assessment

- Assessment is easily done.
- In-office testing is cost-effective.
- Dental assistants can perform assessments.
- Plans for prevention can be individualized.
- Patients are motivated to undergo treatment.

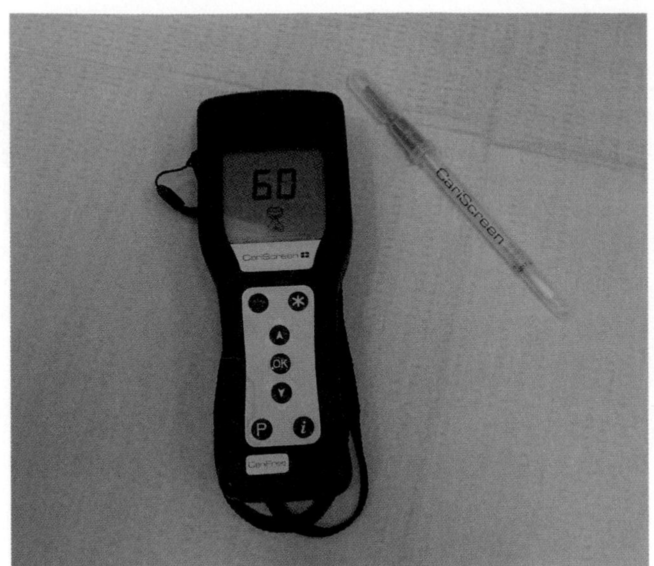


**FIG. 13.19** Hand-held meter used at chairside to identify the bacterial load of the saliva for assessing caries risk. *(Courtesy Dr. Allen Wong.)*

### Risk Factors for Future Dental Caries

- History of dental caries
- Presence of white spot lesions
- Poor oral hygiene
- High mutans streptococci count (test results)
- Lower socioeconomic status
- High daily consumption of sucrose

### Who Should Be Tested for Caries Risk?

- New patients with signs of caries activity
- Pregnant patients
- Patients experiencing a sudden increase in incidence of caries
- Individuals taking medications that may affect the flow of saliva
- Patients with xerostomia
- Patients with upcoming chemotherapy
- Patients who frequently consume fermentable carbohydrates
- Patients with disease of the immune system

**■ Legal and Ethical Implications** When should a carious lesion be observed, or treated with some preventive measure, or actually restored? This question has no single answer. This is an individual decision that the dentist must make for each patient, and it is based on sound professional judgment.

The dentist must analyze the patient's diet, dental history, and oral hygiene regimen to determine which approach to tooth restoration is necessary. People with a high caries rate may need immediate restoration of lesions. On the other hand, for lesions that have been dormant for many years, the dentist may choose to watch for an additional time without dental intervention.

Professional opinions vary about whether small initial carious lesions in the teeth should be restored. Opinions range from the conservative preference for remineralizing initial lesions to a more aggressive approach of restoring all carious lesions. Each dentist must make his or her own decisions on the basis of the individual patient's history and needs. ■

**■ Eye to the Future** Diagnosis of dental caries has become more challenging as knowledge of the disease has increased. More factors involved in the caries process have been identified. Risk factors are better understood, and better methods for detection are being developed. Better methods are needed that can detect occlusal caries while it is still in the enamel and can be arrested by remineralization. It is important that strategies for the prevention of dental caries become part of comprehensive dental care.

It is anticipated that in the future, advances in molecular biology will provide dental professionals with a rapid method of assessing a patient's risk for dental caries before the patient leaves the dental chair. It is likely that a vaccine will someday become available that will prevent dental caries. ■

### ■ Critical Thinking

1. Mr. Johnstone comes into your office reporting pain in a lower right first molar. The tooth has a large amalgam restoration that was placed 10 years ago. As you begin to take the radiograph, you do not see any visible decay. What is a possible cause for his pain?
2. The Williams twins are in your dental office for a routine checkup. Mrs. Williams informs you that they both eat the same quantity of sweets. However, Jeanne eats her sweets all at once, whereas Carol divides her sweets throughout the day. Which of the twins is most likely to have tooth decay? Why?
3. As a dental assistant, you have been asked to speak to a group of pregnant women regarding their dental health. Why is it important for pregnant women to have excellent dental health before their babies are born? ■

CAMBRA for Dental Providers (0-5) Assessment Tool

Caries Risk Assessment Form for Age 0 to 5

Patient Name:________________ I.D.#________ Age________ Date________

Initial/base line exam date________________ Caries recall date________________

| Respond to each question in sections 1, 2, 3, and 4 with a check mark in the "Yes" or "No" column | Yes | No | Notes |
|---|---|---|---|
| **1. Caries Risk Indicators — Parent Interview**** | | | |
| (a) Mother or primary caregiver has had active dental decay in the past 12 months | | | |
| (b) Child has recent dental restorations (see 5b below) | | | |
| (c) Parent and/or caregiver has low SES (socioeconomic status) and/or low health literacy | | | |
| (d) Child has developmental problems | | | |
| (e) No dental home/episodic dental care | | | |
| **2. Caries Risk Factors (Biological) — Parent Interview**** | | | |
| (a) Child has frequent (greater than 3 times daily) between-meal snacks of sugars/cooked starch/sugared beverages | | | |
| (b) Child has saliva-reducing factors present, including:<br>1. Medications (e.g., some for asthma or hyperactivity)<br>2. Medical (cancer treatment) or genetic factors | | | |
| (c) Child continually uses bottle — contains fluids other than water | | | |
| (d) Child sleeps with a bottle or nurses on demand | | | |
| **3. Protective Factors (Nonbiological) — Parent Interview** | | | |
| (a) Mother/caregiver decay-free past 3 years | | | |
| (b) Child has a dental home and regular dental care | | | |
| **4. Protective Factors (Biological) — Parent Interview** | | | |
| (a) Child lives in a fluoridated community or takes fluoride supplements by slowly dissolving or as chewable tablets | | | |
| (b) Child's teeth are cleaned with fluoridated toothpaste (pea-size) daily | | | |
| (c) Mother/caregiver chews/sucks xylitol chewing gum/lozenges 4-5 times daily | | | |
| **5. Caries Risk Indicators/Factors — Clinical Examination of Child**** | | | |
| (a) Obvious white spots, decalcifications, or obvious decay present on the child's teeth | | | |
| (b) Restorations placed in the past 2 years in/on child's teeth | | | |
| (c) Plaque is obvious on the child's teeth and/or gums bleed easily | | | |
| (d) Child has dental or orthodontic appliances present, fixed or removable (e.g., braces, space maintainers, obturators) | | | |
| (e) Risk Factor: Visually inadequate saliva flow — dry mouth | | | |

| ****If yes to any one of 1(a), 1(b), 5(a), or 5(b) or any two in categories 1, 2, 5, consider performing bacterial culture on mother or caregiver and child. Use this as a base line to follow results of antibacterial intervention.** | Parent/Caregiver<br>Date: | Child<br>Date: |
|---|---|---|
| (a) Mutans streptococci (indicate bacterial level: high, medium, low) | | |
| (b) *Lactobacillus* species (indicate bacterial level: high, medium, low) | | |

| **Child's overall caries risk status: (CIRCLE) Extreme** | Low | Moderate | High |
|---|---|---|---|

Recommendations given: Yes________ No________ Date given:________ Date follow up:________

**SELF-MANAGEMENT GOALS** 1)________________ 2)________________

Practitioner signature________________ Date________________

**FIG. 13.20** Caries risk assessment form for ages 0 to 5. *(Redrawn from Ramos-Gomez FJ, Crall J, Gansky SA, et al: Caries risk assessment appropriate for the age 1 visit [infants and toddlers], J Calif Dent Assoc 35:687, 2007.)*

**PROCEDURE 13.1**

# Performing Caries Detection Using the KaVo DIAGNOdent Caries Detection Device (Expanded Function)

## PREREQUISITES FOR PERFORMING THIS PROCEDURE

- ✔ Infection control protocol
- ✔ Patient communication skills
- ✔ Knowledge of oral anatomy
- ✔ Operator positioning
- ✔ Fulcrum positioning

## EQUIPMENT AND SUPPLIES

- ✔ KaVo DIAGNOdent Caries Detection Device
- ✔ Disposable sleeve
- ✔ Prophy angle, bristle brush
- ✔ Sodium bicarbonate powder
- ✔ Pencil and patient's record

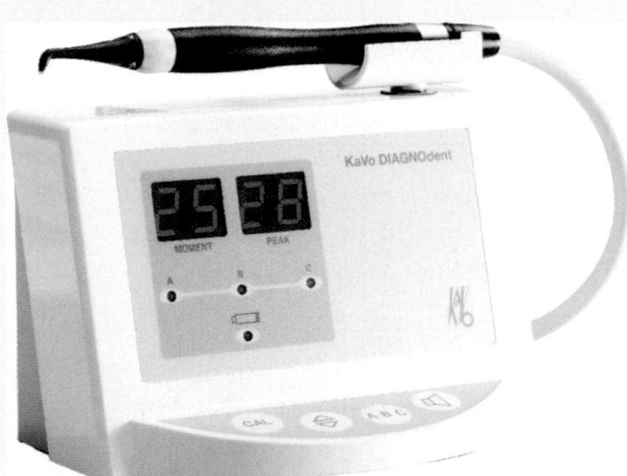


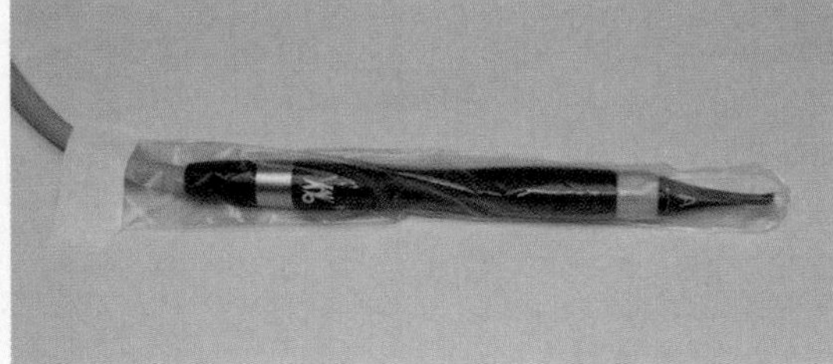

*Courtesy KaVo Kerr, Orange, CA.*

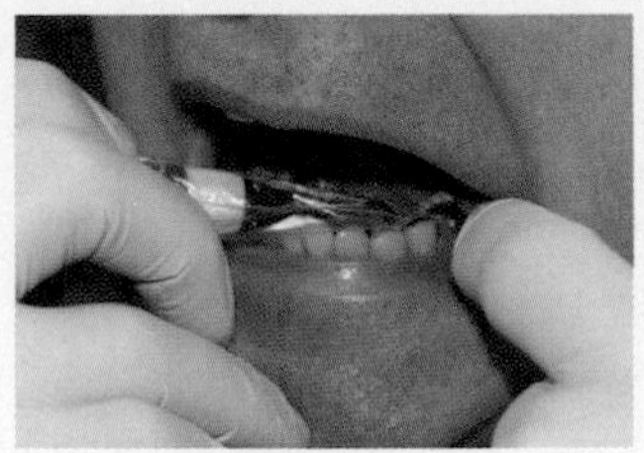

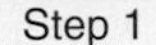

Step 1

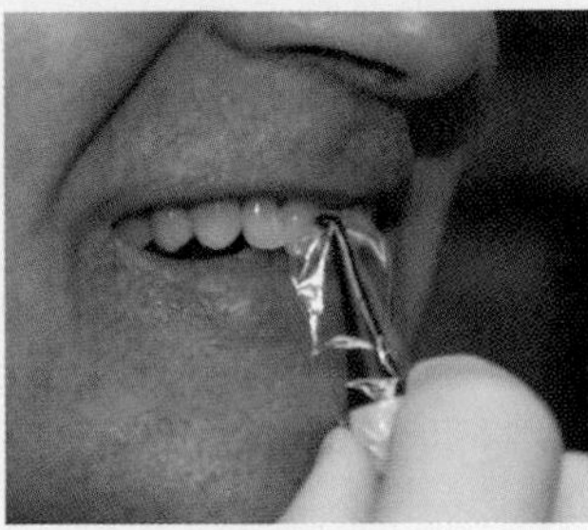

Step 2

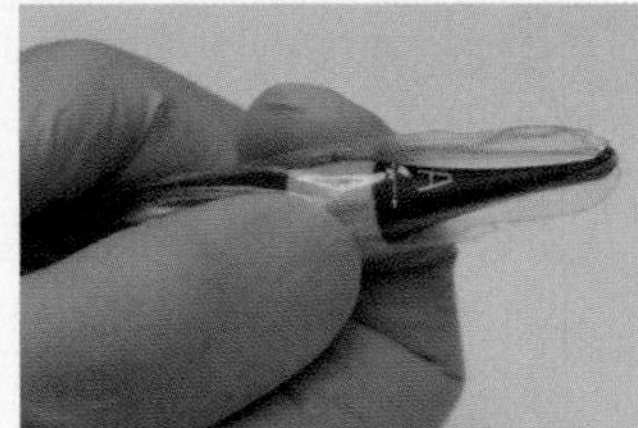

Step 3

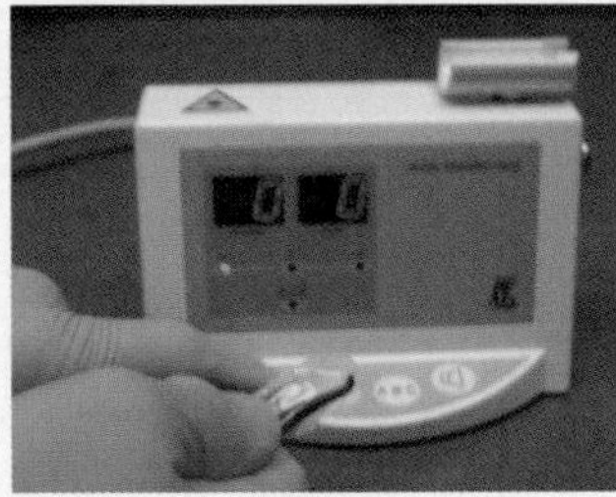

Step 4

## PROCEDURAL STEPS

### Establish Zero Baseline

1 Before scanning, select an anatomical reference point on a healthy nonrestored tooth. The middle third facial surface is ideal.

2 Hold the probe tip against the tooth at right angles to the surface.

3 Gently squeeze the gray ring switch of the handpiece.

4 "Set 0" will appear on the display, confirmed by an audible beep. This indicates that the zero baseline is established.

5 Record the anatomical location where the zero baseline was established in the patient's dental record for future reference.

**EXAMPLE** DIAGNOdent zero baseline: midfacial #8

### Scanning Procedure

6 Clean and dry the teeth using a prophy brush, or other acceptable means.

**PURPOSE** If debris remains, false-positive readings can occur. If this occurs, further cleaning is necessary.

7 Identify tooth surfaces to be tested.

8 During examination of suspicious sites, the tip of the handpiece should be in light contact with the surface of the tooth.

9 Place the probe tip directly on the pits and fissures, making sure the tip is in contact with the long axis of the tooth.

10 When the tip is in contact with the fissure, slowly rotate or rock the handpiece in a pendulum-like manner.

**NOTE** Areas of discoloration and enamel defects or areas may produce a sharp change in the audible signal.

11 Record the readings.

**NOTE** Very high readings (e.g., greater than 80) may indicate that the teeth have not been thoroughly cleaned or are not free of debris. In such situations, the teeth may be recleaned, dried, and reexamined.

12 After the scanning has been completed, hold the tip in the air and hold the gray ring switch until "Set 0" appears on the display.

**PURPOSE** This eliminates the previous patient-specific zero baseline from the unit.

### Documentation

13 Document the procedure and the results in the patient's chart.

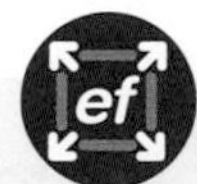

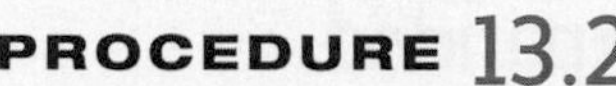

PROCEDURE 13.2

## Performing Caries Risk Assessment (Expanded Function)

### PREREQUISITES FOR PERFORMING THIS PROCEDURE

- ✔ Infection control protocol
- ✔ Patient communication skills

### EQUIPMENT AND SUPPLIES

- ✔ Caries risk assessment kit
- ✔ Paraffin pellet
- ✔ $NaHCO_3$ tablet (sodium, hydrogen, carbonate)
- ✔ Pipette
- ✔ Agar carrier
- ✔ Test vial
- ✔ Evaluation chart
- ✔ Paper cup
- ✔ Pen with waterproof ink
- ✔ Culture incubator

### PROCEDURAL STEPS

1 Explain the procedure to the patient.
**PURPOSE** To educate the patient about the process of caries risk assessment.

2 Have the patient chew the paraffin wax pellet.
**PURPOSE** To stimulate salivation.

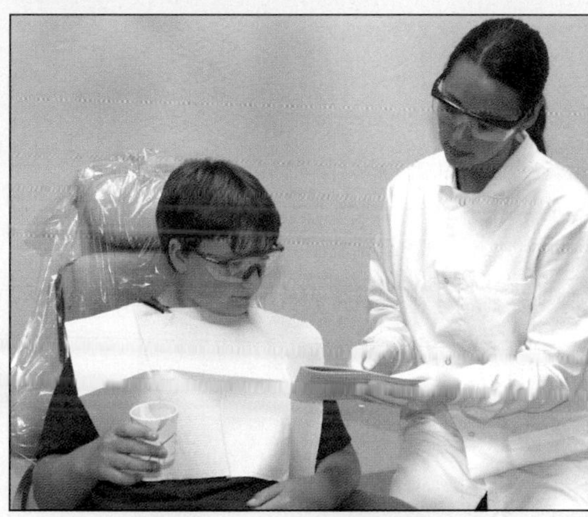

3 Have the patient expectorate into the paper cup.
**PURPOSE** To collect the saliva sample.

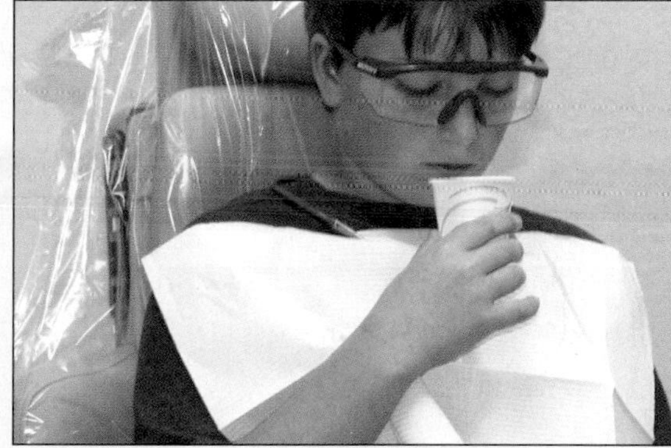

4 Remove the agar carrier from the test vial, and place an $NaHCO_3$ tablet at the bottom of the vial.
**PURPOSE** The $NaHCO_3$ tablet will determine the buffer capacity of the saliva.

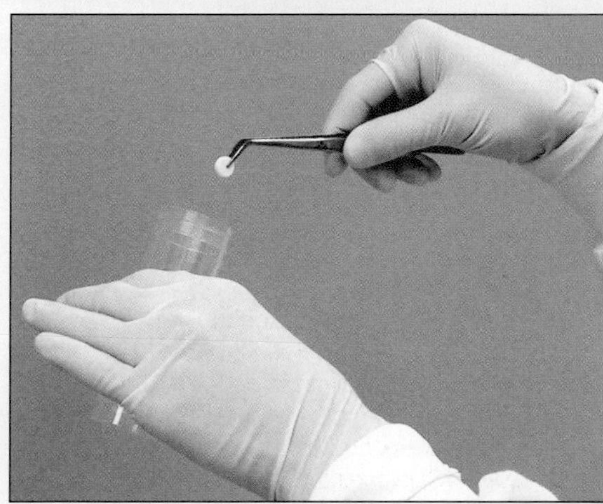

**(Continued)**

## PROCEDURE 13.2 Performing Caries Risk Assessment (Expanded Function)—cont'd

5 Carefully remove the protective foils from the two agar surfaces. Do not touch the agar.
**PURPOSE** To prevent contamination of the agar surfaces.

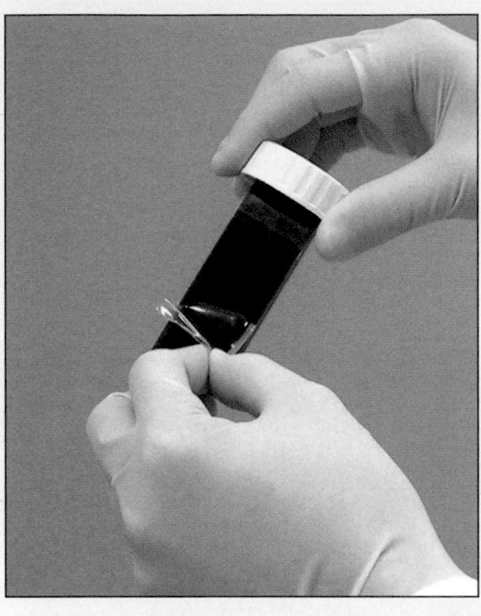

6 Thoroughly wet both agar surfaces using a pipette. Avoid scratching the agar surface. Hold the carrier at an angle while wetting.
**PURPOSE** One side is sensitive to MS, and the other side is sensitive to LB.

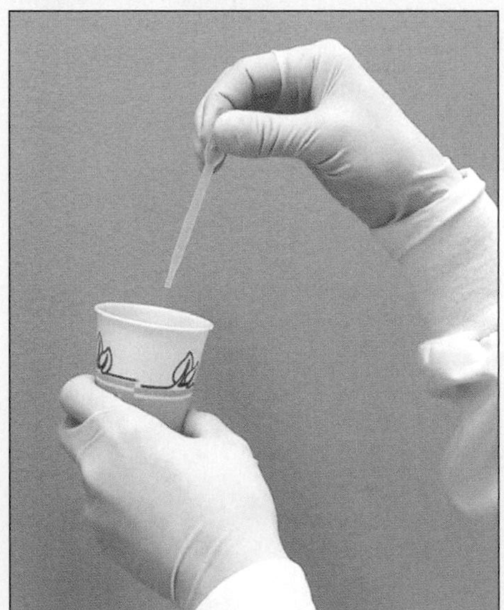

7 Slide the agar carrier back into the vial, and close the vial tightly.
**PURPOSE** To prevent cross-contamination of the sample.

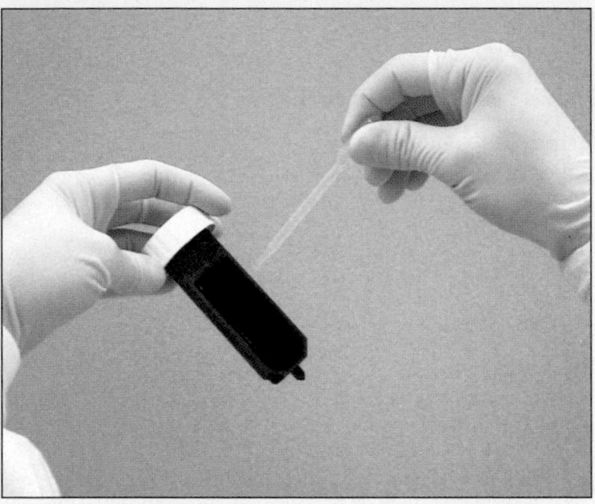

8 Use a waterproof pen to note the name of the patient and the date on the vial.

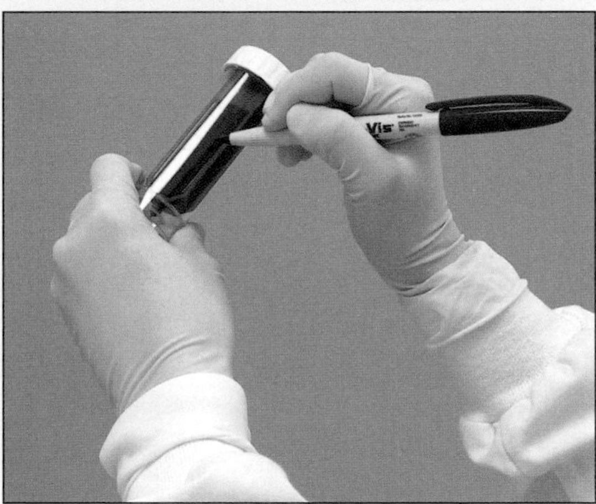

9 Place the test vial upright in the incubator. Incubate at 37° C (99° F) for 49 hours.
**PURPOSE** To allow bacteria on the agar strips to grow.

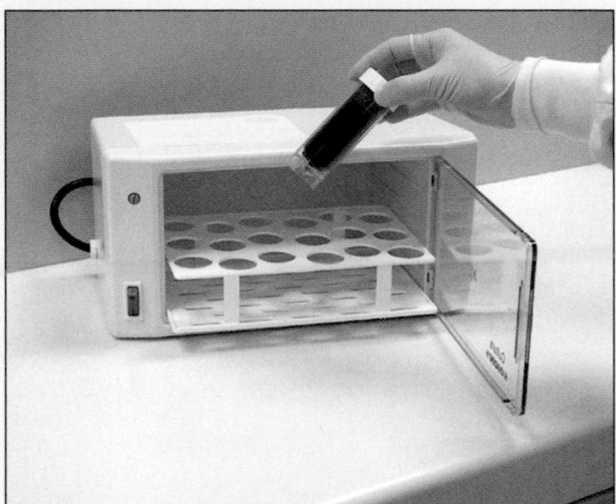

# PROCEDURE 13.2 Performing Caries Risk Assessment (Expanded Function)—cont'd

**10** Remove the vial from the incubator.

**11** Compare the density of the bacterial colonies versus corresponding evaluation pictures on the chart included in the caries risk assessment kit.

**TIP** Hold the agar carrier at a slight angle under a light source, so colonies can be seen clearly.

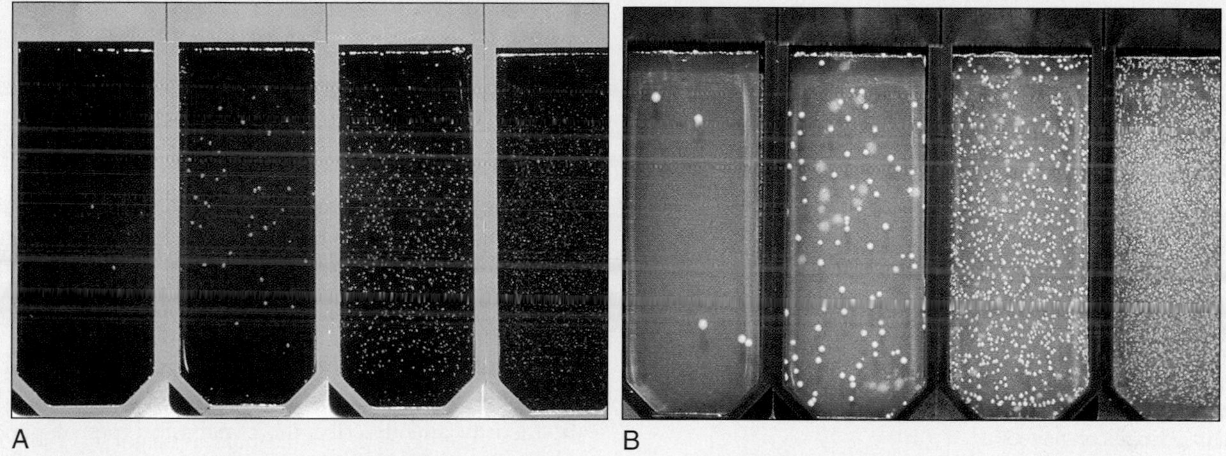


A, Compare the density of the mutans streptococci (MS) colonies. B, Compare the density of the lactobacilli (LB) colonies.

## Documentation

| Date | Tooth Surface | Charting Notes | Signature |
|---|---|---|---|
| 7/18/17 | | Caries risk assessment<br>Incubate vial<br>Evaluate in 49 hours | P. Landry CDA |
| 7/20/17 | | Caries risk assessment test indicates low colony counts for both mutans streptococci (MS) and lactobacilli (LB). Low risk for dental caries. | P. Landry CDA |

# Periodontal Diseases

14

## KEY TERMS

**Biofilm** Also known as *plaque,* oral biofilm is a colorless, soft, sticky coating made up of communities of microorganisms adhering to oral structures.

**Calculus (KAL-kyoo-lus)** Calcium and phosphate salts in saliva that become mineralized and adhere to tooth surfaces.

**Gingivitis (jin-ji-VYE-tis)** Inflammation of the gingival tissue.

**Oral biofilm** Also known as *plaque* or *biofilm,* a colorless, soft, sticky coating made up of communities of microorganisms adhering to oral structures.

**Periodontal (per-ee-oe-DON-tul)** Referring to the periodontium.

**Periodontitis (per-ee-oe-don-TYE-tis)** Inflammatory disease of the supporting tissues of the teeth.

**Periodontium (per-ee-oe-DON-shee-um)** Structures that surround, support, and are attached to the teeth.

**Perioscopy (per-ee-OS-kuh-pee)** Procedure in which a dental endoscope is used subgingivally.

**Plaque (plak)** Also known as *biofilm,* plaque is a colorless, soft, sticky coating made up of communities of microorganisms adhering to oral structures.

**Subgingival (sub-JIN-ji-vul)** Referring to the area below the gingiva.

**Supragingival (soo-pruh-JIN-ji-vul)** Referring to the area above the gingiva.

## LEARNING OUTCOMES

*On completion of this chapter, the student will be able to achieve the following objectives:*

1. Pronounce, define, and spell the key terms.
2. Discuss the periodontium, including the following:
   - Name and describe the structures and tissues of the periodontium.
   - Describe the prevalence of periodontal disease.
3. Identify systemic factors that may cause periodontal disease.
4. Discuss the causes and risk factors of periodontal disease.
5. Identify and describe the two basic types of periodontal disease and explain the significance of biofilm and calculus in periodontal disease.
6. List the seven basic case types and signs and symptoms of periodontal disease.
7. Discuss the use of dental perioscopy in the use of periodontal therapy.

## ELECTRONIC RESOURCES

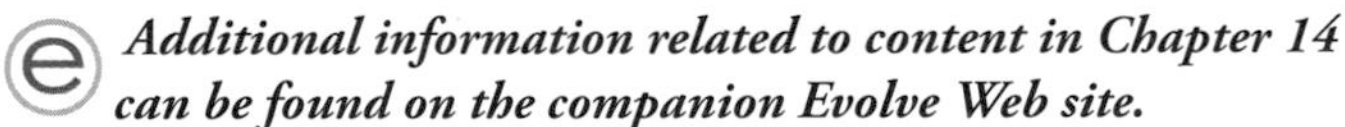

***Additional information related to content in Chapter 14 can be found on the companion Evolve Web site.***

- Practice Quiz

## Definition and Prevalence of Periodontal Disease

This chapter presents the *scientific basis* of periodontal disease. It includes the following:

- The relationship of periodontal disease and several systemic diseases
- The causes of periodontal disease
- Risk factors for periodontal disease
- Types of periodontal disease
- Signs and symptoms of periodontal diseases

Chapter 55 presents the role of the dental assistant in the clinical practice of periodontics, including the periodontal examination, charting, instruments, surgical and nonsurgical techniques, and laser techniques.

**Periodontal** disease is an infectious disease process that involves inflammation of the structures of the **periodontium** (Table 14.1). The periodontium is made up of structures that surround, support, and are attached to the teeth (Fig. 14.1). Periodontal disease causes a breakdown of the periodontium, resulting in loss of tissue attachment and destruction of alveolar bone.

Periodontal diseases are the leading cause of tooth loss in adults. Almost 75 percent of American adults have some form of periodontal disease, and most are unaware of the condition. Almost all adults and many children have calculus on their teeth. Fortunately, with early detection and treatment of periodontal disease, most people can keep their teeth for life.

## The Systemic Connection

Periodontal science has proven a connection with several systemic diseases, including coronary artery disease, diabetes, and stroke, as well as delivery of low-birth-weight infants. This relationship is not likely to affect everyone, but certainly affects many. In these patients, periodontal infection is thought to be a risk factor for systemic disease just as high cholesterol is a risk factor for coronary heart disease (Box 14.1). Chronic inflammation is recognized to do harm to the entire body.

**TABLE 14.1** Structures of the Periodontium

| Name | Description |
|---|---|
| Gingivae | Commonly referred to as gums. This mucosa covers the alveolar process of the jaws and surrounds the necks of the teeth. |
| Epithelial attachment | Tissue at the base of the sulcus where the gingiva attaches to the tooth. |
| Sulcus | Space between the tooth and the free gingiva. |
| Periodontal ligaments | Dense connective fibers that connect the cementum covering the root of the tooth with the alveolar bone of the socket wall. |
| Cementum | Covers the root of the tooth. The primary function of the cementum is to anchor the tooth to the bony socket with attachments of the periodontal ligaments. |
| Alveolar bone | Bone that supports the tooth in its position within the jaw. The alveolar socket is the cavity in the bone that surrounds the tooth. |

From Robinson D, Bird D: Essentials of dental assisting, ed 5, St Louis, 2013, Saunders.

## Cardiovascular Disease

Individuals with periodontal disease have a greater incidence of coronary heart disease. This results in an increased occurrence of strokes and heart attacks. Individuals with severe periodontal

**BOX 14.1** Potential Associations Between Periodontal Infection and Systemic Health

Heart disease
- Infective endocarditis
- Coronary heart disease (atherosclerosis)

Arthritis and failure of artificial joints

Neurologic disease
- Nonhemorrhagic (ischemic) stroke
- Brain abscesses
- Alzheimer's disease
- Meningitis

Pregnancy complications and outcomes
- Preterm birth
- Low birth weight
- Preeclampsia
- Fetal growth restriction

Diabetes mellitus

Pulmonary disease
- Aspiration and ventilator-associated pneumonias
- Chronic obstructive pulmonary disease

Gastrointestinal disease (including cancer)
- Gastric ulcers
- Stomach cancer
- Pancreatic cancer

From Darby ML, Walsh MM: Dental hygiene: theory and practice, ed 4, St Louis, 2015, Saunders.

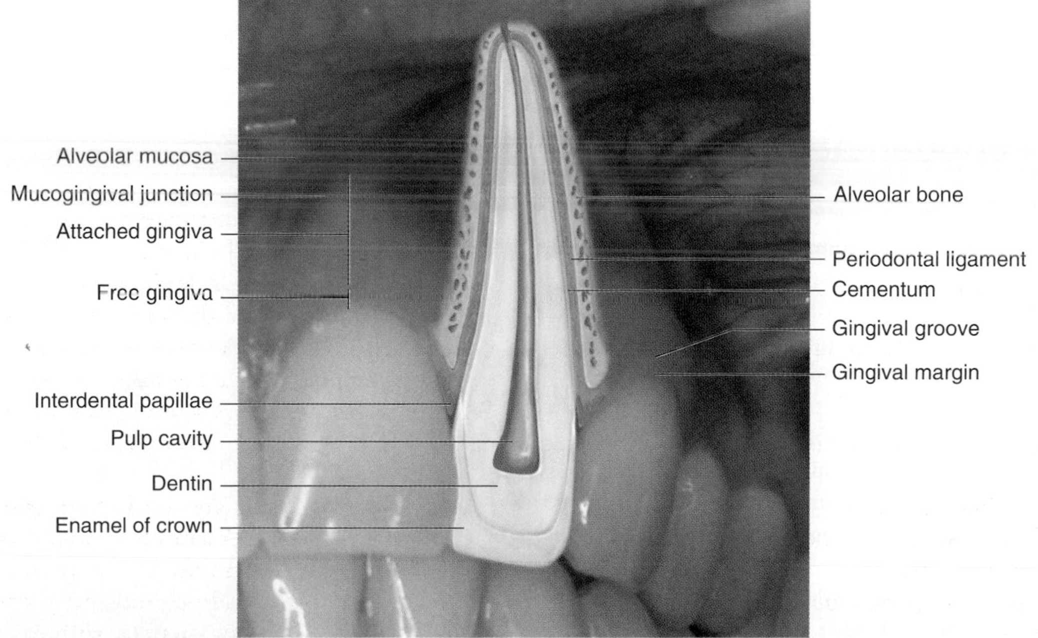


**FIG. 14.1** Anatomic relationship of the normal gingivae. Gingival tissues include the alveolar mucosa, mucogingival junction, attached gingiva, free gingiva, and interdental papilla. *(From Darby ML, Walsh MM: Dental hygiene: theory and practice, ed 4, St Louis, 2015, Saunders.)*

disease have 3 times the risk for stroke and 3.6 times the risk for coronary heart disease compared with individuals without periodontal disease. Studies show that oral bacteria can easily spread into the bloodstream, attach to fatty plaques in the coronary arteries, and contribute to clot formation and heart attacks.

## Preterm/Low Birth Weight

*Preterm birth* is defined as birth that follows a pregnancy that is shorter than 37 weeks; *low birth weight* is defined as less than 5.5 pounds. Preterm birth and low birth weight are the two most significant predictors of the health and survival of an infant. Other risk factors such as smoking, alcohol use, and drug use also contribute to preterm low-birth-weight (PLBW) infants. Women with severe periodontal disease have 7 times the risk for PLBW babies compared with women with little or no periodontal disease. This association may be linked to particular biochemicals that are produced with periodontal disease, such as *prostaglandin* $E_2$, which may create hormones that cause early uterine contraction and labor.

## Respiratory Disease

Individuals with periodontal disease may be at increased risk for respiratory infection. It appears that bacteria that have colonized in the mouth may alter the respiratory epithelium, leaving it more susceptible to pneumonia. In addition, in patients who already have chronic bronchitis, emphysema, or chronic obstructive pulmonary disease, existing conditions may be aggravated by inhalation of bacteria from the mouth into the lungs. These bacteria multiply in the respiratory tract and cause infection.

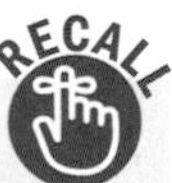


1 What is the leading cause of tooth loss in adults?
2 What systemic diseases have a connection to periodontal disease?
3 Name the structures of the periodontium.

# Causes of Periodontal Disease

## Biofilm

**Biofilm** (also known as **plaque**, **dental plaque, oral biofilm,** and **microbial biofilm**) is a colorless, soft, sticky coating made up of communities of microorganisms that adheres to tooth surfaces, dental appliances, restorations of the teeth, the oral mucosa, the tongue, and alveolar bone.

Dental caries and gingival and periodontal infections are caused by microorganisms in dental biofilm. When the biofilm layer is thin, it is not visible, but it stains pink when a disclosing agent (erythrosine stain) is applied (staining biofilm is discussed further in Chapter 15). If it is not removed, biofilm will continue to build up and will appear as a sticky white material (Fig. 14.2).

Although biofilm is the primary factor causing periodontal disease, type of bacteria, length of time bacteria are left undisturbed on the teeth, and patient response to bacteria are all critical factors in the risk for periodontal disease. Biofilm cannot be removed simply by rinsing the mouth. Bacteria in biofilm cause inflammation by producing enzymes and toxins that destroy periodontal tissues and lower host defenses.

## Calculus

Calcium and phosphate salts in the saliva form **calculus**, which is commonly called "tartar." Calculus is a hard, stonelike material that attaches to the tooth surface. The surface of calculus is porous and rough and provides an excellent surface on which additional plaque can grow. Calculus can penetrate into the cementum on root surfaces. It cannot be removed by the patient and must be removed by the dentist or the dental hygienist with the use of scaling instruments. Regular, effective plaque/biofilm control measures can minimize or eliminate the buildup of calculus. Biofilm control measures are discussed in Chapter 15.

Calculus is usually divided into **supragingival** and **subgingival** types, even though these types often occur together.

### *Supragingival Calculus*

Supragingival calculus is found on the clinical crowns of the teeth, above the margin of the gingiva. It is readily visible as a yellowish-white deposit that may darken over time (Fig. 14.3).

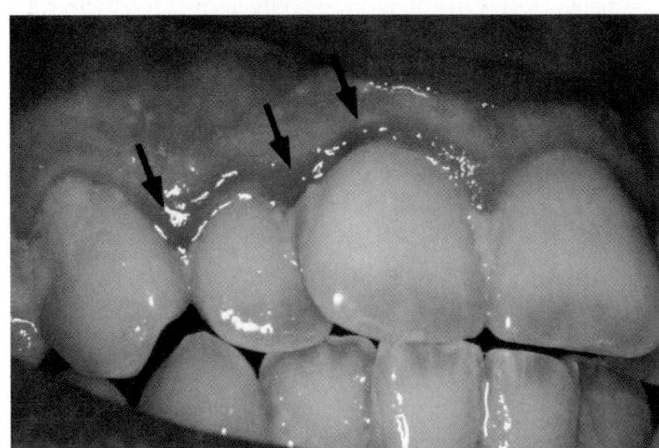

**FIG. 14.2** Clinical photo of 10-day-old supragingival biofilm. The first symptoms of gingival inflammation *(arrows)* are becoming visible. *(From Newman M, Takei T, Klokkevold P et al, editors: Carranza's clinical periodontology, ed 12, St Louis, 2015, Saunders.)*

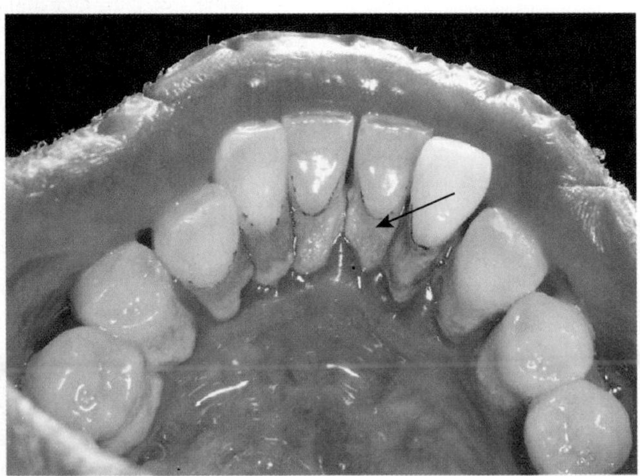

**FIG. 14.3** Heavy calculus deposits on the lingual surfaces of the lower anterior teeth. *(Courtesy Dr. Edward J. Taggart, San Francisco, CA.)*

Supragingival calculus occurs frequently near the openings of Wharton's ducts (on the lingual surfaces of the lower anterior teeth) and Stensen's ducts (on the buccal surfaces of the maxillary molars).

### *Subgingival Calculus*

Subgingival calculus forms on root surfaces below the gingival margin and can extend into the periodontal pockets. It can be dark green or black. The color is caused by stain that results from subgingival bleeding.

Unlike supragingival calculus, the location of subgingival calculus is not site specific. It is found throughout the mouth. Subgingival calculus provides a reservoir for bacteria and endotoxins. Subgingival calculus covered by plaque can cause greater disease than can be produced by biofilm alone.

#### Tooth Deposits

**Acquired pellicle**—Thin film of protein that quickly forms on teeth. It can be removed by coronal polishing with an abrasive agent such as "prophy" paste.

**Materia alba**—Soft mixture of bacteria and salivary proteins, also known as "white material." It is visible without the use of a disclosing agent and is common in individuals with poor oral hygiene.

**Food debris**—Particles of food that are impacted between the teeth after eating. Food debris does not simply become biofilm. If fermentable carbohydrates are present, however, food debris may contribute to dental caries.

## Other Risk Factors

A vast majority of periodontal diseases begin as inflammation caused by an accumulation of bacteria in the biofilm. However, periodontal diseases may be triggered by other factors such as malocclusion, some medications (such as those used for control of blood pressure), and serious nutritional deficiencies.

Disease-causing bacteria are necessary for periodontal disease to occur, but they are not totally responsible for destruction of the periodontium. Other risk factors alter the body's response to bacteria that are present in the mouth. Risk factors involved will determine the onset, degree, and severity of periodontal disease. This is why there is a great deal of variability in the susceptibility of individuals to periodontal disease and in successful outcomes of treatment.

Periodontal disease results from the complex interaction of bacterial infection and risk factors. As the number of risk factors increases, the patient's susceptibility to periodontal disease also increases (Table 14.2).

## Types of Periodontal Disease

The term *periodontal disease* includes both gingivitis and periodontitis, and these two basic forms of periodontal disease each has a variety of forms. It is important for the dental assistant to have a clear understanding of the characteristics of the healthy periodontium, which will serve as

**TABLE 14.2 Common Risk Factors for Periodontal Disease**

| Risk Factor | Rationale |
|---|---|
| Smoking | Smokers have greater loss of attachment, bone loss, periodontal pocket depths, calculus formation, and tooth loss. Periodontal treatments are less effective in smokers than in nonsmokers. |
| Diabetes mellitus | Diabetes is a strong risk factor for periodontal disease. Individuals with diabetes are 3 times more likely to have attachment and bone loss. Persons who have their diabetes under control have less attachment and bone loss than do those with poor control. |
| Poor oral hygiene | Lack of good oral hygiene increases the risk of periodontal disease in all age groups. Excellent oral hygiene greatly reduces the risk of severe periodontal disease. |
| Osteoporosis | An association has been reported between alveolar bone loss and osteoporosis. Women with osteoporosis have increased alveolar bone resorption, attachment loss, and tooth loss compared with women without osteoporosis. Estrogen deficiency also has been linked to decreases in alveolar bone. |
| Human immunodeficiency virus/acquired immunodeficiency syndrome (HIV/AIDS) | Increased gingival inflammation is noted around the margins of all teeth. Often, patients with HIV/AIDS develop necrotizing ulcerative periodontitis. |
| Stress | Psychological stress is associated with depression of the immune system, and studies show a link between stress and periodontal attachment loss. Research is ongoing to identify the link between psychological stress and periodontal disease. |
| Medications | Some medications, such as tetracycline and nonsteroidal anti-inflammatory drugs, have a beneficial effect on the periodontium, and others have a negative effect. Decreased salivary flow (xerostomia) can be caused by more than 400 medications, including diuretics, antihistamines, antipsychotics, antihypertensive agents, and analgesics. Antiseizure drugs and hormones such as estrogen and progesterone can cause gingival enlargement. |
| Local factors | Overhanging restorations, subgingival placement of crown margins, orthodontic appliances, and removable partial dentures also may contribute to the progression of periodontal disease. |

**TABLE 14.3 Clinical Gingival Characteristics in Health and Disease**

| Characteristic | Health | Disease |
|---|---|---|
| Color | Uniformly pale pink with or without generalized dark brown pigmentation | Bright red<br>Dark red, blue-red<br>Pink if fibrotic |
| Consistency | Firm, resilient | Soft, spongy, dents easily when pressed with probe<br>Bleeds readily to probing |
| Surface texture | Free gingival—smooth<br>Attached—stippled | Loss of stippling, shiny<br>Fibrotic with stippling<br>Nodular<br>Hyperkeratotic |
| Contour | Gingival margin is 1–2 mm above CEJ in fully erupted teeth<br>Marginal gingiva is knife-edge, flat; follows a curved line around the tooth and fits snugly around the tooth<br>Papilla is pointed and pyramidal; fills interproximal spaces | Irregular margins from edema, fibrosis, clefting, and/or festooning<br>May be rounded, rolled, or bulbous; therefore more coronal to CEJ<br>May show recessions so that the anatomical root is exposed<br>Bulbous, flattened, blunted, cratered |
| Size | Free marginal gingiva is near CEJ and adheres closely to the tooth | Enlarged from excess fluid in tissues or fibrotic from the formation of excess collagen fibers. Free marginal gingiva may be highly retractable with air |
| Probing depth | 0–4 mm; no apical migration of JE | More than 4 mm with or without apical migration of JE |

*CEJ,* Cementoenamel junction; *JE,* junctional epithelium.

From Darby ML, Walsh MM: Dental hygiene: theory and practice, ed 4, St Louis, 2015, Saunders.

a foundation from which signs of disease can be identified. You may wish to review the appearance of healthy oral tissues as presented in Chapter 10.

## Signs and Symptoms

The following signs and symptoms are most often seen in patients with periodontal disease:

- Red, swollen, or tender gingiva
- Bleeding gingiva while brushing or flossing
- Loose or separating teeth
- Pain or pressure when chewing
- Pus around the teeth or gingival tissues

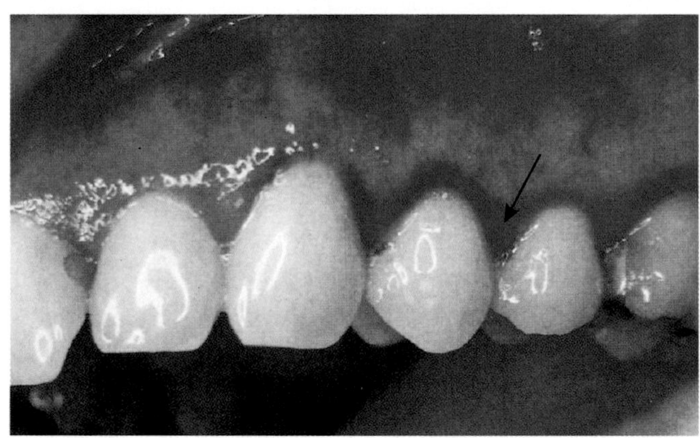

**FIG. 14.4** Gingivitis type I.

## Gingivitis

**Gingivitis** is inflammation of the gingival tissue. It may be the most common human disease and is one of the easiest to treat and control. Areas of redness and swelling characterize gingivitis, and the gingiva tends to bleed easily. In addition, there may be changes in gingival contour and loss of tissue adaptation to the teeth (Table 14.3).

Gingivitis is found only in the epithelium and in gingival connective tissues. *No* tissue recession or loss of connective tissue or bone is associated with gingivitis (Fig. 14.4). Other types of gingivitis are associated with puberty, pregnancy, and the use of birth control medications (Box 14.2 and Fig. 14.5).

Orthodontic appliances tend to retain bacterial plaque and food debris, resulting in gingivitis (Fig. 14.6). Instruction regarding proper home care is a critical part of orthodontic treatment (see Chapter 60).

Gingivitis is painless and often remains unrecognized until a dental professional emphasizes its importance. Improved daily oral hygiene practices may reverse gingivitis.

4 Name two types of calculus.
5 What are the signs of gingivitis?

**BOX 14.2** Characteristics of Plaque-Induced Gingival Disease

**I. Dental Plaque–Induced Gingivitis***

Inflammation of the gingiva with plaque present at the gingival margin. Characterized by absence of attachment loss; clinical redness; bleeding on provocation; and changes in contour, color, and consistency. No radiographic evidence of crestal bone loss is found. Local contributing factors may enhance susceptibility.

**II. Plaque-Induced Gingival Disease Modified by Systemic Factors**

Endogenous Sex Steroid Hormone Gingival Disease

Includes puberty-associated gingivitis, pregnancy-associated gingivitis, and menstrual cycle gingivitis; characterized by an exaggerated response to plaque, reflected by intense inflammation, redness, edema, and enlargement with absence of bone and attachment loss; in pregnancy, may progress to a pyogenic granuloma (pregnancy tumor).

Diabetes Mellitus–Associated Gingivitis

Found in children with poorly controlled type 1 diabetes mellitus. Characteristics similar to plaque-induced gingivitis, but severity is related to control of blood glucose levels rather than to plaque control.

Hematologic (Leukemic) Gingival Disease

Swollen, glazed, and spongy gingival tissues that are red to deep purple; enlargement is first observed in the interdental papilla; plaque may exacerbate condition but is not necessary for it to occur.

Drug-Influenced Gingival Enlargement

Occurs as a result of the use of phenytoin, cyclosporine, and calcium channel blockers such as nifedipine and verapamil. Onset usually occurs within 3 months of drug use and is more common in younger age groups. Characterized by an exaggerated response to plaque that results in gingival overgrowth (most commonly occurring in the anterior area and beginning in the interdental papilla); found in gingiva with or without bone loss but not associated with loss of attachment.

Gingival Disease Associated with Nutrition

Associated with a severe vitamin C deficiency and scurvy. Gingiva appears red, bulbous, spongy, and hemorrhagic.

* Williams R: Periodontal disease: the emergence of a new paradigm, Compendium 19(suppl):4, 1999.

Data from Papapanou PN: Periodontal diseases: epidemiology, Ann Periodontol 1:1, 1996. Data reproduced with permission from the American Academy of Periodontology.

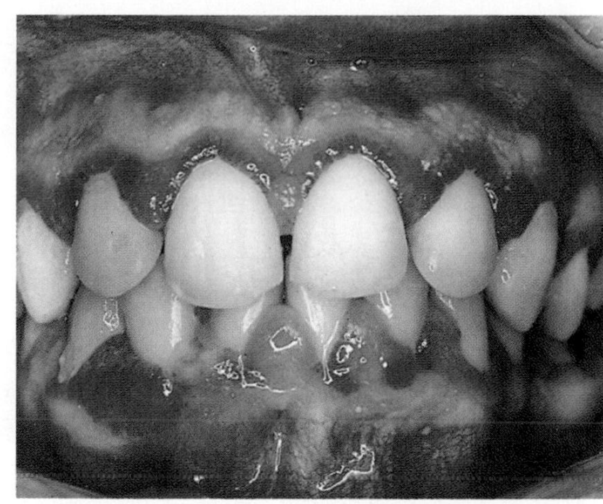

**FIG. 14.5** Medication-induced gingivitis. *(From Perry D, Beemsterboer P: Periodontology for the dental hygienist, ed 4, St Louis, 2014, Saunders.)*

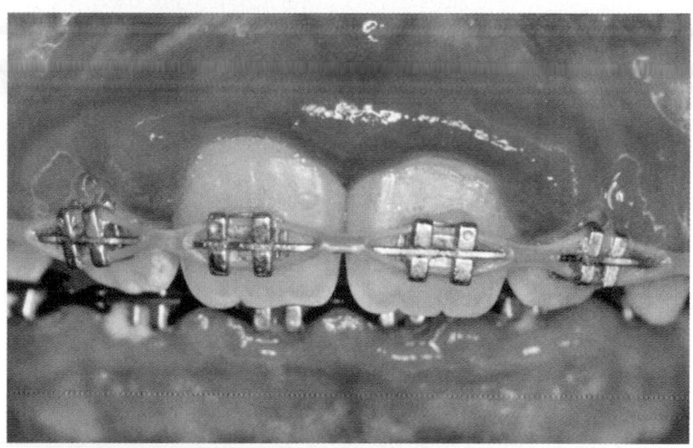

**FIG. 14.6** Gingival inflammation and enlargement associated with orthodontic appliance and poor oral hygiene. *(From Newman M, Takei T, Klokkevold P et al, editors: Carranza's clinical periodontology, ed 12, St Louis, 2015, Saunders.)*

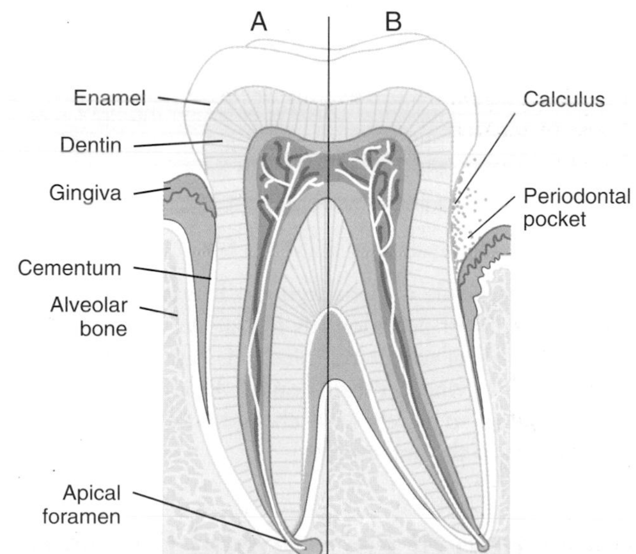


**FIG. 14.7** Cross section of a tooth and associated anatomic structures. A, Illustrates the depth of a normal gingival sulcus. B, Illustrates a periodontal pocket.

## Periodontitis

**Periodontitis** is inflammation of the supporting tissues of the teeth. The inflammatory process progresses from the gingiva into the connective tissue and alveolar bone that support the teeth (Fig. 14.7). The connective tissue attachment at the base of a periodontal pocket is destroyed as the disease progresses.

At one time, it was believed that periodontitis progressed slowly and at a constant rate. All individuals were thought to

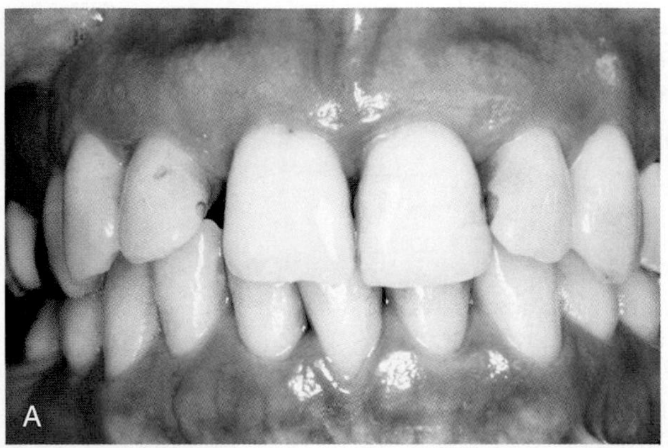

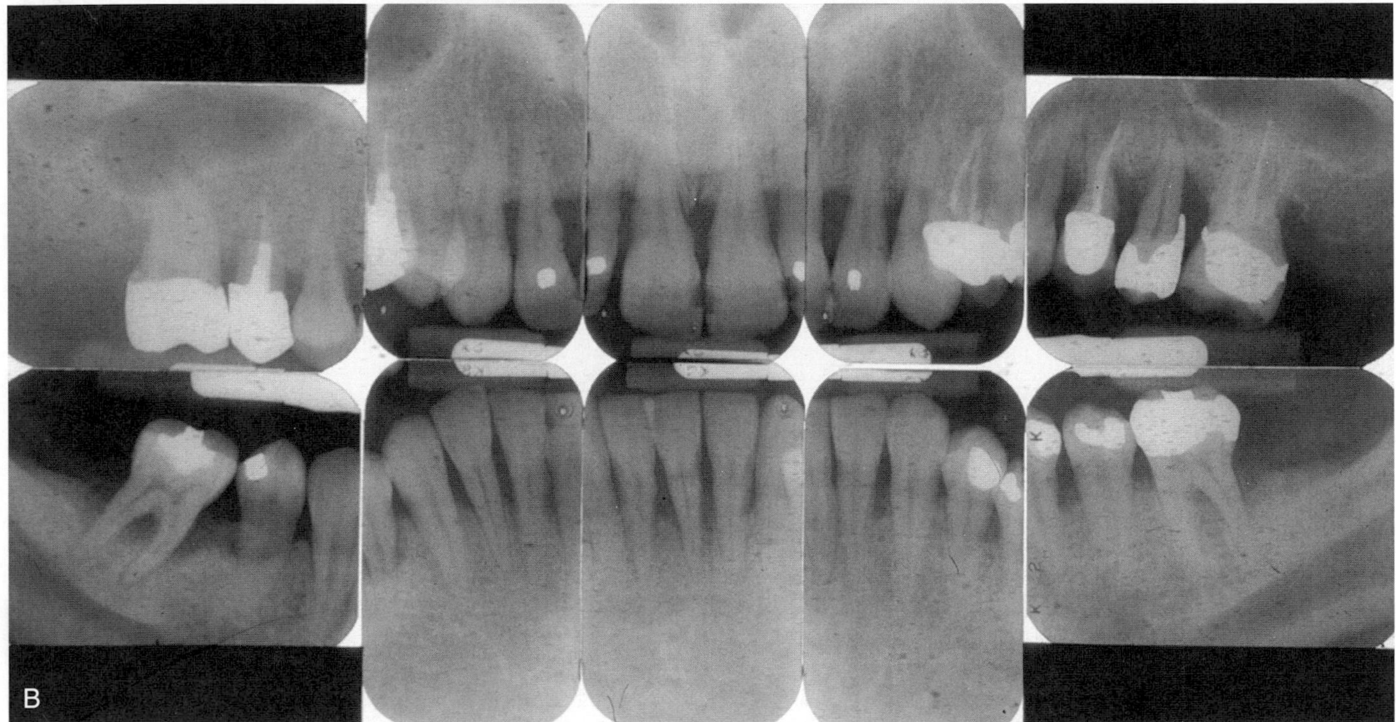

**FIG. 14.8** Generalized chronic periodontitis in a 38-year-old woman with a 20-year history of smoking at least one pack of cigarettes per day. A, Clinical view shows minimal biofilm and inflammation. Probing produced negligible bleeding, which is common with smokers. Patient reported spacing between the right maxillary incisors, which was associated with advanced attachment bone loss. B, Radiographs show severe, generalized, horizontal pattern of bone loss. Maxillary and mandibular molars have already been lost through advanced disease and furcation involvement. *(From Newman M, Takei T, Klokkevold P et al, editors: Carranza's clinical periodontology, ed 11, St Louis, 2012, Saunders.)*

be equally susceptible to periodontitis. This is no longer true. The current view of periodontitis is that the disease can take several forms, all of which are infections caused by groups of microorganisms living in the oral cavity. All forms of periodontal disease appear to be related to changes in the many types of bacteria found in the oral cavity.

## Description of Periodontal Disease

Periodontal disease is described in terms of disease severity and how much of the mouth is affected:

- If less than 30 percent of sites in the mouth are affected, the disease is considered *localized.*
- If more than 30 percent of sites in the mouth are affected, the disease is considered *generalized* (Fig. 14.8).

The severity of the disease is determined by assessment of the amount of lost attachment, as follows:

- Slight or early
- Moderate
- Severe or advanced

On the basis of disease severity and the amount of tissue destruction that has occurred by the time of examination (Box 14.3), the American Academy of Periodontology has identified seven basic case types of periodontal disease.

## Dental Perioscopy

The goal of periodontal therapy is to get the root surfaces as clean as possible so that tissues can heal; now, with the use of dental **perioscopy**, the clinician can actually see any remaining subgingival calculus on root surfaces (Fig. 14.9). With magnification up to 46 times, the clinician can also see initial decay and/or cracks on root surfaces that were previously undiagnosed.

A disposable sterile sheath is placed around the perioscope before each patient use. A miniature camera is attached to a tiny probe (Fig. 14.10) and then is gently inserted into the sulcus. Images are immediately displayed on a chairside video screen for the operator and patient to see (Fig. 14.11).

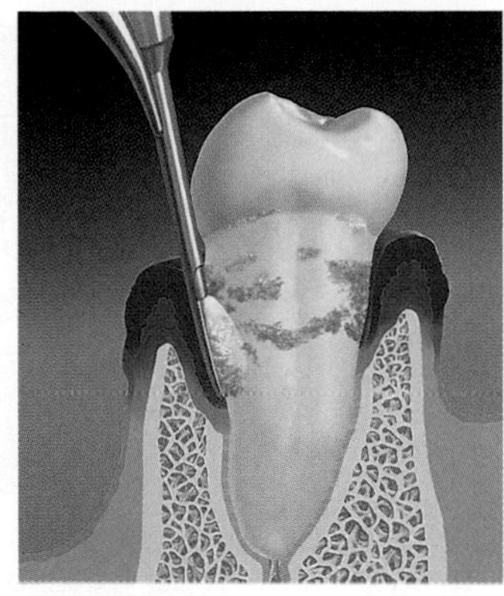

**FIG. 14.9** Diagrammatic illustration of the endoscope's explorer examining the subgingival root surface and calculus deposits. *(Courtesy Danville Materials, Inc., Carlsbad, CA.)*

There is very little discomfort during the procedure, and often the patient does not require the use of local anesthesia. Although costly, this device may one day become a new standard of care in the diagnosis and treatment of patients with periodontal disease worldwide.

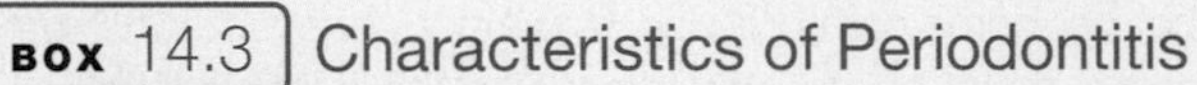

**BOX 14.3** Characteristics of Periodontitis

**I. Chronic Periodontitis***

Onset at any age but most prevalent in adults. Characterized by inflammation of the supporting structures of the teeth, loss of clinical attachment due to destruction of the periodontal ligament, and loss of adjacent bone. Prevalence and severity increase with age. The following levels of chronic periodontal classification have been identified:

- *Slight or early periodontitis:* Progression of gingival inflammation into the alveolar bone crest and early bone loss that results in slight attachment loss of 1 to 2 mm with periodontal probing depths of 3 to 4 mm.
- *Moderate periodontitis:* A more advanced state of the previous condition, with increased destruction of periodontal structures, clinical attachment loss of up to 4 mm, moderate to deep pockets (5–7 mm), moderate bone loss, tooth mobility, and furcation involvement not exceeding class I in molars.
- *Severe or advanced periodontitis:* Further progression of periodontitis with severe destruction of periodontal structures, clinical attachment loss greater than 5 mm, increased bone loss, increased pocket depth (usually 7 mm or greater), increased tooth mobility, and furcation involvement greater than class I in molars.

**II. Aggressive Periodontitis†**

Occurs before age 35 and is associated with rapid rate of progression of tissue destruction, host defense defects, and composition of subgingival flora. The following subclassifications have been identified:

- *Prepubertal periodontitis:* Onset occurs between eruption of the primary teeth and puberty; occurs in localized forms usually not associated with a systemic disease and generalized forms usually accompanied by alterations in neutrophil functioning; clinically manifests as attachment loss around primary and/or permanent teeth.
- *Juvenile periodontitis:* Localized and generalized forms. The generalized form occurs late in the teenage years with a variable microbial origin that may include *Actinobacillus actinomycetemcomitans* and *Porphyromonas gingivalis* and affects most teeth. The localized form is associated with less-acute clinical signs of inflammation than would be expected on the basis of severity of destruction. The localized form is associated with bone and attachment loss that is most often confined to permanent first molars and/or incisors. Onset occurs at or around puberty; associated with *Actinobacillus actinomycetemcomitans* and neutrophil dysfunction.

**III. Necrotizing Periodontal Disease‡**

- *Necrotizing ulcerative gingivitis:* A gingival infection of complex origin (e.g., plaque, temporary depression of polymorphonuclear neutrophil functioning, stress, poor diet) that is characterized by sudden onset of pain, necrosis of the tips of the gingival papillae (punched out appearance), and bleeding. Secondary features include fetid breath and a pseudomembrane covering. Fusiform bacteria, *Prevetella intermedia,* and spirochetes have been associated with gingival lesions.
- *Necrotizing ulcerative periodontitis:* Characterized by necrosis of gingival tissues, periodontal ligament, and alveolar bone. Associated with immune disorders such as HIV infection and immunosuppressive therapies; characteristics include severe and rapid periodontal destruction. Extensive necrosis of the soft tissue occurs simultaneously with alveolar bone loss, resulting in lack of deep pocket formation.

*Slavkin HC: Building a better mousetrap: toward an understanding of osteoporosis, J Am Dent Assoc 150:1632, 1999.

†Fedi P, Vernino A, Gray J: The periodontic syllabus, Philadelphia, 2000, Lippincott Williams and Wilkins.

‡Armitage G: Development of a classification system for periodontal diseases and conditions, Ann Periodontol 4:1, 1999.

From Darby M, Walsh M: Dental hygiene theory and practice, ed 4, St Louis, 2015, Saunders.

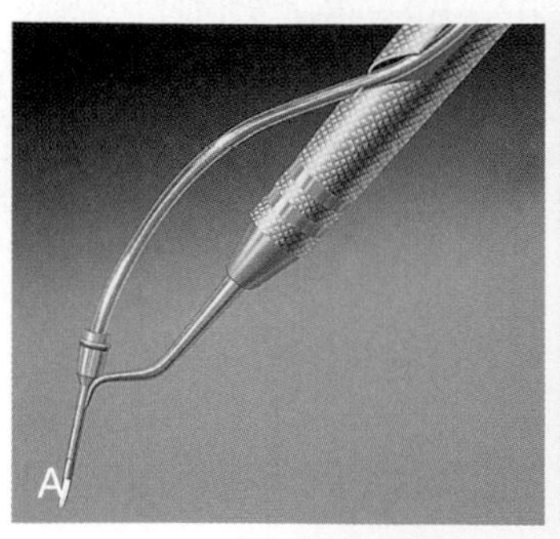


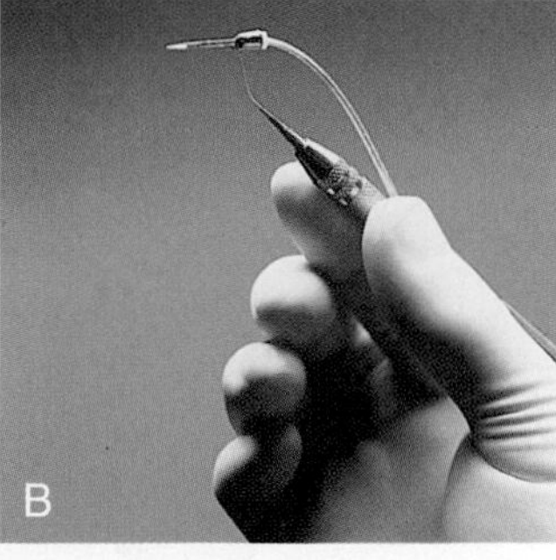


**FIG. 14.10** A, The endoscope explorer with sheath and fiberoptic bundle in the "thistle" adapter. B, Proper grasp for the endoscope explorer. *(Courtesy Danville Materials, Inc., Carlsbad, CA.)*

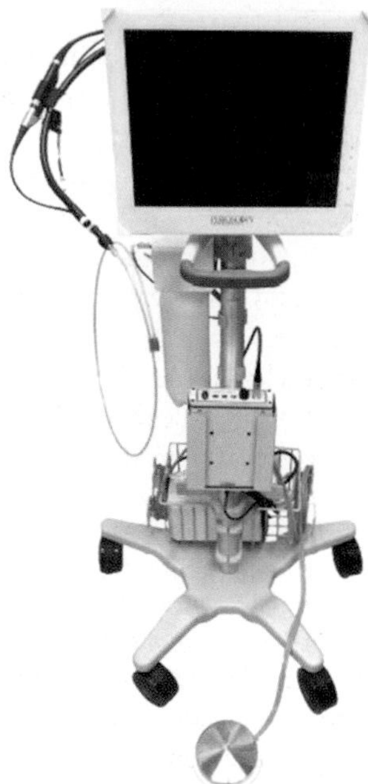

**FIG. 14.11** The Perioscopy endoscope. *(Courtesy Danville Materials Inc., Carlsbad, CA.)*

RECALL

6 What is the definition of periodontitis?
7 What are signs and symptoms of periodontitis?
8 How many basic types of periodontal disease have been identified by the American Academy of Periodontology?
9 How is the severity of periodontal disease determined?
10 What are the advantages of perioscopy?

**■ Legal and Ethical Implications** One of the most common types of malpractice lawsuits alleges that the dentist failed to diagnose the condition and inform a patient that he or she had periodontal disease.

A common scenario is that the dentist had discussed the need for improved oral hygiene care with the patient at every visit but did not document those conversations. Years later, when the resulting periodontal disease became a serious problem, the patient did not recall these instructions and denied being told about the causes of periodontal disease. It is important to observe and chart the patient's oral hygiene status. Be certain to document all home care instructions that have been given to the patient. In addition, it is important to document that the patient has been clearly informed about the potential for future periodontal disease if home care does not improve. ■

## ■ Critical Thinking

1. Laura Sinclair is a 24-year-old patient in your dental practice. During her routine checkup, the dentist notices that Laura has some slight bleeding around the molars and slightly reddish gingival margins around other teeth. Laura insists that her home care practices have not changed. What other factors might be involved in causing this mild gingivitis in Laura?
2. Roger Fernandez is a 63-year-old man who has come into your office for a new patient examination. His medical history indicates that he is taking medications for his type 1 diabetes mellitus. On the basis of this information, do you think you might see any unusual conditions in his oral tissues? If so, what and why?
3. A pregnant patient has been scheduled to come into your office for an emergency appointment. The receptionist tells you and the dentist that this patient is very concerned about her painful and bleeding gums, which she never had before. What is your first impression as to the possible cause of this pregnant patient's problems?
4. Karyn Mentr is a 28-year-old woman who is pregnant with her first child. She has moderate early signs of periodontal disease. This is her first visit to your office, and the dentist wants to begin periodontal treatment immediately, but Mrs. Mentr wants to wait until after her baby is born. Why do you think the dentist wants to begin periodontal treatment immediately? ■

15

# Preventive Dentistry

## KEY TERMS

**Dental sealant** Coating that covers the occlusal pits and fissures of teeth.

**Disclosing agent** Coloring agent that makes plaque visible when applied to teeth.

**Fluoride varnish** Method of administration of topical fluoride.

**Pontic (PON-tik)** Artificial tooth that replaces a missing natural tooth.

**Preventive dentistry** Program of patient education, use of fluorides, application of dental sealants, proper nutrition, and plaque control.

**Systemic fluoride** Fluoride that is ingested and then circulated throughout the body.

**Topical fluoride** Fluoride that is applied directly to the tooth.

## LEARNING OUTCOMES

*On completion of this chapter, the student will be able to achieve the following objectives:*

1. Pronounce, define, and spell the key terms.
2. Discuss preventive dentistry, including the following:
   - Explain the goal of preventive dentistry.
   - Describe the components of a preventive dentistry program.
   - List the guidelines for preventive patient education.
3. Discuss the benefits of early dental care, including the following:
   - Describe why dental care is important for pregnant women.
   - Describe the method used to clean a baby's mouth.
   - Describe when children should first visit the dentist.
   - Explain the purpose of dental sealants.
4. Describe age-related changes in oral health.
5. Describe the effects of water fluoridation on the teeth, including the following:
   - Explain how fluoride works.
   - Discuss safe and toxic levels of fluoride.
   - Explain the precautions to protect patients from receiving too much fluoride.
   - Describe the purpose of a fluoride needs assessment.
   - Identify sources of systemic and topical fluoride.
6. Describe the relationship between nutrition and dental caries, including the steps involved in analyzing a food diary.
7. List the oral hygiene products available to aid in a plaque control program, including the following:
   - Compare and contrast toothbrushing techniques.
   - Describe the process required for cleaning a denture.

## PERFORMANCE OUTCOMES

*On completion of this chapter, the student will be able to meet competency standards in the following skills:*

- Apply a topical fluoride gel or foam competently and effectively.
- Apply fluoride varnish competently and effectively.
- Teach a patient how to use dental floss effectively.

## ELECTRONIC RESOURCES

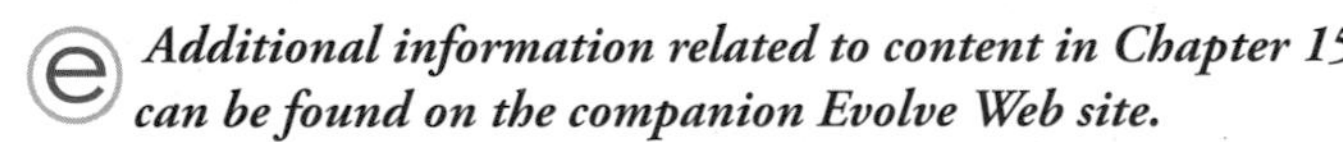

***Additional information related to content in Chapter 15 can be found on the companion Evolve Web site.***

- Practice Quiz
- Videos: Applying Topical Fluoride Gel or Foam, Toothbrushing Methods, Flossing Techniques
- Canadian Content Corner

The goal of **preventive dentistry** is to help people of all ages attain optimal oral health throughout their lives. To achieve this goal, dental professionals must work together with their patients to prevent new and recurring disease. As was discussed in Chapters 13 and 14, various types of bacteria found in dental plaque are responsible for *dental caries* and *periodontal disease,* the two most common dental diseases.

The information provided in this chapter will help you to educate patients on how to achieve and maintain their oral health.

## Partners in Prevention

To prevent dental disease, a *partnership* must be formed between the patient and the dental healthcare team. As a dental assistant, your first step is to help patients understand what causes dental disease and how to prevent it. The next step that you must follow is to motivate patients to change their behaviors and become partners in recognizing and preventing dental disease in themselves and their families. For example, mothers can be taught to simply lift their children's lips to look for any stains, white spots, or dark areas on the teeth (Fig. 15.1).

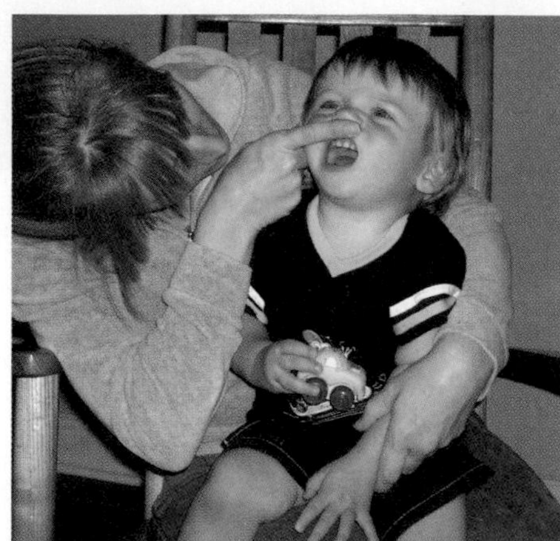

**FIG. 15.1** The mother lifts the child's lip to look for early signs of decay.

Optimal oral health can become a reality when partners work together in a comprehensive preventive dentistry program that includes the following (Table 15.1):

- Patient education
- Use of fluorides
- Application of dental sealants
- Proper nutrition
- Plaque control program

### Patient Education Guidelines

*Listen carefully* to learn how patients perceive their dental healthcare needs. Each patient will have different needs. Because you are so aware of the importance of good dental health, the patient's perception and your perception of the patient's dental needs may be very different.

*Instruct the patient on how to remove plaque.* This is the initial instruction for most patients. Because plaque is not visible on most teeth, you must use a disclosing agent. This is a very effective aid that allows a patient to actually see plaque on the teeth. Disclosing agents are available in tablet or liquid form. This is the time to explain the relationship of plaque to dental disease (caries and periodontal disease). You must customize the message for each patient.

*Assess the patient's motivations and needs.* Then combine the patient's motivating factors with the patient's needs to make recommendations for oral healthcare. For instance, when a patient's immediate concern is staining on the front teeth, it is not effective to emphasize the plaque on the lingual surface of the molars.

*Select home care aids.* With the patient's needs identified, select a toothbrush, a toothbrushing method, interproximal cleaning aids (such as dental floss), and a dentifrice (toothpaste).

*Keep the instruction simple.* If you select a style of communication that is comfortable for the individual patient, you are more likely to have the desired impact. Help the patient make any necessary improvements in his or her technique. Comment positively on the patient's efforts.

*Reinforce home care* during the patient's return visits for dental treatment. People tend to regress in their home care efforts, so expect periodic setbacks. When these occur, help patients achieve their goals in a positive and helpful manner.

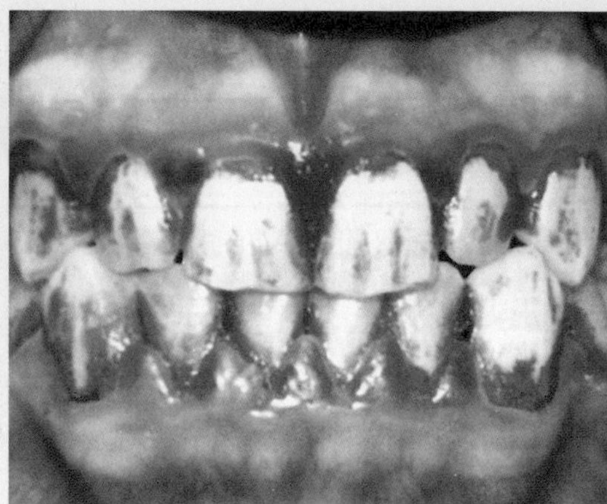

Disclosing solution shows heavy plaque formation throughout the mouth.

RECALL

1 What is the goal of preventive dentistry?
2 What are the two most common dental diseases?
3 What are the guidelines of patient education programs?
4 What is the initial step in a patient education program?

# Early Dental Care

## Pregnancy and Dental Care

The American Academy of Pediatric Dentistry (AAPD) guidelines advise all pregnant women to receive counseling and oral healthcare during pregnancy, and advise that infants undergo oral health assessment by their first birthday. Many women are not aware of these guidelines and do not seek dental care during their pregnancy because they believe that they do not have any dental problems. However, dental care is an important aspect of total prenatal care. When the mother has a healthy mouth and teeth, she is protecting her unborn child. Untreated tooth and periodontal disease can increase the risk of giving birth to a preterm, low-birth-weight baby. Pregnant women should ask their dentist about using an antibacterial mouth rinse and chewing gum or eating mints that contain xylitol to reduce the bacteria in their mouth that cause tooth decay. This is very important because tooth decay is caused by bacteria that a new mother can transfer to her infant.

## Dental Care for 0 to 5 Years

Good oral health for a lifetime begins at birth. Even before the baby has teeth, the parent should wipe the gums gently with a clean wet cloth after each feeding. To avoid spreading bacteria that cause caries, the parent should not put anything into the baby's mouth that has been in his or her own mouth, including spoons, cups, and so forth.

As soon as the first tooth appears, the parent can begin brushing the baby's teeth in the morning and before bedtime

**TABLE 15.1 Comprehensive Preventive Dentistry Program**

| Component | Description |
|---|---|
| Nutrition | Dietary counseling extends beyond the narrow scope of limiting sugar consumption and may include a discussion of nutrition from the standpoint of oral health and general health. |
| Patient education | Education motivates patients, provides them with information, and assists them in developing the skills necessary to practice good oral hygiene. |
| Plaque control | Daily removal of bacterial plaque from the teeth and adjacent oral tissues. |
| Fluoride therapy | Includes professionally applied fluorides, at-home fluoride therapy, and the consumption of fluoridated community water. |
| Sealants | Sealants are most frequently applied to the difficult-to-clean occlusal surfaces of the teeth. Decay-causing bacteria are then prevented from reaching into occlusal pits and fissures. |

(Fig. 15.2, *A*). A pea-sized dab of toothpaste across a small soft brush can be used. Excess toothpaste should be wiped off. The baby should never be put to bed at naptime or at bedtime with a bottle or sippy cup unless it has *only* water in it, because milk and juices cause early childhood caries, which is also known as "baby bottle tooth decay."

A baby should visit the dentist by the time of his or her first birthday and thereafter as often as the dentist recommends (Fig. 15.2, *B*).

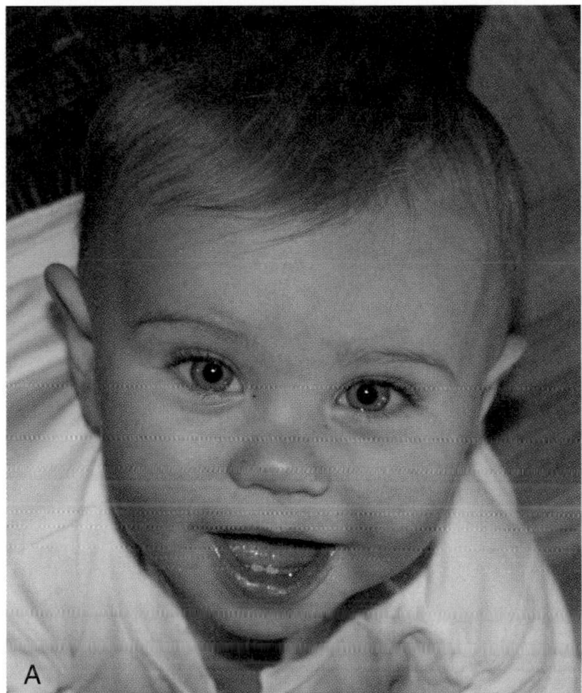


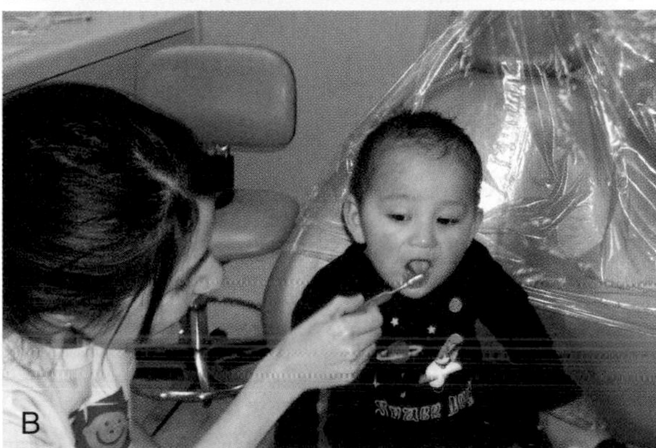


**FIG. 15.2** A, Toothbrushing should begin as soon as the first tooth appears. B, This is the first dental visit for this 15-month-old boy. The dental assistant is showing the mother how to brush her son's teeth.

## Dental Sealants

A **dental sealant** is a plastic-like coating that is applied over the occlusal pits and grooves of the teeth. Sealants are used to protect difficult-to-clean occlusal surfaces of the teeth from the bacteria that cause decay (Fig. 15.3).

Dental sealants are an important component in preventive dentistry. In several states, the application of dental sealants is delegated to the dental assistant as an expanded function (see Chapter 59).

**5** What are dental sealants?

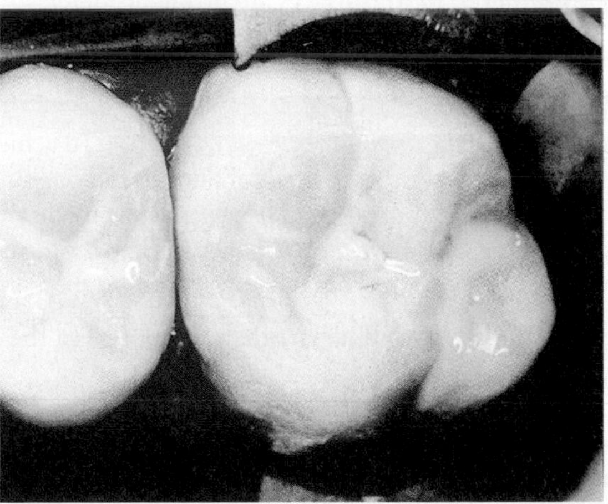

**FIG. 15.3** This molar is protected from decay with the use of a dental sealant. *(Copyright © 3M 2017. All rights reserved.)*

## Oral Health and Aging

The numbers of adults age 65 years old and older are increasing at a faster rate than the general population. This increase is due primarily to an increase in life expectancy. There has also been a significant decrease in the number of edentulous people. This means that more adults are committed to taking care of their teeth and are going to the dentist to seek routine dental care.

## Age-Related Dental Changes

With age, teeth normally undergo several changes, including changes in the enamel, cementum, dentin, and pulp. Many of today's older adults may have used a stiff toothbrush and abrasive toothpaste in the past, which resulted in tooth abrasion. The dental assistant can assist patients to learn proper oral hygiene techniques.

### Age-Related Dental Changes

- The enamel becomes darker in color
- The enamel surface develops numerous cracks
- The vitality of the dentin is greatly decreased
- Cementum has compositional changes
- Pulpal blood supply decreases
- The size of the pulp chamber is reduced
- Abrasion and attrition occur in the crowns of the teeth

## Age-Related Pathology-Related Conditions

Older adults are more likely to develop new coronal and root caries at a greater rate than the younger population. In addition, there are a number of other conditions common in the older adult population.

### Age-Related Pathology Conditions

- Both coronal and root caries
- Alveolar bone becomes more porous
- Increase of gingival recession
- Systemic disease and medications causing dry mouth
- Salivary gland changes causing reduced saliva flow
- Older adults frequently have anemia caused by iron deficiencies resulting in red and burning tongue

# Fluoride

Since the 1950s, fluoride has been the primary weapon used to combat dental caries. *Slowing demineralization* and *enhancing remineralization* of tooth surfaces are now considered to be the most important ways that fluoride controls the caries process (see Chapter 13).

Fluoride, sometimes referred to as "nature's cavity fighter," is a mineral that occurs naturally in food and water. To achieve the maximum cavity prevention benefit of fluoride, an ongoing supply of both systemic and topical fluoride must be made available throughout life. According to the patient's needs, various ways are available to receive fluoride therapy, including the following:

- Prescription-strength fluorides that are applied in the dental office
- Nonprescription-strength, over-the-counter products for home use
- Consumption of fluoridated bottled water or community water

**Systemic fluoride** is ingested in water, food, beverages, or supplements. The fluoride is absorbed through the intestine into the bloodstream and is transported to the tissues where it is needed. The body excretes excess systemic fluoride through the skin, kidneys, and feces.

**Topical fluoride** is applied in direct contact with the teeth through the use of fluoridated toothpaste, fluoride mouth rinses, and topical applications of rinses, gels, foams, and varnishes (Fig. 15.4).

### Oral Health Educational Materials and Web Sites

- Healthy Teeth Begin at Birth
  www.first5oralhealth.org
- A Healthy Mouth for Your Baby
  www.nohic.nidcr.nih.gov
- Taking Care of Your Child's Baby Teeth
  www.deltadentalksfoundation.org
- One Tooth, Two Teeth, Clean Teeth, Good Teeth (Un Diente, Spanish version)
  Log on to www.sugar.org to order a publication (#501) from the Sugar Association
- National Maternal and Child Oral Health Resource Center
  www.mchoralhealth.org

RECALL

6 What is the process by which fluoride prevents decay?
7 What are the two routes or means by which the body receives fluoride?

## How Fluoride Works

### *Preeruptive Development*

Before a tooth erupts, it is surrounded by a fluid-filled sac. The fluoride present in this fluid strengthens the enamel of the developing tooth and makes it more acid resistant.

Before birth, the source of systemic fluoride is the mother's diet. After birth and before the teeth erupt, the child ingests systemic fluoride.

### *Posteruptive Development*

After eruption of teeth, fluoride continues to enter the enamel and strengthen the structure of the enamel crystals. These fluoride-enriched crystals are *less acid soluble* than is the original structure of the enamel.

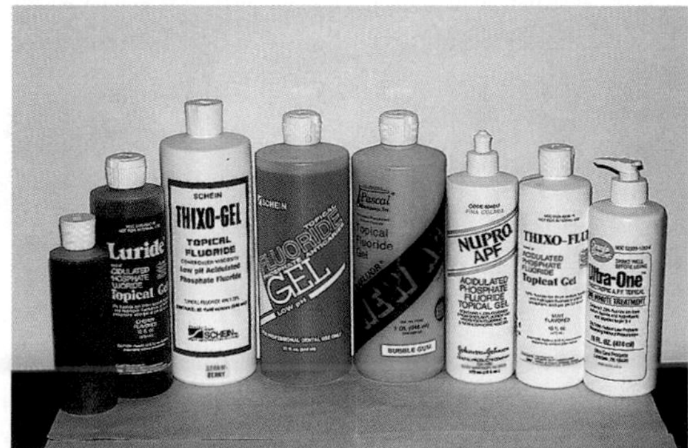


**FIG. 15.4** Topical fluoride gels for professional application. *(From Darby ML, Walsh MM: Dental hygiene: theory and practice, ed 4, St Louis, 2015, Saunders.)*

After eruption, an ongoing supply of fluoride from both systemic and topical sources is important for the remineralization process.

## Safe and Toxic Levels

Fluorides used in the dental office have been proved to be safe and effective *when used as recommended.* Chronic overexposure to fluoride, even at low concentrations, can result in dental *fluorosis* in children younger than 6 years with developing teeth (Fig. 15.5). Abuse of high-concentration gels or solutions of fluoride or accidental ingestion of a concentrated fluoride preparation can lead to a toxic reaction. Acute fluoride poisoning is rare.

## Precautions

To protect patients from receiving too much fluoride, current fluoride intake should be evaluated. For example, a child may live in an area with community water fluoridation, attend a preschool with a fluoride rinse program, and use a fluoride toothpaste at home. The dentist will consider these multiple sources of fluoride before prescribing additional fluoride supplements or office treatments for this child.

A particular area of concern involves young children, who may consume excessive fluoride by swallowing fluoridated toothpaste, which may cause fluorosis. Adult supervision of young children during toothbrushing is necessary, and the child should be instructed not to swallow the toothpaste. Fluoride in drinking water, fluoride toothpaste, fluoride rinses, and professionally applied treatments provide a cumulative effect, and the amount taken in should be monitored.

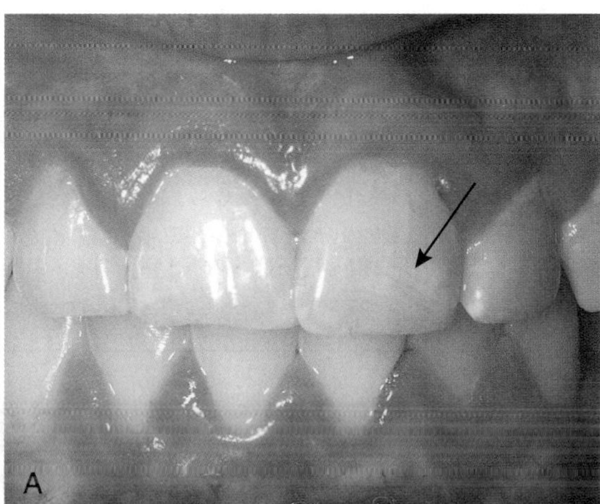


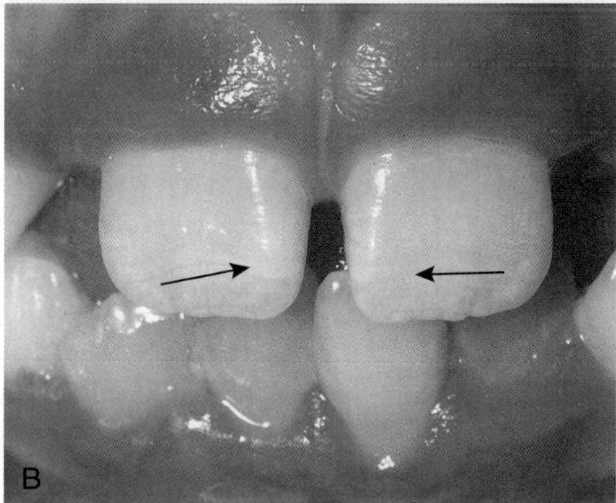


**FIG. 15.5** A, Mild fluorosis. B, Moderate fluorosis.

**8** What is the name of the dental condition that results from too much fluoride?
**9** What precautions are necessary for children who use fluoridated toothpaste?

## Fluoride Needs Assessment

A "fluoride needs assessment" is often used to help patients become more involved in their caries prevention program. The clinician who performs this assessment strengthens the dental partnership process by gathering relevant information from the patient and then helping the patient understand why fluoride is important and how it plays a role in the risk for future caries. Use of the fluoride needs assessment provides the following advantages:

- Saves time by identifying risk factors
- Opens communication between the dental professional and the patient
- Helps "individualize" patient fluoride therapies
- Allows the dentist to more accurately select the appropriate fluoride therapy

### Fluoride Needs Assessment

This assessment will help us determine your individual need for a specific fluoride therapeutic program that can help you keep your teeth for life.

Please put a check mark in front of any of the following statements that apply to you:

___ No fluoride in your drinking water as a child.
___ No fluoride in your drinking water now.
___ Drink filtered or bottled water.
___ Have receding gums or history of gum disease.
___ Have multiple fillings or crowns.
___ Strong family history of dental decay.
___ Currently wear orthodontic braces.
___ Have sensitivity to hot, cold, or touch.
___ Use home care whitening products.
___ Limited hand dexterity.
___ Use strong breath mints or sugar-containing chewing gum, lozenges, or hard candy between meals.
___ Visit dental office regularly.
___ Currently undergoing (or history of) chemotherapy.
___ Suffer from acid reflux.
___ Teeth that do not feel clean or that trap food.
___ Dental work done in the past year.
___ Snack frequently between meals.
___ Sip on beverages throughout the day (other than water).
___ Use tobacco products of any type.
___ Grind teeth frequently.
___ Brush less often than twice daily.
___ Floss less often than once daily.

Modified from Oral-B Laboratories, Boston, MA.

## Sources of Fluoride

### *Fluoridated Water*

Until recently, it was believed that water fluoridation was effective in preventing tooth decay through systemic uptake and incorporation into the enamel of developing teeth. It has now been proved that the major effects of water fluoridation are *topical* and not systemic. Topical uptake means that the fluoride diffuses into the surface of the enamel of an *erupted tooth* rather than only being incorporated into unerupted teeth during development.

For more than 50 years, fluoride has been safely added to communal water supplies. Most major cities in the United States have fluoridated water, and efforts to fluoridate water in communities without fluoridation are ongoing. From a public health standpoint, fluoridation of public water supplies is a good way to deliver fluoride to lower socioeconomic populations that may not otherwise have access to topical fluoride products such as fluoridated toothpaste and mouth rinses.

Approximately *1 part per million* (ppm) of fluoride in drinking water has been specified as the safe and recommended concentration to aid in the control of dental decay. In January 2011 the U.S. Department of Health and Human Services (HHS) recommended lowering the recommended concentration of fluoride from a range of 0.7 to 1.2 mg/L to a flat 0.7 mg/L. This concentration will provide the best balance of protection from dental caries while limiting the risk of dental fluorosis. This is the first change in HHS's position on fluoride in nearly 50 years.

Levels of fluoride provided through controlled water fluoridation are so low that there is *no danger* that an individual will ingest an acutely toxic quantity of fluoride in water. Communities in some states, however, have water that naturally contains more than twice the optimal level of fluoride, and fluorosis is often seen in patients who live in these areas (see Chapter 17).

### *Bottled Water*

Although many people consume bottled water, they may not realize that bottled water may not be equal to tap water with regard to dental health. The reason is the level of fluoride in bottled water. Some bottled waters may contain fluoride; however, most are below the optimum level of fluoride (0.7–1.2 ppm). The amount of fluoride in bottled water depends on the fluoride content of the source water, the treatment the source water receives before bottling (such as reverse osmosis or distillation), and whether fluoride additives were used. Currently the U.S. Food and Drug Administration (FDA) does not require the bottler to list the amount of fluoride content on bottled water.

## Sources of Systemic Fluoride

### *Foods and Beverages*

Because many processed foods and beverages are prepared with fluoridated water, they must be considered a source of dietary fluoride in children who drink them regularly. In addition, many brands of bottled water contain fluoride.

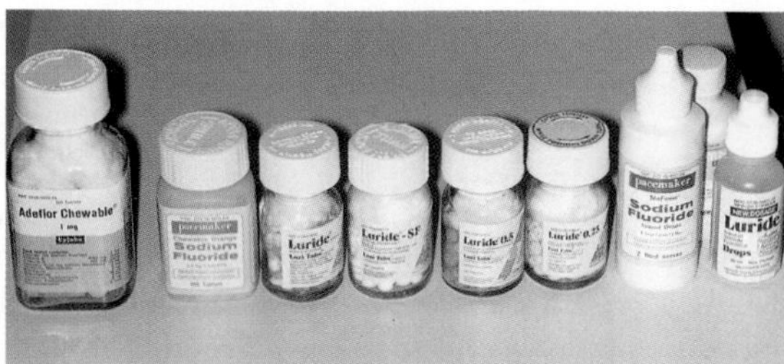


**FIG. 15.6** Fluoride can be dispensed by the dentist in tablet form.

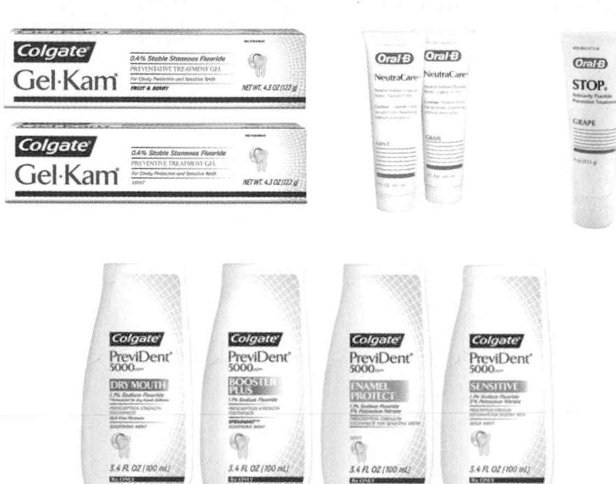


**FIG. 15.7** Examples of 0.4% stable stannous fluoride gels and pastes, and 1.1% sodium fluoride prescription toothpastes. *(Colgate products courtesy Colgate Palmolive Company, New York; Oral-B products courtesy Procter & Gamble, Cincinnati, OH.)*

Persons who want the benefits of fluoride must be sure to check labels.

### *Prescribed Dietary Supplements*

The dentist may prescribe dietary fluoride supplements in the form of tablets, drops, or lozenges for children ages 6 months to 16 years who live in areas with no source of fluoridated water (Fig. 15.6). Before prescribing supplements, the dentist considers the following factors:

- Fluoride level of the child's drinking water
- The child's exposure to multiple water sources (e.g., a child whose home water source is not fluoridated but whose day-care center or school is located in a fluoridated area)
- All potential sources of fluoride, because many juice products and prepared foods marketed for young children contain fluoride
- Whether the parents and the patient are willing to cooperate on an ongoing basis, because supplementation is recommended until age 16

## Sources of Topical Fluoride

Topical fluoride is available in home care products such as fluoridated toothpastes and mouth rinses, as well as in professional topical fluoride applications used in the dental office (Fig. 15.7; Tables 15.2 and 15.3).

**TABLE 15.2 Types of Professionally Applied Fluorides**

| Type | Form | Application Technique | Comments |
|---|---|---|---|
| Sodium fluoride (NaF) pH = neutral | Solution 2% | Paint-on | Use cotton rolls to absorb excess solution. |
| Sodium fluoride (NaF) pH = neutral | Gel 2% | Tray | Do not allow the patient to swallow the gel. |
| Sodium fluoride (NaF) pH = neutral | Foam 2% | Tray | Patients are less likely to swallow this because of the consistency. Use less in the tray than is used for the gel. |
| Acidulated phosphate fluoride (APF) pH 3.0–3.5 | Solution 1.23% | Paint-on | Avoid use in patients with ceramic and composite restorations. Use cotton rolls to absorb excess solution. |
| Acidulated phosphate fluoride (APF) pH 3.0–3.5 | Gel 1.23% | Paint-on or tray | Avoid use in patients with ceramic and composite restorations. Take care not to overfill tray. |
| Acidulated phosphate fluoride (APF) pH 3.0–3.5 | Foam | Tray | Avoid use in patients with ceramic and composite restorations. Smaller amounts are needed for tray. |

**TABLE 15.3 Fluoride Therapies for Home Use**

| Patient Problem | Type of Therapy | Active Ingredient | Benefits |
|---|---|---|---|
| **Adult Caries** | | | |
| Patient compliance | Toothpaste | 1.1% neutral sodium fluoride (NaF) | Helps prevent tooth decay |
| Exposed roots | Prescription therapy | | Safe for restorations and ceramic crowns |
| Root caries | | | Applies fluoride while brushing |
| Xerostomia (dry mouth) | | | Alcohol free |
| Exposed roots | Brush-on gel | 1.1% neutral NaF | Arrests 91% of early root caries |
| Root caries | Prescription therapy | | Helps prevent tooth decay |
| Xerostomia (dry mouth) | | | Safe for restorations and ceramics<br>Alcohol free |
| **Caries** | | | |
| Requires high concentration of fluoride | Dental rinse | 0.2% neutral NaF | Up to 55% reduction in caries with weekly use |
| Difficulty brushing | Prescription therapy | | Highest concentration home fluoride rinse |
| Patient compliance | | | Safe for restorations<br>Once a week |
| **Dentinal Sensitivity and Decay** | | | |
| Exposed dentin | Home care gel | 0.4% stannous fluoride (SnF) | Reduces hypersensitivity |
| Caries risk | | | Prevents caries<br>Available without a prescription |
| **Exposed Roots** | | | |
| After scaling | Home care rinse | 0.63% SnF (dilutes to 0.1%) | Helps prevent demineralization of exposed roots |
| After root planing | | Prescription (Rx) | Helps prevent plaque accumulation |
| After periodontal surgery | | | Reduces *Streptococcus mutans* count in saliva<br>Reduces caries<br>Alcohol free |

Continued

TABLE 15.3 Fluoride Therapies for Home Use—cont'd

| Patient Problem | Type of Therapy | Active Ingredient | Benefits |
|---|---|---|---|
| **Hypersensitivity** | | | |
| Temporary sensitivity during whitening | Dentin desensitizer | 1.09% NaF | Rapid temporary relief at home |
| Sensitivity due to loss of temporary crowns | Rx | 0.4% SnF | One-minute applications |
| Temporary sensitivity at home | | 0.14% hydrogen fluoride | |
| **Orthodontic Calcification** | | | |
| Caries in children | Oral rinse | 0.044% NaF and acidulated phosphate topical solution | Helps prevent demineralization<br>Enhances remineralization<br>Alcohol free<br>Available over the counter |
| | Gel | 1.1% NaF and acidulated phosphate | Safe, effective against white spots |
| | Rx | | Helps reduce decalcification<br>Promotes remineralization<br>Safe for orthodontic appliances |
| **Caries Prevention** | | | |
| Children | Anticavity fluoride rinse | 0.05% neutral NaF | Up to 71% less adult root caries |
| Adolescents | | | Up to 40% fewer cavities in children |
| Adults | | | Freshens breath<br>Available over the counter |

## Toothpastes

Toothpaste containing fluoride is the *primary source* of topical fluoride. A major benefit of this source of fluoride is the brushing action that brings it into close contact with the surfaces of the teeth.

Daily brushing with fluoride-containing toothpaste is of benefit to patients of all age groups. Children younger than 6 or 7 years should be carefully supervised because ingestion of fluoride-containing toothpaste may cause dental fluorosis. Training toothpastes that do not contain fluoride are now available for very young children (Fig. 15.8).

Additional types of toothpastes are available on the market, including some that contain whitening and desensitizing agents.

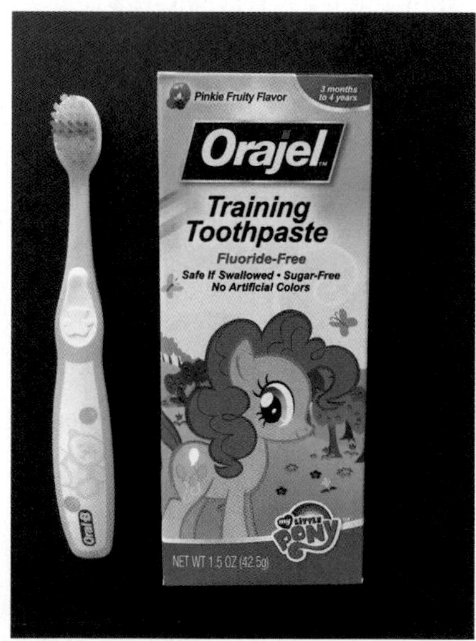


FIG. 15.8 Training toothpaste for young children.

## Mouth Rinses

Mouth rinses that contain fluoride may be recommended as an additional source of topical fluoride for high-risk patients. *Over-the-counter nonprescription rinses* generally contain 0.05% sodium fluoride and are designed for daily use. *Prescription rinses* generally contain 0.63% stannous fluoride or 0.2% sodium fluoride. Fluoride rinses are often used for their antiplaque properties. Stannous fluoride is also effective in decreasing dental *hypersensitivity* (extreme sensitivity of the tooth, such as to hot and cold).

Fluoride mouth rinses are most effective when used after brushing and flossing. Approximately 10 ml of solution should be swished vigorously for 1 minute and then spit out. The patient should be instructed not to eat or drink for 30 minutes after using the mouth rinse. Because of the chance that excessive fluoride could be ingested, the adult patient must be cautioned not to swallow the mouth rinse, and children should be closely supervised.

Also available on the market are mouth rinses that contain antimicrobial properties, which show promise for the prevention and control of periodontal disease (Fig. 15.9).

**High concentration 5000 ppm fluoride toothpaste/gel for caries high-risk clients from age 6 years and older**

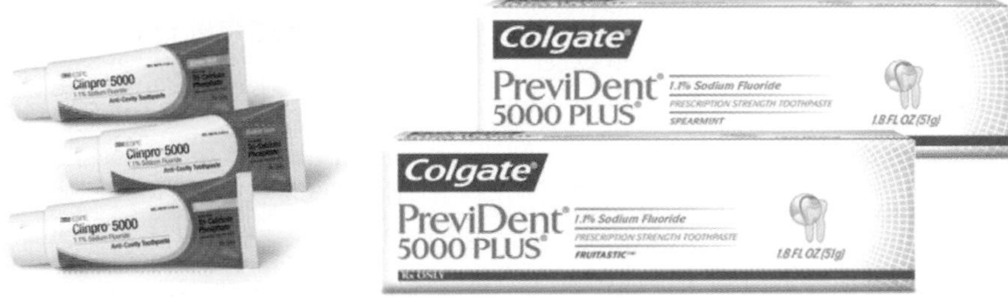


FIG. 15.9 Sample prescription fluoride products. *(Courtesy Dr. Mark Dillenges.)*

### *Gels*

Gels that contain varying concentrations of sodium fluoride are available for home use. Gels with a higher concentration (2%) require a prescription, and those products that contain a lower concentration (1.1%) may be purchased over the counter.

High-risk patients can use these at home by brushing or applying with a reusable custom tray. The patient is instructed to use the tray at bedtime. A small amount of the brush-on gel is placed in the tray, and the tray is placed over the teeth for 5 minutes.

*Note:* If water in the area is fluoridated, the patient is instructed to rinse out the mouth with water, to prevent swallowing any remaining fluoride gel. If the water is not fluoridated, the patient is told to spit out the excess gel but not to rinse with water after the application. Any small amounts of fluoride swallowed provide extra dietary fluoride. It is not the fluoride in the rinse water that is the problem, it is swallowing any remaining gel if the patient is already getting systemic fluoride.

### *Varnish*

**Fluoride varnish** is a concentrated topical fluoride within a resin or synthetic base that is painted on the teeth to prolong fluoride exposure. It can be used instead of a fluoride gel, and two to three professional applications a year are effective in preventing decay.

The efficacy of fluoride varnish in preventing dental caries is comparable with professional gel application, but the advantage is in the ease of application and patient acceptance. Also, less ingestion of fluoride occurs compared with other methods of application. Fluoride varnish is used with patients of all ages to treat hypersensitivity and prevent decay. Currently the FDA approves fluoride varnish only as a hypersensitivity agent, although it is currently being used in caries prevention. Fluoride varnish contains 5% sodium fluoride and is available in single-unit dosing (Fig. 15.10).

### *Professional Applications*

Professional applications of fluoride gels or varnishes may be recommended for some children soon after eruption of the permanent teeth and for some high-risk patients. These treatments can be performed by the dentist, hygienist, or qualified dental assistant (Procedure 15.1: Applying Topical Fluoride Gel or Foam [Expanded Function] and Procedure 15.2: Applying Fluoride Varnish [Expanded Function]).

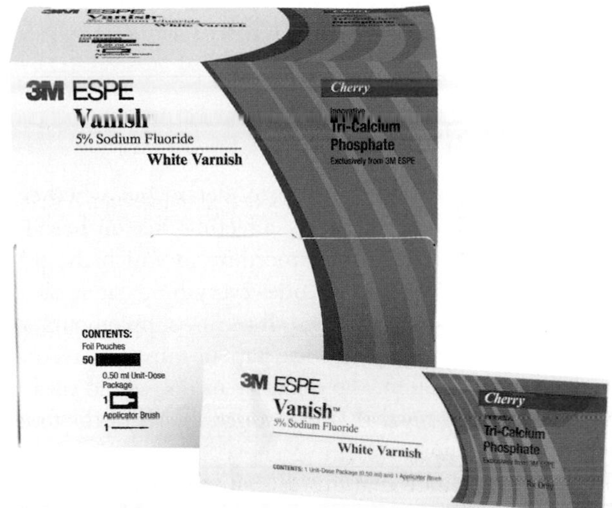


FIG. 15.10 Fluoride varnish with tricalcium phosphate *(Copyright © 3M 2017. All rights reserved.)*

## Nutrition and Dental Caries

Dental caries cannot occur without dietary sugars. Sucrose is more *cariogenic* (caries-causing) than other types of sugars, although maltose, lactose, glucose, and fructose also have high caries-producing abilities. Flour and starches alone are not highly cariogenic, but when starch is mixed with sugar, as in cookies, the chance that dental decay will occur increases dramatically.

### Sugar Substitutes

Initially, artificial sweeteners were developed for the 10 million patients with diabetes in the United States and for people who struggle with obesity. In recent years, the use of artificial sweeteners has significantly increased. The principal sugar substitutes available are *saccharine* (Sweet'N Low), *aspartame* (NutraSweet and Equal), *sorbitol, xylitol,* and *mannitol.*

Of these sugar substitutes, saccharine, aspartame, sorbitol, and mannitol are *noncariogenic,* which means that they do not *cause* dental caries. Xylitol is the only one of the artificial sweeteners that actually *prevents caries* (anticariogenic).

### Xylitol

The exact mechanism by which xylitol prevents tooth decay is under investigation, but it is believed that bacteria cannot use xylitol to produce acid, and that it may inhibit the growth of *Streptococcus mutans.* Xylitol is derived from birch trees, corn cobs, oats, bananas, and some mushrooms. Its cost is about 10 times that of sucrose. Therefore although products that contain xylitol are significantly better, they are more expensive than products made with other types of artificial sweeteners (Fig. 15.11).

### Hard Facts about Soft Drinks

- Large sizes mean more calories, more sugar, and more acid in a single serving. A 64-ounce "big cup" contains more than five 12-ounce cans in a single serving.
- Soft drinks have no nutritional value. In regular sodas, all the calories come from sugar.
- Sugar in sodas combines with bacteria in the mouth to form acid.
- Diet or "sugar-free" sodas contain their own acid. This acid attacks the teeth. Each acid attack lasts about 20 minutes.
- In addition to tooth decay, heavy soda consumption has been linked to diabetes, obesity, and osteoporosis.
- Teenagers today drink 3 times more soda than teenagers 20 years ago did, often as a substitute for milk.
- One fifth of all 1- and 2-year-old children drink sodas.
- Sealants protect only the chewing surfaces of teeth. Decay caused by sodas tends to occur on smooth tooth surfaces, where sealants cannot reach.

Modified from the Minnesota Dental Association, Minneapolis, MN.

## Dietary Analysis

A dietary analysis is performed to determine whether the patient's current food intake is affecting his or her dental health. It is a quick and easy procedure in which the patient maintains a *food diary* that includes everything eaten each day for 1 week. This listing includes all meals, supplements, gum, snacks, and fluoridated water. The patient must also record the time the food was eaten, the quantity in household measures, and the amount of sugar that was added to any of the foods or beverages (see Chapter 16).

If the patient's food diary reveals any diet-related oral problems such as high sugar intake or frequent snacks, some form of dietary counseling is indicated.

### Steps for Analyzing a Food Diary

1. Note the time when meals and snacks were eaten.
2. Note the foods sweetened with added sugar, including soft drinks, sugar added to coffee or tea, candy, pastry, cough drops, and fruits. Note *all* carbonated beverages, including soft drinks and beer (even those considered "diet" drinks), because of their acidity.
3. Note any dried fruit, such as berries, dates, prunes, and raisins, because they are highly concentrated sweets. However, fresh fruits such as apples or oranges are not concentrated sweets because of their high water content.

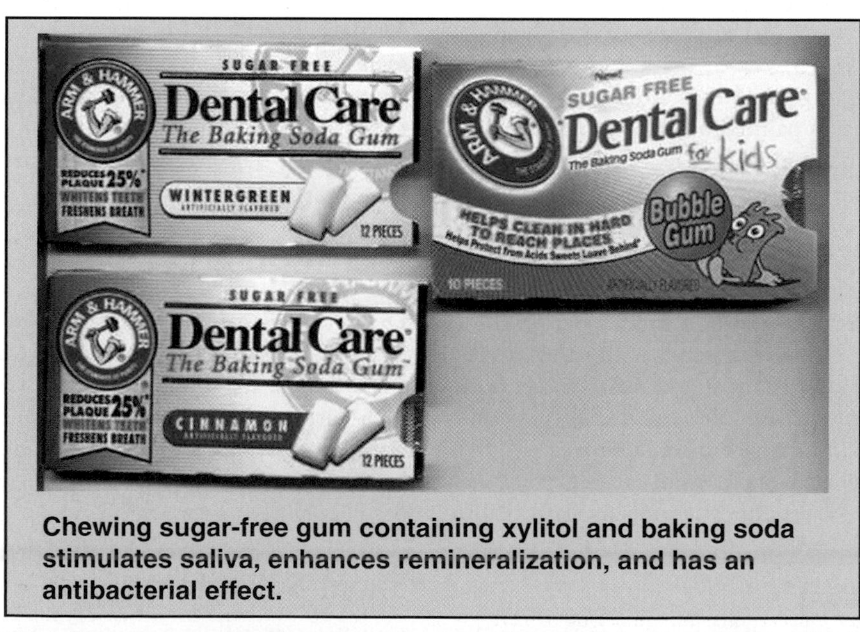


**FIG. 15.11** Sugar-free sodium bicarbonate gum containing xylitol. *(From Darby ML, Walsh MM: Dental hygiene: theory and practice, ed 4, St Louis, 2015, Saunders.)*

4. Arrange the remaining foods into the appropriate food groups.
5. Evaluate the adequacy of the diet by comparing the servings from each food group with the servings recommended in the dietary guide.
6. Assess the frequency and consistency (sticky or nonretentive) of the presweetened foods, and determine the likelihood of their contributing to the patient's oral health problems.
7. From information provided in the food diary, determine the patient's need for dietary counseling. For example, a patient with rampant caries and a diet high in sweets is in need of comprehensive dietary counseling. Conversely, a patient with slight caries and minimal sugar intake would likely need only minimal dietary counseling.

RECALL

**10** What is the key dietary factor that relates to dental caries?
**11** What information must a patient include in a food diary?
**12** How do sugar-free sodas relate to dental caries?

## Plaque Control Program

Patients cannot remove all the plaque on their teeth every day, but they can keep plaque under control by brushing, flossing, using interdental cleaning aids, and using antimicrobial solutions. The dental assistant can work with the patient to develop a program of oral hygiene strategies to be followed routinely at home.

The goal is to thoroughly remove plaque *at least* once daily. After plaque has been thoroughly removed, it takes about 24 hours for it to form again. Techniques selected must be based on the needs and abilities of the individual patient. Children younger than 8 years of age generally do not have the manual dexterity to thoroughly clean all surfaces of their teeth and usually require the help of an adult (Fig. 15.12).

A wide variety of oral hygiene products are currently available. It is important for dental assistants to remain up to date on the newest products on the market, so that they can advise patients, make recommendations, and answer questions.

## Toothbrushes and Toothbrushing

Choosing the size and style of a toothbrush is a personal decision. The two basic types of toothbrushes are *manual* and *automatic*. When used properly, both types are effective in the removal of dental plaque.

### Baby Toothbrushes

Baby and infant toothbrushes are very small and very soft, and should be used as soon as the baby's first tooth appears in the mouth. Finger brushes, which fit over the parent's finger, are another way to clean the baby's teeth (Fig. 15.13). Brushing the teeth is an excellent way to introduce infants and toddlers to dental care.

### Manual Toothbrushes

Toothbrushes come in many styles of head size, tuft shape, and angle and shape of handle (Fig. 15.14). There is no one "ideal" toothbrush for everyone.

In general, dental professionals recommend soft-bristled brushes, because these bristles are gentler to the soft tissues and to any exposed cementum or dentin. Soft bristles also adapt to the contours of the tooth better than hard bristles do.

The bristles may be nylon or natural. *Nylon* is preferred because the ends are rounded and polished, which makes the toothbrush safer.

The most important factor that should be ensured is that the toothbrush readily removes plaque without causing tissue damage. Toothbrushes should be replaced as soon as the bristles show signs of wear or begin to splay outward, usually after about 8 to 12 weeks (Fig. 15.15). Some people choose to discard their toothbrush after an illness; however, no scientific basis has been found for this practice.

### Automatic Toothbrushes

Automatic, or powered, toothbrushes are gaining in popularity. As with manual toothbrushes, various types of automatic brushes are available.

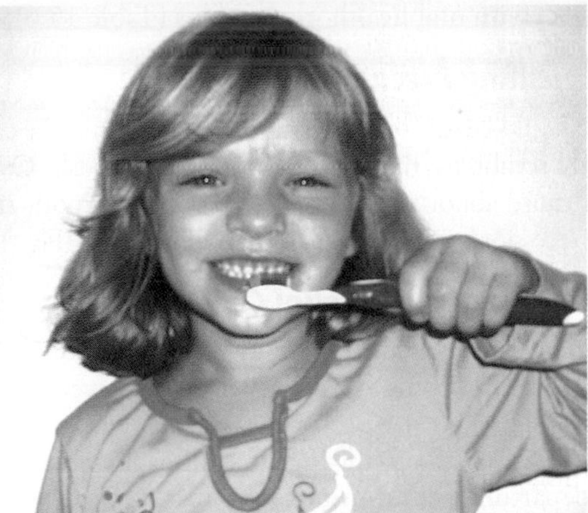

**FIG. 15.12** Children younger than 8 years of age should be supervised while brushing to ensure that all areas of the teeth have been thoroughly cleaned.

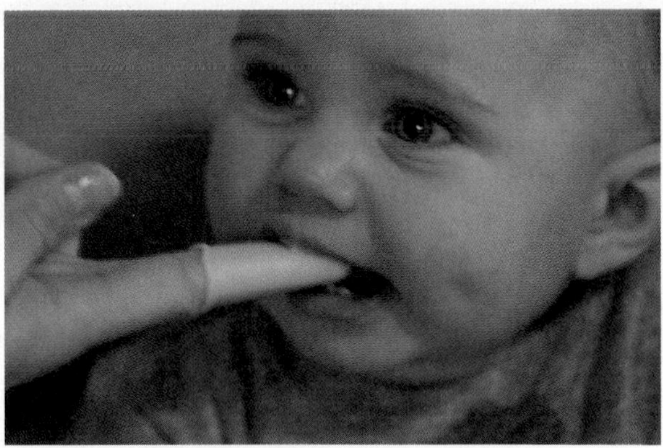

**FIG. 15.13** The "finger brush" should be used as soon as teeth appear in the baby's mouth.

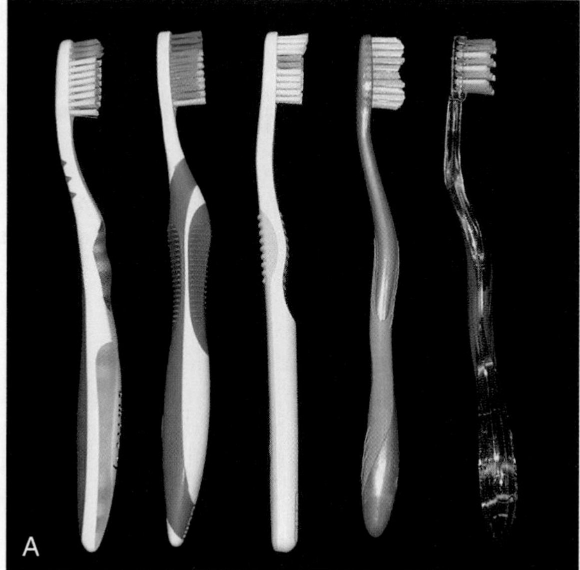


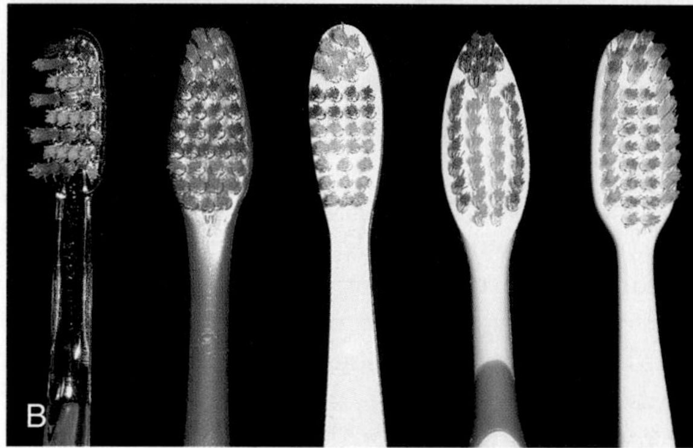


**FIG. 15.14** Examples of manual toothbrushes. *(From Newman M, Takei T, Klokkevold P, et al, editors: Carranza's clinical periodontology, ed 12, St Louis, 2015, Saunders.)*

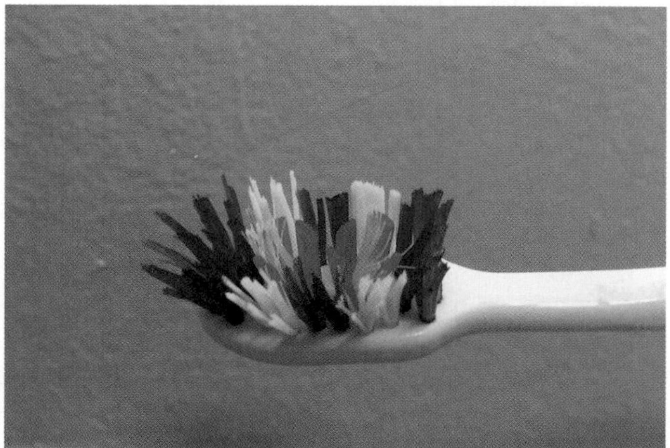

**FIG. 15.15** Worn-out toothbrush.

Automatic brushes have larger handles that contain a rechargeable battery. The larger handle also makes them useful for patients with physical disabilities. In addition, automatic toothbrushes may have some motivational value for children.

Automatic toothbrushes use one of several motions, including back and forth, up and down, or circular. Some models of automatic toothbrushes feature pulsating and ultrasonic action (Fig. 15.16). Some types have a timing device that sounds every 30 seconds to remind the user to change quadrants in the mouth (Tables 15.4 and 15.5).

## Toothbrushing

Regardless of the type of toothbrush a patient chooses, it can remove plaque thoroughly only when it is used properly. Toothbrushing requires instruction specific to each individual. Things to consider when teaching a patient how to brush most effectively include the patient's age, dexterity, and personal preferences. You should teach the patient to clean the mouth and tongue thoroughly using a systematic approach and to understand the importance of controlling plaque and inflammation. The Bass method is a frequently recommended brushing technique (Fig. 15.17).

When reviewing toothbrushing with patients, observe their toothbrushing technique before recommending a particular brushing method. When patients have healthy gingivae and few plaque deposits, you should not recommend a totally new brushing technique but should merely coach them to continue their safe, effective pattern of brushing. You may be able to offer tips to patients on how to better reach a specific area of the mouth if they have plaque retention in that area. Many patients require only minor modifications to the technique they are using.

Ask patients to demonstrate their brushing technique for you. It is helpful to have a large hand mirror so that patients can observe their own technique. You can provide tips while they are brushing (Fig. 15.18). Whenever possible, give patients written materials that reinforce the concepts you presented in the oral health lesson. Patients will frequently ask, "How often should I brush?" The most commonly accepted answer among dental professionals is to brush twice a day. Patients will also ask about the proper length of time to brush. Often, patients will brush for only 1 minute or less. Some dental professionals recommend at least 3 minutes, whereas others recommend five to ten strokes in each area. It is best to customize your instructions according to the patient's oral health status and history of compliance with oral health instructions (Table 15.6).

## Toothbrushing Precautions

Patients should be cautioned about damage that may be caused by vigorously scrubbing the teeth with any toothbrush. Over time, this can cause abnormal *abrasion* (wear) of the tooth structure, gingival recession, and exposure of the root surface (Fig. 15.19).

## Toothbrushing for Unusual Conditions

Even when an unusual or painful oral condition exists, the patient must be encouraged to brush wherever possible. It is inadvisable to go for prolonged periods without removing plaque. However, the following conditions may require a temporary departure from routine oral care:

- *Acute oral inflammation* or a *traumatic lesion* may make brushing painful. Patients should be instructed to brush all areas of the mouth that are not affected and to resume

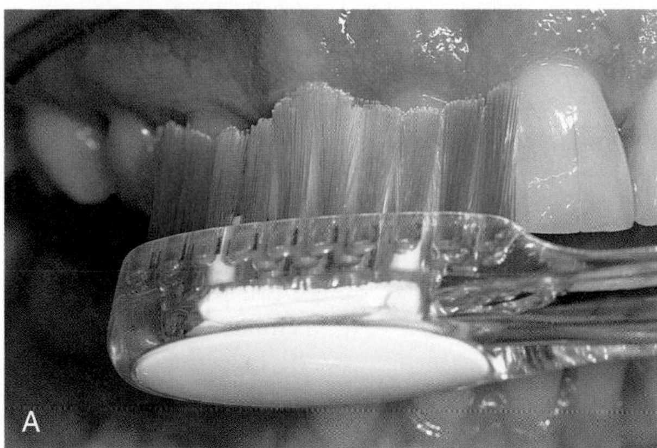


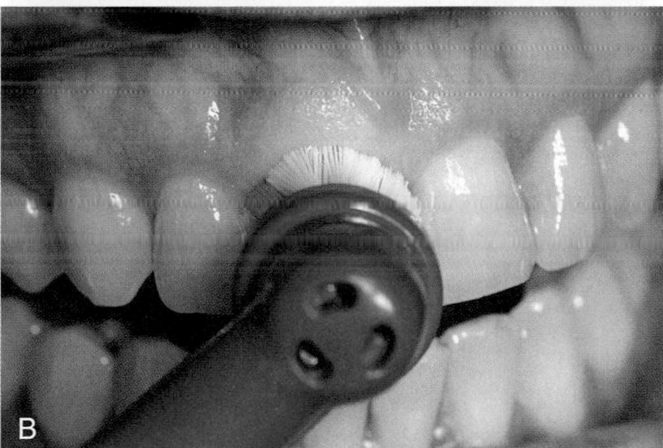


**FIG. 15.16** Positioning the toothbrush head and bristle tips so that they reach the gingival margin is critical for achieving the most effective cleaning results. A, Straight head placement. B, Round head placement. *(From Newman M, Takei I, Klokkevold P, et al, editors: Carranza's clinical periodontology, ed 12, St Louis, 2015, Saunders.)*

regular oral hygiene practices as soon as possible. Rinsing with a warm, mild saline solution can encourage healing and remove debris.

- *After periodontal surgery,* patients are given instructions regarding brushing where sutures or dressings are placed. Direct or vigorous brushing of a periodontal dressing could dislodge it. Patients may be instructed to brush only the occlusal surfaces and to use *very light* strokes over the dressing. The other teeth and gingiva should be brushed as usual.
- *After dental extractions,* patients are often reluctant to brush their teeth. However, the teeth adjacent to the extraction site need cleaning as soon as possible to reduce bacterial collections and to promote healing. Patients are usually instructed to avoid the surgical site but to brush the other teeth as usual.
- *After dental restorations,* patients are often reluctant to brush a new crown or a new fixed bridge. Specific oral hygiene instructions should be given to the patient at the time of the visit. Most often, patients are instructed to brush all areas of their mouth normally.

**13** What can patients do daily to remove plaque?
**14** Which type of toothbrush bristle is usually recommended?
**15** Which method of toothbrushing is generally recommended?

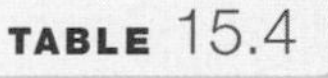


**TABLE 15.4 Examples of Powered Toothbrushes**

| Product and Company | Description |
|---|---|
| **Oral-B Braun**<br>3-D Plaque Remover<br>Oral-B Laboratories<br>Iowa City, IA | Oscillating, small circulating brush head; some units include dual oscillating and back-and-forth motions. |
| **Butler GUM**<br>Pulse Plaque Remover<br>John O. Butler Co.<br>A Sunstar Company<br>Chicago, IL | Brush tufts move up and down; uses disposable AA batteries rather than rechargeable battery. |
| **Colgate Actibrush**<br>Colgate-Palmolive Co.<br>New York, NY | Small, round, soft-bristle head with oscillating movement. |
| **Crest Spin Brush**<br>Procter & Gamble<br>Cincinnati, OH | The brush head is a combination of stationary bristles on the posterior two thirds and small, round oscillating bristles on the anterior one third of the head; disposable AA batteries are used to operate the brush. |
| **Interplak**<br>Powered Brush<br>Bausch & Lomb<br>Tucker, GA | Individual brush tufts rotate and counterrotate; choice of large or small brush head. |
| **Rotadent**<br>Prodentec<br>Batesville, AR | Small rotating brush; choice of flat or pointed brush head. |
| **SynchroSonic**<br>Water Pik Technologies<br>Fort Collins, CO | Brush head vibrates with sound. |
| **Sonicare**<br>Philips Oral Healthcare<br>Snoqualmie, WA | Brush head vibrates with sound. |

From Daniel SJ, Harfst SA: Mosby's dental hygiene: concepts, cases, and competencies—2004 update, St Louis, 2004, Mosby.

## Dental Floss or Tape

When used properly, dental floss or tape removes bacterial plaque and thus reduces interproximal bleeding (Fig. 15.20 and Procedure 15.3: Assisting the Patient with Dental Floss [Expanded Function]). Dental floss is circular in shape, and dental tape is flat. Dental floss can be purchased in various colors and flavors, although these types do not perform better than plain floss.

Floss and tape are available in waxed and unwaxed varieties, and patients should be encouraged to use the type they prefer. Some patients dislike unwaxed floss because it is thinner and tends to shred or tear on older dental restorations. Research has revealed no difference in the effectiveness of waxed or unwaxed floss for plaque removal.

**TABLE 15.5 Powered Toothbrushes: General Modes of Action**

| Action | Description | Examples | Diagram |
|---|---|---|---|
| Side-to-side | Brush head that moves laterally. | Early power models | |
| Counter oscillation | Adjacent tufts rotate in one direction, then the other independently; each tuft rotates in the opposite direction to adjacent tufts. | Interplak | 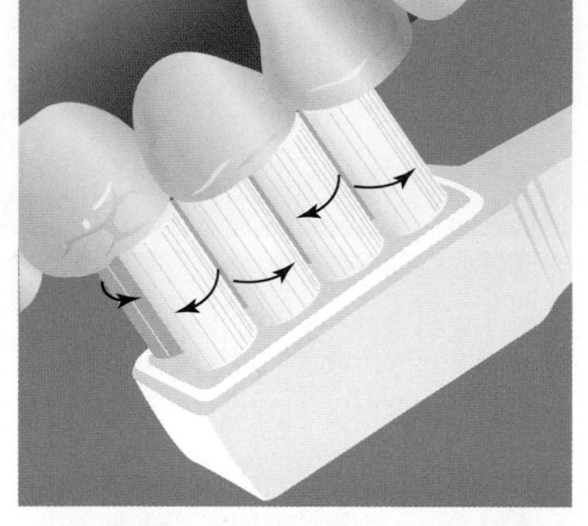 |
| Rotation oscillation | Entire brush head rotates in one direction and then the other and also pulsates in and out. | Braun Oral-B | 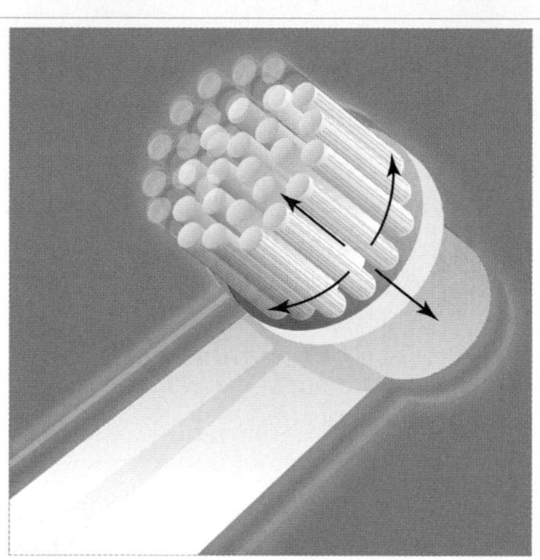 |
| Circular | Entire brush head rotates in one direction. | Rota-Dent | 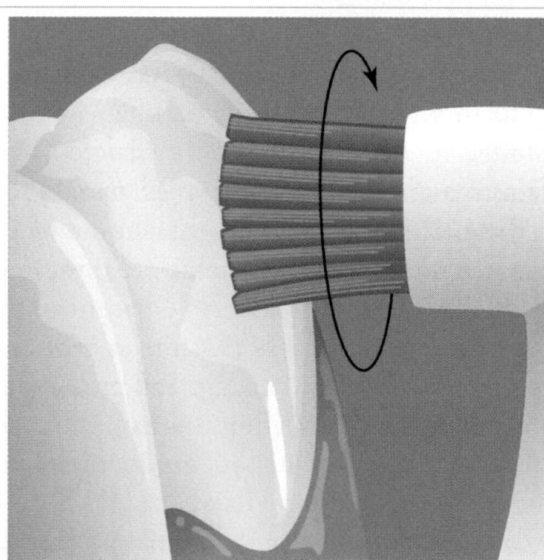 |

**TABLE 15.5 Powered Toothbrushes: General Modes of Action—cont'd**

| Action | Description | Examples | Diagram |
|---|---|---|---|
| Sonic | Bristles move with high amplitude and high frequency; sound waves cause fluid motion. | Philips Sonicare | |
| Ultrasonic | Bristles vibrate at ultrasonic frequencies. | Ultreo | |

Data from Darby ML, Walsh MM: Dental hygiene: theory and practice, ed 4, St Louis, 2015, Saunders.

### When to Floss

Dental floss should be used *before* toothbrushing for the following reasons:

- When plaque has been removed from proximal surfaces, the fluoride in the dentifrice used during brushing is able to reach the proximal surfaces for prevention of dental caries.
- When brushing is done first, the mouth may feel "clean." Thus the patient may see no need to floss or may not want to take the additional time to floss.

RECALL

**16** What is the difference between dental floss and dental tape?
**17** Which is more effective: waxed or unwaxed dental floss?

## Interdental Aids

Special devices are recommended as aids for cleaning between teeth with large or open interdental spaces and under fixed bridges (Fig. 15.21). These are aids to flossing but do not replace it in all areas of the oral cavity (Fig. 15.22).

### End-Tuft Brushes

Interdental brushes are made from soft nylon filaments formed into a narrow cone shape. They are useful for cleaning areas that are difficult to reach with a regular toothbrush, such as those affected by orthodontic appliances, fixed bridges and space maintainers, and proximal tooth surfaces next to open embrasures.

### Bridge Threaders

Bridge threaders are used to pass dental floss under the **pontic** ("false" tooth) of a fixed bridge (Fig. 15.23). They are used with regular dental floss. A piece of dental floss is looped through the circular part of the bridge threader. Then the straight part of the threader is slipped under the pontic, and the floss is pulled through.

### Automatic Flossers

Automatic flossers are designed for patients who have difficulty manipulating dental floss (Fig. 15.24). These battery-operated

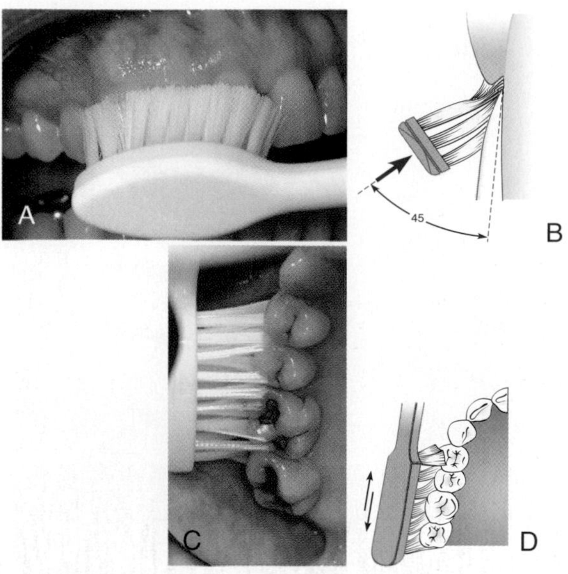


FIG. 15.17 Bass method. A, Place the toothbrush so that the bristles are angled at approximately 45 degrees from the tooth surfaces. B, Start at the most distal tooth in the arch and use a vibrating, back-and-forth motion to brush. C, Place the toothbrush so that the filaments are angled at approximately 45 degrees from the long axis of the tooth. D, Start at the most distal tooth in the arch and use a vibrating, back-and-forth motion to brush. *(A and C from Darby ML, Walsh MM: Dental hygiene: theory and practice, ed 4, St Louis, 2015, Saunders. B and D from Newman M, Takei T, Klokkevold P, et al, editors: Carranza's clinical periodontology, ed 12, St Louis, 2015, Saunders.)*

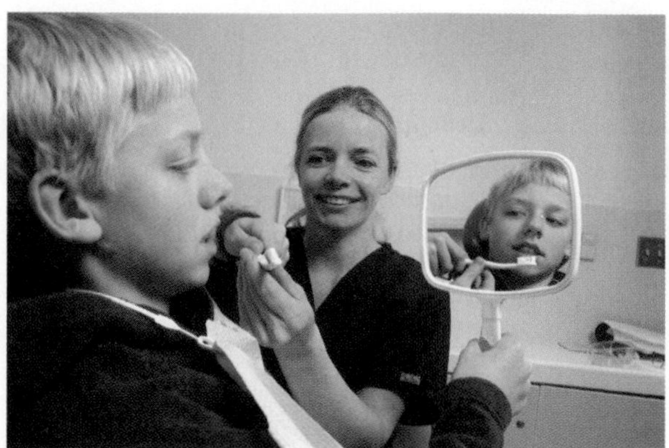

FIG. 15.18 Observing toothbrushing technique.

devices have one-use, replaceable, thin rubber filament tips. The tip is inserted into the interproximal space. When the button on the handle is pressed, the rubber tip vibrates against the interproximal tooth surfaces to remove plaque.

### Perio-Aid

A perio-aid is a handle with holes in the end designed to hold toothpicks (Fig. 15.25). The patient can clean difficult-to-reach areas of the mouth with the toothpick. This device is especially useful in interproximal areas of gingival recession or after periodontal surgery.

To use a perio-aid, a firm, round toothpick is inserted into an opening at either end of the handle, and the excess length is broken off. The end of the toothpick is then carried to the area to be cleansed by simply holding the device with one hand.

**TABLE 15.6 Types of Toothpastes**

| Type | Active Ingredient | How It Works | Comments |
|---|---|---|---|
| Fluoride/anticaries | Sodium fluoride | Assists in remineralization of the teeth. | Excellent choice for caries prevention.<br>Young children must be supervised to keep them from swallowing the toothpaste. |
| Antigingivitis | Triclosan and sodium fluoride | Antimicrobial action on bacteria in the plaque. | ADA-approved as a decay-preventive dentifrice that also helps to reduce gingivitis, plaque, and calculus. |
| Desensitizing | Potassium nitrate | Blocks the openings to exposed dentinal tubules. | These take several weeks to work. |
| Whitening | Hydrogen peroxide or carbamide peroxide | Mild abrasive that removes surface stain and provides a gentle polish. | Some patients notice tissue irritation. Degree of whitening varies among patients. |
| Baking soda | Sodium bicarbonate | Mild abrasive. | May provide some antimicrobial effect. |
| Tartar control | Sodium hexametaphosphate or pyrophosphate | Inhibits calcification of deposits on the teeth. | Major effect is on supragingival calculus. |

*ADA*, American Dental Association.

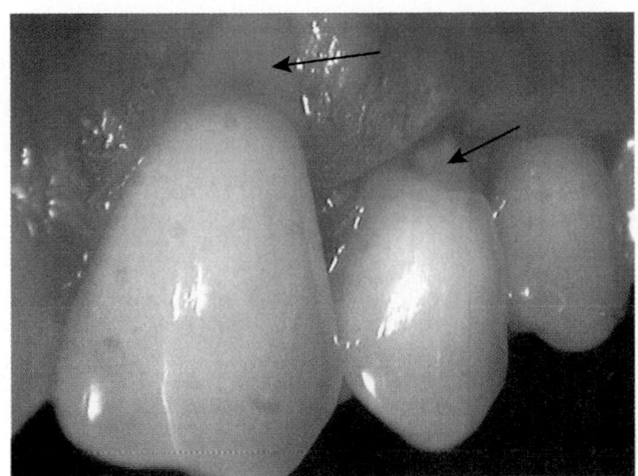

FIG. 15.19 Improper brushing techniques can result in abrasion of the tooth surface and can cause gingival recession. *(Courtesy Dr. Robert Meckstroth, Santa Rosa, CA.)*

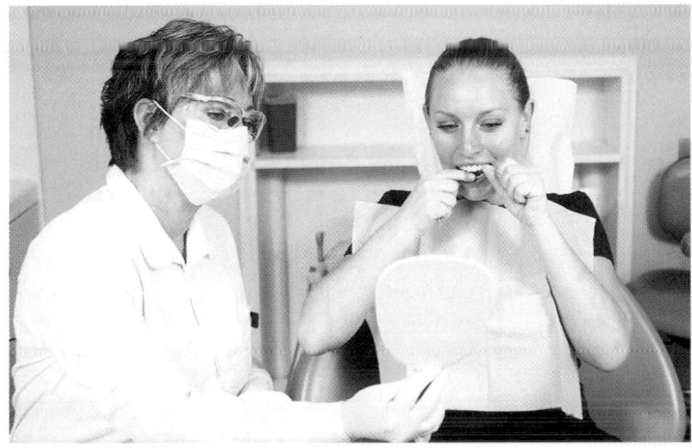

FIG. 15.20 The dental assistant helps the patient with flossing.

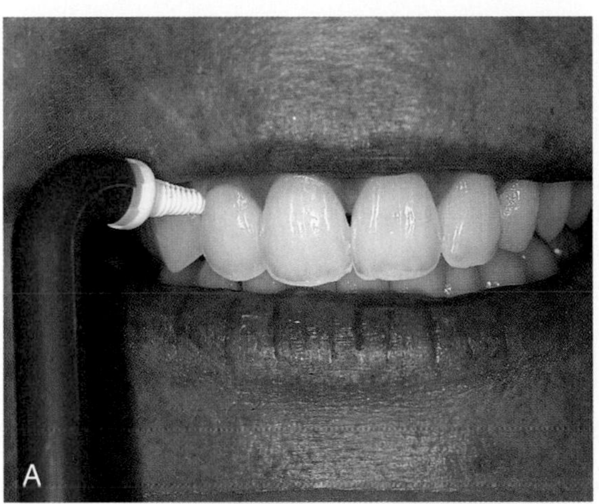


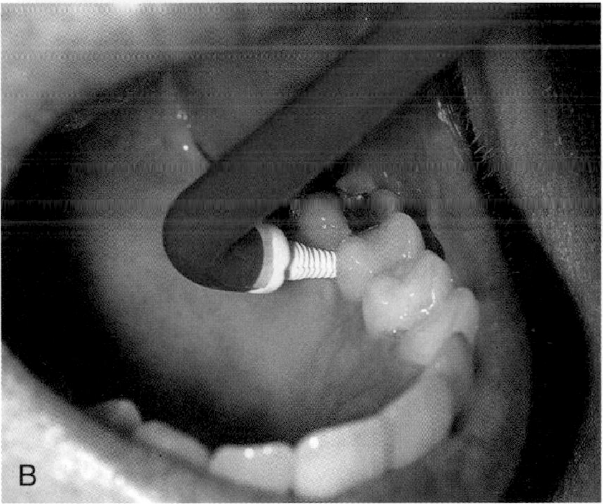


FIG. 15.22 An interdental hygienic aid. A, Anterior teeth. B, Cleaning the posterior interproximal areas that are difficult to reach.

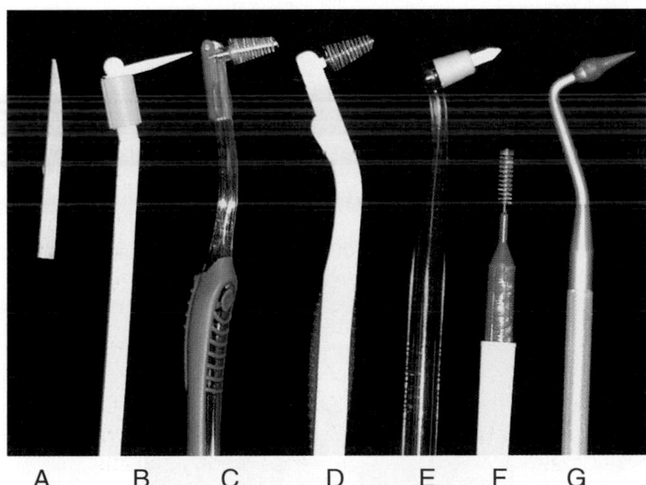


FIG. 15.21 Interproximal cleaning devices include wooden tips (A and B), interproximal brushes (C–F), and rubber-tipped stimulators (G). *(From Newman M, Takei T, Klokkevold P, et al, editors: Carranza's clinical periodontology, ed 12, St Louis, 2015, Saunders.)*

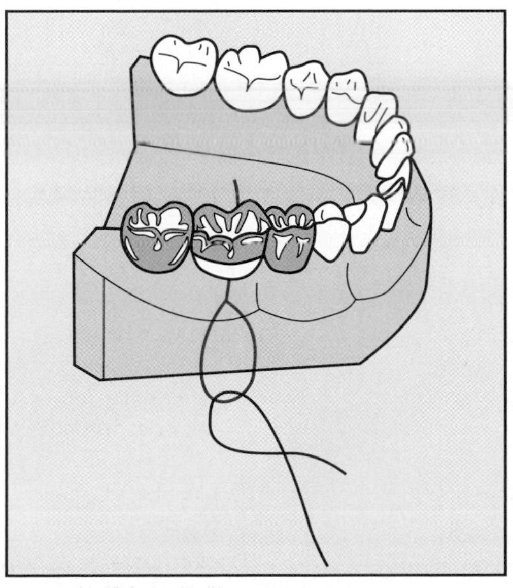

FIG. 15.23 A bridge threader is used as an aid to clean under a fixed bridge.

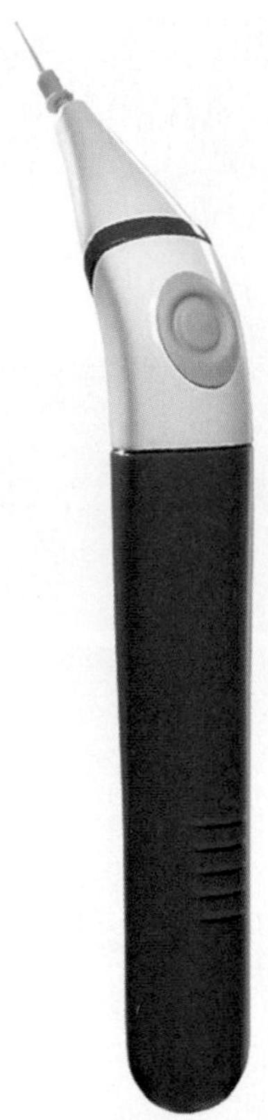

FIG. 15.24 This battery-powered flossing device enables single-handed flossing with a disposable nylon flexible tip, which offers convenience for some patients. *(Courtesy Water Pik, Inc., Fort Collins, CO.)*

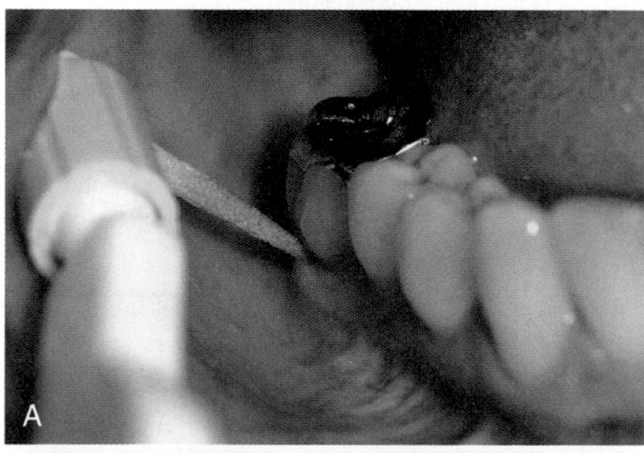

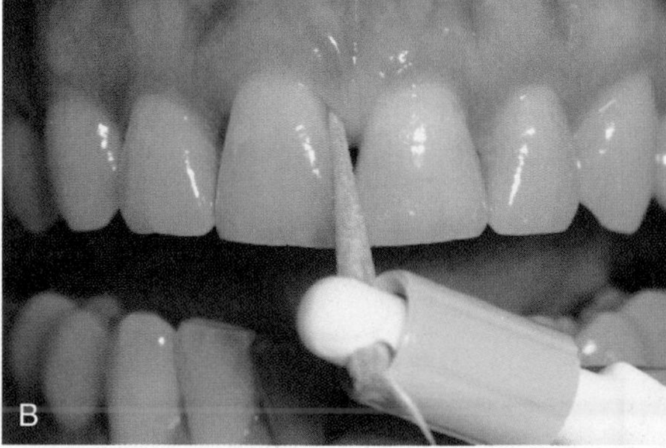

FIG. 15.25 A, Toothpick placed at the gingival margin. B, Gentle up-and-down motion keeping tip on tooth. *(From Newman M, Takei T, Klokkevold P, et al, editors: Carranza's clinical periodontology, ed 12, St Louis, 2015, Saunders.)*

## Dentures

Patients who have full or partial dentures will need to use a denture brush to clean all areas of the denture (Fig. 15.26). A nonabrasive cleanser such as a commercial denture cleanser, a mild soap, dishwashing liquid, or a mild toothpaste should be used on the brush. The denture should be brushed with short strokes. It is always a good idea to put water or a towel in the sink so that the dentures will not break if they are dropped.

## Toothpaste

Toothpaste (dentifrice) contains ingredients designed to remove food residue and includes abrasives to remove stain. Highly polished tooth surfaces will stain less readily and remain clean longer. In addition, most brands of toothpaste now contain fluoride. Many also contain flavoring agents provided to give the mouth a fresh and clean feeling (Fig. 15.27).

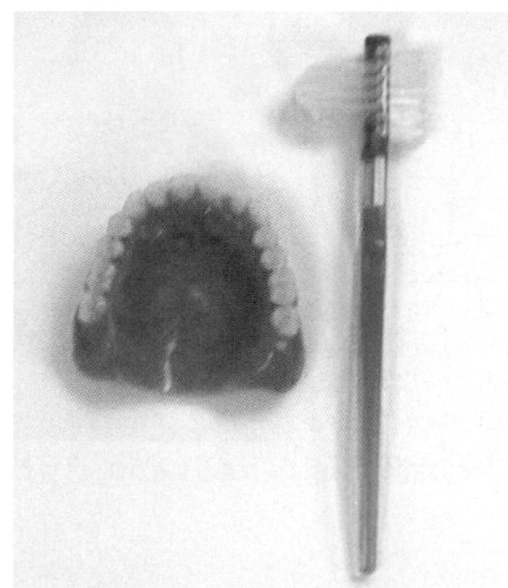

FIG. 15.26 Denture and denture brush.

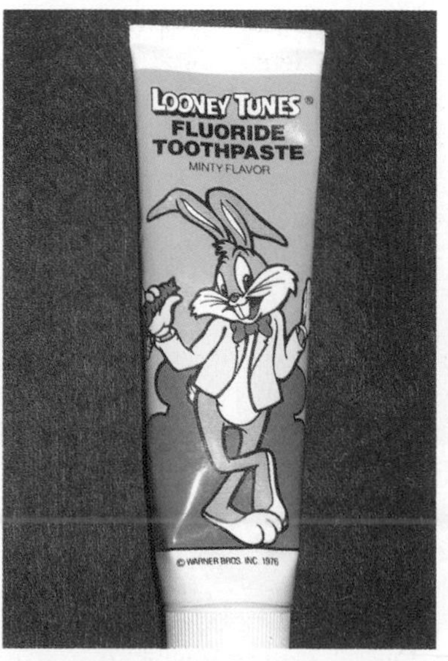


FIG. 15.27 Toothpaste for children.

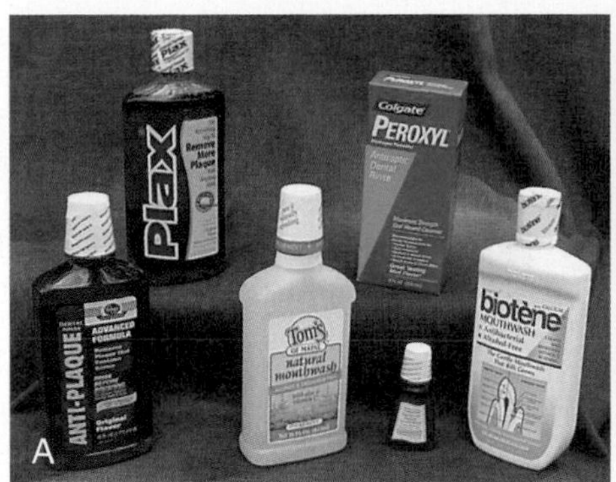


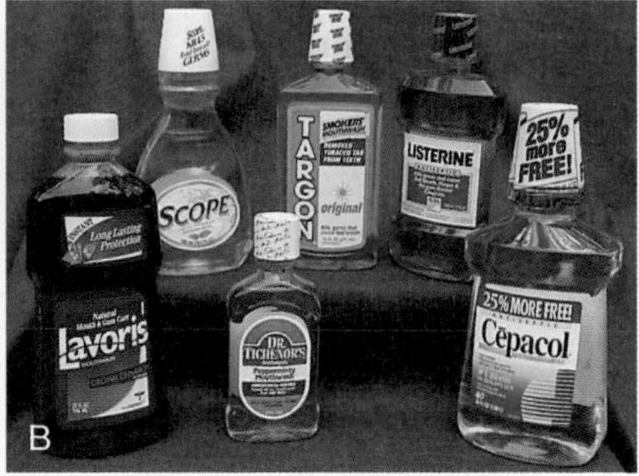


**FIG. 15.28** Mouth rinses. A, Two prerinses (left) and several alcohol-free mouth rinses (right). B, Familiar brands of mouth rinses contain alcohol in amounts ranging from 8% to 27%. *(Courtesy Dr. W. B. Stilley II, Brandon, MS.)*

Some toothpastes now contain a compound that reduces calculus formation when they are used regularly after dental prophylaxis. However, this compound will not remove existing calculus. This "tartar control" toothpaste may be helpful for those individuals who accumulate excessive calculus between regular cleaning appointments (see Table 15.6).

## Mouth Rinses

Many patients like the feeling of freshness provided by a mouth rinse. A wide variety of mouth rinses are currently available, and some also contain fluoride. Because many mouth rinses contain alcohol as an ingredient, recovering alcoholics are advised to read the label and select a mouth rinse that does not contain alcohol (Fig. 15.28).

Rinsing the mouth with water is recommended after meals and snacks when toothbrushing and interdental cleaning are not possible.

## Oral Irrigation Devices

Oral irrigators (also known as dental water jets) deliver a pulsating stream of water or chemical agent through a nozzle to the teeth and gingivae. Oral irrigation can be applied at home by the patient or in the dental office (Fig. 15.29).

Oral irrigation helps to reduce bacterial levels in subgingival and interproximal areas. Using an oral irrigator as part of an oral hygiene program can benefit people with gingivitis, implants, orthodontic appliances, or diabetes, and those who will not or are unable to floss.

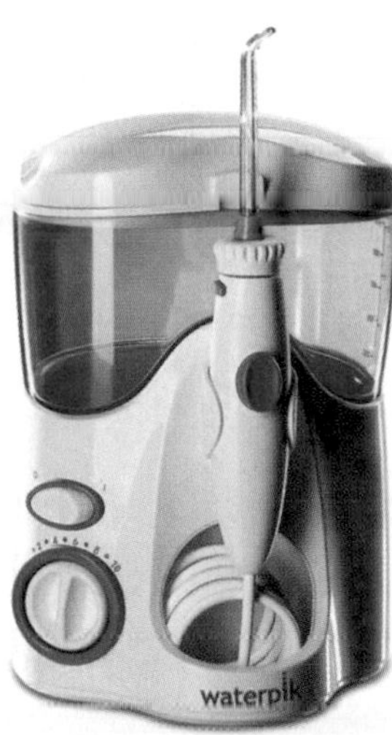


**FIG. 15.29** Waterpik Water Flosser. This unit also comes with six tips or attachments: the classic tip, a subgingival tip, an orthodontic tip, the Plaque Seeker tip, a toothbrush tip, and a tongue cleaner. *(Courtesy Water Pik, Inc., Fort Collins, CO.)*

RECALL

**18** What cleaners can be used to clean dentures?
**19** Will "tartar control" toothpaste remove calculus?
**20** If you cannot brush and floss after lunch, what should you do?

## General Guidelines for Home Care Products

The American Dental Association (ADA) Council on Dental Therapeutics conducts an independent review of the scientific evidence for research claims and evaluation of home care products. When a product meets the appropriate standards, it is given the ADA Seal of Acceptance (Fig. 15.30). The ADA Seal of Acceptance provides a quality assurance guarantee for consumers and professionals.

You can check the ADA's Web site (www.ada.org) to obtain current information on toothbrushes, dentifrices, interproximal aids, and products for the prevention of gingivitis and caries.

■ **Patient Education** As a dental professional, your job is to help patients develop and maintain sound dental habits throughout their lives. To accomplish this, you must educate, encourage, and assist patients to change attitudes and modify behaviors that work against good oral health.

The dental assistant can be a dynamic force in creating the desire for preventive dental care. Most patients have a high regard for their dentist and dental assistant. If you make the patient an active and responsible partner rather than a passive object, you can set the stage for the patient's acquiring more responsible behaviors.

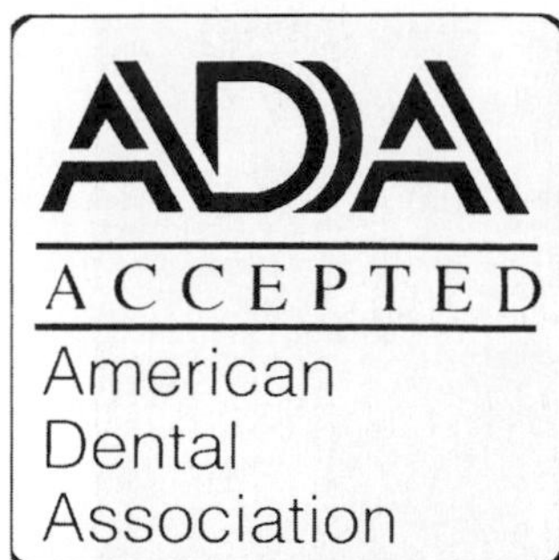


**FIG. 15.30** The American Dental Association Seal of Acceptance.

For a preventive program to be effective, patient education must be reinforced and repeated periodically. Very few people master a skill after just one lesson. On subsequent visits, review the patient's new oral health practices, and be sure to compliment the patient on his or her successes (no matter how small). When you relate well with your patients and communicate effectively in a calm and nonthreatening manner, you can win their trust and confidence. Most important, you will influence another person to adopt healthy behaviors.

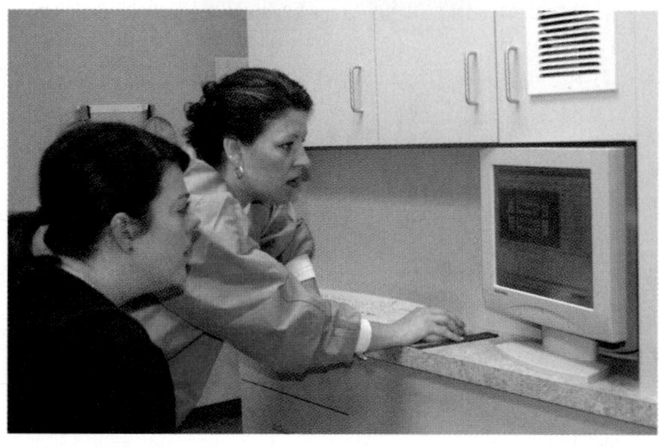

The dental assistant uses the intraoral camera to assist with patient education. ■

**■ Legal and Ethical Implications** Despite powerful evidence in support of water fluoridation, it is frequently the subject of vigorous opposition. The issue of water fluoridation gives dental professionals the chance to promote oral health at the community level. The ADA has a long-standing policy that dentists should work to promote fluoridation in their communities. However, not all dental professionals are comfortable in this role.

Dentists, dental assistants, and dental hygienists should at least educate their patients about what fluoridation is and who benefits from it. They can encourage patients to support the issue with a vote. Dental professionals should know the concentration of fluoride in their community's drinking water supply. This information may be obtained from the state or local health department.

Remember, fluoridation is a political issue as well as a public health issue. Success in a fluoridation campaign requires the use of the media, publicity, education, door-to-door canvassing, telephone calls, and "getting out the vote" on election day. ■

## ■ Critical Thinking

1. Corey Kendall is a 16-year-old patient in your office. Corey is very conscientious about her health and weight. She has a moderately high rate of decay but insists she does not eat candy. When you review her food diary, you notice that she consumes large quantities of diet colas and eats dried fruit for snacks. What recommendations would you make for Corey? What information would you give her regarding diet colas?
2. Mr. Hahn Tran is a 62-year-old patient in your office. He has several older restorations in his mouth that need to be replaced. Mr. Tran does not floss now because the unwaxed floss he previously used shredded and got caught between his teeth. What suggestions do you have for Mr. Tran?
3. Recently several patients have been asking about the benefits of an automatic toothbrush compared with the manual brushes they currently use. How will you respond to these inquiries? ■

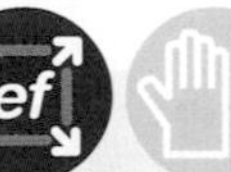

PROCEDURE 15.1 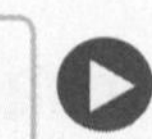

# Applying Topical Fluoride Gel or Foam (Expanded Function)

## PREREQUISITES FOR PERFORMING THIS PROCEDURE

- Infection control protocol
- Patient communication skills
- Knowledge of oral anatomy
- Moisture control techniques

## EQUIPMENT AND SUPPLIES

- Fluoride gel or foam
- Disposable trays of appropriate size
- Saliva ejector
- Cotton rolls
- Air-water syringe
- Timer

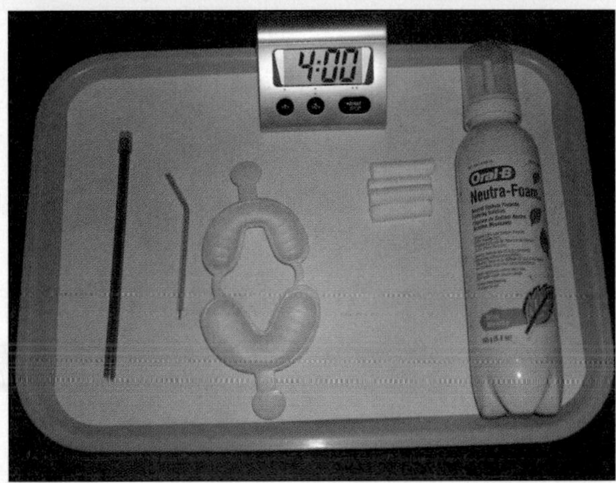


## PROCEDURAL STEPS

### Selecting the Tray

1 Select a disposable tray that is of the appropriate size for the patient's mouth. The tray must be long and sufficiently deep to cover all erupted teeth completely without extending beyond the distal surface of the most posterior tooth.

**PURPOSE** Trays are available in sizes to fit primary, mixed, and adult dentition. If the patient's mouth can accommodate it, you may use a double-arch tray. This saves time by treating both arches at the same time. Remember, trays are discarded after a single use, and if you try a tray in the mouth but do not use it, that tray must be discarded.

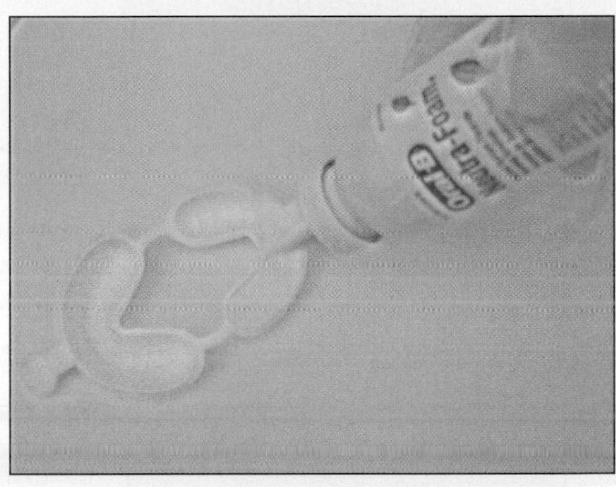


## PREPARING THE TEETH

2 Check to see whether calculus is present; if it is not, no preparation is required.

**PURPOSE** Fluoride diffuses easily through the acquired pellicle and bacterial plaque.

3 If calculus is present, request that the dentist or dental hygienist remove it.

**PURPOSE** Calculus prevents fluoride from reaching the enamel of the tooth.

**NOTE** The presence of plaque will not affect the uptake of fluoride.

## APPLYING THE TOPICAL FLUORIDE

4 Seat the patient in an upright position, and explain the procedure.

**PURPOSE** Having the patient upright prevents the gel from going into the throat.

5 Instruct the patient not to swallow the fluoride.

6 Select the appropriate tray, and load it with a minimal amount of fluoride, following guidelines according to the patient's age.

**REMINDER** Containers that are handled with gloved hands during the appointment should be surface-disinfected during treatment room cleanup.

(Continued)

## PROCEDURE 15.1 Applying Topical Fluoride Gel or Foam (Expanded Function)–cont'd

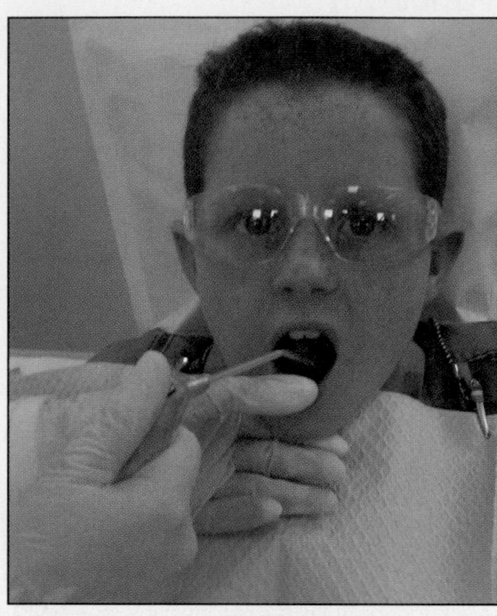

**7** Dry the teeth using air from the air-water syringe.

**PURPOSE** For fluoride to be maximally effective, the teeth must be dry when the fluoride is applied.

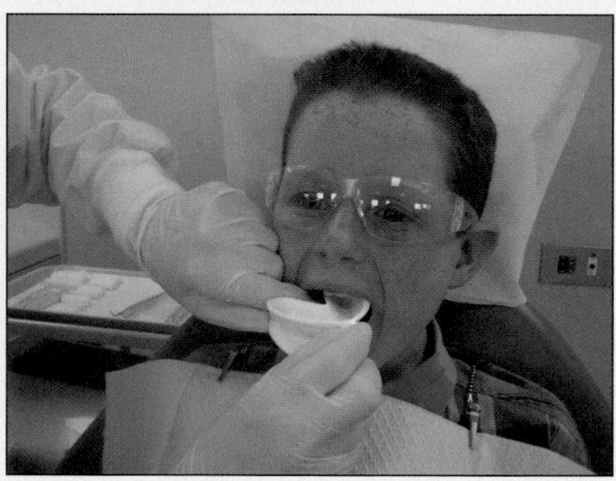

**8** Insert the tray, and place cotton rolls between the arches. Ask the patient to bite up and down gently on the cotton rolls.

**PURPOSE** To squeeze the fluoride over all tooth surfaces.

**9** Promptly place the saliva ejector, and tilt the patient's head forward.

**PURPOSE** To prevent the patient from swallowing the fluoride.

**10** Set the timer for the appropriate amount of time in accordance with the manufacturer's instructions. During this time, do not leave the patient unattended.

**11** On completion, remove the tray, but do not allow the patient to rinse or swallow. Promptly use the saliva ejector or the high-volume oral evacuator tip to remove excess saliva and solution. Do not allow the patient to close the lips tightly around the saliva ejector.

**PURPOSE** Removing excess saliva and fluoride solution will make the patient more comfortable and less likely to rinse with water.

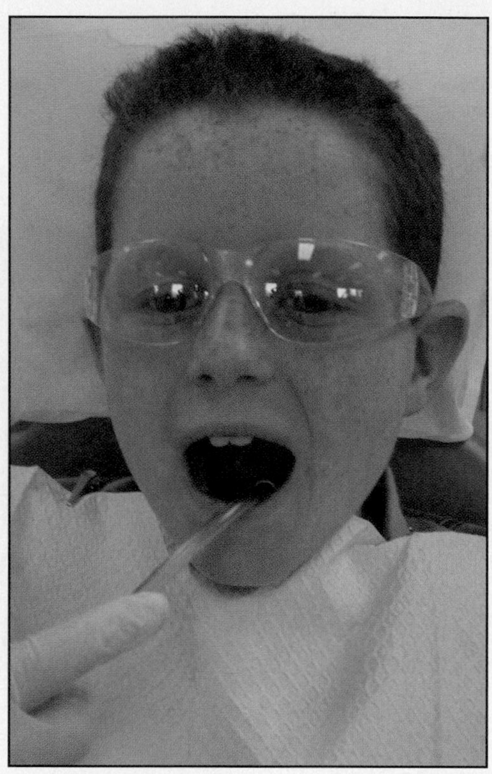

**12** Instruct the patient not to rinse, eat, drink, or brush the teeth for at least 30 minutes.

**PURPOSE** These activities could disturb the action of the fluoride.

### Documentation

| Date | Procedure | Operator |
|---|---|---|
| 8/15/17 | Applied APF fluoride gel. Instructed patient not to eat for 30 min. | PJL46 |

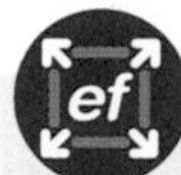

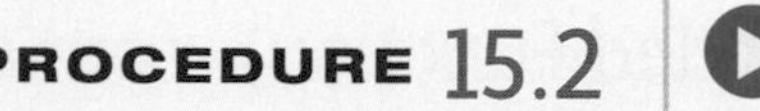


# Applying Fluoride Varnish (Expanded Function)

## PREREQUISITES FOR PERFORMING THIS PROCEDURE

- ✓ Infection control protocol
- ✓ Patient communication skills
- ✓ Knowledge of oral anatomy

## EQUIPMENT AND SUPPLIES

- ✓ 5% sodium fluoride varnish (unit dosage)
- ✓ Cotton-tip applicator or syringe applicator
- ✓ 2 × 2 gauze squares/cotton rolls
- ✓ Saliva ejector

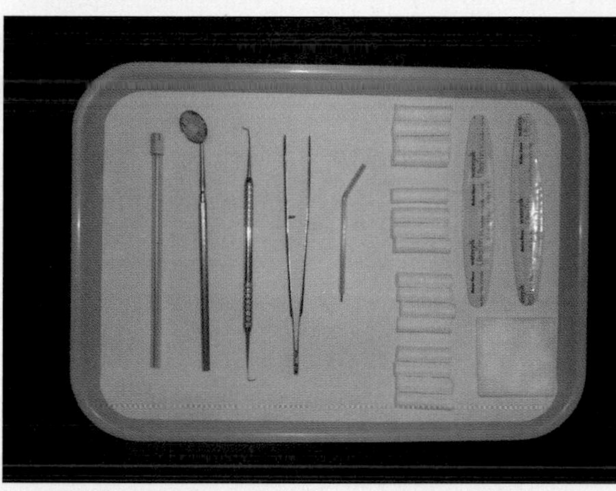

## PROCEDURAL STEPS

1 Obtain informed consent from the patient, or parent/legal guardian in the case of a minor patient.

**PURPOSE** Informed consent is a legal requirement for the provision of any dental treatment.

2 Gather supplies and single-unit dose for application.

**PURPOSE** Once you begin the procedure, you will not be able to stop in the middle to get something you forgot to set out.

3 Recline the patient to an ergonomically correct position.

**PURPOSE** You will have better access to the oral cavity and will be in a comfortable position.

4 Wipe the teeth to be varnished with the gauze or cotton roll, and insert the saliva ejector.

**NOTE** The varnish is not moisture sensitive and can be applied in the presence of saliva.

**PURPOSE** The saliva ejector is for patient comfort only.

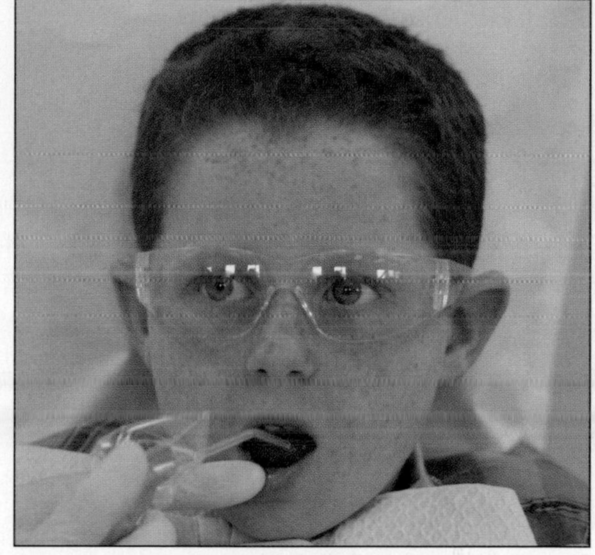

5 Using a cotton-tip applicator, brush, or syringe-style applicator, apply 0.3 to 0.5 ml of varnish (unit dose) to clinical crown of teeth; application time is 1 to 3 minutes.

**NOTE** Refer to manufacturer's instructions for specific application time.

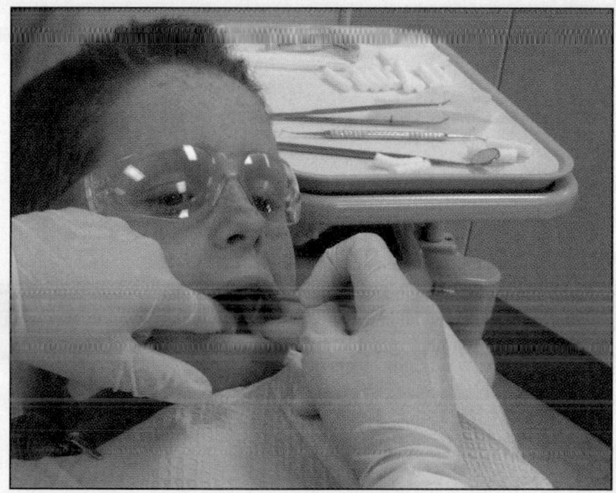

6 Dental floss may be used to draw the varnish interproximally.

**PURPOSE** To provide varnish protection for hard-to-reach surfaces.

**(Continued)**

## PROCEDURE 15.2 Applying Fluoride Varnish (Expanded Function)–cont'd

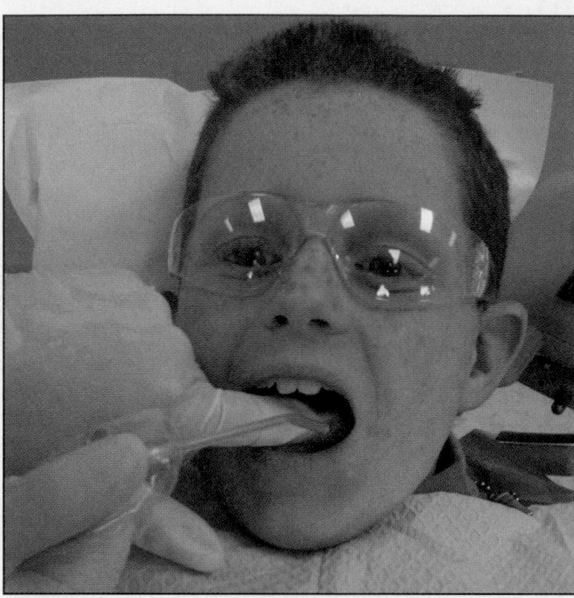

7 Allow your patient to rinse after the procedure has been completed.
**PURPOSE** To remove any residual taste.

8 Remind the patient to avoid eating hard foods, drinking hot or alcoholic beverages, brushing, and flossing for at least 4 to 6 hours, or preferably until the next day after the application. Drink through a straw for the first few hours after application.
**PURPOSE** To prolong the contact of the varnish. Varnish can be removed the next day with toothbrushing and flossing.

### Documentation

| Date | Procedure | Operator |
|---|---|---|
| 8/15/17 | Applied 0.3 ml of 5% sodium fluoride varnish (insert brand name) on facial and lingual surfaces of teeth #'s 6–14, and 19–30. | PJL 46 |

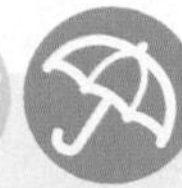

PROCEDURE 15.3 

# Assisting the Patient with Dental Floss (Expanded Function)

## PREREQUISITES FOR PERFORMING THIS PROCEDURE

- Infection control protocol
- Patient communication skills
- Understanding of tooth morphology
- Understanding of oral anatomy
- Manual dexterity

## EQUIPMENT AND SUPPLIES

- Hand mirror for patient
- Dental floss

## PROCEDURAL STEPS

### Preparing the Floss

1 Cut a piece of floss about 18 inches long. Wrap the excess floss around the middle or index fingers of both of your hands, leaving 2 to 3 inches of working space exposed.

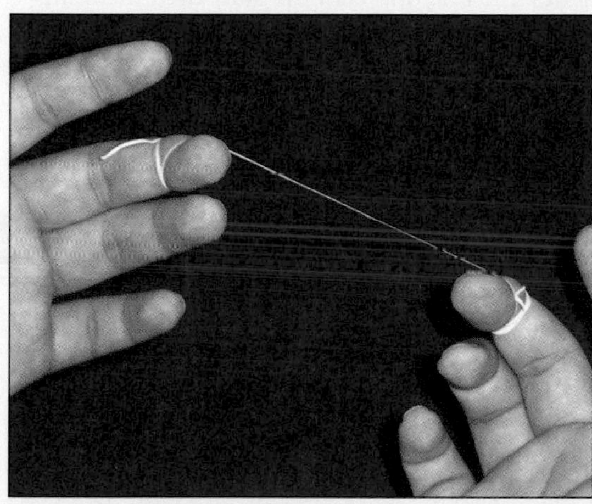

2 Stretch the floss tightly between your fingers, and use your thumb and index finger to guide the floss into place.

3 Hold the floss tightly between the thumb and forefinger of each hand. These fingers control the floss, and they should be no farther than ½ inch apart.

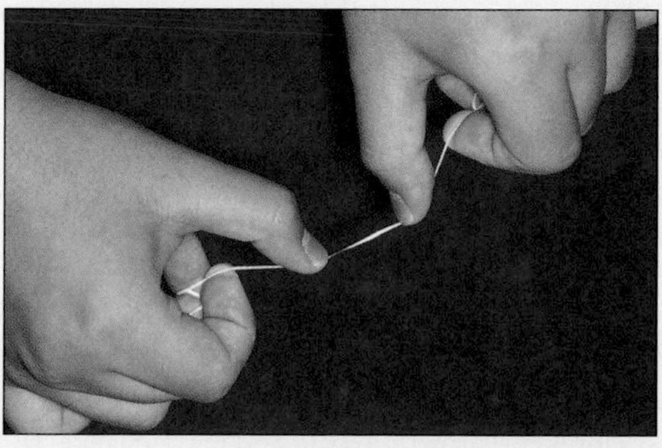

### Flossing the Teeth

4 Pass the floss gently between the patient's teeth, using a sawing motion. Guide the floss to the gumline. Do not force or snap the floss past the contact area.

**PURPOSE** The floss may cut or injure the tissue.

5 Curve the floss into a C shape against one tooth. Slide it gently into the space between the gingiva and the tooth. Use both hands to move the floss up and down on one side of the tooth.

**PURPOSE** To remove plaque from difficult-to-reach proximal areas.

6 Repeat these steps on each side of all the teeth in both arches, including the posterior surface of the last tooth in each quadrant.

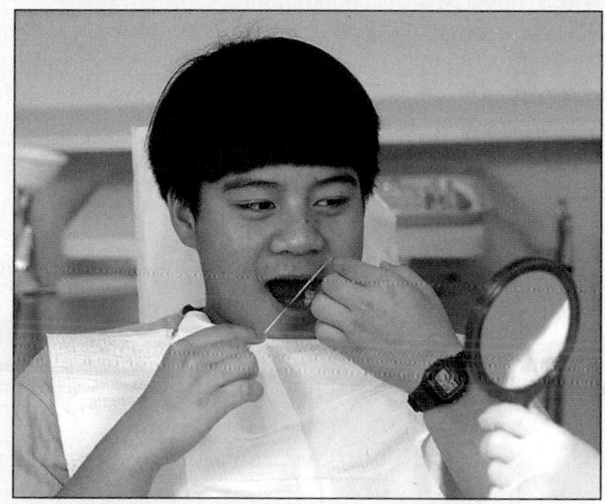

7 As the floss becomes frayed or soiled, move a fresh area into the working position.

**NOTE** This procedure is described as it would be performed by the patient at home.

### Documentation

| Date | Procedure | Operator |
|---|---|---|
| 2/25/17 | Provided flossing demonstration and instruction. Patient practiced technique and did well. | PJL 46 |

16

# Nutrition

## KEY TERMS

**Amino (uh-MEE-noe) acids** Compounds in proteins used by the body to build and repair tissue.
**Anorexia nervosa (an-uh-REK-see-uh nur-VOE-suh)** Eating disorder caused by an altered self-image.
**Bulimia (buh-LEE-mee-uh)** Eating disorder characterized by binge eating and self-induced vomiting.
**Cariogenic** Producing or promoting tooth decay.
**Fats** Lipids.
**MyPlate** The U.S. government's primary food group symbol.
**Nutrients (NOO-tree-ents)** Organic and inorganic chemicals in food that supply energy.
**Organic (or-GAN-ik)** Describes food products that have been grown without the use of chemical pesticides, herbicides, or fertilizers.
**Triglycerides** Neutral fats.

## LEARNING OUTCOMES

*On completion of this chapter, the student will be able to achieve the following objectives:*

1. Pronounce, define, and spell the key terms.
2. Discuss the link between nutrition and dental assisting, including the following:
   - Explain how diet and nutrition can affect oral conditions.
   - Explain why the study of nutrition is important to the dental assistant.
3. Do the following regarding national recommendations and guidelines for nutrition:
   - Discuss the components of the *Healthy People 2020* report.
   - Describe the difference between recommended dietary allowances (RDAs), Dietary Reference Intakes (DRIs), and Dietary Guidelines for Americans.
   - List the five areas of MyPlate.
   - Explain Canada's food guide rainbow.
4. Do the following regarding nutrient components:
   - Describe the role of carbohydrates in the daily diet, and explain the relationship between frequency and quantity of cariogenic foods in causing tooth decay.
   - List the three types of proteins.
   - Describe the role of fats in the daily diet, including cholesterol and antioxidants.
   - Describe the difference between vitamins and minerals, and explain the need for each in the daily diet.
   - Explain the importance of water in the daily diet.
5. Explain the difference between diet modification and dietary analysis.
6. Explain how to interpret food labels, including the criteria that must be met for a food to be considered "organic."
7. Discuss the health and oral implications of eating disorders.
8. List the five healthy habits for a long life.

## ELECTRONIC RESOURCES

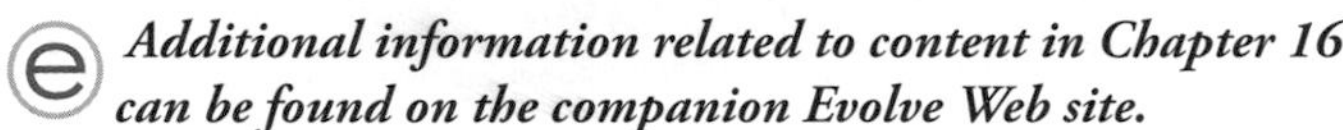
***Additional information related to content in Chapter 16 can be found on the companion Evolve Web site.***

- Practice Quiz
- Canadian Content Corner

## Nutrition and the Dental Assistant

You probably have heard the expression, "You are what you eat." This is true, because food is used to build and repair the body. Food choices therefore must be based on sound information and knowledge.

Although good nutrition is important for everyone, it is particularly critical for pregnant women, young children, and elderly persons. Malnutrition during these crucial periods may result in physical or mental disabilities. Well-nourished persons usually are better able to heal and ward off infection than are poorly nourished individuals.

As a dental assistant, you will be discussing nutrition and food choices with patients in a variety of circumstances (Fig. 16.1), including the following situations:

- Counseling patients about the prevention of tooth decay
- Counseling patients regarding their diet after oral surgery or other dental procedures
- Performing dietary analysis with patients
- Counseling patients who have orthodontic appliances regarding food choices

The study of *nutrition* is the science of how the body uses food for development, growth, repair, and maintenance. **Nutrients** are the components of food that are needed by the body.

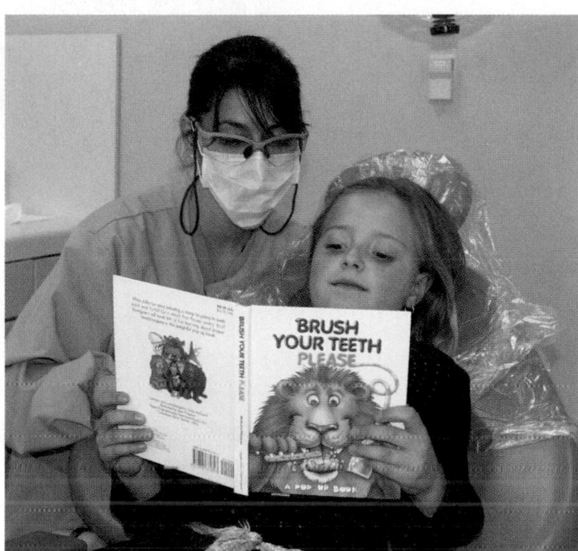


**FIG. 16.1** The dental assistant discusses dental health with her patient.

This chapter discusses the six primary nutrients, new dietary guidelines, antioxidants, food labels, and "right" eating habits for your patients and yourself (Box 16.1).

**BOX 16.1 Functions of Five Major Nutrients**

**Carbohydrates**
- Energy
- Bulk
- Make other compounds

**Proteins**
- Provide structure
- Regulate body processes:
  Enzymes
  Hormones
  Carrier molecules
  Fluid and electrolyte balance
  Energy

**Fats/Lipids**
- Energy
- Essential fatty acids
- Transport for fat-soluble vitamins
- Structure components
- Insulation
- Cushion organs

**Vitamins**
- Function with enzymes

**Minerals**
- Component of body structures
- Part of enzyme molecules
- Part of organic molecules (hemoglobin)
- Fluid and electrolyte balance

From Applegate E: The anatomy and physiology learning system, ed 4, St Louis, 2011, Saunders.

# *Healthy People 2020* Report

Every 10 years, the U.S. Department of Health and Human Services provides science-based *Healthy People* reports. These reports describe the national goals and objectives for improving the health of all Americans. The *Healthy People 2010* report focused on promoting health and disease prevention and improve the disparities in health between diverse population groups (Box 16.2).

The *Healthy People 2020* report focuses attention to the root causes of health disparities, specifically general health status, health-related quality of life and well-being, and disparities in health. See www.healthypeople.gov for details.

# Nutrient Recommendations

Today, there are fewer people with a healthy weight and an increase in adults, children, and adolescents who are overweight. There is also an increase in children with dental caries. The current recommendations for amounts of required nutrients have undergone significant changes in recent years, and the revised set of nutrient-based reference values is collectively referred to as the *Dietary Reference Intakes (DRIs).*

## Dietary Reference Intakes (DRIs)

The DRIs are developed by an expert group of scientists and registered dietitians from the United States and Canada working with the Food and Nutrition Board of the Institute of Medicine, National Academy of Sciences. The goal of the current DRIs is to improve long-term health by *reducing the risk of chronic diseases,* such as heart disease, osteoporosis, and cancer that are affected by nutrition. The DRIs include recommended intakes and tolerable upper intake levels. There are four categories of nutrient-based reference values for various stages of life.

The DRIs are intended for planning and assessing diets of healthy Americans and Canadians. The DRIs are inappropriate for individuals who are malnourished or patients who have diseases that require special nutrition. The DRIs represent a shift in emphasis from preventing deficiencies to reducing the risk of chronic disease through nutrition.

## Recommended Dietary Allowances (RDAs)

The *recommended dietary allowances (RDAs)* focus on the amount of essential nutrients needed on a daily basis to prevent deficiency diseases. The RDA value of a nutrient is based on the amount of that particular nutrient necessary to *prevent a deficiency.*

## Dietary Guidelines for Americans

The U.S. Department of Agriculture (USDA) issues Dietary Guidelines that are important in helping to find ways to

**BOX 16.2** *Healthy People 2020* Report: An Overview

**Vision**

A society in which all people live long, healthy lives.

**Mission**

*Healthy People 2020* strives to:

- Identify nationwide health improvement priorities
- Increase public awareness and understanding of the determinants of health, disease, and disability and the opportunities for progress
- Provide measurable objectives and goals that are applicable at the national, state, and local levels
- Engage multiple sectors to take actions to strengthen policies and improve practices that are driven by the best available evidence and knowledge
- Identify critical research, evaluation, and data collection needs

**Overarching Goals**

- Attain high-quality, longer lives free of preventable disease, disability, injury, and premature death
- Achieve health equity, eliminate disparities, and improve the health of all groups
- Create social and physical environments that promote good health for all
- Promote quality of life, healthy development, and healthy behaviors across all life stages

From U.S. Department of Health and Human Services: About Healthy People (online), Washington, DC, 2010, Healthy People (www.healthypeople.gov).

reduce rates of death and disease related to obesity, diabetes, cardiovascular disease, cancer, and other chronic illnesses.

## MyPlate

In June 2011 **MyPlate** replaced *MyPyramid* as the USDA's familiar guide to primary food groups. MyPlate is an easy-to-understand visual cue to help consumers adopt healthy eating habits by encouraging them to build a healthy plate, consistent with the 2010 Dietary Guidelines for Americans. The new MyPlate icon emphasized the fruit, vegetable, grains, protein, and dairy food groups (Fig. 16.2). Understanding these guidelines is important in planning your own dietary intake and in providing nutrition counseling to your patients.

**USDA MyPlate Resources**

- Ethnic/Cultural Food Pyramids
- MyPlate for Children
- Food Plans for Pregnancy and Breastfeeding
- 10 Tips Nutrition Education Series
- MiPlato—MyPlate materials in Spanish
- MyPlate e-catalog

Accessed at www.guidance/myplatefood-pyramid-resources/usda.

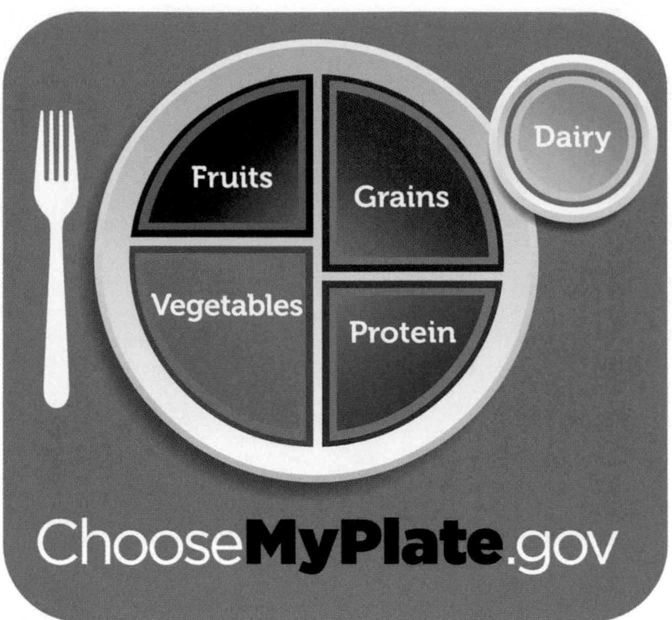


**FIG. 16.2** MyPlate. *(Courtesy the U.S. Department of Agriculture.)*

**Six Key Nutrients**

- Carbohydrates
- Proteins
- Fats
- Water
- Vitamins
- Minerals

The USDA has a Web page (www.myplate.gov) that gives consumers basic messages about healthful eating and physical activity that apply to everyone. The site allows you to enter your age, gender, and activity level. You can then print out a personalized miniposter of your own plan at the appropriate calorie level. The food plan includes specific daily quantities from each food group and a limit for discretionary calories (fats, sugars, alcohol). You can also print out a worksheet that you can use to track your progress and choose goals for tomorrow and the future.

You can discuss MyPlate with patients to help them understand how to achieve healthful eating habits. Eating a healthful diet is necessary for looking better, feeling better, having more energy, and developing a more positive outlook on life.

## Canada's Food Guide

Canada has developed a pictorial food guide to assist Canadians to choose food wisely (Fig. 16.3). *Eating Well with Canada's Food Guide* uses a rainbow graphic which displays the four food groups: grain, vegetables and fruits, milk, and meat and alternatives. The Web site (www.healthcanada.gc.ca/foodguide) allows consumers to personalize the food guide, providing recipes, tips for healthy eating and physical activity, and other educational materials.

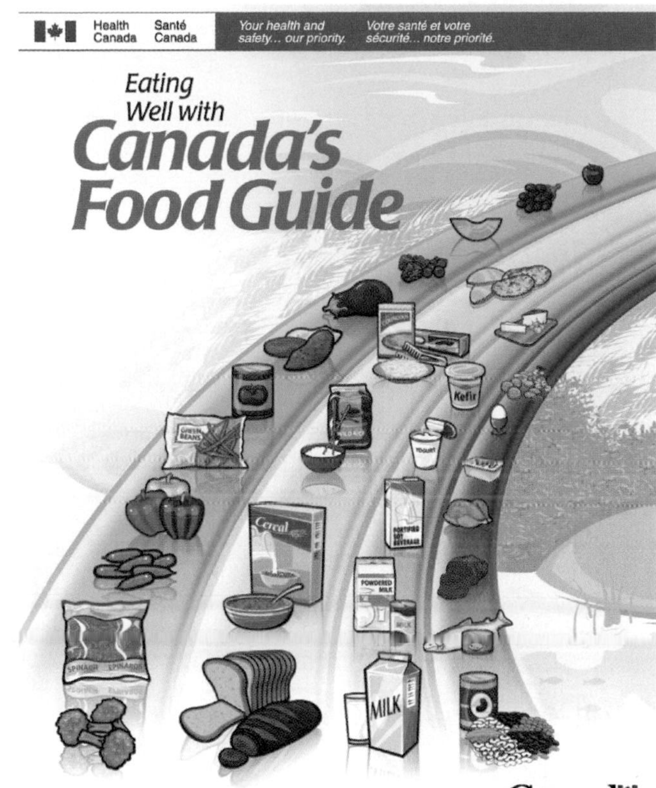


***Recommended Number of Food Guide Servings per Day***

| | Children | | | Teens | | Adults | | | |
|---|---|---|---|---|---|---|---|---|---|
| **Age in Years** | 2-3 | 4-8 | 9-13 | 14-18 | | 19-50 | | 51+ | |
| **Sex** | Girls and Boys | | | Females | Males | Females | Males | Females | Males |
| ***Vegetables and Fruit*** | 4 | 5 | 6 | 7 | 8 | 7-8 | 8-10 | 7 | 7 |
| ***Grain Products*** | 3 | 4 | 6 | 6 | 7 | 6-7 | 8 | 6 | 7 |
| ***Milk and Alternatives*** | 2 | 2 | 3-4 | 3-4 | 3-4 | 2 | 2 | 3 | 3 |
| ***Meat and Alternatives*** | 1 | 1 | 1-2 | 2 | 3 | 2 | 3 | 2 | 3 |

The chart above shows how many Food Guide Servings you need from each of the four food groups every day.

**Having the amount and type of food recommended and following the tips in *Canada's Food Guide* will help:**

- **Meet your needs for vitamins, minerals and other nutrients.**
- **Reduce your risk of obesity, type 2 diabetes, heart disease, certain types of cancer and osteoporosis.**
- **Contribute to your overall health and vitality.**

***What is One Food Guide Serving?***
***Look at the examples below.***

**Fresh, frozen or canned vegetables**
125 mL (½ cup)

**Leafy vegetables**
Cooked: 125 mL (½ cup)
Raw: 250 mL (1 cup)

**Fresh, frozen or canned fruits**
1 fruit or 125 mL (½ cup)

**100% Juice**
125 mL (½ cup)

**Bread**
1 slice (35 g)

**Bagel**
½ bagel (45 g)

**Flat breads**
½ pita or ½ tortilla (35 g)

**Cooked rice, bulgur or quinoa**
125 mL (½ cup)

**Cereal**
Cold: 30 g
Hot: 175 mL (¾ cup)

**Cooked pasta or couscous**
125 mL (½ cup)

**Milk or powdered milk (reconstituted)**
250 mL (1 cup)

**Canned milk (evaporated)**
125 mL (½ cup)

**Fortified soy beverage**
250 mL (1 cup)

**Yogurt**
175 g (¾ cup)

**Kefir**
175 g (¾ cup)

**Cheese**
50 g (1½ oz.)

**Cooked fish, shellfish, poultry, lean meat**
75 g (2 ½ oz.)/125 mL (½ cup)

**Cooked legumes**
175 mL (¾ cup)

**Tofu**
150 g or 175 mL (¾ cup)

**Eggs**
2 eggs

**Peanut or nut butters**
30 mL (2 Tbsp)

**Shelled nuts and seeds**
60 mL (¼ cup)

***Oils and Fats***

- Include a small amount – 30 to 45 mL (2 to 3 Tbsp) – of unsaturated fat each day. This includes oil used for cooking, salad dressings, margarine and mayonnaise.
- Use vegetable oils such as canola, olive and soybean.
- Choose soft margarines that are low in saturated and trans fats.
- Limit butter, hard margarine, lard and shortening.

A

**FIG. 16.3** Eating Well with Canada's Food Guide. *(© All rights reserved. Eating Well with Canada's Food Guide. Health Canada, 2011. Reproduced with permission from the Minister of Health, 2014.)*

## Make each Food Guide Serving count...
*wherever you are – at home, at school, at work or when eating out!*

- **Eat at least one dark green and one orange vegetable each day.**
  - Go for dark green vegetables such as broccoli, romaine lettuce and spinach.
  - Go for orange vegetables such as carrots, sweet potatoes and winter squash.
- **Choose vegetables and fruit prepared with little or no added fat, sugar or salt.**
  - Enjoy vegetables steamed, baked or stir-fried instead of deep-fried.
- **Have vegetables and fruit more often than juice.**

- **Make at least half of your grain products whole grain each day.**
  - Eat a variety of whole grains such as barley, brown rice, oats, quinoa and wild rice.
  - Enjoy whole grain breads, oatmeal or whole wheat pasta.
- **Choose grain products that are lower in fat, sugar or salt.**
  - Compare the Nutrition Facts table on labels to make wise choices.
  - Enjoy the true taste of grain products. When adding sauces or spreads, use small amounts.

- **Drink skim, 1%, or 2% milk each day.**
  - Have 500 mL (2 cups) of milk every day for adequate vitamin D.
  - Drink fortified soy beverages if you do not drink milk.
- **Select lower fat milk alternatives.**
  - Compare the Nutrition Facts table on yogurts or cheeses to make wise choices.

- **Have meat alternatives such as beans, lentils and tofu often.**
- **Eat at least two Food Guide Servings of fish each week.***
  - Choose fish such as char, herring, mackerel, salmon, sardines and trout.
- **Select lean meat and alternatives prepared with little or no added fat or salt.**
  - Trim the visible fat from meats. Remove the skin on poultry.
  - Use cooking methods such as roasting, baking or poaching that require little or no added fat.
  - If you eat luncheon meats, sausages or prepackaged meats, choose those lower in salt (sodium) and fat.

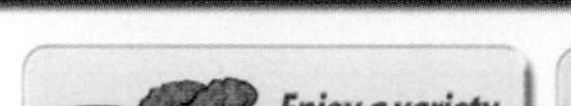

*Enjoy a variety of foods from the four food groups.*

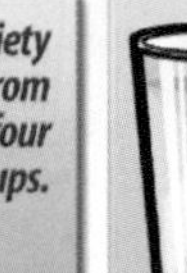

*Satisfy your thirst with water!*

Drink water regularly. It's a calorie-free way to quench your thirst. Drink more water in hot weather or when you are very active.

* Health Canada provides advice for limiting exposure to mercury from certain types of fish. Refer to www.healthcanada.gc.ca for the latest information.

## Advice for different ages and stages...

### Children

Following *Canada's Food Guide* helps children grow and thrive.

Young children have small appetites and need calories for growth and development.

- Serve small nutritious meals and snacks each day.
- Do not restrict nutritious foods because of their fat content. Offer a variety of foods from the four food groups.
- Most of all... be a good role model.

### Women of childbearing age

All women who could become pregnant and those who are pregnant or breastfeeding need a multivitamin containing **folic acid** every day. Pregnant women need to ensure that their multivitamin also contains **iron**. A health care professional can help you find the multivitamin that's right for you.

Pregnant and breastfeeding women need more calories. Include an extra 2 to 3 Food Guide Servings each day.

**Here are two examples:**

- Have fruit and yogurt for a snack, or
- Have an extra slice of toast at breakfast and an extra glass of milk at supper.

### Men and women over 50

The need for **vitamin D** increases after the age of 50.

In addition to following *Canada's Food Guide*, everyone over the age of 50 should take a daily vitamin D supplement of 10 μg (400 IU).

## How do I count Food Guide Servings in a meal?

**Here is an example:**

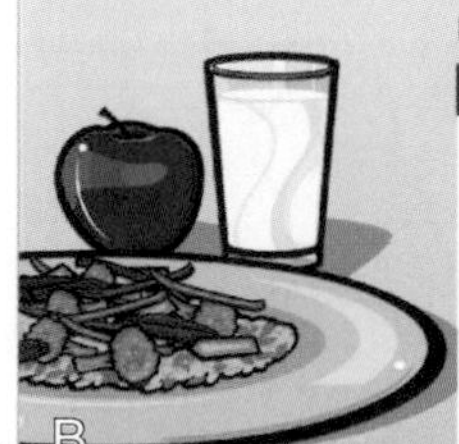

| Vegetable and beef stir-fry with rice, a glass of milk and an apple for dessert | | |
|---|---|---|
| 250 mL (1 cup) mixed broccoli, carrot and sweet red pepper | = | 2 **Vegetables and Fruit** Food Guide Servings |
| 75 g (2½ oz.) lean beef | = | 1 **Meat and Alternatives** Food Guide Serving |
| 250 mL (1 cup) brown rice | = | 2 **Grain Products** Food Guide Servings |
| 5 mL (1 tsp) canola oil | = | part of your **Oils and Fats** intake for the day |
| 250 mL (1 cup) 1% milk | = | 1 **Milk and Alternatives** Food Guide Serving |
| 1 apple | = | 1 **Vegetables and Fruit** Food Guide Serving |

B

## Eat well and be active today and every day!

### The benefits of eating well and being active include:

- Better overall health.
- Lower risk of disease.
- A healthy body weight.
- Feeling and looking better.
- More energy.
- Stronger muscles and bones.

### Be active

To be active every day is a step towards better health and a healthy body weight.

*Canada's Physical Activity Guide* recommends building 30 to 60 minutes of moderate physical activity into daily life for adults and at least 90 minutes a day for children and youth. You don't have to do it all at once. Add it up in periods of at least 10 minutes at a time for adults and five minutes at a time for children and youth.

***Start slowly and build up.***

### Eat well

Another important step towards better health and a healthy body weight is to follow *Canada's Food Guide* by:

- Eating the recommended amount and type of food each day.
- Limiting foods and beverages high in calories, fat, sugar or salt (sodium) such as cakes and pastries, chocolate and candies, cookies and granola bars, doughnuts and muffins, ice cream and frozen desserts, french fries, potato chips, nachos and other salty snacks, alcohol, fruit flavoured drinks, soft drinks, sports and energy drinks, and sweetened hot or cold drinks.

### Read the label

- Compare the Nutrition Facts table on food labels to choose products that contain less fat, saturated fat, trans fat, sugar and sodium.
- Keep in mind that the calories and nutrients listed are for the amount of food found at the top of the Nutrition Facts table.

**Nutrition Facts**

Per 0 mL (0 g)

| Amount | % Daily Value |
|---|---|
| Calories 0 | |
| Fat 0 g | 0 % |
| Saturates 0 g + Trans 0 g | 0 % |
| Cholesterol 0 mg | |
| Sodium 0 mg | 0 % |
| Carbohydrate 0 g | 0 % |
| Fibre 0 g | 0 % |
| Sugars 0 g | |
| Protein 0 g | |
| Vitamin A 0 % | Vitamin C 0 % |
| Calcium 0 % | Iron 0 % |

### Limit trans fat

When a Nutrition Facts table is not available, ask for nutrition information to choose foods lower in trans and saturated fats.

### Take a step today...

- ✓ Have breakfast every day. It may help control your hunger later in the day.
- ✓ Walk wherever you can – get off the bus early, use the stairs.
- ✓ Benefit from eating vegetables and fruit at all meals and as snacks.
- ✓ Spend less time being inactive such as watching TV or playing computer games.
- ✓ Request nutrition information about menu items when eating out to help you make healthier choices.
- ✓ Enjoy eating with family and friends!
- ✓ Take time to eat and savour every bite!

***For more information, interactive tools, or additional copies visit Canada's Food Guide on-line at:***
***www.healthcanada.gc.ca/foodguide***

***or contact:***

Publications
Health Canada
Ottawa, Ontario K1A 0K9
**E-Mail:** publications@hc-sc.gc.ca
**Tel.:** 1-866-225-0709
**Fax:** (613) 941-5366
**TTY:** 1-800-267-1245

Également disponible en français sous le titre : Bien manger avec le Guide alimentaire canadien

This publication can be made available on request on diskette, large print, audio-cassette and braille.

FIG. 16.3, cont'd

## Carbohydrates

Carbohydrates are primarily plant products in origin. No animal sources are available that provide adequate carbohydrates. Carbohydrates are easily converted to energy, and the body uses them as the chief source of energy.

Carbohydrates are divided into three groups according to the complexity of their molecules: *simple sugars, complex carbohydrates* (starch), and *dietary fiber.* With the exception of fiber, carbohydrates are easily digested and absorbed into the body. Simple sugars are absorbed first; complex sugars must be processed before they can be absorbed into the intestinal tract. Dietary fiber is indigestible and passes through the intestinal tract unchanged. Each group has a specific function in health.

*Dietary fiber* is commonly called *roughage.* It is the portion of the plant that is eaten but cannot be absorbed. Fiber is classified by its water solubility. Roughage adds bulk to the intestinal tract and is beneficial for normal gastrointestinal functioning. *Water-soluble fiber,* which is found in oat bran, fruits, and vegetables, helps to lower cholesterol. *Insoluble fiber,* which is found in whole grains and beans, helps to prevent colon cancer and may reduce risk of heart attack (Table 16.1).

*Complex carbohydrates,* which are found mainly in grains, vegetables, and fruits, are important because they provide energy. Foods high in complex carbohydrates also supply vitamins, minerals, and fiber. Although fiber is not classified as a nutrient, it is essential for good health.

**TABLE 16.1** Dietary Fiber in Some Common Foods

| Food | Amount | Weight (g) | Calories | Dietary Fiber (g) |
|---|---|---|---|---|
| **Fruit** | | | | |
| Apple, with peel | 1 medium | 138 | 80 | 3.9 |
| Apple juice | 1 cup | 228 | 116 | 0.7 |
| Banana, peeled | 1 medium | 110 | 100 | 2.5 |
| Orange, peeled | 1 medium | 145 | 67 | 3.1 |
| Prunes, dried | 3 medium | 8 | 60 | 3.5 |
| **Vegetables, Cooked** | | | | |
| Potato with skin, baked | 1 large | 200 | 220 | 3.9 |
| Carrots, sliced | 1 cup | 150 | 60 | 5.0 |
| Broccoli | 1 spear | 180 | 53 | 6.2 |
| Green beans | 1 cup | 130 | 40 | 3.3 |
| Corn | 1 cup | 164 | 134 | 7.7 |
| Peas | 1 cup | 160 | 130 | 7.4 |
| **Vegetables, Raw** | | | | |
| Celery | 1 cup | 120 | 19 | 2.0 |
| Carrots | 1 medium | 72 | 31 | 2.0 |
| Tomato | 1 medium | 120 | 24 | 2.0 |
| Lettuce, chopped | 1 cup | 56 | 53 | 0.8 |
| Cauliflower | 1 cup | 100 | 24 | 2.7 |
| **Legumes and Nuts** | | | | |
| Navy beans, cooked | 1 cup | 190 | 225 | 13.0 |
| Lima beans, cooked | 1 cup | 170 | 170 | 9.2 |
| Lentils, cooked | 1 cup | 200 | 215 | 8.7 |
| Pecans, dried, halves | 1 cup | 108 | 720 | 6.5 |
| Walnuts, English, chopped | 1 cup | 120 | 770 | 8.4 |
| Peanut butter, regular | 1 tablespoon | 16 | 95 | 1.0 |
| **Bread and Pasta** | | | | |
| White bread | 1 slice | 28 | 75 | 0.5 |
| Whole wheat bread | 1 slice | 28 | 70 | 2.4 |
| Spaghetti, cooked | 1 cup | 130 | 190 | 1.0 |
| Brown rice, cooked | 1 cup | 195 | 232 | 2.8 |
| White rice, cooked | 1 cup | 205 | 223 | 0.6 |

From Applegate E: The anatomy and physiology learning system, ed 4, St Louis, 2011, Saunders.

*Simple sugars* are formed in the mouth from refined carbohydrates that are found in processed foods such as sugar, syrup, jelly, bread, crackers, cookies, candy, cake, and soft drinks. In contrast to complex carbohydrates, most refined carbohydrates supply only "empty" calories, and many are high in fat. *Empty calories* are those that provide only calories and no other nutrients or fiber.

Although it may be wise to lower dietary fat, consumers should be cautioned to read food labels carefully. In many low-fat or reduced-fat foods, fat is replaced with sugars. As a result, although the fat content of a food may be less, the calorie count may be the same as or higher than that in the original higher-fat version of the food.

### Sources of Carbohydrates

- Cereal grains: wheat, corn, oat, rice, barley, buckwheat
- Sweets: table sugar, honey, maple and corn syrups
- Vegetables: green leafy vegetables, dried beans, and peas

## Foods That Cause Tooth Decay

Any food that contains sugars or other carbohydrates that can be metabolized by bacteria in plaque is described as **cariogenic** (producing or promoting dental decay). For instance, refined carbohydrates, such as candy and other sweets, are cariogenic (Table 16.2).

A major factor in determining the cariogenicity of a carbohydrate is how long the food stays in the mouth. Sugary liquids such as soft drinks leave the mouth quickly and are not as cariogenic as sticky foods, such as raisins or caramels, which adhere to the teeth and stay in the mouth longer. Furthermore, the frequency with which cariogenic foods are eaten is more important than the amount. The child who snacks all day on small amounts of cariogenic food is far more likely to develop decay than is the child who eats a larger amount of cariogenic food, but only once a day.

Foods such as crackers, although not sweet, are cariogenic because they contain refined carbohydrates that stick to the teeth. They remain in the mouth long enough to be broken down into sugars that can be used by the bacteria in plaque. Complex carbohydrates, such as fruits and vegetables, are less cariogenic because they clear the mouth before they are converted into simple sugars that can be used by bacteria.

Another important factor in determining cariogenicity is whether or not the food stimulates the flow of saliva. *Salivary flow* serves two functions: (1) It speeds clearance of food from the mouth, and (2) it provides a source of dietary fluoride to strengthen the tooth and assist in remineralization. The complete process of tooth decay is described in Chapter 13.

1 What are nutrients?
2 What are the three types of carbohydrates?
3 What is meant by cariogenicity?

## Proteins

Proteins are the only nutrients that can build and repair body tissues, and this is their primary function. Proteins are composed of **amino acids**, which are used in the building and repair process. A total of 20 amino acids have been identified, 8 of which are essential in the adult for normal growth and maintenance of tissues. These *essential* amino acids must come from food.

Proteins are classified as complete, partially complete, or incomplete.

- A *complete protein* contains a well-balanced mixture of all eight essential amino acids. If it is the sole source of protein in the diet, a complete protein will support life and normal growth.

**TABLE 16.2 Diet Recommendations for Common Dental Conditions**

| Dental Condition | Diet Recommendations |
|---|---|
| Dental caries | Limit frequency of eating cariogenic foods.<br>Avoid crackers, donuts, potato chips between meals.<br>Eat fruits for dessert and snacks.<br>Eat raw vegetables for snacks.<br>Avoid sticky or retentive foods.<br>Avoid slowly dissolving candies.<br>Chew sugar-free gum. |
| Periodontal disease | Avoid soft, mushy foods.<br>Avoid popcorn.<br>Eat plenty of fruits high in vitamin C.<br>Eat plenty of dairy products for calcium for bone health.<br>Eat fresh rather than canned, mushy vegetables.<br>Avoid nuts. |
| New dentures | Encourage chewing.<br>Begin by chewing on molar teeth.<br>Work up to biting with incisors.<br>Cut food into smaller pieces.<br>Nuts may be difficult to chew.<br>Eat plenty of dairy products for calcium for bone health.<br>Eat casseroles, lasagna, and other soft foods to increase intake of nutrients. |
| Oral surgery | Eat soft foods, or process foods in a blender if needed.<br>Avoid spicy foods.<br>Maintain nutrient levels to promote healing.<br>Eat hot cereals, rice, pasta, soft bread, soups with rice. |
| Orthodontics | Avoid chewy or sticky foods.<br>Eat soft foods.<br>Avoid hard foods such as apples, raw carrots, etc.<br>Eat plenty of dairy products for calcium for bone health. |

- A *partially complete* protein supplies an unbalanced mixture of essential amino acids. If it is the sole source of protein, a partially complete protein will maintain life but will not support normal growth.
- An *incomplete protein* does not support life or normal growth. It must not be the sole source of protein because the protein is missing or is extremely low in one or more of the essential amino acids.

Each gram of protein supplies 4 calories.

### Sources of Protein

- Complete proteins: meat, fish, poultry, eggs, dairy products
- Partially complete proteins: grains, vegetables
- Incomplete proteins: corn, gelatin

4 What is an amino acid?
5 How many of the amino acids are essential?
6 What is a complete protein?

# Fats (Lipids)

Most fats in the diet are **triglycerides**, or *neutral fats,* which occur in food from both animals and plants. **Fats**, also called *lipids,* have six important functions in the body:

- Fats are important sources of energy.
- Fats provide essential fatty acids.
- Fats transport vitamins.
- Fats provide heat insulation.
- Fats are components of cell membranes and *myelin,* the covering around nerve fibers.
- Fats form protective cushions around body organs.

Although fats are essential components of a healthful diet, excessive amounts are not desirable. Most Americans need to reduce their intake of dietary fat. The American Heart Association recommends that no more than 30 percent of the daily calorie intake should be in the form of fats.

In general, however, 40 percent or more of the calories in the average American diet comes from fat. This overconsumption of fats is unhealthy and is related to cardiovascular disease, obesity, diabetes, and some cancers.

## Cholesterol

Cholesterol is a fat that is typically found in saturated fats (from animal sources). It is also manufactured within the body. Confusion often exists between "good fat" and "bad fat." The *good* fats in our diet are *polyunsaturated* and *monounsaturated* fats. The *bad* dietary fats are *cholesterol* and *saturated* fats.

Body fat is also divided into two categories. The "good" fat is *high-density lipoprotein (HDL);* the "bad" fat is *low-density lipoprotein (LDL).* Levels of HDL and LDL can often be successfully changed through diet.

It is important to understand the differences between types of fat and the meaning of numbers used to identify fat content. Many foods that are high in saturated fats are also high in cholesterol. The recommendation is that cholesterol should be limited to less than 250 mg per day, which is the amount present in one egg yolk. Table 16.3 compares some common sources of fats and cholesterol.

## Antioxidants

Recent research indicates that cholesterol itself may not be the problem in the development of heart disease. Rather, the problem may be the way in which cholesterol reacts with the oxygen *(oxidizes)* in blood.

In addition to lowering the dietary intake of cholesterol, increasing the intake of antioxidants may be beneficial. The antioxidant vitamins E and C and beta-carotene can prevent cholesterol from oxidizing and damaging the arteries. Many fruits and vegetables and some seasonings contain naturally occurring antioxidants.

### Sources of Antioxidants

- Vitamin E: soy beans, almonds, oatmeal, chick peas (garbanzo beans), hazel nuts, rye flour, wheat germ, sunflower seeds
- Vitamin C: peppers, oranges, brussels sprouts, strawberries, tangerines, broccoli, lemons, raspberries, cabbage, grapefruit, black currants, cauliflower
- Beta-carotene: carrots, sweet potatoes, pumpkin, kale, winter squash, spinach, cantaloupe, apricots, mustard greens
- Seasonings: nutmeg, thyme, rosemary, sesame, cloves, green tea, oregano, pepper

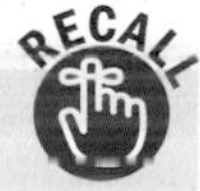


7 Which systemic diseases are related to excess fat in the diet?
8 Which cholesterol is "good" and which is "bad"?

# Vitamins

Vitamins are organic substances that occur in plant and animal tissues. They are essential in minute amounts for the human body to maintain growth and good health. Vitamins do not *supply* energy, but they are needed to *release* energy from carbohydrates, fats, and proteins.

Many vitamins function with enzymes in chemical reactions within the body. To date, 13 vitamins have been discovered. Of these, four are *fat soluble* and nine are *water soluble.* The *fat-soluble vitamins* (A, D, E, and K) are stored in body fat and are not destroyed by cooking.

TABLE 16.3 Common Sources of Fats and Cholesterol

| Food | Amount | Weight (g) | Total Calories | Total Fat (g)* | Saturated Fat (g)* | Cholesterol (mg) |
|---|---|---|---|---|---|---|
| Milk, nonfat | 1 cup | 244 | 86 | 0.4 (4%) | 0.3 (3%) | 4 |
| Milk, 2% | 1 cup | 244 | 121 | 4.8 (36%) | 2.9 (2%) | 22 |
| Milk, whole | 1 cup | 244 | 151 | 8.2 (49%) | 5.0 (30%) | 33 |
| Egg, hard boiled | 1 whole | 50 | 79 | 5.6 (64%) | 1.7 (19%) | 274 |
| Cream cheese | 1 ounce | 28.3 | 100 | 10.0 (90%) | 6.3 (57%) | 31.4 |
| Mayonnaise | 1 tablespoon | 13.8 | 99 | 10.9 (99%) | 1.7 (15%) | 8.1 |
| Butter | 1 tablespoon | 14.2 | 102 | 11.5 (100%) | 7.2 (63%) | 31.1 |
| Cheese, American | 1 ounce | 28.3 | 107 | 9.0 (76%) | 5.7 (48%) | 27.3 |
| Cheese, cheddar | 1 ounce | 28.3 | 115 | 9.2 (72%) | 5.8 (45%) | 27.3 |
| Sirloin steak | 3 ounces | 85 | 240 | 15.0 (66%) | 6.4 (24%) | 74 |
| Ground beef | 3 ounces | 85 | 230 | 16.0 (63%) | 6.2 (24%) | 74 |
| Chicken breast (no skin) | 3 ounces | 86 | 142 | 3.0 (19%) | 0.9 (6%) | 73 |
| Fried chicken | 3 ounces | 85 | 187 | 7.8 (38%) | 2.1 (10%) | 79.6 |
| Frankfurter | 2 ounces | 57 | 183 | 16.6 (82%) | 6.1 (30%) | 29 |
| Turkey, roasted | 3 ounces | 85 | 145 | 4.2 (26%) | 1.4 (9%) | 65 |
| Cod, broiled | 3 ounces | 85 | 97 | 0.9 (8%) | 0.8 (7%) | 51 |
| Tuna salad | ½ cup | 102 | 188 | 9.5 (45%) | 1.6 (8%) | 40 |
| Avocado | 1 medium | 201 | 324 | 30.8 (86%) | 4.9 (14%) | 0 |

*Percentage of total calories represented by fat.

From Applegate E: The anatomy and physiology learning system, ed 4, St Louis, 2011, Saunders.

The *water-soluble vitamins* (B and C), which are naturally present in food, are easily destroyed during food preparation. These water-soluble vitamins are not stored in the body and therefore must be consumed each day. Because of their similar functions, all water-soluble vitamins except vitamin C are often grouped together and are referred to as the *B-complex vitamins* (Table 16.4).

RECALL

9 Which type of vitamin is stored in the body and is not destroyed by cooking?
10 Which vitamins are referred to as the B-complex vitamins?
11 Which vitamins are fat soluble?

## Minerals

Minerals are essential elements that are needed in small amounts to maintain health and function and must be supplied by the diet. Minerals and vitamins are found in all foods except those that are highly refined. They are found in all tissues and fluids, and they account for 4 percent of body weight. Of the many minerals used by the body, 14 are considered to be essential.

Minerals are the components of bones and teeth that make them rigid and strong. They also play an important part in maintaining the body's water-electrolyte balance.

Minerals are usually classified according to the amounts required by the body. The minerals that are needed in larger amounts (100 mg/day or more) are *sodium, potassium, calcium, chloride, phosphorus,* and *magnesium.* The *trace elements,* which are needed in smaller amounts (no more than a few milligrams a day), include iron, zinc, copper, selenium, chromium, manganese, iodine, and fluorine (Table 16.5).

## Water

Water, often called "the forgotten nutrient," is a significant component of saliva. Saliva contains supersaturated concentrations of calcium and phosphate and can promote remineralization of the early carious lesion. Water is also important because it helps to build tissue, aids in regulating body temperature, and acts as a lubricant for joints and mucous membranes.

The body is approximately 80 percent water, and humans can live longer without food than without water. Approximately two thirds of body weight is water. The body loses water daily in urine, feces, sweat, and expiration (exhaling). Life-threatening electrolyte imbalances can result from extensive water loss caused by vomiting, diarrhea, burns, or excessive perspiration.

The daily requirement of water is about 91 ounces of total water for adult women, and 125 ounces of total water for adult men. About 80 percent of total water comes from drinking fluids, and the other 20 percent comes from food. Vegetables and fruits are more than 80 percent water, and meats are 40 to 60 percent water.

**TABLE 16.4** Vitamins: Best Sources, Primary Functions, Deficiency Symptoms, and Toxicity

| Vitamin* | Sources | Functions | Deficiency Symptoms† | Toxicity |
|---|---|---|---|---|
| Vitamin A (carotene) | Yellow or orange fruits and vegetables, green leafy vegetables, oatmeal, liver, dairy products | Formation and maintenance of skin, hair, and mucous membranes; sight in dim light; bone and tooth growth | Night blindness, dry scaly skin, frequent fatigue | Toxic in high doses, although beta-carotene is nontoxic |
| Vitamin $B_1$ (thiamine) | Cereal, oatmeal, meat, rice, pasta, whole grains, liver | Release of energy from carbohydrates, growth, and metabolism | Heart irregularities, fatigue, nerve disorders, mental confusion | Not toxic; high doses excreted by kidneys |
| Vitamin $B_2$ (riboflavin) | Whole grains, green leafy vegetables, organ meats, milk, eggs | Release of energy from proteins, fats, and carbohydrates | Cracks in corners of mouth, rash, anemia | No toxic effects reported |
| Vitamin $B_6$ (pyridoxine) | Fish, poultry, lean meats, bananas, prunes, dried beans, whole grains, avocados | Building of body tissue, metabolism of proteins | Convulsions, dermatitis, muscular weakness, skin cracks, anemia | Possible nerve damage in hands and feet with long-term megadoses |
| Vitamin $B_{12}$ (cobalamin) | Meats, milk products, seafood | Cell development, nervous system functioning, metabolism of proteins and fats | Anemia, nervousness, fatigue | No toxic effects reported |
| Biotin | Cereal/grain products, yeast, legumes, liver | Metabolism of proteins, fats, and carbohydrates | Nausea, vomiting, depression, hair loss, dry scaly skin | No toxic effects reported |
| Folate (folic acid, folacin) | Green leafy vegetables, organ meats, dried peas, beans, and lentils | Genetic material development, red blood cell production | Gastrointestinal disorders, anemia, cracks on lips | Some evidence of toxicity in large doses |
| Niacin | Meat, poultry, fish, cereal, peanuts, potatoes, dairy products, eggs | Metabolism of proteins, fats, and carbohydrates | Skin disorders, diarrhea, indigestion, general fatigue | Physician's care for nicotinic acid form |
| Pantothenic acid | Lean meats, whole grains, legumes, vegetables, fruits | Release of energy from fats and carbohydrates | Fatigue, vomiting, stomach distress, infection, muscle cramps | No toxic effects reported |
| Vitamin C (ascorbic acid) | Citrus fruits, berries, vegetables, peppers | Structure of bone, cartilage, muscle, and blood vessels; maintenance of capillaries and gums; absorption of iron | Swollen or bleeding gums, slow wound healing, fatigue, depression, poor digestion | Nausea, cramps, and diarrhea with 1 g or more |
| Vitamin D | Fortified milk/margarine, butter, eggs, fish, sunlight | Bone and tooth formation; maintenance of cardiac and nervous system function | *Children:* rickets and other bone deformities *Adults:* calcium loss from bones | Diarrhea and weight loss possible with high intake |
| Vitamin E | Multigrain cereals, nuts, wheat germ, vegetable oils, green leafy vegetables | Protection of blood cells, body tissues, and essential fatty acids | Muscular wasting, nerve damage, anemia, reproductive failure | Relatively nontoxic |
| Vitamin K | Green leafy vegetables, fruit, dairy, and grain products | Blood clotting | Bleeding disorders in newborns and patients taking blood-thinning medications | Not toxic as found in food |

*Specifics for each vitamin (recommended intakes and tolerable upper intake levels) vary by life-stage group and are available through the individual Dietary Reference Intake (DRIs) products developed by the Food and Nutrition Board of the Institute of Medicine and published by the National Academies Press. For more information, visit www.nap.edu.

†Many of these symptoms can also be attributed to problems other than vitamin deficiency. If you have these symptoms and they persist, see your physician.

## TABLE 16.5 Minerals: Best Sources, Primary Functions, Deficiency Symptoms, and Toxicity

| Mineral* | Sources | Functions | Deficiency Symptoms† | Toxicity Symptoms |
|---|---|---|---|---|
| Calcium ($Ca^{2+}$, $Ca^{++}$) | Milk and milk products, green leafy vegetables, soy products, sardines, salmon | Muscle and nervous system function, blood coagulation, bone and tooth formation | Poor bone growth and tooth development<br>*Children:* dental caries, rickets<br>*Adults:* soft and brittle bones | Kidney stones |
| Chloride ($Cl^-$) | Salt, fish, vegetables | Fluid and acid-base balance, activation of gastric enzymes | Growth retardation, psychomotor deficits, memory loss | Disturbances in acid-base balance |
| Magnesium ($Mg^{2+}$, $Mg^{++}$) | Dark green vegetables, nuts, soybeans, whole grains, bananas, apricots, seafood | Bone and tooth formation, protein synthesis, lipid metabolism | Rare except in disease states<br>Confusion, hallucinations, poor memory, muscle weakness, cramps | Drowsiness, weakness, lethargy<br>*Severe:* skeletal paralysis, respiratory depression, coma, death |
| Phosphorus ($PO_4$) | Milk and milk products, eggs, meats, legumes, whole grains | Bone and tooth formation, energy metabolism, acid-base balance | *Malabsorption (rare):* anorexia, weakness, stiff joints, fragile bones | Muscle spasms |
| Potassium ($K^+$) | Milk and milk products, apricots, oranges, bananas, greens, meats, legumes | Fluid and acid-base balance, transmission of nerve impulses, enzyme reactions | Impaired growth, hypertension, bone fragility, central nervous system changes | Hyperkalemia (excess potassium in blood), cardiac disturbances |
| Sodium ($Na^+$) | *Major:* salt (sodium chloride)<br>*Minor:* milk, vegetables | Acid-base balance, cell membrane permeability, impulse transmission | Weight loss, central nervous system abnormalities | Hypertension, leading to cardiovascular and kidney diseases |
| Chromium ($Cr^{3+}$) | Liver, whole grains, cheese, legumes | Enzyme activation, glucose removal | Weight loss, central nervous system abnormalities | Inhibited insulin activity |
| Copper ($Cu^{2+}$, $Cu^{++}$) | Shellfish, liver, nuts, whole grains, raisins | Red blood cell production, lipid metabolism | Anemia, bone fragility, impaired immune response | Neuron and liver cell damage from copper accumulation |
| Fluorine ($F^-$) | Foods cooked in fluoridated water, fish, gelatin | Bone and tooth formation | Increased susceptibility to caries | Fluorosis, mottling of teeth |
| Iodine ($I^-$) | *Major:* iodized salt<br>*Minor:* fish, seaweed, vegetables | Energy metabolism, normal cell functioning | Goiter, cretinism (infants of iodine-deficient mothers) | Minimal toxic effect with normal thyroid functioning |
| Iron ($Fe^{3+}$) | Organ meats, cereals, green leafy vegetables, whole grains | Hemoglobin formation, growth and development | Iron deficiency anemia, behavioral changes | Cirrhosis, diabetes, pigmentation, joint pain |
| Manganese ($Mn^{2+}$) | Nuts, whole grains, vegetables and fruits, coffee, tea, cocoa, egg yolk | Normal bone structure, reproduction, normal functioning of cells and central nervous system | None observed in humans | Iron deficiency anemia through inhibiting effect on iron absorption; pulmonary changes, anorexia, apathy, impotence, headache, leg cramps, speech impairment; resembles Parkinson's disease at advanced stages of toxicity |
| Selenium (Se) | Protein-rich foods (meat, eggs, milk), whole grains, seafood, liver and other meats, egg yolks, garlic | Part of an enzyme system; acts as an antioxidant with vitamin E to protect the cell from oxygen | Keshan disease (a human cardiomyopathy) and Kashin-Bek disease (an endemic human osteoarthropathy) | Physical defects of the fingernails and toenails, hair loss |
| Zinc ($Zn^{2+}$) | Whole grains, wheat germ, crabmeat, oyster, liver and other meats, brewer's yeast | Involvement in protein synthesis; essential for normal growth and sexual development, wound healing, cell division and differentiation, smell acuity | Depressed immune function, poor growth, dwarfism, impaired skeletal growth, delayed sexual maturation, acrodermatitis | Severe anemia, nausea, vomiting, abdominal cramps, diarrhea, fever, hypocupremia (low blood serum copper), malaise, fatigue |

*Specifics for each mineral (recommended intakes and tolerable upper intake levels) vary by life-stage group and are available through the individual Dietary Reference Intake (DRIs) products developed by the Food and Nutrition Board of the Institute of Medicine and published by the National Academies Press. For more information, visit www.nap.edu.

†Many of these symptoms can also be attributed to problems other than mineral deficiency. If you have these symptoms and they persist, see your physician.

**12** Which minerals are required by the body in the largest quantities?
**13** What is often called "the forgotten nutrient"?

## Diet Modification

Diet modification provided by members of the dental team is usually focused on dental health and is not intended to replace the services of a registered dietitian. Patients with dietary issues related to underlying medical conditions must be referred to a physician and to a registered dietitian.

The patient's lifestyle and background must be considered when one is making recommendations. Remember, if your dietary recommendations are compatible with the patient's normal diet, the patient is more likely to comply.

## Dietary Analysis

A dietary analysis is used to help patients understand the role of nutrition in their dental and general health. To do this, ask the patient to keep a diet diary for about 3 days. The patient's cooperation is essential in performing this analysis because the patient must record *every* food eaten, including the amount, how it was prepared, and when it was eaten.

The dental team then reviews the completed diary with the patient, using a dietary analysis form (Fig. 16.4). Information from the diet diary is divided into groups on the analysis form and is compared with the recommended numbers of servings per day. Empty calories and cariogenic foods are highlighted.

Always suggest modifications in a *positive* manner. The review of the dietary analysis should *never* be phrased in critical terms or stated in any way to make the patient uncomfortable. A collection of nutrition labels from food boxes is helpful in making the patient aware of how much sugar and fat is consumed.

## Reading Food Labels

In 1995 the U.S. Department of Agriculture (USDA) required that all food products must contain a nutrition facts label

Food Diary

Day ______

| Time | Place | Food Eaten | Amount Eaten | How Prepared |
|---|---|---|---|---|
| Example:<br>6:00 AM | Kitchen | Orange juice<br>Whole wheat bread<br>Diet margarine<br>Egg | ½ c<br>2 slices<br>1 tsp<br>1 | Unsweetened<br>Toasted<br>Tub<br>Fried in oil |
| | | | | |
| | | | | |
| | | | | |
| | | | | |
| | | | | |
| | | | | |

Instructions:
1. List EVERYTHING you eat or drink on 3 consecutive, typical days.
2. Use 2 weekdays and 1 weekend day.
3. Include extras such as chewing gum, sugar and cream in coffee, or mustard on a sandwich.

**FIG. 16.4** Food diary. Typically used for 1 to 7 days. (A customizable version is available on Evolve.) *(From Stegeman CA, Ratcliff Davis J: The dental hygienist's guide to nutritional care, ed 4, St Louis, 2014, Saunders.)*

(Fig. 16.5). These labels are an excellent source of nutrition information. Every food label must include the following nutrition facts:

- Individual serving size
- Number of servings per container
- Total calories
- Calories derived from fat content
- Percentage of daily value (% of RDA)

## Product Label Information

Begin with the *serving size.* This information is given in both common household units and metric units. The serving size is uniform across product lines so that you can easily compare similar foods.

The *amount* of each nutrient in the food is expressed in two ways: as a percentage of the DRI and by weight of the serving size. By using the percentage of daily values, you can easily determine whether a food contributes a large or a small amount of a particular nutrient. Remember, if you eat more or less than the serving size on the label, you will need to adjust the quantities of nutrients accordingly. For example, the label on ice cream indicates 150 calories per serving, but the serving size is only cup. The average dish of ice cream actually eaten may contain 500 or 600 calories.

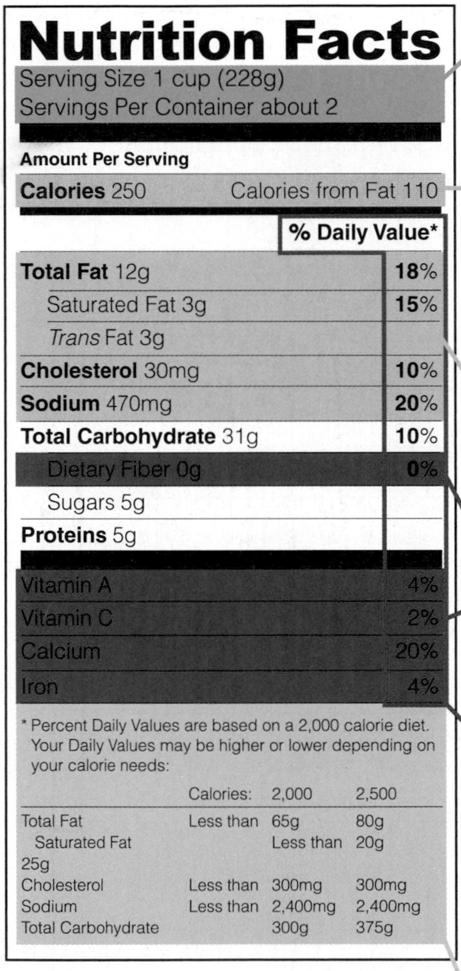

**Nutrition Facts**

Serving Size 1 cup (228g)
Servings Per Container about 2

**Amount Per Serving**

| **Calories** 250 | Calories from Fat 110 |
|---|---|
| | **% Daily Value*** |
| **Total Fat** 12g | **18%** |
| Saturated Fat 3g | **15%** |
| *Trans* Fat 3g | |
| **Cholesterol** 30mg | **10%** |
| **Sodium** 470mg | **20%** |
| **Total Carbohydrate** 31g | **10%** |
| Dietary Fiber 0g | **0%** |
| Sugars 5g | |
| **Proteins** 5g | |
| Vitamin A | 4% |
| Vitamin C | 2% |
| Calcium | 20% |
| Iron | 4% |

* Percent Daily Values are based on a 2,000 calorie diet. Your Daily Values may be higher or lower depending on your calorie needs:

| | Calories: | 2,000 | 2,500 |
|---|---|---|---|
| Total Fat | Less than | 65g | 80g |
| Saturated Fat | | Less than | 20g |
| 25g | | | |
| Cholesterol | Less than | 300mg | 300mg |
| Sodium | Less than | 2,400mg | 2,400mg |
| Total Carbohydrate | | 300g | 375g |

For educational purposes only. This label does not meet the labeling requirements described in 21 CFR 101.9.

**1 Serving Size**
This section is the basis for determining number of calories, amount of each nutrient, and %DVs of a food. Use it to compare a serving size to how much you actually eat. Serving sizes are given in familiar units, such as cups or pieces, followed by the metric amount, e.g., number of grams.

**2 Amount of Calories**
If you want to manage your weight (lose, gain, or maintain), this section is especially helpful. The amount of calories is listed on the left side. The right side shows how many calories in one serving come from fat. In this example, there are 250 calories, 110 of which come from fat. The key is to balance how many calories you eat with how many calories your body uses. ***Tip:*** *Remember that a product that's fat-free isn't necessarily calorie-free.*

**3 Limit these Nutrients**
Eating too much total fat (including saturated fat and trans fat), cholesterol, or sodium may increase your risk of certain chronic diseases, such as heart disease, some cancers, or high blood pressure. The goal is to stay below 100%DV for each of these nutrients per day.

**4 Get Enough of these Nutrients**
Americans often don't get enough dietary fiber, vitamin A, vitamin C, calcium, and iron in their diets. Eating enough of these nutrients may improve your health and help reduce the risk of some diseases and conditions.

**5 Percent (%) Daily Value**
This section tells you whether the nutrients (total fat, sodium, dietary fiber, etc.) in one serving of food contribute a little or a lot to your total daily diet.

The %DVs are based on a 2,000-calorie diet. Each listed nutrient is based on 100% of the recommended amounts for that nutrient. For example, 18% for total fat means that one serving furnishes 18% of the total amount of fat that you could eat in a day and stay within public health recommendations. Use the Quick Guide to Percent DV (%DV): 5%DV or less is low and 20%DV or more is high.

**6 Footnote with Daily Values (DVs)**
The footnote provides information about the DVs for important nutrients, including fats, sodium and fiber. The DVs are listed for people who eat 2,000 or 2,500 calories each day.

– The amounts for total fat, saturated fat, cholesterol, and sodium are maximum amounts. That means you should try to stay below the amounts listed.

**FIG. 16.5** Nutrition facts label. *(From U.S. Department of Health and Human Services, Food and Drug Administration. Available at* http://www.fda.gov/. *Accessed August 22, 2013.)*

## Labeling Ingredients

Almost all foods are required to have the ingredients listed on the package. Ingredients are listed in descending order of weight to indicate the proportion of any ingredient. For example, by reading a label on a fruit drink, you may find that only 5 percent of the drink is fruit juice (see Fig. 16.5).

Artificial coloring must also be named in the list of ingredients. It is no longer acceptable to simply state "color added." The government has set strict conditions under which statements such as "low-fat" and "a good source of fiber" can be used as part of the front label on the product.

## Label Claims

Examples of nutrient claims include "high fiber," "reduced calorie," and "cholesterol free." Usually, these claims are based on a comparison with the "regular" version of the product. For example, a *reduced fat* claim on a jar of peanut butter means that the peanut butter has at least 25 percent less fat than the regular peanut butter. A *light* salad dressing has at least 50 percent less fat or one third fewer calories than the regular dressing.

Other labels show that a food is high or low in a particular nutrient. For example, *low-fat* Italian salad dressing has 3 g of fat or less per 2-tablespoon (30-g) serving, and *fat-free* Italian salad dressing has less than 0.5 g of fat per serving (Box 16.3).

## Organic Foods

In 1990 the USDA put forth rules regarding the labeling of food that was "organically grown." Now, foods with the **organic** label must have been grown without the use of

### BOX 16.3 Food Label Terminology

**Calories**

- *Calorie free:* Fewer than 5 calories per serving
- *Low calorie:* 40 calories or fewer per serving, or per 50 g of the food
- *Reduced or fewer calories:* At least 25% fewer calories per serving than reference food

**Fat**

- *Fat free:* Less than 0.5 g of fat per serving
- *Saturated fat free:* Less than 0.5 g per serving and the level of *trans*-fatty acids does not exceed 1% of total fat
- *Low fat:* 3 g or less per serving, or per 50 g of the food
- *Low saturated fat:* 1 g or less per serving and not more than 15% of calories from saturated fatty acids
- *Reduced or less fat:* At least 25% less per serving than reference food
- *Reduced or less saturated fat:* At least 25% less per serving than reference food

**Cholesterol**

- *Cholesterol free:* Less than 2 mg of cholesterol and 2 g or less of saturated fat per serving
- *Low cholesterol:* 20 mg or less and 2 g or less of saturated fat per serving, or per 50 g of the food
- *Reduced or less cholesterol:* At least 25% less and 2 g or less of saturated fat per serving than reference food

**Sodium**

- *Sodium free:* Less than 5 mg per serving
- *Low sodium:* 140 mg or less per serving, or per 50 g of the food
- *Very low sodium:* 35 mg or less per serving, or per 50 g of the food
- *Reduced or less sodium:* At least 50% less per serving than reference food

**Fiber**

- *High fiber:* 5 g or more per serving (Foods with high-fiber claims must meet the definition for low fat, or the level of total fat must appear next to the high-fiber claim.)
- *Good source of fiber:* 2.5 to 4.9 g per serving
- *More* or *added fiber:* At least 2.5 g more per serving than reference food

**Sugar**

- *Sugar free:* Less than 0.5 g per serving
- *No added sugar, without added sugar,* or *no sugar added:* No sugars are added during processing or packaging, including ingredients that contain sugars (e.g., fruit juices, applesauce, dried fruit)
- Processing does not increase the sugar content to an amount higher than is naturally present in the ingredients (A functionally insignificant increase in sugars is acceptable from processes used for purposes other than increasing sugar content.)
- The food that resembles it and for which it substitutes normally contains added sugars
- If it does not meet the requirements for a low- or reduced-calorie food, that product bears a statement that the food is not low calorie or reduced calorie and that directs consumers' attention to the nutritional panel for additional information on sugar and calorie content
- *Reduced sugar:* At least 25% less sugar per serving than reference food

**Healthy**

Products using the term "healthy" in the product name or as a claim on the label must contain, per serving, no more than 3 g of fat, 1 g of saturated fat, 350 mg of sodium, or 60 mg of cholesterol. They must supply at least 10% of the daily value for at least one of six nutrients: vitamins A and C, calcium, iron, protein, and fiber. Raw meat, poultry, and fish can be labeled "healthy" if they contain, per serving, no more than 5 g of fat, 2 g of saturated fat, and 95 mg of cholesterol.

From Stegeman CA, Ratcliff Davis J: The dental hygienist's guide to nutritional care, ed 4, St Louis, 2015, Saunders; modified from U.S. Food and Drug Administration: Food labeling guide. September 1994; revised October 2009. Accessed August 22, 2013, at: www.fda.gov/FoodLabelingGuide.

TABLE 16.6 Common Diet-Related Disorders

| Disorders | Major Dietary Components | Corrective Dietary Measures |
|---|---|---|
| Allergies | Wide variety of foods are possible allergens: wheat, milk, eggs, chocolate most common | Eliminate or restrict food sources of allergen. |
| Anemia | Deficiency of iron, vitamin $B_{12}$, or folacin | Increase intake of deficient nutrient. |
| Anorexia nervosa | Starvation, fear of becoming fat, altered body image | Recommend a high-calorie diet, psychotherapy, behavior modification. |
| Atherosclerosis | High cholesterol, high saturated fat, excessive calories | Control calories; decrease total fat in diet to 30%–35% of calories; change to increased unsaturated fats, lower cholesterol content of diet; stress complex carbohydrates rather than simple sugars. |
| Bulimia | Binge eating, self-induced vomiting | Recommend regular diet, behavior modification, psychotherapy. |
| Cancer of the colon | Low fiber | Increase dietary fiber and fluids. |
| Cirrhosis of the liver | Excessive ingestion of alcohol or nutrients | Reduce dietary level of excessive nutrient or substance. |
| Constipation/diverticulosis | Poor fiber intake, poor fluid intake | Increase dietary fiber and fluids. |
| Diabetes mellitus | Obesity, excessive sugar consumption | Control calories and carbohydrates. |
| Hypertension | Obesity, high salt intake | Control calories, decrease sodium intake. |
| Obesity | Excessive calorie intake, inadequate physical activity | Decrease calories, increase activity, recommend behavior modification and group therapy. |

From Proctor DB et al: Kinn's the medical assistant, ed 13, St Louis, 2017, Elsevier.

chemical pesticides, herbicides, or fertilizers. Also, the use of hormones in organic seed preparation is prohibited.

In addition, regulations have been provided regarding meat, poultry, and milk. As with plants, the use of hormones is prohibited during the organic animal's growth or the product's preparation for consumption. Organic milk must contain no added vitamins or chemicals, and preparations are closely monitored.

Regulations regarding labeling of organic products protect the consumer by ensuring that products are in fact "organic."

## Eating Disorders

On the flip side of the obesity epidemic in the United States is the serious threat caused by eating disorders. Influences of the media and the fashion industry and perceived cultural values have led to a preoccupation with being thin. Such influences have contributed to a society of weight-conscious adolescents and adults and an increase in eating disorders. Eating disorders have serious medical, oral, and psychological implications and can be life threatening. Eating disorders commonly occur during adolescence and adulthood and include *anorexia nervosa* and *bulimia* (the two most common), as well as other related disorders such as *binge eating, compulsive overeating, female athlete triad,* and *chronic dieting syndrome.* Most of those who suffer from eating disorders are 14 to 25 years old, white, and affluent. The occurrence of eating disorders is much more common among females; the ratio of affected females to males is 10:1 (Table 16.6).

### Bulimia

**Bulimia** is often referred to as "bingeing and purging" disorder. Often, this pattern occurs when an individual is only slightly overweight and tries to lose weight by dieting but fails to achieve the desired results. This person believes that self-worth is related to being thin.

Usually, the pattern begins with some form of upset or stress, after which the individual finds comfort in eating a huge amount of high-calorie food. The eating binge is followed by guilt and behaviors that may include self-induced vomiting, food abstinence, the use of laxatives and enemas, and excessive exercise.

Most bulimic individuals want help and often make attempts to get into a treatment program. In the dental office, bulimic individuals are easily recognized because they often have severe wear on the lingual surfaces of their teeth caused by stomach acid produced by repeated vomiting (Fig. 16.6).

### Anorexia Nervosa

**Anorexia nervosa** is characterized by self-starvation. Affected individuals are usually female and in their early to middle twenties. They have an abnormal fear of becoming fat and have a severely distorted image of their body. Without medical intervention, persons with anorexia nervosa become extremely malnourished, lose excessive amounts of weight, and die.

Physical signs of possible anorexia nervosa include muscle wasting, amenorrhea (stopping menstruation), dry skin, constipation, brittle nails, and thin brittle hair. Because calcium intake is usually decreased, the strength of the teeth and the health of the periodontal tissues are reduced.

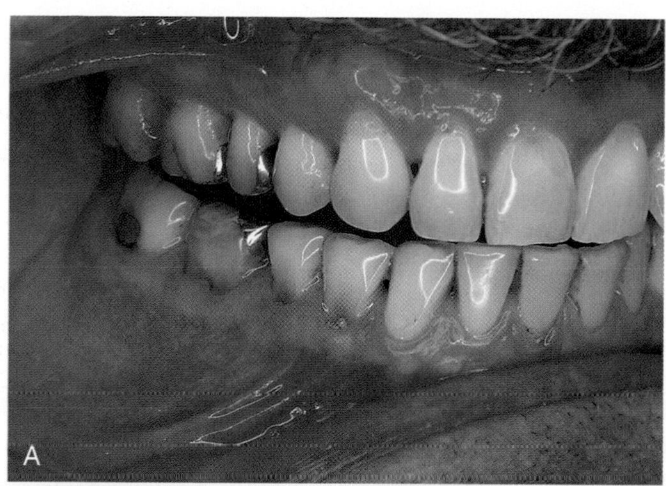


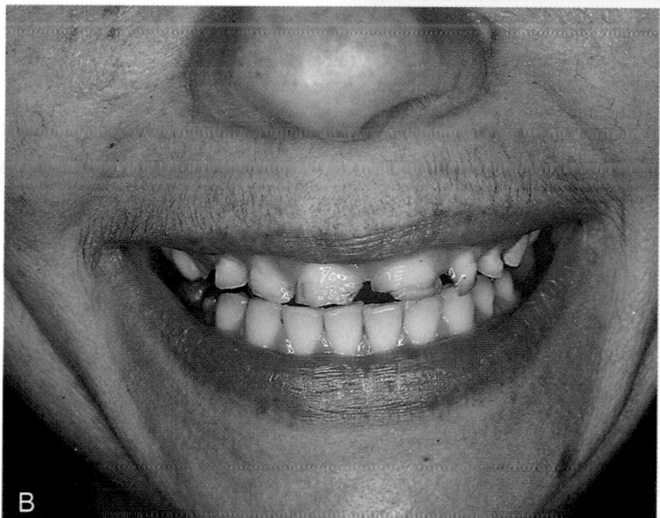


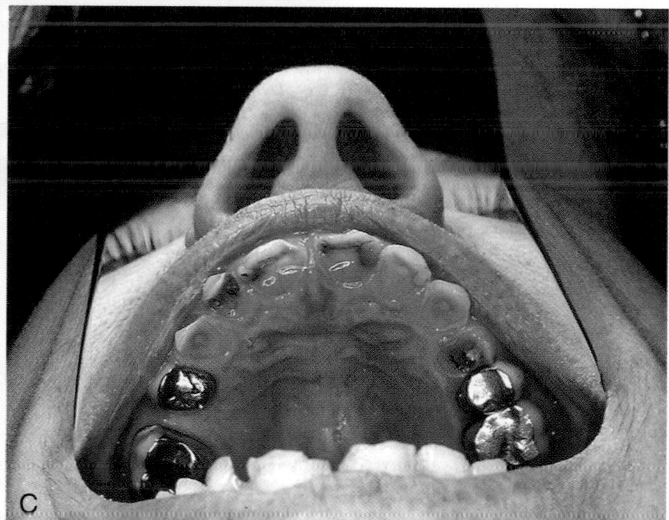


**FIG. 16.6** A, Erosion of buccal and lingual surfaces that occurred as a result of accidental exposure to sulfuric acid. Erosion caused by bulimia. B, Decreased tooth size. C, Erosion of maxillary lingual surfaces. *(From Ibsen OA, Phelan JA: Oral pathology for the dental hygienist, ed 6, St Louis, 2014, Saunders.)*

## Female Athlete Triad

This condition affects young female athletes and is characterized by an eating disorder that includes restrictive dieting, overexercising, weight loss, and lack of body fat. It results in osteoporosis (bone thinning) and amenorrhea. Dental risks include enamel decalcification, increased caries, and increased periodontal and soft tissue inflammation.

## Management of Eating Disorders

Anorexia nervosa and bulimia are considered psychiatric diseases with serious medical, dental, and nutritional complications. Dental professionals are often the first healthcare providers to diagnose an eating disorder. In addition to providing dental care and education, the dentist is obligated to assist the patient in obtaining psychotherapy and medical care.

Successful management of these disorders requires a team approach that includes the involvement of psychiatrists, psychologists, physicians, nurses, dietitians, social workers, and dentists. The road to recovery is often long and expensive.

RECALL

**14** Which governmental agency regulates the labeling of food products?
**15** What criteria are used to determine whether a product is "organic"?
**16** What are the two most serious eating disorders?

## Healthy Habits

As a dental assistant, you can educate your patients regarding the following five healthy habits for a long life:

- *Eat right.* Consume five servings of fruits and vegetables daily, plus generous portions of grains, beans, and dairy products.
- *Keep bones strong.* Include sufficient calcium in your diet. If you do not receive enough direct sunlight, take a daily supplement of vitamin D, which helps your body absorb calcium more effectively.
- *Protect the immune system.* Be sure to eat whole grains, green leafy vegetables, seafood, lean meats, and moderate amounts

of vegetable oils to receive vitamins E and $B_6$ and the trace mineral zinc. These substances help your body to fight infection and chronic disease.

- *Maintain a healthy body weight.* Excess fat can hasten the onset of diabetes, heart disease, arthritis, and other problems.
- *Exercise.* Combine aerobic exercises such as walking or running with simple stretch training to strengthen your muscles.

■ **Patient Education** As a dental assistant, you can help your patients prevent dental disease. You can teach them how to adjust their diet and make more healthful food choices.
For your teaching to be effective, you must have a thorough understanding of the material you are going to discuss and the rationale behind it. The following tips are helpful when you are providing nutrition information to patients:

- Use pictures and charts to illustrate your points
- Remember that ethnic and cultural foods are important to patients
- Encourage patients to play an active role in the learning process
- Invite patients to call the office whenever questions or concerns arise
- Use resources such as the USDA MyPlate ■

■ **Legal and Ethical Implications** Information you provide to the patient during dietary counseling should be documented in the patient's record.

Dental assistants should not counsel patients beyond the scope of dentistry (e.g., weight control, eating disorders). If you see signs of nutrition-related diseases or deficiencies, notify the dentist so that the patient may be referred to a physician for diagnosis and treatment. ■

■ **Eye to the Future** Research today is focusing on nutrition as a tool that can be used to help prevent chronic disease and prolong life. Already, advances in genetic engineering have resulted in lower-fat meats, tomatoes with good flavor year round, and virus-resistant vegetables. Fortification is being used to boost the quantities of nutrients in foods and to add nutrients to foods that do not usually contain them. For example, orange juice is now being fortified with calcium and vitamin D. The science of nutrition will continue to evolve in this direction. ■

## ■ Critical Thinking

1. Access the MyPlate Web site and analyze your own dietary habits. Are there any areas in which you need to improve?
2. Linda Hines is a 17-year-old patient in your dental office. While sitting in the reception area, Linda notices a poster of MyPlate on the wall and asks you what it means. How would you explain the concept of the plate?
3. Leanne is an energetic cheerleader who attends a local high school. She is very conscious about her appearance, especially her weight. She does not appear malnourished and does not exhibit any oral manifestations of bulimia. She tells you that she tries to "watch her diet." Would you have any suggestions or recommendations for Leanne?
4. The label on a bag of "light" potato chips indicates that only 100 calories are included per serving. What is the other important piece of information that you should know before you eat that bag of potato chips? ■

17

# Oral Pathology

## KEY TERMS

**Abscess (AB-ses)** Localized area of pus originating from an infection.
**Acute inflammation** Minimal and short-lasting injury to tissue.
**Biopsy (BYE-op-see)** Removal of tissue from living patients for diagnostic examination.
**Candidiasis (kan-di-DYE-i-sis)** Superficial infection caused by a yeastlike fungus.
**Carcinoma (kahr-si-NOE-muh)** Malignant tumor in epithelial tissue.
**Cellulitis (sel-yoo-LYE-tis)** Inflammation of cellular or connective tissue.
**Chronic inflammation** Continuous injury or irritation to tissue.
**Congenital (kun-JEN-i-tul) disorders** Disorders that are present at birth.
**Cyst (sist)** Closed cell or pouch with a definite wall.
**Ecchymosis (ek-i-MOE-sis)** Technical term for bruising.
**Erosion** Wearing away of tissue.
**Glossitis (glos-EYE-tis)** Inflammation of the tongue.
**Granuloma (gran-yoo-LOE-muh)** A granular tumor or growth.
**Hematoma (hee-muh-TOE-muh)** Swelling or mass of blood collected in one area or organ.
**Inflammation** Protective response of the tissues to irritation or injury.
**Lesion (LEE-zhun)** An area of pathology.
**Leukemia (loo-KEE-mee-uh)** A progressive disease in which the bone marrow produces an increased number of immature or abnormal white cells.
**Leukoplakia (loo-koe-PLAY-kee-ah)** Formation of white spots or patches on the oral mucosa.
**Lichen (LI-kun) planus** Benign, chronic disease that affects the skin and oral mucosa.
**Lymphadenopathy (lim-fad-uh-NOP-uh-thee)** Disease or swelling of the lymph nodes.
**Lymphoma (lim-FOE-muh)** Malignant disorder of the lymphoid tissue.
**Metastasize (muh-TAS-tuh-size)** To spread (disease) from one part of the body to another.
**Methamphetamine** Potent central nervous system stimulant.
**Meth mouth** Informal name for the rampant tooth decay caused by heavy methamphetamine use.
**Pathology (pa-THOL-uh-jee)** The study of disease.
**Petechiae (pe-TEE-kee-uh)** Small, pinpoint red spots on the skin or mucous membrane.
**Sarcoma (sahr-KOE-muh)** Malignant tumor in connective tissue such as muscle or bone.
**Tori (TOR-eye, TOR-ee)** Abnormal growths of bone in a specific area.
**Xerostomia (zeer-oe-STOE-mee-uh)** Dryness of the mouth caused by reduction of saliva.

## LEARNING OUTCOMES

*On completion of this chapter, the student will be able to achieve the following objectives:*

1. Pronounce, define, and spell the key terms.
2. Explain why oral pathology is important for the dental assistant.
3. Describe the steps necessary to make a diagnosis.
4. Describe the difference between acute and chronic inflammation, including the classic signs of inflammation.
5. Describe the types of oral lesions.
6. Name three types of diseases of the oral soft tissues.
7. Describe three conditions associated with the tongue.
8. Discuss oral cancer, including the following:
   - Describe the warning symptoms of oral cancer.
   - Describe leukemia.
   - Describe the appearance of lesions associated with the use of smokeless tobacco.
   - Name three types of therapy for oral cancer.
9. Discuss HIV/AIDS and its oral manifestations, including five lesions that are associated with HIV/AIDS.
10. Recognize developmental disorders of the jaws and dentition, including the following:
    - List and define three anomalies that affect jaw development.
    - List and define an anomaly that affects lip, palate, and tongue development.
    - List and define three anomalies that affect the number of teeth.
    - List and define five anomalies related to the shape of the teeth.
    - Explain the conditions associated with abnormal eruption of the teeth.
11. Discuss other types of disorders that can occur, including the following:
    - Identify two oral conditions related to nutritional factors.
    - Describe bruxism.
    - Describe the oral conditions of a patient with bulimia.
    - Describe the dental complications of oral piercings.
    - Identify the oral effects of methamphetamine use.

## ELECTRONIC RESOURCES

e ***Additional information related to content in Chapter 17 can be found on the companion Evolve Web site.***

- Practice Quiz

Oral **pathology** is the study of diseases in the oral cavity. Only a dentist or a physician may diagnose pathologic *(disease)* conditions, but it is important for the dental assistant to be able to recognize the differences between normal and abnormal conditions that appear in the mouth. For example, while taking radiographs or impressions, the dental assistant might notice a lesion in the patient's mouth that appears abnormal. The dental assistant would then inform the dentist so that a diagnosis could be made.

Many *systemic diseases,* as well as *infectious diseases,* have oral manifestations (signs and symptoms). The dental assistant should understand how oral abnormalities affect the patient's general health and planned dental treatment.

Before you can recognize abnormal conditions in the mouth, you must have a solid understanding of the appearance of normal oral conditions. You might want to review the appearance of normal oral tissues in Chapter 10.

As a dental assistant, you should understand the terms used to describe pathologic conditions and should record preliminary identification and descriptions of lesions. You should use these terms in the clinical setting so that they become part of your everyday professional vocabulary. You then can communicate effectively with other professionals.

In addition to pathologic conditions, this chapter presents conditions that are variations of normal but are not considered pathologic.

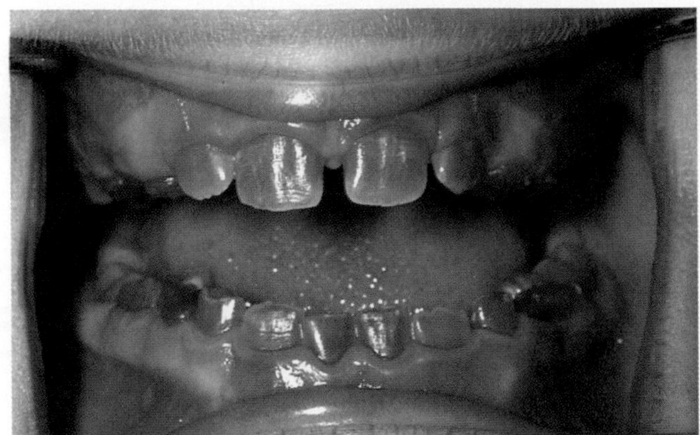

**FIG. 17.1** Dentinogenesis imperfecta. *(From Dean J, Avery DR, McDonald RE: McDonald & avery's dentistry for the child and adolescent, ed 10, St Louis, 2016, Elsevier.)*

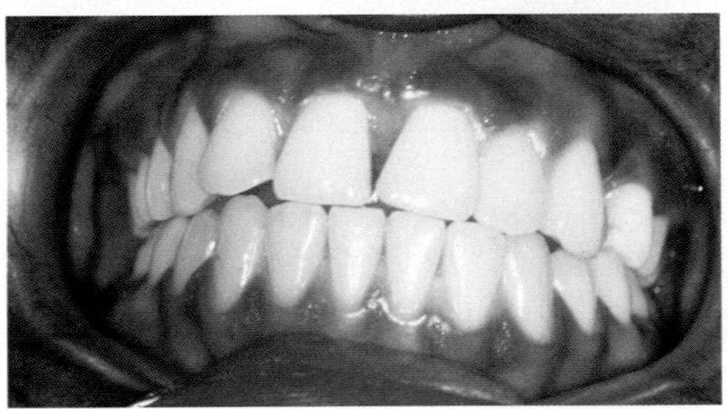

**FIG. 17.2** Melanin pigmentation. *(From Ibsen O, Phelan JA: Oral pathology for the dental hygienist, ed 6, St Louis, 2014, Saunders.)*

## Making a Diagnosis

Making an accurate diagnosis is much like putting a puzzle together—many pieces are necessary. To make an accurate diagnosis, the dentist must rely on a variety of types of information. Remember, one piece of information alone usually is not enough to make a diagnosis. Eight sources of information can be used to make a final diagnosis. These include *historical, clinical, radiographic, microscopic, laboratory, therapeutic, surgical,* and *differential findings.* Imagine each of these findings as a piece of a puzzle that leads to diagnosis.

### Historical Diagnosis

Personal history, family history, medical and dental histories, and history of the lesion are often useful in making a diagnosis. Family histories are important because of genetic disorders such as dentinogenesis imperfecta (Fig. 17.1). Melanin pigmentation of the gingiva is common in dark-skinned individuals (Fig. 17.2). Medical histories can provide information about medication the patient may be taking that could have an effect on the oral tissues.

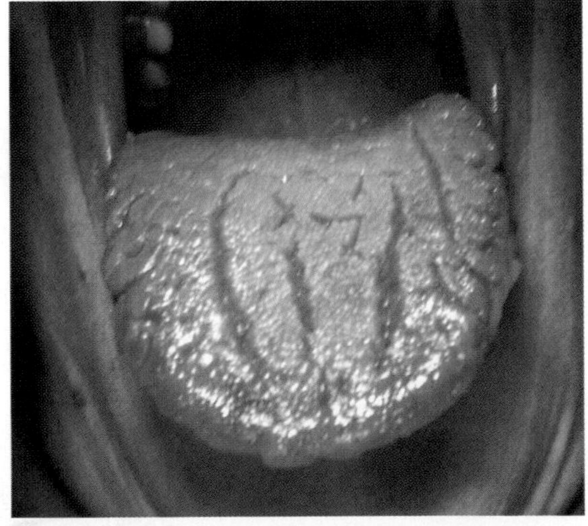

**FIG. 17.3** Fissured tongue. *(From Ibsen O, Phelan JA: Oral pathology for the dental hygienist, ed 6, St Louis, 2014, Saunders.)*

### Clinical Diagnosis

A clinical diagnosis is based on the clinical appearance of the lesion, including the color, size, shape, and location. Examples of conditions diagnosed on the basis of clinical appearance are fissured tongue (Fig. 17.3), maxillary and mandibular **tori** and torus palatinus (Fig. 17.4), and median rhomboid glossitis (Fig. 17.5).

### Radiographic Diagnosis

Radiographs are excellent in providing information about periapical pathology (Fig. 17.6), internal resorption (Fig. 17.7), and impacted teeth (Fig. 17.8).

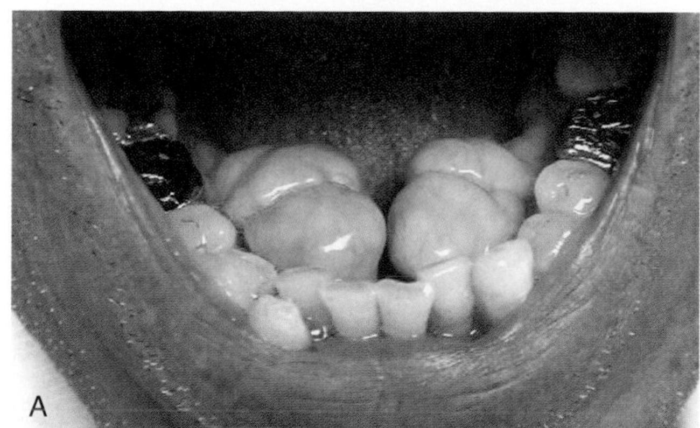


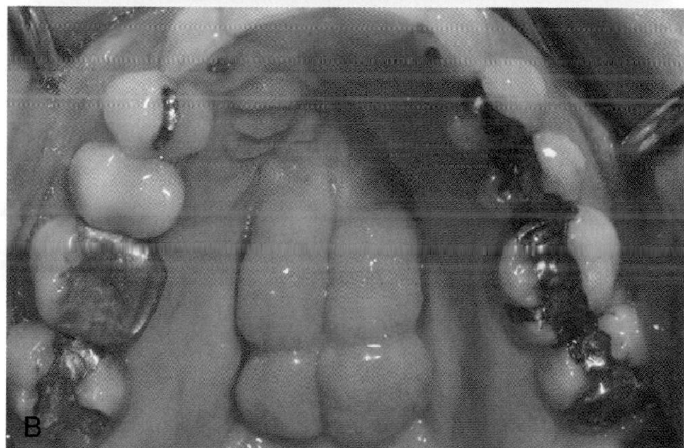


**FIG. 17.4** A, Clinical appearance of bilateral mandibular tori. B, Clinical appearance of lobulated torus palatinus. *(A, From Swartz MH: Textbook of physical diagnosis, ed 7, Philadelphia, 2014, Saunders. B, From Neville BW, et al: Oral and maxillofacial pathology, ed 4, St Louis, 2016, Elsevier.)*

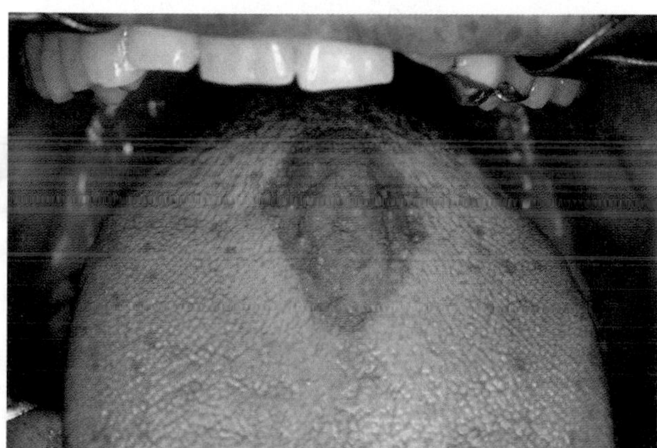

**FIG. 17.5** Median rhomboid glossitis *(arrow)*. *(From Regezi JA, Sciubba JJ, Jordan RCK: Oral pathology: clinical pathologic correlations, ed 7, St Louis, 2017, Elsevier.)*

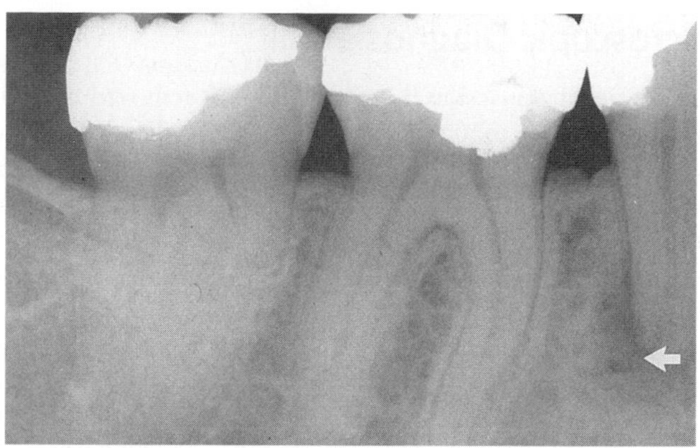

**FIG. 17.6** Periapical pathology. *(From Ibsen O, Phelan JA: Oral pathology for the dental hygienist, ed 6, St Louis, 2014, Saunders.)*

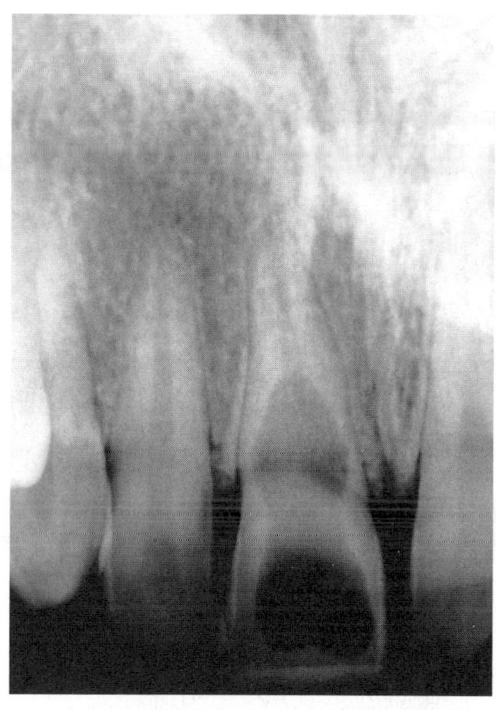

**FIG. 17.7** Internal resorption. *(From Regezi JA, Sciubba JJ, Jordan RCK: Oral pathology: clinical pathologic correlations, ed 7, St Louis, 2017, Elsevier.)*

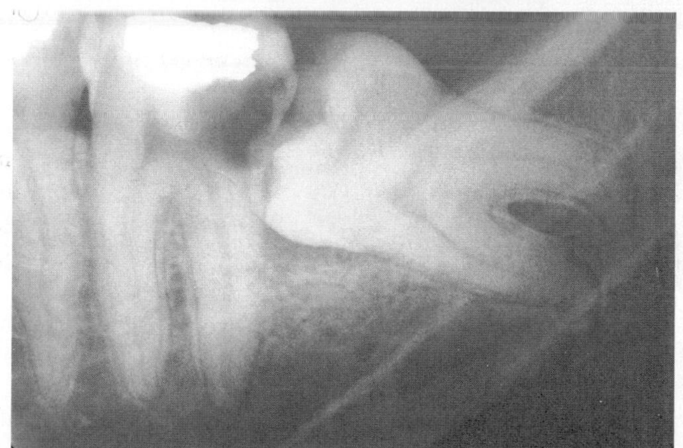

**FIG. 17.8** Horizontal impaction of the third molar. *(From Sapp JP, Eversole LR, Wysocki GP: Contemporary oral and maxillofacial pathology, ed 2, St Louis, 2002, Mosby.)*

## Microscopic Diagnosis

When a suspicious lesion is present, tissue is removed from the lesion and is sent to a pathology laboratory, where it is evaluated microscopically (called **biopsy**). This procedure is very often used to make the definitive (final) diagnosis. For example, a white lesion cannot be diagnosed on the basis of clinical appearance alone. A biopsy must be performed to determine whether or not the lesion is malignant.

## Laboratory Diagnosis

Blood chemistries and other laboratory tests, including urinalysis, can provide information that leads to a diagnosis. Cultures done in the laboratory can be used to diagnose types of oral infection.

## Therapeutic Diagnosis

Therapeutic diagnosis is made by providing a treatment (therapy) and seeing how the condition responds. For example, angular cheilitis (Fig. 17.9) may be caused by lack of the B-complex vitamins, or it could simply be a fungal infection. If angular cheilitis improves after the patient is given an antifungal cream, the vitamin deficiency theory can be ruled out.

## Surgical Diagnosis

A diagnosis is made on the basis of findings from a surgical procedure. For example, on a radiograph, a traumatic bone cyst (Fig. 17.10) looks like a static bone cyst (Fig. 17.11). However, one condition would require treatment, whereas the other would not. Surgically opening the area and inspecting it would reveal whether the radiolucency on the radiograph was indeed a condition that required further treatment.

## Differential Diagnosis

When two or more possible causes of a condition are identified, a differential diagnosis must be made. The dentist will determine which tests or procedures should be done to rule out the incorrect cause and make a final diagnosis.

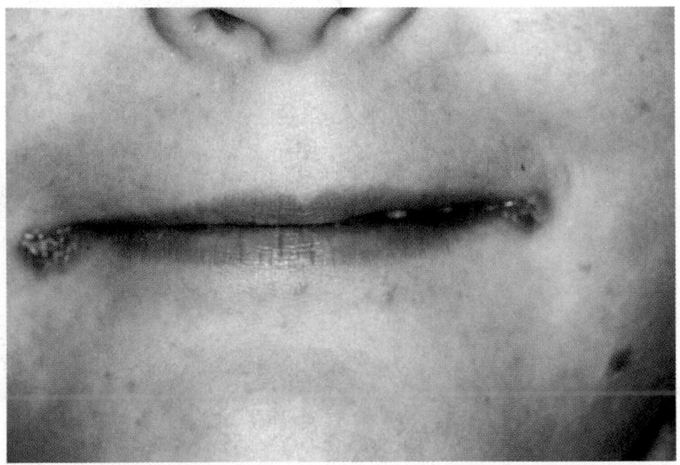

**FIG. 17.9** Angular cheilitis. *(From Kliegman RM, et al: Nelson textbook of pediatrics, ed 20, Philadelphia, 2016, Elsevier.)*

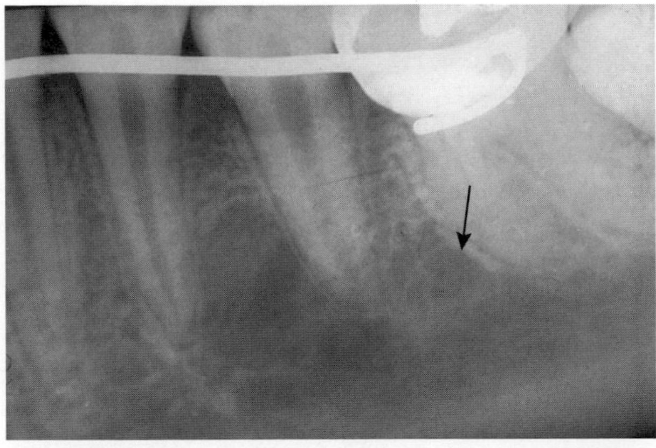

**FIG. 17.10** The *arrow* points to a traumatic bone cyst. *(Courtesy Dr. Edward V. Zegarelli.)*

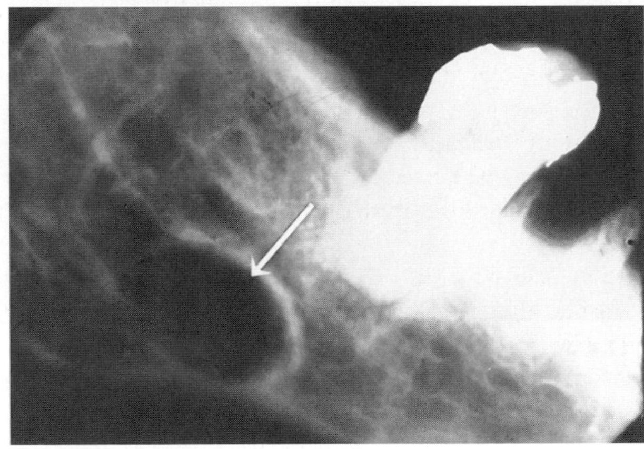

**FIG. 17.11** The *arrow* points to static bone cyst. *(Courtesy Dr. Edward V. Zegarelli.)*

# Acute/Chronic Inflammation

**Inflammation** is the body's protective response to irritation or injury. The inflammatory response is determined by the extent and duration of the injury. Inflammation can be acute or chronic. For example, **acute inflammation** occurs if injury to the tissue is minimal and short-lasting and the tissue begins to repair quickly. **Chronic inflammation** occurs when injury or irritation to the tissue continues. Inflammation of a specific tissue is described by the suffix *-itis* added to the name of the tissue (e.g., gingivitis, periodontitis, pulpitis). Refer to Chapter 14 for a discussion of gingival and periodontal inflammatory diseases.

### Classic Signs of Inflammation

- Redness
- Swelling
- Heat
- Pain

## Oral Lesions

**Lesion** is a broad term for abnormal tissues in the oral cavity. A lesion can be a wound, a sore, or any other tissue damage caused by injury or disease. It is important for the clinician to identify the type of lesion to make a diagnosis. Lesions of the oral mucosa are classified as to whether they extend below or extend above the mucosal surface, and whether they lie flat or even with the mucosal surface.

### Lesions Extending Below Mucosal Surface

An *ulcer* is a break in the mucosa that looks like a punched-out area, similar to a crater. An ulcer may be as small as 2 mm or as large as several centimeters.

An **erosion** of the soft tissue is a shallow injury in the mucosa caused by mechanical trauma, such as chewing. (*Trauma* means wound or injury.) The margins may be ragged and red and quite painful.

An **abscess** is a collection of pus in a specific area. Abscesses are commonly found at the apex of a tooth (periapical abscess). An abscess may be caused by bacteria in a badly decayed tooth or by bacteria resulting from a severe periodontal infection (see Chapter 14).

A **cyst** is a fluid or semisolid, fluid-filled sac. The material within the cyst is not always infectious. In dentistry, a cyst may form around the crown of an unerupted tooth (Fig. 17.12).

### Lesions Extending Above the Mucosal Surface

*Blisters,* also known as *vesicles,* are filled with a watery fluid. (They look like the blisters that appear on feet as a result of poorly fitting shoes.) They are rarely seen in the oral cavity because they tend to rupture, leaving ulcers with ragged edges.

A *pustule* looks like a blister, but it contains pus. A **hematoma** is also similar to a blister, but it contains blood.

A *plaque* is any patch or flat area that is slightly raised from the surface. (*Note.* This is *not* the same as dental plaque, which is discussed in Chapter 13.)

### Lesions Even with the Mucosal Surface

These lesions lie flat or even with the surface of the oral mucosa and are well-defined areas of discoloration. An **ecchymosis**, which is the medical term for *bruising,* is an example of this type of lesion.

### Raised or Flat Lesions

*Nodules,* which may appear below the surface or may be slightly elevated, are small, round, solid lesions. When palpated, a nodule feels like a pea beneath the surface.

**Granuloma** is a term with many meanings. In dentistry, it is often used to describe a type of nodule that contains granulation tissue. (The suffix *-oma* means tumor or neoplasm.) A granuloma may appear on the gingival surface as a swollen mass. It also may be located within the bone as a periapical granuloma at the apex of a nonvital tooth.

Tumors are also known as *neoplasms.* A tumor is any mass of tissue that grows beyond the normal size and serves no useful purpose. A tumor may be *benign* (not life threatening) or *malignant* (life threatening).

1 Which lesions are below the mucosal surface?
2 Which lesions extend above the mucosal surface?
3 What lesion is even with the mucosal surface?

## Diseases of the Oral Soft Tissues

### Leukoplakia

**Leukoplakia** is a general term that means "white patch." It may occur anywhere in the mouth. Very little pain is associated with leukoplakia unless ulceration and secondary infection are also present.

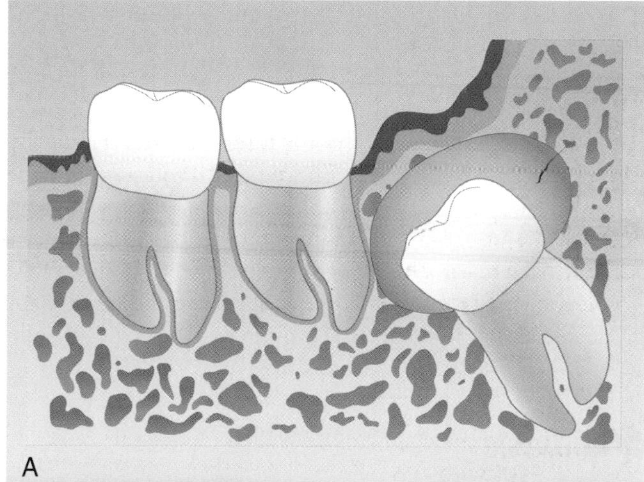


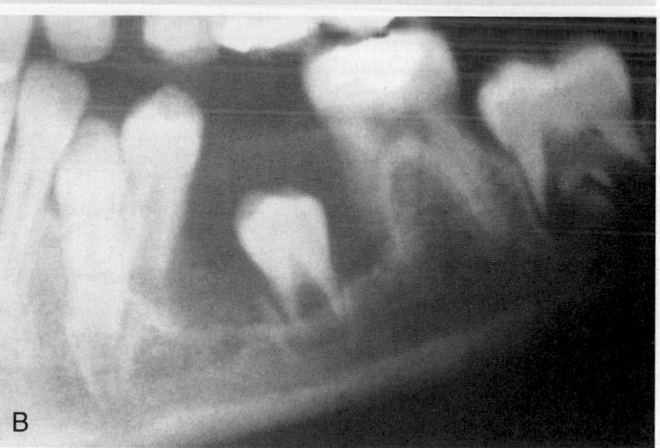


**FIG. 17.12** Dentigerous cysts around the crown of an unerupted bicuspid (A) and an impacted third molar (B). *(From Sapp JP, Eversole LR, Wysocki GP: Contemporary oral and maxillofacial pathology, ed 2, St Louis, 2002, Mosby.)*

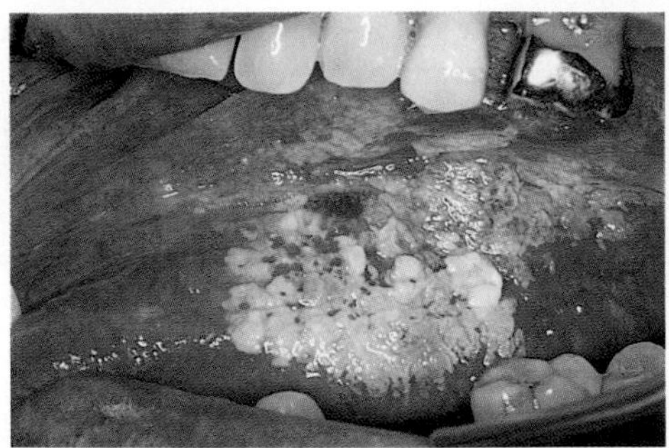

**FIG. 17.13** Leukoplakia. *(From Eisen D, Lynch DP: The mouth: diagnosis and treatment, St Louis, 1998, Mosby.)*

The lesions vary in appearance and texture from a fine, white transparency to a heavy, thick, warty plaque. To be classified as leukoplakia, the lesion should be firmly attached to the underlying tissue, and rubbing or scraping with an instrument should not remove it.

The cause of leukoplakia is unknown, but the presence of this disease is often linked to chronic irritation or trauma. Such injury may result from the use of smokeless tobacco, poorly fitting dentures, or cheek biting (Fig. 17.13).

Leukoplakia often appears before a malignant lesion develops, so early diagnosis and treatment are important.

## Lichen Planus

**Lichen planus** is a benign, chronic disease that affects the skin and oral mucosa. Many factors have been implicated in lichen planus, but the cause remains unknown.

On the oral mucosa, the patchy white lesions exhibit a characteristic pattern of circles and interconnecting lines called *Wickham's striae* (Fig. 17.14). A second type of lichen planus can cause erosive lesions on the gingiva. This type of lesion tends to worsen with emotional stress.

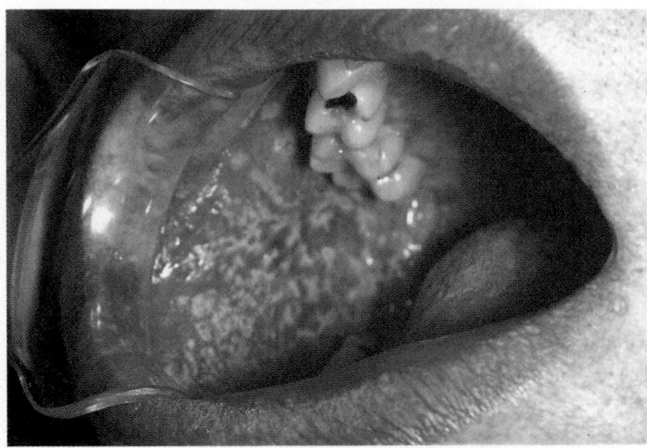

**FIG. 17.14** Lichen planus on the buccal mucosa. *(Courtesy Dr. Edward V. Zegarelli.)*

## Candidiasis

**Candidiasis** is a superficial infection caused by the yeastlike fungus *Candida albicans.* It is the most common oral fungal infection, but it does not usually occur in the healthy general population.

Candidiasis can result from antibiotic therapy, diabetes, xerostomia (dry mouth), and weakened immunologic reactions. It also may be the initial clinical manifestation for patients with acquired immunodeficiency syndrome (AIDS; see later discussion in this chapter).

Candidiasis is accompanied by discomfort or pain, *halitosis* (unpleasant breath odor), and *dysgeusia* (distorted sense of taste). Diaper rash, vaginitis, and thrush are other common types of candidiasis.

## Pseudomembranous Candidiasis

In pseudomembranous candidiasis, also known as *thrush,* creamy white plaques (resembling cottage cheese or curdled milk) form in the mouth (Fig. 17.15). The patient frequently describes a burning sensation, an unpleasant taste, or the feeling of "blisters forming in the mouth." These "blisters" generally prove to be the pseudomembranous plaques. (*Pseudomembranous* is a term that describes a false membrane or tissue.)

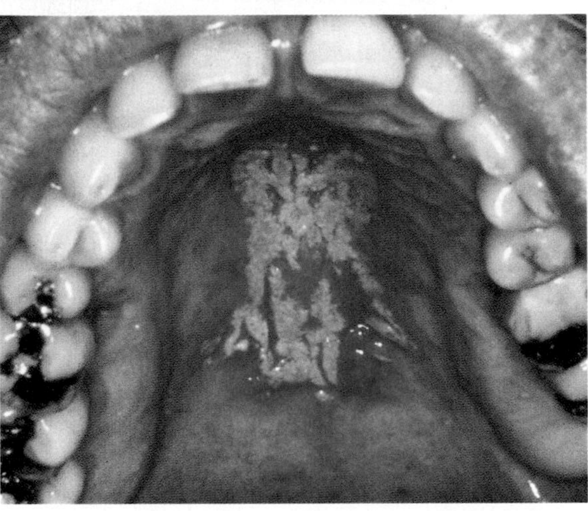

**FIG. 17.15** Pseudomembranous candidiasis. *(From Ibsen O, Phelan JA: Oral pathology for the dental hygienist, ed 6, St Louis, 2014, Saunders.)*

The plaques can be scraped off, and they rarely bleed when they are removed. When bleeding does occur, the patient likely has an additional mucosal problem. When this condition is seen in babies, it is called *infantile candidiasis.*

### Hyperplastic Candidiasis

Hyperplastic candidiasis appears as a white plaque that cannot be removed by scraping. This form is most often found on the buccal mucosa in patients infected with human immunodeficiency virus (HIV) (Fig. 17.16).

In most patients, antifungal therapy begins to resolve the infection within 2 to 3 days, with complete clearing noted after 10 to 14 days. If the lesions are still present after this time, or if they recur quickly, further investigation is necessary to rule out endocrine disturbances or immunologic deficiencies.

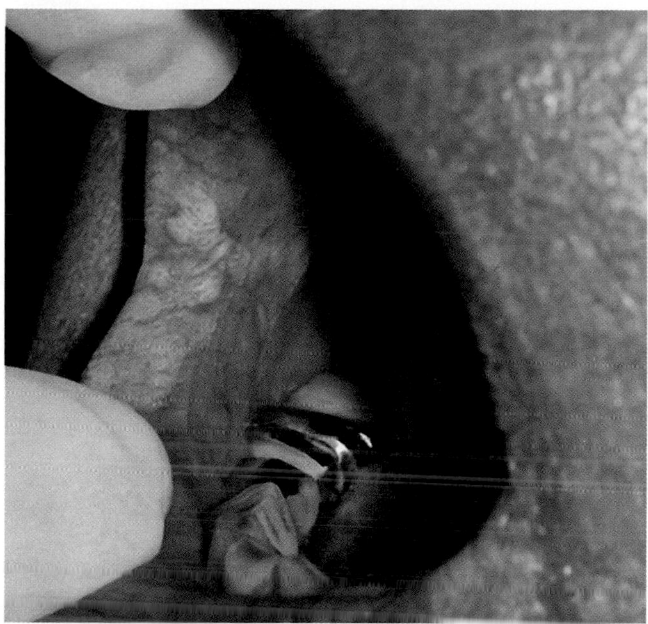

**FIG. 17.16** Chronic hyperplastic candidiasis. The white appearance of the tongue did not wipe off, and it disappeared with antifungal treatment. *(From Sapp JP, Eversole LR, Wysocki GP: Contemporary oral and maxillofacial pathology, ed 2, St Louis, 2002, Mosby.)*

### Atrophic Candidiasis

In atrophic candidiasis, also known as *erythematous candidiasis,* smooth red patches may appear on the dorsal areas of the tongue and palate. Atrophic candidiasis usually appears after the patient has been taking a broad-spectrum antibiotic. The patient may report that the mouth feels scalded or burned, "like swallowing something too hot."

In most patients, antifungal therapy begins to resolve the infection within 2 to 3 days, with complete clearing occurring after 10 to 14 days. If the lesions are still present after this time, or if they recur quickly, further investigation is necessary to rule out endocrine disturbances or immunologic deficiencies.

## Aphthous Ulcers

Aphthous ulcers, also known as "canker sores," occur as a common form of oral mucosal ulceration.

Recurrent aphthous ulcer (RAU) is a disease that causes recurring outbreaks of blister-like sores inside the mouth and on the lips. These sores appear on the lining mucosa of the cheeks; edge of the tongue; floor of the mouth; palates; and soft, red portion of the lip.

In the early stages of an outbreak, the patient experiences a burning sensation, followed by the formation of small blisters. When the blister breaks, a typical ulcer forms. The ulcer is small and oval, and the center is yellow to gray and is surrounded by a red margin.

*Minor RAU,* the mildest form of involvement, represents 90 percent of all cases. Patients usually experience recurring episodes fewer than six times a year, and the lesions typically heal within 7 to 10 days (Fig. 17.17).

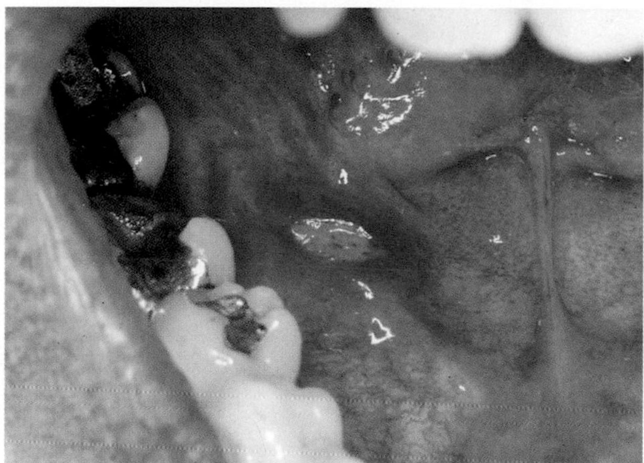

**FIG. 17.17** Minor aphthous ulcer. *(From Ibsen O, Phelan JA: Oral pathology for the dental hygienist, ed 6, St Louis, 2014, Saunders.)*

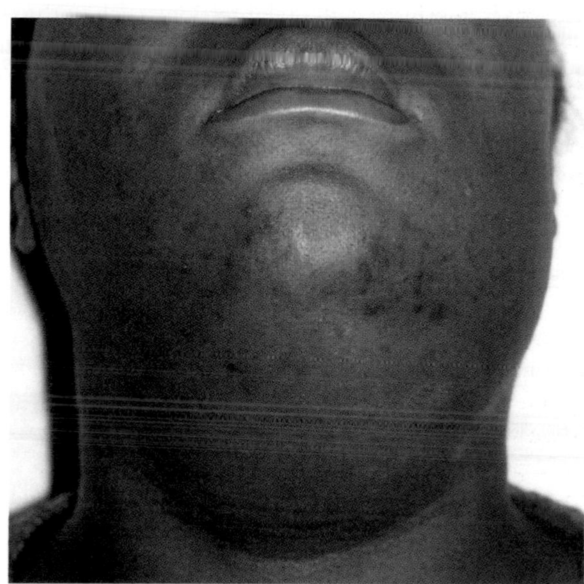

**FIG. 17.18** Cellulitis. Swelling is caused by increased local edema associated with a dental infection. The patient was hospitalized for treatment of the swelling. *(From Flynn TR: Surgical management of orofacial infections, Atlas Oral Maxillofac Surg Clin North Am 8:79, 2000.)*

*Major RAU,* which occurs in only about 10 percent of cases, is characterized by more frequent outbreaks of larger, deeper ulcers that take longer to heal. This is found most often in patients with a compromised immune system.

The patient with RAU is often debilitated (weakened) because these sores make eating and drinking difficult. Various agents, such as topical anesthetic agents for pain control and drugs to promote healing, may be prescribed.

## Cellulitis

**Cellulitis** is a condition in which an inflammation is *uncontrolled* within a localized area. It spreads throughout the soft tissue or organ (Fig. 17.18).

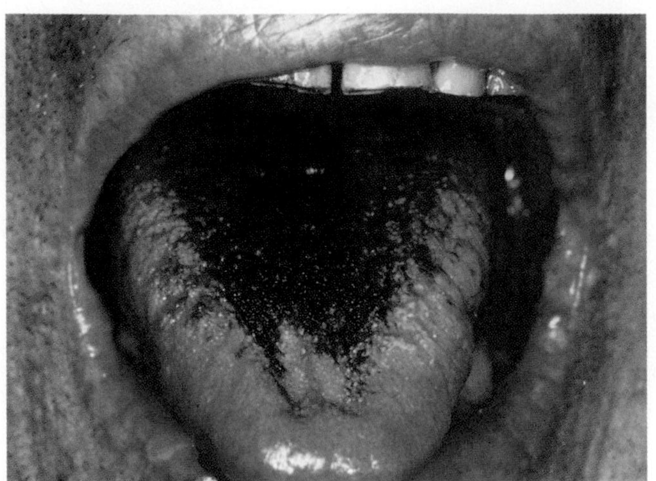

FIG. 17.19 Black hairy tongue. *(From Swartz MH: Textbook of physical diagnosis, ed 7, Philadelphia, 2014, Saunders.)*

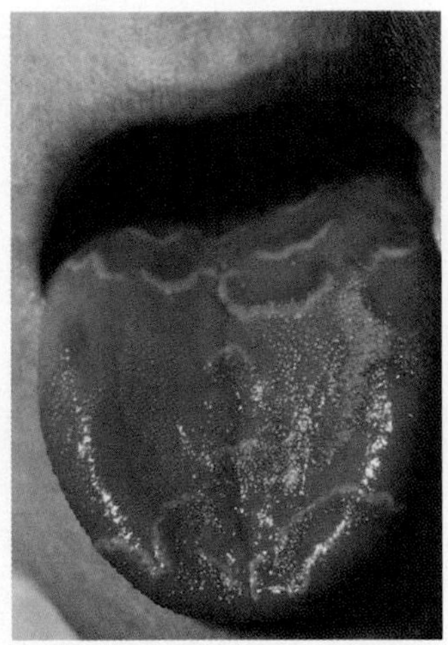

FIG. 17.20 Geographic tongue. *(From Swartz MH: Textbook of physical diagnosis, ed 7, Philadelphia, 2014, Saunders.)*

Cellulitis is associated with oral infections, such as abscessed teeth. Swelling usually develops rapidly. The patient has a high fever, the skin usually becomes very red, and the area is characterized by severe throbbing pain as the inflammation localizes.

Cellulitis can be dangerous because it can travel quickly to sensitive tissues such as the eye or the brain.

RECALL

4 What type of condition appears as a white patch or area?
5 What condition is caused by yeastlike fungal infection?
6 What is another term for "canker sore"?
7 What is the condition in which inflammation causes severe pain and high fever?

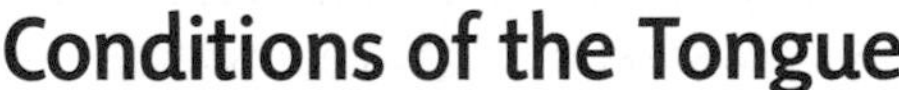

## Conditions of the Tongue

**Glossitis** is a general term that is used to describe inflammation and changes to the tongue. A condition called *black hairy tongue* may be caused by an oral flora imbalance after antibiotics are administered. In this condition, the filiform papillae become elongated so that they resemble hairs. These elongated papillae become stained by food and tobacco, producing the name "black hairy tongue" (Fig. 17.19).

In *geographic tongue,* the surface of the tongue loses areas of the filiform papillae in irregularly shaped patterns. The smooth areas resemble a map, thus the name "geographic tongue." Over days or weeks, the smooth areas and the whitish margins seem to change locations across the surface of the tongue by healing on one border and extending on another (Fig. 17.20). Geographic tongue affects 1 to 3 percent of the population. The condition occurs at all ages, and women are affected almost twice as often as men.

*Fissured tongue* is considered a variation of normal, and its cause is unknown (Fig. 17.21). Theories include a vitamin deficiency or chronic trauma over a long period. The top of the tongue appears to have deep fissures or grooves that become irritated if food debris collects in them. The patient with a fissured tongue is advised to brush the tongue gently with a soft toothbrush to keep the fissures clean of debris and irritants. No treatment is indicated for this condition.

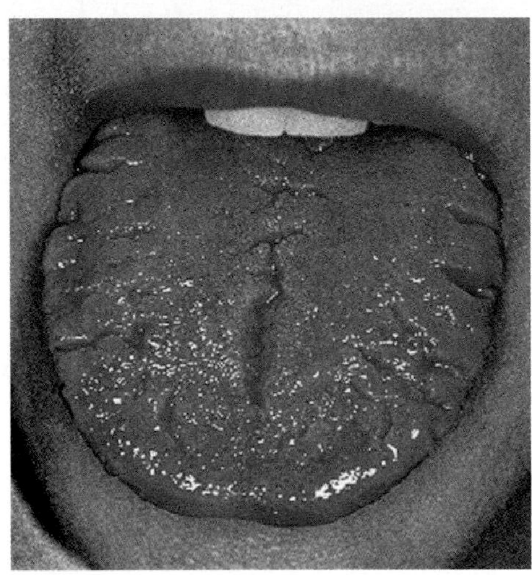

FIG. 17.21 Fissured tongue. *(From Casamassimo PS, et al: Pediatric dentistry: infancy through adolescence, ed 5, St Louis, Saunders.)*

*Pernicious anemia* is a condition in which the body does not absorb vitamin $B_{12}$. People who have this condition show signs of anemia, weakness, pallor, and fatigue on exertion. Other signs include nausea, diarrhea, abdominal pain, and loss of appetite.

Oral manifestations of pernicious anemia include *angular cheilitis* (ulceration and redness at the corners of the lips), mucosal ulceration, loss of papillae on the tongue, and a burning and painful tongue (Fig. 17.22).

RECALL

8 What is the term for an inflammation of the tongue?
9 What is the condition in which a pattern on the tongue changes?
10 What is the condition in which the body does not absorb vitamin $B_{12}$?

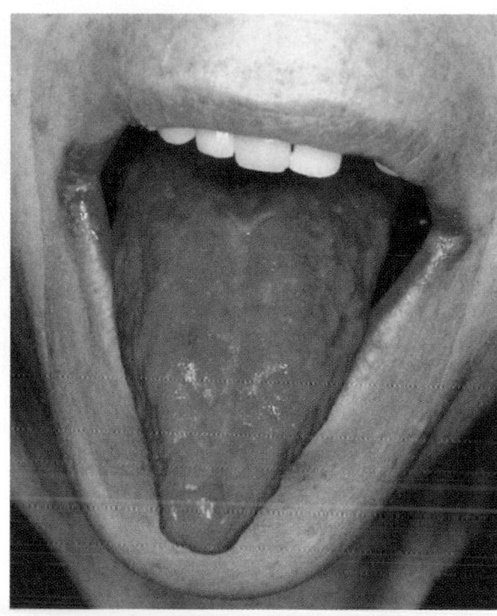

**FIG. 17.22** Pernicious anemia. Angular cheilitis and depapillation of the tongue in a patient with pernicious anemia. *(From Ibsen O, Phelan JA: Oral pathology for the dental hygienist, ed 6, St Louis, 2014, Saunders.)*

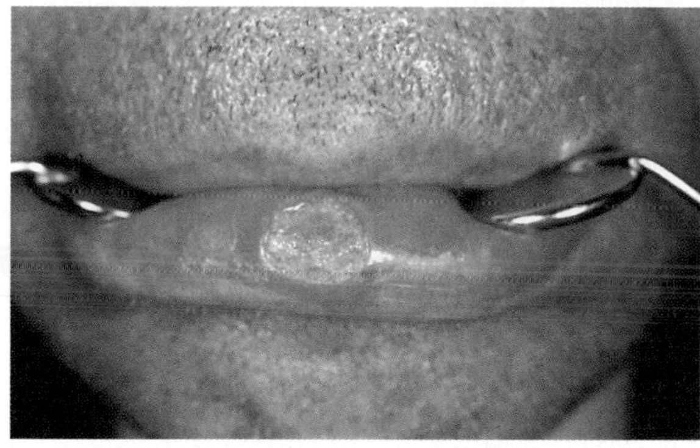

**FIG. 17.23** Clinical appearance of squamous cell carcinoma of the lower lip. *(From Ibsen O, Phelan JA: Oral pathology for the dental hygienist, ed 6, St Louis, 2014, Saunders.)*

## Oral Cancer

Oral cancer is one of the 10 most frequently occurring cancers in the world. In the United States the site most often affected is the vermilion border of the lip (Fig. 17.23).

In the early stages, most oral cancers are not painful; therefore they frequently go undetected. Oral cancers are frequently fatal if not detected early enough or if left untreated (Table 17.1).

A **carcinoma** is a malignant neoplasm (growth) of the epithelium (tissue lining the mouth) that tends to invade surrounding bone and connective tissue. These cancers quickly **metastasize** (spread) to other regions of the body, usually the neck and cervical lymph nodes.

Carcinomas occur on the lips, tongue, cheeks, and floor of the mouth. The lesions usually appear first as a white or ulcerated area, although some types may also appear as a velvety smooth red lesion.

**TABLE 17.1 Appearance of Early Cancer**

| Type of Lesion | Clinical Appearance |
|---|---|
| White areas | Lesions may vary from a filmy, barely visible change in the mucosa to a heavy, thick area of white tissue. Fissures or ulcers in a white area are most indicative of a malignancy. *Leukoplakia,* a white patch that cannot be wiped off, may be associated with chemical agents or tobacco. |
| Red areas | Lesions may have a velvety texture, sometimes with small ulcers. The term *erythroplakia* is used to designate lesions that appear as bright red patches. |
| Ulcers | Lesions may have flat or raised margins. Palpation may reveal *induration* (hardening). |
| Masses | Papillary masses, sometimes with ulcerated areas, occur as elevations above the surrounding tissues. Other masses may develop below the normal mucosa and may be found only by palpation. |
| Pigmentation | Black or brown pigmented areas may be located on the mucosa, where pigmentation does not normally occur. |

An *adenocarcinoma* is a malignant tumor that comes from the glands underlying the oral mucosa (the prefix *adeno-* means "gland"). This tumor first appears clinically as a lump or a bulge beneath overlying normal mucosa.

A **sarcoma** is a malignant neoplasm that comes from supportive and connective tissue such as bone. An *osteosarcoma* is a malignant tumor that involves the bone. In the mouth, the affected bones are those of the jaws. Although the cancer may start in the bone, it often spreads and involves surrounding soft tissues (Fig. 17.24).

### Oral Cancer Warning Signs

- Any sore in the mouth that does not heal
- Any lump or swelling on the neck, lips, or oral cavity
- White or rough-textured lesions on the lips or oral cavity
- Numbness in or around the oral cavity
- Dryness in the mouth for no apparent reason
- Burning sensation or soreness in the oral cavity for no apparent reason
- Repeated bleeding in a specific area of the oral cavity for no apparent reason
- Difficulty speaking, chewing, or swallowing

## Leukemia

**Leukemia** is a cancer of the blood-forming organs that is characterized by rapid growth of immature *leukocytes* (white blood cells). Oral symptoms may be among the first indications of leukemia. These symptoms include hemorrhage,

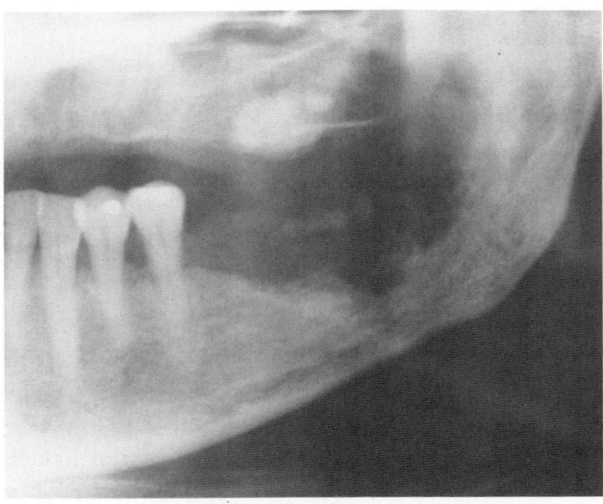

FIG. 17.24 Left side of a panoramic radiograph shows destruction of the mandible by squamous cell carcinoma. *(From Ibsen O, Phelan JA: Oral pathology for the dental hygienist, ed 6, St Louis, 2014, Saunders.)*

ulceration, enlargement, spongy texture, and magenta coloration of the gingiva (Fig. 17.25). Enlargement of lymph nodes, symptoms of anemia, and general bleeding tendencies also are typical.

## Smokeless Tobacco

Smokeless tobacco, in the form of chewing tobacco or snuff, presents a serious health hazard. It is a major concern because of the high rates of precancerous leukoplakia and oral cancer that occur among users of smokeless tobacco. In addition, cancers of the pharynx, larynx, and esophagus occur 400 to 500 times more frequently among users than among nonusers.

Smokeless tobacco is also linked to serious irritation of the oral mucosa and an increased incidence of tooth loss from periodontal disease (Fig. 17.26).

RECALL

11 What type of cancer affects the blood-forming organs?
12 What is a common precancerous lesion among users of smokeless tobacco?
13 What is the term for a malignant lesion in the epithelial tissue of the oral cavity?

## Therapy for Oral Cancer

Oral cancers are treated by surgery, radiation therapy, or chemotherapy. Often, a combination of these three is used.

## Dental Implications of Radiation Therapy

Because radiation for treatment of head and neck cancer affects the salivary glands, blood vessels, and bones of the jaws, patients who receive this treatment can be expected to develop specific dental problems, such as radiation mucositis and post-radiation **xerostomia** (Fig. 17.27).

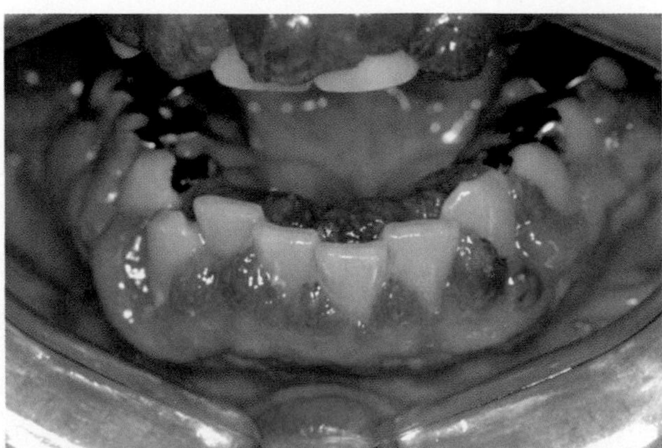

FIG. 17.25 Leukemia. *(From Regezi JA, Sciubba JJ, Jordan RCK: Oral pathology: clinical pathologic correlations, ed 7, St Louis, 2017, Elsevier.)*

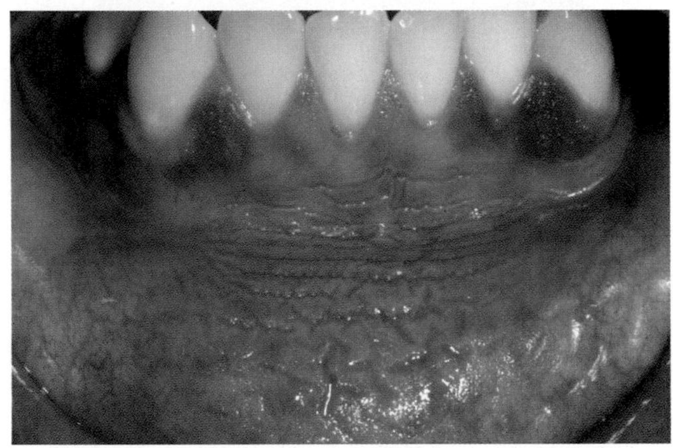

FIG. 17.26 Tobacco chewer's lesion. Note the rough texture of the surface. *(From Neville BW, et al: Oral and maxillofacial pathology, ed 4, St Louis, 2016, Elsevier.)*

### Xerostomia

If radiation affects the major salivary glands, irreversible destruction of these glands may be observed. When this occurs, saliva can no longer be produced, and the patient will suffer from severe xerostomia (dry mouth). Lack of adequate saliva and reduced blood supply to the tissues also can precipitate oral infection, delay healing, and make it difficult to wear dentures. Saliva substitutes may be used by the patient for some relief.

### Radiation Caries

Caused by the lack of saliva, caries usually appears first in the cervical areas of the teeth. The teeth also may become extremely sensitive to hot and cold stimuli.

### Osteoradionecrosis

*Radiation* also causes a decreased blood supply to the bones of the jaw. This can result in osteonecrosis (death of the bone). Patients should not have teeth extracted after they have been treated with head or neck radiation, because the jaw could be fractured and the wound may fail to heal as a result of

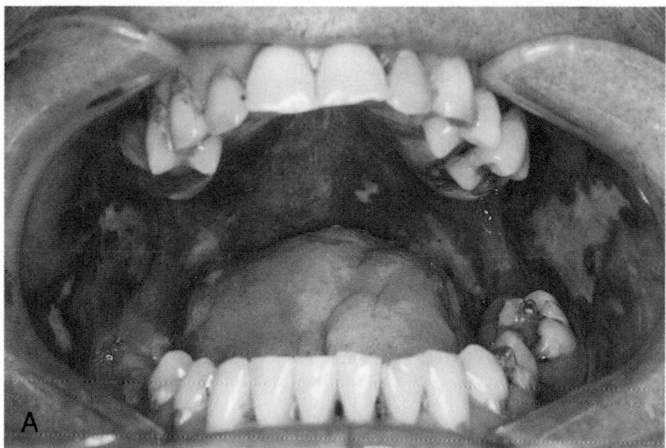


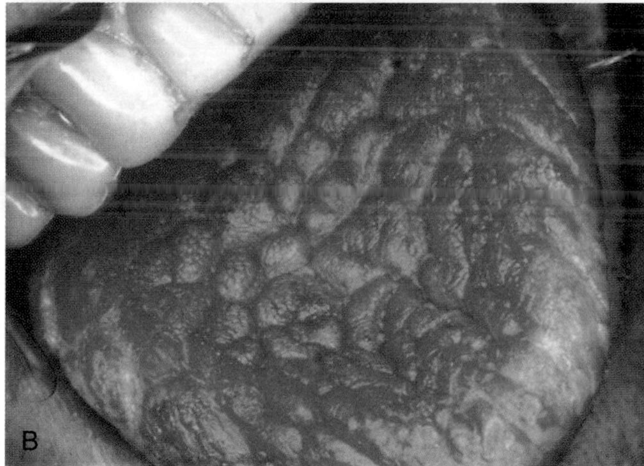


**FIG. 17.27** A, Radiation mucositis. B, Postradiation xerostomia. *(A, From Regezi JA, Sciubba JJ, Jordan RCK: Oral pathology: clinical pathologic correlations, ed 7, St Louis, 2017, Elsevier. B, Courtesy JE Bouquot, DDS, Morgantown, WV.)*

osteoradionecrosis. To avoid osteoradionecrosis, it may be necessary to extract the patient's teeth before providing radiation treatment.

## Dental Implications of Chemotherapy

Chemotherapeutic agents are powerful drugs that destroy or deactivate rapidly dividing cancer cells. The significant adverse effects of these drugs frequently involve the oral tissues (Table 17.2).

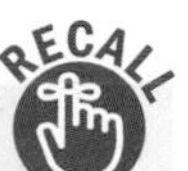


**14** What causes radiation caries?
**15** What is the term for lack of saliva?

**TABLE 17.2** Dental Implications of Chemotherapy

| Adverse Effect | Appearance |
|---|---|
| Mucositis | In this inflammatory change in the oral mucosa, the mucosa takes on a whitish appearance. |
| Aphthous ulcers | These are a common adverse effect of most chemotherapeutic agents. |
| Transient reactions | Cheilitis (inflammation of corners of the lips), glossitis (inflammation of the tongue), and paresthesia (abnormal burning or tingling sensation or loss of sensation) are less common, transient reactions. (*Transient* means the condition will disappear without additional treatment.) |
| Xerostomia | Dryness of the mouth caused by the lack of normal salivary secretions is another transient phenomenon in chemotherapy. Recovery usually occurs within 10 days. |
| Delayed healing | Because chemotherapeutic drugs act on all dividing cells, interference with healing may be anticipated when the drug is administered during the healing period. |
| Dentinal malformation | Chemotherapy administered to children during dentinal development can be expected to produce dental defects. |

## Human Immunodeficiency Virus and Acquired Immunodeficiency Syndrome

Acquired immunodeficiency syndrome (AIDS) is the end-stage disease for an individual infected with human immunodeficiency virus (HIV). Oral lesions are prominent features of AIDS and HIV infections.

Some of these lesions are known to be indicators of developing immunodeficiency and predictors of the development of AIDS in individuals who are HIV positive. Lesions appear because the immune system is compromised when T-helper cells become depleted as a result of the disease. Causes of oral lesions include opportunistic infections, tumors, and autoimmune-like diseases.

## Oral Manifestations

Because the patient's immune system is severely damaged, death is usually caused by an opportunistic infection. An opportunistic infection is one that normally would be controlled by the immune system but that cannot be controlled because the immune system is not functioning properly because of HIV/AIDS or other causes.

It is important to remember that some of the lesions that look like those that occur commonly with HIV and AIDS infection may also be caused by other disorders.

### *HIV Gingivitis*

A bright red line along the border of the free gingival margin characterizes HIV gingivitis, also known as *atypical gingivitis.* In some patients, the bright red line may progress from the free gingival margin over the attached gingival and alveolar mucosa. Other patients have petechia-like patches over the gingiva. (**Petechiae** are small, pinpoint bruises.)

### Oral Lesions Associated with HIV Infection

- Candidiasis
- Herpes simplex infection
- Herpes zoster
- Hairy leukoplakia
- Human papillomavirus lesions
- Atypical gingivitis and periodontitis
- Other opportunistic infections reported:
  - *Mycobacterium avium, Mycobacterium intracellulare*
  - Cytomegalovirus
  - *Cryptococcus neoformans*
  - *Klebsiella pneumoniae*
  - *Enterobacter cloacae*
  - *Histoplasma capsulatum*
- Kaposi's sarcoma
- Non-Hodgkin's lymphoma
- Aphthous ulcers
- Mucosal pigmentation
- Bilateral salivary gland enlargement and xerostomia
- Spontaneous gingival bleeding resulting from thrombocytopenia

From Ibsen O, Phelan J: Oral pathology for the dental hygienist, ed 6, St Louis, 2014, Saunders.

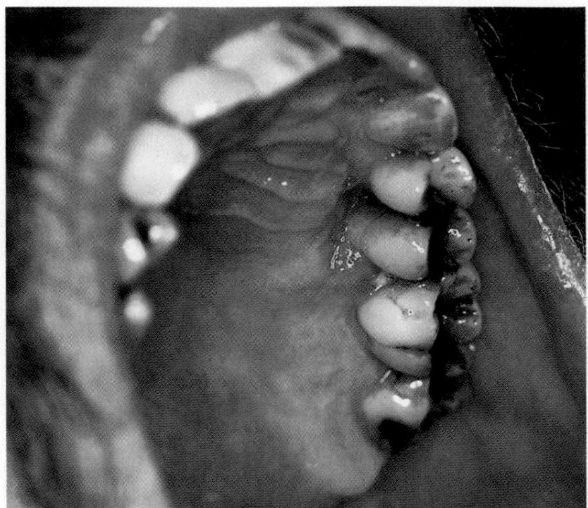

**FIG. 17.28** Atypical periodontal disease in a patient with human immunodeficiency virus (HIV) infection. *(From Ibsen O, Phelan JA: Oral pathology for the dental hygienist, ed 6, St Louis, 2014, Saunders.)*

## HIV Periodontitis

The periodontal lesions of HIV periodontitis, also known as *AIDS virus–associated periodontitis,* resemble those observed in acute necrotizing gingivitis superimposed on rapidly progressive periodontitis (Fig. 17.28). Other symptoms include interproximal necrosis and cratering, marked swelling and intense erythema over the free and attached gingiva, intense pain, and spontaneous bleeding and bad breath.

## Cervical Lymphadenopathy

Cervical **lymphadenopathy** is the enlargement of the cervical (neck) nodes (Fig. 17.29). Lymphadenopathy, meaning disease or swelling of the lymph nodes, is indicative of a systemic problem and is frequently seen in association with AIDS.

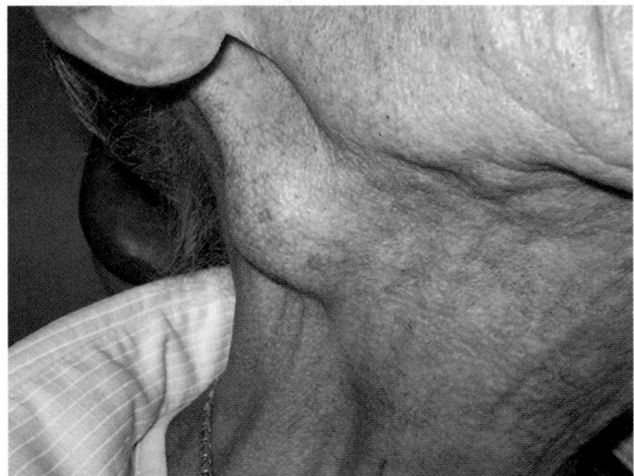

**FIG. 17.29** Lymphadenopathy. *(From Scully C: Scully's Medical Problems in Dentistry, ed 7, Edinburgh, 2014, Churchill Livingstone/Elsevier Ltd.)*

## Candidiasis

Candidiasis, as discussed earlier, is often the initial oral sign of progression from HIV-positive status to AIDS. In a patient with a compromised immune system, candidiasis can be a very debilitating and serious disorder (Fig. 17.30).

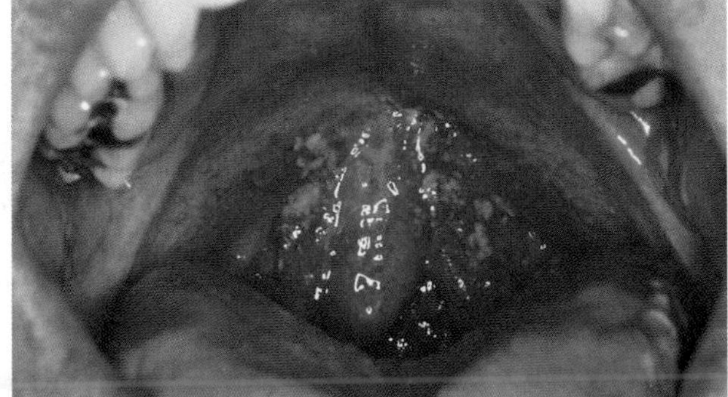

**FIG. 17.30** Candidiasis in a patient with human immunodeficiency virus (HIV) infection. Removable plaques are present on the mucosa of the soft palate. *(From Ibsen O, Phelan JA: Oral pathology for the dental hygienist, ed 6, St Louis, 2014, Saunders.)*

## Lymphoma

**Lymphoma** is the general term used to describe malignant disorders of the lymphoid tissue. In the immunocompromised individual, lymphoma may occur as a solitary lump or nodule, a swelling, or a nonhealing ulcer that appears anywhere in the oral cavity. The swelling may be ulcerated or may be covered with intact, normal-appearing mucosa.

Usually painful, the lesion grows rapidly in size and may be the first evidence of lymphoma. Diagnosis must be made from a biopsy because this condition closely resembles other oral diseases (Fig. 17.31).

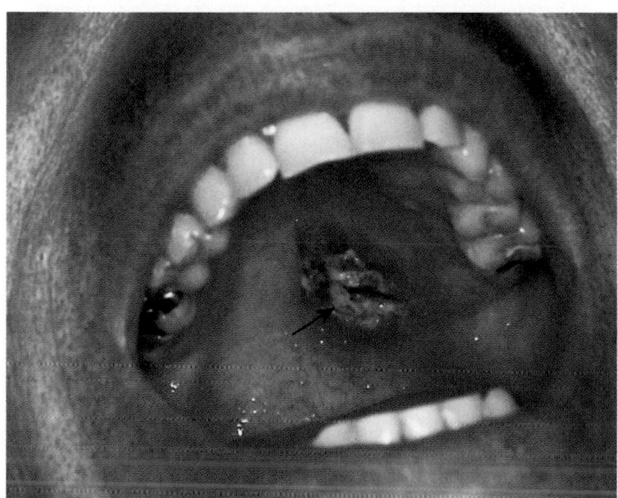

**FIG. 17.31** Intraoral lymphoma *(arrow)* in a patient with acquired immunodeficiency syndrome (AIDS). *(From Ibsen O, Phelan JA: Oral pathology for the dental hygienist, ed 6, St Louis, 2014, Saunders.)*

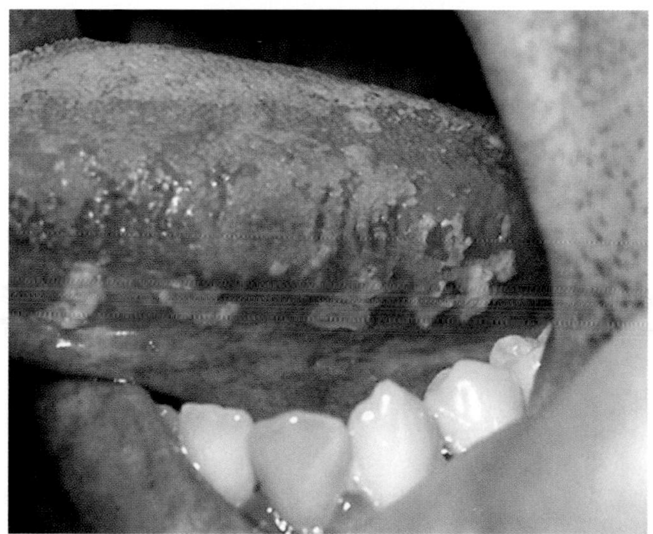

**FIG. 17.32** Hairy leukoplakia on the lateral borders of the tongue. *(From Sapp JP, Eversole LR, Wysocki GP: Contemporary oral and maxillofacial pathology, ed 2, St Louis, 2002, Mosby.)*

## Hairy Leukoplakia

Most individuals with hairy leukoplakia are positive for HIV, and it can be an important *early* sign of the change to AIDS status. Hairy leukoplakia is a white plaque that is usually found on one side or sometimes on both sides on the lateral borders (sides) of the tongue (Fig. 17.32).

Hairy leukoplakia may spread to cover the entire dorsal surface of the tongue. It can also develop on the buccal mucosa, where it generally has a flat appearance.

## Kaposi's Sarcoma

Kaposi's sarcoma is one of the opportunistic infections that occur in patients with HIV infection. Oral lesions of Kaposi's

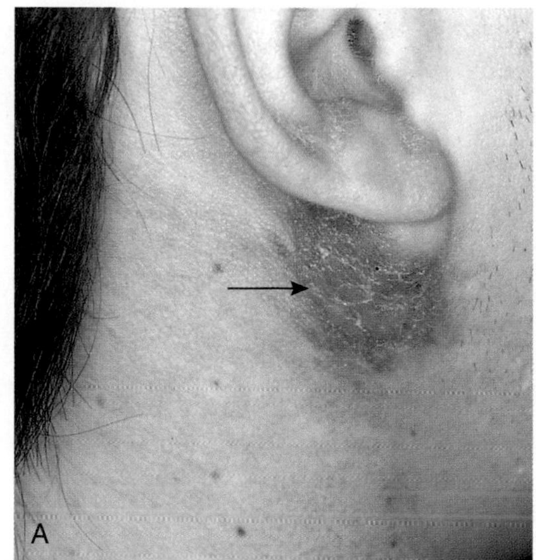


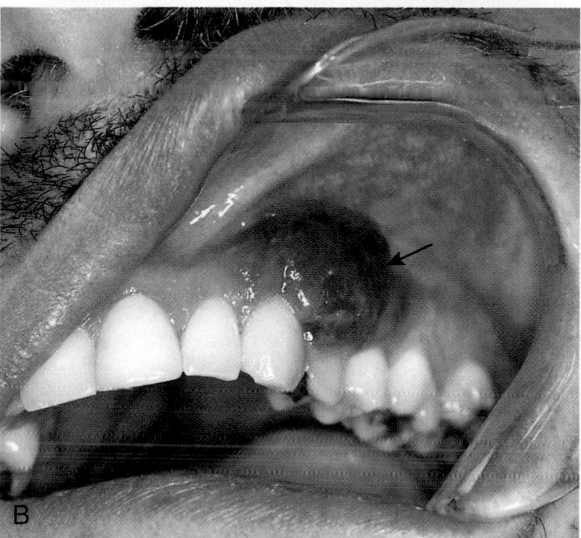


**FIG. 17.33** Kaposi's sarcoma *(arrows)* in a patient with acquired immunodeficiency syndrome (AIDS). A, Skin. B, Gingivae. *(From Ibsen O, Phelan JA: Oral pathology for the dental hygienist, ed 6, St Louis, 2014, Saunders.)*

sarcoma may appear as multiple bluish, blackish, or reddish blotches that are usually flat in the early stages.

At present, no effective treatment is available for Kaposi's sarcoma. Surgical excision to decrease the size of the lesion is sometimes attempted, as are radiation treatment and chemotherapy.

Kaposi's sarcoma is one of the intraoral lesions used to diagnose AIDS (Fig. 17.33).

## Herpes Simplex

Herpes simplex lesions usually occur on the lip. In immunocompromised patients, however, the lesions may be noted throughout the mouth (Fig. 17.34).

The herpes virus causes an ulcer-like lesion. A lesion that persists for longer than 1 month is particularly significant as an indicator of AIDS. Patients who do *not* have HIV or AIDS may develop herpes.

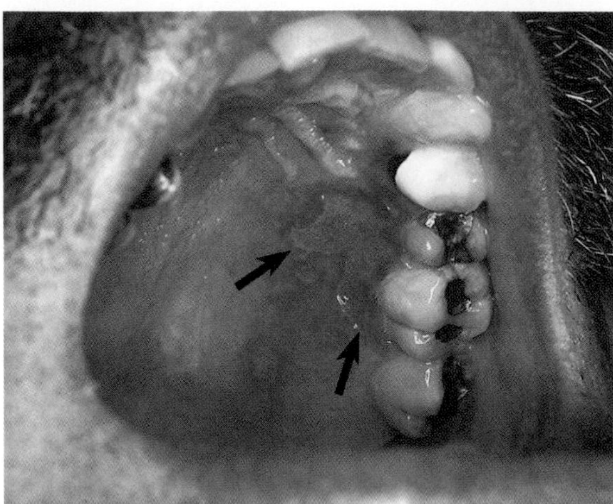

**FIG. 17.34** Herpes simplex ulceration of the hard palate in a patient with human immunodeficiency virus (HIV) infection. *Arrows* point to the periphery of the ulcer. *(From Ibsen O, Phelan JA: Oral pathology for the dental hygienist, ed 6, St Louis, 2014, Saunders.)*

## Herpes Zoster

In the immunocompromised patient, the latent herpes zoster virus, also known as *shingles,* may cause intraoral manifestations in the form of blisters. These blisters break and form ulcers.

The lesions are generally present on both sides of the mouth and are very painful. A complaint of pain coming from the teeth, without apparent dental cause, is an early symptom of herpes zoster.

## Human Papillomavirus

Human papillomaviruses are responsible for warts such as oral papillomas. These appear most often in immunocompromised individuals. The warts are a common finding in patients with early HIV infection.

Diagnosis is made on the basis of history, clinical appearance, and biopsy. The warts appear spiky, and some have a raised, cauliflower-like appearance. Other lesions are well defined, have a flat surface, and essentially disappear when the mucosa is stretched.

Although surgery or carbon dioxide laser excision can be performed to remove these warts, they frequently recur after removal (Fig. 17.35).

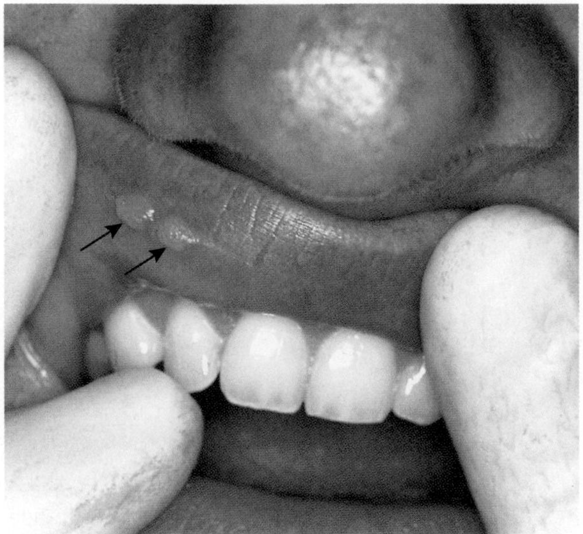

**FIG. 17.35** Papillary lesion *(arrows)* of the upper lip caused by human papillomavirus in a patient with human immunodeficiency virus (HIV) infection. *(From Ibsen O, Phelan JA: Oral pathology for the dental hygienist, ed 6, St Louis, 2014, Saunders.)*

RECALL

**16** What is the condition that is frequently seen on the lateral border of the tongue of patients with HIV/AIDS?

**17** Which opportunistic infection is seen as bluish lesions on the skin or oral mucosa of patients with HIV/AIDS?

**18** What is the malignant condition that involves the lymph nodes of patients with HIV/AIDS?

# Developmental Disorders

The development of the human body is an extremely complex process. When cells in the body divide, developmental disorders may occur. The result is usually a deformity of part of the body.

*Inherited disorders* are different from developmental disorders because they are caused by an *abnormal gene* in an individual and are transmitted from parent to child through the egg or sperm.

**Congenital disorders** are present at birth. They can be inherited or developmental, but the exact cause of most congenital abnormalities is unknown.

Developmental disturbances are influenced by *genetic* and *environmental* factors (Table 17.3).

## Genetic Factors

Malformations are often caused by genetic factors, such as abnormalities in the chromosomes. The size of the teeth and the size of the jaw are common genetic factors. A child can inherit large teeth from one parent and a small jaw from the other, or a child may inherit small teeth and a large jaw.

## Environmental Factors

Environmental factors that have a negative effect on development are called *teratogens.* Examples of teratogens are infections, drugs, and exposure to radiation. Women of childbearing age should avoid teratogens from the time of their first missed menstrual period if they could be pregnant.

During the pregnancy, fever and disease in the mother affect the developing teeth of the fetus. Some drugs taken during pregnancy may cause birth defects. Such drugs include certain prescribed medications, over-the-counter remedies such as aspirin and cold tablets, and drugs of abuse, including alcohol.

Antibiotics, particularly tetracycline, taken during pregnancy may produce a yellow-gray-brown stain on the primary teeth (Fig. 17.36) (see Chapter 58).

## TABLE 17.3 Dental Developmental Disturbances

| Disturbance | Stage | Description | Etiologic Factors | Clinical Ramifications |
|---|---|---|---|---|
| Anodontia | Initiation stage | Absence of single or multiple teeth | Hereditary, endocrine dysfunction, systemic disease, excessive radiation exposure | May cause disruption of occlusion and esthetic problems. Partial or full dentures, bridges, and/or implants may be needed to replace teeth. |
| Supernumerary teeth | Initiation stage | Development of one or more extra teeth | Hereditary | Occurs commonly between the maxillary centrals, distal to third molars, and the premolar region. May cause crowding, failure of normal eruption, and disruption of occlusion. |
| Macrodontia/ microdontia | Bud stage | Abnormally large or small teeth | Developmental or hereditary | Commonly involves permanent maxillary lateral incisor and third molars. |
| Dens in dente | Cap stage | Enamel organ invaginates into the dental papilla | Hereditary | Commonly affects the permanent maxillary lateral incisor. Tooth may have a deep lingual pit, and endodontic therapy may be needed. |
| Gemination | Cap stage | Tooth germ tries to divide | Hereditary | Large, single-rooted tooth with one pulp cavity exhibits "twinning" in crown area. Normal number of teeth in dentition. May cause problems in appearance and spacing. |
| Fusion | Cap stage | Union of two adjacent tooth germs | Pressure on area | Large tooth with two pulp cavities. Extra tooth in dentition. May cause problems in appearance and spacing. |
| Tubercle | Cap stage | Extra cusp due to effects on enamel organ | Trauma, pressure, or metabolic disease | Common or permanent molars or cingulum of anterior teeth. |
| Enamel pearl | Apposition and maturation stages | Sphere of enamel on root | Displacement of ameloblasts to root surface | May be confused with calculus deposit on root. |
| Enamel dysplasia | Apposition and maturation stages | Faulty development of enamel from interference involving ameloblasts | Local or systemic or hereditary | Pitting and intrinsic color changes in enamel. |
| Dentinal dysplasia | Apposition and maturation stages | Faulty development of dentin from interference with odontoblasts | Local or systemic or hereditary | Intrinsic color changes and changes in thickness of dentin possible. Problems in function or esthetics. |
| Concrescence | Apposition and maturation stages | Union of root structure of two or more teeth by cementum | Traumatic injury or crowding of teeth | Common with permanent maxillary molars. |

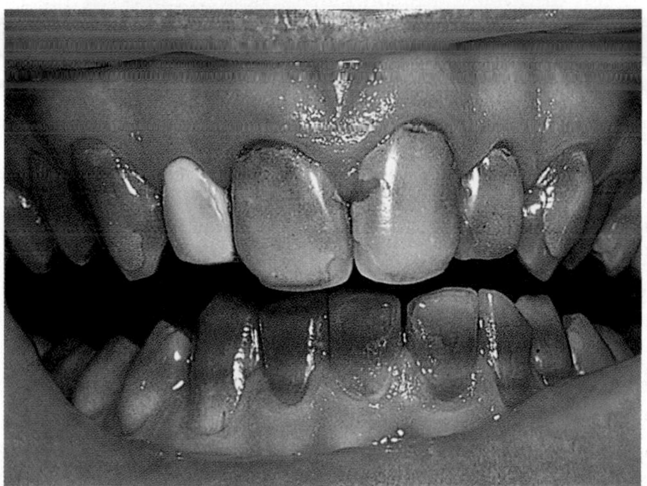

**FIG. 17.36** Tetracycline staining of the dentition. This patient was treated with tetracycline during formation of the teeth. *(Courtesy Dr. George Taybos, University of Mississippi Medical Center, Jackson, Miss.)*

### Known Teratogens Involved in Congenital Malformations

**Drugs**

Ethanol, tetracycline, phenytoin (Dilantin), lithium, methotrexate, aminopterin, diethylstilbestrol, warfarin, thalidomide, isotretinoin (retinoic acid), androgens, progesterone

**Chemicals**

Methylmercury, polychlorinated biphenyls

Infections

Rubella virus, herpes simplex virus, human immunodeficiency virus, syphilis microbe

**Radiation**

High levels of ionizing type*

*Note that diagnostic levels of radiation should be avoided but have not been directly linked to congenital malformations.

From Fehrenbach MJ, Popowics T: Illustrated dental embryology, histology, and anatomy, ed 4, St Louis, 2016, Saunders.

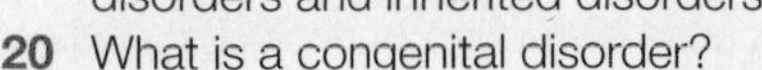

19 What is the difference between developmental disorders and inherited disorders?
20 What is a congenital disorder?

## Disturbances in Jaw Development

*Macrognathia* is a condition that is characterized by abnormally large jaws. This occurs most often in the mandible, and the result is a class III malocclusion (see Chapter 60).

*Micrognathia* is a condition that is characterized by abnormally small jaws. This occurs most often in the mandible, and the result is a class II malocclusion.

An *exostosis* (*plural,* exostoses) is a benign bony growth that projects outward from the surface of a bone. An exostosis also may be referred to as a *torus* (*plural,* tori), which is defined as a bulging projection.

A *torus palatinus* is a bony overgrowth at the midline of the hard palate (see Fig. 17.4). A *torus mandibularis* is a bony overgrowth on the lingual surface of the mandible near the premolar and molar areas. These growths are not harmful; however, it may be necessary to remove them so that a full or a partial denture may be placed and worn comfortably (see Fig. 17.4).

## Disturbances in Lip, Palate, and Tongue Development

A *cleft lip* results when the maxillary and medial nasal processes fail to fuse (Fig. 17.37).

A *cleft palate* results when the palatal shelves fail to fuse with the primary palate. This disturbance may be hereditary or environmental. A *cleft uvula* is the mildest form of cleft palate. Cleft palate, with or without cleft lip, occurs in 1 per 2500 live births.

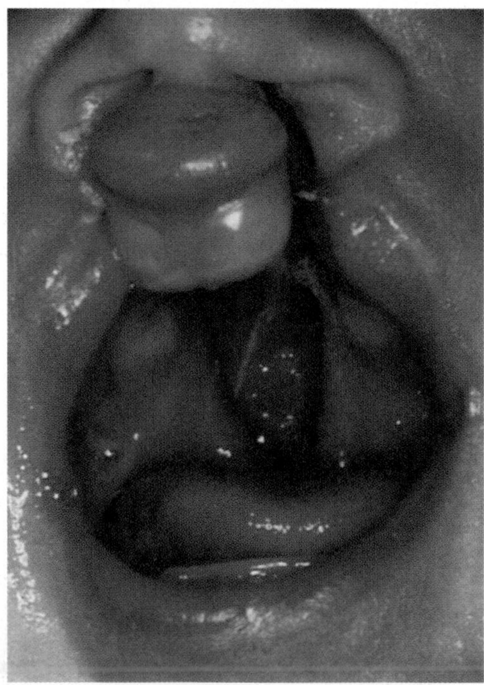

**FIG. 17.37** A newborn with bilateral complete cleft lip and palate. Note severe angulation of the premaxillary segment. *(From Zitelli BJ, McIntire SC, Nowalk AJ: Zitelli and Davis' Atlas of Pediatric Physical Diagnosis, ed 6, 2012, Mosby.)*

*Ankyloglossia,* also known as *tongue-tie,* results in a short lingual frenum that extends to the apex of the tongue. This limits the movement of the tongue (Fig. 17.38).

21 What is the term for abnormally large jaws?
22 What is the term for bony growths in the palate?
23 What is a more common term for ankyloglossia?

## Disturbances in Tooth Development and Eruption

An *ameloblastoma* is a tumor composed of remnants of the dental lamina that failed to disintegrate after the tooth buds were formed.

*Anodontia* is the congenital absence of teeth. It may be partial or total and may affect the primary or permanent dentition or both. The teeth most often involved are third molars, followed by maxillary lateral incisors and second premolars (Fig. 17.39).

*Supernumerary teeth* are any teeth in excess of the 32 normal permanent teeth. These teeth may be normal in size and shape, but they are most frequently small and poorly developed (Fig. 17.40).

*Macrodontia* is the term used to describe abnormally large teeth. It may affect the entire dentition or may appear in only two teeth, such as the maxillary central incisors.

*Microdontia* is the term used to describe abnormally small teeth. When microdontia affects an entire dentition, it is frequently associated with other defects, such as congenital heart disease or Down syndrome.

*Dens in dente,* or "a tooth within a tooth," is a developmental anomaly that results in the formation of a small, toothlike mass of enamel and dentin within the pulp (Fig. 17.41). On a radiograph, this resembles a tooth within another tooth.

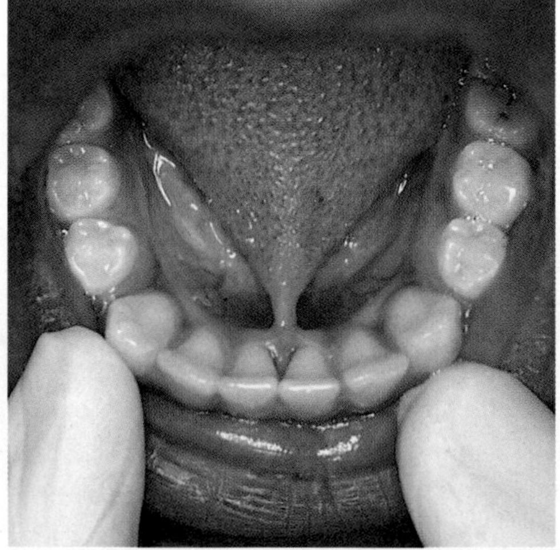

**FIG. 17.38** Ankyloglossia. Restriction of movement of the tongue due to a lingual frenum that is abnormally short or is attached too close to the tip of the tongue. *(From Zitelli BJ, McIntire SC, Nowalk AJ: Zitelli and Davis' atlas of pediatric physical diagnosis, ed 6, St Louis, 2013, Saunders.)*

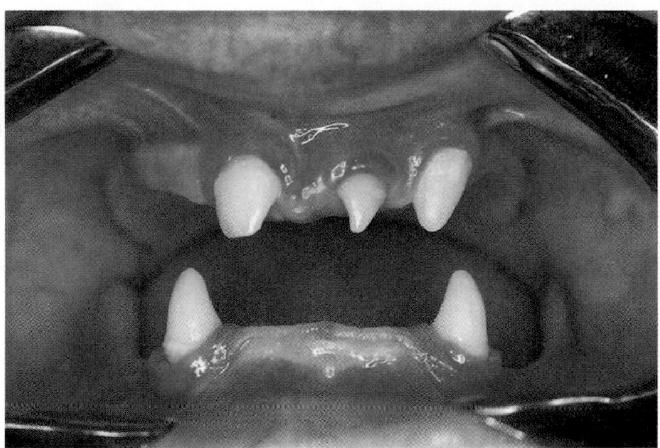

**FIG. 17.39** Partial anodontia. *(From Regezi JA, Sciubba JJ, Jordan RCK: Oral pathology: clinical pathologic correlations, ed 7, St Louis, 2017, Elsevier.)*

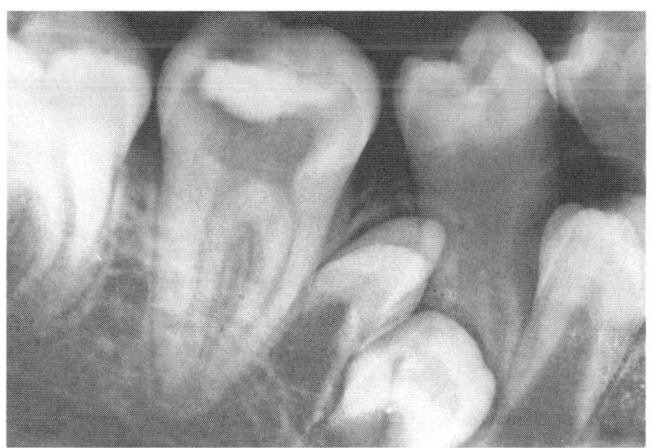

**FIG. 17.40** Radiograph shows unerupted supernumerary teeth. *(Courtesy Dr. George Blozis.)*

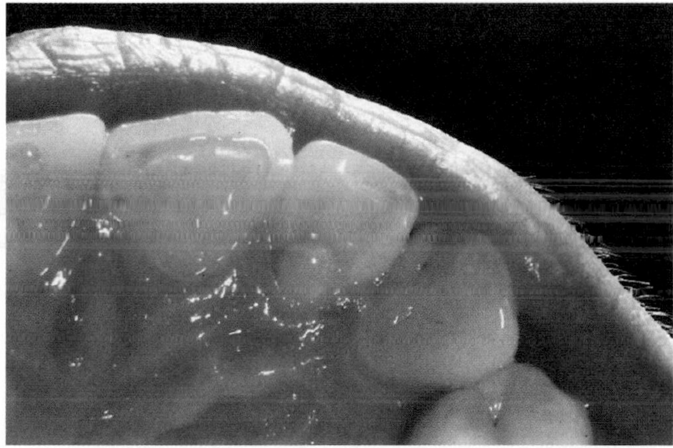

**FIG. 17.41** Dens in dente.

*Variation in form* may include extra, missing, or fused cusps or anomalies of roots. The most common variations, however, take the form of peg-shaped teeth. *Hutchinson's incisors,* a variety of peg-shaped teeth, are usually associated with maternal syphilis (Fig. 17.42).

*Fusion* is the joining together of the dentin and the enamel of two or more separate developing teeth. Fusion of teeth leads to a reduced number of teeth in the dental arch (Fig. 17.43).

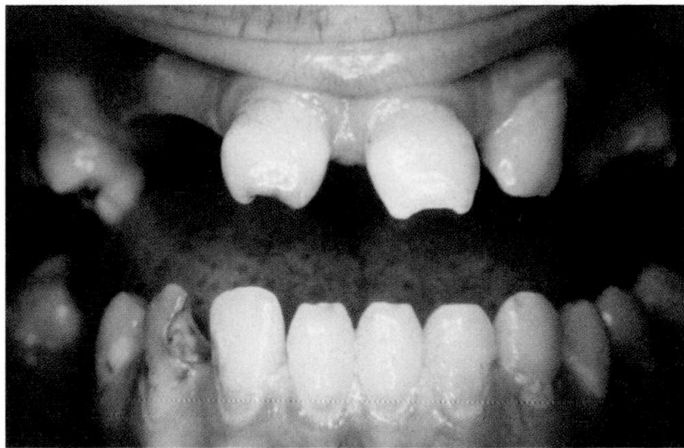

**FIG. 17.42** Hutchinson's incisors. *(From Halstead CL, Blozis GG, Drinnan AJ, et al: Physical Evaluation of the Dental Patient, St Louis, 1982, Mosby.)*

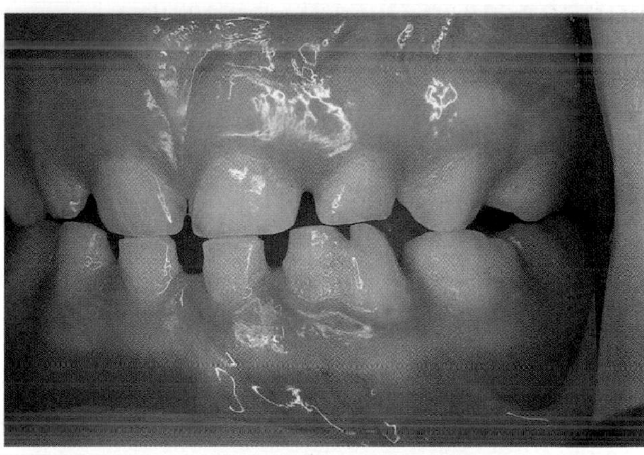

**FIG. 17.43** Clinical picture of fusion involving a permanent lateral incisor. *(From Regezi JA, Sciubba JJ, Jordan RCK: Oral pathology: clinical pathologic correlations, ed 7, St Louis, 2017, Elsevier.)*

*Gemination* is an attempt by the tooth bud to divide. An incisal notch indicates when this attempt is not successful.

*Twinning* means that tooth bud division is complete, and the result is the formation of an extra tooth. This tooth is usually a mirror image of its adjacent partner in the dental arch.

RECALL

**24** What is the dental term for "tooth within a tooth"?
**25** What is the term used for abnormally small teeth?
**26** What term is used to describe two teeth that are joined together?

## Disturbances in Enamel Formation

*Amelogenesis imperfecta* is a hereditary abnormality characterized by defects in the formation of enamel (Fig. 17.44).

*Hypocalcification* is the incomplete calcification or hardening of the enamel of a tooth.

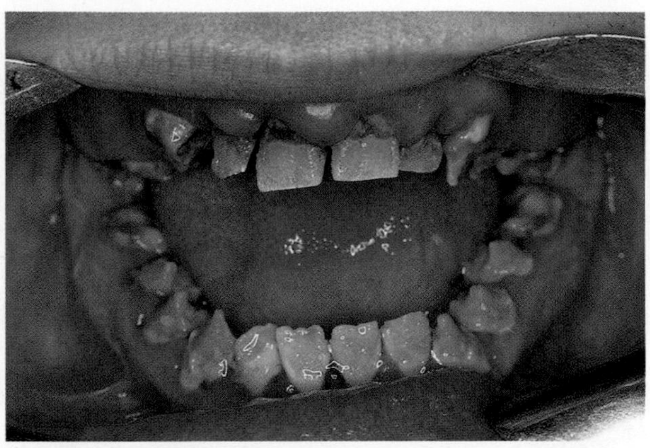

**FIG. 17.44** Note loss of enamel in these teeth in a patient with hypocalcified amelogenesis imperfecta. *(From Regezi JA, Sciubba JJ, Jordan RCK: Oral pathology: clinical pathologic correlations, ed 7, St Louis, 2017, Elsevier.)*

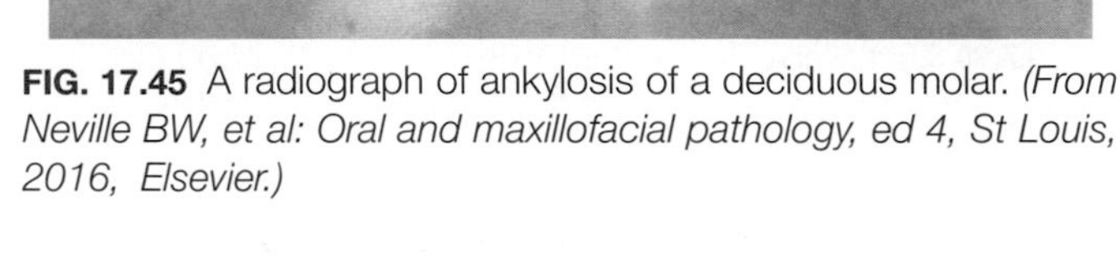

**FIG. 17.45** A radiograph of ankylosis of a deciduous molar. *(From Neville BW, et al: Oral and maxillofacial pathology, ed 4, St Louis, 2016, Elsevier.)*

## Disturbances in Dentin Formation

*Dentinogenesis imperfecta* is a hereditary condition that affects the formation of dentin. It is found in both the primary and the permanent dentition. Teeth that have dentinogenesis imperfecta are opalescent and have an almost amber color. Soon, however, the enamel tends to chip away from the dentin, and the weakened teeth become worn down (see Fig. 17.1).

## Abnormal Eruption of the Teeth

### Premature Eruption

*Natal teeth* are the teeth that are present at birth. Neonatal teeth erupt within the first 30 days of life. The teeth most often involved are the mandibular incisors. Because of the lack of root formation, these teeth are soon shed. Often, they will be removed so that the infant does not swallow them if they are shed.

### Ankylosis

Ankylosed teeth are deciduous teeth in which the bone has fused to cementum and dentin. This prevents exfoliation of the deciduous tooth and eruption of the underlying permanent tooth. Deciduous molars are most often affected by ankylosis (Fig. 17.45).

### Impaction

*Impaction* is the term used to describe any tooth that remains unerupted in the jaws beyond the time at which it should normally erupt (Fig. 17.46). The following three processes may cause impaction:

- Premature loss of primary teeth
- Shifting of the developing tooth into a horizontal or other abnormal position
- Shifting of the developing tooth into a position from which it cannot erupt because of the presence of other teeth, lack of jaw space, or abnormally large tooth crowns

Impactions and their treatment are discussed further in Chapter 56.

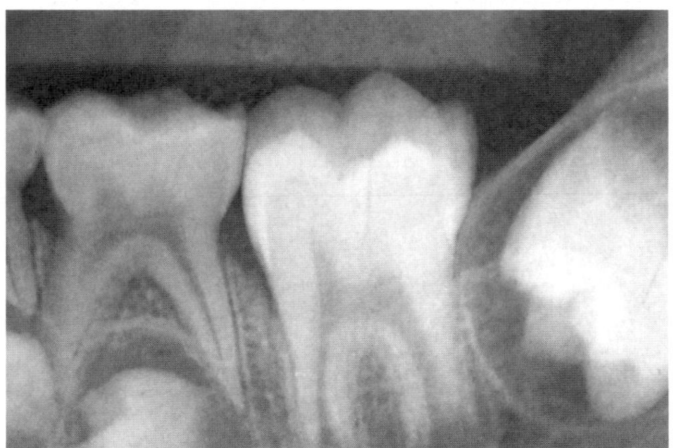

**FIG. 17.46** Impactions in mixed dentition visible on a dental radiograph.

RECALL

**27** Which teeth are most often affected by ankylosis?
**28** What is the hereditary condition that affects the dentin?

# Miscellaneous Disorders

## Abrasion

Abrasion, the abnormal wearing away of tooth structure, is caused by a repetitive habit, such as improper toothbrushing, most often a back-and-forth scrubbing motion that involves excessive pressure. The use of an abrasive dentifrice or a hard-bristled toothbrush may also cause abrasion (Fig. 17.47).

## Attrition

Attrition is the normal wearing away of tooth structure during chewing (Fig. 17.48). Attrition is normal and occurs with age on the incisal, occlusal, and proximal surfaces of the teeth. It is reported in both deciduous and permanent dentitions.

A diet of more fibrous food causes a greater rate of attrition. Attrition is made worse by bruxism, as well as by the use of

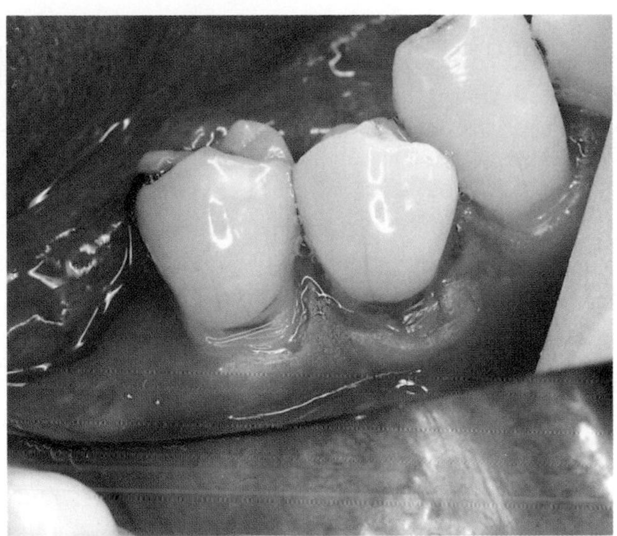

**FIG. 17.47** Abrasion at the cervical area of mandibular premolars caused by toothbrushing. *(From Ibsen O, Phelan JA: Oral pathology for the dental hygienist, ed 6, St Louis, 2014, Saunders.)*

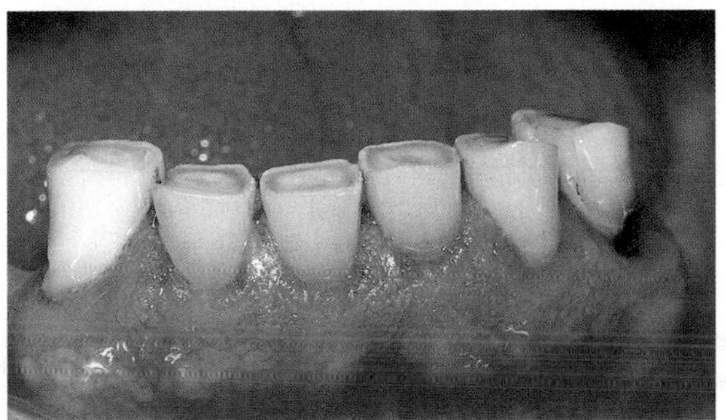

**FIG. 17.48** Attrition of adult dentition *(incisal view)*. *(Courtesy Margaret J. Fehrenbach, RDH, MS.)*

chewing tobacco. The rate of attrition appears to be greater in men than in women.

## Bruxism

Bruxism is an oral habit that is characterized by involuntary gnashing, grinding, and clenching of the teeth. It is usually performed during sleep and is often associated with stress or tension. Bruxism causes abnormal wear of the teeth (Fig. 17.49).

Bruxism also damages the periodontal ligament and associated supporting structures and is a major factor contributing to temporomandibular joint disorders.

In addition to stress reduction techniques, a night guard or a removable splint is frequently used as a temporary aid in the treatment of bruxism. The purpose of this splint is to reduce the damage caused by grinding while the patient is asleep.

## Bulimia

Bulimia is an eating disorder that is characterized by food bingeing followed by self-induced vomiting. The dental

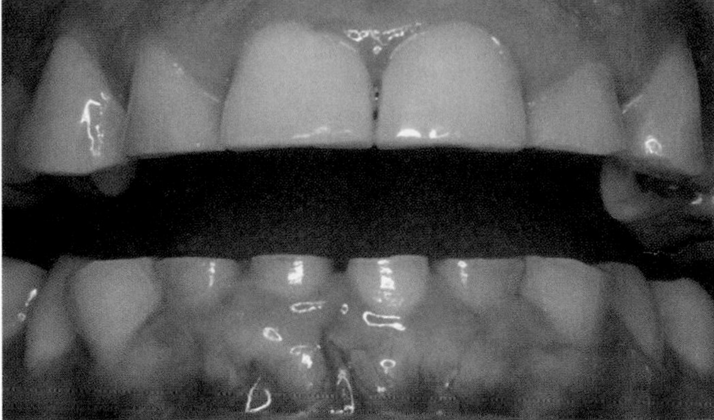

**FIG. 17.49** Attrition of the mandibular anterior teeth resulting from bruxism. *(From Perry DA, Beemsterboer PL, Essex G: Periodontology for the dental hygienist, ed 4, St Louis, 2014, Saunders.)*

professional is often the first healthcare professional to identify a patient with bulimia, because of the pattern of erosion that becomes apparent on the lingual surfaces of the teeth.

Generally, the person with bulimia maintains a normal body weight but is secretive about eating habits. Vomiting after eating is a component of bulimia but not of anorexia nervosa, another eating disorder. Generalized erosion of the lingual surfaces of the teeth is common and results from the acid produced by frequent vomiting (see Chapter 16).

Dental management of the patient with bulimia requires minimizing the effects of stomach acids on tooth enamel by encouraging the daily use of a fluoride rinse and fluoridated toothpaste. Rinsing the mouth with water and thoroughly cleaning the teeth immediately after vomiting also lessens the effects of the acid. However, the patient should be encouraged to seek professional treatment to eliminate the eating disorder.

## Orofacial Piercings

Piercing of parts of the face and oral cavity followed by the insertion of various objects has recently become popular among some segments of the population. The dental complications of this practice can include chipped teeth, broken teeth, and serious infection at the sites of the piercings. Infection can spread throughout the head and neck area with serious results.

RECALL

**29** What is the difference between attrition and abrasion?
**30** What is an oral indication of bulimia?
**31** What are three potential complications of orofacial piercing?

## Meth Mouth

The illegal use of **methamphetamine** is on the rise in the United States. This is partly because the drug is cheap and easy to make, and the high lasts up to 12 hours—much

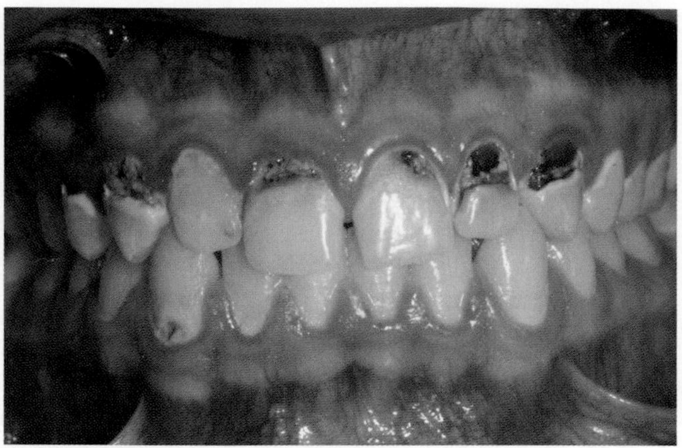

**FIG. 17.50** Meth mouth. *(From Neville B, Damm DD, Allen CM, et al: Oral and maxillofacial pathology, ed 3, St Louis, 2008, Mosby.)*

longer than crack cocaine. Although methamphetamine use occurs throughout society, most users are males between the ages of 19 and 40. Methamphetamine is a potent central nervous system stimulant that can cause brain damage and severe oral health effects. Methamphetamine can be smoked, snorted, injected, or taken orally. Street names for methamphetamine include *meth, speed, ice, chalk, crank, fire,* and *glass.* One reason for the tremendous growth in meth labs is the easy and legal availability of the components. When users smoke, inject, or ingest meth, they are sending highly toxic chemicals to their brain and cardiovascular system, and throughout their bodies.

## Some Common Meth Ingredients

- Alcohol
- Gasoline additives
- Benzene
- Paint thinner
- Freon
- Campfire stove fuel
- Toluene (found in brake cleaners)
- Drain cleaner
- Muriatic acid
- Battery acid
- Lithium from batteries
- Chloroform

The oral effects of methamphetamine use are devastating and are referred to as "**meth mouth.**" The pattern of rampant caries is most often seen on the buccal smooth surface of the teeth and the interproximal surfaces of the anterior teeth (Fig. 17.50). Drug-related xerostomia (dry mouth), poor oral hygiene, frequent consumption of highly sugared soft drinks, and clenching and grinding of the teeth all contribute to the rampant caries. Speculation suggests that the acidic nature of the drug is also a contributing factor; however, other reports dispute the role of "chemical" or "contaminant" factors in causing meth mouth. Dental professionals must be aware of the signs and symptoms of methamphetamine use.

## Signs and Symptoms of Meth Use

**Early Meth Use**

- Incessant talking
- Euphoric "high" state
- Decreased appetite
- Dilated pupils
- Violent behavior

**Continued Meth Use**

- Weight loss
- Shadows under the eyes
- Dry or itchy skin
- Irritability and moodiness
- Aggressiveness

**Advanced Meth Use**

- Discolored, decayed teeth
- Extreme weight loss
- Severe mental illness symptoms
- Paranoia; hallucinations
- Insomnia

**Meth Overdose**

- High fever
- Chest pain
- Profuse sweating
- Chances of heart attack, stroke, or coma
- Liver and kidney disorders

■ **Patient Education** You will probably see patients with piercings of the tongue, lip, or other oral areas. As a dental assistant, you may have the opportunity to educate patients about how piercing can be dangerous.

The mouth contains millions of bacteria, and infection is a common complication of oral piercing. Pain and swelling are other adverse effects of piercing. The tongue, the most popular piercing site in the mouth, could swell large enough to close off the airway. Piercing can also cause uncontrollable bleeding or nerve damage.

Even if the piercing injury itself does not cause problems, other hazards are created by the jewelry inserted. People can choke on studs, barbells, or hoops that come loose in the mouth. Chipped or cracked teeth can result from contact with the jewelry.

Educate patients that this fashion statement involves more than just deciding on the style or placement of jewelry. The decision to pierce oral structures could have major consequences for oral health as well. ■

■ **Legal and Ethical Implications** Always carefully check the medical histories of all your patients before each appointment. Many patients take medications that can cause changes in the oral tissues. For example, antianxiety medications, antipsychotic medications, and antihistamines can cause xerostomia. Drugs such as prednisone can increase the risks for candidiasis and other oral infections. Other medications can cause gingival hyperplasia. By being alert, you can play an important role in patient care. ■

**■ Eye to the Future** Today, surgery, radiation therapy, and chemotherapy are used to treat oral cancer. Unfortunately, radiation therapy and chemotherapy can cause several serious oral conditions. Perhaps in the future, more effective and less damaging therapies will be developed. Better yet, perhaps a significant reduction in the number of oral cancers will result from reduced smoking and alcohol use, along with improved treatment technologies. An oral cancer examination should be part of every routine dental examination. The key to long-term survival is early recognition and diagnosis. ■

## ■ Critical Thinking

1. Tyler Hansen is a 32-year-old man in your practice. His medical history indicates that he is HIV positive. While exposing radiographs, you note several purplish areas on his neck and also on his palate. What do you think these purplish areas could be?
2. Blanche Jones is an 82-year-old woman who lives alone. She is very thin and sometimes appears weak. She is in your office describing her burning tongue. While the dentist is examining the patient, you note that her tongue is smooth and very red. What could be the problem?
3. Jason is a 16-year-old patient who comes to your office for his annual dental checkup. He is a pitcher on his high school baseball team. He admits to using smokeless tobacco. What type of lesions do you expect to see in his mouth? ■

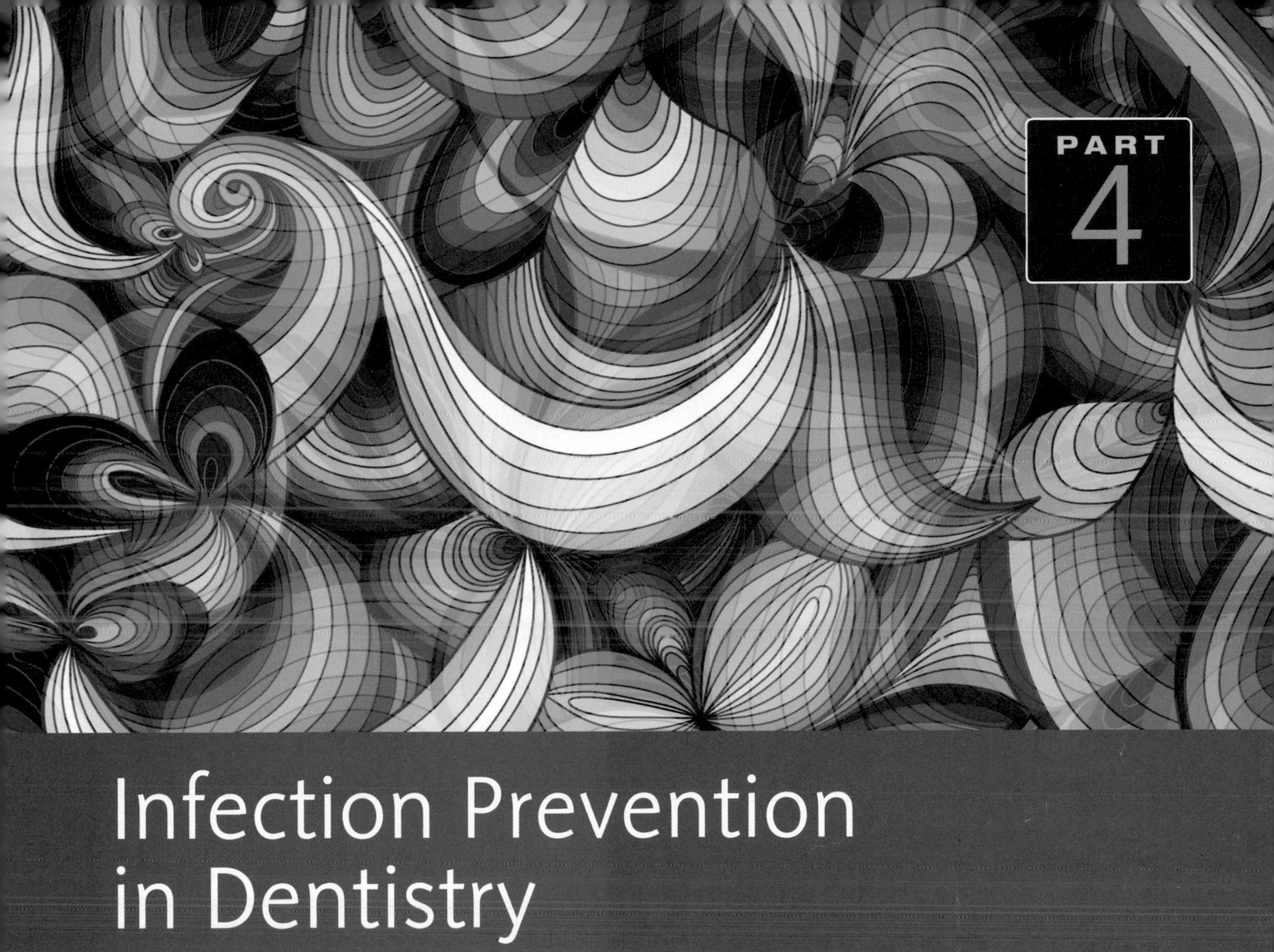


# Infection Prevention in Dentistry

On a daily basis, dental health professionals and patients alike are exposed to a wide variety of disease-causing microorganisms that may be transmitted in the dental office. When you master the information in this section, you will feel confident in your ability to understand the rationale for proper infection control and you will know that you have the knowledge and ability to implement all of the infection control policies and procedures necessary to protect yourself and to prevent the transmission of disease in the dental office.

The microbiology chapter in this section will provide you with the necessary foundation, so you can understand the organisms that cause disease and the approaches necessary to destroy them. Of special interest are diseases that are of concern for dentistry, such as herpes, the various forms of hepatitis, and the human immunodeficiency virus (HIV).

The Centers for Disease Control and Prevention (CDC) has issued *Guidelines for Infection Control in Dental Health Care Settings*. These guidelines are the gold standard for infection prevention in dentistry. The Blood-Borne Pathogens Standard (BBP) of the Occupational Safety and Health Administration (OSHA), the most important infection control law in dentistry, was issued to protect employees from exposure to blood-borne diseases. Together, the CDC guidelines and the OSHA requirements outline *what* dental professionals need to do to comply, but not *how* they should do what is needed. The guidelines tell you to clean and heat-sterilize instruments and to maintain a safe environment, but they do not tell you specifically *how* to do these things. New products and materials are continually appearing on the market. Therefore, as a dental healthcare professional, it is your responsibility to seek current evidence-based information to determine the best products, safest methods, and most effective techniques to maintain a safe environment for yourself and your patients.

The step-by-step procedures described in the following chapters will help you put into daily practice information provided in the OSHA requirements and in the CDC guidelines. You will be able to base your day-to-day infection control decisions on sound scientific information.

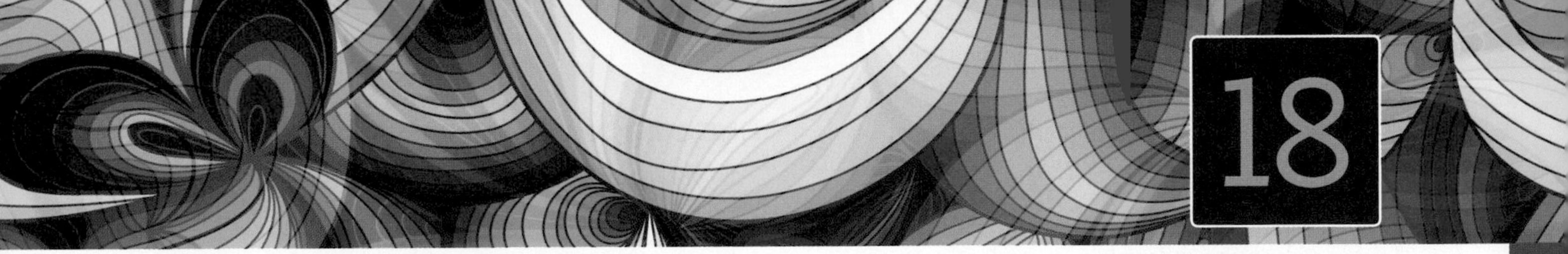

18

# Microbiology

## KEY TERMS

**Aerobes (AYR-oebz)** Bacteria that require oxygen to grow.

**Anaerobes (AN-uh-roebz)** Bacteria that grow in the absence of oxygen and are destroyed by oxygen.

**Bacilli (singular, bacillus)** Rod-shaped bacteria that cause tuberculosis and other diseases.

***Candida*** A yeast commonly found in the oral cavity, gastrointestinal tract, and female genital tract, and sometimes in the skin.

**Chancre** A painless ulcerating sore.

**Cocci (singular, coccus)** Spherical bacterial cells that reproduce by dividing into two.

**Creutzfeldt-Jakob (KROITS-felt YAH-koeb) disease** Rare chronic brain disease with onset in middle to late life (40 to 60 years).

**Ebola** A rare but deadly virus that causes bleeding inside and outside the body.

**Endospores** A resistant, dormant structure formed inside of some bacteria that can withstand adverse conditions.

**Facultative anaerobes** Organisms that can grow with or without oxygen.

**Fungi (singular, fungus)** Plants, such as mushrooms, yeasts, and molds that lack chlorophyll.

**Gram negative** Classification of bacteria that do not hold a dye stain under a microscope.

**Gram positive** Classification of bacteria that hold a dye stain and appear dark purple under a microscope.

**Gram's stain** Four-step staining process developed by Hans Christian Gram and used to separate bacteria into groups.

**Gram variable** Classification of bacteria that are not consistently stained.

**H1N1** A form of swine influenza virus.

**Herpesvirus** A virus that causes infections in humans, such as herpes, cytomegalovirus, chickenpox, shingles, mononucleosis, measles, and Kaposi's sarcoma.

**Latent** Dormant

**Microbiology** The study of microorganisms.

**Microcephaly** Abnormal smallness of the head, a congenital condition associated with incomplete brain development.

**Methicillin-resistant *Staphylococcus aureus*** Type of staph infection that is resistant to several common antibiotics.

**Nonpathogenic (non-path-oe-JEN-ik)** Pertaining to microorganisms that do *not* produce disease.

**Oral candidiasis (kan-di-DYE-uh-sis)** *Candida* yeast infection of the oral mucosa.

**Pandemic (pan-DEM-ik)** A condition that occurs throughout the people of a country or the world.

**Pathogens (PATH-uh-jenz)** Disease-producing microorganisms.

**Percutaneous (pur-kyoo-TAY-nee-us)** Through the skin, such as a needle stick, a cut, or a human bite.

**Petri plate** A small, flat dish made of thin glass or plastic that contains sterile solid medium for the culture of microorganisms; also called *Petri dish.*

**Prions (PRYE-ons)** Infectious particles of proteins that lack nucleic acids.

**Protozoa (proe-toe-ZOE-uh)** Single-celled microscopic animals without a rigid cell wall.

**Provirus** Virus that is hidden during the latency period.

**Spirochetes** Spiral-shaped bacteria.

**Staphylococci** Cocci that form irregular groups or clusters.

**Streptococci** Cocci that form chains as they divide.

**Tyndallization (tin-duhl-i-ZAY-shun)** Intermittent, or fractional, sterilization.

**Virulent (VIR-yoo-lent)** Capable of causing serious disease.

**Viruses** Ultramicroscopic infectious agents that contain DNA or RNA.

**Zika** A virus that is spread to people primarily through the bite of an infected *Aedes* species mosquito.

## LEARNING OUTCOMES

*On completion of this chapter, the student will be able to achieve the following objectives:*

1. Pronounce, define, and spell the key terms.
2. Explain why the study of microbiology is important for the dental assistant.
3. Discuss the contributions of early pioneers in microbiology.
4. List the four criteria of Koch's postulates.
5. Identify and explain the five major groups of microorganisms, including the following:
   - Identify the three basic types of bacteria according to their shape.
   - Explain the Gram's stain classification system used to identify bacteria.
   - Describe the differences among aerobes, anaerobes, and facultative anaerobes.
   - Identify the most resistant form of life known, and explain how it survives.
   - Describe how prions differ from viruses and bacteria and name two diseases caused by prions.
   - Compare viruses with bacteria, and name diseases caused by each.
   - Explain why specificity in viruses is important.
6. Discuss viral diseases, including the following:
   - Identify five types of viral hepatitis and explain how each one is transmitted.
   - Identify methods of HIV transmission and explain the effect of HIV on the human body.
   - Explain the difference between the five types of herpes virus, including type 1 and type 2 herpes simplex virus.
   - Describe the symptoms of an infection of West Nile virus.
   - Describe the symptoms of influenza and how it is spread.

7 Discuss bacterial diseases, including the following:
- Name the disease that is the leading cause of death from infectious diseases worldwide.
- Identify the bacterium discovered during an American Legion convention and explain its mode of transmission.
- Explain how tetanus can be prevented.
- Describe the three stages of syphilis.
- Identify the method of transmission of methicillin-resistant *Staphylococcus aureus* (MRSA) and explain the best methods to prevent its spread.

8 Describe the possible effects of a pandemic disease.

## ELECTRONIC RESOURCES

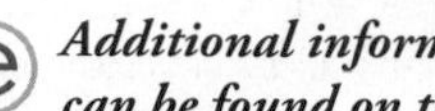

***Additional information related to content in Chapter 18 can be found on the companion Evolve Web site.***

- Practice Quiz

The dental assistant must acquire a foundation in microbiology to understand the nature of **pathogens** (disease-producing microorganisms) and ways to prevent the transmission of disease in the dental office. This knowledge helps the assistant to make important decisions regarding infection control products and procedures (see Chapter 19). It is important to note that the two most common oral diseases, *dental caries* (decay) and *periodontal disease,* are caused by bacterial infections.

**Microbiology** is the study of microorganisms (*micro-* means microscopically small, and *bio-* means living organisms). Because of their microscopic size, the existence of microorganisms usually goes unnoticed unless they cause illness. Most people experience common colds in the winter months, and many others experience life-threatening illnesses caused by microorganisms.

Fortunately, most microorganisms are **nonpathogenic** (i.e., they do not produce human illness). In fact, microorganisms are valuable allies in many ways. Microorganisms used in the production of flavorful cheeses and yogurt, for example, are particularly beneficial. Other microorganisms are used in the disposal of waste products, the fertilization of soil, and the production of lifesaving drugs.

# Pioneers in Microbiology

Aristotle (384–322 BC) introduced the earliest belief that life was "spontaneously generated" from nonliving matter. This theory remained unchallenged for more than 2000 years. According to this theory, living things arose from muck, decaying food, warm rain, or even dirty shirts.

Antony van Leeuwenhoek (LAY-vuhn-hoak) (1632–1723) was a Dutch merchant and an amateur scientist. He used a primitive microscope to observe stagnant water and scrapings from the teeth. His microscope was simple; it consisted of a small lens that was mounted between two thin plates of metal. Through the lens at about 300× magnification, van Leeuwenhoek could see small life-forms he called "animalcules." After 20 years of careful observation, he reported his findings to the Royal Society of London.

John Tyndall (TIN-duhl) (1820–1893) was an English physicist who explained the need for prolonged heating to destroy microbial life in broth. He discovered that bacteria existed in heat-stable and heat-sensitive forms. Prolonged or intermittent heating was needed to destroy the heat-stable form. Intermittent heating, now called **tyndallization**, killed both forms. Almost simultaneously, German botanist Ferdinand Cohn (1828–1898) described the heat-stable forms as **endospores**, which are formed during the life cycle of certain bacteria (see Chapter 21).

Joseph Lister (1827–1912) was an English surgeon who recognized the role of airborne microorganisms in postsurgical infection. By applying carbolic acid to dressings and using an aerosol of carbolic acid during surgery, he lowered the risk of infection after surgery.

Robert Koch (1843–1910) was a German physician who provided the techniques and discipline necessary to guide future microbiologists. He developed a two-part dish that was used for growing bacteria and a technique used for isolating pure colonies of bacteria (Fig. 18.1). The two-part dishes were named **Petri plates** after Julius Petri (1852–1921), a German bacteriologist. Petri plates are still used in microbiology laboratories today. To prove that a specific microorganism caused a particular disease, Koch applied guidelines that are still in use today.

Louis Pasteur (1822–1895) was the famous French chemist who disproved the theory of spontaneous generation of life and

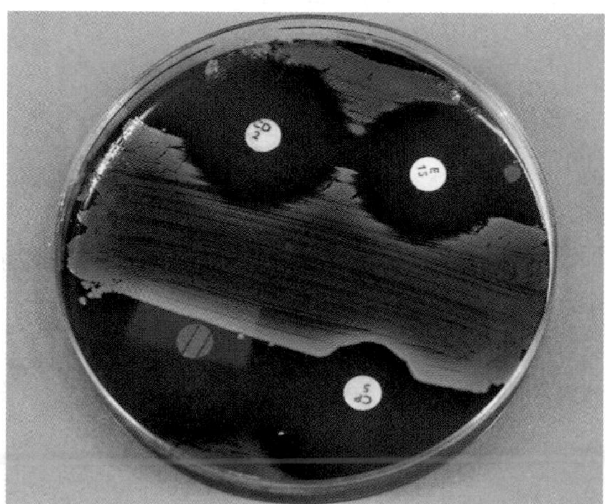

**FIG. 18.1** Colonies of bacteria are growing in the culture medium in this Petri plate. *(From Samaranayake LP: Essential microbiology in dentistry, ed 4, New York, 2012, Churchill Livingstone.)*

associated living microorganisms with disease. Pasteur designed flasks shaped like swan necks (S-shaped) for heating broths. The curved pathway caused by bends in the glass prevented dust particles, which contained microorganisms from the air, from entering the heated broth. Instead, the dust particles settled in the bends of the long-necked flasks, even over an extended period. When the top of a flask was removed, microorganisms once again appeared in the liquid. Pasteur's experiments put an end to the theory of spontaneous generation of life.

## Koch's Postulates

- The microbial agent must be found in every case of the disease.
- The microorganism must be isolated and grown in pure culture.
- The microorganism must cause the same disease when inoculated into a susceptible animal.
- The same microbial agent must be recovered from the inoculated animal.

Pasteur's ongoing contributions to the emerging germ theory of disease earned him the title "Father of Microbiology." At the request of Napoleon III in 1863, Pasteur saved the French wine industry by showing that vats of spoiled wine contained acid-producing bacteria. Contaminants could be destroyed in a short time at temperatures of 50° F to 60° F. The process of heating grape juice to reduce microorganisms became known as *pasteurization.* Today, pathogens in milk are destroyed through pasteurization.

Pasteur prepared the first vaccine for the fatal animal disease *rabies.* Although he never isolated the actual rabies virus, he infected rabbits by inoculating them with a preparation from the medulla (a portion of the brain stem and spinal cord) of rabid dogs. The virus migrated to the spinal cord and the brain of rabbits. Pasteur maintained the organism through successive inoculations in rabbits (Fig. 18.2). He inoculated dogs with dried, powdered rabbit medulla, suspended in broth, to prevent rabies.

The French government built the Pasteur Institute in 1888 to honor Pasteur, whose last words reportedly were, "There is still a great deal to do" (Fig. 18.3).

RECALL

1 Why is microbiology important to the dental assistant?
2 Who is referred to as the "Father of Microbiology"?
3 Who recognized that airborne microorganisms were responsible for postsurgical infections?
4 Who was responsible for discovering the rabies vaccine?

## Major Groups of Microorganisms

The five major groups of microorganisms are (1) bacteria, (2) algae, (3) protozoa, (4) fungi, and (5) viruses. Members of the first four groups are easily recognized with the aid of a light microscope, which is used in most laboratories. Viruses, however, are so tiny that they can be seen only with a powerful electron microscope.

**Viruses** often have been described as "perfect parasites" because they live inside cells of the host and use the resources of the cells to produce up to 10,000 offspring as quickly as within 7 hours. Today, viruses are responsible for most of the emerging microbial diseases. Cells in which invading viruses live and replicate are called *host cells.*

Although it is not a member of the major groups, a recently discovered infectious particle is known as a *prion.* **Prions** are unique agents in that they contain abnormal protein with *no* DNA or RNA (deoxyribonucleic or ribonucleic acid). Prions are responsible for a group of chronic diseases with long incubation periods (see later discussion in the section about prions).

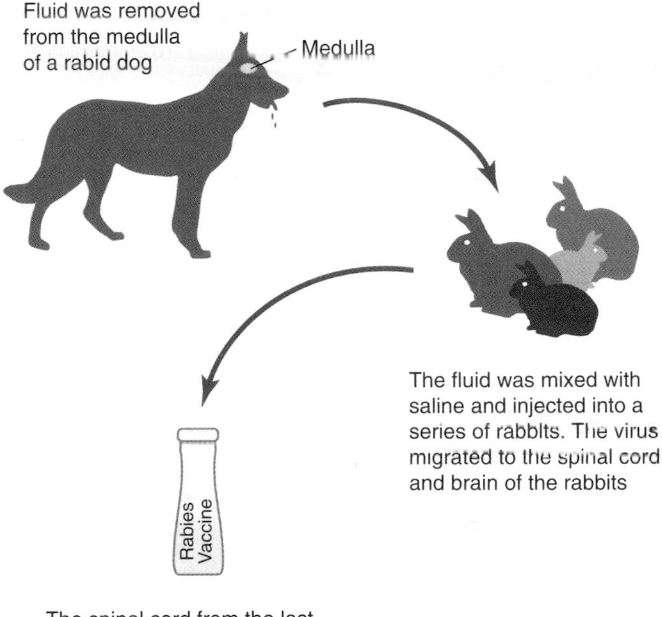


**FIG. 18.2** Discovery of rabies vaccine by Louis Pasteur, 1885.

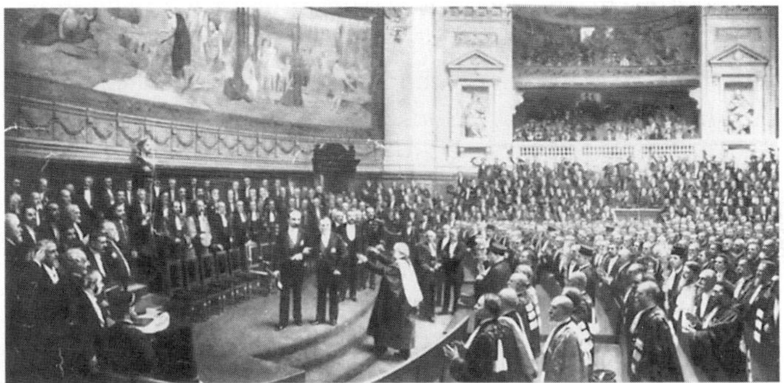

**FIG. 18.3** Louis Pasteur is honored at the Sorbonne. *(Courtesy National Library of Medicine, Bethesda, MD.)*

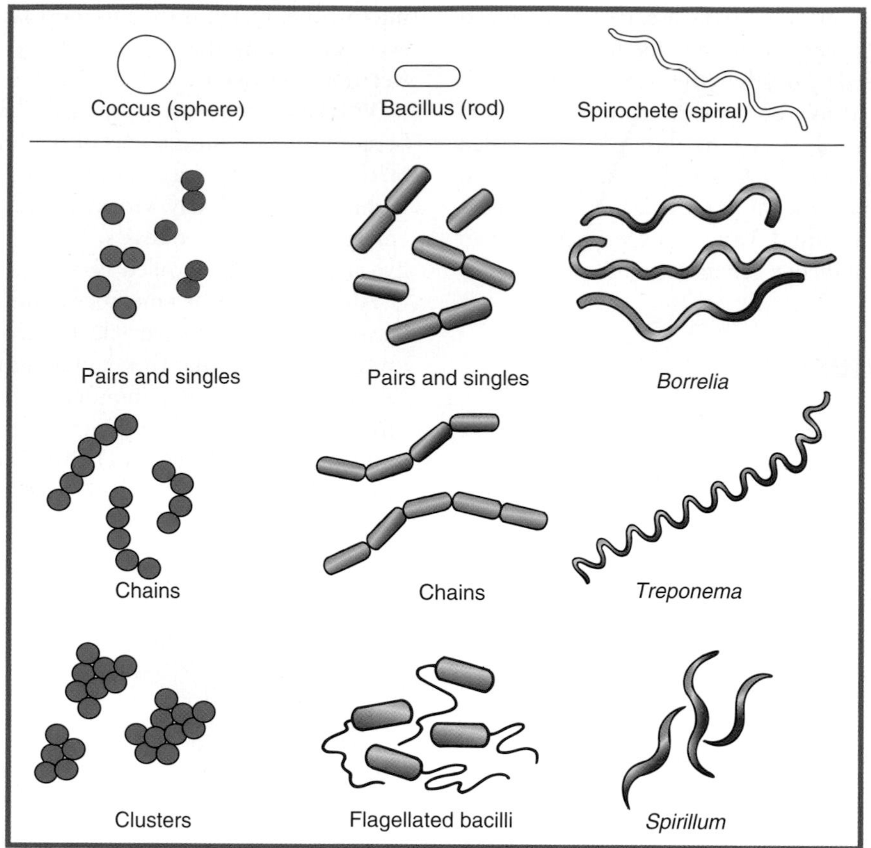


**FIG. 18.4** Three basic shapes of bacteria. *(From Stepp CA, Woods M: Laboratory procedures for medical office personnel, Philadelphia, 1998, Saunders.)*

## Bacteria

**Bacteria** (singular, *bacterium*) make up a large group of one-celled microorganisms that vary in size, shape, and arrangement of cells. Most bacteria are capable of living independently under favorable environmental conditions. Pathogenic bacteria usually grow best at 98.6° F (37° C) in a moist, dark environment.

Bacterial infection can be spread through various means (see Chapter 19). Humans host a variety of bacteria at all times. The skin, respiratory tract, and gastrointestinal tract are inhabited by a great variety of harmless bacteria, called *normal flora.* These bacteria are beneficial and protect the human host by aiding in metabolism and preventing entrance of harmful bacteria.

Infection occurs when bacteria that occur naturally in one part of the body invade another part of the body and become harmful. When this occurs, normal florae are considered *opportunistic,* or causing infection. For example, the urinary tract infection called *cystitis* is caused by contamination with *Escherichia coli,* a bacterium that is found in normal flora in the intestine.

### *Shape*

Most bacteria can be classified according to their shape. When viewed under a microscope, bacteria can be seen to have three shapes: (1) spherical (cocci), (2) rod (bacilli), and (3) spiral (spirochetes) (Fig. 18.4).

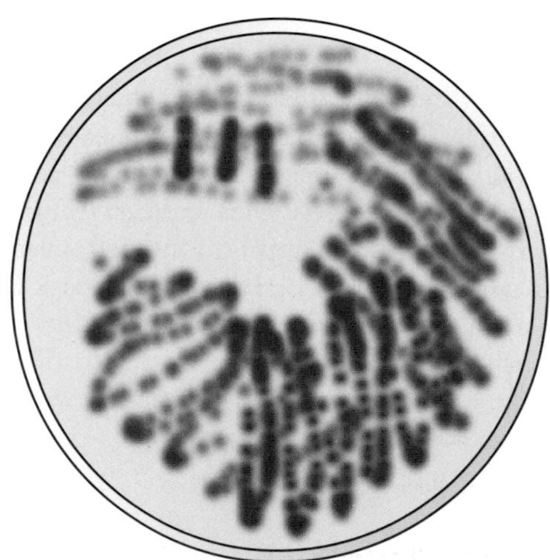

**FIG. 18.5** Colonies of streptococci growing on agar medium are diagnostic for strep throat. *(From Stepp CA, Woods M: Laboratory procedures for medical office personnel, Philadelphia, 1998, Saunders.)*

**Cocci** reproduce by dividing into two. Cocci that form chains as they divide are called **streptococci**. Examples of infections caused by streptococci include pharyngitis (a severe sore throat commonly known as "strep throat"), tonsillitis, pneumonia, and endocarditis (Fig. 18.5). Cocci that form irregular groups or clusters are called **staphylococci**. Examples of infections caused by staphylococci include boils

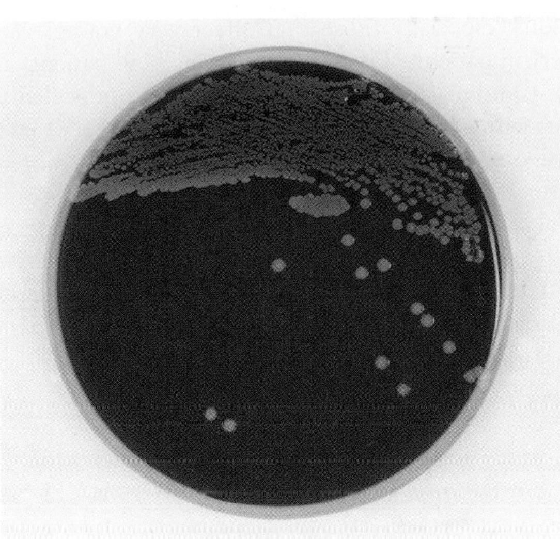

**FIG. 18.6** Golden-yellow colonies of staphylococci. *(From Samaranayake LP: Essential microbiology in dentistry, ed 4, New York, 2012, Churchill Livingstone.)*

and other skin infections, endocarditis, and pneumonia (Fig. 18.6).

**Bacilli** (singular, *bacillus*) are rod-shaped bacteria. Tuberculosis is a disease that is caused by a bacillus.

**Spirochetes** are spiral-shaped bacteria that have flexible cell walls and are capable of movement. Lyme disease, which is transmitted to humans through the bite of an infected deer tick, is caused by a spirochete. Syphilis is also caused by a spirochete (see later discussion in the section about syphilis under Bacterial Diseases).

## Gram-Positive and Gram-Negative Bacteria

In 1884 Hans Christian Gram, a Danish bacteriologist, developed a four-step staining process for separating bacteria into two groups. **Gram's stain** requires the sequential use of a crystal violet dye, iodine solution, alcohol solution, and safranin dye. A physician may make a diagnosis on the basis of Gram's stain and begin appropriate antimicrobial therapy. The classification follows:

- Bacteria that are stained by the dye are classified as **Gram positive**. They appear dark purple under the microscope (Fig. 18.7).
- Bacteria that do not hold the stain are classified as **Gram negative**. They are almost colorless and nearly invisible under the microscope (Fig. 18.8).
- Bacteria that are not consistently stained are classified as **gram variable**. An example is the organism called *Mycobacterium tuberculosis*.

## Need for Oxygen

**Aerobes** are a variety of bacteria that require oxygen to grow. **Anaerobes** are bacteria that grow in the absence of oxygen and are destroyed by oxygen. **Facultative anaerobes** are organisms that can grow in the presence or the absence of oxygen.

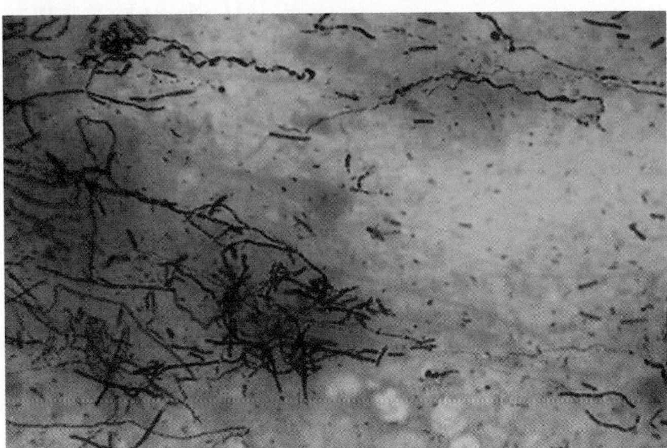

**FIG. 18.7** Gram-positive stain. *(Mahon CR, Lehman DC, Manuselis G: Textbook of diagnostic microbiology, ed 4, Philadelphia, 2011, Saunders.)*

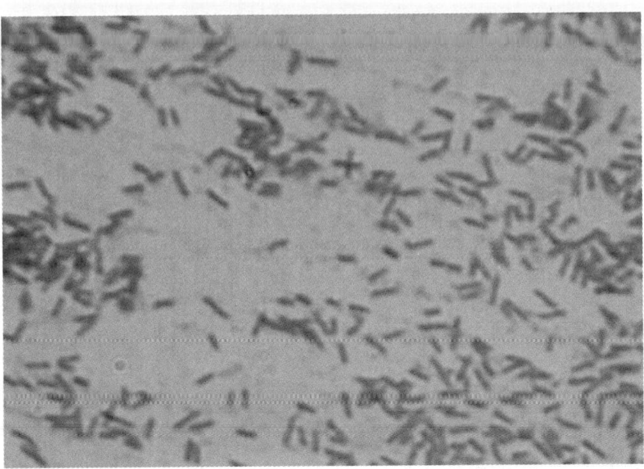

**FIG. 18.8** Gram-negative stain. *(From VanMeter KC, VanMeter WG, Hubert RJ: Microbiology for the healthcare professional, St Louis, 2010, Mosby.)*

## Capsules

Some types of bacteria form a capsule that serves as a protective layer that covers the cell wall. *Streptococcus mutans*, which is a causative factor in dental caries, forms such a capsule.

Bacteria with this protective coating are generally **virulent** (capable of causing serious disease) because the capsule enhances their ability to resist the body's defense mechanisms. The capsule may also prevent antibiotic agents from affecting the bacteria.

## Spores

Under unfavorable conditions, some bacteria change into a highly resistant form called *spores*. Tetanus is an example of a disease caused by a spore-forming bacillus.

Bacteria remain alive in the spore form but are inactive. As spores, they cannot reproduce or cause disease. When conditions are again favorable, these bacteria become active and capable of causing disease.

Spores represent the *most resistant form* of life known. They can survive extremes of heat and dryness and even the presence of disinfectants and radiation. Because of this incredible resistance, harmless spores are used to test the effectiveness of techniques used to sterilize dental instruments (see Chapter 21).

RECALL

5 What are the three primary shapes of bacteria?
6 What is the staining process for separating bacteria?
7 What is the term for bacteria that require oxygen to grow?
8 What is the most resistant form of bacterial life?

## Rickettsiae

Rickettsiae are short, nonmotile (nonmovable) rods that normally live in the intestinal tract of insects such as lice, fleas, ticks, and mosquitoes. These organisms are very small and require host cells to reproduce.

Diseases caused by rickettsiae include typhus and Rocky Mountain spotted fever. These diseases are transmitted to humans through the bite of an infected insect.

## Algae

Algae range from microscopic single-cell organisms to larger multiple-cell organisms such as seaweed and kelp. All algae contain chlorophyll, as well as pigments that cause them to appear yellow-green, brown, or red. Algae are found in abundance in freshwater and marine habitats. Most algae do not produce human disease.

## Protozoa

**Protozoa** (singular, *protozoon* or *protozoan*) consist of a large group of one-cell organisms that do not have a rigid cell wall. Protozoa are found in freshwater and marine habitats and in moist soil. Their diet includes bacteria, small algae, and other protozoa.

Some protozoa can remain viable as cysts outside their hosts for long periods. The thick walls of the cyst make them resistant to drying. Most protozoa do not cause disease, but some live in hosts and do cause damage. A small number of protozoa are responsible for intestinal infections of humans; others invade the blood, lungs, liver, or brain.

## Fungi

**Fungi** (singular, *fungus*) are organisms such as mushrooms, yeasts, and molds that lack *chlorophyll,* the substance that makes plants green. Fungi are not green.

***Candida*** is a common yeast that is found in the oral cavity of about half the patient population. It also is found in the gastrointestinal tract, the female genital tract, and sometimes the skin. Cross-infection may occur from mother to baby and among infant siblings.

**Oral candidiasis** is caused by the yeast *Candida albicans.* All forms of candidiasis are considered to be opportunistic infections, especially those that affect very young, very old, and very ill patients. Infants and terminally ill patients also are at risk. Candidiasis infections are common under dentures in patients with human immunodeficiency virus (HIV) infection.

Oral candidiasis is characterized by white membranes on the surface of the oral mucosa, on the tongue, and elsewhere in the oral cavity. The lesions may resemble thin cottage cheese; wiping reveals a raw, red, and sometimes bleeding base (Fig. 18.9). Candidiasis is treated with topical antifungal preparations such as nystatin, administered in the form of lozenges.

## Prions

Prions were discovered by Dr. Stanley Prusiner while he was doing research into **Creutzfeldt-Jakob disease** (a rare central nervous system disease causing dementia) and other degenerative disorders. Prions are defined as "small proteinaceous infectious particles," thus their name. Prions are composed entirely of proteins that lack nucleic acids (DNA or RNA).

The recent discovery that proteins alone can transmit an infectious disease came as a great surprise to the scientific community. Until the discovery of prions, it was believed that any agent capable of transmitting disease had to be made up of genetic material composed of nucleic acids.

Prions convert normal protein molecules into dangerous ones simply by causing the normal ones *to change their shape.*

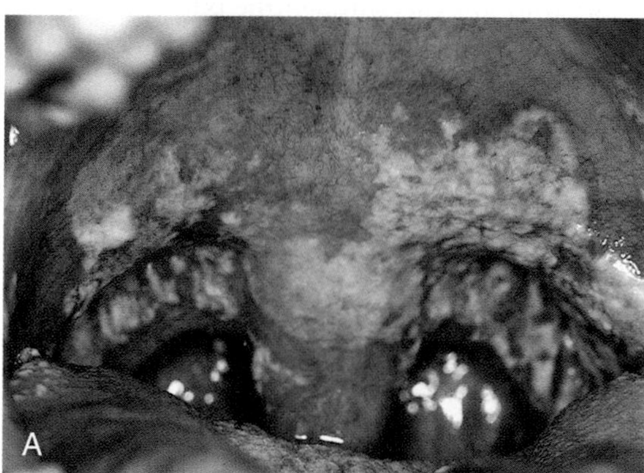


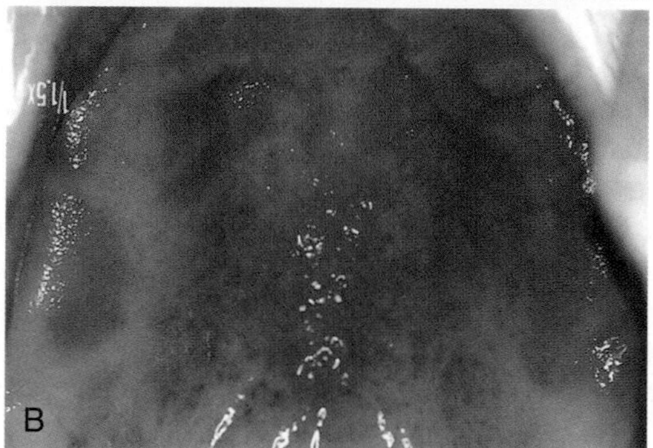


**FIG. 18.9** A, Multiple white plaques of pseudomembranous candidiasis (thrush) in an individual infected with human immunodeficiency virus (HIV). B, *Candida*-associated denture stomatitis with the edentulous maxillary arch. *(From Regezi JA, Sciubba JJ, Pogrel MA: Atlas of oral and maxillofacial pathology, St Louis, 2000, Saunders.)*

Therefore prions are a new and separate class, different from bacteria, fungi, viruses, and all other known pathogens.

### Prion Diseases

Prions are responsible for mad cow disease and are linked to human diseases such as Creutzfeldt-Jakob disease and possibly Alzheimer's disease. The known prion diseases are all fatal. These diseases are sometimes referred to as *spongiform encephalopathies.* They are so named because they frequently cause holes in the brain.

Prion diseases in humans are rare; all affect the brain and can be dormant for years. Disease has been transmitted by corneal transplant, contaminated surgical instruments, and injections of growth hormone derived from human pituitaries (before artificial hormone became available).

In animals, prions cause *scrapie* (a disease in sheep) and *bovine spongiform encephalopathy* (mad cow disease). Prion diseases may be hereditary *or* transmissible; this is of particular interest to scientists and infection control experts. Prions are highly resistant to heat, chemical agents, and irradiation. No treatment or vaccine is available to protect against prion diseases. The only known preventive measure consists of not eating suspected foods, especially those that contain *neural* (nerve) tissue.

**9** How are prions different from other microorganisms? 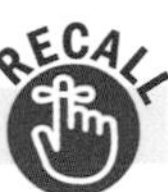


### Future Research

Research is ongoing to determine whether prions that consist of other proteins play a part in more common neurodegenerative conditions such as Alzheimer's disease, Parkinson's disease, and amyotrophic lateral sclerosis (Lou Gehrig's disease). These three disorders have marked similarities. As with all prion diseases, these neuropathologic diseases occur sporadically but sometimes run in families. All are usually diseases of middle to later life, and they share similar pathologies.

## Viruses

Viruses are much smaller than bacteria. Despite their tiny size, many viruses cause fatal disease. New and increasingly destructive viruses are being discovered, and this event has caused the creation of a special area within microbiology called *virology* (the study of viruses and their effects).

Viruses can live and multiply only *inside* an appropriate host cell. The host cells may be human, animal, plant, or bacteria. A virus invades a host cell, *replicates* (produces copies of itself), and then destroys the host cell so that viruses are released into the body. The various forms of viral hepatitis and HIV are discussed in greater detail later in this chapter.

### Specificity

Viruses must have *specificity* (preference) for particular cell types to replicate. Some viruses have a high degree of specificity. For example, HIV infects cells known as CD4 cells, and hepatitis virus infects only liver cells. Other viruses are able to cause disease in more than one organ. For example, the mumps virus can infect the thyroid, pancreas, testicles, and ovaries.

Unfortunately, some viruses can cross the placenta and infect the fetus. One fourth of HIV-infected mothers pass the infection on to the infant. Cytomegalovirus (CMV) infection during pregnancy is a major cause of intellectual disability, blindness, and impaired hearing in children.

### Latency

Some viruses establish a **latent** (dormant) state in host cells. The virus becomes integrated into the nucleic acid of the host cell and is known as a **provirus**. A latent virus can be reactivated in the future to produce additional infective viral particles, followed by signs and symptoms of the disease.

Stress, infection with another virus, and exposure to ultraviolet light can reactivate the virus. Some patients with HIV have experienced prolonged periods of latency and have remained in good health for many years. For example, hepatitis C is known to have a latency period of 15 to 25 years.

### Treatment of Viral Diseases

Viruses cause many clinically significant diseases in humans. Unfortunately, most viral diseases can be treated only *symptomatically,* that is, treatment targets the *symptom,* not the infective cause.

Viruses cannot be grown on artificial culture media and *cannot* be destroyed by antibiotic drugs. General antibiotics are ineffective in preventing or curtailing viral infections. Even the few drugs that are effective against specific viruses have limitations because viruses often produce different types of infection, have different host cells, or the drugs themselves may cause serious effects.

Viruses are also capable of *mutation* (changing). Viruses can change in such a way that they become better suited to survive current conditions and to resist efforts to kill them. It is very difficult to develop vaccines against viruses because of their ability to change their genetic code.

### Transmission of Viral Diseases

Viral diseases are transmitted by (1) direct contact, (2) insects, (3) **percutaneous** injury, (4) blood transfusions, (5) contaminated food or water, and (6) inhalation of droplets expelled by coughing or sneezing.

### Viruses in the Environment

Viruses can be destroyed easily in the external environment. Widely used chemicals such as chlorine (bleach), iodine, phenol, and formaldehyde effectively destroy viruses on surfaces and objects coming into contact with the infected patient. These agents, however, are too toxic to be used internally (see Chapter 21).

## Viral Diseases

## Viral Hepatitis

At least five types of viral hepatitis are known, each of which is caused by a different virus: hepatitis A virus (HAV), hepatitis B virus (HBV), hepatitis C virus (HCV), hepatitis D virus (HDV), and hepatitis E virus (HEV) (Table 18.1).

**TABLE 18.1** Primary Types of Hepatitis

| | A | B | C | D | E |
|---|---|---|---|---|---|
| Source of virus | Fecal-oral | Blood and body fluids | Blood and body fluids | Blood and body fluids | Fecal-oral |
| Route of transmission | Fecal-oral | Percutaneous and mucosal tissues | Percutaneous and mucosal tissues | Percutaneous and mucosal tissues | Fecal-oral |
| Chronic infection | No | Yes | Yes | Yes | No |
| Prevention | Vaccine | Immunization | Perform blood donor screening; modify risky behavior | HBV vaccine | Ensure safe drinking water |

### Hepatitis A

Hepatitis A virus (HAV) can affect anyone. It is spread from person to person by putting something in the mouth that has been contaminated through the stool of a person with hepatitis A. This type of transmission is called "fecal-oral." Good personal hygiene and proper sanitation can help prevent hepatitis A. Always wash your hands after changing a diaper or using the bathroom. Hepatitis A is the least serious form of viral hepatitis. A vaccine is available that provides long-term prevention in persons older than 2 years of age.

### Hepatitis B

Hepatitis B virus (HBV) causes a very serious disease that may result in prolonged illness, liver cancer, cirrhosis of the liver, liver failure, and even death. It is a blood-borne disease that may also be transmitted by other body fluids, including saliva.

Anyone who has ever had the disease, and some persons who have been exposed but have not actually been ill, may be carriers of HBV. This means that patients who appear to be healthy and have no history of the disease may actually be spreading the infection to others. HBV is responsible for 34 percent of all types of acute viral hepatitis. This presents a high risk for dental personnel because dental treatment brings them into contact with saliva and blood.

For more information on hepatitis and other blood-borne diseases, go to http://www.cdc.gov/ncidod/diseases/hepatitis. Information presented here has been modified from the Top 11 Most Frequently Asked Questions about Viral Hepatitis, found on the CDC Web site.

In addition, dental personnel may unknowingly be carriers of the disease. This situation always presents the risk that the infection may be transmitted to the patient during treatment.

#### Questions Frequently Asked About Viral Hepatitis

Q. What is viral hepatitis?

A. Hepatitis is inflammation of the liver caused by a virus. Five types of hepatitis have been identified, and each one is caused by a different virus. In the United States hepatitis A virus (HAV), hepatitis B virus (HBV), and hepatitis C virus (HCV) are the most common types.

Q. What are the symptoms of viral hepatitis?

A. The symptoms of newly acquired hepatitis A, B, and C are the same. If symptoms occur, they might include the following:

- Tiredness
- Loss of appetite
- Nausea
- Abdominal discomfort
- Dark urine
- Clay-colored bowel movements
- Yellowing of the skin and eyes (jaundice)

Q. How long can HAV, HBV, and HCV survive outside the body?

A. HAV can live outside the body for months, depending on environmental conditions. HBV can survive outside the body for at least 7 days and still be capable of transmitting infection. HCV can survive outside the body and continue to transmit infection for 16 hours, but not longer than 4 days.

Q. How long is the HBV vaccine effective?

A. The HBV vaccine protects against chronic HBV infection for at least 15 years, even though antibodies may drop to below detectable levels.

Q. Are booster doses of the HBV vaccine needed?

A. No, booster doses of the vaccine are not recommended routinely.

#### Who Should Get the HBV Vaccine?

- All babies at birth
- All children from birth to 18 years of age who have not been vaccinated
- Persons of any age whose behavior puts them at risk for HBV infection
- Persons whose jobs expose them to human blood and/or body fluids

*HBV,* Hepatitis B virus.

**HEPATITIS B VIRUS IMMUNIZATION.** A highly effective vaccine is available to prevent HBV. All dental personnel with a chance of occupational exposure should be vaccinated against HBV. The Occupational Safety and Health Administration (OSHA) Blood-Borne Pathogens Standard (BBP) (see Chapter 19) requires that an employer offer the hepatitis B vaccination, at no cost to the employee, within 10 days of initial assignment to a position in which an employee may be occupationally exposed to blood or other body fluids. The employee has the right to refuse the offer of vaccination; however, that employee must sign a release form that states that the employer offered the vaccine, and that the employee understands the potential risks of contracting HBV. Should the employee decide at a later date to receive the vaccine, the employer is responsible to provide the vaccine at no cost.

Postvaccination testing is recommended 1 to 6 months after the third injection, to ensure that the individual has developed the antibodies necessary for immunity. Should antibodies not be present, the three-dose series should be repeated. The HBV vaccine is considered safe for pregnant women.

### Hepatitis C

Hepatitis C virus (HCV) is most efficiently transmitted through blood transfusion or by percutaneous exposure to blood. The carrier rate associated with HCV is higher than that associated with HBV. Currently, there is no vaccine against HCV.

Up to 75 percent of people with HCV are unaware that they have the disease; however, their livers are slowly being damaged. Often, by the time symptoms appear, liver damage is already advanced.

Before 2011 treatment for HCV could last as long as a year, often with cure rates of only 40 to 50 percent. (Note: *Cure* means that the virus is not detected in the blood when measured 3 months after treatment is completed.) Today HCV treatments are more effective than in previous years. Advances in science provide more treatment options that are shorter and injection free with higher cure rates for most patients with HCV.

The risk of occupational exposure to HCV for dental professionals involves needle sticks or other percutaneous injuries.

#### Updated CDC Guidelines

The CDC guidelines now recommend a one-time HCV screening for all baby boomers (persons born between 1945 and 1965).

Testing can save lives. As baby boomers are 5 times more likely to have HCV than other adults, it is estimated that this recommendation will save over 120,000 lives.

*CDC,* Centers for Disease Control and Prevention.

### Hepatitis D

Hepatitis D virus (HDV) is a defective virus that cannot replicate itself without the presence of HBV. Therefore infection with HDV may occur simultaneously as a coinfection with HBV, or it may occur in an HBV carrier. Persons with a coinfection of HBV and HDV often have more severe acute disease and a greater risk of death than those infected with HBV alone. Vaccination against HBV also prevents infection with HDV.

### Hepatitis E

Hepatitis E virus (HEV) is not transmitted through bloodborne contact. It is most frequently transmitted via the fecal-oral route through contaminated food or water. The disease is most frequently seen in the form of an epidemic in developing countries, and transmission is not a major concern in a standard dental setting.

#### Tips for Remembering Types of Hepatitis

- Consonants refer to the blood-borne strains (B, C, and D).
- Vowels refer to fecal-oral transmission (A and E).

Additional resource: Dental Infection Control Educators and Trainers Toolkit. Available at www.osap.org.

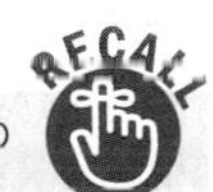


**10** Which types of hepatitis are spread by exposure to blood?

## Human Immunodeficiency Virus

Human immunodeficiency virus (HIV) infection is a bloodborne viral disease in which the body's immune system breaks down. Acquired immunodeficiency syndrome (AIDS) is caused by HIV. When HIV enters the body, it infects special *T cells* and slowly kills them. T cells have special receptors on their surfaces and are primarily responsible for immunity. As more and more T cells die, the body's ability to fight infection weakens.

A person with HIV infection may remain healthy for many years. HIV-positive people develop AIDS when they become sick with serious illnesses and infections that can occur with HIV. See Chapter 17 for the oral conditions that are frequently associated with HIV infection.

HIV is spread through sexual contact with an infected person and by needle sharing among drug users. Before blood donor screening for HIV was instituted, the virus was also transmitted by blood transfusion. Now that blood is screened for HIV antibodies, the blood supply in this country is safe. Babies born to HIV-infected mothers may become infected before or during birth, or through breastfeeding after birth.

In (nondental) healthcare settings, workers have been infected with HIV after they were stuck with needles containing HIV-infected blood or, less frequently, after infected blood entered the worker's bloodstream through an open cut or through splashes into a mucous membrane (e.g., eyes, inside of the nose).

## Herpesviruses

A **herpesvirus** is a double-stranded DNA virus that causes infection in humans such as herpes, CMV, chickenpox, shingles, mononucleosis, measles, and Kaposi's sarcoma. This virus may be dormant for years and then may become activated and cause disease.

Four major herpesviruses are known to affect humans (Table 18.2):

- Herpes simplex virus (HSV) is divided into two types: herpes simplex virus type 1 (HSV 1) and herpes simplex virus type 2 (HSV 2)
- Herpes zoster virus (HZV) or varicella-zoster virus
- Cytomegalovirus (CMV)
- Epstein-Barr virus (EBV)

### *Herpes Simplex Virus Type 1*

Herpes simplex virus type 1 is a viral infection that causes recurrent sores on lips. Because these sores frequently develop when the patient has a cold or fever of other origin, the disease is now commonly known as *fever blisters* or *cold sore* (see Chapter 17).

**PRIMARY HERPES.** This disease, which is highly contagious, makes its first appearance in very young children (1 to 3 years of age) and is known as *primary herpes.* The child may have a slight fever, pain in the mouth, increased salivation, bad breath, and a general feeling of illness. The inside of the mouth becomes swollen, and the gingivae are inflamed.

Healing begins naturally within 3 days, and the illness usually lasts 7 to 14 days. During this time, supportive measures can be taken to make the child more comfortable, relieve pain, and prevent secondary infection.

**RECURRENT HERPES LABIALIS.** After this initial childhood infection occurs, the virus of herpes simplex lies dormant and reappears later in life as the familiar recurring fever blister or cold sore (Fig. 18.10).

**TABLE 18.2 Types of Human Herpesviruses**

| Virus | Description |
|---|---|
| Herpes simplex virus (HSV) | |
| • Herpes simplex virus type 1 | Causes primarily oral lesions |
| • Herpes simplex virus type 2 | Causes primarily genital lesions |
| Herpes zoster virus (HZV) | Causes herpes zoster, shingles, and chickenpox |
| Cytomegalovirus (CMV) | Normally latent (does not cause disease) but may become active when the immune system is damaged; once active, it is highly contagious and is transmitted through most body fluids |
| Epstein-Barr virus (EBV) | Causes infectious mononucleosis and Burkitt's lymphoma, which is a malignancy of the lymph tissues |

For more information about these conditions, go to www.cdc/gov, and search for the specific condition.

Recurrences tend to take place when the patient's general resistance is lowered as a result of stress, fever, illness, injury, and exposure to the sun. The use of sunscreen with a sun protection factor of 15 helps to prevent sun-induced recurrences of herpes. Attacks may recur as infrequently as once a year or as often as weekly or even daily. As in the case of primary herpes, recurrent herpes labialis sores heal by themselves in 7 to 10 days, leaving no scar.

### *Herpes Simplex Virus Type 2*

Herpes simplex virus type 2, also known as *genital herpes,* is one of the most common sexually transmitted diseases (STDs) in the United States. Initial symptoms, which generally appear 2 to 10 days after infection, include tingling, itching, and a burning sensation during urination.

Once a person is infected with the virus, outbreaks will recur. The disease can be transmitted only during these recurrences.

A mother with active vaginal or cervical herpetic lesions at the time of delivery can pass the virus to her newborn. About 50 percent of such newborns will be infected as they pass through the birth canal. At least 85 percent of infected infants will be severely damaged or will be killed by the virus.

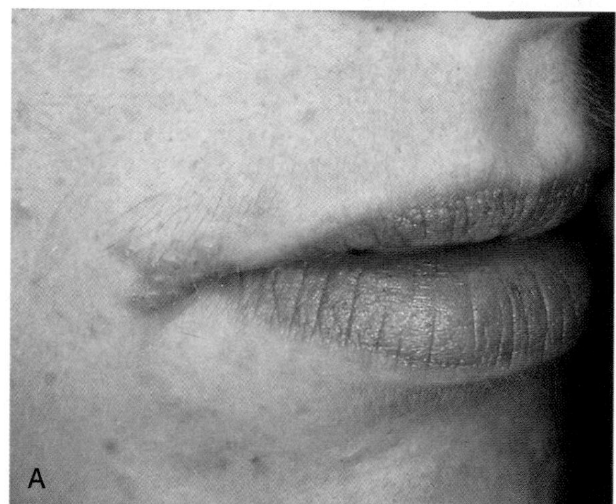


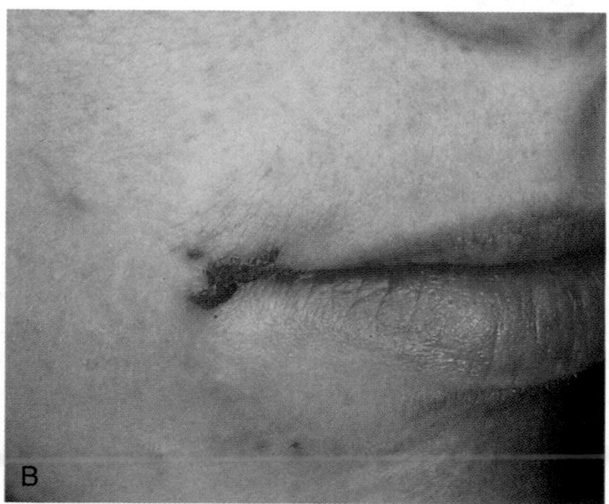


**FIG. 18.10** Herpes labialis. A, 12 hours after onset. B, 48 hours after onset. *(From Ibsen OAC, Phelan JA: Oral pathology for the dental hygienist, ed 6, Philadelphia, 2014, Saunders.)*

### Herpes Zoster Virus

HZV (human herpesvirus type 3) causes both varicella (chickenpox) and herpes zoster (shingles). These two different diseases are caused by the identical organism. Chickenpox is the primary infection, and zoster represents reactivation of the illness. It is a highly contagious infection in individuals who have not been previously exposed to the virus. Transmission occurs through direct contact with skin lesions or through droplet infection from infectious saliva.

### Cytomegalovirus

CMV (human herpesvirus type 5) rarely causes disease unless other factors such as a compromised immune system are present. However, it can infect the fetus during pregnancy. In some cases, infants are born deaf or are intellectually disabled. The route of transmission of CMV is unclear.

### Epstein-Barr Virus

EBV (human herpesvirus type 4) is responsible for various infections, including infectious mononucleosis, nasopharyngeal cancer, lymphoma, and oral hairy leukoplakia (see Chapter 17). Infectious mononucleosis is an acute infectious disease that primarily affects people between the ages of 15 and 20 years. EBV is present in the saliva and is transmitted by kissing; hence it is often called the "kissing disease."

### Herpes Transmission

The major transmission route for the herpesvirus is through direct contact with lesions or with infectious saliva. When oral lesions are present, the patient may be asked to reschedule his or her appointment for a time after the lesions have healed. Even when no active lesions are present, viral transmission through saliva or through aerosol spray from the dental handpiece may occur.

Because no preventive vaccine is available to protect against herpes, it is essential that precautions be taken to prevent exposure. Protective eyewear is particularly important because a herpes infection in the eye may cause blindness. Gloves protect against infection that may be passed through lesions or abrasions on the hands.

## West Nile Virus

The West Nile virus is commonly found in Africa, West Asia, and the Middle East. It is believed to have been present in the United States since the early summer of 1999. This virus is carried by mosquitoes and can infect humans, birds, horses, and some other mammals. It affects a person's nervous system, causing inflammation of the brain and spinal cord. Symptoms include fever, headache, tiredness, aches, and sometimes rash. Cases occur primarily in late summer or early fall. In southern climates, where temperatures are milder, West Nile virus can be transmitted year-round.

## H1N1 Flu Virus (Swine Flu)

The H1N1 is a respiratory disease of pigs caused by type A viruses (Fig. 18.11). The **H1N1** flu virus (also called swine flu) is a virus that until recently has not been known to attack humans. This virus is not related to human seasonal influenza viruses (Table 18.3).

The H1N1 virus spreads very easily from person to person. Infected people may be contagious 1 day before symptoms appear and up to 7 days or longer. Younger children might be contagious for an even longer period. Remember, bacteria can be spread when a person touches something that is contaminated with the virus and then touches the eyes, nose, or mouth before washing hands. Contaminated droplets from the cough or sneeze of an infected person can move through the air and remain on surfaces such as door knobs, shopping carts, telephones, and other objects.

The most effective way to protect yourself is to receive the H1N1 vaccine and practice meticulous hand hygiene. For additional resources on hepatitis, other blood-borne diseases, and H1N1 flu, go to www.osap.org.

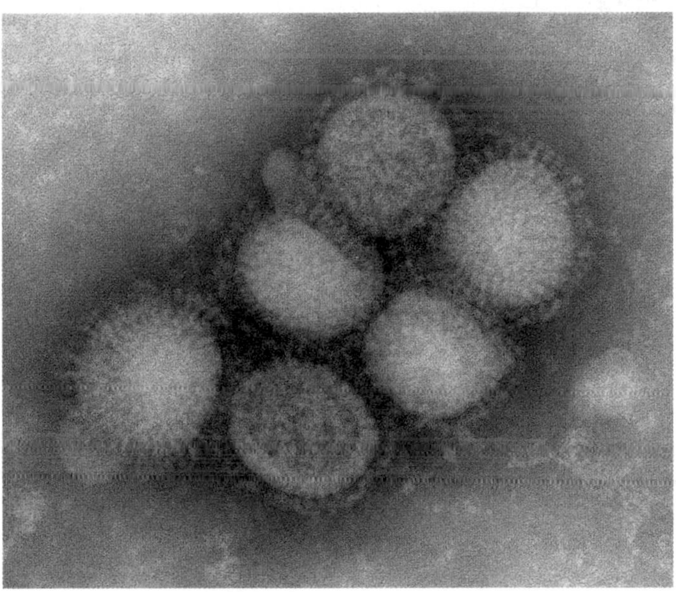

**FIG. 18.11** A colonized transmission electron micrograph (TEM) image showing the presence of a number of novel H1N1 virus virons in a tissue sample. *(Courtesy Centers for Disease Control and Prevention, Atlanta, GA.)*

**TABLE 18.3 Types of Influenza**

| Type | Description |
|---|---|
| Seasonal (or common) flu | Respiratory illness that is easily transmitted from person to person. Most people have some immunity, and a vaccine is available. |
| H1N1 (or swine) flu | Caused by viruses that occur naturally among pigs. The H1N1 variant is deadly to domestic pigs, and the virus can now be transmitted from person to person. A vaccine is available. |
| Pandemic flu | A virulent human flu that causes a global outbreak of serious illness. Because little natural immunity occurs, the disease can spread easily from person to person. |

## Ebola Virus

**Ebola** is a rare but often deadly virus that causes bleeding inside and outside the body (Fig. 18.12). Ebola virus disease (EVD) first occurred in 1976 in remote villages in Central Africa, near tropical rainforests, but the more recent outbreaks in West Africa have involved major urban as well as rural areas. The disease kills up to 90% of people who are infected. Ebola is not as contagious as viruses such as colds, influenza, or measles, and it is not spread from air, water, or food. It is spread through **direct contact** (through broken skin or mucous membranes) with blood and body fluids (urine, feces, saliva, vomit, and semen) of a person who is sick with Ebola. A person infected with Ebola is not considered contagious until symptoms appear.

### *Guideline for Dental Professionals on the Ebola Virus*

Due to the virulent nature of the disease, it is highly unlikely that someone with Ebola symptoms will seek dental care when they are severely ill. However, the Centers for Disease Control and Prevention (CDC) and the American Dental Association (ADA) Division of Science advise dental professionals to take a medical history, including a travel history, from their patients. Any person within 21 days of returning from the West African countries Liberia, Sierra Leone, or Guinea may be at risk of having contacted persons infected with Ebola and may not exhibit symptoms. If this is the case, dental professionals are advised to delay routine dental care of the patient until 21 days have elapsed from their trip. Palliative care for serious oral health conditions, dental infections, and pain can be provided if necessary after consulting with the patient's physician and following standard precautions.

## Zika Virus

Zika virus disease (**Zika**) is a disease caused by the Zika virus that is spread to people primarily through the bite of an infected *Aedes* species mosquito. The most common symptoms of Zika are fever, rash, joint pain, and conjunctivitis (red eyes). The illness is usually mild with symptoms lasting for several days to a week after being bitten by an infected mosquito. People usually do not get sick enough to go to the hospital, and they very rarely die of Zika.

Zika virus can be spread from a pregnant woman to her fetus and has been linked to a serious birth defect of the brain called **microcephaly** (Fig. 18.13) in babies of mothers who had Zika virus while pregnant. Other problems have been detected among fetuses and infants infected with Zika virus before birth, such as absent or poorly developed brain structures, defects of the eye, hearing deficits, and impaired growth. CDC recommends special precautions for pregnant women. Women who are pregnant should not travel to areas with Zika. If you must travel to one of these areas, talk to your healthcare provider first and strictly follow steps to prevent mosquito bites during your trip. There is no vaccine to prevent Zika infection; therefore prevention of mosquito bites is necessary.

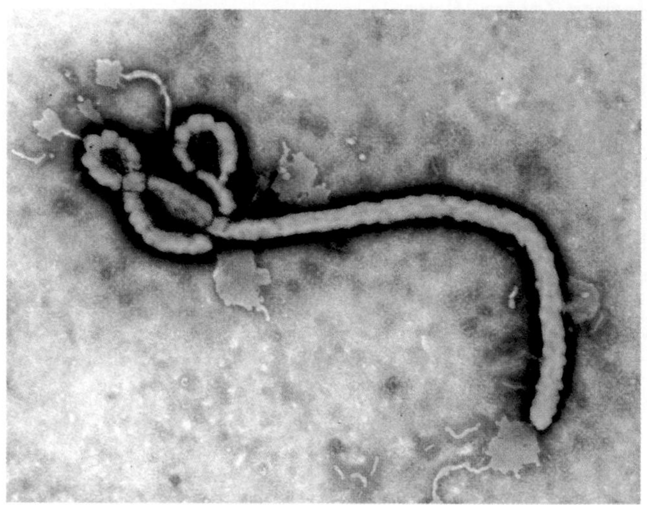

**FIG. 18.12** The Ebola virus is a single-stranded RNA virus that causes the deadly Ebola virus disease. *(From Frederick A. Murphy/Centers for Disease Control and Prevention. http://phil.cdc.gov/phil/home.asp. Accessed March 28, 2016.)*

RECALL

**11** How is HIV spread?
**12** What tissues are affected by the West Nile virus?
**13** How is the H1N1 virus spread?
**14** How is the Ebola virus spread?
**15** How is the Zika virus spread?
**16** What birth defect can be caused by the Zika virus?

# Bacterial Diseases

## Tuberculosis

Tuberculosis, which is caused by the bacterium *Mycobacterium tuberculosis,* is the leading cause of death from infectious diseases worldwide.

Because HIV-infected patients have a weakened immune system, they are highly susceptible to tuberculosis; therefore HIV and tuberculosis often occur together. Of the two, tuberculosis presents a greater health risk for healthcare workers. One reason for this is that the rod-shaped tubercle bacillus is able to withstand disinfectants that kill many other bacteria. Tuberculosis kill time is the benchmark for the effectiveness of a surface disinfectant (see Chapter 20).

## Legionnaires' Disease

The *Legionella pneumophila* bacterium (named after an epidemic of this disease that was reported during an American Legion convention in Philadelphia) is responsible for two acute bacterial diseases: *Pontiac fever* and *Legionnaires' disease.* Bacteria are transmitted through aerosolization and aspiration of contaminated water. (Chapter 24 discusses dental unit waterlines.)

No person-to-person transmission is involved. *L. pneumophila* bacteria have been found to thrive in lakes, creeks, hot tubs, spas, air conditioning systems, shower heads, water distillation systems, and the biofilm found in dental unit waterlines (Fig. 18.14). Dental personnel have higher levels of antibodies

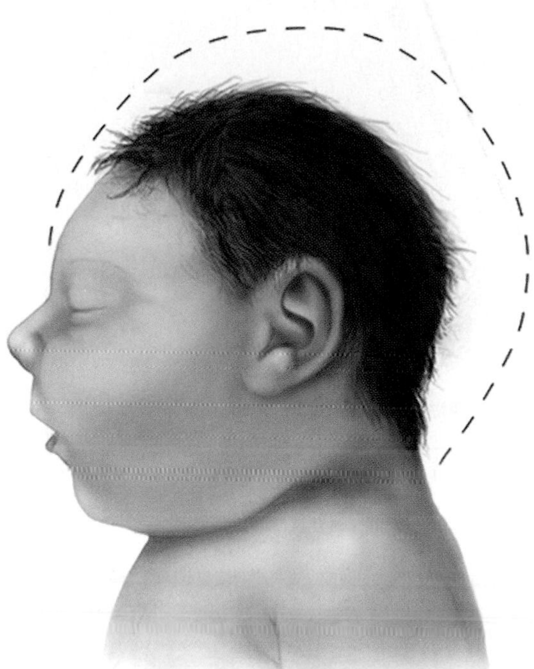

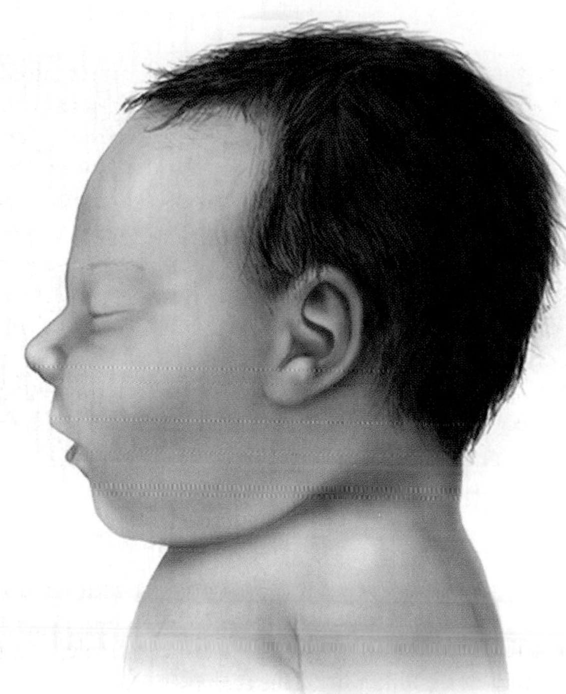

**FIG. 18.13** A baby with microcephaly (left) compared with a baby with a typical head size. (By Centers for Disease Control and Prevention, via Wikimedia Commons.)

against *L. pneumophila* than the general public, indicating occupational exposure and resistance to this organism.

The less serious form of infection, called *Pontiac fever,* causes acute flulike symptoms with headache, high fever, dry cough, chills, diarrhea, chest pain, and abdominal pain. The more serious form of infection, called *Legionnaires' disease,* causes a very severe pneumonia. In immunocompromised or elderly individuals, the disease can be fatal.

## Tetanus

Tetanus, which is also known as *lockjaw,* is an extremely dangerous and often fatal disease that is caused by a spore-forming bacillus found in soil, dust, or animal or human feces. This microbe is usually introduced into the body through a wound or a break in the skin (as is seen in a puncture wound from a soiled instrument).

The organism that causes tetanus produces the severe muscle spasms and rigidity that give the disease its popular name of lockjaw. The disease can be prevented by the administration of a vaccine; however, immunity must be kept current through booster doses. (It is important that dental personnel keep all immunizations current.)

## Syphilis

Syphilis, an STD, is caused by *Treponema pallidum* spirochetes. Although these bacteria are fragile outside of the body, direct cross-infection may occur in the dental operatory through contact with oral lesions.

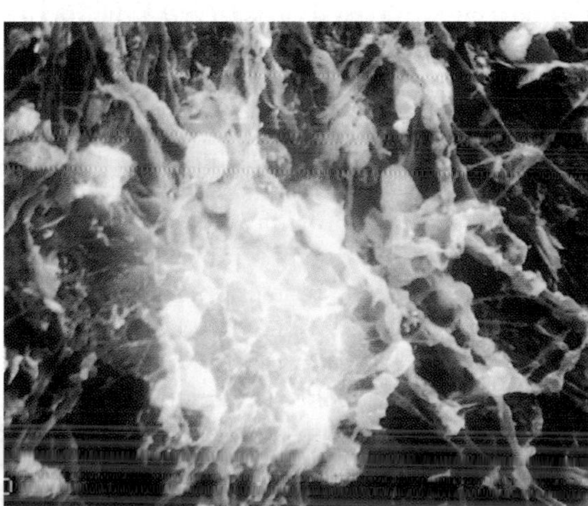

**FIG. 18.14** Bacteria in biofilm taken from dental unit waterlines. *(Courtesy Dr. Shannon Mills/United States Air Force.)*

The first stage of syphilis is characterized by the presence of a painless ulcerating sore, known as a **chancre**, which is infectious *on contact.* When it occurs on the lip, it may resemble herpes, but the crusting is darker (Fig. 18.15).

The second stage is also infectious, and immediate infection may occur through contact with an open sore. Signs of special interest to dental personnel include the following:

- Split papules at the corners of the mouth
- Grayish-white, moist, "mucous patches" on the tongue, roof of the mouth, tonsils, or inner surfaces of the lips (these are *highly infectious*)

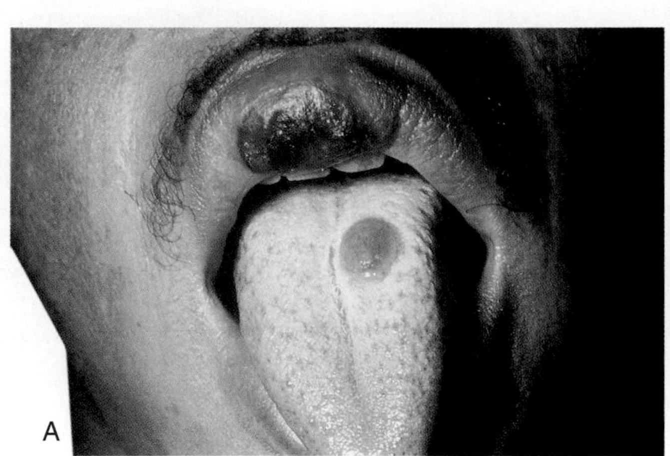


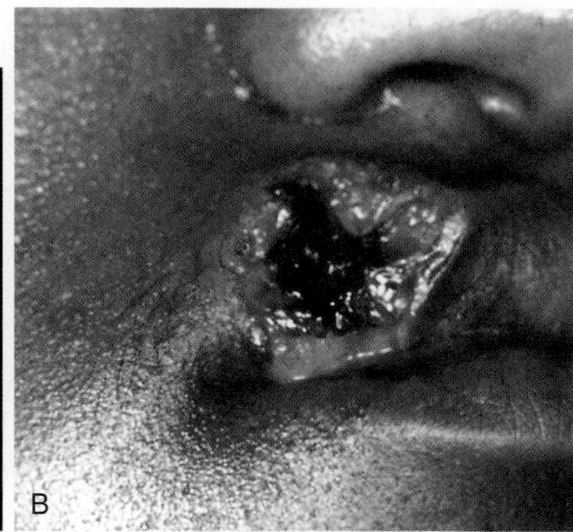


**FIG. 18.15** A, Chancre on tongue seen in primary syphilis. B, Chancre on lip. *(A, From Schachner LA, Hansen RC, eds: Pediatric dermatology, ed 4, London, 2011, Mosby; B, Courtesy Dr. Edward V. Zegarelli.)*

- Generalized measles-type rash, poxlike pustules, oozing sores, and hair falling out of the scalp

The third stage, known as *latent syphilis,* is usually fatal and may occur after the disease has been dormant for 20 years.

## Methicillin-Resistant *Staphylococcus aureus* (MRSA)

**Methicillin-resistant** *Staphylococcus aureus*, commonly referred to as MRSA, is a bacterium that is resistant to some antibiotics. This type of *S. aureus* has evolved through the excessive use of penicillin antibiotics over the years. It causes an infection that is resistant to some antibiotics such as methicillin and other penicillin-type antibiotics such as amoxicillin and the cephalosporins.

*S. aureus* (known as staph) is a common bacterium that is carried on the skin or in the nose of healthy people. It is estimated that 30% of people worldwide carry this bacterium, and most never develop symptoms or illness. Health experts say that MRSA is a version of an everyday bacterium that causes pimples, boils, sinus infection, and, in rare cases, meningitis and blood infection; MRSA is resistant to methicillin. MRSA infections can occur on the surface of the skin or may go into the soft tissue and form a boil or abscess (Fig. 18.16). This infection is common in places where people are in close contact, including schools, dormitories, military barracks, and daycare facilities.

Because MRSA is easily passed to others, you should follow these prevention tips:

- Always maintain good hand hygiene practices
- Never squeeze or try to drain any sore
- Keep any wound covered until it has healed
- Do not share personal items such as towels, razors, sheets, and clothes

Experts say that the key to dealing with MRSA is early diagnosis followed by completion of a full course of antibiotic treatment. The public needs to watch for wounds that do not heal and are not helped by normal antibiotic treatment. Hand hygiene is the best means to prevent the spread of MRSA and all other diseases.

You may obtain additional information from the Centers for Disease Control and Prevention, Environmental Management of Staph and MRSA in Community Settings 8.

## Pandemic Diseases

A **pandemic** disease is a global disease outbreak. A pandemic occurs when a new virus or disease emerges for which people have little or no immunity and for which no vaccine is available. The disease spreads easily from person to person, causes serious illness, and can sweep across the country and around the world in a very short time. In addition to illness and death, an especially severe influenza pandemic may cause severe disruption resulting from school and business closings and interruption of public transportation and food services. Refer to the CDC Web site to learn about the preparations that are available for use in case of a pandemic (www.pandemicflu.gov).

**17** What microorganism is used as the benchmark for the effectiveness of a surface disinfectant?
**18** What disease is also known as lockjaw?
**19** What is a sign of the first stage of syphilis?
**20** What is a pandemic?

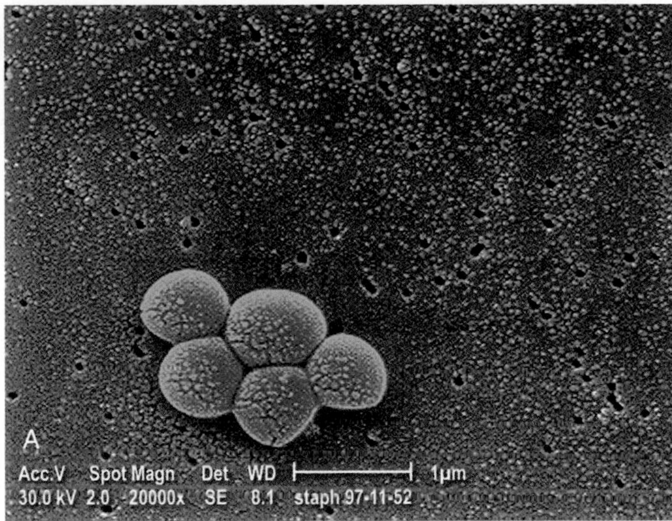


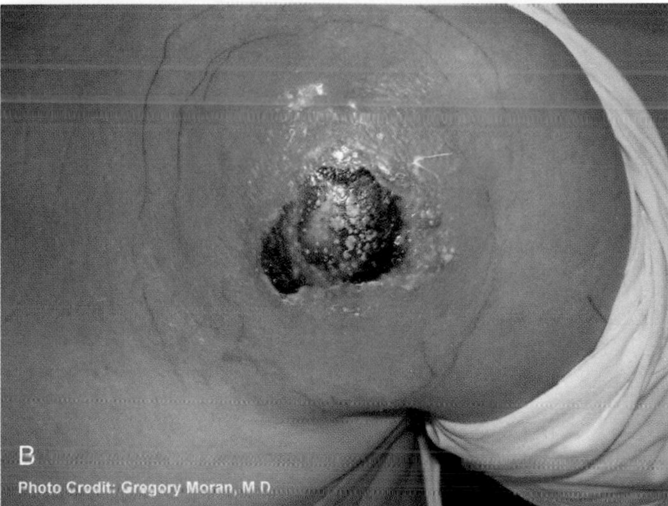


**FIG. 18.16** A, Magnified 20,000×, the colorized scanning electron micrograph (SEM) depicts a grouping of methicillin-resistant *Staphylococcus aureus* (MRSA) bacteria. B, MRSA-caused skin infection depicting a cutaneous abscess on the back of the shoulder. *(A, From Janice Carr, Public Health Image Library [PHIL]. Courtesy Centers for Disease Control and Prevention, Atlanta, GA.* B, *From Gregory Moran, MD. Courtesy Centers for Disease Control and Prevention, Atlanta, GA.)*

**■ Legal and Ethical Implications** As people travel across the country and around the world, the microorganisms they carry travel with them. The patients you see in the office bring with them a variety of microorganisms.

Dental assistants must be especially aware of their daily encounters with microorganisms and the possible consequences. Understanding the microbial world is part of the dental assistant's personal and professional responsibility. Today, many patients are concerned about possible disease transmission in the dental office. To assure patients, the dental assistant should be prepared to discuss all aspects of the infection control procedures followed in the office. To do this, one must have an understanding of microbiology and the characteristics of microorganisms. ■

**■ Eye to the Future** Progress in developing drugs to treat viral diseases such as HIV infection and hepatitis has been slow and difficult because it is difficult to find drugs that are capable of killing viruses without hurting host cells. Antiviral agents must reach target organs without disturbing the cell functions of the host. Progress is being made in the development of drugs for the management of HIV and HCV.

Research continues in the search for antiviral agents that will target only the enzymes responsible for replication of the virus in infected cells. Often, drugs used in combinations can delay or prevent disease. The hope for a cure or for prevention of all forms of hepatitis and HIV infection through vaccines lies with drugs that have not yet been developed. ■

Additional information and resources on Ebola, Zika, and other diseases are available on the CDC's Web site at cdc.gov.

## ■ Critical Thinking

1. On your next trip to the supermarket, look for foods that have been treated through the process of pasteurization.
2. How would you answer a friend who asked, "Why are you studying microbiology to be a dental assistant?"
3. Do you think the world would be a better place if there were no bacteria? Why or why not?
4. Should physicians prescribe antibiotics for viral infections? Why or why not? ■

19

# Disease Transmission and Infection Prevention

## KEY TERMS

**Acquired immunity** Immunity that is developed during a person's lifetime.
**Acute infection** An infection of short duration that is often severe.
**Anaphylaxis (an-uh-fi-LAK-sis)** Extreme hypersensitivity to a substance that can lead to shock and life-threatening respiratory collapse.
**Artificially acquired immunity** Immunity that results from a vaccination.
**Blood-borne disease** Disease that is caused by microorganisms such as viruses or bacteria that are carried in blood.
**Blood-borne pathogens** Disease-causing organisms transferred through contact with blood or other body fluids.
**Chain of infection** Conditions that all must be present for infection to occur.
**Chronic infection** An infection of long duration.
**Communicable disease** Condition caused by an infection that can be spread from person to person or through contact with body fluids.
**Contaminated waste** Items such as gloves and patient napkins that may contain potentially infectious body fluids of patients.
**Direct contact** Touching or contact with a patient's blood or saliva.
**Droplet infection** An infection that occurs through mucosal surfaces of the eyes, nose, or mouth.
**Epidemiologic (ep-i-dee-mee-oe-LOJ-ic) studies** Studies of the patterns and causes of diseases.
**Hazardous waste** Waste that poses a danger to humans or to the environment.
**Immunity (i-MYOO-ni-tee)** Ability of the body to resist disease.
**Indirect contact** Touching or contact with a contaminated surface or instrument.
**Infection control** Policies and practices designed to prevent the spread of infectious agents.
**Infection prevention** Ultimate goal of all infection control procedures and policies.
**Infectious disease** Disease that is communicable.
**Infectious waste** Waste that is capable of transmitting an infectious disease.
**Inherited immunity** Immunity that is present at birth.
**Latent (LAY-tent) infection** Persistent infection with recurrent symptoms that "come and go."
**Naturally acquired immunity** Immunity that occurs when a person has contracted and is recovering from a disease.
**Occupational exposure** Any reasonably anticipated skin, eye, or mucous membrane contact or percutaneous injury involving blood or any other potentially infectious materials.
**OSHA Blood-Borne Pathogens (BBP) Standard** Guidelines designed to protect employees against occupational exposure to blood-borne pathogens.
**Pathogen (PA-thuh-jen)** Disease-causing organism.
**Percutaneous (pur-kyoo-TAY-nee-us)** Through the skin, such as with a needle stick, cut, or human bite.
**Permucosal (per-myoo-KOE-sul)** Contact with mucous membranes, such as the eyes or mouth.
**Personal protective equipment (PPE)** Items such as protective clothing, masks, gloves, and eyewear used to protect employees.
**Sharps** Pointed or cutting instruments, including needles, scalpel blades, orthodontic wires, and endodontic instruments.
**Standard Precautions** Standard of care designed to protect health-care providers from pathogens that can be spread by blood or any other body fluid via excretion or secretion; expands on the concept of Universal Precautions.
**Universal Precautions** Guidelines based on treating all human blood and body fluids (including saliva) as potentially infectious.
**Virulence (VIR-yoo-luhns)** Strength of a pathogen's ability to cause disease; also known as *pathogenicity.*

## LEARNING OUTCOMES

*On completion of this chapter, the student will be able to achieve the following objectives:*

1 Pronounce, define, and spell the key terms.
2 Name the links in the chain of infection.
3 Describe the four types of infections.
4 Describe the modes of disease transmission.
5 Describe the types of immunity, and give examples of each.
6 Describe the five ways disease can be transmitted in a dental office.
7 Describe the roles of the CDC and OSHA in infection control, including the following:
  - Describe the importance of the OSHA Blood-Borne Pathogens Standard.
  - Describe the components of an OSHA exposure control plan.
  - Explain the difference between Standard Precautions and Universal Precautions.
  - Identify the OSHA categories of risk for occupational exposure.
  - Describe the first aid necessary after an exposure incident.

- Discuss the rationale for hepatitis B vaccination for dental assistants.
- Describe the employer's responsibility regarding employee medical records.
- Identify the objects that must be placed in the sharps container.
- Describe ways to prevent needle stick injuries.

**8** Explain the importance of infection control practices for dental assistants, including the following:
- Explain proper hand hygiene for dental assistants.
- Explain the advantages of alcohol-based hand rubs.
- Discuss the types of PPE needed for dental assistants and demonstrate the proper sequence for donning and removing personal protective equipment.
- Identify the various types of masks, eyewear, and gloves used in a dental office.

**9** Give examples of the infection control considerations needed to protect high-tech equipment in the dental office.

**10** Explain the types and symptoms of latex reactions.

**11** Describe waste management in the dental office, including the proper handling and disposal methods for contaminated waste, biohazard waste, and extracted teeth.

**12** Discuss additional infection control practices in the dental office, including the following:
- Explain the CDC recommendations regarding the use of a saliva ejector.
- Describe procedures to prevent cross-contamination in the dental laboratory.
- Explain the precautions necessary when a patient with active tuberculosis is treated.
- Explain the use of preprocedural mouth rinses.
- Describe the rationale of CDC recommendations regarding Creutzfeldt-Jakob disease and other prion-related diseases.
- Describe the rationale of CDC recommendations regarding laser plumes.

## PERFORMANCE OUTCOMES

*On completion of this chapter, the student will be able to meet competency standards in the following skills:*
- To perform appropriate first aid after an exposure incident.
- To wash hands properly before gloving.
- To apply an alcohol-based hand rub.
- To properly put on and remove personal protective equipment.
- To disinfect an alginate impression

## ELECTRONIC RESOURCES

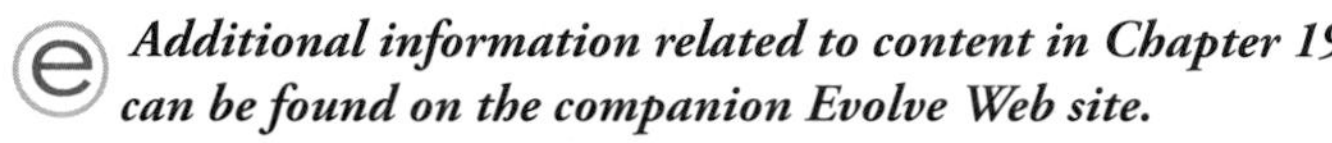
***Additional information related to content in Chapter 19 can be found on the companion Evolve Web site.***

- Practice Quiz
- Video: Handwashing Techniques

As a dental assistant you are at risk of exposure to disease causing agents in a variety of ways. It could be through contact with blood or saliva, contaminated instruments, or airborne infectious agents. In this chapter, you will learn how to break the chain of infection, identify methods of disease transmission, and explain how the immune system provides the body with resistance to infection.

This chapter discusses the Centers for Disease Control and Prevention (CDC) **Infection Control** Guidelines and the requirements of the Occupational Safety and Health Administration **(OSHA) Blood-Borne Pathogens (BBP) Standard**. By carefully following the infection control recommendations and safety information provided in this chapter, you will minimize the risks of disease transmission to yourself, your patients, and other members of the dental team.

## The Chain of Infection

To understand how infection can occur, imagine a chain that has six links. Each link is a condition that *must be present* for infection or disease to occur. The links in the **chain of infection** are (1) an infectious agent, (2) a reservoir, (3) a portal of exit, (4) a mode of transmission, (5) a portal of entry, and (6) a susceptible host (Fig. 19.1). Infection control strategies are intended to break one or more links in the imaginary chain of infection. Break any one link in the chain, and you break the infectious process.

### Overview of the CDC Infection Control Recommendations for Dentistry

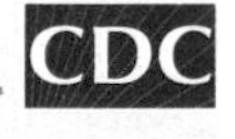

- Personal Health Elements of an Infection Control Program
- Prevention of Transmission of Blood-borne Pathogens
- Prevention of Exposure to Blood and Other Potentially Infectious Materials
- Hand Hygiene
- Personal Protective Equipment
- Contact Dermatitis and Latex Sensitivity
- Environmental Infection Control
- Dental Unit Waterlines, Biofilms, and Water Quality
- Boil Water Notices
- Dental Handpieces and Other Devices Attached to Airlines and Waterlines
- Dental Radiology
- Aseptic Technique for Parenteral Medications
- Single-Use Disposable Devices
- Oral Surgical Procedures
- Handling of Extracted Teeth
- Dental Laboratory
- *Mycobacterium tuberculosis* Program Evaluation

*Note:* These recommendations are summarized in Chapters 19, 20, and 21, and are available in total from the CDC at oralhealth@cdc.gov, by phone at 770-488-6054, or by fax at 770-488-6080.

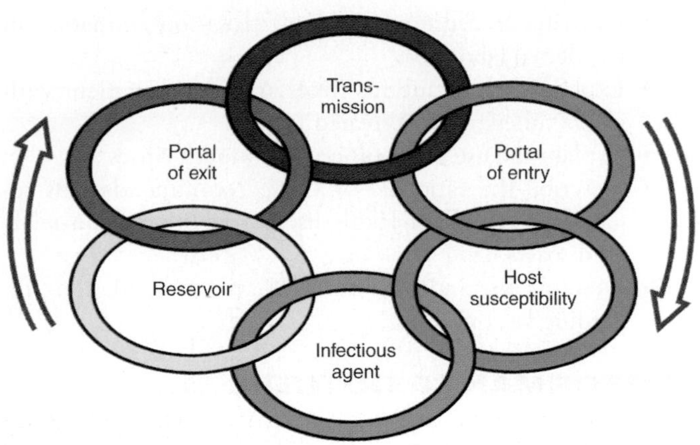


**FIG. 19.1** At least one part must be removed to break the chain of infection. *(From Potter PA, Perry AG, Stockert P, et al: Mosby's basic nursing, ed 7, St Louis, 2013, Mosby.)*

## Infectious Agent

A **pathogen** (e.g., bacterium, virus, fungus, parasite, prion) must be present in sufficient numbers to cause infection. In addition to the numbers, the organism must be virulent. **Virulence** means the degree of pathogenicity, or the strength of that organism in its ability to cause disease. If an organism is not very virulent, it may be incapable of causing disease. On the other hand, if an organism is very virulent, it can cause a serious disease. Because the body cannot change the virulence of microorganisms, this task is left to the body defenses and to specific immunizations, such as the vaccine for hepatitis B virus (HBV). Another defense is to avoid coming in contact with microorganisms by always following the infection control techniques described in this chapter.

## Reservoir

A **reservoir** is a place where microorganisms normally live and reproduce. Examples of reservoirs could include humans, animals, water, food, contaminated surfaces, and bioburden. *Bioburden* refers to organic materials such as blood and saliva. The use of the dental dam and high-volume evacuation help to minimize the number of microorganisms in the aerosol. Maintaining excellent hand hygiene and through cleaning and disinfection of contaminated surfaces will minimize reservoirs for microorganisms.

## Portal of Entry

To cause infection, pathogens must have a **portal of entry**, or a means of entering the body. The portals of entry for *airborne pathogens* are the mouth and the nose. **Blood-borne pathogens** must have access to the blood supply as a means of entry into the body. This can occur through a break in the skin caused by a needle stick, a cut, or even a human bite that breaks the skin. It can also occur through the mucous membranes of the nose and mouth.

## Susceptible Host

A susceptible host is a person who is unable to resist infection by a particular pathogen. An individual who is in poor health, is chronically fatigued and under extreme stress, or has a weakened immune system is more likely to become infected. Therefore staying healthy, washing the hands frequently, and keeping immunizations up to date will help members of the dental team to resist infection and stay healthy.

# Types of Infections

## Acute Infection

In **acute infection**, symptoms often are severe and usually appear soon after the initial infection occurs. Acute infections are of *short duration.* For example, with a viral infection such as the common cold, the body's defense mechanisms usually eliminate the virus within 2 to 3 weeks.

## Chronic Infection

**Chronic infections** are those in which the microorganism is present for a *long duration;* some may persist for life. The person may be *asymptomatic* (not showing symptoms of the disease) but may still be a carrier of the disease, as with hepatitis C virus (HCV) or human immunodeficiency virus (HIV) infection.

## Latent Infection

A **latent infection** is a persistent infection in which the symptoms "come and go." Cold sores (oral herpes simplex) and genital herpes are latent viral infections.

The virus first enters the body and causes the original lesion. It then lies dormant, away from the surface, within a nerve cell, until certain conditions (such as illness with fever, sunburn, and stress) cause the virus to leave the nerve cell and seek the surface again. Once the virus reaches the surface, it becomes detectable for a short time and causes another outbreak at that site.

Another herpesvirus, *herpes zoster,* causes chickenpox. This virus may lie dormant and later may erupt as the painful disease shingles.

## Opportunistic Infection

Opportunistic infections, which are caused by normally nonpathogenic organisms, occur in individuals whose resistance is decreased or compromised. For example, in an individual who is recovering from influenza, pneumonia or an ear infection may develop. Opportunistic infections are common in patients with autoimmune disease or diabetes and in elderly persons.

# Modes of Disease Transmission

Before you can prevent disease transmission in the dental office, you must first understand how infectious diseases are spread.

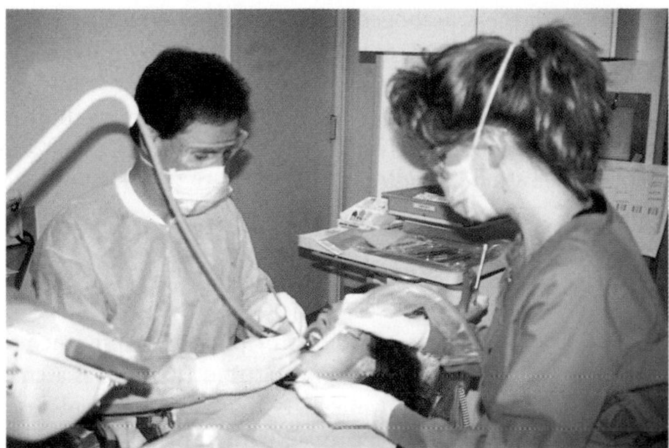

**FIG. 19.2** Pathogens can be transferred from staff to patient, patient to staff, and patient to patient through contaminated equipment.

An **infectious disease** is one that is *communicable* or *contagious.* These terms mean that the disease can be transmitted (spread) in some way from one host to another (Fig. 19.2)

## Primary Modes of Disease Transmission in Dentistry

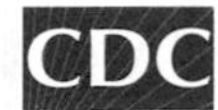



- *Direct contact:* Touching or contact with the patient's blood or other body fluids
- *Indirect contact:* Touching or contact with a contaminated surface or instrument
- *Droplet infection:* An infection that occurs through mucosal surfaces of the eyes, nose, or mouth
- *Parenteral transmission:* Needle stick injuries, human bites, cuts, abrasions, or any break in the skin
- *Immunizations strongly recommended for healthcare personnel:*
  - Hepatitis B
  - Influenza
  - Measles
  - Mumps
  - Rubella
  - Varicella-zoster

Modified from CDC Guidelines for Infection Control in Dental Healthcare Settings—2003.

## Direct Transmission

Direct transmission of pathogens occurs through person-to-person contact. An example would be droplets that are spread through sneezing or coughing, or even by spatter produced during dental treatment. Direct transmission also can occur through unprotected contact with an infectious lesion or infected body fluids, such as blood, saliva, semen, and vaginal secretions. Diseases such as hepatitis, herpes infection, HIV infection, and tuberculosis are spread through **direct contact**.

Exposure to blood and saliva is a matter of particular concern for dental workers during dental treatment. Although blood may not be visible in the saliva, it often is present.

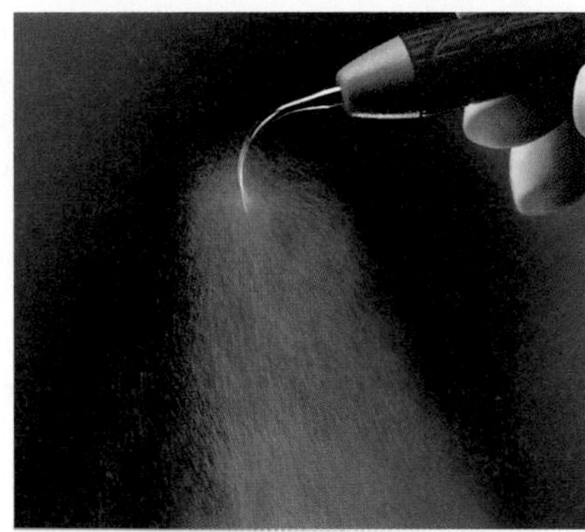

**FIG. 19.3** Aerosol from an ultrasonic scaler. *(Courtesy Hu-Friedy Mfg. Co. LLC, Chicago, IL.)*

## Indirect Transmission

Indirect transmission occurs when microorganisms first are transmitted to an object or surface, and then are transferred to another person who touches those objects or surfaces. An example would be a dental chart that is handled by a dental assistant while wearing contaminated gloves that is then handled by the receptionist with bare hands. It is important to wash your hands frequently and to carefully disinfect or cover surfaces that can become contaminated to prevent indirect transmission of microorganisms.

## Airborne Transmission

Airborne transmission, also known as **droplet infection**, refers to the spread of disease through droplets of moisture that contain bacteria or viruses. Most of the contagious respiratory diseases are caused by pathogens that are carried in droplets of moisture. Some of these pathogens are carried long distances through the air and through ventilation systems. Airborne transmission also can occur when someone coughs or sneezes.

## Aerosol, Spray, or Spatter

*Aerosols, sprays,* and *spatter* that are generated during dental treatment can contain blood, saliva, and nasopharyngeal (nasal) secretions. The difference between aerosols, sprays, and spatter is simply the size of the particles. These terms are often used interchangeably to describe droplets of potentially infectious materials.

The finest are the mistlike aerosols. Aerosols can remain airborne for extended periods and can be inhaled. They are not typically visible to the naked eye. Aerosols are created by the use of the high-speed handpiece and the ultrasonic scaler during dental procedures (Fig. 19.3). Inhaling the bacteria in the aerosol (without the protection of a face mask) is comparable to having someone sneeze in your face twice a minute, at a distance of 1 foot. Aerosols can transmit respiratory infections, but they do not transmit HBV or HIV despite the fact that they are inhaled.

Sprays and spatter are also created by the use of the handpiece and the ultrasonic scaler, as well as the air-water syringe, during dental procedures. Spatter consists of larger droplet particles that are contaminated by blood, saliva, and other debris (e.g., calculus, tooth particles).

Spray and spatter droplets travel farther than aerosol mist does and tend to land on the upper surfaces of the wrist and forearms, upper arms, and chest. Droplets also may reach the necktie/collar area of the dentist, assistant, or hygienist.

*Intact skin,* which is not broken in any way, acts as a natural protective barrier. *Nonintact skin,* in which a cut, a scrape, or a needle stick injury has occurred, provides a means of entrance for pathogens into the body.

Good work practices such as the use of dental dams and high-velocity air evacuation will help minimize splashes, spatter, and aerosols. In addition, wearing of gloves, masks, eyewear, and protective clothing will reduce the risk of exposure to pathogens.

### Parenteral Transmission

*Parenteral* means through the skin, as with cuts or punctures. Parenteral transmission of blood-borne pathogens (i.e., disease-causing organisms transferred through contact with blood or other body fluids) can occur through needle stick injuries, human bites, cuts, abrasions, or any break in the skin.

### Blood-Borne Transmission

Certain pathogens, referred to as *blood-borne pathogens,* are carried in the blood and body fluids of infected individuals and can be transmitted to others. Blood-borne transmission occurs through direct or **indirect contact** with blood and other body fluids. Saliva is of particular concern during dental treatment because it frequently is contaminated with blood. Remember, although blood may not be visible in the saliva, it still may be present.

Improperly sterilized instruments and equipment can transfer all blood-borne diseases. Individuals who share needles while using illegal drugs easily transmit these diseases to each other. Unprotected sex is another common method of transmission of blood-borne disease.

Common blood-borne microorganisms of concern in dentistry include HCV, HBV, and HIV. Because dental treatment often involves contact with blood and always with saliva, blood-borne diseases are of major concern in the dental office.

### Food and Water Transmission

Many diseases are transmitted by contaminated food that has not been cooked or refrigerated properly and by water that has been contaminated with human or animal fecal material. For example, tuberculosis, botulism, and staphylococcal and streptococcal infections are spread by contaminated food or water.

### Fecal-Oral Transmission

Many pathogens are present in fecal matter. If proper sanitation procedures, such as handwashing after use of the toilet, are not followed, these pathogens may be transmitted directly by touching another person, or they may be transmitted indirectly through contact with contaminated surfaces or food.

Fecal-oral transmission occurs most often among health-care and daycare workers (who frequently change diapers) and among careless food handlers.

## The Immune System

The immune system is responsible for providing resistance to communicable diseases. A **communicable disease** is a condition that is caused by an infection that can be spread from person to person or through contact with body fluids.

**Immunity** allows the body to resist disease and prevents foreign bodies from causing infection. When immunity is present at birth, it is called **inherited immunity**. Immunity that is developed during a person's lifetime is called **acquired immunity**. Acquired immunity can occur naturally or artificially (Fig. 19.4).

### Naturally Acquired Immunity

**Naturally acquired immunity** occurs when a person has previously contracted a disease and recovered. When the body was fighting the invading pathogen, it formed antibodies that provide future resistance against that particular pathogen. This form of immunity is called *active immunity* because the body of the host is actively involved in the process.

Another type, *passive immunity,* occurs during pregnancy when the fetus receives antibodies from the mother's placenta. Passive immunity also occurs when the mother breastfeeds the infant. It is called "passive" immunity because the antibodies are acquired from an outside source.

### Artificially Acquired Immunity

When the human body has not been exposed to a disease, it has not developed antibodies and is completely defenseless against the disease. However, antibodies can be introduced into the body artificially by *immunization* or *vaccination.*

A vaccine that contains weakened disease-causing organisms or genetically engineered organisms is injected into the body. Harmful characteristics of the disease-producing organisms are eliminated from the vaccine to make them less likely to cause disease. The body then forms antibodies in response to the vaccine, resulting in **artificially acquired immunity**.

## Disease Transmission in the Dental Office

Disease transmission in the dental office can occur in a variety of ways:

- Patient to dental team
- Dental team to patient

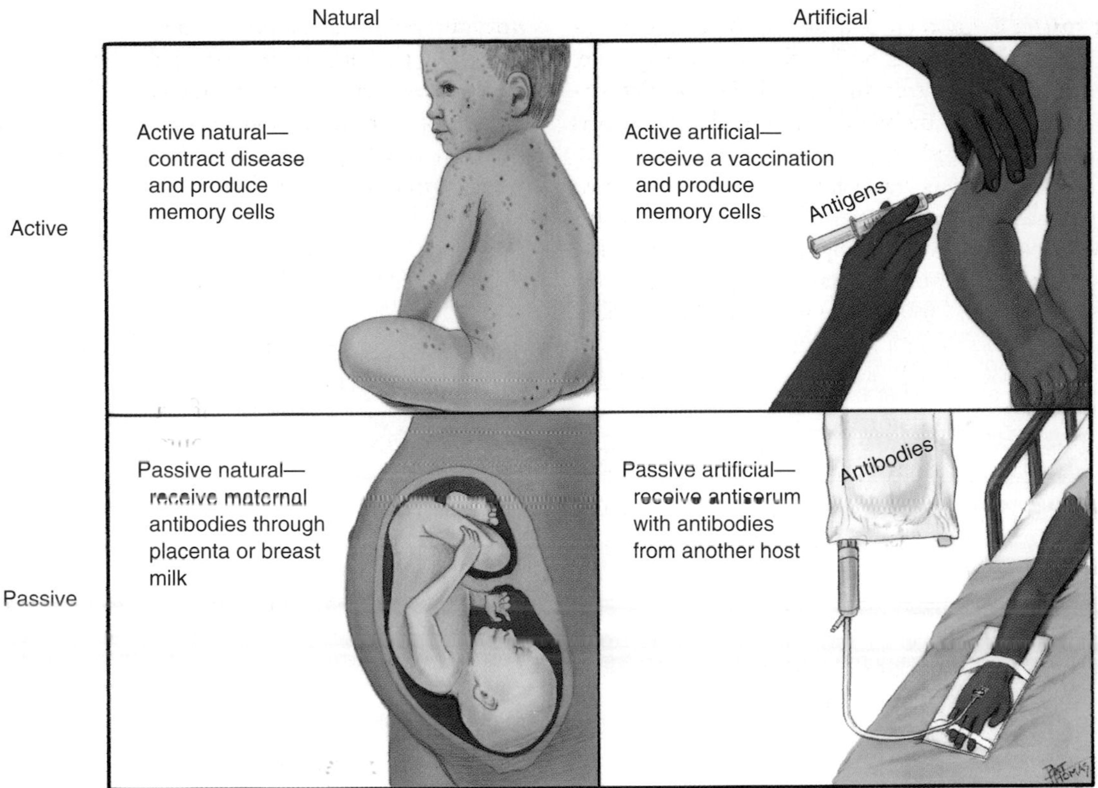


**FIG. 19.4** Acquired immunity. *(From Applegate EJ: The anatomy and physiology learning system, ed 4, St Louis, 2011, Saunders.)*

- Patient to patient
- Dental office to community (includes dental team's family)
- Community to dental office to patient

## Patient to Dental Team

Microorganisms from the patient's mouth can be passed to the dental team through the following routes:

- The most common route is through direct contact (touching) with the patient's blood or saliva. If the dental team member has cuts, abrasions, or breaks in the skin around the fingernails, microorganisms may gain entrance.
- Droplet infection affects mucosal surfaces of the eyes, nose, and mouth. It can occur when the dental team member inhales aerosol generated by the dental handpiece or the air-water syringe.
- Indirect contact can occur when the team member touches a contaminated surface or instrument. Cuts or punctures with contaminated needles, burs, instruments, or files may also result in disease transmission.

Infection control measures that help prevent disease transmission from the patient to the dental team member include (1) gloves, (2) handwashing, (3) masks, (4) rubber dams, and (5) patient mouth rinses.

Always remember, a patient may be a carrier of a disease. Carrier-transmitted diseases include certain types of viral hepatitis, herpes, tuberculosis, typhoid fever, and HIV, among others.

## Dental Team to Patient

Fortunately, the spread of disease from a member of the dental team to a patient is very unlikely to happen. If proper procedures are not followed, however, disease transmission could occur.

Team-to-patient transmission can result if the dental team member has lesions on the hands, or if the hands are cut while in the patient's mouth, permitting the transfer of microorganisms. Droplet infection of the patient can occur if the dental team member has a cold, but this can also occur outside the dental office.

Infection control measures that help to prevent team-to-patient transmission include (1) masks, (2) gloves, (3) handwashing, and (4) immunization.

## Patient to Patient

Patient-to-patient disease transmission has occurred in the medical field, but only two cases of this type of transmission have been documented in dentistry. For this type of transmission to occur, contamination from instruments used on one patient would need to be transferred to another patient.

Infection control measures that can prevent patient-to-patient transmission include (1) instrument sterilization, (2) surface barriers, (3) handwashing, (4) gloves, and (5) use of sterile instruments (Boxes 19.1 and 19.2).

**BOX 19.1 Rare Case of Hepatitis B Patient-to-Patient Transmission in a Dental Office**

An article in the *Journal of Infectious Disease* describes a patient-to-patient transmission of hepatitis B virus (HBV) in a dental setting. The event occurred in 2001, when a person with acute hepatitis B was reported to a state health department. The state health department's epidemiologic investigation found that the patient had none of the traditional hepatitis B risk factors, but reported having recent oral surgery. An investigation of the oral surgery practice where the patient received dental treatment revealed that another surgical patient seen earlier on that same day was on the state's reportable disease registry for HBV. Molecular epidemiologic techniques concluded that transmission of HBV between the two patients had occurred.

When investigators later visited the office and monitored its operation, they found that the office followed standard infection control procedures, and that all staff had been previously vaccinated and were negative for HBV. The investigators could only speculate that a lapse in cleanup procedures had occurred after treatment of the source patient, leaving an area contaminated with blood.

This is the only known case of patient-to-patient hepatitis B transmission in a dental setting.

Data from Redd JY, Baumback J, Kohn W, et al: *Journal Infectious Disease* 195(9):1245–1247, 2007.

**BOX 19.2 Patient-to-Patient Transmission of Hepatitis C in a Dental Office**

The first documented instance of patient-to-patient transmission of hepatitis C in a dental office was reported by the Oklahoma State Department and the Tulsa Health Department in September 2013. The Oklahoma State Epidemiologist reported that the CDC conducted genetic-based testing of patient specimens to confirm the patient-to-patient transmission of the hepatitis C virus.

The Oklahoma Health Department notified thousands of the dentist's former patients of the potential hepatitis C exposure and recommended the patients have hepatitis C testing at free and private clinics. The state epidemiologist emphasized that U.S. dental procedures are generally safe, but the hepatitis C incident emphasized the importance of strict infection control procedures in dental practices. The patient-to-patient transmission of the hepatitis C virus in this case resulted from improper infection control procedures.

The CDC recommends one-time screening of hepatitis C for all persons born between 1945 and 1965, even if they do not have symptoms of the disease or feel sick. Among the former dental patients in the Oklahoma dental office that were screened and newly identified as having hepatitis C, 56% were over age 50. Early identification and treatment of hepatitis C is important to prevent liver damage, cirrhosis, and even liver cancer and can prevent the further spread of disease.

## Dental Office to Community

Microorganisms can leave the dental office and enter the community in a variety of ways. For example, contaminated impressions may be sent to the dental laboratory, or contaminated equipment may be sent out for repair. Office-to-community transmission also can occur if members of the dental team transport microorganisms out of the office on their clothing or in their hair.

Infection control measures that help prevent organisms from leaving the dental office include (1) handwashing, (2) changing clothes before leaving the office, and (3) disinfecting impressions and contaminated equipment before such items leave the office.

## Community to Dental Office to Patient

In this type of disease transmission, microorganisms enter the dental office through the municipal water that supplies the dental unit. Waterborne organisms colonize the inside of dental unit waterlines and form *biofilm.* As water flows through the handpiece, air-water syringe, and ultrasonic scaler, a patient can swallow contaminated water (see Chapter 24).

**RECALL**

1 What is the most common route of contamination?
2 What type of infection transmission occurs through mucosal tissues?
3 What infection control measures help prevent disease transmission from the dental team to the patient?

# Roles and Responsibilities of the CDC and OSHA in Infection Control

The CDC and the OSHA are federal agencies that play very important roles in infection control for dentistry (see Chapter 22).

The CDC is *not* a regulatory agency. Its role is to issue specific *recommendations* that are based on sound scientific evidence for health-related matters. In 1986 the CDC issued the first recommendations for the dental profession to prevent the transmission of blood-borne disease. OSHA *is* a regulatory agency. Its role is to issue specific *standards* designed to protect the health of employees in the United States. In 1991, on the basis of CDC guidelines, OSHA issued the BBP Standard. Failure to comply with OSHA requirements can result in serious consequences, including heavy fines.

As a dental assistant, it is important to follow *all* of these guidelines and recommendations.

# *CDC Guidelines for Infection Control in Dental Health-Care Settings*

In December 2003, the CDC released its *Guidelines for Infection Control in Dental Health-Care Settings—2003* (Fig. 19.5).

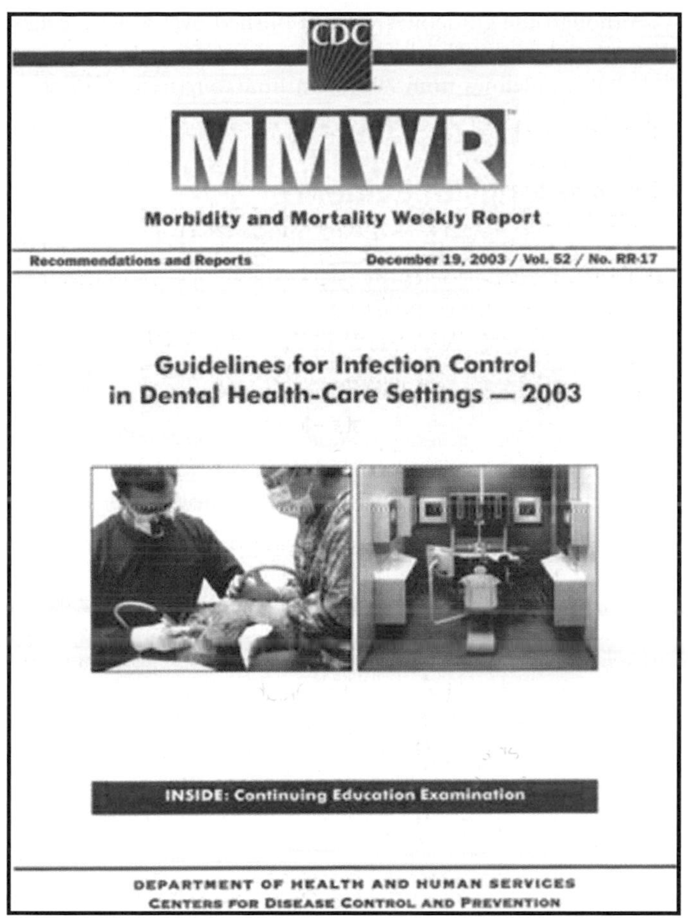


**FIG. 19.5** CDC *Guidelines for Infection Control in Dental Health-Care Settings—2003. (From Centers for Disease Control and Prevention, Atlanta, GA.)*

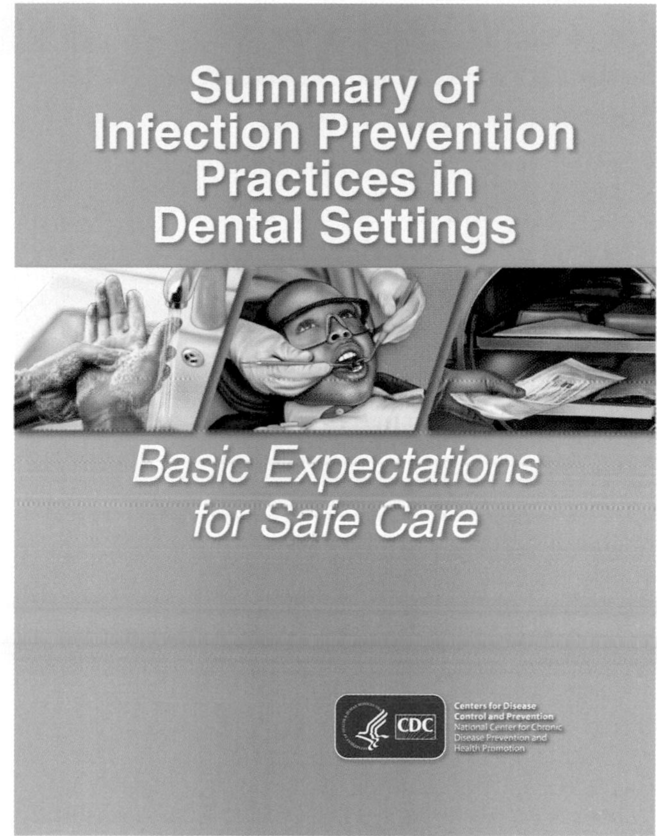


**FIG. 19.6** Summary of Infection Prevention Practices in Dental Settings: Basic Expectations for Safe Care. Atlanta, GA: US Department of Health and Human Services, Centers for Disease Control and Prevention, National Center for Chronic Disease Prevention and Health Promotion, Division of Oral Health; March 2016. *(From Centers for Disease Control and Prevention, Atlanta, GA.)*

The 2003 guidelines expanded on the existing OSHA BBP Standard and added some information. The guidelines were developed in collaboration with experts on infection control from the CDC and other public agencies; input was also sought from private and professional organizations. These guidelines are based on scientific evidence and are categorized on the basis of existing scientific data, theoretical rationale, and applicability.

The guidelines apply to *all* paid and unpaid dental health professionals who might be occupationally exposed to blood and body fluids by direct contact or through contact with contaminated environmental surfaces, water, or air.

Although it is not law, the CDC *Guidelines for Infection Control in Dental Health-Care Settings* represents the standard of care for the dental profession.

## 2016 CDC Dental Infection Prevention Summary

In March 2016 the CDC issued the *2016 CDC Dental Infection Prevention Summary.* It is an easy to read and understand summary of the *Guidelines for Infection Control in Dental Health-Care Settings—2003* (Fig. 19.6). The *2016 CDC Dental Infection Prevention Summary* is *not* a replacement for CDC's *Guidelines for Infection Control in Dental Health-Care Settings—2003.*

The *Summary* includes additional topics and information relevant to dental infection prevention and control published by the CDC since 2003, including the following:

- Infection prevention program administrative measures
- Infection prevention education and training
- Respiratory hygiene and cough etiquette
- Updated safe injection practices
- Administrative measures for instrument processing

The *Summary* is intended for use by anyone needing information about basic infection prevention measures in dental healthcare settings, but is *not* a replacement for the *Guidelines for Infection Control in Dental Health-Care Settings—2003,* which provides additional background, rationales, and scientific evidence behind each recommendation. All guidelines are available at http://www.cdc.gov/HAI/prevent/prevent_pubs.html.

### CDC Recommendations for Respiratory Hygiene and Cough Etiquette in Dental Settings

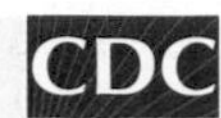

- Implement measures to contain respiratory secretions in patients and accompanying individuals who have signs and symptoms of a respiratory infection, beginning at point of entry to the facility and continuing throughout the visit.
- Post signs at entrances with instructions to patients with symptoms of respiratory infection to:
  - Cover their mouths/noses when coughing or sneezing.
  - Use and dispose of tissues.
  - Perform hand hygiene after hands have been in contact with respiratory secretions.
- Provide tissues and no-touch receptacles for disposal of tissues.
- Provide resources for performing hand hygiene in or near waiting areas.
- Offer masks to coughing patients and other symptomatic persons when they enter the dental setting.
- Provide space and encourage persons with symptoms of respiratory infections to sit as far away from others as possible. If available, facilities may wish to place these patients in a separate area while waiting for care.
- Educate dental healthcare providers on the importance of infection prevention measures to contain respiratory secretions to prevent the spread of respiratory pathogens when examining and caring for patients with signs and symptoms of a respiratory infection.

### CDC Recommendations for Sterilization and Disinfection of Patient-Care Devices for Dental Settings

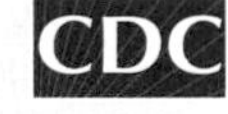

- Clean and reprocess (disinfect or sterilize) reusable dental equipment appropriately before use on another patient.
- Clean and reprocess reusable dental equipment according to manufacturer instructions. If the manufacturer does not provide such instructions, the device may not be suitable for multipatient use.
- Have manufacturer instructions for reprocessing reusable dental instruments/equipment readily available, ideally in or near the reprocessing area.
- Assign responsibilities for reprocessing of dental equipment to dental healthcare providers with appropriate training.
- Wear appropriate personal protective equipment when handling and reprocessing contaminated patient equipment.
- Use mechanical, chemical, and biological monitors according to manufacturer instructions to ensure the effectiveness of the sterilization process; maintain sterilization records in accordance with state and local regulations.
- Label sterilized items with the sterilizer used, the cycle or load number, the date of sterilization, and, if applicable, the expiration date.
- Ensure routine maintenance for sterilization equipment is performed according to manufacturer instructions and maintenance records are available.

Although the guidelines were published over a decade ago, the basic principles of infection control have not changed, and the CDC guidelines from 2003 continue to represent the standard of care for dental infection control.

## CDC Rankings of Evidence

Each recommendation made by the CDC is categorized on the basis of existing scientific data, theoretical rationale, and applicability. Rankings are based on the following categories.

### CDC Rankings of Evidence

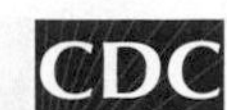

| | |
|---|---|
| Category IA | Strongly recommended for implementation and strongly supported by well-designed experimental, clinical, or **epidemiologic studies** |
| Category IB | Strongly recommended for implementation and supported by experimental, clinical, or epidemiologic studies and a strong theoretical rationale |
| Category IC | Required for implementation, as mandated by federal or state regulation or standard |
| Category II | Suggested for implementation and supported by suggestive clinical or epidemiologic studies or a theoretical rationale |
| Unresolved Issue | No recommendation—practices for which insufficient evidence or no consensus regarding efficacy exists |

# OSHA Blood-Borne Pathogens Standard

OSHA's BBP Standard is the most important infection control law in dentistry. It is designed to protect employees against occupational exposure to blood-borne, disease-causing organisms, such as HBV, HCV, and HIV.

The BBP requires employers to protect their employees from exposure to blood and *other potentially infectious material* (OPIM) in the workplace and to provide proper care to the employee if an exposure should occur. This standard applies to any type of facility in which employees might be exposed to blood and other body fluids, including dental and medical offices, hospitals, funeral homes, emergency medical services, and nursing homes.

OSHA requires that a copy of the BBP Standard be present in every dental office and clinic. A copy of the OSHA BBP Standard is available at http://www.osha.gov/SLTC/bloodbornepathogens/index/html.

## Exposure Control Plan

Each dental office must have a written exposure control plan that clearly describes how that office complies with the BBP Standard. This exposure control plan must be reviewed and updated at least annually. A copy must be made available to all employees.

### Written Exposure Control Plan Required by OSHA

General policy of implementing Centers for Disease Control and Prevention guidelines and American Dental Association infection control recommendations:

- Use of Standard Precautions
- Required use of personal protective equipment
- Standardized housekeeping
- Laundering of contaminated protective clothing
- Standardized policy on cleaning and disinfection
- Policy on general waste disposal
- Labeling procedure (secondary labeling)
- Policy on sterilization (including monitoring) and disinfection
- Use of sharps containers and disposal system
- Standardized handwashing protocol
- Hepatitis B virus vaccination
- Postexposure evaluation and medical follow-up

*OSHA,* Occupational Safety and Health Administration.

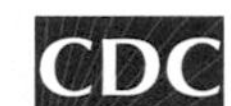

### Overview of CDC *Guidelines for Infection Control in Dental Health-Care Settings—2003*

- Use of Standard Precautions rather than Universal Precautions
- Work restrictions for healthcare personnel infected with infectious diseases
- Postexposure management of occupational exposures to blood-borne pathogens (hepatitis B virus, human immunodeficiency virus, hepatitis C virus)
- Selection of devices with sharps injury–prevention features
- Hand hygiene products and surgical hand asepsis
- Contact dermatitis and latex hypersensitivity
- Sterilization of unwrapped instruments
- Dental unit waterline concerns
- Dental radiology infection control
- Aseptic technique for injectable medications
- Preprocedural mouth rinses for patients
- Oral surgical procedures
- Laser/electrosurgery plumes
- Tuberculosis
- Creutzfeldt-Jakob disease and other prion-related diseases
- Infection control program evaluation
- Research considerations

Modified from CDC Guidelines for Infection Control in Dental Healthcare Settings—2003.
Copies of these guidelines may be requested at oralhealth@cdc.gov, by phone at 770-488-6054, or by fax at 770-488-6080.

## Standard and Universal Precautions

The term *Universal Precautions* is still referred to in the OSHA BBP Standard. **Universal Precautions** is based on the concept that all human blood and body fluids (including saliva) are to be treated as if known to be infected with a **blood-borne disease** such as HBV, HCV, or HIV infection. The rationale for this concept is that it is not possible to identify those individuals who are infectious, so Universal Precautions are to be used for all healthcare personnel and their patients.

The CDC expanded the concept and changed the term to *Standard Precautions.* **Standard Precautions** integrate and expand the elements of Universal Precautions into a standard of care that is designed to protect healthcare providers from pathogens that can be spread by *blood or any other body fluid, excretion, or secretion.* Saliva has always been considered a potentially infectious material in dental infection control; therefore no difference in clinical dental practices is noted between Universal Precautions and Standard Precautions. Standard Precautions apply to contact with the following:

- Blood
- All body fluids, secretions, and excretions except sweat, regardless of whether or not they contain blood
- Nonintact skin
- Mucous membranes

### Standard Precautions

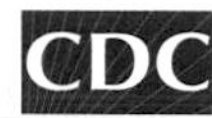

- Wash hands before and after every patient (Categories IA and IC)
- Wear gloves when touching blood, body fluids, secretions, and contaminated items
- Use care when handling sharps (Categories IA and IC)
- Wear a mask and eye protection, or a face shield, during procedures likely to generate splashes or sprays (Categories IA and IC)
- Carefully handle contaminated patient care items to prevent the transfer of microorganisms to people or equipment (Categories IA and IC)
- Use a mouthpiece or another ventilation device as an alternative to mouth-to-mouth resuscitation when practical (Categories IA and IC)
- Standard Precautions must be used in the treatment of all patients (Categories IA and IC)

### OSHA Blood-Borne Pathogens Standard Training Requirements

- Epidemiology, modes of transmission, and prevention of hepatitis B virus (HBV) and human immunodeficiency virus (HIV)
- Risks to the fetus from HBV and HIV
- Location and proper use of all protective equipment
- Proper work practices using Universal Precautions
- Meaning of color codes, biohazard symbol, and precautions to follow in handling infectious waste
- Procedures to follow if needle stick or other injury occurs

From Robinson D, Bird D: Essentials of dental assisting, ed 5, St Louis, 2013, Saunders.

## Categories of Employees

The OSHA BBP Standard requires employers to categorize tasks and procedures during which an employee might experience occupational exposure (Table 19.1).

The BBP defines an **occupational exposure** as "any reasonably anticipated skin, eye, mucous membrane contact, or percutaneous injury with blood or any other potentially infectious materials." **Percutaneous** (through the skin, such as needle sticks, cuts, and human bites) and **permucosal** (contact with mucous membranes, such as the eyes or mouth) exposures to blood, saliva, and other body fluids pose the greatest risk for transmission of HIV, HBV, and HCV.

## Postexposure Management

Despite efforts to prevent occupational exposure incidents, accidents happen. Therefore before an accident occurs, the BBP Standard requires the employer to have a written plan. This plan explains exactly what steps the employee must follow after the exposure incident occurs and the type of medical follow-up that will be provided to the employee at no charge.

The employer must provide training to employees on the proper response to an exposure incident. See Procedure 19.1: Applying First Aid After an Exposure Incident.

### Management of an Exposure Incident*

- Document the route(s) of exposure and the circumstances in which the incident occurred (e.g., cut, needle stick, or blood splash).
- Identify and document the *source individual* (patient whose blood or body fluid is involved in the exposure incident), unless the employer can establish that identification is not possible or is prohibited by state or local law.
- Request that the source individual have his or her blood tested for human immunodeficiency virus (HIV) and hepatitis B virus (HBV) (the source individual can refuse this request).
- Advise the employee to have his or her blood tested for HIV and HBV. (The employee has the right to refuse to be tested.) By law, the employee's blood test results are held confidential from the employer.
- Provide medically indicated prophylactic treatment, such as necessary injections of gamma globulin, HBV vaccine booster, tetanus booster, or a combination.
- Provide appropriate counseling.
- Evaluate reported illnesses after the incident.

*Employer actions as required by the OSHA Blood-Borne Pathogens (BBP) Standard.

### Follow-up Measures for Exposed Worker

The following services must be offered to the employee without charge:

- Confidential medical counseling
- Human immunodeficiency virus (HIV) test series immediately and at 6 weeks, 12 weeks, and 6 months
- Hepatitis B virus (HBV) immune globulin (if no prior HBV vaccination)
- Tetanus booster
- Documentation of incident on appropriate Occupational Safety and Health Administration (OSHA) form

From Robinson D, Bird D: Essentials of dental assisting, ed 5, St Louis, 2013, Saunders.

## Employee Training

The BBP Standard requires the dentist/employer to provide training in infection control procedures and safety issues to all personnel who may come in contact with blood, saliva, or contaminated instruments or surfaces. The employer must keep records of all training sessions. The record of each training session must include the date of the session, the name of the presenter, the topic, and the names of all employees who attended.

## Hepatitis B Immunization

The BBP Standard requires the dentist/employer to offer the HBV vaccination series to all employees whose jobs include category I and II tasks. The vaccine must be offered within 10 days of assignment to a category I or II job. To document compliance, the dentist/employer must obtain proof from the physician who administered the vaccination to the employee.

The employee has the right to refuse the HBV vaccine for any reason. The employee is then required to sign an *informed refusal* form that is kept on file in the dental office (Fig. 19.7). Even if the employee originally signed the refusal form, the employee always has the right to reverse the decision and receive the vaccine at a later date at no charge.

The CDC does *not* recommend routine booster doses of the HBV vaccine, nor does it recommend routine blood testing to monitor the HBV antibody level in individuals who have already had the vaccine. This assumes that the individual was tested after receiving the vaccine and was known to have initially developed antibodies. An exception is the immunized

**TABLE 19.1 Occupational Exposure Determination**

| Category | Definition | Example |
|---|---|---|
| I | Routinely exposed to blood, saliva, or both | Dentist, dental hygienist, dental assistant, sterilization assistant, dental laboratory technician |
| II | May on occasion be exposed to blood, saliva, or both | Receptionist or office manager who may occasionally clean a treatment room or handle instruments or impressions |
| III | Never exposed to blood, saliva, or both | Financial manager, insurance clerk, or computer operator |

**OSHA Blood-borne Pathogens Standard (29CFR 1910.1030)**
**Hepatitis B Vaccine Declination**

I understand that due to my occupational exposure to blood and other potentially infectious materials I may be at risk of acquiring hepatitis B virus (HBV) infection. I have been given the opportunity to be vaccinated with the hepatitis B vaccine, at no charge to myself. However, I decline hepatitis B vaccination at this time. I understand that by declining this vaccine, I continue to be at risk of acquiring hepatitis B, a serious disease. If in the future I continue to have occupational exposure to blood or other potentially infectious materials and I want to be vaccinated with hepatitis B vaccine, I can receive the vaccination series at no charge to me.

__________________ ________
Employee signature Date

__________________ ________
Witness signature Date

**FIG. 19.7** Standard hepatitis B virus (HBV) informed refusal.

individual who has a documented exposure incident for whom the attending physician orders a booster dose.

### Postvaccine Testing

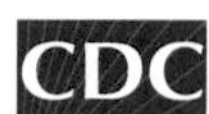

Between 1 and 2 months after the series has been completed, a blood test should be performed to ensure that the individual has developed immunity. Individuals who have not developed immunity should be evaluated by their physician to determine the need for an additional dose of hepatitis B virus (HBV) vaccine. Individuals who do not respond to the second three-dose series of the vaccine should be counseled regarding their susceptibility to HBV infection and precautions to take. (Categories IA and IC)

## Employee Medical Records

The dentist/employer must keep a confidential medical record for each employee. The employer must store these records in a locked file for the duration of employment plus 30 years.

### Requirements for Employee Medical Records

1. Employee's name and Social Security number
2. Proof of employee's hepatitis B virus (HBV) vaccination or signed refusal
3. Circumstances of any exposure incident (such as a needle stick) involving the employee and the name of the source individual (e.g., a patient whose blood or bodily fluid was involved in the incident)
4. A copy of the postexposure follow-up procedures for any injuries sustained by that employee
5. These records must be retained by the employer for the duration of employment plus 30 years

From Robinson D, Bird D: Essentials of dental assisting, ed 5, St Louis, 2013, Saunders.

## Managing Contaminated Sharps

Contaminated needles and other disposable **sharps**, such as scalpel blades, orthodontic wires, and broken glass, must be placed into a sharps container. The *sharps container* must be puncture-resistant, closable, leakproof, and color-coded or labeled with the biohazard symbol (Fig. 19.8).

Sharps containers must be located as close as possible to the place of immediate disposal. Do not cut, bend, or break the needles before disposal. Never attempt to remove a needle from a *disposable-type device.*

### Guidelines for Needles

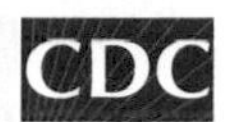

Never recap used needles by using both hands or any other technique that involves directing the point of a needle toward any part of the body. (Categories IA and IC)

### *Preventing Needle Sticks*

Some needles on the market have safety guards to prevent accidental needle sticks (Fig. 19.9). Do not bend or break needles before disposal. Always use the single-handed scoop technique or some type of safety device (Fig. 19.10).

RECALL

4 What is the purpose of the BBP?
5 How often should an exposure control plan be reviewed and updated?
6 What does the term *Standard Precautions* include?
7 What information must be included in the employee training record?
8 What must the employee do if he or she does not want the hepatitis B vaccine?

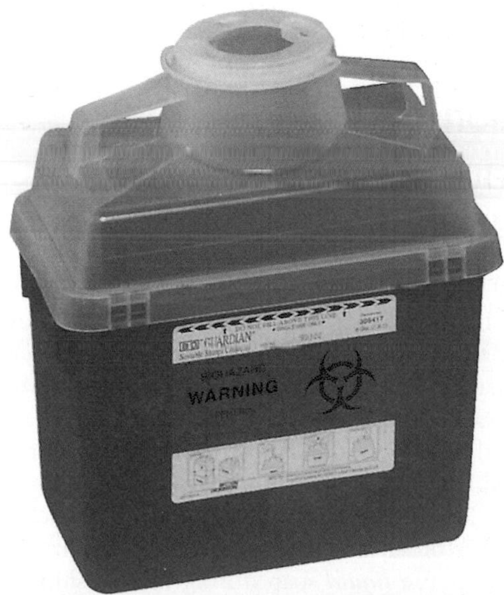


**FIG. 19.8** A puncture-resistant sharps disposal container should be located as close as possible to the area where the disposal of sharps takes place.

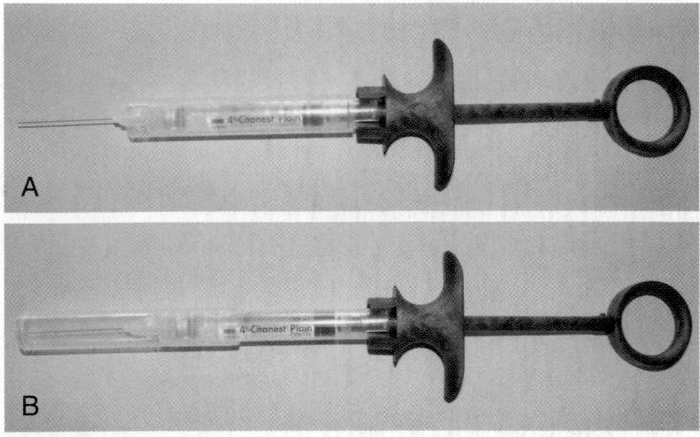


FIG. 19.9 A, UltraSafety Plus XL aspirating syringe, ready for injection. B, UltraSafety Plus XL aspirating syringe; needle sheathed to prevent needle-stick injury. *(From Logothetis DD: Local anesthesia for the dental hygienist, ed 2, St Louis, 2017, Elsevier.)*

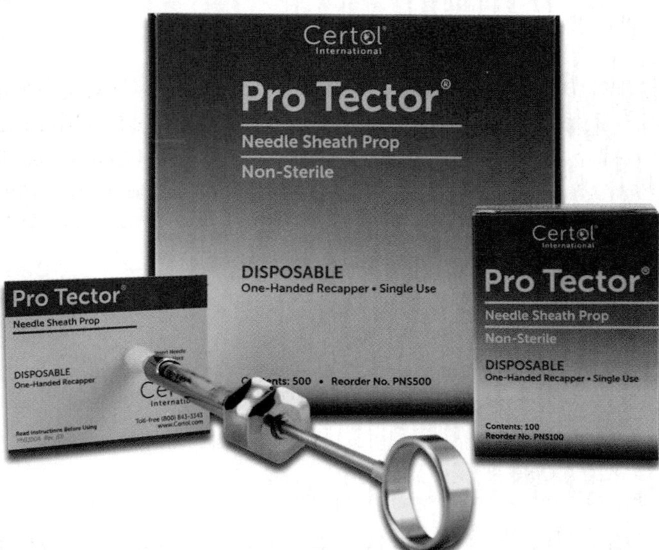


FIG. 19.10 ProTector disposable needle guard. *(Courtesy Certol, Commerce City, CO.)*

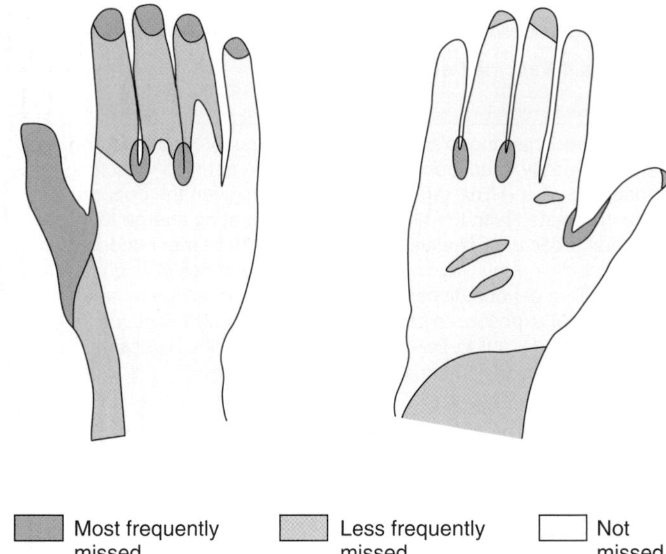


FIG. 19.11 Areas of the hand not thoroughly washed because of poor handwashing technique. *(From Samaranayake LP: Essential microbiology for dentistry, ed 4, New York, 2014, Churchill Livingstone.)*

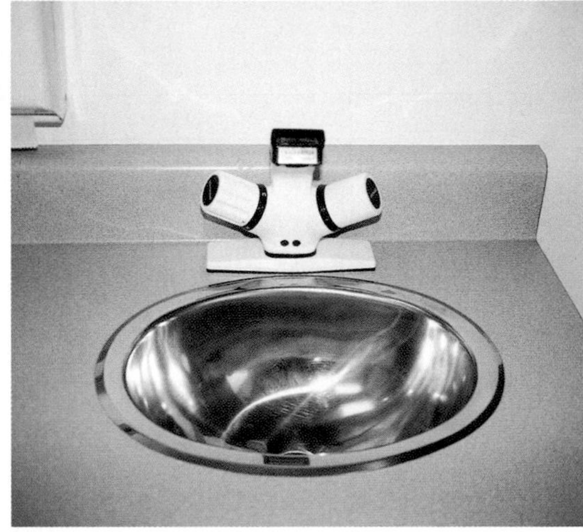

FIG. 19.12 Sensing device automatically turns the water on and off with hands-free operation.

# Infection Control Practices

## Hand Hygiene

### Handwashing Guidelines

You must wash your hands before you put on gloves (see Procedure 19.2: Handwashing Before Gloving) and immediately after you remove gloves. Gloves may have small, unapparent defects or may be torn during use, and your hands can become contaminated during glove removal. In addition, bacteria can multiply rapidly in moist environments underneath gloves; thus you should dry your hands thoroughly before donning gloves and wash immediately after removing gloves. Handwashing is also required if you inadvertently touch contaminated objects or surfaces while barehanded (Fig. 19.11). You should always use *liquid* soap during handwashing. Bar soap should never be used because it may transmit contamination.

To minimize cross-contamination, it is preferable that treatment room sinks be equipped with "hands-free" faucets that are activated electronically or with foot pedals (Fig. 19.12).

### Alcohol-Based Hand Rubs

A new category of antiseptic products for hand hygiene is now on the market. Waterless antiseptic agents are alcohol-based products that are available in gels, foams, or rinses (Fig. 19.13). They do not require the use of water. The product is simply applied to the hands, which are then rubbed together to allow the product to cover all surfaces.

These products are more effective than plain soap, or even an antimicrobial hand wash, at reducing microbial flora. Concentrations of 60 to 95 percent are most effective. Higher concentrations are actually *less effective.* In addition, these products are actually good for your skin. They contain emollients that reduce incidences of chapping, irritation, and drying of the skin. These products are very "dose sensitive." This means that you must use the amount that is recommended. Using a smaller amount seriously decreases the effectiveness of the product.

Alcohol-based hand rubs are *not* indicated if your hands are visibly soiled or are contaminated with organic matter, such as blood

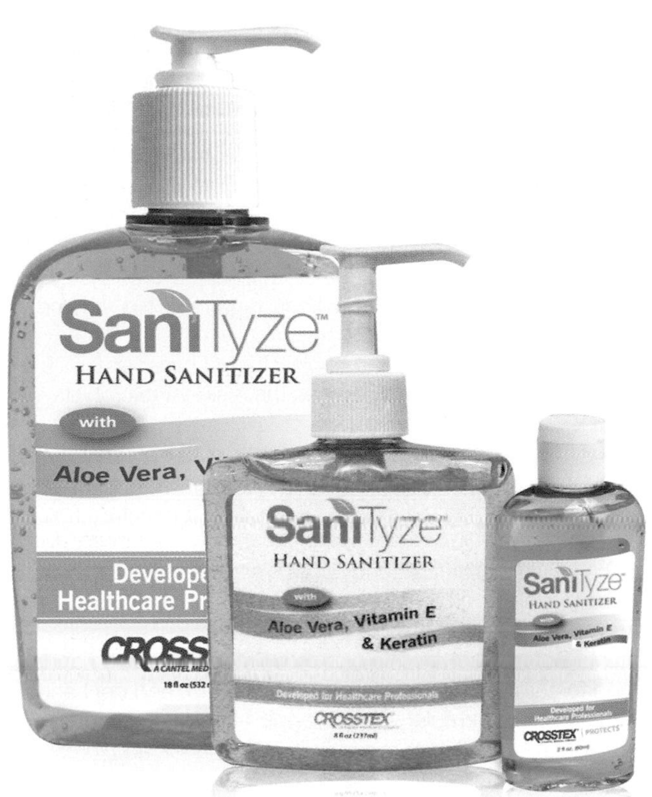


FIG. 19.13 Alcohol-based hand rub agents are available for refillable wall-mounted containers, in counter size, and in purse size. (© 2017 Crosstex International, Inc.)

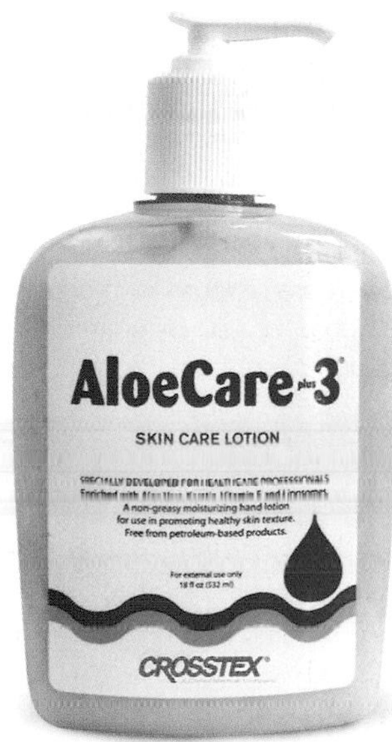


FIG. 19.14 Water-based hand products will not break down latex gloves. (© 2017 Crosstex International, Inc.)

or saliva. In these cases, you would need to first wash your hands with soap and water, and then follow with use of the alcohol-based product. See Procedure 19.3: Applying Alcohol-Based Hand Rubs.

### *Hand Care Recommendations*

Healthy skin is better able to withstand the damaging effects of repeated washing and of wearing gloves. It is important to dry your hands well before donning gloves. The use of skin cream can help relieve dry, chapped hands caused by the use of latex gloves and frequent handwashing. Select water-based hand care products because petroleum-based products will break down the latex in the glove and compromise its effectiveness (Fig. 19.14).

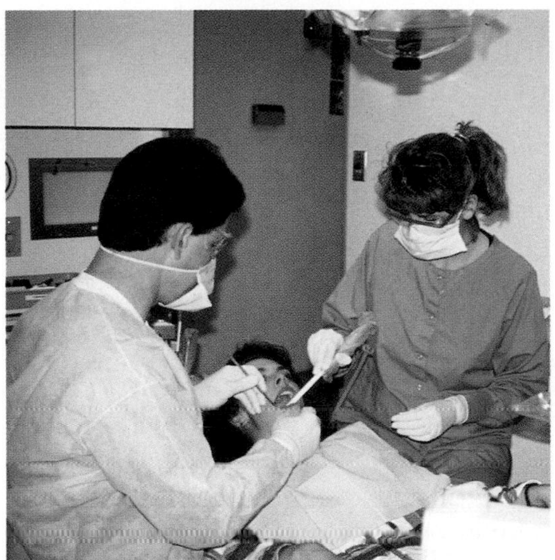

FIG. 19.15 Appropriate clinical attire consists of long-sleeved gowns, gloves, and eyewear.

RECALL

9 What is the most effective hand product on the market for use on clean hands?

10 Why should long or artificial nails and rings be avoided when you are working in a dental office?

## Personal Protective Equipment

OSHA's BBP Standard requires the employer to provide employees with appropriate **personal protective equipment (PPE)** without charge to the employee. Examples of PPE include protective clothing, surgical masks, face shields, protective eyewear, disposable patient treatment gloves, and heavy-duty utility gloves.

Because dental assistants are likely to come in contact with blood and saliva, you must wear PPE whenever you are performing tasks that could produce splash, spatter, aerosol, or other contact with body fluids (Fig. 19.15).

You must also wear appropriate PPE when you perform other clinical activities that require handling of items contaminated with patient secretions. Examples include processing dental radiographs and handling laboratory cases, dentures, and other prosthetic appliances, or contaminated equipment and surfaces.

You put on your PPE in the reverse order of what you change most frequently during the day. Gloves are changed most often, face protection less often, and protective clothing least often (see Procedure 19.4: Putting on Personal Protective Equipment). You remove your PPE in a manner that prevents contaminating hands, clothing, skin, and mucous membranes (see Procedure 19.5: Removing Personal Protective Equipment).

## Hand Hygiene in Dental Healthcare Settings

CDC

For most routine dental procedures, such as examinations and nonsurgical procedures, wash your hands with antimicrobial or non-antimicrobial soap and water. If your hands are not visibly soiled, you may use an alcohol-based, waterless hand rub. For surgical procedures, you should perform a surgical scrub using antimicrobial or non-antimicrobial soap and water, dry your hands, and apply an alcohol-based surgical hand rub with persistent activity. (Category IA)

### Overview of 2002 CDC Hand Hygiene Guidelines

In 2002 the Centers for Disease Control and Prevention released new recommendations for hand hygiene in healthcare settings. *Hand hygiene* is a term that applies to handwashing, use of an antiseptic hand rub, or surgical hand antisepsis. Evidence suggests that hand antisepsis, the cleansing of hands with an antiseptic hand rub, is more effective in reducing nosocomial infections than is plain handwashing.

Follow these guidelines in the care of all patients:

- Continue to wash hands with antimicrobial or non-antimicrobial soap and water whenever the hands are visibly soiled.
- Use an alcohol-based hand rub to routinely decontaminate the hands in the following clinical situations (if alcohol-based hand rubs are not available, the alternative is handwashing):
  - Before and after client contact
  - Before donning sterile gloves when inserting central intravascular catheters
  - Before performing nonsurgical invasive procedures (e.g., urinary catheter insertion, nasotracheal suctioning)
  - After contact with body fluids or excretions, mucous membranes, nonintact skin, and wound dressings
  - When moving from a contaminated body site (rectal area or mouth) to a clean body site (surgical wound, urinary meatus) during client care
  - After contact with inanimate objects (including medical equipment) in the immediate vicinity of the client
  - After removing gloves
- Before eating and after using a restroom, wash hands with a non-antimicrobial or antimicrobial soap and water.
- Antimicrobial-impregnated wipes (i.e., towelettes) are not a substitute for using an alcohol-based hand rub or antimicrobial soap.
- If exposure to *Bacillus anthracis* is suspected or proven, wash hands with non-antimicrobial or antimicrobial soap and water. The physical action of washing and rinsing hands is

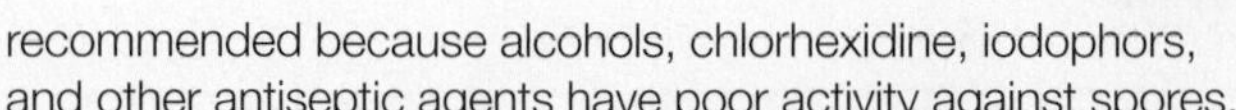

recommended because alcohols, chlorhexidine, iodophors, and other antiseptic agents have poor activity against spores.

### Method for Decontaminating Hands

When using an alcohol-based hand rub, apply the product to the palm of one hand and rub the hands together, covering all surfaces of the hands and fingers, until hands are dry. Follow the manufacturer's recommendations regarding the volume of product to use.

Follow these guidelines for surgical hand antisepsis:

- Surgical hand antisepsis reduces the resident microbial count on the hands to a minimum.
- The CDC recommends using an antimicrobial soap and scrubbing hands and forearms for the length of time recommended by the manufacturer, usually 2 to 6 minutes. The Association of Operating Room Nurses recommends 5 to 10 minutes. Refer to agency policy for time required.
- When using an alcohol-based surgical hand rub product with persistent activity, follow the manufacturer's instructions. Before applying the alcohol solution, prewash hands and forearms with a non-antimicrobial soap, and dry hands and forearms completely. After application of the alcohol-based product as recommended, allow hands and forearms to dry thoroughly before donning sterile gloves.

### General Recommendations for Hand Hygiene

- Use hand lotions or creams to minimize the occurrence of irritant contact dermatitis associated with hand antisepsis or handwashing.
- Do not wear artificial fingernails or extenders when having direct contact with clients at high risk (e.g., those in intensive care units or operating rooms).
- Keep natural nail tips less than ¼-inch long.
- Wear gloves when contact with blood or other potentially infectious materials, mucous membranes, and nonintact skin could occur.
- Remove gloves after caring for a client. Do not wear the same pair of gloves for the care of more than one client, and do not wash gloves between uses with different clients.
- Change gloves during client care if moving from a contaminated body site to a clean body site.

From Morbidity and Mortality Weekly Report 51(RR16):1–44, October 25, 2002. Centers for Disease Control and Prevention. Available at www.cdc.gov/handhygiene.

## Special Considerations for Hand Hygiene

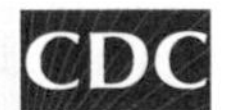

Because rings and long fingernails can harbor pathogens, nails should be kept short and well manicured. Rings, long nails, and artificial nails are likely to puncture examination gloves and may poke a patient during an examination. In addition, microorganisms thrive around rough cuticles and can enter the body through any break in the skin. The CDC Guidelines recommend that rings, fingernail polish, and artificial nails should not be worn at work. (Category II)

## Hand Care Products

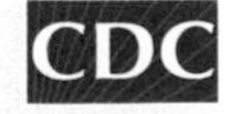

Use hand lotions to prevent skin dryness associated with handwashing (Category IA). Check the compatibility of the lotion with your gloves (see Fig. 19.14). (Petroleum or other oil emollients can have a harmful effect on the integrity of the gloves.)

Store liquid hand care products in disposable closed containers or closed containers that can be washed and dried before refilling. Do not add soap or lotion to a partially empty dispenser (Category IA). Refilling partially empty containers can lead to bacterial contamination.

## Protective Clothing

The purpose of protective clothing is to protect the skin and underclothing from exposure to saliva, blood, aerosol, and other contaminated materials. Types of protective clothing can include smocks, pants, skirts, laboratory coats, surgical scrubs (hospital operating room clothing), scrub (surgical) hats, and shoe covers. Technically, clinic shoes and hosiery also are part of PPE.

The decision regarding the type of protective clothing you should wear is based on the degree of anticipated exposure to infectious materials (Fig. 19.16). For example, assisting with use of the high-speed handpiece during a cavity preparation carries a high risk of exposure to contaminated aerosol. Charting during an oral examination, on the other hand, carries a lower risk of exposure because it does not involve use of the handpiece or the air-water syringe, which creates contaminated aerosol.

The BBP Standard prohibits an employee from taking protective clothing home to be laundered. Laundering contaminated protective clothing is the responsibility of the employer, and many offices have a laundry service that will pick up contaminated laundry from the dental office.

### Protective Clothing Requirements

- Protective clothing should be made of fluid-resistant material. Cotton, cotton/polyester, or disposable jackets or gowns usually are satisfactory for routine dental procedures.
- To minimize the amount of uncovered skin, clothing should have long sleeves and a high neckline.
- The design of the sleeve should allow the cuff to be tucked inside the band of the glove.
- During high-risk procedures, protective clothing must cover dental personnel at least to the knees when seated.
- Buttons, trim, zippers, and other ornamentation (which may harbor pathogens) should be kept to a minimum.

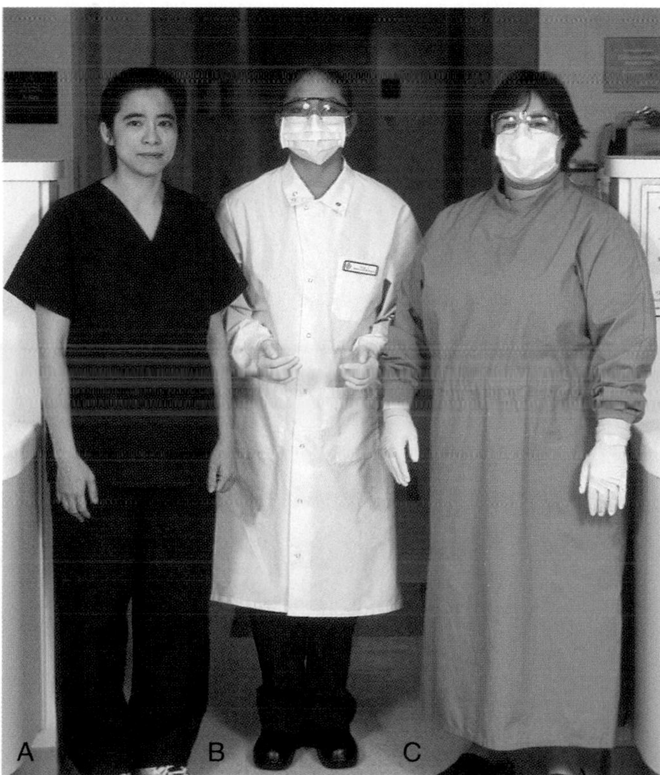


**FIG. 19.16** Depending on the task, the dental assistant's attire might consist of scrubs, laboratory coats, or surgical gowns. A, Dental assistant in scrubs. B, Dental assistant in laboratory coat. C, Dental assistant in surgical gown.

*Note:* The type and characteristics of protective clothing depend on the anticipated degree of exposure.

### Handling Contaminated Laundry

As mentioned, the BBP Standard states that protective clothing may not be taken home and washed by employees. It may be laundered in the office if the equipment is available and if Universal Precautions are followed for handling and laundering the contaminated clothing.

Contaminated linens that are removed from the office for laundering should be placed in a leakproof bag with a biohazard label or an appropriately color-coded label (Fig. 19.17). Disposable gowns must be discarded daily and more often if visibly soiled (Fig. 19.18).

#### Guidelines for the Use of Protective Clothing

- Because protective clothing can spread contamination, it is *not* worn out of the office for any reason, including travel to and from the office.
- Protective clothing should be changed at least daily and more often if visibly soiled.
- If a protective garment becomes visibly soiled or saturated with chemicals or body fluids, it should be changed immediately.
- Protective clothing must *not* be worn in staff lounge areas or when workers are eating or consuming beverages.

**FIG. 19.17** Containers of contaminated laundry must be labeled with the universal biohazard symbol.

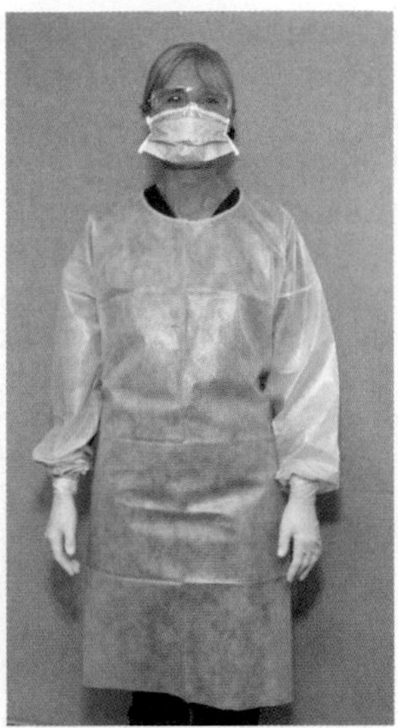

**FIG. 19.18** Fluid-impervious gown. *(Courtesy Crosstex, Hauppauge, NY.)*

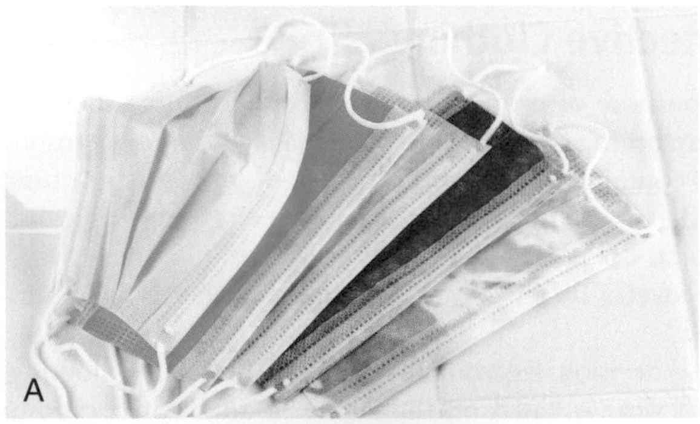


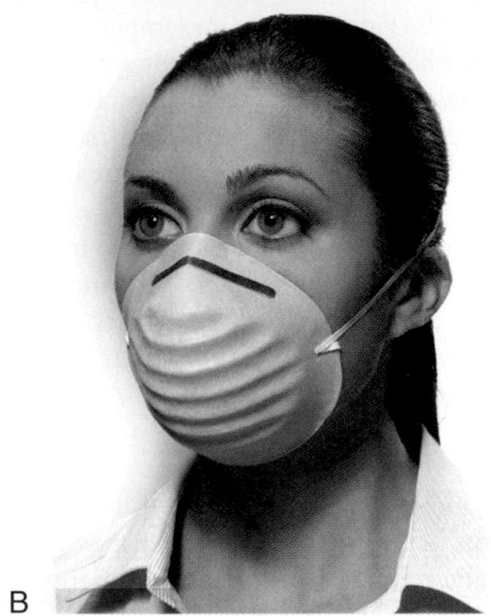


**FIG. 19.19** Flat (A) and dome-shaped or molded (B) types of face masks. *(A, Courtesy Practicon Dental, Greenville, NC; B, © 2017 Crosstex International, Inc.)*

## Protective Masks

A mask is worn over the nose and mouth to protect the person from inhaling infectious organisms spread by the aerosol spray of the handpiece or air-water syringe and by accidental splashes. A mask with at least 95 percent filtration efficiency for particles 3 to 5 micrometers (μm) in diameter should be worn whenever splash or spatter is likely. Masks do not provide a perfect seal around the edges; therefore unfiltered air can pass through the edges. For that reason, it is important to select a mask that fits your face well. Masks should be changed between patients, or during patient treatment if the mask becomes wet.

The two most common types of masks are the *dome-shaped* and *flat* types. Some operators prefer the dome-shaped type, particularly during lengthy procedures, because it *conforms* ("molds") more effectively to the face and creates an air space between the mask and the wearer (Fig. 19.19).

When not in use, face masks should *never* be worn below the nose or on the chin. Remember, the outer surface of the mask is highly contaminated (Fig. 19.20).

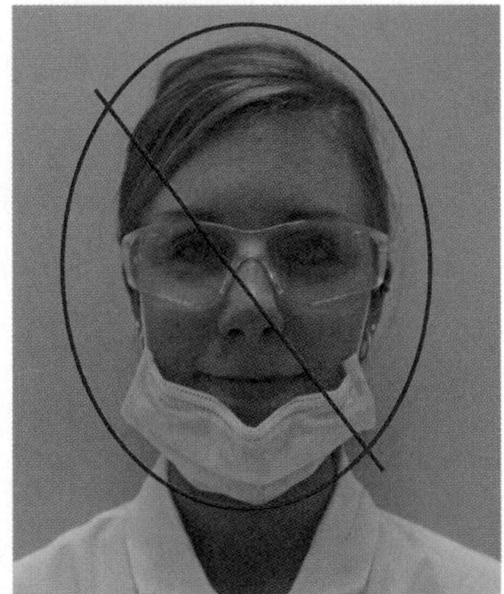

**FIG. 19.20** Face masks should never be worn below the nose or on the chin.

## Protective Eyewear

Eyewear is worn to protect the eyes against damage from aerosolized pathogens such as herpes simplex viruses and *Staphylococcus* and from flying debris such as scrap amalgam and tooth fragments. Protective eyewear also prevents injury from splattered solutions and caustic chemicals. Such damage may be irreparable and may lead to permanent visual impairment or blindness.

The BBP Standard requires the use of eyewear with both front and side protection (solid side shields) during exposure-prone procedures. If you wear prescription glasses, you must add protective side and bottom shields. Protective eyewear that can be worn over prescription glasses is also available. If you wear contact lenses, you must also wear protective eyewear with side shields or a face shield.

The CDC *Guidelines* recommend that you clean your eyewear with soap and water, or, if visibly soiled, you can clean and disinfect reusable facial protective wear between patients.

The two types of protective eyewear used during patient care are (1) glasses with protective side shields, and (2) clear face shields (Fig. 19.21).

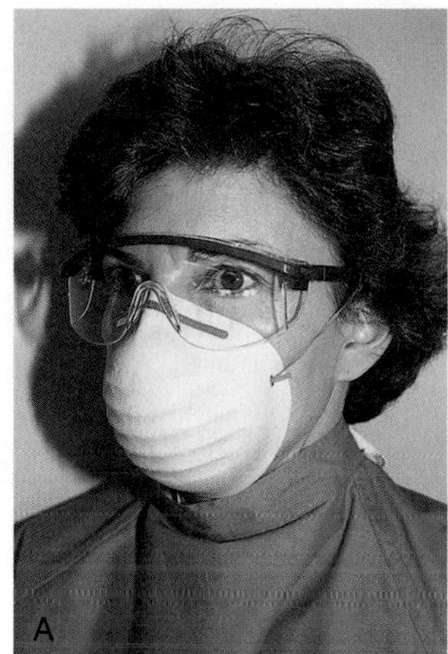


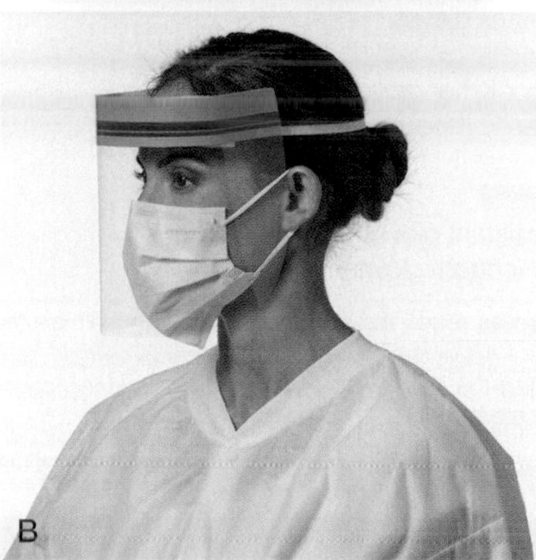


FIG. 19.21 A, Face mask and safety glasses. B, Face mask and disposable face shield. *(A, From Darby ML, Walsh MM: Dental hygiene: theory and practice, ed 4, St Louis, 2015, Saunders; B, © 2017 Crosstex International, Inc.)*

### Guidelines for the Use of Protective Masks

- Masks should be changed for every patient or more often, particularly if heavy spatter is generated during treatment, or if the mask becomes damp.
- Masks should be handled by touching only the side edges to avoid contact with the more heavily contaminated body of the mask.
- Masks should conform to the shape of the face.
- Masks should not contact the mouth when worn because the moisture generated will decrease the mask filtration efficiency. A damp or wet mask is *not* an effective mask.
- Masks should *not* be worn below the nose or mouth.

### Face Shields

A chin-length plastic face shield may be worn as an alternative to protective eyewear. However, a shield cannot replace a face mask because the shield does not protect against inhalation of contaminated aerosols (Fig. 19.22).

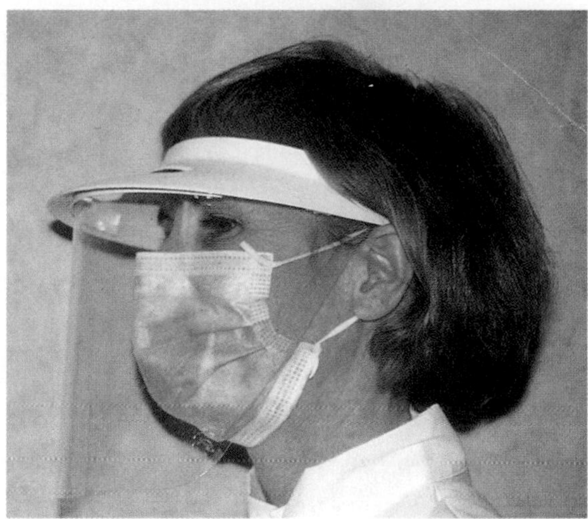

FIG. 19.22 Face shields provide adequate eye protection, but a face mask is still required when one is assisting with aerosol-generating procedures.

When splashing or spattering of blood or other body fluids is likely to occur during a procedure such as surgery, a face shield is often worn *in addition to* a protective mask.

### Patient Eyewear

Patients should be provided with protective eyewear because they also may be subject to eye damage from (1) handpiece spatter, (2) spilled or splashed dental materials such as caustic chemical agents, and (3) airborne bits of acrylic or tooth fragments (Fig. 19.23).

When certain laser treatments are performed, patients must be supplied with special filtered-lens glasses.

RECALL

11 What are four examples of PPE?
12 What determines the types of PPE to be worn?
13 What are the two types of protective eyewear?

## Gloves

Different types of gloves are used in a dental office. The type of glove you use should be based on the type of procedure to be performed (e.g., surgical vs. nonsurgical, housekeeping procedures). Medical grade nonsterile examination gloves and sterile surgical gloves are medical devices that are regulated by the U.S. Food and Drug Administration (FDA).

### Guidelines for the Use of Gloves

- *All* gloves used in patient care must be discarded after a single use. These gloves may not be washed, disinfected, or sterilized, although they may be rinsed with water to remove excess powder.
- Latex, vinyl, or other disposable medical quality gloves may be used for patient examinations and dental procedures.
- Replace torn or damaged gloves immediately.
- Do not wear jewelry under gloves. (Rings harbor pathogens and may tear the glove.)
- Change gloves frequently. (If the procedure is long, change gloves about once each hour.)

- Remove contaminated gloves before leaving the chairside during patient care, and replace them with new gloves before returning to patient care (see "Guidelines for the Use of Overgloves").
- Wash hands after glove removal and before regloving.

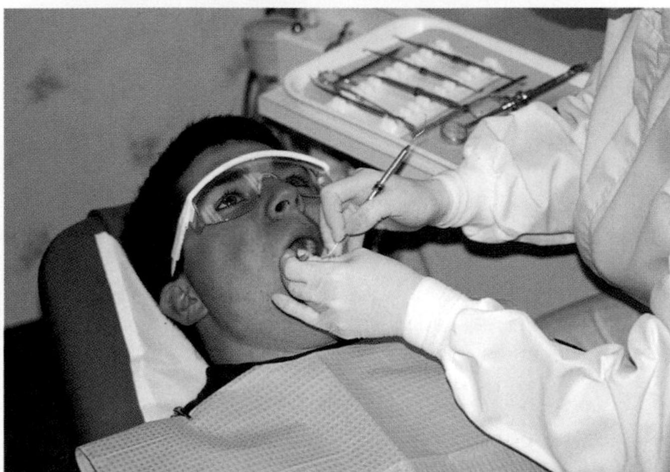

**FIG. 19.23** Patients should be provided with protective eyewear.

The FDA does not regulate utility gloves because these are not promoted for medical use. Sterile surgical gloves must meet standards for sterility assurance as established by the FDA (Box 19.3).

## Gloves Damaged During Treatment

Gloves are effective only when they are *intact* (not damaged, torn, ripped, or punctured). If gloves are damaged during treatment, change them immediately and wash your hands before regloving. The procedure for regloving in this situation is as follows:

- Excuse yourself and leave the chairside.
- Remove and discard the damaged gloves.
- Wash your hands thoroughly.
- Reglove before returning to the chairside to resume the dental procedure.

If you leave the chairside for any reason during the treatment of a patient, overgloves should be used. You must remove your contaminated examination gloves and wash your hands

### Gloves

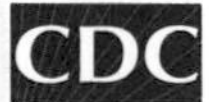


Because dental personnel are most likely to contact blood or contaminated items with their hands, gloves may be the most critical personal protective equipment. The dentist, dental assistant, and dental hygienist must wear medical gloves during all treatments that may involve contact with the patient's blood, saliva, or mucous membranes, or with contaminated items or surfaces. Wear a new pair of gloves for each patient, remove them promptly after use, and wash your hands immediately to avoid transfer

### BOX 19.3 Types of Gloves in Dentistry

**Patient Care Gloves**

- Sterile latex surgical gloves
- Sterile neoprene surgical gloves*
- Sterile styrene surgical gloves*
- Sterile synthetic copolymer gloves*
- Sterile reduced-protein latex surgeon's gloves
- Latex examination gloves
- Synthetic copolymer examination gloves*
- Nitrile examination gloves*
- Styrene-butadiene examination gloves*
- Polyurethane gloves*
- Powderless gloves
- Flavored gloves
- Low-protein gloves

**Utility Gloves**

- Heavy latex gloves
- Heavy nitrile gloves
- Thin copolymer gloves
- Thin plastic ("food handler") gloves

**Other Gloves**

- Heat-resistant gloves
- Dermal (cotton) gloves

* Nonlatex gloves; review the labeling or check with the manufacturer to confirm.

Data from Miller CH, Palenik CJ: Infection control and management of hazardous material, ed 5, St Louis, 2014, Mosby.

of microorganisms to other patients or to the environment. (Category IB)

Consult with the glove manufacturer regarding the chemical compatibility of the glove material and the dental materials you use. (Category II)

*before* you leave the chairside. When you return, you should wash and dry your hands and use fresh examination gloves.

## Gloves Damaged by Dental Materials

The chemicals you come in contact with on a daily basis may damage your gloves. For example, exposure to glutaraldehyde, hydrogen peroxide, and alcohol preparations may weaken latex, vinyl, nitrile, and other synthetic glove materials. Other chemicals in dental materials that may weaken gloves include acrylic monomer, chloroform, orange solvent, eugenol, cavity varnish, and acid etch.

Because so many dental materials are available on the market, you should consult the glove manufacturer about the compatibility of the glove material with various chemicals.

## Examination Gloves

Medical examination gloves usually are latex or vinyl and often are referred to as "examination gloves" or "procedure gloves." These gloves are most frequently worn by dental personnel during patient care (Fig. 19.24).

Examination gloves are inexpensive, are available in a range of sizes from extra small to extra large, and fit either hand. These gloves are *nonsterile* and serve strictly as a protective barrier for the wearer.

### Overgloves

Overgloves, also known as "food handler gloves," are made of lightweight, inexpensive, clear plastic. These may be worn over contaminated treatment gloves *(overgloving)* to prevent the contamination of clean objects handled during treatment (Fig. 19.25).

Infection control procedures for use in the mixing and passing of dental materials are discussed in greater detail in Chapter 47.

#### Guidelines for the Use of Overgloves

- Overgloves are *not* acceptable alone as a hand barrier or for intraoral procedures.
- Overgloves must be worn carefully to avoid contamination during handling with contaminated procedure gloves.
- Overgloves are placed before the secondary procedure is performed and are removed *before* patient treatment is resumed.
- Overgloves are discarded after a single use.

### Sterile Surgical Gloves

Sterile gloves, which are the type used in hospital operating rooms, should be worn for invasive procedures involving the cutting of bone or significant amounts of blood or saliva, such as oral surgery or periodontal treatment.

Sterile gloves are supplied in prepackaged units to maintain sterility before use. They are provided in specific sizes and are fitted to the left or right hand. Hand preparation and the use of surgical gloves are discussed in Chapter 56.

#### Sterile Surgeon's Gloves

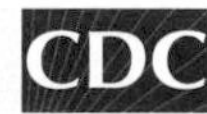


The CDC Guidelines offer no recommendations regarding the effectiveness of wearing two pairs of gloves to prevent disease transmission during oral surgical procedures. (Unresolved issue)

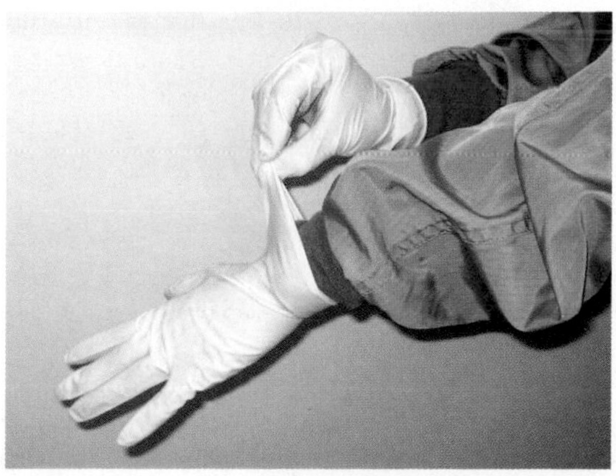

**FIG. 19.24** Nonsterile examination gloves. *(Courtesy Crosstex, Hauppauge, NY.)*

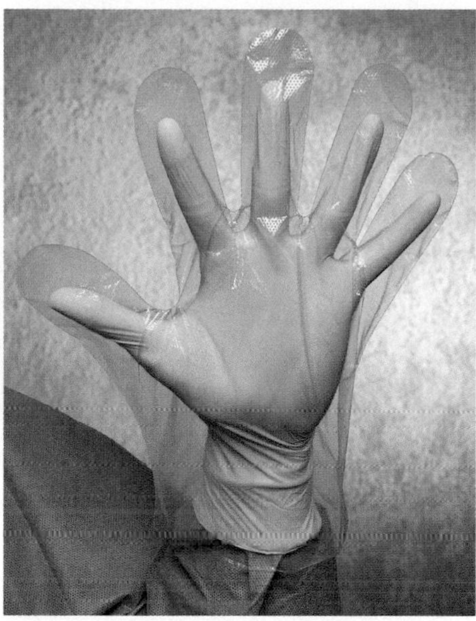

**FIG. 19.25** Overglove worn over an examination glove. *(From Boyd LRB: Dental instruments: a pocket guide, ed 6, St. Louis, 2018, Elsevier.)*

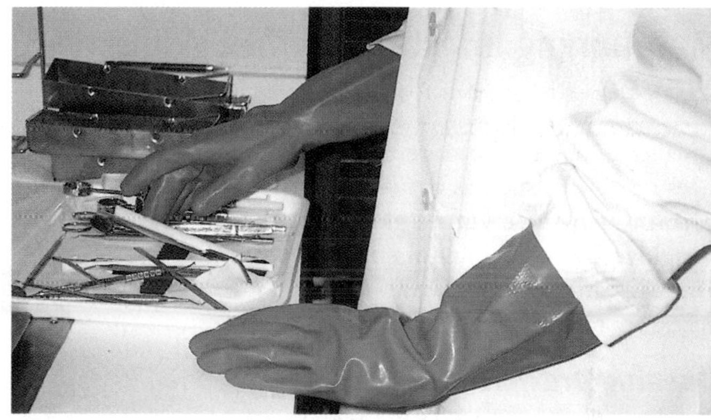

**FIG. 19.26** Utility gloves are used when instruments are prepared for sterilization.

### Utility Gloves

Utility gloves are *not* used for direct patient care. Utility gloves are worn (1) when the treatment room is cleaned and disinfected between patients, (2) while contaminated instruments are being cleaned or handled, and (3) for surface cleaning and disinfecting (Fig. 19.26). Utility gloves may be washed, disinfected, or sterilized and reused. Utility gloves must be discarded, however, when they become worn and no longer have the ability to provide barrier protection. After use, utility gloves must be considered contaminated and must be handled appropriately until they have been properly disinfected or sterilized. Each staff member responsible for cleanup procedures must have his or her own designated pair of utility gloves.

### Non–Latex-Containing Gloves

Occasionally, healthcare providers or patients may experience serious allergic reactions to latex (see Latex Allergies

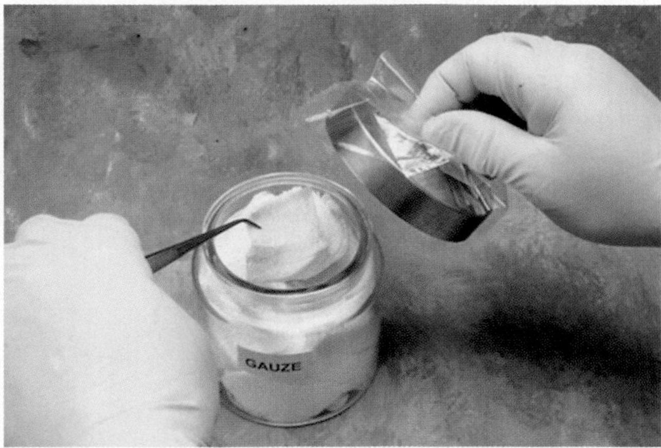


**FIG. 19.27** Aseptic retrieval using sterilized cotton pliers issued for each patient. *(From Miller CH: Infection control and management of hazardous materials for the dental team, ed 6, St Louis, 2018, Elsevier.)*

section). The person who is sensitive to latex can substitute with gloves made from vinyl, nitrile, and other non–latex-containing materials.

## Maintaining Infection Control While Gloved

During a dental procedure, it may be necessary to touch surfaces or objects such as drawer handles or material containers. If you touch these with a gloved hand, both the surface and the glove become contaminated. To minimize the possibility of cross-contamination, you can use an overglove when it is necessary to touch a surface.

### Opening Drawers and Cabinets

If you anticipate what materials you will need and have those items ready and easily accessible for each procedure, you will save time and minimize cross-contamination. Each surface you touch with contaminated gloves also becomes contaminated. By eliminating the need to open drawers and cabinets, you limit operatory contamination.

Set up instruments, medications, and impression materials ahead of time, and use disposable and unit-dose items whenever possible. Keep a pair of salad tongs or forceps within reach in the operatory. These simple tools can be used to open cabinets, pull out drawers, and obtain any unanticipated yet necessary items without contaminating additional items and surfaces. Appropriately disinfect the tongs or forceps between patients.

### Opening Containers

During the procedure, it may become necessary to open containers of materials or supplies. When opening a container, you may use overgloves, a paper towel, or sterile gauze to remove the lid or cap. In doing this, take care not to touch any surface of the container.

Use sterile cotton pliers to remove an item from the container (Fig. 19.27). If the container or bottle is touched, it becomes contaminated and must be disinfected at the end of the procedure.

RECALL

14 What may be the most critical PPE?
15 When should sterile gloves be worn?
16 When should utility gloves be worn?
17 What type of glove should be worn to open drawers during a dental procedure?

## High-Tech Equipment

Every aspect of dentistry is entering the arena of high-technology equipment and devices. You must carefully consider what infection control procedures are needed to make each piece of equipment safe for use. Some devices become contaminated from use in a patient's mouth. Other types may not be used in the mouth but may be held or touched with contaminated gloved hands (Fig. 19.28).

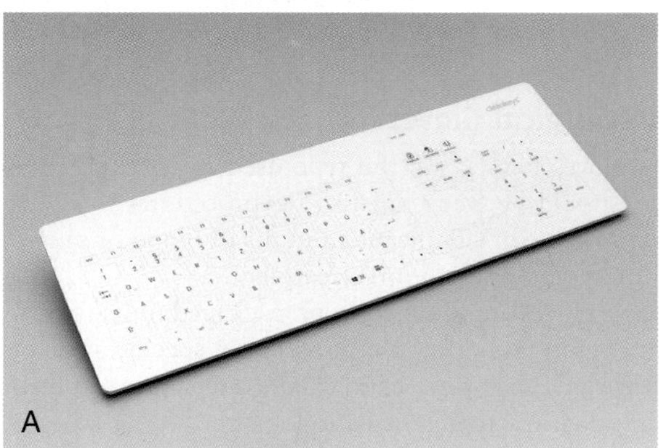


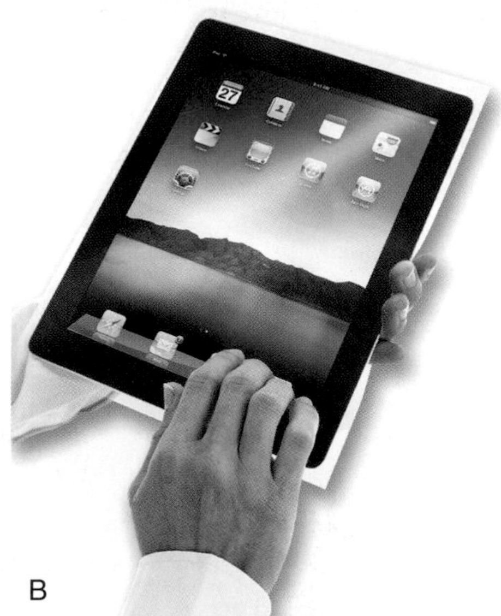


**FIG. 19.28** A, Computer keyboard with a smooth surface that allows for effective cleaning and disinfection. B, Disposable sleeve for high-tech devices, such as iPads or remotes. *(A, Courtesy Cleankeys Inc., Edmonton, Alberta, Canada; B, © 2017 Crosstex International, Inc.)*

### Examples of High-Tech Equipment

- Caries detection devices
- Intraoral cameras
- Extraoral cameras
- Microscopes
- Lasers
- Ultrasonic and piezo scalers
- Electric handpieces
- Optical illumination devices
- Computer keyboards
- CAD/CAM systems
- Curing lights
- Digital sensors
- Air-abrasion units
- Magnification loupes
- X-ray scanners

Always follow the manufacturer's infection control recommendations for every device and piece of equipment. If these procedures are not followed carefully, the equipment warranty and patient and office staff may be jeopardized.

Some infection control considerations when working with high-tech equipment and devices are provided in Box 19.4.

## Latex Allergies

The use of natural rubber latex gloves has proved to be one of the most effective means of protecting the dental worker and the patient from transmission of disease. However, increased use of latex gloves and other products that contain latex in the dental office and other healthcare settings has created other problems. The numbers of healthcare workers and patients who have become hypersensitive to latex have increased dramatically (Box 19.5).

Three common types of allergic reactions to latex have been identified. Irritant dermatitis involves only a surface irritation. Type I and type IV allergies involve an immune reaction.

### BOX 19.4 Infection Control Considerations for High-Tech Equipment

- Can it be protected with a barrier during use?
- Will barrier covers interfere with the operation or function of the equipment?
- Are detailed instructions for cleaning and sterilization provided?
- Can it withstand ultrasonic cleaning?
- Can it withstand heat sterilization?
- Can it withstand immersion with liquid chemical sterilants or high-level disinfectants?
- Do you have the type of sterilizer recommended for sterilization (steam, saturated chemical vapor, or dry heat sterilizer)?

Data from OSAP: Infection control in practice, volume 8, no. 5, November 2009.

### CDC Guidelines for Contact Dermatitis and Latex Hypersensitivity

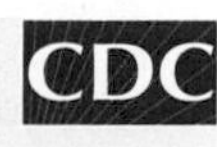


- Educate dental healthcare workers regarding the signs, symptoms, and diagnoses of skin reactions associated with frequent hand hygiene and glove use. (Category IB)
- Screen all patients for latex allergy (e.g., take health history and refer patient for medical consultation when latex allergy is suspected). (Category IB)
- Ensure a latex-safe environment for patients and dental healthcare personnel. (Category IB)
- Have emergency treatment kits with latex-free products available at all times. (Category II)

### BOX 19.5 Recommendations From NIOSH for Preventing Latex Allergies in the Workplace

**What Workers Should Do**

- Use nonlatex gloves when appropriate.
- If one uses latex gloves, use powder-free gloves with reduced protein content.
- If one uses latex gloves, do not use oil- or petroleum-based hand lotions.
- After removing latex gloves, wash hands with a mild detergent and dry thoroughly.
- Frequently clean areas that may be contaminated with latex powder (upholstery, carpets, ventilation ducts, and plenums).
- Frequently change ventilation filters and vacuum bags used in latex-contaminated areas.
- Take advantage of latex allergy training provided by your employer and learn about procedures for preventing latex allergies and about latex allergy symptoms (skin rash; hives; flushing; itching; nasal, eye, or sinus symptoms; asthma; and shock).
- If symptoms of latex allergy develop, avoid direct contact with latex-containing gloves and other items until after seeing a physician.
- If a latex allergy develops, consult a physician regarding the following precautions: avoid contact with latex-containing products; avoid areas where powder may be inhaled from latex gloves; tell employer about the latex allergy; and wear a medical alert bracelet.
- Carefully follow physician's instructions for dealing with allergic reactions to latex.

**What Employers Should Do**

- Provide workers with nonlatex gloves.
- If workers choose latex gloves, provide reduced-protein powder-free gloves.
- Ensure that workers use good housekeeping practices to remove latex-containing dust from the workplace: identify areas contaminated with latex dust for frequent cleaning (upholstery, carpets, ventilation ducts, and plenums), and make sure that workers change ventilation filters and vacuum bags frequently in latex-containing areas.

- Provide workers with education programs and training materials about latex allergy.
- Periodically screen high-risk workers for latex allergy symptoms. Detecting symptoms early and removing symptomatic workers from latex exposure are essential to preventing long-term health effects.
- Evaluate current prevention strategies whenever a worker is diagnosed with latex allergy.

From Centers for Disease Control and Prevention, National Institute for Occupational Safety and Health. *NIOSH alert: Preventing allergic reactions to natural rubber latex in the workplace*, Cincinnati, OH, 1997, U.S. Department of Health and Human Services, Public Health Service, CDC, National Institute for Occupational Safety and Health, Pub No 97-135.

## Irritant Dermatitis

Irritant dermatitis is a *nonimmunologic* process (does *not* involve the body's immune system). It is caused by contact with a substance that produces a chemical irritation to the skin. The skin becomes reddened, dry, irritated, and, in severe cases, cracked (Fig. 19.29).

Identifying and correcting the causes, which include the following, can reverse irritant dermatitis:

- Frequent handwashing with soaps or antimicrobial agents
- Failure to rinse soaps or microbial agents completely from the hands
- Irritation caused by the cornstarch powder in gloves
- Excessive perspiration on the hands while wearing gloves
- Failure to dry hands thoroughly after rinsing

## Type IV Allergic Reaction

Type IV allergic reaction, the most common type of latex allergy, is a delayed contact reaction that involves the immune system. It may take 48 to 72 hours for the red, itchy rash to appear. Reactions are limited to the areas of contact and do not involve the entire body. The chemicals used to process the latex in these gloves cause an immune response; the proteins in the latex do not cause it.

*Note:* Chemicals such as glutaraldehyde and acrylates readily permeate (pass through) latex gloves and can irritate the skin. This irritation may be mistaken for an allergic reaction to the chemicals in the latex glove. Thus latex gloves should never be worn when handling chemicals.

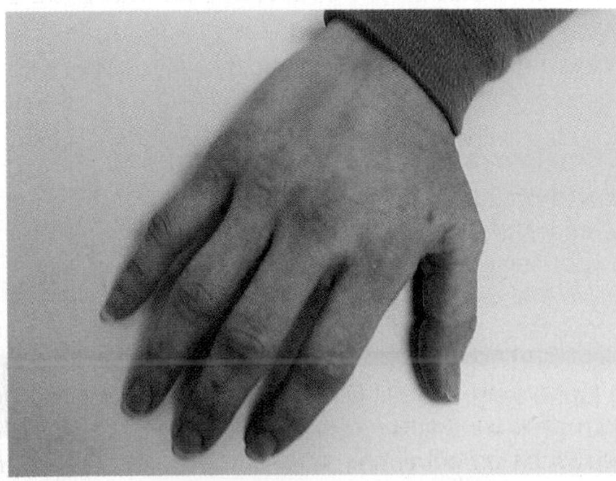

**FIG. 19.29** Irritant dermatitis.

## Type I Allergic Reaction

Type I allergic reaction is the most serious type of latex allergy and can result in death. This reaction occurs in response to the latex *proteins* in the glove, in contrast to the reaction to chemical additives in type IV. A severe immunologic response occurs, usually 2 to 3 minutes after latex allergens contact the skin or mucous membranes.

Proteins from the latex adhere to the cornstarch powder particles inside the gloves. Frequent handling of powdered latex gloves, such as during donning and frequent removal of powdered gloves from boxes during the day, cause the proteins, which are bound to the powder, to remain suspended in the air for prolonged periods. Sensitized persons can experience coughing, wheezing, runny eyes and nose, shortness of breath, and respiratory distress.

The primary cause of death associated with latex allergies is anaphylaxis. **Anaphylaxis** is the most severe form of immediate allergic reaction. Death results from closure of the airway caused by swelling (see Chapter 31).

## Treatment

No specific cure has been identified for latex allergy. The only options are prevention, avoidance of latex-containing products, and treatment of the symptoms. Persons who suspect that they are allergic to latex should see a qualified healthcare provider for a test to confirm the allergy. Once diagnosed as having a latex allergy, patients should avoid latex in all aspects of their personal and professional lives.

*Note:* When one employee in the dental office has been diagnosed as having a latex allergy, all staff members should follow practices to minimize the use of latex-containing products. These measures include use of powderless gloves by all dental staff members to minimize the risk of airborne latex particles.

## Latex-Sensitive Patients

In the healthcare setting, patients with latex allergies should be treated with alternatives to latex. Vinyl gloves and a nonlatex rubber dam should be available in all dental offices.

RECALL

**18** What type of response is irritant dermatitis?
**19** What is the most common type of latex allergy?
**20** What is the most serious type of latex allergy?
**21** What type of gloves should be used for a latex-sensitive patient?

# Waste Management in the Dental Office

Dental practices are subject to a wide variety of federal, state, and local regulations regarding waste management issues. Waste management can be confusing because agencies do not always use a consistent glossary of terms and definitions (Table 19.2). For example, the Environmental Protection Agency (EPA) and

**TABLE 19.2** Classification of Waste

| Type | Examples | Handling Requirements |
|---|---|---|
| General waste | Paper towels, paper mixing pads, empty food containers | Discard in covered containers made of durable materials such as plastic or metal. |
| Hazardous waste | Waste that presents a danger to humans or to the environment (toxic chemicals) | Follow your specific state and local regulations. |
| Contaminated waste | Waste that has been in contact with blood or other body fluids (used barriers, patient napkins) | In most states, dispose of with the general waste. |
| Infectious or regulated waste (biohazard) | Waste that is capable of transmitting an infectious disease | Follow your specific state and local regulations. |
| Blood and blood-soaked materials | Blood or saliva that can be squeezed out, or dried blood that may flake off of an item | Containers for all three types of infectious waste must be labeled with the biohazard label. |
| Pathologic waste | Soft tissue and extracted teeth | Follow your specific state and local regulations. |
| Sharps | Contaminated needles, scalpel blades, orthodontic wires, endodontic instruments (reamers and files) | Closable, leakproof, puncture-resistant containers. Containers should be color-coded red and marked with the biohazard symbol. Sharps containers should be located as close as possible to the work area. |

most state and local regulations do not categorize saliva or saliva-soaked items as infectious waste. However, because of the high probability that blood may be carried in saliva during dental procedures, CDC *Guidelines* and OSHA BBP Standard regulations consider saliva in dentistry to be a potentially infectious body fluid. As such, saliva-coated items should be treated as *potentially infectious waste* and disposed of as contaminated waste. The OSHA BBP Standard requires that all waste be disposed of according to applicable federal, state, and local regulations.

## CDC Guidelines for Regulated Medical Waste

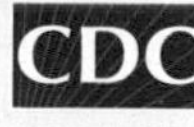


- Develop a medical waste management program. Disposal of regulated medical waste must follow federal, state, and local regulations. (Category IC)
- Ensure that dental healthcare personnel who handle and dispose of regulated medical waste are trained in appropriate handling and disposal methods and are informed of the possible health and safety hazards. (Category IC)
- Pour blood, suctioned fluids, or other liquid waste carefully into a drain connected to a sanitary sewer system, if local sewage discharge requirements are met and the state has declared this an appropriate method of disposal. Wear appropriate personal protective equipment while performing this task. (Category IC)

## Classification of Waste

The handling, storage, labeling, and disposal of waste depend entirely on the type of waste. For example, when a dental treatment room is reprocessed, the waste should be separated into general waste containers and hazardous waste containers. The dental assistant must understand the types of waste to know what items are discarded in which container.

### General Waste

General waste consists of all nonhazardous, nonregulated waste and should be discarded in covered containers made of durable material such as plastic or metal. For ease in handling, general waste receptacles should be lined with plastic bags. General waste includes disposable paper towels, paper mixing pads, and empty food containers.

### Contaminated Waste

Waste that has been in contact with blood or other body fluids is considered **contaminated waste**; this includes used barriers and patient napkins. In most states, contaminated waste is disposed of as general waste (regular household-type waste). In a few states, however, it may be considered and defined as regulated, or infectious, waste.

Appropriate PPE should be worn when handling or disposing of contaminated waste.

### Hazardous Waste

**Hazardous waste** poses a risk to humans and to the environment. Toxic chemicals and materials are hazardous waste. Examples include scrap amalgam, spent fixer solution, and lead foil from x-ray film packets. Some items, such as extracted teeth with amalgam restorations, may be both hazardous waste (because of the amalgam) and infectious waste (because of the blood).

### Infectious or Regulated Waste (Biohazard)

**Infectious waste**, also called *regulated waste* or *biohazardous waste,* is contaminated waste that is capable of transmitting an infectious disease. For waste to be infectious, pathogens must be strong enough and must be present in sufficient numbers to infect a susceptible individual.

Infectious waste is never disposed of as general waste. It requires special handling and disposal. Most dental offices are exposed to the following three types of infectious waste:

1. *Blood and blood-soaked materials.* Blood or saliva can be squeezed out, or dried blood may flake off from the item. Gauze dripping with blood is such an item.
2. *Pathologic waste.* Soft tissue and extracted teeth are examples.
3. *Sharps.* Examples include all contaminated sharp objects used for patient care.

## Handling Extracted Teeth

Dispose of extracted teeth as regulated medical waste unless returned to the patient. When teeth are returned to the patient, the provisions of the standard no longer apply. Do not dispose of extracted teeth that contain amalgam with regulated medical waste that will be incinerated. Because of the mercury that is present in amalgam fillings, you should check your state and local regulations regarding disposal of teeth that contain amalgam.

### CDC Guidelines for Handling Extracted Teeth CDC

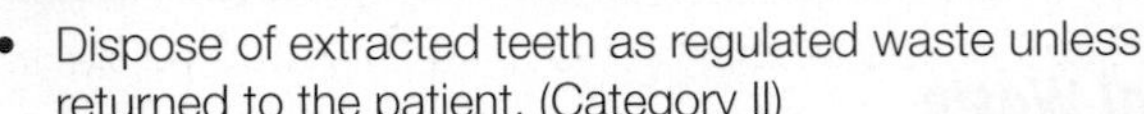

- Dispose of extracted teeth as regulated waste unless returned to the patient. (Category II)
- Do not dispose of extracted teeth that contain amalgam as regulated medical waste intended for incineration. (Category II)
- Heat-sterilize teeth that do not contain amalgam before they are used for educational purposes. (Category IB)

## Handling Contaminated Waste

Contaminated items that may contain the body fluids of patients, such as gloves and patient napkins, should be placed in a lined trash receptacle. Receptacles for contaminated waste should be covered with a properly fitted lid that can be opened with a foot pedal. Keeping the lid closed prevents air movement and the spread of contaminants. This receptacle should not be overfilled, and it should be emptied at least once daily.

Red bags or containers should *not* be used for unregulated waste. Check the specific requirements of your local state or county health department (Fig. 19.30).

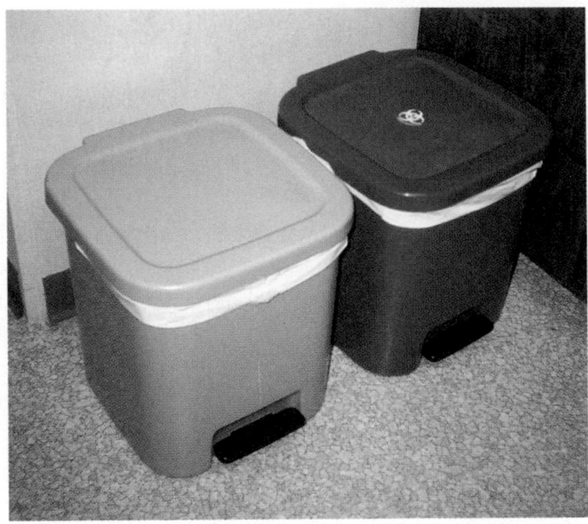

**FIG. 19.30** Waste is separated into clearly marked containers. *Left,* Unregulated waste. *Right,* Regulated waste.

## Handling Medical Waste

Medical waste is any solid waste that is generated in the diagnosis, treatment, or immunization of humans or animals in research. Infectious waste is a subset of medical waste. Only a small percentage of medical waste is infectious and has to be regulated.

### *Infectious Waste*

Containers of infectious waste (regulated waste), as defined earlier, must be labeled with the universal biohazard symbol, identified in compliance with local regulations, or both. Local regulations may vary regarding the return of extracted teeth to patients, especially for young children who give their tooth to the "tooth fairy."

*Note:* Containers used for holding contaminated items also must be labeled. Examples of such containers are contaminated sharps containers, pans or trays used for holding contaminated instruments, bags of contaminated laundry, specimen containers, and storage containers.

### *Disposal of Medical Waste*

Once contaminated waste leaves the office, it is then regulated by the EPA and by state and local laws. Under most regulations, the manner of disposal is determined by the quantity (weight) of infectious materials for disposal.

The average dental practice is categorized as a "small producer" of infectious waste, and disposal is regulated accordingly. The law requires the dentist to maintain records of the final disposal of this medical waste, including documentation of how, when, and where it was disposed.

RECALL

22 What are two examples of contaminated waste?
23 What are three examples of general waste?
24 What is another term for infectious waste?
25 Which type of waste must be identified with the biohazard label?

# Additional Infection Control Practices

## OSHA Blood-Borne Pathogens Standard

Never eat, drink, smoke, apply cosmetics or lip balm, or handle contact lenses in any area of the dental office where possible contamination is present, such as dental treatment rooms, dental laboratory, sterilization area, or x-ray processing area.

Never store food or drink in refrigerators that contain potentially contaminated items.

## CDC Guidelines: Special Considerations

### *Saliva Ejectors*

Backflow from low-volume saliva ejectors occurs when the pressure in the patient's mouth is less than that in the evacuator. This backflow can be a potential source of cross-contamination between patients. Although no adverse health effects associated with the saliva ejector have been reported, you should be aware that in certain situations, backflow could occur when a saliva ejector is used.

## Saliva Ejector

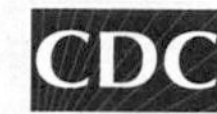

Do not advise patients to close their lips tightly around the tip of the saliva ejector to evacuate oral fluids. (Category II)

### Dental Laboratory

Items that are commonly used in a dental laboratory (e.g., dentures, partials, impressions, bite registrations) are potential sources of cross-contamination. Dental prostheses or impressions can be contaminated with bacteria, viruses, and fungi. These items should be handled in a manner to prevent exposure to dental team members, patients, and the office environment.

When cases are sent to a commercial dental laboratory, effective communication between the laboratory and dental office is needed. Written information should be provided to the laboratory regarding the type of cleaning and disinfecting solutions that were used on the impressions, models, etc. Follow the manufacturer's recommendations to ensure that the materials are not damaged or distorted as a result of disinfectant exposure (Fig. 19.31).

Dental prostheses or impressions should be thoroughly cleaned and disinfected before they are handled in an in-office laboratory (see Procedure 19.6: Disinfecting an Alginate Impression). The best time to clean and disinfect impressions, prostheses, or appliances is as soon as possible after removal from the patient's mouth, before the blood or saliva can dry (Fig. 19.32). Always check the manufacturer's recommendations regarding the stability of specific materials during disinfection. The majority of items can be disinfected with an EPA-registered hospital disinfectant.

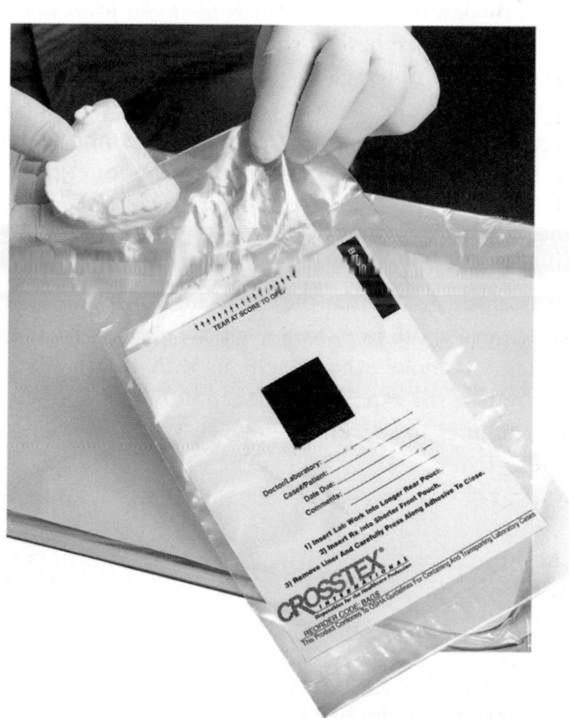


FIG. 19.31 Pouch for laboratory cases with the biohazard label. (© 2017 Crosstex International, Inc.)

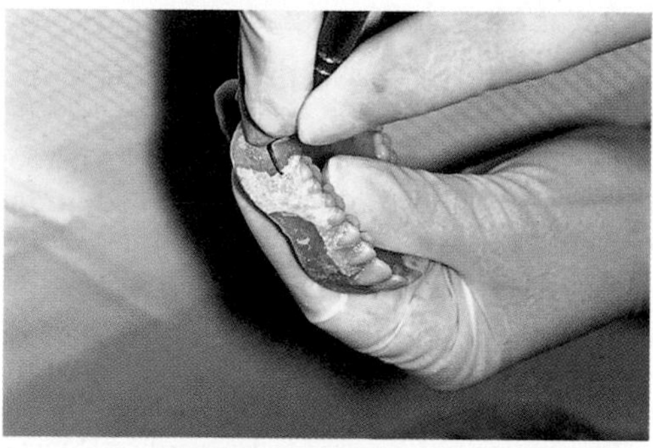

FIG. 19.32 This denture has large amounts of calculus adhering to it. *(Courtesy Bertha Chan, RHD, BS. From Darby ML, Walsh MM: Dental hygiene: theory and practice, ed 4, St Louis, 2015, Saunders.)*

Environmental surfaces in the laboratory should be barrier-protected or cleaned and disinfected in the same way that is done for the dental operatory.

Laboratory items (e.g., burs, polishing points, rag wheels, laboratory knives) that have been used on contaminated appliances or prostheses should be heat-sterilized, disinfected between patients, or discarded (disposable products).

## CDC Guidelines for Dental Laboratories

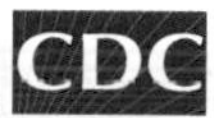

- Use personal protective equipment when handling items received in the laboratory until they have been decontaminated. (Categories IA and IC)
- Before they are handled in the laboratory, clean, disinfect, and rinse all dental prostheses and prosthodontic materials (e.g., impressions, bite registrations, occlusal rims, extracted teeth) by using an Environmental Protection Agency (EPA)–registered hospital disinfectant that has at least intermediate-level activity. (Category IB)
- Consult with manufacturers regarding the stability of specific materials (e.g., impression materials) relative to disinfection procedures. (Category II)
- Include specific information regarding disinfection techniques when laboratory cases are sent off-site and on their return. (Category II)
- Clean and heat-sterilize heat-tolerant items used in the mouth (e.g., metal impression trays, face-bow forks). (Category IB)
- Follow manufacturers' instructions for cleaning, sterilizing, or disinfecting items that become contaminated but do not normally contact the patient (e.g., burs, polishing points, rag wheels, articulators, case pans, lathes). If manufacturers' instructions are unavailable, clean and sterilize heat-stable items and disinfect with an EPA-registered hospital disinfectant with low- to intermediate-level activity. (Category II)

### Preprocedural Mouth Rinses

Some dental practitioners have their patients rinse with an antimicrobial mouth rinse before dental procedures. This procedure is intended to reduce the number of microorganisms released in the form of aerosol or spatter. In addition, preprocedural mouth rinsing can decrease the number of microorganisms introduced into the patient's bloodstream during invasive dental procedures. The scientific evidence is inconclusive that preprocedural mouth rinsing prevents clinical infection among dental health professionals or patients. Therefore the CDC identifies the use of a preprocedural mouth rinse as an unresolved issue.

### *Mycobacterium tuberculosis*

Patients infected with *M. tuberculosis* (the microorganism that causes tuberculosis [TB]) may seek dental treatment in private offices. It is important for the dental assistant to understand how to manage these patients. *M. tuberculosis* is a bacterium that is spread by airborne infective particles when the patient sneezes, coughs, or even speaks. The small particles can remain airborne for hours. Infection occurs when a susceptible person inhales the bacteria, which then travel to the lungs. TB bacteria can remain alive in the lungs for years, a condition called *latent TB infection.* Persons with latent TB usually have a reactive tuberculin skin test (TST), but they have no symptoms of active disease and are not infectious. However, they can develop disease later in life if they do not receive treatment for their latent infection. For patients with known or suspected active TB, the CDC recommends that elective dental treatment be delayed until the patient is noninfectious. For patients who require urgent dental care, the CDC recommends referring the patient to a facility with TB engineering controls and a respiratory protection program.

#### CDC Guidelines for *Mycobacterium tuberculosis*

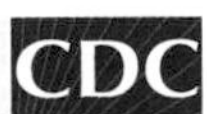

- All dental healthcare professionals (DHCPs) should be educated regarding the signs, symptoms, and transmission of tuberculosis (TB). (Category IB)
- All DHCPs who could have contact with persons with suspected or confirmed cases of TB should have a baseline tuberculosis skin test (TST). (Category IB)
- Assess each patient for a history of TB, and document it on the medical history. (Category IB)
- Follow CDC recommendations for developing, maintaining, and implementing a TB infection control plan. (Category IB)
- The following applies to patients known or suspected to have active TB:
  - The patient should be evaluated away from other patients and personnel. (Category IB)
  - Elective dental treatment should be deferred until the patient is noninfectious. (Category IB)
  - Patients who require urgent dental treatment should be referred to a facility with TB engineering controls and a respiratory protection program. (Category IB)

### Creutzfeldt-Jakob Disease and Other Prion Diseases

Creutzfeldt-Jakob disease (CJD) belongs to a group of rapidly progressive, invariably fatal, degenerative neurologic disorders. The disease can affect both humans and animals. It is thought that the disease is caused by a prion infection (see Chapter 18). Prion diseases have an incubation period (time between infection and signs of disease) of years and are usually fatal within 1 year of diagnosis. The CDC offers no recommendation regarding the use of special precautions in addition to Standard Precautions when one is treating known patients with CJD. This remains an unresolved issue.

#### Creutzfeldt-Jakob Disease

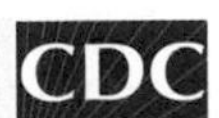

Potential infectivity of oral tissues in patients with Creutzfeldt-Jakob disease is an unresolved issue. Scientific data indicate that the risk, if any, of sporadic transmission of the disease during dental and oral surgical procedures is low to nil. No recommendation is offered regarding use of special precautions in addition to Standard Precautions when treating patients known to have Creutzfeldt-Jakob disease. (Unresolved issue)

### Laser/Electrosurgery Plumes or Surgical Smoke

During surgical procedures in which a laser or an electrosurgical unit is used, a smoke by-product is created through thermal destruction of the tissue. Laser plumes and surgical smoke create additional potential risks for dental healthcare professionals. One concern is that aerosolized infectious material in the laser plume may reach the nasal mucosa of the operator or other members of the dental team. However, the presence of an infectious agent within a laser plume might not be enough to cause disease from airborne exposure, especially if the agent's normal mode of transmission is not airborne. Because the effect of exposure on dental personnel from the use of dental lasers has not yet been adequately evaluated, the CDC offers no recommendations, and this remains an unresolved issue.

It has been suggested that the use of high-filtration surgical masks and possible full face shields, central room suction units, and mechanical smoke exhaust systems with a high-efficiency filter may reduce the exposure of dental healthcare professionals to laser plumes and surgical smoke.

#### Laser/Electrosurgery Plumes/Surgical Smoke

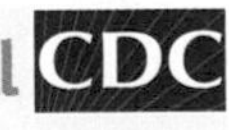

The effect of exposure (e.g., disease transmission, adverse respiratory effects) on dental healthcare professionals from the use of lasers in dentistry has not been adequately evaluated. (Unresolved issue)

RECALL

26 What is the BBP Standard rule regarding refrigerators in dental offices?
27 What is the CDC guideline for using saliva ejectors?
28 How does tuberculosis infection occur?
29 What is the CDC recommendation on the use of preprocedural mouth rinses?
30 Did the CDC make a recommendation regarding the effects of exposure to laser plumes on dental healthcare professionals? Why or why not?

## ■ Legal and Ethical Implications

The CDC *Guidelines for Infection Control in Dental Health-Care Settings—2003* apply to approximately 168,000 dentists, 218,000 dental assistants, 112,000 dental hygienists, and 53,000 dental laboratory technicians. They also apply to students, trainees, and other persons not directly involved in patient care but who are potentially exposed to infectious agents (e.g., administrative, clerical, housekeeping, maintenance, volunteers). Refer to the CDC 2016 Summary of Infection Prevention Practices in Dental Settings for checklists you will find helpful. Remember that these guidelines are the established standard of care for infection control in dentistry.

**Infection prevention** is also an ethical issue for the dental assistant. Often, the dental assistant is alone when performing infection control procedures; if cross-contamination occurs, no one else may know. Always following proper infection prevention procedures is a matter of personal commitment and integrity.

Patients should have absolute confidence that the infection prevention procedures followed in the office are never compromised. This confidence is as important for the protection of dental team members as it is for the patient. ■

## ■ Eye to the Future

The area of infection prevention in dentistry is continually evolving, and as new diseases are identified, new practices and techniques will be developed to prevent their spread. Although some concepts of dental infection control may seem confusing, the basic principles serve as the cornerstone for preventing disease transmission in the dental setting.

Dental professionals must remain vigilant and must keep current on the latest information to ensure the health of patients, their families, and themselves. ■

## ■ Critical Thinking

1. How would you handle a situation in which you knew that a coworker was not routinely following infection control policies?
2. Mrs. James becomes offended when you put on gloves before taking her radiographs. She insists that she does not have a disease, and that her previous dental assistant never wore gloves. What would you explain to her?
3. What precautions would you take if a new patient in your office said that he was allergic to latex?
4. How would you explain the CDC *Guidelines* and the OSHA Blood-borne Pathogens Standard to a new employee who has no formal dental-assisting education? ■

PROCEDURE 19.1

## Applying First Aid After an Exposure Incident

### GOAL

To perform appropriate first aid after an exposure incident

### EQUIPMENT AND SUPPLIES

- ✓ Soap and water
- ✓ Paper towels
- ✓ Antiseptic cream or ointment
- ✓ Adhesive bandage
- ✓ Exposure incident report form

### PROCEDURAL STEPS

1 Stop operations immediately.
2 Remove your gloves.
3 Wash your hands thoroughly, using antimicrobial soap and warm water.
4 Dry your hands.
5 Apply a small amount of antiseptic to the affected area.
**NOTE** Do not apply caustic agents such as bleach or disinfectant solutions to the wound.
6 Apply an adhesive bandage to the area.
7 Complete applicable postexposure follow-up steps.
**NOTE** The employer should be notified of the injury immediately after initial first aid is provided.

PROCEDURE 19.2 

## Handwashing Before Gloving

### GOAL

To wash hands properly before gloving

### EQUIPMENT AND SUPPLIES

- ✓ Sink with running water
- ✓ Liquid soap in a dispenser
- ✓ Nailbrush or orange stick
- ✓ Paper towels in a dispenser

### PROCEDURAL STEPS

1 Remove all jewelry, including watch and rings.
**PURPOSE** Jewelry is difficult to clean, can harbor microbes, and can puncture the gloves.

2 Use the foot or electronic control to regulate water flow. If this is not available, use a paper towel to grasp the faucets to turn them on and off. Discard the towel after use. Allow your hands to become wet.
**PURPOSE** Faucets may have been contaminated by being touched with soiled or contaminated hands.

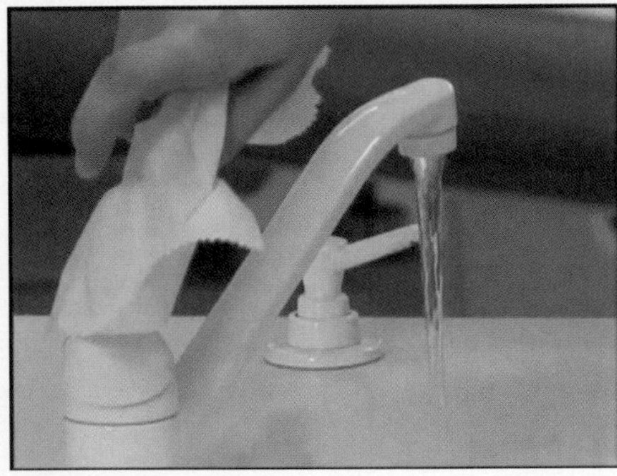

3 Apply soap, and lather using a circular motion with friction while holding your fingertips downward. Rub well between your fingers. If this is the first handwashing of the day, use a nailbrush or an orange stick. Inspect and clean under every fingernail during this step.
**PURPOSE** Friction removes soil and contaminants from your hands and wrists.

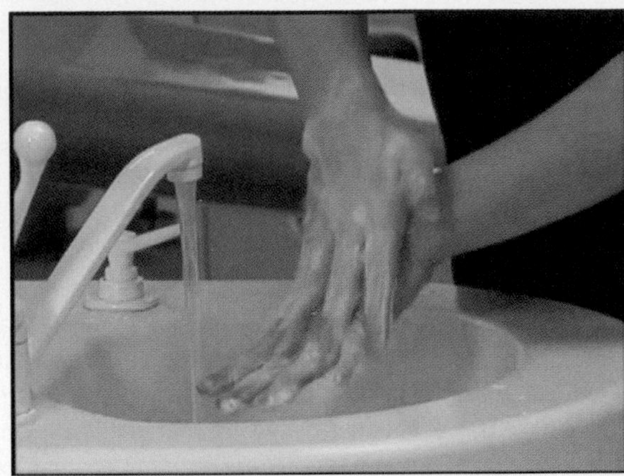

4 Vigorously rub together the lathered hands under a stream of water to remove surface debris.
**PURPOSE** Scrubbing the first time removes gross debris.

5 Apply more soap, and vigorously rub together lathered hands for a minimum of 10 seconds under a stream of water.
**PURPOSE** Secondary scrubbing removes residual debris and tenacious microorganisms, which thrive under the free edges of the fingernails.

6 Rinse the hands with cool water.
**PURPOSE** Cool water closes the pores.

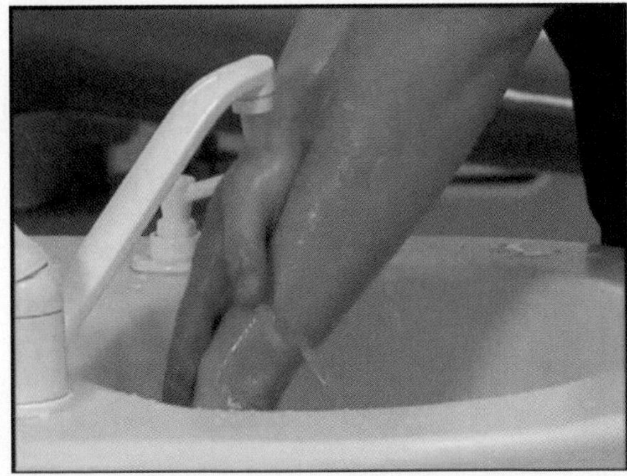

## PROCEDURE 19.2 Handwashing Before Gloving—cont'd.

7 Use a paper towel to dry the hands thoroughly, and then dry the forearms.

**PURPOSE** Reusable cloth towels remain moist, contribute to microbial growth, and spread contamination.

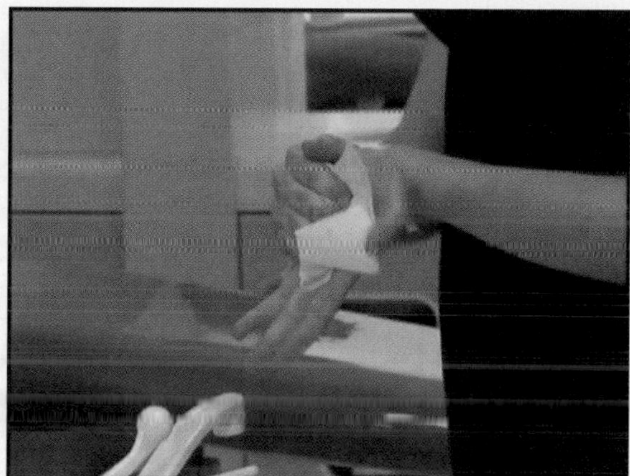

8 If water faucets are not foot-operated, turn off the faucet with a clean paper towel.

**PURPOSE** The faucet is dirty and will contaminate your clean hands.

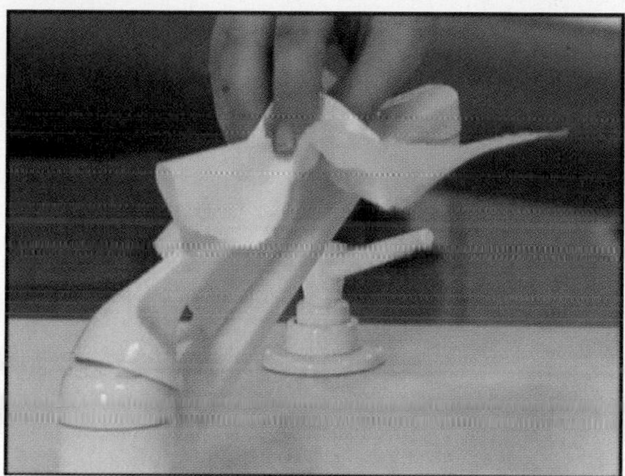

## PROCEDURE 19.3

# Applying Alcohol-based Hand Rubs

### GOAL

To apply an alcohol-based hand rub

### EQUIPMENT AND SUPPLIES

- ✓ Alcohol-based hand rub (60 to 95 percent concentration)

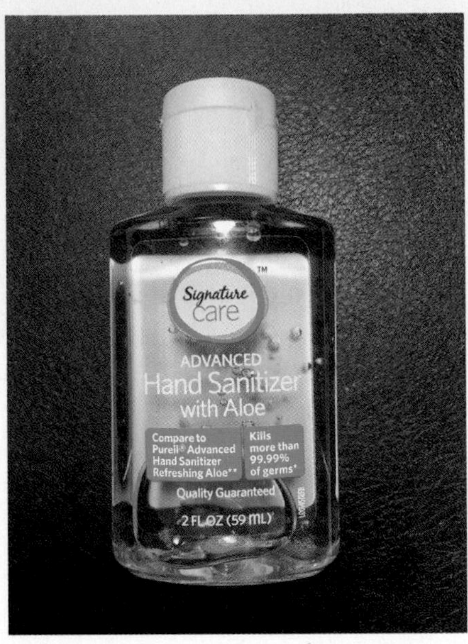


### PROCEDURAL STEPS

1 Check your hands to be sure they are not visibly soiled or contaminated with organic matter, such as blood or saliva. If necessary, wash your hands with soap and water, and dry them thoroughly.

**PURPOSE** Alcohol-based hand rubs are not effective in the presence of organic matter.

2 Read directions carefully to determine the proper amount to dispense.

**PURPOSE** These products are very dose sensitive. If you use a smaller amount than is recommended, effectiveness will be seriously decreased.

3 Dispense the proper amount of the product into the palm of one hand.

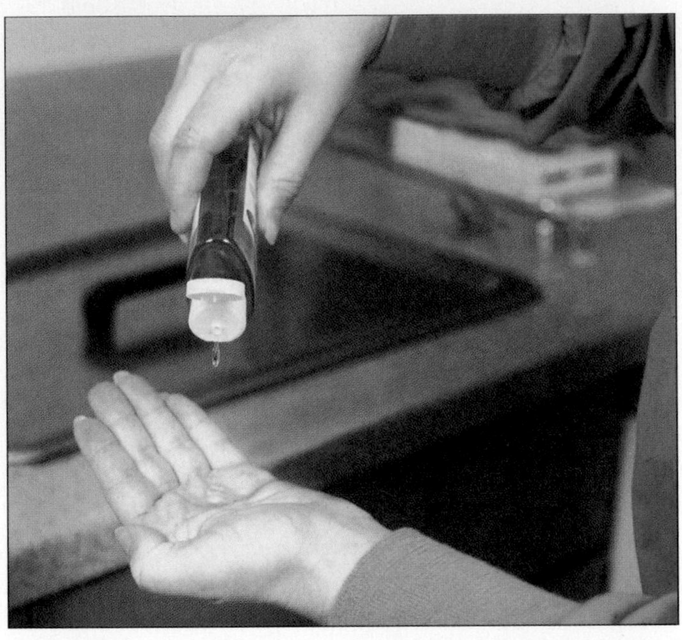

4 Rub the palms of your hands together.

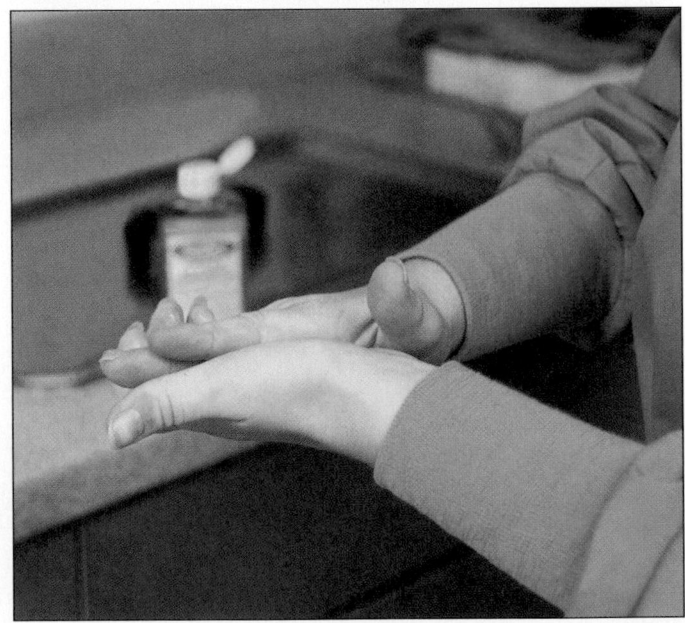

## PROCEDURE 19.3 Applying Alcohol-based Hand Rubs—cont'd.

5 Rub the product between your fingers.

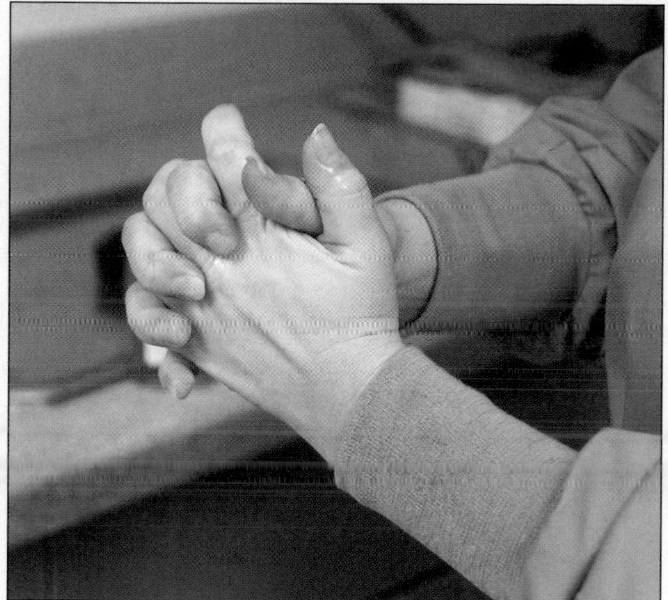

6 Rub the product over the back of your hands.

**PURPOSE** It is important to thoroughly cover both of your hands.

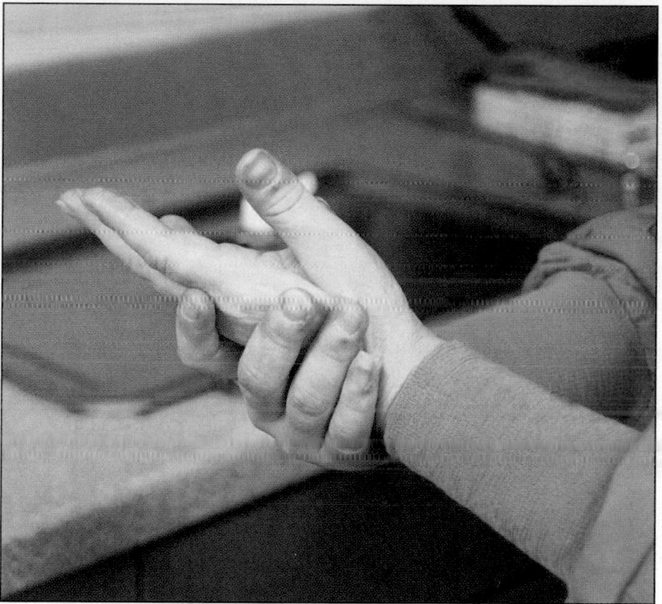

## PROCEDURE 19.4

# Putting on Personal Protective Equipment

### GOAL

To put on PPE before providing patient care

### EQUIPMENT AND SUPPLIES

- ✓ Protective clothing
- ✓ Protective eyewear
- ✓ Surgical mask
- ✓ Gloves

### PROCEDURAL STEPS

1 Put on your protective clothing over your uniform, street clothes, or scrubs.

**NOTE** Protective clothing could be long-sleeved laboratory coats, clinic jackets, or gowns.

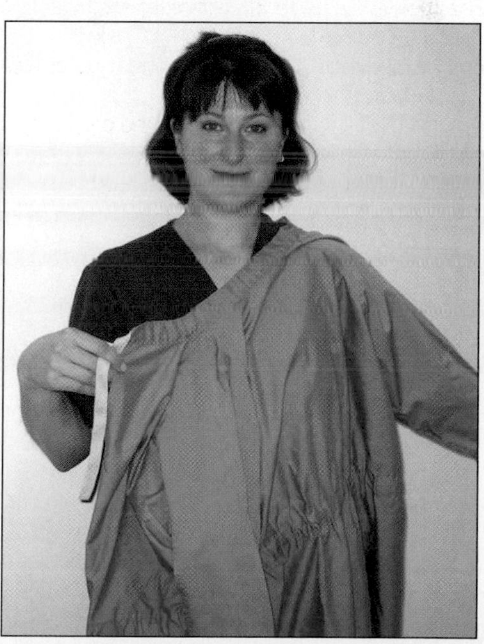

(Continued)

## PROCEDURE 19.4 Putting on Personal Protective Equipment—cont'd.

**2** Put on your surgical mask, and adjust the fit.

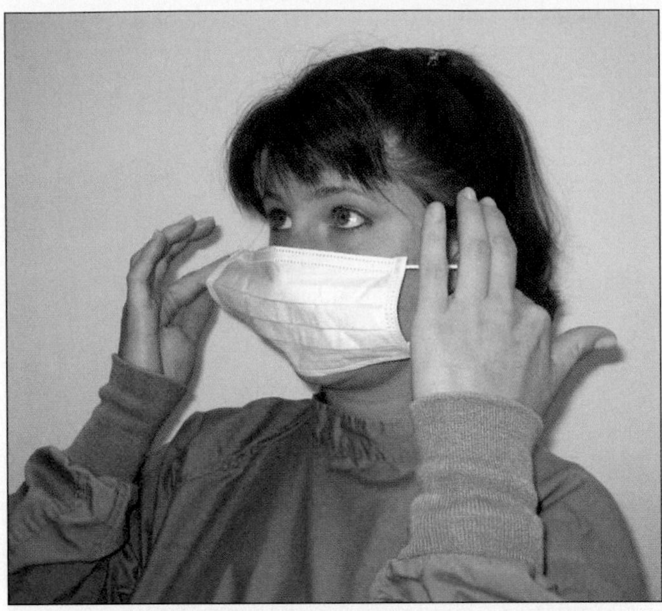

**3** Put on your protective eyewear.

**NOTE** Eyewear should be impact-resistant and have side protection. Goggles or face shields are also acceptable.

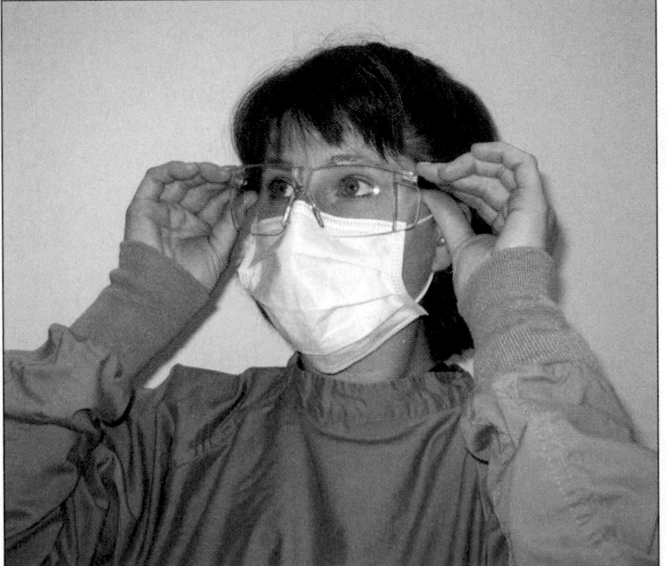

**4** Thoroughly wash and dry your hands.

**NOTE** If your hands are not visibly soiled, you may use an alcohol-based hand rub.

**5** Hold one glove at the cuff, place your opposite hand inside the glove, and pull it onto your hand. Repeat with a new glove for your other hand.

**IMPORTANT NOTE** Regarding the sequence of putting on PPE, the *most important* step is to put on the gloves last to avoid contaminating them before they are placed in the patient's mouth.

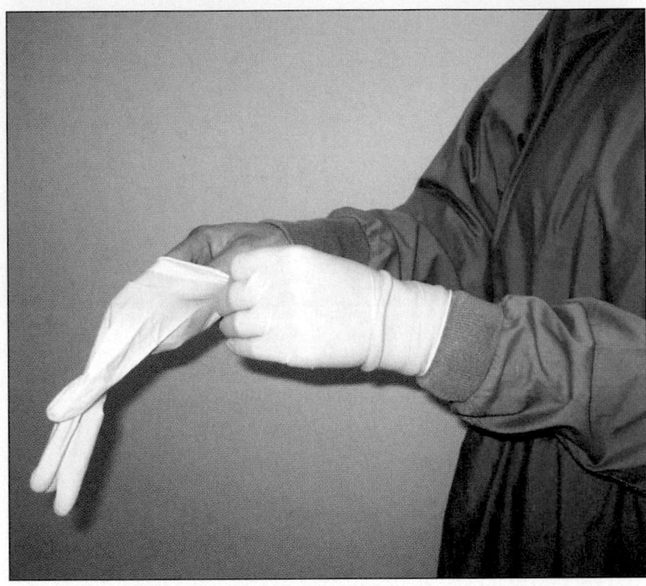

*PPE,* Personal protective equipment.

Modified from Policy to practice: OSAP's guide to the guidelines, Annapolis, MD, 2016, OSAP.

PROCEDURE 19.5

# Removing Personal Protective Equipment

## GOAL

To remove PPE after providing patient care

## EQUIPMENT AND SUPPLIES

- Protective clothing
- Surgical mask
- Protective eyewear
- Gloves

## PROCEDURAL STEPS

1 Use your gloved hand to grasp the other glove at the outside cuff. Pull downward, turning the glove inside out as it pulls away from your hand.

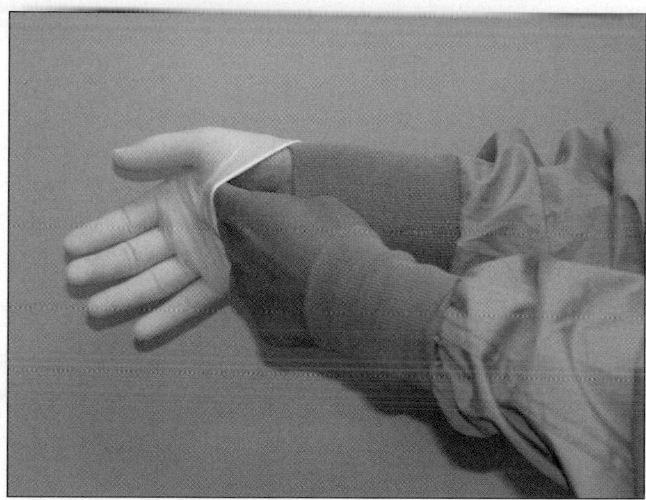

2 For the other hand, use your ungloved fingers to grasp the inside (uncontaminated area) of the cuff of the remaining glove. Pull downward to remove the glove, turning it inside out. Discard the gloves into the waste receptacle.

3 Wash and thoroughly dry hands.

**NOTE** If no visible contamination exists and gloves have not been torn or punctured during the procedure, you may use an alcohol-based hand rub in place of handwashing. However, if your hands are damp from perspiration or have glove powder, you may prefer to wash them with soap and water.

## EYEWEAR

4 Remove eyewear by touching it only on the ear rests (which are not contaminated).

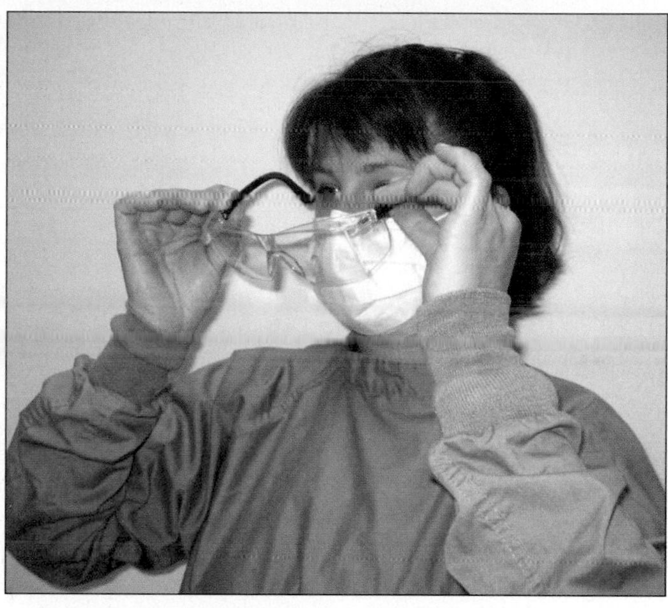

5 Place the eyewear on a disposable towel until it can be properly cleaned and disinfected.

## MASKS

6 Slide the fingers of each hand under the elastic strap in front of your ears and remove the mask. Discard the mask into the waste receptacle.

**NOTE** Be sure your fingers contact only the mask's ties or elastic strap.

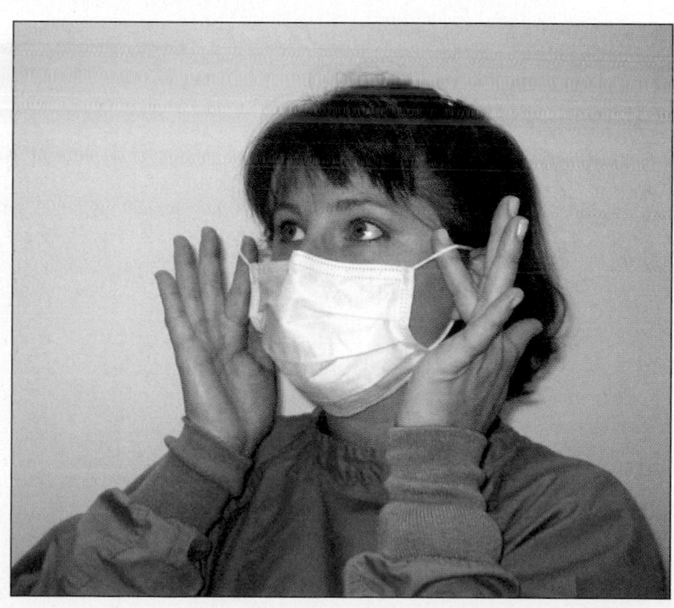

(Continued)

## PROCEDURE 19.5 Removing Personal Protective Equipment—cont'd.

### PROTECTIVE CLOTHING

7 Pull the gown off, turning it inside out as it comes off.
**NOTE** Be careful not to allow the gown to touch underlying clothes or skin.

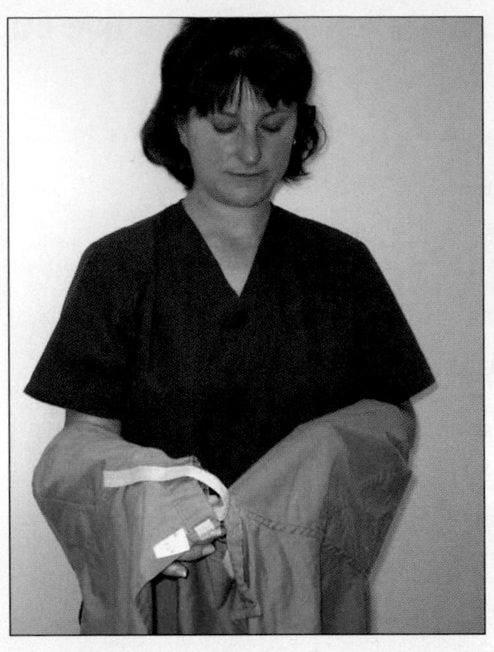

*PPE,* Personal protective equipment.

Modified from Policy to practice: OSAP's guide to the guidelines, Annapolis, MD, 2016, OSAP.

## PROCEDURE 19.6

# Disinfecting an Alginate Impression

### GOAL

To disinfect an alginate impression

### EQUIPMENT AND SUPPLIES

- ✓ Protective clothing
- ✓ Surgical mask
- ✓ Protective eyewear
- ✓ Chemical-resistant utility gloves
- ✓ EPA-registered disinfectant solution

### PROCEDURAL STEPS

1 Rinse the impression under running tap water to clean it. If necessary, use a soft, camel-hair brush to remove debris.
**PURPOSE** To remove any blood and/or saliva.

2 Disinfect the impression using an intermediate-level (tuberculocidal claim) hospital disinfectant for the time recommended by the manufacturer.
**NOTE** Follow the manufacturer's recommendations for disinfection. Spraying uses less solution, and often you can use the same disinfectant that you use for the operatory. However, sprayed disinfectants may pool, which may prevent some surfaces from being adequately exposed to the germicide.

3 If spraying is used, spray the impression thoroughly and wrap it with well-moistened paper towels. Unwrap the impression after the manufacturer's recommended contact time has elapsed.

4 If immersion is used, remove the impression after the manufacturer's recommended contact time has elapsed.

5 Rinse the disinfected impression under tap water to remove any residual germicide.

6 After a thorough rinse, gently shake the impression within the sink basin to remove the remaining water with minimal spatter.
**NOTE** Always check the recommendations of the impression manufacturer as to the stability of the impression material during disinfection.

Modified from Policy to practice: OSAP's guide to the guidelines, Annapolis, MD, 2016, OSAP.

20

# Principles and Techniques of Disinfection

## KEY TERMS

**Antiseptic** Substance for killing microorganisms on the skin.

**Bioburden** Blood, saliva, and other body fluids.

**Broad-spectrum activity** Capable of killing a wide range of microbes.

**Chlorine dioxide** Effective, rapid-acting environmental surface disinfectant or chemical sterilant.

**Clinical contact surface** Surface touched by contaminated hands, instruments, or spatter during dental treatment.

**Disinfectant** Chemical used to reduce or lower the numbers of microorganisms on inanimate objects.

**Environmental surface** Surface within a healthcare facility that is not directly involved in patient care, but that may become contaminated during the course of treatment (e.g., countertops, floors, walls, instrument control panels).

**Fungicidal (fun-ja-SI-dal)** A product that is capable of killing fungi.

**Glutaraldehyde (gloo-tuh-RAL-duh-hide)** Environmental Protection Agency (EPA)–registered high-level disinfectant.

**Greener infection control** Minimizing the environmental impact of infection control products and procedures.

**High-level disinfectant** Hospital disinfectant with tuberculocidal activity.

**Hospital disinfectant** Disinfectant with the ability to kill *Staphylococcus aureus, Salmonella choleraesuis,* and *Pseudomonas aeruginosa.*

**Housekeeping surface** Surface that is not contaminated during dental treatment (e.g., floors, walls).

**Immersion disinfectant** Disinfectant used for immersion (soaking) of heat-sensitive instruments.

**Intermediate-level disinfectant** Liquid disinfectant with EPA registration as a hospital disinfectant with tuberculocidal activity. It is used for disinfecting operatory surfaces.

**Iodophor (eye-oe-doe-FOR)** EPA-registered, intermediate-level hospital disinfectant.

**Liquid sterilant (STER-i-lunt)** Chemical used at room temperature for items that are damaged by heat sterilization.

**Low-level disinfectant** Disinfectant that destroys certain viruses and fungi; used for general housecleaning (e.g., walls, floors).

**Precleaning** Removal of bioburden before disinfection.

**Residual activity** Action that continues long after initial application, as with disinfectants.

**Reuse life** Time period that a disinfectant should remain effective during use and reuse.

**Shelf life** How long a product may be stored before use.

**Single-use items** Items that are used on only one patient and then are thrown away.

**Sodium hypochlorite (hye-poe-KLOR-ite)** Surface disinfectant commonly known as *household bleach.*

**Splash, spatter, and droplet surface** Surface that does not contact members of the dental team or contaminated instruments or supplies.

**Sporicidal** Capable of killing bacterial spores.

**Sterilization (ster-i-li-ZAY-shun)** Process that kills all microorganisms.

**Surface barrier** Fluid-resistant material used to cover surfaces likely to become contaminated.

**Synthetic phenol (sin-THEH-tik FEE-nol) compound** EPA-registered intermediate-level hospital disinfectant with broad-spectrum disinfecting action.

**Touch surface** Surface directly touched and contaminated during procedures.

**Transfer surface** Surface not directly touched but often contacted by contaminated instruments.

**Tuberculocidal (too-bur-kyoo-loe-SYE-dul)** Capable of inactivating tuberculosis-causing microorganisms.

**Virucidal** Capable of killing some viruses.

## LEARNING OUTCOMES

*On completion of this chapter, the student will be able to achieve the following objectives:*

1 Pronounce, define, and spell the key terms.

2 Discuss environmental infection control of clinical contact surfaces, including the following:
- Explain why dental treatment room surfaces need barriers or disinfection.
- Describe two methods to deal with surface contamination.
- Demonstrate how to place and remove surface barriers.
- Describe the CDC guidelines for disinfecting clinical contact surfaces.
- List the types of surfaces in the dental office that are typically covered with barriers.

3 Name types of items that are single-use only and types of items that are single-use or reusable.

4 Discuss precleaning and disinfection, including the following:
- Explain the process of precleaning contaminated dental instruments.
- Explain the difference between disinfection and sterilization.

- Explain the difference between a disinfectant and an antiseptic.
- Name the government agency that is responsible for registering disinfectants.
- Explain the precautions that should be taken when chemical sterilants/disinfectants are used.
- Identify chemical products used for intermediate-level and low-level surface disinfection, and explain the advantages and disadvantages of each.
- Demonstrate the process of cleaning and disinfecting a treatment room.

5 Discuss how use of a high-volume evacuation system reduces contamination of the dental team and clinical surfaces.

6 Describe the CDC guidelines for disinfecting housekeeping surfaces.

7 Discuss green infection control measures that can be taken in the dental office.

## PERFORMANCE OUTCOMES

On completion of this chapter, the student will be able to meet competency standards in the following skills:

- Place and remove surface barriers.
- Clean and disinfect a treatment room.

## ELECTRONIC RESOURCES

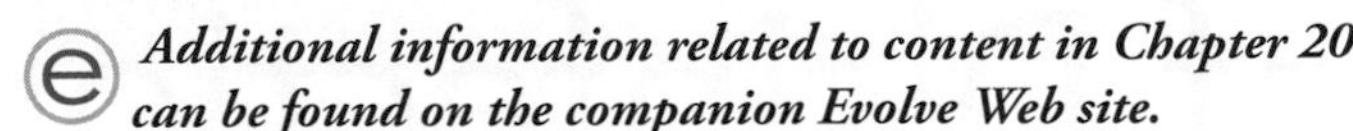

***Additional information related to content in Chapter 20 can be found on the companion Evolve Web site.***

- Practice Quiz
- Videos: Placing and Removing Surface Barriers; Performing Treatment Room Cleaning and Disinfection

During patient treatment, dental equipment and treatment room surfaces are likely to become contaminated with saliva or aerosol containing blood and saliva. Surfaces that are touched frequently (e.g., light handles, unit controls, drawer handles) can act as reservoirs for microorganisms. When these surfaces are touched, microbial agents can be transferred to instruments; to charts; or to the nose, mouth, or eyes of dental team members or of other patients. A primary source of cross-contamination occurs when a member of the dental team touches surfaces with contaminated gloved hands.

Laboratory studies have determined that microorganisms may survive on **environmental surfaces** for different lengths of time. For example, *Mycobacterium tuberculosis* may survive for weeks, whereas the herpes simplex virus dies in a matter of minutes. It is impossible to predict accurately the life span of microorganisms on the surfaces of dental equipment. Therefore the safest approach for avoiding contamination is to assume that if the surface has had contact with saliva, blood, or other potentially infectious material, live microorganisms are present.

*Note:* Throughout this chapter, specific recommendations of the Centers for Disease Control and Prevention (CDC) are shown in boxes with the CDC logo in the corner of the box, and the category of scientific evidence is noted at the end of each recommendation.

### Rankings of Evidence

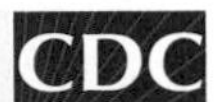


Each recommendation made by the CDC is categorized on the basis of existing scientific data, theoretical rationale, and applicability. Rankings are based on the following categories:

| | |
|---|---|
| Category IA | Strongly recommended for implementation and strongly supported by well-designed experimental, clinical, or epidemiologic studies (studies of patterns and causes of diseases) |
| Category IB | Strongly recommended for implementation and supported by experimental, clinical, or epidemiologic studies and a strong theoretical rationale |
| Category IC | Required for implementation, as mandated by federal or state regulation or standard |
| Category II | Suggested for implementation and supported by suggestive clinical or epidemiologic studies or a theoretical rationale |
| Unresolved Issue | No recommendation—practices for which insufficient evidence or no consensus regarding efficacy exists |

# Environmental Infection Control

The CDC *Guidelines for Infection Control in Dental Healthcare Settings—2003* divide environmental surfaces into **clinical contact surfaces** and **housekeeping surfaces.** Housekeeping surfaces include floors, walls, and sinks. Because these have a much lower risk for disease transmission, cleaning and decontamination techniques are not as rigorous as those used for clinical areas and for patient treatment items.

Things to consider when planning for cleaning and disinfection of patient treatment areas include the following:

- Amount of direct patient contact
- Type and frequency of hand contact
- Potential amount of contamination by aerosol and/or spray
- Other sources of microorganisms (e.g., dust, soil, water)

## Clinical Contact Surfaces

Clinical contact surfaces can be directly contaminated by direct spray or spatter generated during dental procedures, or by contact with the dental professional's gloved hands. Current infection control guidelines of the Organization for Safety, Asepsis and Prevention (OSAP) recommend that clinical surfaces should be classified and maintained under three categories: (1) touch; (2) transfer; and (3) splash, spatter, and droplet (Fig. 20.1).

**Touch surfaces** are directly touched and contaminated during treatment procedures. Touch surfaces include dental light handles, dental unit controls, chair switches, chairside computers, pens, telephones, containers of dental materials, and drawer handles.

**Transfer surfaces** are not directly touched but often are touched by contaminated instruments. Transfer surfaces include instrument trays and handpiece holders.

**Splash, spatter, and droplet surfaces** do not actually contact members of the dental team or contaminated instruments or supplies. Countertops are a major example.

Touch and transfer surfaces should be barrier protected or cleaned and disinfected between patients. Splash, spatter, and droplet surfaces should be cleaned at least once daily (Table 20.1).

## CDC Recommendations for Environmental Infection Control

CDC

### General Recommendations

- Follow the manufacturers' instructions for correct use of cleaning and EPA-registered hospital disinfecting products. (Categories IB, IC)
- Do not use liquid chemical sterilants/high-level disinfectants for disinfection of environmental surfaces (clinical contact or housekeeping). (Categories IB, IC)
- Use PPE, as appropriate, when cleaning and disinfecting environmental surfaces. (Category IC)

### Clinical Contact Surfaces

- Use surface barriers to protect clinical contact surfaces, particularly those that are difficult to clean, and change barriers between patients. (Category II)
- Clean and disinfect clinical contact surfaces that are not barrier protected by using an EPA-registered hospital disinfectant with low-level (i.e., HIV and HBV label claims) to intermediate-level (i.e., tuberculocidal claim) activity after each patient. Use an intermediate-level disinfectant if visibly soiled with blood. (Category IB)

### Housekeeping Surfaces

- Clean housekeeping surfaces (e.g., floors, walls, sinks) with a detergent and water or an EPA-registered hospital disinfectant/detergent on a routine basis, depending on the nature of the surface and the type and degree of contamination, and as appropriate according to location within the facility, and when visibly soiled. (Category IB)
- Clean mops and cloths after use and allow to dry before reuse, or use single-use disposable mop heads or cloths. (Category II)
- Prepare fresh cleaning or EPA-registered disinfecting solutions daily and as instructed by the manufacturer. (Category II)
- Clean walls, blinds, and window curtains in patient care areas when they are visibly dusty or soiled. (Category II)

*EPA,* Environmental Protection Agency; *HBV,* hepatitis B virus; *HIV,* human immunodeficiency virus; *PPE,* personal protective equipment.

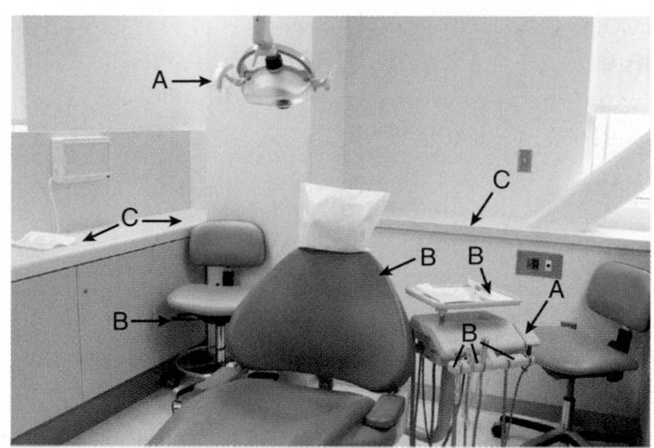


**FIG. 20.1** Touch surfaces (A); transfer surfaces (B); and splash, spatter, and droplet surfaces (C).

## Surface Contamination

Two methods that may be used to deal with surface contamination are (1) to prevent the surface from becoming contaminated with the use of a **surface barrier**, and (2) to preclean and disinfect the surface between patients (Fig. 20.2). Each has advantages and disadvantages, and most dental offices use a combination of surface disinfection and surface barriers.

Smooth, hard surfaces such as countertops, trays, handles, supply containers, and bottles can be quickly and easily cleaned. Surfaces with crevices, knobs, or other difficult-to-clean features, such as light handles, air-water syringe handles, and electrical switches (which can short-circuit), are better protected with surface barriers.

It is the responsibility of the dental assistant to make certain that equipment and treatment room surfaces are properly managed to prevent patient-to-patient disease transmission.

### *Surface Barriers*

Placing barriers on surfaces and equipment can prevent contamination of clinical contact areas, but barriers are especially important for those areas that are difficult to clean (Fig. 20.3).

All surface barriers should be resistant to fluids. Fluid-resistant barriers prevent microorganisms in saliva, blood, and other liquids from soaking through the barrier material to contact the surface underneath (Fig. 20.4). Some plastic bags are specially designed to fit the shapes of dental chairs, air-water syringes, hoses, pens, and light handles (Fig. 20.5). Other types of barrier materials include clear plastic wrap, bags, tubing, plastic tape, and plastic-backed paper, and sticky tape is frequently used as a plastic barrier to protect smooth surfaces, such as touch pads on equipment or electrical switches on chairs and x-ray equipment. Aluminum foil can also be used because it is easily formed around any shape. See Procedure 20.1: Placing and Removing Surface Barriers.

Between patients, while you are still gloved, you should remove and discard contaminated barriers. If, when removing contaminated barriers, you are careful not to touch the surface below, you do not have to clean and disinfect the surface. However, if you do inadvertently touch a surface, you will have to clean and disinfect that surface.

Even though surfaces have been covered with barriers, the surfaces should still be cleaned and disinfected at the beginning and at the end of each workday.

**TABLE 20.1** Comparison of Surface Barriers and Precleaning/Disinfection

| | Advantages | Disadvantages |
|---|---|---|
| Surface barrier | Protects surfaces that are not easily cleaned and disinfected<br>Prevents contamination when properly placed<br>Less time consuming<br>Reduces handling and storage of chemicals<br>Provides patient with visual assurance of cleanliness<br>Does not damage equipment or surfaces | Adds plastics to the environment after disposal<br>May be more expensive than precleaning and disinfecting<br>Requires a variety of sizes and shapes<br>May become dislodged during treatment |
| Precleaning and disinfecting | May be less expensive than surface barriers<br>Does not add plastic to the environment<br>Some dentists do not like the appearance of plastic barriers | Requires more time and therefore may not be done properly<br>Not all surfaces can be adequately precleaned<br>Over time, some chemicals are destructive to dental equipment surfaces<br>No method to determine whether the microbes have been removed or killed<br>Some disinfectants must be prepared fresh daily<br>Chemicals are added to the environment upon disposal |

## Surfaces Typically Protected with Barriers*

- Headrest on dental chair
- Control buttons on dental chair
- Light handles
- Light switches
- Evacuator hoses and controls
- X-ray control switches
- Air-water syringe handles
- Dental unit control touch pads
- Patient mirror handles
- Handle on light-curing device
- Switch on amalgamators or other automatic mixing devices
- Drawer handles
- Adjustment handles on operator and assistant stools
- Bracket table
- Computer keyboards
- Electronic devices

*If a surface cannot be easily and thoroughly cleaned and disinfected or damaged by moisture, it should have barrier protection.

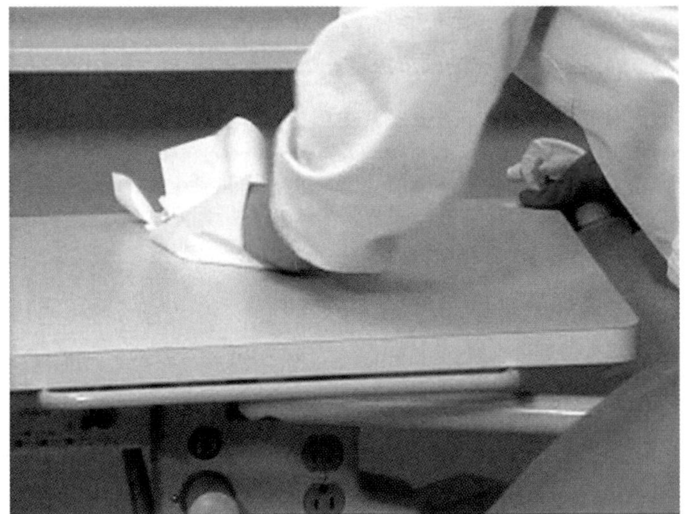

**FIG. 20.2** Smooth surfaces are easily sprayed and wiped.

## Clinical Contact Surfaces

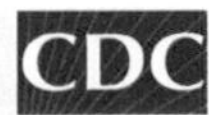


If barriers are not used, surfaces should be cleaned and disinfected between patients with an EPA-registered hospital disinfectant with an HIV, HBV claim.

*EPA,* Environmental Protection Agency; *HBV,* hepatitis B virus; *HIV,* human immunodeficiency virus.
*Note:* Under the new CDC *Guidelines,* only commercially available EPA-registered agents should be used on clinical contact surfaces in dental healthcare facilities.

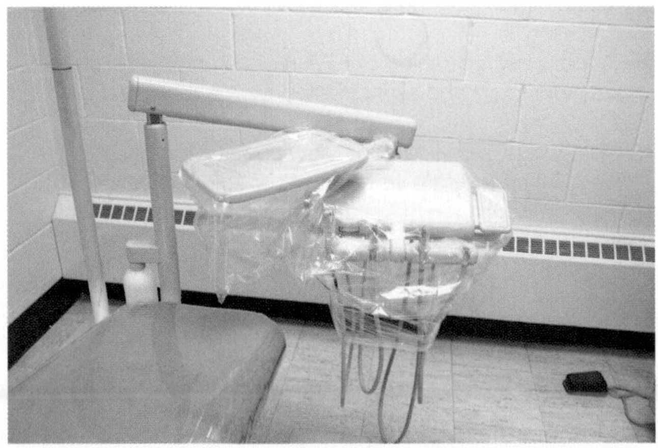

**FIG. 20.3** Barriers on control unit and instrument tray holder. *(From Miller CH: Infection control and management of hazardous materials for the dental team, ed 6, St Louis, 2018, Elsevier.)*

## Single-Use (Disposable) Items

Numerous **single-use items**, also called disposable items, are used in dentistry. Because these items are used on only one patient and then discarded, they help to reduce the chance for patient-to-patient contamination. Single-use items are often made of plastic or less expensive metals, and they are not intended to withstand cleaning, disinfection, or **sterilization**. Single-use items save time because they do not have to be cleaned and sterilized. *Never* process (clean, disinfect/sterilize) single-use items for use on another patient.

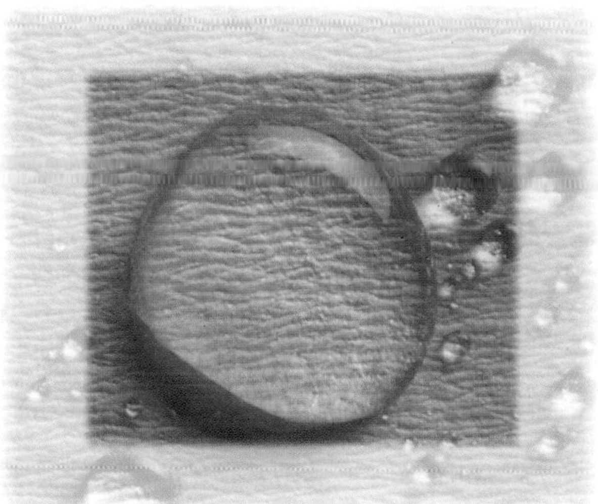

**FIG. 20.4** An example of water on a fluid-resistant material. *(Courtesy Crosstex, Hauppauge, NY.)*

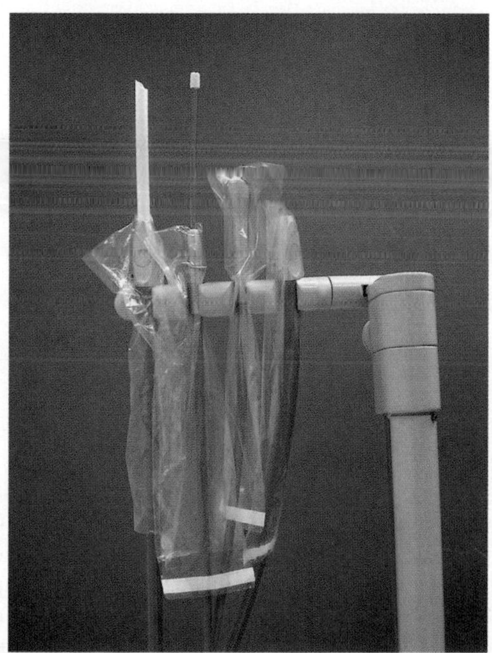

**FIG. 20.5** Tube socks provide barrier protection for difficult-to-clean areas. *(Courtesy Certol, Commerce City, CO.)*

Some items are manufactured to be *either* disposable or reusable. If an item is difficult to clean, it may be more efficient to switch to a disposable type (Fig. 20.6).

### Single-Use (Disposable) Devices

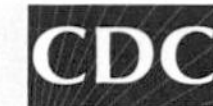


Use single-use devices for one patient only, and dispose of them properly. (Category IC)

### Disposable or Not?

**Always Single-Use-Only Items**

- Prophy cups and brushes
- Sterilization pouches
- Irrigating syringes
- Patient napkins
- Surface barriers
- Face masks
- Examination and surgical gloves
- Syringe needles
- Suture needles
- Plastic orthodontic brackets
- Sharps containers (dispose of when fill-to line is reached; *never* empty and reuse)

**Either Disposable or Reusable**

- Air-water syringe tips
- High-volume evacuator tips
- Impression trays
- Mirrors
- Prophy angles
- Burs/diamonds
- Vacuum line traps

In most areas, contaminated disposable items that are not sharps and are not soaked or caked with blood may be discarded with the regular office trash; there is no need to discard these items in a

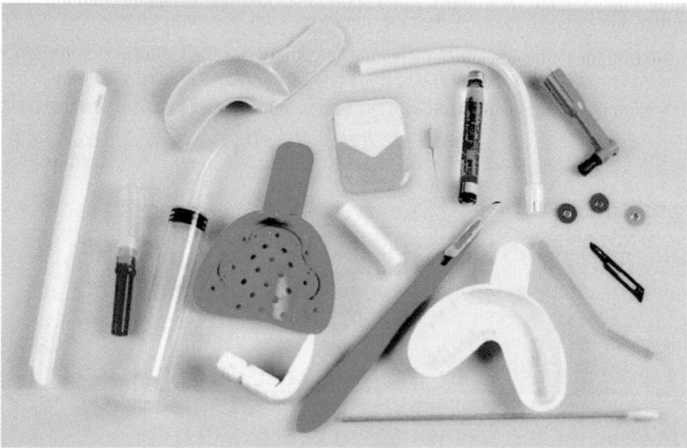

**FIG. 20.6** Examples of disposable items. *(From Miller CH: Infection control and management of hazardous materials for the dental team, ed 6, St Louis, 2018, Elsevier.)*

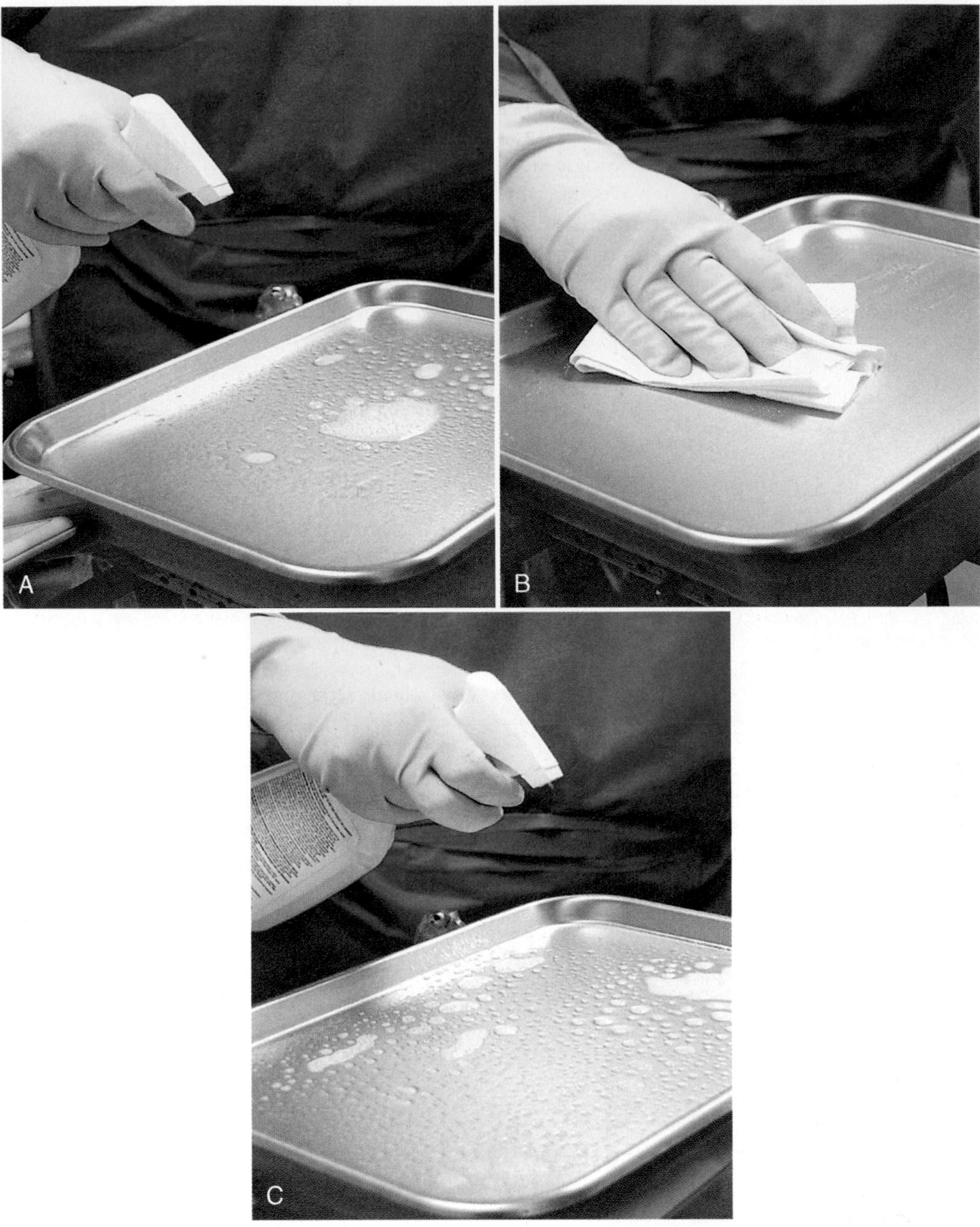

**FIG. 20.7** Surface precleaning and disinfecting by the spray-wipe-spray technique. Precleaning consists of (A) spraying with surface disinfectant, (B) wiping the surface to clean it, and (C) reapplying the disinfectant followed by the appropriate contact time. The surface may then be dried if needed. *(From Miller CH: Infection control and management of hazardous materials for the dental team, ed 6, St Louis, 2018, Elsevier.)*

medical waste or biohazard container. State and local regulations may vary, so always consult the regulatory agency for your area.

RECALL

1 Why must surfaces in dental treatment rooms be disinfected or protected with barriers?
2 What are the two methods that deal with surface contamination?
3 Why is it recommended to use single-use items?
4 What should you do if the barrier becomes torn?

## Precleaning and Disinfection

Although no cases of cross-infection have been linked to dental treatment room surfaces, cleaning and disinfection of these surfaces are important components of an effective infection control program. In addition, the Occupational Safety and Health Administration (OSHA) Blood-Borne Pathogens Standard requires that contaminated work surfaces be disinfected between patient visits (Fig. 20.7) (see Chapter 19).

**TABLE 20.2 Categories of Disinfecting/Sterilizing Chemicals**

| Category | Definition | Examples | Use |
|---|---|---|---|
| Sterilant | Destroys all microorganisms, including high numbers of bacterial spores | Glutaraldehyde, glutaraldehyde phenate, hydrogen peroxide, hydrogen peroxide with peracetic acid, peracetic acid | Heat-sensitive reusable items: immersion only |
| High-level disinfectant | Destroys all microorganisms, but not necessarily high numbers of bacterial spores | Glutaraldehyde, glutaraldehyde phenate, hydrogen peroxide, hydrogen peroxide with peracetic acid, peracetic acid, ortho-phthalaldehyde | Heat-sensitive reusable items: immersion only |
| Intermediate-level disinfectant | Destroys vegetative bacteria, most fungi, and most viruses; inactivates *Mycobacterium tuberculosis* var. *bovis* (is tuberculocidal) | EPA-registered hospital disinfectant with label claim of tuberculocidal activity (e.g., chlorine-based products, phenolics, iodophors, quaternary ammonium compounds with alcohol, bromides) | Clinical contact surfaces; noncritical surfaces with visible blood |
| Low-level disinfectant | Destroys vegetative bacteria, some fungi, and some viruses; does not inactivate *M. tuberculosis* var. *bovis* (is not tuberculocidal) | EPA-registered hospital disinfectant with no label claim of tuberculocidal activity (e.g., quaternary ammonium compounds) | Housekeeping surfaces (e.g., floors, walls); noncritical surfaces without visible blood; clinical contact surfaces |

Adapted from Kohn WG, Collins AS, Cleveland JL, et al: Centers for Disease Control and Prevention: Guideline for infection control in dental health-care settings—2003, *MMWR Recomm Rep* 52 (No. RR-17):66, 2003.

## Personal Protective Equipment (PPE) 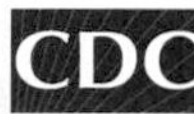

- Use PPE, as appropriate, when cleaning and disinfecting environmental surfaces. Such equipment might include gloves (e.g., puncture- and chemical-resistant utility), protective clothing, protective eyewear/face shield, and mask. (Category IC)
- Because of the risks associated with exposure to chemical disinfectants and contaminated surfaces, always wear PPE to prevent occupational exposure to infectious agents and hazardous chemicals.

**PRECLEANING. Precleaning** means to clean before disinfecting. All contaminated surfaces must be precleaned before they can be disinfected. Even if no blood is visible on the surface, it must be precleaned because even a thin layer of saliva on the surface can decrease the effectiveness of the disinfectant. Precleaning reduces the number of microbes and removes blood, saliva, and other body fluids, called **bioburden**. *Remember: If a surface is not clean, it cannot be disinfected.*

Precleaning techniques are most effective when used on contaminated surfaces that are *smooth* and *easily accessible* for cleaning. Irregular or textured surfaces are difficult or impossible to clean and therefore interfere with disinfection.

Regular soap and water may be used for precleaning. If you select a disinfectant that cleans as well as disinfects, however, you can save time and limit the number of products you need (Table 20.2).

RECALL

5 Which regulation requires the use of surface disinfection?
6 Why must surfaces be precleaned?
7 For which types of surfaces must barriers be placed?

**DISINFECTION.** *Disinfection* is intended to kill disease-causing microorganisms that remain on the surface *after* precleaning. Spores are not killed during disinfecting procedures (Figs. 20.8 and 20.9).

The term **disinfectant** is used for chemicals that are applied to inanimate surfaces, such as countertops and dental equipment. The term **antiseptic** is used for *antimicrobial* (organism-killing) agents that are applied to living tissue. Disinfectants and antiseptics should never be used interchangeably because tissue toxicity and damage to equipment can result.

Do not confuse disinfection with sterilization. Sterilization is the process in which all forms of life are destroyed (see Chapter 21).

### *Disinfectants*

Disinfectants are chemicals that destroy or inactivate most species of *pathogenic* (disease-causing) microorganisms. The Environmental Protection Agency (EPA) registers and regulates disinfectants and chemical sterilants according to chemical classification (Table 20.3). A sterilant kills all microorganisms.

In dentistry, *only* those products that are registered with the EPA as **hospital disinfectants** with **tuberculocidal** claims (kills the organism *Mycobacterium tuberculosis*) should be used to disinfect dental treatment areas. *M. tuberculosis* is highly resistant to disinfectants. If a disinfectant inactivates *M. tuberculosis,* it will certainly inactivate less resistant microbial families (such as bacteria, viruses, and most fungi) on treated surfaces. A product that is capable of killing spores would be labeled as **sporicidal**. A product that is capable of killing some viruses would be labeled as **virucidal**. A product that is capable of killing fungi would be labeled as **fungicidal**.

A variety of chemical agents are currently marketed as surface disinfectants and instrument-immersion disinfectants. It is important to carefully read the label of every disinfectant

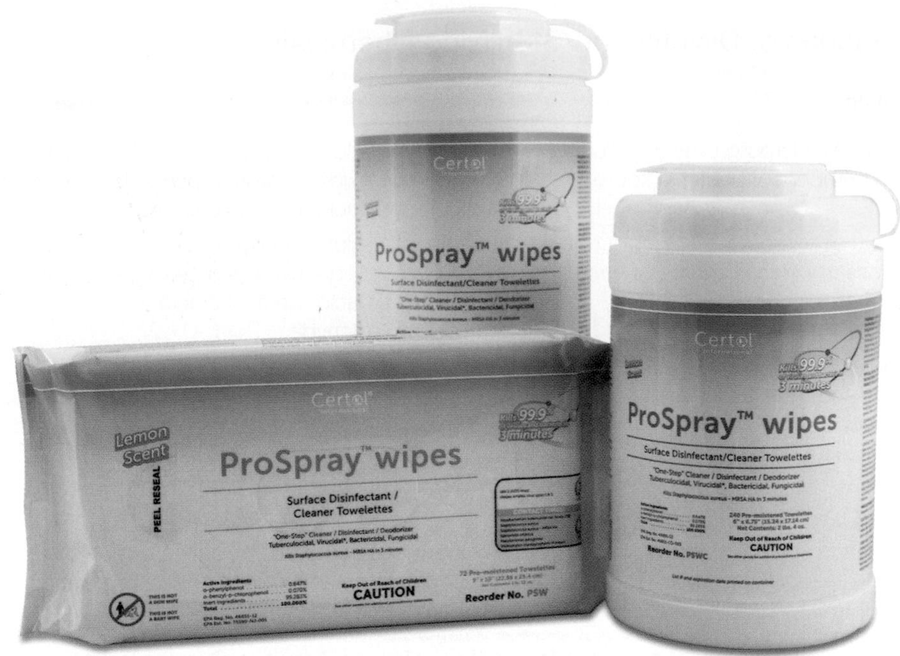


**FIG. 20.8** Germicidal disposable wipes with tuberculocidal activity. *(Courtesy Certol, Commerce City, CO.)*

product before you use it. Labels commonly include information about the product such as **shelf life**, **reuse life**, directions for use, precautionary statements on handling the product, and storage and disposal information (Table 20.4).

**IDEAL SURFACE DISINFECTANT.** The ideal surface disinfectant would rapidly kill a broad spectrum (range) of bacteria, would exhibit residual activity and minimal toxicity, and would not damage surfaces to be treated. If a disinfectant has **residual activity**, its action continues long after initial application. The ideal disinfectant would also be odorless and inexpensive, would work on surfaces with remaining bioburden, and would be simple to use. Unfortunately, no surface disinfectant is ideal. No current disinfectant product meets all of these criteria. Therefore when selecting a surface disinfectant, you must carefully consider the advantages and disadvantages of various products. Often the manufacturers of dental equipment will recommend the type of surface disinfectant that is most appropriate for their dental chairs and units (Table 20.5).

### *Disinfectant Precautions*

Follow the manufacturers' recommendations for the following:

- Mixing and diluting
- Application technique
- Shelf life
- Activated use life
- All safety warnings

8 How are antiseptics different from disinfectants?
9 Which agency regulates disinfectants?
10 What is the ideal disinfectant?

**IODOPHORS.** **Iodophors** are EPA-registered intermediate-level hospital disinfectants with tuberculocidal action. Iodophors are recommended for disinfecting surfaces that have been soiled with potentially infectious patient material. When used according to the manufacturer's instructions, iodophors are usually effective within 5 to 10 minutes. They also may be used as an immersion disinfectant for nonhydrocolloid impressions.

Because iodophors are inactivated by hard water, they must be mixed with soft or distilled water. Because they contain iodine, iodophors may corrode or discolor certain metals or may temporarily cause red or yellow stains on clothing and other surfaces.

**SYNTHETIC PHENOL COMPOUNDS.** **Synthetic phenol compounds** are EPA-registered intermediate-level hospital disinfectants with **broad-spectrum activity**, meaning that they can kill a wide range of microbes. When diluted properly, phenols are used for surface disinfection, provided the surface has been thoroughly cleaned first (Fig. 20.10).

Phenols can be used on metal, glass, rubber, or plastic. They also can be used as a holding solution for instruments; however, phenols leave a residual film on treated surfaces. Synthetic phenol compound is prepared daily. Phenols may also be used to disinfect impressions; however, always check with the manufacturer of the impression material.

**SODIUM HYPOCHLORITE.** **Sodium hypochlorite** is classified as an **intermediate-level disinfectant** and is the main ingredient in household bleach. Sodium hypochlorite is a fast-acting, economical, and broad-spectrum disinfectant. Under the 1993 CDC *Guidelines,* it was a recommended disinfectant. However, under the new CDC *Guidelines,* because it is *not* an EPA-registered disinfectant, household bleach alone is *no longer* a recommended product for use in dental settings as a disinfectant.

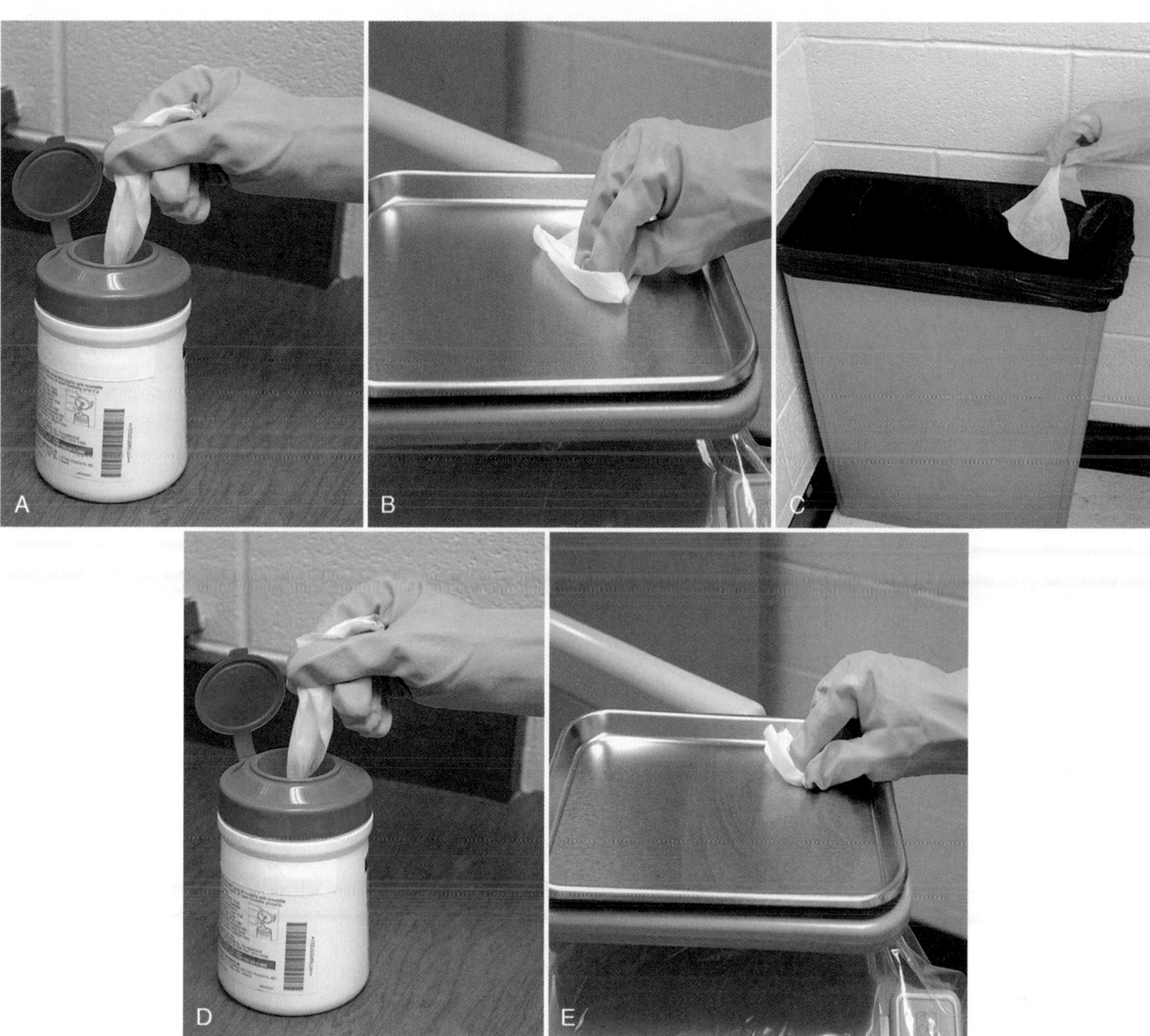

**FIG. 20.9** Surface precleaning and disinfecting by the wipe-discard-wipe technique. Precleaning consists of (A) obtaining a fresh surface wipe, (B) wiping the surface to clean it, and, (C) discarding the wipe. Disinfection is (D) obtaining a fresh surface wipe and (E) wiping the surface again, followed by the appropriate contact time. *(From Miller CH: Infection control and management of hazardous materials for the dental team, ed 6, St Louis, 2018, Elsevier.)*

**TABLE 20.3** Chemical Classification of Disinfectants

| Level of Disinfection | EPA Classification | Use |
|---|---|---|
| High level | High-level disinfectant with a relatively short contact time and a sterilant when used with a prolonged contact time | Semicritical items that cannot tolerate heat sterilization |
| Intermediate level | Hospital disinfectant with tuberculocidal activity | Noncritical items or surfaces that have been contaminated with blood or saliva |
| Low level | Nontuberculocidal | Surfaces not contaminated with blood |

*EPA,* Environmental Protection Agency.

**TABLE 20.4** OSAP Surface Disinfectant Reference Chart—2014

| Product Classification | Product Brand Information | | | | |
|---|---|---|---|---|---|
| **Category** | **Brand (packaged as)** | **EPA No.** | **Dilution** | **TB Claim** | **Manufacturer or Distributor** |
| Accelerated Hydrogen Peroxide | Optim 33 TB | 74559-1-83259 | RTU | 5 min | SciCan |
| **Phenolics (Dual) Water-Based** | Birex SE Concentrate | 1043-92-51003 | 1:256 | 10 min | Biotrol |
| Phenylphenol and benzylchlorophenol or tertiary amylphenol | Birex Disinfectant Wipes | 46851-10-51003 | RTU | 10 min | Biotrol |
| | DisCide Germicidal Foaming Cleaner | 33176-6 | RTU | 10 min | Palmero Health Care |
| | ProSpray C-60 Conc. Surface Disinfectant | 46851-1-50611 | 1:32 | 10 min | Certol International |
| | ProSpray Surface Disinfectant Spray | 46851-5-50611 | RTU | 10 min | Certol International |
| | ProSpray Wipes | 46851-10 | RTU | 10 min | Certol International |
| **Phenolics (Dual) Alcohol-Based** Tertiary amylphenol and/or phenylphenol + ethyl alcohol or isopropyl alcohol | DisCide Disinfectant Spray | 706-69-10492 | RTU | 10 min | Palmero Health Care |
| **Quaternaries Dual or Synergized Plus Alcohol** | CaviCide Spray | 46781-6 | RTU | 3 min | TotalCare/Pinnacle/Metrex |
| Diisobutylphenoxyethoxy-ethyl dimethylbenzyl ammonium chloride; isopropanol or ethanol; alkyldimethyl benzyl ammonium chloride | CaviWipes | 46781-8 | RTU | 3 min | TotalCare/Pinnacle/Metrex |
| | Cetylcide II Broad Spectrum Disinfectant | 61178-1-3150 | 2 oz/gal | NOL | Cetylite Industries |
| | Clorox Disinfecting Spray | 67619-3 | RTU | 10 min | Harry J. Bosworth Company |
| | DisCide ULTRA Spray | 10492-5 | RTU | 1 min | Palmero Health Care |
| | DisCide ULTRA Wipes | 10492-4 | RTU | 1 min | Palmero Health Care |
| | DisCide V Detergent Disinfectant | 1839-83-10492 | RTU | 5 min | Palmero Health Care |
| | Lysol IC Disinfectant Spray | 777-72-675 | RTU | 10 min | Sultan Healthcare |
| | Maxispray Plus | 46781-6-10597 | RTU | 5 min | Henry Schein Dental |
| | Maxiwipe Germicidal Cloth | 9480-4-10597 | RTU | 5 min | Henry Schein Dental |
| | Opti-Cide-3 Spray | 70144-1-51003 | RTU | 3 min | Biotrol |
| | OptiCide-3 Wipes | 70144-2-51003 | RTU | 3 min | Biotrol |
| | PDCare Surface Disinfectant Spray | 46781-6-43100 | RTU | 3 min | Patterson Dental |
| | PDCare Wipes | 46781-8-43100 | RTU | 5 min | Patterson Dental |
| | Sanitex Plus Spray | 1130-150-64285 | RTU | 6 min | Crosstex International |
| | Sanitex Plus Wipes | 9480-4-64285 | RTU | 5 min | Crosstex International |
| | Sani-Cloth HB Wipes | 61178-4-9480 | RTU | 10 min | PDI (Professional Disposables International) |
| | Sani-Cloth Plus Wipes | 9480-6 | RTU | 5 min | PDI (Professional Disposables International) |
| | Super Sani-Cloth Wipes | 9480-4 | RTU | 2 min | PDI (Professional Disposables International) |
| | Z3 Surface Disinfectant/ Decontaminant Cleaner | 46781-6-35659 | RTU | 3 min | Benco Dental Co. |
| | Z3 Wipes | 59894-10-67454 | RTU | 2 min | Benco Dental Co. |

TABLE 20.4 OSAP Surface Disinfectant Reference Chart—2014—cont'd

| Product Classification | Product Brand Information | | | | |
|---|---|---|---|---|---|
| **Quaternary Ammonium** | Lysol IC Disinfectant Wipes | 1839–174–675 | RTU | 10 min | Sultan Healthcare |
| No alcohol | Sani-Cloth AF (Wipes) | 9480–5 | RTU | 3 min | PDI (Professional Disposables International) |
| Sodium Hypochlorite | Clorox Germicidal Spray | 67619–13 | RTU | 30 sec | Harry J. Bosworth Company |
| | Clorox Germicidal Wipes | 67619–12 | RTU | 2 min | Harry J. Bosworth Company |
| Sodium Bromide and Chlorine | Microstat 2 Tablets | 70369–1 | 2 tabs/qt water | 5 min | Septodont |

**IMPORTANT INFORMATION:** Listing does not imply endorsement, recommendation, or warranty. Other products are available. Only OSAP member *Hospital Disinfectants* are represented in this chart. Purchasers are legally required to consult label and package insert for changes in formulation and recommended use. Check compatibility of material before use on dental/medical equipment.

**Key:** RTU = Ready to use, NOL = not on label, e.g., one or both of the HIV/HBV claims is not provided on the label. OSAP is using the CDC guidelines. Be sure to use a disinfectant with a TB claim if there is any blood or OPIM present.

This chart is a publication of the Organization for Safety, Asepsis and Prevention (OSAP). OSAP assumes no liability for actions taken based on the information herein. 

TABLE 20.5 Categories of Disinfecting/Sterilizing Chemicals

| Category | Definition | Examples | Use |
|---|---|---|---|
| Sterilant* | Destroys all microorganisms, including high numbers of bacterial spores | Glutaraldehyde, glutaraldehyde phenate, hydrogen peroxide, hydrogen peroxide with peracetic acid, peracetic acid | Heat-sensitive reusable items: immersion only |
| High-level disinfectant* | Destroys all microorganisms, but not necessarily high numbers of bacterial spores | Glutaraldehyde, glutaraldehyde phenate, hydrogen peroxide, hydrogen peroxide with peracetic acid, peracetic acid, orthophthalaldehyde | Heat-sensitive reusable items: immersion only |
| Intermediate-level disinfectant | Destroys vegetative bacteria, most fungi, and most viruses; inactivates *Mycobacterium tuberculosis* var. *bovis* (is tuberculocidal) | EPA-registered hospital disinfectant† with label claim of tuberculocidal activity (e.g., chlorine-based products, phenolics, iodophors, hydrogen peroxide, quaternary ammonium compounds with alcohol, bromides) | Clinical contact surfaces; noncritical surfaces with visible blood |
| Low-level disinfectant | Destroys vegetative bacteria, some fungi, and some viruses; does not inactivate *M. tuberculosis* var. *bovis* (is not tuberculocidal) | EPA-registered hospital disinfectant with no label claim of tuberculocidal activity (e.g., quaternary ammonium compounds) | Housekeeping surfaces (e.g., floors, walls); noncritical surfaces without visible blood; clinical contact surfaces‡ |

*Some, but not all, of these products can serve as high-level disinfectants and sterilants depending on the immersion time used.

†A hospital disinfectant is one that has been shown to kill *Staphylococcus aureus, Pseudomonas aeruginosa,* and *Salmonella choleraesuis*.

‡The Centers for Disease Control and Prevention indicates that low-level disinfectants can be used on clinical contact surfaces if the product has a label claim of killing human immunodeficiency virus (HIV) and hepatitis B virus (HBV) in addition to being an EPA-registered hospital disinfectant.

From Miller CH: Infection control and management of hazardous materials for the dental team, ed 6, St Louis, 2018, Elsevier. Adapted from Kohn WG, Collins AS, Cleveland JL, et al: Centers for Disease Control and Prevention: Guideline for infection control in dental health-care settings—2003, *MMWR Recomm Rep* 52 (No. RR-17):66, 2003.

EPA-approved disinfectant products now on the market may contain sodium hypochlorite or other chlorine compounds. Always check the product label for the EPA registration number.

The disadvantages of sodium hypochlorite are as follows:

- It is unstable and needs daily preparation.
- It has a strong odor and is corrosive to some metals.
- It is destructive to fabrics and may eventually cause plastic chair covers to crack.
- It is irritating to the eyes and skin.

**ALCOHOL.** Ethyl alcohol and isopropyl alcohol have been used over the years as skin antiseptics and surface disinfectants. However, alcohols are *not* effective in the presence of bioburden such as blood and saliva, and its rapid rate of evaporation limits the antimicrobial activity of alcohol. In addition, alcohols are damaging to certain materials, such as plastics and vinyl, which are prevalent.

The American Dental Association (ADA), CDC, and OSAP do *not* recommend alcohol as an environmental surface disinfectant.

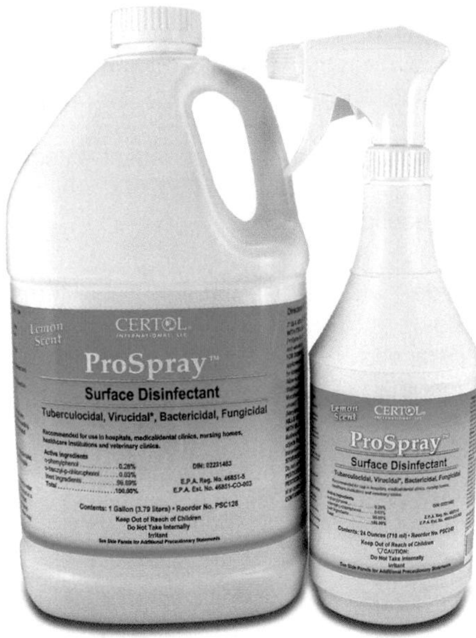


**FIG. 20.10** Synthetic phenol disinfectant. *(Courtesy Certol, Commerce City, CO.)*

See Procedure 20.2: Performing Treatment Room Cleaning and Disinfection.

**IMMERSION DISINFECTANTS. Immersion disinfectants** are chemicals on the market that can be used for sterilization or high-level disinfection. When used as a sterilant, they destroy all microbial life, including bacterial endospores. Depending on the type, the time for sterilization can range from 6 hours to 30 hours. At weaker dilutions or at shorter contact time, these chemicals provide high-level disinfection, which inactivates all microorganisms *except* endospores (Table 20.6).

Most of these chemicals are toxic and can irritate the eyes, skin, and lungs. Personal protective equipment (PPE) must always be worn when these chemicals are used. They are to be used for immersion (soaking) of heat-sensitive instruments and should never be used as surface disinfectants.

Always keep the container lid closed to minimize fumes (Fig. 20.11).

### Glutaraldehyde

**Glutaraldehyde** is classified as a high-level disinfectant/sterilant. It can also be used as a **liquid sterilant** when the immersion time is greatly increased (see Chapter 21). Times for disinfection range from 10 to 90 minutes; always read the manufacturer's recommendations. Glutaraldehyde products are useful for plastics and other items that cannot withstand heat sterilization. Some glutaraldehyde products are effective for only 28 days after activation.

Glutaraldehyde is very toxic and should be handled carefully to avoid the fumes. Glutaraldehyde-treated instruments should never be used on patients without thorough rinsing with water. Prolonged contact of certain types of instruments with glutaraldehyde solutions can lead to discoloration and corrosion of instrument surfaces and cutting edges.

### Chlorine Dioxide

**Chlorine dioxide** is classified as a high-level disinfectant/sterilant. Products that contain chlorine dioxide can be used as effective, rapid-acting, environmental surface disinfectants (3 minutes) or as chemical sterilants (6 hours). However, chlorine dioxide products do not readily

**TABLE 20.6** FDA-Cleared Instrument-Immersion Disinfectants for Dentistry

| Category or Active Ingredient | Sterilant Contact Time | High-Level Disinfectant Time |
|---|---|---|
| Glutaraldehyde 2.4%–3.4% alkaline and acidic formulations* | 6-10 hr at 20° C, 22° C, or 25° C* | 20-90 min at 20° C, 22° C, or 25° C* |
| Hydrogen peroxide, 7.3% | 6 hr at 20° C | 30 min at 20° C |
| Ortho-phthalaldehyde, 0.55% | Not indicated for sterilization | 12 min at 20° C |

*FDA,* U.S. Food and Drug Administration.
*Note:* Glutaraldehydes and simple quaternary ammonium compounds should not be used for surface disinfection in dentistry.
*Varies by active ingredient or disinfectant brand.

penetrate organic debris and must be used with a separate cleaner.

Other disadvantages of chlorine dioxide are (1) it must be prepared fresh daily, (2) it must be used with good ventilation, and (3) it is corrosive to aluminum containers.

### Ortho-Phthalaldehyde

Ortho-phthalaldehyde (OPA) is a chemical that is used as a **high-level disinfectant**. It is effective in achieving high-level disinfection within 12 minutes at room temperature. It is more expensive than glutaraldehydes, but it may be a good alternative for healthcare workers who have a sensitivity to glutaraldehyde. It has very little odor and does not require activation or mixing (Fig. 20.12).

Disadvantages include (1) the cost, (2) that it can be used in dentistry only half as long as most glutaraldehydes, (3) that it may stain skin and fabrics, (4) that plastics turn a blue-green color when proteins have not been removed, and (5) that it does not have a sterilization claim.

RECALL

11 What disinfectant can leave a reddish or yellow stain?
12 What is a disadvantage of synthetic phenols?
13 What is a more common term for sodium hypochlorite?
14 Are alcohol disinfectants effective when blood or saliva is present?
15 What are two uses of chlorine dioxide?

## Evacuator System

High-volume evacuation (HVE) greatly reduces the escape of saliva and spatter from the patient's mouth, which reduces contamination of the dental team and nearby clinical surfaces. Regular cleaning of the evacuation system keeps the tubing, piping, and pumps free-flowing. The HVE system should be cleaned at the end of the day by flushing a detergent or water-based detergent-disinfectant through the system (Fig. 20.13). *Never use a sodium hypochlorite (bleach) product because it may cause corrosion of the metal parts of the system.*

### Traps

Periodically, the traps in the evacuation system must be removed and cleaned. A safer approach is to use a disposable trap. These traps typically contain bits of organic tissue, fluoride gel, coagulated blood, and impression material, and may contain scrap amalgam that should be disposed of properly (see Chapter 42). While changing or cleaning the traps, be certain to wear gloves, masks, protective eyewear, and protective clothing to avoid splashing and direct contact with contaminated materials in the lines.

## Housekeeping Surfaces

No scientific evidence shows that housekeeping surfaces (e.g., floors, walls, sinks) pose a risk for disease transmission in dental healthcare settings. Most housekeeping surfaces need to be cleaned only with a detergent or a **low-level disinfectant** (disinfectant that destroys certain viruses and fungi) and water or with an EPA-registered hospital disinfectant/detergent.

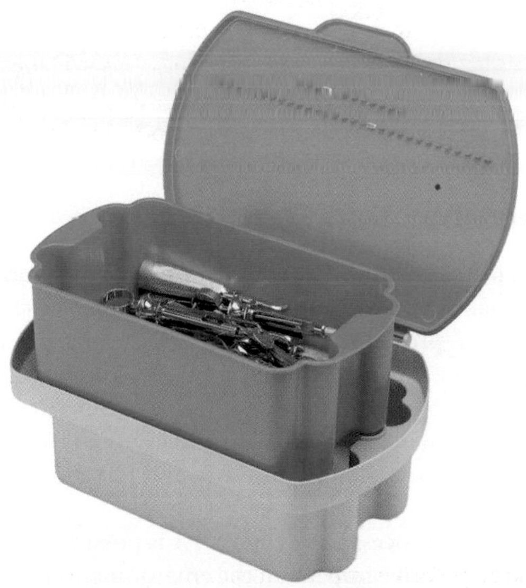

**FIG. 20.11** Covered instrument tray for use with immersion disinfectants. *(Courtesy Zirc Company, Buffalo, MN.)*

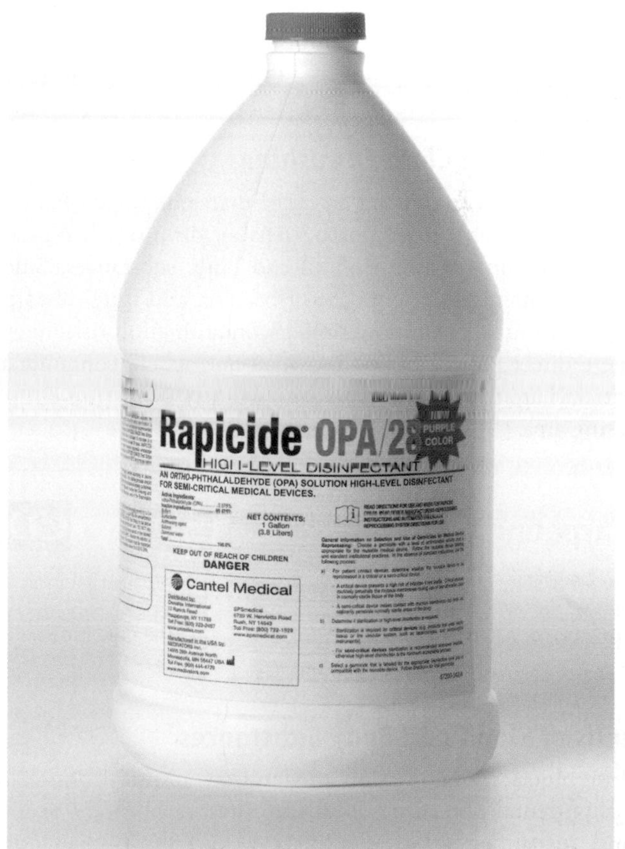


**FIG. 20.12** OPA is classified as a high-level disinfectant. *(© 2017 Crosstex International, Inc.)*

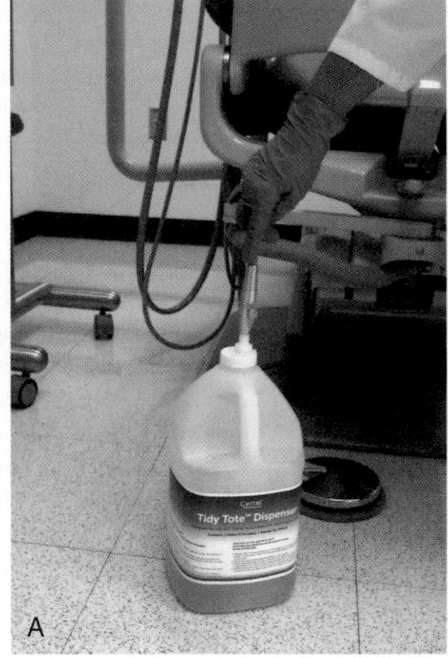

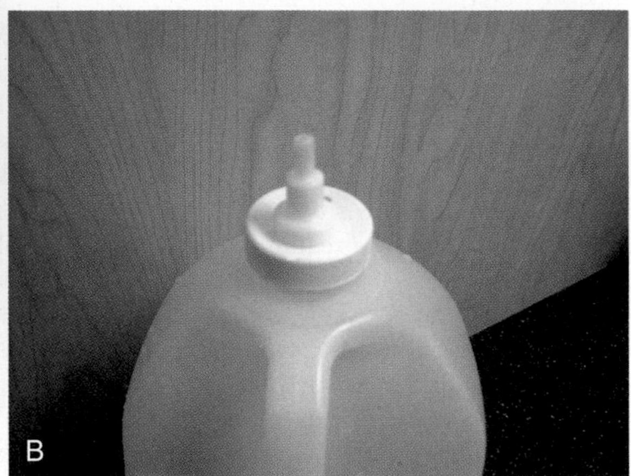

**FIG. 20.13** A, ProE-Vac liquid evacuation system cleaner. B, Convenient closed container for transporting solution between units. *(Courtesy Certol, Commerce City, CO.)*

However, in the cleaning process, used solutions of detergents or disinfectants can serve as a reservoir for microorganisms, especially if prepared in dirty containers, stored for long periods of time, or prepared incorrectly. Make fresh cleaning solution each day, discard any remaining solution, and let the container dry. This will minimize bacterial contamination. When cleaning, avoid producing mists and aerosols or dispersing dust in patient care areas.

### *Carpeting and Cloth Furnishings*

Carpeting is more difficult to clean than nonporous hard-surface flooring, and it cannot be reliably disinfected, especially after contamination with blood and body substances. Studies have documented the presence of bacteria and fungi in carpeting. Cloth furnishings pose similar contamination risks in areas where direct patient care is provided and where contaminated materials are handled, such as an operatory or instrument-processing area.

#### Carpeting

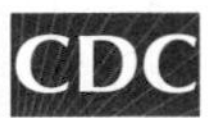


Avoid using carpeting and cloth-upholstered furnishings in dental operatories, laboratories, and instrument-processing areas. (Category II)

### *Spills of Blood and Body Substances*

Most blood contamination in dentistry results from spatter during dental procedures and from the use of rotary or ultrasonic instruments. No scientific evidence shows that human immunodeficiency virus (HIV), hepatitis B virus (HBV), or hepatitis C virus (HCV) has been transmitted from a housekeeping surface.

However, good infection control practices and OSHA require that blood spills and other body fluids be removed and surfaces disinfected. Always wear gloves and other PPE when you are decontaminating areas of spills.

#### Managing Spills

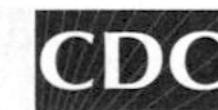


Clean spills of blood or other potentially infectious materials, and decontaminate surface with an EPA-registered hospital disinfectant with low-level (i.e., HBV and HIV label claims) to intermediate-level (i.e., tuberculocidal claims) activity, depending on the size of the spill and the surface porosity. (Categories IB, IC)

*EPA,* Environmental Protection Agency; *HBV,* hepatitis B virus; *HIV,* human immunodeficiency virus.

## Greener Infection Control

Protecting the environment has become an important part of our personal lives and in our homes, and that responsibility extends to the provision of dental care. Unfortunately, many of the infection control products and procedures we must use to protect our patients and ourselves have a negative impact on the environment. Many of our infection control practices lead to an increased volume of waste and the spread of harmful chemicals.

By altering a process or a material, it is possible to minimize a potentially negative impact on the environment. For example, using disinfectant wipes instead of spraying disinfectants could reduce the quantity of chemicals in the air. Practicing **greener infection control** requires thoughtful planning, research, and experimentation.

### Greener Infection Control

- Reduce the volume of waste
- Reduce adding excess chemicals to the environment
- Conserve water and energy
- Use products with recyclable packaging
- Go paperless
- Use digital radiography
- Continue to use only EPA-registered disinfectants

**Green Resources**

- Green Seal: www.greenseal.org (U.S. green certification program)
- EcoLogo: www.ecologo.org/en (Canadian "green" certification program)

## Paper

A typical patient's chart contains 12.8 pages of paper. If pages were reduced to only 6 pages, a practice with 2000 charts could save 12,600 pieces of paper per year. All paper that can be recycled should be. Digital patient records could have a significant impact on the amount of paper that is used.

## Radiology

Digital radiology is rapidly becoming the state-of-the-art. Traditional film-based radiology requires the use of chemicals, recycling fixer and developer solutions, and lead foil from film packets (see Chapter 39).

## Personal Protective Attire

Protective barriers present more of a challenge in the attempt to go greener. Much PPE consists of single-use, disposable items. Gloves and masks are not reusable. Some single-use paper gowns are recyclable. Washable gowns are an alternative to disposable gowns, but this uses energy, chemicals, and water. Energy Star washers and dryers are more efficient and use less energy.

## Surface Barriers and Precleaning/ Disinfection

When applied and removed properly, surface barriers will prevent contamination. They are single-use and disposable and therefore increase the amount of waste.

Precleaning and disinfection involves the use of chemicals and PPE. Disinfectant wipes release fewer chemicals into the environment. An acceptable surface disinfectant should be able to kill *M. tuberculosis* in 10 minutes or less. No disinfectant is perfect.

Most dental offices use a combination of surface barriers and disinfection (see Table 20.1).

RECALL

16 How can you help your dental office go greener?
17 What are the CDC's recommendations regarding carpeting and cloth furnishings in dental operatories, laboratories, and instrument processing areas?
18 With what should most housekeeping surfaces be cleaned?

■ **Legal and Ethical Implications** Today, more than at any time in history, patients are concerned about the risk of disease transmission in the dental office. Malpractice lawsuits have resulted from improper infection control techniques.

All healthcare team members in the dental office must understand the importance of good infection control. Most important, they must follow all infection control procedures. The best approach is to use a combination of barriers and between-patient disinfection to maintain the highest level of safety for both patients and the dental team. ■

■ **Eye to the Future** Currently, no legal "green-labeled" EPA-registered disinfectants are sold in the United States. In the past, the EPA did not allow manufacturers to place any type of environmental claim or seal on any EPA-registered product, including disinfectants. However, the EPA is currently relaxing this policy to allow valid claims of "environmental preferability." Never compromise an infection control procedure so you can "go green." You must continue to use only EPA-registered disinfectants.

Every day, new surface disinfectants appear on the market. Yet no single perfect disinfectant is available for all dental practices.

Although no products on the market today meet your every need, make a list of what is important to you and what you expect in a disinfectant. Then compare your list with the advantages and disadvantages of each product. With the rapidly changing array of products on the market, it is important that you stay up-to-date with new information as it becomes available. By becoming a member of OSAP (Organization for Safety, Asepsis and Prevention), you will receive monthly updates on important infection control information (www.osap.org). ■

■ **Critical Thinking**

1. How can you protect the electrical switches on an x-ray unit while keeping the switches free from contamination and electrical short circuits?
2. The label on a new disinfectant states in large print that the product "will kill HIV in 30 seconds," and in smaller print, it states that the tuberculocidal time is "10 minutes." How long should you leave this product on the surface to be disinfected?
3. What precautions must you take when using immersion-type disinfectants?
4. As you are removing plastic barriers from the light handle, you notice that one of the barriers has a tear in it. No blood is visible on the handle. What would you do, and why?
5. You begin a new job in Dr. Landry's office and discover that the dental assistant is using a 1:100 solution of household bleach for surface disinfection. What would you suggest to the assistant, and why? ■

PROCEDURE 20.1 

# Placing and Removing Surface Barriers

## GOAL

To place surface barriers before patient treatment and remove barriers at the end of the procedure

## EQUIPMENT AND SUPPLIES

- ✔ Liquid antimicrobial hand soap
- ✔ Utility gloves
- ✔ Plastic surface barriers
- ✔ Noncontaminated surfaces in dental treatment room

## PROCEDURAL STEPS

1 Wash and dry hands.

2 Select the appropriate surface barrier to be placed over the clean surface.

**NOTE** If the surfaces to be covered have been previously contaminated, put on your utility gloves, and preclean and disinfect the surface. Then wash, disinfect, and remove your utility gloves. Wash and dry your hands before applying the surface barriers.

3 Place each barrier over the entire surface to be protected. Check that the barrier is secure and will not come off.

**PURPOSE** If the barrier slips out of position, the underlying surface will become contaminated and will require precleaning and disinfection, negating the barrier's purpose.

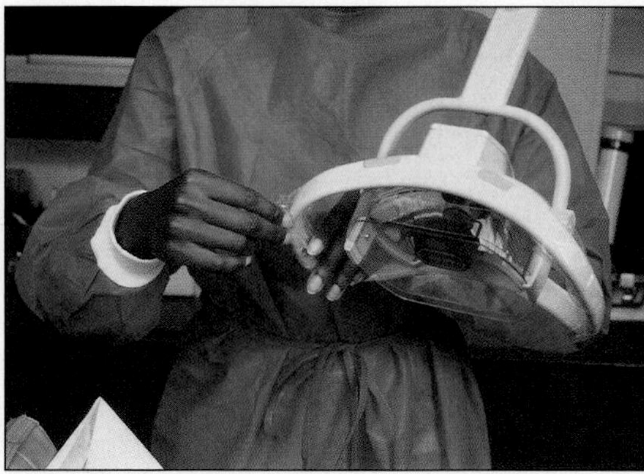

4 Wear your utility gloves to remove contaminated surface barriers after dental treatment.

**PURPOSE** Utility gloves protect the skin from contamination.

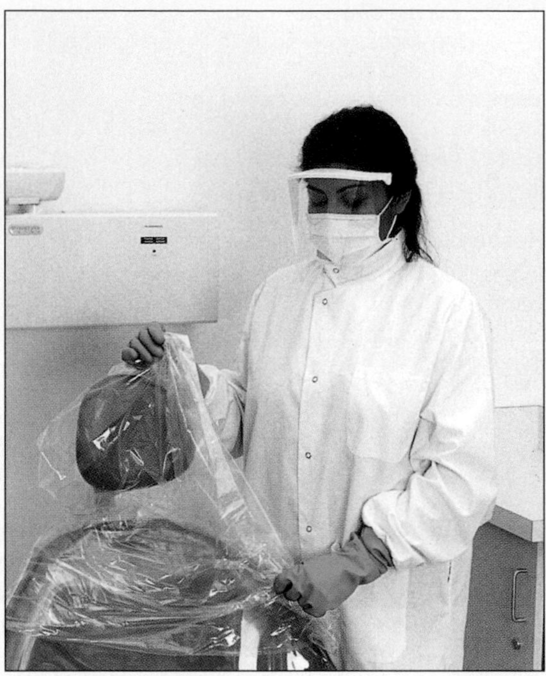

5 Very carefully remove each cover without touching the underlying surface with either the utility glove or the contaminated outside surface of the barrier.

**PURPOSE** If a surface is accidentally touched during removal of the cover, the surface must be precleaned and disinfected.

6 Discard the used covers in the regular waste trash. (Check disposal laws in your state.)

**PURPOSE** Most states do not consider barriers to be regulated waste (requiring special disposal) unless an item is soaked or caked with blood or saliva that would be released if the item was compressed.

7 Wash, disinfect, and remove your utility gloves. Wash and dry your hands, then apply fresh surface covers for the next patient.

**PURPOSE** Your utility gloves are contaminated from handling the used barriers. By washing, drying, and disinfecting your utility gloves, you will know they are ready for the next use.

PROCEDURE 20.2

# Performing Treatment Room Cleaning and Disinfection

## GOAL

To clean and disinfect dental treatment rooms effectively

## EQUIPMENT AND SUPPLIES

- Personal protective equipment (PPE), including utility gloves, goggles, and a mask
- Intermediate-level surface cleaner/disinfectant
- Paper towels

## PROCEDURAL STEPS

1 Put on utility gloves, protective eyewear, and protective clothing.

**PURPOSE** To prevent contact with contaminated surfaces and chemicals.

**NOTE** The latex examination gloves used in patient care should *not* be used for precleaning and disinfecting procedures. The chemicals will degrade the latex glove and will allow chemicals and contaminants to penetrate to the skin.

2 Make sure that the precleaning/disinfecting product has been prepared correctly and is fresh. Be certain to read and follow the manufacturer's instructions.

**PURPOSE** Some products are concentrated and must be diluted for use. In addition, some products must be prepared daily.

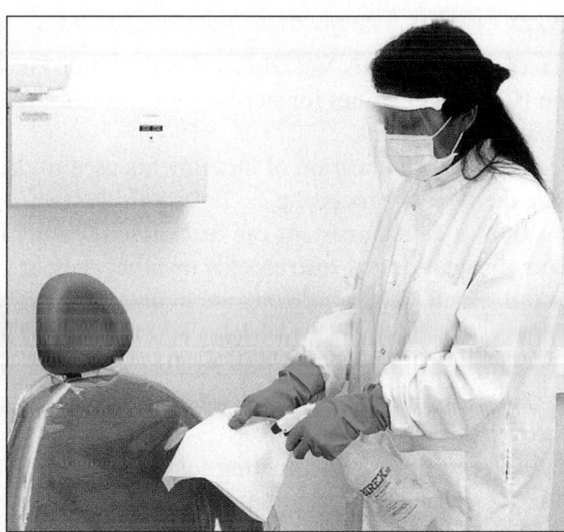

3 To preclean, spray the paper towel or gauze pad with the product and vigorously wipe the surface. You may use a small brush for surfaces that do not become visibly clean from wiping. If you are cleaning a large area, use several towels or gauze pads.

**PURPOSE** Overspray is reduced by spraying the product onto the towel or gauze pad. Large areas require more towels or pads to avoid spreading bioburden instead of removing it.

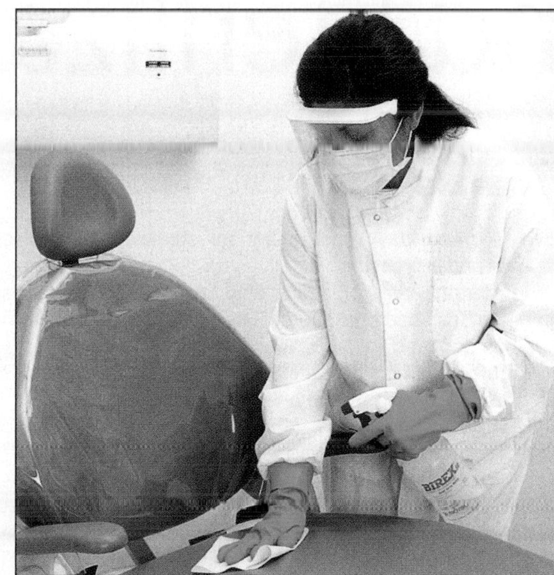

4 To disinfect, spray a fresh paper towel or gauze pad with the product. Let the surface remain moist for the manufacturer's recommended time for tuberculocidal action (usually 10 minutes).

5 If the surface is still moist after the kill time and you are ready to seat another patient, you may wipe the surface dry. Use water to rinse any residual disinfectant from surfaces that will come in contact with the patient's skin or mouth.

**PURPOSE** The chemicals used for precleaning and disinfecting may irritate the patient's skin or damage the patient's clothing.

21

# Principles and Techniques of Instrument Processing and Sterilization

## KEY TERMS

**Autoclave (AW-toe-klayv)** Instrument for sterilization by means of moist heat under pressure.

**Biologic indicators** Vials or strips, also known as *spore tests,* that contain harmless bacterial spores; used to determine whether sterilization has occurred.

**Biologic monitoring** Verifies sterilization by confirming that all spore-forming microorganisms have been destroyed.

**Chemical vapor sterilization (ster-i-li-ZAY-shun)** Sterilization by means of hot formaldehyde vapors under pressure.

**Clean area** Place where sterilized instruments, fresh disposable supplies, and prepared trays are stored.

**Contaminated area** Place where contaminated items are brought for precleaning.

**Critical instrument** Item used to penetrate soft tissue or bone.

**Dry heat sterilizer** Instrument for sterilization by means of heated air.

**Endospore** A resistant, dormant structure formed inside of some bacteria that can withstand adverse conditions.

**Event-related packaging** Instruments in packages should remain sterile indefinitely unless an event causes them to become contaminated (e.g., torn or wet packaging).

**Multiparameter indicators** Strips placed in packages that change color when exposed to a combination of heat, temperature, and time. Also known as *process integrators.*

**Noncritical instrument** Item that comes in contact with intact skin only.

**Process indicators** Tapes, strips, or tabs with heat-sensitive chemicals that change color when exposed to a certain temperature.

**Process integrators** Strips placed in packages that change color when exposed to a combination of heat, temperature, and time.

**Safety Data Sheet** OSHA's newer term for material data sheets. Safety Data Sheets are required for each hazardous chemical in a facility.

**Semicritical instrument** Item that comes in contact with oral tissues but does not penetrate soft tissue or bone.

**Single-parameter indicators** Tapes, strips, or tabs with heat-sensitive chemicals that change color when exposed to a particular temperature. Also known as *process indicators.*

**Ultrasonic cleaner** Instrument that loosens and removes debris by sound waves traveling through a liquid.

**Use-life** Period of time during which a germicidal solution is effective after it has been prepared for use.

**Wicking** Process of microorganisms being drawn through wet or damp paper packaging contaminating the instruments inside.

## LEARNING OUTCOMES

*On completion of this chapter, the student will be able to achieve the following objectives:*

1. Pronounce, define, and spell the key terms.
2. Discuss the classification of patient care items, including the following:
   - List the seven steps involved in processing dental instruments.
   - Describe the Centers for Disease Control and Prevention (CDC) guidelines for sterilization and disinfection of patient care items.
   - Describe the classification of instruments used to determine the type of processing.
3. Discuss how a dental assistant can be exposed to microorganisms through dental instruments or other patient care items and which CDC guidelines are in place to limit that exposure.
4. Describe the ideal instrument processing area.
5. Discuss precleaning and packaging of instruments, including the following:
   - Explain the purpose of a holding solution.
   - Describe the safety precautions that are necessary when one is operating an ultrasonic cleaner.
   - Describe the precautions that are necessary when one is packaging materials for sterilization.
   - Describe the CDC guidelines for preparing and packaging instruments for sterilization.
   - Describe the CDC guidelines for sterilization of unwrapped instruments.
6. Discuss methods of sterilization, including the following:
   - Describe the three most common methods of heat sterilization and the advantages and disadvantages of each.

- Explain the primary disadvantage of flash sterilization.
- Explain the limitations of liquid chemical sterilants.
- Explain how sterilization failures can occur.

7 Discuss sterilization monitoring, including the following:
- Describe the three forms of sterilization monitoring.
- Explain the differences between process indicators and process integrators.
- Describe when and how biologic monitoring is done.

8 Describe the steps involved in cleaning and sterilizing the high-speed dental handpiece.

## PERFORMANCE OUTCOMES

*On completion of this chapter, the student will be able to meet competency standards for the following skills:*

- Operate the ultrasonic cleaner.
- Perform biologic monitoring.
- Perform follow-up on sterilization failure.
- Use autoclave instruments.
- Sterilize instruments with chemical vapor.
- Sterilize instruments with dry heat.
- Sterilize instruments with chemical liquid.
- Sterilize the dental handpiece.

## ELECTRONIC RESOURCES

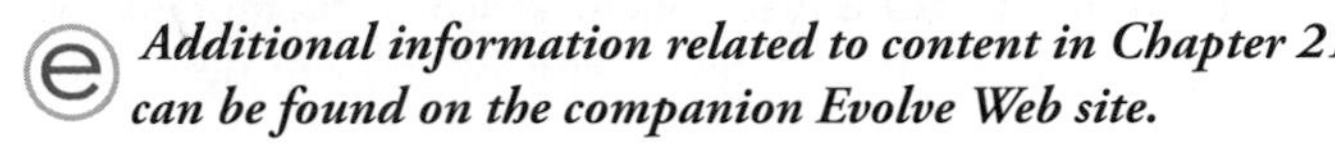
***Additional information related to content in Chapter 21 can be found on the companion Evolve Web site.***

- Practice Quiz
- Videos: Operating the Ultrasonic Cleaner; Autoclaving Instruments

One of the most important responsibilities of the dental assistant is to process contaminated instruments and other patient care items for reuse (Box 21.1).

Instrument processing involves much more than sterilization. Proper processing of contaminated dental instruments is actually a seven-step process (Table 21.1). Although the seven steps are not difficult to learn, it is very important for you to have a clear understanding of how and why each step is performed.

*Note:* Throughout this chapter, Centers for Disease Control and Prevention (CDC) recommendations are indicated, and the category of scientific evidence is noted at the end of each recommendation.

### Rankings of Evidence

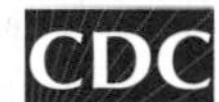


Each recommendation made by the CDC is categorized on the basis of existing scientific data, theoretical rationale, and applicability. Rankings are based on the following categories:

| | |
|---|---|
| Category IA | Strongly recommended for implementation and strongly supported by well-designed experimental, clinical, or epidemiologic studies (studies of patterns and causes of diseases) |
| Category IB | Strongly recommended for implementation and supported by experimental, clinical, or epidemiologic studies and a strong theoretical rationale |
| Category IC | Required for implementation, as mandated by federal or state regulation or standard |
| Category II | Suggested for implementation and supported by suggestive clinical or epidemiologic studies or a theoretical rationale |
| Unresolved Issue | No recommendation—practices for which insufficient evidence or no consensus regarding efficacy exists |

# Classification of Patient Care Items

Patient care items are categorized into three classifications: *critical, semicritical,* and *noncritical.* These categories are based on the potential risk for infection associated with their intended use. The classifications are used to determine the *minimum* type of posttreatment processing that is required (Table 21.2).

### CDC Guidelines for Sterilization and Disinfection of Patient Care Items

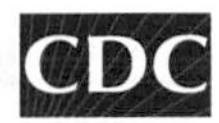


#### General Recommendations

- Use only U.S. Food and Drug Administration (FDA)–cleared medical devices for sterilization, and follow the manufacturer's instructions for correct use. (Category IB)
- Clean and heat-sterilize critical dental instruments before each use. (Category IA)
- Clean and heat-sterilize semicritical items before each use. (Category IB)
- Allow packages to dry in the sterilizer before they are handled to avoid contamination. (Category IB)
- Reprocess heat-sensitive critical and semicritical instruments by using FDA-cleared sterilants/high-level disinfectants or an FDA-cleared low-temperature sterilization method (e.g., ethylene oxide). Follow manufacturers' instructions for use of chemical sterilants/high-level disinfectants. (Category IB)
- Single-use disposable instruments are acceptable alternatives if they are used only once and are disposed of correctly. (Categories IB, IC)
- Do not use liquid chemical sterilants/high-level disinfectants for environmental surface disinfection or as holding solutions. (Categories IB, IC)
- Ensure that noncritical patient care items are barrier protected or cleaned or, if visibly soiled, are cleaned and disinfected after each use with an Environmental Protection Agency (EPA)–registered hospital disinfectant. If visibly contaminated with blood, use an EPA-registered hospital disinfectant with a tuberculocidal claim (i.e., intermediate level). (Category IB)
- Inform dental healthcare personnel of all Occupational Safety and Health Administration (OSHA) guidelines for exposure to chemical agents used for disinfection and sterilization.

## Critical Instruments

**Critical instruments** are items that are used to penetrate soft tissue or bone. They have the greatest risk of transmitting infection and are to be sterilized by heat. Examples of critical instruments include forceps, scalpels, bone chisels, scalers, and burs.

## Semicritical Instruments

**Semicritical instruments** touch mucous membranes or nonintact skin and have a lower risk of transmission. Most semicritical items in dentistry are heat tolerant, and they should be sterilized. If the item will be damaged by heat, it should receive minimum high-level disinfection (see Chapter 20). Examples of semicritical items include plastic-handled brushes, high-volume evacuator (HVE) tips, rubber dam forceps, x-ray film holders, and amalgam carriers.

In dental offices today, most items that are used intraorally are capable of withstanding the heat of sterilization. A fundamental rule of infection control states, *"If an item can be heat-sterilized, it should be heat-sterilized."*

### BOX 21.1 Instrument Processing

1. Holding (presoaking): facilitates the cleaning process by preventing debris from drying.
2. Precleaning: removes as much of the bioburden as possible to give the subsequent sterilization step the best change to work.
3. Corrosion control, drying, lubrication: reduces damages to instruments and helps ensure proper functioning of the instruments.
4. Packaging: helps maintain sterility of instruments after sterilization and before they are presented to a subsequent patient.
5. Sterilization or high-level disinfection: kills all microbes remaining on the instruments to help ensure patient safety.
6. Sterilization monitoring: measures the use and functioning of the sterilizer.
7. Handling process instruments: helps maintain the sterility of the instruments during storage until they are used on a subsequent patient.

From Miller CH: Infection control and management of hazardous materials for the dental team, ed 6, St Louis, 2018, Elsevier.

## Noncritical Instruments

**Noncritical instruments** pose the least risk of transmission of infection because they contact only intact skin, which is an effective barrier to microorganisms. These items should be cleaned and processed with an Environmental Protection Agency (EPA)–registered intermediate-level or low-level disinfectant after each patient use.

Noncritical clinical devices include the position indicator device of the x-ray unit tube head, the lead apron, and the curing light that comes into contact only with intact skin.

## Personal Protective Equipment

To prevent disease agents from a previous patient from being transferred to you, another dental team member, or the next patient, instrument processing must be performed in a consistent and disciplined manner. You must *always* use personal protective equipment (PPE), including utility gloves, mask, eyewear, and protective clothing, when processing instruments (Fig. 21.1).

### TABLE 21.1 Seven Steps for Instrument Processing

| Step | Technique |
|---|---|
| 1. Transport | Transport contaminated instruments to the processing area in a manner that minimizes the risk of exposure to persons and the environment. Use appropriate PPE and a rigid, leakproof container. |
| 2. Cleaning | Clean instruments with a hands-free, mechanical process such as use of an ultrasonic cleaner or instrument washer. If instruments cannot be cleaned immediately, use a holding solution. |
| 3. Packaging | In the clean area, wrap/package instruments in appropriate materials. Place a chemical indicator inside the package next to the instruments. If an indicator is not visible on the outside of the package, place an external process indicator on the package. |
| 4. Sterilization | Load the sterilizer according to the manufacturer's instructions. Label packages. Do not overload the sterilizer. Place packages on their edges in single layers or on racks to increase circulation of the sterilizing agent around the instruments. Operate the sterilizer according to the manufacturer's instructions. Allow packages to cool before removing them from the sterilizer. Allow packages to cool before handling. |
| 5. Storage | Store instruments in a clean, dry environment in a manner that maintains the integrity of the package. Rotate packages so that those with the oldest sterilization dates will be used first. |
| 6. Delivery | Deliver packages to point of use in a manner that maintains sterility of the instruments until they are used. Inspect each package for damage. Open package aseptically. |
| 7. Quality | An effective quality assurance program should incorporate training, record keeping, maintenance, and the use of biologic indicators. |

*PPE,* Personal protective equipment.

**TABLE 21.2** CDC Classification of Instruments and Procedures

| Category | Functions and Examples | Intraoral Use | Risk of Disease Transmission | Procedure |
|---|---|---|---|---|
| Critical | *Function:* Touch bone or penetrate soft tissue<br>*Examples:* Surgical and other instruments used to penetrate soft tissue or bone, including forceps, scalpels, bone chisels, scalers, and burs | Yes | Very high | Sterilization |
| Semicritical | *Function:* Touch mucous membranes but will not touch bone or penetrate soft tissue<br>*Examples:* Mouth mirrors and amalgam condensers | Yes | Moderate | Sterilization or high-level disinfection |
| Noncritical | *Function:* Contact only with intact skin<br>*Examples:* External dental x-ray head | No | Very low or none | Intermediate- to low-level disinfection or basic cleaning |

*CDC,* Centers for Disease Control and Prevention.

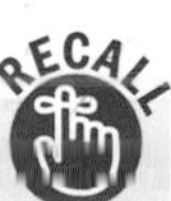


1 What are the three instrument classifications that are used to determine the method of sterilization?
2 What PPE is necessary when one is processing instruments?

## Transporting and Processing Contaminated Patient Care Items

The dental assistant can be exposed to microorganisms through contact with contaminated instruments or other patient care items. Exposure can occur through percutaneous injury (i.e., needle sticks or cuts) or by contact with the mucous membranes of the eyes, nose, or mouth.

### CDC Guidelines for Receiving, Cleaning, and Decontamination Procedures

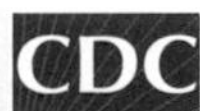


- Minimize handling of loose contaminated instruments during transport to the instrument-processing area. Use work practice controls (e.g., carry instruments in a covered container) to minimize exposure potential. (Category II)
- Clean all visible blood and other contamination from dental instruments and devices before sterilization or disinfection procedures. (Category IA)
- Use automated cleaning equipment (e.g., ultrasonic cleaner, washer/disinfector) to remove debris to improve cleaning effectiveness and decrease worker exposure to blood. (Category IB)
- Use work practice controls that minimize contact with sharp instruments if manual cleaning is necessary (e.g., long-handled brush). (Category IC)
- Wear puncture- and chemical-resistant/heavy-duty utility gloves for instrument cleaning and decontamination procedures. (Category IB)
- Wear appropriate personal protective equipment (PPE) (e.g., mask, protective eyewear, gown) when splashing or spraying is anticipated during cleaning. (Category IC)
- Do not store critical instruments unwrapped. (Category IB)

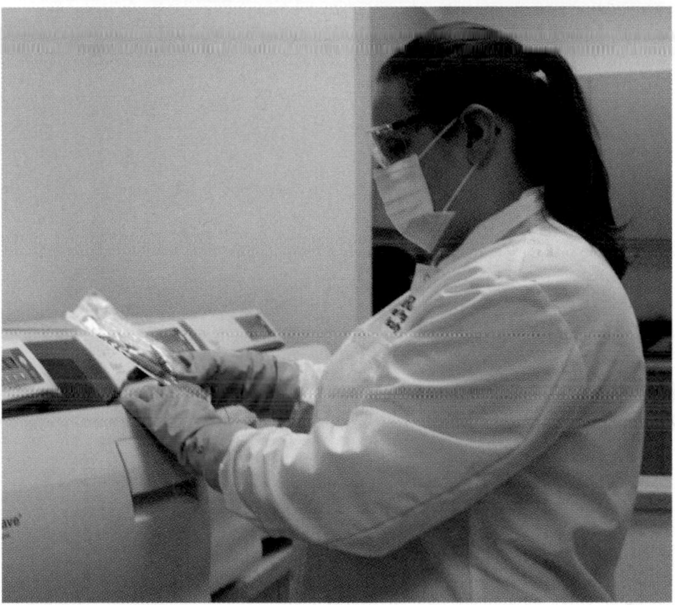

**FIG. 21.1** Personal protective equipment (PPE) must be worn while instruments are prepared for sterilization.

## Instrument-Processing Area

The instrument-processing area, or *sterilization area,* should be centrally located in the office to allow easy access from all patient care areas. This minimizes the need to carry contaminated items through **clean areas** of the office, where sterilized instruments, fresh disposable supplies, and prepared trays are stored.

The "ideal" instrument-processing area (1) should be dedicated only to instrument processing, (2) should be physically separated from the operatories and the dental laboratory, and (3) should *not* be a part of a common walkway. The area should *not* have a door or windows that open to the outside, because dust can enter the area.

The processing area should have good air circulation to control the heat generated by the sterilizers. The size of the area should accommodate all equipment and supplies necessary for instrument processing, with multiple outlets and proper

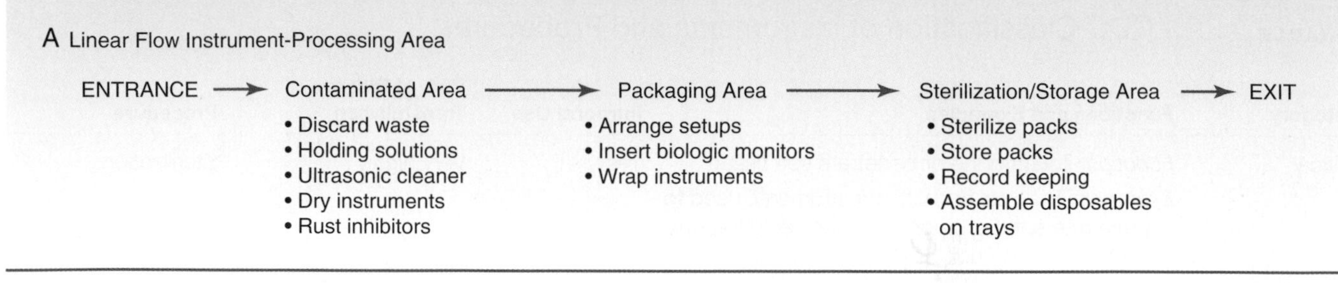


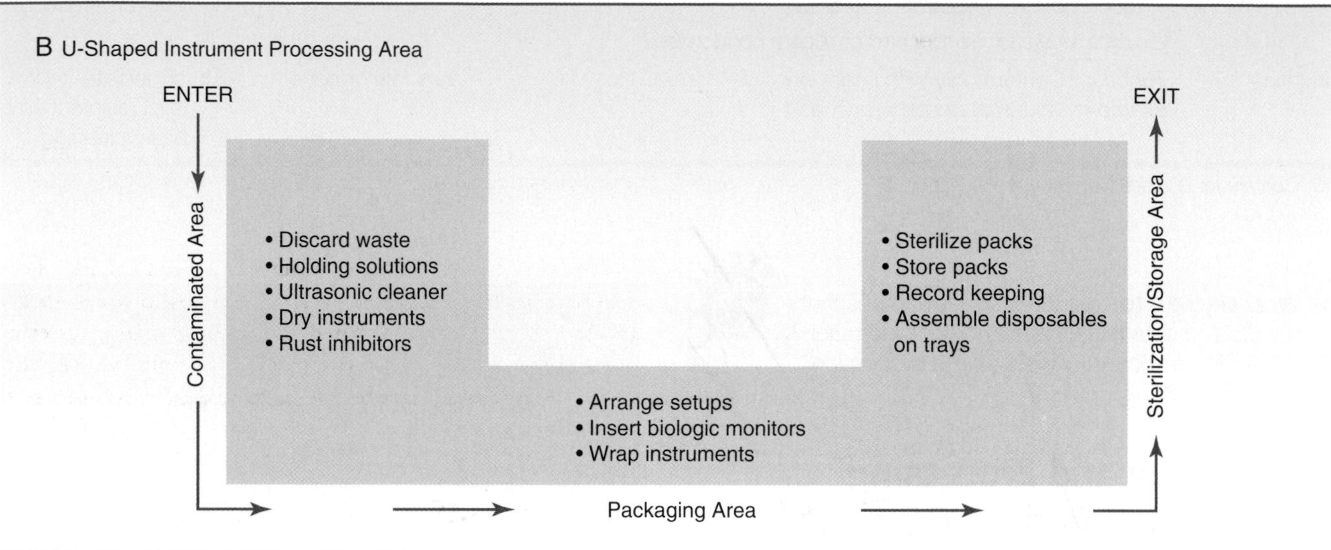


**FIG. 21.2** Instrument-processing areas. A, Linear. B, U-shaped.

lighting, water, and an air line and a vacuum line for flushing high-speed handpieces.

A deep sink should provide hands-free controls for instrument rinsing and (if space permits) a foot-operated or other hands-free trash receptacle. The flooring should be an uncarpeted, seamless, hard surface. The size, shape, and accessories of the instrument-processing area vary among dental offices.

## Terms Used in Instrument Processing

- **Precleaning:** Reducing the number of microorganisms that are present by physically removing debris.
- **Sterilization:** Process that inactivates all microbial life, including bacterial spores, viruses, bacteria, and fungi.
- **Disinfection:** Process that kills disease-causing microorganisms, but not necessarily all microbial life.
- **High-level disinfection:** Process that kills some but not all bacterial endospores and inactivates *Mycobacterium tuberculosis*.
- **Intermediate-level disinfection:** Inactivates *Mycobacterium tuberculosis* and destroys less-resistant organisms such as hepatitis B virus and human immunodeficiency virus.
- **Low-level disinfection:** Ineffective against *M. tuberculosis* and should be used only in the dental office for housekeeping purposes.

## CDC Guidelines for Instrument-Processing Area

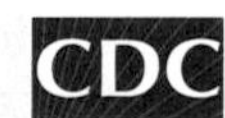


- Designate a central processing area. Divide the instrument-processing area—physically or, at a minimum, spatially—into distinct areas for (1) receiving, cleaning, and decontamination, (2) preparation and packaging, (3) sterilization, and (4) storage. Do not store instruments in an area where contaminated instruments are held or cleaned. (Category II)
- Train dental healthcare personnel to employ work practices that prevent contamination of clean areas. (Category II)

# Workflow Pattern

Regardless of the size or shape of the instrument-processing area, four basic rules govern the pattern of workflow. Processing of instruments should proceed in a single loop, from dirty, to clean, to sterile, to storage, without ever "doubling back" (Fig. 21.2).

If the instrument-processing area is small, you can use signs that read, "Contaminated items only," "Precleaning area," "Cleaned items only," "Sterile items only," or "Sterilization area," to separate contaminated and clean areas. This method works well to prevent mixing of contaminated and sterile items in a small sterilization area.

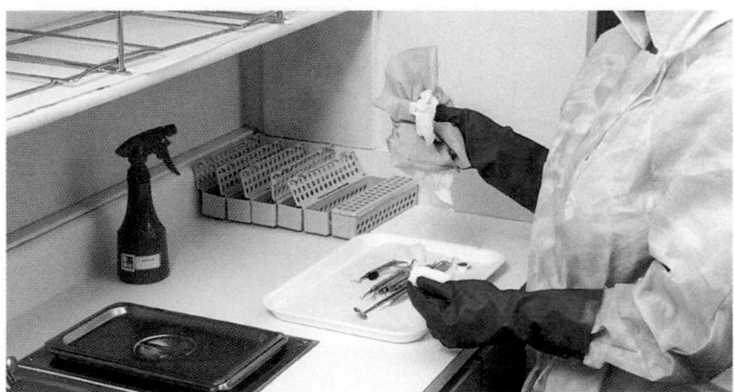

**FIG. 21.3** Waste items are properly discarded.

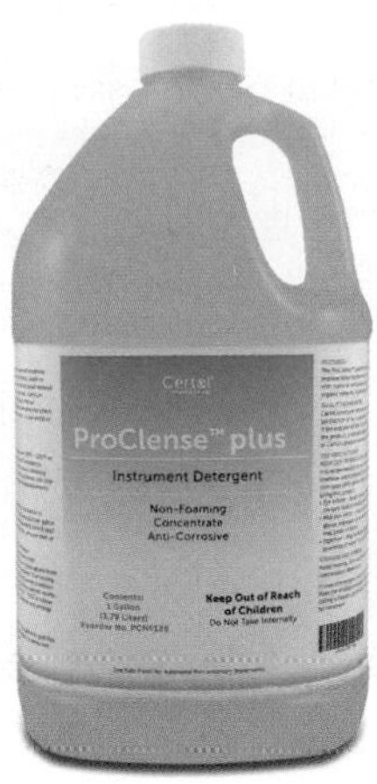


**FIG. 21.5** Commercial holding solutions are available for use in precleaning. *(Courtesy Certol, Commerce City, CO.)*

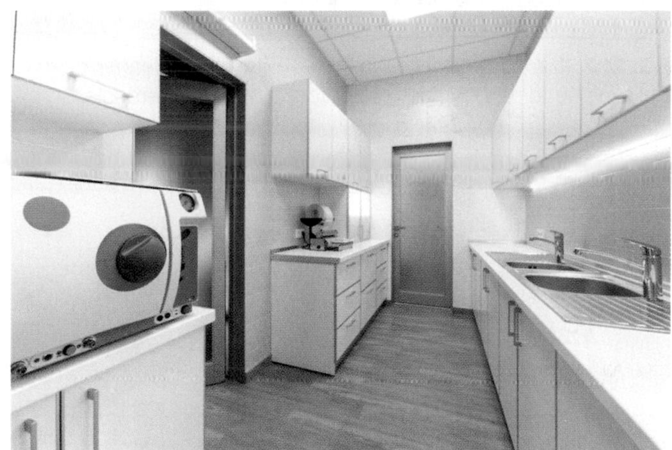

**FIG. 21.4** A modern sterilization center. *(Copyright © luckyraccoon/iStock/Getty Images.)*

## Contaminated Area

All soiled instruments are brought into the **contaminated area**—the *initial receiving area,* where they are held for processing. Any disposable items not already discarded in the treatment room are removed from the instrument tray and disposed of as contaminated waste.

Thorough cleaning should be done before all disinfection and sterilization processes. This should involve removal of all debris and organic materials (e.g., blood, saliva). Methods of cleaning are described later in this chapter.

The contaminated area contains clean protective eyewear and utility gloves, counter space, a sink, a waste disposal container, holding solution, an ultrasonic cleaner, an eyewash station, and supplies for wrapping instruments before sterilization (Fig. 21.3).

*Note:* Soiled and clean instruments are never stored in the same cabinet.

## Preparation and Packaging Area

In the preparation and packaging area, cleaned instruments and other dental supplies should be inspected, assembled into sets or trays, and wrapped or placed in packages for sterilization (Fig. 21.4).

The preparation and packaging area should consist of counter space and storage space for sterilized instruments, fresh disposable supplies, and prepared trays or instrument cassettes.

*Clean* instruments are not sterile and could harbor pathogens. Instruments must be packaged and sterilized before they are used on a patient.

# Precleaning and Packaging Instruments

Instruments may be precleaned in one of three ways: hand scrubbing, *ultrasonic cleaning,* or *instrument washing machines.*

## Holding Solution

If instruments cannot be cleaned immediately after a procedure is performed, they should be placed in a holding solution to prevent the drying of blood and debris on the instruments.

The holding solution may be any noncorrosive liquid. A commercial enzymatic solution that partially dissolves organic debris may be used (Fig. 21.5). Dishwasher detergent also makes a good holding solution because it is a low-cost, low foaming, and readily available product. It is neither cost-effective nor desirable to use a disinfectant alone as a holding solution.

The container must have a lid and be labeled with both a *biohazard* label (because of the contaminated instruments) and a *chemical* label (because of the cleaner/detergent). The holding solution should be changed at least twice daily, and more frequently if it becomes clouded.

Remember, a holding solution is necessary *only* when contaminated instruments cannot be processed immediately.

## Hand Scrubbing

Hand scrubbing is the *least* desirable method of cleaning instruments because it requires direct hand contact with the

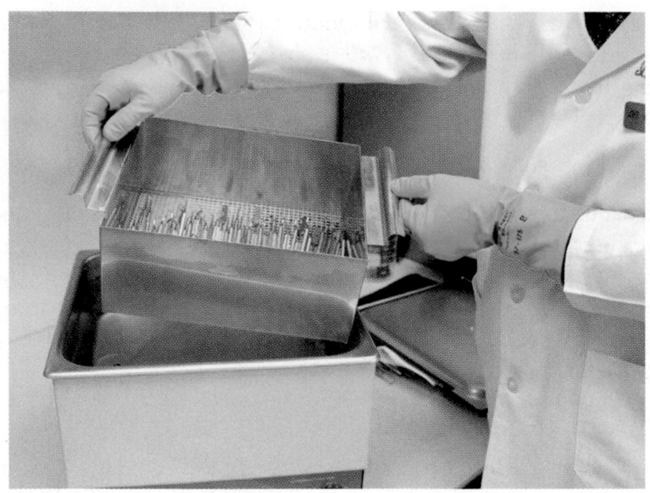

**FIG. 21.6** Ultrasonic cleaning. Instruments are placed in an ultrasonic cleaning basket, and the basket is placed in the cleaning solution. *(From Miller CH: Infection control and management of hazardous materials for the dental team, ed 6, St Louis, 2018, Elsevier.)*

contaminated instrument. If you absolutely must hand-scrub instruments, follow these precautions:

- Wear goggle-type eyewear and puncture-resistant gloves, as well as your protective clothing.
- Clean only one or two instruments at a time.
- Use only a long-handled brush, preferably one with a hand guard or a wide surface.
- Keep items above the waterline; fully immersing them in a basin of soapy water interferes with one's ability to see the sharp ends.
- Allow instruments to air-dry, or carefully pat them with thick toweling. *Never* rub or roll the instruments while they are in the towel, because of the risk of accidental injury.

*Note:* Some states have specific infection control guidelines or state Occupational Safety and Health Administration (OSHA) plans that prohibit hand scrubbing of instruments. In these states, you must use an ultrasonic cleaner or machine cleaning.

## Ultrasonic Cleaning

**Ultrasonic cleaners** are used to loosen and remove debris from instruments. These cleaners also reduce the risk of hand injury from cuts and punctures that occur during the cleaning process (Fig. 21.6). See Procedure 21.1: Operating the Ultrasonic Cleaner.

Puncture-resistant utility gloves, a mask, protective eyewear, and a protective gown should always be worn when the ultrasonic cleaner is used. To further limit contact with contaminated instruments, keep a set of tongs near the ultrasonic unit; these can be used to remove instruments after the cleaning cycle has been completed.

The ultrasonic cleaner works by producing sound waves beyond the range of human hearing. These sound waves, which

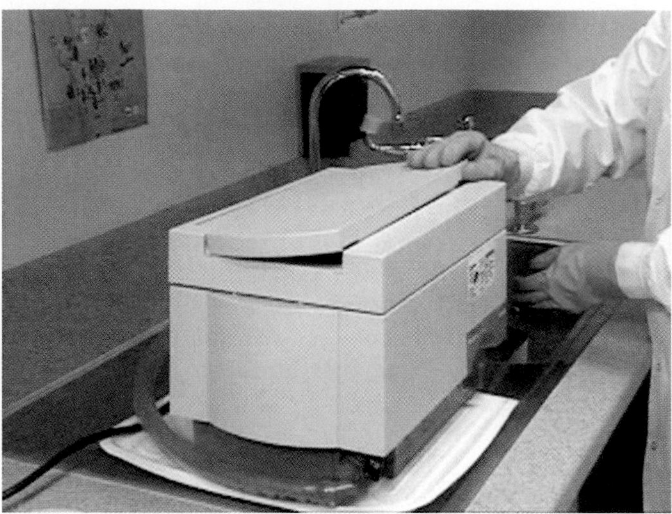

**FIG. 21.7** It is important to keep the ultrasonic cleaner covered while in use to reduce spatter and contaminated aerosols.

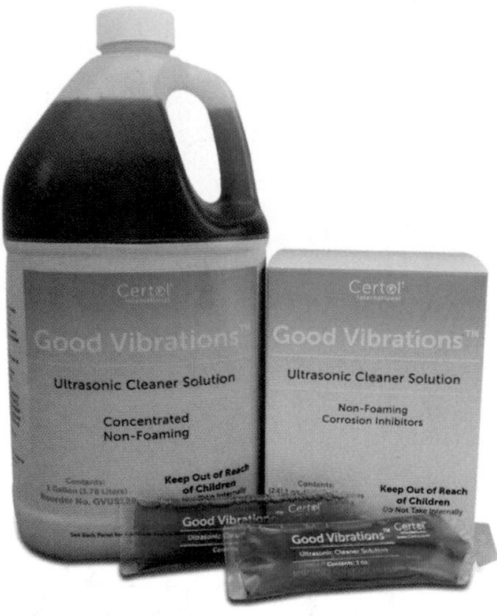


**FIG. 21.8** A commercial all-purpose ultrasonic cleaner. *(Courtesy Certol, Commerce City, CO.)*

can travel through metal and glass containers, cause *cavitation* (formation of bubbles in liquid). The bubbles, which are too small to be seen, burst by *implosion* (bursting inward—the opposite of an explosion). The mechanical cleaning action of the bursting bubbles combined with the chemical action of the ultrasonic solution removes the debris from the instruments.

Instruments should be processed in the ultrasonic cleaner until they are visibly clean. The time may vary from 5 to 15 minutes, depending on the amount and type of material on the instruments and the efficiency of the ultrasonic unit (Fig. 21.7). Instruments in plastic or resin cassettes require slightly longer cleaning time because the cassette material absorbs some of the ultrasonic energy.

### Ultrasonic Cleaning Solutions

You should use only ultrasonic solutions that are specially formulated for use in the ultrasonic cleaner (Fig. 21.8). Some

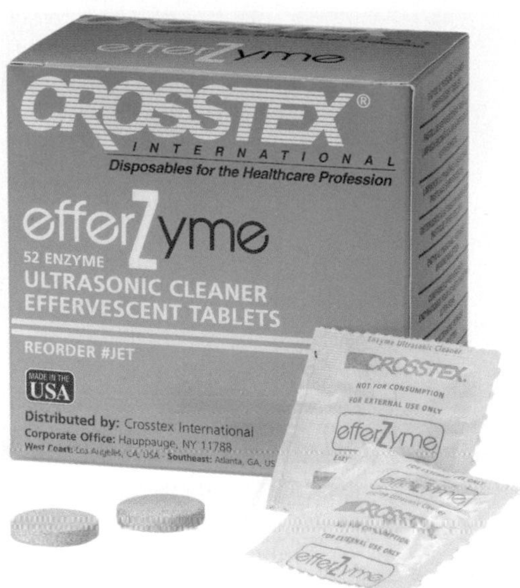


FIG. 21.9 An enzyme ultrasonic cleaner in tablet form. *(© 2017 Crosstex International, Inc.)*

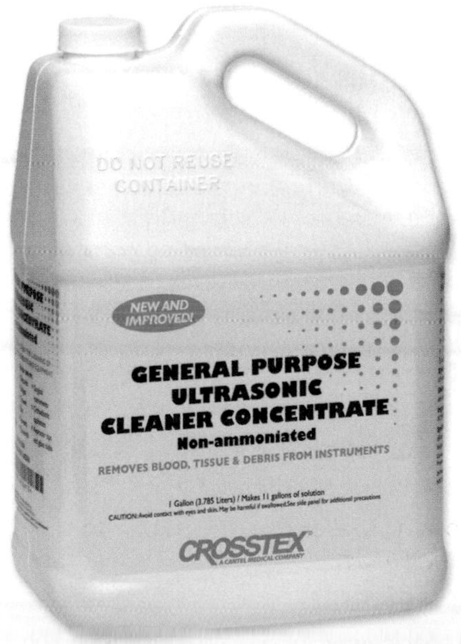


FIG. 21.10 Special tartar and stain remover ultrasonic solution. *(© 2017 Crosstex International, Inc.)*

ultrasonic cleaning products have enzyme activity (Fig. 21.9). Other ultrasonic cleaning products have antimicrobial activity, which reduces the buildup of microbes in solutions with repeated use. The antimicrobial activity *does not disinfect* the instruments; it merely prevents microorganisms from increasing in number.

Do *not* use other chemicals such as plain disinfectants in the ultrasonic cleaner. Some disinfectants can "fix" the blood and debris onto the instruments, making subsequent cleaning more difficult. Specific ultrasonic solutions are available that remove difficult materials, such as cements, tartar, stains, plaster, and alginate (Fig. 21.10). Refer to the ultrasonic unit manufacturer's instructions regarding the specific solution to be used.

As with the holding solution, the ultrasonic cleaning unit should be labeled with *both* a chemical label and a biohazard label because it contains a chemical *and* contaminated instruments.

### Care of the Ultrasonic Cleaner

The ultrasonic cleaner solution is *highly contaminated* and must be discarded at least once a day, or sooner if it becomes visibly cloudy. When the solution is changed, the inside of the pan and the lid should be rinsed with water, disinfected, rinsed again, and dried. All PPE should be worn while one is changing solutions in the ultrasonic cleaner.

### Testing the Ultrasonic Cleaner

If you notice that the instruments are not being cleaned completely after they have been processed in the ultrasonic cleaner, the unit may not be functioning properly.

To determine whether the ultrasonic cleaner is working properly, hold a 5 × 5–inch sheet of lightweight aluminum foil vertically (like a curtain) half-submerged in the fresh, unused solution. Run the unit for 20 seconds, and then hold the foil up toward the light. Surfaces that were submerged into the solution should be evenly marked with a tiny pebbling effect over the entire surface (Fig. 21.11). An area on the foil that is greater than an inch without pebbling suggests a problem with the unit and indicates that it needs to be serviced by the manufacturer.

RECALL

3 What is the basic rule of the workflow pattern in an instrument-processing area?
4 If instruments cannot be processed immediately, what should be done with them?
5 Name the three methods of precleaning instruments.
6 Which method of precleaning instruments is the least desirable?
7 How does an ultrasonic cleaner work?

## Automated Washers/Disinfectors

Automated instrument washers/disinfectors look and work similar to a household dishwasher. However, the U.S. Food and Drug Administration (FDA) must approve them for use with dental instruments (Fig. 21.12).

Automated washing/disinfecting units use a combination of very hot water recirculation and detergents to remove organic material. Then the instruments are automatically dried. These units are classified as *thermal* disinfectors because they have a disinfecting cycle that subjects instruments to a *level of heat* that kills most vegetative microorganisms.

Instruments processed in automatic washers/disinfectors must be wrapped and sterilized before they are used on a patient.

## Drying, Lubrication, and Corrosion Control

Instruments and burs made of carbon steel will rust during steam sterilization. Rust inhibitors such as sodium nitrate or

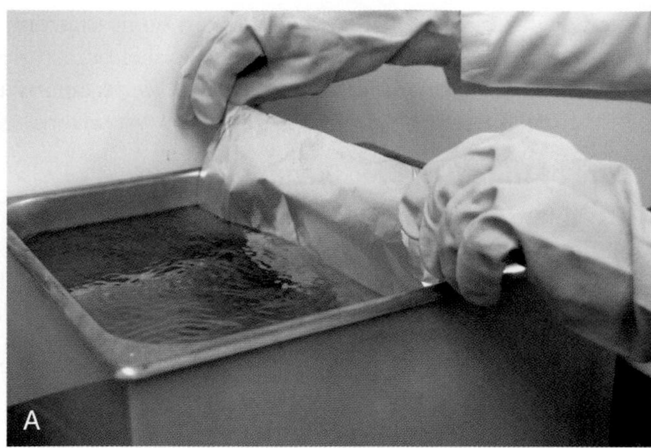


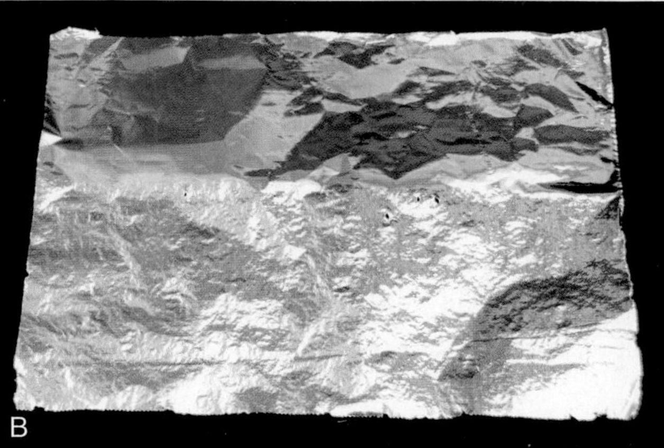


**FIG. 21.11** Aluminum foil test for ultrasonic cleaners. A, The lower half of the foil is submerged in the cleaning solution for 20 seconds of operation. B, Note the indentations and some holes evenly distributed over the submerged portion of the foil. *(From Miller CH: Infection control and management of hazardous materials for the dental team, ed 6, St Louis, 2018, Elsevier.)*

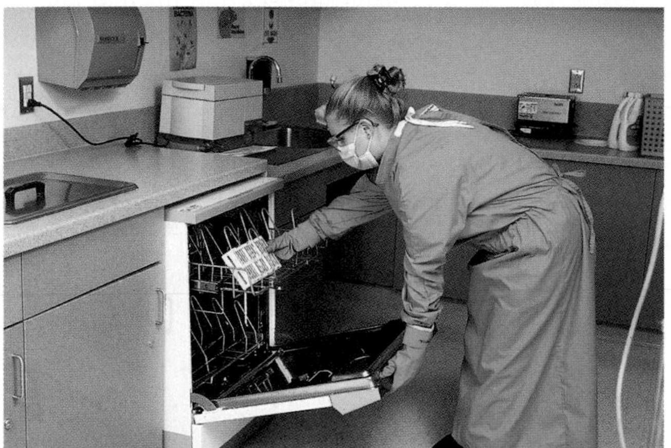

**FIG. 21.12** A Miele thermal disinfector provides safe and thorough instrument cleaning, disinfecting, and drying. Instruments must be packaged and sterilized after the cycle.

commercial products are available as a spray or dip solution and help to reduce rust and corrosion.

An alternative to using rust inhibitors is to dry the instrument thoroughly with dry heat or unsaturated chemical vapor sterilization (see Unsaturated Chemical Vapor Sterilization later in this chapter), which does not cause rusting.

Hinged instruments may have to be lubricated to maintain proper opening. Take care to remove all excess lubricant before performing heat sterilization.

## Packaging Instruments

Before sterilization, the instruments should be wrapped or packaged to protect them from becoming contaminated *after* sterilization. When instruments are sterilized without being packaged, they are immediately exposed to the environment as soon as the sterilizer door is opened. They can be contaminated by aerosols in the air, dust, improper handling, or contact with nonsterile surfaces.

An additional advantage to packaging instruments is that they can be grouped into special setups, such as crown/bridge, amalgam, prophy, or composite.

### CDC Guidelines for Preparation and Packaging

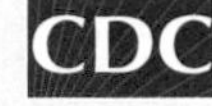

- Use an internal chemical indicator from inside each package. If the internal indicator cannot be seen from outside the package, also use an external indicator. (Category II)
- Use a container system or wrapping compatible with the type of sterilization process used and that has received FDA clearance. (Category IB)
- Before sterilization of critical and semicritical instruments, inspect instruments for cleanliness, then wrap or place them in containers designed to maintain sterility during storage (e.g., cassettes, organizing trays). (Category IA)

*FDA,* U.S. Food and Drug Administration.

### *Packaging Materials*

Sterilization packaging materials and cassettes are medical devices and therefore must be approved by the FDA. It is critical to use *only* products and materials that are labeled as "sterilization" packaging. Never substitute products such as plastic wraps, paper, or zipper-lock freezer bags that are not registered for this purpose. These products may melt or may prevent the sterilizing agent from reaching the instruments inside.

Specific types of packaging material are available for each method of sterilization. You should use *only* the type of packaging material designed for the particular method of sterilization that you are using (Table 21.3).

A wide variety of sterilization packaging materials are available. Self-sealing or heat-sealed "poly" bags or tubes provide an excellent wrap (Fig. 21.13). In addition, paper wraps and cloth wraps are available. If the package is not the self-sealing type, you should use only sterilization indicator tape to seal the package. *Never* use safety pins, staples, paper clips, or other sharp objects that could penetrate the packaging material. Label the package with the date of sterilization, and if there is more than one sterilizer used in the office, indicate which sterilizer is used. This is important in the event of a sterilization failure.

The instruments are now ready for the sterilization process.

## Sterilization of Unwrapped Instruments

An unwrapped cycle (sometimes called *flash sterilization*) is a method used to sterilize unwrapped patient care items for immediate use. The time required for unwrapped sterilization cycles depends on the type of sterilizer and the type of item (i.e., porous or nonporous) to be sterilized. Unwrapped sterilization should be used only under certain conditions. Flash sterilization is discussed later in this chapter.

**TABLE 21.3 Packaging Materials and Types of Sterilization**

| Packaging Material | Tips |
|---|---|
| **Steam Sterilization** | |
| Paper wrap | Do not use closed containers. |
| Nylon tubing | Do not use thick cloth. |
| Paper/plastic peel pouches | Some plastics melt. |
| Thin cloth | |
| Wrapped perforated cassettes | |
| **Dry Heat Sterilizers** | |
| Paper wrap | Some paper may char. |
| Appropriate type of nylon "plastic" tube | Some plastics melt. |
| Closed containers (use biologic indicator) | Use only materials approved for dry heat. |
| **Unsaturated Chemical Vapor** | |
| Paper wrap | Do not use closed containers. |
| Paper/plastic peel pouches | Do not use cloth (absorbs too much chemical vapor). |
| Wrapped perforated cassettes | Some plastics melt. |
| | Use only materials approved for chemical vapor. |

### CDC Guidelines for Sterilization of Unwrapped Instruments

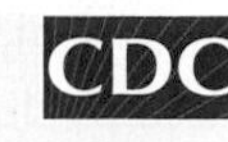


- Instruments are thoroughly cleaned and dried before sterilization.
- Mechanical monitors are checked, and chemical indicators are used for each cycle.
- Care is taken to avoid thermal injury to the dental professional or patients.
- Items are aseptically transported to the point of use to maintain sterility.
- Critical instruments that were sterilized unwrapped should not be stored unwrapped, and semicritical instruments should be used within a short period of time. Do not sterilize implantable devices unwrapped.

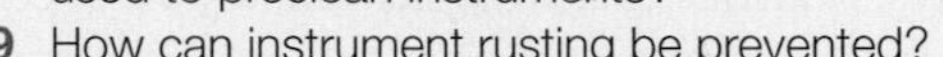

RECALL

8 What prevents kitchen dishwashers from being used to preclean instruments?
9 How can instrument rusting be prevented?
10 Why should instruments be packaged before sterilization?
11 Why should you never use pins, staples, or paper clips on instrument packages?

## Methods of Sterilization

Sterilization destroys all microbial forms, including bacterial spores. *Sterile* is an absolute term; there is no "partially sterile" or "almost sterile."

All reusable items (i.e., critical and semicritical instruments) that come in contact with the patient's blood, saliva, or mucous membranes must be heat-sterilized. The most common forms

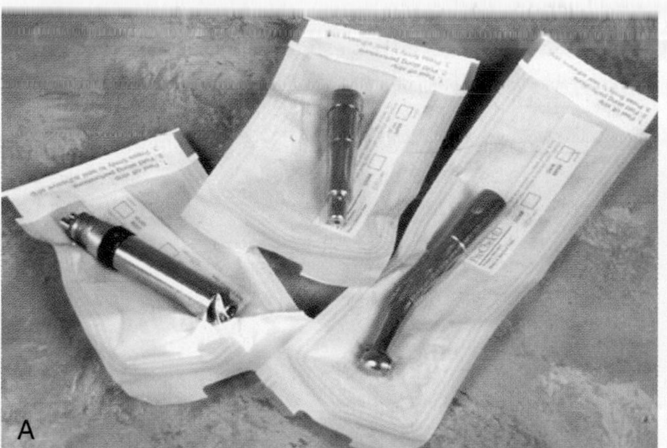


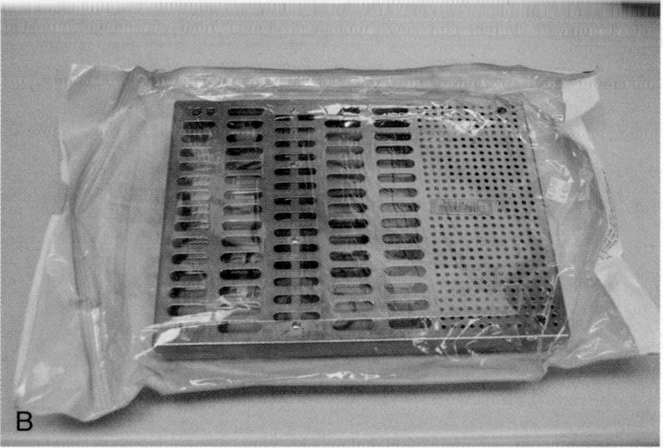


**FIG. 21.13** Instrument packing using a self-sealing, paper/plastic peel pouch. A, Packaged handpieces. B, Packaged instrument cassette. *(From Miller CH: Infection control and management of hazardous materials for the dental team, ed 6, St Louis, 2018, Elsevier.)*

of heat sterilization in the dental office are (1) steam sterilization, (2) chemical vapor sterilization, and (3) dry heat sterilization (Table 21.4).

Although most reusable items can withstand heat processing, a few plastic items, such as rubber dam frames, shade guides, and x-ray film–holding devices, may be damaged by heat. For such items, a liquid sterilant must be used. A liquid sterilant is not recommended for use on any item that can withstand heat sterilization or is disposable (Table 21.5).

## Steam Autoclave

An **autoclave** is used to sterilize dental instruments and other items by means of steam under pressure (Fig. 21.14). This involves heating water to generate steam to produce a moist heat that rapidly kills microorganisms. Autoclaves usually operate through four cycles: (1) heat-up cycle, (2) sterilizing cycle, (3) depressurization cycle, and (4) drying cycle.

As steam completely fills the sterilizing chamber, cooler air is pushed out of an escape valve, which then closes and allows pressure to increase. It is the heat, not the pressure, that actually kills the microorganisms. All autoclaves operate in a similar manner, but different manufacturers provide different features. Various sizes of chambers and mechanisms of air removal, steam generation, drying, temperature displays, and recording devices are available. Some manufacturers have added a presterilization vacuum cycle to their units to remove any air pockets from the chamber before steam enters the chamber. Other manufacturers provide several surges of steam to help force the air out before the sterilizing portion of the cycle begins. The temperature is maintained for the set time, usually ranging from 3 to 30 minutes (Table 21.6).

The autoclave is used for sterilization of a variety of dental instruments and accessories, including heat-resistant plastics, dental handpieces, instruments, cotton rolls, and gauze. Packaging material for steam sterilization must be porous enough to permit the steam to penetrate to the instruments inside. The packaging material may be fabric but most often consists of sealed film or paper pouches, nylon tubing, sterilizing wrap, or paper-wrapped cassettes.

Solid closed metal trays, capped glass vials, and aluminum foil cannot be used in an autoclave because they prevent the steam from reaching the inside of the pack.

See Procedure 21.2: Autoclaving Instruments.

### *Drying and Unloading Instruments*

To maintain sterility, it is important to allow the packages to dry while inside the steam sterilizer. Packages that are wet or damp can easily be torn or damaged. When wet or damp packages are allowed to dry outside of the sterilizer wicking can occur. **Wicking** is when bacteria from the air or contaminated surfaces are drawn through the wet packaging material and contaminates the instruments inside (Fig. 21.15).

## Flash Sterilization

Flash sterilization refers to sterilizing *unpackaged instruments* with the use of short exposure times. The disadvantage of this method of sterilization is that unwrapped instruments are no longer sterile once they are removed from the sterilizer and before they are used on the next patient.

Flash sterilization should be used only for instruments that are to be used promptly upon removal from the sterilizer. It is always the best policy to use a method of sterilization in which the instruments can be packaged before use and can remain packaged until the time of use.

**TABLE 21.4 Advantages and Disadvantages of Sterilization Methods**

| Method of Sterilization | Advantages | Disadvantages |
|---|---|---|
| Steam autoclave | Short time<br>No corrosion<br>Instruments dry quickly following cycle | Damages some plastic and rubber items<br>Requires use of distilled water<br>May rust non–stainless steel instruments and burs<br>Cannot use closed containers |
| Unsaturated chemical vapor | Short time<br>Good penetration of steam<br>Commonly used in dental offices | Instruments must be dry<br>Damages some plastic and rubber items<br>Requires special solution<br>Requires good ventilation<br>Cannot sterilize liquids<br>Cannot use closed containers<br>Cloth wrap may absorb chemicals |
| Dry heat oven type (static air) | No corrosion<br>Can use closed containers<br>Items are dry after cycle | Long sterilization time<br>Instruments must be predried<br>Damages some plastic and rubber items<br>Cannot sterilize liquids |
| Rapid heat transfer (forced air) | Very fast<br>No corrosion<br>Items are dry after cycle | Damages some plastic and rubber items<br>Instruments must be predried<br>Cannot sterilize liquids |

## TABLE 21.5 Sterilization and Disinfection Guide for Common Dental Items

| | Steam Autoclave | Dry Heat Oven | Chemiclave | Chemical Disinfection/ Sterilization | Disposable |
|---|---|---|---|---|---|
| Angle attachments | + | + | + | + | * |
| **Burs** | | | | | |
| Carbon steel | – | + | + | – | ++ |
| Steel | + | + | + | – | ++ |
| Tungsten-carbide | + | ++ | + | + | * |
| Condensers | ++ | ++ | ++ | + | * |
| Dappen dishes | ++ | + | + | + | * |
| **Endodontic Instruments** | | | | | |
| Broaches, files, reamers | + | ++ | ++ | –– | * |
| Non–stainless steel metal handles | –– | ++ | ++ | –– | * |
| Stainless steel handles | ++ | ++ | ++ | + | * |
| Stainless steel with plastic handles | – | – | – | + | * |
| **Fluoride Gel Trays** | | | | | |
| Heat-resistant plastic | ++ | –– | – | – | * |
| Non–heat-resistant plastic | | | | – | ++ |
| Glass slabs | ++ | ++ | ++ | + | * |
| **Hand Instruments** | | | | | |
| Carbon steel | – | ++ | ++ | – | * |
| Stainless steel | ++ | ++ | ++ | + | * |
| **Handpieces** | | | | | |
| Autoclavable | ++ | – | – | – | * |
| Contra-angles | – | – | – | + | * |
| Nonautoclavable | – | – | – | + | * |
| Prophylaxis angles | + | + | + | + | * |
| **Impression Trays** | | | | | |
| Aluminum metal: chrome-plated | ++ | ++ | ++ | + | * |
| Custom acrylic resin | –– | –– | –– | + | * |
| Plastic | –– | –– | –– | + | ++ |
| Instruments in packs | ++ | + | ++ | * | * |
| **Instrument Tray Setups** | | | | | |
| Restorative or surgical | + | + | + | * | * |
| Mirrors | – | ++ | ++ | + | * |
| Needles | –– | –– | –– | – | ++ |
| **Orthodontic Pliers** | | | | | |
| High-quality stainless steel | ++ | ++ | ++ | + | * |
| Low-quality stainless steel | – | ++ | ++ | – | * |
| With plastic parts | –– | –– | –– | + | * |
| Pluggers | ++ | ++ | ++ | + | * |
| **Polishing Wheels and Discs** | | | | | |
| Garnet and cuttle | –– | – | – | –– | + |
| Rag | ++ | – | + | –– | * |
| Rubber | + | – | – | + | + |
| **Prostheses, Removable** | | | | | |
| Rubber dam equipment | – | – | – | + | * |
| Carbon steel clamps | – | ++ | ++ | – | * |
| Metal frames | ++ | ++ | ++ | + | * |

*Continued*

TABLE 21.5 Sterilization and Disinfection Guide for Common Dental Items—cont'd

| | Steam Autoclave | Dry Heat Oven | Chemiclave | Chemical Disinfection/ Sterilization | Disposable |
|---|---|---|---|---|---|
| Plastic frames | – | –– | –– | + | * |
| Punches | – | ++ | ++ | + | * |
| **Radiographic Equipment** | | | | | |
| Plastic film holders | – | – | – | – | ++ |
| Collimating devices | –– | –– | –– | + | * |
| **Rubber Items** | | | | | |
| Prophylaxis cups | + | – | – | + | ++ |
| **Saliva Evacuators, Ejectors** | | | | | |
| High-melting plastic | ++ | + | + | + | * |
| Low-melting plastic | – | – | – | + | ++ |
| Stainless steel clamps | ++ | ++ | ++ | + | * |
| **Stones** | | | | | |
| Diamond | + | ++ | ++ | + | * |
| Polishing | ++ | + | ++ | – | * |
| Sharpening | ++ | ++ | ++ | – | * |
| **Surgical Instruments** | | | | | |
| Stainless steel | ++ | ++ | ++ | + | * |
| Ultrasonic scaling tips | + | –– | –– | + | * |

From Samaranayake LP: Essential microbiology for dentistry, ed 4, New York, 2012, Churchill Livingstone.

+, Effective and preferred method; ++, effective and acceptable method; –, effective method, but risk of damage to materials; ––, ineffective method with risk of damage to materials; *, not applicable.

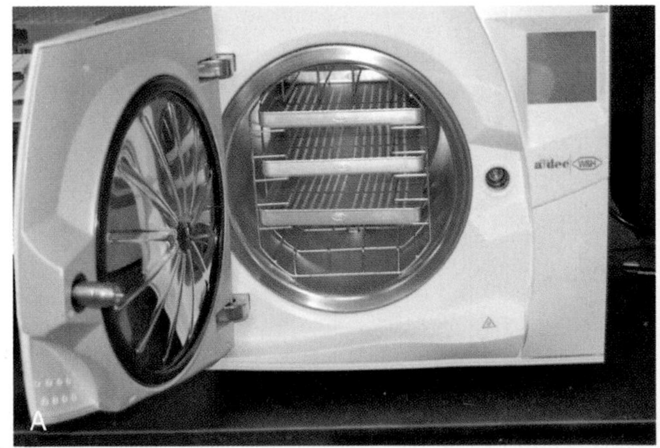

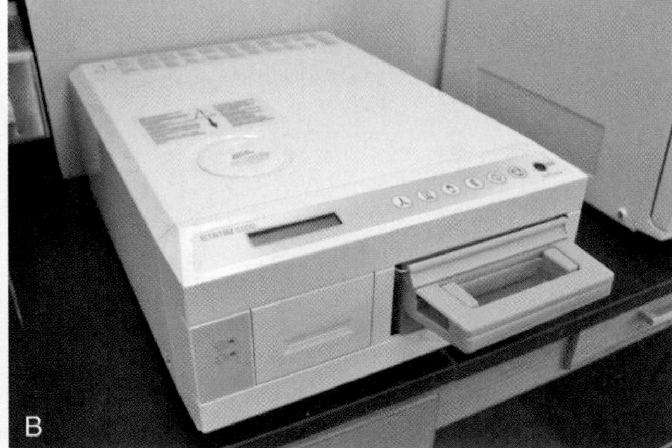

**FIG. 21.14** Examples of steam sterilizers. A, Unit with cylindrical chamber. B, Unit with a removable chamber (cassette). *(From Miller CH: Infection control and management of hazardous materials for the dental team, ed 6, St Louis, 2018, Elsevier.)*

## Unsaturated Chemical Vapor Sterilization

Unsaturated **chemical vapor sterilization** is very similar to autoclaving, except that a combination of chemicals (alcohol, formaldehyde, ketone, acetone, and water) is used instead of water to create a vapor for sterilizing (Fig. 21.16 and see Procedure 21.3: Sterilizing Instruments with Unsaturated Chemical Vapor). OSHA requires a **Safety Data Sheet** (SDS) on the chemical vapor solution because of the toxicity of the chemicals (see Chapter 23).

### Advantages

The major advantage of the chemical vapor sterilizer is that it does not rust, dull, or corrode dry metal instruments.

**TABLE 21.6** Typical Steam Temperatures in Sterilizing Cycle

| Temperature | Time |
|---|---|
| 250° F (121° C) | 30 minutes |
| 250° F (121° C) | 15 minutes |
| 273° F (134° C) | 10 minutes |
| 273° F (134° C) | 3 minutes |

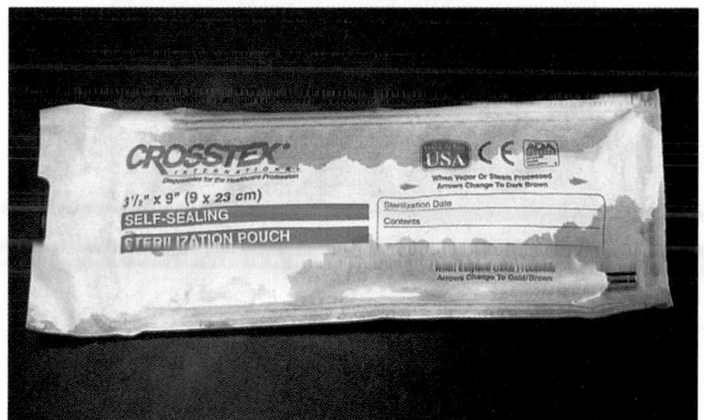


**FIG. 21.15** A package that was taken out of the steam sterilizer before it was dry. Note the tear allowing an instrument to protrude and breach sterility. *(From Miller CH: Infection control and management of hazardous materials for the dental team, ed 6, St Louis, 2018, Elsevier.)*

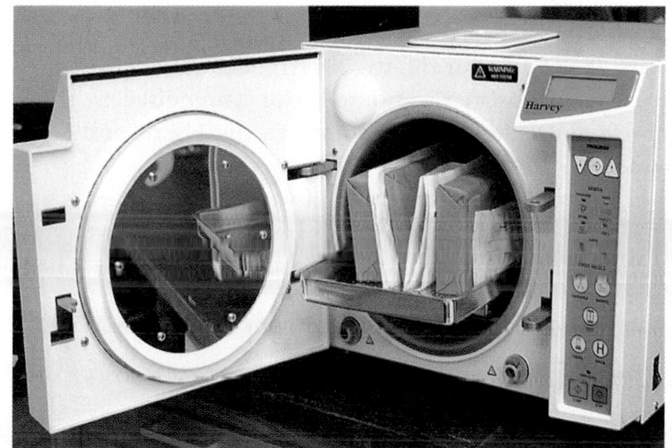


**FIG. 21.16** The unsaturated chemical vapor sterilizer. *(From Miller CH: Infection control and management of hazardous materials for the dental team, ed 6, St Louis, 2018, Elsevier.)*

The low water content of the vapor prevents destruction of items such as endodontic files, orthodontic pliers, wires, bands, and burs. A wide range of items can be sterilized routinely without damage. Other advantages include the short cycle time and the availability of a dry instrument after the cycle.

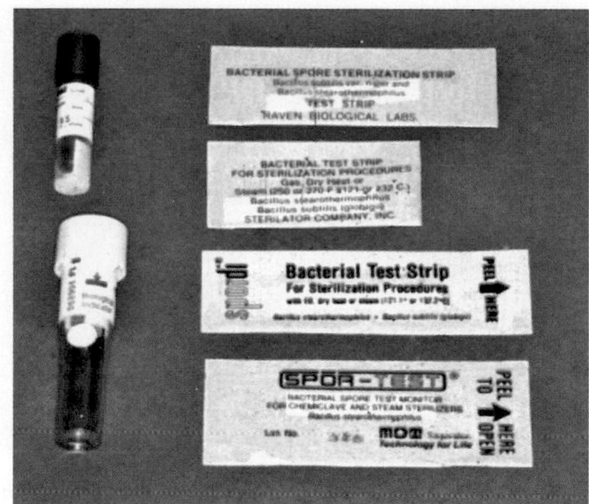


**FIG. 21.17** Chemical vapor sterilant. *(From Miller CH: Infection control and management of hazardous materials for the dental team, ed 6, St Louis, 2018, Elsevier.)*

### Disadvantages

The primary disadvantage is that adequate ventilation is essential because residual chemical vapors containing formaldehyde and methyl alcohol can be released when the chamber door is opened at the end of the cycle. These vapors can temporarily leave an unpleasant odor in the area and may be irritating to the eyes. An improved formula in some products has reduced the odor-causing agents (Fig. 21.17).

### Filtration and Monitoring of Chemical Vapors

Newer sterilizers are equipped with a special filtration device that reduces the amount of chemical vapor remaining in the chamber at the end of the cycle. Older models usually can be retrofitted.

*Formaldehyde monitoring badges,* similar to radiation monitoring devices, also are available for employees. The monitoring badge measures personal exposure to formaldehyde for a specified period; the badge is mailed to the monitoring service, and a laboratory analysis is sent to the employee.

### Packaging

Standard packaging for chemical vapor sterilization includes film pouches or paper bags, nylon see-through tubing, sterilization wrap, and wrapped cassettes. Thick or tightly wrapped items require longer exposure because unsaturated chemical vapors are unable to penetrate as well as saturated chemical vapors under pressure.

As in autoclaving, closed containers (such as solid metal trays and capped glass vials) and aluminum foil *cannot* be used in a chemical vapor sterilizer because they prevent the sterilizing agent from reaching the instruments inside.

### Pressure, Temperature, and Time

The three major factors involved in chemical vapor sterilization consist of (1) pressure, which should measure 20 psi; (2) temperature, which should measure 270° F (131° C); and (3) time, which should measure 20 to 40 minutes.

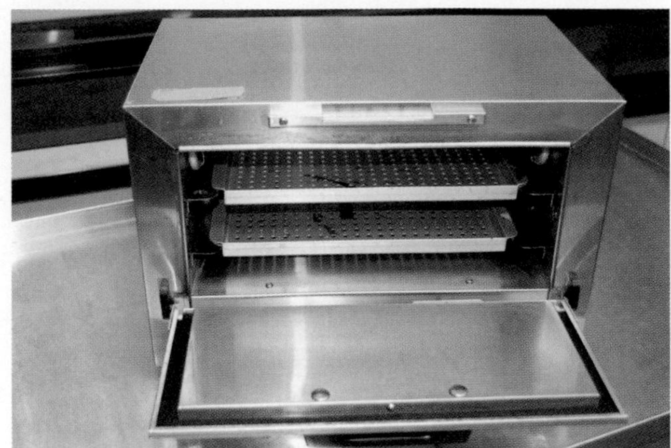

FIG. 21.18 Example of a static air dry heat sterilizer. *(From Miller CH: Infection control and management of hazardous materials for the dental team, ed 6, St Louis, 2018, Elsevier.)*

## Dry Heat Sterilization

**Dry heat sterilizers** operate by heating up air and transferring that heat from the air to the instruments. This form of sterilization requires higher temperatures than are required for steam or chemical vapor sterilization. Dry heat sterilizers operate at approximately 320° F to 375° F (160° C to 190° C) and operate for variable lengths of time, depending on the manufacturer's instructions. See Procedure 21.4: Sterilizing Instruments with Dry Heat.

The advantage of dry heat is that the instruments will not rust *if* they are thoroughly dry before they are placed in the sterilizer. Two types of dry heat sterilizers that are currently available are *static air* and *forced air.*

### Static Air Sterilizers

Static air sterilizers are similar to an oven: The heating coils are on the bottom of the chamber, and the hot air rises inside through natural convection. Heat is transferred from the *static* (nonmoving) air to the instruments in about 1 to 2 hours. Disadvantages of static dry heat are that (1) the sterilization process is time consuming, and (2) it may not be effective if the operatory makes errors in calculating the optimum processing time. The wrapping material must be heat resistant. Aluminum foil, metal, and glass containers may be used. Paper and cloth packs should be avoided because they may burn or discolor as a result of the intense heat (Fig. 21.18).

### Forced Air Sterilizers

Forced air sterilizers, also called *rapid heat transfer sterilizers,* circulate hot air throughout the chamber at a high velocity. This action permits rapid transfer of heat energy from the air to the instruments, reducing the time needed for sterilization. Exposure time in forced air sterilizers, after the sterilizing temperature has been reached, ranges from 6 minutes for unpackaged items to 12 minutes for packaged items (Fig. 21.19).

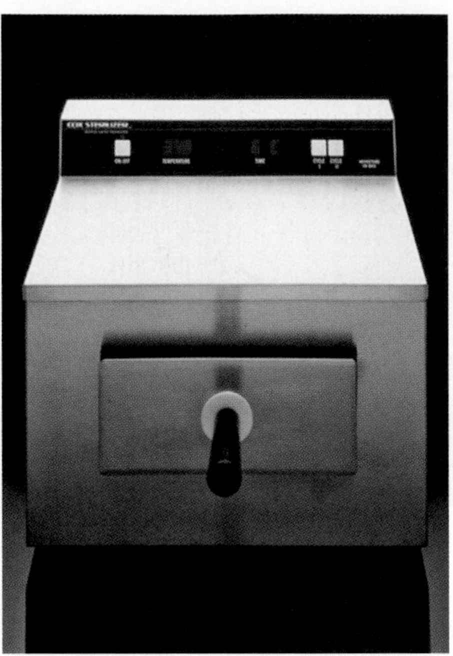

FIG. 21.19 Example of a forced-air rapid heat dry heat sterilizer. *(From Miller CH: Infection control and management of hazardous materials for the dental team, ed 6, St Louis, 2018, Elsevier.)*

## Ethylene Oxide Sterilization

Ethylene oxide gas is a recognized method of sterilization. This method is performed at low temperatures, which offers an advantage for plastic and rubber items that would melt in heat sterilizers.

However, ethylene oxide sterilization requires 4 to 12 hours, depending on the sterilizer model used. Also, at least 16 hours of poststerilization aeration is required to remove the gas molecules that are bound to the plastic and rubber surfaces.

Ethylene oxide is ineffective on wet items. Toxicity is a risk if the gas is not handled properly. These units are used often in large clinics or in hospital settings but rarely in private dental practices.

## Liquid Chemical Sterilants

Not all items can withstand heat sterilization. Some types of plastics, such as some rubber dam frames, shade guides, and x-ray film–holding devices, are damaged by heat sterilization. Thus a liquid sterilant such as 2 to 3.4 percent glutaraldehyde must be used for sterilization of these items (see Procedure 21.5: Sterilizing Instruments with Liquid Chemical Sterilants). Sterilization in glutaraldehyde requires a 10-hour contact time; anything shorter than 10 hours is disinfection, *not* sterilization (Fig. 21.20).

Be sure that you have an SDS for these products. All employees should be properly trained on how to handle such materials.

## Liquid Chemical Sterilants/ High-Level Disinfectants CDC

- When a liquid chemical germicide is used for sterilization, certain poststerilization procedures are essential: (1) Rinse with sterile water after removal to remove toxic or irritating residues, (2) handle with sterile gloves and dry with sterile towels, and (3) deliver to the point of use in an aseptic manner.
- If stored before use, the instrument should not be considered sterile and should be sterilized again just before use. The sterilization process with liquid chemical sterilant cannot be verified with biologic indicators.
- In addition, these products must be used full strength (not diluted) on precleaned instruments. Liquid sterilants may *not* be used as surface disinfectants because of the toxicity of the fumes. (Category IB)

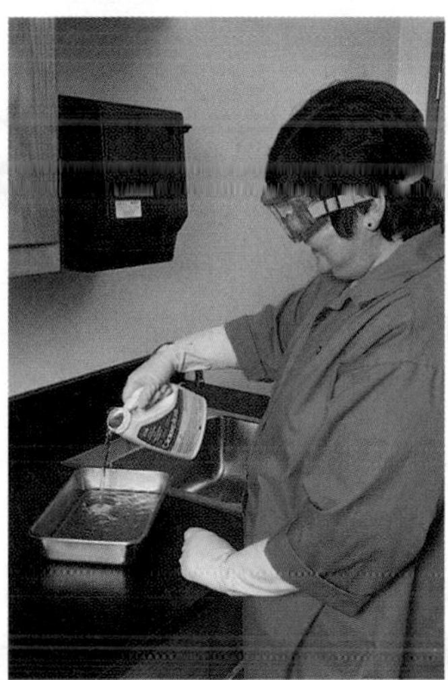

**FIG. 21.20** Preparing the high-level disinfectant/sterilizer, used for immersion of instruments that cannot tolerate heat sterilization. *(From Bonewit-West K, Hunt SA, Applegate E: Today's medical assistant: clinical & administrative procedures, ed 3, St Louis, 2016, Elsevier.)*

RECALL

12 What are the most common forms of heat sterilization?
13 What is a primary disadvantage of flash sterilization?
14 What is a major advantage of chemical vapor sterilization?
15 What are the two types of dry heat sterilization?
16 What is the primary disadvantage of liquid chemical sterilization?
17 How should instruments processed in a liquid chemical sterilant be rinsed?

## Sterilization Failures

A load may fail to become sterilized when direct contact for the required time between the sterilizing agent (chemical or steam) and all surfaces of the items being processed is insufficient. Several factors can cause the sterilization process to fail, including improper instrument cleaning or packaging and sterilizer malfunction (Table 21.7).

The monitoring service will generally report a sterilization failure *(positive result)* to the dental office immediately by phone. (A positive report indicates that sterilization did *not* occur.) If the culture is negative *(negative result),* the monitoring service will mail a report to the dental office to document that the cultures were read at 24, 48, and 72 hours. (A negative report indicates that sterilization *did* occur.) See Procedure 21.6: Following a Sterilization Failure.

## Sterilization Monitoring

It is critical that dental instruments are properly sterilized. Because microorganisms cannot be seen with the naked eye, the major difficulty associated with sterilization is determining *when* an item is sterile.

**TABLE 21.7** Results of Sterilization Errors

| Errors | Examples | Results |
|---|---|---|
| Inadequate instrument cleaning | Dried blood and/or cement remains on instruments | Organisms may be insulated from sterilizing agents. |
| Improper packaging | Excessive wrap (too thick) | Prevents sterilizing agent from reaching instruments. |
| | Packaging material is not compatible with type of sterilizer | Wrap may melt or sterilizing agent may not penetrate wrap. |
| | Closed container in chemical vapor or autoclave | Sterilizing agent cannot reach inside surfaces. |
| Improper loading of sterilizer | Overloading | Increases time to reach proper temperature and can slow the penetration to the center of the load. |
| | No separation between packages (too close together) | May prevent sterilizing agent from reaching all items and surfaces. |
| Improper timing | Operator error in timing | Insufficient time to sterilize. |
| | Timing started before reaching proper temperature (in nonautomatic units) | Insufficient time to sterilize. |
| | Dry heat sterilizer door opened during cycle without restarting time | Insufficient time to sterilize. |
| Improper temperature | Error in operation of sterilizer | Insufficient heat to sterilize. |
| | Malfunction of sterilizer | Insufficient heat to sterilize. |

In the early days of sterilization, a raw potato sometimes was placed in the sterilizer with the instruments and was examined later to see whether it was cooked. If the potato was cooked, the load was considered sterile. As sterilization processes became more sophisticated, more scientific monitoring practices replaced the potato.

Currently, three forms of sterilization monitoring are used: *physical, chemical,* and *biologic.* All three processes are unique, have different functions, and must be used consistently to ensure sterility.

## CDC Guidelines for Sterilization Monitoring

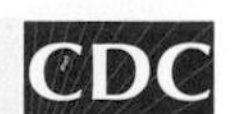


- Use mechanical, chemical, and biologic monitors according to the manufacturer's instructions to ensure the effectiveness of the sterilization process. (Category IB)
- Monitor each load with mechanical (e.g., time, temperature, pressure) and chemical indicators. (Category II)
- Place a chemical indicator on the inside of each package. If the internal indicator is not visible from the outside, also place an exterior chemical indicator on the package. (Category II)
- Place items/packages correctly and loosely into the sterilizer so as not to impede penetration of the sterilant. (Category IB)
- Do not use instrument packs if mechanical or chemical indicators indicate inadequate processing.
- Monitor sterilizers at least weekly by using a biologic indicator with a matching control (e.g., biologic indicator and control from the same lot number). (Category IB)
- Use a biologic indicator for every sterilizer load that contains an implantable device. Verify results before using the implantable device, whenever possible. (Category IB)
- Maintain sterilization records (i.e., mechanical, chemical, and biologic) in compliance with state and local regulations. (Category I)

## Physical Monitoring

Physical monitoring of the sterilization process involves looking at the gauges and readings on the sterilizer and recording the temperatures, pressure, and exposure time. Although correct readings do not guarantee sterilization, an incorrect reading gives you the first signal of a problem.

Remember that the temperature recorded is for the chamber, *not* for the inside of the pack. Therefore problems with overloading or improper packaging would not be detected from readings on the gauges.

## Chemical Monitoring

Chemical monitoring (external and internal) involves the use of a heat-sensitive chemical that changes color when exposed to certain conditions. The two types of chemical indicators are process indicators and process integrators.

### Process Indicators

Process indicators (external) are placed *outside* of instrument packages before sterilization. Examples include autoclave tape and color-change markings on packages or bags (Fig. 21.21).

**Process indicators** simply identify instrument packs that have been exposed to a certain temperature; they *do not* measure the duration or the pressure. Process indicators are also known as **single-parameter indicators.** Process indicators are useful in distinguishing between packages that were processed and those that were not processed. They can be used to prevent accidental use of unprocessed instruments.

### Process Integrators

**Process integrators** (internal) are placed *inside* instrument packages. They respond to a combination of pressure, temperature, and time. Process integrators are also known as **multiparameter indicators.** All sterilization factors are *integrated* (Fig. 21.22).

Examples of process integrators include strips, tabs, and tubes of colored liquid. The advantage of placing integrators

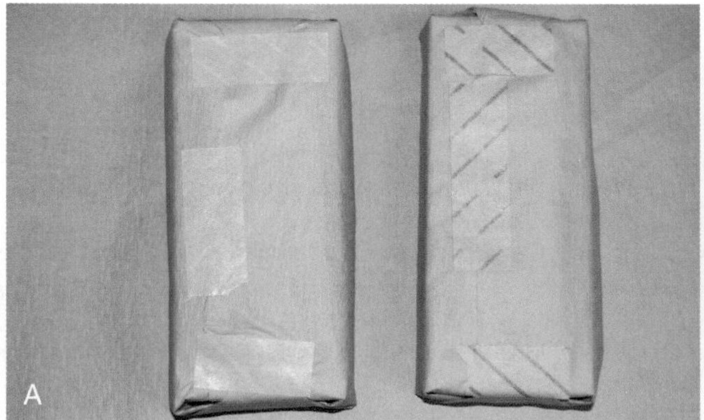


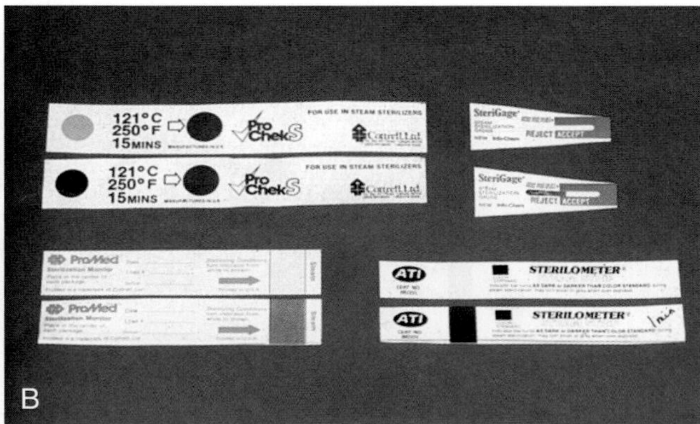


**FIG. 21.21** Examples of chemical indicators. A, Autoclave tape before being heat processed (left), and autoclave tape after being heat processed (right). B, Other chemical indicators. The top of each pair shows appearance before being heat processed, and the bottom shows the color change after heat processing. *(From Miller CH: Infection control and management of hazardous materials for the dental team, ed 6, St Louis, 2018, Elsevier.)*

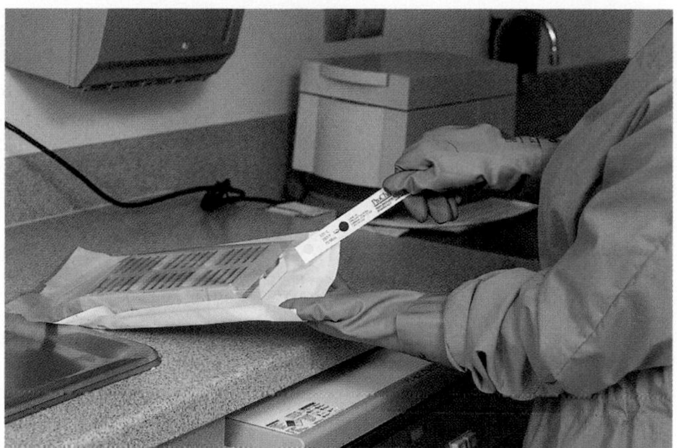

FIG. 21.22 The dental assistant inserts the integrator strip into the sterilization pouch with the instruments.

inside each package is that penetration of the packaging by the sterilizing agent is ensured.

### Limitations

Process indicators and integrators provide immediate, visual control of sterilizing conditions. They *do not indicate sterility* and are not a replacement for biologic monitoring.

## Biologic Monitoring

**Biologic monitoring**, or *spore testing,* is the only way to determine whether sterilization has occurred and to confirm that all bacteria and **endospores** have been killed. The CDC, the American Dental Association (ADA), and the Organization for Safety, Asepsis and Prevention (OSAP) recommend at least *weekly* biologic monitoring of sterilization equipment.

Several states also require routine biologic monitoring at weekly, monthly, or cycle-specific intervals, such as spore testing after every 40 hours of use or every 30 days, whichever comes first. (Check the requirements in your state.) In addition to the recommended weekly guidelines, biologic monitoring should be done at other times. See Procedure 21.7: Performing Biologic Monitoring.

**Biologic indicators** (BIs), also known as *spore tests,* are vials or strips of paper that contain harmless bacterial spores (spores are highly resistant to heat).

Three BIs are used in testing. Two BIs are placed inside instrument packs, and the sterilizer is operated under normal conditions. The third strip is set aside as a control.

After the load has been sterilized, all BIs are cultured. If the spores survive the sterilization cycle *(a positive culture),* a sterilization failure has occurred. If the spores are killed *(a negative culture),* the sterilization cycle was successful.

Culturing of the spore test is usually handled through the use of a mail-in monitoring service (Fig. 21.23). If in-office culturing is done, the manufacturer's instructions must be followed carefully to prevent errors (Fig. 21.24).

You must use the type of BI that is compatible with the method of sterilization you are using. Spores used to test the steam autoclave and the chemical vapor sterilizer are different from bacteria used to test dry heat and ethylene oxide sterilizers. *Dual-species* BIs contain spores of both organisms and can be used with dry heat, ethylene oxide, autoclave, or chemical vapor sterilization.

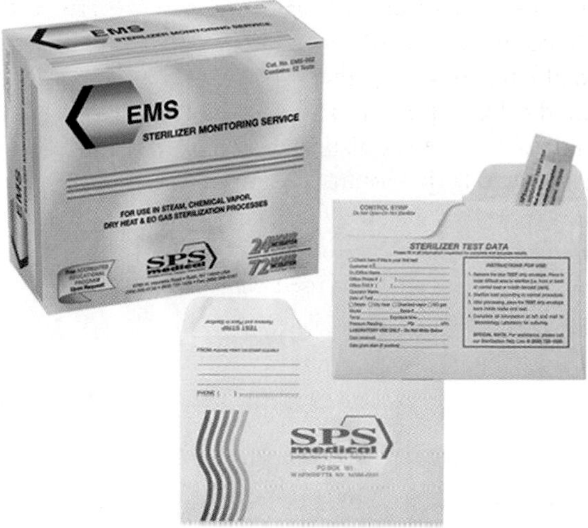


FIG. 21.23 Use of a mail-in service is a convenient method of biologic monitoring. *(Courtesy SPS Medical Supply Corp., Rush, NY.)*

### Additional Reasons for Biologic Monitoring

CDC

- Once each week, as recommended by the CDC, ADA, and OSAP
- After the sterilizer has been serviced, to verify proper functioning
- When you change packaging materials, to be sure the sterilizing agent is reaching the instruments
- After an electrical or power source failure, to verify proper functioning of the sterilizer
- After training new employees, to be sure they are following proper procedures
- For all cycles that contain any device to be implanted*

*ADA,* American Dental Association; *CDC,* Centers for Disease Control and Prevention; *OSAP,* Organization for Safety, Asepsis and Prevention.

* The implant should not be placed until sterilization has been biologically monitored.

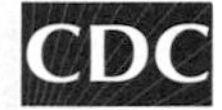


18 What causes sterilization failure?
19 What are the three forms of sterilization monitoring?
20 What is a process indicator, and where is it placed?
21 What is a process integrator, and where is it placed?
22 Do process indicators and integrators ensure that an item is sterile?
23 What is the best way to determine whether sterilization has occurred?

## Handpiece Sterilization

High-speed dental handpieces rotate at speeds up to 400,000 revolutions per minute. Blood, saliva, and tooth fragments,

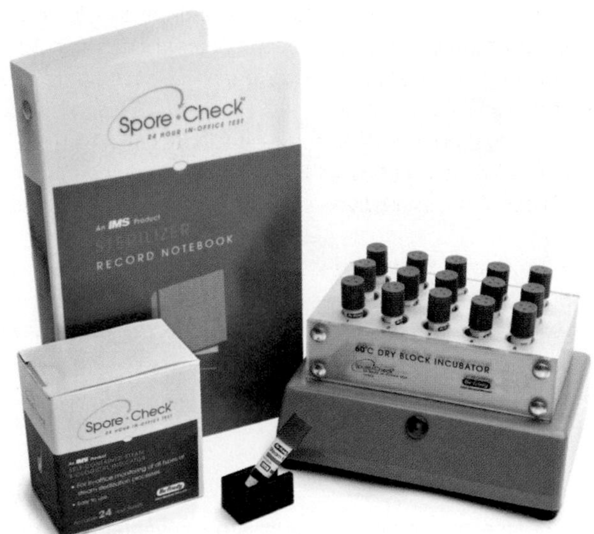


**FIG. 21.24** In-office biologic monitoring system.

as well as restorative materials, may lodge in the head of the handpiece, where they may be retained and transferred to another patient. Therefore dental handpieces must be properly cleaned and heat-sterilized according to the manufacturer's recommendations. See Procedure 21.8: Sterilizing the Dental Handpiece.

## Flushing Techniques

The life expectancy of the dental handpiece depends on its frequency of use and how it is used and maintained. If debris is not removed before heat sterilization, it will bake onto the turbine and bearings. Flushing the handpiece is the best way to remove debris from the head of the handpiece.

To flush a dental handpiece, attach a pressurized handpiece cleaner to the intake tube of the handpiece (where the air passes through), and flush the head of the handpiece to remove debris. Afterward, blow out the handpiece using compressed air to remove debris before sterilization. Most handpieces should not be run without a bur in place (see Chapter 35).

Running coolant water from the dental unit through the handpiece at chairside is insufficient. Coolant water does not run through the turbine chamber, where debris can collect.

## Sterilizing Techniques

Only steam sterilization and chemical vapor sterilizers are recommended, because handpiece sterilization temperatures should not exceed 275° F (135° C). Unless they will be used immediately after sterilization, handpieces should be packaged in bags, wraps, or packs to protect them from contamination before use.

Never run a handpiece "hot" out of the sterilizer, and avoid rapid cool-downs, such as running the handpiece under cold water. Handpieces use very small metal components; extreme cold changes stress the metal.

### Storage Area for Sterilized Items and Clean Dental Supplies

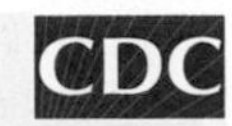


The storage area should provide enclosed storage for sterile items and disposable (single-use) items. Storage practices for wrapped sterilized instruments can be date or event related. Event-related packaging means that it is assumed the contents will remain sterile indefinitely unless some event (e.g., a torn or wet package) occurs to contaminate the contents. For event-related packaging, minimally, the date of sterilization should be placed on the package, and if multiple sterilizers are used in the facility, the sterilizer used should be indicated on the outside of the packaging material. If packaging is compromised, the instruments should be recleaned, packaged in a new wrap, and sterilized again. (Category IB)

Clean supplies and instruments should be stored in closed or covered cabinets, if possible. Dental supplies and instruments should not be stored under sinks or in other locations where they might become wet. (Category II)

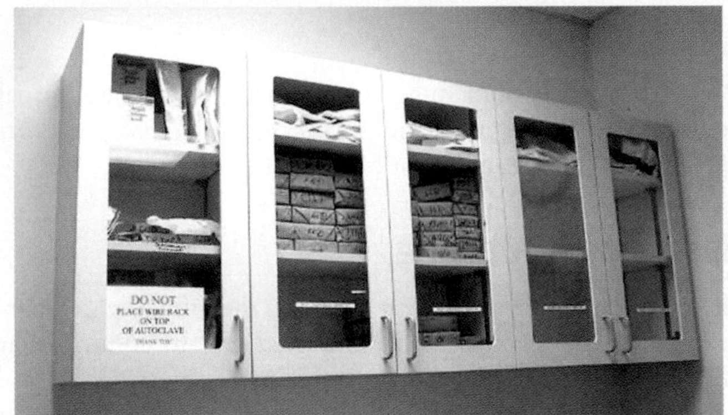


Instruments and supplies stored in a closed cabinet.

RECALL

24 How should high-speed handpieces be processed before sterilization?
25 What types of heat sterilization are appropriate for high-speed handpieces?
26 What does event-related packaging mean?
27 How should clean supplies and instruments be stored?

■ **Legal and Ethical Implications** The CDC *Guidelines for Infection Control in Dental Health-Care Settings—2003* were written to protect patients and members of the dental healthcare team from transmission of disease in the dental office. The Occupational Safety and Health Administration (OSHA) Blood-Borne Pathogens Standard requires biologic monitoring of sterilizers and maintenance of records of the results. In addition, many states have adopted infection control regulations that are based on the CDC *Guidelines for Infection Control.*

As a dental assistant, you are legally and ethically responsible for performing the procedures described in this chapter in a thorough and careful manner. Remember, proper instrument processing is necessary to prevent the transfer of microorganisms from a previous patient to the next patient or to you. ■

**■ Eye to the Future** Visible light, ionizing radiation, microwave radiation, and ultraviolet (UV) rays are among the technologies that are being studied and applied in the areas of disinfection and sterilization. Presently, *ionizing radiation* technology is being used in sterilization of heat-sensitive items and in food processing, thus reducing the number of foodborne illnesses.

*UV lamps* are used in surgical or inoculating hoods to reduce the numbers of microorganisms on surfaces. In the future, a light approved by the U.S. Food and Drug Administration may destroy aerosols in dental operatories and may sterilize all surfaces as well. ■

## ■ Critical Thinking

1. The dentist you work with is building a new dental office with all new equipment. She asks you to plan, design, and equip the instrument-processing area. What factors should you consider about the physical layout? What pieces of equipment should you order? What supplies will you want to have available?
2. You receive a phone call from the sterilization monitoring company informing you that the last spore test you sent in has failed. What should you check to determine the possible cause?
3. Your friend who is not a dental assistant asks why you have to follow the CDC *Guidelines for Infection Control in Dental Health-Care Settings—2003* if these guidelines are not laws. How would you answer your friend? ■

PROCEDURE 21.1 

# Operating the Ultrasonic Cleaner

### GOAL

To prepare and use effectively the ultrasonic cleaner

### EQUIPMENT AND SUPPLIES

- ✓ Ultrasonic cleaning unit
- ✓ Instruments
- ✓ Ultrasonic solution
- ✓ Clean towel

### PROCEDURAL STEPS

**1** Put on protective clothing, mask, eyewear, and utility gloves.

**PURPOSE** You will be handling sharp, contaminated instruments and using a chemical ultrasonic solution that could splash in your eyes.

**2** Remove the lid from the container.

**PURPOSE** The lid should remain on the ultrasonic device when not in use to prevent evaporation of the solution and to minimize airborne contamination.

**3** Be certain the container has been filled with solution to the level recommended by the manufacturer.

**PURPOSE** The instruments that are being cleaned must be completely submerged in the solution.

**4** Place loose instruments in the basket, or, if using cassettes, place the cassette in the basket.

**5** Replace the lid, and turn the cycle to "On." The time of the cycle may vary depending on the efficiency of the ultrasonic unit. The time ranges from 5 to 15 minutes.

**PURPOSE** Instruments in resin or plastic cassettes require longer cleaning times because resin and plastic absorb some of the ultrasonic energy.

**6** After the cleaning cycle, remove the basket and thoroughly rinse the instruments in a sink under tap water with minimal splashing. Hold the basket at an angle to allow water to run off into the sink to minimize splashing.

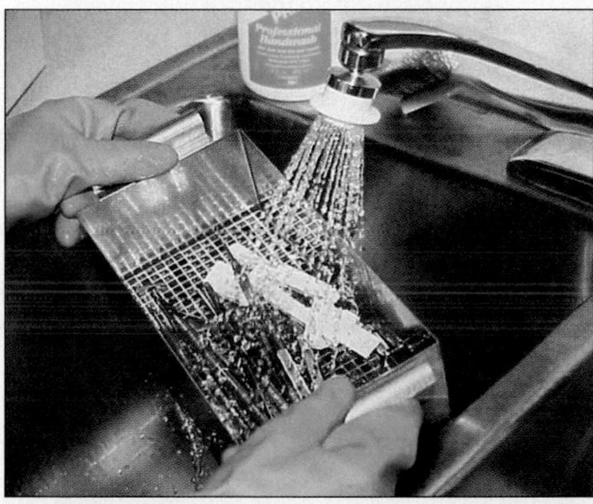

**7** Gently turn the basket onto a towel, and remove the instruments or cassettes. Replace the lid on the ultrasonic cleaner.

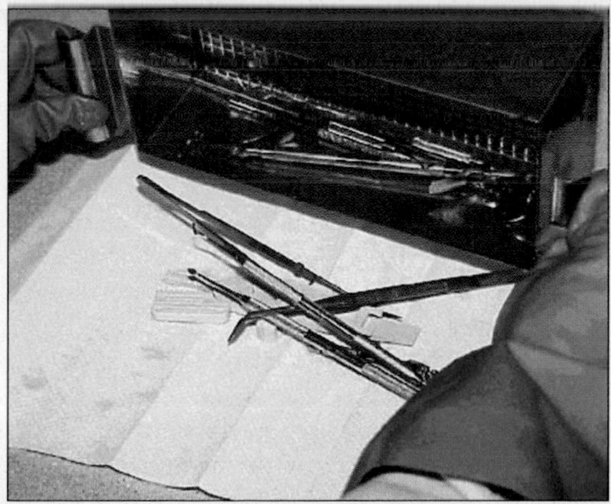

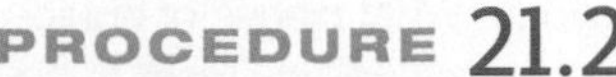
PROCEDURE 21.2

# Autoclaving Instruments

## GOAL

To prepare and use autoclave instruments

## EQUIPMENT AND SUPPLIES

- ✓ Appropriate personal protective equipment (PPE)
- ✓ Autoclaving wrapping materials
- ✓ Process integrator
- ✓ Corrosion inhibitor solution (1 percent sodium nitrate)
- ✓ Tape to seal packages
- ✓ Pen or pencil to label packages
- ✓ Oven mitt

## PROCEDURAL STEPS

1 Instruments must be clean, but not necessarily dry, before they are wrapped for autoclaving.

**NOTE** Exceptions are glass slabs and dishes, rubber items, and stones. These objects must be dry before they are autoclaved.

2 Nonstainless instruments and burs may be dipped in a corrosion inhibitor solution (1 percent sodium nitrate) before they are wrapped.

**NOTE** An alternative for these instruments is sterilization by dry heat.

3 Insert the process integrator into the package.

4 Package, seal, and label the instruments.

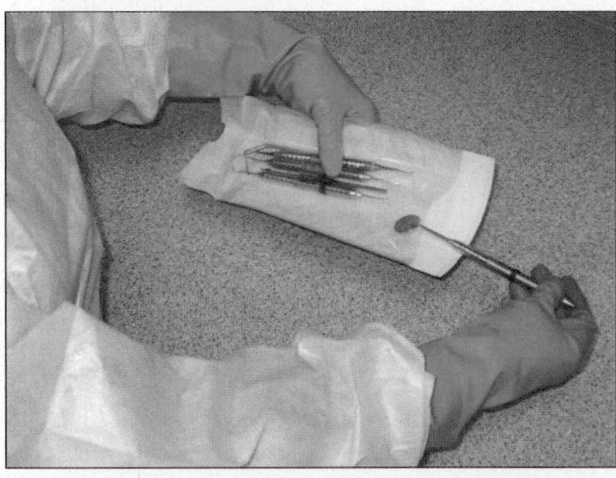

## LOAD THE AUTOCLAVE

5 Place bagged and sealed items in the autoclave.

6 Separate articles and packs from each other by a reasonable space. Tilt glass or metal canisters at an angle.

**PURPOSE** To permit a free flow of steam within and around all instrument packs.

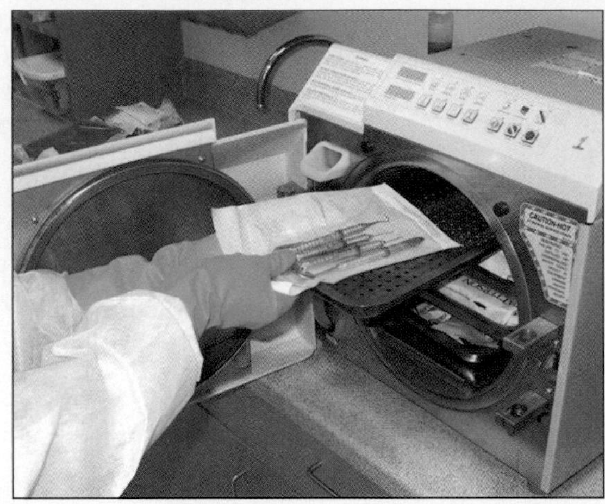

7 Place larger packs, which might block the flow of steam, at the bottom of the chamber.

**PURPOSE** Large loads prevent the autoclave from reaching the correct temperature and pressure and make it difficult for the steam to flow properly.

8 Never overload the autoclave.

**PURPOSE** Trapped air in the autoclave will inhibit the top-to-bottom flow of steam.

## OPERATE THE AUTOCLAVE

9 Read and follow the manufacturer's instructions. Most autoclaves require distilled water.

**PURPOSE** Tap water often contains minerals that can damage the autoclave by forming deposits on the chamber's inner surfaces, and that can corrode metals.

10 Ensure that an adequate supply of water is available. If not, add distilled water.

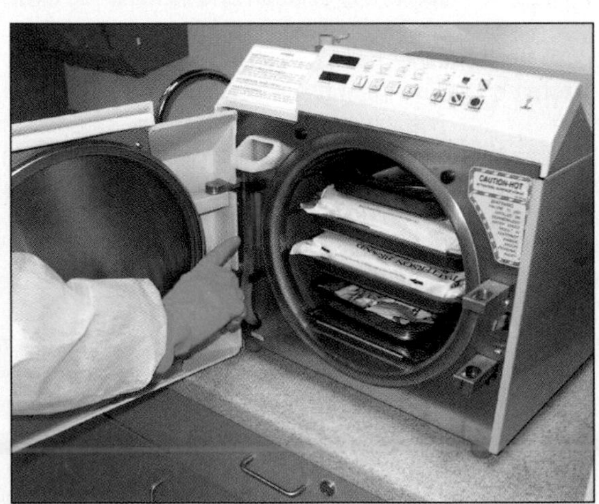

## PROCEDURE 21.2 Autoclaving Instruments–cont'd

11 Set autoclave controls for the appropriate time, temperature, and pressure.

**NOTE** Pressure and temperature must be reached before timing begins. Duration of this warm-up time depends on the autoclave and the size of the load.

12 At the end of the sterilization cycle, vent the steam into the room. Allow the contents of the autoclave to dry and cool.

**NOTE** Most models vent and cool automatically. If the machine is not so equipped, open the door of the autoclave slightly after the pressure has dropped within the chamber. Do this with *extreme caution* because the contents and remaining steam are scalding. The contents should be allowed to dry and cool before they are removed.

### REASSEMBLE AND STORE THE TRAYS

13 Wash your hands and put on clean examination gloves for handling sterile packs and reassembling trays.

14 Remove sealed packs from the sterilizer, and place them in the clean area.

**IMPORTANT NOTE** Work only in the clean area of the sterilization center.

15 Place the sealed packs on the tray, and add the supplies necessary to perform the procedure.

**OPTIONAL** In some practices, the necessary gloves and masks are added to the tray at this time. In other practices, these items are stored in the treatment room.

16 Store the prepared tray in the clean area until it is needed in the treatment room.

## PROCEDURE 21.3

# Sterilizing Instruments with Unsaturated Chemical Vapor

### GOAL

To prepare and sterilize instruments by chemical vapor sterilization

### EQUIPMENT AND SUPPLIES

- ✔ Appropriate personal protective equipment (PPE)
- ✔ Chemical vapor wrapping materials
- ✔ Precleaned and dried instruments
- ✔ Process integrator
- ✔ Tape to seal packages
- ✔ Pen or pencil to label packages

### PROCEDURAL STEPS

#### Wrap the Instruments

1 Ensure that the instruments are clean and *dry* before wrapping them for chemical vapor sterilization.

**PURPOSE** If instruments are not absolutely dry, they will rust.

2 Insert the appropriate process integrator into the test load instrument package.

3 Take care not to create packs that are too large to be sterilized throughout.

**PURPOSE** Chemical vapor sterilization is not recommended for large loads or tightly wrapped instruments.

#### Load and Operate the Chemical Vapor Sterilizer

4 Read and follow the manufacturer's instructions.

**IMPORTANT NOTE** Always follow the precautions in the Safety Data Sheet (SDS).

5 Load the sterilizer according to the manufacturer's instructions.

**NOTE** This step is similar to loading an autoclave.

6 Set the controls for the appropriate time, temperature, and pressure.

**NOTE** Pressure and temperature must be reached before timing begins.

7 Follow the manufacturer's instructions for venting and cooling.

8 When the instruments are cool and dry, reassemble and store the preset tray.

PROCEDURE 21.4

# Sterilizing Instruments with Dry Heat

## GOAL

To prepare and sterilize instruments by dry heat sterilization

## EQUIPMENT AND SUPPLIES

- ✓ Wrapping materials
- ✓ Precleaned instruments
- ✓ Process integrator for dry heat
- ✓ Tape to seal packages
- ✓ Pen or pencil to label packages

## PROCEDURAL STEPS

### Wrap Instruments

1 Clean and dry instruments before wrapping.

**PURPOSE** Wet instruments can rust during dry heat sterilization.

2 Prepare hinged instruments, such as surgical forceps, hemostats, and scissors, with their hinges opened.

**PURPOSE** To allow heat to reach all areas during sterilization.

### Load and Operate the Dry Heat Sterilizer

3 Read and follow the manufacturer's instructions.

4 Insert the process integrator into the test load package.

5 Load the dry heat chamber to permit adequate circulation of air around the packages.

**PURPOSE** Sterilization does not occur unless heat reaches all areas of the instruments.

6 Set the time and temperature according to the manufacturer's instructions. Allow time for the entire load to reach the desired temperature.

**PURPOSE** Timing does not start until the desired temperature has been reached throughout the entire load.

7 Do not place additional instruments in the load once the sterilization cycle has begun.

**PURPOSE** Cooler instruments will significantly lower the temperature of the oven.

8 At the end of the sterilization cycle, allow the packs to cool, then handle them very carefully.

**PURPOSE** Packs are very hot and could cause injury.

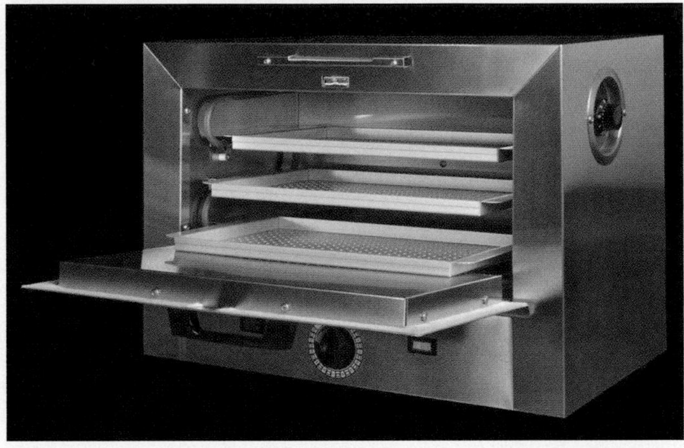

Courtesy Wayne Metal Products Inc., Sanford, FL.

9 When the packs are cool, reassemble and store the preset tray.

PROCEDURE 21.5

# Sterilizing Instruments with Liquid Chemical Sterilants

## GOAL

To prepare and sterilize instruments with a chemical sterilant

## EQUIPMENT AND SUPPLIES

- ✓ Appropriate personal protective equipment (PPE)
- ✓ Precleaned and dried items that cannot be heat-sterilized
- ✓ Liquid chemical sterilant
- ✓ Sterile instrument tongs
- ✓ Sterile rinse water

## PROCEDURAL STEPS

### Prepare the Solution

1 Use utility gloves, mask, eyewear, and protective clothing when preparing, using, and discarding the solution.

**PURPOSE** Liquid sterilants are highly toxic and can lead to respiratory problems if not handled properly.

2 Follow the manufacturer's instructions for preparing/activating, using, and disposing of the solution.

**PURPOSE** In many areas, glutaraldehyde is considered a hazardous material, requires special disposal methods, and may not be dumped down the sink.

3 Prepare the solution for use as a sterilant. Label the containers with the name of the chemical, the date of preparation (to indicate the use-life), and any other information that relates to the hazards of this product.

**PURPOSE** Some brands remain active for 30 days; others may have a longer or shorter life.

## PROCEDURE 21.5 Sterilizing Instruments with Liquid Chemical Sterilants–cont'd

4 Cover the container and keep it closed unless you are putting instruments in or taking them out.

**PURPOSE** Glutaraldehyde produces toxic fumes.

### Use the Solution

5 Preclean, rinse, and dry items to be processed.

6 Place the items in a perforated tray or pan. Place the pan in the solution, and cover the container. An alternative method is to use tongs and avoid splashing.

7 Be certain that all items are fully submerged in the solution for the entire contact time.

**PURPOSE** The solution must remain in contact with the items for the recommended contact time.

8 Thoroughly rinse processed items with water, and dry. Place items in clean package.

**NOTE** Sterility is best maintained by rinsing with sterile water, drying with a sterile towel, and placing in a sterile container.

### Maintain the Solution

9 Periodically test the glutaraldehyde concentration of the solution with a chemical test kit (available from the manufacturer).

10 Replace the solution as indicated on the instructions, or when the level of the solution is low or the solution is visibly dirty.

11 When you replace the used solution, discard all of the used solution, clean the container with a detergent, rinse with water, dry, and fill the container with a fresh solution.

Modified from Miller CH: Infection control and management of hazardous materials for the dental team, ed 6, St Louis, 2018, Elsevier.

## PROCEDURE 21.6

# Following a Sterilization Failure

### GOAL

To identify and correct the cause of a sterilization failure

### EQUIPMENT AND SUPPLIES

- Records of the monitoring service
- Sterilizer operating manual
- Biologic and chemical indicators
- Backup sterilizer

### PROCEDURAL STEPS

1 Take the sterilizer out of service immediately.

**NOTE** Items that have been processed since the last spore test, and have not been used since, must be resterilized.

**PURPOSE** The sterilizer cannot be considered safe for patient care items until the cause of the failure is determined and the appropriate corrections are made.

2 Using the manufacturer's manual, review the proper loading and operating procedures. Determine if the times and temperatures were correct. Was a new staff member involved with the instrument processing?

**RATIONALE** Many sterilization failures are a result of improper procedures being performed, and not due to malfunction of the sterilizer.

3 Retest and monitor the cycle. Place a chemical indicator next to the biologic indicator on the inside of a package. Check the sterilization gauges, lights, and/or the digital readouts to determine if they reach the proper sterilizing conditions.

**RATIONALE** To determine if the problem has been corrected or whether the sterilizer has malfunctioned.

4 Make a decision regarding the proper operation of the sterilizer.

**RATIONALE** To determine if the problem was caused by human error and has been resolved, or the sterilizer is malfunctioning and needs to be repaired.

**NOTE** Before a repaired or new sterilizer is placed into service, it should be spore tested in three consecutive empty-chamber cycles and receive a negative result before being used to sterilize patient care items.

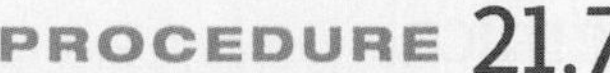

PROCEDURE 21.7

# Performing Biologic Monitoring

## GOAL

To assess sterilization using biologic indicators (BIs) (spore tests)

## EQUIPMENT AND SUPPLIES

- Appropriate personal protective equipment (PPE)
- Instruments
- Pencil
- Dual-species BI
- Sterilization log
- Mail-in envelope

## PROCEDURAL STEPS

1 While wearing all PPE, place the BI strip in the bundle of instruments and seal the package.

**PURPOSE** Although the instruments have been pre-cleaned, they are still contaminated.

2 Place the pack with the BI in the center of the sterilizer load.

**PURPOSE** The center of the load is the most difficult for the sterilizing agent to penetrate.

3 Place the remainder of the packaged instruments into the sterilizer, and process the load through a normal sterilization cycle.

**PURPOSE** Monitoring evaluates what is considered the "normal" cycle.

4 Remove utility gloves, mask, and eyewear. Wash and dry hands.

**PURPOSE** To avoid contamination of the sterilization log.

5 In the sterilization log, record the date of the test, the type of sterilizer, cycle, temperature, time, and the name of the person operating the sterilizer.

**PURPOSE** Maintaining records is part of the exposure control program, and specific information is necessary in the event of a sterilization failure.

6 After the load has been sterilized, remove the processed BI strip.

**PURPOSE** The BI has been exposed to the same sterilizing conditions as the instruments.

7 Mail the processed spore test strips and the control BI to the monitoring service.

**PURPOSE** It is important to obtain and maintain the results as part of the exposure control program.

PROCEDURE 21.8

# Sterilizing the Dental Handpiece

## GOAL

To sterilize the dental handpiece according to the manufacturer's recommendations.

## EQUIPMENT AND SUPPLIES

- Sterilizable handpiece
- Bur
- Ultrasonic cleaner (if recommended by the manufacturer)
- Lubrication (if recommended by the manufacturer)
- Cotton swab
- Alcohol
- Biological indicators
- Chemical indicators
- Heat Sterilizer

**NOTE** Always be certain to follow the manufacturer's instructions for cleaning, lubricating, and sterilizing dental handpieces.

## PROCEDURAL STEPS

1 With the handpiece still attached to the hose, and the bur still in the chuck, wipe away visible debris on the handpiece. Operate the handpiece for approximately 10 to 20 seconds to flush water and air into the lines.

**PURPOSE** This will remove any loose debris that has become lodged in the head.

2 Remove the bur from the handpiece and then the handpiece from the hose.

3 If the manufacturer recommends ultrasonic cleaning, follow those instructions, then thoroughly drain the handpiece, attach the hose, and briefly operate the handpiece to expel debris.

4 If ultrasonic cleaning is not expressly recommended, scrub the handpiece thoroughly under running water with a brush and soap/detergent cleaner.

5 If the handpiece requires presterilization lubrication, use a handpiece cleaner recommended by the manufacturer to remove internal debris, and lubricate the handpiece.

6 If the handpiece does not require presterilization lubrication, *do not* use a cleaner that contains a lubricant.

7 Follow the manufacturer's instructions for each type of handpiece used.

**PURPOSE** To avoid overlubricating the handpiece.

8 Reattach the handpiece to an air hose, and blow out the excess lubricant from the rotating parts. With most handpieces, a bur must be inserted before it is operated.

**PURPOSE** Failure to do this can result in accumulation of excess lubricant in the head and "stickiness" of the excess during the heat cycle.

## PROCEDURE 21.8 Sterilizing the Dental Handpiece–cont'd

9 Use a cotton-tip applicator dampened (not soaked) with isopropyl alcohol to remove all excess lubricant from fiber optic interfaces and exposed optical surfaces. Never use strong solvents on fiber optics.

**PURPOSE** Strong solvents can dissolve the epoxy binding between the fibers.

10 Be sure the handpiece is clean; then dry it and package it for sterilization. Sterilize according to the manufacturer's instructions. After the heat cycle, allow the bagged handpiece to cool and dry. Keep sterilization packaging sealed until the handpiece is to be prepared for use on a patient.

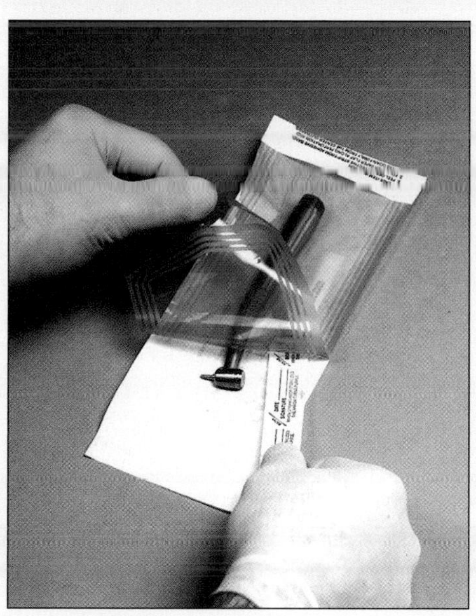

11 Flush water and air into the lines for 20 to 30 seconds before attaching the handpiece.

**PURPOSE** To remove any residual debris and free-floating bacteria.

12 If the handpiece does not require poststerilization measures, open the sterilized bag at chairside in front of the patient to demonstrate that a fresh handpiece is being used.

13 If the handpiece requires poststerilization lubrication, keep a separate lubricant container for use on sterilized handpieces. Lubricate the handpiece as close as possible to the actual time of use.

**PURPOSE** To reduce the risk of cross-contamination.

14 Open only the *end* of the sterilization packaging. Spray the lubricant into the handpiece air drive to reduce the amount of overspray and help control excess lubricant.

**NOTE** The dental handpiece is now ready for use.

# Procedure 21-3 Sterilizing the Dental Handpiece—cont'd

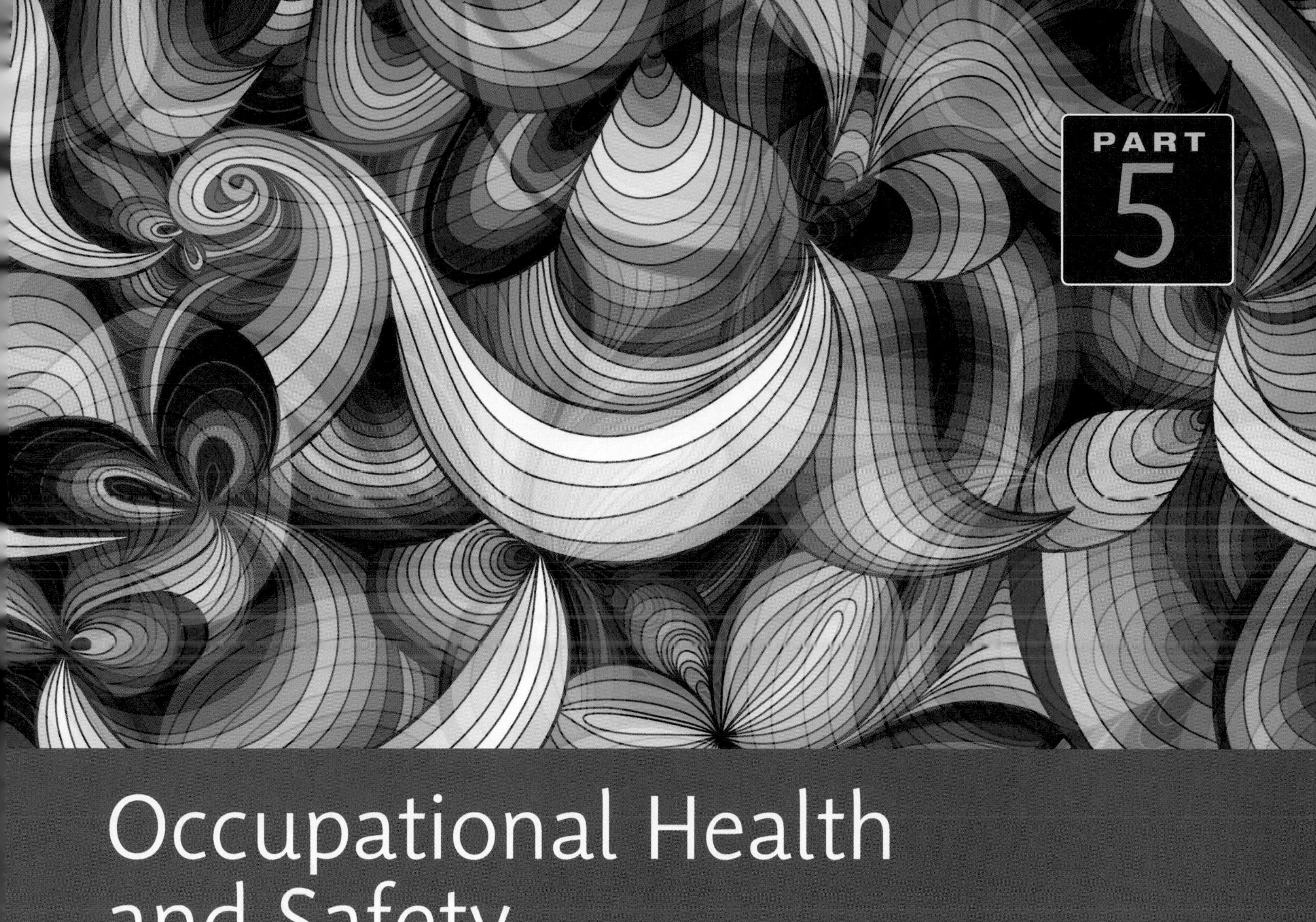


# Occupational Health and Safety

Occupational health and safety, as it relates to careers in dentistry, is receiving increased attention. Agencies are developing new rules and regulations to prevent workplace hazards and injuries to dental personnel. The dental assistant is very often the person who is responsible for ensuring that the dental office is in compliance with a wide variety of federal, state, and local regulations. These regulations deal with the handling of hazardous chemicals, prevention of employee injuries, and management of dental waste.

In this section, you will learn the roles and responsibilities of the various agencies and how they affect the dental office. You will learn how to handle chemicals safely in the dental office, how to identify and correctly dispose of waste materials, and why it is so important to maintain the dental unit waterlines. In addition, you will learn how to protect yourself against workplace injuries. Injuries commonly associated with the clinical practice of dental assisting include headaches; back, neck, and shoulder pain; and other musculoskeletal disorders.

22

# Regulatory and Advisory Agencies

## KEY TERMS

**American Dental Assistants Association (ADAA)** The professional organization for dental assistants in the United States.

**American Dental Association (ADA)** The professional organization for dentists.

**American Dental Hygienists' Association (ADHA)** The professional organization for dental hygienists.

**Canadian Dental Assistants Association (CDAA)** The professional organization for dental assistants in Canada.

**Centers for Disease Control and Prevention (CDC)** Federal agency that is nonregulatory and that issues recommendations on health and safety.

**Environmental Protection Agency (EPA)** Federal regulatory agency responsible for protecting and restoring the environment and public health through environmental laws.

**Food and Drug Administration (FDA)** Federal regulatory agency that regulates food, drugs, medical devices, animal feed and drugs, cosmetics, and radiation-emitting products (cell phones, lasers, microwaves, etc.).

**National Institute for Occupational Safety and Health (NIOSH)** Federal agency that is nonregulatory and provides national and worldwide leadership to prevent work-related illnesses and injuries.

**National Institute of Dental and Craniofacial Research (NIDCR)** Federal agency with the mission to improve oral, dental, and craniofacial health through research, research training, and the dissemination of health information.

**National Institutes of Health (NIH)** One of the world's foremost research centers.

**Occupational Safety and Health Administration (OSHA)** Federal regulatory agency with the mission to ensure the safety and health of America's workers by setting and enforcing standards.

**Organization for Safety, Asepsis and Prevention (OSAP)** The premier infection control agency in the United States.

**Public Health Agency of Canada (PHAC)** The main federal agency responsible for public health in Canada.

## LEARNING OUTCOMES

*On completion of this chapter, the student will be able to achieve the following objectives:*

1 Pronounce, define, and spell the key terms.
2 Explain the difference between regulations and recommendations.
3 Discuss professional organizations and associations, including the following:
   - Identify four professional sources for dental information.
   - Name the professional organizations for dentists, dental assistants, and dental hygienists.
   - Name the premier infection control educational organization in dentistry.
4 Discuss the role of government agencies in relation to dentistry, including the following:
   - Explain a primary difference between OSHA and NIOSH.
   - Describe the role of the Public Health Agency of Canada.

## ELECTRONIC RESOURCES

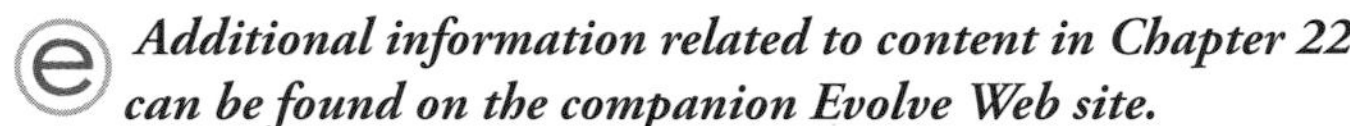
***Additional information related to content in Chapter 22 can be found on the companion Evolve Web site.***

- Practice Quiz
- Canadian Content Corner

It is important for the dental assistant to recognize and understand the roles of the government agencies and professional organizations that have a direct influence on the practice of dentistry. This is especially true in the areas of infection control, chemicals, and other occupational health and safety issues. Some agencies are *regulatory* and issue rules and regulations with which dental offices must comply. Penalties for not complying with regulations may include fines, imprisonment, or suspension or revocation of licenses. Other agencies are *advisory* and have no authority for enforcement. These *nonregulatory* agencies issue recommendations that are based on strong scientific evidence and are the standard of care for dentistry today.

The governmental agencies and organizations described in this chapter are huge, and this chapter is intended to serve only as an introduction to them. When you are in practice as a dental assistant, these agencies will be excellent resources for information for you, and they are easily accessed on the Internet.

## Associations and Organizations

Professional organizations are a valuable resource for current infection control and other professional information (Table 22.1). Many dental professionals choose to become a member of their professional organizations.

## American Dental Association

The **American Dental Association (ADA)** is the national professional organization for dentists. The ADA was established in 1859. Today, more than 161,000 dentists are members. It is the world's largest and oldest national

**TABLE 22.1 Professional Organizations**

| Organization | Logo |
|---|---|
| **American Dental Association (ADA)**<br>211 E. Chicago Ave.<br>Chicago, IL 60611<br>(312) 440-2500<br>www.ada.org | ADA American Dental Association®<br>America's leading advocate for oral health |
| **American Dental Assistants Association (ADAA)**<br>35 East Wacker Drive, Suite 1730<br>Chicago, IL 60601<br>(312) 541-1550<br>www.dentalassistant.org | 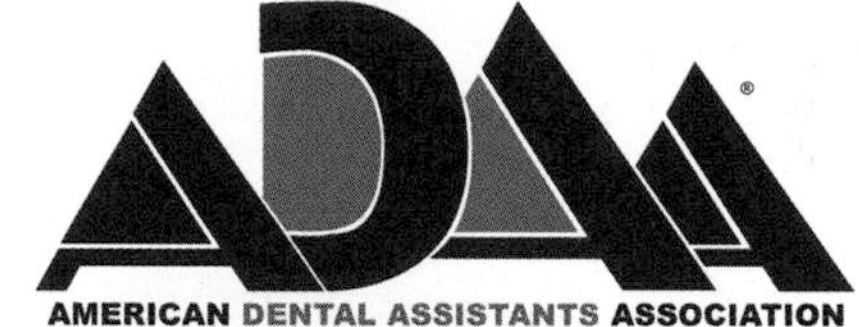 |
| **American Dental Hygienists' Association**<br>444 North Michigan Ave., Suite 3400<br>Chicago, IL 60611<br>(312) 440-8900<br>www.adha.org | 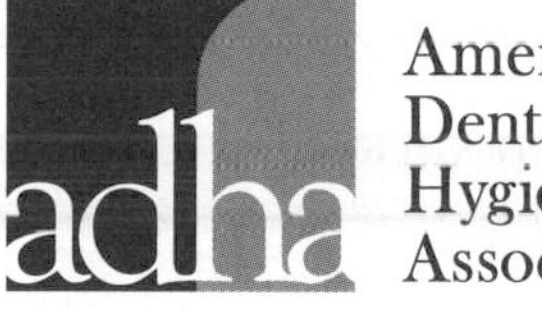 |
| **Canadian Dental Assistants Association**<br>2255 St. Laurent Blvd., Suite 203<br>Ottawa, ON K1G 4K3<br>www.info@cdaa.ca | 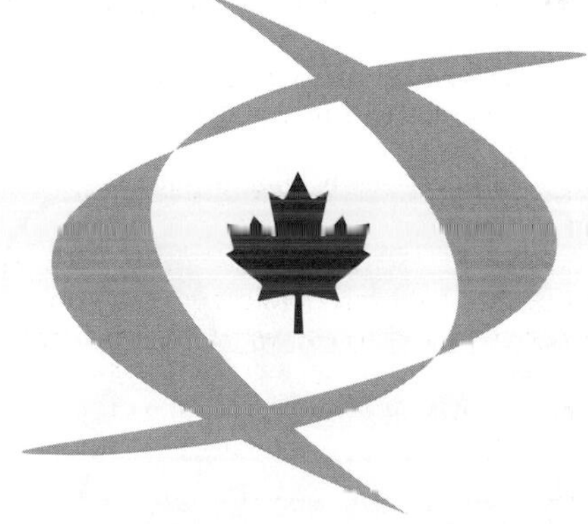 |
| **Organization for Safety, Asepsis and Prevention (OSAP)**<br>P.O. Box 6297<br>Annapolis, MD 21401<br>(410) 571-0003<br>www.osap.org | 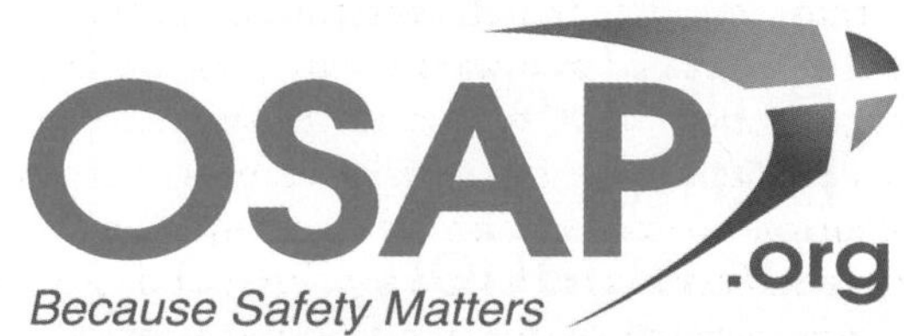 |

dental association. The ADA provides information on best practice and emerging issues of interest to the dental community.

Dentists and consumers have long recognized the American Dental Association (ADA) Seal of Acceptance as an important symbol of a dental product's safety and effectiveness. This is a voluntary program, and participating companies commit significant resources to test products to earn the ADA Seal of Acceptance (Fig. 22.1).

## American Dental Assistants Association

The **American Dental Assistants Association (ADAA)** is the oldest, largest group that represents professional dental assistants. Its members include clinical personnel who work chairside with the dentist, as well as the receptionist, the office manager, and those working behind the scenes in dental product sales, insurance, and education. The ADAA encourages education, registration, and certification for dental-assisting professionals.

In Canada, the **Canadian Dental Assistants Association (CDAA)** operates under similar principles with professional dental assistants.

### ADAA Creed for Dental Assistants

- To be loyal to my employer, my calling, and myself.
- To develop initiative—having the courage to assume responsibility and the imagination to create ideas and develop them.
- To be prepared to visualize, take advantage of, and fulfill the opportunities of my calling.
- To be a coworker—creating a spirit of cooperation and friendliness rather than one of fault-finding and criticism.
- To be enthusiastic—for therein lies the easiest way to accomplishment.
- To be generous, not alone of my name but of my praise and my time.
- To be tolerant with my associates, for at times I too make mistakes.
- To be friendly, realizing that friendship bestows and receives happiness.
- To be respectful of the other person's viewpoint and condition.
- To be systematic, believing that system makes for efficiency.
- To know the value of time for both my employer and myself.
- To safeguard my health, for good health is necessary for the achievement of a successful career.
- To be tactful—always doing the right thing at the right time.
- To be courteous—for this is the badge of good breeding.
- To walk on the sunny side of the street, seeing the beautiful things in life rather than fearing the shadows.
- To keep smiling always.

***Juliette A. Southard, Founder of the ADAA***

From American Dental Assistants Association, Chicago, IL.

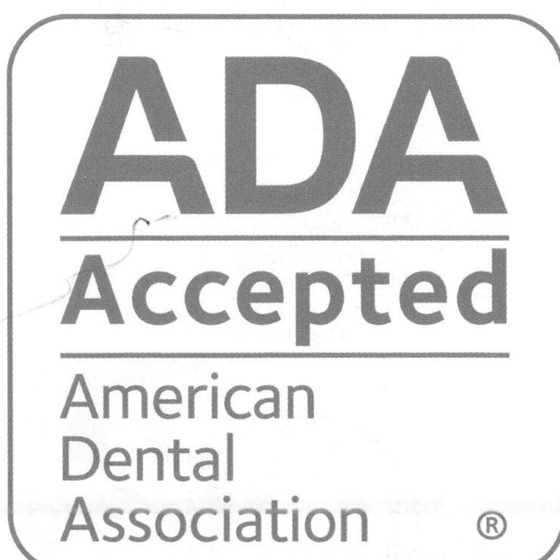


**FIG. 22.1** ADA Seal of Acceptance. *(Courtesy American Dental Association, Chicago, IL.)*

## American Dental Hygienists' Association

The **American Dental Hygienists' Association (ADHA)** is the national professional organization for dental hygienists. The ADHA provides its members with professional support, educational programs, and opportunities to participate in the organization. The mission of the organization is to advance the art and science of dental hygiene and to promote the highest standards of education and practice.

## Organization for Safety, Asepsis and Prevention

The **Organization for Safety, Asepsis and Prevention (OSAP)** is dentistry's resource for infection control and safety. It is a not-for-profit organization composed of dentists, dental hygienists, dental assistants, government representatives, dental manufacturers, university professors, researchers, and dental consultants, along with other interested persons with a collective mission to promote infection control and related science-based health and safety policies and practices.

OSAP is a valuable resource that provides practical, scientifically sound information and recommendations on specific issues such as instrument processing, surface asepsis, dental unit waterline management, and so forth. OSAP members receive a monthly newsletter on a specific issue of interest and an opportunity to receive an hour of continuing education for each newsletter reviewed.

OSAP is the premier infection control educational organization in dentistry, and all members of the dental team should consider becoming members to keep up to date in the areas of infection control and dental office safety.

1 What is the main difference between a recommendation and a regulation?
2 What is OSAP?

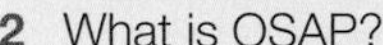

## State and Local Dental Societies

State and local dental societies can be helpful to you in complying with regulatory issues in your specific area. State and local dental and dental-assisting societies can often answer questions and work with you or act as liaisons to the regulatory agencies.

# Government Agencies

Several agencies run by the federal government interact with the dental industry (Table 22.2).

## Centers for Disease Control and Prevention

The **Centers for Disease Control and Prevention (CDC)** is an agency of the U.S. Department of Health and Human Services. It is recognized as the lead federal agency for protecting the health and safety of people at home and abroad. The CDC bases its public health *recommendations* on scientific data of the highest quality.

The infection control procedures practiced in dentistry today are based on the *Guidelines for Infection Control in Dental Healthcare Settings—2003* issued by the CDC. The CDC also has an Oral Health Services section that studies oral diseases, fluoride application, and infection control in dentistry. The CDC does *not* have the authority to make laws, but many local, state, and federal agencies use CDC recommendations to formulate laws.

**TABLE 22.2** Government Agencies

| Agency | Logo |
|---|---|
| **Centers for Disease Control and Prevention (CDC)**<br>1600 Clifton Rd.<br>Atlanta, GA 30333<br>(404) 639-3311<br>Division of Oral Health: (770) 488-6054<br>Surveillance and Research: (770) 488-6055<br>www.cdc.gov | 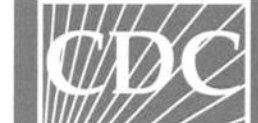 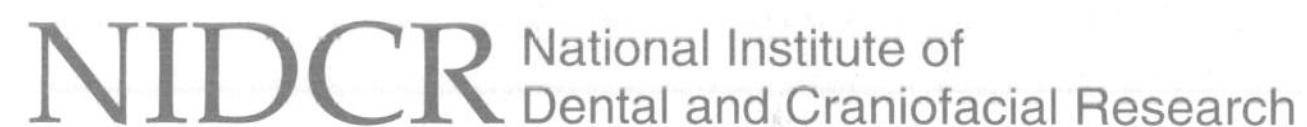  |
| **National Institute for Dental and Craniofacial Research (NIDCR)**<br>31 Center Drive<br>Bethesda, MD 20892<br>(301) 402-2185<br>www.nidcr.gov | NIDCR National Institute of Dental and Craniofacial Research |
| **National Institute for Occupational Safety and Health (NIOSH)**<br>Education and Information Division<br>4676 Columbia Parkway<br>Cincinnati, OH 45226<br>(513) 533-8377<br>www.cdc.gov/niosh | 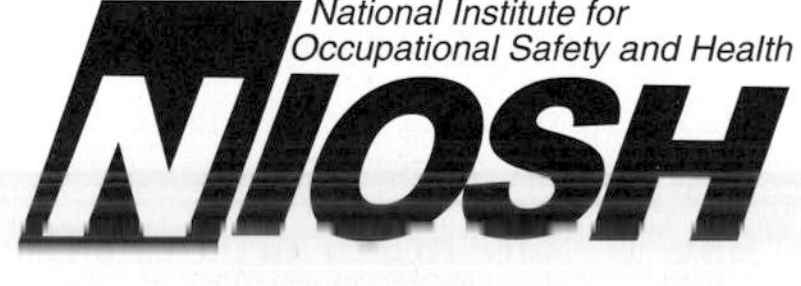  |
| **National Institutes of Health (NIH)**<br>9000 Rockville Pike<br>Bethesda, MD 20892<br>(301) 496-4000<br>www.nih.gov | 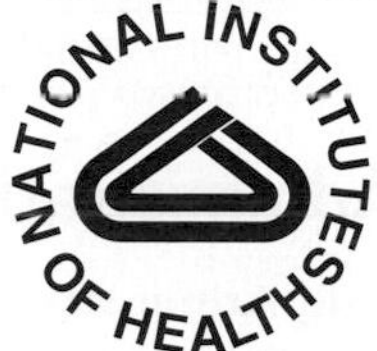  |
| **U.S. Environmental Protection Agency (EPA)**<br>Ariel Rios Building<br>1200 Pennsylvania Ave., N.W.<br>Washington, DC 20460<br>(202) 272-0167<br>www.epa.gov | 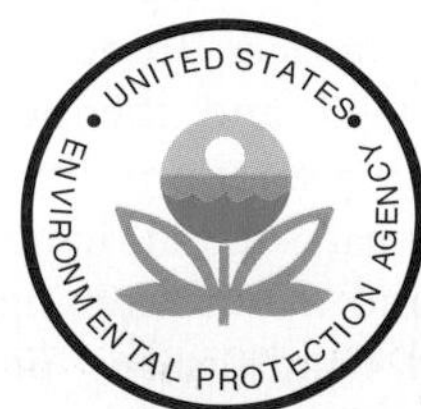  |

Continued

**TABLE 22.2 Government Agencies—cont'd**

| Agency | Logo |
|---|---|
| **U.S. Food and Drug Administration (FDA)**<br>5600 Fishers Lane<br>Rockville, MD 20857<br>Center for Devices and Radiologic Health: (800) 638-2041<br>MEDwatch: (800) FDA-1088<br>www.fda.gov | 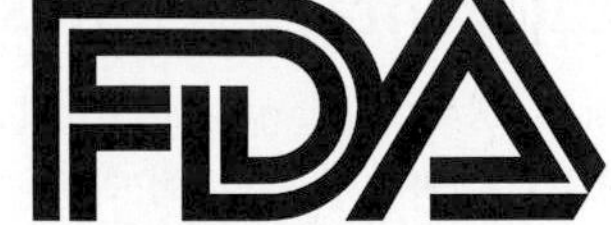  |
| **U.S. Occupational Safety and Health Administration (OSHA)**<br>200 Constitutional Ave., N.W.<br>Washington, DC 20210<br>(202) 693-1299<br>www.osha.gov<br>*Check online to see whether your state operates its own OSHA.* | 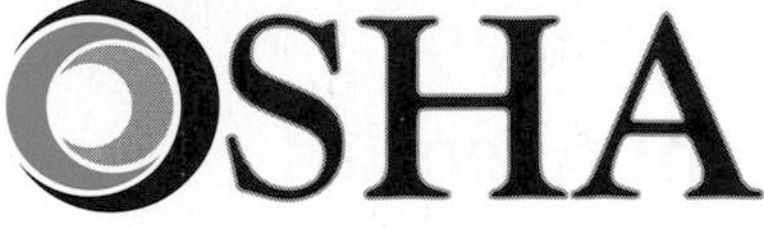  |
| **Public Health Agency of Canada***<br>Chief Public Health Officer<br>Public Health Agency of Canada<br>130 Colonnade Road<br>A.L. 6501H<br>Ottawa, ON K1A 0K9<br>or<br>Chief Public Health Officer<br>Public Health Agency of Canada<br>1015 Arlington Street<br>Winnipeg, MB R3E 3R2<br>www.phac-aspc.gc.ca<br>(613) 957-2991 | 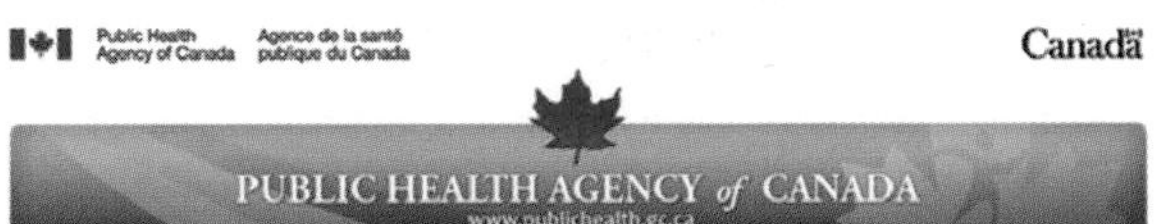  |

*PHAC is run by the Canadian government.

The CDC has published guidelines on preventing transmission of tuberculosis in healthcare settings, including dental offices. It publishes the *Morbidity and Mortality Weekly Report,* which provides data on health and disease trends based on reports by state health departments.

Although the CDC's national headquarters are in Atlanta, Georgia, more than 2000 CDC employees work at other locations, including 47 state health departments. About 120 employees are assigned overseas in 45 countries.

The CDC is an excellent resource for health information for the public and for all dental professionals.

## Food and Drug Administration

The U.S. **Food and Drug Administration (FDA)** is a *regulatory* agency and is part of the U.S. Department of Health and Human Services. The FDA regulates the manufacturing and labeling of medical devices. In dentistry, the FDA must approve sterilizers, biologic and chemical indicators, ultrasonic cleaners and cleaning solutions, liquid sterilants, gloves, masks, protective eyewear, dental handpieces and instruments, dental chairs, and dental unit lights. The FDA also regulates antimicrobial handwashing products and mouth rinses (Fig. 22.2).

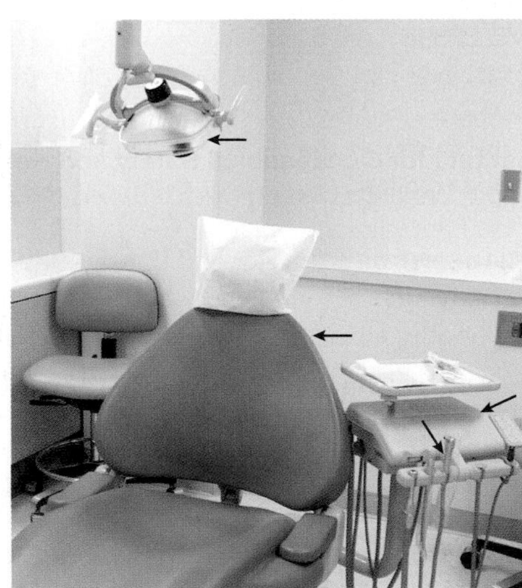

**FIG. 22.2** Overview of a dental operatory showing items *(arrows)* regulated by the U.S. Food and Drug Administration (FDA).

The FDA requires "good manufacturing practices" and reviews the safety and effectiveness of drugs and medical devices. The agency also reviews claims on the labels of products to be certain that those claims are true. All medical and dental devices to be sold in the United

States must first be cleared by the FDA before they can be marketed.

## Environmental Protection Agency

The U.S. **Environmental Protection Agency (EPA)** is a *regulatory* agency. The EPA is associated with dentistry in ensuring the safety and effectiveness of disinfectants. Manufacturers of disinfectants must submit information about the safety and effectiveness of their products. The EPA reviews the manufacturer's antimicrobial claims to ensure that they are supported by scientific evidence. If the manufacturer's claims meet the EPA criteria, the product receives an EPA registration number. That number must appear on the product label.

The EPA is also involved in regulating waste materials, such as chemicals and medical waste, after they are sent from the dental office to a final disposal site.

## Occupational Safety and Health Administration

The U.S. **Occupational Safety and Health Administration (OSHA)** is a federal *regulatory* agency that is a division of the U.S. Department of Labor. The responsibility of OSHA is to ensure the safety and health of America's workers. To do this, OSHA sets and enforces protective standards that employers *must* follow so as to provide a safe workplace for their employees. In addition, OSHA provides training and outreach education and encourages continual improvement in workplace safety and health. In dentistry, the two most important OSHA standards are the Blood-Borne Pathogens Standard (see Chapter 19) and the Hazard Communication Standard (see Chapter 23).

All states are regulated by the federal OSHA. In addition, 22 states administer their own state-operated OSHA programs. In those states that administer their own OSHA programs, the state standards *must* meet or exceed federal OSHA standards.

OSHA monitors compliance with its standards through a process of investigation of the workplace. If the workplace fails to meet safety requirements, a citation may be issued for each violation. Citations usually result in a fine. If a workplace fails to correct the unsafe conditions, OSHA has the legal authority to close the workplace until the problem is corrected. OSHA provides hazard information, record-keeping guidelines, and copies of standards at no cost.

### OSHA Inspections

Dental inspections may occur at the following times:

- When an employee or patient complaint is made
- Randomly in an office with 11 or more employees
- On request of the dentist for a consultation visit

*OSHA,* Occupational Safety and Health Administration.

## National Institutes of Health

The **National Institutes of Health (NIH)** is part of the U.S. Department of Health and Human Services. It is the primary federal agency for conducting and supporting medical research. NIH scientists investigate ways to prevent disease, and they research the causes, treatments, and even cures for common and rare diseases. This agency provides leadership and financial support to researchers in every state and nation throughout the world.

The NIH supports a wide spectrum of research, from learning how the brain becomes addicted to alcohol to combating heart disease. The agency is at the forefront of new progress in medical research. Indeed, many important health and medical discoveries of the past century resulted from research supported by the NIH. The NIH translates research results into practice and communicates research findings to patients and their families, healthcare providers, and the general public.

## National Institute of Dental and Craniofacial Research

The **National Institute of Dental and Craniofacial Research (NIDCR)** is the dental research institute of the NIH. Its mission is to promote the general health of the American people by improving their oral, dental, and craniofacial health. Through research and the training of researchers, the NIDCR promotes health, prevents diseases and pathologic conditions, and develops new diagnostic and therapeutic techniques.

## National Institute for Occupational Safety and Health

In contrast to OSHA, the **National Institute for Occupational Safety and Health (NIOSH)** does *not* have regulatory authority. NIOSH is the only federal institute responsible for conducting research and making *recommendations* for the prevention of work-related disease and injury. NIOSH, which is part of the CDC, conducts research on the full scope of occupational disease and injury, ranging from lung diseases in miners to carpal tunnel syndrome (see Chapter 25) and allergic reactions to latex.

### Duties of NIOSH

In addition to conducting research, NIOSH performs the following duties:

- Investigates potentially hazardous conditions when requested by employees or employers
- Makes recommendations and disseminates information on preventing workplace disease, injury, and disability
- Provides training to occupational safety and health professionals

*NIOSH,* National Institute for Occupational Safety and Health.

## Public Health Agency of Canada

As the main Canadian federal agency responsible for public health, the **Public Health Agency of Canada (PHAC)** supports approximately 2400 researchers and staff, as well as a wide variety of programs and services offered by both federal government and nongovernment agencies across Canada.

### Roles of the PHAC

- Promote health
- Prevent and control chronic diseases and injuries
- Prevent and control infectious diseases
- Prepare for and respond to public health emergencies

*PHAC,* Public Health Agency of Canada.

RECALL

3 What is the primary role of the CDC in dentistry?
4 What is the primary role of the FDA in dentistry?
5 What is the primary role of the EPA in dentistry?
6 What is the primary role of OSHA in dentistry?
7 What is the primary role of the NIH?
8 What is the primary role of the NIDCR?
9 What is the responsibility of the PHAC?

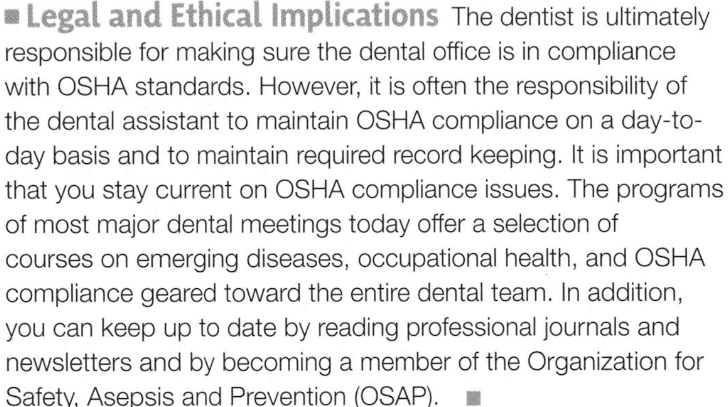

**■ Legal and Ethical Implications** The dentist is ultimately responsible for making sure the dental office is in compliance with OSHA standards. However, it is often the responsibility of the dental assistant to maintain OSHA compliance on a day-to-day basis and to maintain required record keeping. It is important that you stay current on OSHA compliance issues. The programs of most major dental meetings today offer a selection of courses on emerging diseases, occupational health, and OSHA compliance geared toward the entire dental team. In addition, you can keep up to date by reading professional journals and newsletters and by becoming a member of the Organization for Safety, Asepsis and Prevention (OSAP). ■

**■ Eye to the Future** Staying current with the literature will always be important to the educated dental assistant. The Internet will continue to be an excellent resource through which you can obtain information on any dentistry-related topic. All of the professional societies and government agencies are listed on the Internet. These agencies' Web sites make their guidelines, recommendations, or regulations available to you with just a few keystrokes and clicks of the mouse. You can download most information directly from these Web sites.

*PubMed* is an Internet search tool that can make staying current easier and more efficient. Developed by the National Library of Medicine, PubMed provides access to more than 10 million citations, research articles, and literature reviews from journals around the world in several languages. The Web address at which you can find PubMed is www.pubmed.gov. ■

### ■ Critical Thinking

1. At a local dental-assisting society meeting, the conversation turned to infection control. Several of the dental assistants had different opinions regarding local dental waste disposal regulations. How would you obtain accurate information regarding local regulations about dental waste removal?
2. You have been asked by a local women's group to speak about children's dental health. Where can you obtain current information on this topic to prepare for your presentation?
3. When you become a certified dental assistant or a registered dental assistant, you will need to maintain your credential with continuing education. Where will you find sources of continuing education?
4. Visit each of the federal agencies online, and see the vast resources, services, and information available to you—at no cost. ■

23

# Chemical and Waste Management

## KEY TERMS

**Acute exposure** High levels of exposure over a short period.

**Chemical** Any substance or mixture of substances.

**Chemical inventory** A list of every product used in the office that contains chemicals.

**Chronic exposure** Repeated exposures, generally to lower levels, over a long time.

**Contaminated waste** Items such as gloves and patient napkins that may contain the potentially infectious body fluids of patients.

**Flammable** Readily capable of catching fire.

**Globally Harmonized System of Classification and Labeling of Chemicals (GHS)** An international approach to hazard communication.

**Hazard class** The nature of the physical or health hazards (e.g., flammable solid, carcinogen, oral acute toxicity).

**Hazard classification** To identify the properties of a chemical to determine the degree of hazard.

**Hazard Communication Standard (HCS)** Revised Occupational Safety and Health Administration (OSHA) standard regarding employees' "right to know" about hazardous chemicals in the workplace.

**Hazard statement** A statement assigned to a hazard class and category that describes the nature of the hazard(s) of a chemical, including, where appropriate, the degree of hazard.

**Hazardous waste** Waste that poses a risk to humans or to the environment.

**Health hazard** A chemical for which acute or chronic health effects may occur in an exposed employee.

**Infectious waste** Waste that is capable of transmitting an infectious disease.

**Label elements** The pictogram, hazard statement, signal word, and precautionary statement for each hazard class and category.

**Oxidizers** Substances that react or cause a chemical to react with oxygen.

**Physical hazard** A chemical that is a combustible liquid, a compressed gas, or an explosive material or is flammable-reactive or water-reactive.

**Pictograms** Graphic elements used on a hazard label, used to identify the specific hazard class and category.

**Precautionary statement** A phrase that describes recommended measures to be taken to minimize or prevent adverse effects resulting from exposure to a hazardous chemical, or improper storage or handling of a hazardous chemical.

**Product identifier** The name or number used for a hazardous chemical on a label or in the Safety Data Sheet (SDS).

**Regulated waste** Infectious waste that requires special handling, neutralization, and disposal.

**Safety Data Sheet (SDS)** Form provided by the chemical manufacturer that provides printed information regarding the hazards of materials and products that contain chemicals.

**Signal word** Two words used on the SDS: "Warning" for less severe hazard categories, and "Danger" for more severe hazard categories.

**Toxic chemicals** Chemicals that can have a fatal or toxic effect to humans.

**Toxic waste** Waste that can have a toxic effect to humans.

## LEARNING OUTCOMES

*On completion of this chapter, the student will be able to achieve the following objectives:*

1. Pronounce, define, and spell the key terms.
2. Discuss the proper use and handling of hazardous chemicals, including the following:
   - Explain why the dental assistant must be well informed about exposure to chemicals in the workplace.
   - Describe the dental assistant's duties that could result in exposure to chemicals.
   - Explain how chemicals enter the human body.
   - Explain the difference between chronic and acute chemical exposure, including the potential long-term and short-term effects of exposure.
   - Identify the personal protection methods against chemical exposure.
   - Describe the necessary precautions when working with mercury.
   - Describe methods to minimize exposure to chemical hazards in the dental office.
   - Describe in general how chemicals should be stored.
3. Describe the components of an OSHA Hazard Communication Program, including the following:
   - Explain the concept of "Global Harmonization" regarding chemical labeling.
   - Recognize the nine Hazard Communication Standard (HCS) pictograms.
   - Describe the record-keeping requirements of the Hazard Communication Standard.
   - Explain the purpose of a Safety Data Sheet (SDS).
   - State the date by which employers must train employees regarding the new label elements and SDSs.
   - Demonstrate how to create a label for a secondary container.

4 Discuss dental office waste management, including the following:
- Name the three classifications of dental waste.
- Name types of regulated waste generated in a dental office.
- Name types of toxic waste generated in a dental office.
- Describe precautions to take with photochemical waste.
- Describe the responsibilities of the dentist regarding waste disposal.

## PERFORMANCE OUTCOME

*On completion of this chapter, the student will be able to meet competency standards in the following skill:*
- Identify an appropriate label for a secondary container according to the SDS.

## ELECTRONIC RESOURCES

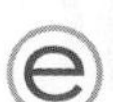
***Additional information related to content in Chapter 23 can be found on the companion Evolve Web site.***

- Practice Quiz
- Canadian Content Corner

In the day-to-day practice of dentistry, the dental assistant is exposed to a wide variety of **chemicals**. All chemicals that are used for treatment procedures, cleaning of instruments and surfaces, disinfection and sterilization, laboratory procedures, and dental x-ray processing are capable of causing serious health consequences if they are handled improperly and are absorbed into the body in sufficiently large amounts.

Chemicals can also seriously damage the heart, kidney, liver, and lung tissues. Results range from short-term discomfort, such as burns or rashes, to life-threatening conditions, such as cancer or organ failure.

As a dental assistant, it is important for you to understand the proper use, storage, handling, spill cleanup, and disposal methods for all the chemicals you use in the dental office. In addition, you should know the first aid procedures associated with chemicals. You must be aware of the hazardous materials that may be regulated under federal, state, or local guidelines and the requirements associated with the disposal of these hazardous materials. Common examples of items that require special disposal procedures include x-ray processing solutions, lead foil backing from film packets, scrap dental amalgam, and elemental mercury.

This chapter also includes the Occupational Safety and Health Administration (OSHA) Hazard Communication Standard, the recent revisions to these regulations, and the dates for implementation. OSHA is the agency responsible for safety in the workplace (see Chapter 22).

# Hazardous Chemicals

A **hazardous chemical** is defined as any chemical that can cause a **physical hazard** or a **health hazard**. A chemical is considered hazardous if it (1) can ignite (catch fire), (2) can react or explode when mixed with other substances, (3) is corrosive, or (4) is toxic (Fig. 23.1).

## Exposure to Chemicals

The three primary methods of chemical exposure are inhalation, skin contact, and ingestion.

Inhalation of the gases, vapors, or dusts of chemicals can cause direct damage to the lungs. Some chemicals may not affect the lungs but are absorbed by them and are then sent through the blood to other organs, such as the brain, liver, or kidneys, where they may cause damage.

Skin is an effective barrier against many chemicals, but some chemicals can be absorbed through the skin. In general, you must have *direct skin contact* with the chemical for absorption to occur. Sometimes, after repeated contact with a chemical, a skin condition called *dermatitis* may develop.

Ingestion *(swallowing)* is another way in which chemicals can enter the body. Common ways of ingesting harmful chemicals in the workplace include eating lunch in an area in which chemicals are used or eating with hands that are contaminated with chemicals. It is important to wash your hands thoroughly after contact with any chemical.

### How Chemicals Enter the Body

- Inhalation of chemical vapor
- Absorption of chemical through the skin
- Ingestion of chemical (eating or drinking)

# Acute and Chronic Chemical Toxicity

The potential for a chemical to cause harm and the extent of harm depend on the amount of the dose and the duration of exposure to the chemical. Chemical toxicity may be acute or chronic.

Acute chemical toxicity results from high levels of exposure over a short period. Acute toxicity is often caused by a chemical spill, in which exposure is sudden and often involves a large amount of the chemical.

The victim of acute toxicity feels the effects immediately. Dizziness, fainting, headache, nausea, and vomiting are symptoms of acute overexposure to chemicals.

Chronic chemical toxicity results from many repeated exposures, generally to lower levels, over a much longer time (months or even years). Many effects of chronic toxicity are possible, including liver disease, brain disorders, cancer, and infertility. Always check the **Safety Data Sheet (SDS)** and the product label for information on potential dangers associated with the chemicals included in the products you use.

*Note:* In the newly revised OSHA Hazard Communication Standard, the term *Material Safety Data Sheet (MSDS)* has been replaced with the term *Safety Data Sheet (SDS).*

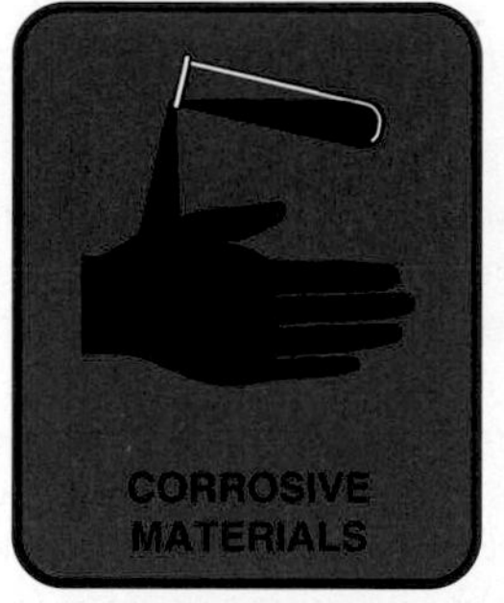

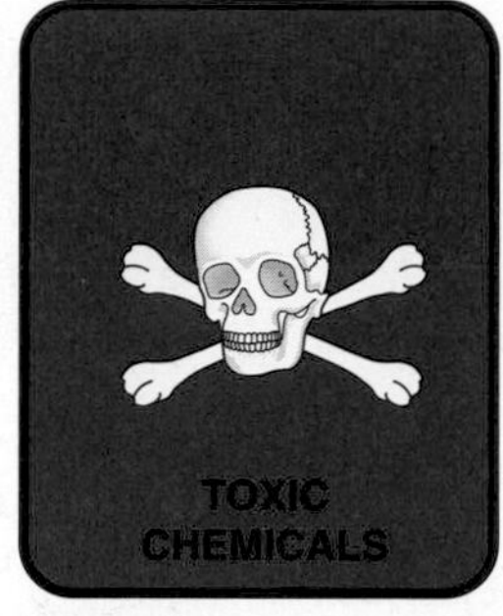

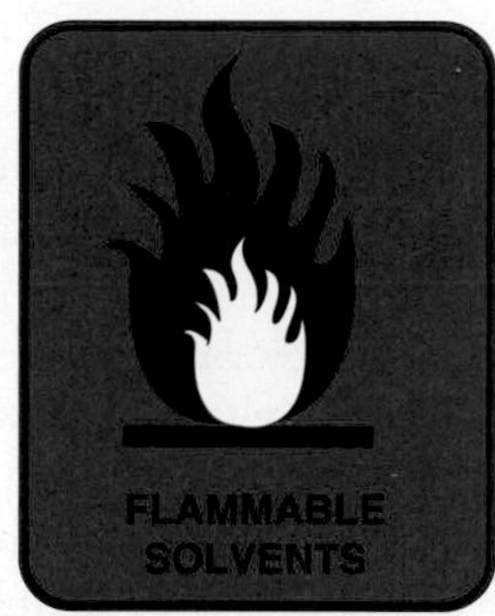


**FIG. 23.1** Chemical hazard warning labels.

The difference between acute and chronic toxicity can be illustrated by considering the effects of **acute exposure** and **chronic exposure** to the same chemical. For example, a single exposure to a high concentration of benzene (acute toxicity) may cause dizziness, headache, and unconsciousness, whereas long-term daily exposure to low levels of benzene (chronic toxicity) may eventually cause leukemia.

## Hand Protection

When using chemicals, be certain to wear utility gloves made from a *chemical-resistant* material, such as natural rubber, neoprene, or industrial-grade nitrile (Fig. 23.2). These chemical-resistant gloves are essential because the latex gloves worn during patient care do *not* provide adequate protection when one is handling chemicals. When exposed to chemical disinfectants, the latex in the glove degrades and creates a *wicking* (sucking) action that will actually pull contaminants and chemicals through the glove and onto the hands.

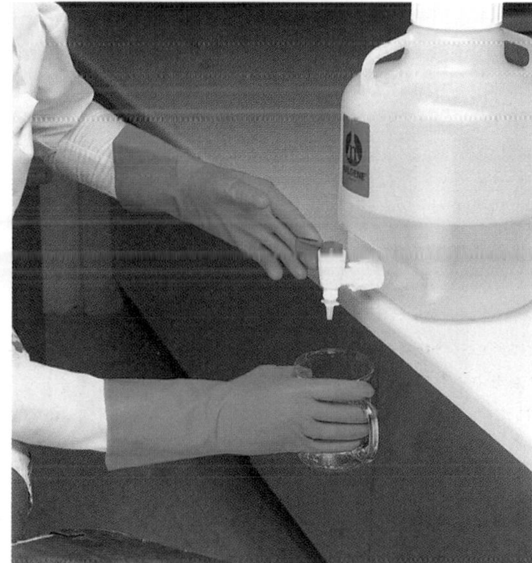

**FIG. 23.2** Clean room nitrile gloves provide protection and dexterity when handling chemicals. *(Courtesy Lab Safety Supply, Janesville, WI.)*

## Eye Protection

Serious damage to the eyes, even blindness, can result from chemical accidents. It is crucial to protect the eyes from fumes and splashes while pouring chemicals such as x-ray processing solutions, ultrasonic solutions, disinfectants, and sterilants.

A variety of safety eyewear is available. The ideal goggles have soft, vinyl flanges (rims) at the top and bottom and fit the face snugly (Fig. 23.3).

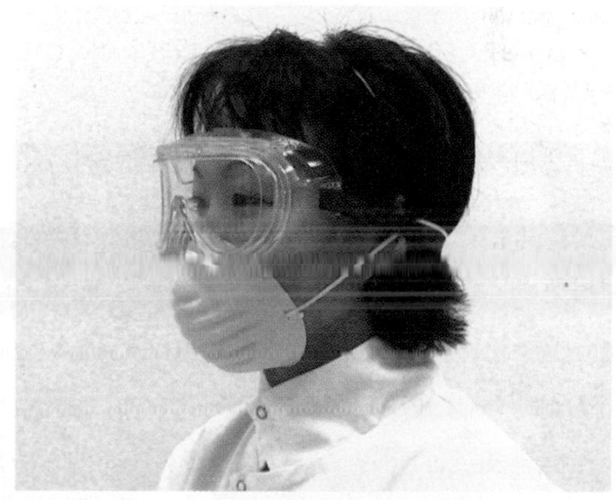

**FIG. 23.3** Dental assistant wearing chemical goggles.

## Protective Clothing

When caustic or staining chemicals are used, it is best to wear a rubber or neoprene apron when mixing or pouring the chemical. The SDS for each product provides specific information regarding the need for additional personal protective equipment (PPE).

## Inhalation Protection

Depending on the quality, the masks worn during patient care may or may not provide adequate protection when one is working with chemicals. The proper face mask should be fluid repellent and should provide respiratory protection.

If your job requires you to pour or mix chemicals frequently, or if you are sensitive or allergic to substances, you might require a mist respirator face mask approved by the National Institute of Occupational Safety and Health (NIOSH) (Fig. 23.4).

RECALL

1. What are the three primary methods of chemical exposure?
2. What is the difference between acute and chronic chemical toxicity?
3. What is the best way to protect your hands from chemicals?
4. What types of personal protection should be worn when handling toxic chemicals?

## Control of Chemical Spills

Accidents and spills should not be common occurrences. Planning and practice in dealing with such spills should minimize accidents and the employee exposure to harmful chemicals. Refer to the SDS (formerly MSDS) or the specific product label for accurate information on how to manage spills.

*Mercury spill kits* should be available in all dental offices in which amalgam is used. Exposure to even small amounts of mercury is very hazardous to the health of dental personnel. Mercury can be absorbed through the skin or through inhalation of mercury vapors. The spill kit for small amounts of mercury should contain mercury-absorbing powder, mercury-absorbing sponges, and a disposal bag (Fig. 23.5). A mask and utility gloves should be worn whenever one is cleaning up a mercury spill.

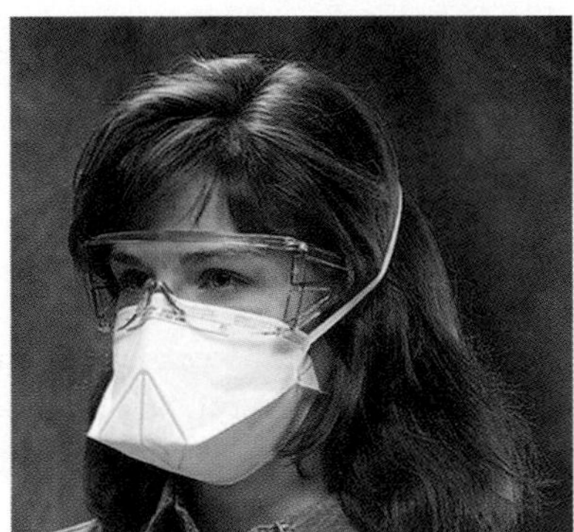

**FIG. 23.4** Disposable respirator has tapered angle to fit facial contours around nose and chin to protect against dusts and chemical mists. *(Courtesy Grainger Industrial Supply, Lake Forest, IL.)*

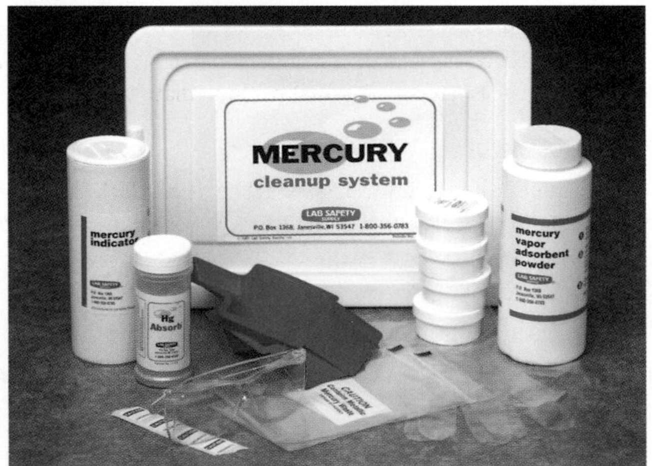


**FIG. 23.5** Mercury spill kit, with aspirator to pick up larger drops of mercury, labeled bottle for recovered mercury, base/activator product to absorb small amounts of mercury, product to absorb mercury vapors, gloves, scoop, sponge, mixing cups, spatulas, and labeled polyethylene bag for disposal. *(Courtesy Grainger Industrial Supply, Lake Forest, IL.)*

### Precautions When Working with Mercury

- Work in a well-ventilated space.
- Avoid direct skin contact with mercury.
- Avoid inhaling mercury vapor.
- Store mercury in unbreakable, tightly sealed containers, away from heat.
- When preparing amalgam for restorations, use preloaded capsules. (This avoids exposure while measuring mercury.)
- When mixing amalgam, always close the cover before starting the amalgamator.
- Reassemble amalgam capsules immediately after dispensing the amalgam mass. (The used amalgam capsule is highly contaminated with mercury and is a significant source of mercury vapor if left open.)
- Leftover scrap amalgam (that was not used) is stored dry in a tightly closed container.
- Scrap amalgam (that has been retrieved from dental unit traps) is disinfected in a solution of bleach and water. Then it is placed in the container with other scrap amalgam. *Never* rinse a dental unit trap in the sink. (Wastewater plants are not equipped to remove mercury from waste, and the mercury will enter the environment via the waterways.)
- Clean spills using appropriate procedures and equipment. *Do not use a household vacuum cleaner or the high-volume evacuator.* (Dangerous fumes from the mercury can be released into the air.)
- Place contaminated disposable materials into polyethylene bags and seal. Dispose according to the regulations specific to your area.

## Eyewash Units

OSHA regulations require eyewash units to be installed in every workplace where chemicals are used. A variety of styles are available. The standard eyewash unit attaches directly to existing faucets for emergencies but still allows normal faucet use. When turned on, the eyewash unit will irrigate the eyes with a soft, wide flow of water, which is necessary to bathe away contaminants without causing additional damage. Wall-mounted eyewash stations offer an alternative to the sink-mounted style. OSHA requires that all eyewash stations be inspected monthly to ensure that they are functioning properly. A record of the date of each inspection must be maintained (Fig. 23.6).

Employees must be trained in the proper use of the eyewash station. The unit should be inspected frequently to ensure that it is functional. Some manufacturers of eyewash units recommend a weekly 3-minute flushing to reduce microbial content in the waterline. Always follow the manufacturer's instructions regarding proper maintenance of the eyewash unit in your office.

## Ventilation

Good ventilation is necessary when you are dealing with any type of chemical. Many dental offices are equipped with special

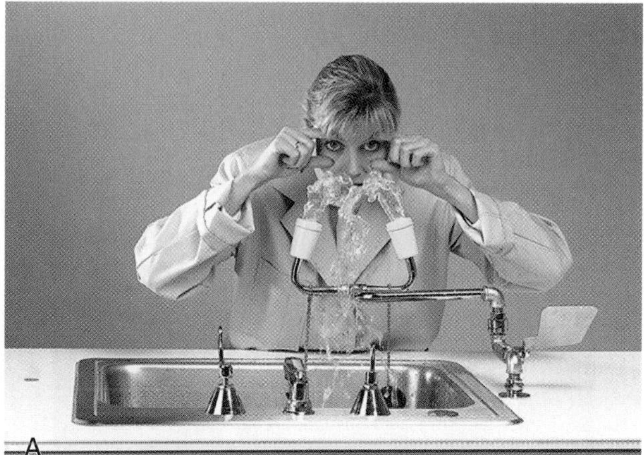

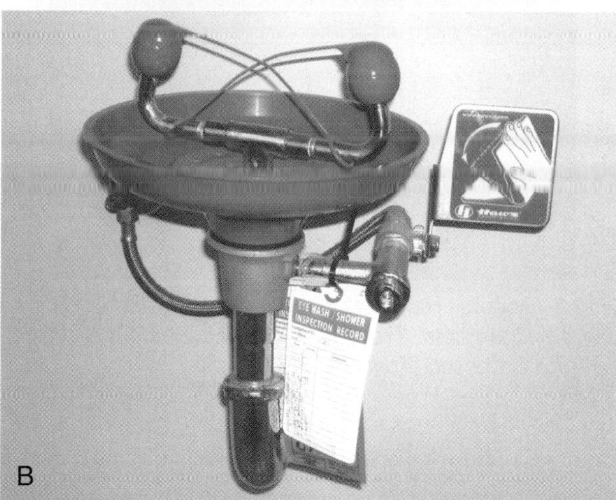


**FIG. 23.6** A, Countertop eyewash and eye/face washes provide water to the face and eyes to gently wash away contaminants. B, A wall-mounted style of eyewash station with a card attached on which to record inspection dates. *(A, Courtesy Grainger Industrial Supply, Lake Forest, IL.)*

exhaust systems for fumes and dust in the laboratory, sterilization areas, and darkroom areas. For example, radiographic processing chemicals can cause contact dermatitis and irritation of the eyes, nose, throat, and respiratory system produced by chemical vapors and fine particles. Be sure to keep processing tanks covered to help contain the fumes.

## General Precautions for Storing Chemicals

All dental materials contain chemicals, and some chemical components are more hazardous than others. Careful use and storage of dental materials are important to ensure that these preparations retain their effectiveness.

The chemical composition of materials can change for many reasons. When changes take place, the product may no longer retain its effectiveness. A basic "safe" policy for the storage of dental medications and chemicals is to keep them in a dry, cool, dark place where they are not exposed to direct sunlight.

### Guidelines for Minimizing Exposure to Chemical Hazards in the Dental Office

- Keep a minimum of hazardous chemicals in the office.
- Read the labels and use only as directed.
- Store according to the manufacturer's directions.
- Keep containers tightly covered.
- Avoid mixing chemicals unless consequences are known.
- Wear appropriate personal protective equipment (PPE) when handling hazardous substances.
- Wash hands immediately after removing gloves.
- Avoid skin contact with chemicals; immediately wash skin that has come in contact with chemicals.
- Maintain good ventilation.
- Do not eat, drink, smoke, apply lip balm, or insert contact lenses in areas in which chemicals are used.
- Keep chemicals away from open flames and heat sources.
- Always have on hand an operational fire extinguisher.
- Know and use proper cleanup procedures.
- Keep neutralizing agents available for strong acid and alkaline solutions.
- Dispose of all hazardous chemicals according to Safety Data Sheet (SDS) instructions.

### Follow Instructions

The manufacturer has determined the best methods for packaging and storage. The manufacturer's instructions for storage can be found on the SDS and should be followed.

### Avoid Exposure to Light

Light is the primary cause of the deterioration of sodium hypochlorite (household bleach), epinephrine, and hydrogen peroxide. This is why many chemicals are sold in dark or opaque containers. Change in color is a common sign that the chemical has deteriorated.

### Check Expiration Date

The expiration date, which may be listed on the container, should be checked frequently. Products that have outlived their expiration date should be disposed of immediately.

### Rotate Inventory

Fresh supplies should always be stocked behind the current inventory to ensure that the oldest product is used first. This is the same method that is used to stock milk and other perishable items in a grocery store.

RECALL

5 Describe the necessary precautions when working with mercury.
6 What are the OSHA requirements regarding an eyewash unit?
7 Describe guidelines for minimizing exposure to chemical hazards in the dental office.
8 What could be the effects of exposure to radiographic processing solutions kept in a poorly ventilated area?
9 In general, how should chemicals be stored?

## Disposal of Empty Containers

Even empty containers can be hazardous because they often hold residues that can burn or explode. *Never* fill an empty container with another substance, because a dangerous chemical reaction could occur. Always follow the instructions on the label and on the SDS on how to dispose of empty containers.

## Hazardous Waste Disposal

Substances are considered **hazardous waste** if they have certain properties or contain chemicals that could pose dangers to human health and the environment after they are discarded. Regulations for proper disposal of hazardous waste vary widely among states, provinces, or territories. Even within the same state, regulations often vary among counties or even cities. To be safe, always check the regulations specific to the area in which you work. In general, wastes are classified as "hazardous" if they have the following characteristics:

- *Ignitable:* **Flammable** or combustible
- *Corrosive:* Highly acidic (pH less than 2.0) or extremely basic (pH greater than 12.5) (pH is a measure of the solution's hydrogen ion concentration; water has a pH of 7.0)
- *Reactive:* Chemically unstable or explosive, violent reaction with water, or capable of giving off toxic fumes when mixed with water
- *Toxic:* Contains arsenic, barium, chromium, mercury, lead, silver, or certain pesticides
- *Listed by Environmental Protection Agency (EPA):* Several hundred chemicals are listed as hazardous

RECALL

**10** In general, how are chemicals determined to be hazardous?
**11** How could an empty container be considered to be hazardous?

# Hazard Communication Program

In 1983 OSHA issued the **Hazard Communication Standard (HCS)**, also known as the Employee Right-to-Know Law. It requires employers to inform their employees about the identity and hazards of all chemicals that they are exposed to in the workplace.

## Revision of the HCS Standard

In 2012 OSHA revised the HCS and adopted the **Globally Harmonized System of Classification and Labeling of Chemicals (GHS)** (Fig. 23.7). Under the international GHS, each chemical will be classified and labeled the same regardless of where in the global market the chemical is manufactured or used. It will end confusion and eliminate the need for different labels.

The new hazard communication standard will still require chemical manufacturers and importers to evaluate the chemicals they produce or import and provide hazard information to employers and workers by putting labels on containers and preparing SDSs.

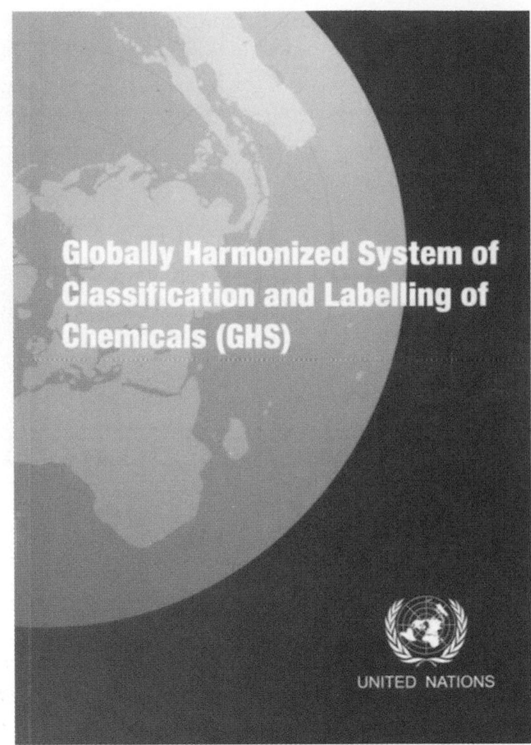


**FIG. 23.7** Globally Harmonized System of Classification and Labeling of Chemicals. *(From http://www.osha.gov/dsg/hazcom/index.html; accessed April 26, 2013.)*

Employers will still be required to have a written program with the same components, provide training, and identify hazards by using labels and SDS. What has changed is the way that chemical hazards are identified and the way information is communicated by standardized information on the labels and SDS. The new system is being implemented throughout the world by countries including Canada, the European Union, China, Australia, and Japan.

The revised HCS is a modification to the existing standard. Those parts of the existing standard that do not relate to the GHS or are already consistent with it remain unchanged. Although much of it remains unchanged, there have been some modifications to terminology. For example, the term *hazard determination* has been changed to **hazard classification** and *Material Safety Data Sheet* has been changed to *Safety Data Sheet* (as noted earlier in this chapter). The new standards will improve the quality and consistency of the information available to employees using chemicals in the workplace.

## Major Changes to the Hazard Communication Standard

The three major areas of change are in hazard classification, labels, and SDSs.

### *Hazard Classification*

Specific criteria for hazards have been developed, and chemicals are classified into categories that compare hazard severity within a **hazard class**. Once a chemical is classified, warnings are automatically assigned so each chemical that falls into the same category will have the same label requirements and language. This will help to ensure that evaluations of the hazardous effects are consistent for all manufacturers and that labels and SDSs are also consistent.

### *Labels*

All labels will now include a harmonized **signal word**, **pictogram**, and **hazard statement** for each hazard class and category (Fig. 23.8).

### *Safety Data Sheets*

SDSs will now have a specified 16-section format.

### *Information and Training*

Employers are required to train workers on the new **label elements** and safety data sheets by June 1, 2016.

### *Phase-in Period*

There is a phase-in period in which employers are required to be in compliance with either the existing HCS or the revised HCS, or a combination of both. OSHA understands that there will be a period of time where both the previous types of labels and MSDSs will be used in the workplace, as well as the new GHS pictograms and SDSs. This will be acceptable, and employers are not required to maintain two sets of labels and SDSs.

## Written Program

The written program must identify, by name, all the employees in the office who are exposed to hazardous chemicals. It must also identify the individual who is responsible for the program. This is often a dental assistant. The written program must describe (1) staff training; (2) how chemicals are handled in the office, including information on all labeling and safety measures; and (3) how to respond to chemical emergencies such as spills or exposures.

If several dentists are working in one clinic or practice, all employers must be aware of hazards and protective measures so that they can train their employees.

### Responsibilities of Dental Assistant as Coordinator of Hazard Communication Program

- Read and understand the OSHA Hazard Communication Standard.
- Implement the written hazard communication program.
- Compile a list (chemical inventory) of products in the office that contain hazardous chemicals.
- Obtain Safety Data Sheets (SDSs).
- Update the SDS file as new products are added to the office inventory.
- Inform other employees of the location of SDSs.
- Label appropriate containers.
- Assist in training other employees.

## Chemical Inventory

The **chemical inventory** is a list of all products used in the office that contain chemicals. It includes amalgam, composites, bonding materials, etching agents, disinfectants, sterilants, and impression materials, among others. Each time a new product that contains a chemical is brought into the office, it must be added to the chemical inventory. The SDS for that product must be placed in the SDS file. The manufacturer or distributor must provide an updated SDS when appropriate.

The dentist will often appoint the dental assistant to be the program coordinator and to take responsibility for maintaining the chemical inventory and updating the SDS file.

## Safety Data Sheets

SDSs contain health and safety information about every chemical in the office. SDSs provide comprehensive technical information and are an important resource for employees who work with chemicals. They describe the physical and chemical properties of a material, health hazards, routes of exposure, precautions for safe handling and use, emergency and first aid procedures, and spill control measures.

The manufacturer of a product that contains chemicals is required to supply the dental office with an SDS for the product. However, it is the responsibility of the dental office to make sure that an SDS is available for every chemical used in the office. SDSs often are enclosed in the package with the product. These sheets should be organized in binders so that employees have ready access to them and can easily locate a particular SDS (Fig. 23.9, Table 23.1, and Box 23.1).

RECALL

12 What is purpose of the OSHA Hazard Communication Standard?
13 Why was the OSHA Hazard Communication Standard Revised?
14 What information is contained on the SDS?

## Employee Training

Employee training is essential for a successful hazard communication program. Staff training is required (1) when a new employee is hired, (2) when a new chemical product is introduced to the office, and (3) once a year for all continuing employees. Records of each training session must be kept on file for at least 5 years.

Although the dentist is responsible for providing the training, the dental assistant may assist in the training of new employees and is also responsible for routinely following safety precautions. The chemical training program for employees must provide information on the following:

- How to safely use hazardous chemicals
- Understanding information on the SDS
- All safety practices, including all warnings
- How to use required PPE
- Safe handling and disposal methods

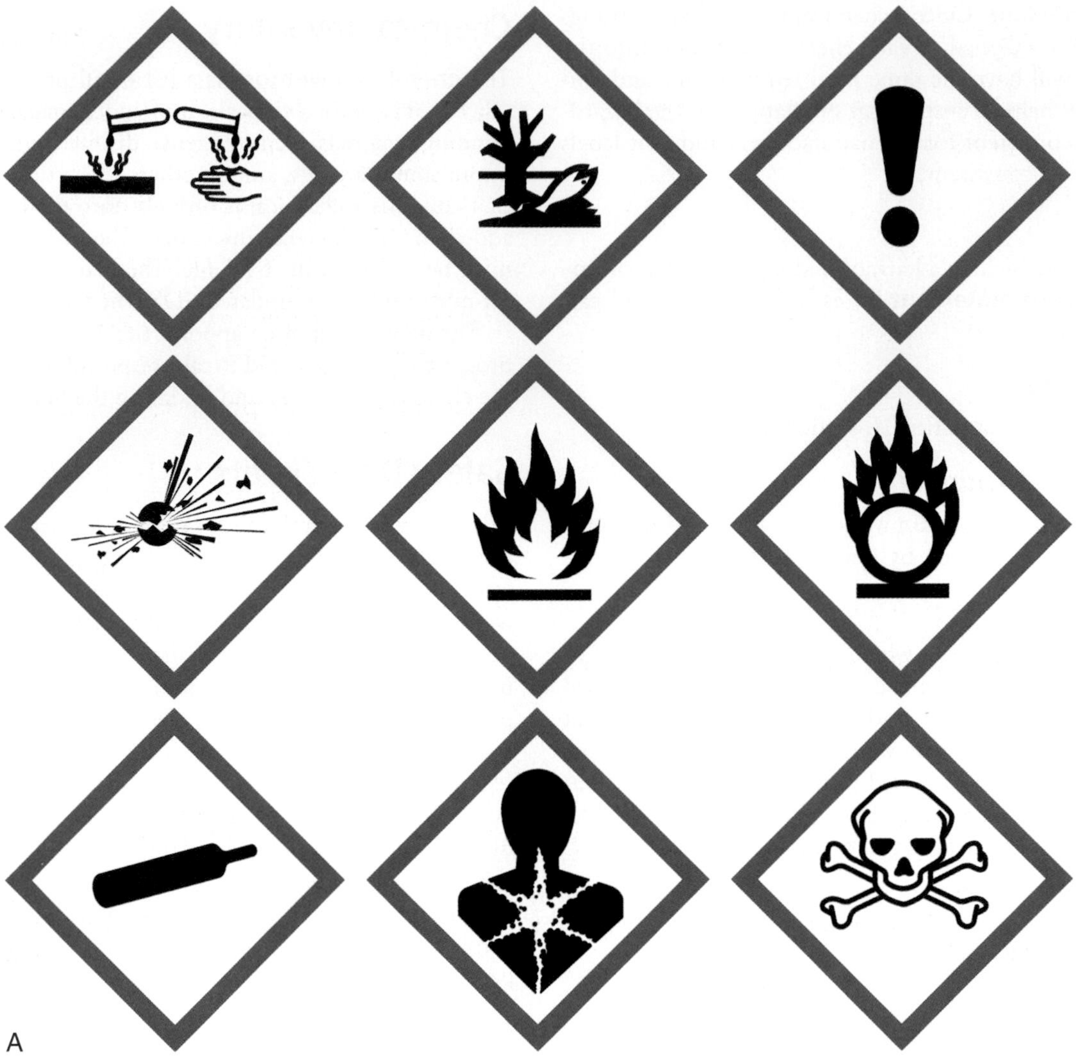

A

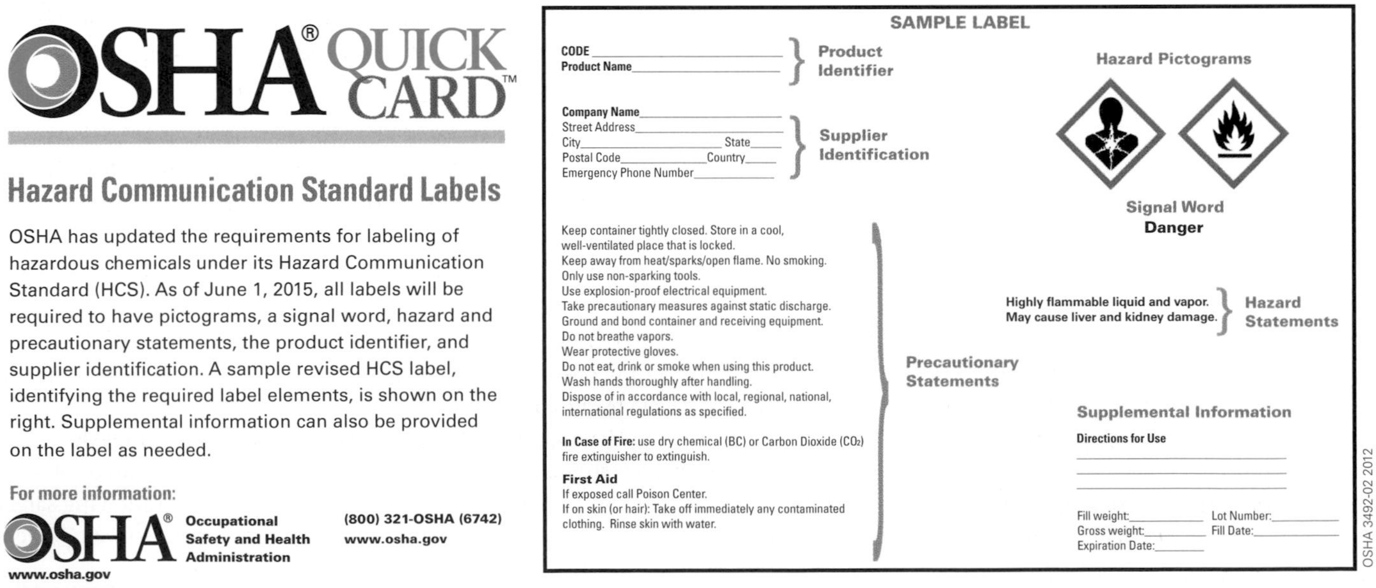

OSHA® QUICK CARD™

## Hazard Communication Standard Labels

OSHA has updated the requirements for labeling of hazardous chemicals under its Hazard Communication Standard (HCS). As of June 1, 2015, all labels will be required to have pictograms, a signal word, hazard and precautionary statements, the product identifier, and supplier identification. A sample revised HCS label, identifying the required label elements, is shown on the right. Supplemental information can also be provided on the label as needed.

For more information:

OSHA® Occupational Safety and Health Administration
(800) 321-OSHA (6742)
www.osha.gov

www.osha.gov

SAMPLE LABEL

CODE ______
Product Name ______
} Product Identifier

Company Name ______
Street Address ______
City ______ State ______
Postal Code ______ Country ______
Emergency Phone Number ______
} Supplier Identification

Hazard Pictograms

Signal Word
**Danger**

Highly flammable liquid and vapor.
May cause liver and kidney damage.
} Hazard Statements

Keep container tightly closed. Store in a cool, well-ventilated place that is locked.
Keep away from heat/sparks/open flame. No smoking.
Only use non-sparking tools.
Use explosion-proof electrical equipment.
Take precautionary measures against static discharge.
Ground and bond container and receiving equipment.
Do not breathe vapors.
Wear protective gloves.
Do not eat, drink or smoke when using this product.
Wash hands thoroughly after handling.
Dispose of in accordance with local, regional, national, international regulations as specified.

**In Case of Fire:** use dry chemical (BC) or Carbon Dioxide ($CO_2$) fire extinguisher to extinguish.

**First Aid**
If exposed call Poison Center.
If on skin (or hair): Take off immediately any contaminated clothing. Rinse skin with water.
} Precautionary Statements

Supplemental Information

Directions for Use
______

Fill weight: ______ Lot Number: ______
Gross weight: ______ Fill Date: ______
Expiration Date: ______

OSHA 3492-02 2012

B

**FIG. 23.8** A, Hazard Communication Standard pictograms. B, Sample label. *(From http://www.osha.gov/dsg/hazcom/index.html; accessed April 26, 2013.)*

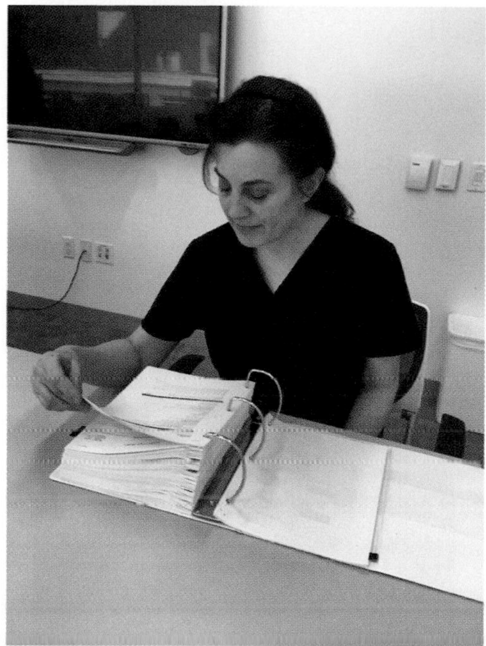

**FIG. 23.9** Example of a dental assistant referring to Safety Data Sheets.

## Guide for Hazard Communication Employee Training Program*

- Requirements of the Hazard Communication Standard
- Written communication plan for the office (location, use, etc.)
- Understanding of the hazards of the chemicals with which employees work
- Ability to interpret warning pictograms and SDSs
- Knowledge of where to obtain additional information
- Measures to protect employees and others:
  - Office safety procedures
  - Available PPE
  - Instructions for reporting accidents and emergencies
  - Information about first aid
  - Methods and observations to detect the presence or release of a hazardous chemical
- Question and answer opportunity

*On completion, employees are asked to sign a training record that will be kept in the personnel file.

*PPE*, Personal protective equipment; *SDSs*, Safety Data Sheets.

## TABLE 23.1 Sections of Hazard Communication Standard Safety Data Sheets

The Hazard Communication Standard (HCS) requires chemical manufacturers, distributors, or importers to provide Safety Data Sheets (SDSs) (formerly known as Material Safety Data Sheets [MSDSs]) to communicate the hazards of hazardous chemical products. As of June 1, 2015, the HCS will require new SDSs to be in a uniform format and include the section numbers, the headings, and associated information under the headings below:

| Section | Description | Explanation |
|---|---|---|
| 1 | Identification | Includes product identifier; manufacturer or distributor name, address, phone number; emergency phone number; recommended use; restrictions on use. |
| 2 | Hazard(s) identification | Includes all hazards regarding the chemical; required label elements. |
| 3 | Composition/information on ingredients | Includes information on chemical ingredients; trade secret claims. |
| 4 | First-aid measures | Includes important symptoms/effects, acute, delayed; required treatment. |
| 5 | Fire-fighting measures | Lists suitable extinguishing techniques, equipment; chemical hazards from fire. |
| 6 | Accidental release measures | Lists emergency procedures; protective equipment; proper methods of containment and cleanup. |
| 7 | Handling and storage | Lists precautions for safe handling and storage, including incompatibilities. |
| 8 | Exposure controls/personal protection | Lists OSHA's Permissible Exposure Limits (PELs); Threshold Limit Values (TLVs); appropriate engineering controls; personal protective equipment (PPE). |
| 9 | Physical and chemical properties | Lists the chemical's characteristics. |
| 10 | Stability and reactivity | Lists chemical stability and possibility of hazardous reactions. |
| 11 | Toxicological information | Includes routes of exposure; related symptoms, acute and chronic effects; numerical measures of toxicity. |
| 12 | Ecological information* | |
| 13 | Disposal considerations* | |
| 14 | Transport information* | |
| 15 | Regulatory information* | |
| 16 | Other information | Includes the date of preparation or last revision. |

*Note:* Because other agencies regulate this information, OSHA will not be enforcing Sections 12 through 15 (29 CFR 1910.1200(g)(2)).

For more information: www.osha.gov; (800) 321-OSHA (6742); U.S. Department of Labor.

**BOX 23.1 Required Format of Safety Data Sheets**

- Section 1. Identification
- Section 2. Hazard(s) identification
- Section 3. Composition/information on ingredients
- Section 4. First-aid measures
- Section 5. Fire-fighting measures
- Section 6. Accidental release measures
- Section 7. Handling and storage
- Section 8. Exposure controls/personal protection
- Section 9. Physical and chemical properties
- Section 10. Stability and reactivity
- Section 11. Toxicological information
- *Section 12. Ecological information*
- *Section 13. Disposal considerations*
- *Section 14. Transport information*
- *Section 15. Regulatory information*
- Section 16. Other information, including date of preparation or last revision

*Note:* Although the headings for Sections 12 to 15 are mandatory for the SDS, OSHA will not enforce the content of these four sections because these sections are within other agencies' jurisdictions.

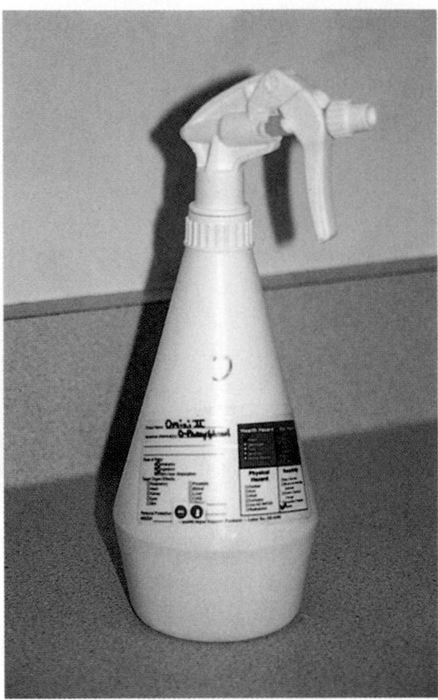

**FIG. 23.10** Chemical disinfectants not in their original container must be clearly labeled.

## Labeling of Chemical Containers

Containers must be labeled to indicate what chemicals they contain and any hazards that may be associated. The important considerations are that (1) the labeling system includes all required information and (2) all employees are properly trained to understand and read the label.

When the chemical is transferred to a different container, however, the secondary container also must be labeled. For example, when a concentrated chemical disinfectant is mixed fresh and is placed into a spray bottle or tub *(secondary containers),* the spray bottle or tub must be labeled (Fig. 23.10). Other examples of secondary containers that hold chemicals and require labeling are automatic x-ray film processors and manual processing tanks, ultrasonic cleaning tanks, and chemical vapor sterilizers.

All labels are required to have pictograms, a signal word, hazard statement and **precautionary statement**, the **product identifier**, and supplier. Supplier information must include the name, address, and phone number of manufacturer, importer, or distributor. Precautionary statements must also be provided. In addition to labeling, the SDSs must be available to employees.

OSHA has not changed the general requirements for workplace labeling. Employers still have the option to create their own workplace labels. The labels can either provide all of the required information from the chemical manufacturer, or the product identifier and words, pictures, symbols, or a combination of these. It is most important that employees have information immediately available regarding the hazards of the chemicals. Employees must be informed about where to obtain that information within the office.

### National Fire Protection Association Labels

The National Fire Protection Association (NFPA) has a labeling system that has long been used to label containers of hazardous chemicals. Under the revised Standard, the NFPA system may still be used. This system involves the use of four diamonds (blue, red, yellow, and white) that are filled with numeric ratings from 0 to 4. The categories are health hazard (blue), flammability (red), reactivity (yellow), and special hazard symbols, such as OX for **oxidizers** (white). See Procedure 23.1: Creating an Appropriate Label for a Secondary Container.

### Exemptions to Labeling Requirements

Certain chemicals, including tobacco and tobacco products, wood and wood products, food, drugs, cosmetics, and alcoholic beverages sold and packaged for consumer use, are exempted from the standard. Drugs dispensed by a pharmacy to a healthcare provider for direct administration to a patient also are exempt from the labeling requirement, as are over-the-counter drugs and drugs intended for personal consumption by employees while in the workplace, such as aspirin and first aid supplies.

**RECALL**

15 Which employees must receive training about hazardous chemicals?
16 What should be included in employee training for the hazard communication program?
17 What is a secondary container?
18 What is a pictogram?
19 Using the National Fire Protection Association labeling system, what is the meaning of each color in the triangle?

**TABLE 23.2** Types of Dental Waste

| Category | Definition | Examples |
|---|---|---|
| Medical waste | Waste generated as part of treatment; can be contaminated or infectious | Contaminated barriers |
| Contaminated waste | Waste that has been in contact with blood or other body fluids; in most states, disposed of as general waste | Contaminated patient bibs |
| Infectious waste | Contaminated waste that is capable of causing an infectious disease | Blood and blood-saturated materials |
| Chemical waste | Waste that poses a threat to humans or the environment | Pathologic waste: tissue, extracted teeth* |
| Hazardous waste | Usually refers to **toxic chemicals** or materials | Sharps: needles, burs |
| Toxic waste | | Scrap amalgam |
| General waste | Nonhazardous, nonregulated waste | Lead foil<br>Radiographic solutions†<br>Paper waste generated at front desk<br>Discarded lunch bags or wraps |

*If teeth contain amalgam restorations, they are hazardous waste as well.

†Some states consider only fixer as toxic waste; others consider both fixer and developer as toxic.

## Dental Office Waste Management

Dental offices use some substances that may be regulated under federal, state, or local environmental regulations (Table 23.2). When discharged into a sewer system, these materials may affect the wastewater treatment plant or may bypass the treatment plant and enter a bay, ocean, river, or other waters. The environmental impact is minimized when these materials are handled, recycled, treated, or disposed of properly. Regulations vary from state to state, and many states *require* dental offices to have specific types of waste hauled away by a licensed carrier. The dental assistant should know the types of dental waste, how to comply with regulations, and ways to minimize the costs associated with disposal.

### Dental Materials That May Be Regulated

- Mercury and dental amalgam
- Elemental mercury
- Amalgam capsules
- Scrap amalgam
- Amalgam traps
- Lead foil and shields
- Disinfectant solutions
- X-ray fixer solution
- X-ray developer solution

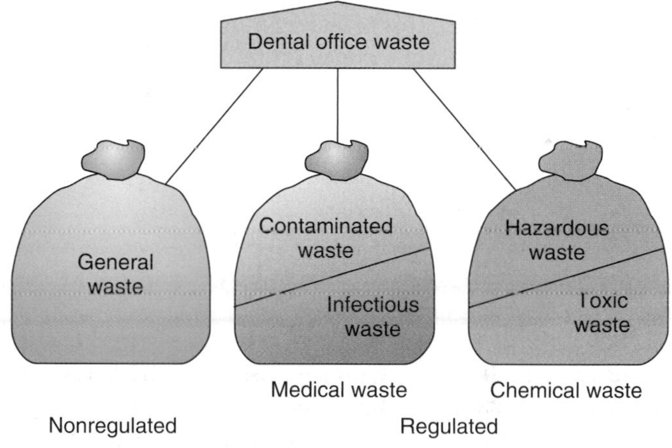


*NOTE:* Contaminated waste is disposed of as general waste.

**FIG. 23.11** Classification of dental waste.

## Classification of Waste

OSHA regulations apply to the handling of waste in the dental office for the protection of employees. When waste *leaves* the dental office, Environmental Protection Agency (EPA) regulations apply to the disposal. All dental waste should be classified according to EPA guidelines as regulated or nonregulated (Fig. 23.11).

**Regulated waste** includes *sharps,* such as disposable needles, scalpel blades, contaminated broken glass, disposable dental burs, and endodontic files and reamers. Other regulated waste includes blood, blood-soaked and blood-caked items, human tissue, and pathologic waste. Regulated waste requires special disposal.

Nonregulated waste includes **contaminated waste** materials, as well as saliva-soaked gauze, used patient bibs, and surface barriers.

**Toxic waste** is waste that can have a poisonous effect.

All waste containers that hold *potentially infectious materials* (whether regulated or nonregulated) must be labeled with the *biohazard* symbol. OSHA requires this label to protect the employees, and the EPA requires this label to inform the public.

## Extracted Teeth

Extracted teeth are considered to be potentially infectious materials and thus are *regulated waste* if they are not disinfected and returned to the patient. Many states allow the dental office to sterilize the extracted teeth. Teeth that do not contain amalgam and are going to be used for educational purposes must be heat-sterilized first.

Extracted teeth that contain amalgam restorations should *never* be heat-sterilized because the high temperatures may create toxic mercury vapors. For teeth that contain amalgam restorations, immersion in fresh, full-strength glutaraldehyde for at least 30 minutes is recommended for disinfection. After the tooth is rinsed, it can be disposed of according to local regulations.

RECALL

**20** Name dental materials that would be regulated waste.
**21** Name four materials that would be contaminated waste.
**22** What type of waste are extracted teeth?

## Sharps

OSHA, the Centers for Disease Control and Prevention (CDC), and the EPA classify sharps as **infectious waste.** According to OSHA regulations, disposable sharps must be placed in a closable, leakproof, puncture-resistant container immediately after use. This container must be labeled with the biohazard symbol and color coded for ready identification (Fig. 23.12). State regulations may differ regarding how frequently sharps containers must be picked up. Check the regulations in your state.

## Scrap Amalgam

Scrap dental amalgam should be collected and stored in a designated, dry, airtight container. Scrap amalgam that is *not* recycled must be managed as hazardous waste. The container of scrap amalgam that *is* recycled must be labeled with the name, address, and telephone number of the dental office and the date on which you first started collecting material in the container. Check with the mercury recycling company for any additional requirements.

In the past, scrap dental amalgam may have been kept under photographic fixer, water, or other liquid. If you encounter amalgam stored in this manner, do *not* pour the liquid down the drain under any circumstances. Contact a mercury recycler or a hazardous waste hauler for more information on how to dispose of this material properly.

## Photochemical Waste

Dental offices generate two separate types of waste from x-ray processing solutions: radiographic fixer and radiographic developer (Fig. 23.13).

### Radiographic Fixer

Radiographic fixer is considered a hazardous waste because of its high silver content. The two basic options for its management in the dental office are *on-site* treatment and *off-site* treatment. On-site treatment requires the installation of silver recovery systems to remove the toxic silver from the solution. Off-site treatment involves storing the used fixer and contracting with a disposal company to have it picked up. Contact your local wastewater treatment plant for specific requirements in your area.

### Radiographic Developer

The developer solution may exceed the pH standard set by the local wastewater treatment plant. Products with a high or a low pH are likely to be considered hazardous waste and must be managed according to local regulations.

## Lead Contamination

### Lead Foil

Lead foil from x-ray film packages is easily recyclable but cannot be disposed of in the garbage. Lead foil is exempt from regulation as a hazardous waste when recycled as a scrap metal, but it must be recycled through a licensed recovery facility. Eastman Kodak offers a mail-in service for recycling this material.

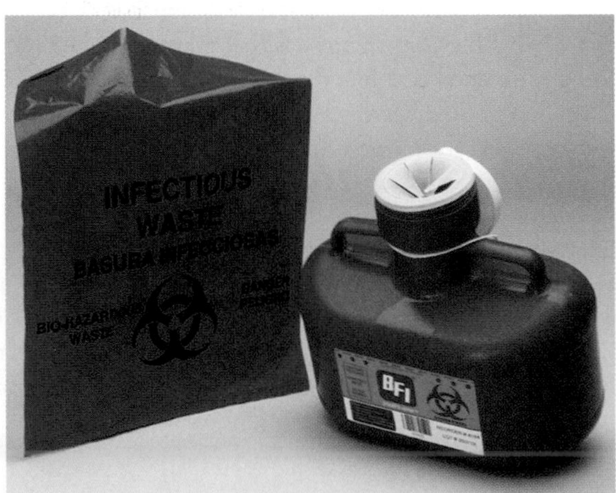


**FIG. 23.12** Biohazard bag and biohazard sharps containers. *(From Proctor DB, et al: Kinn's the medical assistant: an applied learning approach, ed 13, St Louis, 2017, Elsevier.)*

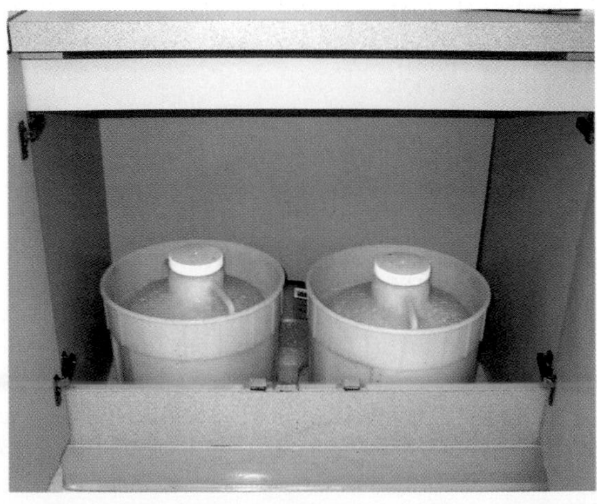

**FIG. 23.13** Radiographic solutions in holding containers.

## Disinfectants

Small quantities of spent germicidal solutions that contain 2 percent or less glutaraldehyde can usually be poured down the drain. Germicidal solutions with greater than 2 percent glutaraldehyde may need to be managed as a hazardous waste. Check with local authorities on disposal methods for these chemicals.

Used or unused disinfectant with a high concentration of formaldehyde or a *flash point* less than 140° F is a hazardous waste that cannot be discharged into the sewer. Products with a red flammable label have a flash point lower than 100° F. Always check the SDS for the flash points of other materials.

## Nonhazardous Waste Management

Regular dental office waste should be recycled whenever possible. This includes aluminum, glass, newspapers, corrugated fiber, office paper, and mixed paper. The local sanitation department or garbage collection service is a source of recycling information.

**23** Describe the requirements for sharps containers.
**24** What is the best method to store scrap amalgam?
**25** Why is radiographic fixer considered to be hazardous waste?
**26** Where could you find information about the flash point of a disinfectant?

## Waste Disposal

The EPA enforces the disposal of regulated waste. If state and local regulations are more stringent than federal rules, state and local regulations must be followed.

The dentist is responsible for proper packaging, labeling, transportation, and ultimate disposal of waste generated in the dental office. All containers should be rigid, leak resistant, impervious to moisture, and strong enough to prevent damage and leakage during handling. All containers must be labeled according to state law.

Many dental offices choose to use a licensed transporter, a disposal source, or a recycling company. However, the dentist is always responsible for the waste until it is rendered nonhazardous or is destroyed; therefore choosing a reputable disposal service is important.

■ **Legal and Ethical Implications** The dental health professional cannot anticipate or prevent every health and safety risk, but the risks are greatly reduced when all dental office personnel are aware of chemical safety and infectious waste guidelines.

Use good common sense. If you are ever in doubt about the safety of a chemical product, read the SDS, ask the dentist, or contact the manufacturer. All regulated waste must be disposed of in a manner consistent with the local regulations. Always check your local and state regulations for management of dental waste if you are uncertain about disposal methods.

Your health, the health of your coworkers, and the health of the community may depend on your commitment to chemical safety. ■

■ **Eye to the Future** The dental assistant who is responsible for the hazard communication program must clearly understand the basic concepts of chemical management. If you become the hazard communication coordinator in your office, you must stay current with the increasing number and complexity of products in the dental office. You must also be vigilant and watch for changes in your state and federal regulations. ■

### ■ Critical Thinking

1. One of your coworkers frequently eats her lunch in an area of the office in which chemicals are used. What can you say to her to convince her that this is a bad habit?
2. If you were using a chemical that had the number 4 in the red triangle on the chemical label, what would this indicate to you?
3. You have just been placed in charge of putting chemical labels on secondary containers in your dental office. What are some types of containers that should be labeled?
4. Look at the SDS for products usually found in the dental office. What products contain chemicals that pose hazards for (a) inhalation, (b) skin contact, and (c) flammability?
5. Go online to research regulations regarding disposal of hazardous waste in your area. ■

PROCEDURE 23.1

# Creating an Appropriate Label for a Secondary Container

## GOAL

To create a label for a secondary container according to OSHA regulations and standards for hazardous chemicals.

## EQUIPMENT AND SUPPLIES

- Safety Data Sheet (SDS) for product to be labeled
- Pen
- National Fire Protection Association (NFPA) chemical label

## PROCEDURAL STEPS

1. Write the manufacturer's name and address on the label. (This information is found in the Product Information section of the SDS.)
2. Write the name of the chemical(s) and the "target organ" on the label. (This information is also found in the Product Information section.)
3. Write the appropriate health hazard code in the blue diamond. (This information is found in the Health Hazard Data section of the SDS.)
4. Write the appropriate flammability and explosion code in the red diamond. (This information is found in the Fire and Explosion section of the SDS.)
5. Write the appropriate reactivity code in the yellow diamond. (This information is found in the Reactivity Data section of the SDS.)
6. Write the appropriate specific hazard warning in the white diamond. (This information is found in the Precautions for Safe Handling and Use section of the SDS.)
7. Attach the chemical label to the secondary container.

24

# Dental Unit Waterlines

## KEY TERMS

**Antiretraction device** A mechanism that prevents entry of fluids and microorganisms into waterlines as a result of negative water pressure; also called "suck back."

**Biofilm (BYE-oe-film)** Slime-producing bacterial communities that may also harbor fungi, algae, and protozoa.

**Colony-forming units (CFUs)** A number of separable cells on the surface of a semisolid agar medium that create a visible colony.

**Dental unit waterline (DUWL)** Small bore tubing usually made of plastic, used to deliver dental treatment water through a dental unit.

**Heterotrophic (het-ur-oe-TROF-ik) bacteria** Bacteria that use organic carbon as a source of nutrients. Protozoa, fungi, and most bacteria fall into this category.

**Immunocompromised** Having an immune system that is weakened.

***Legionella*** **(lee-juh-NEL-uh)** Genus of bacteria responsible for the disease legionellosis.

**Microfiltration** Use of membrane filters to trap microorganisms suspended in water.

**Planktonic (plank-TON-ik)** Describes bacteria that are freely floating in water.

**Self-contained water reservoir** Container attached to a dental unit that is used to hold and supply water or other solutions to handpieces and air-water syringes.

## LEARNING OUTCOMES

*On completion of this chapter, the student will be able to achieve the following objectives:*

1. Pronounce, define, and spell the key terms.
2. Discuss microorganisms in dental unit waterlines (DUWLs), including the following:
   - Explain why dental unit waterlines contain more bacteria than faucets.
   - Discuss why there is a renewed interest in DUWL contamination.
   - Identify the primary source of microorganisms in dental unit water.
   - Explain the role of biofilm in DUWL contamination.
   - List the factors involved in bacterial contamination of dental unit water.
3. Describe methods used to reduce bacterial contamination in DUWLs.
4. Discuss infection control and dental unit water, including the following:
   - Describe the Centers for Disease Control and Prevention (CDC) recommendations for dental unit water quality.
   - Explain the CDC recommendation for the use of dental handpieces and other devices attached to air and waterlines, including saliva ejectors.

## PERFORMANCE OUTCOME

*On completion of this chapter, the student will be able to meet competency standards in the following skill:*

- Testing a DUWL.

## ELECTRONIC RESOURCES

***Additional information related to content in Chapter 24 can be found on the companion Evolve Web site.***

- Practice Quiz

Outbreaks of waterborne disease have occurred in a broad range of facilities, including hospitals, nursing homes, schools, restaurants, community water supplies, swimming pools, and spas. Although no evidence suggests a widespread public health problem, published reports have associated illness with exposure to water from dental units. Bacteria capable of causing disease in some humans are found in dental unit waterlines (DUWLs); this is reason for concern (Fig. 24.1). In addition, exposing patients or dental professionals to water with extremely high bacterial counts is not in line with currently accepted infection control principles.

In community water, the number of waterborne bacteria is kept below 500 **colony-forming units (CFUs)** per milliliter (ml). Water from air-water syringes and dental handpieces frequently has levels that are hundreds or thousands of times *greater* than are permissible in drinking water. The types of bacteria found in dental unit water are frequently the same as those found in community water, but the quantity of bacteria found in dental units is almost always higher. Research has shown that microbial counts in DUWLs can reach 200,000 CFUs/ml within 5 days of installation of new lines. Counts greater than 1,000,000 CFUs/ml have been reported.

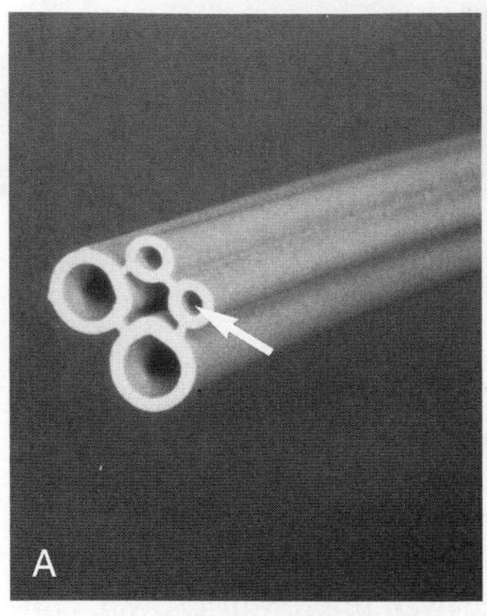


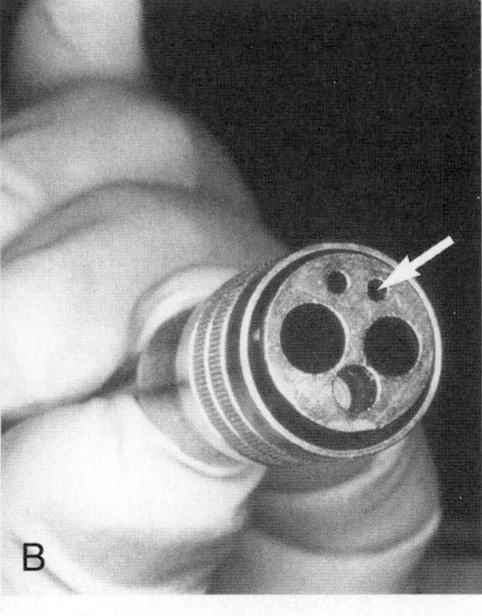


**FIG. 24.1** Dental unit waterline. A, The four-hole high-speed handpiece hose. B, The connector at the end of the hose to which a high-speed handpiece is attached. (*Arrows* indicate the water lines.) *(From Miller CH: Infection control and management of hazardous materials for the dental team, ed 6, St Louis, 2018, Elsevier.*

**TABLE 24.1** Sample Amounts of Bacteria in Dental Unit Water at Various U.S. Sites

| Source | CFUs/ml* |
|---|---|
| 10 dental units from three offices | 180,000 |
| Tap water from three offices above | 15 |
| 54 air-water syringe hoses | 165,000 |
| 22 high-speed handpiece hoses | 739,000 |
| 10 faucets | <30 |
| 4 water coolers | <30 |
| 11 rivers and streams | 28,200 |
| 8 dental units | 110,000 |

Modified from Miller CH: Infection control and management of hazardous materials for the dental team, ed 6, St Louis, 2018, Elsevier.
*Colony-forming units per milliliter.

This chapter provides an overview of the problem of **dental unit waterline (DUWL)** contamination, the potential health risks to patients and dental personnel, and the steps that you can take to lower the risk for DUWL contamination. You will also learn how to comply with Centers for Disease Control and Prevention (CDC) recommendations related to DUWLs, biofilm, and water quality.

# Microorganisms in Dental Unit Waterlines

## Background

The presence of bacteria in DUWLs was first reported more than 30 years ago. This issue is now attracting renewed attention because of increased awareness of occupational hazards in the dental office, as well as concern about the increasing number of dental patients who have a weakened immune system. Elderly patients, patients who smoke or who are alcoholic, and patients who have received organ transplants or blood transfusions are among the types of patients with weakened immune systems.

Studies have demonstrated that DUWLs (i.e., tubing that carries water to the high-speed handpiece, air-water syringe, and ultrasonic scaler) can become colonized with microorganisms, including bacteria, fungi, and protozoa. These microorganisms colonize and multiply on the interior surfaces of the waterline tubing and form a biofilm. (Biofilms are discussed later in this chapter.)

Several studies reveal that dental healthcare workers are exposed to *Legionella* bacteria at a much higher rate than the general public. ***Legionella*** species are harmful bacteria often found in water and moist places that are responsible for the disease *legionellosis.* Dental personnel are exposed to *Legionella* by inhaling the contaminated aerosol generated by the handpiece and the air-water syringe.

Fortunately, most dental healthcare workers are healthy and do not develop the disease. However, one dentist's death has been linked to legionellosis. **Immunocompromised** patients have also developed postoperative infection caused by contaminated dental water.

## Sources of Microorganisms

Waterborne and human oral microorganisms have been found in dental unit water. This indicates that *both* incoming community water and the patient's mouth are sources of these microorganisms.

The *primary source* of microorganisms in DUWLs is the public water supply. However, saliva may be retracted back into the waterlines during treatment, a process called "backflow." The installation of **antiretraction devices** on dental units and thorough flushing of DUWLs between patients minimize this risk. The risk for backflow from saliva ejectors is discussed later in this chapter.

When community water enters the dental office, it contains fewer than 500 CFUs/ml. However, once that water enters DUWLs, and existing bacteria colonize and multiply within the biofilm, the CFU count greatly increases (Table 24.1).

Two "communities" of bacteria have been detected in DUWLs. The bacterial community in the water itself is referred to as **planktonic**. The other community exists in the biofilm attached to DUWL walls.

RECALL

1. Are waterborne diseases limited to dentistry?
2. Is the presence of bacteria in DUWLs a recent finding?
3. Has a widespread public health problem regarding contaminated dental water been reported?
4. What bacteria cause the disease legionellosis?

## Biofilm

**Biofilm** consists of bacterial cells and other microbes that adhere to surfaces and form a protective slime layer. You may

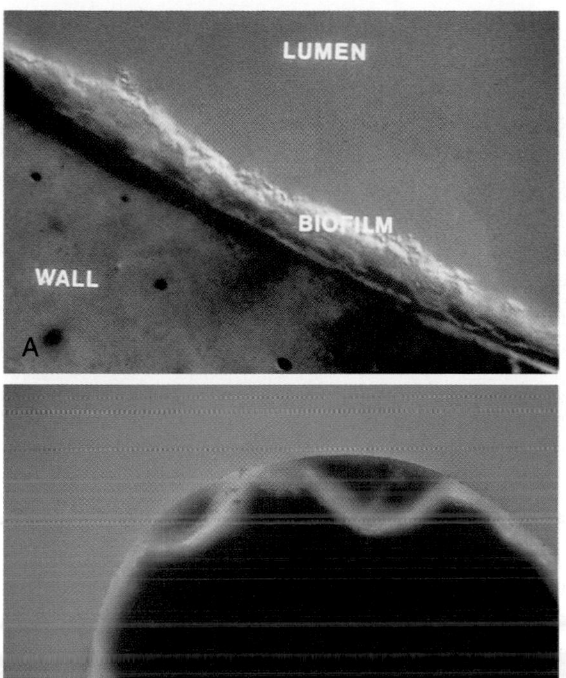


FIG. 24.2 A, Magnification of biofilm formation on the walls of the tube. B, Magnification of cross section of biofilm formation in DUWL. *(Courtesy Dr. Shannon Mills/United States Air Force.)*

have seen or felt the biofilm slime layer that forms on the inside surface of a flower vase or a pet's water bowl.

Biofilm is found in virtually all places where moisture and a suitable surface exist. The inside of dental tubing is an especially favorable environment for formation of biofilm (Fig. 24.2).

The best example of biofilm in dentistry is *dental plaque.* Biofilm is a type of "plaque" that develops inside DUWLs and causes "infection" of the water delivery system. Biofilm can contain many types of bacteria, as well as fungi, algae, and protozoa.

*Note:* Viruses, such as the human immunodeficiency virus (HIV), *cannot* multiply within the DUWL.

## Biofilm in Dental Waterlines

Water enters the dental office from municipal supplies or from wells. It is then routed to various sites within the office, including sink faucets, toilets, air conditioners, and the dental unit.

At the dental unit, the water enters plastic waterlines, which pass through a multichannel control box that allows the water to be distributed to the hoses that feed various attachments, such as high-speed handpieces, air-water syringes, and ultrasonic scalers. Thus the water that enters the dental unit is the same water that supplies the entire office.

DUWLs have a narrow tube (⅛ to 1⁄16 inch). Biofilm forms on the inside of DUWLs as water flows through the unit.

### Growth-Promoting Factors

Several factors contribute to the formation of biofilm in DUWLs. Water moves at normal line pressure (slowly). Intermittent stagnation of water inside the units typically occurs between patients, overnight, and over weekends, allowing the planktonic community of bacteria to attach to the walls of the tube. The bacteria become stabilized on a surface, and the nutrients in the water feed them (Fig. 24.3).

Some dental offices have water heaters in the dental units that warm the water for the patient's comfort. The use of water heaters also may contribute to increased levels of bacterial colonization. Heating water to near body temperature for patient comfort may enhance the growth of microorganisms. Another factor in biofilm formation within DUWLs is the maze of waterlines in which water can accumulate and become stagnant.

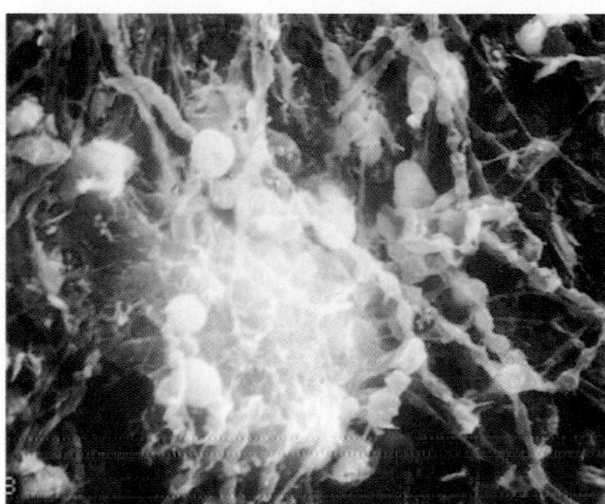

FIG. 24.3 Bacteria in biofilm taken from DUWLs. *(Courtesy Dr. Shannon Mills/United States Air Force.)*

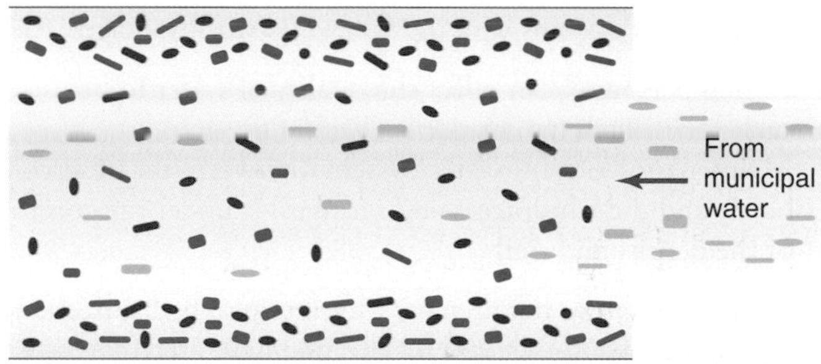


FIG. 24.4 Bacteria in biofilm dropping into waterlines. Some bacteria are planktonic and enter directly from the municipal water supply.

### Bacterial Characteristics

When bacteria are embedded in the protective biofilm (slime layer), they are extremely difficult to remove or kill. Bacteria in the biofilm are up to 1500 times more resistant to chemical germicides than are planktonic (free-floating) bacteria.

During use of the dental handpiece or air-water syringe, some bacteria already present in the incoming public water, as well as bacteria dropping off the biofilm, are carried out (Fig. 24.4).

RECALL

5 Where is biofilm found?
6 What is the disadvantage of heating the dental unit water?

## Methods for Reducing Bacterial Contamination

Complete elimination of biofilms and bacteria would be the ideal solution to the problem of DUWL contamination. Although this is not yet possible, methods for greatly reducing the level of bacterial contamination in waterlines are listed in Box 24.1.

## Self-Contained Water Reservoirs

Many manufacturers of dental units offer optional **self-contained water reservoir** systems. These systems work by supplying air pressure to the water bottle *(reservoir)*. The air pressure in the bottle forces the water from the bottle up into the DUWL and out to the handpiece and air-water syringe (Fig. 24.5). Self-contained water systems have the following two advantages:

- Dental personnel can select the quality of water to be used, such as distilled, tap, or sterile (Fig. 24.6).
- Maintenance of the water system (between the reservoir bottle and the handpieces and syringes) is under the control of the dentist and staff.

Failure to follow maintenance (cleaning and disinfection) procedures as recommended by the manufacturer may cause the water to become contaminated with even *higher than normal* counts of waterborne pathogens.

*Note:* Because the inside parts of the dental unit cannot be sterilized, the use of sterile water in the reservoir provides water of drinking quality, but it will not be sterile at the point of delivery.

**BOX 24.1 Methods to Reduce Bacterial Contamination of Dental Unit Waterlines (DUWLS)**

- Flush waterlines for several minutes at the beginning of the day and longer after weekends.
    - *Note:* Biofilms cannot be removed by flushing alone. Flushing for 20 to 30 seconds between patients is recommended to eliminate material retracted from the previous patient.
- Use a self-contained water reservoir system.
- Use a self-contained water reservoir system combined with periodic or continuous application of chemical germicides, as recommended by the equipment manufacturer.
- Use a separate (sterile water) system for surgical procedures.
- Purge the water from the dental lines and dry them with air at the end of each day.
- Use microfiltration cartridges in the waterlines.
- Stay current with new techniques and manufacturing technology for DUWLs.
- Follow the recommendations for monitoring water quality provided by the manufacturer of the dental unit or waterline treatment product.

## Microfiltration Cartridges

A disposable in-line **microfiltration** cartridge can dramatically reduce bacterial contamination within the dental unit water. This device must be inserted as close to the handpiece or air-water syringe as possible. The use of filtration cartridges combined with water reservoirs ensures improved water quality. Depending on the amount of use, the cartridges must be changed according to the manufacturer's recommendations (Fig. 24.7).

*Note:* Microfilters reduce the bacterial contamination of the water but *do not affect* the biofilms that colonize the DUWLs.

## Chemical Agents

Chemicals can be used to help control biofilm in two ways:

1. Periodic or "shock" treatment with *biocidal* levels (levels that will kill microorganisms) of chemicals
2. Continuous application of chemicals to the system (at biocidal levels but not levels that harm humans)

Because biofilms are extremely resistant to chemical destruction, chemical treatments must be provided regularly, usually

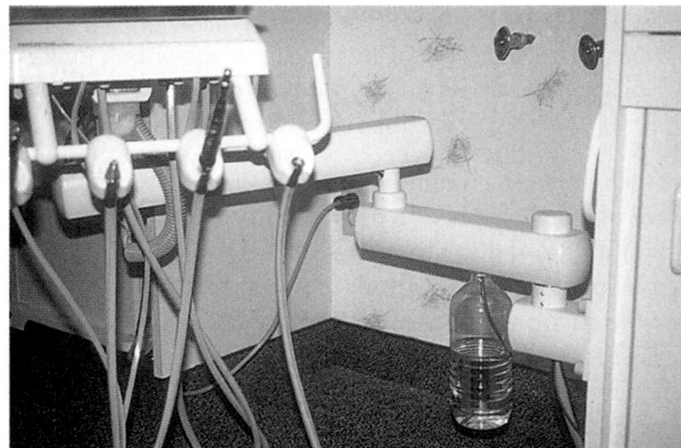

**FIG. 24.5** Self-contained dental water unit. *(Courtesy Dr. Ronald Johns.)*

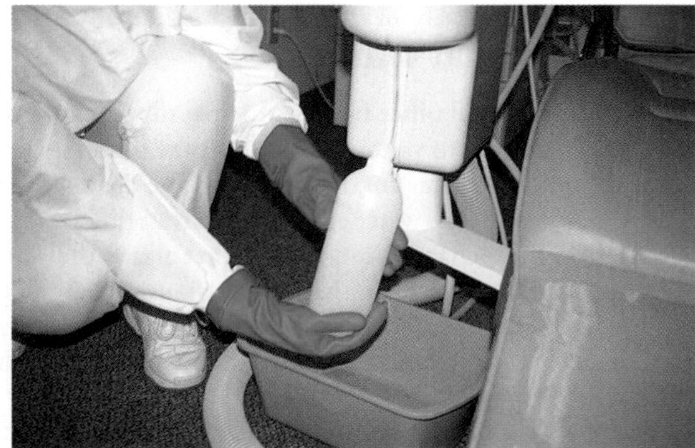

**FIG. 24.6** Reservoir water bottles and lines in self-contained water systems must be cleaned and disinfected according to the manufacturer's instructions. The container under the water bottle will catch any solution drips. Note that the dental assistant is careful not to touch and contaminate the neck of the bottle. *(Courtesy Pamela Landry, RDA.)*

once a week. Some products now on the market provide excellent cleaning and bacterial control properties. You must take care in selecting the best product to use, because some chemicals can cause damage to the dental units (Fig. 24.8).

*Always* check with the manufacturer of the dental equipment to determine the recommended chemical product and maintenance protocol.

RECALL

7 Is it possible to eliminate biofilm completely?
8 If sterile water is used in the self-contained reservoir, will the water that enters the patient's mouth be sterile?
9 How often should microfilters be changed?
10 What precautions should you take when selecting a chemical for the dental unit?

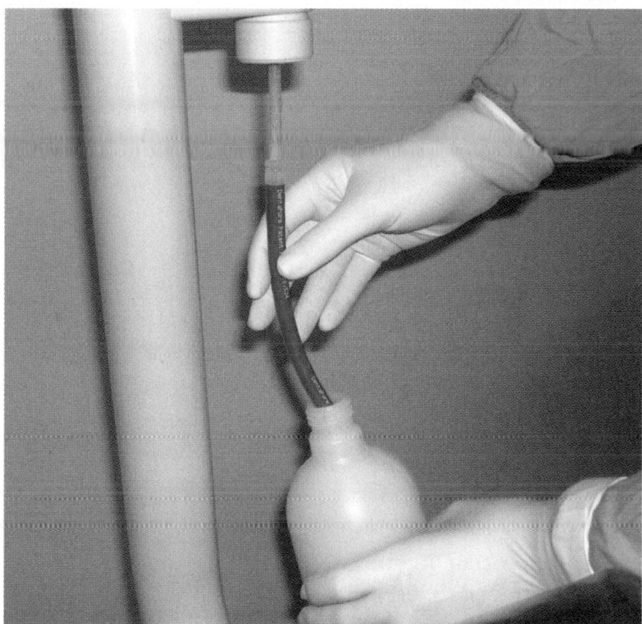

**FIG. 24.7** The DentaPure (blue) cartridge is attached to the tube in the unit that draws the water from the bottle. As the water is drawn from the bottle and passes through the cartridge, 2 to 6 parts per million of iodine are released into the water. Then the water that is delivered to the handpiece, three-way water syringe, and ultrasonic scaler is treated.

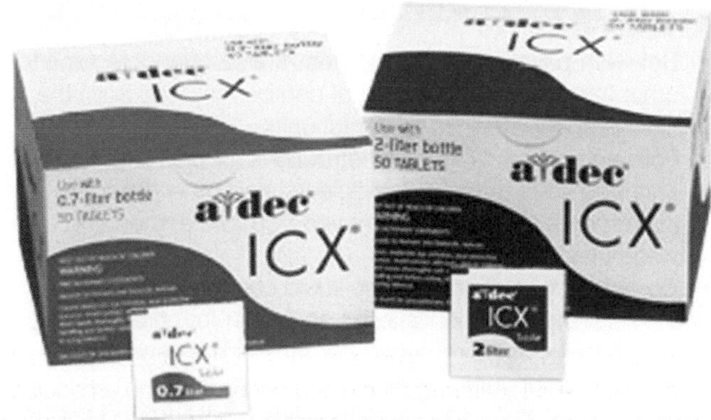


**FIG. 24.8** A-dec ICX waterline treatment tablets help protect waterlines from contamination. *(Courtesy A-dec Inc., Newberg, OR.)*

# Infection Control and Dental Unit Water

## Using the Proper Water

Dental unit water should *not* be used as an irrigant for surgery involving exposure of bone. Only sterile water from special sterile water delivery systems or hand irrigation with sterile water in a sterile disposable syringe should be used in these types of surgeries.

## Flushing Waterlines

All DUWLs and handpieces should be flushed every morning and from 20 to 30 seconds after each patient treatment. Flushing temporarily reduces the microbial count in the water and helps clean the handpiece waterlines of materials that may have entered from the patient's mouth. Flushing also brings a fresh supply of chlorinated water from the main waterlines into the dental unit.

*Note:* Flushing will not remove biofilm from the lines; biofilm can form while water is moving through the lines.

## Minimizing Aerosol

Always use the high-volume evacuator when assisting with use of the high-speed handpiece, ultrasonic scaler, and air-water syringe. This will reduce contamination from the aerosol and spatter from the patient's saliva, and from contact with the water spray. High-volume evacuation may reduce exposure of the patient, as well as the dental team, to these waterborne microorganisms (Fig. 24.9).

## Using Protective Barriers

The rubber dam serves as a protective barrier for the patient from dental unit water. The dam not only eliminates exposure, it also greatly reduces direct contact. The dam reduces the aerosolizing and spattering of patient microorganisms onto the dental team, but it does not reduce exposure of the dental team to dental unit water.

Protective barriers, including masks, eye protection, and face shields, also serve as barriers for the dental team against microorganisms coming from the patient's mouth and from the aerosols and sprays of dental unit water.

## Monitoring Water Quality

The only way to know whether the waterline cleaning regimen is effective is to test the water coming out of the unit. Two options are available for testing dental unit water. The first is to use a commercial testing service, by which you send samples of the unit water, and results are mailed or faxed back to the dental office. A certificate is issued if the sample is below 500 CFUs. This is similar to the procedure used for monitoring the sterilizers. The second method is to use an in-office test kit (see Procedure 24.1: Testing Dental Unit Waterlines). Testing is usually done with three samples of water taken from the same dental unit. Dental handpieces should be removed before

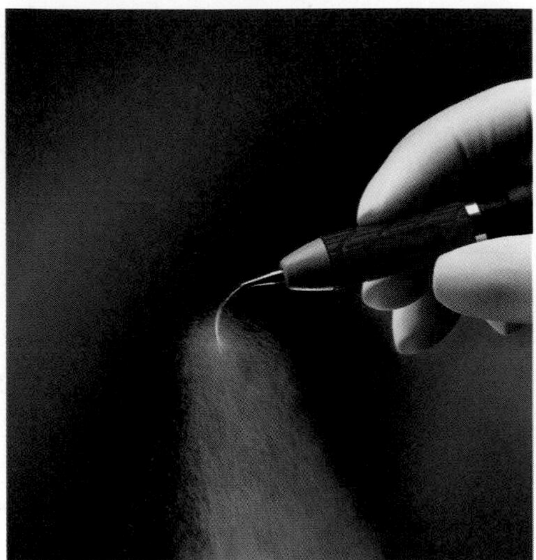

**FIG. 24.9** Water spray from ultrasonic scaler tip. *(Courtesy Hu-Friedy Mfg. Co. LLC, Chicago, IL.)*

the samples are taken. With either method of monitoring, it is important that you do not contaminate the water during sampling; you should wear gloves and very carefully follow the directions of the service or the test kit. *It is important for quality assurance to maintain records of the testing results when using either a commercial testing service or an in-office system.*

The CDC recommends that dental offices follow the recommendations of the manufacturer of the dental unit or the treatment product to monitor the quality of the dental unit water.

## Recommendations for Dental Unit Waterlines, Biofilm, and Water Quality CDC

- For routine dental treatment output water, use water that meets the regulatory standards of the Environmental Protection Agency (EPA) for drinking water (i.e., fewer than 500 CFUs/ml of **heterotrophic bacteria**).
- Consult with the dental manufacturer for appropriate methods and equipment to maintain the recommended quality of dental water.
- Follow recommendations for monitoring water quality provided by the manufacturer of the unit or waterline treatment product.
- After each patient treatment, discharge water and air for a minimum of 20 to 30 seconds from any device connected to the dental water system that enters the patient's mouth (e.g., handpieces, ultrasonic scalers, air-water syringes).
- Consult with the dental unit manufacturer on the need for periodic maintenance of antiretraction devices.

## Use of Saliva Ejectors

Backflow from low-volume saliva ejectors occurs when the pressure in the patient's mouth is less than that in the evacuator. When a patient closes his or her lips around the tip of a saliva ejector, a partial vacuum is created, which can cause backflow to occur. This backflow is a potential source of cross-contamination.

Furthermore, studies have demonstrated that gravity pulls fluid back toward the patient's mouth whenever the suction tubing holding the tip is positioned above the patient's mouth. This can also occur if you are using high-volume evacuation while using the saliva ejector.

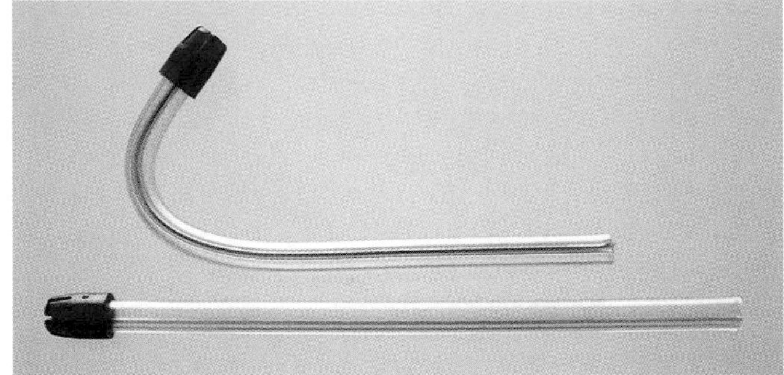

**FIG. 24.10** Low-volume saliva ejectors can cause backflow to occur. *(From Boyd LB: Dental instruments: a pocket guide, ed 6, St Louis, 2018, Elsevier.)*

Although no adverse health effects associated with the saliva ejector have been reported, you should be aware that in certain situations, backflow may occur when a saliva ejector is used (Fig. 24.10).

## Recommendations for Dental Handpieces and Other Devices Attached to Airlines and Waterlines

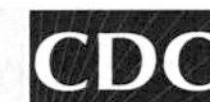

- Between patients, clean and heat-sterilize handpieces and other intraoral instruments that can be removed from the airlines and waterlines of dental units.
- Follow the manufacturer's instructions for cleaning, lubrication, and sterilization of handpieces and other intraoral instruments that can be removed from the airlines and waterlines of dental units.
- Do not surface-disinfect; use liquid chemical sterilants or ethylene oxide on handpieces and other intraoral instruments that can be removed from the airlines and waterlines of dental units.
- Advise patients not to close their lips tightly around the tip of the saliva ejector to evacuate oral fluids.

RECALL

11 What type of water must be used as an irrigant for surgery involving bone?
12 Will flushing DUWLs remove biofilm?
13 When should the high-volume evacuator be used to minimize aerosol?
14 Will the use of a rubber dam totally eliminate exposure to microorganisms?
15 What methods are available to test the quality of dental unit water?

**Legal and Ethical Implications** As a dental assistant, you will be exposed to countless types of microorganisms. However, having exposure to these common microbes does *not* mean that you will develop an infection or disease.

When a person's immune system is compromised because of age, smoking, heavy drinking, an organ transplant, cancer, or human immunodeficiency virus (HIV) infection, that person may have more difficulty fighting off invading pathogens. It is therefore important for patients who have weakened immune systems to inform dental personnel so that the right treatment decisions can be made. Patients should always feel free to ask questions about water quality or any other aspect of dental practice.

To date, no published scientific evidence has been reported regarding serious health problems for either patients or dental personnel caused by contact with dental unit water. Nonetheless, exposing patients or dental personnel to water of poor microbiologic quality violates standard infection control principles. ■

**Eye to the Future** Although the research community and dental equipment manufacturers have been working diligently on the issue of dental waterline contamination, additional research is needed in the following areas:

- Improved understanding of biofilm formation so that new means of prevention, control, and removal can be developed
- Identification of health implications for patients, practitioners, and allied dental personnel resulting from exposure to aerosols generated during dental procedures
- Simple, reliable, cost-effective devices for monitoring the microbial quality of water used during dental treatment ■

## Critical Thinking

1. Mrs. Kato is coming in next week for dental treatment. She has not been to the dental office for some time because she has been receiving chemotherapy treatment for breast cancer. Should you discuss any special considerations with the dentist before beginning Mrs. Kato's treatment?
2. Mr. Torrence is a patient in your practice who has teeth that are extremely sensitive to cold water. On his last visit, Mr. Torrence suggested that you heat the water in the dental unit so it would be more comfortable. Do you think this is a good idea? Why or why not?
3. The staff in your dental office have decided to develop a patient information sheet to help patients understand about DUWL issues. What do you think should be included on this patient information sheet? ■

PROCEDURE 24.1

# Testing Dental Unit Waterlines

### GOAL

To obtain a water sample and prepare it for shipping.

### EQUIPMENT AND SUPPLIES

- ✓ Testing service kit and instructions
- ✓ Clean gloves

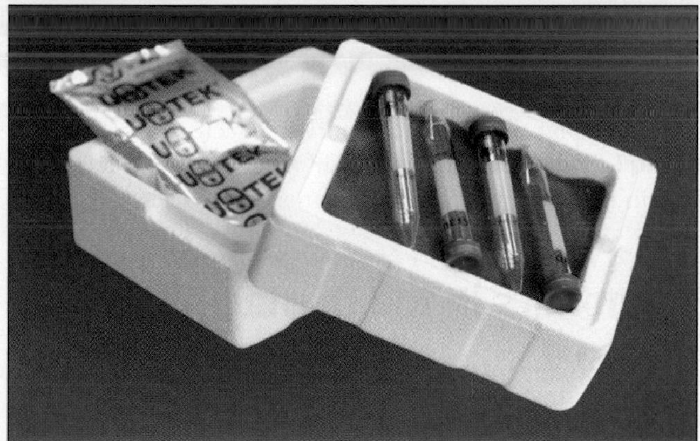


*Courtesy Confirm Monitoring Systems, Inc., Englewood, CO (www.BluTab.com).*

### PROCEDURAL STEPS

1 Place refrigerant pack in the Styrofoam lid, and place in freezer overnight.

2 Flush waterlines for a minimum of 2 minutes before taking samples.

**NOTE** Sampling should always be conducted just before any scheduled waterline maintenance or treatment.

**PURPOSE** To ensure that the sample is accurate.

3 Fill sterile collection vials until they are approximately full. Do not touch the outlet of the waterline or the interior of the collection vial.

**NOTE** The collection tubes contain a dehydrated chlorine neutralizer that is visible in the bottom of the vial.

**PURPOSE** You must not contaminate the vial.

4 Use a permanent marker to label each water sample.

5 Indicate the sample location and type (e.g., Operatory 3, air-water syringe [Op3, a/w]).

6 Fill out the sample submission form, and enclose it with the samples.

7 Place refrigerant pack and water samples in Styrofoam shipper.

8 Place Styrofoam shipper in mailer box.

9 Complete U.S. Express Mail shipping label, and affix to box.

**NOTE** U.S. Express Mail can be picked up by your U.S. Post Office mail carrier or taken to a post office. It must be picked up or mailed on the same day the sample was taken.

10 Documentation of the results should be maintained for either in-house or commercial testing.

25

# Ergonomics

## KEY TERMS

**Carpal tunnel syndrome (CTS)** Pain associated with continued flexion and extension of the wrist.

**Cumulative (KYU-myeh-luh-tiv) trauma disorders (CTDs)** Painful conditions that result from ongoing stresses to muscles, tendons, nerves, and joints.

**Ergonomics (er-guh-NAH-miks)** Adaptation of work environment and tasks to the human body.

**Maximum horizontal reach** Reach created when the upper arm is fully extended.

**Maximum vertical reach** Reach created by a vertical sweep of the forearm while the elbow is kept at midtorso level.

**Musculoskeletal (mus-kyu-loh-SKEH-leh-tul) disorders (MSDs)** Painful conditions that affect both muscles and bones, such as neck or back pain and carpal tunnel syndrome.

**Neutral position** Position when the body is properly aligned and the distribution of weight throughout the spine is equal.

**Normal horizontal reach** Reach created by a sweep of the forearm with the upper arm held at the side.

**Sprains** Injuries caused by sudden twisting or wrenching of a joint with stretching or tearing of ligaments.

**Strains** Injuries caused by extreme stretching of muscles or ligaments.

**Thenar eminence (THEE-nar EH-meh-nents)** Fleshy mound on the palm at the base of the thumb.

## LEARNING OUTCOMES

*On completion of this chapter, the student will be able to achieve the following objectives:*

1. Pronounce, define, and spell the key terms.
2. Discuss ergonomics in the dental office, including the following:
   - Describe the goal of ergonomics.
   - Identify common symptoms of musculoskeletal disorders.
   - Identify three categories of risk factors that contribute to increased risk for injury.
3. Demonstrate proper posture and the neutral working position, and discuss guidelines for reaching movements.
4. Discuss cumulative trauma disorders, including the following:
   - Describe the symptoms of carpal tunnel syndrome.
   - Explain the importance of properly fitting gloves to the dental assistant.
5. Demonstrate the exercises that can reduce muscle fatigue and strengthen muscles, including exercises to reduce eyestrain and neck strain.

## ELECTRONIC RESOURCES

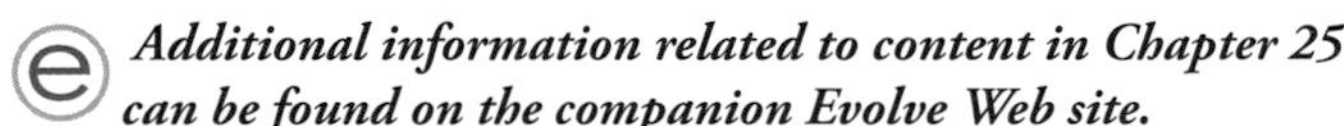
***Additional information related to content in Chapter 25 can be found on the companion Evolve Web site.***

- Practice Quiz
- Video: Body Strengthening Exercises

Many dental assistants have had to give up the career they love because of acute pain. Dental assistants frequently suffer with ongoing headaches, pain in the neck and shoulders, or numbness and tingling in the hands and wrists. Too often, when the dental assistant finally seeks help, the pain is severe and structural damage may be irreversible. You do not have to accept these hazards as part of your job. The key to preventing injury is to recognize and address the causes.

**Ergonomics** (from the Greek *ergon,* meaning "work," and *nomos,* meaning "law") deals with adaptation of the work environment to the human body. The goal of ergonomics is to help people stay healthy while performing their work more effectively. This can be done by changing workplace design, modifying instruments, strengthening muscles, taking breaks, using certain products, and providing proper training (Fig. 25.1).

This chapter discusses common risk factors for **musculoskeletal disorders (MSDs)**, their symptoms, and techniques you can use to protect yourself from such injuries.

## Ergonomics in the Dental Office

Ergonomics designs the work area and the task around the human body, rather than requiring the human to adapt to poorly designed equipment and working environments. Members of the dental team most frequently perform their work in a seated position, and they often use excessive motion and have unbalanced posture (Fig. 25.2). Many dental professionals

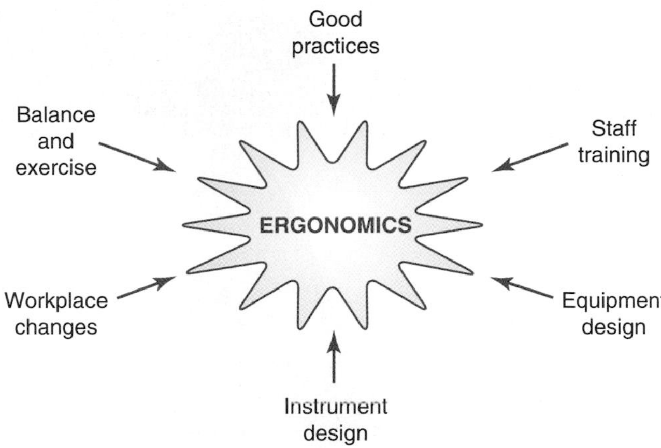


FIG. 25.1 Ergonomic factors in dentistry.

experience pain associated with MSDs. Work-related symptoms range from back and joint pain to neck and shoulder pain, hand and wrist pain, and headaches.

The *early onset* of pain should alert the worker that (1) an imbalance exists, and (2) if it is ignored, serious damage can occur over time. When you first experience pain, you should inform your employer, and take steps to reduce musculoskeletal inflammation and to facilitate healing. If you ignore the early symptoms of pain and stiffness, chronic disease may develop. It is important for the dental assistant to understand how to implement ergonomic changes and methods to prevent MSDs.

Three categories of risk factors contribute to MSDs: *posture, repetition,* and *force.*

## Ergonomic Chairside Tips

- Use muscles to remain balanced for ease of movement.
- Avoid prolonged, awkward positions.
- Do not remain in one position for an extended time.
- Do not constantly lean forward or to the side.
- Remain in good physical condition.
- Take breaks to stretch the neck, shoulders, and hands.
- Avoid repetitive, forceful movements.
- Rearrange items in the operatory for easy use.

RECALL

1. What is meant by ergonomics?
2. What is the goal of ergonomics?
3. What types of disorders are considered to be MSDs?
4. What three categories of risk factors contribute to MSDs?

# Posture

Posture affects the ability of the dental assistant to reach, hold, and use equipment. Positioning also influences how long the assistant can perform a task without suffering adverse health effects.

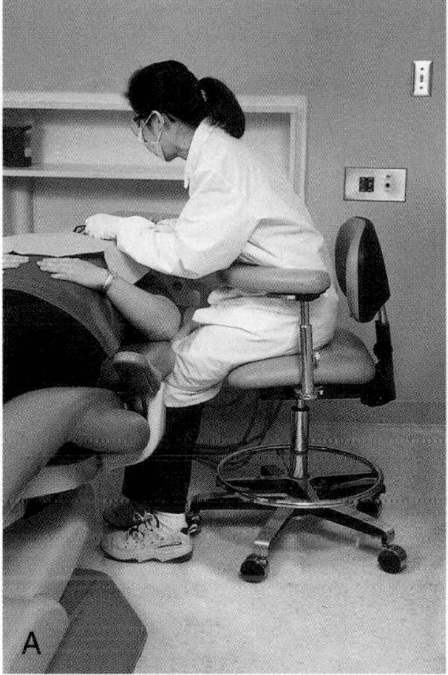


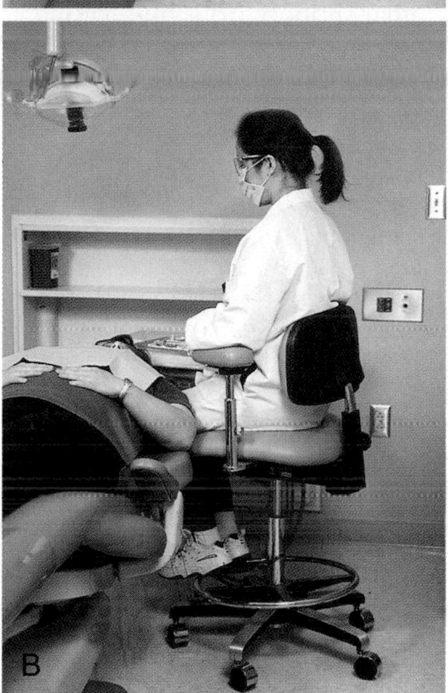


FIG. 25.2 A, Dental assistant in poor position. B, Dental assistant in proper position.

Most dental assistants are seated while working on patients. Although sitting is generally less fatiguing than standing, any position eventually will become fatiguing over time. This may lead to low back pain.

## Dental Assistant Positioning

- Sit at the patient's shoulder.
- Knees even with the edge of the patient headrest.
- Head in an upright position.
- Back straight and supported with a backrest.
- Thighs parallel to the floor.
- Elbows kept close to your body.
- Avoid sitting on the edge of your chair.
- Keep your eye level about 6 inches above the dentist's.

### Operator Positioning

- Head in an upright position.
- Elbows kept close to your body.
- Thighs parallel to the floor.
- Work in a neutral position.
- Reposition the patient as necessary. Do not reach, lean, or bend for better access.

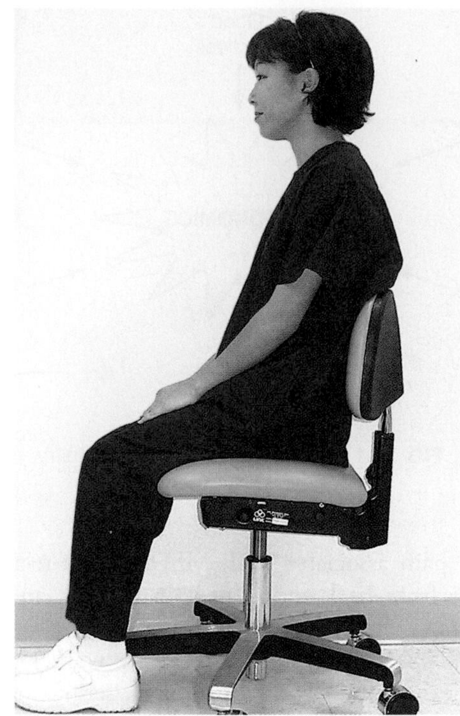

**FIG. 25.3** Configuration of spine in seated dental assistant.

## Neutral Position

The ideal way to work is from a "neutral" position. You can establish a **neutral position** by sitting upright with your weight evenly distributed. Your legs should be separated with your feet flat on the floor when you are working as an operator—or they should be flat on the footrest of the assistant's stool when you are assisting. Your back should be pressed against the back of the chair for lumbar support. Your hips should lean forward to rotate the pelvis backward.

The properly aligned spine resembles a gentle "S." When the spine is properly aligned, the ears, shoulders, and hips are in straight vertical alignment, providing balance, support, and equal distribution of weight throughout the spine (Fig. 25.3).

## Deviations and Problems

Unfortunately, while assisting the dentist, the dental assistant tends to deviate from the neutral position. Such deviations include leaning forward, twisting, overbending the back, and reaching. These poor postures can lead to aches, pains, numbness, and tingling. Ideally, the assistant alternates sitting and standing whenever possible.

Frequent reaching, twisting, and working with the arms in awkward positions can cause strains and sprains. **Strains** result from extreme stretching of muscles or ligaments. **Sprains** usually involve a sudden twist or wrenching of a joint with stretching or tearing of ligaments. Shoulder problems can result when one repeatedly reaches behind the body for instruments or supplies (Fig. 25.4).

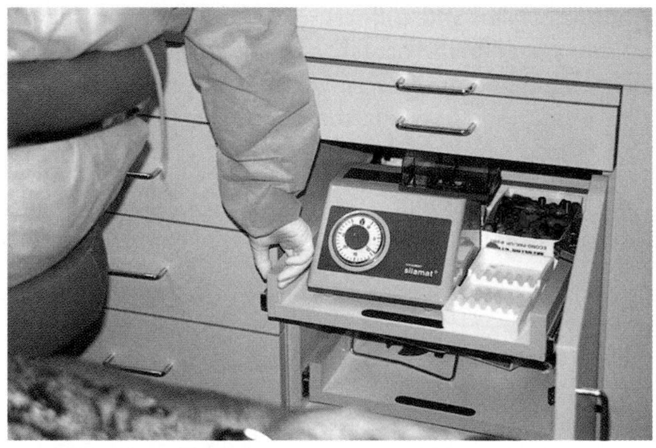

**FIG. 25.4** Small pieces of equipment should be kept in a location that does not require twisting or bending.

## Reaching Movements

Keep frequently used items, such as the air-water syringe, handpiece, saliva ejector, and high-volume oral evacuator, within a comfortable distance—*not* above shoulder level or below the waist. Adjust the instrument tray and equipment so that items are within **normal horizontal reach**, that is, the reach created by a sweep of your forearm with the upper arm held at your side.

Keep the operatory light within a safe **maximum vertical reach**, that is, the reach created by a vertical sweep of your forearm while your elbow is kept at midtorso level. Other supplies used less frequently should be placed within **maximum horizontal reach**, that is, the reach created when your upper arm is fully extended.

Reaches should be made to the front only. Reaching behind your back and lifting can cause shoulder injury. When turning is necessary, rotate the chair to avoid twisting your body.

# Repetition and Force

Repetitive motion, overflexion, and overextension of the wrist can significantly increase the risk for **cumulative trauma disorders (CTDs)**, particularly when the task requires force (Fig. 25.5). To help prevent common CTDs such as carpal tunnel syndrome, take periodic breaks, and when scheduling patients, alternate difficult procedures with less stressful procedures.

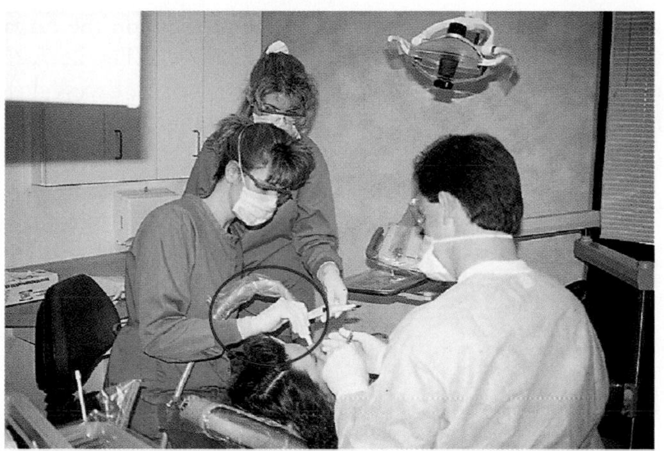

**FIG. 25.5** Repetitive stress on the bend in the wrist over long periods can lead to carpal tendon injury. This dental assistant should periodically change her grasp on the oral evacuator to straighten out her wrist. She also should use the back support on her chair.

## Carpal Tunnel Syndrome

The term *carpal tunnel* refers to an anatomic area of the hand and wrist. Eight carpal bones arranged as a tunnel form this area. Inside the tunnel are nine flexor tendons and the median nerve. With improper motion, the tendons swell and exert pressure on the median nerve (Fig. 25.6). Repetitive and forceful motion can lead to **carpal tunnel syndrome (CTS)**.

Often, the first symptom of CTS is a painful tingling in one or both hands that occurs at night. A decrease in ability and power to squeeze objects or make a tight fist may follow. In advanced cases, the thenar muscle (located at the base of the thumb) may weaken, causing a feeling of decreased strength in the handgrip.

Other repetitive hand and wrist movements, such as knitting, gardening, or using a keyboard, may also cause CTS. Patients who are pregnant, taking oral contraceptives, or given a diagnosis of premenstrual syndrome or rheumatoid arthritis may be more prone to develop CTS.

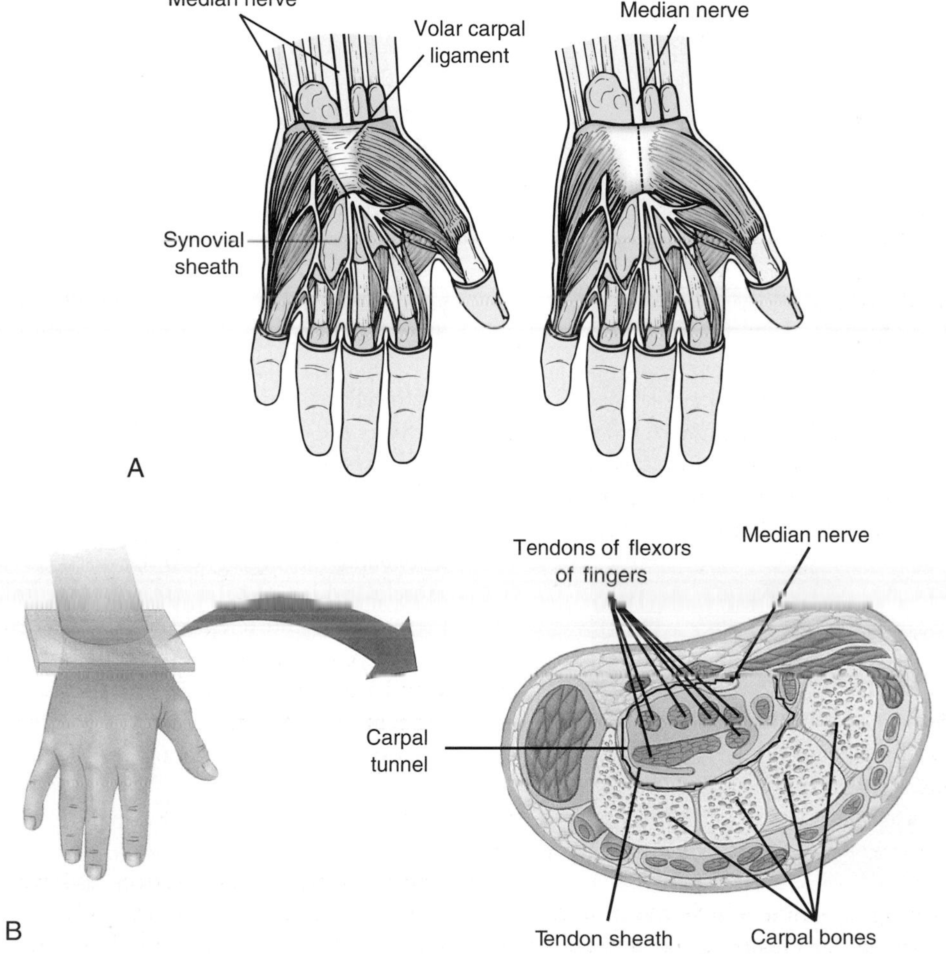


**FIG. 25.6** A, Cross section of the wrist. B, Schematic view of the carpal tunnel. *(B, From Patton KT, Thibodeau GA: Anatomy and physiology, ed 8, St Louis, 2013, Mosby.)*

## Gloves

The use of *ambidextrous gloves* (gloves designed to be worn on either hand) can place excessive tension on the **thenar eminence** (the fleshy elevation on the palm at the base of the thumb) (Fig. 25.7, *A*) and the hypothenar eminence by forcing the hand to work against the vertical alignment of the glove form. *Right-left gloves* that are properly sized support the hands naturally and properly position the thumb, index finger, and middle finger.

### Properly Fitting Gloves

It is important to wear gloves that fit you properly. Gloves that are *too tight* (Fig. 25.7, *B*) can cause circulation problems to your fingers and hands, and also place pressure on the carpal tunnel across the wrist. Gloves that are *too loose* (Fig. 25.7, *C*) make it difficult to grasp and transfer instruments. Excess glove material at the fingertips hinders your ability to roll instruments or the oral evacuators while assisting.

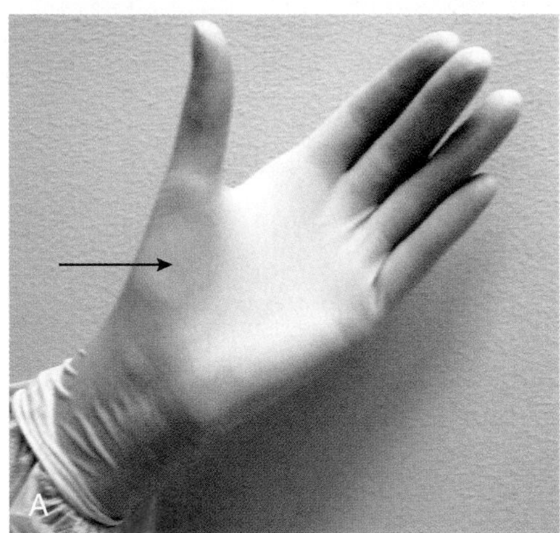


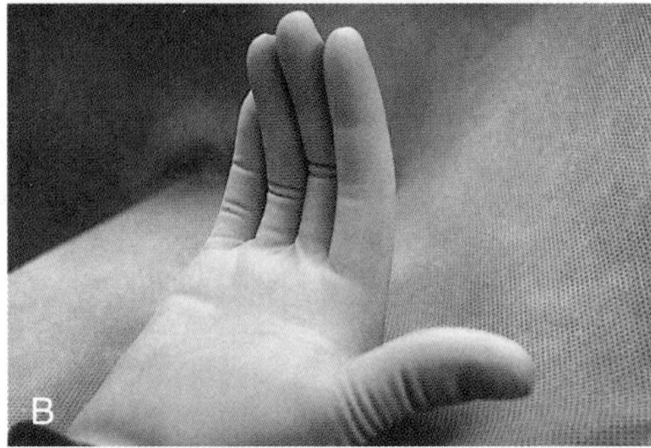


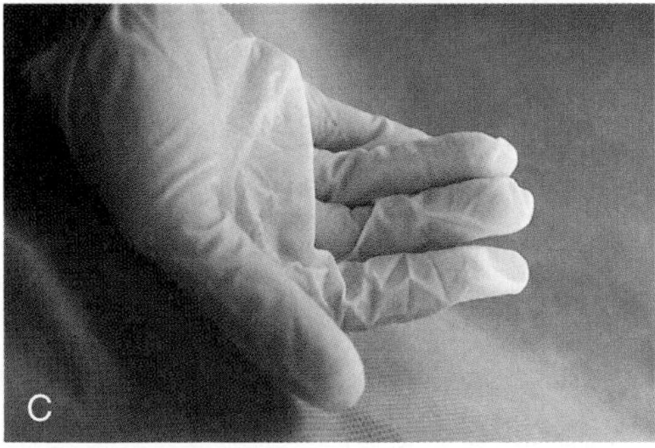


**FIG. 25.7** A, *Arrow* indicates the location of the thenar eminence on a gloved hand. B, *Glove is too tight.* C, *Glove* is too loose. *(B and C, From Darby ML, Walsh MM: Dental hygiene: theory and practice, ed 4, St Louis, 2015, Saunders.)*

5 What is the neutral position?
6 What is meant by normal horizontal reach?
7 What factors increase the risk of CTS?

## Muscle-Strengthening Exercises

Stretching and strengthening the muscles that support your back and neck and those used in the forearm, wrist, and hand help to keep these muscles strong and healthy. You should do periodic stretching throughout the workday (Box 25.1).

*Frequently resting the hands* is one of the most important factors in prevention of CTS. To warm the muscles and joints of your hands, slowly open and close your hands, moving from a completely open position to a completely closed position, which ends with your fingers tucked into your palm (Fig. 25.8, *A* and *B*). Also, press your palms together, and then relax them (Fig. 25.8, *C* and *D*).

Another recommended stretching exercise is to hold one arm out in front of your body with your hand extended. With the fingers of your other hand, gently pull back on your extended fingers to increase the stretch (Fig. 25.8, *E*).

To relieve *eyestrain* caused by focusing intensely at one depth of vision for long periods, look up from the task, and focus your eyes at a distance for about 20 seconds. Practice this frequently throughout the day to use your full range of vision and to lessen eyestrain.

To relieve stresses placed on the back, neck, and shoulders, perform the *full back release* (Fig. 25.9). Do head rotations for neck stiffness. *Head rotations* involve tilting the head from right to left and from forward to backward without forcing the motion beyond a range of comfort.

*Shoulder shrugging* can be used to stretch the shoulder muscles, which may be stressed from holding oral evacuators, instruments, and telephone handsets. Pull your shoulders up toward your ears, and then roll them backward and forward in a circular motion (Fig. 25.10). Before you begin any exercise program, you should check with your physician, particularly if you experience pain with any movements.

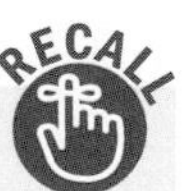


8 How can you reduce eyestrain?
9 What exercise relieves neck strain?
10 What is one of the most important factors in preventing CTS?

## BOX 25.1 Strengthening Exercises

**Pelvic Tilt: Strengthens Lumbar Spine**

1. Lie on your back (ideally); or, if at work, stand flat against the wall.
2. Keep knees slightly bent.
3. Flatten and press back into floor (or wall).
4. Hold briefly.
5. Repeat.

**Hyperextension: Safeguards Lumbar Curve**

1. Lie on your stomach.
2. Arch body backward, in an upward direction.
3. Hold briefly.
4. Repeat.

**Knee-to-Chest: Stretches Lumbar Spine**

1. Lie on your back.
2. Bring both knees to your chest.
3. Hold briefly.
4. Return to original position; avoid straightening legs.
5. Repeat.

**Sit-ups: Strengthen Abdominal Muscles**

1. Lie on your back.
2. Bend knees.
3. Support neck.
4. Gently raise shoulders toward knees.
5. Hold briefly and return.
6. Repeat.

**Suspend from a Bar: Relieves Lower Back Pain**

1. Firmly grasp bar.
2. Suspend your body from bar; lift feet slowly.
3. Hold for a short time.
4. Repeat.

**Doorway Stretch: Reverses Poor Posture**

1. Stand in front of an open doorway.
2. Place hands on either side of doorframe.
3. Gently allow your body to lean forward through doorway.
4. Hold briefly and return.
5. Repeat.

**Neck Isometric: Stretches Cervical Spine and Relieves Neck Muscle Strain**

1. Grasp hands behind head.
2. Gently press your head back.
3. Do not allow any backward movement.
4. Hold briefly.
5. Repeat.

**Rubber Ball Squeeze: Strengthens Hand and Finger Muscles**

1. Grasp a rubber ball firmly in your hand.
2. Gently squeeze.
3. Hold briefly.
4. Repeat.

**Rubber Band Stretch: Strengthens Hand and Finger Muscles**

1. Extend rubber band between fingers of hand.
2. Gently stretch rubber band until you feel resistance.
3. Hold briefly.
4. Release rubber band.
5. Repeat.

From Darby ML, Walsh M: Dental hygiene: theory and practice, ed 4, St Louis, 2015, Saunders.

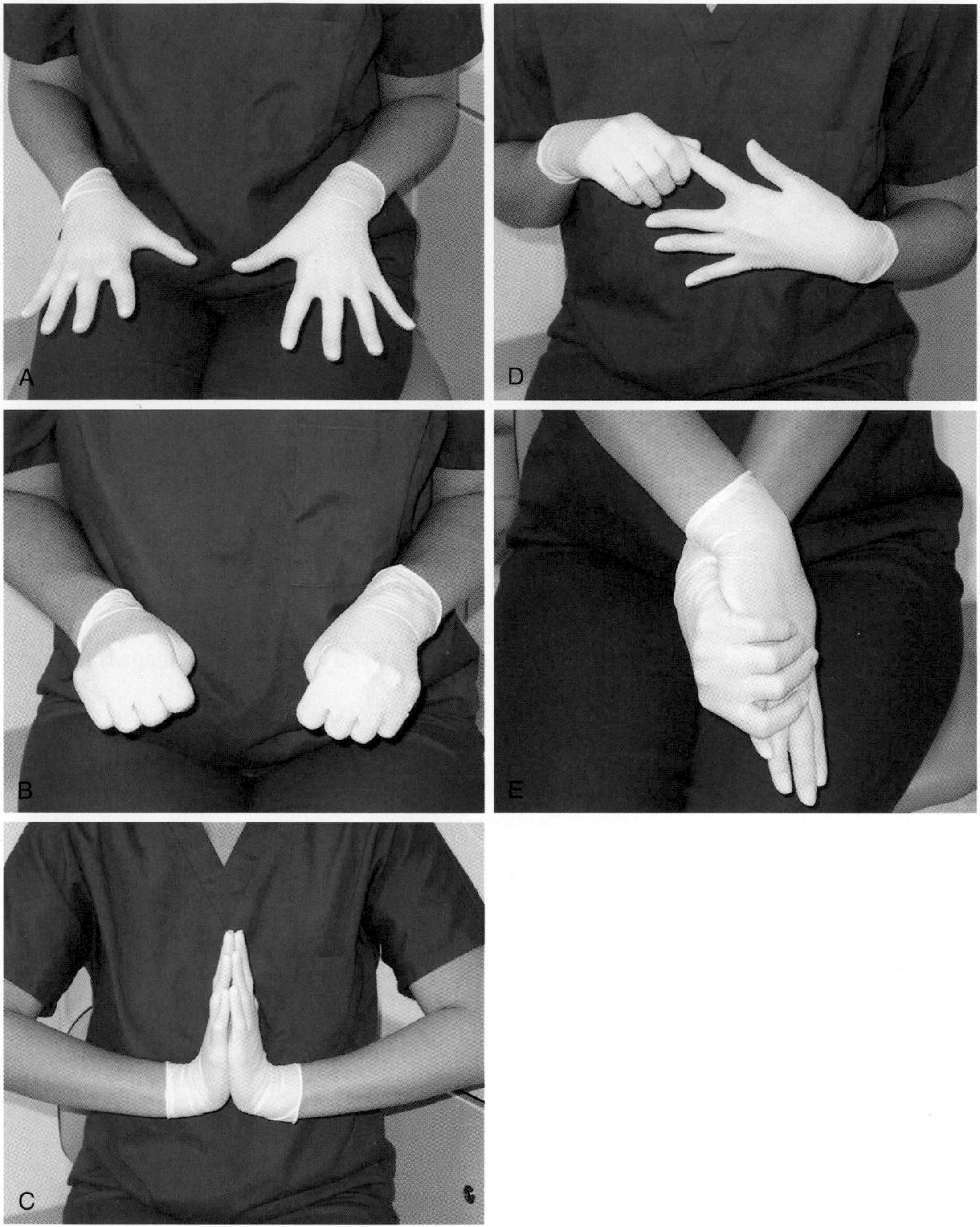

**FIG. 25.8** Hand exercises. A and B, Slowly open and close the hands from a completely open position to a completely closed position, ending with the fingers tucked into the palms. C, Press the palms of the hands together and then relax. D, Gently pull on and relax each finger on each hand separately. E, Cross the wrists and gently stretch and relax.

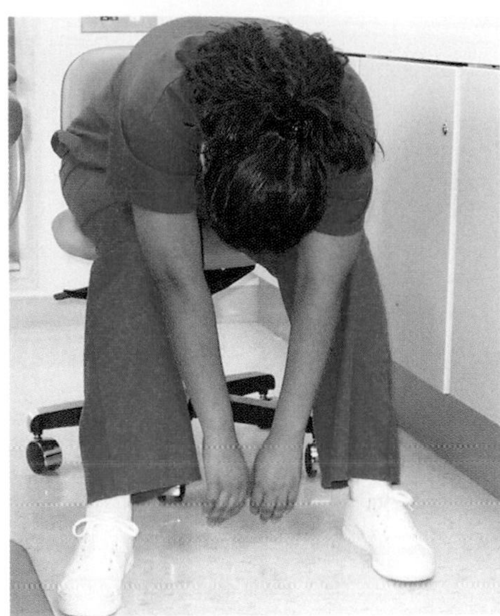

**FIG. 25.9** Full back release. Let the head move down slowly, allow the arms and head to fall between the knees, hold for a few seconds, and then raise slowly by contracting the stomach muscles and rolling up. Bring the head up last.

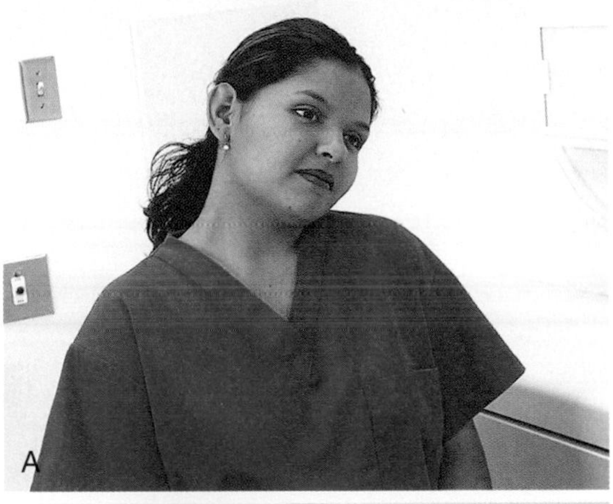

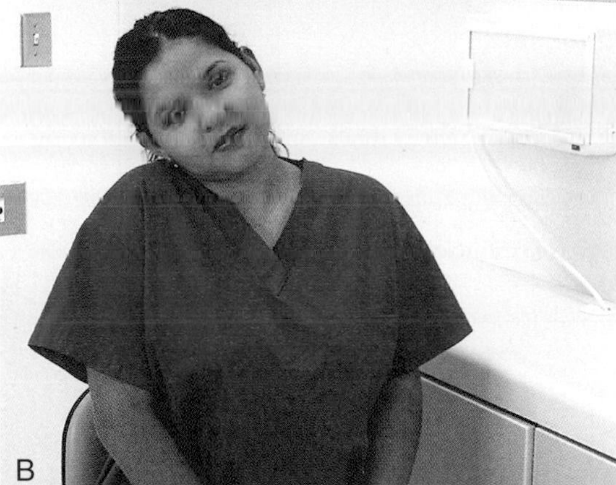

**FIG. 25.10** Shoulder shrugging.

■ **Legal and Ethical Implications** The Occupational Safety and Health Administration (OSHA) requires employers to ensure a safe and healthy working environment for the employees. The best way for a dental employer to protect employees from musculoskeletal injury is to make ergonomics an important part of the practice for everyone. Many dental offices include ergonomics as an important topic for discussion during staff meetings. Other offices choose to incorporate ergonomics into the existing health and safety program. Regardless of how it is accomplished, practicing good ergonomics is critical for avoiding potential career-ending injuries. ■

■ **Eye to the Future** To enjoy a healthy and pain-free career as a dental assistant, you must keep your muscles, tendons, nerves, and joints healthy. Remember to apply ergonomic principles in all of your daily activities. Do not ignore early signals of pain and stiffness. The longer symptoms are ignored, the more severe the damage will be. Dentistry can be a physically stressful profession, but it is also a very rewarding profession that benefits both practitioners and patients. ■

## ■ Critical Thinking

1. How would you describe good posture and chairside position to a newly hired dental assistant who has not had formal training in ergonomics?
2. What exercises would you perform throughout the day to minimize the risk for MSDs?
3. What changes would you make to create a more ergonomic operatory?
4. Can you make any changes to your own home and/or school environment to make it more "worker friendly"? ■

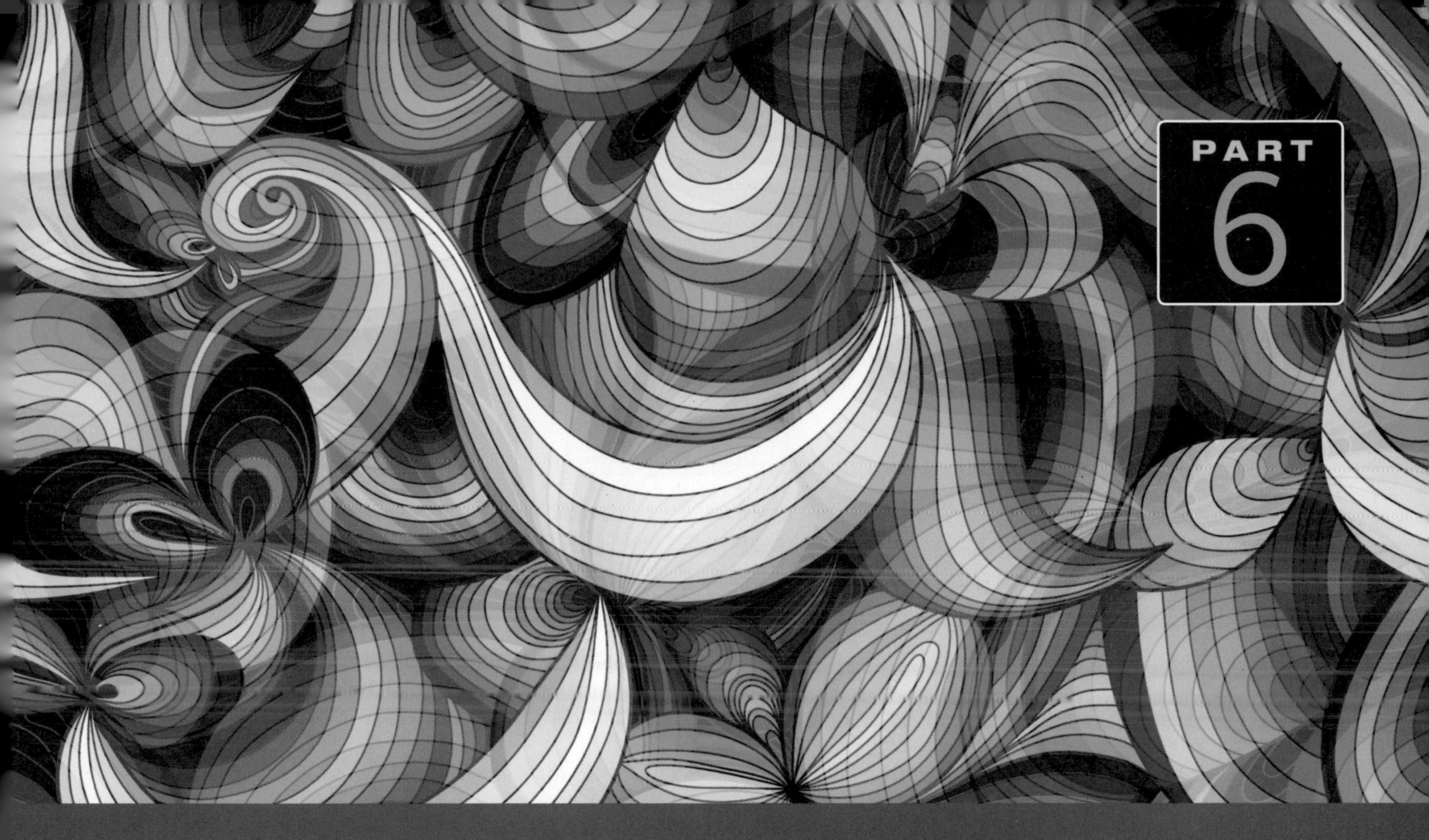

PART 6

# Patient Information and Assessment

As you begin your preclinical phase, you will discover early on the importance of learning as much as you can about your patient before treatment begins. From the first phone call to the moment a patient walks into the dental practice, the dental team must take on the shared responsibility of providing total patient care.

The chapters within Part 6 will provide you with the background knowledge and skills you will use to assist the dentist in assessing a patient's overall health and dental health status. Whether you are collecting personal information from a new or returning patient, obtaining diagnostic information, working with a medically compromised patient, or assisting the team in a medical emergency, you are a valuable resource and an integral part of the dental team.

26

# The Patient's Dental Record

## KEY TERMS

**Alert** To bring attention to a specific medical or clinical condition.
**Assessment** The process of collecting data and then evaluating or drawing conclusions from the findings.
**Chronic** Persisting over a long time.
**Chronologic** Arranged according to the time of occurrence; earliest to most recent.
**Demographics** Personal information that can include address, phone, and work information; also, statistical characteristics of populations.
**Diagnosis** Identification or determination of the nature and cause of a disease or injury through evaluation of a patient's history and examination findings.
**Forensic (fuh-REN-zik)** Pertaining to the identity of an individual on the basis of scientific methods.
**HIPAA** The Health Insurance Portability and Accountability Act of 1996 describes the federal regulations that ensure privacy regarding a patient's healthcare information.
**Litigation (li-ti-GAY-shun)** Act of initiating legal proceedings, as in a lawsuit.
**Quality assurance** Program in place for monitoring and evaluating a project, service, or facility to ensure that standards of quality are being met.
**Registration** Act of completing forms by providing personal information.

## LEARNING OUTCOMES

*On completion of this chapter, the student will be able to achieve the following objectives:*

1. Pronounce, define, and spell the key terms.
2. Explain the importance of a patient's dental record, including patient compliance, its legal significance, and how the dentist uses the record to manage patient treatment.
3. Discuss how electronic dental records have changed the dental industry, including the four benefits of going paperless.
4. Discuss and describe patient record forms, including the following:
   - Rationale for using electronic dental records.
   - Describe each form in the dental record.
   - Discuss the importance of the patient's medical-dental health history and explain its relevance to dental treatment.
   - Explain the standards and criteria for data entered in a dental record.

## PERFORMANCE OUTCOMES

*On completion of this chapter, the student will be able to meet competency standards in the following skills:*

- Oversee the completion of a new patient registration form.
- Obtain a completed medical-dental health history form for a new patient.
- Record a completed dental treatment.
- Demonstrate how to make corrections on a patient's record.

## ELECTRONIC RESOURCES

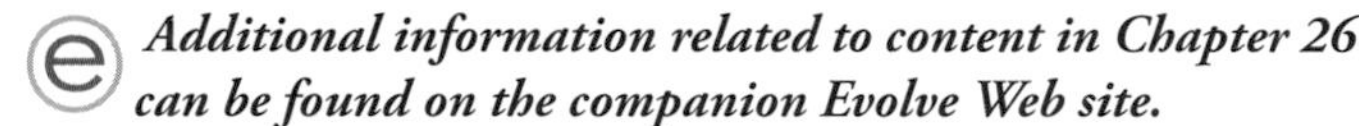
***Additional information related to content in Chapter 26 can be found on the companion Evolve Web site.***

- Dentrix Exercise
- Practice Quiz

The dental record is the most important document maintained for each patient in a dental practice (Fig. 26.1). Whether you are communicating with a patient by phone or in person, speaking to a dental laboratory about a prescription, speaking to an insurance company regarding treatment, or referring a patient to a specialist, the patient's dental record must be available to refer to.

A dental record consists of several components, which can include the patient's medical/dental history, the clinical examination, diagnosis, radiographs, referral letters, drug prescriptions, laboratory prescriptions, and treatment and prognosis of a patient's dental health.

## Patient Compliance

A patient's dental record contains confidential information related to that patient's personal background. It is important for the dental team to follow a standard when documenting and handling this information. Chapter 5 introduces legal guidelines to follow when working with patient records and confidential information.

Besides its use in the clinical care of a patient, the dental record can have legal significance, of which the dentist and staff must be aware.

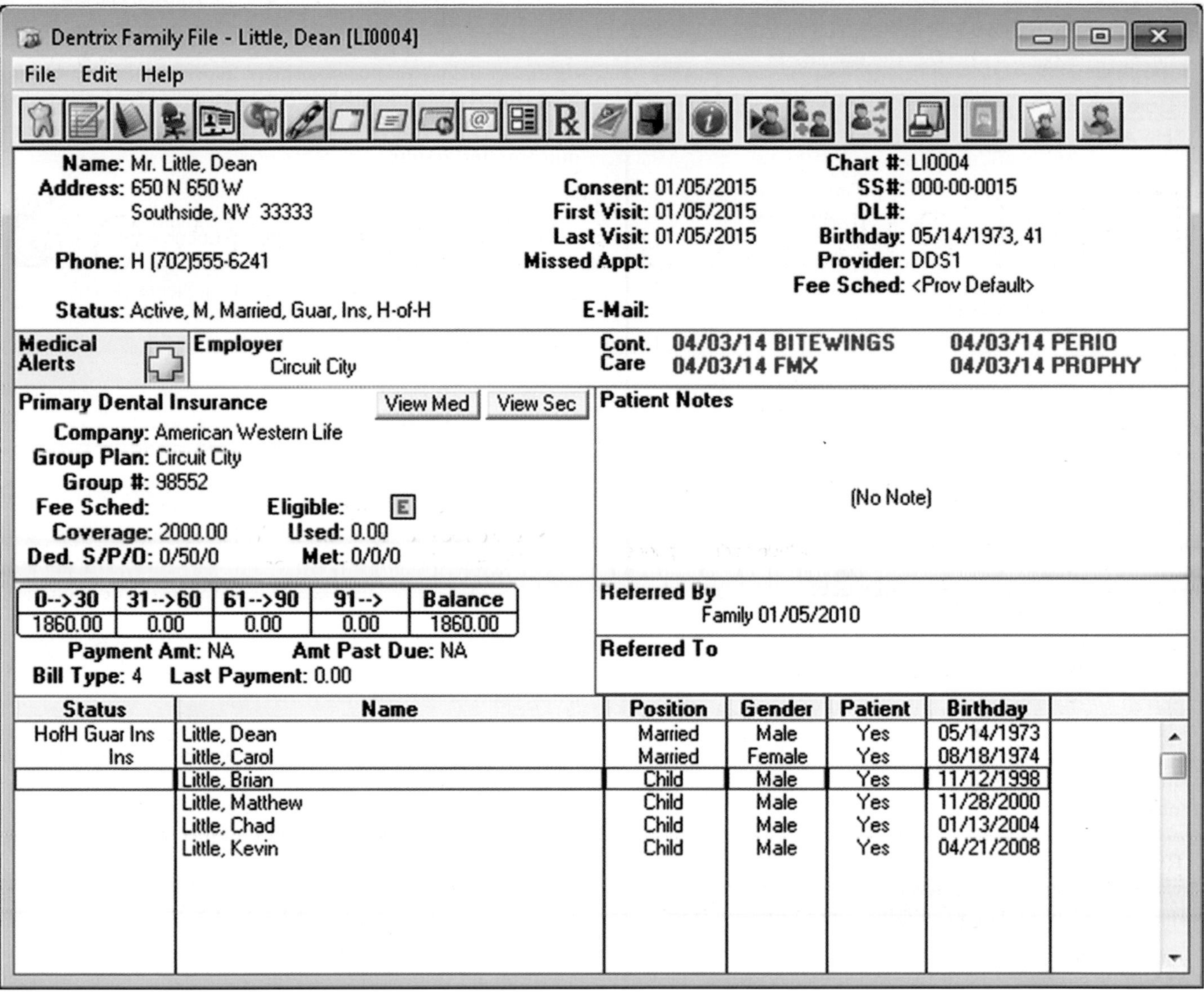


**FIG. 26.1** Example of the patient record electronic form. *(Courtesy Henry Schein Practice Solutions, American Fork, UT.)*

## Permanent Record

The dental record is a **permanent document** of the dentist. This permanent document, also considered a **legal document,** can be used as (1) evidence in a legal settlement or lawsuit; (2) a reference tool in a **forensic** case for identification of an individual with the use of a patient's radiographs or study casts; or (3) a reference for appropriate third parties, such as dental insurance companies and government-aided programs.

## Privacy

**HIPAA** requires that all dental practices today have a written privacy policy. This written policy must inform the patient that the office will not use or disclose protected health information (PHI) for any purpose other than treatment, diagnosis, and billing. The privacy policy is prepared in a written format and must be provided to every patient; all patients must review and sign an acknowledgment that they have received notice of privacy practices (Fig. 26.2). This signed acknowledgment is kept in the patient's record for a minimum of 6 years. See Chapter 5 for additional legal information regarding HIPAA.

## Quality Assurance

The dentist will use the patient record as the primary source of information in determining the overall quality of care that a patient receives. *Quality* is the key word to remember when a patient is receiving dental care.

Does the patient believe that the best and timeliest treatment is being provided? This question can be particularly important if the clinical setting is a larger practice with multiple practitioners, or a community dental clinic or teaching institution, where patients may be seen by different dentists and clinical professionals. Each dental setting must promote an efficient and effective quality assurance program. The following

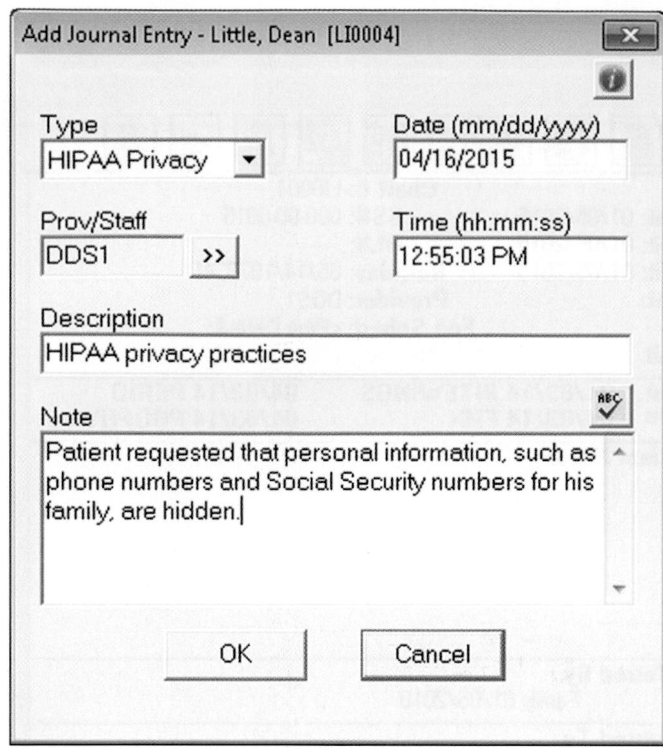
Add Journal Entry - Little, Dean [LI0004]

| Type | Date (mm/dd/yyyy) |
| --- | --- |
| HIPAA Privacy | 04/16/2015 |
| **Prov/Staff** | **Time (hh:mm:ss)** |
| DDS1 | 12:55:03 PM |

Description: HIPAA privacy practices

Note: Patient requested that personal information, such as phone numbers and Social Security numbers for his family, are hidden.

OK Cancel

**FIG. 26.2** Notice of HIPAA privacy practices form. *(Courtesy Henry Schein Practice Solutions, American Fork, UT.)*

examples are ways to provide **quality assurance** in your dental office:

- Routine forms are completed for each patient and verified with his or her signature and date.
- Timely "recall" of patients is followed to address their dental needs.
- A completed dental record is kept for each "active" patient in the dental practice.
- Documentation includes information when radiographs are taken.
- Current and up-to-date emergency protocols are adhered to by the dental team.
- Current and up-to-date licenses, registrations, and certifications and training of dental team members are maintained.

## Risk Management

As noted earlier, the dental record provides documentation regarding a patient's clinical findings, diagnosis, treatment plan, and response to treatment. For the dentist to avoid **litigation** such as a malpractice suit in the process or outcome of treating a patient, patient records must be kept organized and complete.

## Research

A complete and **chronologic** order of a dental record, or of a specific dental condition that has been diagnosed, could provide data to be used for research purposes. In an educational or public health setting, patients may be asked to participate in a research study. When a new research study begins, the steps taken to inform the patient and to clarify all steps in patient treatment or in the specific use of a new dental product must be accurately documented. If documentation is not complete, data could be eliminated from the study, which could affect the outcome and results.

RECALL

1. The patient record is a permanent document for whom?
2. How can quality assurance affect a patient's dental care?
3. What is PHI the abbreviation for?

# Electronic Dental Record

The most dramatic change in the dental practice over the past 20 years has been the integration of the electronic dental record (EDR). This type of system parallels the electronic health record (EHR) from the medical community. The software is designed to capture, store, present, import, and export relevant information from a patient's personal and clinical record.

For the majority of dental practices today, the benefits of going paperless include the following:

- Access to the dental record is safeguarded in many locations of the office.
- To perform practice management tasks such as patient registration, scheduling, billing, and inquiry about an insurance status.
- To allow the dental team to enter relevant clinical documentation, charting, complete a laboratory prescription, and electronically prescribe medication.
- To share health information with authorized providers across more than one healthcare organization.

The dentist and the office manager will decide on the type of software and the design of the forms to be used, and the order in which they are to be assembled and accessed. Each staff member must learn this sequence to ensure that all materials are accessible and can be easily found.

# Patient Record Forms

**Information-gathering forms** are to be completed by the patient before any treatment is provided. It is common in dental practices today that these forms are available for patients to complete either online before their scheduled appointment or by having the forms downloaded onto an iPad to complete on arrival to the office.

Examples of these types of forms include the following:

- Patient registration form (personal patient information)
- Medical-dental health history form (patient's overall health and dental status)
- Medical alert information (any medical concerns that need to alert the dental team before treatment)

PATIENT INFORMATION (CONFIDENTIAL)

NAME ______ FIRST ______ MI ______ LAST ______ DATE ______
ADDRESS ______ CITY ______ STATE/PROV. ______ ZIP/P.C. ______
E-MAIL ______ CELL PHONE ______ HOME PHONE ______
SS#/SIN ______ BIRTHDATE ______
CHECK APPROPRIATE BOX: ☐ MINOR ☐ SINGLE ☐ MARRIED ☐ DIVORCED ☐ WIDOWED ☐ SEPARATED
IF COLLEGE STUDENT, F.T. / P.T., NAME OF SCHOOL ______ CITY ______ STATE/PROV. ______
PATIENT'S OR PARENT'S/GUARDIAN'S EMPLOYER ______ WORK PHONE ______
BUSINESS ADDRESS ______ CITY ______ STATE/PROV. ______ ZIP/P.C. ______
SPOUSE OR PARENT'S/GUARDIAN'S NAME ______ EMPLOYER ______ WORK PHONE ______
WHOM MAY WE THANK FOR REFERRING YOU? ______
PERSON TO CONTACT IN CASE OF AN EMERGENCY ______ PHONE ______

RESPONSIBLE PARTY

NAME OF PERSON RESPONSIBLE FOR THIS ACCOUNT ______ RELATIONSHIP TO PATIENT ______
ADDRESS ______ HOME PHONE ______
DRIVER'S LICENSE # ______ BIRTHDATE ______ SS#/SIN ______
EMPLOYER ______ WORK PHONE ______
IS THIS PERSON CURRENTLY A PATIENT IN OUR OFFICE? ☐ YES ☐ NO

INSURANCE INFORMATION

NAME OF INSURED ______ RELATIONSHIP TO PATIENT ______
BIRTHDATE ______ SS#/SIN ______ DATE EMPLOYED ______
NAME OF EMPLOYER ______ UNION OR LOCAL # ______ WORK PHONE ______
EMPLOYER ADDRESS ______ CITY ______ STATE/PROV. ______ ZIP/P.C. ______
INSURANCE CO. ______ TEL. # ______ GRP # ______ POLICY / I.D. # ______
INS. CO. ADDRESS ______ CITY ______ STATE/PROV. ______ ZIP/P.C. ______
HOW MUCH IS YOUR DEDUCTIBLE? ______ HOW MUCH HAVE YOU USED? ______ MAX ANNUAL BENEFIT? ______

DO YOU HAVE ANY ADDITIONAL INSURANCE? ☐ YES ☐ NO IF YES, COMPLETE THE FOLLOWING:

NAME OF INSURED ______ RELATIONSHIP TO PATIENT ______
BIRTHDATE ______ SS#/SIN ______ DATE EMPLOYED ______
NAME OF EMPLOYER ______ UNION OR LOCAL # ______ WORK PHONE ______
EMPLOYER ADDRESS ______ CITY ______ STATE/PROV. ______ ZIP/P.C. ______
INSURANCE CO. ______ TEL. # ______ GRP # ______ POLICY / I.D. # ______
INS. CO. ADDRESS ______ CITY ______ STATE/PROV. ______ ZIP/P.C. ______
HOW MUCH IS YOUR DEDUCTIBLE? ______ HOW MUCH HAVE YOU USED? ______ MAX ANNUAL BENEFIT? ______

X ______
SIGNATURE OF PATIENT OR PARENT/GUARDIAN IF MINOR ______ PATIENT NUMBER

REGISTRATION

**FIG. 26.3** Example of a patient registration form. *(Courtesy Patterson Dental, St Paul, MN.)*

- Consent forms (Health Insurance Portability and Accountability Act [HIPAA], verification of accuracy, insurance)

Once the preliminary information is gathered, the business assistant will either prepare the dental record in paper form or enter the information into the electronic patient record, and alert the clinical staff that the patient is ready to be escorted to the clinical setting.

## Patient Registration

The patient registration form contains information related to patient **demographics** and financial responsibility (Fig. 26.3). The patient is asked to provide the following information on the **registration** form (see Procedure 26.1: Registering a New Patient):

- *Patient information:* Full name, date of birth, address, email address, telephone numbers (home, cell, work), employment information, spousal information, and emergency contact (a patient's social security number should no longer be included in this area because of the privacy act).
- *Insurance information:* Dental insurance company name and policy number; name of employee, date of birth; employer's name, address, and telephone number. Many practices will ask the patient for their insurance card to make a copy for their records.
- *Responsible party:* Person responsible for payment of the account (patient, spouse, parent, or legal guardian).
- *Signature and date:* The patient verifies the accuracy of the information.

## Medical-Dental Health History

The patient must complete a medical-dental health history form (Fig. 26.4; Procedure 26.2: Obtaining a Medical-Dental Health History). The health history form should be regarded as minimal information from a patient. The responsibility of the dental team is to review the form and initiate conversation and ask questions to gain greater insight into the patient's

# Health History Form

ADA. American Dental Association www.ada.org

E-mail: Today's Date:

As required by law, our office adheres to written policies and procedures to protect the privacy of information about you that we create, receive or maintain. Your answers are for our records only and will be kept confidential subject to applicable laws. Please note that you will be asked some questions about your responses to this questionnaire and there may be additional questions concerning your health. This information is vital to allow us to provide appropriate care for you. This office does not use this information to discriminate.

Name: (Last, First, Middle) Home Phone: Include area code ( ) Business/Cell Phone: Include area code ( )
Address: (Mailing address) City: State: Zip:
Occupation: Height: Weight: Date of birth: Sex: M F
SS# or Patient ID: Emergency Contact: Relationship: Home Phone: ( ) Cell Phone: ( ) Include area codes
If you are completing this form for another person, what is your relationship to that person? (Your Name, Relationship)

**Do you have any of the following diseases or problems:** *(Check DK if you Don't Know the answer to the question)* Yes No DK
- Active Tuberculosis
- Persistent cough greater than a 3 week duration
- Cough that produces blood
- Been exposed to anyone with tuberculosis

***If you answer yes to any of the 4 items above, please stop and return this form to the receptionist.***

## Dental Information *For the following questions, please mark (X) your responses to the following questions.*

Yes No DK
- Do your gums bleed when you brush or floss?
- Are your teeth sensitive to cold, hot, sweets or pressure?
- Does food or floss catch between your teeth?
- Is your mouth dry?
- Have you had any periodontal (gum) treatments?
- Have you ever had orthodontic (braces) treatment?
- Have you had any problems associated with previous dental treatment?
- Is your home water supply fluoridated?
- Do you drink bottled or filtered water?
- If yes, how often? Circle one: DAILY / WEEKLY / OCCASIONALLY
- Are you currently experiencing dental pain or discomfort?
- Do you have earaches or neck pains?
- Do you have any clicking, popping or discomfort in the jaw?
- Do you brux or grind your teeth?
- Do you have sores or ulcers in your mouth?
- Do you wear dentures or partials?
- Do you participate in active recreational activities?
- Have you ever had a serious injury to your head or mouth?

Date of your last dental exam:
What was done at that time?
Date of last dental x-rays:
What is the reason for your dental visit today?
How do you feel about your smile?

## Medical Information *Please mark (X) your response to indicate if you have or have not had any of the following diseases or problems.*

Yes No DK
- Are you now under the care of a physician?
- Physician Name: Phone: Include area code ( )
- Address/City/State/Zip:
- Are you in good health?
- Has there been any change in your general health within the past year?
- If yes, what condition is being treated?
- Date of last physical exam:
- Have you had a serious illness, operation or been hospitalized in the past 5 years?
- If yes, what was the illness or problem?
- Are you taking or have you recently taken any prescription or over the counter medicine(s)?
- If so, please list all, including vitamins, natural or herbal preparations and/or diet supplements:



A

## Medical Information *Please mark (X) your response to indicate if you have or have not had any of the following diseases or problems.*

*(Check DK if you Don't Know the answer to the question)* Yes No DK
- Do you wear contact lenses?
- **Joint Replacement.** Have you had an orthopedic total joint (hip, knee, elbow, finger) replacement? Date: ____ If yes, have you had any complications?____
- Are you taking or scheduled to begin taking either of the medications, alendronate (Fosamax®) or risedronate (Actonel®) for osteoporosis or Paget's disease?
- Since 2001, were you treated or are you presently scheduled to begin treatment with the intravenous bisphosphonates (Aredia® or Zometa®) for bone pain, hypercalcemia or skeletal complications resulting from Paget's disease, multiple myeloma or metastatic cancer? Date Treatment began:
- Do you use controlled substances (drugs)?
- Do you use tobacco (smoking, snuff, chew, bidis)? If so, how interested are you in stopping? (Circle one) VERY / SOMEWHAT / NOT INTERESTED
- Do you drink alcoholic beverages? If yes, how much alcohol did you drink in the last 24 hours? ____ If yes, how much do you typically drink in a week? ____
- **WOMEN ONLY** Are you: Pregnant? Number of weeks: ____ Taking birth control pills or hormonal replacement? Nursing?

**Allergies** - Are you allergic to or have you had a reaction to: To all **yes** responses, specify type of reaction. Yes No DK
- Local anesthetics
- Aspirin
- Penicillin or other antibiotics
- Barbiturates, sedatives, or sleeping pills
- Sulfa drugs
- Codeine or other narcotics
- Metals
- Latex (rubber)
- Iodine
- Hay fever/seasonal
- Animals
- Food
- Other

***Please mark (X) your response to indicate if you have or have not had any of the following diseases or problems.*** Yes No DK
- Artificial (prosthetic) heart valve
- Previous infective endocarditis
- Damaged valves in transplanted heart
- Congenital heart disease (CHD)
  - Unrepaired, cyanotic CHD
  - Repaired (completely) in last 6 months
  - Repaired CHD with residual defects

*Except for the conditions listed above, antibiotic prophylaxis is no longer recommended for any other form of CHD.*

- Cardiovascular disease
- Angina
- Arteriosclerosis
- Congestive heart failure
- Damaged heart valves
- Heart attack
- Heart murmur
- Low blood pressure
- High blood pressure
- Other congenital heart defects
- Mitral valve prolapse
- Pacemaker
- Rheumatic fever
- Rheumatic heart disease
- Abnormal bleeding
- Anemia
- Blood transfusion
  - If yes, date:
- Hemophilia
- AIDS or HIV infection
- Arthritis
- Autoimmune disease
- Rheumatoid arthritis
- Systemic lupus erythematosus
- Asthma
- Bronchitis
- Emphysema
- Sinus trouble
- Tuberculosis
- Cancer/Chemotherapy/Radiation Treatment
- Chest pain upon exertion
- Chronic pain
- Diabetes Type I or II
- Eating disorder
- Malnutrition
- Gastrointestinal disease
- G.E. Reflux/persistent heartburn
- Ulcers
- Thyroid problems
- Stroke
- Glaucoma
- Hepatitis, jaundice or liver disease
- Epilepsy
- Fainting spells or seizures
- Neurological disorders
  - If yes, specify:
- Sleep disorder
- Mental health disorders
  - Specify:
- Recurrent Infections
  - Type of infection:
- Kidney problems
- Night sweats
- Osteoporosis
- Persistent swollen glands in neck
- Severe headaches/migraines
- Severe or rapid weight loss
- Sexually transmitted disease
- Excessive urination

Has a physician or previous dentist recommended that you take antibiotics prior to your dental treatment?
Name of physician or dentist making recommendation: Phone:
Do you have any disease, condition, or problem not listed above that you think I should know about? Please explain:

**NOTE: Both Doctor and patient are encouraged to discuss any and all relevant patient health issues prior to treatment.**
I certify that I have read and understand the above and that the information given on this form is accurate. I understand the importance of a truthful health history and that my dentist and his/her staff will rely on this information for treating me. I acknowledge that my questions, if any, about inquiries set forth above have been answered to my satisfaction. I will not hold my dentist, or any other member of his/her staff, responsible for any action they take or do not take because of errors or omissions that I may have made in the completion of this form.

Signature of Patient/Legal Guardian: Date:

**FOR COMPLETION BY DENTIST**
Comments:

B

**FIG. 26.4** Example of a medical-dental health history form. A, Dental history. B, Medical history. *(Courtesy American Dental Association, Chicago, IL.)*

well-being. Once the form has been completed, the adult patient who completed the form or the patient's legal guardian must sign and date the form to confirm that the information is correct. The health history form is divided into medical assessment and dental assessment sections.

### *Medical History*

The medical history section includes questions regarding the patient's past medical history, present physical conditions, **chronic** conditions, allergies, and current medications. This information (1) alerts the dentist to possible medical conditions and medications that could complicate or interfere with dental treatment; (2) aids the dentist in anticipating any potential medical emergencies based on the patient's medical background; and (3) identifies special treatment needs that a patient may require.

If specific medical conditions are a matter of concern to the dentist, the dentist will consult with the patient's physician regarding treatment. The patient will be required to sign a release-of-information form to give consent before a consultation can take place.

### *Dental History*

The dental history section of the form is used to obtain information about the patient's previous dental treatment and care. By asking questions about oral home care and previous dental experiences, the dental team can gain insight into the patient's feelings toward dentistry and information about the patient's own dental care.

## Medical Alert

When you receive a completed medical-dental health history form, one of your first priorities is to review indications of health conditions, allergic reactions, and medications that could interfere with or be life-threatening to the patient during dental treatment. An example of this would be a reaction to a specific antibiotic that is prescribed for a specific dental treatment. The dental team would inquire with further questions and then would make note with an alert listing the antibiotic this patient cannot be prescribed (Fig. 26.5).

In the dental record, medical **alerts** and other precautions should be entered so that safe care is provided to the patient. When you receive this information, an "alert" entry will be noted in the EDR. If you are using paper forms, the alert sticker is to be placed inside the record to maintaining dentist/patient confidentiality. The alert sticker should never be placed on the outside for others to see.

## Medical-Dental Health History Update

Returning patients are to be asked to update their medical-dental health history at every appointment (Fig. 26.6). Even if a patient was seen by the dentist 2 weeks ago, the dentist may not be aware of any changes to a patient's medication regimen or medical diagnosis if the history was not updated. A slight change in a medical condition could cause a reaction when anesthesia or pain control methods are used by the dentist. The patient's initial medical-dental health history form should be given to the patient for review. If any changes are needed, a patient should record these on an additional form or on a separate line in the treatment section of the patient record. The patient or parent/guardian must indicate in writing "No change," or must write in any changes to the patient's health status. The patient or parent/guardian is then instructed to sign and date the form to indicate that the information is accurate and up to date.

RECALL

4 What forms would the business assistant ask a new patient to complete before he or she is seen for treatment?
5 What type of demographics would be included in the patient registration form?
6 To verify that the information is accurate, what must a patient provide after completing a health history form?
7 What does the dental history section of the form provide for the dentist?
8 Give an example of a medical alert.

## Diagnostic Information–Gathering Forms

- Physical examination form (posture and gait, vital signs, cognition, and communication skills)
- Radiographic examination (this can include any of the following exposures: periapical, bitewing, occlusal, panoramic)
- Clinical examination form (extraoral examination, intraoral examination, periodontal examination)

At the completion of a patient's visit, the diagnostic information–gathering process will have been completed, and at that time the dentist will formulate an assessment of the patient's oral health status from the findings. An **assessment** is the process of collecting data and then evaluating or drawing conclusions from the findings. The dentist will do the following:

- Assess a patient's intraoral and extraoral conditions by completing a comprehensive clinical examination.
- Review all significant findings.
- Present a **diagnosis** to the patient.
- Develop and document a treatment plan with input from the patient.
- Schedule a sequence of appointments to complete treatment in a timely manner.
- Follow through with maintenance appointments in the patient care process.

## Clinical Examination

The clinical examination and recall examination form is the most detailed document in the dental record (Fig. 26.7). This form provides the dental team with past, present, and future examination data, analysis, and charting needs of the patient. This form is completed for every new patient of the practice

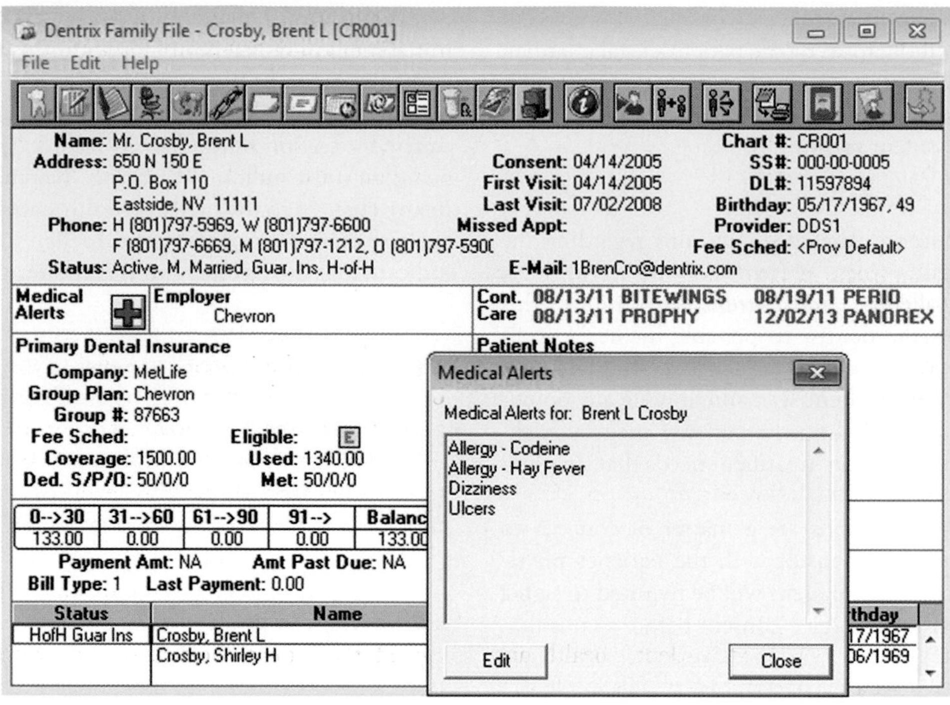


**FIG. 26.5** Examples of medical alert in an electronic patient record. *(Dentrix screenshot courtesy Henry Schein Practice Solutions, American Fork, UT.)*

## MEDICAL HISTORY UPDATE

GENERAL HEALTH: EXCELLENT ____ GOOD ____ FAIR ____ POOR ____

YES ___ NO ___ HAS THERE BEEN ANY CHANGES IN YOUR HEALTH SINCE YOUR LAST DENTAL APPOINTMENT?

IF YES, PLEASE DESCRIBE: ______________________________________________

______________________________________________________________

YES ___ NO ___ HAS THERE BEEN ANY CHANGES IN YOUR MEDICATIONS?

IF YES, PLEASE DESCRIBE:

______________________________________________________________

______________________________________________________________

YES ___ NO ___ IS THERE ANY REASON THAT RECEIVING DENTAL CARE MIGHT POSE A RISK TO YOU, OUR STAFF, OR OTHER PATIENTS

IF YES, PLEASE DESCRIBE:

______________________________________________________________

______________________________________________________________

____________________ ________________________________

Date Patient Signature

____________________ ________________________________

Date Dentist Signature

**FIG. 26.6** Example of the medical-dental health history update form.

and is updated at every appointment including recall appointments with the dental hygienist thereafter.

The dentist will examine the patient and dictate the findings to the dental assistant to chart or record. Specific areas on the clinical examination form include the following (see Chapter 28 for detailed explanations of charting symbols):

- Patient's name and date of examination
- Charting system for existing restorations and present conditions
- Charting system for periodontal conditions
- Patient's chief complaint
- Occlusal evaluations
- Temporomandibular joint (TMJ) evaluations
- Comments

Specific guidelines must be followed for proper patient record management.

## Treatment Plan

Once the dentist has reviewed the medical-dental health history form and has dictated any charting or updates needed on the clinical examination form, he or she then records the plan of care on the treatment plan form (Fig. 26.8). The treatment plan for a patient is properly sequenced to address all problems that were identified during the examination and diagnosis portions of the patient visit.

The treatment plan may change course if financial arrangements become a factor. For example, a patient's treatment plan that indicates the need for an implant might change if the patient has limited income and cannot afford the cost of the implant. A second option of a fixed bridge or a removable partial would then be discussed with the patient to accommodate financial limitations.

## Informed Consent

The informed consent form pertains to a specific treatment or procedure that has been presented to the patient as part of his or her treatment needs (Fig. 26.9). This document provides the patient with expected outcomes of treatment and describes possible complications. These individualized forms are more commonly used when invasive or extensive treatment is required, such as surgical procedures, orthodontics, endodontics, prosthodontics, periodontics, and implants.

The dentist will review the treatment plan with the patient and address any questions or concerns. Once both parties have agreed, the patient, the dentist, and a witness will sign and date the forms.

## Progress Notes

At the conclusion of a procedure, the details of what was accomplished will be entered in the "Progress notes" section

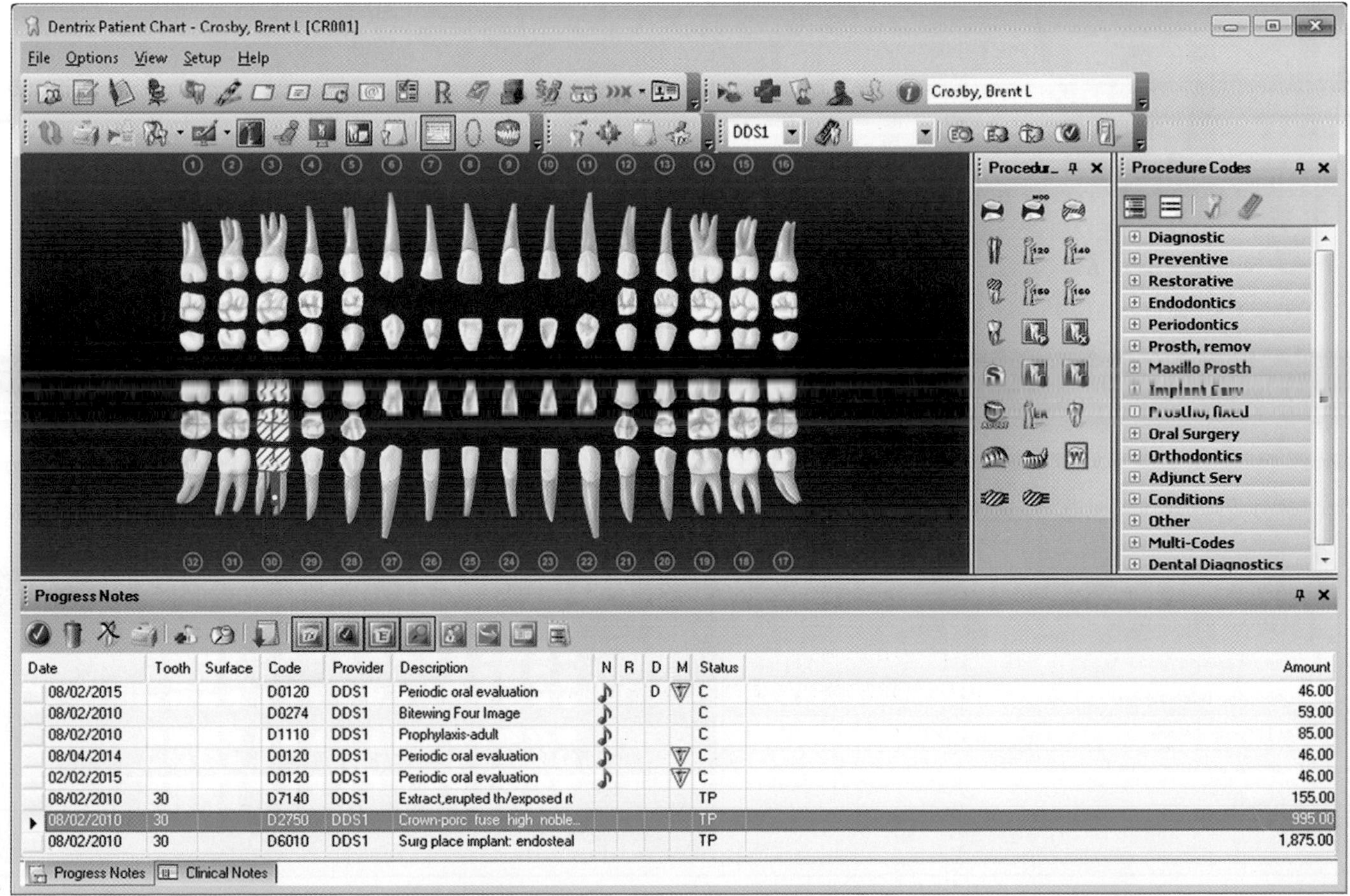


FIG. 26.7 A, Example of a clinical examination form.

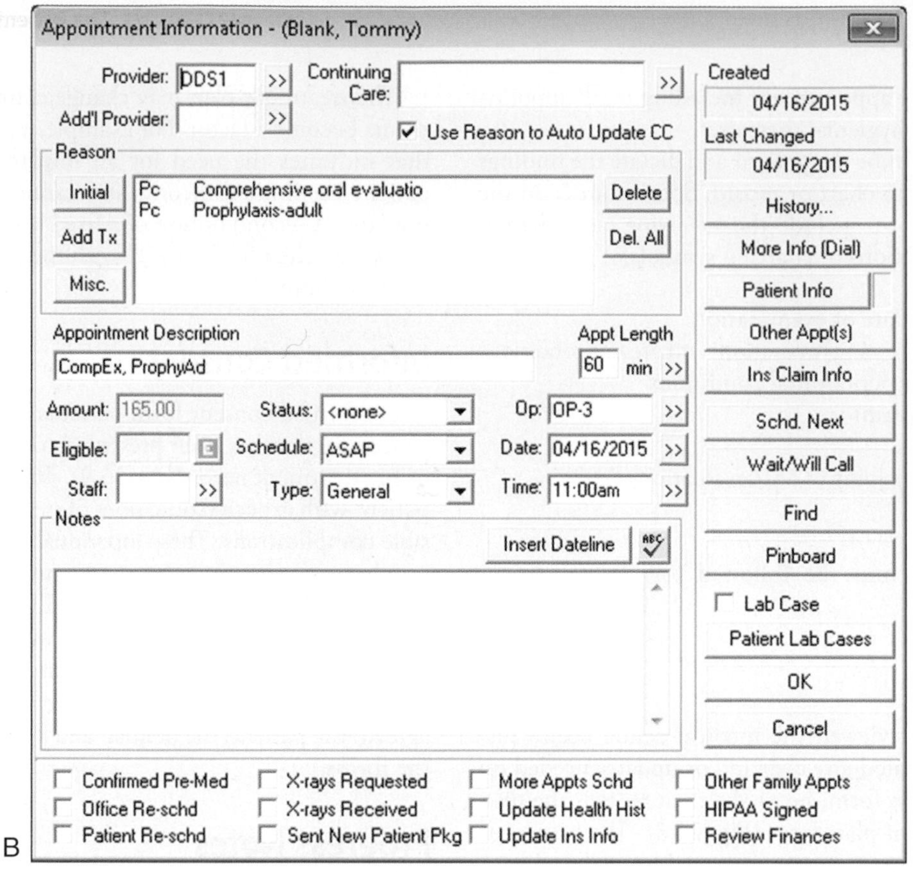


**FIG. 26.7, cont'd** B, Example of a recall examination form. *(Courtesy Henry Schein Practice Solutions, American Fork, UT.)*

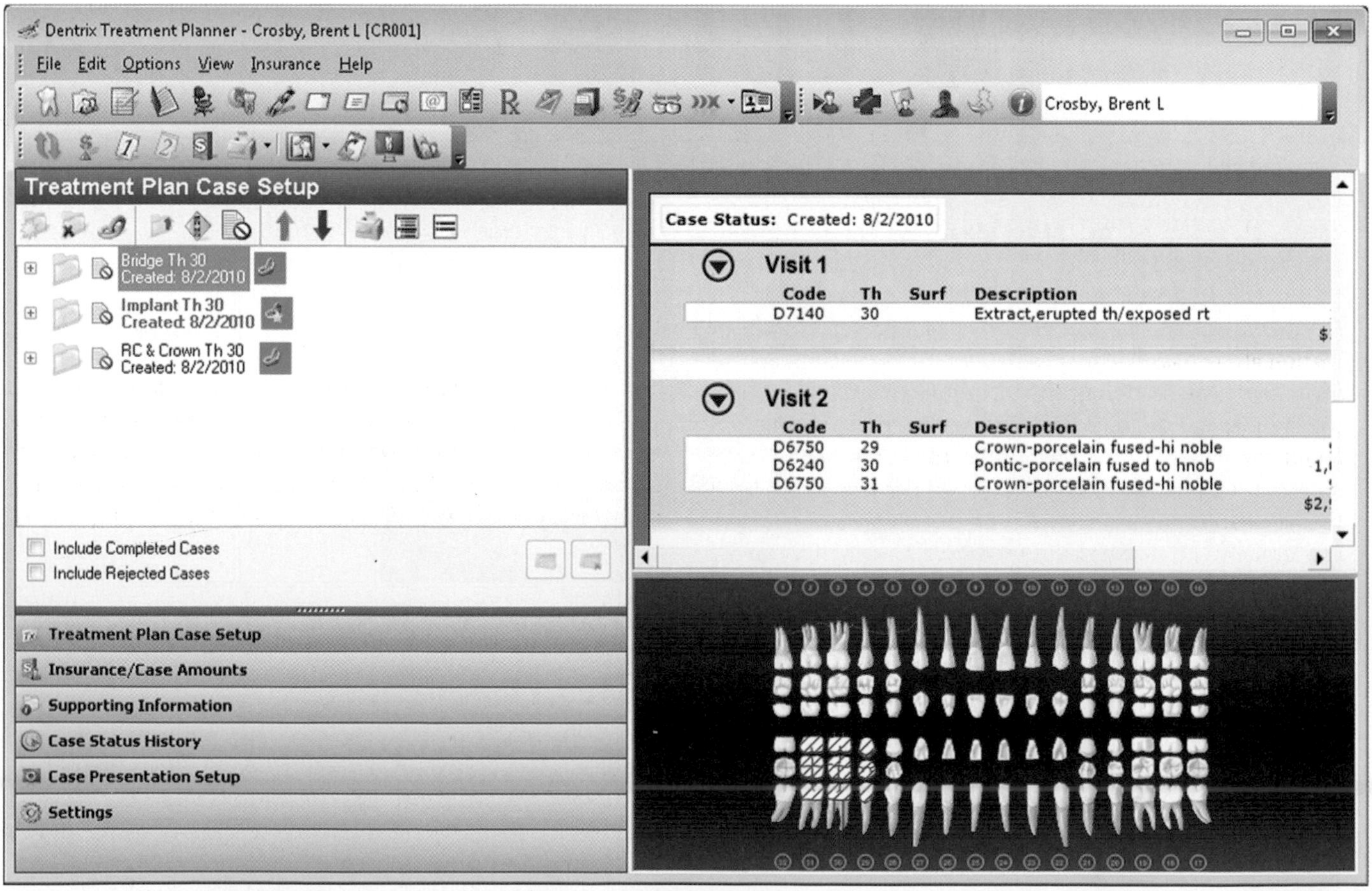

**FIG. 26.8** Example of a treatment plan form. *(Courtesy Henry Schein Practice Solutions, American Fork, UT.)*

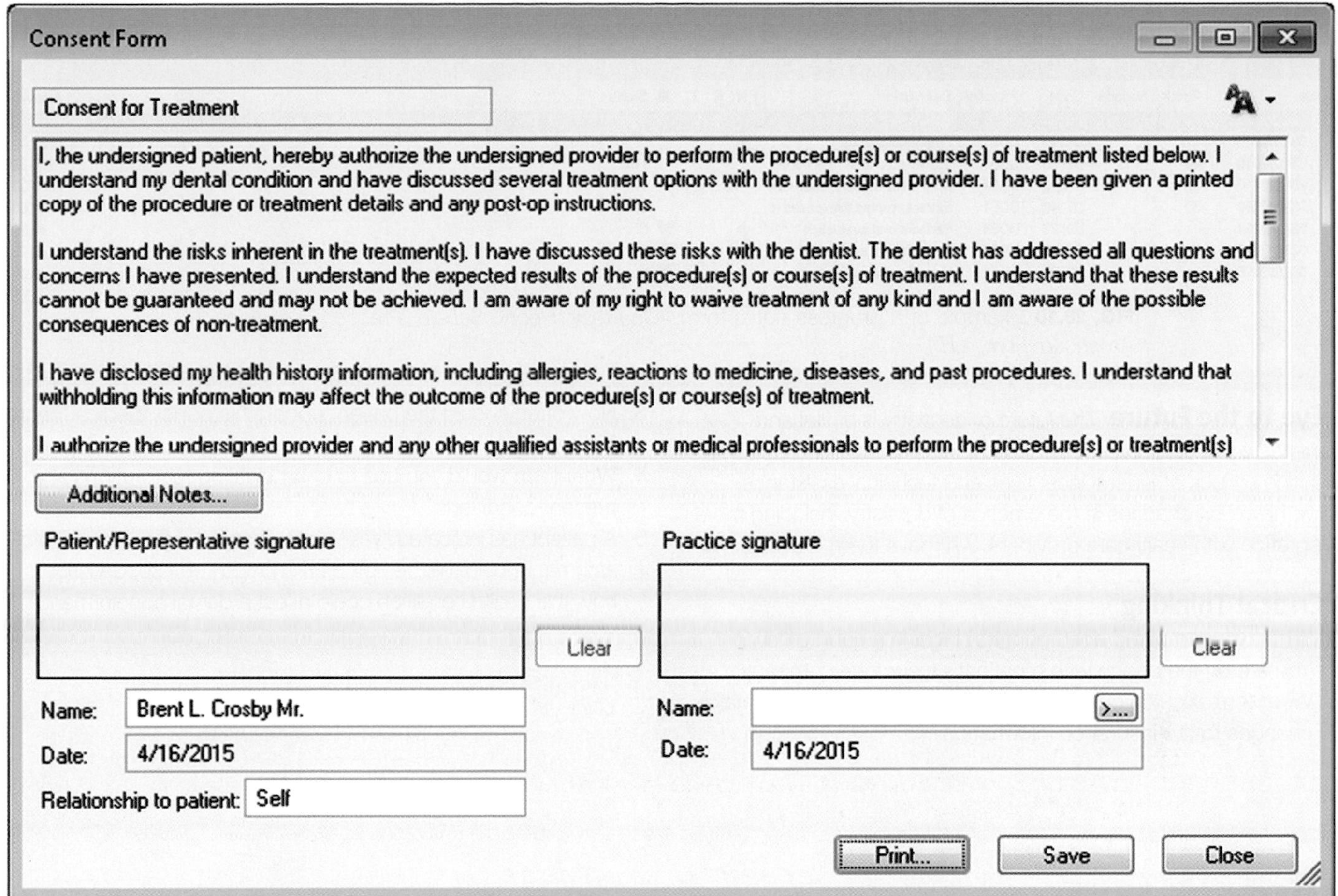

Consent Form

Consent for Treatment

I, the undersigned patient, hereby authorize the undersigned provider to perform the procedure(s) or course(s) of treatment listed below. I understand my dental condition and have discussed several treatment options with the undersigned provider. I have been given a printed copy of the procedure or treatment details and any post-op instructions.

I understand the risks inherent in the treatment(s). I have discussed these risks with the dentist. The dentist has addressed all questions and concerns I have presented. I understand the expected results of the procedure(s) or course(s) of treatment. I understand that these results cannot be guaranteed and may not be achieved. I am aware of my right to waive treatment of any kind and I am aware of the possible consequences of non-treatment.

I have disclosed my health history information, including allergies, reactions to medicine, diseases, and past procedures. I understand that withholding this information may affect the outcome of the procedure(s) or course(s) of treatment.

I authorize the undersigned provider and any other qualified assistants or medical professionals to perform the procedure(s) or treatment(s)

Additional Notes...

Patient/Representative signature | Clear

Practice signature | Clear

Name: Brent L. Crosby Mr.

Date: 4/16/2015

Relationship to patient: Self

Name:

Date: 4/16/2015

Print... | Save | Close

**FIG. 26.9** Example of the informed consent form. *(Courtesy Henry Schein Practice Solutions, American Fork, UT.)*

(Fig. 26.10). Specific information that should be noted on this form includes the following:

- *Date:* This shows the month/day/year of treatment/communication.
- *Tooth number:* If a specific tooth is being treated/discussed, it should be indicated by the number in this section. This information allows faster reference to previous appointments.
- *Treatment:* This section of the form must be filled out completely and accurately. This should include information about the patient's vital signs, scheduled treatment for the day, and the procedure performed, with the surface related to the procedure. All pertinent information, such as type and amount of anesthesia, dental materials used, how the patient tolerated the procedure, and postoperative instructions, must be recorded.
- *Communication with patient:* This documentation can include anything from the patient scheduling/canceling the appointment, to a follow-up call, communicating with a dental laboratory, or communication with a specialist involved in treatment care.

It is important to make note that, following each entry, the dentist and clinical staff involved in treatment must sign and date the entry.

RECALL

**9** What term describes the collection of data used to make a correct diagnosis?

**10** What form in the patient record would provide knowledge to the dental team of an existing restoration?

## Entering Data in a Patient's Dental Record

Every entry in a paper or electronic chart should be made as if the chart will be seen in a court of law. Specific guidelines must be followed when any type of entry is made in a patient record. See Procedure 26.3: Entering Treatment in a Patient Record and Procedure 26.4: Correcting a Chart Entry.

**■ Legal and Ethical Implications** The patient record is the most confidential document that exists between the dentist and the patient. The information shared between the dental healthcare team and the patient is private and must remain private.

Do not discuss patient information, specific treatments, or patient discussions with anyone. Information talked about outside the office and then reported could have serious consequences for the dentist, the assistant, and the entire practice. All members of the dental team should be familiar with HIPAA (the Health Insurance Portability and Accountability Act). ■

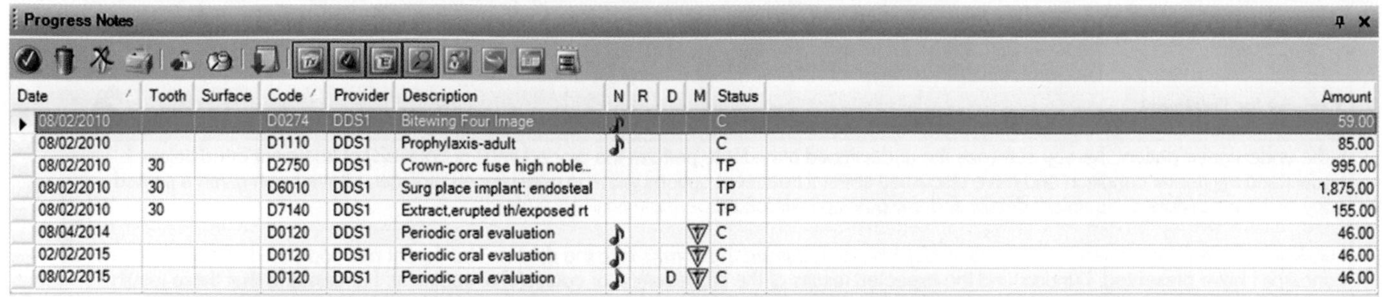

Progress Notes

| Date | Tooth | Surface | Code | Provider | Description | N | R | D | M | Status | Amount |
|---|---|---|---|---|---|---|---|---|---|---|---|
| 08/02/2010 | | | D0274 | DDS1 | Bitewing Four Image | | | | | C | 59.00 |
| 08/02/2010 | | | D1110 | DDS1 | Prophylaxis-adult | | | | | C | 85.00 |
| 08/02/2010 | 30 | | D2750 | DDS1 | Crown-porc fuse high noble... | | | | | TP | 995.00 |
| 08/02/2010 | 30 | | D6010 | DDS1 | Surg place implant: endosteal | | | | | TP | 1,875.00 |
| 08/02/2010 | 30 | | D7140 | DDS1 | Extract,erupted th/exposed rt | | | | | TP | 155.00 |
| 08/04/2014 | | | D0120 | DDS1 | Periodic oral evaluation | | | | | C | 46.00 |
| 02/02/2015 | | | D0120 | DDS1 | Periodic oral evaluation | | | | | C | 46.00 |
| 08/02/2015 | | | D0120 | DDS1 | Periodic oral evaluation | | | D | | C | 46.00 |

**FIG. 26.10** Example of a progress notes form. *(Courtesy Henry Schein Practice Solutions, American Fork, UT.)*

**■ Eye to the Future** The future of dentistry is digital and paperless. Dentists have been slow to transition in the digital practice by lack of federal incentives and technical assistance. Now, however, changes in the practice of dentistry, including more integration with healthcare providers, will move them forward. ■

## ■ Critical Thinking

1. What would make a document *not* legal in a court of law?
2. You are on the phone with a patient's insurance company. What form would you refer to from the patient record to make changes to the insurance information?
3. How often should the patient update his or her medical-dental history?
4. What form would you use to chart existing restorations and present conditions?
5. A patient has indicated "yes" on the health history that he has asthma. Should this be noted as an ALERT? If so, describe how this health condition could affect a dental appointment. ■

## Standards and Criteria for Data Entered in a Clinical Record

- All entries must be dated and legible. To be completed in *black* ink if using a paper chart.
- The individual who documents the information must provide a signature or entry of initials.
- Inaccurate entries should *never* be corrected with correction fluid or other methods of "blocking out" the original entry. Crossing through an entry should be done only to make corrections of errors in documentation and should be marked with a single line followed by the initials of the individual who corrected the entry.
- The patient's response to treatment (outcomes) should be routinely recorded.
- All appointment cancellations, broken appointments, late arrivals, and changes of appointment should be documented, whether patient or provider generated.
- All conversations with the patient and with other healthcare providers regarding the patient should be documented.
- Evaluations and statements of "opinion" that the dentist is not professionally qualified to make should not be documented in the record (e.g., patient's mental health status). For example, instead of "Suspected drug abuser," document that "Patient requested narcotic meds after routine simple restorative procedure."
- All individuals who have access to the patient record must maintain the confidentiality of the information contained in the document. Information in the record may not be shared with anyone outside of the healthcare team without the patient's written authorization.
- A patient's record must never be altered once it is possible that legal action may be taken by the patient.
- The patient's treatment record is the property of the dentist and may not be removed from the dental practice. Original records and radiographs may not be given to anyone except through a court order.
- Patients have a right to access the information contained within their record and are entitled to receive a copy of their record. Release of a copy of the record, in part or in its entirety, to anyone requires a written request from the patient.
- The original entry is readable with only a line through it when a charting error is corrected.

Standards and Criteria for Data Entered in a Clinical Record—Cont'd

| DATE | TOOTH | SERVICE RENDERED |
|---|---|---|
| ~~2/10/xx~~ | | ~~exam, adult prophy 2/15/xx DDA~~ |
| 2/10/xx | 3 | X-ray, remove amal restoration. Place |
| | | sedative treatment. If pain persists, |
| | | refer to endodontist. 2/15/xx DDA |
| | | |
| | | |

PROCEDURE 26.1

# Registering a New Patient

## EQUIPMENT AND SUPPLIES

- Registration form
- Black ink pen
- Clipboard

## PROCEDURAL STEPS

1 Explain the need for the form. Hand the registration form on a clipboard with a black pen to the patient, or instruct patient on using the computer, and provide instructions on how to complete and where to return the document when finished.

2 The business assistant will review the completed form for the necessary information:
   - Full name, birth date, name of spouse or parent
   - Home address and telephone numbers (home, cell, work)
   - Employment, name of employer, business address, and telephone number
   - Name and address of person responsible for payment
   - Method of payment (cash, check, credit, assignment of benefits)
   - Dental insurance information (photocopy of both sides of insurance ID card)

   **PURPOSE** This information is necessary for processing financial arrangements and insurance claims.
   - Name of primary insurance carrier
   - Referral to the practice
   - Emergency contact
   - Verification that the patient has provided a signature and a date on the form

## PROCEDURE 26.2

# Obtaining a Medical-Dental Health History

### EQUIPMENT AND SUPPLIES

- Medical-dental health history form
- Black ink pen
- Clipboard

### PROCEDURAL STEPS

1 Explain the need for the information and the importance of the patient fully completing the form.
2 Provide the patient with a black ink pen and the form on a clipboard, or access to the electronic version.
3 Offer assistance to the patient when completing the form.
**PURPOSE** The patient may not understand the terminology or may have a language barrier.
4 Ask the patient to return the form and clipboard to you after he or she has answered all questions.
5 Thank the patient for completing the form, and request that the patient take a seat in the reception area.
6 Review the form for errors and/or any questions that may arise before you hand it to the clinical assistant.
7 Use information from the patient's medical-dental health history form to complete additional documents. Remember, the information provided to you by the patient is confidential and must be maintained as such.

## PROCEDURE 26.3

# Entering Treatment in a Patient Record

### EQUIPMENT AND SUPPLIES

- Black ink pen
- Patient's record or electronic record

### PROCEDURAL STEPS

1 In the Date column, record the date the treatment was provided, using numbers in a month/date/year format, such as 2/27/17.
2 In the Progress Notes column, record all aspects of the dental procedure, such as the tooth, the surfaces of the tooth restored, the type and amount of anesthetic agent given, the dental materials used, and information on patient tolerance of the treatment.
3 If appropriate, describe the procedure that was performed with appropriate details, such as whether the tooth was prepared for a crown.
**PURPOSE** The treatment is documented, and this serves as a reference for future appointments.
4 After entering the completed treatment, sign the entry.
**NOTE** Always make sure to have the dentist sign. This verifies that the entry is accurate.
5 Return the completed dental record to the business office.
**PURPOSE** The patient returns to the business office area to make payment for services and to schedule any additional appointments.

## PROCEDURE 26.4

# Correcting a Chart Entry

### GOAL

To gain competency in correcting an error on a patient's record.

### PROCEDURAL STEPS

1 Using a black ink pen, draw a single line through the previous entry. Initial and date the correction.
**PURPOSE** To ensure that the original entry is still readable and that the change is permanent.
2 Write the corrected entry in ink on the next available line.
3 Initial and date the new entry.
**PURPOSE** To identify the individual responsible for the chart entry.

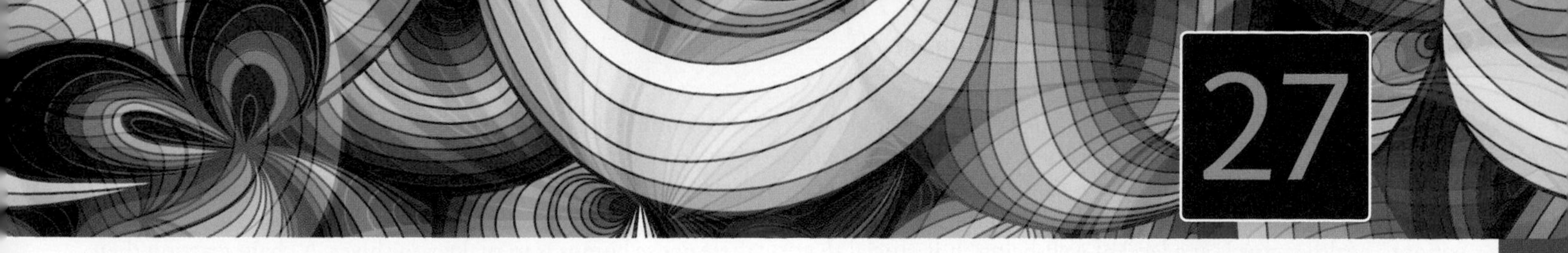


# Vital Signs

## KEY TERMS

**Antecubital (an-tee-KYOO-bi-tul) space** Small groove or fold in the inner arm, at or "in front of" *(ante)* the elbow *(cubitus).*

**Arrhythmia (uh-RITH-mee-uh)** Abnormality and irregularity in the force or rhythm of the heartbeat.

**Blood pressure (BP)** Pressure exerted by the blood against the walls of the blood vessels.

**Brachial (BRAY-kee-uhl)** Relating to the arm (brachium), as in *brachial artery.*

**Carotid (kuh-ROT-id)** Relating to either of the two major arteries on each side of the neck that carry blood to the head.

**Depth** In respiration, the amount of air in a breath.

**Diastolic (dye-uh-STOL-ik, dye-uh-STAHL-ik)** The normal rhythmic relaxation and dilation of the heart chambers.

**Electrocardiogram (ee-lek-tro-KAHR-dee-oe-gram)** Instrument used in the detection and diagnosis of heart abnormalities. It generates a record of the electrical currents associated with heart muscle activity.

**Korotkoff (kuh-ROT-kof) sounds** Specific sounds heard when one is taking a blood pressure.

**Metabolism (muh-TAB-uh-liz-um)** Physical and chemical processes that occur within a living cell or organism and are necessary for the maintenance of life.

**Oximetry (ok-SIM-uh-tree)** Measurement of oxygen concentration in the blood.

**Palpate (PAL-payt)** To examine or explore by touching.

**Pulse** Rhythmic throbbing of the arteries produced by regular contractions of the heart.

**Radial** Related to the radius *(bone)* or forearm *(antebrachium),* as in *radial artery.*

**Rate** A quantity measured, as in breaths and heartbeats.

**Respiration** Act or process of inhaling and exhaling; breathing.

**Rhythm** A sequence or pattern, such as the heartbeat or breathing.

**Sphygmomanometer (sfig-moe-muh-NOM-e-ter)** Instrument for measuring blood pressure in the arteries.

**Stethoscope** Instrument used for listening to sounds produced within the body.

**Systolic (sis-TOL-ik)** Rhythmic contraction of the heart, especially of the ventricles.

**Temperature** Degree of hotness or coldness of a body or an environment.

**Thermometer** Instrument for measuring temperature.

**Tympanic (tim-PAN-ik)** Related to or resembling a drum, as in the *tympanic membrane,* or eardrum.

**Volume** Quantity or amount, as in force of a heartbeat.

## LEARNING OUTCOMES

*On completion of this chapter, the student will be able to achieve the following objectives:*

1. Pronounce, define, and spell the key terms.
2. List the four vital signs routinely taken in the dental office.
3. Discuss temperature, including the following:
   - Describe how metabolism affects a patient's vital signs.
   - List the average temperature readings and areas of the body used to obtain a temperature reading.
   - Discuss three types of thermometers.
4. Discuss pulse, including the following:
   - List common pulse sites used for taking a pulse.
   - Describe the characteristics of the pulse and normal pulse readings that you would look for in taking a patient's pulse.
5. Discuss respiration, including the following:
   - Describe the characteristics of respiration, and explain how they affect a patient's breathing.
   - Describe the best way to obtain accurate readings of respiration.
6. Discuss blood pressure, including the following:
   - Classify blood pressure readings according to normal values and stages of hypertension.
   - Differentiate the Korotkoff sounds heard when one is taking a patient's blood pressure.
   - Explain the importance of taking a patient's blood pressure.
7. Discuss additional techniques used to assess a patient's health status.

## PERFORMANCE OUTCOMES

*On completion of this chapter, the student will be able to meet competency standards in the following skills:*

- Take an oral temperature reading with a digital thermometer.
- Take a patient's pulse.
- Take a patient's respiration.
- Take a patient's blood pressure.
- Take a patient's pulse oximetry.
- Take a patient's electrocardiogram

## ELECTRONIC RESOURCES

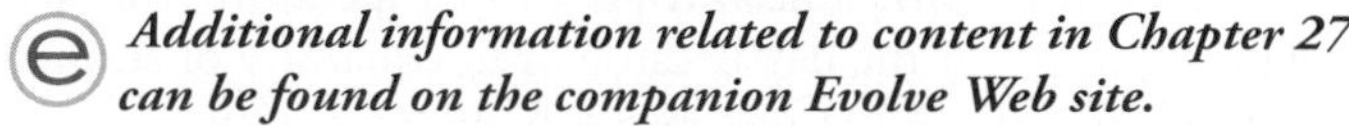
***Additional information related to content in Chapter 27 can be found on the companion Evolve Web site.***

- Animation: Pulse Oximetry
- Canadian Content Corner
- Practice Quiz
- Video: Taking a Patient's Blood Pressure

Attention toward a patient's immediate health should be the first priority of every healthcare provider. By taking a patient's basic vital signs on a routine basis before providing dental treatment, the dental team is confirming that the patient's health status is at a level of well-being. It is crucial that you gain confidence in both the background knowledge and the practical application of taking a patient's vital signs.

Vital signs consist of taking and recording a person's temperature, pulse, respiration, and blood pressure. If this is the patient's first visit, 6-month recall, or a medical emergency, the clinical assistant should routinely take and record the vital signs. This type of baseline information provides the dental team with assurance regarding the patient's well-being and health status.

## Factors That Can Affect Vital Sign Readings

The human body is influenced by both emotional and physical factors. Before a dental appointment, for example, the patient may have had a hot or a cold beverage, either of which would alter the oral temperature. Or a patient may be fearful of an upcoming dental appointment; thus his or her blood pressure and respiration may be higher than at a previous reading.

If a patient were to come directly to a dental appointment from a workout at the gym, what changes would you expect to see in the patient's vital signs? If you predicted an elevation in the patient's temperature, pulse, respiration, and blood pressure, you are correct. When an increase in metabolism occurs (such as during strenuous exercise), vital sign measurements also typically increase.

One of your roles as a dental assistant is to inquire about and recognize these situations and help the patient relax before taking his or her vital signs. You may need to take these measurements more than once. If you think the patient is abnormally anxious, provide reassurance, wait several minutes, and then repeat the procedure.

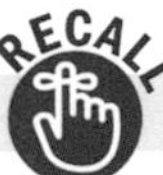


1 Identify the four basic vital signs.

## Temperature

Body **temperature** is the degree of hotness or coldness of the body's internal environment. The process of physical and chemical changes that take place in the production of the body's heat is called **metabolism**. A healthy person's temperature will vary slightly throughout the day because of the quantity of stimuli that it encounters. A person's lowest body temperature occurs in the early morning hours, and the highest temperature occurs in the evening.

During an illness, a person's metabolism increases for the purpose of elevating the body's temperature. Most bacteria and viruses cannot survive in excess heat, and this is the body's way of defending against such diseases. Have you ever wondered why you become chilled when you have a fever? When fever is present, the blood vessels closest to the surface of the skin constrict, producing "goose bumps." The body's reaction to these goose bumps is to make you shiver. A chain reaction then begins, causing the body to produce internal heat for warmth.

### Temperature Readings

The **thermometer** is the instrument used to measure body temperature. Temperature readings are calibrated according to the Fahrenheit (F) or the Celsius (C) scale. The Fahrenheit scale is the reading most frequently used in the United States, and the Celsius scale is used most frequently in Canada and Europe.

The average range of oral temperature of a resting person is 97.6° F to 99° F (36.4–37.3° C). The average body temperature is higher in infants and younger children than in adults.

Several areas of the body can be used to obtain a temperature reading. The thermometer can be placed under the tongue, in the ear, under the arm, in the rectum, or on the forehead.

Average temperature readings vary according to the body site used:

- Oral temperature is 98.6° F or 37° C.
- Rectal temperature is 0.5° F to 1° F or 0.3° C to 0.6° C higher than an oral temperature.
- Ear (tympanic) temperature is 0.5° F to 1° F or 0.3° C to 0.6° C higher than an oral temperature.
- Armpit (axillary) temperature is 0.5° F to 1° F or 0.3° C to 0.6° C lower than an oral temperature.
- Forehead (temporal) scanner is 0.5° F to 1° F or 0.3° C to 0.6° C lower than an oral temperature.

### Types of Thermometers

#### *Digital*

Digital thermometers are popular today because of their convenience (Fig. 27.1). These thermometers are battery operated and function on the same theory as a glass thermometer, except that a timing system shows a digital reading after 30 seconds, rather than a line of mercury that expands ("rises") along a marked scale. It is important to remember that the timed feature of the digital thermometer may attain an inaccurate reading if the battery is low.

A disposable plastic sheath slides over the probe before insertion. Most digital thermometers emit a "beeping" sound that indicates completion, with the reading appearing on the digital screen. See Procedure 27.1: Taking an Oral Temperature Reading with a Digital Thermometer.

#### *Tympanic*

This technique allows you to take a patient's temperature in the ear canal (a **tympanic** reading). The ear canal is a protected cavity, so the tympanic temperature reading is not affected by an open mouth, hot or cold drinks, or nose congestion. The tympanic thermometer has a much smaller probe, which is

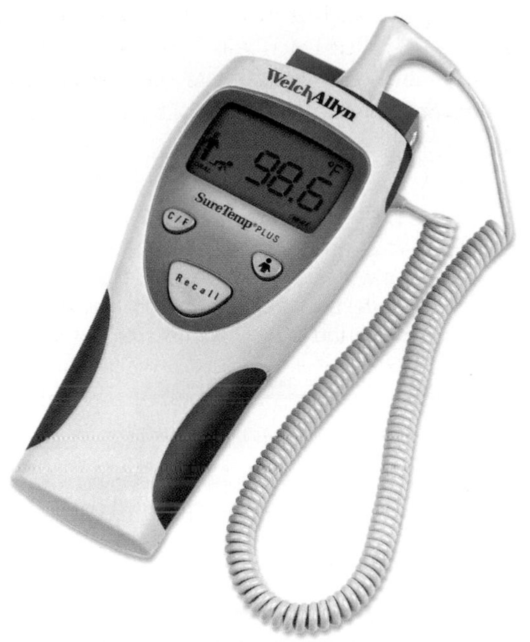


FIG. 27.1 A digital thermometer. (Courtesy Welch Allyn, Inc., Skaneateles, NY.)

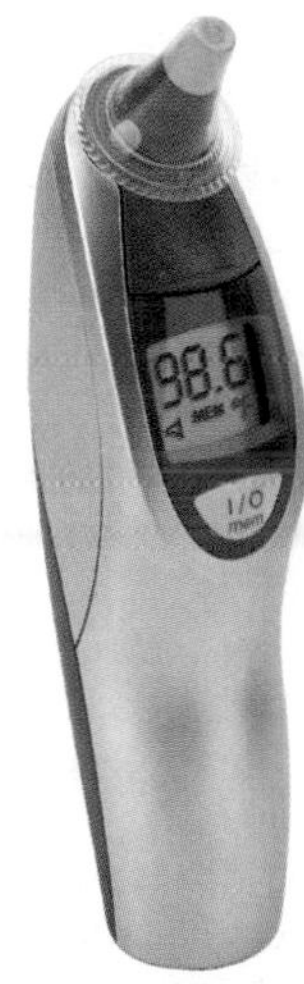


FIG. 27.2 A tympanic thermometer. (Courtesy Welch Allyn, Inc., Skaneateles, NY.)

gently placed into the ear canal (Fig. 27.2). An infrared signal is bounced off the eardrum, and an accurate reading is provided within 2 seconds. The risk of spreading communicable diseases while taking a temperature tympanically is greatly reduced because the covered probe of the thermometer does not actually touch the eardrum. This approach has become very popular in younger children. The rapid measurement may be more accurate because less patient movement occurs.

### Temporal Scanner

The temporal thermometer uses the surface temperature of the artery on the forehead to determine the presence of a fever. The temperature of the forehead (temporal) artery does not change if the person eats or drinks. Proper use of your temporal thermometer ensures you get the most

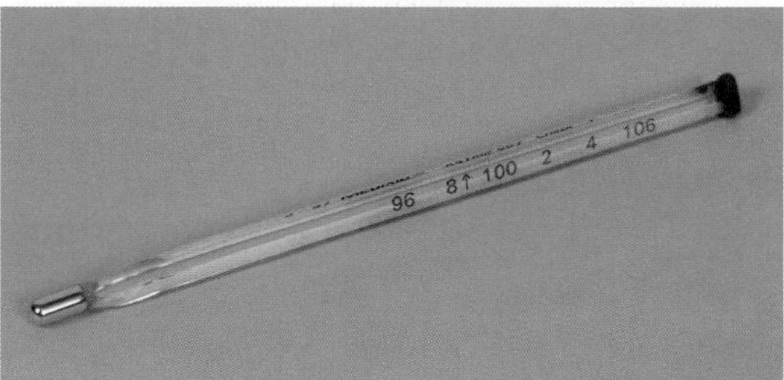


FIG. 27.3 A glass thermometer showing the mercury bulb.

accurate results. The instrument is easy to operate by pressing the button on the temporal thermometer and holding it while you slide the thermometer straight across the forehead in a line parallel to the eyebrows, halfway between the hairline and the eyebrows. Listen for a beeping sound and look for a red light to signal that the thermometer has registered a temperature.

### Glass

The glass thermometer is a glass tube with a small mercury bulb at the end that comes in contact with body tissue (Fig. 27.3). When it touches warm tissues of the body, the mercury expands and "rises" along a marked numeric scale. After 3 minutes, the mercury stops expanding and registers its highest reading.

Mercury thermometers historically proved to be a useful measuring device over many years and can still be found in a few clinical settings. However, mercury is a toxic substance that can harm both humans and wildlife. Many states have banned the use of mercury thermometers because of these health hazards. In 1998 the American Hospital Association (AHA) signed an agreement with the U.S. Environmental Protection Agency (EPA) to commit to the elimination of mercury from hospital waste. Furthermore, in July 2001 the American Academy of Pediatrics urged doctors and parents to stop using mercury thermometers.

RECALL

2 What is the purpose of a thermometer?
3 What locations on the body most often give the highest temperature reading of the body?
4 Where would the tympanic thermometer be placed?

## Pulse

A **pulse** is the rhythmic expansion of an artery each time the heart beats. Every artery throughout the body has a pulse, although many pulses cannot be read because of their location. When an artery is close to the surface of the skin, you can push against it with your fingers as it rests on a tendon or bone and feel the beating. The pulse can be felt in seven areas of the body with slight finger pressure. See Table 27.1 for these locations and descriptions in taking the pulse.

**TABLE 27.1 Pulse Locations**

| Pulse Point | Location | Description for Finding Pulse |
|---|---|---|
| **Radial** artery | 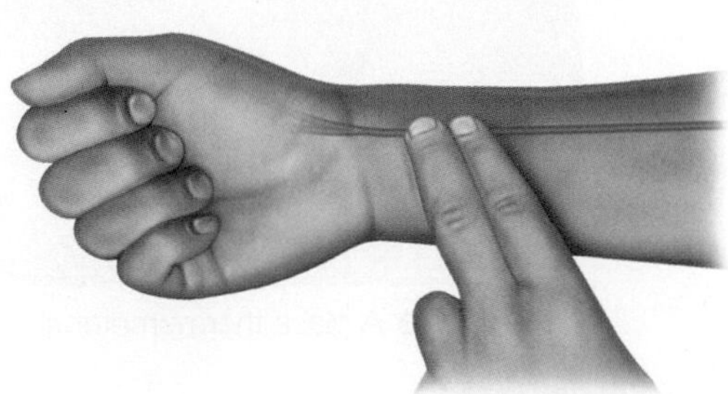 | Located on the inner surface of the wrist (thumb side). It is the most common site for taking a patient's pulse in the dental office. To take the pulse, place your index and middle fingers lightly on the patient's wrist between the radius (bone on the thumb side) and the tendon. This measures about 1 inch from the base of the thumb. |
| **Brachial** artery | 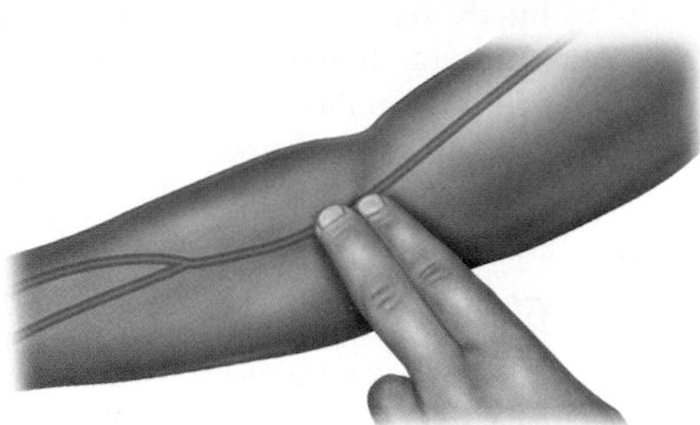 | Located on the inner fold of the arm, it is also referred to as the **antecubital** area of the elbow. This artery is used when a patient's blood pressure is taken. |
| **Carotid** artery | 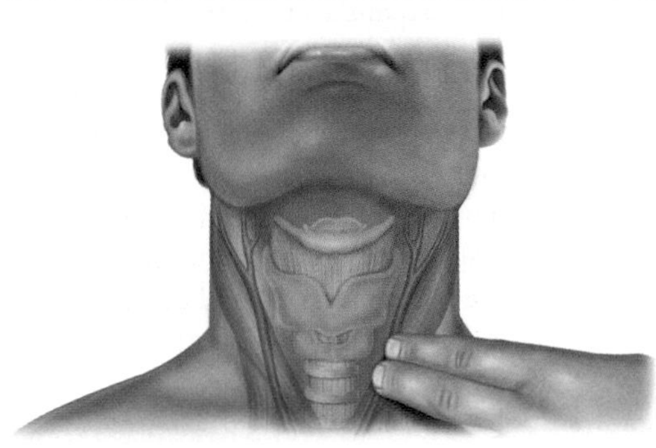 | Locate alongside the patient's larynx (Adam's apple). Taking the carotid pulse is common when performing cardiopulmonary resuscitation (CPR; see Chapter 31). Because CPR is an emergency situation, it is important that you know how to find the carotid artery quickly.<br>To detect the carotid pulse, place two fingers alongside the patient's larynx on the side of the neck nearest you. Move your fingers slowly down the groove to the soft area above the clavicle (collarbone), and then **palpate** this area gently to determine a pulse. |
| Temporal artery | | Located just above the temple, on the sides of the head. |
| Femoral artery | | Located in the inside front of the leg where it joins the pelvic. |
| Posterior tibial artery | | Located on the foot behind the ankle. |
| Dorsalis pedis artery | | Located on the top of the foot running along the vein from the large toe to the ankle. |



## Pulse Characteristics

When taking a patient's pulse, look for any distinct changes. The following characteristics must be noted in the patient's dental record when documenting a patient's pulse:

- **Rate** is the number of beats that occur during the counting period.
- **Rhythm** describes the pattern of the beats, such as an occasional skipping, speeding up, or slowing down of a beat.
- **Volume** is the force of the beat, such as a strong or a weak beat.

## Pulse Readings

When taking a patient's radial pulse, make sure the patient is positioned with his or her arm at the same level as or lower than the heart. The arm should be well supported and extended straight out.

### Resting Heart Rate

Newborns (0–3 months old): 100–150 beats per minute
Infants (3–6 months old): 90–120 beats per minute
Infants (6–12 months old): 80–120 beats per minute
Children 1–10 years: 70–130 beats per minute
Children over 10 through adults (including seniors): 60–100 beats per minute
Well-trained athletes: 40–60 beats per minute

A simple method of timing and counting pulse beats is to observe a watch or a clock with a second hand while palpating the pulse. To minimize counting, you may count for 30 seconds and then double that number for the rate of 1 full minute. However, it is best not to count for less than 30 seconds, because it is difficult to detect any possible **arrhythmia** (irregularity) in the heartbeat in times shorter than 30 seconds. See Procedure 27.2: Taking a Patient's Pulse.

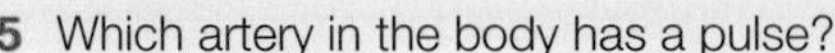

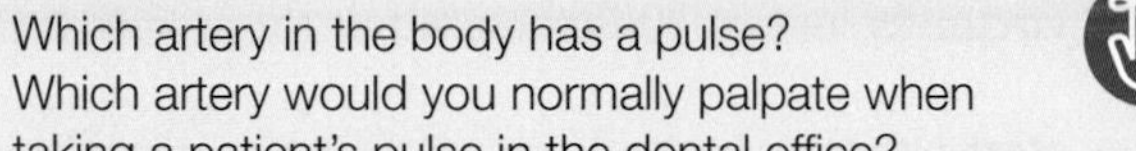

RECALL

**5** Which artery in the body has a pulse?
**6** Which artery would you normally palpate when taking a patient's pulse in the dental office?
**7** What is the normal pulse rate for an adult?
**8** What is the term for the small groove or fold on the inner arm?

## Respiration

**Respiration** is the process of inhaling and exhaling, or breathing. During respiration, oxygen is taken into the body, and carbon dioxide is released as a waste product. Breathing is an automatic response that is controlled by the body's nervous system. Respiration is both an involuntary response and a voluntary function. Breathing is primarily under the control of the brain, which is why people can hold their breath for only a limited period. When the carbon dioxide level increases in the blood, the cells become starved for oxygen, and a stimulus is sent to the brain to breathe again.

### Respiration Characteristics

A person's breathing is usually not noticeable unless that person is having trouble taking a breath. The following characteristics are to be noted in the patient record when taking a patient's respiration (Fig. 27.4):

- *Rate* is the total number of breaths per minute.
- *Rhythm* refers to the breathing pattern.
- **Depth** is the amount of air that is inhaled and exhaled during a breath.

### Respiration Readings

The normal respiration rate for a relaxed adult is 10 to 20 breaths per minute. For children and teenagers, the rate ranges from 18 to 30 breaths. To take the respiratory rate, observe the number of times the patient's chest rises and falls (one count)

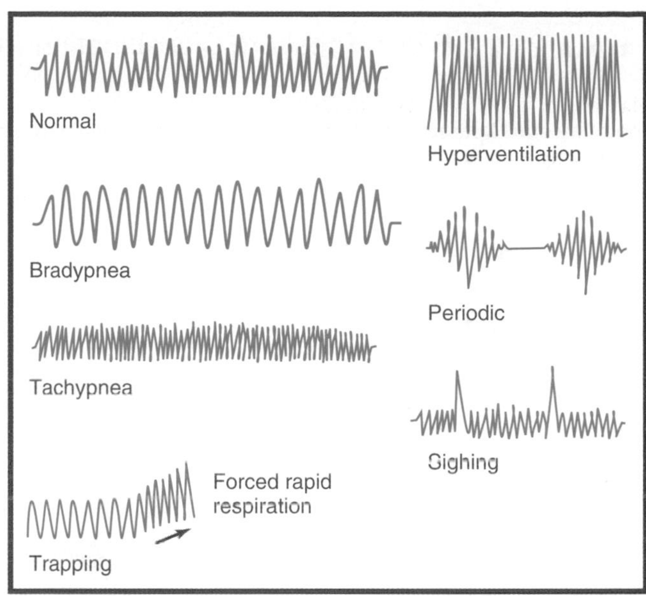


**FIG. 27.4** Respiration patterns. Bradypnea is an abnormally slow respiratory rate. Tachypnea is excessively short, rapid breaths, and hyperventilation is excessively long, rapid breaths. *(From Proctor DB et al: Kinn's the medical assistant, ed 13, St Louis, Elsevier, 2017.)*

for 30 seconds; then double the count to obtain the number of breaths for 1 minute.

If a patient realizes that his or her breaths are being counted, you will probably notice a change in the breathing pattern. Therefore the best way to count a patient's respirations is to do this while your fingers are still positioned on the wrist as if taking the pulse. The patient will assume you are still taking the pulse, but you will refocus your eyes on the patient's chest and count the breaths instead. See Procedure 27.3: Taking a Patient's Respiration.

**9** Respiration is the process of doing what?
**10** What breathing pattern is characteristic of excessively short rapid breaths?
**11** What is the normal respiration rate for an adult?

## Blood Pressure

**Blood pressure (BP)** refers to the amount of labor the heart has to exert to pump blood throughout the body. The heart produces two sounds for a blood pressure reading. The first sound *(systole)* indicates the **systolic** pressure, which is a *sharp* tapping sound and is the first and larger number recorded. This number reflects the amount of pressure that is required for the left ventricle of the heart to compress or push oxygenated blood out into the blood vessels. The last sound *(diastole),* which indicates the **diastolic** pressure, is a *soft* tapping sound; it is the second and lower number recorded. This number reflects the heart muscle at rest, allowing the heart to take in blood to be oxygenated before the next contraction occurs.

TABLE 27.2 Blood Pressure Classification for Adults

| Blood Pressure Category | Systolic mm Hg (Upper Number) | | Diastolic mm Hg (Lower Number) |
|---|---|---|---|
| Normal | Less than 120 | *and* | Less than 80 |
| Prehypertension | 120–139 | *or* | 80–89 |
| High blood pressure (hypertension) stage 1 | 140–159 | *or* | 90–99 |
| High blood pressure (hypertension) stage 2 | 160 or higher | *or* | 100 or higher |
| Hypertensive crisis (emergency care needed) | Higher than 180 | *or* | Higher than 110 |

From the American Health Association.

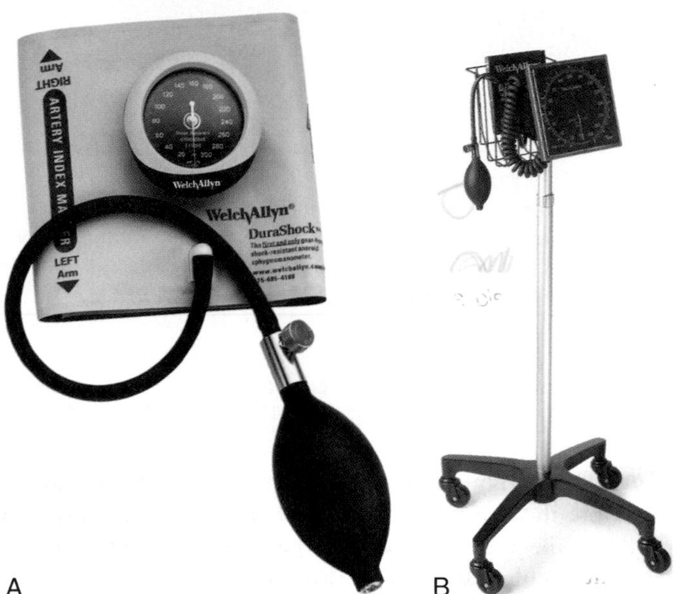


**FIG. 27.5** Types of sphygmomanometers. A, Aneroid (without liquid) dial system. B, Aneroid floor model. *(Courtesy Welch Allyn, Inc., Skaneateles, NY.)*

Systolic and diastolic pressures are measured in millimeters of mercury (mm Hg) above atmospheric pressure. The reading is recorded with the systolic value over the diastolic value. For example, 129/78 ("129 *over* 78") indicates systolic pressure of 129 mm Hg and diastolic pressure of 78 mm Hg. Blood pressure readings for adults are classified according to normal values and stages of hypertension (Table 27.2).

## Blood Pressure Equipment

The equipment used when taking a patient's blood pressure consists of the sphygmomanometer and the stethoscope. The **sphygmomanometer**, which includes the blood pressure cuff and meter, is used to measure blood pressure (Fig. 27.5) and must include specific parts to obtain a correct reading. The *cuff* is a cloth wrap that holds an inflatable rubber bladder (Fig. 27.6). A *rubber bulb* is attached to the cuff with rubber tubing. To get an accurate blood pressure reading, it is important to use the proper size cuff. Using a cuff that is too small or too large can give a false reading. The official guidelines for cuff sizes are as follows:

- Arm circumference 8 to 10 inches: "small adult" cuff
- Arm circumference to 13 inches: "adult" cuff
- Arm circumference to 17 inches: "large adult" cuff
- Arm circumference to 20 inches: "adult thigh" cuff

The **stethoscope** is used to amplify Korotkoff sounds, which are a series of sounds produced by the blood rushing back into the brachial artery, which has been collapsed by the pressure of the blood pressure cuff (**Korotkoff sounds**, named for the man who first described them) (Fig. 27.7). As the pressure in the cuff is slowly released, the stethoscope picks up a distinct thumping sound that grows louder and then softens to a murmur as the flow of blood causes the artery to expand to its former shape. Five phases of Korotkoff sounds occur during deflation of the blood pressure cuff (Table 27.3).

An *automated electronic blood pressure device* is used in many practices today to simplify and speed up the taking of blood pressure (Fig. 27.8). As with the electronic thermometer, batteries operate the electronic blood pressure meter. Weak batteries may lead to an inaccurate reading. Using the electronic blood pressure device is similar to using the sphygmomanometer without the stethoscope.

Wrist blood pressure monitors can be accurate if used exactly as directed. These devices are extremely sensitive to body position. To get an accurate reading when taking a blood pressure with a wrist monitor, the arm and wrist must be at heart level, with the patient quiet and still.

## Blood Pressure Readings

A situation may arise in which it is necessary to take several blood pressure readings to obtain an accurate or average reading. If this occurs, allow the deflated blood pressure cuff to remain on the patient for a minimum of 10 minutes before you obtain another reading. If taken too soon, the reading may be incorrect.

### *Medical Considerations*

The stress and anxiety of a dental procedure could possibly elevate a patient's blood pressure. Review the patient's health history, and discuss the types of medications that he or she is

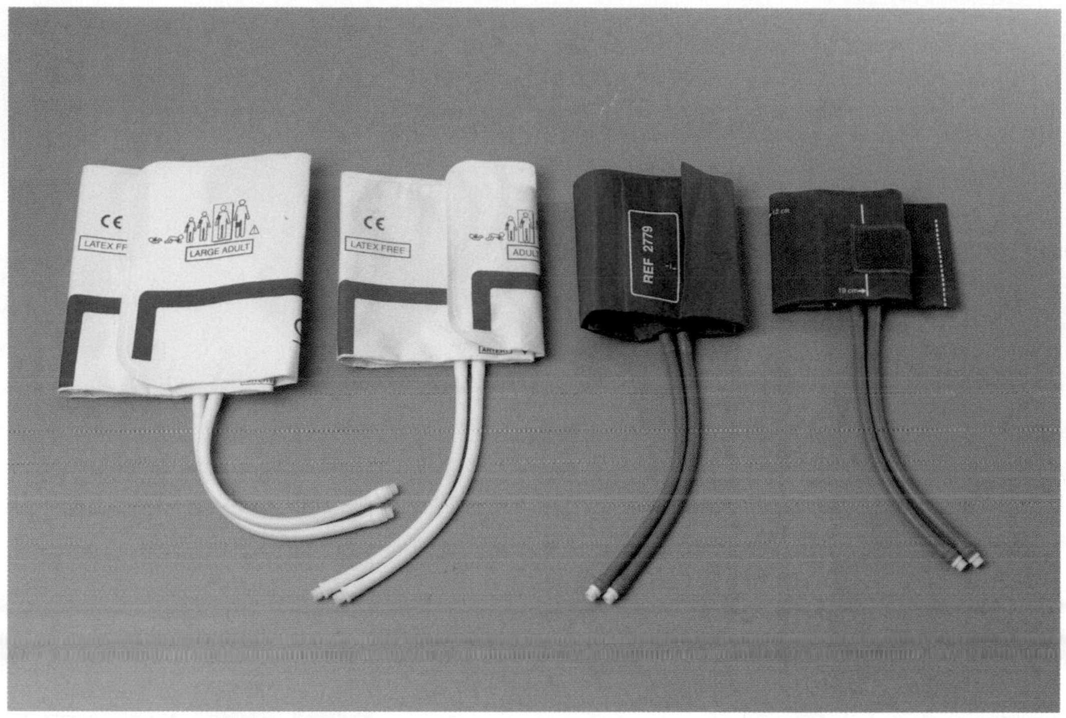


**FIG. 27.6** Sizes of blood pressure cuffs. *(From Dean JA: McDonald and Avery's dentistry for the child and adolescent, ed 10, St Louis, 2015, Mosby.)*

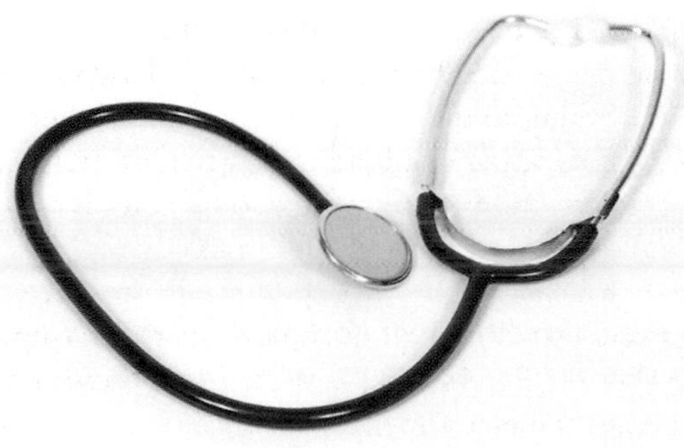

**FIG. 27.7** Stethoscope.

taking. Many drugs have adverse effects that can interfere with dental treatment. A patient who has been diagnosed with hypertension should be under the care of a physician during a treatment regimen. If concern arises about a patient's medical status on the basis of blood pressure readings, the patient may have to reschedule the appointment until after the dentist or the surgeon has had the chance to speak directly to the patient's physician.

See Procedure 27.4: Taking a Patient's Blood Pressure.

RECALL

12 Is the diastolic reading the first or the last sound heard when you are taking a blood pressure?
13 What two instruments are used for taking a patient's blood pressure?
14 Who first described a series of sounds (now named for him) heard during the taking of a blood pressure?
15 What is the range of a normal blood pressure reading for an adult?

## Advanced Monitoring Procedures

Additional patient monitoring techniques have been used successfully for medical procedures and are now being introduced into dental surgical procedures as a standard of monitoring a patient's health status in a noninvasive way.

Monitoring patients during the preoperative, operative, and postoperative phases can occur as an expanded function once the certified dental assistant has completed a board-approved course in these procedures.

### Pulse Oximetry

Pulse **oximetry** is a procedure used for measuring the concentration of oxygen in the blood (Fig. 27.9). This procedure is of particular importance for monitoring oxygenation and pulse rate throughout anesthesia and during the recovery phase.

The pulse oximeter works by passing a beam of red and infrared light through a pulsating capillary bed; it works on the principle that the oxygenated blood is a bright color of red and deoxygenated blood is more blue-purple. The oximeter detects the pulse and then subtracts the intensity of color detected when the pulse is absent. The remaining intensity of color represents only the oxygenated red blood. A fit, healthy person should have an oxygen saturation level between 95% and 99%. See Procedure 27.5: Taking a Patient's Pulse Oximetry (Expanded Function).

### Electrocardiogram

The **electrocardiogram** (ECG; sometimes called EKG) is a procedure that measures the electrical activity of the heartbeat.

**TABLE 27.3 Five Phases of Korotkoff Sounds in Blood Pressure Measurement**

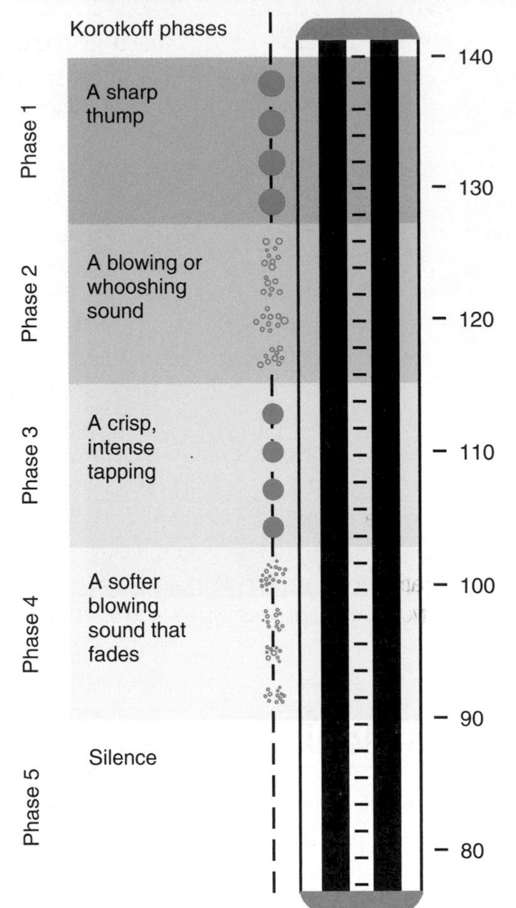


| Phase | Description |
|---|---|
| Phase I | Blood is beginning to flow back into the artery and can be heard as a sharp tapping sound. This is the systolic blood pressure reading. |
| Phase II | The cuff is deflated slowly, with blood flowing. A swishing sound may be heard. This sound is softened and becomes prolonged into a murmur. |
| Phase III | A large amount of blood is flowing into the artery. A distinct, sharp tapping sound returns and continues rhythmically. |
| Phase IV | Blood is flowing easily, and the sound changes to a soft tapping. The sound becomes distinctly muffled and fainter. |
| Phase V | At this point, the artery is fully open, and the sound disappears. This is the diastolic blood pressure reading. |

Figure from Potter PA, Perry AG: Basic nursing, ed 7, St Louis, Mosby, 2011.

In dentistry, the ECG can be used as a preventive measure when a patient is undergoing general anesthesia or intravenous (IV) sedation in a hospital or outpatient setting. The surgeon or dentist will use the ECG to follow the patient's cardiac activity throughout a procedure (see Procedure 27.6: Taking a Patient's ECG [Expanded Function]).

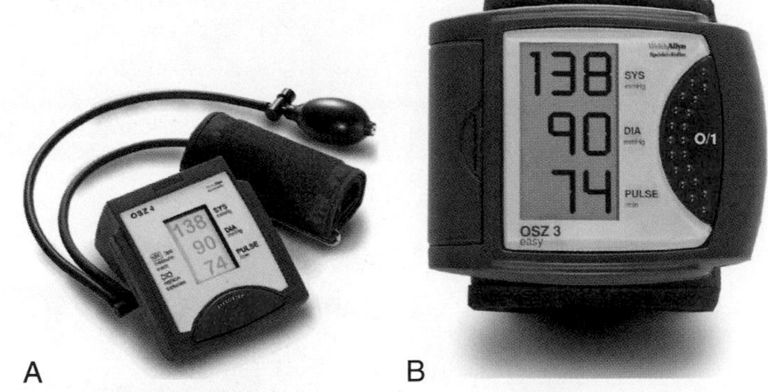


**FIG. 27.8** Automated electronic blood pressure devices. A, Arm-cuff model. B, Wrist-cuff model. *(Courtesy Welch Allyn, Inc., Skaneateles, NY.)*

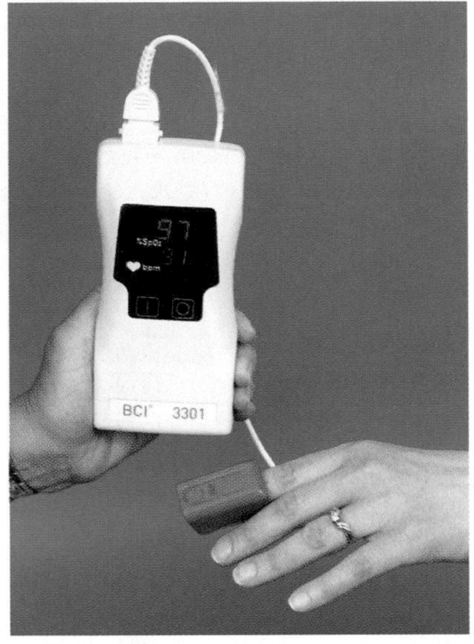


**FIG. 27.9** Pulse oximetry. *(From Kostelnick C: Mosby's textbook for long-term care nursing assistants, ed 7, St Louis, 2015, Mosby.)*

Wires with electrodes are attached to the patient. Most dental surgeons use an electrocardiograph that records six leads. The chest leads are placed on the patient at specific locations (Fig. 27.10). The machine then amplifies the natural electrical currents generated by the electrical impulses of the heart, and the pattern of the heartbeat is traced on graph paper. With each beat, an electrical impulse or wave travels through the heart. The ECG records a series of waves that move above or below a baseline value. Each deflection corresponds to a particular part of the cardiac cycle (Fig. 27.11 and Table 27.4).

- The detection of arrhythmia is the most useful function of the ECG.
- *Sinus arrhythmia* occurs when the rate or rhythm of the heartbeat is altered.
- *Atrial arrhythmia* occurs when the atria contracts before the next cardiac cycle begins. This would be of concern to the surgeon if it is occurring more than 6 times per minute. It is more common to see this with a patient who smokes or consumes a large amount of caffeine.

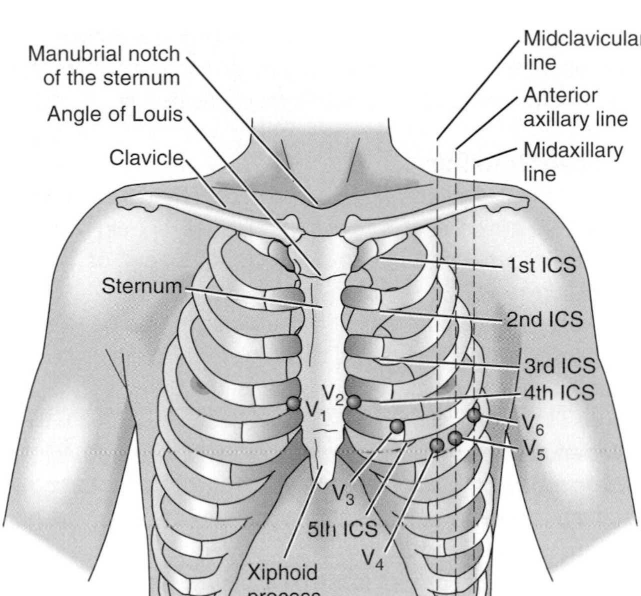


**FIG. 27.10** Chest leads for ECG. *(From Proctor DB et al: Kinn's the medical assistant, ed 13, St Louis, Elsevier, 2017.)*

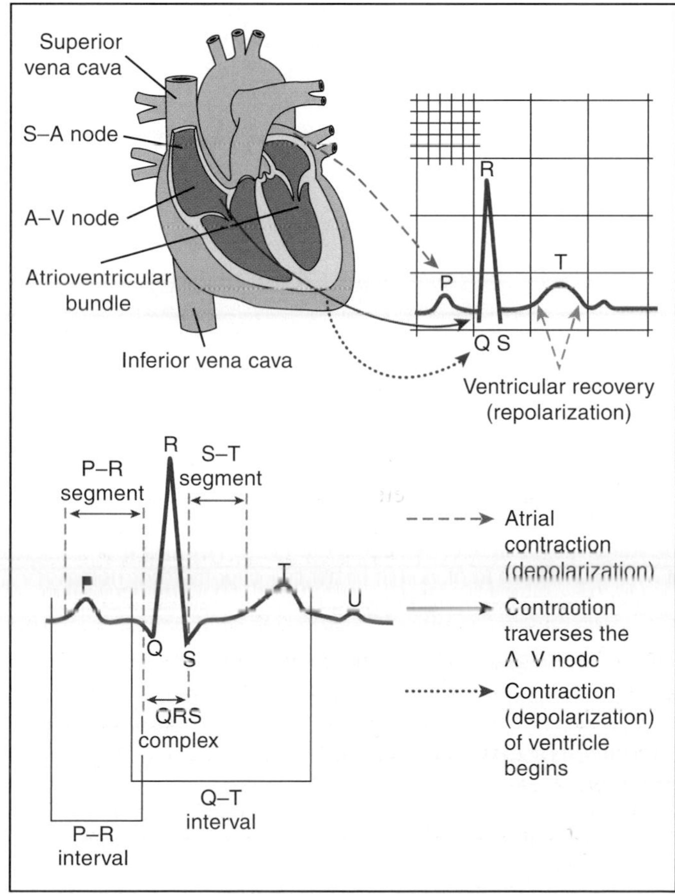


**FIG. 27.11** Recording of ECG.

- *Atrial flutter* is seen when the atria is beating at an extremely rapid rate. An example would be up to 300 beats per minute. This can be reversed with medication to slow the heart.
- *Ventricular arrhythmia,* such as premature ventricular contractions (PVCs), occurs when the ventricles contract before the next cardiac cycle. PVCs are commonly seen when a patient uses tobacco, alcohol, or medications containing epinephrine, and occasionally with anxiety.
- *Ventricular tachycardia,* also referred to as V-tach, occurs when the ventricles are beating at an extremely fast rate. The patient's heart rate will be anywhere from 101 to 250 beats per minute. This can become life threatening if not reversed with drugs or the use of a defibrillator.
- *Ventricular fibrillation,* also referred to as V-fib, is the most critical and life-threatening arrhythmia. This will result in death if not treated. The electrical system of the heart is in total dysfunction. The patient is unresponsive with no pulse and is not breathing. The patient would require a defibrillator to restore normal cardiac function.
- *Asystole* is the result of no heartbeat and a flatline on the ECG.

**TABLE 27.4 The Cardiac Cycle**

| Stage | Heart Activity | Electrical Current |
|---|---|---|
| P wave* | Atrial contraction | Atrial depolarization |
| PR segment† | Contraction traversing the atrioventricular node | Depolarization traversing the atrioventricular node |
| QRS complex‡ | Ventricular contraction | Ventricular depolarization |
| ST segment | Time interval between ventricular contraction and the beginning of ventricular recovery | Time interval between ventricular depolarization and ventricular repolarization |
| T wave | Ventricular contraction subsides | Ventricular repolarization (electrical recovery) |
| U wave (not always present) | Associated with further ventricular relaxation | Associated with further ventricular repolarization |
| Baseline§ | The heart at rest | Polarization |
| PR interval¶ | Time interval between atrial contraction and ventricular contraction | Time interval between atrial depolarization and ventricular depolarization |
| QT interval | Time interval between the beginning of ventricular contraction and the subsiding of ventricular contraction | Time interval between the beginning of ventricular depolarization and ventricular repolarization (electrical recovery) |

From Proctor AB, Adams AP: Kinn's the medical assistant: an applied learning approach, ed 12, St Louis, 2014, Saunders.

*Wave: A uniformly advancing deflection (upward or downward) from a baseline on a recording.

†Segment: A portion of an ECG recording between two consecutive waves. Represents the time needed for an electrical current to move on.

‡Complex: The portion of an ECG tracing that represents the sum of three waves (contraction of the ventricles).

§Baseline: A neutral line against which waves are valued as they deflect upward (positive) or downward (negative) from the line.

¶Interval: The lapse of time between two different electrocardiographic events.

**■ Patient Education** It is estimated that 50 million Americans have high blood pressure, and approximately one fourth of that population are not aware of their medical condition. Unfortunately, many people do not have their blood pressure checked regularly. By taking a patient's blood pressure at every visit, not only are you gathering this vital information for their treatment for that day, but you also may be saving that person's life. ■

**■ Legal and Ethical Implications** As easy as it is to take a patient's vital signs, more than 80 percent of dental offices do not complete this service on a routine basis. The common reason for not taking a blood pressure is "lack of time in the schedule." It is crucial that you are aware of your patient's health before a dental procedure begins. If an emergency were to occur and you did not have a baseline of your patient's health (documented vital sign readings), the dental team would be liable for the type of emergency care provided. ■

**■ Eye to the Future** Radar can catch you if you are speeding, and one day it might save your life if you stop breathing. Engineers from the University of Florida have developed a new system using radar technology to assess a person's vital signs from a few feet away. What it does is emit a radio wave system to detect through the motion of the chest wall a person's heartbeat and respirations. For now, the sensor has a limit of about 6 feet, but one day you might find the system in an ambulance being used to detect life much faster. ■

## ■ Critical Thinking

1. Research "Parkinson's disease" on the Internet. After reading about the clinical description of the disease, explain how it is common for the patient to experience either "low" or "high" blood pressure.
2. Ms. Stewart is a new patient to the practice. You have just reviewed her medical-dental health history. Where in the office would be the best place to take Ms. Stewart's vital signs? In what order would you take them for optimum time efficiency?
3. While reviewing Ms. Stewart's medical history, you notice that she checked "Yes" next to "Hypertension." You take her blood pressure, and the reading is 143/95. Is this considered hypertensive? If so, at what stage is her hypertension?
4. Your next patient would be classified as obese. As you seat him in the dental chair, you do not feel confident about taking his vital signs. What are some of the obstacles that should be considered when taking vital signs on an obese patient?
5. Describe the three types of characteristics you are looking for when taking a patient's pulse. ■

PROCEDURE 27.1

# Taking an Oral Temperature Reading with a Digital Thermometer

### EQUIPMENT AND SUPPLIES

- ✓ Digital thermometer
- ✓ Probe cover
- ✓ Patient record for documenting temperature

### PROCEDURAL STEPS

1. Wash hands and place gloves.
2. Place a new sheath over the probe of the digital thermometer.
3. Turn the thermometer on. When the display indicates "Ready," gently place the tip under the patient's tongue.
4. Tell the patient to close his or her lips over the thermometer and to refrain from talking or removing it from the mouth.
   **PURPOSE** Talking or removing the thermometer can alter the temperature reading.
5. Leave the thermometer in place until the display indicates a final reading and you hear a beeping sound; remove from the patient's mouth.
6. Record the reading in the patient's record.
7. Turn the thermometer off, remove the sheath, and disinfect the thermometer as recommended by the manufacturer.

   Date Temp 99° F Signature

## PROCEDURE 27.2

# Taking a Patient's Pulse

**EQUIPMENT AND SUPPLIES**

- ✔ Watch with second hand
- ✔ Patient record to document findings
- ✔ Black ink pen

**PROCEDURAL STEPS**

1. Seat the patient in an upright position.
2. Extend the patient's arm, resting it on his or her leg or on the armrest of the chair. Have the arm at heart level.
3. Place the tips of your index and middle fingers on the patient's radial artery.
   **NOTE** Indicate in the patient's record whether you are using the right or the left arm.

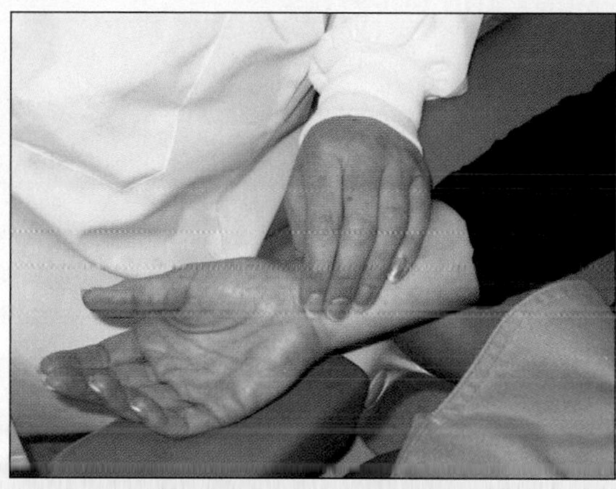

4. Feel for the patient's pulse before you begin to count.
   **PURPOSE** This makes it easier to maintain one position during counting.
5. Count the pulse for 30 seconds; then multiply by 2 to compute the rate for a 1-minute reading.
6. Record the rate, along with any distinct changes in rhythm.

| Date | Pulse rate 77 *(skipping but strong)* | Signature |
|---|---|---|

## PROCEDURE 27.3

# Taking a Patient's Respiration

**EQUIPMENT AND SUPPLIES**

- ✔ Watch with second hand
- ✔ Patient record to document findings

**PROCEDURAL STEPS**

1. With patient seated, maintain the position used while taking the pulse.
   **PURPOSE** The patient should not be aware that you are observing his or her breathing.
2. Count the rise and fall of the patient's chest for 30 seconds; then multiply by 2 to compute the rate for a 1-minute reading.
3. Enter the rate, rhythm, and depth in the patient record.

| Date | Respiration 14 *(slight sighing, depth—moderate)* | Signature |
|---|---|---|

PROCEDURE 27.4 

# Taking a Patient's Blood Pressure

## EQUIPMENT AND SUPPLIES

- ✓ Stethoscope
- ✓ Sphygmomanometer
- ✓ Patient record to document the findings
- ✓ Black ink pen

## PROCEDURAL STEPS

1 Seat the patient with the arm extended at heart level and supported on the chair arm or on a table.
   **PURPOSE** The patient's arm should be at the same level as the heart.

2 If possible, roll up the patient's sleeve.
   **PURPOSE** Tight clothing can interfere with an accurate measurement and reading.

3 If you are taking the patient's blood pressure for the first time and you do not have a previous blood pressure reading to use for reference, you will need to establish a basis from which to determine how high to pump up the cuff. To do this, first palpate the brachial artery to feel for the patient's pulse.

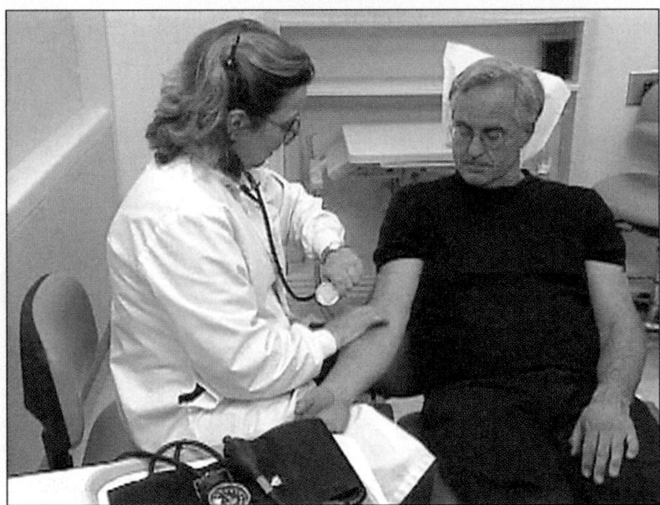

4 Take the patient's brachial pulse for 30 seconds; then double the number for a 1-minute reading. To that number add 40 mm Hg to obtain your inflation level. For example, if the reading was 85, you would add 40, arriving at an inflation level of 125 mm Hg.

5 Expel any air from the cuff by opening the valve and pressing gently on the cuff.

6 Place the blood pressure cuff around the patient's arm approximately 1 inch above the antecubital space, making sure to center the arrow over the brachial artery.
   **PURPOSE** Pressure must be applied directly over the artery for a correct reading.

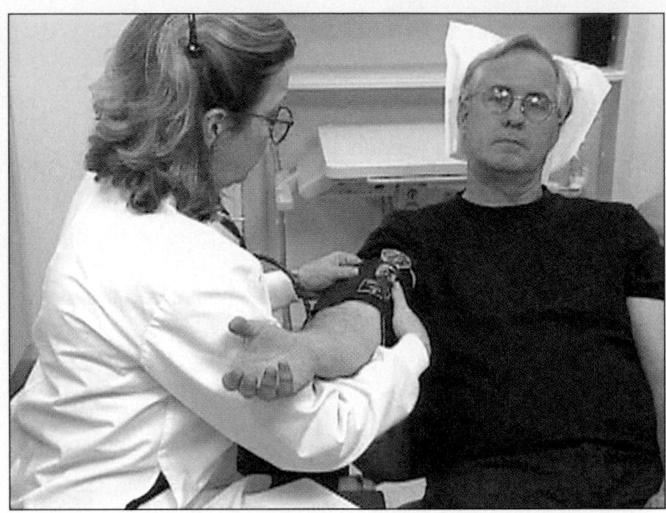

7 Use the Velcro closure to hold it in place to tighten the cuff.
   **NOTE** Make sure that the cuff is tight enough that you can place only a finger between the cuff and the arm.

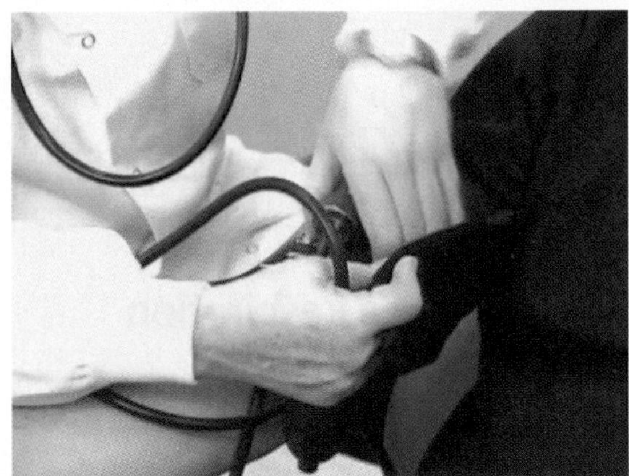

8 Place the earpieces of the stethoscope into your ears so they are facing toward the front.
   **PURPOSE** This position of the earpieces is most comfortable and blocks out distracting noises while you are taking blood pressure.

9 Place the stethoscope disc over the site of the brachial artery, using slight pressure with the fingers.

## PROCEDURE 27.4 Taking a Patient's Blood Pressure—cont'd

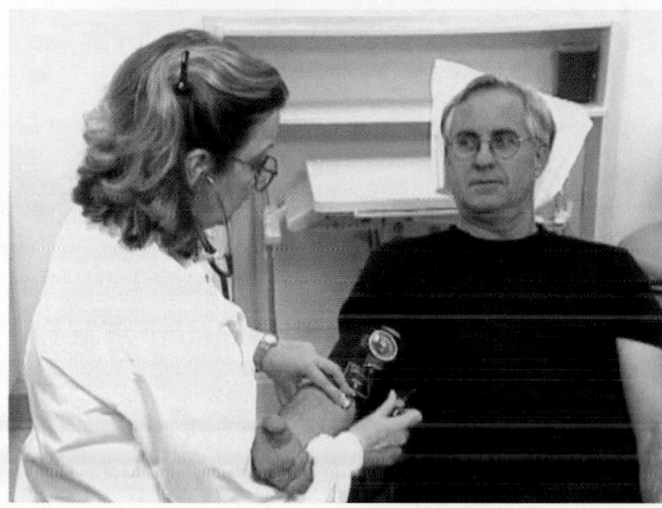

10 Grasp the rubber bulb with the other hand, locking the valve. Inflate the cuff to the noted reading.

**NOTE** You need to inflate the bulb quickly.

11 Slowly release the valve, and listen through the stethoscope.

12 Note the first distinct thumping sound as the cuff deflates. This is the systolic pressure reading.

13 Slowly continue to release the air from the cuff until you hear the last sound. This is the diastolic pressure reading.

14 Record the reading, indicating which arm was used.

15 Disinfect the stethoscope earpieces and diaphragm as recommended by the manufacturer. Return the setup to its proper place.

Date BP 117/68 R Signature/Date

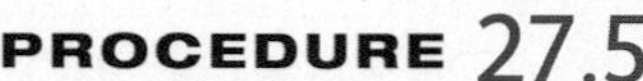

## PROCEDURE 27.5

# Taking a Patient's Pulse Oximetry (Expanded Function)

### EQUIPMENT AND SUPPLIES

- Pulse oximetry machine
- Probe
- Patient record to document the findings
- Black ink pen

### PROCEDURAL STEPS

1 Seat the patient with his or her arm extended on the chair arm.

2 Turn the pulse oximeter machine on, and wait for it to go through its calibration and check tests.

3 Select the probe, with particular attention to correct sizing and to which finger it will be placed on.

**NOTE** The finger should be cleaned, and any nail polish should be removed.

4 Position the probe on the chosen finger, avoiding excess force.

5 Allow several seconds for the pulse oximeter to detect the pulse, and calculate the oxygen saturation.

6 Look for a displayed waveform. Without this, any reading is meaningless.

7 Record the displayed oxygen saturation and pulse rate.

8 If the "Low Oxygen Saturation" alarm sounds, check the patient's airway, and make sure the patient is breathing adequately. Lift the chin or apply other airway maneuvers as appropriate.

9 Ready the oxygen system if necessary. Call for assistance.

10 If the "Pulse Not Detected" alarm sounds, look for the displayed waveform on the pulse oximeter. Feel for a central pulse. If no pulse is felt, call for assistance and start the procedures for basic and advanced life support. If a pulse is felt, try repositioning the probe, or place the probe on a different finger.

11 Do not alter an alarm just to stop it from sounding—it could be telling you something important!

Date Oximetry reading—98 Signature

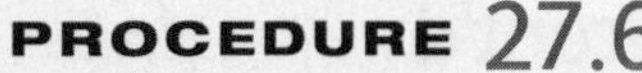

PROCEDURE 27.6

# Taking a Patient's ECG (Expanded Function)

*This procedure is completed only by a certified dental assistant with additional credentials in this technique.*

### EQUIPMENT AND SUPPLIES

- ✓ ECG machine with the patient lead cables
- ✓ 6 disposable, self-adhesive electrodes
- ✓ Patient record to document the readings
- ✓ Black ink pen

### PROCEDURAL STEPS

1. Explain the procedure to your patient.
2. Position the patient in a lying position.
3. Turn on the machine.
4. Label all forms and tracing paper with the patient's name, date, time, and any medication the patient is receiving intravenously or orally.
5. At each location, wipe the patient's chest with an alcohol wipe, and place the electrodes to the six positions on the patient's chest.
6. Connect the lead wires to the correct electrode, making sure the lead wires are not crossed.
7. The surgeon will indicate when to proceed. At that time, press the auto button. The machine will automatically begin the tracing.
8. Continue the tracings until the procedure has been completed.
9. Remove the lead wires and electrodes from the patient's chest.
10. Assist the patient with getting dressed.
11. Shut down the ECG machine; properly disinfect and place in its storage area.
12. Record results of ECG in the patient record.

28

# Oral Diagnosis and Treatment Planning

## KEY TERMS

**Detection** Act or process of discovering tooth imperfections or decay.

**Extraoral** Outside the oral cavity.

**Furcation (fur-KAY-shun)** Area between two or more root branches.

**Intraoral** Within the oral cavity.

**Mobility** To have movement.

**Morphologically (mor-fuh-LOJ-i-kul-lee), morphologic (mor-fuh-LOJ-ik), morphology (mor-FOL-uh-jee)** Branch of biology that deals with form and structure.

**Palpation (pal-PAY-shun)** Touching or feeling for abnormalities within soft tissue.

**Probing** Use of a slender, flexible instrument to explore and measure the periodontal pocket.

**Restoration** The use of a dental material to restore a tooth or teeth to a functional permanent unit.

## LEARNING OUTCOMES

*On completion of this chapter, the student will be able to achieve the following objectives:*

1. Pronounce, define, and spell the key terms.
2. List and describe the examination and diagnostic techniques used for patient assessment, including instrumentation, digital imaging, and digital photography.
3. Discuss documenting the dental examination, including the following:
   - Describe the need for an extraoral examination.
   - Differentiate between an anatomic and a geometric diagram for charting.
   - Identify the three tooth-numbering systems.
   - Explain the color coding of a chart diagram.
   - List the six categories of Black's classification of cavities.
   - Identify the use of charting symbols.
4. Discuss the role of the dental assistant in the clinical examination, including the following:
   - Describe the need for a soft tissue examination.
   - Describe the pocket depth and bleeding index of the gingival tissues and the recording process.
5. Discuss the importance of a treatment plan.

## PERFORMANCE OUTCOMES

*On completion of this chapter, the student will be able to meet competency standards in the following skills:*

- Take intraoral and extraoral photographs of a patient's mouth.
- Chart the periodontal examination correctly, including existing restorations on a required treatment.
- Conduct a soft tissue examination.
- Conduct a periodontal screening.

## ELECTRONIC RESOURCES

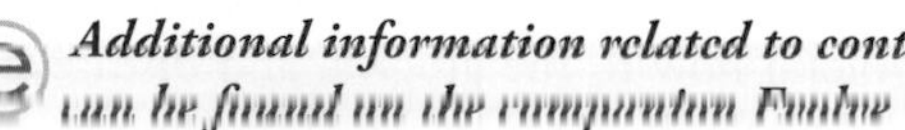

***Additional information related to content in Chapter 28 can be found on the companion Evolve Web site***

- Dentrix Exercise
- Practice Quiz
- Video: Extraoral and Intraoral Photography

Sound dental care begins with a thorough examination of the head, neck, and oral cavity. For the dentist to make an accurate diagnosis, he or she must first review the medical and dental history and discuss all health concerns with the patient; then continue with a thorough **extraoral** and **intraoral** examination; evaluate the radiographic images, photographs, and study models; and finally discuss the plan of treatment.

A patient will seek dental care for the following reasons:

- As a new patient to begin dental care
- As a returning patient, for continued assessment and care
- As an emergency patient when experiencing discomfort, or in pain
- For consultation with a specialist for a specific condition or procedure as a referral

The dental team is involved at every stage of the patient's dental care. Specific areas in which the dental assistant is involved include assisting the patient with completion of patient information forms; taking and recording vital signs;

charting and recording the dentist's findings during the extraoral and intraoral examinations; exposing intraoral and extraoral radiographic images; taking preliminary impressions and preparing the diagnostic models; taking extraoral and intraoral photographs; organizing the patient's dental record; and preparing for the case presentation.

## Examination and Diagnostic Techniques

Today, in the field of dentistry, advanced technology allows the dentist to attain a more accurate conclusion than ever before. The techniques discussed in this chapter are valuable in helping the dentist determine the patient's dental status. Once the required assessments have been completed, the dentist will recommend options in the types of a treatment to the patient.

There are a number of techniques that allow the dental team to acquire the most thorough evaluation depending on the patient's needs.

### Visual Evaluation

The dentist must be able to distinguish between symptoms described by the patient and visual clues. The examination always begins with a visual evaluation of the patient's extraoral and intraoral conditions. This enables the dentist to determine an overall assessment of the type of dental care received previously and reveals any existing conditions that have not been treated. Specific areas to be examined include the face, lymph nodes, temporomandibular joints (TMJs), neck, lips, soft tissue within the mouth, tongue, tooth structure, restorations, and missing teeth.

The *soft tissue*—oral mucosa—should exhibit a uniform color that is described as "coral pink." The evenness of color is more important than the underlying color itself. You may see a variation in this color in individuals from factors such as natural pigmentation, thickness and degree of keratinization of the epithelium, blood flow to the gingiva, and disease and medications.

Other colors such as red, white, or blue can signify inflammation or pathology. If areas of soft tissue appear reddened and not constant in color, this should be noted in the appropriate portion of the clinical examination form and a more extensive evaluation should be completed.

*Tooth structure* should appear **morphologically** sound and intact. The dentist will use a mouth mirror, dental light, and air from the air-water syringe to look for any imperfections in the enamel. Unhealthy tooth structure can appear darkened, discolored, chipped, abraded, or fractured, or may have an abnormal morphologic appearance.

The dentist will evaluate each **restoration** for discrepancies and complete coverage of tooth structure. All missing teeth and abnormalities are noted in the charting section of the clinical examination form.

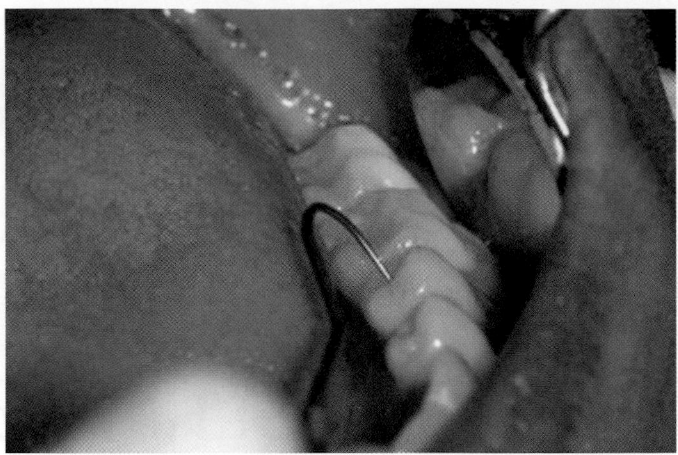

**FIG. 28.1** Detecting decay.

It is essential for the clinical assistant to become competent in knowing the names and numbering systems of the teeth, as well as the type of charting system used during a clinical examination procedure.

### Palpation

**Palpation** is an examination technique in which the examiner uses his or her fingers and hands to feel texture, size, and consistency of the hard and soft tissue (see Chapter 9 for a review of the basic anatomy and physiology of the head and neck). This technique is used extraorally for detecting swelling and is the primary way of detecting swollen lymph glands and nodules that may be in underlying tissue. It can also be used intraorally to determine the health status of the periapical tissues of a tooth.

### Instrumentation

Instrumentation is using a variety of dental instruments to examine the teeth and surrounding tissues. Specialized instruments enable the dentist or the dental hygienist to further evaluate areas that were first examined visually. The standard instrument used to initially examine the teeth is the mouth mirror and explorer, with the periodontal probe used to examine gingival tissues.

The dentist uses the explorer to detect imperfections in all exposed surfaces of the tooth structure (Fig. 28.1). Besides **detection** of carious lesions or disease, the dentist will use the explorer to evaluate existing restorations and all dental work for stability and integrity.

The dentist or dental hygienist will use the periodontal probe to initially assess the gingival sulcus for the presence of periodontal pockets from the loss of gingival attachment or bone (Fig. 28.2). Periodontal **probing** is a technique used to detect periodontal disease.

Percussion is a type of instrumentation used to evaluate the pulpal and periapical tissues of a tooth (see Chapter 54 for further discussion).

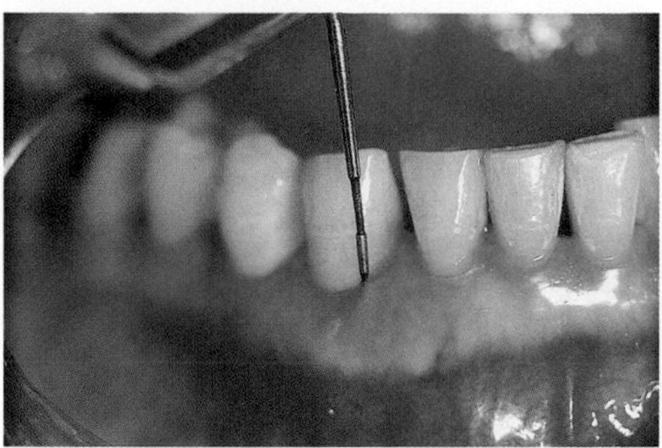

FIG. 28.2 Using a periodontal probe to measure the sulcus. *(From Boyd LRB: Dental instruments: a pocket guide, ed 6, St Louis, 2018, Elsevier.*

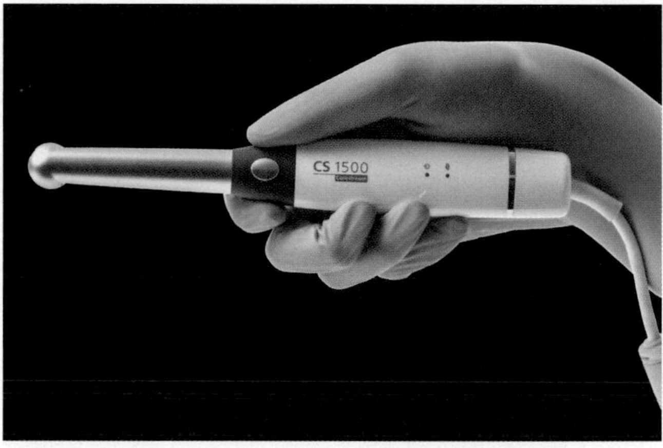


FIG. 28.3 An intraoral imaging system is used to evaluate the condition and educate the patient. *(Courtesy Carestream Health, Inc.)*

## Digital Imaging

Digital imaging in dentistry can be defined as a broad scope of dental technology or devices that incorporates digital or computer-controlled components. Digital imaging has become indispensable for identifying carious lesions, defective restorations, periodontal conditions, pathology, developmental conditions, and other abnormalities. The following list represents some of the areas of digital dentistry.

- Caries diagnosis (see Chapter 13)
- Occlusion and TMJ analysis and diagnosis (see Chapter 42)
- Digital radiography—intraoral and extraoral, including cone beam computed tomography (CBCT) (see Chapters 41 and 42)
- Patient education—similar to a video camera to display an image (Fig. 28.3)
- Shade matching (see Chapter 50)
- CAD/CAM and intraoral imaging—both laboratory and clinician controlled (see Chapter 50)

## Digital Photography

Digital photography is a diagnostic tool used for intraoral and extraoral structures. Photographic images provide the dentist and the patient with a visual means of identifying and understanding a specific problem (Fig. 28.4). For comprehensive treatment such as reconstructive or orthodontic procedures, a patient will have before-and-after photographs taken to illustrate the changed results (see Procedure 28.1: Extraoral and Intraoral Photography [Expanded Function]).

RECALL

1 Identify four reasons why a patient seeks dental care.
2 What diagnostic techniques are used to evaluate a patient's oral conditions?
3 What hand instrument is commonly used by the dentist to detect decay?
4 An intraoral image used for patient education is similar to doing what?

## Documenting the Dental Examination

The documentation of the dental examination is often referred to as "shorthand," which is used to describe the dentist's findings. Charting symbols, abbreviations, and color coding can be used in the recording process to indicate various conditions and existing restorations.

To accurately and quickly chart the information dictated by the dentist, the dental assistant must learn the dentist's preferred system for each of the areas described in this section.

## Tooth Diagrams

Dental charting systems are available in a variety of diagram styles, but anatomic and geometric designs are the most frequently used. In the anatomic diagram, the illustrations resemble the actual crown and root of the tooth (Fig. 28.5). In the geometric diagram, a circle represents each tooth. The circle is divided to represent each tooth surface (Fig. 28.6).

Electronic charting has provided a standardized system whereby all clinical staff members will chart the same way (Fig. 28.7). Charting software has provided new directions for general and specialized dental offices. Software programs can include intraoral and extraoral examination, charting of dental anatomy, current restorations, pathology, and periodontal conditions.

There is a primary dentition diagram that represents 20 primary teeth, and a permanent dentition diagram that represents 32 teeth. When looking at teeth diagrams on the form or electronically, always remember that the teeth are presented from the perspective that you are looking into the patient's mouth. Thus the right side or right quadrants of the mouth are on the left side of the page,

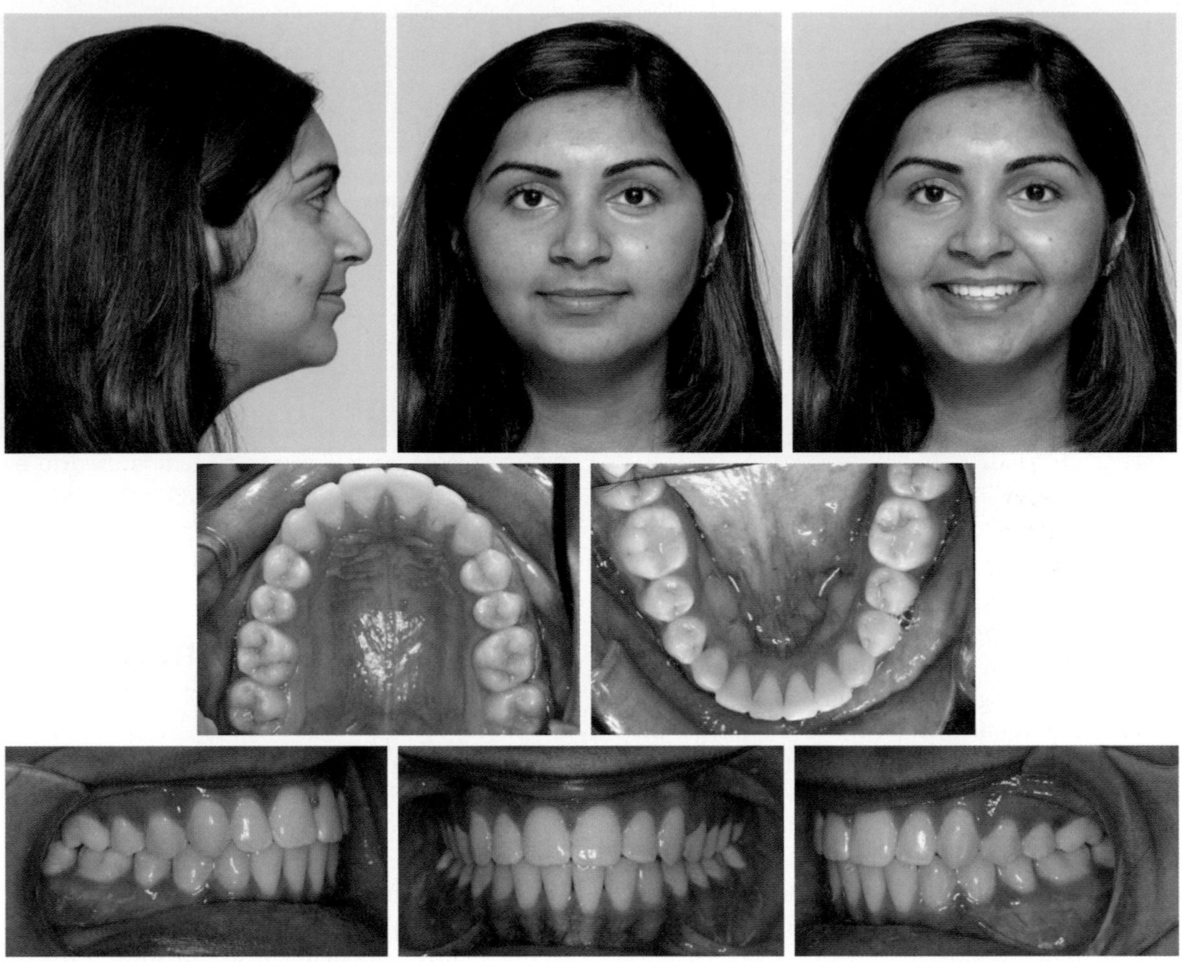

**FIG. 28.4** Photographs are taken to provide a visual evaluation of the patient. *(From Graber LW, Vanarsdall RL, Vig KW: Orthodontics: current principles and techniques, ed 5, Philadelphia, 2012, Mosby.)*

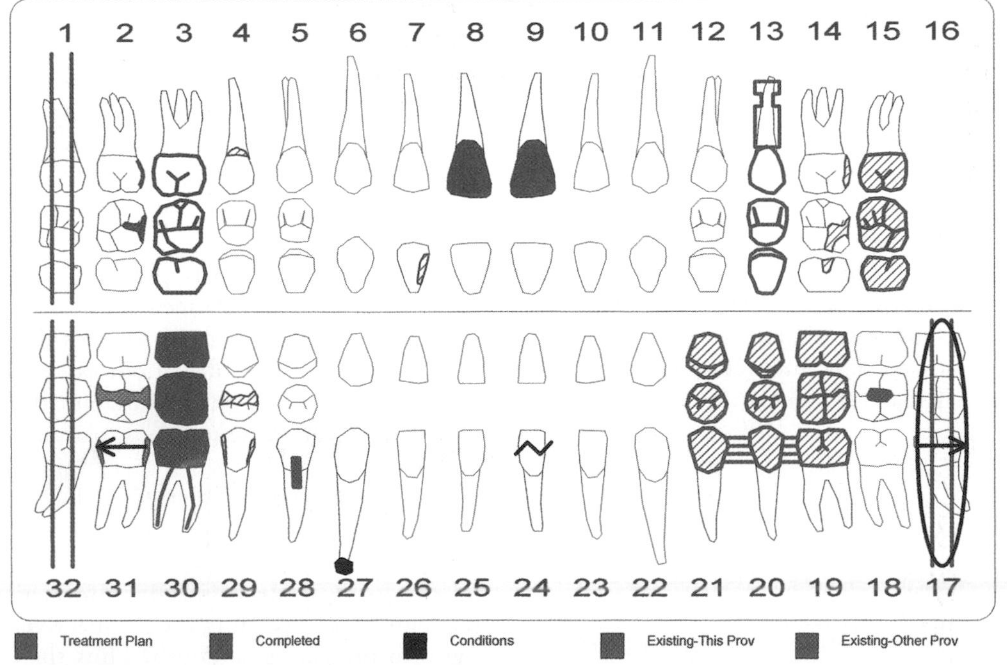


**FIG. 28.5** Example of an anatomic diagram for charting conditions of the mouth. *(From Gaylor LJ: The administrative dental assistant, ed 4, St Louis, 2017, Elsevier.)*

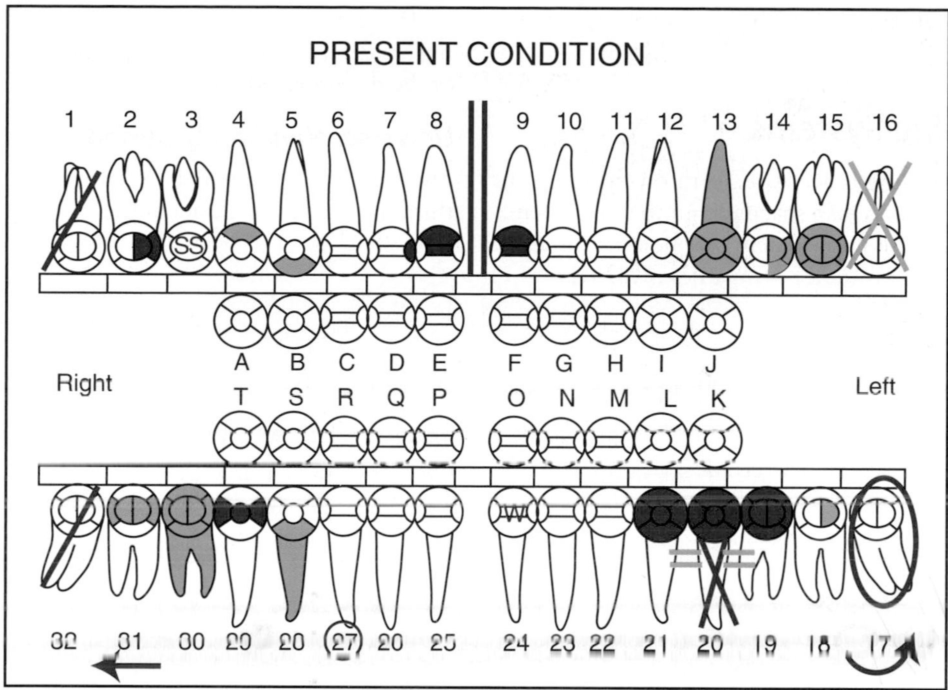


**FIG. 28.6** Example of a geometric diagram for charting conditions of the mouth. *(From Gaylor LJ: The administrative dental assistant, ed 4, St Louis, 2017, Elsevier.)*

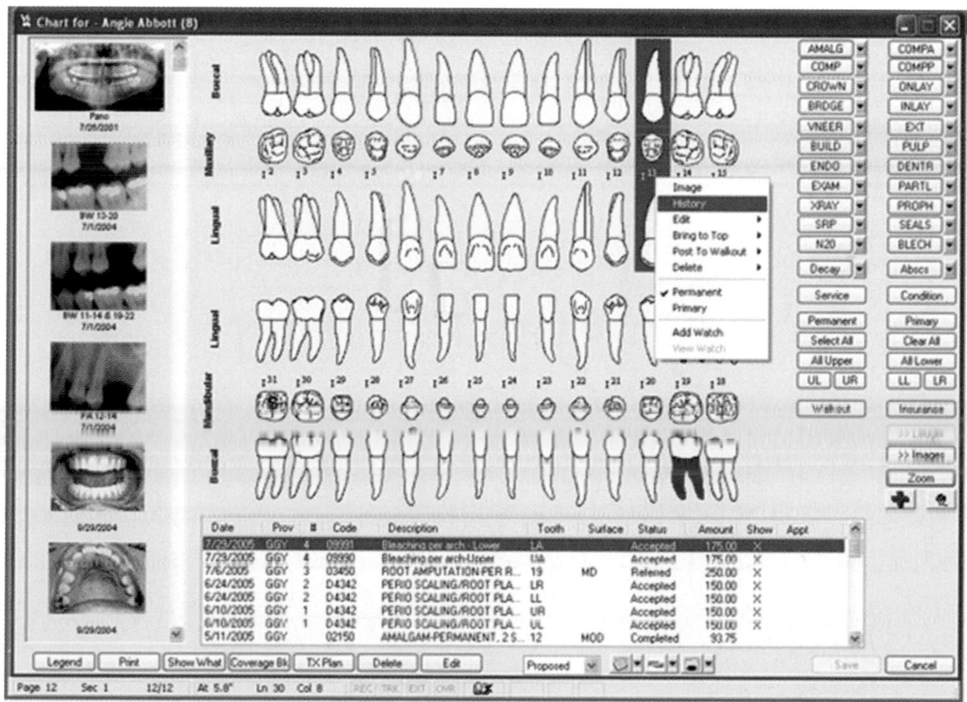


**FIG. 28.7** Electronic charting. *(Courtesy Patterson Dental, St Paul, MN.)*

and the left side or left quadrants are on the right side of the page.

## Tooth-Numbering Systems

To ensure that the recording is accurate, teeth on the diagram are numbered in the sequence of a specified numbering system. The dentist selects the numbering system that best fits the dental practice, as well as the insurance companies involved.

The three most common numbering systems used for charting are described in detail in Chapter 11, but a brief overview of these is provided here.

### *Universal Numbering System*

This numbering system (1–32) begins with the maxillary right third molar and concludes at the mandibular right third molar (Fig. 28.8, *A*).

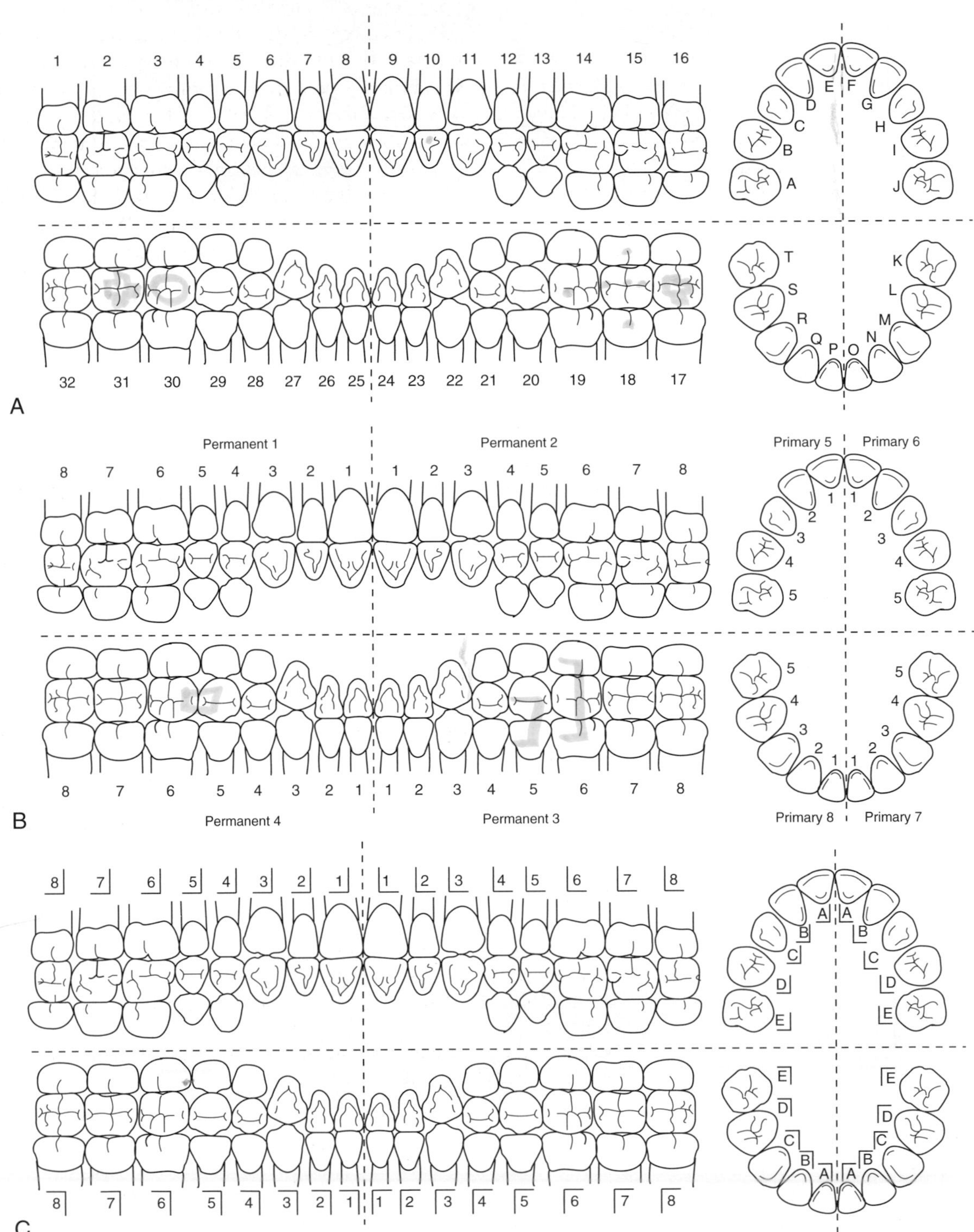


**FIG. 28.8** A, Universal numbering system. B, International Standards Organization System/Fédération Dentaire Internationale numbering system. C, Palmer notation system.

### International Standards Organization System/ Fédération Dentaire Internationale System

This numbering system assigns a two-digit number to each tooth (the first number is the quadrant; the second number is the tooth) (Fig. 28.8, *B*).

### Palmer Notation System

This numbering system uses a bracket to designate the four quadrants of the mouth (Fig. 28.8, *C*).

## Color Coding

Whether you are charting by hand or entering information electronically, color coding is a visual code used to differentiate between treatment that has already been completed and treatment that still needs to be completed.

*Black* or *blue* symbols represent dental work that has been completed. This can indicate dental work completed by another dentist or work completed from previous appointments with the current dentist. *Red* symbols indicate treatment that needs to be completed at future dental appointments. Once this work has been completed, you will update or mark over the red with a blue or black notation to indicate that the work has been completed.

## Black's Classification of Cavities

Before you can master charting methods, you also need to understand the process of how a dentist decides the appropriate type of restoration needed, from one tooth to many teeth. When a dentist detects any deviation from normal, the decision is made to follow through with the best treatment for that area.

Dentists restore teeth according to a method developed by G. V. Black in the early 1900s. This standard classification system is universal to all dentists and is used to describe the location of decay and the best method for restoring a tooth. Black's original classifications included Class I through Class V, with Class VI added at a later date. Table 28.1 provides Black's classifications, the surfaces involved, and a diagram of the cavity classification.

**TABLE 28.1** Black's Classification of Cavities

| Classification | Location and Description |
|---|---|
| Class I 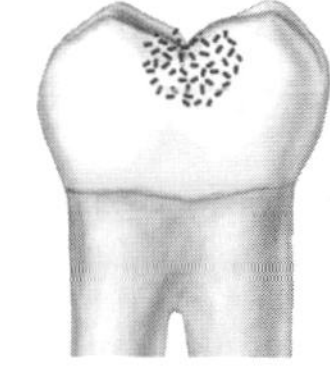 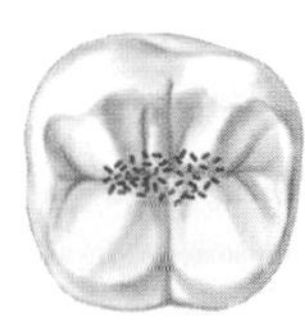 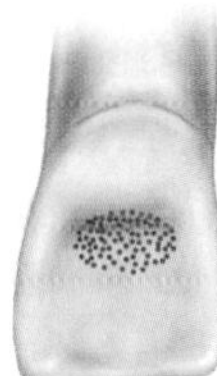 | Decay is diagnosed in the pits and fissures of the occlusal surfaces of molars and premolars, the buccal or lingual pits of molars, and the lingual pits of maxillary incisors.<br>Amalgam or composite resins are the restorative material of choice. Selection will depend primarily on where the lesion is and what type of strength is required from the material. |
| Class II 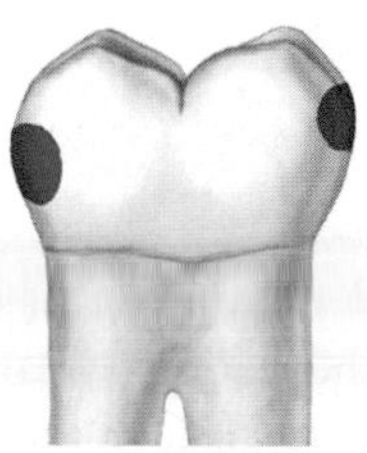 | Decay is diagnosed on the proximal (mesial or distal) surfaces of premolars and molars. Because this surface area is difficult to detect visually, a radiograph is also used to determine the location of decay. The design of the preparation/restoration will include the occlusal surface and involve proximal surfaces.<br>The type of dental material used to restore this classification is silver amalgam (chosen for its strength) or newer composite (tooth colored) resins designed for posterior teeth (chosen for esthetic appeal). If the tooth has extensive decay, the dentist may choose to restore the tooth with a gold or porcelain inlay, onlay, or crown. |
| Class III 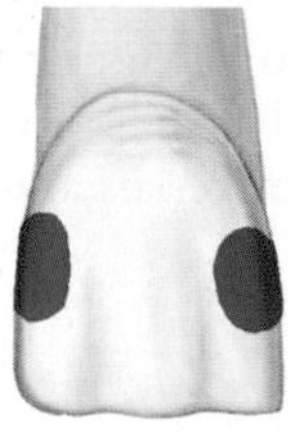 | Decay is diagnosed on the proximal (mesial or distal) surfaces of incisors and canines. This decay is similar to class II, except that it involves the anterior teeth. It is easier for the dentist to access these surfaces with less tooth structure affected.<br>The type of dental material used to restore this classification consists of composite (tooth-colored) resins (for esthetic appearance). |

Continued

**TABLE 28.1** Black's Classification of Cavities—cont'd

| Classification | Location and Description |
|---|---|
| Class IV 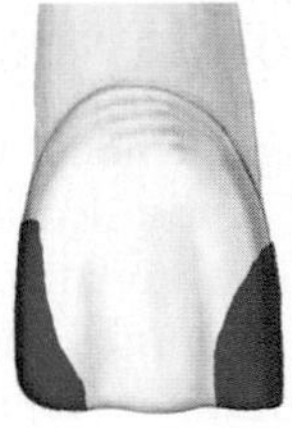 | Decay is diagnosed in the proximal (mesial or distal) surfaces of incisors and canines. The difference between class IV and class III decay is that class IV involves the incisal edge or angle of the tooth.<br>The type of dental material used to restore this classification is composite (tooth-colored) resins (for esthetic appearance). If the tooth has extensive decay, the dentist may choose to restore the tooth with a porcelain crown. |
| Class V 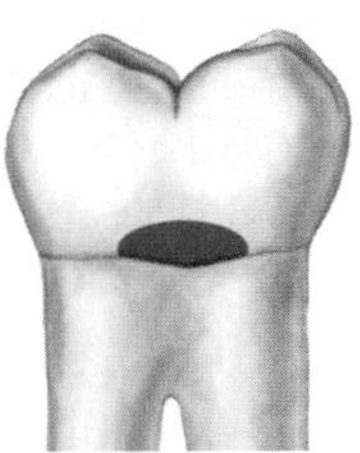 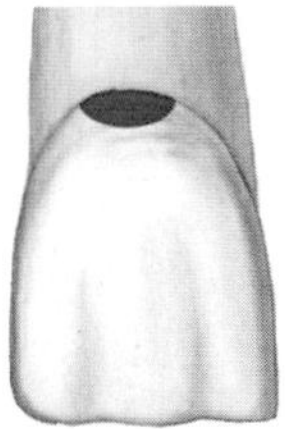 | Decay is diagnosed in the gingival third of the facial or lingual surface of any tooth. This is also referred to as smooth-surface decay.<br>The type of dental material used to restore this classification depends on which teeth are affected. If decay occurs in posterior teeth, the dentist may choose silver amalgam; if anterior teeth are involved, composite (tooth-colored) resin will most likely be used. |
| Class VI 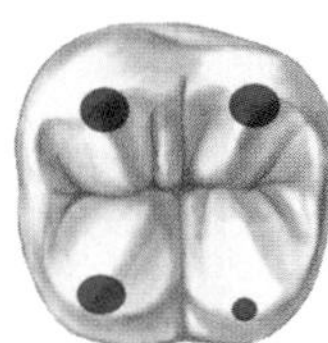 | Decay is diagnosed on the incisal edges of the anterior teeth and the cusp tips of the posterior teeth. Class VI decay is caused by abrasion (wear) and defects.<br>The dental material chosen is composite (tooth-colored) resins (for esthetic appearance). |

## Abbreviations

Because of limited space in the progress notes or chart, it is best to abbreviate certain terms. Abbreviations are used to indicate a single surface or a combination of tooth surfaces.

For single-surface restorations, charting abbreviations are based on the names of the tooth surfaces as follows: buccal—B, distal—D, facial—F, incisal—I, lingual—L, mesial—M, and occlusal—O.

In multiple-surface restorations, two or more surfaces are involved. The combined surfaces become one name on which the abbreviation is based. The rule for combining two surfaces is to substitute the letter "*o*" for the *-al* ending of the first surface. For example, for distal and occlusal, the combined surfaces are referred to as disto-occlusal, or DO. If three surfaces are combined, the same rule applies, for example, mesio-occluso-distal, or MOD. When these combined surfaces are discussed, the letters of the abbreviations are pronounced separately, such as a "dee-oh" (D-O) or an "em-oh-dee" (M-O-D) restoration.

## Charting

Now that you have become familiar with the clinical examination form, Black's classification of cavities, the anatomic diagram, the numbering system, color coding, and abbreviations, the next step is to learn the actual charting symbols that correlate with the dental work that has been completed or is to be provided.

### *Symbols*

Charting symbols are placed on the tooth diagram of the dental record to represent the various treatments and the types of dental material used to restore the tooth or teeth. Charting symbols are used in many styles and ways, and each dentist will have individual preferences. It is important for you to learn the charting symbols for either a paper form or electronic form for treatment to be completed, as well as for treatment already provided. Table 28.2 provides a review of the more common restorative materials and symbols used in charting.

5 Do you chart missing teeth? If so, how?
6 What class(es) in Black's classification involves the premolars and molars?
7 What class(es) in Black's classification involves incisors?
8 How would you chart an MOD amalgam on tooth #4?

**TABLE 28.2 Commonly Used Charting Symbols**

| Conditions | Explanation | Charting Symbol | Procedure |
|---|---|---|---|
| Missing Tooth | Tooth or teeth that are not present or congenitally missing | 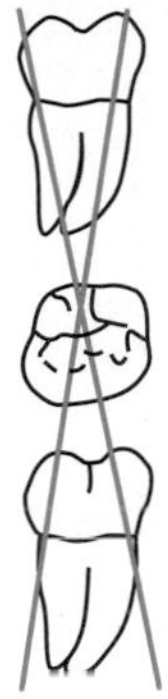 | Draw a black/blue "X" through the tooth. It does not matter whether the tooth was extracted, or is congenitally missing. If a quadrant, or arch, is edentulous, make one "X" over all teeth missing. |
| Impacted or Unerupted Tooth | Tooth or teeth that have not erupted and are not exposed in the mouth | 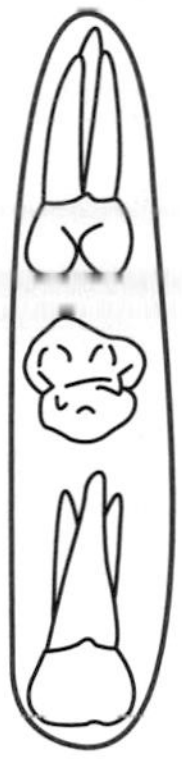 | Draw a red circle around the whole tooth, including the root. |
| Tooth to Be Extracted | Tooth that has been diagnosed to be removed. | 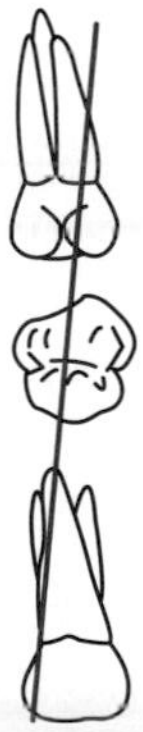 | Draw a red diagonal line through the tooth. An alternative method is to draw two red parallel lines through the tooth. |
| Caries/Restor Class I | Decay affecting the pits and fissure of the occlusal surface | 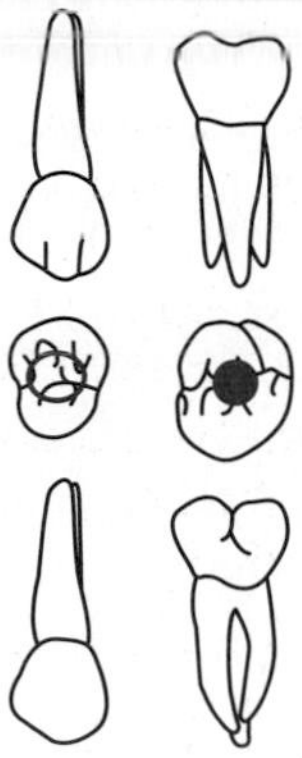 | Outline the area involved if using composite and, if using amalgam, color in the area to complete in red and black/blue for the area already restored. |

*Continued*

**TABLE 28.2 Commonly Used Charting Symbols—cont'd**

| Conditions | Explanation | Charting Symbol | Procedure |
|---|---|---|---|
| **Caries/Restore Class II** | Decay affecting the occlusal and interproximal surfaces of posterior teeth | 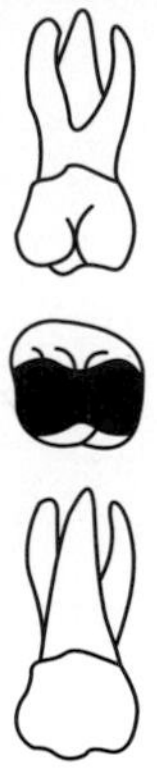 | Outline the area involved if using composite and, if using amalgam, color in the area in red to complete and black/blue for the area already restored. |
| **Caries/Restore Class III** | Decay affecting the occlusal and interproximal surfaces of anterior teeth | 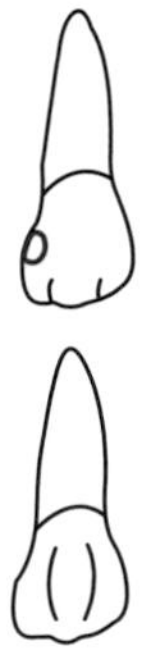 | Outline the area to indicate composite in red to complete and black/blue for the area already restored. |
| **Caries/Restore Class IV** | Decay affecting the interproximal and incisal surface of an anterior tooth | 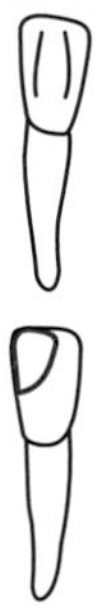 | Outline the area to indicate composite in red to complete and black/blue for the area already restored. |
| **Caries/Restore Class V** | Decay affecting the gingival third of a tooth | 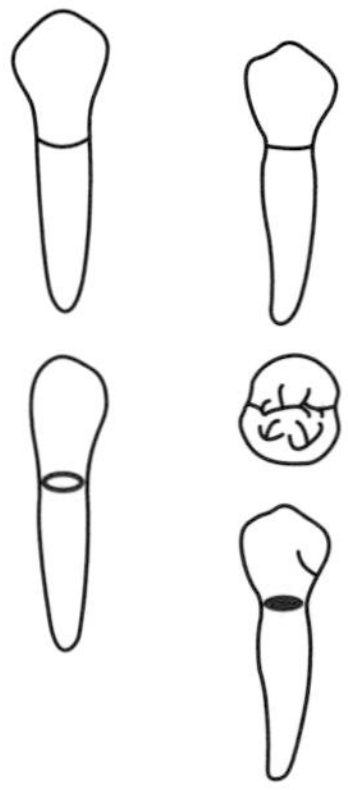 | Outline the area involved if using composite and, if using amalgam, color in the area in red to complete and black/blue for the area already restored. |

**TABLE 28.2 Commonly Used Charting Symbols—cont'd**

| Conditions | Explanation | Charting Symbol | Procedure |
|---|---|---|---|
| Recurrent Decay | Decay is diagnosed from radiograph or from the margin of an existing restoration | 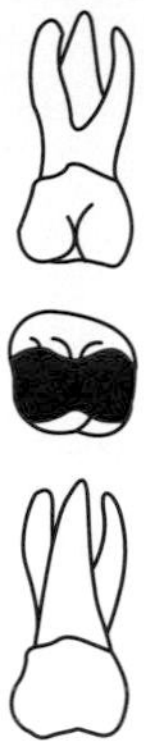 | Outline the existing restoration in red to indicate decay in the area. |
| Sealant | Resin material placed in the pits and fissures of occlusal surface as a preventive means | 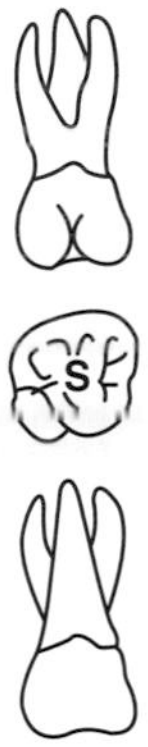 S | Place an "S" on the occlusal surface in red to complete and black/blue for already restored. |
| Periapical Abscess | Infection is within the pulp of a tooth | 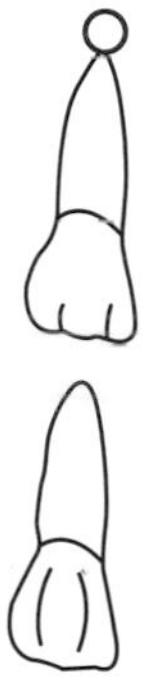 | Draw a red circle at the apex of the root to indicate infection. |
| Root Canal | Disease has affected the pulp of the tooth and requires pulp therapy | 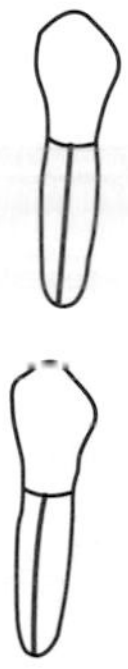 | Draw a line through the center of each root involved in red to be completed and black/blue for already restored. |
| Veneer | Thin shell-like covering made from porcelain or composite to cover the facial aspect of a tooth surface | 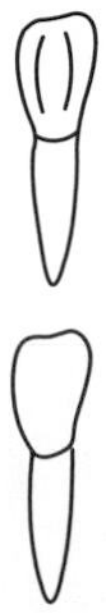 | Outline the facial portion only in red to be completed and black/blue for already restored. |

*Continued*

TABLE 28.2 Commonly Used Charting Symbols—cont'd

| Conditions | Explanation | Charting Symbol | Procedure |
|---|---|---|---|
| Inlay | Cast restoration made from either porcelain or gold for a conservative Class II restoration | 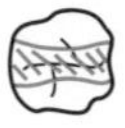 | Outline the shape of the restoration in red or black/blue if using porcelain and place diagonal lines if using gold. |
| Onlay | Cast restoration made from either porcelain or gold for more coverage of the occlusal surface | 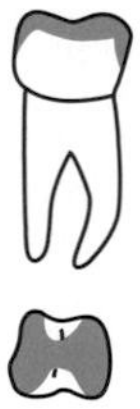 | Outline the shape of the restoration in red or black/blue if using porcelain and place diagonal lines if using gold. |
| Porcelain Fused to Metal (PFM) Crown | Full crown of a single tooth using two types of materials, porcelain for esthetics and metal for strength | 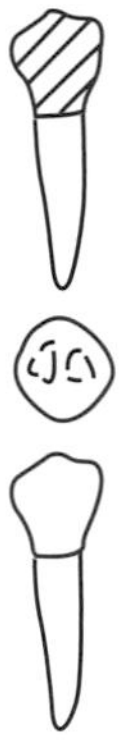 | Outline the coronal portion of the tooth and add diagonal lines to indicate gold on the facial surface, in red to be completed, and black/blue for already restored. |
| Gold Crown | Full crown of a single tooth using gold | 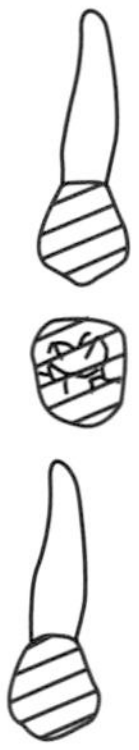 | Outline the crown of the tooth and place diagonal lines in red to be completed and black/blue for already restored. |
| Stainless Steel Crown | Full metal crown used for primary molars | 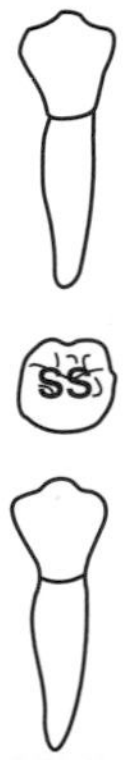 SS | Outline the crown of the tooth and place "SS" on the occlusal surface in red to be completed and black/blue for already restored. |

**TABLE 28.2** Commonly Used Charting Symbols—cont'd

| Conditions | Explanation | Charting Symbol | Procedure |
|---|---|---|---|
| **Post and Pore** | Used for additional strength in an endodontically treated tooth | 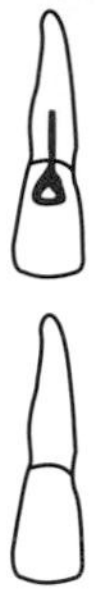 | Draw a line through the root requiring the post; then continue the line into the gingival one third of the crown, making a triangle shape in red to be completed and black/blue for already restored. |
| **Fixed Bridge** | Cast unit to restore an area where one or more teeth are missing | 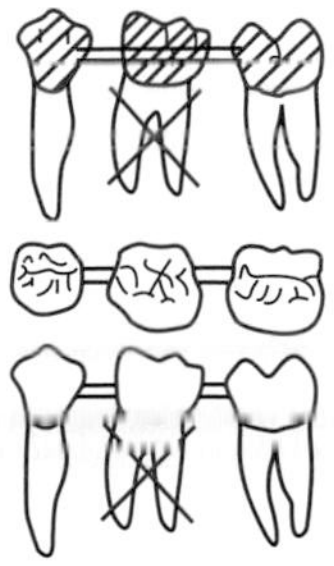 | Draw an "X" through the root(s) of the missing tooth or teeth involved. Then draw a line to connect all teeth that make up the bridge. The type of material used to make the bridge will determine whether you outline the crowns for porcelain, use diagonal lines for gold, or use a combination of the two in red to be completed and black/blue for already restored. |
| **Implant** | Complete replacement of a tooth and root | 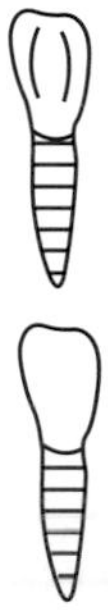 | Draw horizontal lines through the root or roots of a tooth in red to be completed and black/blue for already placed. |
| **Rotated Tooth** | Tooth that has rotated from its normal position | 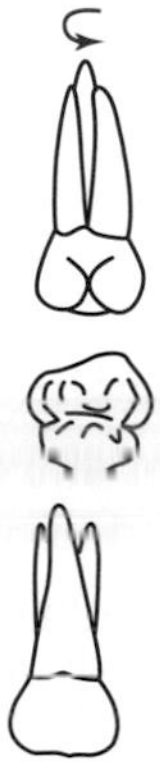 | Indicate the direction the tooth has turned by placing a red arrow above the tooth. |
| **Drifting** | Tooth or teeth that have shifted from their normal position | 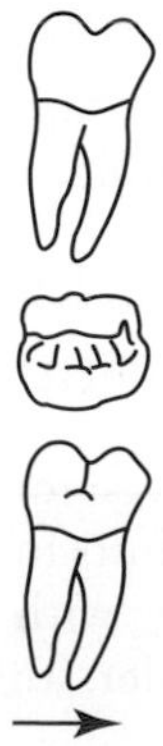 | Place a red arrow that points to the direction in which a tooth is drifting. |

Continued

**TABLE 28.2 Commonly Used Charting Symbols—cont'd**

| Conditions | Explanation | Charting Symbol | Procedure |
|---|---|---|---|
| Diastema | Additional space existing between two teeth with no contact | | Draw two red vertical lines between the teeth. |
| Fractured Tooth or Root | Surface of a tooth that has fractured due to trauma or extensive caries | | If a tooth or a root is fractured, draw a red zigzag line where the fracture occurred. |
| Denture | Removable prosthetic to replace a full arch | CLD<br>PUD PUD | Draw a complete line below the roots of the teeth connecting the teeth in red if denture is to be fabricated, or in blue/black if already fabricated. |

# Clinical Examination of the Patient

As the clinical assistant, you will follow a routine protocol for this procedure. The patient is seated in the dental treatment area, draped with a patient "napkin," and positioned for the dentist to begin the examination.

## Soft Tissue Examination

The soft tissue examination involves a complete examination of the face, neck, TMJ, cheeks, mucosa, lips, lingual and facial alveolar bone, palate, tonsil area, tongue, and floor of the mouth. This examination requires the use of visual assessment and palpation. The purpose of this part of the examination is to detect any abnormalities in the head and neck area of a patient.

See Procedure 28.2: The Soft Tissue Examination (Expanded Function).

## Examination and Charting of the Teeth

A clinical examination of the teeth includes a thorough assessment of each tooth. Using a mirror and explorer, the dentist examines each surface of each tooth and dictates findings to the dental assistant, who records these findings on the clinical examination form of the patient's record. Regardless of whether findings are recorded manually or electronically, it is essential that all entries are recorded correctly and accurately.

See Procedure 28.3: Charting of Teeth for complete details of the charting procedure.

## Examination and Charting of the Periodontium

The Centers for Disease Control and Prevention reports 47% of adults in the United States have a form of periodontal disease, with the rate increasing to 70% for those age 65 and older. This portion of the examination is completed to assess the tissues that support the teeth, which includes the gingiva, cementum, periodontal ligament, and alveolar and supporting bone structures. The alveolar and supporting bone structures cannot be visually evaluated, so updated periapical radiographic images are required for this examination process.

Periodontal findings to be recorded are as follows:

- Overall health of the gingiva
- Signs and location of inflammation
- Location and amount of plaque and calculus
- Areas of unattached gingiva
- Areas of periodontal pockets measuring greater than 3 mm
- Presence of furcation involvement
- **Mobility**

This component of the clinical examination can be completed by either the dentist or dental hygienist. The operator will use the mouth mirror, periodontal probe, and additional supplies. Under gentle pressure, the periodontal probe is inserted into the gingival sulcus until resistance is met. The probe is inserted into six specific sites for each tooth (mesiofacial, facial, distofacial, mesiolingual, lingual, and distolingual). The depth of insertion is read by noting the position of the markings on the probe while in the sulcus (Boxes 28.1 through 28.3; see Chapter 55 for further discussion of the periodontal examination).

**Periodontal screening and recording (PSR)** is a type of periodontal examination that records an overall score or rating for each sextant within the mouth. The PSR is a rapid method of screening patients to decide if a more comprehensive assessment is necessary. A PSR chart can be completed on a routine basis even when a complete periodontal examination is not required (Fig. 28.9).

See Procedure 28.4: Periodontal Screening: Examination of the Gingival Tissues for details related to charting of the periodontium.

**BOX 28.1 Description of Probing Scores**

0: The colored area of the probe remains completely visible in the deepest sulcus in the sextant; no calculus or defective margins are detected.
1: The colored area of the probe remains completely visible during the deepest probing in the sextant; no calculus or defective margins are detected; bleeding occurs after gentle probing.
2: The colored area of the probe remains completely visible during the deepest probing in the sextant; supragingival or subgingival calculus and defective margins are detected.
3: The colored area of the probe remains partially visible at the deepest probing depth in the sextant.
4: The colored area of the probe completely disappears, indicating probing depth greater than 5.5 mm.

Note additional items on the examination form, including sensitivity, calculus, saliva changes, and **furcation** involvement.

RECALL

9 Which members of the dental team can perform the periodontal examination for a patient?
10 If a tooth has movement in any direction, the dentist will have you record what?

## The Treatment Plan

After gathering sufficient information and reviewing everything carefully, the dentist will come to a conclusion as to the patient's dental conditions. On the basis of this diagnosis, the dentist may prepare one or more treatment plans for presentation to the patient.

A written treatment plan states that the dentist has made a thorough study of the patient's condition and is prepared to offer options to help the patient manage dental treatment according to the patient's needs, priorities, and financial resources.

## Types of Treatment Plans

Each treatment plan includes a description of the proposed treatment and an estimate of the fee involved. Many dentists prepare optional treatment plans for the patient's consideration. These plans may represent the following levels of care.

### *Level I: Emergency Care*

The emergency care plan relieves immediate discomfort and provides relief to the patient.

**BOX 28.2 Classification of Furcations**

**Class I Furcation**

Beginning involvement. Furcation can be detected with an explorer or probe, but it cannot be entered. Cannot be detected radiographically.

**Class II Furcation**

Can enter furcation from one aspect with a probe or explorer but is not able to penetrate through to the other side.

**Class III Furcation**

Furcation covered by soft tissue, but has complete involvement from both sides.

**Class IV Furcation**

Furcation not covered by soft tissue and complete involvement from both sides.

**BOX 28.3 Classification of Dental Mobility**

**Class I mobility**: Tooth can be moved up to 1 mm in any direction.
**Class II mobility**: Tooth can be moved greater than 1 mm in any direction but is not depressible into the socket.
Class III mobility: Tooth can be moved in a buccolingual direction and is depressible in socket.

### *Level II: Standard Care*

The standard care plan restores the dentition to normal function. As needed, this includes restoring teeth with composite or amalgam restorations, saving teeth with endodontic treatment, conservatively treating periodontal problems, and replacing missing teeth with either fixed or removable prostheses.

### *Level III: Optimum Care*

The optimum care plan restores the dentition to maximum function and an esthetically pleasing result. When applicable, this includes restoring teeth with cast restorations (crowns, inlays, or onlays); treating periodontal, orthodontic, or endodontic problems; and replacing missing teeth with fixed and removable prosthodontic prostheses or dental implants.

## Treatment Plan Presentation

On completion of a thorough clinical examination, an appointment will be scheduled to present the treatment plan to the patient. Typically, a 30-minute to 1-hour appointment without interruptions is scheduled for the patient.

Rather than seating the patient in a treatment room, the dentist traditionally chooses to conduct the case presentation in a private office setting. It is important to have available the diagnostic tools used to present the case. The dentist should have readied the patient chart, radiographs, diagnostic casts, and treatment plans. Other visual aids might include the following:

- Before-and-after photographs
- Diagnostic casts of similar cases
- Models of proposed appliances, such as full or partial dentures, dental implants, or fixed crowns and bridges
- Anatomic models to demonstrate conditions

The patient is made comfortable, and the dentist takes care to present all information in terms that the patient can understand. The dentist then explains findings regarding the patient's diagnosis and prognosis.

After the presentation has been made, the dentist or finance manager will present the fee estimate for each treatment option. The patient is encouraged to ask questions and to discuss the advantages and disadvantages of each plan. When the patient makes a decision and accepts a treatment plan, he or she is giving informed consent for treatment (Fig. 28.10). At this time, the finance manager will explain the payment plans and will make the necessary financial arrangements with the patient (Fig. 28.11). When all these arrangements have been completed, the patient is scheduled for treatment.

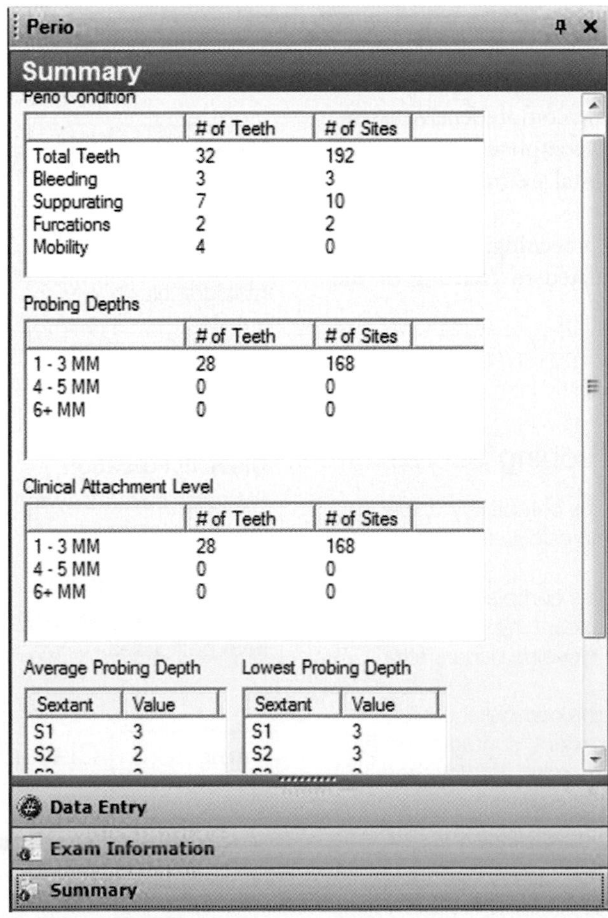


**FIG. 28.9** Charting diagram of the PSR. *(Courtesy Henry Schein Practice Solutions, American Fork, UT.)*

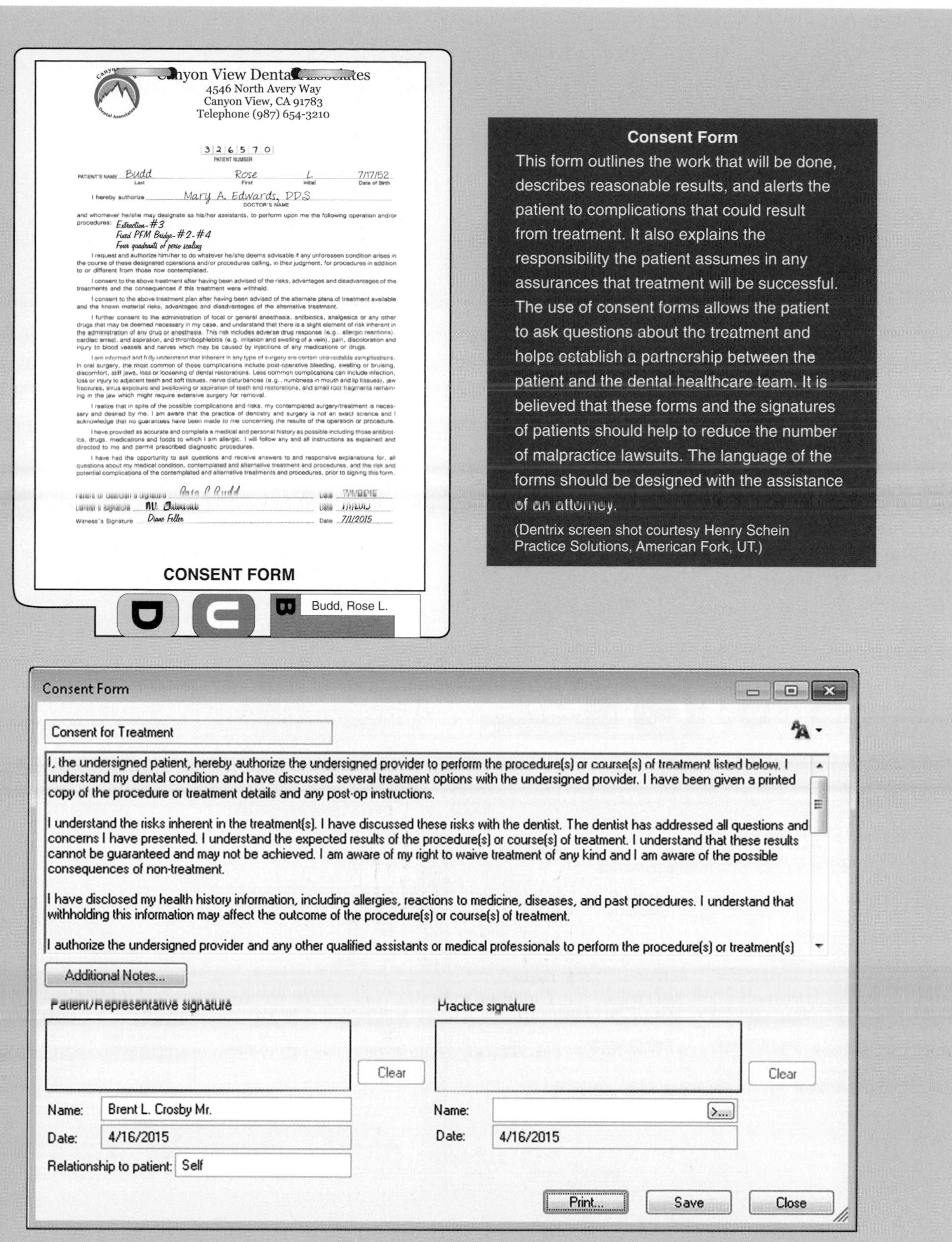


**FIG. 28.10** Treatment plan form presented following treatment plan presentation. *(From Gaylor LJ: The administrative dental assistant, ed 4, St Louis, 2017, Elsevier; Dentrix screenshot courtesy Henry Schein Practice Solutions, American Fork, UT.)*

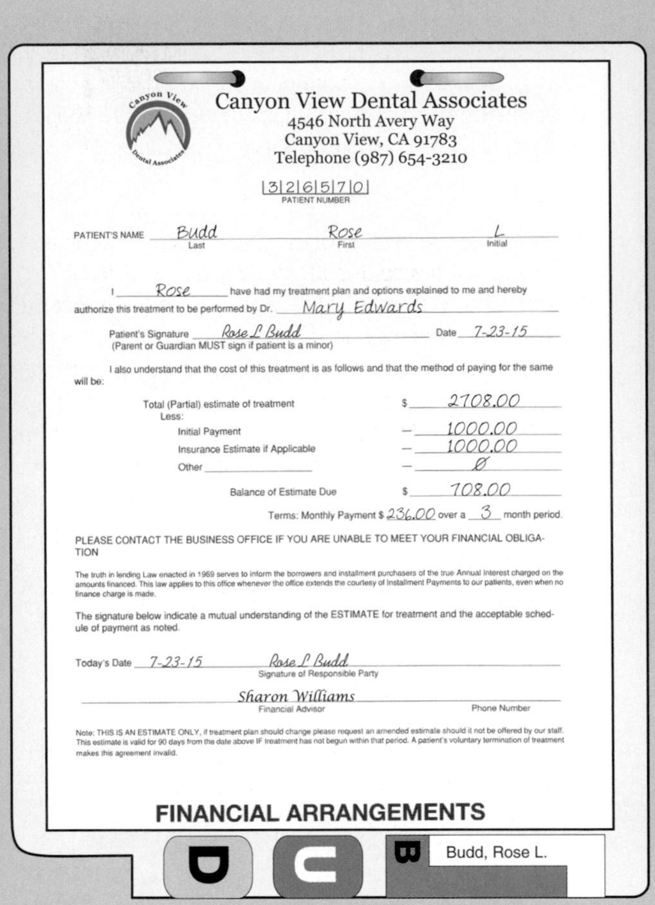

Canyon View Dental Associates
4546 North Avery Way
Canyon View, CA 91783
Telephone (987) 654-3210

3 2 6 5 7 0
PATIENT NUMBER

PATIENT'S NAME Budd (Last) Rose (First) L (Initial)

I Rose have had my treatment plan and options explained to me and hereby authorize this treatment to be performed by Dr. Mary Edwards

Patient's Signature Rose L Budd Date 7-23-15
(Parent or Guardian MUST sign if patient is a minor)

I also understand that the cost of this treatment is as follows and that the method of paying for the same will be:

| | |
|---|---|
| Total (Partial) estimate of treatment | $ 2708.00 |
| Less: | |
| Initial Payment | — 1000.00 |
| Insurance Estimate if Applicable | — 1000.00 |
| Other | — Ø |
| Balance of Estimate Due | $ 708.00 |

Terms: Monthly Payment $ 236.00 over a 3 month period.

PLEASE CONTACT THE BUSINESS OFFICE IF YOU ARE UNABLE TO MEET YOUR FINANCIAL OBLIGATION

The truth in lending Law enacted in 1969 serves to inform the borrowers and installment purchasers of the true Annual Interest charged on the amounts financed. This law applies to this office whenever the office extends the courtesy of Installment Payments to our patients, even when no finance charge is made.

The signature below indicate a mutual understanding of the ESTIMATE for treatment and the acceptable schedule of payment as noted.

Today's Date 7-23-15 Rose L Budd
Signature of Responsible Party

Sharon Williams
Financial Advisor Phone Number

Note: THIS IS AN ESTIMATE ONLY, if treatment plan should change please request an amended estimate should it not be offered by our staff. This estimate is valid for 90 days from the date above IF treatment has not begun within that period. A patient's voluntary termination of treatment makes this agreement invalid.

FINANCIAL ARRANGEMENTS

Budd, Rose L.

**Financial Arrangements Form**

The use of the financial arrangements form places in writing the total estimated cost of the proposed dental treatment, when payments are expected, and the amount of each payment. It meets regulations by providing a "truth-in-lending" statement and gives instructions on what should be done if payment cannot be made. By signing the form, patients state that they understand what is going to be done, agree to the estimated fee, and accept the payment schedule.

Electronic: Practice management systems pull treatment and insurance information and easily generate printable forms.

(Dentrix screen shots courtesy Henry Schein Practice Solutions,American Fork, UT.)

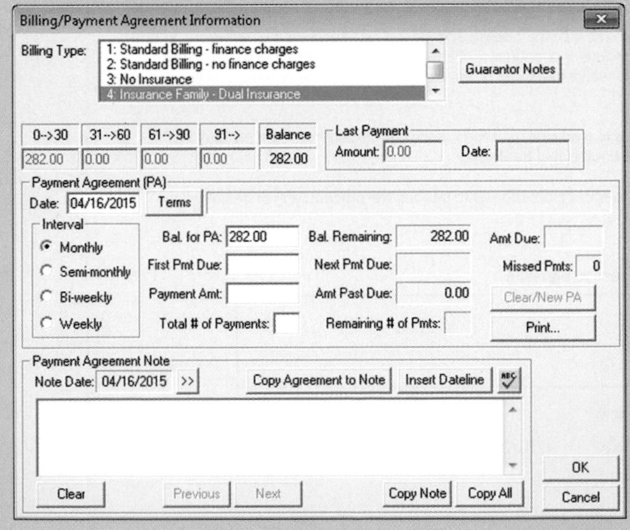


**PRACTICE NAME AND ADDRESS**

Dentrix Dental Practice
1220 South 630 East #100
American Fork, UT 84003
(801)763-9300

**GUARANTOR NAME AND ADDRESS**

Brent L Crosby
650 N 150 E
P.O. Box 110
Eastside, NV 11111
(702)555-5969

| | |
|---|---|
| Date: | 04/16/2015 |
| Chart #: | CR001 |
| SS #: | 000-00-0005 |
| Loan Amount: | $ 282.00 |
| Interest Rate: | 12.000 % |

**FEDERAL TRUTH-IN-LENDING DISCLOSURE STATEMENT**

| ANNUAL PERCENTAGE RATE | FINANCE CHARGE | AMOUNT FINANCED | TOTAL OF PAYMENTS |
|---|---|---|---|
| The cost of your credit as a yearly rate. | The dollar amount the credit will cost you. | The amount of credit provided to you or on your behalf. | The amount you will have paid after you have made all payments as scheduled. |
| 12.683 % | $ 18.71 | $ 282.00 | $ 300.71 |

**PAYMENT SCHEDULE SUMMARY**

| | | |
|---|---|---|
| Num Payments: 13 | Amt Each Payment: $25.00 | First Payment Due: 05/01/2015 |
| | Last Payment Amt: $0.71 | Last Payment Due: 05/01/2016 |

Late Charge: If any payment is thirty (30) days late, you will be charged 1.000% of the installment, or at least $0.50.

**FIG. 28.11** Financial arrangements form. *(From Gaylor LJ: The administrative dental assistant, ed 4, St Louis, 2017, Elsevier; Dentrix screenshot courtesy Henry Schein Practice Solutions, American Fork, UT.)*

**■ Patient Education** Diagnostic procedures are precise and often complex. These services provide the dental team and the patient with a complete and accurate assessment of the patient's oral health condition. When properly informed, a patient is better prepared to continue with home oral health procedures.

It is important to have available the educational materials, diagrams, and consumer information necessary to describe the types of dental conditions and available treatment options for your patients. Patients prefer to have information they can take with them to review personally before making a final decision. When you work as a team, you are putting your patients first and providing them with the best care. ■

**■ Legal and Ethical Implications** The procedures described in this chapter are clinical functions that the dental assistant is asked to perform every day. The techniques used require knowledge and understanding of the clinical examination form and proper charting techniques. When you perform the charting for a patient, you are responsible for what has been documented. You must do the following:

- Understand the diagrams on the clinical examination form.
- Know the numbering system used in your office.
- Know the surfaces of teeth.
- Know charting symbols.

If you chart the wrong tooth or the wrong condition, you initiate a compromising legal situation. ■

**■ Eye to the Future** With increased intake of fluoridation in the population, dentists are finding it challenging to detect decay in areas of the teeth that are more difficult to examine. New devices are being designed that use laser light energy (wavelength) that can be directed to a specific area of a tooth surface. When illuminated, the carious lesion will become fluorescent. These devices will measure the laser fluorescence and calculate a value. Calculated values will be used to determine a course of action ranging from no action, to preventive therapy, to monitoring of caries development, to placement of sealants, and, finally, to restoration of the tooth. ■

## ■ Critical Thinking

1. During which portion of the diagnosis and treatment planning examination would tooth mobility be evaluated?
2. Describe two areas of the face that would be included in the soft tissue examination.
3. What instruments and supplies are included in the tray setup for the charting of teeth?
4. When the periodontium is charted, tooth #4 has a reading of a 5-mm pocket on the mesiofacial surface and a 6-mm pocket on the mesiolingual surface with bleeding. Should these areas be charted? If so, how is the bleeding indicated on the chart?
5. With a charting form in front of you, chart the following conditions:
   - Tooth 1 is missing.
   - Tooth 2 has occlusal decay.
   - Tooth 7 has a PFM crown.
   - Tooth 11 has an MI composite.
   - Tooth 13 has disto-occlusal decay.
   - Tooth 16 is missing.
   - Tooth 19 has a root canal.
   - Tooth 21 has a sealant.
   - Teeth 23 to 26 have a bridge to replace teeth 24 and 25.
   - Tooth 29 has a periapical abscess.
   - Tooth 32 is impacted. ■

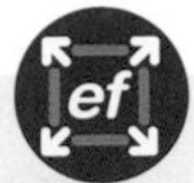

PROCEDURE 28.1 

# Extraoral and Intraoral Photography (Expanded Function)

*In many states, this procedure can be performed by certified dental assistants.*

## EQUIPMENT AND SUPPLIES

- ✔ Camera setup
- ✔ Cheek retractors
- ✔ Mouth mirror
- ✔ Reflection mirror

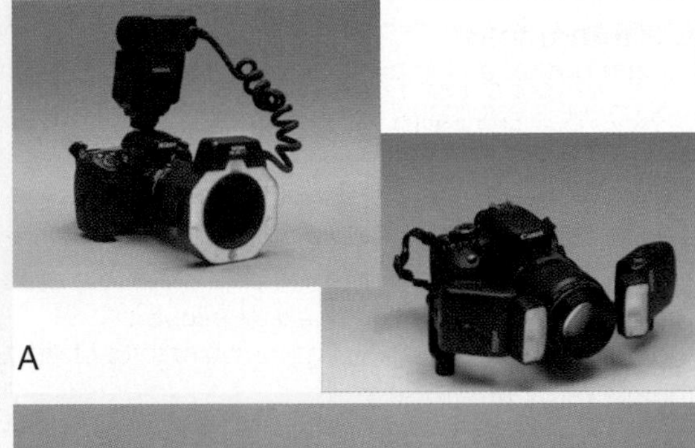

A

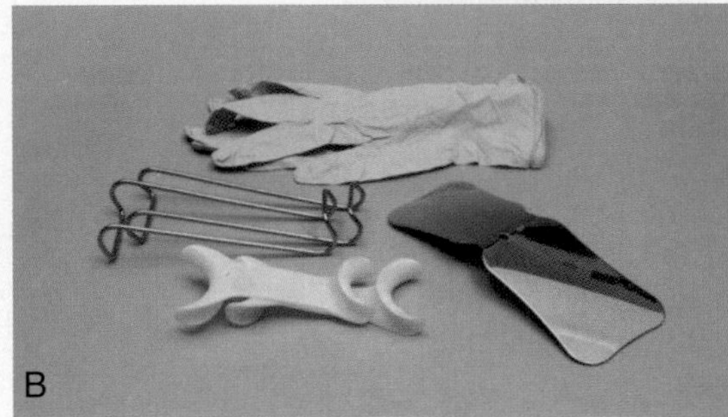

B

## PROCEDURAL STEPS

### Readying Your Camera

1 Calibrate the camera system so that you become familiar with the settings for intraoral and extraoral photographs.

**NOTE** For intraoral photography, set your camera to landscape mode, and for extraoral photography, use the portrait mode.

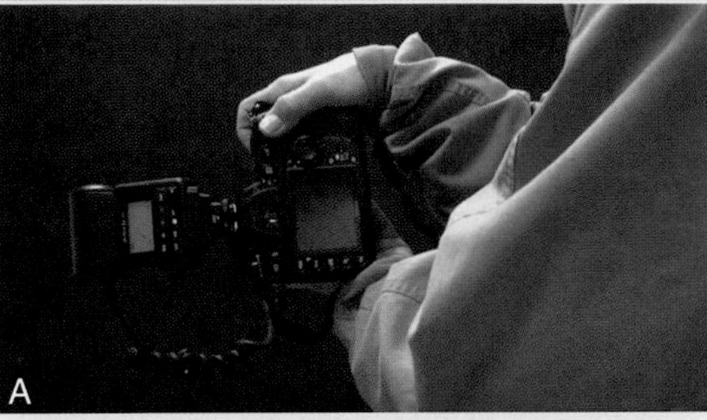

A

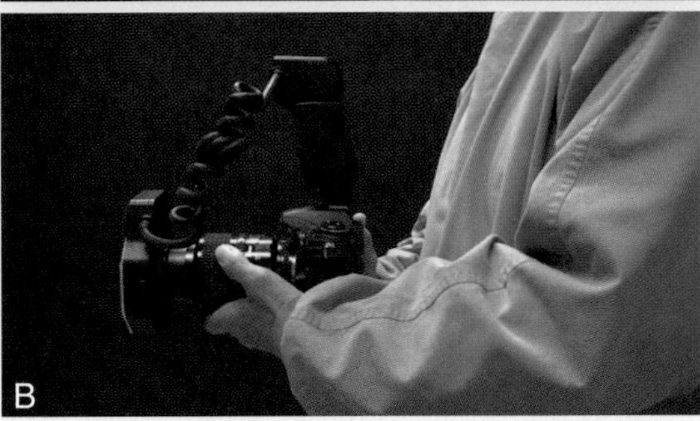

B

2 Use of manual focus is recommended, as autofocus can be unreliable in the oral cavity.

**NOTE** In general, for anterior teeth, focus on the central and lateral incisors to ensure that the maximum number of teeth are in focus.

3 Strive for optimum exposure. Keep in mind that mirrors absorb light, and exposures will have to be adjusted accordingly. Light absorption will vary from one mirror to another.

4 Generally, use an aperture compensation of +1 f-stop to help ensure proper illumination of mirror shots.

5 If using a digital camera, check the overall brightness.

### Readying Your Patient

6 For extraoral photographs, be 5 to 6 feet from your patient with a neutral color background.

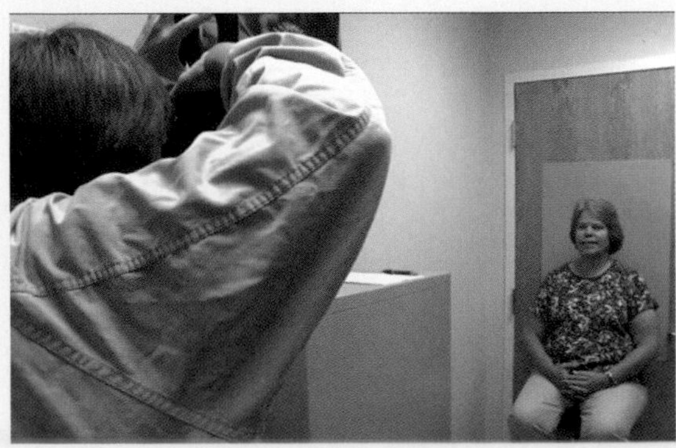

7 For intraoral photographs, clean the area you are photographing of excess saliva, blood, air bubbles, impression material, and cement.

## PROCEDURE 28.1 Extraoral and Intraoral Photography (Expanded Function)–cont'd

**8** The area you are photographing should not be completely dry.

**9** Position retractors symmetrically, and then pull out and away from the mouth.

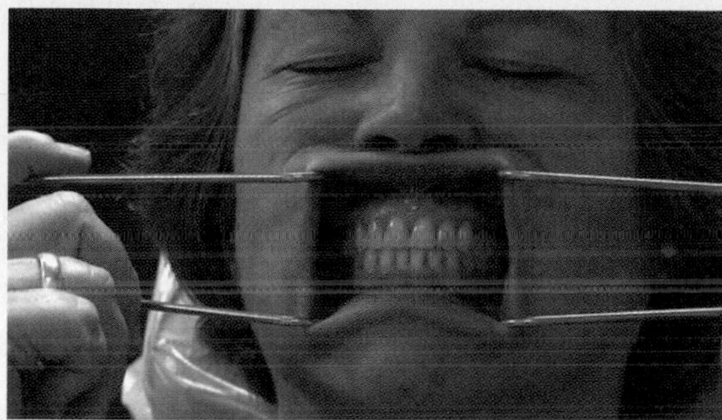

**10** If you are using a mouth mirror or a reflection mirror, you can control fogging by dipping the mirror into hot water or using a stream of air from the air-water syringe to keep the mirror clean.

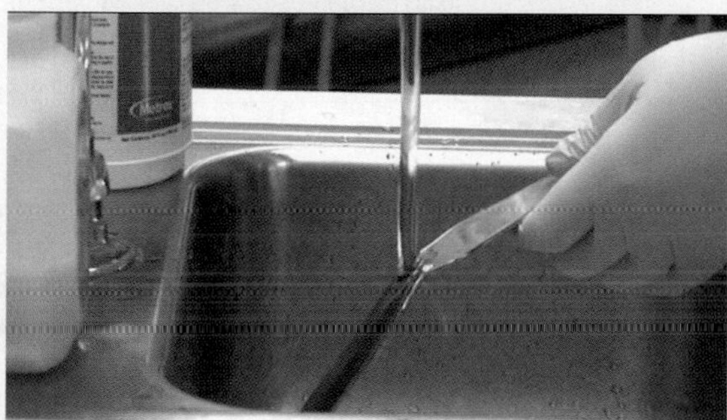

**11** Retract the tongue with a mirror or tongue retractor, or have the patient move the tongue to the posterior so as not to hide the teeth.

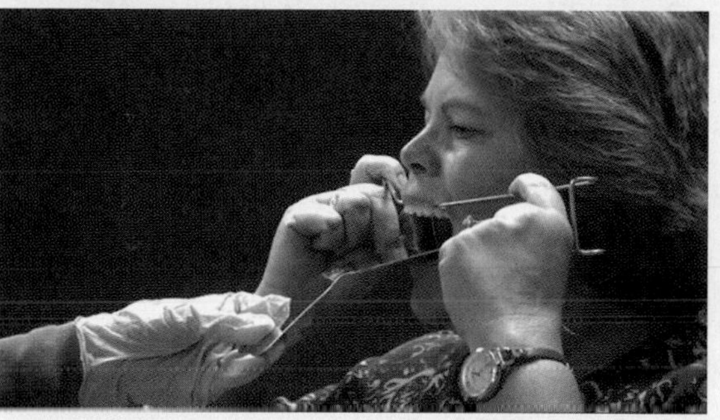

### Taking Photographs

**12** Think about your object. Remember to keep in mind what you are looking at: positioning, lighting, color, magnification, perspective, contrast, and background.

**13** Make sure everyone in the office who will be taking photographs is standardized, so that direct comparisons are possible, especially if successive photographs are to be taken by different photographers over long time intervals.

**14** Keep fingertips, mirror edges, and retractors out of the picture as much as possible.

**15** Photograph the teeth in correct axial alignment (e.g., the occlusal plane should be parallel to the floor, not slanted).

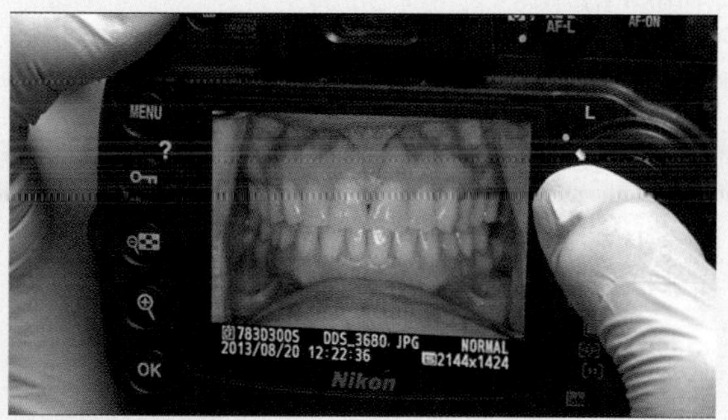


**16** When using a mirror, try to photograph the mirror image only. Having both the direct and mirror image appear in the same photograph can be confusing.

**NOTE** To avoid shadows, when using a flash in combination with a mouth mirror, keep the flash on the mirror side.

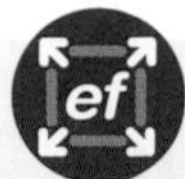

PROCEDURE 28.2

# The Soft Tissue Examination (Expanded Function)

*In certain states, this procedure can be legally completed by certified dental assistants.*

## EQUIPMENT AND SUPPLIES

- ✔ Gauze sponges (2 × 2 and 4 × 4)
- ✔ Tongue depressor (optional)
- ✔ Mouth mirror
- ✔ Patient record to document findings

## PROCEDURAL STEPS

### Patient Preparation

1 When escorting the patient to the treatment area, observe the patient's general appearance, speech, and behavior.

**PURPOSE** Unusual behavior or appearance must be immediately noted or called to the dentist's attention.

2 Seat the patient in the dental chair in an upright position. Drape the patient with a patient napkin.

3 Explain the procedure to the patient.

**PURPOSE** The patient who knows what to expect will be more comfortable and more willing to participate in the examination.

### Extraoral Features

4 Examine the face, neck, and ears for asymmetry or abnormal swelling.

**PURPOSE** The two sides of the face should be symmetric.

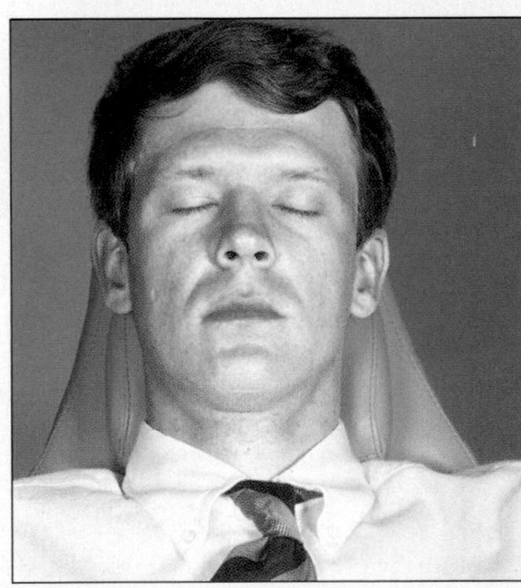

5 Look for abnormal tissue changes, skin abrasions, and discoloration.

**PURPOSE** Unusual bruising, scratches, or cuts may require further evaluation of the area.

6 Evaluate the texture, color, and continuity of the vermilion border, the commissures of the lips, the philtrum, and the smile line.

**PURPOSE** Lumps, dryness, and cracking of the tissues are deviations from normal that may indicate that further evaluation of the area is required.

7 Document all findings in the patient record.

### Cervical Lymph Nodes

8 Position yourself behind the patient so that you can easily place your fingers just below the patient's ears.

9 To examine the right side of the neck, use the left hand to steady the patient's head. The fingers and thumb of the right hand gently follow the chain of lymph nodes downward, starting in front of the right ear and continuing to the clavicle (collarbone).

**PURPOSE** You are looking for swelling, abnormal formation, and tenderness in the area.

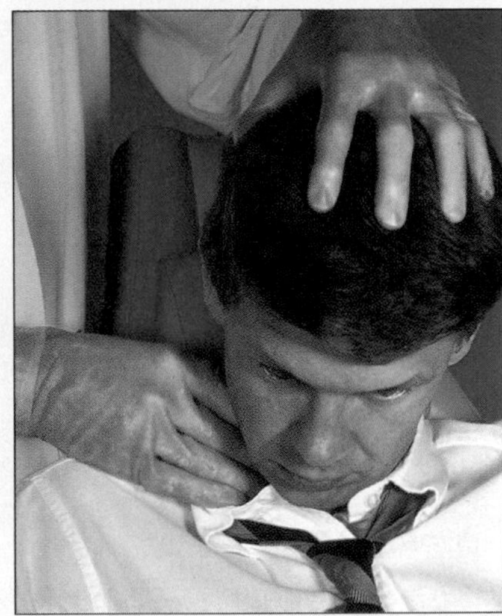

10 To examine the left side of the neck, use the right hand to steady the patient's head. The fingers and thumb of the left hand gently follow the chain of lymph nodes downward, starting in front of the left ear and continuing to the clavicle (collarbone).

11 Document all findings in the patient record.

### Temporomandibular Joint

12 To evaluate temporomandibular joint (TMJ) movements during centric, lateral, protrusive, and retrusive movements, ask the patient to open and close the mouth normally and then to move the jaw from side to side.

13 To further evaluate movement of the TMJ, gently place your fingers into the external opening of the ear. Ask the patient to open and close the mouth normally.

# PROCEDURE 28.2 The Soft Tissue Examination (Expanded Function)–cont'd

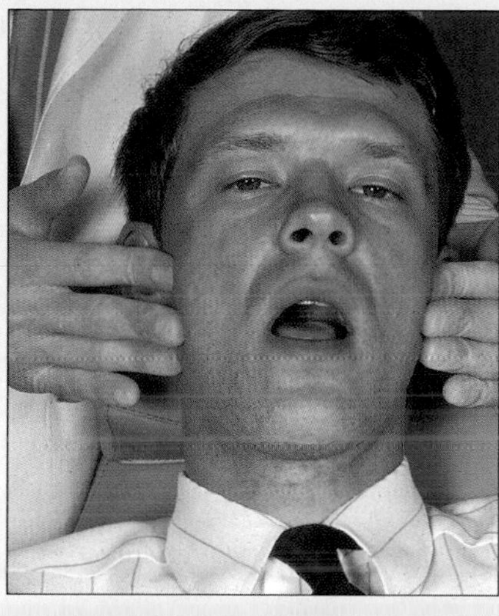

14 To determine whether noise occurs in the TMJ during movement, listen as the patient opens and closes the mouth. A stethoscope may be placed on the joint.

15 Note in the patient record any abnormalities or patient comments regarding pain, tenderness, or other problems related to opening and closing of the mouth.

## Indications of Oral Habits

16 Look for indications of oral habits such as thumb sucking, tongue-thrust swallow, mouth breathing, and tobacco use.
**PURPOSE** These habits can affect the patient's oral health.

17 Look for signs of other oral habits such as bruxism, grinding, and clenching. Indications include abnormal wear on the teeth and problems in the TMJ.

## Interior of the Lips

18 Ask the patient to open his or her mouth slightly.

19 Examine the mucosa and the labial frenum of the upper lip by gently retracting the lip with the thumbs and index fingers.

20 Examine the mucosa and the labial frenum of the lower lip by gently retracting the lip with the thumbs and index fingers.

21 Palpate the tissues gently to detect lumps or other abnormalities.

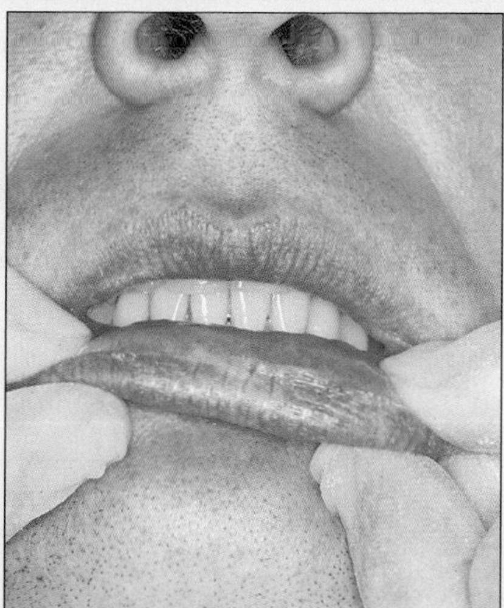

## Oral Mucosa and Tongue

22 Palpate the tissue of the buccal mucosa gently by placing the thumb of one hand inside the mouth and the index and third fingers of the other hand on the exterior of the cheek.

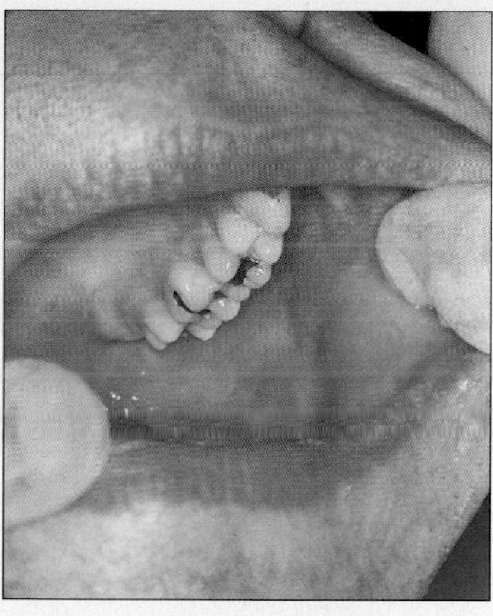

23 Examine the tissue that covers the hard palate.

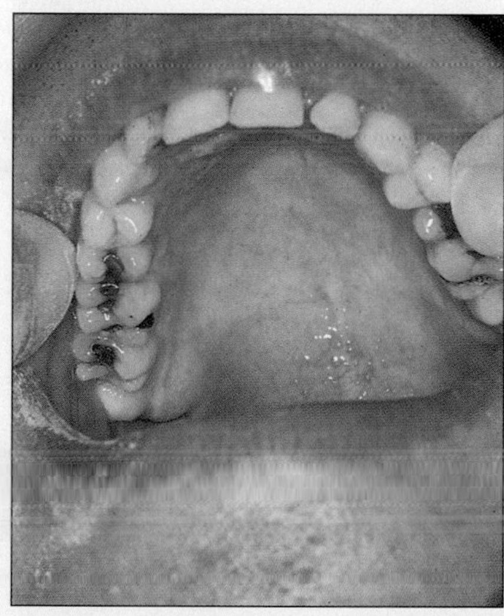

24 Visually examine the buccal mucosa and the opening of Stensen's duct. A warm mouth mirror may also be used to view the flow of saliva from the duct.
**PURPOSE** The mouth mirror is warmed to prevent fogging.

25 Ask the patient to extend the tongue and to relax it. Using sterile gauze, gently grasp the tip of the tongue, and pull it forward.

26 Observe the dorsum (top) of the tongue for color, papillae, presence or lack of a coating, and abnormalities.

27 Gently move the tongue from side to side to examine the lateral (side) and ventral (underneath) surfaces.

(Continued)

## PROCEDURE 28.2 The Soft Tissue Examination (Expanded Function)–cont'd

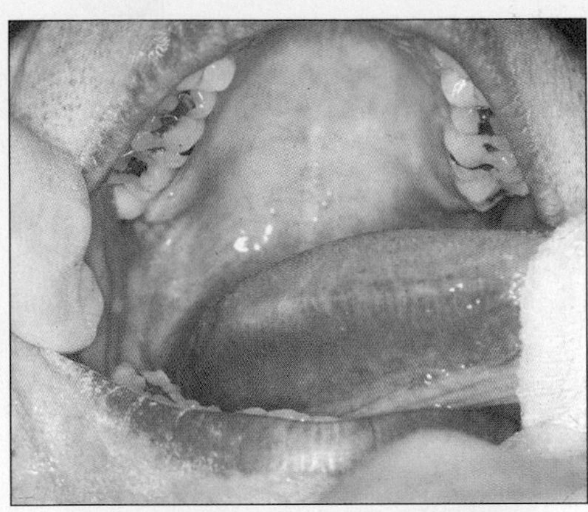

28 Use a warm mouth mirror to observe the posterior area.
**CAUTION** To avoid triggering the gag reflex, this mirror is placed very carefully and is moved very little.

29 Examine the uvula, the base of the tongue, and the posterior area of the mouth by placing a mouth mirror or a tongue depressor firmly at the base of the tongue.
**CAUTION** Firm but gentle placement reduces the possibility of triggering the gag reflex.

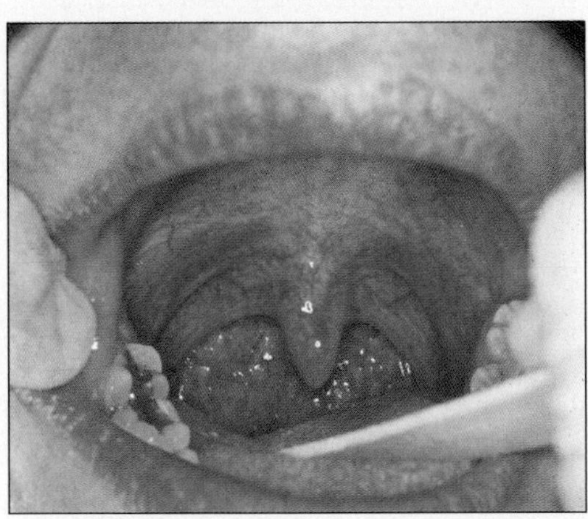

30 With the mouth mirror firmly depressing the base of the tongue, have the patient say, "Ahh."
**PURPOSE** The oropharynx expands, providing a better view of the upper portion of the throat.

### Floor of the Mouth

31 With the patient's mouth closed, palpate the soft tissues of the face above and below the mandible.
**PURPOSE** Tori and other abnormalities can be detected.

32 Gently palpate the interior of the floor of the mouth by placing the index finger of one hand on the floor of the mouth and by placing the fingers of the other hand on the outer surface under the chin.

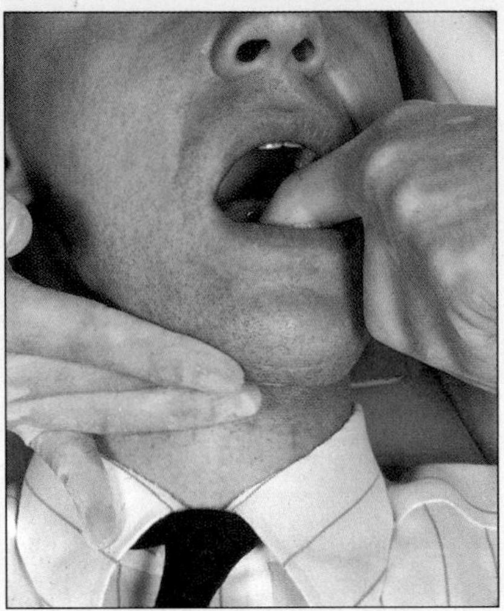

33 Instruct the patient to touch the tongue to the hard palate.
**PURPOSE** The floor of the mouth, the lingual frenum, and the salivary ducts can be visually examined.

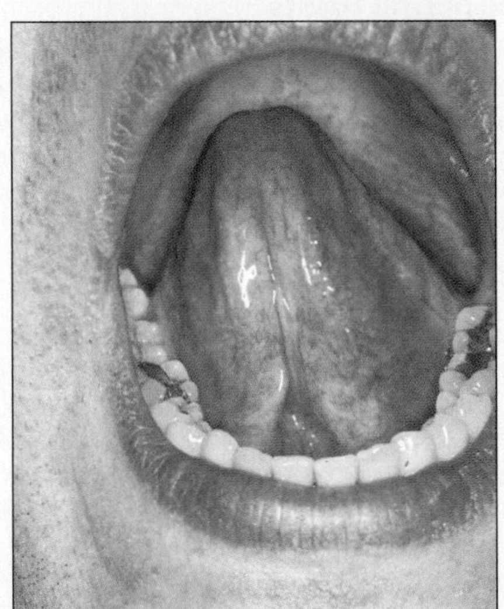

34 Observe the quantity and consistency of the flow of saliva. Depending on the patient's general health, diet, and medications, the saliva may vary in consistency from watery to thick and ropy.

35 Document all information accurately in the patient record.

| Date | Extraoral examination; no changes since last examination | Signature/Date |
|---|---|---|

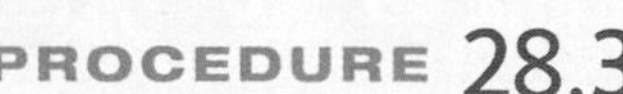

PROCEDURE 28.3

# Charting of Teeth

## EQUIPMENT AND SUPPLIES

- Mouth mirror
- Explorer
- Cotton pliers
- Periodontal probe
- Gauze sponges (2 × 2)
- Dental floss
- Articulating paper
- Articulating paper holder
- Air-water syringe
- Colored pencils (red and blue/black)
- Eraser
- Clinical examination form

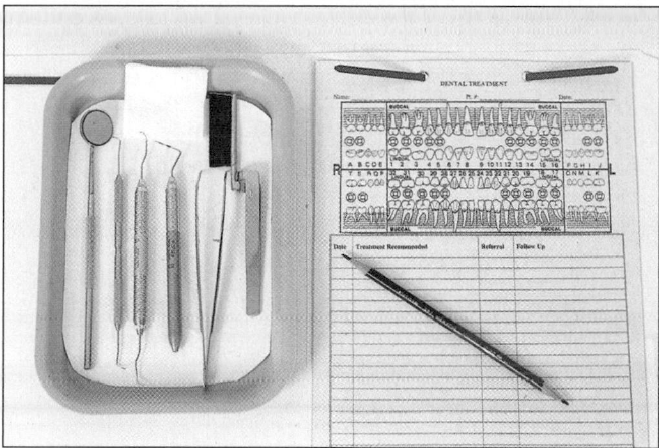

## PROCEDURAL STEPS

### Patient Preparation

1 The patient is already seated and has been draped with a patient napkin.

2 Reposition the patient in a supine position.

**PURPOSE** The dentist can use instruments more easily and has better intraoral vision with the patient in the supine position.

### Examination of the Teeth and Occlusion

3 Ensure that colored pencils, an eraser, the clinical examination form, and a flat surface are readily available.

**NOTE** If charting electronically, you will not need pencils. Make sure the keyboard is covered properly for infection control.

**PURPOSE** The more organized you are, the fewer errors and stops will be made.

4 Throughout the procedure, use the air syringe to clear the mouth mirror, and adjust the operating light as necessary.

**PURPOSE** Better visualization is provided for the dentist as the teeth are examined.

5 Transfer the mirror and the explorer to the dentist. The dentist will begin with tooth #1 and will continue to tooth #32. The dentist will examine every surface of each tooth.

6 Record the specific notations as the dentist calls them out.

7 The dentist will examine the patient's occlusion (bite). Place the articulating paper within the holder, and transfer the instrument with the paper positioned correctly for that side of the mouth.

**NOTE** The holder is positioned closest to the cheek and the paper between the teeth.

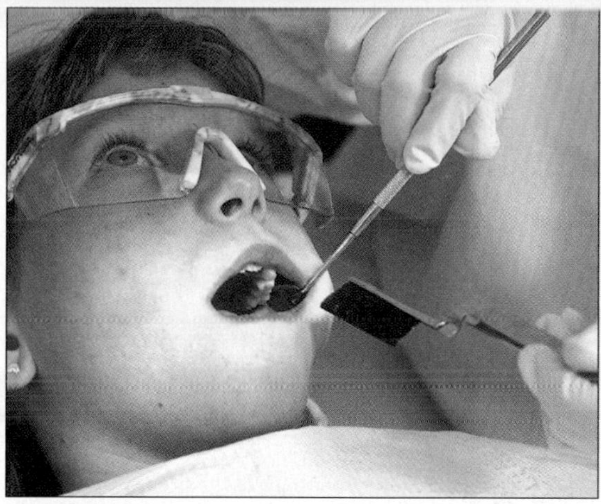

8 Any marks made by the paper will remain on the patient's occlusal and incisal surfaces.

**PURPOSE** The dentist will look for any abnormal markings to indicate improper occlusion.

9 At the completion of the procedure, rinse and dry the patient's mouth.

10 Document all information accurately in the patient record, and sign.

| Date | Intraoral examination: mo decay on tooth #5<br>Reschedule pt for a 2-unit appt. for MO posterior composite on #5 | Signature/Date |
|---|---|---|

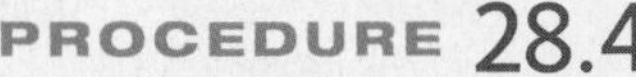

PROCEDURE 28.4

# Periodontal Screening: Examination of the Gingival Tissues

## EQUIPMENT AND SUPPLIES

- ✔ Mouth mirror
- ✔ Air-water syringe
- ✔ Explorer
- ✔ Periodontal probe
- ✔ Dental floss
- ✔ Gauze sponges (2 × 2)
- ✔ Black ink pen
- ✔ Red pencil
- ✔ Clinical examination form

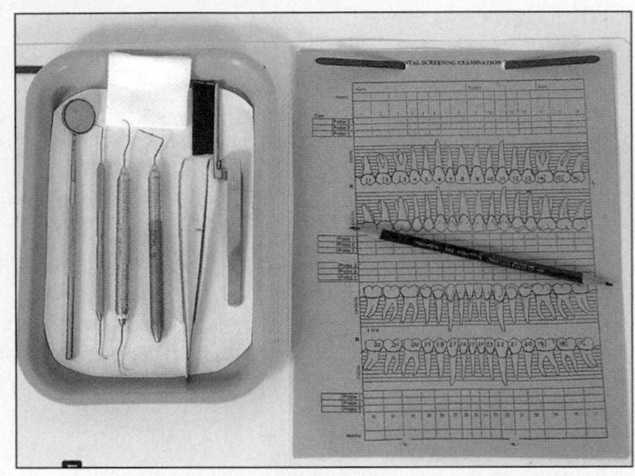

## PROCEDURAL STEPS

1 The dentist or the dental hygienist observes gingival status throughout the mouth using a mouth mirror. Assistant should provide a slight, continuous flow of air on the mirror from the air-water syringe.

**PURPOSE** This keeps the mirror from becoming fogged.

2 Transfer the periodontal probe.

**PURPOSE** This instrument can reveal the health of the gingiva by indicating firmness of the tissue and the presence of inflammation or bleeding.

3 The periodontal probe is used to measure the depth of the gingival sulcus for each tooth. Beginning at tooth #1, each tooth will have six measurements: three from the facial side and three from the lingual side.

**NOTE** The dentist or the dental hygienist will follow a pattern or sequence when measuring the pocket depth.

4 Record every reading greater than 3 mm on the examination form.

5 If bleeding is detected during the probing, this should be noted by circling the recorded reading. See Box 28.1, Description of Probing Scores.

Date Perio charting, distofacial of
14–16 recession w/pockets +5
Refer to periodontist for consult. Signature/Date

29

# The Special Needs and Medically Compromised Patient

## KEY TERMS

**Alzheimer's (AHLTS-hie-merz) disease** A form of progressive mental deterioration that occurs in middle to older age.

**Anemia (uh-NEE-mee-uh)** A shortage of red blood cells or hemoglobin in the blood, resulting in paleness and weakness.

**Angina (an-JYE-nah)** Severe chest pain associated with an insufficient supply of blood to the heart.

**Arthritis (ahr-THRYE-tis)** Inflammation of a joint or many joints, resulting in pain and swelling.

**Asthma (AZ-muh)** Respiratory disease often associated with allergies and characterized by sudden recurring attacks of labored breathing, chest constriction, and coughing.

**Atrophy (AT-ruh-fee)** A wasting away or deterioration.

**Bacteremia (bak-tur-EE-mee-uh)** Presence of bacteria in the blood.

**Bronchitis (bron-KYE-tis)** Inflammation of the mucous membranes of the bronchial tubes.

**Dementia (duh-MEN-shuh)** A mental disorder characterized by loss of memory, concentration, and judgment.

**Diabetes mellitus (dye-uh-BEE-teez MEL-e-tus, me-LYE-tus) (DM)** Metabolic disorder characterized by high blood glucose and insufficient insulin.

**Emphysema (em-fi-ZEE-muh)** Abnormal increase in the size of the air spaces in the lungs, resulting in labored breathing and an increased susceptibility to infection.

**Endocarditis (en-doe-kahr-DYE-tus)** Inflammation of the endocardium.

**Epilepsy (EH-pi-lep-see)** Neurologic disorder with sudden recurring seizures of motor, sensory, or psychic malfunction.

**Hemophilia (hee-moe-FIL-ee-uh)** Blood coagulation disorder in which the blood fails to clot normally.

**Hyperthyroidism (hye-pur-THYE-roid-iz-em, hye-pur-THYE-roi-dizem)** Condition that results from excessive activity of the thyroid gland.

**Hypothyroidism (hye-poe-THYE-roid-iz-em, hi-poe-THYE-roi-dizem)** Condition that results from severe thyroid hormone insufficiency.

**Leukemia (loo-KEE-mee-uh)** A progressive disease in which the bone marrow produces an increased number of immature or abnormal white cells.

**Myocardial infarction (mye-oe-KAHR-dee-ul in-FAHRK-shun)** Condition in which damage occurs to the muscular tissue of the heart, commonly caused by obstructed circulation; also referred to as a *heart attack.*

**Rheumatoid arthritis (RA)** A disease that causes pain, stiffness, swelling, and loss of function in the joints.

**Seizure** A sudden attack, spasm, or convulsion that occurs in specific disorders.

**Stroke** A sudden loss of brain function caused by blockage or rupture of a blood vessel to the brain; also called *cerebrovascular accident.*

**Xerostomia (zeer-oe-STOE-mee-uh)** Loss of saliva production causing a dry mouth.

## LEARNING OUTCOMES

*On completion of this chapter, the student will be able to achieve the following objectives:*

1. Pronounce, define, and spell the key terms.
2. Discuss the role of the dental assistant in caring for the special care patient.
3. Describe the stages of aging in the older population and the orally related conditions that affect this population.
4. Describe the importance of the medical history for the special needs/medically compromised patient.
5. Describe the major medical disorders that can affect a patient's oral health, including the type of dental management a medically compromised patient would receive.

## PERFORMANCE OUTCOME

*On completion of this chapter, the student will be able to meet competency standards in the following skill:*

- Demonstrate the correct transfer of a wheelchair-bound patient.

## ELECTRONIC RESOURCES

***Additional information related to content in Chapter 29 can be found on the companion Evolve Web site.***

- Practice Quiz

Today, just about every dental practice cares for patients with special needs. Because of the major advances in medicine, people are living longer and are surviving medical disorders that in the past would have resulted in disability or premature death. According to the U.S. Department of Commerce, statistics show that nearly 1 in 2 people (133 million) have a chronic condition. This could be an illness such as heart disease or diabetes, or a condition such as arthritis, migraines, or back pain from a car accident. Additionally, it is estimated that 2% have some type of disabling disorder, such as developmental disabilities, neuromuscular disorders, immunocompromising conditions, cognitive impairment, mental disorders, and trauma.

It is the responsibility of the dentist and the dental team to become knowledgeable and to identify the challenges that face these patients. Patients who enter your dental practice may be ill, in pain, or physically challenged. Your job is to use good judgment when working with these patients, which may mean bypassing some of the usual routines that take place during an appointment. The dental team and the patient's medical team must work together to modify dental treatment according to the patient's needs.

## Role of the Dental Assistant

The dental assistant's role in caring for the special care patient can be divided into three major areas:

1. *Aiding the dentist in providing treatment.* The chairside assistant must be familiar with specialized techniques and equipment used in treating the medically and physically compromised patient. The efficiency of all dental team members is important to the speed and ease of treatment.
2. *Serving as a source of information to the patient and the family.* Preventive dentistry is particularly important and may prove difficult for the physically and medically challenged patient. The assistant may be asked to work with the patient and family to develop and implement a preventive program that is tailored to the needs of the patient.
3. *Making the patient more comfortable and reducing anxiety.* The patient may be particularly apprehensive because of extensive past painful experiences with medical treatment. It is the job of the dental team to help alleviate anxiety and provide a comfortable environment.

## The Aging Population

With a declining birth rate and increased longevity, the aging population is the fastest-growing segment of the U.S. population. People age 65 and older make up 13.7 percent of the population and represent about one in every eight persons in the United States. It is estimated that by 2050, people age 65 and older will make up 21 percent of the U.S. population.

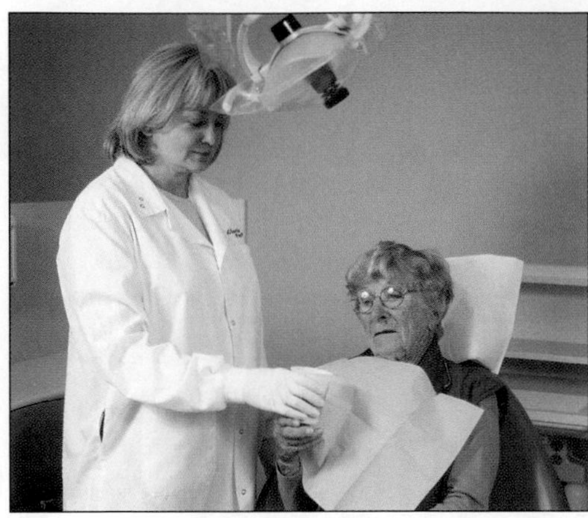

**FIG. 29.1** Aging person.

## Stages of Aging

*Aging* refers to the irreversible and inevitable changes that occur with time. Most oral conditions that develop in older adults were once believed to be the result of aging, not of disease. Current science is showing that this is not the case. In diagnosis and treatment planning, it is helpful to differentiate signs and symptoms caused by aging from those caused by *disease.*

Older adults, or persons older than age 65, vary in their psychological and physiologic stages. In agreement with their varying attitudes, characteristics, and needs, older adults can be divided into three categories:

- *Functionally independent older adults* are better educated and are more demanding of health services than in the past. This group has retained most of their natural teeth and expects to maintain them throughout their lives.
- *Frail older adults* are beginning to have multiple health problems. Some have maintained their natural teeth, but more of them have fixed and removable prostheses.
- *Dependent older adults* have fewer natural teeth and believe that tooth loss is an inevitable part of aging. This segment of the population tends to have medical conditions that are reflected in their oral health.

RECALL

1 What role does the dental assistant have with the medically and physically compromised patient?
2 What is the fastest-growing segment of the population?

## Oral Health of the Aging

The aging population is faced with special oral health issues, and the goal of the dental team for these patients is to factor this into the treatment planning phase (Fig. 29.1). The condition of a patient's mouth can affect self-esteem, esthetics, nutrition, social interaction, and personal comfort. A person's general health can actually deteriorate because of poor oral health.

Along with the medical history, it is essential that a *medication profile* be completed for each patient. One of the hallmarks of disease is the list of prescriptions a patient is taking. These drugs not only indicate the patient's disease state; they

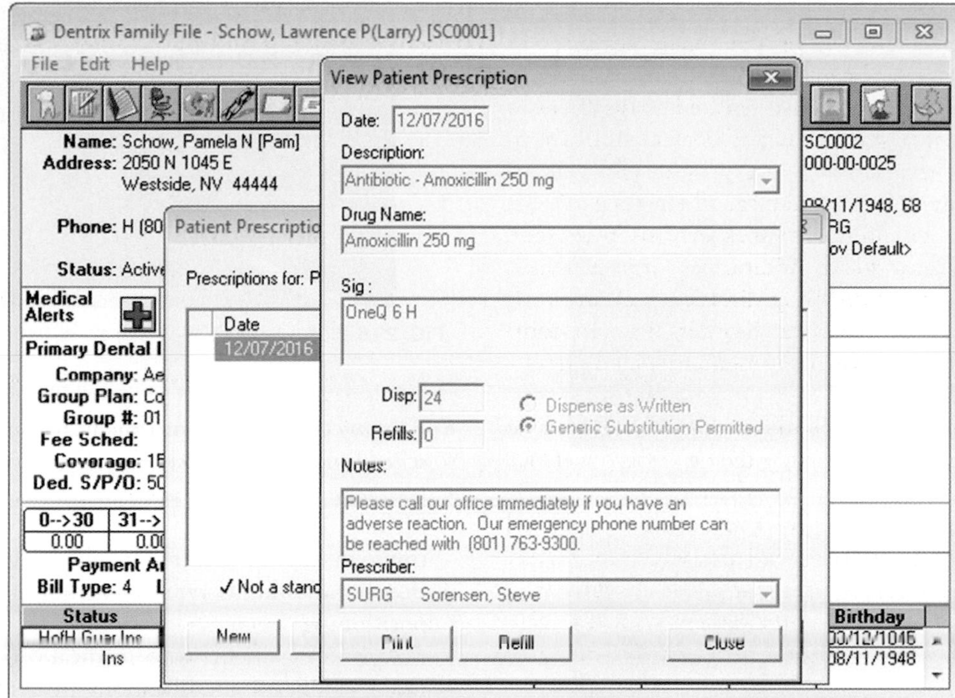


FIG. 29.2 Example of a medication profile for a patient. *(Courtesy Henry Schein Practice Solutions, American Fork, UT.)*

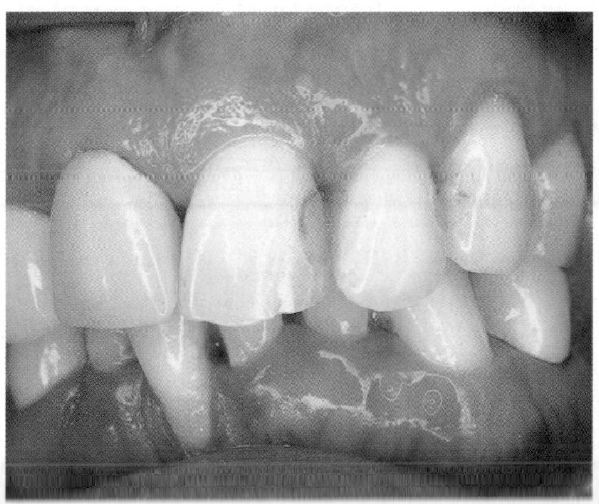

FIG. 29.3 Periodontal conditions of an older patient.

also have potential adverse effects that, along with drug interactions, must be taken into consideration during treatment planning. A medication profile can indicate the severity of a patient's medical condition (Fig. 29.2).

## Oral Health Conditions

The most commonly reported oral health–related conditions that affect the aging population are xerostomia, periodontal disease, tooth decay, dark and brittle teeth, and bone resorption.

### Xerostomia

Also known as *dry mouth,* **xerostomia** is the result of medical disorders and medications that cause a decreased flow of saliva. Hundreds of medications, including many over-the-counter drugs, produce dry mouth as a side effect. In addition to drug adverse effects, xerostomia is frequently associated with alcoholism, autoimmune disorders, Parkinson's disease, psychological disorders, dehydration, radiation to the salivary glands, diabetes, Sjögren's syndrome, and oral breathing.

### Periodontal Disease

Periodontal conditions are an increasing problem in the aging population. More than 50 percent of older people may be affected by periodontal disease, and most are unaware of it. As a larger number of older people retain their teeth, periodontal disease will increase (Fig. 29.3). Periodontal disease can be prevented by better oral hygiene and more frequent visits to the hygienist.

### Tooth Decay

Studies have shown that older patients have a higher risk of root caries and recurrent decay around old or worn restorations. With aging, often the gums recede, exposing the roots of the teeth. In contrast to the crowns, the roots of the teeth are not protected by enamel, so decay can quickly develop on root surfaces (Fig. 29.4). Root caries can sometimes be prevented by dietary adjustments and changes in oral hygiene care.

### Dark and Brittle Teeth

As we age, teeth may darken and become more brittle. This is a result of deposits of secondary dentin that have gradually reduced the size of the pulp chamber. These teeth can then become more susceptible to fracture (Fig. 29.5).

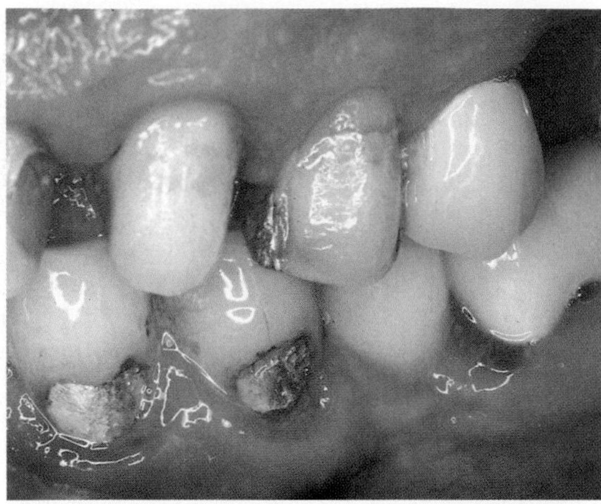

FIG. 29.4 Root caries of a tooth in an older patient.

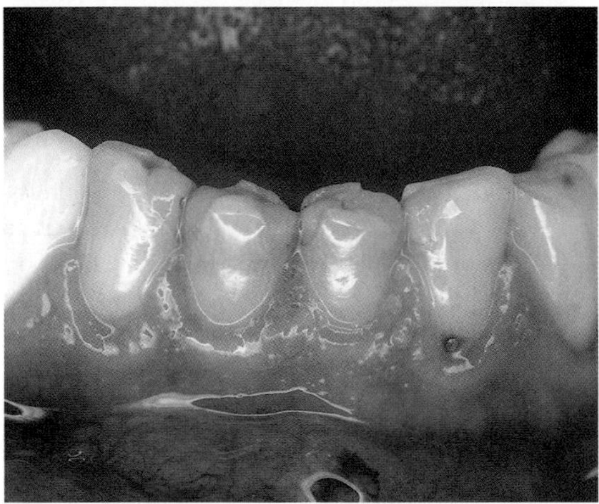

FIG. 29.5 Darkened teeth associated with secondary dentin and aging.

### Bone Resorption

When teeth are missing, the patient is partially to fully edentulous. Portions of the alveolar ridge will become compromised and lost (Fig. 29.6). Bone resorption can affect whether the patient will wear a removable prosthesis, as well as the patient's speech and diet (see Chapter 52).

## The Special Needs Patient

Providing dental care to patients with a physical or medical disorder will require increased awareness and attention, and possibly modification of clinical care by the dentist and dental staff. Once the health and medication histories have been obtained from the patient, this information must be used effectively. Each patient should be assessed before treatment can be provided.

An easy technique to use with your patients is to categorize each patient according to how treatment is anticipated to proceed, and what changes are to be made by the dental team:

- *Category I:* healthy patients who require no special modifications

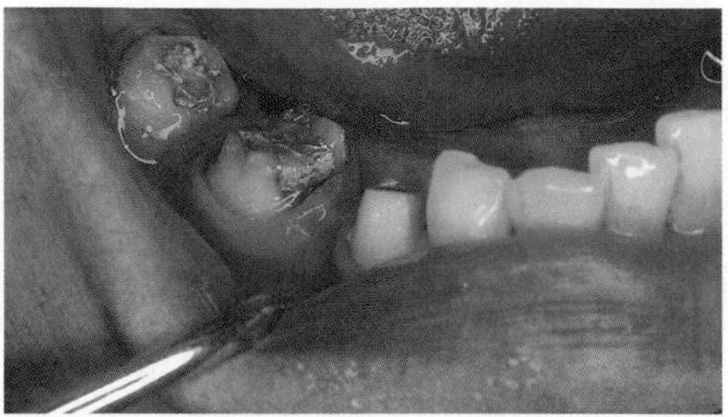

FIG. 29.6 Bone resorption with loss of teeth and alveolar ridge.

- *Category II:* patients with medical conditions who require scheduling changes or shorter appointments
- *Category III:* patients with medical conditions that have lifelong implications; these patients require modifications in dental treatment planning, including alterations in anesthetic, types of dental materials, and patient positioning
- *Category IV:* patients with medical conditions who require more significant modifications in dental treatment planning, including treatment to meet dental needs within the operating room
- *Category V:* patients with serious medical conditions who require only limited care to eliminate serious acute oral disease; includes patients who must be kept free of pain and discomfort

## Assistance from Organizations

Many organizations can provide information to assist you in updating and educating the dental staff. To better prepare you, the patient, and the family, seek out guided assistance from these groups.

The American Speech-Language-Hearing Association, for example, offers information on hearing loss and communication problems in older people and provides a list of certified audiologists and speech pathologists.

RECALL

3 In what category would you assess a patient that has experienced a stroke and is wheelchair bound?
4 What is xerostomia?
5 What are the most common oral health conditions that affect the aging population?

## Specific Disorders of the Medically Compromised Patient

A basic understanding of how a disorder can affect a person's oral health is important to prevent tooth loss or other complications. Symptoms of more than 100 diseases can indirectly affect a patient by causing a person to be less capable of caring for his or her mouth.

Specific medical and physical disorders are categorized to help you learn and understand each disease and how to care for that specific patient in your practice.

## Developmental Disorders

Developmental disorders are the result of an impairment that occurred during the developmental phase (prenatal through age 18) of a person. This impairment can occur prenatally, during birth, or postnatally. Disorders causing a developmental disability can be chromosomal abnormalities such as intellectual disability and Down syndrome, autism, cerebral palsy, fetal alcohol syndrome, postnatal infection, or birth anoxia. Many patients with developmental disorders are routinely seen in a pediatric dental office. The pediatric dentist receives extensive education and training on seeing and treating these types of special patients. For more information on oral conditions and clinical management, refer to Chapter 57.

### *Intellectual Disability*

Intellectual disability is impairment in intellectual and adaptive functioning. The cause is not always known; rarely, a single cause is identified. Some of the known causes are chromosomal abnormalities, prenatal conditions (rubella, alcohol use, and drug use), perinatal events (anoxia), and postnatal conditions (meningitis, encephalitis, trauma, cultural deprivation, severe malnutrition).

Intellectual disability occurs at many levels, and it is important to understand each patient's level of communication.

### *Down Syndrome*

*Down syndrome,* also termed *trisomy 21,* is probably the most known developmental disorder. It is associated with an extra chromosome of the twenty-first group. These individuals have 47 chromosomes rather than the normal complement of 46. The overall incidence of Down syndrome is 1 in 700 live births. However, incidence increases with the age of the mother; at age 54, the incidence is 1 in 54.

The typical facial appearance includes slanted eyes and a broad, flat nose; short stature is also noted. This disorder brings along multiple medical conditions that need to be considered when treating the patient, including intellectual disability, congenital cardiac anomalies, seizure disorders, upper respiratory disease, leukemia, and hepatitis.

### *Autism*

Autism affects how information is processed in the brain by altering how nerve cells and their synapses connect and organize. Individuals with autism disorders demonstrate difficulties in three main areas: social interaction, communication, and repetitive behaviors or restricted interests.

The aspects of social interaction in individuals with autism may alter how a patient will interact at the dental office. They may have difficulties with poor eye contact, an inability to read facial expressions, and difficulties with social exchange and interactions.

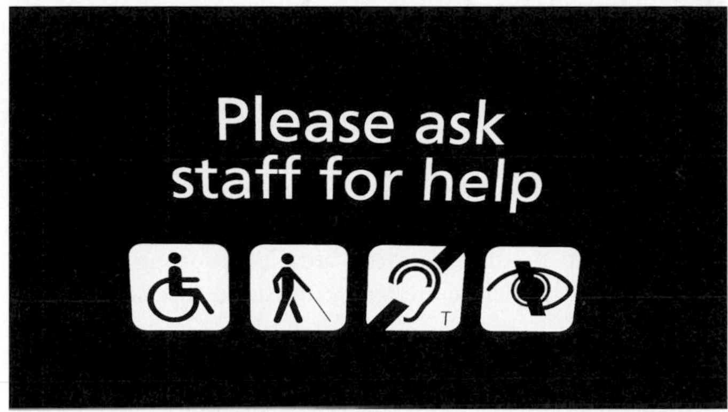


**FIG. 29.7** Handicapped sticker. *(Copyright © 2009 Mila Dragonfly, United Kingdom. Image from BigstockPhoto.com.)*

## Physical Disorders

The patient who is physically challenged must adapt to a very fast-paced and mobile world. A wheelchair-bound, vision-impaired, or hearing-impaired patient who is entering the dental office can alter the daily routine if the office is not prepared. This patient may need more time for the appointment, and the dental unit may have to be arranged differently. However, the best way to prepare is through teamwork and communication.

### *The Patient in a Wheelchair*

Accessibility to the dental office is necessary if you are going to provide dental care to individuals with physical disabilities (Fig. 29.7). Failure to provide access such as wheelchair ramps could be considered discrimination. Specific considerations should be included when an office is being designed for all patients:

- Walkways, sidewalks, and parking facilities
- Entrance ramps, handrails, hallways, and elevators
- Door width and door pressure or ease of opening
- Adequate space around door to maneuver a wheelchair, and elevator accessibility
- Floor surfaces, carpets, and rugs
- Restroom facilities
- Reception room design, furniture style, and lighting
- Operatory design to allow for wheelchair transfer or in-wheelchair treatment

A wheelchair provides mobility to an individual who is paralyzed, has had an amputation, or has a debilitating disease that produces weakness in the lower half of the body. Many dental units now are designed to accommodate a wheelchair, so the patient may remain seated in the chair rather than having to be moved. If the circumstance arises for the patient to be transferred to the dental chair, you must follow a routine procedure for transferring a patient (see Procedure 29.1: Transferring a Patient from a Wheelchair).

### Vision Impairment

Visual impairments vary from total blindness to limitations in color perception, distance perception, recognition of shapes, and size of visual field (Fig. 29.8). The vision-impaired person has learned to rely on the sense of touch and on verbal communication with others. For patients who cannot see their surroundings, all procedures should be thoroughly explained first. The trip to the treatment area, positioning, and even smells from the dental materials must be discussed before treatment.

#### Clinical Considerations for Visually Impaired Patients

- When guiding the visually impaired patient, offer your arm and let the patient hold your arm; do not push the patient.
- Describe obstacles as you guide the patient.
- If a guide dog is being used, do not pet or interfere with the dog; ask the patient first how to handle the dog.

### Hearing Impairment

The patient who is hearing impaired should be treated with extra care and courtesy. Hearing-impaired patients may show no visible evidence of hearing loss and may not respond to questions and instructions or may respond inappropriately.

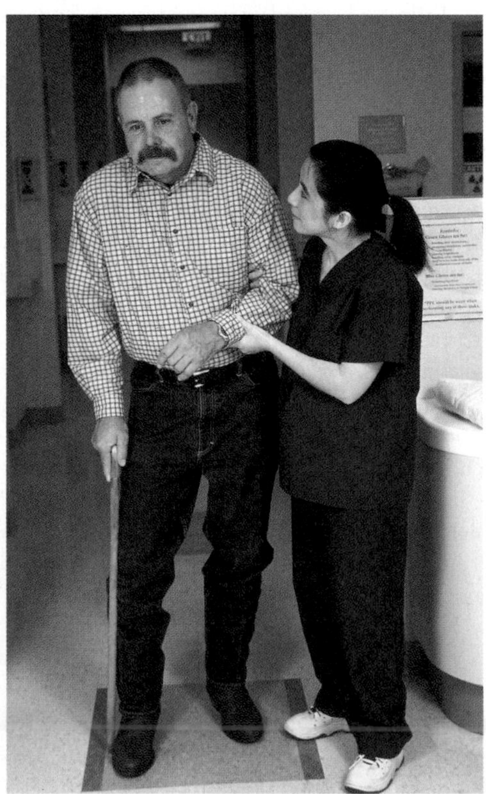

**FIG. 29.8** Escorting a vision-impaired patient.

#### Clinical Considerations for Hearing-Impaired Patients

- Remove extraneous noise such as suction and music when communicating.
- Remove your mask when speaking to expose your lips.
- Use mirrors, models, drawings, and written information to supplement communication.
- Keep directions simple, and provide written copies for the patient to take home.
- A sign language interpreter can be very valuable.

## Neurologic Disorders

A neurologic disorder involves the nervous system, beginning in the brain. Specifically, it covers all categories of diseases involving the central, peripheral, and autonomic nervous systems, which include the coverings, blood vessels, and tissues such as muscle.

### Alzheimer's Disease

**Alzheimer's disease** is a disorder that begins at middle age and is marked by deterioration of mental capacity (**dementia**). This disease is the fourth-leading cause of death in adults older than age 65 in the United States. The patient starts by showing loss of memory and impairment of judgment, comprehension, and intellect. Anxiety, depression, and emotional disturbances can occur as well. Over time, the person becomes totally dependent and unable to perform activities of daily living without assistance.

#### Clinical Considerations for Alzheimer's Disease

- Complete a thorough dental examination in the early stages of the disease. Dental treatment can be tolerated easily in the early stages.
- Pay special attention to prevention. Regular oral hygiene and the use of fluoride supplements and salivary substitutes are important in preserving dental health.
- In advanced stages of the disease, many patients are not able to tolerate dentures.
- Patients may experience xerostomia, which is caused by prescribed psychoactive drugs.
- Dental visits should be scheduled with an awareness of the patient's best time of day.
- The presence of a familiar caregiver, such as a family member, in the treatment room often eases the patient's fear.

### Seizures

Seizure disorders are a symptom of brain damage that causes abnormal electrical brain activity, which can manifest in several ways. A patient with a history of **seizures** can have an abrupt suspension of motor, sensory, behavioral, or bodily function at any time. Patients who have a seizure disorder may be receiving antiepileptic medication such as Dilantin, which may cause increased bleeding tendencies, drowsiness, lack of coordination, drug-induced gingival overgrowth, and xerostomia.

**Epilepsy** is a neurologic disorder characterized by clusters of nerve cells, or neurons in the brain, that signal abnormally and cause recurrent episodes of seizures. In most patients, epileptic seizures are controlled with medication; however, under stressful conditions, a seizure may still occur.

There are many different types of seizures. Generally, seizures are categorized based on what part of the brain is involved in a seizure. People might experience one type or more than one type of seizure. There are four main categories of seizures:

- *Generalized seizures,* having been referred to *grand mal seizures,* affect the entire brain.
- *Partial seizures,* having been referred to *petit mal seizures,* affect a part of the brain. A person experiencing a partial seizure will often stay awake and aware throughout the seizure; however, although the person knows what is happening, he or she may be unable to speak and/or move until the seizure is over.
- *Nonepileptic seizures* are not related to epilepsy but are caused by other things, such as diabetes, a high fever, or some other cause.
- *Status epilepticus* is a continuing seizure and one of the few reasons emergency personnel should be contacted.

## Types of Generalized Seizures

- **Absence seizures** may cause the person to appear to be staring into space with or without slight twitching of the muscles.
- **Tonic seizures** cause stiffening of muscles of the body, generally those in the back, legs, and arms.
- **Clonic seizures** cause repeated jerking movements of muscles on both sides of the body.
- **Myoclonic seizures** cause jerks or twitches of the upper body, arms, or legs.
- **Atonic seizures** cause a loss of normal muscle tone, which often leads the affected person to fall down or drop the head involuntarily.
- **Tonic-clonic seizures** cause a combination of symptoms, including stiffening of the body and repeated jerks of the arms and/or legs, as well as loss of consciousness.

## Clinical Considerations for Seizures

- Be aware of trigger factors.
- Be aware of the presence of an aura.
- Sedation may help to prevent a seizure during a stressful dental visit.
- Staff should be prepared to handle an emergency.
- Severe cases may require treatment under general anesthesia.
- Maintain oral hygiene.
- Before treatment, question patients about (1) skipping medications or meals, (2) stress and fatigue, (3) pain, and (4) alcohol consumption.

### Multiple Sclerosis

Multiple sclerosis is one of the most common neurologic disorders that affects adults between the ages of 30 and 50. As the disorder advances, the patient experiences progressive weakening of the lower extremities, causing muscle weakness, unsteady gait, and paralysis. In the treatment of patients with multiple sclerosis, adrenal suppressants such as prednisone and muscle relaxants such as diazepam may be prescribed to control muscle spasms.

## Clinical Considerations for Multiple Sclerosis

- Schedule shorter appointments.
- Patient may have to be transferred from wheelchair to dental chair.
- Patient may have difficulty in localizing intraoral pain and discomfort.
- Some patients develop trigeminal neuralgia.
- Respiratory problems may be caused by the effect of the disease on the muscles that control breathing. A rubber dam may be useful only if the patient is able to breathe through the nose.
- Do not position the patient in a supine position (to protect airway); 45 degrees is better.
- Sedation may be required before treatment is provided.

### Cerebrovascular Accident

A patient who has had a cerebrovascular accident (CVA), or **stroke**, has experienced minor to severe loss of central nervous system function caused by a sudden vascular lesion of the brain. This can be attributed to hemorrhage, embolism, thrombosis, or ruptured aneurysm (Fig. 29.9). The clinical presentation of a patient can vary, depending on the area and extent of injury to the brain. The patient may have unilateral weakness or paralysis of the eyes and facial muscles, as well as slurring or loss of speech. Numbness, vertigo, visual disturbances, sweating, headache, and nausea can often be present.

## Clinical Considerations for a Patient with History of Stroke

- Schedule for the midmorning, with an average of 10 minutes added to the appointment for additional communication and explanation of instructions.
- Modified oral hygiene aids may have to be introduced.

6 What is dementia?
7 What adverse effects can occur as the result of taking Dilantin?
8 What is another term for cerebrovascular accident?
9 What are two examples of neurologic disorders?

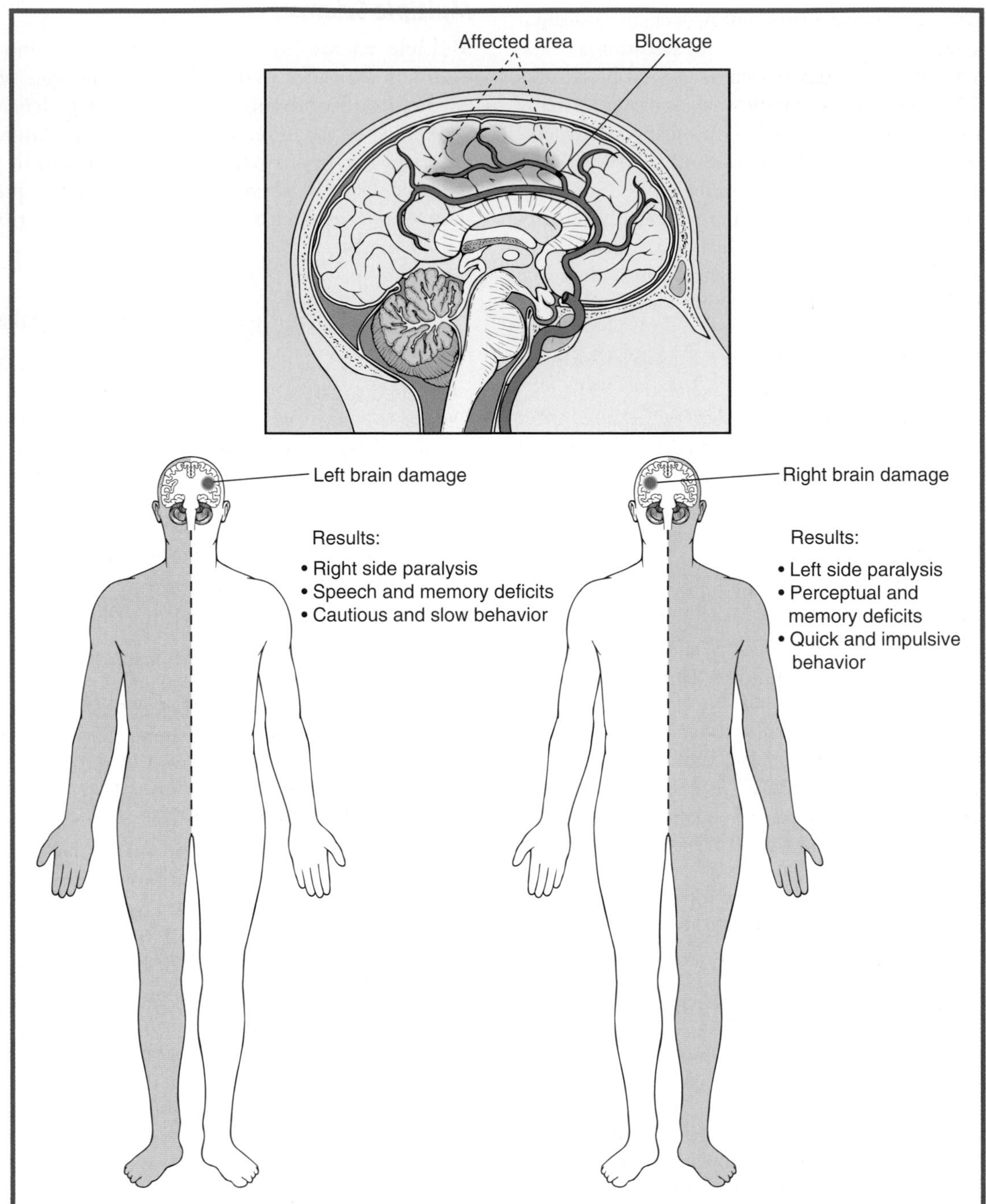


**FIG. 29.9** Effects of a cerebrovascular accident (stroke). *(From Frasier MS, Drzymkowski J: Essentials of human disease and conditions, ed 6, St Louis, 2016, Elsevier.)*

## Neuromuscular Disorders

Neuromuscular disorders affect the nerves that control your voluntary muscles. Voluntary muscles are the ones you can control, such as those in your arms and legs. Your nerve cells, also called neurons, send messages that control these muscles. When neurons become unhealthy or die, communication between your nervous system and muscles breaks down. As a result, your muscles weaken and waste away. Weakness can lead to twitching, cramps, aches and pains, and joint and movement problems. Sometimes it also affects heart function and your ability to breathe. The neuromuscular disorders listed involve the same type of clinical considerations needed when treating this type of patient.

### Clinical Considerations for Neuromuscular Disorders

- Patients require short appointments.
- A patient may have to be transferred from wheelchair to dental chair.

- A dental dam may be useful if the patient is able to breathe through the nose.
- Do not place patient in a supine position (to protect airway), but the patient can be placed at 45 degrees.
- Nitrous oxide, sedation, and general anesthesia should be avoided because of impaired pulmonary (breathing) function.

### Muscular Dystrophy

Muscular dystrophy is a group of diseases characterized by progressive **atrophy** and weakness of the skeletal muscles with increasing disability and deformity. The muscle fibers degenerate and are replaced by fatty and fibrous tissue. This disease is eventually fatal because of the onset of infectious and respiratory diseases, as well as pulmonary dysfunction. Atrophy of the muscles involved in respiration reduces the vital capacity of the lungs and interferes with the ability to cough.

### Parkinson's Disease

Parkinson's disease (PD) is a motor system disorder that is the result of loss of dopamine-producing brain cells. The four primary symptoms of PD are tremor, or trembling in hands, arms, legs, jaw, and face; rigidity, or stiffness of the limbs and trunk; slowness of movement; and impaired balance and coordination. As these symptoms become more pronounced, patients may have difficulty walking, talking, or completing other simple tasks. PD usually affects people older than age 50.

### Cerebral Palsy

Cerebral palsy is a group of nonprogressive neuromuscular disorders caused by brain damage (usually resulting from anoxia) sustained during the prenatal or perinatal period or during infancy. This condition affects 1 to 4 individuals in 1000 live births.

### Amyotrophic Lateral Sclerosis

Commonly referred to as Lou Gehrig's disease, amyotrophic lateral sclerosis (ALS) is a degenerative nervous system disease that causes loss of motor neurons in the cerebral cortex, brainstem, and spinal cord, resulting in muscular atrophy, weakness, and spasticity. The disease is progressive, with patient survival of 3 to 5 years or less. The origin is unknown, and no cure is known.

### Arthritis

There are several types of **arthritis**, but the two most commonly seen in the dental office are **rheumatoid arthritis** (RA) and osteoarthritis.

**RHEUMATOID ARTHRITIS.** RA is a chronic disease that causes pain, stiffness, swelling, and loss of function in the joints. It occurs when the immune system, the system that protects the body from outside harm, mistakenly starts attacking healthy tissue. This causes inflammation that leads

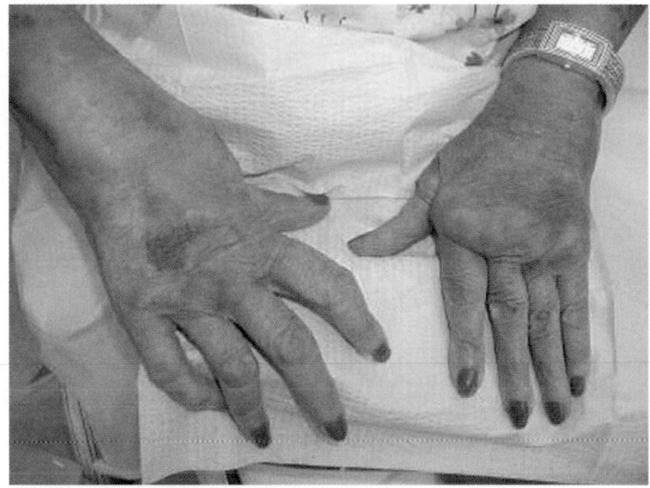

FIG. 29.10 Effects of rheumatoid arthritis on the body. *(Courtesy Kathleen Muzzin and Bobi Robles, Dallas, TX.)*

to swelling in the joints, making them progressively less mobile (Fig. 29.10). If not managed properly, over time RA can cause joint damage and can even result in permanent joint destruction.

**OSTEOARTHRITIS.** Older patients are likely to have chronic progressive arthritis with stiffening of joints called osteoarthritis. This disorder causes the joints to become inflamed and painful. Physicians prescribe aspirin and corticosteroids to reduce the symptoms of arthritis.

#### Clinical Considerations for Arthritis

- Schedule patients with arthritis in the morning, and keep appointments short.
- The disease can limit the patient's ability to hold and use a toothbrush. Modified oral hygiene aids may have to be introduced.
- Arthritis of the jaw joints limits the patient's ability to open the mouth or chew comfortably.

## Cardiovascular Disorders

It is estimated that 20 million Americans today have some form of cardiovascular disease. Heart disease continues to be one of the most serious threats to the health of an individual; it is the leading cause of death among men over age 40 and among women over age 65. Heart disease can manifest in many ways, such as hypertension, stable or unstable angina, congestive heart failure, and **myocardial infarction**. The dentist initiates communication with the patient's cardiologist and acquires a background on how the patient's heart disease is being managed and what medications the patient is taking.

The cardiovascular disorders listed involve the similar types of clinical considerations needed when treating this type of patient.

### Clinical Considerations for Cardiovascular Disorders

- Avoid stressful, lengthy appointments.
- Assess vital signs before treatment; consider monitoring throughout the procedure.
- The dentist may use psychotropic premedication and nitrous oxide to help relieve stress.
- Consider the use of supplemental oxygen throughout the procedure.
- The dentist may consult with the patient's cardiologist about the use of prophylactic sublingual nitroglycerin immediately before treatment.
- Epinephrine and other vasoconstrictors can be administered within limits to patients with mild to moderate cardiovascular disease.
- Seated patients are more comfortable in a semisupine rather than a supine position.

### *Congestive Heart Failure*

Congestive heart failure is a condition in which the heart cannot pump enough blood to the body's other organs. People with heart failure cannot exert themselves because they become short of breath and tired. This lack of circulation throughout the body can result from any of the following: narrowed arteries, scar tissue from a past heart attack that interferes with function of the heart muscle, high blood pressure, heart valve disease, heart defect, or infection of the heart valve or muscle (endocarditis or myocarditis).

### *Hypertension*

Also referred to as *high blood pressure,* hypertension is the result of the heart's having to work harder as it pumps against resistance such as that provided by a blocked artery (Fig. 29.11). According to the American Heart Association, about **80 million U.S. adults** have been diagnosed with high blood pressure. Age, heredity, smoking, obesity, and stress are considered to be contributing factors in the disease.

Most patients with a diagnosis of hypertension are on a program of drug therapy to help relieve the high blood pressure. In addition, patients are instructed to limit salt intake, follow a particular diet, increase their exercise regimen, and reduce stress in their lives.

### *Angina*

Angina pectoris is a coronary disease in which a decrease in blood supply to the heart muscle causes a sharp pain in the chest. **Angina** can be "stable," in which case the pain is usually predictable, or "unstable," in which case the pain is unpredictable. Patients in whom angina has been diagnosed usually also have been given a diagnosis of coronary atherosclerotic heart disease. Angina is a sign that a patient is at risk for a heart attack.

Patients with a history of angina pectoris should be on a program of drug therapy, exercise, weight control, salt restriction, and smoking cessation.

### *Endocarditis*

Cardiac disease and prosthetic replacements convey an increased risk for bacteria to be carried in the blood system (**bacteremia**); this is called **endocarditis**. Infective endocarditis is a severe infection of the cardiac valves and supporting structures that is caused by blood-borne pathogens that gain entry to the bloodstream from such places as the mouth and the gastrointestinal tract. Refer to Chapter 30 for information on the use of antibiotic therapy if a patient requires premedication.

RECALL

**10** What is the leading cause of death of men over 40 and women over 65 in the United States?
**11** Is epinephrine recommended for use in patients with heart disease?
**12** Provide another term for hypertension.

## Pulmonary Disorders

Pulmonary disorders affect the lungs and are characterized by airway obstruction. Patients can be diagnosed with a pulmonary disorder with symptoms from several disease categories.

### *Allergies*

It is estimated that one in every four individuals is allergic to something. An allergy is a condition in which the body reacts to an antigen. Common antigens include dust, mites, pollen, animal dander, food, and drugs. Most reactions can be managed by having the patient take an over-the-counter medication or a prescribed medication that reduces the symptoms of the allergy. If the reaction goes beyond this type of management, the allergy becomes a life-threatening emergency (see Chapter 31).

### Clinical Considerations for Allergies

- Complete a thorough medical history to determine specific allergens.
- Pay special attention to latex and dental material use.
- Have epinephrine stick available for possible emergency.

### *Bronchial Asthma*

Asthma is a chronic lung disease that inflames and narrows the airways. Asthma causes recurring periods of wheezing, chest tightness, shortness of breath, and coughing. Coughing often occurs at night or early in the morning. Bronchial **asthma** often arises from allergies and is characterized by an increased hypersensitivity to various stimuli, resulting in bronchial edema and widespread narrowing of the bronchial airways.

The disease affects people of all ages, but it most often starts in childhood. In the United States more than 22 million people are known to have asthma. Nearly 6 million of these people are children.

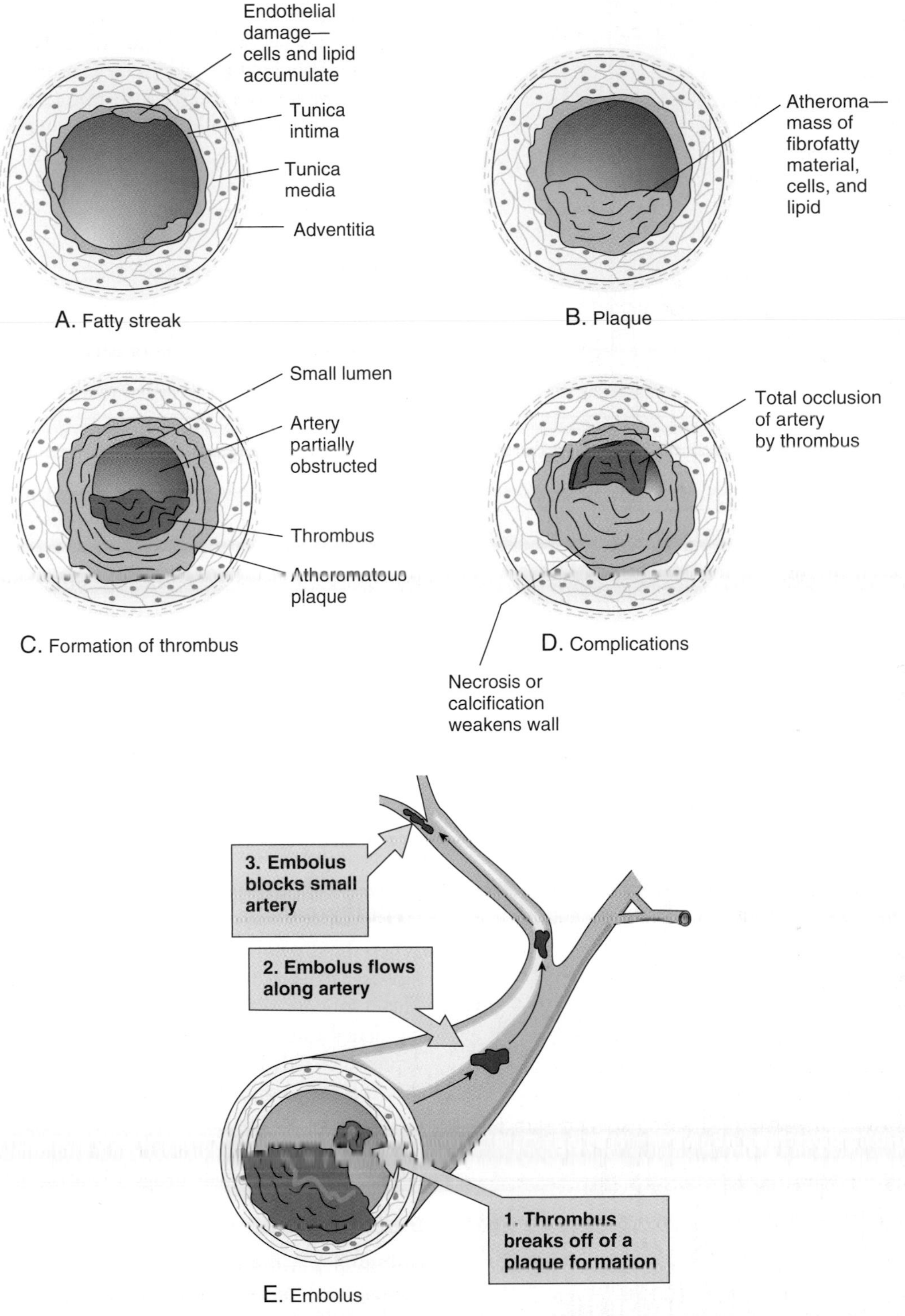


**FIG. 29.11** Effects of increased blood pressure. *(From Gould BA: Pathophysiology for the health professions, ed 5, St Louis, 2015, Saunders.)*

## Clinical Considerations for Bronchial Asthma

- Every effort should be made to minimize stress.
- It is best to schedule short appointments and to use sedation techniques.
- The use of epinephrine and aspirin should be minimized. Epinephrine can enhance the adverse effects of bronchodilators, and aspirin may cause a laryngospasm or attack.

### Chronic Obstructive Pulmonary Disease

Chronic obstructive pulmonary disease (COPD) is a general term for pulmonary diseases characterized by blocked airflow during respiration. Chronic **bronchitis** and **emphysema** are the two most common diseases classified as COPD.

*Chronic bronchitis* is a disorder that results in irreversible narrowing of the bronchial airways caused by chronic

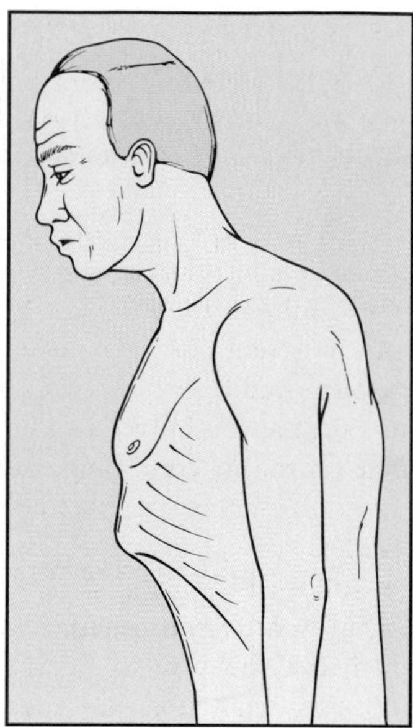

**FIG. 29.12** Appearance of a patient with chronic obstructive pulmonary disease (COPD). *(From Frasier MS, Drzymkowski J: Essentials of human disease and condition, ed 6, St Louis, 2016, Elsevier.)*

inflammation, increased production of mucus, edema of the bronchial mucosa, and reduced ciliary activity (Fig. 29.12).

*Emphysema* is the irreversible enlargement of the size of the air spaces that results in labored breathing and an increased susceptibility to infection. This interferes with expiration, and the lungs become overinflated as a result of the trapping of air.

### Clinical Considerations for COPD

- Minimize stress by keeping appointments short and scheduling them in the morning.
- Consider using sedation techniques in low-risk to moderate-risk patients.
- Consider using humidified oxygen given by nasal cannula.
- Avoid the use of nitrous oxide.
- Do not treat patients in a fully reclined chair.
- Avoid anticholinergic drugs, which dry bronchial secretions.
- Do not schedule elective treatment during hot and humid weather.

**13** What organs of the body do pulmonary disorders affect?

**14** What does the abbreviation COPD stand for?

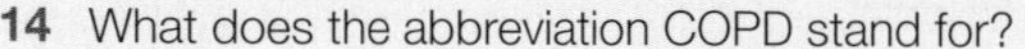

## Blood Disorders

Blood disorders can involve cellular elements of the body. The bone marrow can be susceptible to malignant cells, which can cause tumors of the bone marrow. **Anemia** is a condition that develops when your blood lacks enough healthy red blood cells or hemoglobin. An excessive increase in white blood cells may indicate infection or **leukemia**. Excessive bleeding caused by congenital lack of a protein substance necessary for blood clotting can occur in patients with **hemophilia**.

### Clinical Considerations for Blood Disorders

- The important factor for patients with a blood disorder is their *susceptibility to bacterial infection.*
- Treatment modifications have to be made for any surgical procedure.
- Antibiotic prophylaxis may need to be prescribed for high-risk procedures.

## Endocrine Disorders

The endocrine system is composed of glands located in many different regions of the body, all of which release hormones into the bloodstream. The *thyroid gland* regulates metabolism in body cells and stimulates passage of calcium into the bones from the blood.

### Hyperthyroidism

A patient with an overactive thyroid gland has *Graves' disease,* the most common form of **hyperthyroidism**. This disorder affects women 4 to 7 times more often than men. The average age of onset is before 40. Infection, physical or emotional stress, trauma, pain, or surgery may precipitate a *hyperthyroid crisis,* which can be fatal.

### Clinical Considerations for Hyperthyroidism

- An accurate and current patient history and medical consultation are essential.
- Hyperthyroid patients who are not being treated are highly sensitive to epinephrine and other amine anesthetics.

### Hypothyroidism

When the thyroid gland is underactive and produces fewer hormones than usual, the patient is diagnosed with **hypothyroidism**. These patients are not in any danger associated with receiving dental care. Patients with mild hypothyroidism can receive depressants, sedatives, or narcotic analgesics before treatment, but they may show signs of an exaggerated response to these drugs. Patients who are not under a physician's care may be sensitive to narcotic analgesics, barbiturates, and tranquilizers because of the depressant effects of these drugs on the central nervous system.

### Diabetes Mellitus

**Diabetes** is a disorder of the metabolism, the way the body uses digested food for energy. With the help of a hormone called insulin, cells throughout the body absorb glucose and use it for energy. Diabetes develops when the body does not make enough insulin or is not able to use insulin effectively, in which blood glucose (a type of sugar in the blood) levels become too high.

The disease is classified in two categories:

- **Type 1 diabetes**, previously known as juvenile diabetes, is usually diagnosed in children and young adults. The body does not make insulin and the patient is insulin dependent.
- **Type 2 diabetes** was previously known as adult-onset diabetes as it was commonly diagnosed in adults. Because of an

increase in obesity in children, type 2 diabetes is increasing in children and young adults. The patient is treated with lifestyle changes, oral medications (pills), and possibly insulin.

When the balance shifts, with too much or too little food ingested, insulin levels change, resulting in **hyperglycemia** (too much blood sugar) or **hypoglycemia** (too little blood sugar).

Hyperglycemia is a condition where there is an abnormal increase in the glucose (sugar) level in the blood. (*Hyperglycemia* means blood sugar that is abnormally high.) If untreated, hyperglycemia may progress to diabetic ketoacidosis and a life-threatening diabetic coma.

Hypoglycemia, also known as *insulin shock,* is an abnormal decrease in glucose level in the blood. (*Hypoglycemia* means blood sugar that is abnormally low.) Hypoglycemia can manifest itself rapidly. The most common causes of hypoglycemia are missing a meal, taking an overdose of insulin without adequate food intake, and exercising excessively without appropriate adjustment of insulin and food intake.

### Clinical Considerations for Diabetes Mellitus

- Minimize stress by keeping appointments short and scheduling them in the midmorning.
- Use sedation techniques such as administration of nitrous oxide or oral diazepam.
- Instruct patient to maintain normal dietary intake before dental appointments; the most common cause of hypoglycemia is failure to eat.
- Minimize the risk for infection.

RECALL

**15** What disorder is associated with an overactive thyroid gland?

**16** What treatment is prescribed for a patient with type 2 diabetes?

## Behavioral and Psychiatric Disorders

Biologic, genetic, psychological, and social components can contribute to many types of behavioral and mental disorders. Psychiatric disorders can affect the treatment of dental patients because of the drugs prescribed, which influence the function of the brain. The disorders listed include the same types of clinical consideration when treating this type of patient.

*Anxiety* is a feeling that "all is not well," including a sense of impending disaster. Treatment may involve counseling, stress reduction therapy, and antianxiety medications.

*Depression* is a condition of general emotional rejection and withdrawal. The disorder may lead to a lack of interest in personal hygiene. Patients with depression are most often treated with antidepressant agents.

*Eating disorders* are marked by extremes. These are present when a person experiences severe disturbances in eating behavior, such as extreme reduction of food intake or extreme overeating, or feelings of extreme distress or concern about body weight or shape. Chapters 16 and 17 provide additional information regarding nutritional and pathologic aspects of these disorders.

*Anorexia nervosa* is a serious, potentially life-threatening eating disorder characterized by self-starvation and excessive weight loss.

*Binge eating disorder* is a type of eating disorder characterized by recurrent binge eating without the regular use of compensatory measures to counter the binge eating.

*Bulimia nervosa* is a serious, potentially life-threatening eating disorder characterized by a cycle of bingeing and compensatory behaviors such as self-induced vomiting designed to undo or compensate for the effects of binge eating.

*Bipolar disorder* is also known as manic-depressive disorder. The patient suffers from alternating, prolonged episodes of extreme elation followed by depression. Periods of mania are characterized by hyperactivity involving excessive participation in multiple activities; this is unrecognized by the patient. Speech is often pressured, loud, rapid, theatrical, dramatic, and difficult to interpret, with abrupt changes in topics.

*Substance abuse* with alcoholism and drug dependence is a serious problem in the United States. Chemical dependency is a chronic progressive disease that can affect all aspects of a person's life.

*Posttraumatic stress disorder* is characterized by the "reexperiencing" of a psychologically traumatic event. It is most commonly associated with veterans of war. It can also be seen in patients who experience trauma such as natural disasters, airplane crashes, and rape. The traumatic event is experienced as recurring disruptive intrusive thoughts of past experiences and nightmares.

*Schizophrenia* is a psychotic disorder characterized by varying degrees of personality disorganization. The individual's thought processes are disrupted by bizarre delusions and perceptual disturbances such as hallucinations. This decreases the individual's ability to communicate and work with others. Therefore routine daily functions such as work, social relationships, and self-care are impaired. The therapy of choice involves antipsychotic agents and phenothiazines.

### Clinical Considerations for Behavioral and Psychiatric Disorders

- Understand that xerostomia may result from the psychoactive drugs prescribed.
- Regular hygiene and the use of fluoride supplements and salivary substitutes are important for preserving dental health.
- Patient cooperation and informed consent may cause problems, particularly in the patient with anxiety.

**Legal and Ethical Implications** All patients, whether healthy or diagnosed with a compromising medical or physical condition, have the right to know about treatment plans and available alternative procedures. Patients have rights regarding privacy of personal and medical information and informed consent. The dentist is accountable for obtaining a physical and medical background on every patient, and then presenting the method of treatment that would best suit a patient with a medical or compromising condition. ■

■ **Eye to the Future** The use of adult stem cells in research and therapy is not as controversial as embryonic stem cells because the production of adult stem cells does not require the destruction of an embryo. Official licensed clinics today throughout the world are treating patients with their own adult stem cells. They extract and select stem cell material for self-treatment. They are already focusing on therapy for diabetes, stroke, spinal injury, multiple sclerosis, Parkinson's disease, and Alzheimer's disease, as well as arthritis, heart disease, and eye disease. ■

## ■ Critical Thinking

1. One of your patients, Ms. Smith, has submitted an updated health history, and you notice that she has checked "Yes" for recently being diagnosed with a blood disorder. When you ask her about this, Ms. Smith tells you that tests showed she was positive for leukemia. What is one of your main considerations regarding how Ms. Smith will now be treated in the dental office?
2. Mr. Jones, a patient of the practice, has diabetes but does not take insulin. How would Mr. Jones' type of diabetes be classified? What dental considerations might apply to Mr. Jones?
3. You are preparing Mrs. Rodriguez for a dental procedure when she mentions that pollen has been bothering her lately. You review her medical-dental history and notice that she has asthma. What type of drugs should be minimized for an asthmatic patient such as Mrs. Rodriguez?
4. Describe three ways to help treat a patient with coronary artery disease in the dental office.
5. Describe your thoughts and personal experiences about working with a medically or physically compromised patient. ■

PROCEDURE 29.1

# Transferring a Patient from a Wheelchair

### EQUIPMENT

- ✓ Gait belt

### PROCEDURAL STEPS

1 Clear all items from the pathway of the wheelchair to the dental chair.

2 When entering the treatment room, determine whether it is best to go forward or to back the patient into the area.

**PURPOSE** You want the patient to be positioned the same way he or she would be seated in the dental chair.

3 Move the wheelchair as close to the dental chair as possible so that it is at a 45-degree angle to the dental chair.

**PURPOSE** Allows the patient to move closer to the chair without having to pivot as much.

4 Lock the wheelchair, and raise the footrests.

5 Ask the patient to scoot forward in the wheelchair so a gait belt can be placed around the waist. Make sure the belt is positioned over the clothing and that the clip is in front. This will allow for easier belt adjustments and removal. Bring the patient to the edge of the wheelchair if possible.

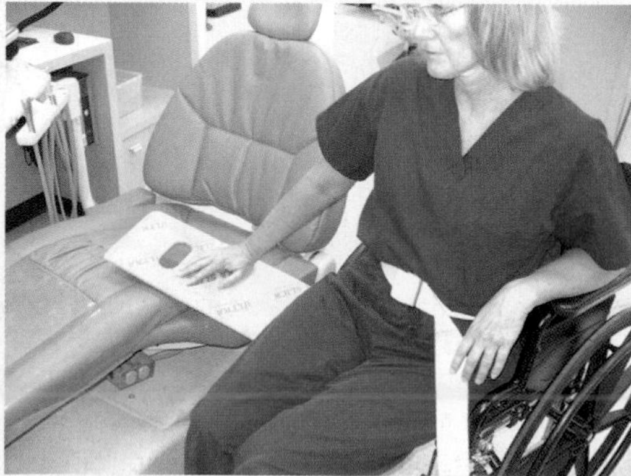

6 Ask the patient to slide forward to the edge of the wheelchair seat, making sure the patient's feet are placed flat on the floor.

7 Stand facing the patient with your feet slightly apart and knees bent.

8 Place your fingers between the gait belt and the patient, using an underhand motion to grasp the gait belt. Ask the patient to stand as you lift him or her with the belt and guide the patient to the transfer location.

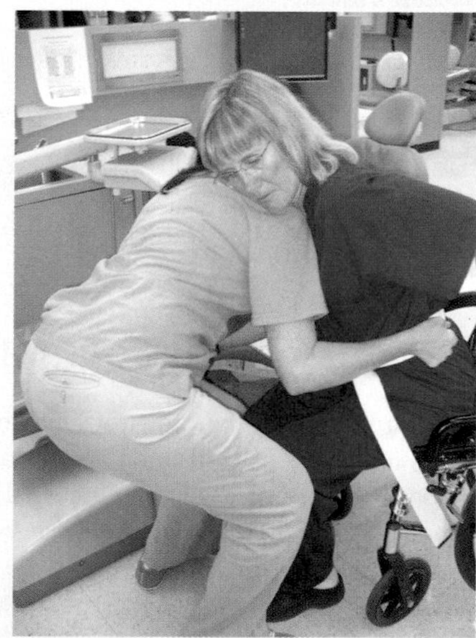

9 Help the patient stand slowly.

10 Pivot the patient so that the patient's backside is where the patient should be seated in the dental chair.

11 Help the patient to safely sit down. Ask the patient to slide back a bit, so not in danger of falling from the seated location. Once the patient is safely seated on the transfer location, remove the gait belt.

12 Swing the patient's legs over and onto the dental chair.

Photos courtesy Kathleen Muzzin and Bobi Robles, Dallas, TX.

30

# Principles of Pharmacology

## KEY TERMS

**Absorption** Process by which the body takes in or receives (absorbs) a drug.
**Distribution** Action by which a drug is released throughout the body.
**Dosage** Amount of drug to be administered in a specific time, often according to body weight.
**Dose** A specified quantity of a drug or medicine.
**Drug** A substance used in the diagnosis, treatment, or prevention of a disease.
**Ethical drug** A drug that requires a prescription.
**Excretion (ek-SKREE-shun)** Action by which a drug leaves the body.
**Generic (jeh-NAIR-ik)** Drug sold without a brand name or trademark.
**Inscription** The name and quantity of a drug listed on the prescription.
**Metabolism (me-TAB-eh-liz-um)** Physical and chemical processes that occur within a living cell or organism and are necessary for the maintenance of life.
**Patent medicine** Drug that can be obtained without a prescription; also called *over-the-counter drug.*
**Pharmacology** A branch of medicine concerned with the uses, effects, and actions of drugs.
**Prescription** A written order for a specific drug.
**Prophylaxis (pro-fah-LAK-sus)** Administration of drugs to prevent disease or protect a patient.
**Signature** Instructions on a prescription explaining how to take a specific medicine.
**Subscription** Directions to the pharmacist for mixing the medication; this is seldom done by the pharmacist anymore.
**Superscription** The patient's name, address, date, and Rx symbol on a prescription.
**Systemic (sis-TE-mik)** Referring to a drug that affects a specific system (or multiple systems) of the body.

## LEARNING OUTCOMES

*On completion of this chapter, the student will be able to achieve the following objectives:*

1 Pronounce, define, and spell the key terms.
2 Differentiate between a drug's chemical, generic, and brand or trade names.
3 Discuss the dispensing of drugs, including the following:
- Define the DEA, and explain why drugs are categorized in five schedules of the Controlled Substances Act.
- List each part of a prescription.

4 Describe the use of drug reference materials.
5 Describe relevant factors in determining the dosage of a drug, how medications are administered, and the stages a drug goes through in the body.
6 List the commonly prescribed drugs in dentistry.
7 List the commonly prescribed drugs in medicine.
8 Describe the negative effects of drug use.

## ELECTRONIC RESOURCES

e ***Additional information related to content in Chapter 30 can be found on the companion Evolve Web site.***

- Practice Quiz

**Pharmacology** is the science or branch of medicine that includes the research, development, and manufacture of drugs. A **drug** is a substance that can be taken for the prevention, diagnosis, and treatment of a disease. All drugs must be recognized and defined by the U.S. Food, Drug, and Cosmetic Act before they can be marketed for public use in the United States.

A vast variety of drugs are available on the market, and each drug produces a different effect. The most probable situations where the dental assistant will be required to identify drug types include (1) when reviewing a patient's medication history; (2) when assisting in dental procedures that require premedication; (3) when assisting in a specific dental procedure for which pain control is required; and (4) when assisting in a medical emergency.

Your role in understanding pharmacology is to become familiar with the drugs used in dentistry, the drugs your patients are taking for a specific medical condition, the terminology and use of prescriptions, and the drug reference materials that are available.

## Overview of Drugs

Drugs are derived from many sources. *Organic* drugs are derived from living organisms such as plants or animals, and *inorganic* drugs are synthesized in the laboratory or extracted from inorganic compounds. Most drugs today are derived from a chemical source, which makes them purer in form than those derived from an original natural source that may be contaminated or polluted. The manufacturing of drugs takes place in a pharmaceutical laboratory.

A drug can be identified by three names:

1. **Chemical name** is the atomic or molecular structure of the drug. *N*-(4-hydroxyphenyl) acetamid is the chemical formula for acetaminophen.
2. **Generic name** is the shorthand version of the drug's chemical name, structure, or formula, which may be used by any company; acetaminophen is an example of a generic name.
3. **Brand name,** or **trade name,** is controlled by a pharmaceutical company as a registered trademark; for example, Tylenol is the brand name for acetaminophen.

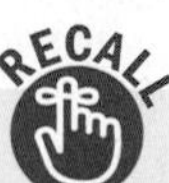


1 Identify three sources of drugs.
2 What type of drug name is Motrin?

## Dispensing of Drugs

Drugs are classified into two categories according to the way an individual can purchase them: patent medicines and prescription drugs. **Patent medicines** are drugs that can be obtained without a prescription; these are also referred to as *over-the-counter (OTC) drugs.* The U.S. Food and Drug Administration (FDA) regulates the sale of patent medicines and evaluates their safety and effectiveness for daily use. *Prescription drugs,* also termed **ethical drugs**, are licensed medicines that are regulated by legislation; a prescription is required before they can be obtained from a pharmacist. An understanding of the term *ethical* is important in that these types of drugs can be harmful to the patient if they are not used correctly (i.e., it would not be ethical to prescribe or supply these drugs improperly). A patient who is taking a prescribed drug must be under the guidance of a physician or dentist.

## Controlled Substances Act

The drugs and drug products covered under the *Federal Comprehensive Drug Abuse Prevention and Control Act* are divided into five schedules. The drugs included in this Act, also referred to as *schedule drugs,* are classified on the basis of their potential for abuse, their medical usefulness, and the extent to which they may lead to physical and psychological dependence.

Each level of control has specific requirements for ordering, storing, prescribing, dispensing, and destroying the scheduled drugs within its definition. Many individual states have their own controlled substances acts, which are patterned after the federal law. Some state laws are more restrictive, but none may be less restrictive than the federal law. The dentist must comply with the provisions of the federal law and those of the state, province, or territory in which he or she practices (always following the most restrictive guidelines when the laws differ). Under these laws, any professional who is authorized to prescribe these medications is issued a federal Drug Enforcement Agency (DEA) identification number, which is to be printed on the dentist's prescription pad.

### Schedule I Drugs

Schedule I drugs have no current accepted medical usefulness and have a high potential for abuse. Normally, Schedule I drugs cannot be prescribed. Examples of substances listed in Schedule I include the following:

- Heroin (diacetylmorphine)
- LSD (lysergic acid diethylamide)
- Marijuana (cannabis, THC)
- Mescaline (Peyote)
- MDMA (ecstasy)
- GHB (gamma-hydroxybutyric acid)
- Methaqualone (Quaalude)

### Schedule II Drugs

Schedule II drugs have limited medical use, high risk for abuse, and high risk for physical or psychological dependence. Prescriptions for these drugs are only given in writing and cannot be renewed. Examples of Schedule II narcotics include the following:

- Vicodin
- Cocaine
- Methamphetamine
- Dolophine (Methadone)
- Hydromorphone (Dilaudid)
- Meperidine (Demerol)
- OxyContin (Percocet)
- Fentanyl
- Dexedrine
- Adderall
- Ritalin

### Schedule III Drugs

Schedule III drugs have less abuse potential than the drugs in Schedules I and II and also have accepted medical usefulness. Prescriptions for Schedule III drugs may be renewed. Examples of Schedule III narcotic drugs include a combination of products containing less than 15 milligrams of hydrocodone per dosage unit (Vicodin), products containing not more than 90 milligrams of codeine per dosage unit (Tylenol with Codeine), and buprenorphine (Suboxone).

Examples of Schedule III nonnarcotics include the following:

- Benzphetamine (Didrex)
- Phendimetrazine, ketamine
- Anabolic steroids such as Depo-Testosterone

### Schedule IV Drugs

Schedule IV drugs have low abuse potential and have accepted medical usefulness. Prescriptions for Schedule IV drugs may be renewed. A patient may have up to five refills of these drugs in a 6-month period. Examples of Schedule IV substances include the following:

- Alprazolam (Xanax)
- Carisoprodol (Soma)
- Clonazepam (Klonopin)
- Clorazepate (Tranxene)
- Diazepam (Valium)

- Lorazepam (Ativan)
- Midazolam (Versed)
- Temazepam (Restoril)
- Triazolam (Halcion)

### *Schedule V Drugs*

Schedule V drugs have the lowest abuse potential and have accepted medical usefulness. Some states do require that these drugs be dispensed only by prescription. Under federal law, however, they are available only under controlled circumstances. Examples of Schedule V drugs include cough medicines with codeine. With the misuse and illicit distribution of methamphetamine (pseudoephedrine), many states have passed a law requiring a prescription, or requiring customers to show a photo ID and sign a log book, before pharmacies can dispense any cold remedy containing pseudoephedrine.

## Prescriptions

A **prescription** is a written order provided by a physician or dentist for the preparation and administration of a medicine. Only a professional who is legally authorized to prescribe medications may write a prescription. A professional who is authorized to prescribe medications is issued a DEA identification number.

Under no circumstances can any member of the dental team prescribe medications, except the dentist. The dental assistant may dispense medicine according to explicit instructions and under direct supervision of the dentist.

### *Prescription Terminology*

Prescriptions are handwritten on a preprinted prescription form that is assembled into pads. Prescription pads are to be kept in a locked drawer and should never be visible or available to use as notepaper. Individual state laws regulate the format and information to be included on a prescription. There are many abbreviations that can be used in a prescription. Table 30.1 provides some of the common abbreviations used in dentistry.

For a prescription to be valid it must contain the following information (Fig. 30.1):

- Dentist's name, address, and phone number
- **Superscription**: patient's name, address, date, and the symbol from the Latin *recipe* (meaning "take")
- **Inscription**: main body of the prescription—name and quantity of the drug
- **Subscription**: directions to the pharmacist for mixing the medication (this is seldom done by the pharmacist anymore, so you do not see this routinely on a prescription)
- **Signature**: instructions for the patient on how to take the medicine, when to take it, and how much to take
- Dentist's signature
- Dentist's DEA number

### *Recording Prescriptions*

Each drug prescribed must be documented in the patient record. The dentist will write the prescription in duplicate so a copy can be retained for future reference.

**TABLE 30.1 Common Prescription Abbreviations**

| Abbreviation | Meaning |
|---|---|
| a.a. | of each |
| a.c. | before meals |
| a.m. | morning |
| b.i.d. | twice a day |
| disp. | dispense |
| H | hour |
| h.s. | at bedtime |
| NPO | nothing by mouth |
| p.c. | after meals |
| prn | as needed |
| q. | every |
| q.d. | once a day |
| q.i.d. | four times a day |
| SL | sublingual |
| t, tsp | teaspoon |
| T, tbs | tablespoon |
| t.i.d. | three times a day |

### *Telephone Guidelines*

The following guidelines apply to the dental assistant regarding telephone interaction with a pharmacy:

- Controlled substances cannot be prescribed over the phone. Under DEA law, for these substances—which include opioid pain medications and amphetamines—a written prescription must be presented to the pharmacist with a valid medical license number, DEA number, and signature, in order to be filled.
- It is illegal for a dental assistant to "call in" a prescription.
- When a pharmacist calls, notify the dentist immediately. Do not try to relay information between them.
- If the dentist is unable to come to the telephone, take the pharmacist's name and telephone number so the dentist can return the call.
- Never attempt to evaluate a patient's reaction to a drug. Only the dentist or pharmacist is qualified to evaluate drug effects.

RECALL

3 What type of scheduled drug is Tylenol with codeine?
4 What agency regulates how drugs are sold and how safe they are?
5 Who is allowed to write prescriptions in the dental office?
6 What part of the prescription includes the name and quantity of the drug?
7 What does the abbreviation b.i.d. mean?

## Drug Reference Materials

Because of constant change in the pharmaceutical industry, it is important that your dental office have several sources on hand

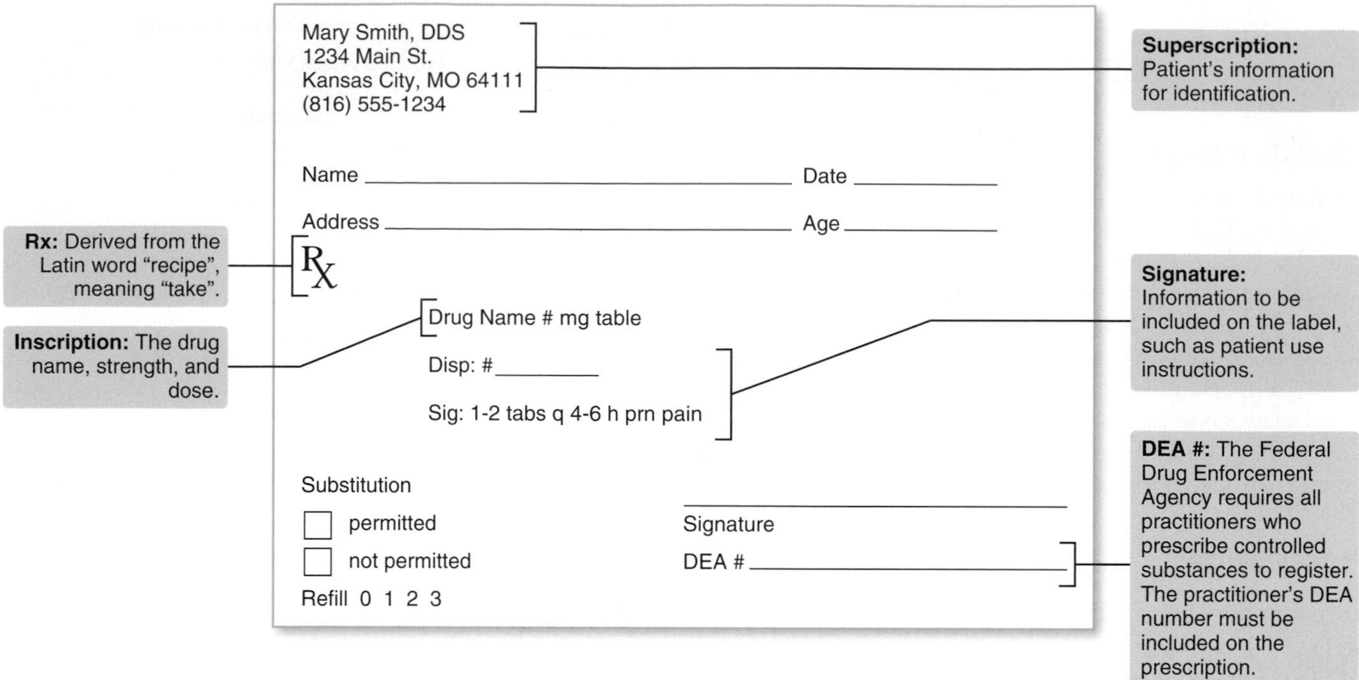


**FIG. 30.1** Example of a prescription pad. (© Elsevier Collection.)

for reference purposes. It is essential that a dental office stay up to date with its drug reference materials. Printed drug references such as the *Physicians' Desk Reference* and dental-specific sources such as Mosby's *Dental Drug Reference* are comprehensive. Drug reference information is also available electronically through software programs, which can be downloaded, allowing all staff to connect to the Internet for easy reference.

Pharmaceutical companies that visit the office to speak with the dentist are also a resource for acquiring the latest information on existing drugs or new agents that have gained approval from the FDA.

### Package Inserts

Every prescription filled by a pharmacist includes an insert, or information sheet, that describes the drug. Specific information commonly listed includes the following:

- How the drug will affect the body (e.g., relieve itchy, scratchy throat and eyes)
- For what condition the drug is being prescribed (e.g., allergies)
- Any adverse effects (e.g., drowsiness)
- Any adverse or long-term effects (e.g., possible liver damage)
- Special precautions to follow when taking the drug (e.g., do not drink alcohol)
- Contraindications to taking the drug (e.g., if taking blood pressure medication, consult physician)
- Dosage and route for the drug (e.g., take one tablet each day, orally)

## Drug Dosage

The amount of a drug that a patient takes is termed a **dose**. The manufacturer of the drug has calculated the exact time required for the drug to take effect and compiles the **dosage**, or the dose administered during a specified period. Specific factors must be considered when the dentist and pharmacy determine the dosage of a drug:

- Age of the patient, with this affecting newborns and the aged the most. This is because the person's body system may be immature or weakening.
- Weight of the patient has a direct relation to the effect of the medication.
- Time of day the drug is to be taken is important because the body's rhythm plays an important part in the effects of some drugs.
- Patient tolerance to the drug can take place, especially if the patient has taken a specific drug over a period of time.

## Administration of Medications

Drugs are manufactured in different forms, which include pills, capsules, liquids, drops, ointments, sprays, gases, and lotions (Table 30.2). The way a drug is administered determines how quickly or how slowly the drug will take effect. If a drug is applied directly to the site of use, it is considered a *local-action drug,* or simply a *local drug.* This type of drug affects only the specific area of the body to which it is applied. An example in the dental office would be topical anesthetic ointment, which is applied directly where the injection is to take place. If a drug is taken internally, it is considered a *systemic-action drug,* or simply a *systemic drug.* A **systemic** drug can affect the whole body by way of the circulatory system. An example is the antibiotic, which will eliminate an infection throughout the body when taken for the specified period.

## TABLE 30.2 Routes of Drug Administration

| Route of Drug | Description of Type | Photo |
|---|---|---|
| **Oral route** | Form of pills, tablets, capsules, or liquids | 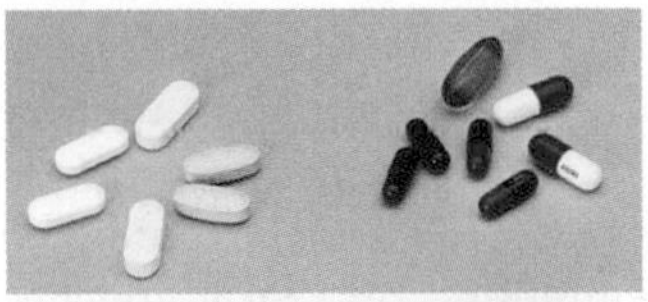 |
| **Topical route** | Application on the surface of the mucosa or skin | 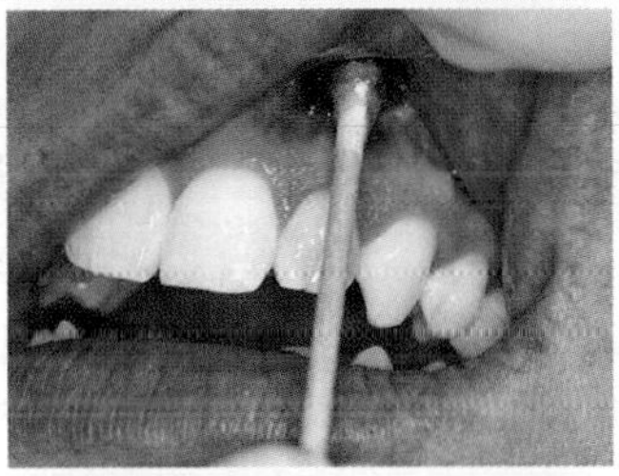 |
| **Transdermal route** | Through a patch that continuously releases a controlled quantity of a medication through the skin | 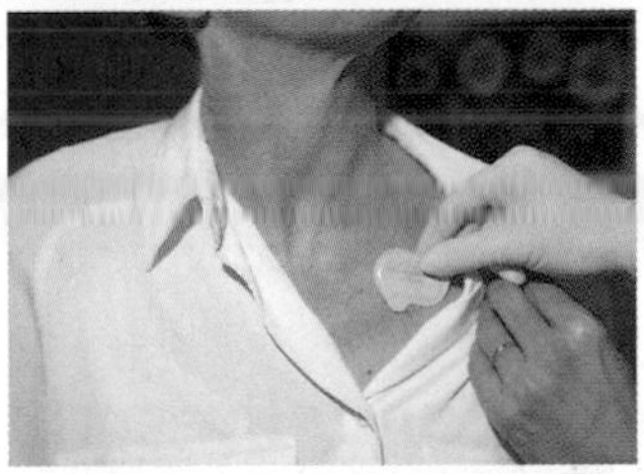 |
| **Inhalation route** | By breathing in a gaseous substance through the mouth, or inhaling an aerosol through the nose | 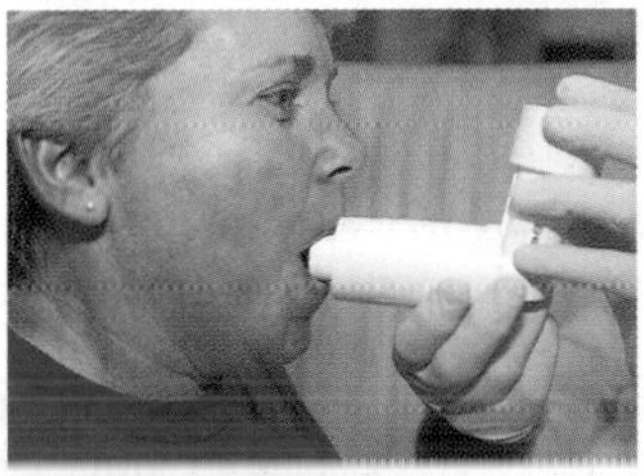 |
| **Sublingual route** | Placing medication under the tongue (absorption takes place through the oral mucosa) | 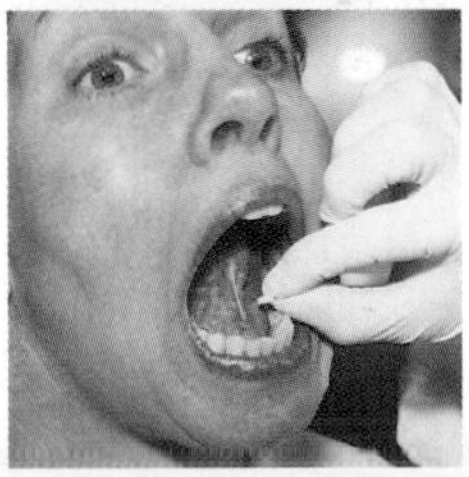 |
| **Injection route** | The type of drug determines how the injection is given: *subcutaneous*, directly under the skin; *intramuscular*, into a muscle; *intradermal*, into the skin | 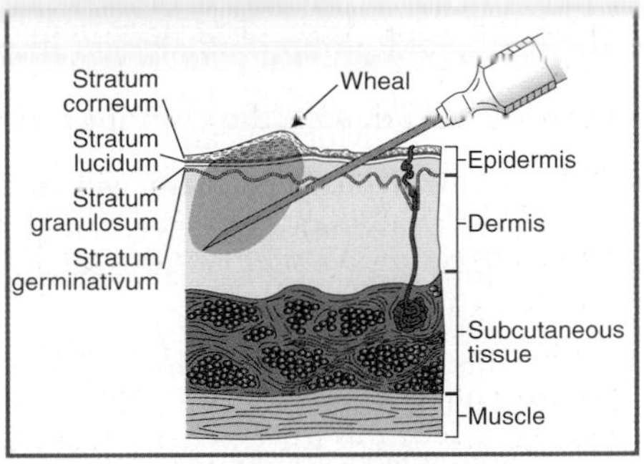 |

Oral and injection route figures from Proctor DB, et al: Kinn's the medical assistant: an applied learning approach, ed 13, St Louis, 2017, Elsevier. Topical route figure from Daniel SJ, Harfst SA, Wilder R: Mosby's dental hygiene: concepts, cases, and competencies, ed 2, St Louis, 2008, Mosby. Transdermal, inhalation, and sublingual route figures from Chester GA: Modern medical assisting, Philadelphia, 1998, Saunders.

## Stages of Drug Action in the Body

When a drug enters the body, it undergoes four stages:

1. **Absorption**: The drug is absorbed from the site of entry. (Sites of entry are described in Table 30.2.) The speed of absorption varies depending on the way a drug is administered. The slowest route of absorption is by mouth (orally).
2. **Distribution**: Once a drug has entered the bloodstream, the chemical compound of a drug attaches to proteins within the blood. It is then circulated throughout the body to be released and take effect where it is meant to act.
3. **Metabolism**: Once the chemical compound is released, the drug becomes metabolized and is then excreted through the liver or kidneys.
4. **Excretion**: The drug leaves the body by way of kidneys, liver, saliva, breast milk, and sweat.

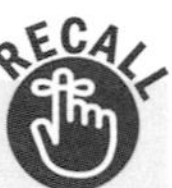


8 Where is a sublingual drug administered?
9 Where is a subcutaneous drug administered?
10 What is the slowest route of absorption for a drug?

# Drugs Commonly Prescribed in Dentistry

A series of drugs listed in this section are the types of drugs that would be routinely prescribed for patients by the dentist. The drugs that are prescribed in dentistry are to be taken by the patient before a clinical procedure, following a clinical procedure, or in relation to a condition that has affected the oral cavity.

## Analgesics

Analgesic medications are prescribed for the relief of acute pain, postoperative pain, and/or chronic pain. This type of drug lessens the sensory function of the brain by blocking pain receptors. Analgesic medications belong in two major categories: nonopioid and opioid.

The nonopioid group of analgesics includes the nonsteroidal anti-inflammatory drugs such as acetaminophen (Tylenol), ibuprofen (Advil, Motrin), and aspirin. This group is indicated for mild to moderate pain, which can include pain of dental origin, or for postoperative dental pain. It may also be prescribed for chronic oral-facial pain caused by an inflamed temporomandibular joint (TMJ). These drugs decrease the prostaglandin concentration, which raises the level of a person's pain threshold.

The opioid analgesics are prescribed for moderate to moderately severe pain. The most common type of drug prescribed is codeine. This type of drug is always prescribed as a combination preparation, meaning that codeine would be given in combination with aspirin, acetaminophen, or ibuprofen. It would be common for a dentist or surgeon to prescribe this after endodontic treatment or a surgical procedure.

## Antibiotics

An antibiotic can be classified as bactericidal or bacteriostatic. Bactericidal antibiotics such as penicillin directly kill an infecting organism; bacteriostatic antibiotics such as tetracycline and erythromycin inhibit the production of bacteria by interfering with their metabolic process, and the bacteria are then eliminated by the person's immune defense system. In most cases with antibiotics, the dentist will select an antibiotic that best combats a particular type of bacteria. For example, if the patient were diagnosed with an abscessed tooth, four to six different types of bacteria could be involved. An antibiotic would be selected to combat that type of bacteria.

Dental antibiotics come in a variety of forms, including gels, threadlike fibers, microspheres (tiny round particles), and mouth rinses. More than 100 different types of antibiotics are available; the following listed antibiotics are the most common types found in the dental setting:

- Penicillin is one of the most important antibiotics. It is derived from a number of penicillium molds commonly found on breads and fruits. It is one of the most effective and one of the least toxic of the antimicrobial agents used in dentistry. Amoxicillin (Amoxil) and ampicillin are examples.
- Cephalosporins consist of a group of antibiotics that are structurally and pharmacologically related to penicillin. Because cephalosporins are structurally similar to penicillins, some patients who are allergic to penicillin may be allergic to a cephalosporin drug. An example is a cephalosporin such as cephalexin (Keflex).
- Erythromycin is one of the drugs of choice when penicillin is contraindicated. Many patients cannot tolerate the nausea and stomach upset commonly associated with erythromycin, so the dentist may have to prescribe an alternative drug. Examples include macrolides such as erythromycin (E-Mycin), clarithromycin (Biaxin), and azithromycin (Zithromax).
- Chlorhexidine is an antibiotic that is used to control plaque and gingivitis in the mouth or in periodontal pockets. This medication is available as a mouth rinse and as a gelatin-filled chip that is placed in the deep gum pockets next to the teeth after root planing.
- Tetracyclines such as demeclocycline, doxycycline, minocycline, oxytetracycline, and tetracycline can be used in combination with surgery and other therapies, or may be given alone, to reduce or temporarily eliminate the bacteria associated with periodontal disease, to suppress the destruction of the tooth's attachment to the bone, or to reduce the pain and irritation of canker sores.

### *Antibiotic Prophylaxis*

Antibiotic **prophylaxis** is the prescribing of an antibiotic to a patient to prevent bacterial colonization. For many years, patients with certain heart conditions were prescribed an antibiotic to be taken before their dental treatment. It was believed that the antibiotic would prevent infective endocarditis.

In 2008 the American Heart Association updated its recommendations for the use of preventive antibiotics before certain dental procedures, including teeth cleaning and extractions, for people with specific heart problems. The use of preventive antibiotics before certain dental procedures is recommended for patients with any of the following:

- Artificial heart valves
- A history of infective endocarditis (an infection of the lining inside the heart or the heart valves)
- A cardiac (heart) transplant that develops a heart valve problem
- A congenital (present from birth) heart condition
- Unrepaired or incompletely repaired cyanotic congenital heart disease, including those with palliative shunts and conduits
- A completely repaired congenital heart defect with prosthetic material or device, whether placed by surgery or by catheter intervention, during the first 6 months after the procedure
- Any repaired congenital heart defect with residual defect at the site or adjacent to the site of a prosthetic patch or a prosthetic device

In 2012 the American Dental Association and the American Academy of Orthopaedic Surgeons (AAOS) released the first codeveloped evidence-based guideline on the *Prevention of Orthopaedic Implant Infection in Patients Undergoing Dental Procedures.* Before some dental treatments, patients with artificial joints are advised to take antibiotics. The rationale is that they could be at risk of developing an infection. Premedication (antibiotic prophylaxis) may reduce this risk. If a patient has had a total joint replacement, the dentist should communicate with the patient's orthopedist before undergoing dental treatment (Box 30.1).

In 2007 the American Heart Association provided recommendations specifically for prescribing antibiotics depending on the tolerance of the patient for medication and the patient's age (Table 30.3).

**BOX 30.1 Management of Patients with Prosthetic Joints Undergoing Dental Procedures**

**Clinical Recommendation**

In general, for patients with prosthetic joint implants, prophylactic antibiotics are *not* recommended before dental procedures to prevent prosthetic joint infection.

For patients with a history of complications associated with their joint replacement surgery who are undergoing dental procedures that include gingival manipulation or mucosal incision, prophylactic antibiotics should only be considered after consultation with the patient and orthopedic surgeon.* To assess a patient's medical status, a complete health history is always recommended when making final decisions regarding the need for antibiotic prophylaxis.

**Clinical Reasoning for the Recommendation**

- There is evidence that dental procedures are not associated with prosthetic joint implant infections.
- There is evidence that antibiotics provided before oral care do not prevent prosthetic joint implant infections.
- There are potential harms of antibiotics including risk for anaphylaxis, antibiotic resistance, and opportunistic infections such as *Clostridium difficile.*
- The benefits of antibiotic prophylaxis may not exceed the harms for most patients.
- The individual patient's circumstances and preferences should be considered when deciding whether to prescribe prophylactic antibiotics before dental procedures.

 From Sollecito T, Abt E, Lockhart P, et al: The use of prophylactic antibiotics prior to dental procedures in patients with prosthetic joints: evidence-based clinical practice guideline for dental practitioners—a report of the American Dental Association Council on Scientific Affairs, JADA 146(1):11–16, 2015.

* In cases where antibiotics are deemed necessary, it is most appropriate that the orthopedic surgeon recommend the appropriate antibiotic regimen and when reasonable write the prescription.

## Antifungal Agents

As with antibiotics, certain types of antifungal drugs are better at fighting certain types of fungi. Fungal infections occur less frequently than bacterial infections, but they can be diagnosed in patients who are immunocompromised, those who have a poorly fitting prosthesis, patients with xerostomia, and those who are taking antibiotics. One of the most commonly prescribed drugs is nystatin (Mycostatin, Nilsat, Nystex).

## Antiviral Agents

Viral infections such as hepatitis, hand-foot-and-mouth disease, primary herpes simplex, recurrent herpes, herpes zoster, and human immunodeficiency virus (HIV) can all affect the oral cavity. With most viral infections, some type of lesion commonly appears in the mouth. Antiviral agents are prescribed in capsule, tablet, liquid, and ointment forms. The most common antiviral agent is acyclovir (Zovirax).

## Antianxiety Agents

Antianxiety drugs have become a large part of "pain-free dentistry." Patients who have hesitated to go to the dentist because of their fear of pain can now receive antianxiety drugs or sedation dentistry to help manage their pain and anxiety during dental appointments. For a more in-depth look at anesthesia and pain control, refer to Chapter 37.

RECALL

**11** An analgesic could be used for what reason in dentistry?

**12** Give an example of a type of antibiotic that would be prescribed for plaque or gingivitis.

# Drugs Commonly Prescribed in Medicine

Many patients who will be seen in the dental office will be taking prescription and/or OTC drugs prescribed by their personal

**TABLE 30.3** American Heart Association Antibiotic Recommendations for a Dental Procedure

| Situation | Agent | Regimen: Single Dose 30–60 Minutes Before Procedure | |
|---|---|---|---|
| | | **Adults** | **Children** |
| **Oral** | Amoxicillin | 2 g | 50 mg/kg |
| **Unable to Take Oral Medication** | Ampicillin<br>*OR*<br>Cefazolin<br>*OR*<br>Ceftriaxone | 2 g IM or IV<br><br>1 g IM or IV | 50 mg/kg IM or IV<br><br>50 mg/kg IM or IV |
| **Allergic to Penicillins or Ampicillin (Oral)** | Cephalexin*†<br>*OR*<br>Clindamycin<br>*OR*<br>Azithromycin<br>*OR*<br>Clarithromycin | 2 g<br><br>600 mg<br><br>500 mg | 50 mg/kg<br><br>20 mg/kg<br><br>15 mg/kg |
| **Allergic to Penicillins or Ampicillin and Unable to Take Oral Medication** | Cefazolin or ceftriaxone†<br>*OR*<br>Clindamycin | 1 g IM or IV<br><br>600 mg IM or IV | 50 mg/kg IM or IV<br><br>20 mg/kg IM or IV |

From Wilson W, Taubert AK, Gewitz M, et al: Prevention of infective endocarditis: guidelines from the American Heart Association, Circulation 116(15):1736–1754, 2007. Copyright 2007 American Heart Association, Inc.

*IM,* Intramuscularly; *IV,* intravenously.

*Or other first- or second-generation oral cephalosporin in equivalent adult or pediatric dosage.

†Cephalosporins should not be used in individuals with a history of anaphylaxis, angioedema, or urticaria with penicillins or ampicillin.

doctor because of a medical condition. It is important to have background knowledge of the drugs that your patients are taking and to know how they affect your patient's total health, as well as how they could interfere with their dental care. The drugs listed are classified according to the body system they affect and their action in the body.

## Cardiovascular Drugs

A series of drug classifications can be prescribed for patients with cardiovascular disorders:

- **Statins** may be better known to people as cholesterol-lowering drugs. When people are unable to control cholesterol levels through diet and exercise, doctors may prescribe different types of statins. Examples include Lipitor, Zocor, Mevacor, and Crestor.
- **Diuretics** are cardiovascular drugs that help to reduce fluid retention. These may also reduce blood pressure. When the body is retaining fluid, this can often make the heart work harder, and the intent with using diuretics is to reduce heart workload. Examples include HCTZ, Thiazide, and Quinapril.
- **Anticoagulants** lengthen the time it takes for blood to clot, which can help prevent formation of blood clots that might cause a stroke. People who have artificial valves, who have had a stroke, or who are at risk for one may need an anticoagulant such as heparin or Coumadin to minimize future risk. This classification of drug can inhibit natural clotting and could interfere with certain dental procedures. It is important for the dentist to be aware when the patient is taking this drug.
- **Antiplatelet** drugs may be preferred to anticoagulants, and simple ones include medications such as aspirin. These also work to keep blood clots from forming, but through a different mechanism than most anticoagulants. Examples of these include aspirin and Plavix.
- **Beta blockers** have numerous uses. They can help control blood pressure, slow fast arrhythmias, and reduce chest pain associated with angina. Use of various beta blockers may result in a slower heartbeat, which may help control numerous heart disease symptoms and may reduce future risk of heart attack. Examples of these include Levatol, Lopressor, Toprol, and Zebeta.
- **Digitalis** provides a good contrast to beta blockers. Medications with digitalis stimulate the heart to beat more forcefully. Some people with arrhythmias may require this medication; at other times, it is used when a person is in congestive heart failure. An example is Digoxin.
- **Vasodilators** such as beta blockers may reduce the work of the heart and are often prescribed to treat chest pain resulting from angina. Examples include Norvasc, nitroglycerin, Apresoline, and Loniten.
- **Calcium channel blockers** make up another group of cardiovascular drugs that are useful in the treatment of some

forms of angina; they may also be prescribed to treat certain arrhythmias or high blood pressure.

- **Angiotensin-converting enzyme (ACE) inhibitors** have been proven to slow the progression of heart failure. They are vasodilators, which are medications that cause the blood vessels to expand, lowering blood pressure and reducing the heart's workload. Examples include Altace, Zestril, and Vasotec.

## Respiratory Drugs

A significant number of individuals have respiratory disorders that require the use of medications. Agents from two drug classifications can be prescribed:

- **Inhibitors or anti-inflammatory drugs** such as beclomethasone dipropionate (Beclovent, Vanceril) are prescribed as inhalers. These drugs stabilize mast cells, which release histamine, leukotrienes, and other inflammatory cells.
- **Bronchodilators** are used for treatment of patients with acute bronchospasm. This type of drug relaxes the smooth muscle of the airway. Examples include albuterol (Proventil, Ventolin) and epinephrine (Bronkaid Mist).

## Gastrointestinal Drugs

Specific diseases that affect the gastrointestinal tract are heartburn, acid reflux disease, peptic ulcer, diarrhea, Crohn's disease, and ulcerative colitis. Most of the drugs in this series are OTC drugs. Those that would be prescribed for a patient include the following:

- **Acid reflux disease and peptic ulcer disease drugs** help to neutralize the stomach contents and reduce gastric acid secretions. Examples include cimetidine (Tagamet) and ranitidine (Zantac).
- **Antidiarrheal drugs** are used to treat diarrhea. Examples include bismuth (Pepto-Bismol), kaolin (Kaopectate), and loperamide (Imodium A-D).
- **Crohn's disease and ulcerative colitis drugs** provide increased resistance to infection and assist in the wound-healing response. Examples include prednisone (Meticorten) and metronidazole (Flagyl).

## Neurologic Drugs

Neurologic conditions include diseases such as seizure disorders, Parkinson's disease, multiple sclerosis, and Alzheimer's disease. Long-term medication management is common and can produce adverse effects. Examples of neurologic drugs include the following:

- **Anticonvulsant drugs** are given to control seizures. Examples of these drugs include diazepam (Apo-Diazepam, Valium) and phenytoin (Dilantin).
- **Antimyasthenic drugs** are used for muscular weakness. An example is ambenonium (Mytelase).
- **Antiparkinsonism drugs** are used to help control tremors; these include benztropine (Apo-Benztropine) and diphenhydramine (Benadryl).
- **Antispastic drugs** are given for spasms. An example is dantrolene (Dantrium).

## Psychoactive Drugs

Psychiatric medications include antidepressants and antianxiety, antipsychotic, and antimanic drugs, as well as sedatives such as sleeping pills and drugs given for attention deficit/hyperactivity disorders. Examples of psychoactive drugs include the following:

- **Antianxiety drugs** are prescribed for patients who are in a state of uneasiness of mind that resembles fear. Examples include chlordiazepoxide (Librium) and diazepam (Valium).
- **Antidepressant drugs** are prescribed to those patients diagnosed with depression. Examples include bupropion (Wellbutrin), fluoxetine (Prozac), paroxetine (Paxil), and sertraline (Zoloft).
- **Antimanic/bipolar disorder drugs** are prescribed for patients who are in a state of hyperactivity or are exhibiting aggressive behavior. Examples of these drugs include carbamazepine (Epitol) and lithium (Carbolith).
- **Antipsychotic drugs** are a group of drugs that are used to treat psychosis. Common conditions include schizophrenia, mania, and delusional disorder. Examples of drugs prescribed are chlorpromazine (Thorazine) and haloperidol (Haldol).

## Endocrine/Hormonal Drugs

Endocrine drugs correct the overproduction or underproduction of the body's natural hormones.

- Specific drugs associated with diabetes are Metformin, commonly prescribed for type 2, and insulin for type 1 diabetes.
- Estrogen and progesterone are used in birth control pills and also are prescribed to women for relief of symptoms of menopause.

RECALL

**13** What type of drug may be prescribed for a patient with angina?
**14** Would a patient be taking a diuretic to treat a cold?

# Adverse Drug Effects

*Adverse drug effects* are the body's negative reactions to a drug. It is important to review the printed insert with the patient and to discuss any of the possible adverse effects that a drug could cause. When drugs are prescribed to prevent a disease, treat a condition, alleviate pain, or suppress fear, they can possibly interfere with normal function and may even create a potentially life-threatening circumstance.

## Common Adverse Effects of Medications

- Hyperexcitability
- Insomnia
- Dizziness
- Drowsiness
- Central nervous system effects
- Gastrointestinal disturbances (nausea, vomiting, diarrhea)
- Changes in bleeding time
- Hypertension
- Hypotension and fainting
- Weight changes
- Appetite changes
- Edema
- Sexual dysfunction
- Sweating
- Opportunistic infections (yeast, fungal)
- Photosensitivity
- Loss of hair
- Blurred vision
- Cardiac arrhythmia
- Skin changes
- Respiratory difficulties

## Drug Complications

An *allergic reaction* will occur if a drug triggers the immune response. Repeated exposure to the same drug can produce this type of allergic response. Reactions can range from a common rash to life-threatening anaphylactic shock. The most common cause of drug-induced anaphylaxis is penicillin.

*Drug toxicity* refers to toxin-induced cell damage and cell death. During the breakdown of a drug, biochemical damage may take place and harm the cell. This, in turn, may cause death or mutation of the cell.

*Drug interaction* takes place when multiple drugs are introduced to the body system. The severity of this interaction can range from minor incidents to life-threatening conditions. These types of reactions can easily be prevented by the dentist who is knowledgeable of proper drug relationships and aware of all drugs a patient is taking.

*Drug tolerance* is the loss of a drug's effectiveness that occurs when a patient has taken the drug over time and no longer receives the drug's beneficial effects. When this occurs, the physician or dentist may need to increase the dosage or prescribe a different drug.

*Drug addiction* is physical dependence on a drug. If the person stops taking the drug, the body undergoes a withdrawal illness and displays physical symptoms associated with stopping use of the drug.

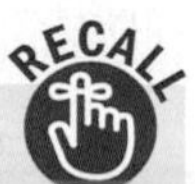


**15** What is the term for the body's negative reaction to a drug?

**■ Patient Education** One of the most important informational tools is the patient's medical history form, which includes a section on medications currently taken. When first reviewing the medication history with the patient, emphasize the importance of your awareness of the types of medications being taken. Educate the patient on how some drugs can negatively interact with drugs used in dentistry or with certain dental procedures.

If patients are unsure of the names of drugs they are taking, ask them to bring their prescriptions with them at their next visit. You can then identify the drugs and list them in the patient record. ■

**■ Legal and Ethical Implications** Under no circumstances may a dental assistant prescribe medication to a patient. The role of the dental assistant is to dispense medicine according to direct instructions and under direct supervision provided by the dentist.

It is your responsibility to become familiar with the drugs and medications that your dentist uses and prescribes. Develop the practice of referring to drug reference materials and researching any drug about which you are unsure. ■

**■ Eye to the Future** According to the FDA, more than one person a day in the United States dies from a medication error. Many of these involve giving a patient the wrong dose of a drug or even the wrong drug. Now, new technology could help put an end to these errors.

A new optical device helps reduce medication errors by recognizing medications in 30 seconds through unique fluorescence fingerprints. Pharmacists now have a new tool called ValiMed. Medications are drawn up and dropped in the unit. Ultraviolet light shines on the drug, giving it a fluorescent glow. Just like a fingerprint, every drug has a unique glow based on its chemistry. In 30 seconds, ValiMed tells pharmacists if they have the right drug. ■

**■ Critical Thinking**

1. A patient has indicated on his medical history that he is taking Allegra-D for the relief of allergy symptoms. Refer to a drug reference source for contraindications to this medication.
2. It is Friday afternoon, and Mrs. Greenville is calling the office complaining of a tooth ache. She is unable to get to the office until Tuesday because of going out of town. Mrs. Greenville has requested a prescription for pain medication until she can get to the office. How would you handle this situation?
3. You notice that a prescription pad is missing from the locked drawer. With whom do you discuss this?
4. An antibiotic has been prescribed for an adult patient who is scheduled for scaling and root planing. The patient reports a history of an artificial heart valve. Why was an antibiotic prescribed?
5. What is the recommended route of administration for the drug nitroglycerin? ■

31

# Assisting in a Medical Emergency

## KEY TERMS

**Acute** Referring to a condition with a rapid onset.

**Allergen (AL-ur-jen)** A substance, such as pollen, that causes an allergy.

**Allergy (AL-ur-jee)** High sensitivity to a certain substance.

**Anaphylaxis (an-uh-fi-LAK-sis)** Extreme hypersensitivity reaction to a substance that can lead to shock and life-threatening respiratory collapse.

**Angina (an-JYE-nuh)** Chest pain caused by inadequate oxygen to the heart.

**Antibodies** Immunoglobulins produced by lymphoid tissue in response to a foreign substance.

**Antigen (AN-ti-jen)** A substance introduced into the body to stimulate the production of an antibody.

**Aspiration (as-pi-RAY-shun)** The act of inhaling or ingesting, as of a foreign object.

**Asthma (AZ-muh)** A respiratory disease often associated with allergies and characterized by sudden recurring attacks of labored breathing, chest constriction, and coughing.

**Cardiopulmonary resuscitation (CPR) (kahr-dee-oe-PUL-muh-nar-ee ree-suh-si-TAY-shun)** A planned action for restoring consciousness or life.

**Convulsion (kun-VUL-shun)** An involuntary muscular contraction.

**Epilepsy (EH-pi-lep-see)** Neurologic disorder with sudden recurring seizures of motor, sensory, or psychic malfunction.

**Erythema (er-i-THEE-muh)** Skin redness, often caused by inflammation or infection.

**Gait** A particular way of walking, or *ambulating*.

**Hyperglycemia (hye-pur-glye-SEE-mee-uh)** Abnormally high blood glucose level.

**Hypersensitivity** State of being excessively sensitive to a substance, often with allergic reactions.

**Hyperventilation** Abnormally fast or deep breathing.

**Hypoglycemia (hye-poe-glye-SEE-mee-uh)** Abnormally low blood glucose level.

**Hypotension (hye-poe-TEN-shun)** Abnormally low blood pressure.

**Myocardial infarction (mye-oe-KAHR-dee-ul in-FAHRK-shun)** Condition in which damage to the muscular tissue of the heart is commonly caused by obstructed circulation; also referred to as a *heart attack*.

**Syncope (SING-kuh-pee)** Loss of consciousness caused by insufficient blood to the brain.

**Ventricular fibrillation (VF) (ven-TRIK-yoo-lur fib-ri-LAY-shun)** Abnormal cardiac rhythm that prevents the heart from pumping blood.

## LEARNING OUTCOMES

*On completion of this chapter, the student will be able to achieve the following objectives:*

1 Pronounce, define, and spell the key terms.
2 Describe the preventive measures taken for a medical emergency that might occur during dental treatment.
3 Describe the elements of emergency preparedness required for successful management of medical emergencies.
4 Describe the common signs and symptoms of an emergency and how to recognize them.
5 Discuss required emergency care standards, including the following:
   - List the credentials and skills that a dental assistant must have for emergency preparedness.
   - List the fundamental aspects of basic life support.
   - Identify when CPR must be initiated and the proper sequence of steps.
   - Describe measures to prevent airway obstruction and choking during dental treatment.
   - Discuss the use of a defibrillator in an emergency situation.
6 List the basic items that must be included in an emergency kit.
7 List the responsibilities of the dental assistant in an emergency.
8 Describe common medical emergencies experienced in the dental office and how one should respond to them.
9 Discuss the importance of proper documentation of medical emergencies.

## PERFORMANCE OUTCOMES

*On completion of this chapter, the student will be able to meet competency standards in the following skills:*

- Accurately perform CPR on a simulated mannequin.
- Accurately perform the Heimlich maneuver on a mannequin.
- Demonstrate use of the automated external defibrillator.
- Demonstrate preparation and placement of oxygen.
- Demonstrate how to respond to an unconscious patient.

- Demonstrate how to respond to a patient with chest pain.
- Demonstrate how to respond to a patient experiencing a stroke.
- Demonstrate how to respond to a patient with a breathing problem.
- Demonstrate how to respond to a patient experiencing an allergic reaction.
- Demonstrate how to respond to a patient experiencing a seizure.
- Demonstrate how to respond to a patient experiencing a diabetic emergency.

## ELECTRONIC RESOURCES

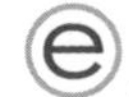

***Additional information related to content in Chapter 31 can be found on the companion Evolve Web site.***

- Practice Quiz

A *medical emergency* is a condition or circumstance that requires immediate attention toward a person who has been injured or has suddenly become ill. When a medical emergency occurs, it is not possible to refer to a medical textbook for answers. You must be prepared to respond immediately. Your knowledge and skills could mean the difference between life and death.

At the time of a medical emergency, you may be the only person in the area. If this happens, you must initiate first response until the dentist or medical assistance arrives. If this is the case, it will be your responsibility to use well-chosen words of support, to show a willingness to help, and to demonstrate capable lifesaving skills.

# Preventing a Medical Emergency

One of the most important ways to prevent a medical emergency is to *know your patient.* This means establishing open communication about the patient's health and having a completed and updated medical history before dental treatment begins.

The front desk assistant (business assistant) is responsible for ensuring that patients update this information as they enter the office. Once they have received the forms, patients should indicate any changes in their health, even if they were seen as recently as the previous week. They should also verify that the information is accurate by dating and signing the form (see Chapter 26 for a review of a medical history update).

Most emergencies that occur in the dental office are initiated by the combined *stress* of a person's daily life and the apprehension of going to the dentist. If a patient has had a negative experience or is nervous about a specific procedure, the patient's stress level could be altered, which may lead to a medical crisis. It is important to recognize the areas of dental treatment that are most stressful for a patient.

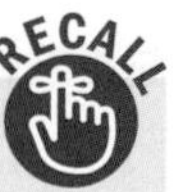


1 What is the best way to prevent an emergency?
2 What is a probable cause of most medical emergencies in the dental office?

# Emergency Preparedness

While the patient is in the dental office, the dentist is responsible for the individual's safety. If a medical emergency involving the patient arises, the dentist and staff members are responsible for providing emergency care until more qualified personnel arrive. Emergency first aid protocols must be established and routinely practiced in the dental office.

Successful management of medical emergencies in the dental office requires preparedness, prompt recognition, and effective treatment. Every member of the dental team must be prepared for an emergency when one occurs in the dental office.

*Ongoing observation* of the patient is an important part of emergency preparedness. A calm, well-functioning staff is capable of handling an emergency in the dental office without complicating the seriousness of the situation by frightening the patient. To prevent added stress and complications, every staff member should know and practice his or her role in emergency protocols before any emergency arises. A standardized procedure for the management of emergencies must be established and followed.

## Assigned Roles

In the management of an emergency, the combined efforts of trained persons are more efficient when each person takes on a specific, assigned role. It is the responsibility of the dentist to define these roles. Most often, dental team members are in charge of specific roles:

- Front desk staff (business assistant) will call emergency services and remain on the telephone until appropriate medical assistance arrives (Fig. 31.1).
- The clinical assistant or dental hygienist will retrieve the oxygen unit and emergency drug kit and prepare for use (Fig. 31.2).
- The dentist, clinical assistant, or dental hygienist will remain with the patient to assist in assessment or with basic life support.
- Additional dental team members will respond to the needs of other patients in the office.

## Routine Drills

Training must be kept current at all times. A "mock emergency" should be created in the dental office monthly, so that dental team members can practice their roles, take on additional roles, and refine the office's emergency plan.

## Emergency Telephone Numbers

A list of emergency numbers should be posted next to each telephone throughout the office. Maintaining a *current* list of

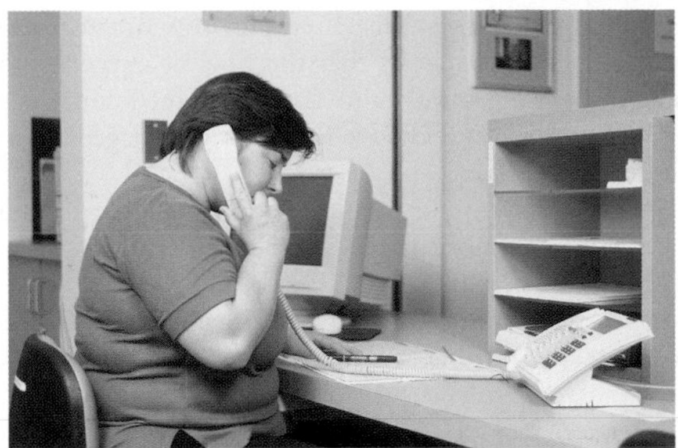

FIG. 31.1 It is important to have open communication with emergency personnel.

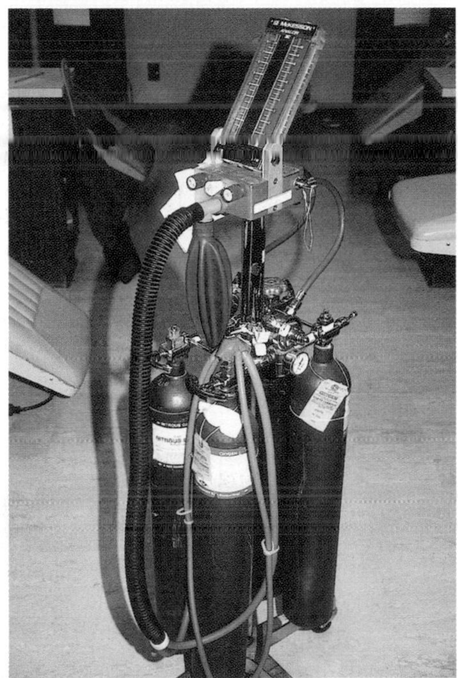

FIG. 31.2 Preparing oxygen for an emergency.

these telephone numbers is an important part of emergency preparedness.

The list should include telephone numbers for emergency medical services (EMS) personnel, local police, and firefighters. In areas of the United States and Canada, all three agencies can be reached by dialing 9-1-1. (Fig. 31.3). The availability of and response time in which these services respond to emergencies vary widely according to the geographic area and the population served. Two important factors in emergency preparedness are to know (1) the time it takes for local EMS personnel to reach the dental office, and (2) the life support capabilities that are available on arrival of the EMS staff (Fig. 31.4). Not all EMS personnel carry the same equipment or provide the same level of lifesaving care.

A list of the telephone numbers of the nearest hospital, physicians, and oral surgeons should also be available. These professionals would be able to offer the life support needed while you wait for EMS personnel or another type of emergency response.

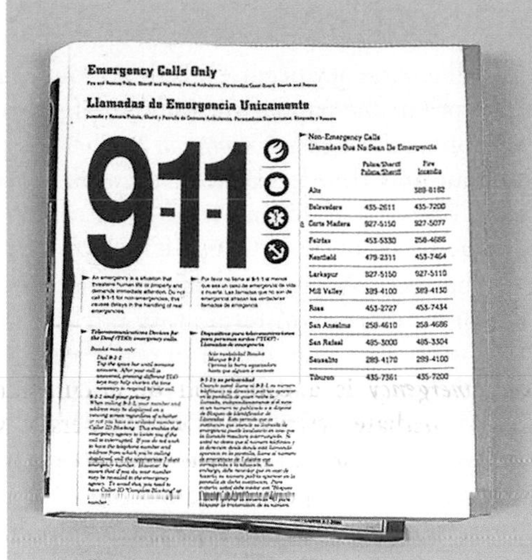


FIG. 31.3 Poster shows the most common number to be dialed for emergency services—911.

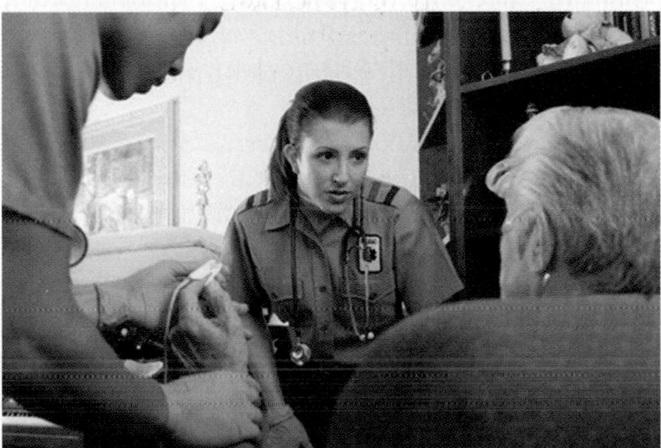

FIG. 31.4 Emergency medical services personnel on the scene. *(Copyright Getty Images.)*

RECALL

3 Who is responsible for a patient's safety in the dental office?
4 Who in the dental office would most likely be in charge of calling the emergency medical services?
5 Where should emergency phone numbers be kept in a dental office?

## Recognizing a Medical Emergency

The dental staff must be aware that a medical emergency can occur at any time. For this reason, ongoing observation of the patient in the reception area, in the dental chair, or leaving the office cannot be overemphasized. The "attentive" dental team observes the patient's general appearance and **gait** as he or she enters the clinical area. Note the patient's response to routine questions. Slow responses and changes in speech patterns from a previous appointment should be noted for the dentist to evaluate. Recognition of a problem is critical.

## Signs and Symptoms

When a medical emergency occurs, it is important to be attentive and take note in the patient's response of a symptom and your observation of the signs. A *symptom* is what the patient is telling you about how they feel or what they are experiencing, such as, "I feel dizzy," "I'm having trouble breathing," or "My arm hurts."

A *sign* is what you observe in a patient, such as a change in skin color or an increase in respiratory rate. Because signs are actually observed by you and/or another member of the dental team, they are considered to be more reliable than symptoms.

# Emergency Care Standards

It is imperative that each member of the dental team have the following credentials and skills:

- Ability to assess and record vital signs accurately (see Chapter 27)
- Basic life support for the health care provider (cardiopulmonary resuscitation [CPR])
- Heimlich maneuver (also known as *abdominal thrusts*)
- Operation of the automated external defibrillator

## Basic Life Support

The fundamental aspects of basic life support include (1) immediate recognition of an emergency, (2) activating the emergency response system, (3) early performance of high-quality CPR, and (4) rapid defibrillation when appropriate.

## Cardiopulmonary Resuscitation

In an emergency in which the patient is not breathing and the heart is not beating, **cardiopulmonary resuscitation (CPR)** must be initiated immediately. The 2010 American Heart Association guidelines for CPR determined that immediate activation of the emergency response system and starting chest compressions for any unresponsive victim with no breathing or abnormal breathing increases CPR effectiveness, and will provide better odds in saving a life. All rescuers, regardless of their training and background, should provide chest compressions to all cardiac arrest victims.

The major change in CPR instruction was from the old sequence of steps, "A-B-C" (Airway, Breathing, Chest compressions), to the new sequence of "C-A-B" (Chest compressions, Airway, Breathing) for adults and pediatric patients (children and infants). By changing the sequence to C-A-B, chest compressions are initiated sooner and ventilation is minimally delayed until completion of the first cycle of chest compressions.

CPR combines external cardiac compressions to stimulate the heart with rescue breathing to ensure that adequate air is entering the lungs. This emergency support system must be initiated immediately so that the flow of oxygen-carrying blood quickly reaches the brain. The cells of the brain, the most sensitive tissue in the body, are irreversibly damaged after 4 to 6 minutes without oxygen.

CPR for children and infants is similar to that for adults, but a few changes must be made to adapt to the anatomy and smaller bodies of children.

See Emergency Procedure 31.1: Performing Cardiopulmonary Resuscitation (One Person).

## Automated External Defibrillator

Most sudden cardiac arrest victims are experiencing what is called **ventricular fibrillation (VF)**. VF is an abnormal, chaotic heart rhythm that prevents the heart from pumping blood. VF causes more cardiac arrests than are caused by any other rhythm (about 80–90 percent of cases).

You must defibrillate a victim immediately to stop VF and allow a normal heart rhythm to resume. The sooner defibrillation begins, the better are the victim's chances of survival. If defibrillation is provided within the first 5 minutes of a cardiac arrest, the chance that the victim's life can be saved is about 50%. For each minute that passes during a cardiac arrest, however, the chance of successful resuscitation is reduced by 7 to 10 percent. After 10 minutes, very little chance of successful rescue remains.

Many places are now equipped with an automated external defibrillator (AED). The AED is attached to the patient, the power is turned on, and the device analyzes and defibrillates the patient without further input from the operator. A standard 110-volt current or battery powers this portable defibrillator. The monitor is equipped with a display and can print a copy of the victim's heart rate.

The AED is basically an advanced computer microprocessor that assesses the patient's cardiac rhythm and identifies any rhythm for which a shock is indicated. The shock is an immense jolt of electricity that is sent to the heart muscle to reestablish the proper rhythm of the heart. The AED (1) monitors the patient's heart rhythm, (2) distinguishes VF from other abnormal heart rhythms through computed analysis, and (3) automatically defibrillates if needed.

See Emergency Procedure 31.2: Operating the Automated External Defibrillator.

## Choking

A sudden coughing spasm or movement by the patient during a dental procedure may cause the accidental **aspiration** of a foreign object. The patient's discomfort is immediate; his or her hands move to the throat as spasms of coughing or choking occur.

The severity of the situation depends on (1) how tightly the item is lodged in the person's throat and (2) how much of the airway is blocked. The airway can become totally or partially blocked if the patient inhales a small object, such as a crown, debris, or a tooth fragment. The three most important measures in preventing airway obstruction during dental treatment consist of the following:

- High-velocity suction
- Use of dental dam during routine procedures
- Placement of a *throat pack* (gauze placed at base of throat)

See Emergency Procedure 31.3: Responding to the Patient with an Obstructed Airway, which reviews the steps that should be taken in response to a choking patient.

RECALL

6 When patients tell you how they feel, what is the term for such a "feeling"?
7 What minimum credentials must you have to meet emergency care standards as a dental assistant?
8 What does the abbreviation CAB stand for in emergency care?
9 What is the proper ratio of chest compressions to breaths for an adult victim when CPR is performed?
10 What does the abbreviation AED stand for?
11 What is the danger of ventricular fibrillation?

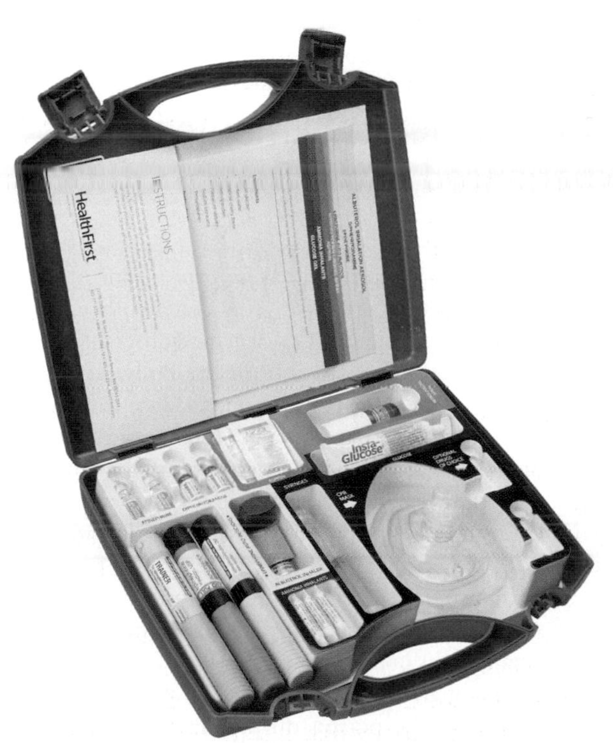


**FIG. 31.5** Standardized color-coded basic emergency kit. *(Courtesy HealthFirst, Mukilteo, WA.)*

## Emergency Equipment and Supplies

In most dental offices, a standardized emergency kit is organized and equipped with emergency supplies (Fig. 31.5). A clinical assistant or hygienist will be assigned the responsibility of maintaining and updating these supplies.

The emergency medical kit must be compliant and prepared for medical emergencies. The contents should meet the basic standard of care, be compliant with state, province, or territory regulations, and consistent with recommendations from the ADA. Table 31.1 lists the most common lifesaving drugs that are included in a basic emergency kit, along with their brand names, uses, routes of administration, and precautions for use.

Maintenance of a drug kit consists of the following:

- Routine check of supplies for quality to determine whether they are in *working condition* (rubber tubing, oxygen masks, tourniquets, intravenous lines, ventilation masks, blood pressure equipment)
- Weekly examination for *expiration* of drugs within the emergency kit (drugs past the expiration date should be replaced immediately)
- Daily check of oxygen tank or tanks

### Oxygen

Oxygen is the most frequently used "drug" in a medical emergency. The ideal agent for resuscitation of a patient

**TABLE 31.1** Recommended Drugs to Be Included in a Basic Emergency Kit

| Drug | Brand or Common Name | Use | Route |
|---|---|---|---|
| **Oxygen** | N/A | Respiratory distress | Inhaled |
| **Ammonia inhalant** | Spirits of ammonia | Fainting | Inhaled |
| **Epinephrine**<br>• Adult 0.3 mg<br>• Pediatric 0.15 mg | Auto-injector<br>EpiPen | Allergic reaction | IM, IV, SC |
| **Diphenhydramine** | Benadryl | Allergic reaction | IV, deep IM |
| **Nitroglycerin (tablet/spray)** | Nitrostat | Angina | Sublingually |
| **Albuterol** | Ventolin | Bronchospasm w/asthma | Inhaled |
| **Aspirin** | Bayer | Myocardial Infarction | Orally |
| **Oral glucose gel** | Glutose | Hypoglycemia | Orally |

*IM*, Intramuscular; *IV*, intravenous; *SC*, subcutaneous.

who is unconscious but is still breathing is 100 percent oxygen. If the patient is not breathing, air must be forced into the lungs through rescue breathing or similar emergency measures.

A portable unit with tanks of oxygen may be stored where it can be moved quickly into a treatment room if needed. A reserve tank of oxygen should be kept available for treatment in emergency situations. Remember, the oxygen cylinder is always color coded green (Fig. 31.6).

See Emergency Procedure 31.4: Preparing the Oxygen System.

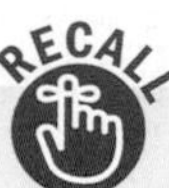


**12** What is the most frequently used "drug" in a medical emergency?

## Emergency Responses

The diagnosis of a specific condition is *not* your responsibility. As a dental assistant, your responsibilities in relation to an emergency are (1) to recognize the signs and symptoms of a significant medical complaint and (2) to provide appropriate support to the dentist in the implementation of emergency procedures.

During assessment of a medical emergency situation, the primary factor in determining the manner of treatment is the *physical change* in the patient. The physical changes most often seen during a dental office emergency include the following:

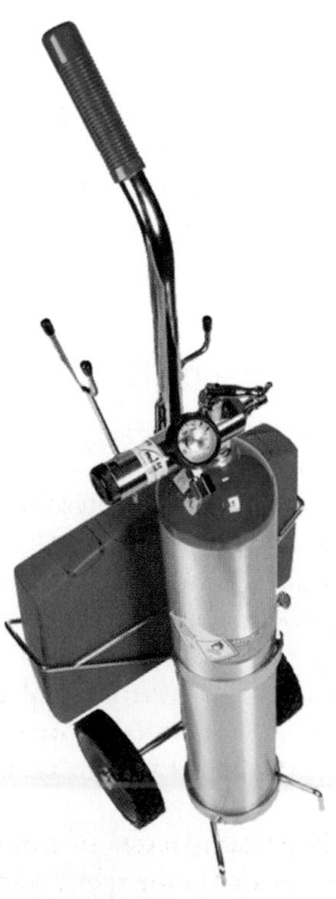

**FIG. 31.6** Mobile oxygen tank. *(Courtesy HealthFirst, Mukilteo, WA.)*

- *Unconsciousness,* the state of unresponsiveness to sensory stimulation
- *Altered consciousness,* with the patient conscious but acting strangely
- *Respiratory distress,* in which the conscious patient has difficulty breathing
- *Convulsions,* which are uncontrolled skeletal muscle contractions
- *Chest pain* in the conscious patient

Most emergencies in the dental office occur during or immediately after the administration of local anesthesia or at the beginning of a procedure. The types of procedures during which medical emergencies most frequently arise in the dental office are *tooth extractions* and *endodontic treatment.* In these two procedures, adequate pain control may be difficult to achieve, and patient anxiety is high.

## Common Medical Emergencies Experienced in the Dental Office

### Syncope

**Syncope**, commonly referred to as *fainting,* is one of the most frequent medical emergencies in the dental office. Syncope is caused by an imbalance in the distribution of blood to the brain and to the larger vessels within the body. This reduced blood flow to the brain causes the patient to lose consciousness.

Psychological factors that can contribute to syncope include stress, apprehension, fear, and the sight of blood or the sight of a certain instrument. Physiologic factors can include remaining in one position for a long time, being in a confined environment, skipping a meal or being hungry, and experiencing fatigue or exhaustion. The patient may complain of symptoms, and the signs may be noticed for several minutes before the patient actually loses consciousness.

Fainting is not harmful to the patient as long as someone is there to protect the person during unconsciousness. Even though it is quite common, syncope is one emergency that may be prevented by close observation of the patient.

### Postural Hypotension

Postural **hypotension**, also referred to as *orthostatic hypotension,* is a level of altered consciousness that may lead to loss of consciousness. This emergency commonly occurs when the patient assumes an upright position too quickly.

Postural hypotension results from insufficient blood flow to the brain and may occur in a patient immediately after a sudden change in positioning. Patients most often affected are those who receive nitrous oxide–oxygen or intravenous sedation and pregnant patients.

The duration of unconsciousness is very brief, usually lasting only seconds to minutes. If unconsciousness persists for a longer time, other causes are probably present, and appropriate action must be taken immediately (see Emergency Procedure 31.5: Responding to the Unconscious Patient).

## The Pregnant Patient

While in a supine position, the pregnant patient may feel dizzy or light-headed and may faint. This reaction results from pressure of the enlarged uterus on the abdominal veins.

In contrast to the procedure for postural hypotension, the patient should be turned onto her left side or moved into an upright sitting position. Change of position relieves pressure on involved blood vessels.

**13** A patient who is unresponsive to sensory stimulation is in what state?

**14** What is the medical term for fainting?

## Cardiac Emergencies

### Angina

The patient with **angina** feels severe *chest pain* because the heart muscle is deprived of adequate oxygen. Although it is painful, angina does not usually lead to death or permanent heart damage. However, such chest pain indicates that the person has some degree of coronary artery disease.

Because the signs and symptoms of angina and those of myocardial infarction are very similar, it is important for the clinician to distinguish angina by using the following criteria:

- Pain from angina usually lasts 3 to 8 minutes.
- Angina pain is relieved or eased promptly by the administration of the drug nitroglycerin.
- A patient with angina should specify this condition on the medical history.
- A patient with a history of angina usually carries some form of nitroglycerin to relieve the symptoms of an attack.
- Even if a patient has a history of angina, when an attack strikes, it is important to remember that the patient could be having a heart attack, and to respond appropriately.

### Acute Myocardial Infarction

During an **acute myocardial infarction**, commonly known as a *heart attack,* the muscles of the heart are damaged because of an insufficient oxygen supply. If this damage is severe enough, the patient will die; however, prompt medical treatment can help to limit damage to the heart.

Although other conditions have similar symptoms, any unexplained chest pain should be treated as a potential acute myocardial infarction. Time is important, and the response of the dental team must be swift and prudent (see Emergency Procedure 31.6: Responding to the Patient with Chest Pain).

## Cerebrovascular Accident

A cerebrovascular accident (CVA), commonly referred to as a *stroke,* is the interruption of blood flow to the brain. If blood flow is interrupted for a sufficient duration, damage to the brain may occur, resulting in loss of brain function. Most CVAs occur in older individuals who have other predisposing diseases, such as arteriosclerosis, heart disease, or uncontrolled high blood pressure (see Emergency Procedure 31.7: Responding to the Patient Who Is Experiencing a Cerebrovascular Accident [Stroke]).

## Hyperventilation

**Hyperventilation**, which is precipitated (initiated) by stress and anxiety, is an increase in the frequency or depth (or both) of respiration. As a result, the patient takes in too much oxygen. The patient will usually remain conscious.

This medical emergency can occur when a patient is extremely anxious or apprehensive before undergoing dental treatment. To prevent or reduce hyperventilation, the dental team should be alert at all times and be prepared to help the patient deal with severe apprehension in a positive manner (see Emergency Procedure 31.8: Responding to the Patient with Breathing Difficulty).

## Asthma Attack

**Asthma** is a pulmonary disorder that is characterized by attacks of sudden onset, during which the patient's airway narrows, causing difficulty in breathing, coughing, and a wheezing sound. An allergic reaction, severe emotional stress, or respiratory infection could cause an asthma attack.

Patients with asthma generally carry an inhaler that contains medication (bronchodilator) to relieve the first symptoms of an attack. It is essential that asthma be identified on the patient's medical history, and that the patient brings his or her inhaler to each dental appointment (see Emergency Procedure 31.8).

**15** What is the medical term for chest pain caused by the heart muscle being deprived of oxygen?

**16** What is the medical term for stroke?

**17** Patients with asthma will usually carry what form of medication?

## Allergic Reaction

An **allergy**, also referred to as **hypersensitivity**, is an altered state of reactivity that occurs in body tissues in response to specific antigens. An **antigen** is a substance that causes an immune response through the production of **antibodies**. An antigen that can trigger the allergic state is known as an **allergen**.

Although the patient's health history is the primary factor in determining risk for allergy, every new drug or dental material introduced to a patient could possibly produce a reaction. Of particular concern is the increasing incidence of allergic reactions to the latex used in examination gloves and dental dams.

The two most important factors to consider when managing an allergic reaction are (1) the speed with which symptoms appear and (2) the severity of the reaction. A *localized* allergic response is usually slow to develop. Mild symptoms typically include itching, **erythema**, and hives.

The symptoms of **anaphylaxis** can be life threatening and may develop very quickly. Without appropriate care, the patient could die within a few minutes (see Emergency Procedure 31.9: Responding to the Patient Who Is Experiencing an Allergic Reaction).

## Epileptic Seizure

**Epilepsy** is a neurologic disorder that is characterized by recurrent episodes of seizures. In most patients, seizures or **convulsions** are controlled with medication. Under stressful conditions, however, a seizure can still occur. As discussed in Chapter 29, there a two main categories of seizures: generalized and partial. It is important to understand the clinical considerations from the different types (see Emergency Procedure 31.10: Responding to the Patient Who Is Experiencing a Convulsive Seizure).

## Diabetes Mellitus

Diabetes mellitus is a metabolic disorder that results from disturbances in the body's normal insulin mechanism. The disease is classified in two categories:

- *Type 1 diabetes mellitus,* in which the patient becomes insulin dependent
- *Type 2 diabetes mellitus,* in which the patient is not insulin dependent but manages the disease by balancing food intake and taking medication

When the balance shifts, with too much or too little food ingested, insulin levels can change, resulting in hyperglycemia (too much blood sugar) or hypoglycemia (too little blood sugar) (see Chapter 29).

### Hyperglycemia

**Hyperglycemia** results from an abnormal *increase* in the glucose (sugar) level in the blood. If untreated, hyperglycemia may progress to diabetic ketoacidosis and a life-threatening diabetic coma.

### Hypoglycemia

**Hypoglycemia** results from an abnormal *decrease* in the glucose level in the blood. This condition can manifest itself rapidly. The most common causes of hypoglycemia are skipping a meal, taking too much insulin without adequate food intake, or exercising excessively without appropriate adjustment of insulin and food intake (see Emergency Procedure 31.11: Responding to the Patient Who Is Experiencing a Diabetic Emergency).

RECALL

**18** What type of allergic reaction can be life threatening?

**19** What condition results from an abnormal increase in blood glucose?

## Documentation of an Emergency

When a medical emergency arises in the dental office, full documentation of the details is essential. After such an emergency, the dentist will make extensive notes in the patient's record to explain exactly what happened, to indicate the treatment provided, and to describe the patient's condition at the time he or she left the office.

If an emergency is not fully resolved while the patient is in the office, the dentist may telephone the patient, the family, or the patient's physician the next day to inquire about the patient's health.

**■ Patient Education** Patients are more aware of their own health status today than ever before. Most patients are able to follow through with their personal care plan and know when to seek professional help.

Throughout the media, such as television and in social media, you may see a report of a child who saved a person's life because the child saw a TV show that discussed CPR or the Heimlich maneuver. The more the healthcare sector discusses the importance of individual awareness through workshops and patient education, the better able patients are to help themselves or others at a time of need. ■

**■ Legal and Ethical Implications** As a dental healthcare professional, you often will be asked for dental and medical advice from your patients, family, and friends. You must be very careful about what you say to people. You are not in the position to diagnose an illness, and you must not do so under any circumstance.

In the case of an emergency, however, the situation is different. You are protected under the "Good Samaritan Law," which states that if you try your best to do what can reasonably be done by others with the same training, the victim cannot legally hold you responsible if something goes wrong. ■

**■ Eye to the Future** New technology is allowing individuals with serious medical conditions to live a normal life with confidence that the emergency medical system will be alerted when the need arises. Furthermore, the Internet has dramatically changed the way America communicates with individuals, emergency systems, and hospitals.

Advances in digital and compression technology mean that vast amounts of information can be stored on ever-smaller chips. Important applications of this technology include the creation of digital medical libraries and medical databases. The potential also exists to develop *electronic medical record systems* and credit card–sized "smart cards" that store personal medical information. ■

### ■ Critical Thinking

1. You are escorting a patient to the treatment area and notice that she appears flushed and is perspiring. You take her vital signs and note a rapid heart rate and a decrease in her blood pressure. What warning sign does this represent regarding a medical emergency?

2. How would the dental team respond to the patient described in question 1?
3. The dentist has just finished administering local anesthesia when a patient complains of shortness of breath and "not feeling well." What medical emergency would you suspect, and how should the dental team respond?
4. What should be kept available in the dental office for a patient with hypoglycemia?
5. Why would you not place anything in a patient's mouth during a grand mal seizure? ■

EMERGENCY PROCEDURE 31.1

# Performing Cardiopulmonary Resuscitation (One Person)

## EQUIPMENT AND SUPPLIES

Mannequin approved by the American Heart Association (AHA) and equipped with a printout for demonstration of proper technique (for instruction purposes and mock emergency drills).

## PROCEDURAL STEPS FOR ADULT, CHILD, INFANT CPR

### Determine Unresponsiveness

Approach the victim and check for signs of circulation, such as normal breathing, coughing, or movement in response to stimulation. Pinch or tap the victim and ask, "Are you OK?"

### Assessment

1 Touch the shoulder and ask, "Are you OK?"
2 Check to see if the person is breathing. If the person is not breathing, activate emergency response.

### Initiate Assistance and get AED

3 If there is no response, **call for assistance** and ask someone to call 911; obtain an AED/defibrillator if available.
4 If you are alone, and your patient is an adult, phone 911 first, and then begin compressions.
5 If the patient is a child, give 2 minutes of compression first, then call 911.

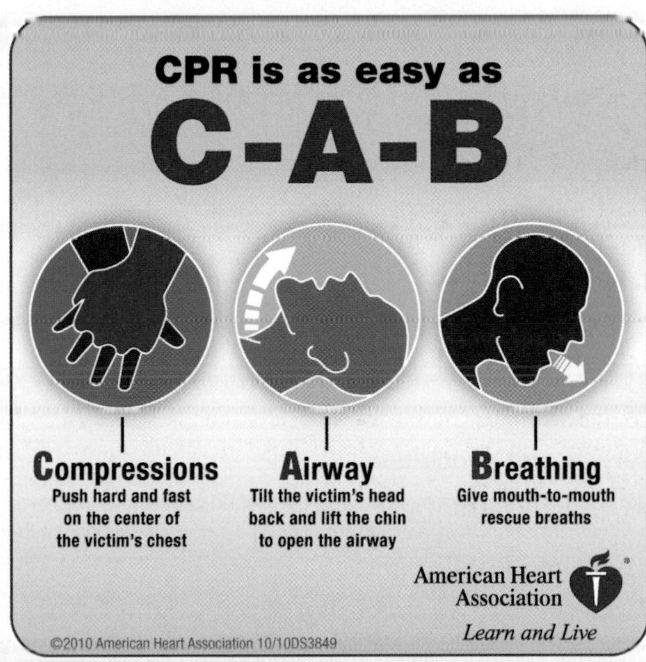


(Copyright American Heart Association.)

### Pulse Check and Initiate Compressions

6 To perform a pulse check, palpate a carotid pulse. If you do not feel a pulse within 10 seconds, start chest compressions.
7 Kneel at the victim's side opposite the chest. Move your fingers up the ribs to the point where the sternum and the ribs join. Your middle finger should fit into the area, and your index finger should be next to it across the sternum.
8 Place the heel of your hand on the chest midline over the sternum, just above your index finger. Place your other hand on top of your first hand, and lift your fingers upward off the chest.

(Continued)

## EMERGENCY PROCEDURE 31.1 Performing Cardiopulmonary Resuscitation (One Person)–cont'd

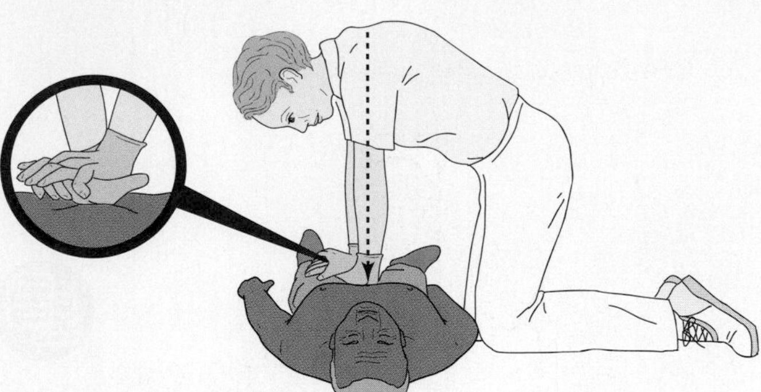

*(From Sorrentino SA, Remmert LN: Mosby 's essentials for nursing assistants, ed 5, St Louis, 2014, Mosby.)*

**9** Bring your shoulders directly over the victim's sternum as you compress downward, and keep your arms straight.

**10** Provide 30 chest compressions at a rate of 100 per minute with adequate depth. Specific techniques to remember during compressions are as follows:

- Push hard and fast.
- Allow complete chest recoil after each compression.
- Minimize interruptions in compressions.
- Avoid excessive ventilation.
- If multiple rescuers are available, they should rotate the task of compressions every 2 minutes.

**11** For adults and children over 8, compress the chest a depth of at least 2 inches (5 cm).

**12** For infants, compress the chest a depth of about 1.5 inches (4 cm).

### Airway and Ventilation

**13** Opening the airway (followed by rescue breaths to improve oxygenation and ventilation) should be completed only if there are two rescuers and one of the rescuers is trained in CPR.

**14** Once chest compressions have been started, a trained rescuer should deliver rescue breaths by mouth-to-mouth or bag-mask to provide oxygenation and ventilation, as follows:

- Deliver each rescue breath over 1 second.
- Give a sufficient tidal volume to produce visible chest rise.
- Use a compression to ventilation ratio of 30 chest compressions to 2 ventilations.

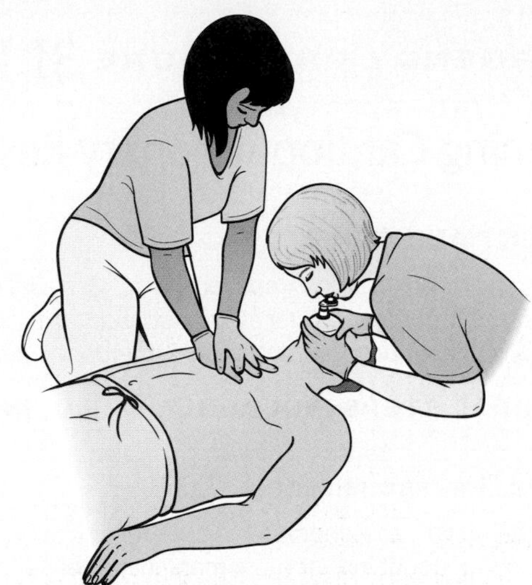

*(From Sorrentino SA, Remmert LN: Mosby 's essentials for nursing assistants, ed 5, St Louis, 2014, Mosby.)*

- Repeat ongoing cycles of CPR until EMS arrives, the person starts breathing, someone comes with an AED, or another trained rescuer takes over.

**15** Document emergency response in the patient record.

EMERGENCY PROCEDURE 31.2

# Operating the Automated External Defibrillator

## EQUIPMENT AND SUPPLIES

- Automated external defibrillator (AED)
- Electrode lines
- Paddles

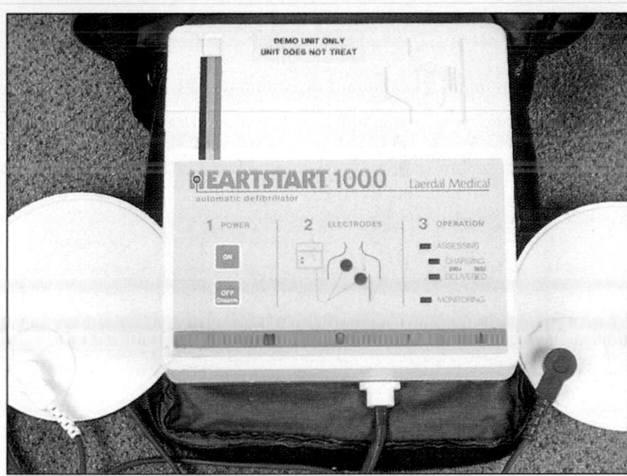


## PROCEDURAL STEPS

1. Activate the emergency response system.
2. Begin providing compressions while second responder readies the AED close to the victim's chest.
3. Turn on the power by lifting the top of the case and turning on the power switch.
4. Position the defibrillator machine on the left side of the patient's head, close to the ear. Turn on the power by lifting the top of the case or turning on the power switch.

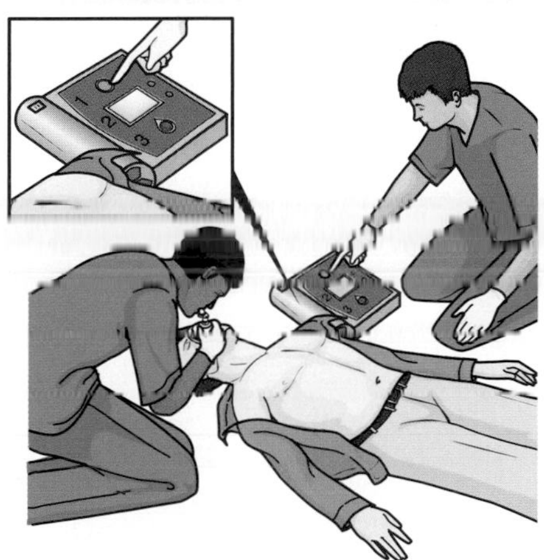

5. Attach the electrode lines to the paddles.

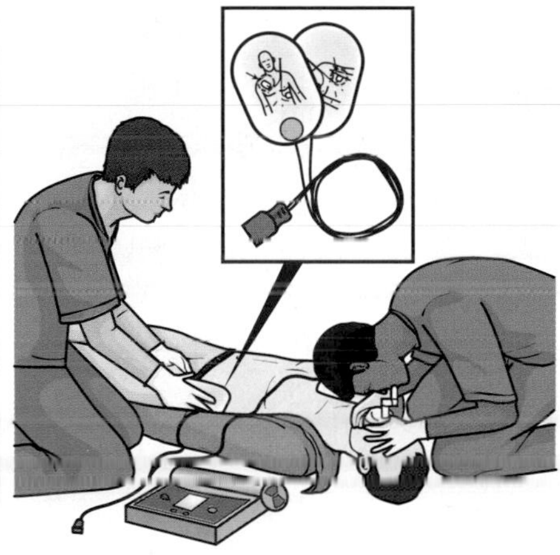

6. Attach the paddles to the patient, one at the left sternal border and the second on the right side above the nipple area.

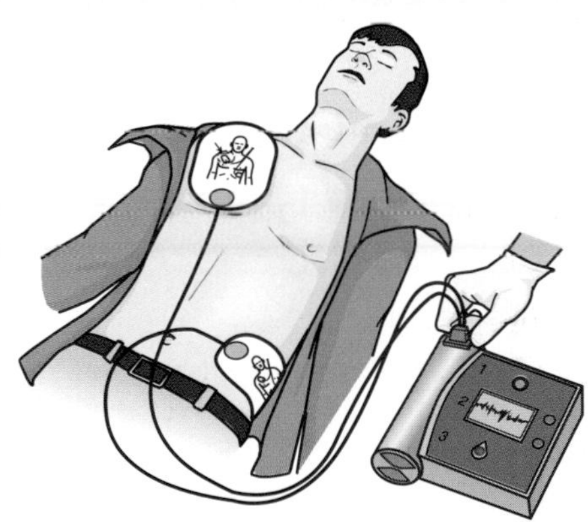

7. Clear the patient (i.e., make sure no one is in direct contact with the patient), and press the analyze button (or let the machine analyze automatically after the pads have been attached).

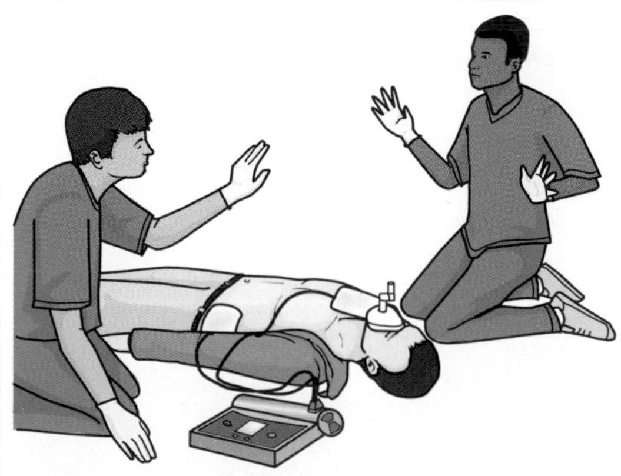

(Continued)

## EMERGENCY PROCEDURE 31.2 Operating the Automated External Defibrillator–cont'd

**8** If the machine advises shock, confirm that everyone present is clear of the patient, and then deliver a shock.

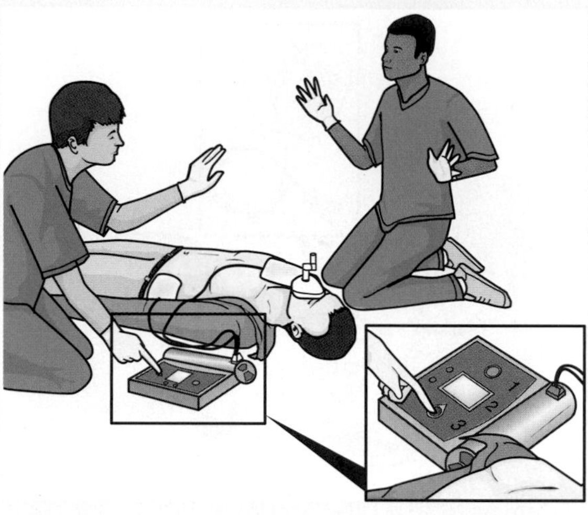


**9** After shock delivery, the rescuer should immediately begin chest compressions followed by checking the pulse.

**10** After 5 cycles of CPR, the AED should then analyze the cardiac rhythm and deliver another shock if indicated.

**11** Document emergency response in the patient record.

Illustrations (except for the photo of the defibrillator) from Kostelnick C: Mosby's textbook for long-term care nursing assistants, ed 7, St Louis, 2015, Mosby.

EMERGENCY PROCEDURE 31.3

# Responding to the Patient with an Obstructed Airway

## SIGNS AND SYMPTOMS

- Patient grasping at throat—the universal sign of choking
- Ineffective cough
- High-pitched breathing sound
- Respiratory difficulty
- Change in skin color

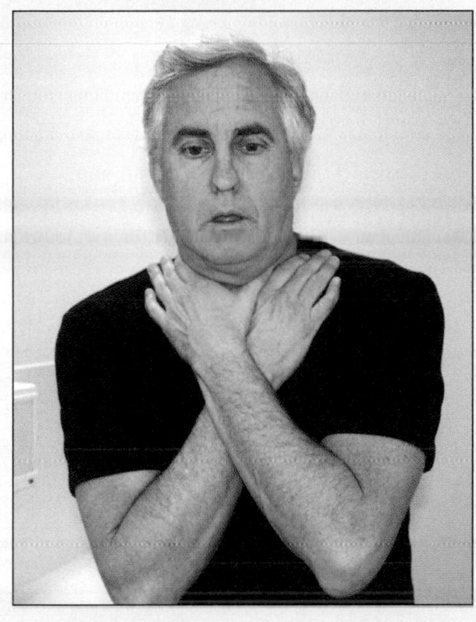

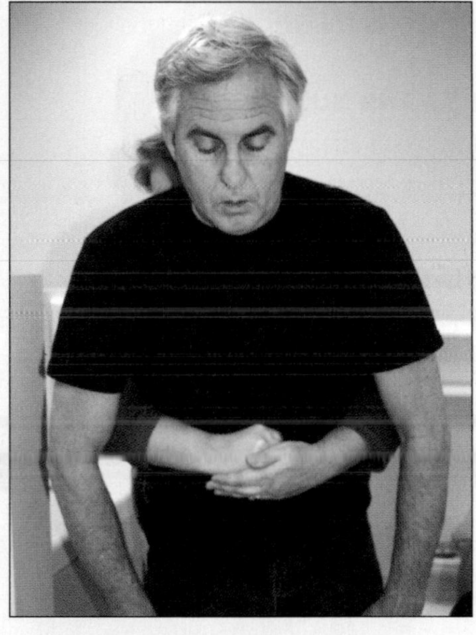

## PROCEDURAL STEPS

### Care of the Patient

1. If the patient cannot speak, cough, or breathe, the airway is completely blocked. Immediately call for assistance and begin administering **abdominal thrusts** (Heimlich maneuver).
2. Make a fist with one hand and place thumb side of hand against the patient's abdomen, just above the navel and below the xiphoid process of the sternum.
3. Grasp the fist with the other hand and forcefully thrust both hands into the abdomen, using an inward and upward motion.
4. Repeat these thrusts until the object is expelled.

### Responding to the Conscious Seated Patient

5. Do not try to move the patient out of the dental chair before you administer the Heimlich maneuver.
   **PURPOSE** Patient movement may cause the lodged item to be swallowed.
6. Place the heel of one hand at the patient's abdomen above the navel and well below the xiphoid process.
7. Place the other hand directly over the first hand. Administer a firm, quick, upward thrust into the patient's diaphragm.
8. Repeat this maneuver 6 to 10 times as needed until the object is dislodged, or until advanced emergency assistance arrives.
9. Document emergency response in the patient record.

EMERGENCY PROCEDURE 31.4

# Preparing the Oxygen System

*Note:* If the dental office is equipped with a nitrous oxide–oxygen unit, the oxygen from these units can be used in emergency situations.

## EQUIPMENT AND SUPPLIES

- ✔ Portable oxygen system
- ✔ Gauge regulator
- ✔ Tubing
- ✔ Face mask

## PROCEDURAL STEPS

1 Confirm that the cylinder contains oxygen by checking the color and the pin index grouping.

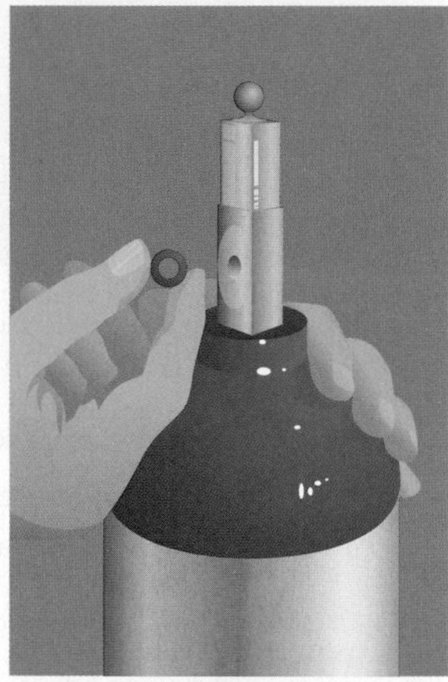

2 Slowly open the main valve at the top of the cylinder until gas starts to come out; then immediately close the valve.

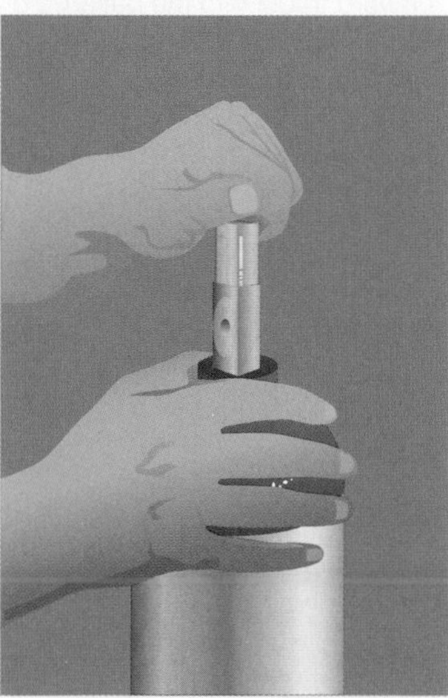

3 Attach the regulator by aligning the pin index into the cylinder holes.

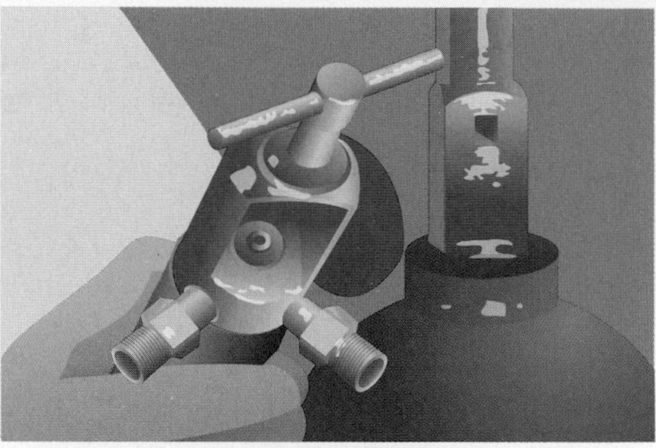

4 Tighten the clamp to ensure an adequate seal.

5 Open the valve two full turns. Check the pressure gauge to make sure that it is showing approximately 2000 pounds per square inch.

**PURPOSE** This much pressure is necessary for the oxygen to flow at a proper rate.

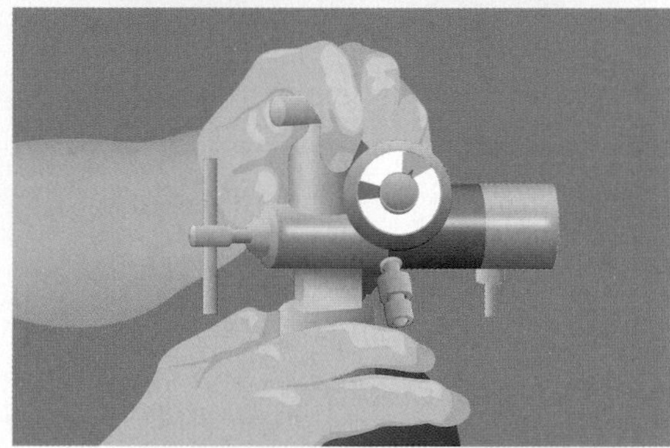

6 Attach the tubing, if it is not already attached.

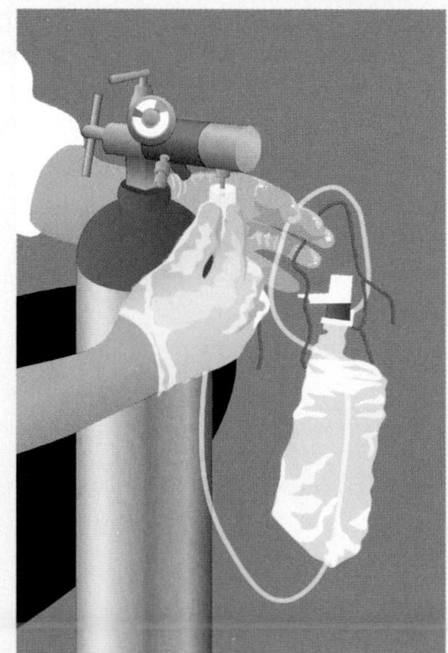

7 Position the mask comfortably over the patient's face.

**NOTE** Make sure that the mask is positioned so that it covers the nose and mouth and forms a good seal.

8 Document emergency response in the patient record.

EMERGENCY PROCEDURE 31.5

# Responding to the Unconscious Patient

## SYNCOPE (FAINTING)

### Signs and Symptoms

- Feeling of warmth or flushing (flushed)
- Nausea
- Rapid heart rate
- Perspiration
- Pallor (pale skin color)
- Lower blood pressure

### Response Steps

1. Place the patient in a subsupine position with the head lower than the feet.
   **PURPOSE** This position causes blood to flow away from the stomach and back toward the brain; this is frequently sufficient to revive the patient.

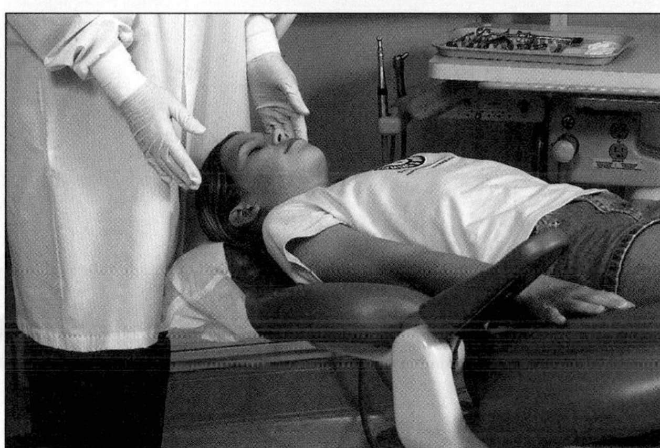

2. Loosen any binding clothes on the patient.
3. Have an ammonia inhalant ready to administer by waving it under the patient's nose several times.
4. Have oxygen ready to administer.
5. Monitor and record the patient's vital signs.
6. If unresponsive, call for emergency assistance (911).

## POSTURAL HYPOTENSION

### Signs and Symptoms

- Low blood pressure
- Altered state of consciousness to possible loss of consciousness

### Response Steps

1. Place the patient in a subsupine position with the head lower than the feet.
   **PURPOSE** This position causes blood to flow away from the stomach and back toward the brain; this is frequently sufficient to revive the patient.
2. Establish an airway.
3. Slowly move the patient into an upright position.
4. Monitor and record vital signs.
5. If unresponsive, call for emergency assistance (911).

EMERGENCY PROCEDURE 31.6

# Responding to the Patient with Chest Pain

## ANGINA ATTACK

### Signs and Symptoms

- Tightness or squeezing sensation in the chest
- Pain radiating to the left shoulder
- Pain radiating to the left side of the face, the jaw, and the teeth

### Response Steps

1. Call for emergency assistance (911).
2. Position the patient upright.
3. Medicate with nitroglycerin (tablets, spray, or topical cream).
4. Administer oxygen.
5. Monitor and record vital signs.

## ACUTE MYOCARDIAL INFARCTION (HEART ATTACK)

### Signs and Symptoms

- Chest pain ranging from mild to severe
- Pain in the left arm, the jaw, and the teeth
- Shortness of breath and sweating
- Nausea and vomiting
- Pressure, aching, or burning feeling of indigestion
- Generalized feeling of weakness

### Response Steps

1. Call for emergency assistance (911).
2. Initiate basic life support (CPR) if the patient becomes unconscious.
3. Ready the nitroglycerin from the office's emergency kit.
4. Administer oxygen.
5. Monitor and record vital signs.

EMERGENCY PROCEDURE 31.7

# Responding to the Patient Who Is Experiencing a Cerebrovascular Accident (Stroke)

## SIGNS AND SYMPTOMS

- Paralysis
- Speech problems
- Vision problems
- Possible seizure
- Difficulty swallowing
- Headache
- Unconsciousness

### Response Steps

1. Call for emergency assistance (911).
2. Initiate basic life support (CPR) if the patient becomes unconscious.
3. Monitor and record vital signs.

**THINK YOU ARE HAVING A STROKE? CALL 9-1-1 IMMEDIATELY!**

*F.A.S.T. is an easy way to remember the sudden signs of stroke. When you can spot the signs, you'll know that* **you need to call 9-1-1 for help right away.** *F.A.S.T. is:*

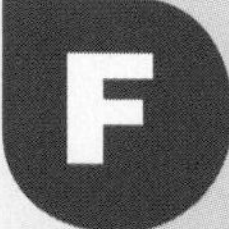


**Face Drooping**
Does one side of the face droop or is numb? Ask the person to smile. Is the person's smile uneven?

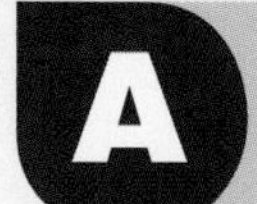


**Arm Weakness**
Is one arm weak or numb? Ask the person to raise both arms. Does one arm drift downward?

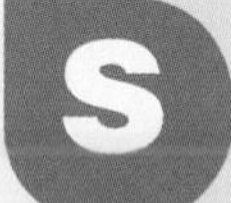


**Speech Difficulty**
Is speech slurred? Is the person unable to speak or hard to understand? Ask the person to repeat a simple sentence, like "The sky is blue." Is the sentence repeated correctly?

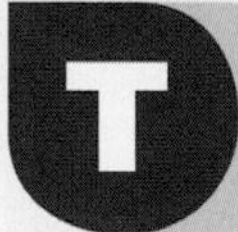


**Time to call 9-1-1**
If someone shows any of these symptoms, even if the symptoms go away, call 9-1-1 and get the person to the hospital immediately. Check the time so you'll know when the first symptoms appeared.

EMERGENCY PROCEDURE 31.8

# Responding to the Patient with Breathing Difficulty

## HYPERVENTILATION

### Signs and Symptoms

- Rapid, shallow breathing
- Light-headedness
- Tightness in the chest
- Rapid heartbeat
- Lump in the throat
- Panic-stricken appearance

### Response Steps

1. Place the patient in a comfortable position.
2. Use a quiet tone of voice to calm and reassure the patient.
3. Have the patient breathe into his cupped hands.

   **NOTE** Some sources will indicate to breathe into a paper bag, but a patient's cupped hands have been found to be better.

   **PURPOSE** This response increases the carbon dioxide supply and restores appropriate oxygen and carbon dioxide levels in the blood.

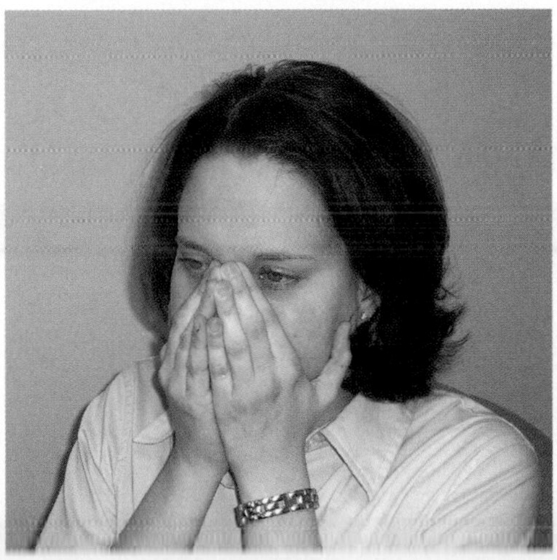

## ASTHMA ATTACK

### Signs and Symptoms

- Coughing
- Wheezing
- Increased anxiety
- Pallor
- Cyanosis (bluish skin around the nails)
- Increased pulse rate

### Response Steps

1. Call for assistance.
2. Position the patient as comfortably as possible (upright is usually best).
3. Have patient self-medicate with an inhaler.
4. Administer oxygen as needed.
5. Assess and record vital signs.

EMERGENCY PROCEDURE 31.9

## Responding to the Patient Who Is Experiencing an Allergic Reaction

### LOCALIZED RASH

#### Signs and Symptoms

- ✔ Itching
- ✔ Erythema (skin redness)
- ✔ Hives

#### Response Steps

1. Identify area of rash.
2. Monitor and record vital signs.
3. Prepare an antihistamine for administration if necessary.
4. Be prepared to administer basic life support (CPR) if necessary.
5. Refer the patient for medical consultation.
   **PURPOSE** If the patient has an allergic reaction once, he or she may become increasingly hypersensitive and may have a life-threatening response the next time.

### ANAPHYLAXIS

#### Signs and Symptoms

- ✔ Feeling physically ill
- ✔ Nausea and vomiting
- ✔ Shortness of breath
- ✔ Heart arrhythmia (irregular heartbeats)
- ✔ Sudden drop in blood pressure
- ✔ Loss of consciousness

#### Response Steps

1. Call for emergency assistance (911).
2. Place the patient in a supine position.
3. Start basic life support (CPR) if the patient becomes unconscious.
4. Prepare EpiPen for administration.
5. Administer oxygen.
6. Monitor and record vital signs.

EMERGENCY PROCEDURE 31.10

## Responding to the Patient Who Is Experiencing a Convulsive Seizure

### GRAND MAL SEIZURE

#### Signs and Symptoms

- ✔ Unconsciousness
- ✔ Increased body temperature
- ✔ Rapid heart rate
- ✔ Increased blood pressure

#### Response Steps

1. Call for emergency assistance (911).
2. If a seizure occurs while the patient is in the dental chair, quickly remove all materials from the mouth, and place the patient in a supine position.
   **PURPOSE** The patient could inflict self-harm if something is in the mouth. Do not place anything in the patient's mouth during a seizure.
3. Protect the patient from self-injury during movements caused by the convulsion.
4. Prepare anticonvulsant (diazepam) from the drug kit if necessary.
5. Initiate basic life support (CPR) if necessary.
6. Monitor and record vital signs.

### PETIT MAL SEIZURE

#### Signs and Symptoms

- ✔ Intermittent blinking
- ✔ Mouth movements
- ✔ Blank stare
- ✔ Not responsive to surroundings; seems to be in his or her "own world"

#### Response Steps

1. Protect patient from self-injury.
2. Monitor and record vital signs.
3. Refer patient for medical consultation.

EMERGENCY PROCEDURE 31.11

# Responding to the Patient Who Is Experiencing a Diabetic Emergency

## HYPERGLYCEMIA

### Signs and Symptoms

- Excessive urination
- Excessive thirst, dry mouth, and dry skin
- Acetone breath (fruity smell)
- Blurred vision and headache
- Rapid pulse
- Lower blood pressure
- Loss of consciousness

### Response Steps

1 If the patient is conscious, ask when he or she last ate, whether the patient has taken insulin, and whether he or she brought insulin along to the dental appointment.

**PURPOSE** If the patient has already eaten but has not taken insulin, he or she needs insulin immediately.

2 Retrieve the patient's insulin if it is available. If able, the patient should self-administer the insulin.

3 Call for emergency assistance (911) if necessary.

4 Provide basic life support (CPR) if the patient becomes unconscious.

5 Monitor and record vital signs.

## HYPOGLYCEMIA

### Signs and Symptoms

- Mood changes
- Hunger
- Perspiration
- Increased anxiety
- Possible unconsciousness

### Response Steps

1 If the patient is conscious, ask when he or she last ate, whether the patient has taken insulin, and whether he or she brought insulin along to the dental appointment.

2 Give a concentrated form of carbohydrate, such as a sugar packet, cake icing, or concentrated orange juice.

**PURPOSE** These substances will be absorbed rapidly into the bloodstream.

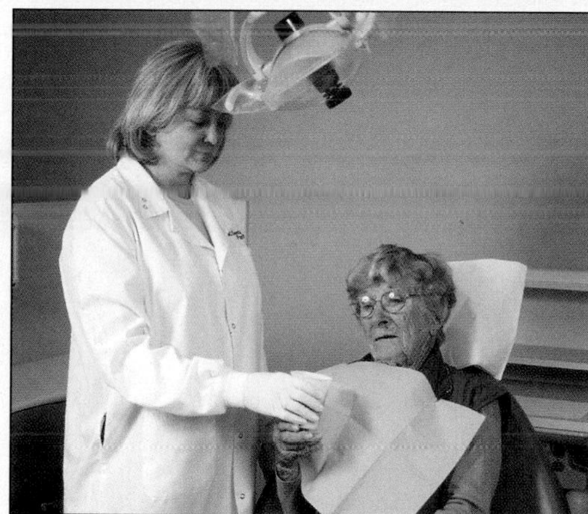

3 Call for emergency assistance (911) if necessary.

4 Provide basic life support (CPR) if the patient becomes unconscious.

5 Monitor and record vital signs.

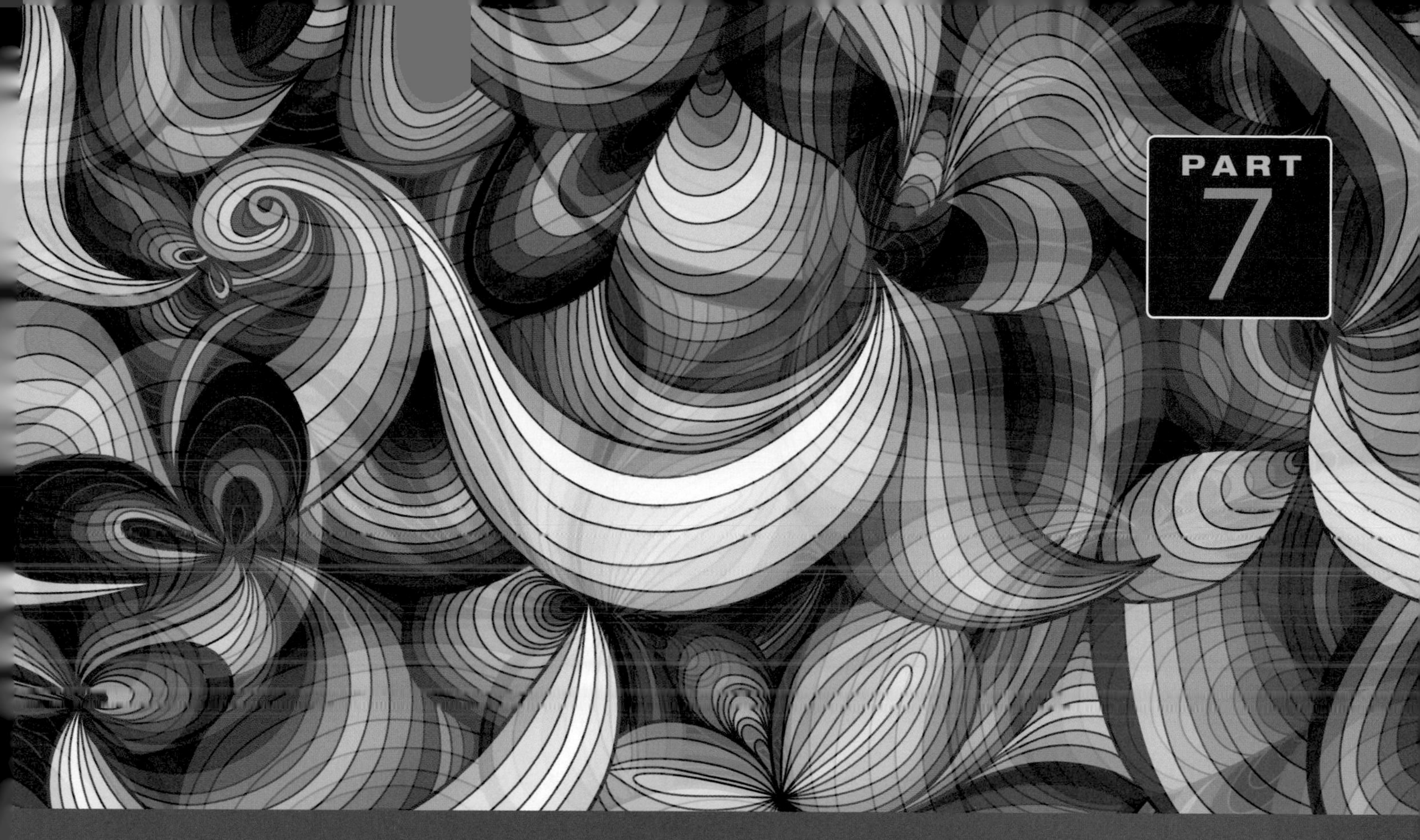


# Foundation of Clinical Dentistry

Before any professional can practice and perfect a skill, he or she must first understand how the skill is performed. As a clinical dental assistant, your role will be ever-changing as the advances of technology advance in the field of dentistry.

The chapters in this section focus on the preclinical skills you will master when learning how dental care is delivered. Areas discussed include the layout and design of the dental office, team dentistry, expanded functions, the specific instruments and supplies used in most general dental procedures, and the importance of patient comfort during dental treatment with the use of moisture control, as well as anesthesia and pain control methods.

32

# The Dental Office

## KEY TERMS

**Condensation (kon-den-SAY-shun)** Process by which liquid is removed from vapor.

**Consultation (kon-sul-TAY-shun) room** Meeting room or specified area where diagnostic and treatment information is discussed with the patient.

**Dental operatory (OP-ur-uh-tor-ee)** Dental treatment room and control center of the clinical area.

**Rheostat (REE-uh-stat)** Foot-controlled device used to operate dental handpieces.

**Subsupine (sub-SOO-pine) position** Lying-down position in which the patient's head is lower than the feet (below the heart); used in emergency situations.

**Supine (SOO-pine) position** Lying-down position in which the patient's head, chest, and knees are at the same level.

**Triturate (TRICH-ur-ayte, TRI-chuh-rayt)** The process of mechanically mixing a material, as when an amalgamator is used to mix an alloy and mercury to create dental amalgam.

**Upright position** Vertical, seated position in which the back of the dental chair is upright at a 90-degree angle.

## LEARNING OUTCOMES

*On completion of this chapter, the student will be able to achieve the following objectives:*

1. Pronounce, define, and spell the key terms.
2. Describe the areas of the dental environment in a professional office, including the important qualities of the reception area and the goals involved in designing the dental treatment area.
3. Describe the qualities necessary to maintain the dental office environment.
4. List the clinical equipment most commonly found in the dental treatment area and their basic functions.
5. Explain the care involved with dental equipment.
6. Describe the morning and evening routines for dental assistants.

## PERFORMANCE OUTCOMES

*On completion of this chapter, the student will be able to meet competency standards in the following skills:*

- Prepare the dental treatment area for patient care in the morning before patients are seen.
- Prepare the dental treatment area for patient care the next day.

## ELECTRONIC RESOURCES

***Additional information related to content in Chapter 32 can be found on the companion Evolve Web site.***

- Practice Quiz
- Canadian Content Corner

"Welcome." Your patients' first opinion of a dental office will be made as soon as they walk through the door. Their first impression of their surroundings and how they are received will initially define the quality of care. Every area of the dental office should portray an organized and professional setting situated for convenience for the patient and the dental team. Attention to detail and organization in the way you receive, treat, and dismiss patients is important when creating a positive experience.

## Design of the Dental Office

A dental office will have designated rooms to accommodate the needs of the dental team to function on a daily basis. The size and design of an office will be determined by the numbers of dentists and clinical and business professionals practicing within the office (Fig. 32.1).

### Reception Area

The goal of a well-planned dental office is to create a reception area that makes patients feel at home, relaxes them, and prepares them for treatment (Fig. 32.2). This area should not be referred to or thought of as the "waiting area," but as an area in which you receive and greet patients. With proper scheduling, patients must be seen on time for their appointments.

Cleanliness should be of utmost concern on a daily basis. You want to provide adequate seating for patients and their families. Keep a selection of up-to-date magazines. Know the preferences of your patients, and have on hand what interests them. For example, if your office is in the business district, have business and financial magazines. Offer wireless service, and have a place to hang coats and umbrellas to help reduce clutter.

If the office sees a notable number of families with children, maintain a section of the reception area for children

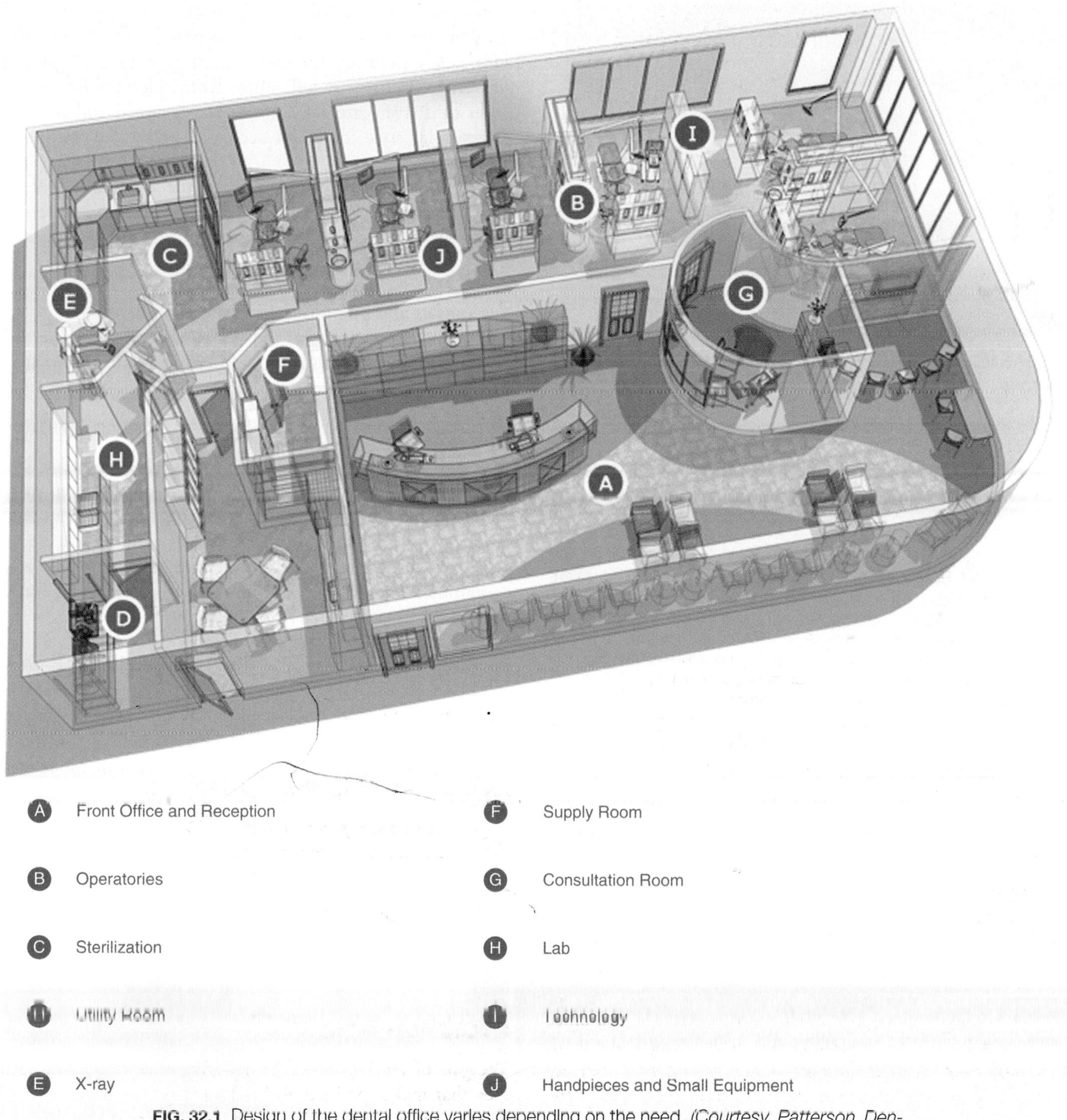


**FIG. 32.1** Design of the dental office varies depending on the need. *(Courtesy Patterson Dental, St Paul, MN.)*

(Fig. 32.3). Items that could be kept in this area include books, toys, and comfortable seating for younger children.

## Administrative Area

The administrative area of the office runs the management or business side of the practice (Fig. 32.4). This area includes a desk, a secured area for patient records and business materials, phone systems, computers, a photocopier, calculators, and fax machines. Additional security measures should be taken in this area because of privacy issues and the need to facilitate discussion and exchange of financial information with patients.

## Treatment Area

All dental treatment provided to patients takes place in the dental treatment area, also referred to as the **dental operatory** (Fig. 32.5). This part of the dental office is the area of concentration, where all clinical procedures take place in the dental practice.

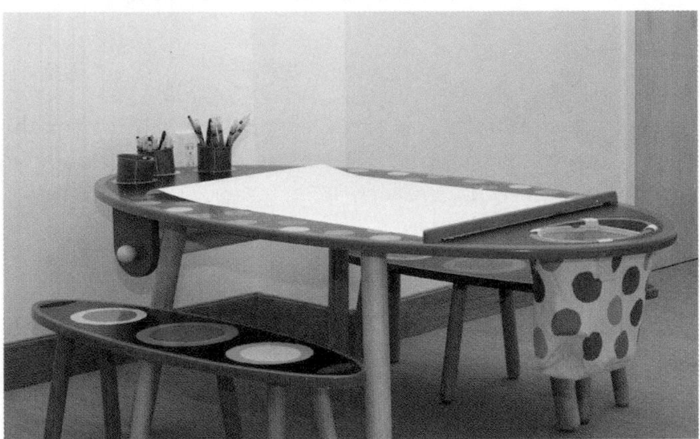

FIG. 32.2 Reception area of a dental office. *(Copyright © 2011 leezsnow, iStock.com. All rights reserved.)*

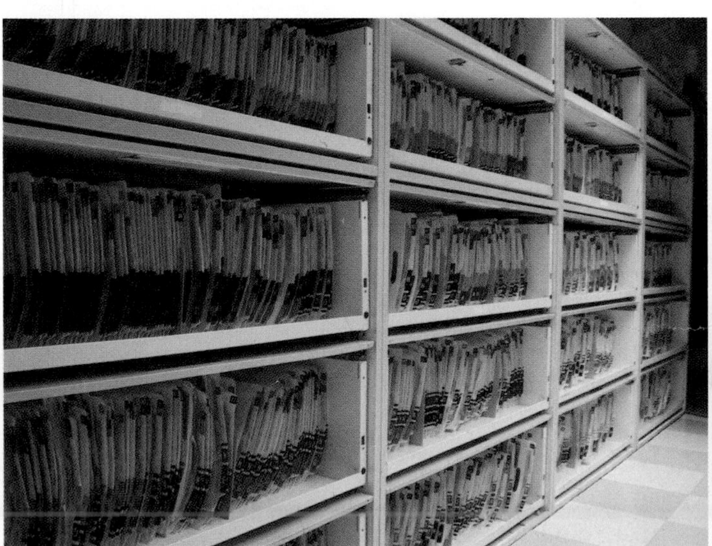

FIG. 32.3 Part of a reception area designed for children. *(From Finkbeiner BL, Finkbeiner CA: Practice management for the dental team, ed 8, St Louis, 2016, Mosby.)*

Most practices will have a minimum of two operatories for the dentist and clinical assistants to practice in, along with an additional operatory for each dental hygienist. To promote efficiency, the dentist will move from one operatory to the other to deliver care. The rooms are designed and furnished in a similar style for easier access to items that are kept in each room.

The design and arrangement of the operatory will vary according to the space available and the dentist's preferences regarding style. The goal in designing the dental treatment area is to achieve the following:

- Comfort and mobility for dental team members
- Privacy and comfort for the dental patient
- Enhanced use of dental equipment through time management and efficient techniques

## Central Sterilization

The sterilization and supply center is the hub where instruments are maintained, cleaned, sterilized, and stored in preparation for reuse. The sterilization center, which must be kept organized and clean at all times, is divided into two areas: the contaminated area and the clean area (see Chapter 21 for further description).

## Dental Laboratory

The dental laboratory is organized around workbenches and wall-mounted storage cabinets. In the laboratory, procedures such as pouring impressions, preparing diagnostic models, and creating custom impression trays can be performed.

During work in the laboratory, infection control and safety are always major concerns. In addition, the entire laboratory must be

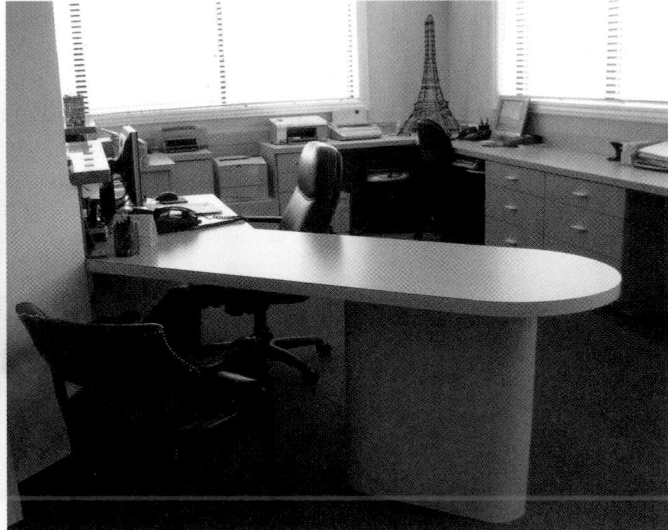

FIG. 32.4 Left, Organization of paper dental records. Right, Design of the business area. *(Left, Copyright © InCommunicado/E+/Getty Images. Right, Courtesy Joseph Ellis, DDS and Lisa Tartaglione, DDS, Grand Rapids, MI.)*

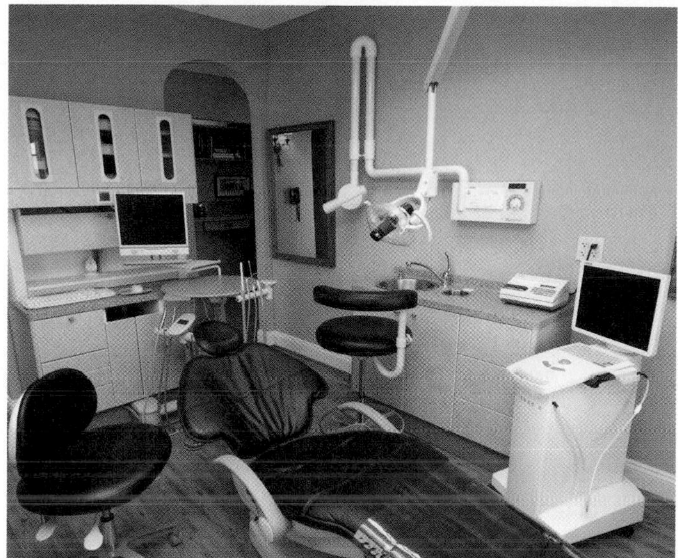

FIG. 32.5 Typical office dental treatment area. *(Courtesy Patterson Dental, St Paul, MN.)*

kept organized and clean at all times. See Chapter 47 for a description of the major equipment found in the dental laboratory.

## Dentist's Private Office

The dentist will have a private office for his or her personal use. Staff members must respect the privacy of this area. The dentist typically has a desk, personal items, a phone system, a computer system, comfortable chairs, and a side table.

It is common for the dentist's private office to be used as a **consultation room** when the dentist is providing a treatment plan to a patient.

## Dental Staff Lounge

A specific area in the dental office should be designated for use by clinical and business staff during breaks or lunchtime. This area may include a table to be used during lunchtime and possibly for staff meetings. Additional items in this area may include a refrigerator or microwave for personal use only and lockers or a locked cabinet for a purse and other personal items. It is customary for the dentist to financially support a coffee service and food vendor.

RECALL

1 What are the important features of the reception area?
2 Where in the dental office are dental procedures performed?
3 What is another term for the treatment area?

# Office Environment

Maintaining a dental office throughout the day involves providing a comfortable, organized, and clean environment. Besides reflecting daily maintenance, the office should have an up-to-date décor and appearance.

## Temperature and Air Exchange

It is important to maintain a comfortable temperature for your patients and staff. The ideal temperature for the reception area should be set at 72° F. The temperature in clinical areas of the office should be lower, from 68° F to 70° F. This area of the office tends to be more hectic and to have more equipment operating, along with additional lighting from overhead and dental units, which can contribute to a warmer environment.

Air exchange should remain constant throughout the office. Have you ever walked into a hospital and thought, "This smells like a hospital"? Then you know that distinct smells can also be associated with a dental office. These odors could be offensive to a patient if the air circulation is not appropriate.

## Lighting

All areas of the office must have appropriate lighting for the task to be completed. In the reception area, more decorative lighting is preferable, such as table and floor lamps that are sufficient for reading.

The business, clinical, laboratory, and sterilization areas frequently used fluorescent lighting, which was more uniform and radiated less heat. Today, as we move toward higher efficiency and green dental office design, there are better options. LED lighting is a great way to reduce energy usage and "green" your office. LEDs generally score higher on the Color Rendering Index than other light sources, giving a "truer" white light.

Additional lighting is provided in the clinical area for procedures and in the laboratory, and is discussed in the Clinical Equipment section later in the chapter.

## Wall and Floor Coverings

Key features in the design of a dental office include the use of colors that should be calming, relaxing, and not too "busy." The wall covering may consist of paint, wallpaper, or both. In terms of a floor covering, a durable high traffic carpet is suitable in the reception area, the administrative area, and the dentist's private office. A more suitable material for infection control, such as linoleum or tile, is appropriate in clinical and laboratory areas.

## Traffic Control

In a dental office, the reception area, front desk, and hallway should be arranged so that traffic flow is efficient to all areas of the office (Fig. 32.6). Separate areas of the front desk should be available for patients to check in and to check out. In the "back" of the office, clinical, sterilization, and laboratory areas should be designed for easy entry into and exit from areas by dental team members without chaos.

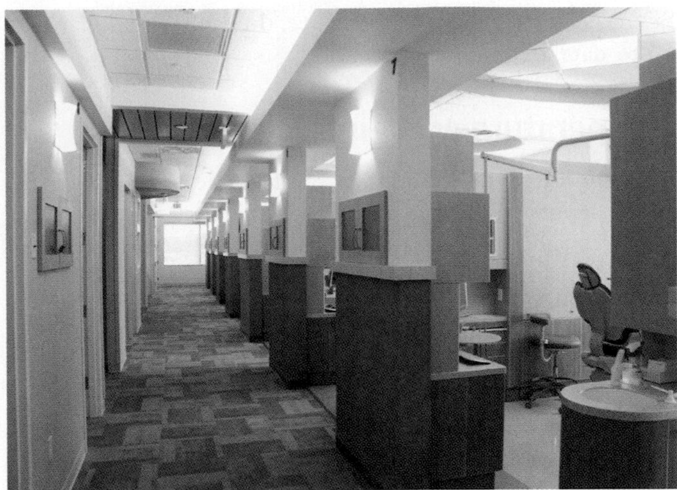

FIG. 32.6 Traffic control. *(Courtesy Patterson Dental, St Paul, MN.)*

## Sound Control

Noise can be a common annoyance in our daily lives, and there are specific sounds associated with a dental office that can present a negative association. The reception area, business office, and clinical areas should be arranged so that minimal sound is carried from one room to another.

Music can provide a distraction from the other sounds. Decide on what type of music will be relaxing and can provide a tranquil environment rather than constant percussion.

## Privacy

Certain areas in the office will require privacy between a patient and staff member. The administrative area should project a professional regard for privacy, especially when the office manager is discussing financial matters with a patient. Clinical areas require privacy to provide the patient and dental team an area in which to complete treatment and talk in privacy without interruption. Finally, the dentist's private office should also ensure privacy away from patient flow.

RECALL

4 What is the ideal temperature for the reception area?
5 What type of flooring should be placed in the clinical area?

# Clinical Equipment

The dentist will work side by side with a representative from a local dental company to select equipment that meets the needs of the practice. The basic equipment found in each operatory includes a patient dental chair, stools for the dentist and assistant to sit on during a procedure, dental units, cabinetry for storage, an operating light, a wall-mounted radiograph unit, a radiograph view box, and a sink.

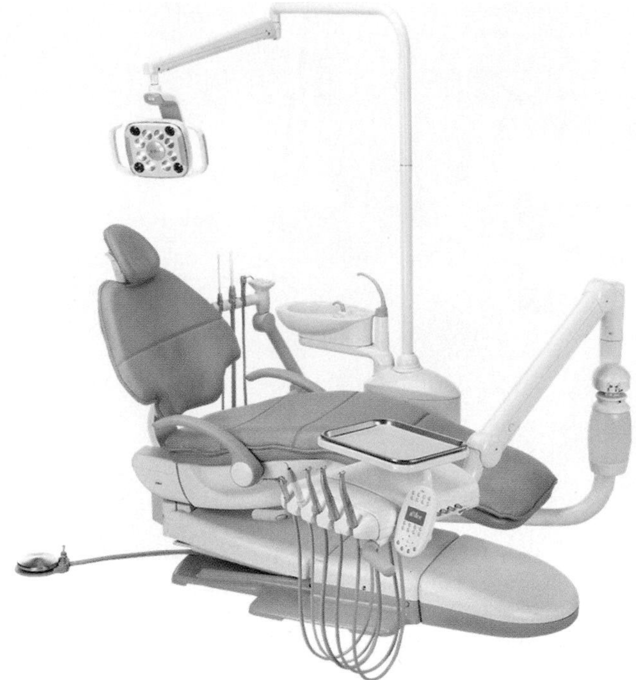

FIG. 32.7 Patient dental chair. *(Courtesy A-dec Inc., Newberg, OR.)*

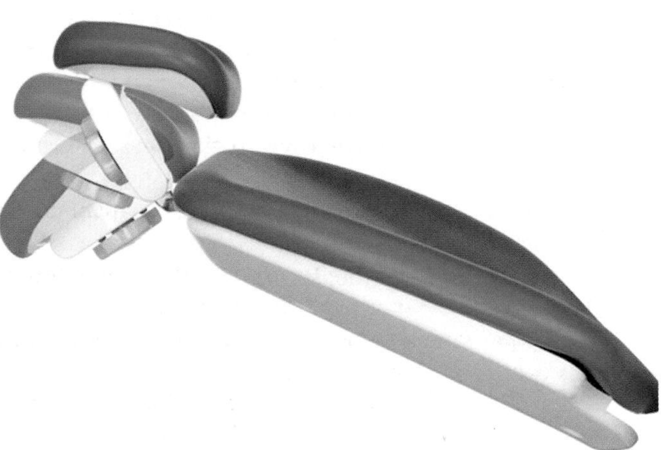

FIG. 32.8 Design of the headrest on a dental chair. *(Courtesy A-dec Inc., Newberg, OR.)*

## Patient Dental Chair

When considering a patient chair, desirable features should be designed for patient comfort and to facilitate a neutral position for the operator. The patient chair should be adjustable to allow the dentist to operate in a neutral seated posture (Fig. 32.7). Patient chairs are designed to be seamless, with few visible mechanical parts for easy cleaning and maintenance. Chairs are available in different sizes for adult practices and for pediatric practices.

When the patient is properly seated, the patient's knees, bottom, and lumbar region of the back should be fully supported. The headrest holds the patient's head securely and comfortably in the appropriate position for the treatment being provided (Fig. 32.8). The headrest can be adjusted to accommodate positioning and height of the patient. The arms of the chair should comfortably support the patient's arms. Chair arms are

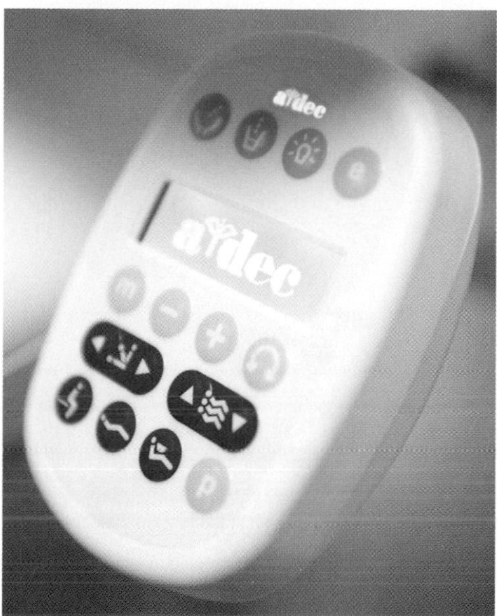

FIG. 32.9 Different parts of the unit may be controlled by buttons on a dental chair. *(Courtesy A-dec Inc., Newberg, OR.)*

designed to be raised or moved aside when seating or dismissing the patient.

The dental chair will have a finger- or foot-operated control system to adjust the chair for dental treatment. These controls allow adjustment of the back of the chair to a lying-down or a sitting-up position. The entire chair can also be adjusted to higher and lower positions for easier patient and oral access (Fig. 32.9).

Adjustment of the dental chair allows the patient to be placed in **upright**, **supine**, and **subsupine positions**. The area of the mouth that is being treated and the type of procedure performed will determine the position selected.

In the upright position, the back of the chair is positioned at a 90-degree angle. The upright position is used for patient entry and dismissal. It provides easy access for the operator when he or she is working on the patient's lower right side (for a right-handed operator). The upright position is also used when radiographs are exposed and when impressions are being taken (Fig. 32.10).

In the supine position, the patient is positioned as if lying down. Because of the contour of the patient chair, however, the patient will not appear flat. The patient's head and knees are at approximately the same level. Most dental treatment is completed with the patient in the supine position (Fig. 32.11).

In the subsupine position, the patient's head is *lower* than the patient's feet. This position can be very uncomfortable for a patient, and it is not used for dental treatment. The subsupine position is recommended for emergency situations and for treatment of the unconscious patient.

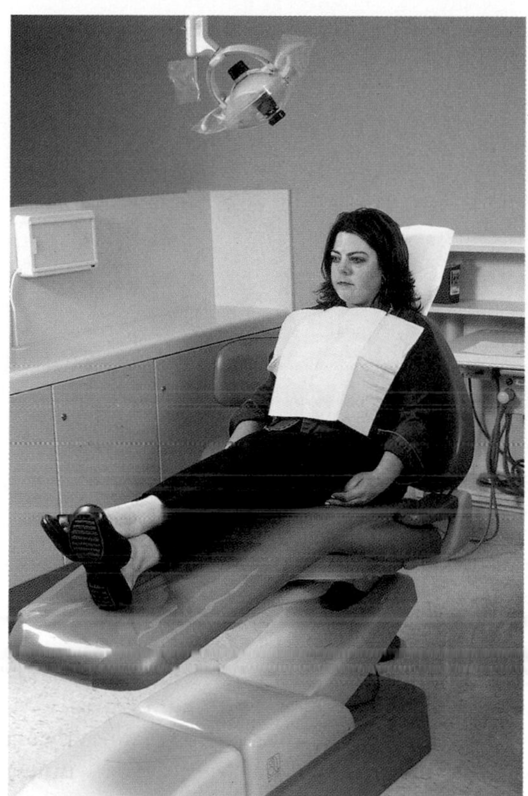

FIG. 32.10 Upright position of a patient in a dental chair.

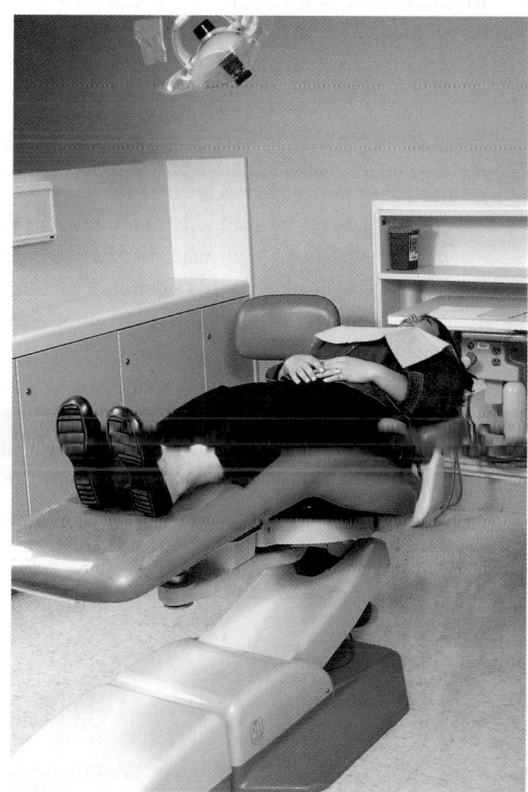

FIG. 32.11 Patient in a supine position in a dental chair.

## Operator's Stool

Depending on the dental procedure being provided, the individual seated as the operator will be the dentist, dental hygienist, or dental assistant. The operator will require a stool to support the body for a prolonged period of fixed muscular activity (Fig. 32.12).

The stool should have a large seat and a back with easily adjustable lumbar support. The seat cushioning should

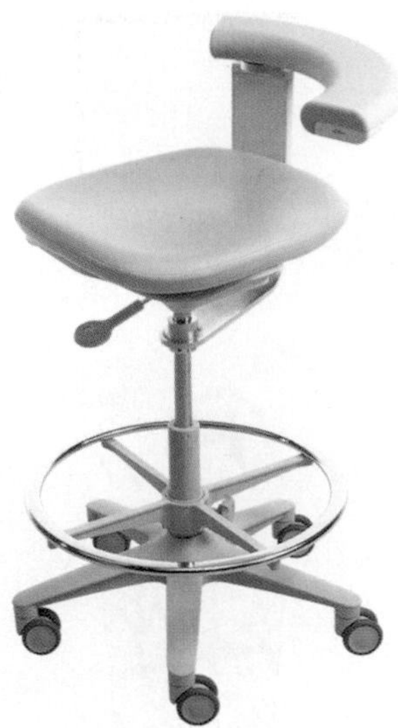

**FIG. 32.12** Dental assistant's stool. *(Courtesy A-dec Inc., Newberg, OR.)*

comfortably support the operator's body for an extended time. The ability of an operator's stool to adjust higher and lower and to move easily around the patient's chair (without tilting for optimal access to the oral cavity) is extremely important in helping to reduce body and eye fatigue.

## Dental Assistant's Stool

The assistant's stool is designed to provide stability, mobility, and comfort and allow the assistant to assist the dentist using proper fatigue-reducing posture. Regardless of the assistant's height or stature, the chair should allow the assistant to twist and turn to reach instruments and equipment located on the countertop.

The dental-assisting stool should minimize fatigue through an adjustable foot platform or foot ring, firm secure cushioning in the seat, and an abdominal support bar. The abdominal bar provides added support for the upper body and arm and allows unobstructed access to the oral cavity. The abdominal bar should be positioned for support, not for resting or leaning. With inappropriate use of the bar, the dental assistant could experience lower back pain caused by continuous leaning over during a dental procedure (Fig. 32.13).

## Dental Unit

The basic function of the dental unit is to provide the necessary electrical and air-operated mechanics to the hoses, handpiece attachments, and working parts of the unit (Fig. 32.14). Dental units are supplied in a range of styles and equipment combinations. The type of dental units selected depends on (1) the space available, (2) the operator's preferred method of delivery, (3) whether the operator is left-handed or right-handed, and (4) whether the operator works primarily with or without a chairside assistant.

The attachments and controls of the dental unit are operated through a master switch. Each attachment has its own control over how much air and water the particular device will receive.

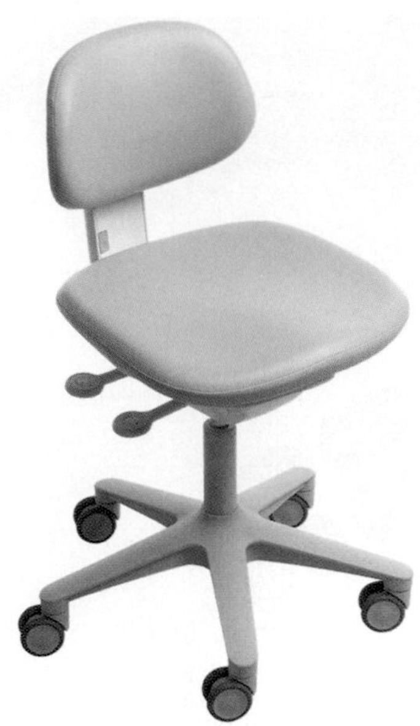

**FIG. 32.13** Operator's stool. *(Courtesy A-dec Inc., Newberg, OR.)*

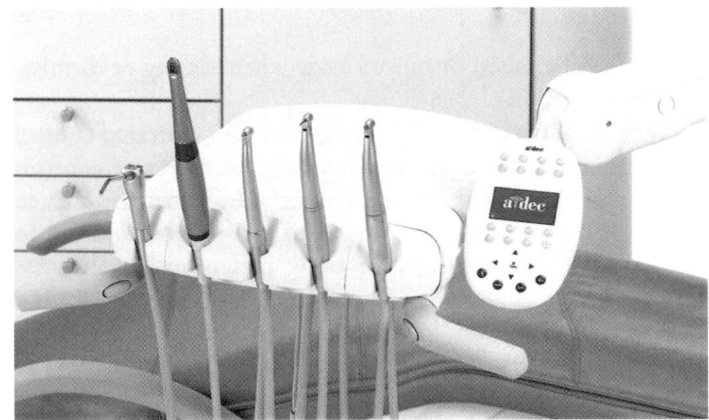

**FIG. 32.14** Dental unit. *(Courtesy A-dec Inc., Newberg, OR.)*

### *Delivery Systems*

The dental unit can be mounted on the floor, the wall, or, most often, the side of the dental chair.

**Front delivery** allows the dental unit to be positioned over the patient's chest. This provides the dentist with easy access to the dental handpieces without twisting of the body (Fig. 32.15, *A*).

**Side delivery** allows the dental unit to be positioned at either side of the patient's chair. The unit provides separate sections for the dentist and the assistant (Fig. 32.15, *B*).

**Rear delivery** allows the dental unit and equipment to be positioned behind the dental chair near the back of the patient's head (Fig. 32.15, *C*).

### *Rheostat*

Each dental handpiece is attached to a specific hose on the dental unit. The dentist or operator will use a **rheostat** to operate and control the speed of the handpieces. A rheostat is a foot-controlled device that is placed on the floor near the operator (Fig. 32.16). With foot pressure, slow-speed and high-speed handpieces are controlled.

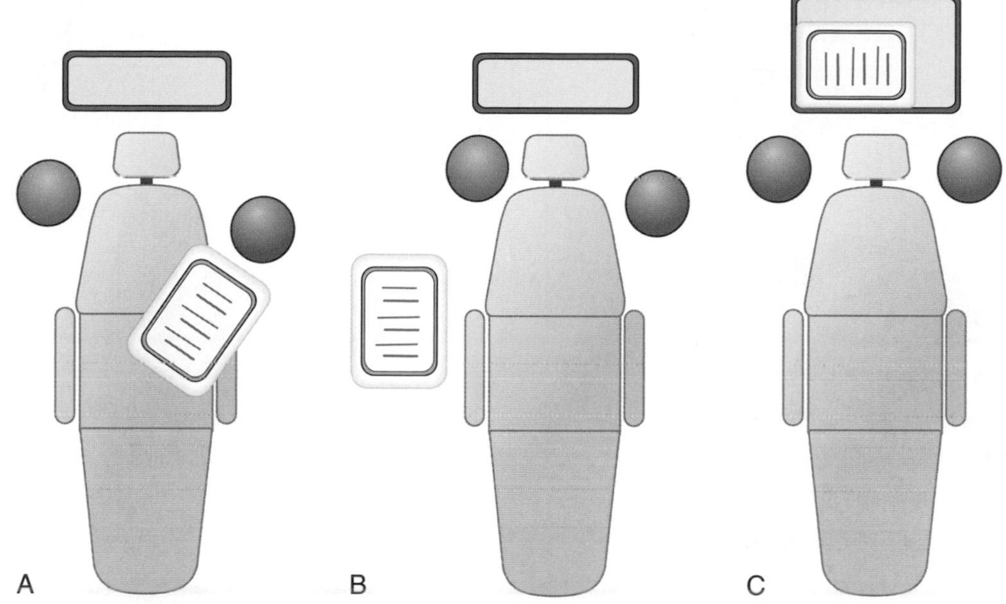


FIG. 32.15 A, Diagram showing front delivery system. B, Diagram showing side delivery system. C, Diagram showing rear delivery system.

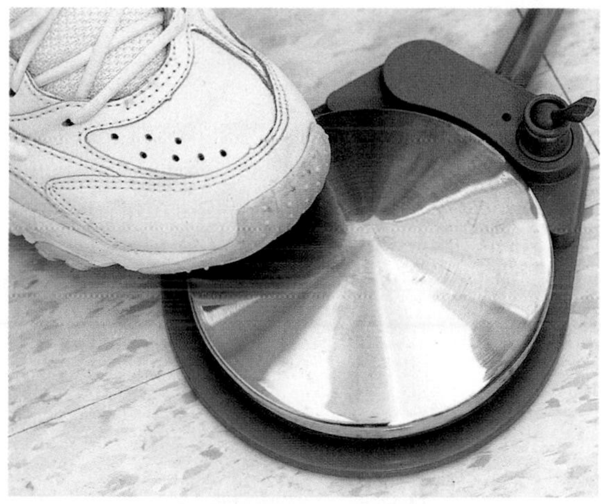

FIG. 32.16 A rheostat controls the handpieces of the dental unit.

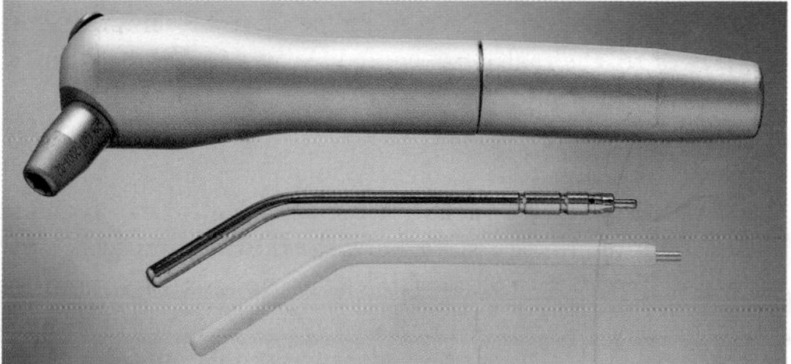

FIG. 32.17 Air-water syringe. *(From Boyd LRB: Dental instruments: a pocket guide, ed 6, St Louis, 2018, Elsevier.)*

## Waterlines

A dental unit is designed with waterlines that carry water through the air-water syringe and dental handpiece. The use of water during a dental procedure is crucial for keeping the tooth clean and cooled against the heat caused by mechanical removal of the tooth structure. Maintenance and cleanliness are high priorities in the use of waterlines (see Chapter 24).

## Air-Water Syringe

The air-water syringe is attached to the dental unit and is essential for every procedure (Fig. 32.17). The air-water syringe functions in three ways:

1. Delivers a stream of water
2. Delivers a stream of air
3. Delivers a combined spray of air and water

The tip of the air-water syringe, which is classified as *semi-critical equipment* under infection control policy, is to be replaced after every procedure. When the air-water syringe is used during patient care, the handle and the tubing are to be covered with a plastic barrier.

## Operating Light

An operating light is used to illuminate the oral cavity during a procedure (Fig. 32.18). Halogen bulbs are used in most operating lights. The light is very bright, and care is taken to avoid shining it into the patient's eyes. The light is attached to a flexible arm, which is track-mounted from the ceiling or attached to the wall or dental chair.

Once the patient is seated and the assistant is gloved, the assistant will position the light on the patient's chest approximately 25 to 30 inches (approximately arm's length) below the patient's chin. The light is turned on and then is slowly adjusted upward to illuminate the oral cavity. When properly positioned, the light illuminates the area to be treated without projecting shadows of the operator's or assistant's hands onto the oral cavity.

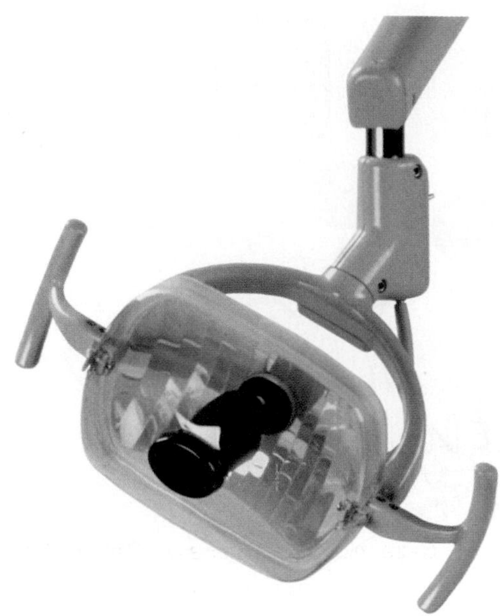

**FIG. 32.18** Operating light. *(Courtesy A-dec Inc., Newberg, OR.)*

The light will become very hot during use. Other than changing the removable barrier on the light handles, the light is cleaned only when it has cooled. When the lens is cool, a mild disinfectant and a soft cloth are used to wipe it free of smudges and debris.

*Note:* Touching a warm lens with a damp cloth can cause the lens to crack.

If a bulb of the operating light needs to be replaced, turn off the light and allow the old bulb to cool before removing it. If you are using a halogen bulb, follow the manufacturer's instructions. Extra bulbs should be kept in inventory to ensure immediate replacement as necessary. *Note:* Halogen bulbs are to be replaced with a gloved hand. The bulb will break if touched with a bare hand.

RECALL

6 What patient chair position is used for most dental procedures?
7 Give two features of the dental assistant's stool that are not seen on the operator's stool.
8 What foot-controlled device is used to operate the dental handpiece?

## Oral Evacuation System

Water is commonly used throughout a dental procedure; when this is the case, you must have some means to remove it. The dental unit contains two evacuation systems: the **saliva ejector** and the **high-volume evacuator** (HVE) (Fig. 32.19) (see Chapter 36).

The disposable saliva ejector has a less-powerful suction system than the HVE. The saliva ejector provides removal of the patient's excess fluids from the mouth. The saliva ejector is used in less-invasive procedures, such as routine cleanings, placement of sealants, and fluoride application.

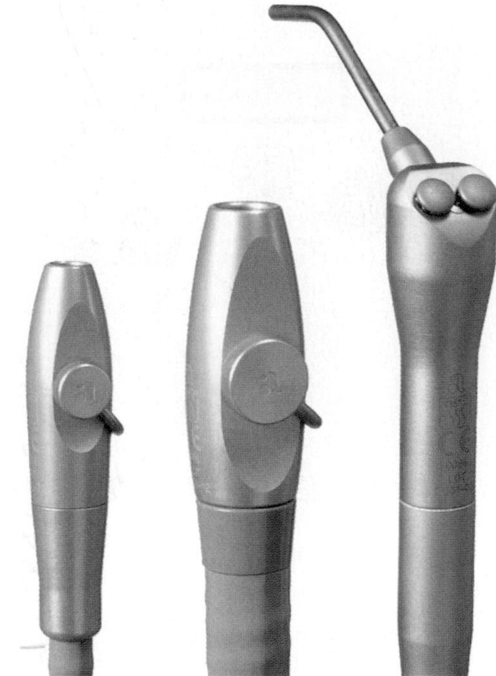

**FIG. 32.19** Oral evacuation system that contains a saliva ejector, a high-volume evacuator, and an air-water syringe. *(Courtesy A-dec Inc., Newberg, OR.)*

The assistant will use the HVE for most procedures. This system is more powerful than the saliva ejector and helps maintain a "clear field" in which the dentist can work. A new HVE tip is used for each patient. During use, the HVE handle and hose are covered with a protective plastic barrier. See Chapter 36 for the types of grasps and positioning of the HVE.

## Curing Light

The curing light is a wandlike attachment used to harden or "cure" light-sensitive dental materials. Components of the light include the protective shield handle and the trigger switch by which it can be turned on and off (Fig. 32.20). Several types of curing units with different light intensities and light sources are available. Light-curing units can use halogen-based, light-emitting diode (LED), plasma-arc, or laser technology. The energy levels of these lights can range from 300 to more than 1000 milliwatts per square centimeter.

Many factors can affect the curing of a dental material. Steps that the clinical assistant can take to maximize the curing process include the following: keep the light tip clean and free of scratches, position the light tip at the correct distance from and the correct orientation to the material, maintain the bulb and filter in good working order, and establish appropriate curing times for each material used in the dental office.

During use, the curing light should be protected with a plastic barrier. If additional cleaning and disinfection are necessary in treatment room preparation, the light should be cooled

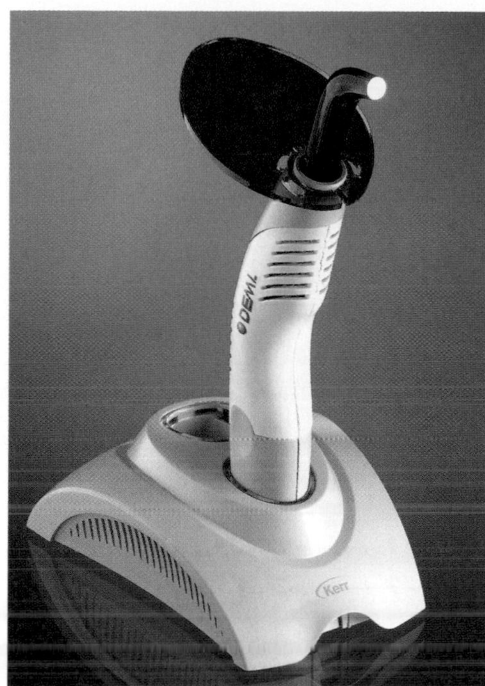


FIG. 32.20 A cordless curing light is used to harden dental materials. *(From Boyd LRB: Dental instruments: a pocket guide, ed 6, St Louis, 2018, Elsevier.)*

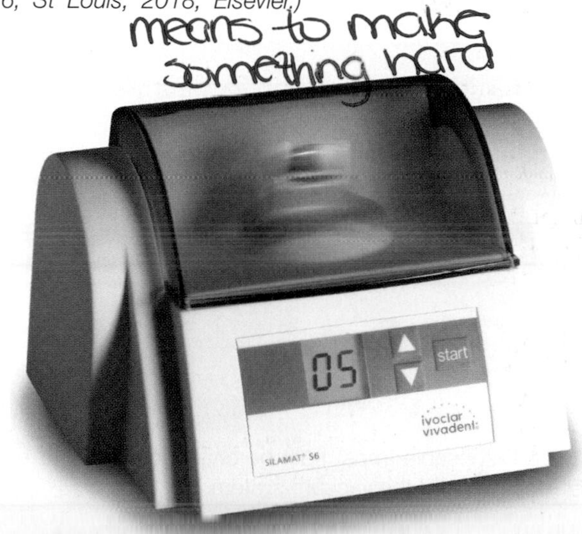


FIG. 32.21 Amalgamator. *(Courtesy Ivoclar Vivadent, Inc., Amherst, NY.)*

before it is wiped with solutions. *Note:* A sudden change in temperature could damage the light system.

## Amalgamator

An **amalgamator** is an electrical machine used to **triturate**, or mechanically mix, dental materials by vigorously shaking the capsule that holds the ingredients. The amalgamator can be mounted under a countertop or placed within a mobile cabinet or stored in the top drawer of a mobile cabinet (Fig. 32.21). Specific settings on the amalgamator will correspond to the manufacturer's directions regarding mixing of that specific dental material.

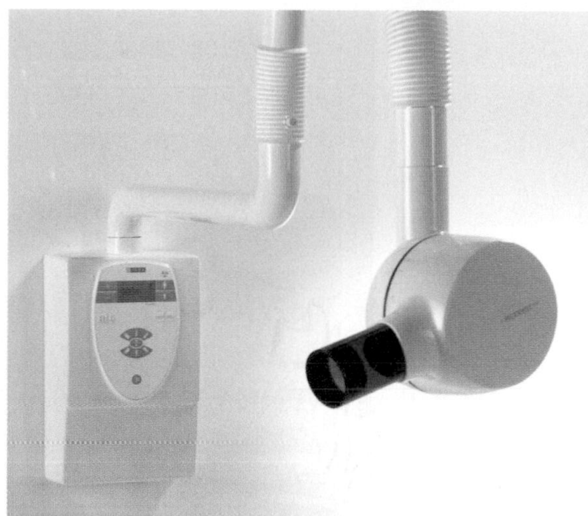

FIG. 32.22 Radiographic unit. *(Courtesy Sirona Dental Inc., Charlotte, NC.)*

## Dental Radiography Unit

Most dental treatment rooms include a dental radiography unit (see Chapter 40). The master switch of the unit may be turned on safely at the beginning of the day and may be left on throughout the day. If the radiography unit requires maintenance, it first must be disconnected from its electrical source (Fig. 32.22).

*Note:* Radiation is emitted from the radiography unit only while the exposure timer switch is depressed.

### *View Box for Radiographs*

A view box consists of a bright white light source with a frosted glass or plastic cover commonly attached to the dental unit or mounted flush on the wall. Radiographic images are displayed on a monitor that is part of the dental unit (Fig. 32.23). Radiographs are uploaded on the view box for evaluation. The light source shines through the radiograph, allowing better visual evaluation by the dentist.

9 What does the abbreviation HVE represent?
10 Where do you place dental materials to be triturated?

## Care of Dental Equipment

Dental equipment is expensive, complex, and delicate. It must be used carefully and maintained properly in accordance with the manufacturer's instructions. Dental assistants who work in the clinical area share responsibility for routine care in this area of the office. Larger practices may contract to have maintenance personnel provide this service.

## Central Vacuum Compressor

A central vacuum compressor provides the suction needed for oral evacuation systems. This equipment actually

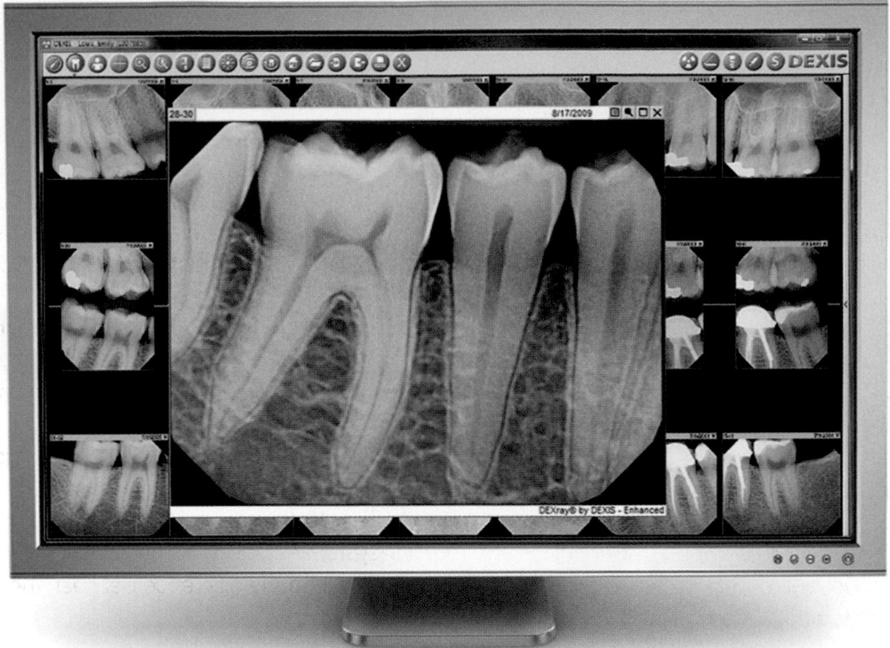


FIG. 32.23 Radiographic image display. *(Courtesy of KaVo Kerr.)*

consists of two parts: the *compressor,* which creates the flow of air, and the *vacuum tank,* which screens the flow of air to create suction. The central vacuum compressor should be serviced regularly, in keeping with the manufacturer's instructions.

## Central Air Compressor

A central air compressor is used to provide compressed air for the air-water syringe and air-driven handpieces. The capacity of the compressor depends on the number of dental units used in the practice. Because of the noise level and for safety reasons, the compressor system is placed away from the clinical setting.

The air compressor must receive routine service according to the manufacturer's instructions. This maintenance includes changing filters and occasionally checking for **condensation** in the lines. Trained maintenance personnel usually handle this service.

Condensation in the airlines may produce moisture, sediment, or algae. These contaminants can ruin handpieces and can cause debris to be ejected into the patient's mouth. If any indication of a condensation problem is noted, the equipment should be serviced immediately.

Disposable traps are located on the dental unit and provide a filtering mechanism for the saliva ejector and the HVE that catches debris drawn from the mouth. These traps are disposable and should be changed weekly. Utility gloves are worn and cotton pliers or utility tongs should be used when these tight, contaminated screens are handled (Fig. 32.24). Chapter 23 discusses removal of amalgam scrap from the traps.

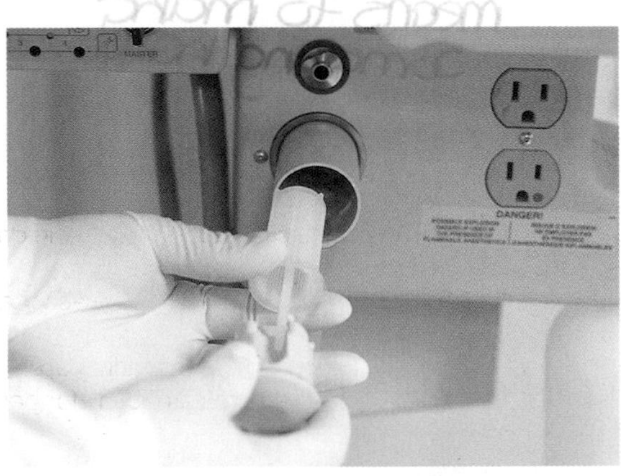


FIG. 32.24 Disposable traps must be changed weekly to ensure proper functioning of the vacuum system.

# Morning and Evening Routines for Dental Assistants

In most practices, the clinical staff will assume the important responsibilities of morning and evening care of the clinical areas. Careful completion of all steps helps ensure the smooth flow of patient care throughout the day.

The goal in the evening is to leave the office ready for patient care the next morning. Failure to complete these steps could result in loss of productive time for the dentist, inconvenience or discomfort for the patient, and unnecessary stress for everyone.

Procedure 32.1: Performing the Morning Routine (Opening the Office) and Procedure 32.2: Performing the Evening Routine (Closing the Office) review steps to be followed during the morning and evening routines of the dental assistant.

**■ Patient Education** When a patient enters the clinical areas of the dental office, the dental equipment will appear foreign and possibly worrisome. When you educate your patients about the environment of the dental equipment, not only will they feel more comfortable, they also may ask questions about new dental procedures and techniques. ■

**■ Eye to the Future** The design and layout of dental offices are keeping up with current interior design trends. You will see more adaptations based on personal style than in the past. Offices are becoming more creative when patient comfort is of utmost importance. You might see a babbling brook running through the reception area to provide the relaxing sound of moving water. Many offices have murals on the ceilings of dental treatment areas for the patient to view.

Additional items for patient use may include personal headphones with a choice of music and televisions with a selection of movies. Remember that the patient is the most important person in the office. Make sure that all of your patients are comfortable. ■

**■ Critical Thinking**

1. The reception area of your dental office was designed in the 1990s, and the furniture and colors are outdated. Your dentist asks you to help in decisions about remodeling. What are some of the thoughts that you would include when decorating the reception area?
2. Your dental office has an open bay structure, where most of the clinical area is open. How could you provide a sense of patient privacy and sound control with this type of office design?
3. What features are important to consider when selecting an operator's stool?
4. The dental unit can be designed to come from three delivery system setups for dental units. List those.
5. Describe the difference between the operating light and the curing light. ■

PROCEDURE 32.1

## Performing the Morning Routine (Opening the Office)

**PROCEDURAL STEPS**

1 Arrive 30 minutes before the first scheduled patient of the day.
**PURPOSE** This allows time to complete tasks so the day can start smoothly and on time.
2 Turn on master switches for the central air compressor and vacuum units.
3 Turn on master switches for the dental and radiography units.
4 Ensure that the dental treatment rooms are ready for patient care.
- Dental chair lowered and positioned in upright position
- All equipment covered with surface barriers for infection control

5 Recheck the appointment schedule of patients for the day to be certain that
- Instruments have been sterilized and readied
- Patient records have been retrieved
- Laboratory cases have been delivered and available for planned treatments

6 Set up the treatment room for the first patient.

PROCEDURE 32.2

## Performing the Evening Routine (Closing the Office)

**PROCEDURAL STEPS**

1 Complete the operatory room exposure control cleanup and preparation protocols.
2 Wear appropriate personal protective equipment (PPE) while emptying waste receptacles and placing fresh plastic liners.
**PURPOSE** Waste must be disposed of safely (see Chapter 23).
3 Turn off all equipment.
4 Ensure that the treatment area is adequately stocked for the next day.
5 In treatment areas, post appointment schedules for the next day.
6 Check appointment schedules to ensure that instruments, patient records, and laboratory work are ready for the next day.
7 Determine that all contaminated instruments have been processed and that the sterilization center has been cleaned.
8 Make sure that treatment rooms are ready for use.
9 Unclutter the reception area.
10 Place any soiled PPE into appropriate containers.
**PURPOSE** Proper handling of contaminated PPE is an important part of exposure control.

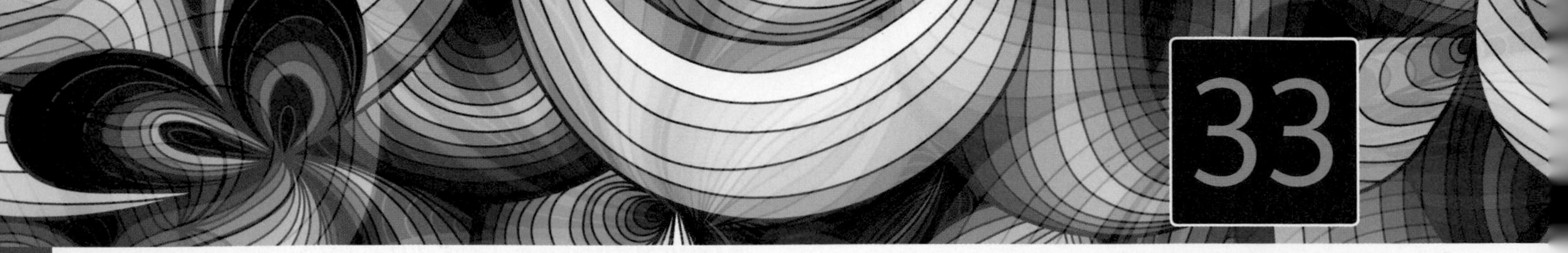

# 33 Delivering Dental Care

## KEY TERMS

**Delegate** To authorize or entrust another person to perform a specific skill or procedure.

**Direct supervision** Level of supervision in which the dentist is physically present when the auxiliary performs delegated functions.

**Expanded function** Specific intraoral function delegated to an auxiliary that requires advanced skill and training.

**Four-handed dentistry** Process by which the operator and the assistant work together to perform clinical procedures in an ergonomically structured environment.

**Fulcrum (FUL-krum)** Finger rest used when one holds an instrument or handpiece for a specified time.

**Grasp** The correct way for an instrument or handpiece to be held.

**Indirect supervision** Overseeing an assistant's work by working in the immediate area.

**Indirect vision** Viewing an object with the use of a mirror.

**Operating zones** Concept by which the face of a clock is used to position the dental team, equipment, and supplies.

## LEARNING OUTCOMES

*On completion of this chapter, the student will be able to achieve the following objectives:*

1. Pronounce, define, and spell the key terms.
2. Discuss knowing your patients, reviewing the patient records, and how to prepare for a patient appointment, including the following:
   - Describe how to prepare the dental treatment area for a patient's arrival.
   - Discuss the importance of preparing a dental treatment room for a procedure.
3. Discuss the concept of team dentistry, and the principles of team positioning, including the following:
   - Describe how the operator is positioned during treatment.
   - Describe how the assistant is positioned during treatment.
4. Explain the classification of motions.
5. Define each of the operating zones.
6. Explain instrument transfer, including the following:
   - Specify three grasps used by the operator.
   - Specify four items that have to be transferred differently because of design or use.
   - Discuss the differences between one-handed and two-handed instrument transfer techniques.
7. Identify five areas in which the assistant must have competency when practicing expanded functions.

## PERFORMANCE OUTCOMES

*On completion of this chapter, the student will be able to meet competency standards in the following skills:*

- Demonstrate admitting and seating of the patient.
- Demonstrate the proper use of a dental mirror.
- Transfer instruments using the single-handed technique.
- Transfer instruments using the two-handed technique.
- Demonstrate the intraoral use of a dental instrument.

## ELECTRONIC RESOURCES

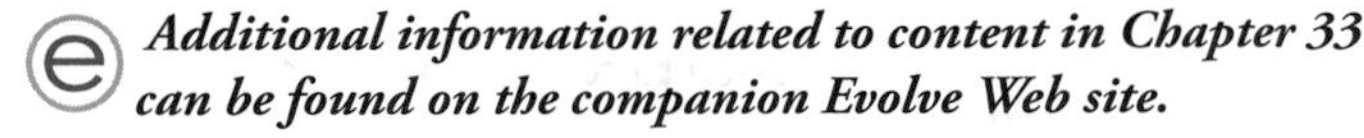

***Additional information related to content in Chapter 33 can be found on the companion Evolve Web site.***

- Practice Quiz
- Video: Transferring Instruments (Single-Handed)

The manner in which dental care is provided is one of the most important responsibilities of the dental team. For a typical day to run smoothly and for the best patient care to be provided, the business assistant, clinical assistant, dental hygienist, and dentist must follow a specific routine.

With advance preparation in reviewing the patient record, with knowledge of the upcoming procedure, and by being ready with the needed supplies and equipment, the dental healthcare professional can prevent the daily routine of clinical care from being hectic and can ensure that the flow of patient care is maintained throughout the day. Failure to meet these standards can result in loss of production for the dentist, inconvenience or discomfort for the patient, and unnecessary stress for everyone.

## Know Your Patients

Once a patient enters the reception area, it is essential that his or her presence be acknowledged immediately. One of the best ways to know your patients and to be better prepared for the day ahead is to have a brief meeting or overview of the day before your patients arrive. Topics that should be discussed among the dental team during this meeting can include the following:

- Change in schedule or procedure
- A patient's health condition or age that could alter dental treatment
- Additional supplies or equipment that may be needed for a procedure
- Preparation for an apprehensive patient in the form of scheduling more time, using premedication, or preparing the setup for the use of nitrous oxide during the procedure
- Assignment of expanded functions to the dental assistant

## Reviewing the Patient Record

Several sections of a patient record are reviewed at each patient visit. The business staff will discuss any changes in the patient's personal information, such as address or phone number change, and make corrections as needed. The clinical staff will discuss any **medical alerts** or changes in medical status and update the health history form. The clinical assistant refers to progress notes for the planned treatment of the day.

## Preparing the Treatment Area

A treatment room preparation checklist should be completed before the patient is seated:

- Is the treatment room clean, disinfected, and ready for the next patient?
- Are the patient's record, radiographs, and laboratory case in place?
- Are the appropriate sterile preset tray and other supplies in place and ready for use?
- Is the dental chair positioned to allow seating of the patient?
- Has additional equipment been moved out of the path of entry for the patient and dental team members?

## Greeting and Seating the Patient

As the clinical assistant, you will enter the reception area to greet and escort your patient to the designated clinical area. Address the patient using his or her title (Mr., Mrs., or Ms.) and last name. Remember that patients must be greeted in a courteous way. When you call out to your patient, make sure to establish eye contact, smile, and introduce yourself.

See Procedure 33.1: Admitting and Seating of the Patient.

## Team Dentistry

Team dentistry, also referred to as **four-handed dentistry**, is a concept that describes the way the dentist and the dental assistant work together to perform clinical procedures in an ergonomically structured environment. The main goal of this concept is to deliver the best and most effective care to patients by increasing productivity and reducing fatigue and stress during the completion of dental procedures.

Team dentistry is a standard of performance that has been taught to dental students and dental-assisting students over the past 40 years. Basic goals of this type of coordination include the following:

- To use ergonomically correct dental equipment
- To use preset trays during dental procedures
- To minimize stress and fatigue during performance of dental procedures by ensuring specific, ergonomically correct positioning of the patient, dentist, and assistant (see Chapter 25)
- To follow the principles of motion economy during the transfer of instruments and dental materials
- To use appropriate moisture control techniques to enhance visualization of the working field in the mouth (see Chapter 36)
- To delegate expanded functions of practice as legally defined within the state

1 State two goals of the dental team that would simplify dental treatment in the dental office.

### Principles of Team Positioning

Correct positioning of the dental team within the clinical area is essential. The dentist and the dental assistant should develop positioning habits that allow access to and visualization of all areas of the oral cavity, while maintaining a position that provides optimal comfort and support (Fig. 33.1).

Whenever the dentist and the assistant must stretch to reach for an instrument or gain access to an area of the mouth, stress is placed on the body. If this occurs daily, the accumulated

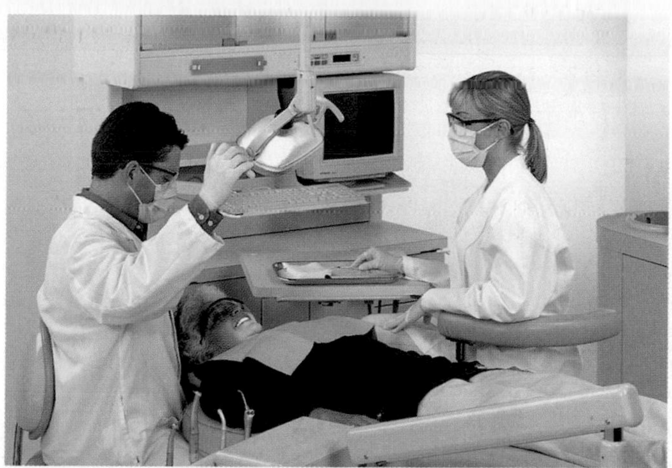

**FIG. 33.1** The concept of four-handed dentistry is shown in the positioning of the patient and dental team members.

strain contributes to lower back pain, circulatory problems, and muscle aches and pain. (Refer to Chapter 25 for more information on ergonomics.)

### Positioning the Patient

After the patient has been escorted to the treatment area and seated, he or she is then lowered to the supine position. The patient is asked to slide up in the chair until the top of the head is even with the top of the headrest. The operator then asks the patient to turn his or her head to the right or the left to allow easier access to a specific area of the mouth.

The operator makes final adjustments to the chair to establish proper working distance. The distance between the patient's face and the operator's face should be approximately 12 to 14 inches (Fig. 33.2). When working in the mandibular area, the back of the chair is raised to a slightly more upright position for better visualization.

### Positioning the Operator

Access and visualization are the most essential qualities for the operator. Chapter 32 describes the unique features of the operator's stool. The positioning of the operator on the stool is important for ensuring comfort and support (Fig. 33.3).

The operator should practice the following guidelines:

- Seated as far back as possible, with front edge of stool just touching the backs of the knees
- Thighs parallel to floor, or knees slightly lower than hips
- Feet kept flat on the floor and not crossed
- Backrest of chair positioned to support lower portion or small of the back
- Height of chair maintained to keep operator's forearms parallel to the floor when bent at the elbow

### Positioning the Dental Assistant

When assisting the dentist, the dental assistant will anticipate what is needed throughout the procedure and must have *access* to the area of the mouth during the procedure (Fig. 33.4). Chapter 32 describes positioning features that are important in ensuring the dental assistant's comfort and support.

The assistant should practice the following guidelines regarding correct positioning on the stool:

- Seated well back on stool
- Feet resting on base or foot ring of stool
- Positioned as close as possible to dental chair
- Legs parallel to patient's chair
- Eye level 4 to 6 inches above the operator

RECALL

2 In relation to the operator, should the assistant be positioned lower or higher when seated properly?
3 How should the operator maintain their forearms when providing dental treatment on a patient?

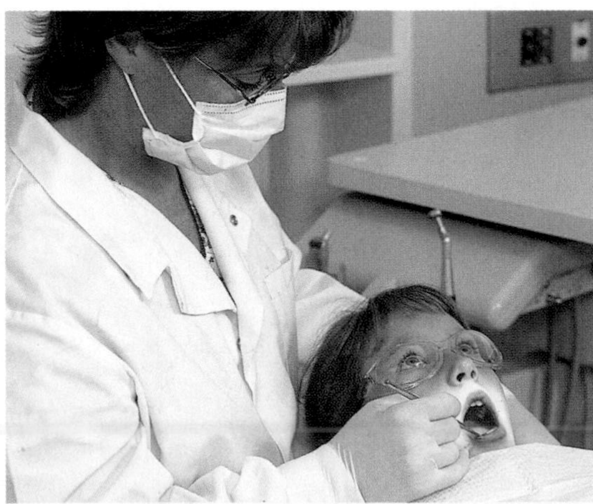

**FIG. 33.2** Distance from the operator's face to the patient's face when positioned correctly.

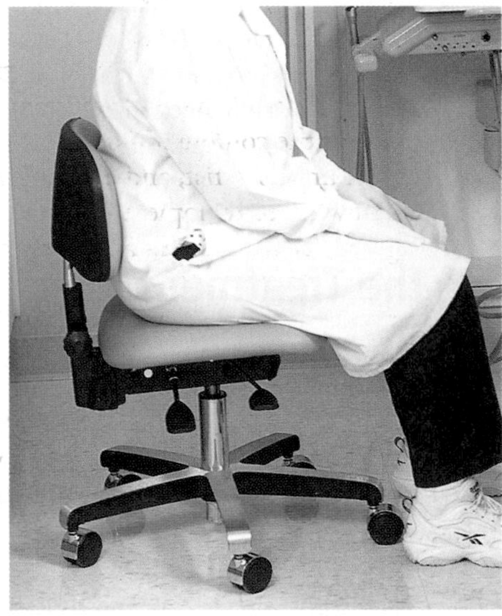

**FIG. 33.3** Position of the operator when seated correctly.

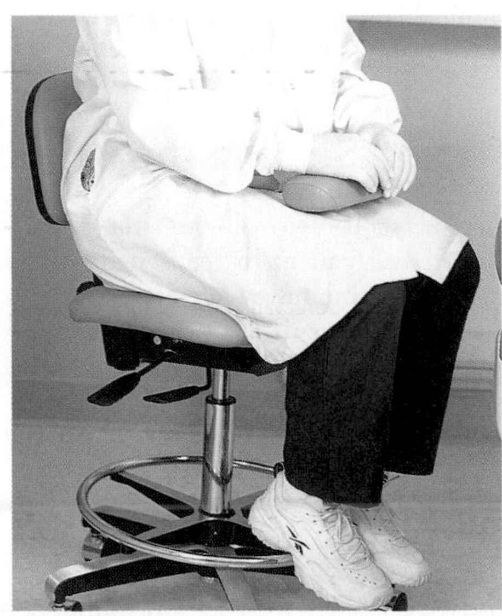

**FIG. 33.4** Position of the dental assistant when seated correctly.

# Motion Economy

If you ask members of the dental team in the business or clinical area what part of the body is most fatigued by the end of the day, they would most likely comment about their lower back. This is because of too much reaching, twisting, and turning while seated in their work position.

## Classification of Motions

Motions are classified into five categories according to extent of movement. By understanding early in your preclinical studies the need to eliminate or reduce Class IV and V motions, you will develop better habits and will truly benefit ergonomically in the long run.

**Class I:** Movement of fingers only. Examples include picking up an instrument or a single object from a flat surface, or picking up a pencil or a pen to write with.

**Class II:** Movement of fingers and wrist. Examples include transferring an instrument with the use of a pen grasp, or mixing a dental material; as the business assistant, typing on a keyboard or using the computer mouse.

**Class III:** Movement of fingers, wrist, and elbow. Examples include using the slow-speed handpiece when performing coronal polishing and, as the business assistant, answering the telephone.

**Class IV:** Use of the entire arm and shoulder. Examples include reaching for items within the mobile unit, moving the radiography unit, and filing patient records.

**Class V:** Use of the entire upper torso. Examples include bending over to see intraorally, retrieving dental materials from a tub or drawer, and reaching to hand patients a form to complete.

# Operating Zones

**Operating zones** are based on a "clock concept" and describe the best way to identify the working position of the dental team, the dental equipment, and the supplies needed to perform a procedure. This basic concept is used in the practice of efficient and comfortable clinical dentistry and can be applied to any dental procedure.

To understand the concept, visualize a circle placed over the dental chair. The patient's face is in the center of the circle, and the top of the patient's head is toward the 12 o'clock position. The face of the clock is divided into four zones. The location of the zones changes according to whether the operator is right-handed or left-handed. The operator's position varies within that zone, depending on the treatment to be delivered (Figs. 33.5 and 33.6).

## Operator's Zone

**The operator's zone** (right-handed—7 o'clock to 12 o'clock; left-handed—12 o'clock to 5 o'clock) is the area where the person who completes the procedure is seated. Most often, the dentist is the operator. However, the dental assistant or the dental hygienist can be referred to as the operator when working individually directly inside the oral cavity.

## Transfer Zone

The **transfer zone** (right-handed—4 o'clock to 7 o'clock; left-handed—5 o'clock to 8 o'clock) is the area where instruments and dental materials are exchanged between the dental assistant and the dentist. This zone is located directly over the patient's chest. In front delivery, the dental unit is located in the transfer zone within easy reach of the dentist and the assistant.

## Assistant's Zone

The **assistant's zone** (right-handed—2 o'clock to 4 o'clock; left-handed—8 o'clock to 10 o'clock) is the area where the dental assistant is positioned. The assistant's mobile cabinet or rear delivery countertop can also be positioned within this zone. To minimize motion, a movable countertop can be positioned over the assistant's lap; this can hold the instrument tray, paper products, and dental materials.

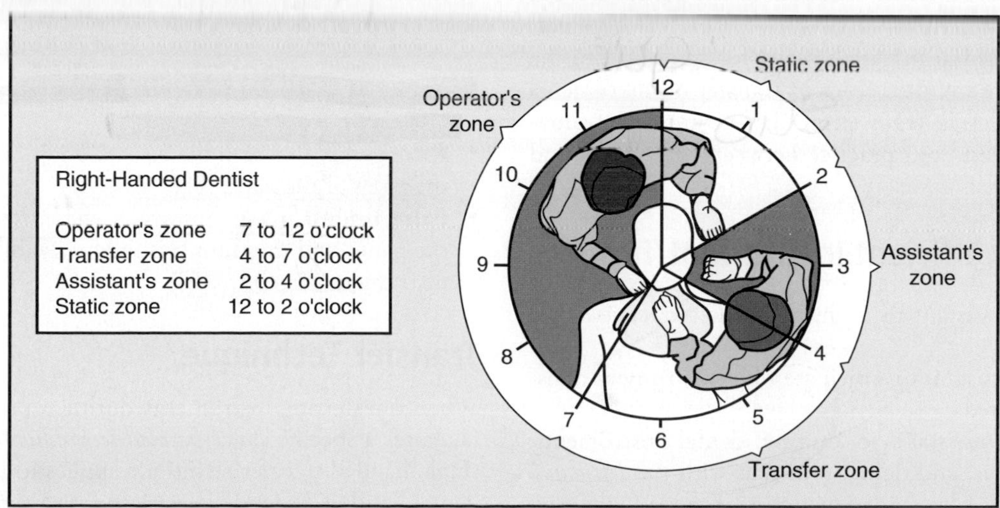


**FIG. 33.5** Operating zones for a right-handed operator.

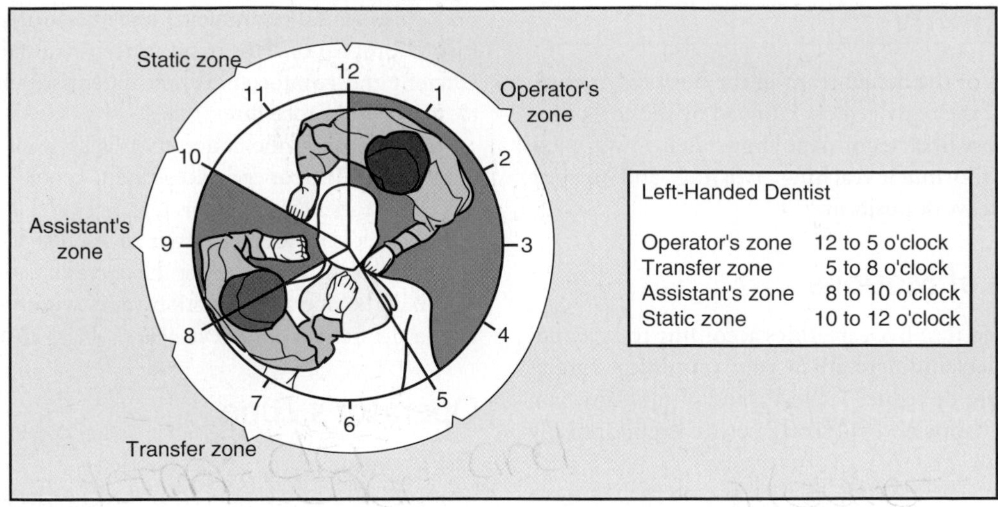


**FIG. 33.6** Operating zones for a left-handed operator.

## Static Zone

The **static zone** (right-handed—12 o'clock to 2 o'clock; left-handed—10 o'clock to 12 o'clock) is located directly behind the patient. If the dental unit has rear delivery, the handpieces, the air-water syringe, and additional countertop space are positioned within the static zone. Portable equipment such as the nitrous oxide unit may also be positioned in the static zone.

RECALL

4 In terms of the clock concept, where is the static zone located for a right-handed operator?
5 Where are instruments exchanged during a procedure?
6 Besides the assistant, what may be located in the assistant's zone?

# Instrument Transfer

Four-handed dentistry is based on the concept that a qualified chairside dental assistant is seated across from the dentist, and they work as a team. Throughout the procedure, the dentist relies on the clinical assistant to have the supplies, instruments, and dental materials ready for transfer into the dentist's hands. The smooth, efficient transfer of instruments and materials reflects a team effort that requires coordination, communication, and practice between the dentist and the dental assistant.

## Objectives of Efficient Instrument Transfer

- For the dental assistant to understand the sequence of the procedure.
- For the dental assistant to anticipate when instrument transfer will be required.
- For the dental assistant to transfer dental instruments, dental handpieces, and dental materials with the *left hand.* The right hand is kept free to suction and to ready the next materials and instruments.
- To transfer instruments with the use of only Class I, Class II, and Class III motions involving only the fingers, wrist, and elbow.
- To transfer instruments in the **position of use,** which refers to directing the working end of the instrument downward for the mandibular arch and upward for the maxillary arch. This is instilled so the dentist does not need to reposition the instrument in his or her hand before use.
- To transfer an instrument so that the dentist can grasp the instrument for its appropriate use.
- To position an instrument in the dentist's hand firmly, so the dentist can receive it without moving his or her eyes from the field of operation.

## Grasping an Instrument

The manner in which the operator grasps and holds an instrument for use varies with the type of instrument, how the instrument is used, and which area of the mouth is being treated. An understanding of instrument **grasp** is essential to smooth instrument transfer and exchange of instruments. The three basic grasps are as follows:

- **Pen grasp,** in which the instrument is held in the same manner as a pen (Fig. 33.7, *A*)
- **Palm grasp,** in which the instrument is held securely within the palm of the hand (Fig. 33.7, *B*)
- **Palm-thumb grasp,** in which the instrument is held in the palm, and the thumb is used to stabilize and guide the instrument (Fig. 33.7, *C*)

## Transfer Technique

When transferring instruments during a procedure, the assistant uses a specific *single-handed technique* for efficiency. This single-handed transfer technique applies to hand instruments, dental handpieces, and air-water syringes (see Procedure 33.2: Transferring Instruments with the Single-Handed Technique).

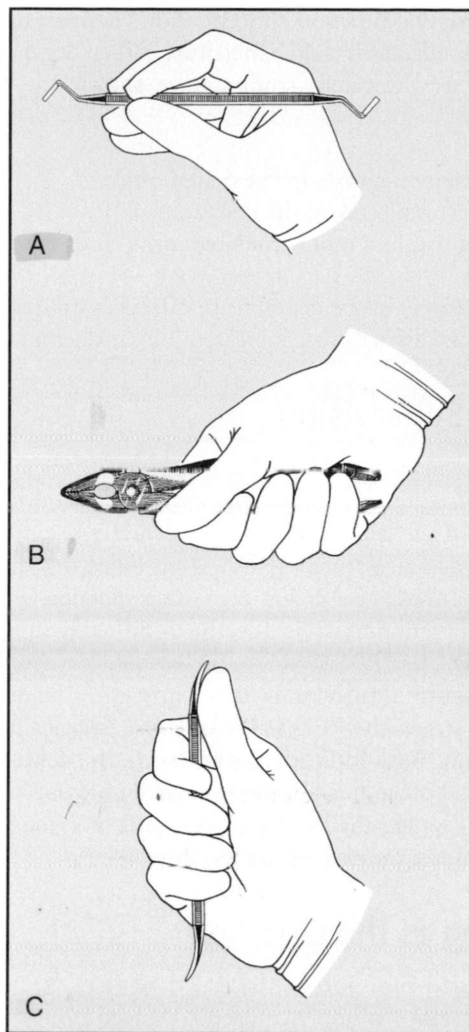


**FIG. 33.7** Basic instrument grasps. A, Pen grasp. B, Palm grasp. C, Palm-thumb grasp.

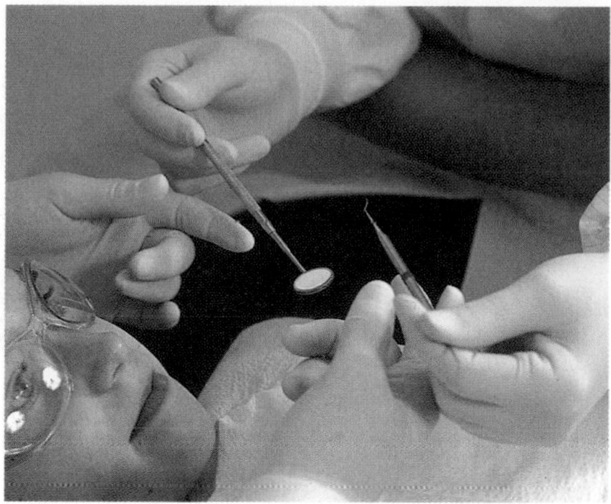

**FIG. 33.8** The dentist prepares to receive the mirror and explorer by positioning the hand on either side of the patient's head.

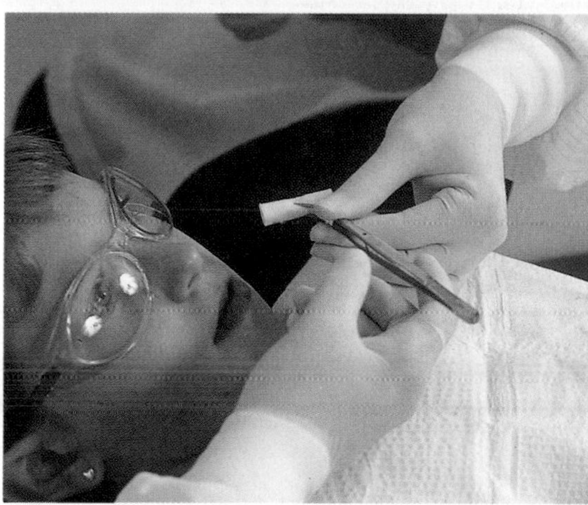

**FIG. 33.9** The assistant transfers the cotton pliers, ensuring that the ends are together so as not to drop the item.

## Variations in Instrument Exchange

Specific items and instruments have to be transferred differently because of their design or use.

### *Mirror and Explorer*

When beginning a procedure, the dentist will immediately use the mouth mirror and the explorer to inspect the area to be treated. The dentist will signal to the assistant by placing one hand on each side of the patient's mouth in a position that indicates readiness to receive the instruments.

The dental assistant delivers the mirror and the explorer simultaneously, using a two-handed exchange. For the right-handed operator, the explorer is transferred with the left hand, and the mirror with the right hand (Fig. 33.8).

### *Cotton Pliers*

When cotton pliers are used to transfer small items to and from the oral cavity, a modification in the single-handed technique must be made. The assistant delivers the pliers to the dentist while pinching together the "beaks" to avoid dropping the item held by the pliers (Fig. 33.9). Grasping the working end of the pliers makes retrieval of the cotton pliers easier. This grasp also prevents the contents of the forceps from slipping out.

### *Handpiece*

The handpiece can be exchanged for an instrument through the same technique used when two instruments are transferred (Fig. 33.10). When you are exchanging the handpiece, take precautions to avoid tangling the hoses during the transfer.

### *Instruments with Hinges*

Instruments with hinges are designed to have an open/closed use. The most common hinged instruments are the rubber dam forceps, surgical forceps, orthodontic pliers, and scissors.

These instruments are held at their hinges and are transferred by directing their handles into the dentist's palm. The handles of scissors are positioned over the dentist's fingers (Fig. 33.11). Because hinged instruments are heavier than single instruments and a steadier hand may be needed, a two-handed transfer technique can be used (see Procedure 33.3: Transferring Instruments with the Two-Handed Technique).

RECALL

7 Should the assistant use one hand or both hands to transfer a single instrument?
8 Which hand is used primarily to transfer instruments to a right-handed dentist?

## Expanded Functions

**Expanded function** is the term used to refer to a specific intraoral skill that is completed as a procedure or as part of a procedure by the clinical dental assistant. The dentist **delegates** expanded functions to the dental assistant.

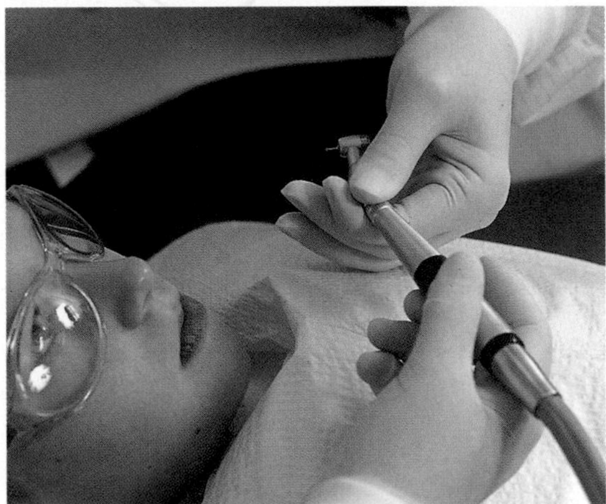

FIG. 33.10 Transferring the handpiece.

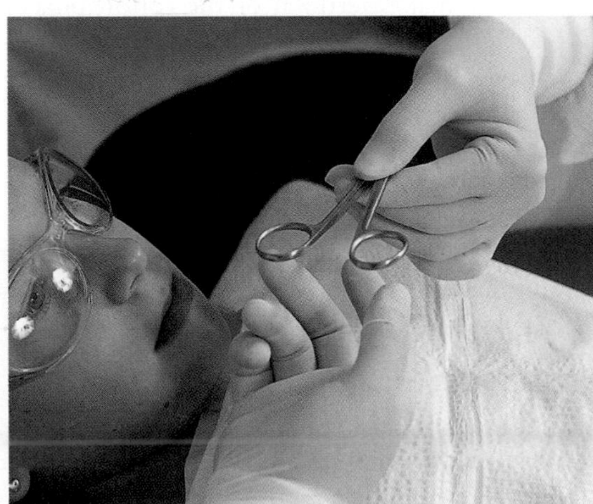

FIG. 33.11 Transferring scissors so the dentist can grasp them correctly.

The expanded function concept allows dentists to use their time more effectively and efficiently. When legal expanded functions are delegated, studies have shown the following results:

- Productivity increases in the dental office.
- Less stress is placed on the dentist.
- The dentist has more available time and can see more patients.
- Each member of the dental team can focus on specific tasks.
- The dental assistant has increased job satisfaction.

### Dental Supervision

The dentist is the person who is *ultimately* responsible for the patient's care and well-being, even if a dental function is delegated to the expanded-function dental assistant (EFDA)/ registered dental assistant (RDA) (see following discussion). The Dental Practice Act for each state dictates whether the expanded function must be directly or indirectly supervised by the dentist.

With **direct supervision**, the dentist must be in the same treatment area as the EFDA/RDA for the assistant to perform the function. With **indirect supervision**, the dentist must be in the dental office area but not necessarily present in the same treatment room as the EFDA/RDA; the dentist must be available to evaluate the assistant's procedure.

### Working as the Operator

An **expanded-function dental assistant (EFDA)** is a clinical dental assistant who has acquired advanced training in clinical functions that have been approved by the Dental Practice Act within the state in which the EFDA is practicing, provided that she or he has met state requirements for these functions.

A **registered dental assistant (RDA)** is a licensed credential. An RDA must graduate from an ADA-accredited dental assisting program, pass a comprehensive written and clinical examination, and maintain his or her license.

Many states require evidence of additional education for advanced functions and mandate completion of a written or clinical examination that is given by the state licensing agency. The Dental Assisting National Board has assembled a comprehensive list of current legislative rulings for the certified or registered dental assistant, and a comprehensive list of the legal functions that is permitted for each state. By going to www.danb.org you can go to your state requirements and view what is allowable or prohibited for each level for the dental assistant in a particular state.

A dental assistant who performs an expanded function assumes the role of the operator. When this transition occurs, it is important for the dental assistant to be prepared and knowledgeable in specific areas such as operator positioning, mirror skills, use of a fulcrum, dental anatomy, cavity preparations, adaptation of instruments, and application of dental materials.

Expanded-function procedures that are most commonly delegated to the dental assistant are presented in their respective chapters throughout *Modern Dental Assisting.* The descriptions of these procedures are designed in a way that allows you to follow the sequence from laboratory to clinical situations. Remember to acquire the appropriate knowledge and skill before you begin the task.

### Operator Positioning

When working intraorally, it is important to follow the guidelines on positioning of the operator, as listed earlier in this chapter. Continued neglect of your own positioning will cause physical problems. Avoid positions that create unnecessary curvature of the spinal column or slumping of the shoulders. Table 33.1 provides information on suggested positioning of the operator when working in different areas of the mouth.

### Developing Mirror Skills

The mouth mirror is a vital instrument that is used when performing specific intraoral expanded functions. Chapter 34 provides a review of the mouth mirror and its uses.

When the mouth mirror is used for indirect vision, it is critical to maintain posture, reduce eyestrain, and complete specific functions. **Indirect vision** describes viewing an object through the use of a mirror (Fig. 33.12). Much trial and error is involved in learning to use a mirror for indirect vision because the object is viewed in reverse (mirror image).

**ESTABLISH A WORKING POSITION.** As the operator, you want to position yourself to gain a "straight-on" visual effect. Once you are positioned, have the patient slightly tip the head back, so the mandibular incisors are perpendicular to the floor. This allows you to position the mirror appropriately in relation to the tooth.

When you and the patient are situated properly, position the light. For the light to be used effectively for indirect vision, it should be placed from your *nondominant* shoulder; that is, if you are right-handed, position the light from your left side.

**ESTABLISH PREFERRED MIRROR-TO-TOOTH POSITION.** The mirror must be kept parallel to the working surface. Remember that you are looking at a mirror reflection, and any angle involved in use of the mirror will create distortion.

To create this parallel position, grasp the distal half of the mirror handle with the thumb, index finger, and middle finger. The farther away you hold the mirror, the more movement will

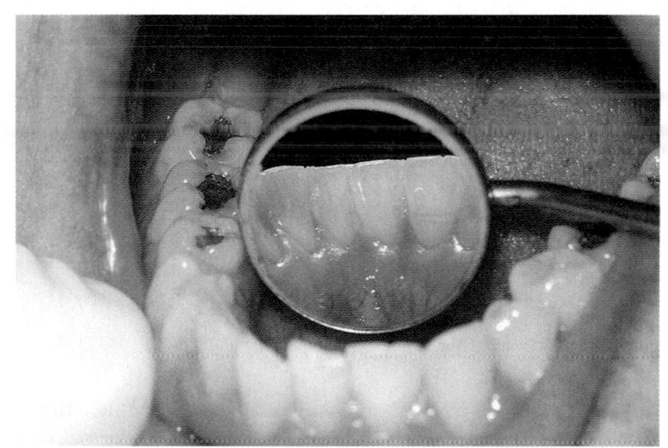

**FIG. 33.12** Positioning the mirror to correctly reflect the image of the tooth.

**TABLE 33.1** Suggested Positioning of the Operator and the Patient According to Areas of the Mouth Being Treated

| Mouth Area | Operator's Position | Type of Vision | Patient's Head Position |
|---|---|---|---|
| Maxillary right buccal | 10–12 o'clock | Direct | Chin up and head turned away from operator |
| Maxillary right occlusal | 11–12 o'clock | Indirect | Chin up and head turned toward operator |
| Maxillary right lingual | 9 o'clock | Direct | Chin up and head turned toward operator |
| Maxillary anterior facial | 11–12 o'clock | Direct | Chin up and head turned toward operator |
| Maxillary anterior lingual | 11 o'clock | Indirect | Chin up and head straight forward |
| Maxillary left buccal | 10 o'clock | Direct | Chin up and head turned toward operator |
| Maxillary left occlusal | 11 o'clock | Indirect | Head turned slightly toward operator |
| Maxillary left lingual | 9 o'clock | Direct | Head turned slightly toward operator |
| Mandibular right buccal | 9–10 o'clock | Direct | Head turned away from operator |
| Mandibular right occlusal | 9 o'clock | Direct | Chin down and head turned toward operator |
| Mandibular right lingual | 9 o'clock | Direct | Chin down and head turned toward operator |
| Mandibular anterior facial | 11–12 o'clock | Direct | Head straight forward |
| Mandibular anterior lingual | 11–12 o'clock | Direct | Head straight forward |
| Mandibular left buccal | 11 o'clock | Direct | Chin up and head turned toward operator |
| Mandibular left occlusal | 11 o'clock | Direct | Chin up and head turned toward operator |
| Mandibular left lingual | 9–10 o'clock | Direct | Chin up and head turned away from operator |

become available for you to position yourself properly (see Procedure 33.4: Using the Dental Mirror Intraorally).

### Using a Fulcrum

The operator will require more than just a proper grasp when using an instrument or a handpiece within the mouth. When you begin to use specific instruments intraorally, you will discover the importance of *stabilizing your hand.*

A **fulcrum** is a "finger rest" that stabilizes the hand (Fig. 33.13). Stabilizing the hand reduces the possibility that slipping or traumatizing of tissues in the mouth will occur. A good fulcrum should provide a stable resting area for the hand and should allow the operator to use *wrist-forearm movement.*

A fulcrum that is established within the mouth is referred to as an *intraoral fulcrum.* Whenever possible, the fulcrum should be positioned on the same arch on which you are working, preferably in the same quadrant. The preferred way to position your finger or hand is with the use of an intraoral fulcrum as close to the working area as possible. Functions that require proper use of a fulcrum include the following:

- Placement of a dental liner and base
- Removal of dental cement
- Placement of retraction cord
- Suture removal
- Coronal polishing
- Placement of sealants
- Placement of separators and the application of ligature and elastomeric ties

### Understanding Dental Anatomy

Knowledge of dental anatomy must be attained if you are to gain an understanding of a dental procedure and a delegated function. (See Chapter 12 for a review of tooth morphology.) The dental assistant must have in-depth knowledge of the following:

- Patient's occlusion of teeth to proper form and function
- Structures of teeth (e.g., enamel, dentin, cementum, pulp)
- Contours of each tooth
- Contact and interproximal surfaces
- Proximal contact area and its importance
- Pits and fissures of each tooth
- Periodontium and its importance

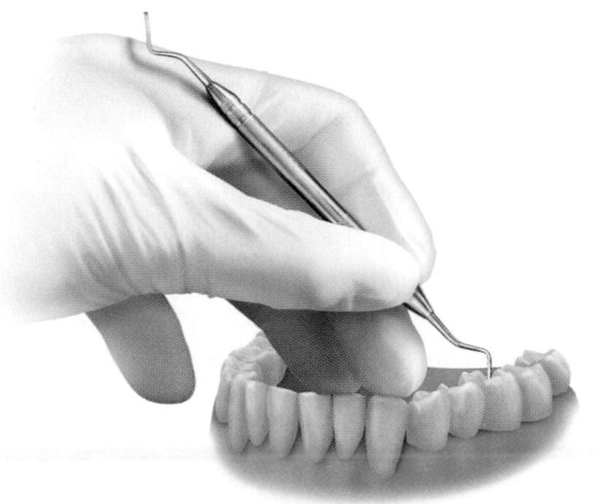

**FIG. 33.13** Using a fulcrum to stabilize the hand and the instrument. (© Elsevier Collection.)

### Understanding Cavity Preparations

Several expanded functions delegated to dental assistants are associated with operative dentistry and restoration of teeth. To know where to place a dental material and how to apply a matrix band and wedge, it is important for the assistant to understand specific cavity terms and classifications (see Chapter 28).

### Adapting Instrumentation

When performing an expanded function, the EFDA/RDA uses instruments to complete the function. When working with instruments, you must be able to *adapt* the working end of the instrument to the tooth surface, and then to go one step further by correctly moving the instrument.

Moving an instrument can be accomplished in two ways: (1) moving the hand, wrist, and forearm as a single unit for enhanced strength, and (2) moving the fingers back and forth in a more confined or precise area (see Procedure 33.5: Using an Instrument Intraorally [Expanded Function]).

### Applying Dental Materials

As a dental assistant, you have the skill to mix dental materials, and you know the materials that should appear before application. When you take on the function of placing a dental material into the mouth or cavity preparation, you also need to know the application process.

Each dental material is unique in how it is used and where it is placed in the mouth. See Chapters 43 through 47, which discuss specific dental materials and review the assistant's role in their application.

## Evaluation of Expanded Functions

An important aspect of acquiring additional responsibilities as an EFDA/RDA is that you are accountable for your skills. It is important that the dentist and the dental assistant have the same expectations and goals in the evaluation process of delegated expanded functions.

You must attain the knowledge and skill needed for an expanded function not only through mastery of course material, but also by talking with the dentist with whom you practice. The dentist will use specific ways to make a temporary tooth, remove a matrix band, or place etchant. To learn the dentist's preferences, engage in open communication with the dentist when new expanded functions are delegated.

**9** What is indirect vision?
**10** What is another term for a finger rest?

**■ Patient Education** Does the dental patient know the role of the dental assistant in the dental office? You and the dentist are responsible for educating patients about the qualifications and responsibilities of the dental team. The best way to do this is to display certificates, diplomas, and additional acknowledgments on walls throughout the dental office as well as in newsletters.

Some offices provide a letter to new patients detailing the professional background of the dental staff. This approach reassures the patient that the clinical team has attained a particular level of competence. ■

**■ Legal and Ethical Implications** Each state has dental practice laws to allow dental assistants to perform expanded functions. Confusion arises because states vary considerably in terms of (1) what duties a dental assistant can perform in the state and (2) what educational requirements must be met if one is to practice expanded functions.

Be sure that you work in an office that maintains a current state-approved expanded-functions list. Display all the credentials that you have earned.

As with all patient treatment, you are responsible for your interventions. The *ultimate* responsibility, however, lies with the dentist. All practices of the dental team should note that the dentist evaluated every procedure, critiqued the work, and communicated findings to the assistant, with documentation provided in the patient record. ■

**■ Eye to the Future** What role will the dental assistant play in the future? It is predicted that a shortage of dentists will occur in this century, and that the dental assistant may take on many roles to compensate for this anticipated shortage.

The dental assistant may take on the role of *preventive assistant.* The EFDA/RDA would be responsible for assisting the dental hygienist in performing supragingival scaling, coronal polishing, application of sealants, and additional preventive procedures for patients.

The EFDA/RDA may also assume the role of *operative assistant.* These expanded functions might include simple and intermediate restorations, final impressions, and additional skills as required by the dentist.

As you will find, states differ in terms of which expanded functions are approved. You will find that dental offices also vary regarding which functions the EFDA/RDA can perform. Stay informed about your profession by keeping up to date with new and approved expanded functions. ■

## ■ Critical Thinking

1. A patient is scheduled today for an extraction. She is very apprehensive about the procedure. What could be discussed among the dental team during the morning meeting to help prepare for this patient?
2. Why do you think the team concept applies to dentistry so well? Is the team concept as prominent in medicine? Why or why not?
3. The operator is positioned a specific way to provide clinical care. Why is it important to follow such guidelines?
4. At this point in your education, what role do you see for yourself as a clinical dental assistant? How can you contribute to the efforts of the dental team in an office?
5. The dentist sees no problem in delegating expanded functions to you because you are a practicing dental assistant. However, you have been asked to complete functions that you are not legally qualified to perform in the state. How should you approach this problem? ■

PROCEDURE 33.1

# Admitting and Seating of the Patient

## PROCEDURAL STEPS

1 Pleasantly greet the patient by name in the reception area. Introduce yourself, and request that the patient follow you to the treatment area.

2 Place the patient's personal items, such as a jacket or a handbag, in a safe place away from the procedure.

**NOTE** Always keep personal items in patient's view for safe keeping.

3 Initiate conversation with the patient.

**PURPOSE** Chatting about things other than the treatment may help the patient feel more comfortable and relaxed.

4 Ask if the patient has any questions that you can answer about treatment for the day. If you do not know the answer, say so and offer to discuss this with the dentist.

**PURPOSE** Patients frequently ask the assistant questions about treatment that they are reluctant to ask the dentist. Your willingness to answer these questions helps reassure the patient.

5 Ask the patient to sit on the side of the dental chair and then to swing his or her legs onto the base of the chair.

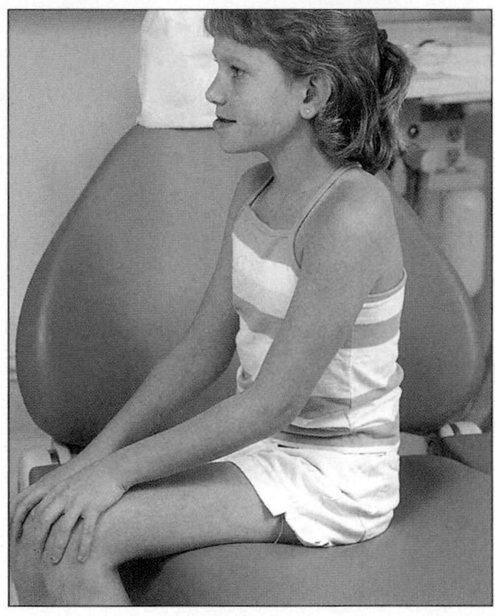

6 Lower or slide the chair arm into position.

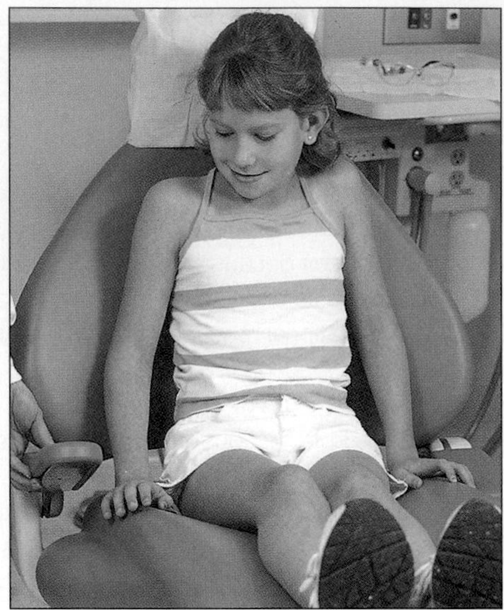

7 Place the disposable patient napkin over the patient's chest, and clasp the corners using a napkin chain.

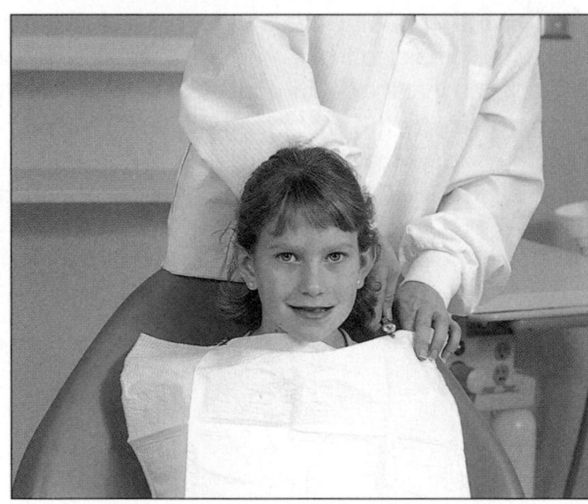

8 Inform the patient before you adjust the chair. Make adjustments slowly until the patient and the chair are in proper position for the planned procedure.

**NOTE** Remember that the most common position for dental procedures is the supine position.

9 Position the operating light over the patient's chest, and turn it on.

## PROCEDURE 33.1 Admitting and Seating of the Patient—cont'd

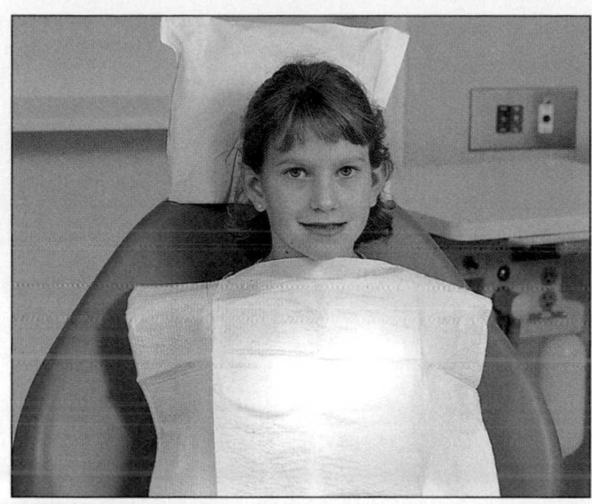

10 Review once again that all treatment room preparations are organized and set out.
11 Wash hands, and put on personal protective equipment.
12 You are now ready to position yourself and begin the procedure.

## PROCEDURE 33.2 

# Transferring Instruments with the Single-Handed Technique

### PROCEDURAL STEPS

1 Pick up the instrument from the tray setup using the thumb, index finger, and middle finger of your left hand.

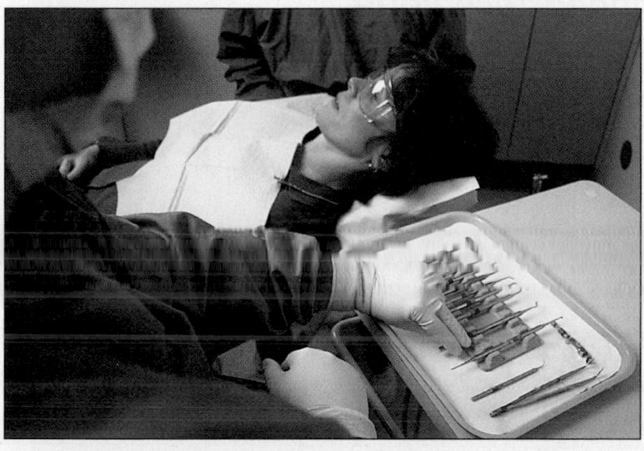

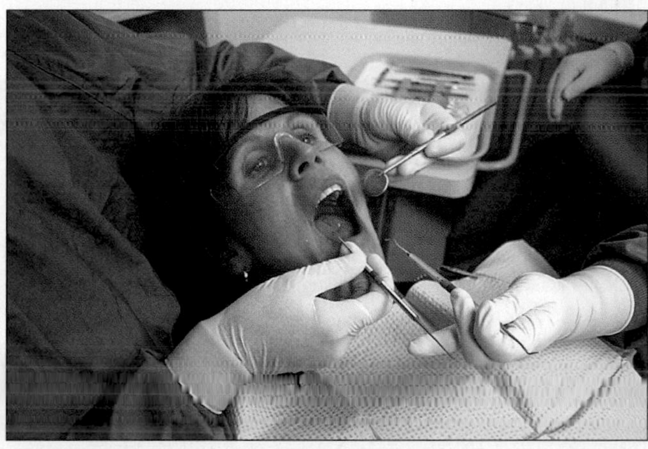

2 Grasp the instrument at the end of the handle or opposite the working end.
**NOTE** Most instruments have two ends (double-ended instruments).
3 Transfer the instrument from the tray into the transfer zone, ensuring that the instrument is parallel to the instrument in the dentist's hand.
4 Using the last two fingers of your left hand, retrieve the used instrument from the dentist, tucking in the instrument toward the palm.

**(Continued)**

## PROCEDURE 33.2 Transferring Instruments with the Single-Handed Technique—cont'd

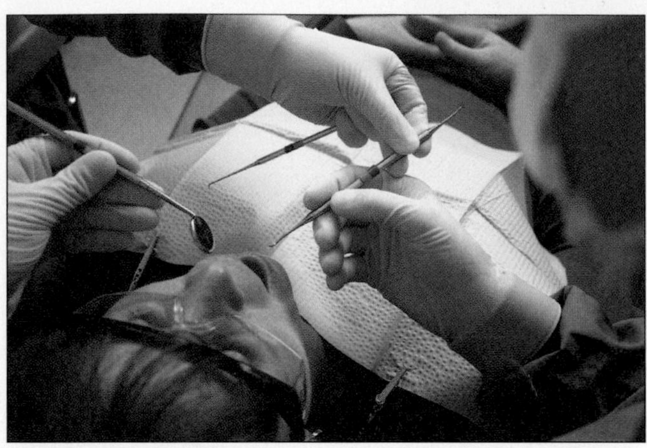

5 Position the new instrument firmly into the operator's fingers.
**NOTE** When placing the instrument, make sure the working end is positioned correctly for the specific arch.

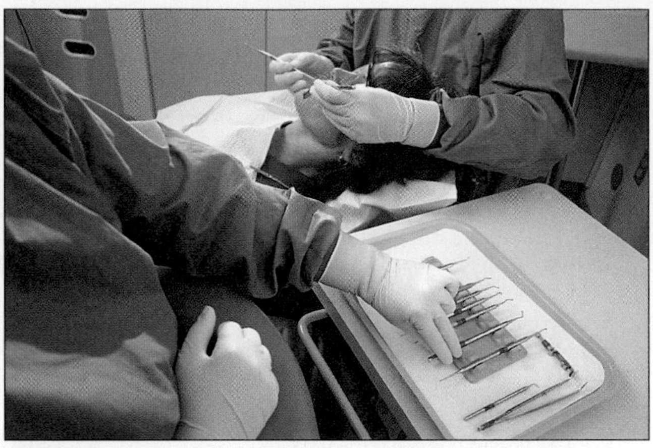

6 Place the used instrument back on the tray setup in its correct position of use.

## PROCEDURE 33.3

# Transferring Instruments with the Two-Handed Technique

### PROCEDURAL STEPS

1 Using your right hand, grasp the instrument on the tray setup closer to the working end with your thumb and first two fingers.
2 With your left hand, retrieve the used instrument from the dentist, using the reverse palm grasp to hold the instrument before placing it back on the tray.
3 Deliver the new instrument to the dentist so that it is oriented with the working end in the appropriate position.
4 Return the used instrument to its proper position on the tray.

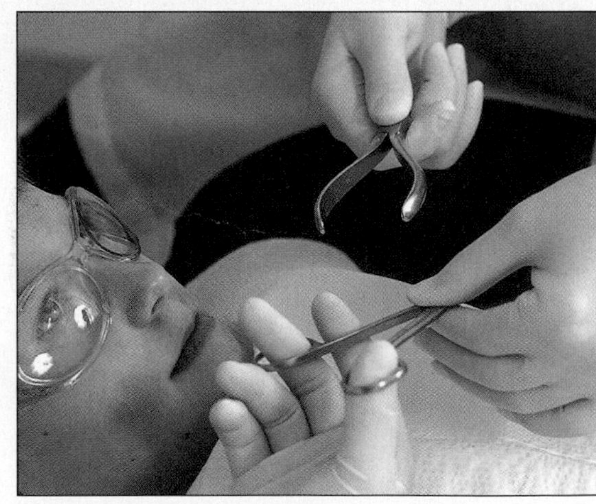

PROCEDURE 33.4

# Using the Dental Mirror Intraorally

## EQUIPMENT AND SUPPLIES

- Dental mirror
- Patient light

## PROCEDURAL STEPS

1 Seat and position the patient in the dental chair in a supine position.

2 Turn on and position the dental light. Keep the light at arm's length away from the oral cavity, and have it coming slightly from your nondominant shoulder.

**PURPOSE** The light is designed to illuminate the oral cavity. If the light is too close, it will not be as effective.

3 Position yourself as the operator.

**NOTE** Remember to follow the guidelines for the operator when seated.

4 Grasp the dental mirror in your left hand (for a right-handed operator) using a pen grasp.

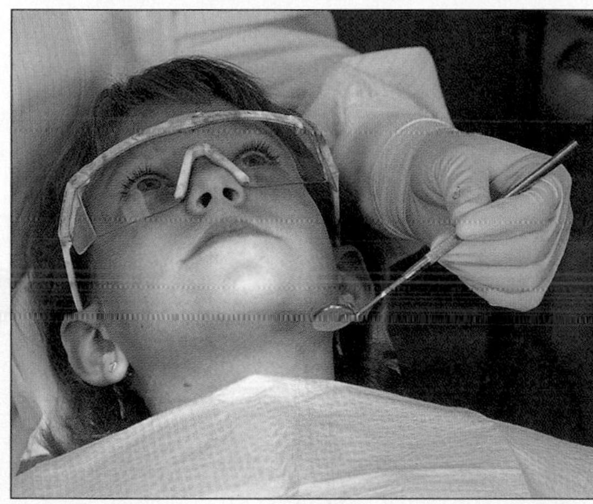

5 Position the dental mirror for indirect vision of the lingual aspect of the maxillary central incisors.

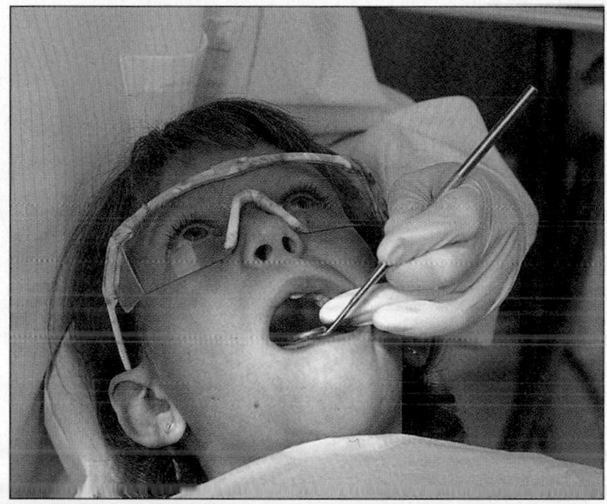

6 Position the dental mirror for light illumination on the lingual aspect of the mandibular central incisors.

7 Position the dental mirror for retraction to obtain better visualization.

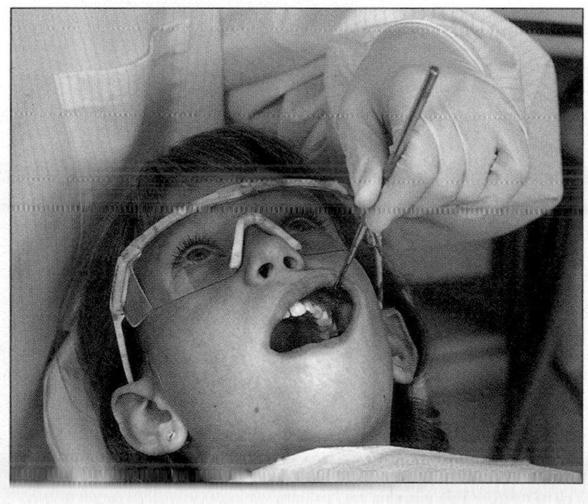

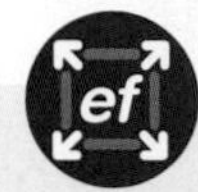

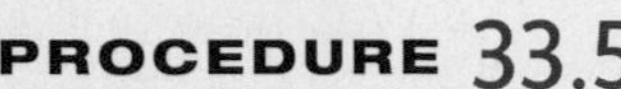

**PROCEDURE 33.5**

# Using an Instrument Intraorally (Expanded Function)

## EQUIPMENT AND SUPPLIES

- ✔ Dental mirror
- ✔ Explorer
- ✔ Cotton pliers

## PROCEDURAL STEPS

1. Seat and place the patient in the supine position.
2. Position yourself as the operator.
3. Adjust the dental light to illuminate the oral cavity.
4. Using a pen grasp, pick up the mirror with your nondominant hand and the explorer with your dominant hand.

   **NOTE** If you are right-handed, use your right hand to grasp the explorer.
5. Instruct your patient to open his or her mouth and turn toward or away from you, depending on the location of the mouth.
6. Establish a fulcrum close to the area that you will be exploring with your instrument.
7. Adapt the explorer to the most posterior tooth in the upper-right quadrant.

   **NOTE** A well-adapted instrument prevents damage to the tooth and surrounding tissue.
8. Follow around the tooth with the mirror and explorer, and examine all surfaces through visualization and touch.

34

# Dental Hand Instruments

## KEY TERMS

**Beveled (BEV-uld)** Characterized by an angle of a surface that meets another angle.

**Blade** Flat edge of instrument, sharp enough to cut.

**Handle** Part of a dental instrument that the operator grasps.

**Nib** Blunt point or tip.

**Plane** Flat or level surface of the working end of an instrument.

**Point** Sharp or tapered end.

**Serrated (sih-RAY-ted)** Having notchlike projections that extend from a flat surface.

**Shank** Part of an instrument where the handle attaches to the working end.

**Tactile (TAK-til)** Having a sense of touch or feeling.

**Working end** Part of a dental instrument that is used on the tooth or when dental materials are mixed.

## LEARNING OUTCOMES

*On completion of this chapter, the student will be able to achieve the following objectives:*

1. Pronounce, define, and spell the key terms.
2. Explain how to identify hand instruments, including the following:
   - Describe the three parts of a dental hand instrument.
   - Describe the instrument formula designed by G. V. Black.
3. Discuss the classification of instruments, including the following:
   - Discuss the theory of placing an instrument in a specific sequence.
   - List the examination instruments and their uses.
   - List the types of hand (manual) cutting instruments and their uses.
   - List the types of restorative instruments and their uses.
   - Describe additional accessory instruments and items used in general dentistry.
   - Describe the use of preset trays, tubs, and color-coding systems in dentistry.

## PERFORMANCE OUTCOMES

*On completion of this chapter, the student will be able to meet competency standards in the following skills:*

- Identify examination instruments.
- Identify hand (manual) cutting instruments.
- Identify restorative instruments.
- Identify accessory instruments and items.

## ELECTRONIC RESOURCES

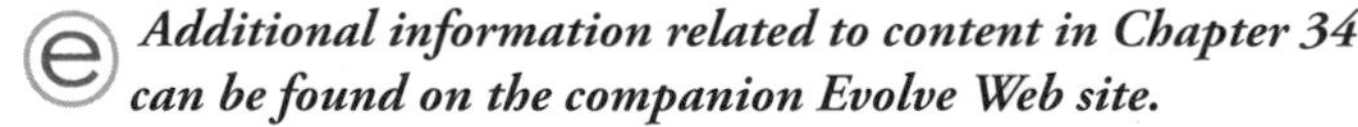

***Additional information related to content in Chapter 34 can be found on the companion Evolve Web site.***

- Practice Quiz
- Tray Setup Drag-and-Drop Exercise: Basic Tray Setup
- Tray Setup Questions

A wide variety of dental instruments are used in dentistry today. This chapter describes the design and purpose of dental instruments that are most commonly used by dentists for general restorative procedures.

Dental supply companies manufacture many variations of instruments for the purpose of accommodating personal preferences. As you study the instruments in this chapter, you will learn that each instrument is designed for a specific area of a tooth, for a specific type of dental material, and for the specific needs of the dentist.

## Identifying Hand Instruments

Each type of dental instrument has a definite purpose in a dental procedure. Knowledge of each instrument is the responsibility of the clinical assistant when setting up for a procedure. The assistant will set up the instruments on the tray in a precise order of use and is expected to transfer from the tray setup when the operator signals for a new instrument.

Instruments are made of stainless steel, carbon steel, plastic, or a specialized metal. Because instruments withstand constant use, they must be able to endure sterilization procedures, as described in Chapter 21.

### Instrument Number

The dental manufacturer assigns a number to most instruments (Fig. 34.1). This number is a universal representation of that instrument. The dentist will often refer to pliers and forceps by their number, rather than by their name. When studying the

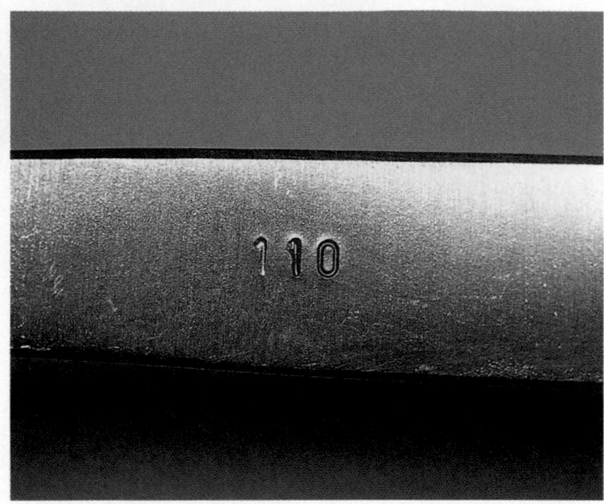


FIG. 34.1 Catalog or call number associated with Howe pliers.

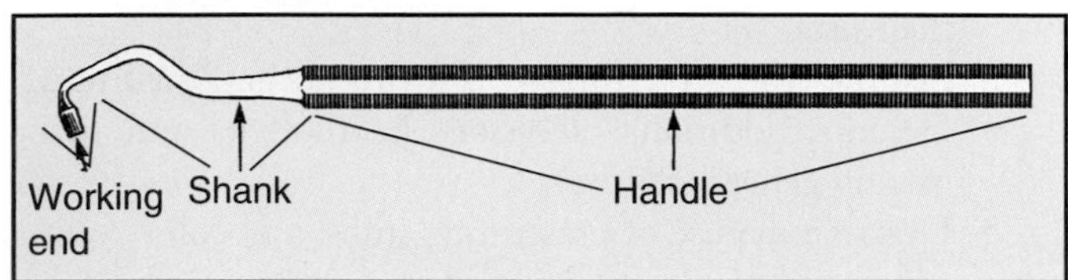


FIG. 34.2 The three parts of a dental hand instrument.

accessory instruments, orthodontic pliers, and surgical forceps, it will be advantageous to learn both the number *and* the name.

## Instrument Design

Hand instruments are designed with three specific parts: the **handle**, the **shank**, and the **working end** (Fig. 34.2).

### Handle

The handle portion of the instrument is where the operator grasps or holds the instrument. Handles are manufactured in various shapes and sizes; some handles are round, and others are hexagonal. They may be smooth or may have a grooved pattern for a better grasp. Instruments are now designed to have a larger handle in circumference, as well as padding for a better grip. As seen in writing instruments, this new padding provides the operator with greater control of the instrument and causes less fatigue on the fingers and the hand muscles.

### Shank

The shank refers to the part of the instrument that attaches the working end to the handle. The bends or angles in the shank are designed so that an instrument can reach specific areas of the tooth. For example, instruments used interproximally have more angles in their shanks, whereas instruments used on the facial or buccal surface of a tooth have a straight shank.

The thickness and strength of the shank dictate the amount of pressure that can be applied to the instrument without breakage.

### Working End

The working end refers to the portion of the instrument with a specific function. This end can have a **point**, **blade**, or **nib**. If the instrument has a nib, the area may be smooth or **serrated**.

Hand instruments are single or double ended. The *double-ended instrument* has a shank and a working end at both ends of the handle. Often, double-ended instruments are mirror images (reverse angles) of each other, allowing adaptation to all surfaces of the tooth. These are referred to as *left and right instruments.*

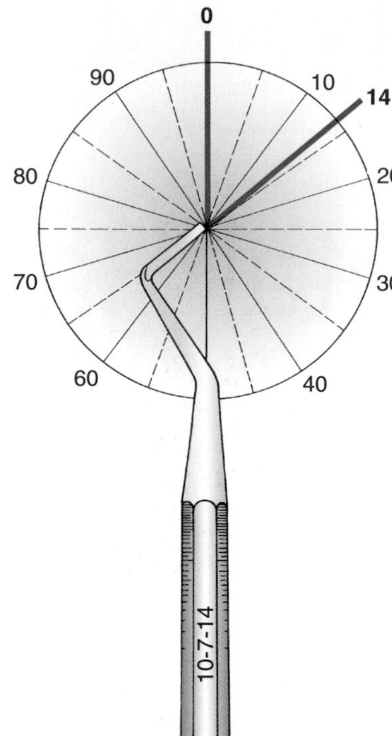


FIG. 34.3 Black's instrument formula. *(From Baum L, Phillips RW, Lund MR: Textbook of operative dentistry, ed 3, Philadelphia, 1995, Saunders.)*

## Black's Instrument Formula

As you have learned in previous chapters, G. V. Black played a significant role in developing many aspects of the way dentistry is practiced today. Black designed a formula that describes the angulations and dimensions of the working end of a hand instrument (Fig. 34.3). Hand cutting and scaling instruments have three sets of numbers that identify the blade's width, length, and angle. Table 34.1 presents the numbers and formulas used in the design of an instrument.

RECALL

1 What types of dental instruments are more often referred to by number than by name?
2 What part of the instrument is located between the handle and the working end?

## Instrument Classification

The instruments used in restorative dental procedures are classified into four categories: examination, hand (manual) cutting,

**TABLE 34.1 Numbers in G. V. Black's Instrument Formula**

| Sequence | Description |
|---|---|
| First number | Width of the blade in tenths of millimeters (e.g., if the number is 10, the width is 1 mm) |
| Second number | Length of the blade in millimeters (e.g., if the number is 7, the length is 7 mm) |
| Third number | Angle of blade in degrees in relation to the handle (e.g., if the number is 90, the working tip [blade] is at a 90-degree angle [right angle] to the handle) |

restorative, and accessory. By learning the instruments by their classification, it will be easier to learn their names, uses, and sequencing for a procedure:

- **Examination instruments** allow the operator to thoroughly examine the health status of the oral cavity.
- **Hand (manual) cutting instruments** allow the operator to remove decay manually and to smooth, finish, and prepare the tooth structure for its final restoration.
- **Restorative instruments** allow the operator to "restore" a tooth by placing, condensing, and carving a dental material to the original anatomy of the tooth structure.
- **Accessory instruments** are miscellaneous instruments and items that are used to complete a procedure.

## Instrument Sequence

A procedure tray is set up from left to right. This sequencing is based on how instruments are transferred and used throughout a dental procedure. Remember that the clinical assistant uses the *left hand* when transferring instruments. Therefore the most frequently used instruments should be placed closer to the dentist for ready availability.

Again, the basic setup will be first on the tray, followed by additional examination instruments, then hand (manual) cutting instruments, and finally restorative instruments. Any accessory items will be situated on the tray or countertop in an organized and sequenced manner (Fig. 34.4).

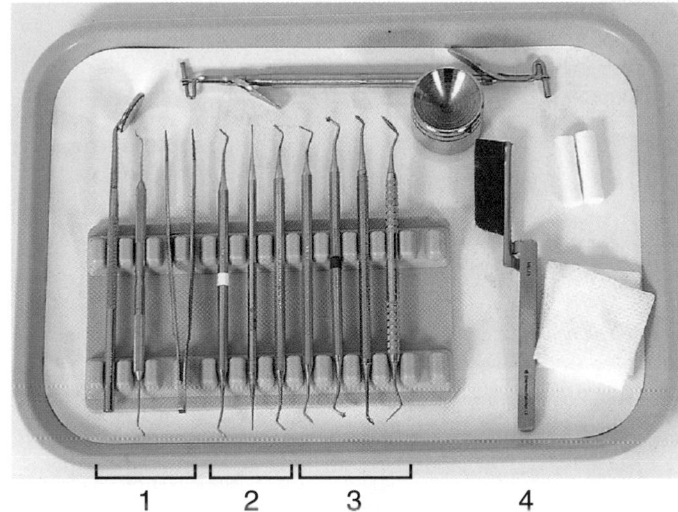


**FIG. 34.4** Tray setup showing appropriate sequence of instruments. *1,* Examination instruments. *2,* Hand cutting instruments. *3,* Restorative instruments. *4,* Accessory instruments.

## Examination Instruments

Examination instruments are the most often used instruments on the tray. They can be used in procedures ranging from the dentist's checking a specific problem, to providing a thorough oral examination, to evaluating a restored tooth. Table 34.2 describes the examination instruments and their uses.

### *Basic Setup*

The mouth mirror, the explorer, and cotton forceps (pliers) are to be "set out" for every procedure. These instruments are referred to as the **basic setup** (Fig. 34.5). Fig. 34.6 provides descriptions of the four major uses of the mouth mirror. When the tray setup is prepared from left to right, the mirror, the explorer, and the cotton forceps (pliers) are the first three instruments.

The mirror and the explorer are to be transferred simultaneously with the use of a two-handed transfer. It is best to position the explorer first and the mirror second on the tray. This setup prevents crossover of your hands when you are transferring the two instruments to the dentist (Fig. 34.7).

See Procedure 34.1: Identifying Examination Instruments.

**RECALL**

3 What classification of instruments is used to remove decay manually?
4 What are the four uses of the mouth mirror?
5 Describe the main feature of the working end of an explorer.
6 What three instruments make up the basic setup?
7 Give the name of the instrument that is used to measure the sulcus of a tooth.

## Hand (Manual) Cutting Instruments

Hand (manual) cutting instruments represent the next group of instruments placed on the tray setup after the examination instruments. These instruments allow the dentist to manually remove decayed tooth structure, to smooth cavity walls and floors of the preparation, and to place any bevels or retention grooves to hold the dental material within the tooth. Table 34.3 shows the excavator, hoe, chisel, hatchet, and gingival margin trimmer and their uses.

Dentists will have a specific preference as to what instruments they want included in this section. The dentist will use a combination of rotary instruments and manual cutting instruments interchangeably throughout a procedure.

**TABLE 34.2** Examination Instruments

| Instrument | Use |
|---|---|
| 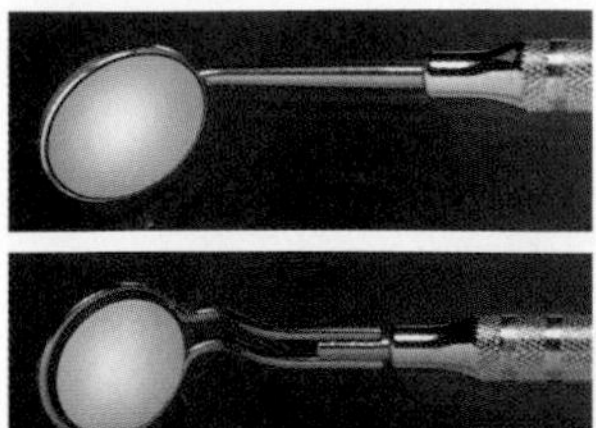 | The **mouth mirror** is designed to have a straight handle, a slight angle to the shank, and a working end, with a round metal disc and a mirror on one side. The mirror can have a flat or a concave (indented) surface. Mouth mirrors are used for a variety of purposes. |
| 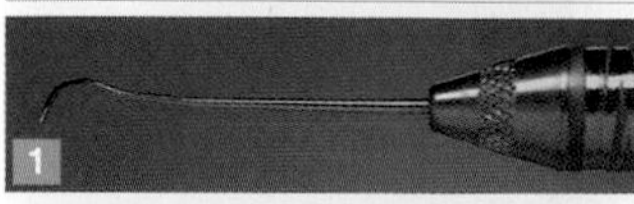 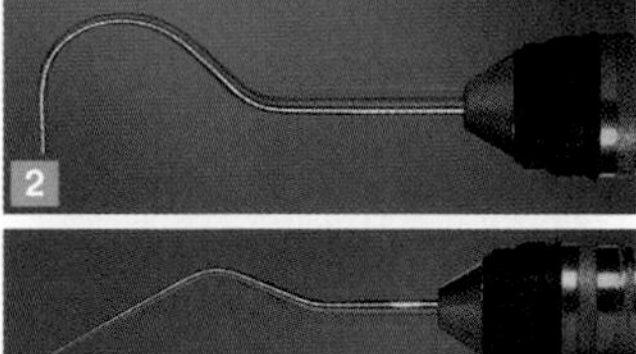 | 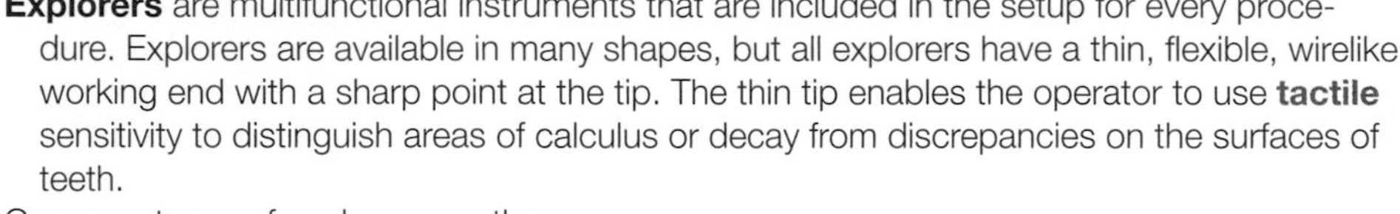 **Explorers** are multifunctional instruments that are included in the setup for every procedure. Explorers are available in many shapes, but all explorers have a thin, flexible, wirelike working end with a sharp point at the tip. The thin tip enables the operator to use **tactile** sensitivity to distinguish areas of calculus or decay from discrepancies on the surfaces of teeth.<br>Common types of explorers are the<br>1. *pig tail*<br>2. *shepherd's hook*<br>3. *orban* |
| 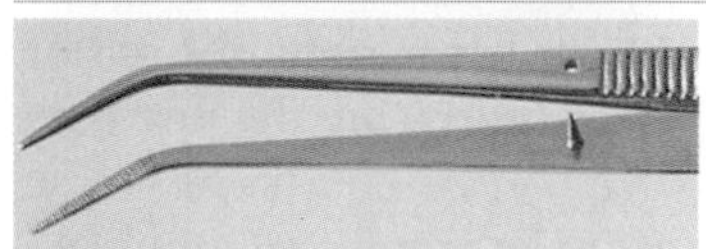 | **Cotton forceps (pliers)** are used to carry, place, and retrieve small objects, such as cotton pellets, gingival retraction cord, matrix bands, and wedges, to and from the mouth. With *nonlocking* cotton forceps (pliers), the handles must be held closed with the fingers. With *locking* pliers, the handles can be locked in a closed position, and the tips do not open until the lock is released. The tips of the cotton forceps (pliers) are available with plain or serrated points, or *beaks.* |
| 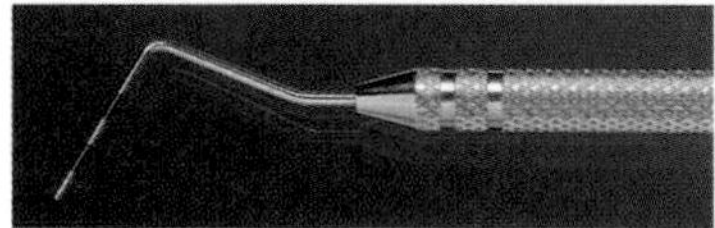 | The **periodontal probe** is used to measure the sulcus or pocket depth of the periodontium of each tooth. This measurement indicates to the clinician the overall gingival health of that area. The working end of the instrument has calibrated markings in millimeters, which are easier to read. Some probes are color coded to enhance reading (see Chapter 55). |

Photos from Boyd LRB: Dental instruments: a pocket guide, ed 6, St Louis, 2018, Elsevier.

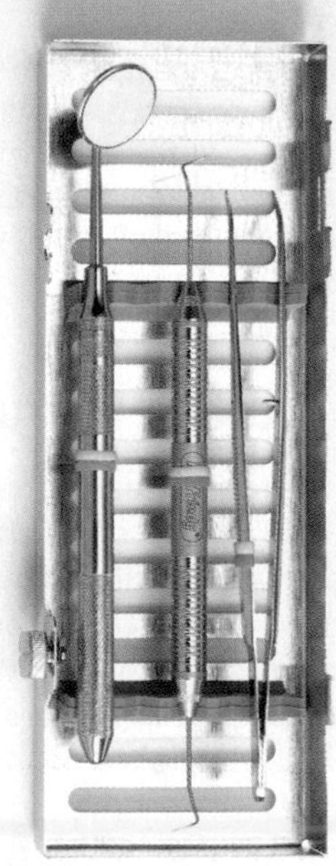

**FIG. 34.5** Basic setup that includes mouth mirror, explorer, and cotton forceps (pliers). *(From Boyd LB: Dental instruments: a pocket guide, ed 6, St Louis, 2018, Elsevier.)*

See Procedure 34.2: Identifying Hand (Manual) Cutting Instruments.

**8** What two excavators are most commonly used in dentistry?

## Restorative Instruments

Restorative instruments are used to place, condense, and carve the restorative dental materials back to reflect the normal anatomy of that tooth. Table 34.4 describes the restorative instruments most commonly used. Most dentists use these instruments in a specific sequence. Instruments selected for the tray setup vary with the dentist's preferences and the type of dental materials selected for the procedure.

See Procedure 34.3: Identifying Restorative Instruments.

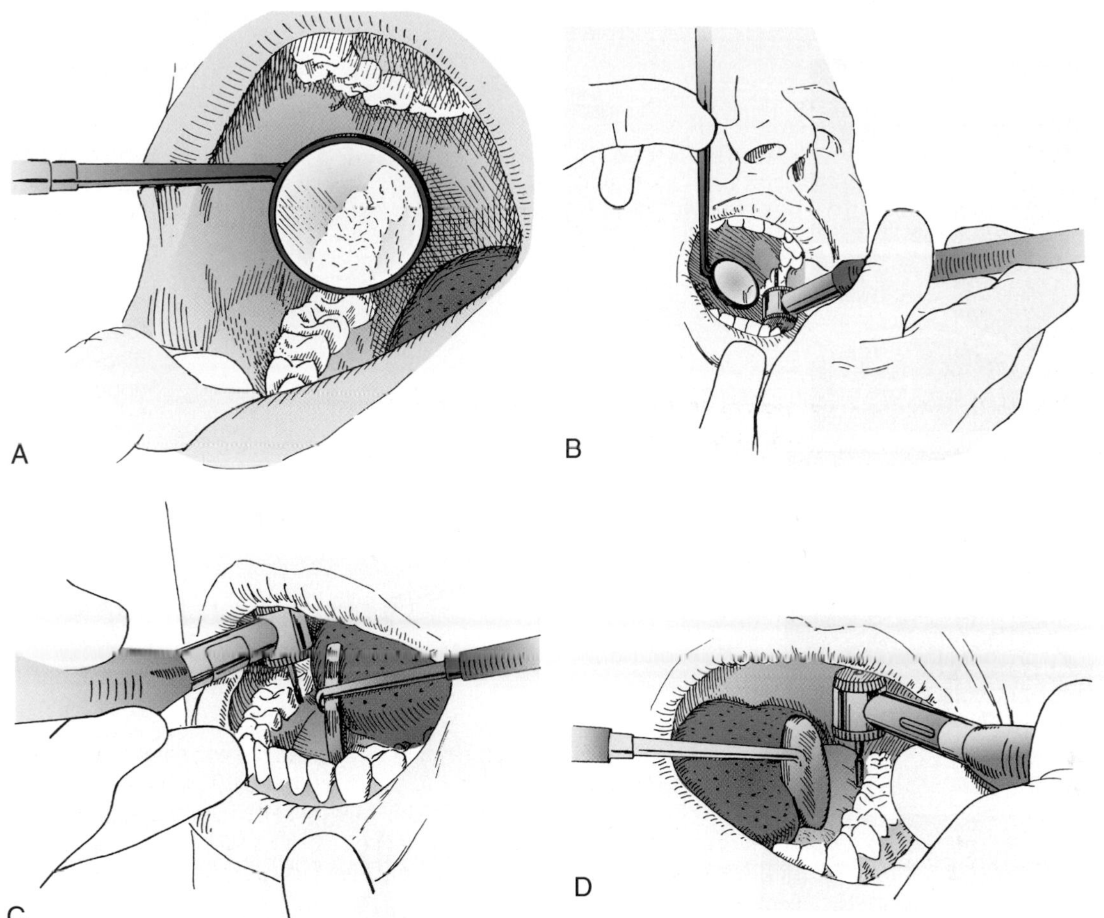


**FIG. 34.6** Uses for the mouth mirror. A, Indirect vision allows the operator to see areas of the mouth that are not visible on direct vision. B, Light reflection directs light into areas of the mouth that are not directly accessible with the operating light. C, Retraction maintains a clear operating field by keeping the tongue or cheek out of the way during a procedure. D, Tissue protection helps guard the tongue or cheek against accidental injury caused by a dental bur.

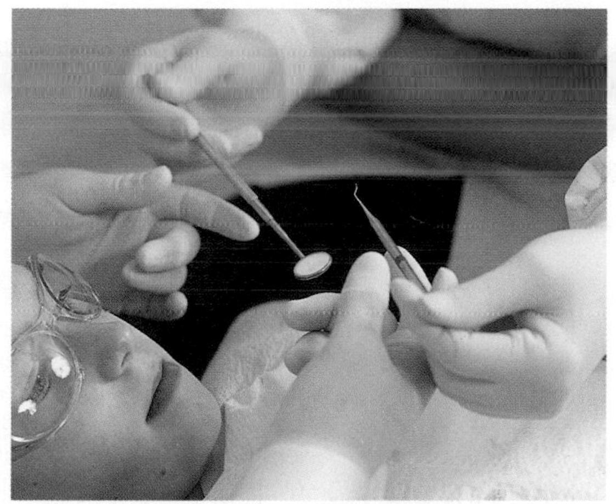

**FIG. 34.7** Transferring mirror and explorer simultaneously to the operator.

RECALL

9 What instrument would you transfer to the dentist to carve anatomy back into the interproximal portion of an amalgam restoration?
10 What instrument is used to pack amalgam during the restoration process?
11 What type of instrument is the discoid-cleoid?

## Accessory Instruments and Items

Accessory items are not necessarily included in the tray setup but can be "pulled" from the dental cabinets or tub to be used for many procedures. Remember that when additional items are used for a procedure, you must follow proper infection control guidelines regarding disinfection or sterilization of the item before you place it back into the cabinet.

Table 34.5 introduces various accessory instruments most commonly used in a restorative procedure.

## TABLE 34.3 Hand (Manual) Cutting Instruments

| Instrument | Instrument in Use | Use |
|---|---|---|
| 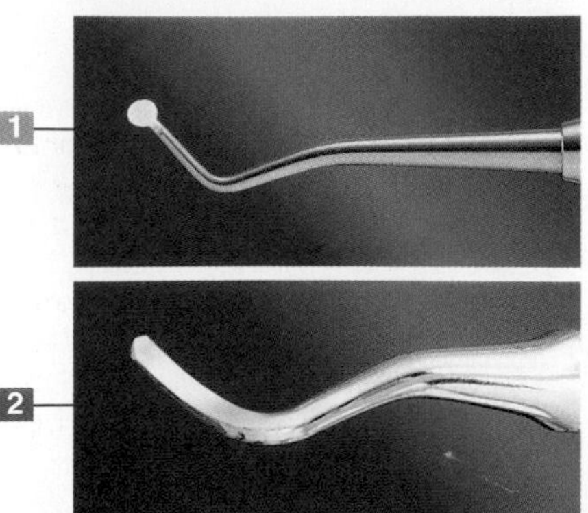  | 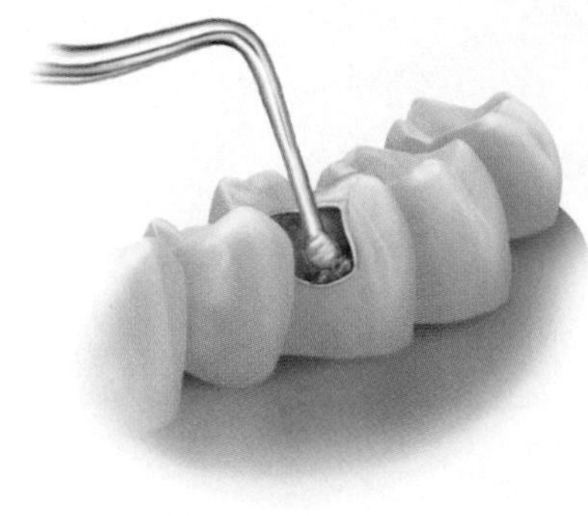 | The **excavator** is one of the most versatile instruments on the tray setup. Excavators have a working end that is circular or elongated. The two most commonly used excavators are:<br>1. spoon excavatoris used for removal of soft dentin, debris, and decay from the tooth<br>2. black spoon has a flat appearance but is used for the same purposes. |
| 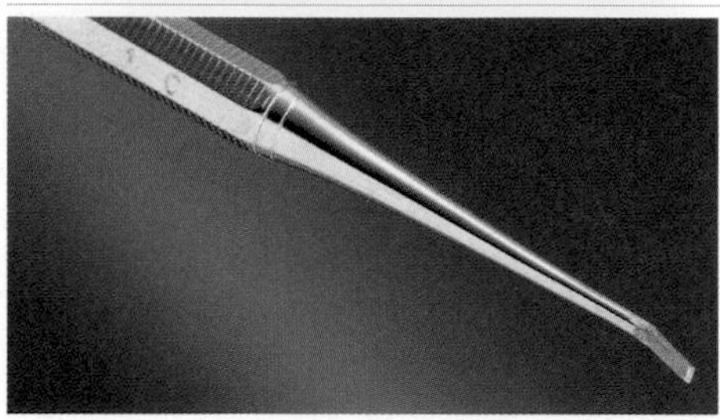 | 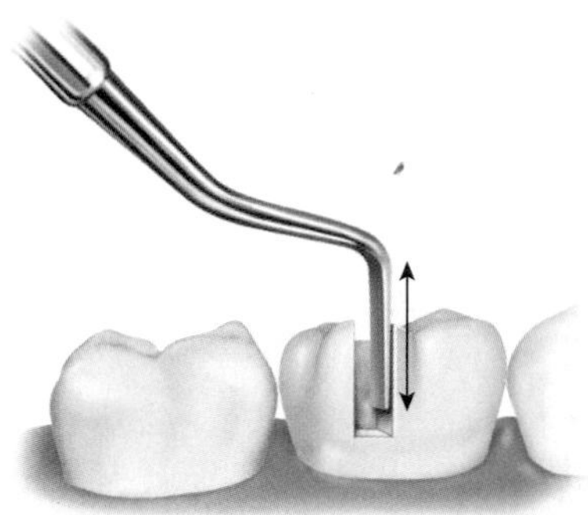 | The **hoe** is similar in appearance to the garden tool. The blade is almost perpendicular to the handle. The *hoe* is used to prepare the tooth and to **plane** the walls and floors of the tooth preparation with a push-pull action. |
| 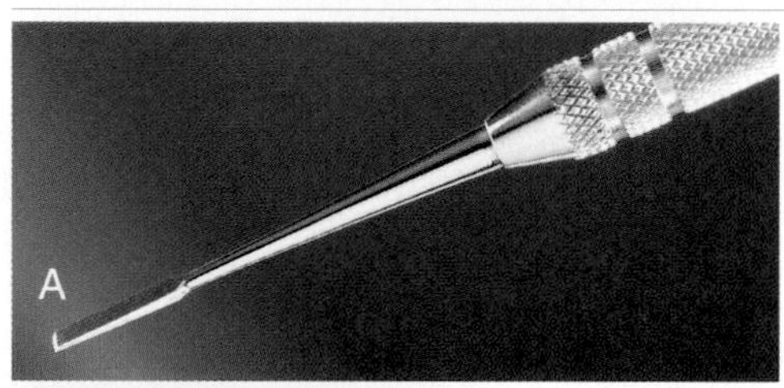  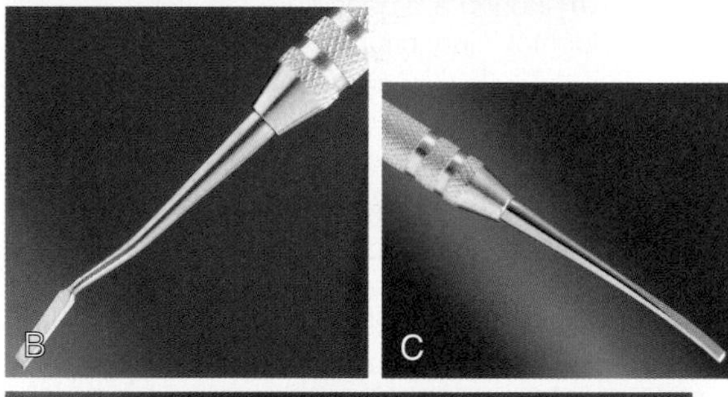  D | 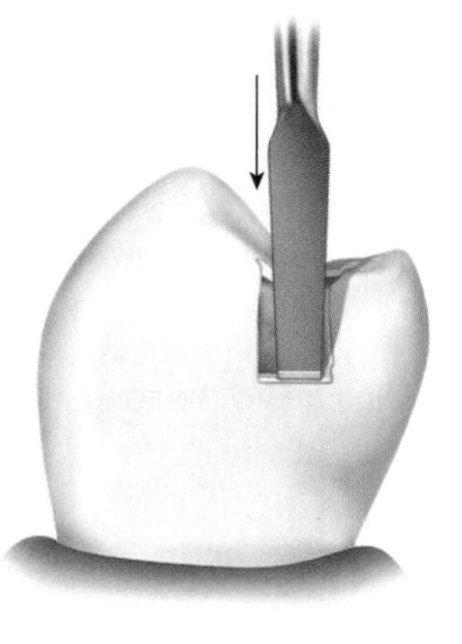 | The **chisel** has a straight or angled shank and a single-**beveled** cutting edge. Chisels are used most often to break down the enamel margin of the tooth preparation, to form sharp lines and **point** angles, and to place retention grooves.<br>Common types include the following:<br>(A) straight chisel<br>(B) bin-angle chisel<br>(C) Wedelstaedt chisel<br>(D) angle-formed chisel |
| 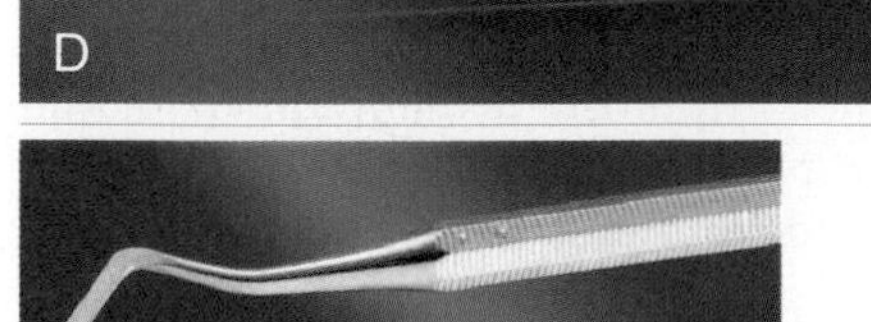 | 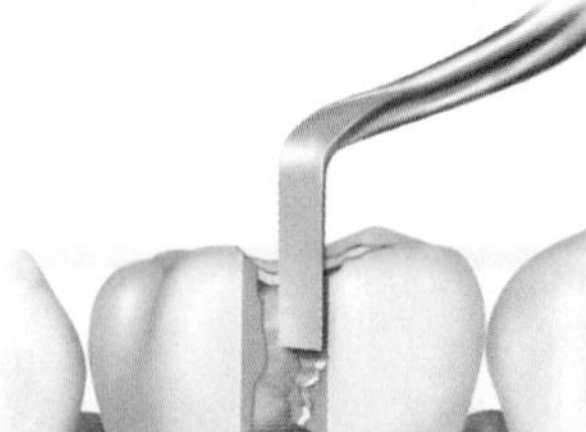 | **Hatchets** are similar in appearance to wood hatchets. The cutting edge is parallel to the long axis of the handle. Hatchets are used to cut enamel and to smooth the walls and floors of the tooth preparation. |

**TABLE 34.3** Hand (Manual) Cutting Instruments—cont'd

| Instrument | Instrument in Use | Use |
|---|---|---|
| 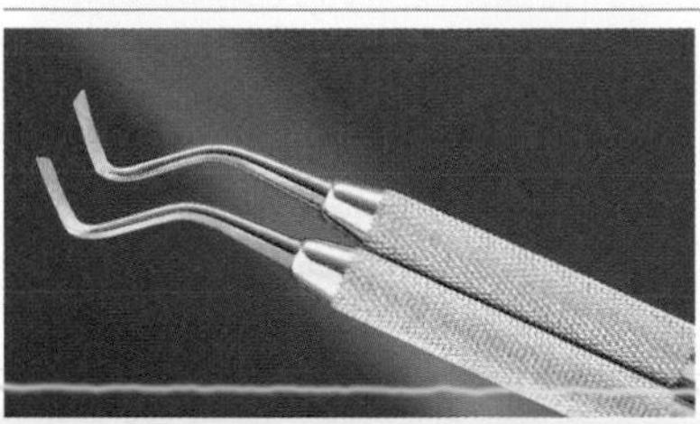 | 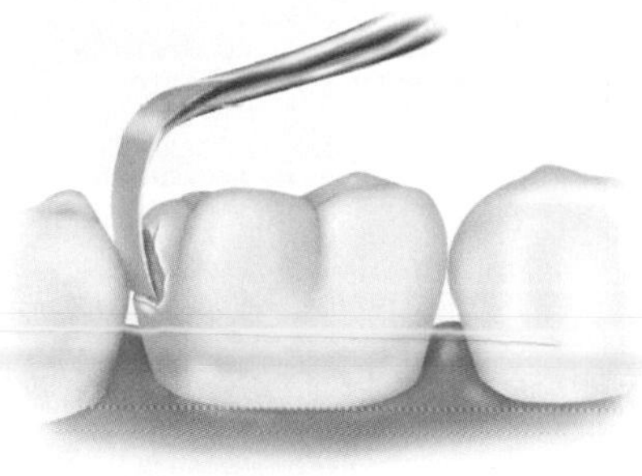 | The **gingival margin trimmer** is a type of chisel that has been modified so that the blade is curved slightly for mesial or distal access into the preparation. Gingival margin trimmers are used to cut enamel and to place bevels along the gingival enamel margins of the preparation. |

Photos from Boyd LRB: Dental instruments: a pocket guide, ed 6, St Louis, 2018, Elsevier; drawings © Elsevier Collection.

**TABLE 34.4** Restorative Instruments

| Instrument | Use |
|---|---|
| 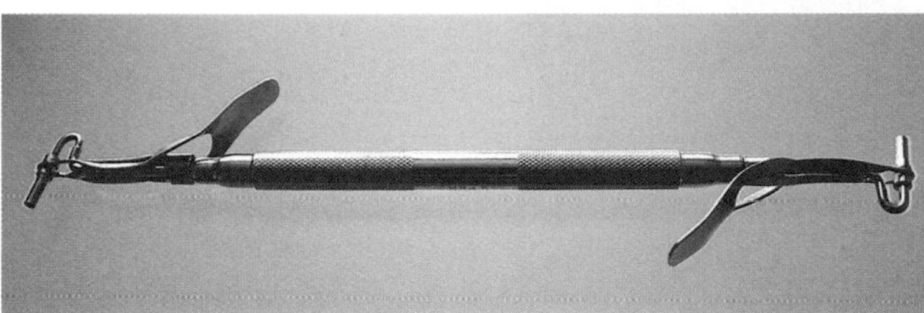 | **Amalgam carrier** is a double-ended instrument designed with wells on either end that is used to pack freshly mixed amalgam and carry it to the prepared tooth. Most amalgam carriers are designed to hold a large increment of amalgam at one end and a smaller increment at the opposite end. The dental assistant uses the amalgam carrier to carry an increment of amalgam, then transfers the carrier to the dentist or directly places the amalgam into the prepared tooth. |
| 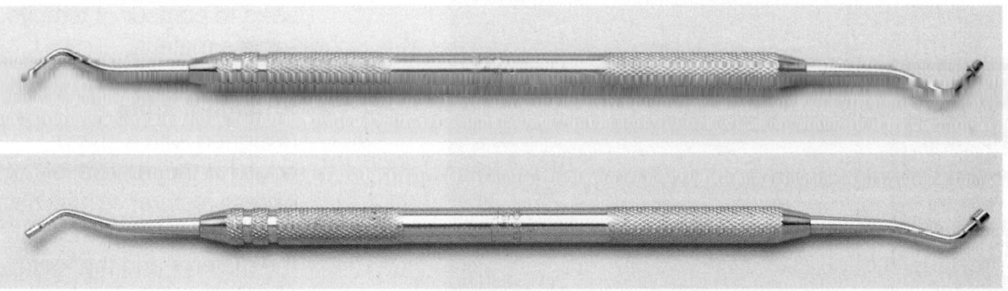 | **Condensers** have a flat working end that can be smooth or serrated; they come in varying sizes to accommodate the size of the preparation. To enable the operator to reach all areas of the preparation, the shank of the instrument is angled. The amalgam condenser, also known as a *plugger,* is used to condense (pack down) freshly placed amalgam into the preparation. |

*Continued*

TABLE 34.4 Restorative Instruments—cont'd

| Instrument | Use |
| --- | --- |
| 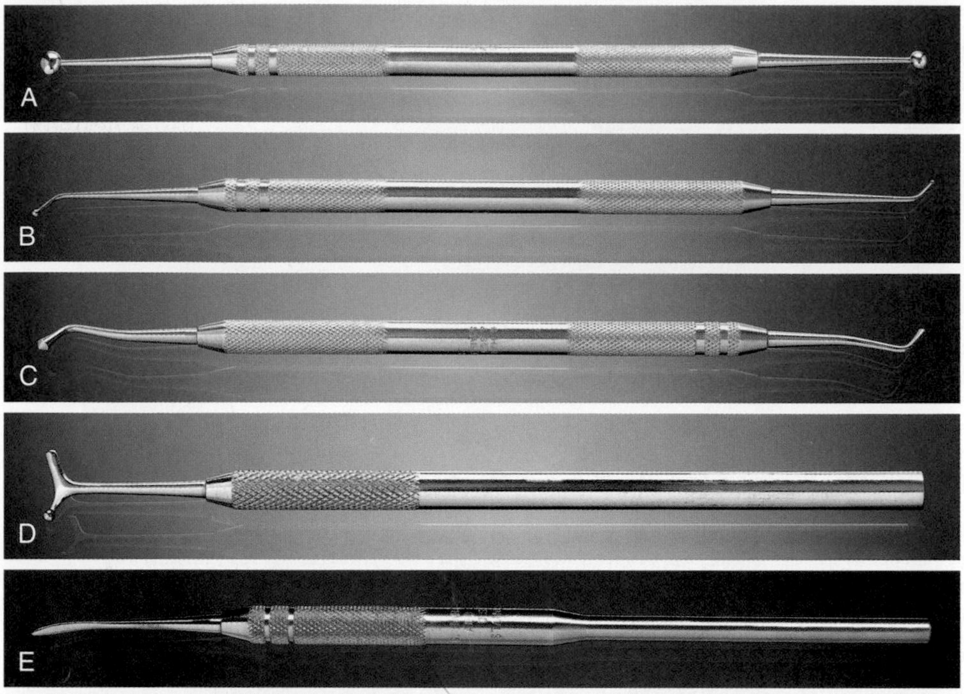 A, B, C, D, E | A **burnisher** is an instrument with a smooth working end. Burnishers are routinely used to smooth the surface of a freshly placed amalgam restoration. The rounded working end is available in many shapes to accomplish different tasks. Common types include the following: A. Football B. Ball C. Acorn D. T-ball E. Beavertail |
| 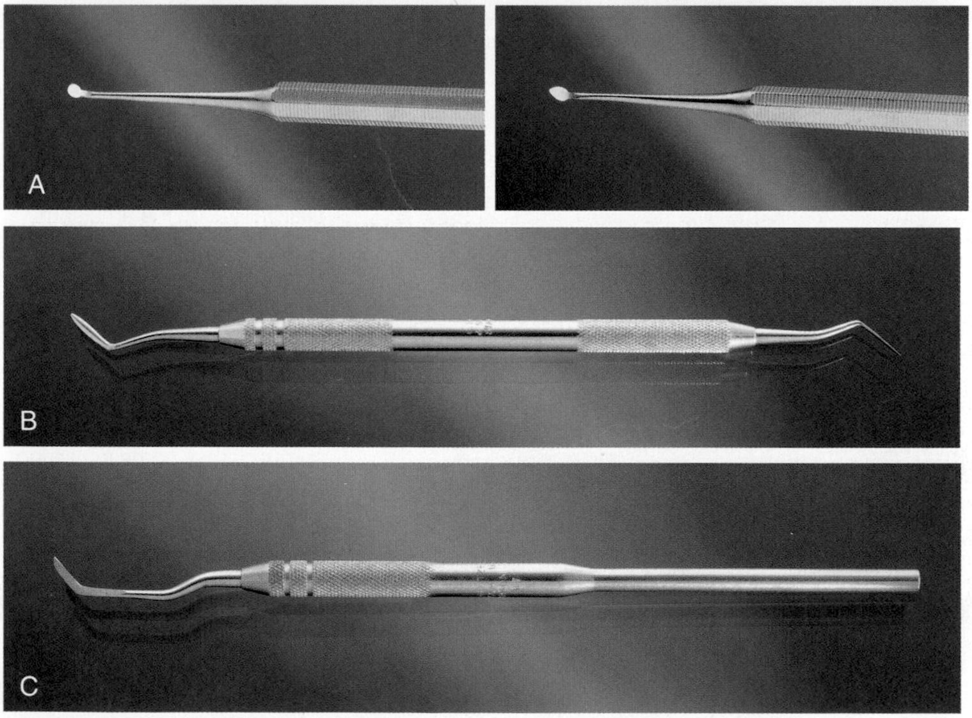 A, B, C | **Carvers** are designed with a sharp edge on the working end to remove excess material, to contour surfaces, and to carve anatomy back into the amalgam or intermediate restoration before it hardens. Various styles of carvers are available: A. **Discoid-cleoid carver** is especially useful for carving of the occlusal surfaces. B. **Hollenback carver** is used to contour or remove excess material interproximally. C. **Amalgam knife** is designed with a sharp edge for the removal of excess restorative material along the margin where the material and the tooth structure meet. The knife has several angles in the shank and working end that enable the operator to reach specific areas of a tooth, most often interproximal areas. |

## TABLE 34.4 Restorative Instruments—cont'd

| Instrument | Use |
|---|---|
| 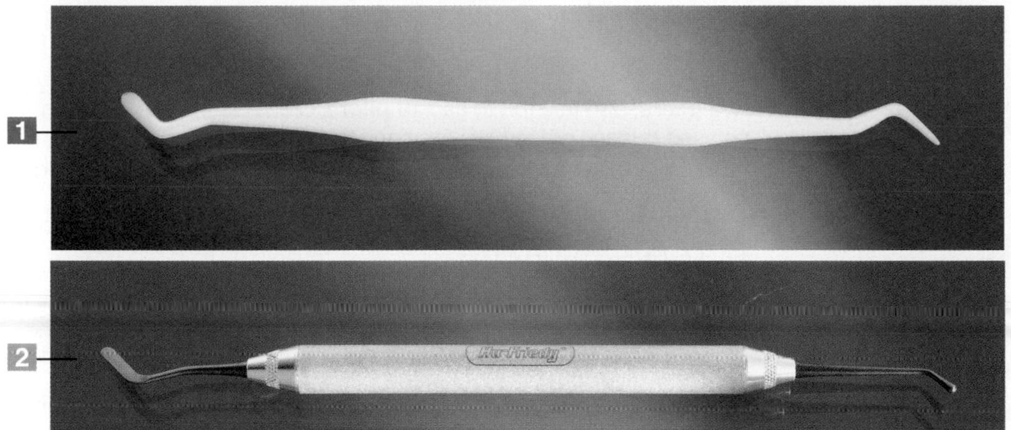 | **Composite placement instruments** are designed specifically for the placement of composite restorative materials. Composite placement instruments are made from anodized aluminum or Teflon. These materials prevent the composite material from being scratched. The instruments do not discolor the composite material, as do stainless steel instruments.<br>1. Teflon composite instrument.<br>2. Aluminum composite instrument. |
| 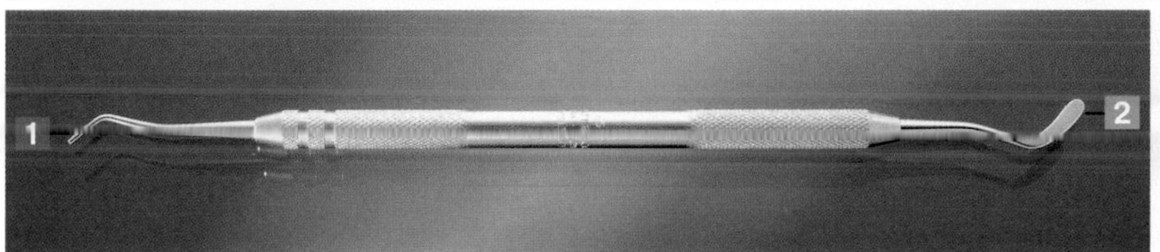 | **Woodson (FP-1)** is a double-ended instrument that is made from hard plastic or stainless steel.<br>1. One end is a **nib,** which resembles a condenser.<br>2. **Paddle** that is used for carrying dental materials to the prepared tooth structure. |

Photos from Boyd LRB: Dental instruments: a pocket guide, ed 6, St Louis, 2018, Elsevier.

## TABLE 34.5 Accessory Instruments and Items

| Instrument/Item | Use |
|---|---|
| 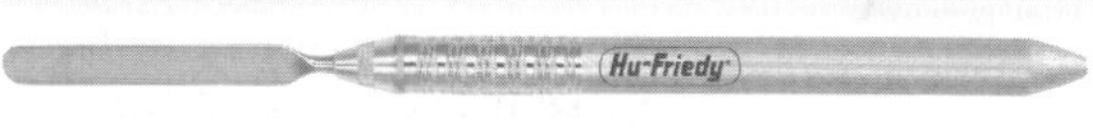 | **Spatulas** are used for most procedures in which a dental material is involved. *Flexible mixing spatula* is single-ended, made of stainless steel, comes in two sizes (#15, #24), and is used to mix liners, bases, and cements. |
| 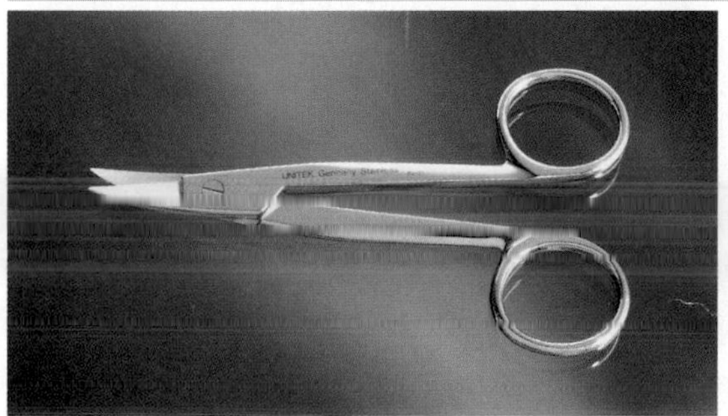 | **Scissors** most often associated with restorative dental procedures are *crown and bridge* scissors, which are available with curved or straight blades. They are useful for many tasks, such as cutting dental dam material, retraction cord, and stainless steel crowns. |
| 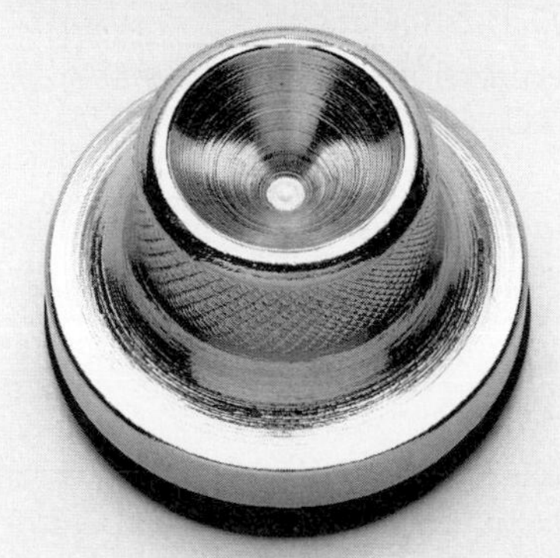 | **Amalgam well** is made of metal and is weighted with a nonskid base. The newly mixed amalgam is placed in the well; it is then picked up in the carrier for transfer to the dentist. |

*Continued*

**TABLE 34.5** Accessory Instruments and Items—cont'd

| Instrument/Item | Use |
|---|---|
| 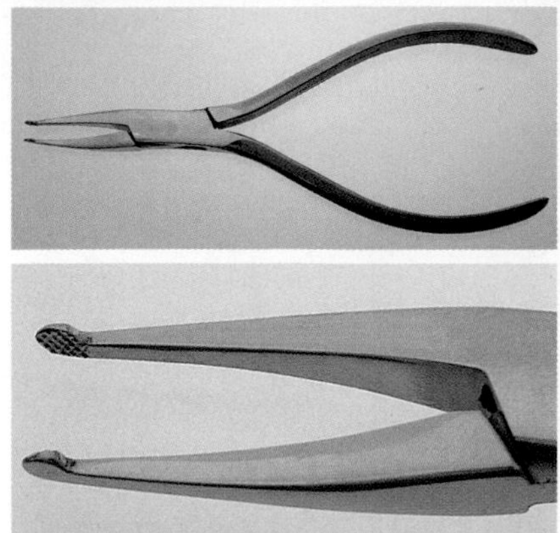 | **Howe pliers**, also referred to as **110 pliers**, are versatile pliers that can be used in many procedures for many tasks. Their design is straight and includes beaks that have a flat rounded end, making them useful for holding items. Howe pliers are useful for carrying cotton products to and from the oral cavity, for removing the matrix band, and for placing and removing the wedge. |
| 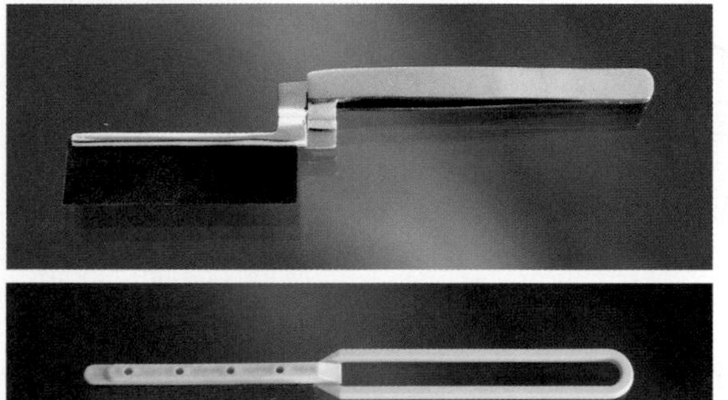 | **Articulating paper holder** is used to hold and carry articulating paper to the mouth. This carbon paper material varies in thickness and color and is used to check a patient's "bite" following placement of a new restoration, crown, bridge, or denture. This mark must appear equal in distribution across the occlusal surface of the tooth. If one area appears lighter or darker, the patient's bite is incorrect and will need to be adjusted. |

Photo of spatula courtesy Hu-Friedy Manufacturing Co., LLC, Chicago, IL. All other photos from Boyd LRB: Dental instruments: a pocket guide, ed 6, St Louis, 2018, Elsevier.

See Procedure 34.4: Identifying Accessory Instruments and Items.

RECALL

12 What types of scissors are commonly placed on the restorative tray setup?
13 What is the numerical name for Howe pliers?
14 Where is the freshly mixed amalgam placed following trituration of the material?

## Preset Cassettes (Trays)

The way to maintain organization and be prepared for a procedure is to have hand instruments in a preset cassette (Fig. 34.8). A dental practice will have sterilized cassettes prepared for most procedures; examples would include restorative, preventive, crown and bridge, surgical. The sterile cassette is taken to the treatment area for preparation before the patient is seated.

If instruments are sterilized and maintained in either pouches or packages, they will need to be set out and organized in a tray for a procedure. Trays are fabricated in metal or plastic and are to be cleaned and disinfected after each use (Fig. 34.9).

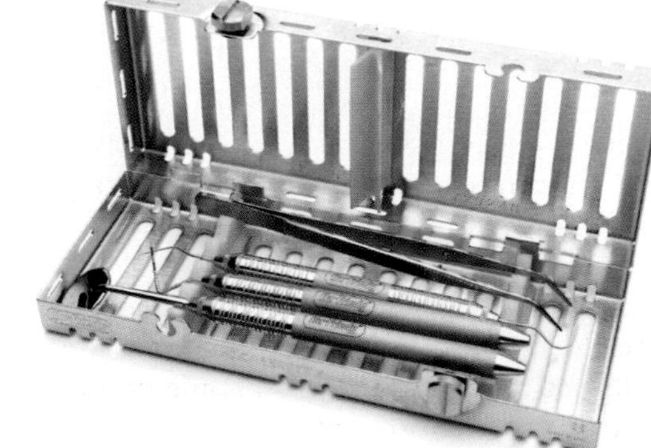

**FIG. 34.8** Cassette for a preventive procedure. *(Courtesy Hu-Friedy Manufacturing Co., LLC, Chicago, IL.)*

## Storage Tubs

Supplies and dental materials for specific procedures can be stored in a covered plastic tub within each operatory

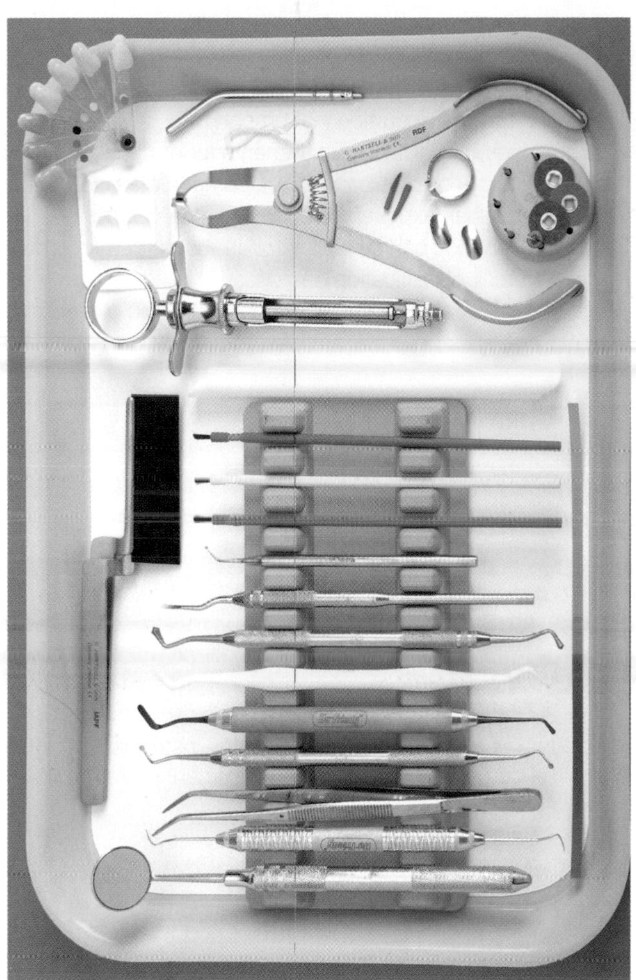

**FIG. 34.9** Preset restorative tray. *(From Boyd LB: Dental instruments: a pocket guide, ed 6, St Louis, 2018, Elsevier.)*

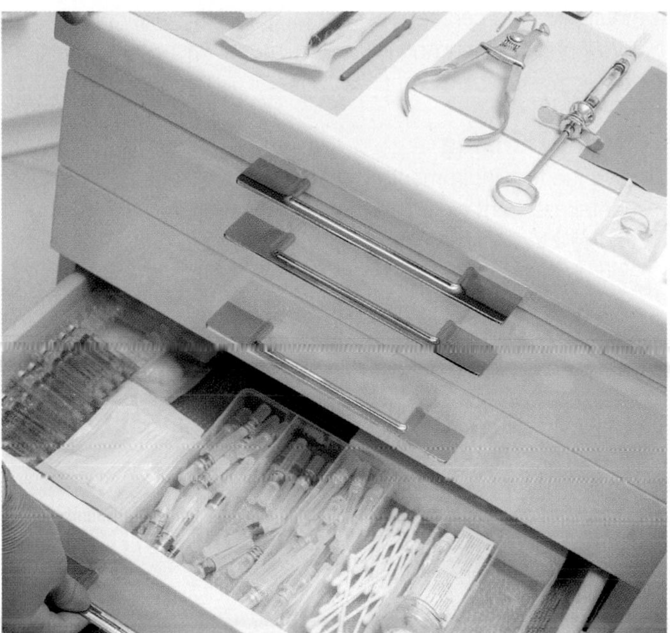

**FIG. 34.10** Storage tub holding additional items needed for a procedure. *(Copyright © Pefostudio/iStock/Getty Images.)*

(Fig. 34.10). The combination is known as the **tub and tray system.**

## Color-Coding Systems

Color coding is one of the most convenient and efficient ways to organize instruments and supplies for specific procedures. The ways in which color coding can be used are limited only by the user's creativity.

The instrument tray and the tub of related materials can be used to indicate the procedure. For example, if yellow is the color chosen to indicate amalgam restorations, each of the instruments has a yellow band, the tray has a yellow label, and a yellow tub is used to transport related materials (Fig. 34.11).

■ **Legal and Ethical Implications** The management and care of instruments and supplies for dental procedure are two of the most important responsibilities as a patient care provider. By carefully following infection control guidelines in the way you package, sterilize, and store instruments, you know you are protecting patients and clinical staff from a possible infectious disease.

Many patients are knowledgeable enough to ask how instruments are maintained. Be certain that you can assure your patients and provide the best answer. ■

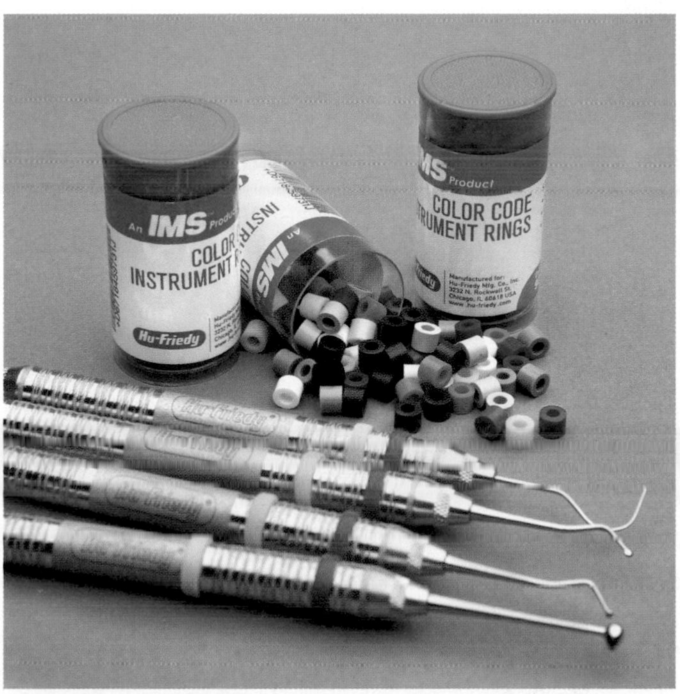


**FIG. 34.11** Color-coding system for instruments. *(Courtesy Hu-Friedy Manufacturing Co., LLC, Chicago, IL.)*

■ **Eye to the Future** Because of greater awareness and concern about the transmission of infectious diseases, you will find that more and more instruments are made of disposable material. This technology has pros and cons. Positive aspects include reduced transmission of disease and less time spent in the sterilization center between patients. Negative concerns involve increased handling of contaminated waste and adding to the ecological problems of today. ■

## ■ Critical Thinking

1. Give the four instrument classifications, and describe how the dental assistant would sequence instruments for the restoration of a tooth.
2. You have just seated your next patient. The dentist sits down and extends her hands on either side of the patient's face. What is she doing, and how do you respond?
3. You are sitting down to assist the dentist in a composite procedure. You note that the enamel hatchet is missing from the setup. Is there anything else that the dentist could use in place of a tooth preparation instrument?
4. You are given the following instruments for an amalgam tray: condenser, spoon excavator, mirror, carrier, cotton forceps (pliers), burnisher, explorer, discoid/cleoid carver, periodontal probe, Hollenback carver, and hatchet. Place them in order in relation to their classification and uses.
5. What accessory instruments or items would you pull from the cabinet or tub for an amalgam procedure? ■

PROCEDURE 34.1

## Identifying Examination Instruments

### EQUIPMENT AND SUPPLIES

See Table 34.2 for examples of instruments.

- ✔ Mouth mirror
- ✔ Explorer
- ✔ Cotton forceps (pliers)
- ✔ Periodontal probe
- ✔ Articulating paper

### PROCEDURAL STEPS

1. Carefully examine the instrument.
2. Consider the general classification of the instrument.
3. Write the complete name of each instrument or item, spell it correctly, and give its uses.

PROCEDURE 34.2

## Identifying Hand (Manual) Cutting Instruments

### EQUIPMENT AND SUPPLIES

See Table 34.3 for examples of instruments.

- ✔ Excavators
- ✔ Hoe
- ✔ Chisels
- ✔ Hatchets
- ✔ Gingival margin trimmer

### PROCEDURAL STEPS

1. Carefully examine the instrument.
2. Consider the general classification of the instrument.
3. Write the complete name of each instrument with its correct spelling, and list its uses.

PROCEDURE 34.3

## Identifying Restorative Instruments

### EQUIPMENT AND SUPPLIES

See Table 34.4 for examples of instruments.

- ✔ Amalgam carrier
- ✔ Condensers
- ✔ Burnishers
- ✔ Carvers
- ✔ Amalgam knife
- ✔ Composite placement instruments
- ✔ Plastic instrument

### PROCEDURAL STEPS

1. Carefully examine the instrument.
2. Consider the general classification of the instrument.
3. Write the complete name of each instrument, spell it correctly, and give its uses.

PROCEDURE 34.4

# Identifying Accessory Instruments and Items

## EQUIPMENT AND SUPPLIES

See Table 34.5 for examples of instruments.

- ✔ Flexible mixing spatula
- ✔ Scissors
- ✔ Amalgam well
- ✔ Howe pliers
- ✔ Articulating paper holder

## PROCEDURAL STEPS

1 Carefully examine the instrument or item.

2 Consider the general classification of the instrument.

3 Write the complete name of each instrument or item, spell it correctly, and give its uses.

35

# Dental Handpieces and Accessories

## KEY TERMS

**Bur** A steel or tungsten carbide rotary cutting instrument.
**Console (KON-soel)** Freestanding cabinet that holds contents or control devices, such as the laser handpiece.
**Dental handpiece** An electrical instrument used to hold rotary instruments.
**Flutes** Blades on the working end of a finishing rotary instrument that resemble pleats.
**Laser** Fiber optic cable that produces a laser light.
**Mandrel (MAN-drul)** Metal shaft on which a sandpaper disc or other abrasive materials are mounted.
**Rotary (ROE-tuh-ree)** Part or device that rotates around an axis.
**Shank** Part of an instrument in which the handle attaches to the working end.
**Torque (tork)** Twisting or turning force.
**Ultrasonic (ul-truh-SON-ik)** Referring to mechanical radiant energy of water and sound vibrations used to break down material or tissue.

## LEARNING OUTCOMES

*On completion of this chapter, the student will be able to achieve the following objectives:*

1. Pronounce, define, and spell the key terms.
2. Discuss the historical importance of the dental handpiece.
3. Discuss dental handpieces, including the following:
   - Describe the low-speed handpiece and its uses in dentistry.
   - Describe the attachments used with the low-speed handpiece.
   - Describe the high-speed handpiece and its uses in dentistry.
   - Review other handpieces used in dentistry.
   - Discuss handpiece maintenance.
4. Describe rotary cutting instruments and how they are used.
5. Do the following regarding burs:
   - List the parts of a bur.
   - Describe the composition, shape, and uses of diamond burs.
   - Explain the difference between a finishing bur and a cutting bur.
6. List the types of abrasive rotary instruments.
7. Explain the difference between laboratory burs and dental burs.

## PERFORMANCE OUTCOMES

*On completion of this chapter, the student will be able to meet competency standards in the following skills:*

- Identify dental handpieces and correctly attach them to the dental unit.
- Identify rotary cutting instruments and correctly attach them to the appropriate dental handpiece or attachment.

## ELECTRONIC RESOURCES

***Additional information related to content in Chapter 35 can be found on the companion Evolve Web site.***

- Practice Quiz
- Video: Identifying and Attaching Handpieces

If you understand the concept of the home power tool, where a drill and a bit are used to create an outline or finish a piece of wood, then you will understand the use of a dental handpiece and its attached rotary instruments. A **rotary** is a part or device that rotates around an axis. When attached to a specific handpiece, rotary instruments operate at different speeds to accomplish different functions in the cutting, polishing, and finishing of tooth structure in the restoration process.

## Evolution of Rotary Equipment

Rotary instruments were introduced to dentistry in the 1940s to complement the use of hand instruments in the cutting, grinding, and polishing procedures of operative dentistry. A significant advancement in the design and construction of the dental handpiece was the addition of electricity as a power source for rotary instruments.

The first **dental handpiece** was operated by a long belt running over a series of pulleys and then back to the motor, continuously moving the inserted rotary instrument. From the 1940s through the 1950s, the development of diamond cutting **burs** and the invention of tungsten carbide burs greatly improved the way dentists could cut into and remove hard tooth structure. Further study of diamond and carbide burs showed that these rotary instruments performed better at higher speeds. The air-driven turbine handpiece was introduced to dentistry in the 1950s.

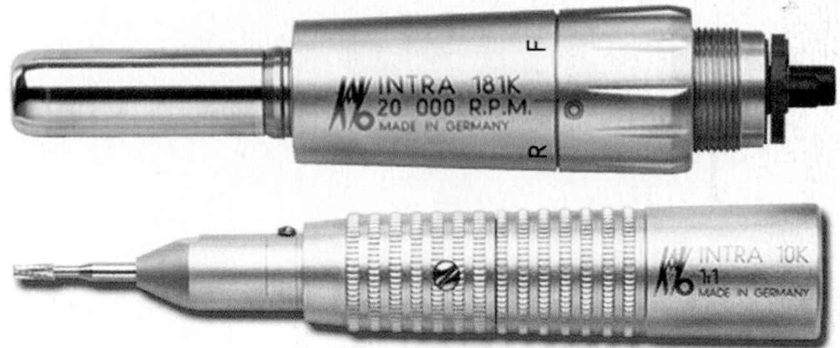


**FIG. 35.1** Low-speed motor. *(Courtesy KaVo Kerr, Orange, CA.)*

## Dental Handpieces

The dental handpiece is the most frequently used instrument in restorative dentistry. The two most common types of dental handpieces are the low-speed handpiece and the high-speed handpiece. The handpiece is a sophisticated device that runs on air pressure. The motor component receptor is attached to a hose housed within the dental unit. As you press on the rheostat, compressed air enters through the back of the handpiece, which rotates the turbine, which then rotates the rotary instrument. It is the turbine that performs all the work of the handpiece. The harder you step on the rheostat, the more air is supplied and the faster the rotary instrument turns.

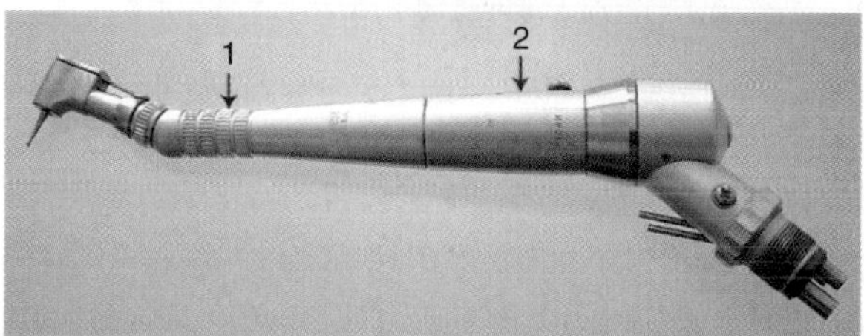


**FIG. 35.2** Low-speed handpiece with contra-angle attachment. *1,* Contra-angle attachment. *2,* Slow-speed motor. *(From Boyd LRB: Dental instruments: a pocket guide, ed 6, St Louis, 2018, Elsevier.)*

## Low-Speed Motor

The low-speed motor (sometimes you will hear it referred to as the "slow"-speed handpiece or **straight handpiece** because of its straight-line design) is one of the most versatile handpieces used by the dental team. The speed for the slow-speed motor ranges from 10,000 up to 40,000 rotations per minute (rpm). Because of its versatility, the low-speed handpiece can be adapted into three basic versions with the addition of attachments:

1. Low-speed motor with straight handpiece attachment (Fig. 35.1)
2. Low-speed motor with contra-angle handpiece attachment (Fig. 35.2)
3. Prophy low-speed, a complete handpiece that only requires the prophy attachment (Fig. 35.3)

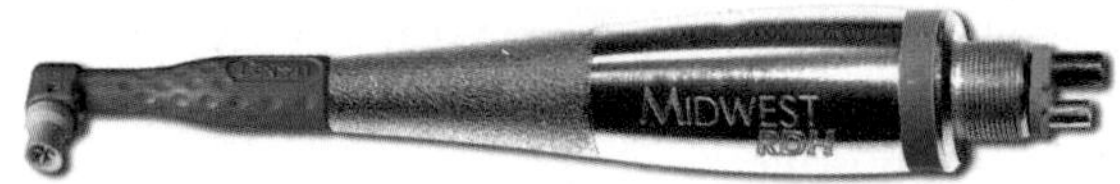


**FIG. 35.3** Prophy slow-speed handpiece motor. *(Courtesy DENTSPLY International, York, PA.)*

### *Low-Speed Motor with Straight Attachment*

The straight attachment slides onto the low-speed motor and locks into place (Fig. 35.4). The straight attachment is most commonly used for laboratory procedures such as the following:

- Trimming and contouring of custom trays
- Trimming and contouring of temporary and provisional appliances
- Trimming and relining of removable partials and dentures
- Trimming and contouring of orthodontic appliances

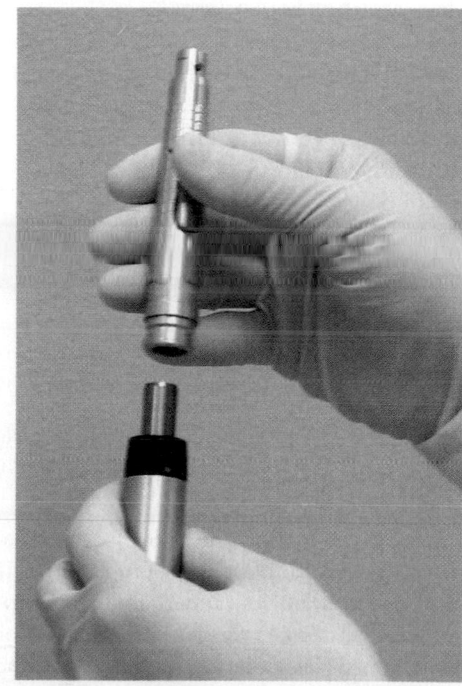

**FIG. 35.4** Straight attachment slides onto the slow-speed motor. *(From Robinson D, Bird D: Essentials of dental assisting, ed 6, St Louis, 2017, Elsevier.)*

### *Low-Speed Motor with Contra-Angle Attachment*

The contra-angle attachment slides directly onto the low-speed motor and locks into place (Fig. 35.5). The angle of

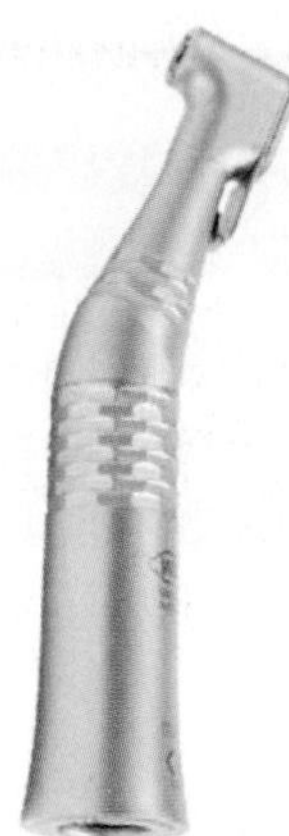

FIG. 35.5 Contra-angle attachment on the low-speed handpiece. *(Courtesy A-dec Inc., Newberg, OR.)*

this attachment is designed to allow the operator intraoral access with easier adaptation to tooth surfaces. This attachment uses a latch type of locking system to hold latch-type rotary instruments, endodontic files, prophylaxis cups, and **mandrels** (discussed later in the chapter). You will use this type of handpiece for clinical procedures such as the following:

- Removal of soft decay and fine finishing of a cavity preparation
- Finishing and polishing of restorations
- Coronal polishing and removal of stains
- Porcelain adjustments
- Root canal treatment

### *Prophylaxis Angle*

The prophylaxis attachments, or "prophy angles," are used during polishing procedures to hold the prophy cup and the bristle brush. The most common type of prophy angle is the plastic disposable prophy angle, which is discarded after a single use (Fig. 35.6). This attachment is available with a rubber cup or a bristle brush already in place.

RECALL

1 How did the first dental handpiece operate?
2 What are the two most common types of dental handpiece?
3 How fast can the low-speed handpiece rotate?
4 Which attachment is used to hold a latch-type bur?

## High-Speed Handpiece

The dentist will use the high-speed handpiece for the majority of restorative procedures, and specialty procedures within endodontics, fixed prosthodontics, and oral surgery. In contrast to the low-speed handpiece, the high-speed handpiece does not have attachments. The only additional item placed in this handpiece is the rotary instrument (bur) itself. The high-speed handpiece operates from air pressure and reaches speeds up to 450,000 rpm (Fig. 35.7).

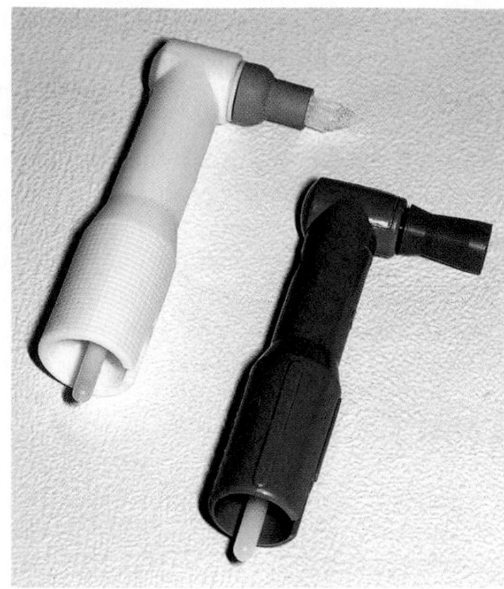

FIG. 35.6 Disposable prophy cup and brush.

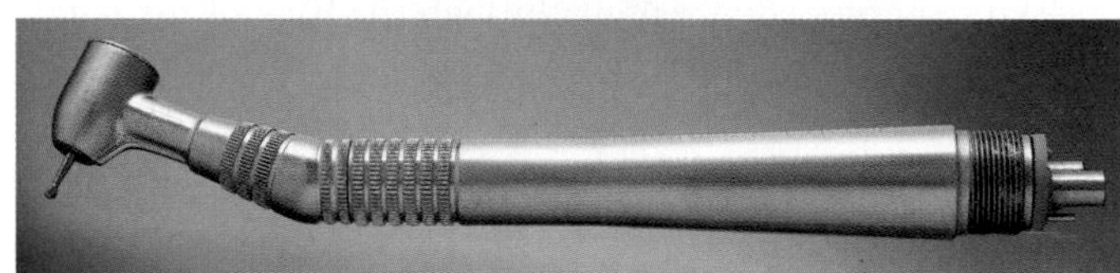

FIG. 35.7 High-speed handpiece. *(From Boyd LRB: Dental instruments: a pocket guide, ed 6, St Louis, 2018, Elsevier.)*

### *Uses of the High-Speed Handpiece*

- Removal of decay
- Removal of an old or faulty restoration
- Reduction in the crown portion of the tooth in preparation for a crown or a bridge
- Preparation of the outline and retention grooves for a new restoration
- Finishing and polishing of restorations
- Sectioning of a tooth during surgery

### *Water Coolant System*

The high speed of the bur rotating in the high-speed handpiece can generate frictional heat on a tooth, which can possibly cause damage to the pulp. To protect against pulp damage, the high-speed handpiece is designed to handle a water coolant system, so that the tooth and the bur are constantly sprayed with cool water while operating. The water spray also helps remove debris from the tooth preparation and allows the operator better visibility.

### *Bur Adaptation*

Burs for high-speed handpieces have a different locking system than those for low-speed handpieces. High-speed handpieces operate with a friction-grip device.

There are multiple designs for how a bur is locked into place in the high-speed handpiece. The method of inserting and removing burs from the handpiece varies according to the manufacturer's design. Regardless of the manufacturer, all high-speed handpieces use the friction-grip method to hold burs, stones, and polishing devices. Some older handpieces require the use of a bur-changing device. For others, with a release built into the head of the handpiece, a bur-changing device is not required (Fig. 35.8).

## Fiber-Optic Lighting

High-speed handpieces are equipped with a fiber-optic light that is placed in the head of the handpiece. Light ports near the bur deliver the proper amount of light directly onto the operating site (Fig. 35.9).

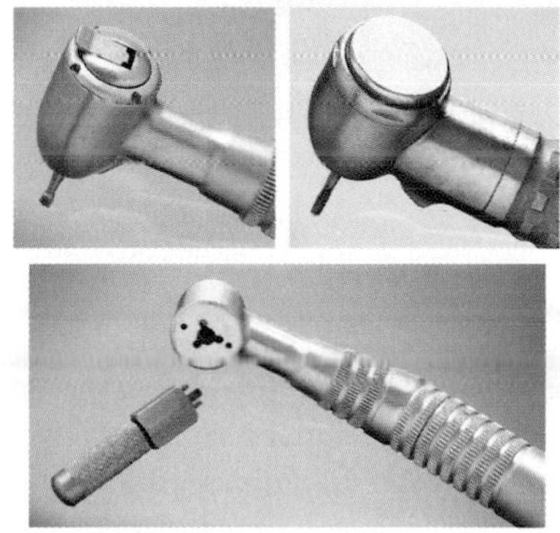

FIG. 35.8 Different styles of securing burs in the handpiece. *(From Boyd LRB: Dental instruments: a pocket guide, ed 6, St Louis, 2018, Elsevier.)*

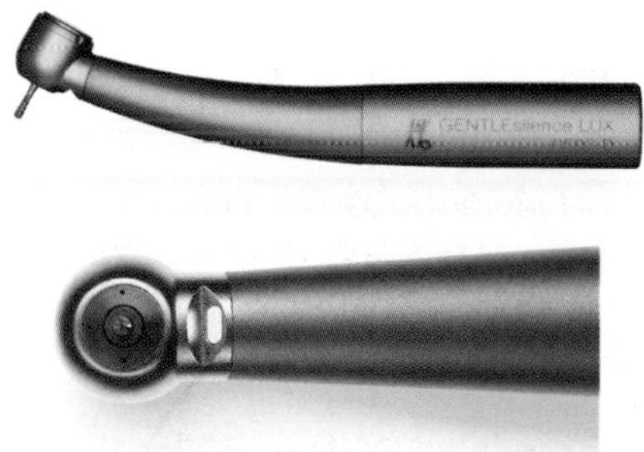


FIG. 35.9 A fiber-optic light provides better illumination of an area for the operator. *(Courtesy KaVo Kerr, Orange, CA.)*

RECALL

5 How fast does the high-speed handpiece operate?
6 How is the tooth kept cool and clean during use of the high-speed handpiece?
7 What type of bur locking system is found on the high-speed handpiece?
8 On the high-speed handpiece, what helps illuminate the working field?

## Ultrasonic Handpiece

The **ultrasonic** handpiece uses mechanical radiant energy of water and sound vibrations to create a pulsating effect on a tooth surface. The ultrasonic handpiece is used primarily for the scaling and root planing procedure (Fig. 35.10). The orthodontist will request it for removal of bonding materials from a tooth surface after orthodontic appliances are removed.

The ultrasonic handpiece is attached to the dental unit and is powered by electricity. Attachments for the ultrasonic handpiece are designed similarly to those for hand (manual) scaling instruments. A specific tip is selected according to the surface and location of use. When activated, the ultrasonic handpiece delivers a pulsating spray of water, which causes the calculus and stain or the bonding agent to break down for easier removal.

## Laser Handpiece

The laser handpiece uses a beam of laser light to cauterize soft tissue or vaporize decayed tooth structure (Fig. 35.11). The handpiece design resembles the standard handpiece and has many similar qualities, such as water and air to cool the tooth and keep the area clean. The **laser**, however, is operated through a fiber-optic cable that extends from the **console** to the laser handpiece.

Use of a laser handpiece offers many benefits over the use of the traditional handpiece or surgical instruments. Laser treatment is painless, so anesthesia is unnecessary. The dentist does not have to wait for the patient to "get numb" before proceeding.

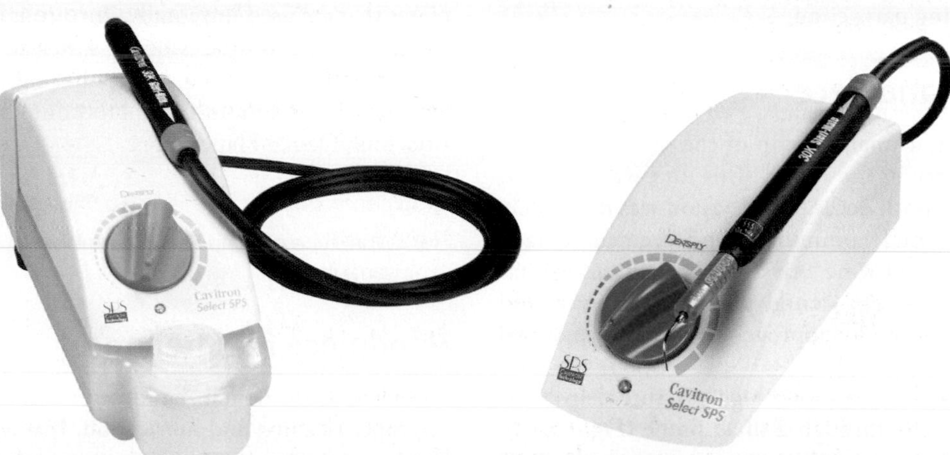


FIG. 35.10 Ultrasonic handpiece. *(Courtesy Dentsply Professional Division, York, PA.)*

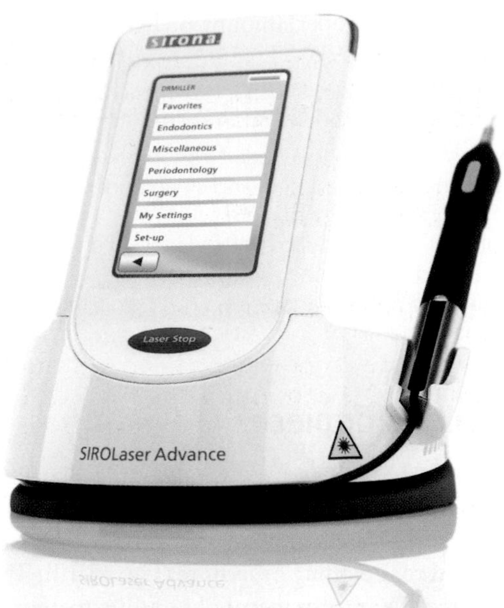


FIG. 35.11 Soft tissue diode laser. *(Courtesy Sirona Dental Systems, Charlotte, NC.)*

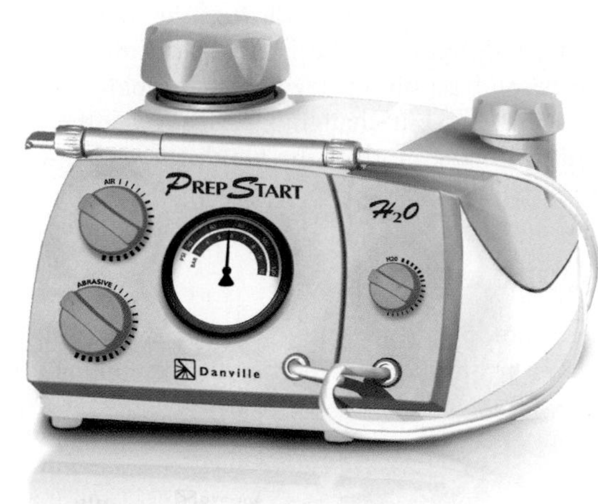


FIG. 35.12 Air abrasion handpiece. *(Courtesy Danville Materials, Inc.)*

Disadvantages of using the laser time include that (1) the laser cannot be used on teeth with restorations already in place, and (2) laser procedures can take longer than conventional methods.

### *Precautions in the Care and Handling of Laser Handpieces*

Follow these precautions to avoid damage to the fiber-optic cables and the laser handpiece:

- Do not sharply bend or twist the fiber-optic cable. The cable could break and burn during use, resulting in injury to the user or the patient.
- Do not touch the exposed fiber-optic cable. Dirt and fingerprints can damage the cable.
- Do not touch the end of the fiber-optic cable connector. The end connector contains a small optical fiber that may degrade if contaminated.
- Keep the connecting parts clean.

## Air Abrasion Handpiece

The air abrasion unit, a small version of the sandblaster, was introduced to dentistry in the 1940s. This unit was designed to remove stains and tooth decay. Air abrasion was not widely recognized by the dental community and seemed to fade out of use for a period of time. Air abrasion technology has been brought back into the dental practice, however, and has become a patient-friendly approach to restorative dental treatment.

The air abrasion technique allows high-pressure delivery of aluminum oxide particles through a small probe (Fig. 35.12). This unique technology is used to remove enamel, dentin, and restorative materials without compromising healthy tooth structure. Dentists can now conservatively remove diseased enamel and dentin without the use of local anesthesia.

Although it was not meant to replace conventional rotary instruments, air abrasion is shifting the way teeth are prepared and treated toward a more conservative approach. The air abrasion technique is most effective when it is used for the following:

- Sealants
- External stain removal
- Class I through class VI preparations
- Endodontic access
- Crown margins
- Preparation of tooth surface for cementation of cast restoration (crown, veneer)

## Laboratory Handpiece

The laboratory handpiece is designed for the dental laboratory. This handpiece operates at speeds up to 20,000 rpm and uses laboratory burs of various shapes and sizes. The laboratory handpiece provides greater torque than is provided by handpieces that are used intraorally. **Torque** is a twisting or turning force. Increased torque is better suited to the heavier pressure required during grinding and polishing procedures that take place outside the mouth. See Procedure 35.1: Identifying and Attaching Dental Handpieces

**9** What type of handpiece resembles a sandblaster?

## Handpiece Maintenance

Problems with dental handpieces most often result from improper cleaning and lubrication. Inadequate cleaning of the handpiece before sterilization can result in the collection of debris in the internal parts of the handpiece.

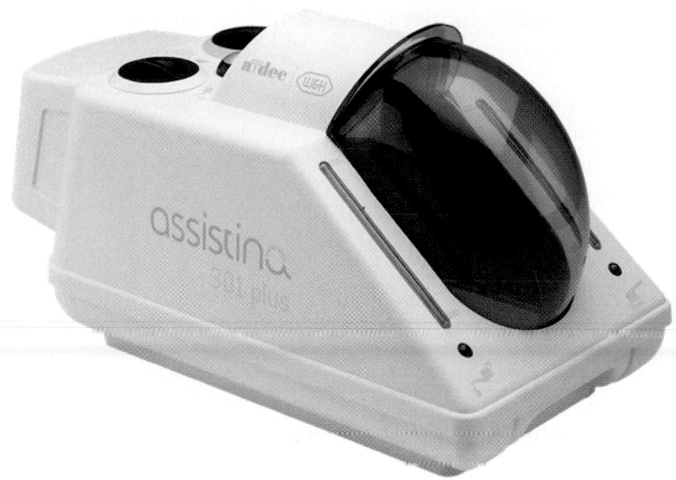


FIG. 35.13 Lubrication system. *(Courtesy A-dec Inc., Newberg, OR.)*

Debris creates wear which is similar to sludge within an automobile engine. Excessive lubrication is as damaging as inadequate lubrication. Handpieces are available with ceramic bearings or heads that require no lubrication. If inappropriate cleaning solutions or techniques are used, the working life of the handpiece is significantly shortened. It is imperative to follow the manufacturer's directions for appropriate maintenance of each handpiece. Failure to do so can result in voiding of the handpiece warranty.

Some types of handpieces require lubrication *before* sterilization, some require lubrication *after* sterilization, and others require lubrication both *before and after* sterilization. You must carefully follow the manufacturer's instructions for sterilization of the handpiece (Fig. 35.13).

### Handpiece Sterilization

The dental handpiece is identified as a **semicritical instrument** (one that comes in contact with blood, saliva, and mucous membrane) that *must* be sterilized before reuse. Dental handpieces require special considerations for sterilization because blood and saliva may be sucked back into the internal portions of the handpiece.

#### GENERAL CONSIDERATIONS FOR HANDPIECE STERILIZATION

- Wear personal protective equipment (PPE), and follow Universal Precautions. The used handpiece is contaminated and must be handled with appropriate care.
- Use mild soap and water, or water alone, to clean debris from the external surface of the handpiece. Certain disinfectants can actually corrode the handpiece and cause more harm.
- Clean the internal components of the handpiece according to the manufacturer's instructions. Some manufacturers recommend ultrasonic cleaning; others do not.
- Ensure that handpieces are dry before they are packaged. Dryness is important to avoid corrosion with autoclave use.
- Wrap the handpiece for sterilization according to the type of sterilization recommended and the manufacturer's care instructions.
- Sterilize the handpiece according to the manufacturer's instructions. Most manufacturers recommend autoclaving or chemical vapor sterilization.
- After sterilization, wipe the light port on the fiber-optic handpiece with an alcohol swab to remove excess lubricant. The light will be dimmed if any lubricant remains.
- Before attaching the sterile handpiece, flush the airlines and waterlines on the handpiece hose for 30 to 60 seconds. Flushing reduces any bioburden that may be sprayed into the patient's oral cavity.

**STERILIZATION PROCEDURE SHEETS.** A dental office may acquire handpieces made by different manufacturers over time as handpieces are replaced or new models become available. Sterilization instructions vary not only between manufacturers but also between different models made by the same manufacturer.

The use of a sterilization procedure sheet is one way to avoid errors in handpiece sterilization. This practice is particularly helpful if several team members are involved in the process. Sterilization procedure sheets can be created for the dental office by using the information found in each manufacturer's instruction book.

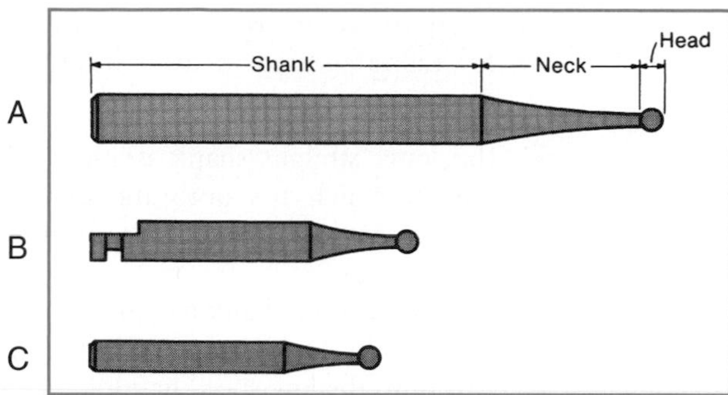


FIG. 35.14 Bur parts and types of shanks. A, Long straight laboratory. B, Latch-type. C, Friction-grip. *(From Robinson D, Bird D: Essentials of dental assisting, ed 6, St Louis, 2017, Elsevier.)*

## Rotary Cutting Instruments

Rotary cutting instruments are accessories that are intended for use with the dental handpiece. Hundreds of different types of rotary instruments are available, and each is designed for a specific use. As with hand instruments, dentists have their preferences and will use only a few rotary instruments for most procedures. Rotary instruments have three basic parts: the shank, the neck, and the head (Fig. 35.14).

### Shank Types

The **shank** of the bur is the portion that fits into the handpiece. Shank length varies according to the specific function of the bur and the handpiece to which it is attached. Rotary instruments are manufactured in three basic shank styles:

- **Straight shank.** The long, straight shank is used in the straight-line attachment, which fits onto the low-speed handpiece. Straight shanks are held in place by a mechanism within the straight attachment.
- **Latch-type shank.** The latch-type shank has a small groove at the end that mechanically locks into the contra-angle attachment, which fits onto the low-speed handpiece.
- **Friction-grip shank.** The friction-grip shank is short and smooth and has no retention grooves in the end. The shank is held in the high-speed handpiece by the creation of friction that grips the entire shank.

## Neck

The neck of the rotary instrument is the narrow portion that connects the shank and the head.

## Head

The head of the rotary instrument is the cutting, polishing, or finishing portion. The head is manufactured in a large variety of sizes, shapes, and materials.

# Dental Burs

The term *bur* is applied to all rotary instruments that have a sharp cutting head. Blades make up these cutting surfaces. Burs are needed in restorative dentistry for the following procedures:

- Preparing the tooth
- Excavating decay
- Finishing cavity walls
- Finishing restoration surfaces
- Removing old fillings
- Finishing crown preparations
- Separating crowns and bridges
- Adjusting and correcting acrylic temporary crowns

Burs were made primarily of steel, but dentists found that the use of steel burs on enamel at high speeds caused the burs to dull rapidly. Since the late 1940s, a tungsten carbide material has replaced the steel in the bur for cavity preparation. Tungsten carbide is stiffer and stronger than steel and remains sharp much longer.

## Bur Shapes

When discussing the "shape" of a bur, you are referring to the *contour* or *design* of the head of the bur. Burs are manufactured in a variety of shapes, and each shape is available in a variety of sizes. A bur will have a name, a series of numbers attached to its shape, and a purpose for use (Table 35.1).

RECALL

10 What type of shank fits into the contra-angle attachment?
11 Restorative burs are made from what material?
12 What design of bur is a 33½?

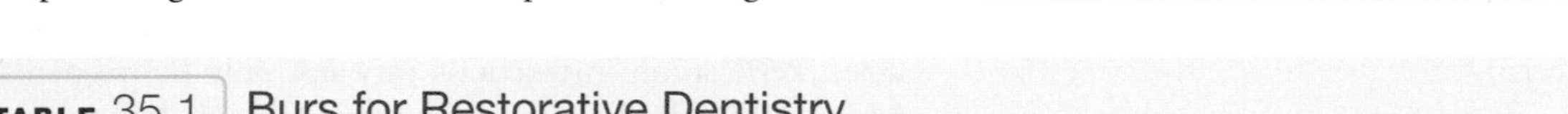

**TABLE 35.1 Burs for Restorative Dentistry**

| Type of Bur | Series of Numbers | Uses | Example |
|---|---|---|---|
| Round | ¼, ½, 1–8, 10 | Initial entry into tooth structure<br>Extends preparation<br>Retention<br>Removes decay | |
| Inverted cone 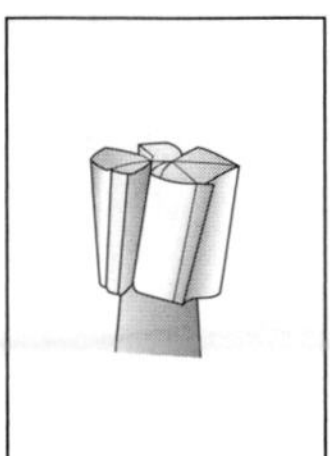 | 33½, 34–39, 36L, 37L | Removes decay<br>Establishes retentive grooves | 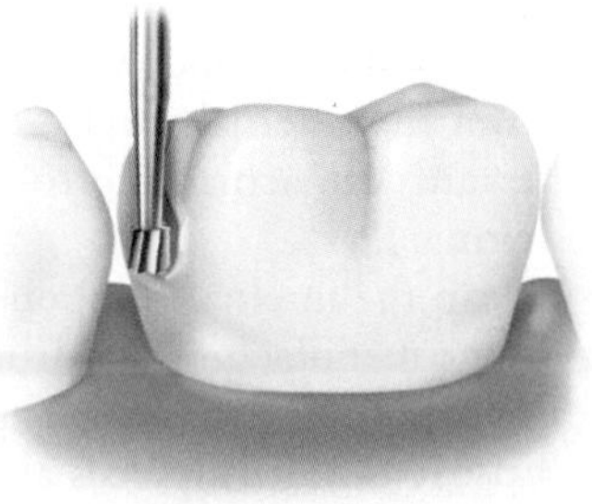 |

**TABLE 35.1** Burs for Restorative Dentistry—cont'd

| Type of Bur | Series of Numbers | Uses | Example |
|---|---|---|---|
| Straight fissure plain cut 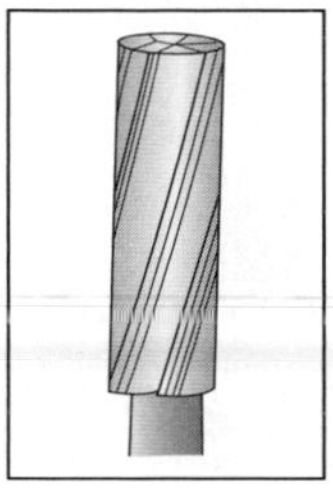 | 55–60, 57L, 58L | Initial entry into tooth<br>Helps in forming the internal walls of the preparation | 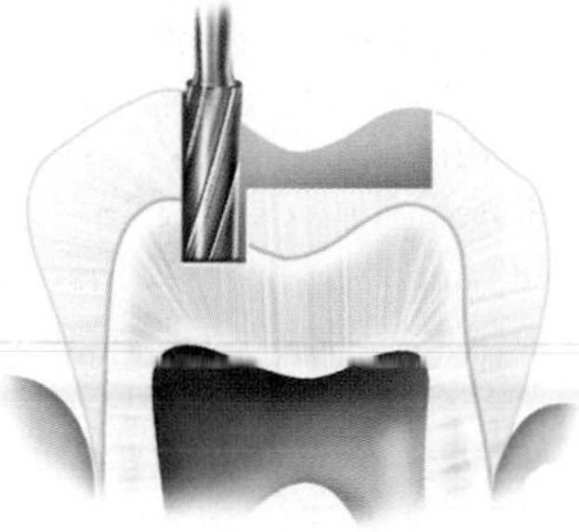 |
| Straight fissure cross-cut 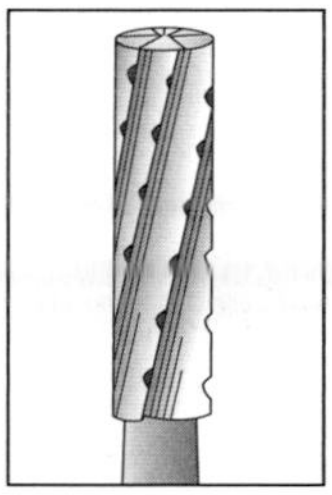 | 556–560, 567L, 568L | Helps in forming the internal walls of the preparation | * 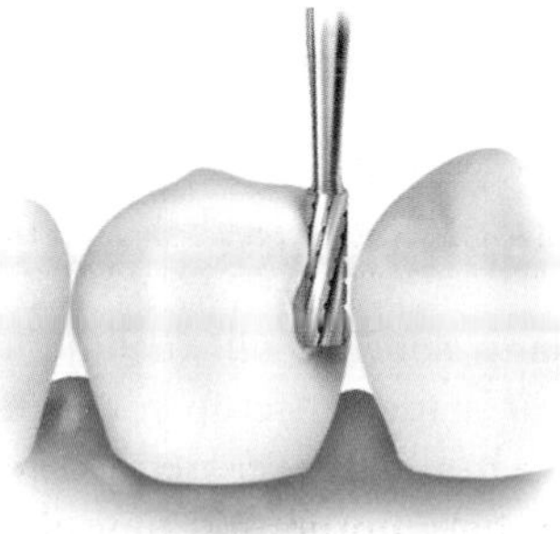 |
| Tapered fissure plain cut 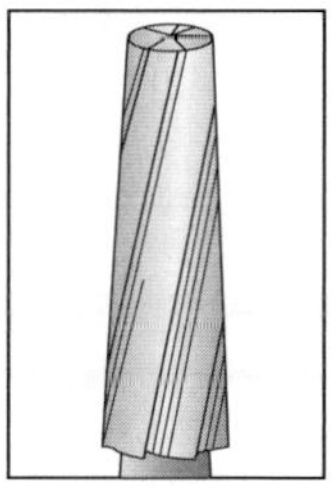 | 169–172, 169L, 170L, 171L | Helps in providing angles to the walls of the prepared tooth | 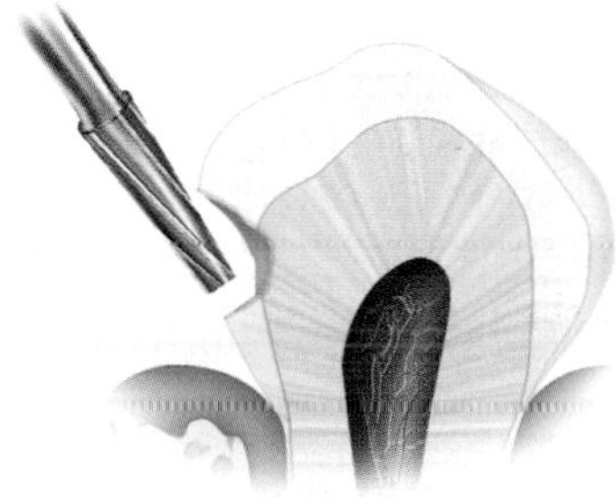 |
| Tapered fissure cross-cut 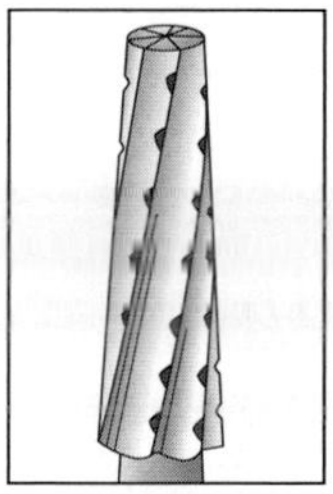 | 699–703, 699L, 700L, 701L | Helps in providing angles to the walls of the prepared tooth | * 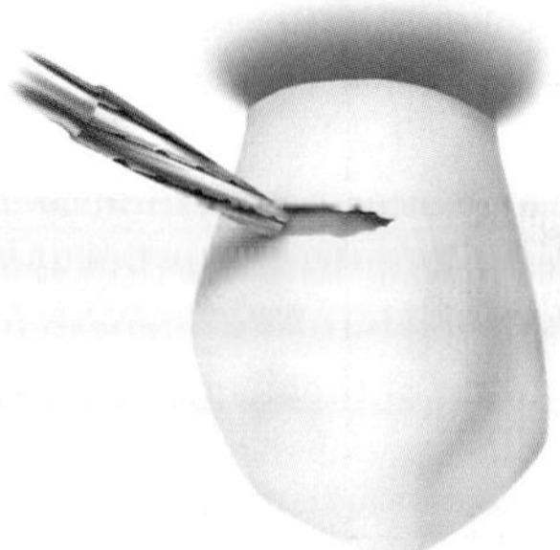 |
| Pear 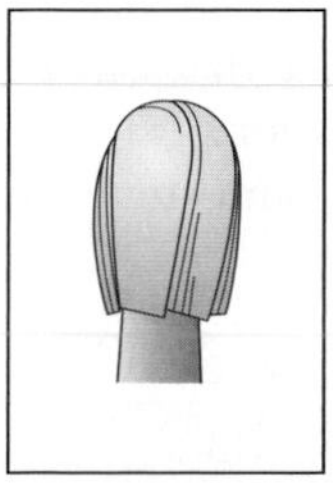 | 330–333, 331L | Initial entry into tooth structure<br>Extends preparation | 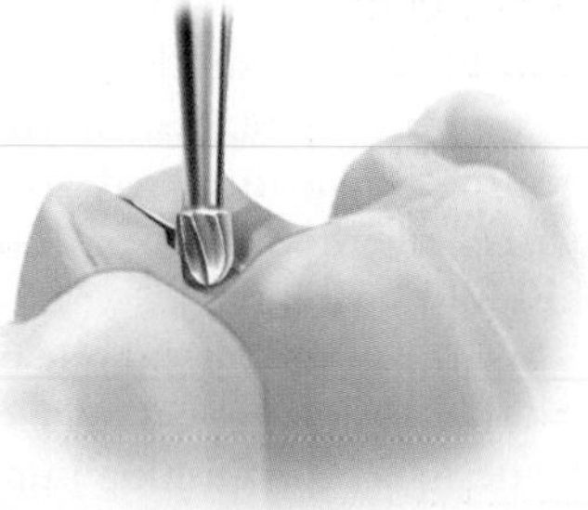 |

*Continued*

**TABLE 35.1 Burs for Restorative Dentistry—cont'd**

| Type of Bur | Series of Numbers | Uses | Example |
|---|---|---|---|
| End cutting | 957, 958 | Initial entry into tooth structure<br>Creates a shoulder for the margin of a crown preparation | |

Illustrations in first column from Finkbeiner BL, Johnson CS: Mosby's comprehensive dental assisting, St Louis, 1995, Mosby. Illustrations in last column © Elsevier Collection.

## Diamond Rotary Instruments

Many dentists will include a diamond rotary instrument in their standard setup for a restorative dental procedure (Box 35.1). This is because the *cutting ability* of a diamond surface shortens preparation time and increases productivity.

Diamond burs have a metal base, with flecks of industrial diamonds embedded into the base. A metallic bonding material holds the bits onto the base. The design or shape of diamond burs varies according to the dentist's need; the most frequently selected diamond burs include the following:

- *Round*—to provide access to the pulp chamber
- *Flat end taper*—to reduce tooth structure during a crown preparation
- *Flame*—to reduce tooth structure in preparation for a crown
- *Wheel*—to make subgingival bevels in a crown preparation

Diamond burs are manufactured in a range of *grit* (coarseness) classifications to allow selection of the proper grit and cutting rate for each phase of restorative dentistry, similar to sandpaper. To identify the various grits, some manufacturers use a letter designation at the end of the bur number to indicate the grit or cutting rate. Others insert a color-coded band on the bur. With repeated use and sterilization, however, debonding of the diamond particles occurs, decreasing the cutting efficiency of the diamond.

**BOX 35.1 Indications for Using Diamond Burs**

- **Round-end taper** bur removes tooth structure and makes mechanical retention grooves.
- **Flat-end taper** bur is used for crown preparation.
- **Cylinder burs** smooth and finish walls in tooth preparations.
- **Flame-shaped bur** makes bevels in crown preparations.
- **Round bur** provides access to the pulp chamber for endodontic treatment and is used to adjust and shape occlusal surfaces.
- **Wheel-shaped bur** is used for anterior crown preparations and can be used to adjust and shape occlusal surfaces.

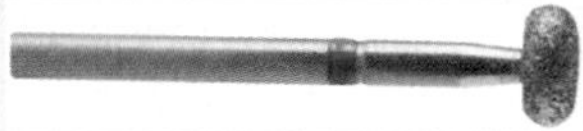

From Robinson D, Bird D: Essentials of dental assisting, ed 6, St Louis, 2017, Elsevier; images courtesy Dentsply International, York, PA.

## Finishing Rotary Instruments

A finishing bur is similar in appearance to a cutting bur, except the number of blades, or **flutes**, on the working end of a finishing bur is increased. The greater the number of cutting surfaces on the head of a bur, the greater is its polishing or finishing capability.

In your studies of esthetic materials, you will find that these materials require a final stage of polishing with a finishing bur. The designs of a finishing bur resemble those of a carbide bur. The most commonly used finishing burs are round, tapered, or flame-shaped (Fig. 35.15).

## Abrasive Rotary Instruments

Abrasive rotary instruments are the most varied of the rotary instruments. Many types of abrasive material are applied to many shapes to create a flexible working surface that can be adapted to the contour of the tooth or restoration. Abrasive materials are made in shapes ranging from discs and stones to points and strips (Fig. 35.16).

### Accessories

Abrasive discs and wheels are supplied separately and are not attached to a shank. Because of this, a **mandrel** (a metal shaft

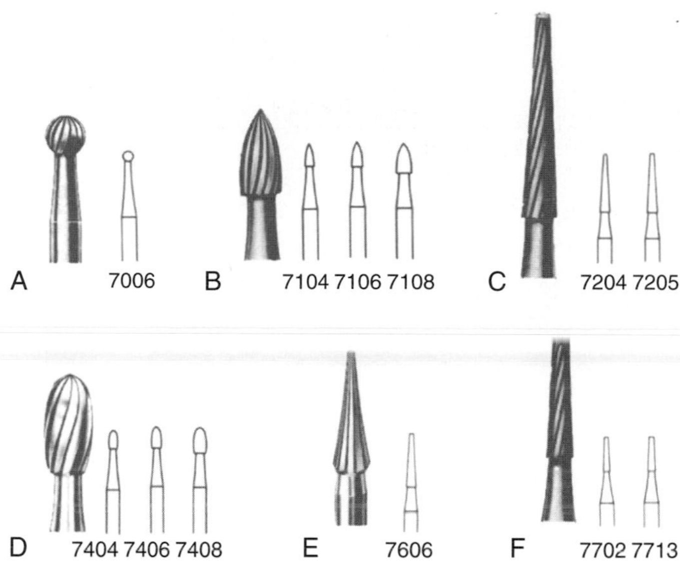


**FIG. 35.15** Finishing burs. A, Round. B, Flame. C, Tapered. D, Pear. E, Cylinder. F, Round end tapered. *(Permission granted by Integra LifeSciences Corporation, Plainsboro, NJ.)*

on which a sandpaper disc or other abrasive materials are mounted) is used to attach these abrasives to the dental handpiece (Fig. 35.17).

Mandrels are designed according to the different types of shank so that they may be used in both low-speed and high-speed handpieces.

## Laboratory Rotary Instruments

Laboratory burs are easy to distinguish from dental burs because of their size (see Procedure 35.2: Identifying and Attaching Burs for Rotary Cutting Instruments). Laboratory burs have a longer shank and a larger head than dental burs.

Laboratory burs are used in the low-speed handpiece for functions such as cutting and polishing of acrylic. The **acrylic bur** is the bur that is most commonly used in the laboratory. As with other types of burs, the heads of the acrylic bur come in various shapes for specific uses (Fig. 35.18).

**13** What gives the diamond bur its advantage?
**14** Finishing burs are used on what type of dental material?
**15** What is used to hold a disc in the handpiece?

**■ Legal and Ethical Implications** By now, you are fully aware of the importance of the sterilization process for instruments that are used intraorally. Dental handpieces and rotary instruments are no exception to the rule. The care that you take in cleaning, packaging, and sterilizing these items is an essential step in preventing the transmission of infectious diseases.

Great emphasis must be placed on the internal makeup of a dental handpiece, when infectious blood and bioburden remain inside a contaminated handpiece and on a rotary instrument. Steps that must be taken to decrease the patient's risk of infection reflect both the legal guidelines for dentistry and the philosophy of the dental practice. ■

**■ Eye to the Future** In the future, patients will have their teeth prepared, finished, and polished exclusively by lasers and air abrasion handpieces. Advancements in technology will allow these handpieces to be used without patient anesthesia.

This new technology will dramatically change the roles of dental team members. The dental assistant and the dental hygienist will perform more traditional and conservative dental treatment, while the dentist will focus on more advanced procedures. ■

**■ Critical Thinking**

1. You are setting up the dental hygiene room for a patient. What dental handpiece and accessories would be assembled for a prophylaxis procedure?
2. While setting up the treatment room in preparation for a restorative appointment, you notice that the #2 round bur has dried blood on it. What do you do with the bur, and how did this happen?
3. The dentist has just finished restoring tooth #7. Because this is an anterior tooth, what rotary instruments could the dentist use to finish and polish a resin material?
4. A patient received her new denture yesterday and has returned to the office with discomfort. The dentist tells the patient that the denture must be adjusted to fit better. Describe how you would set up the low-speed handpiece with a laboratory-type acrylic bur.
5. It is 11:00 AM, and you have a patient seated for a restorative procedure. You notice that you have depleted the supply of clean handpieces while caring for the emergency patients seen earlier in the day. What do you do? ■

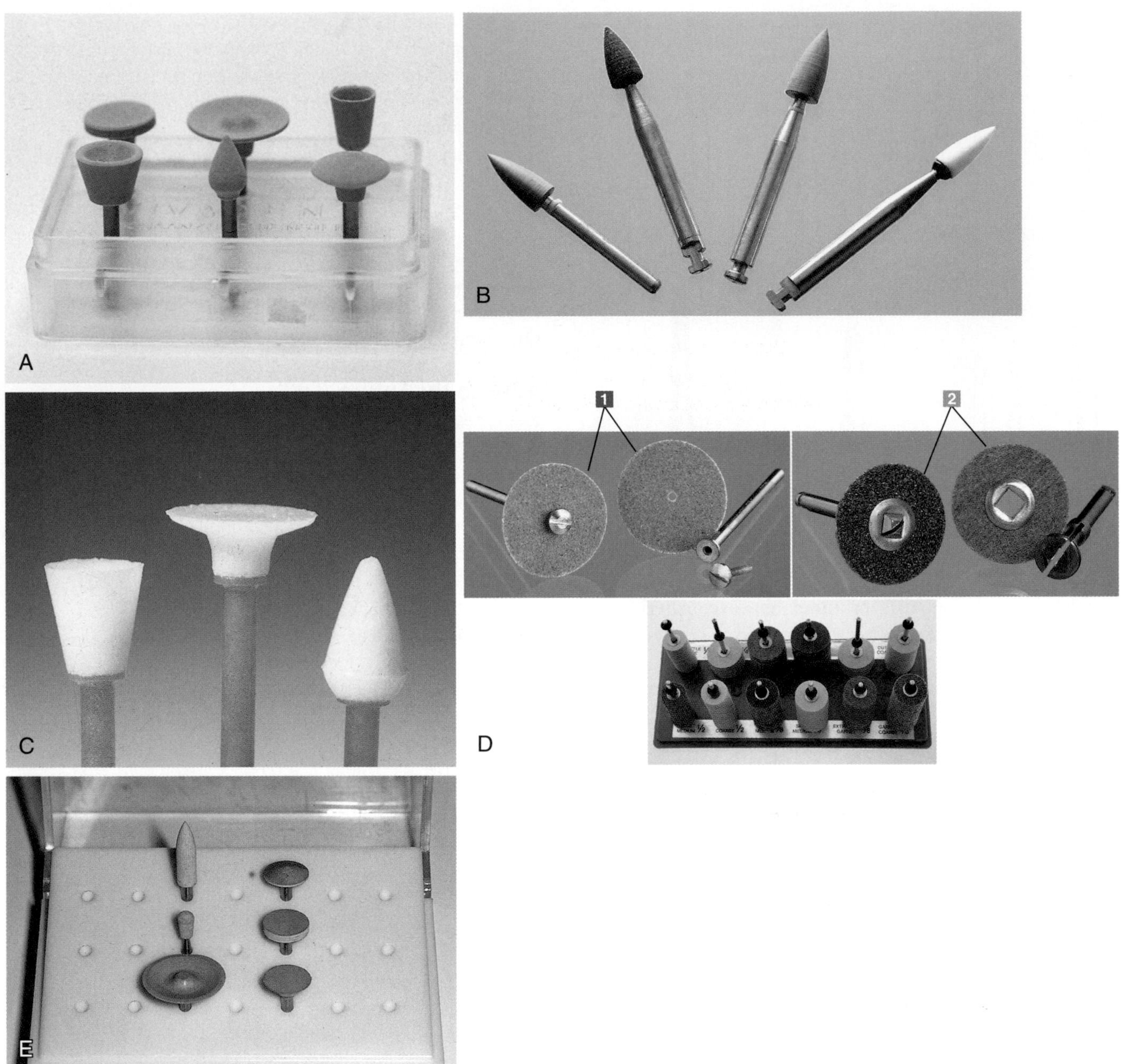


**FIG. 35.16** Accessory attachments for rotary instruments. A, Silicon carbide produces a moderately rough surface. It is available in wheels, points, and stones, and the color varies from gray-green to black. It is used for polishing metal restorations. B, Rubber points come in varying colors, depending on their abrasiveness. The brown is the most abrasive, with green having less abrasiveness, and then white a polishing point. C, Cuttlebone is most often adhered to discs and points. It is used for final finishing and polishing of the restoration. D, Sandpaper discs refer to sand particles adhered to flexible paper discs or strips as a medium abrasive. They are used for finishing and polishing a restoration. *1,* Snap on metal center. *2,* Screw on. E, Carborundum particles adhered to disc. As with carborundum on burs, it is used to cut or separate one structure from another. *(*B *and* D *from Boyd L: Dental instruments: a pocket guide, ed 6, St Louis, 2018, Elsevier.)*

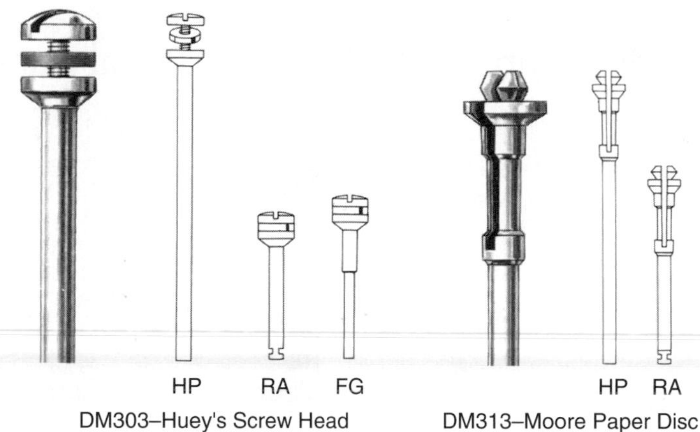


**FIG. 35.17** Types of mandrels. *(Permission granted by Integra LifeSciences Corporation, Plainsboro, NJ.)*

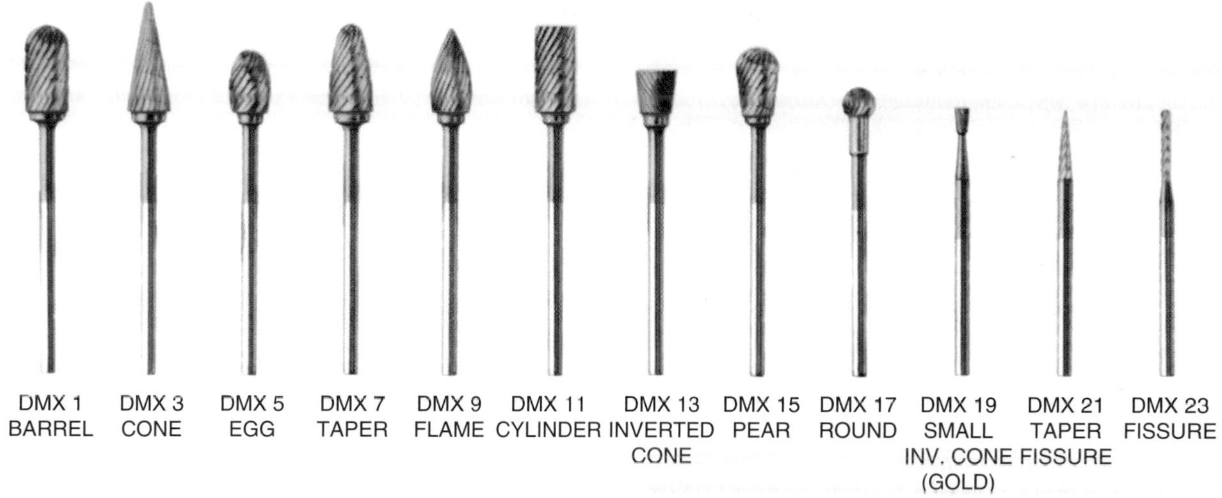


**FIG. 35.18** Varying shapes of laboratory acrylic burs. *(Permission granted by Integra LifeSciences Corporation, Plainsboro, NJ.)*

PROCEDURE 35.1 

# Identifying and Attaching Dental Handpieces

## EQUIPMENT AND SUPPLIES

- ✓ Low-speed handpiece motor
- ✓ Straight attachment
- ✓ Contra-angle attachment
- ✓ Prophylaxis attachment
- ✓ High-speed handpiece
- ✓ Ultrasonic handpiece

## PROCEDURAL STEPS

1 Identify and attach the low-speed handpiece to the dental unit, ensuring that the receptors are aligned and that the handpiece fits correctly onto the correct line.

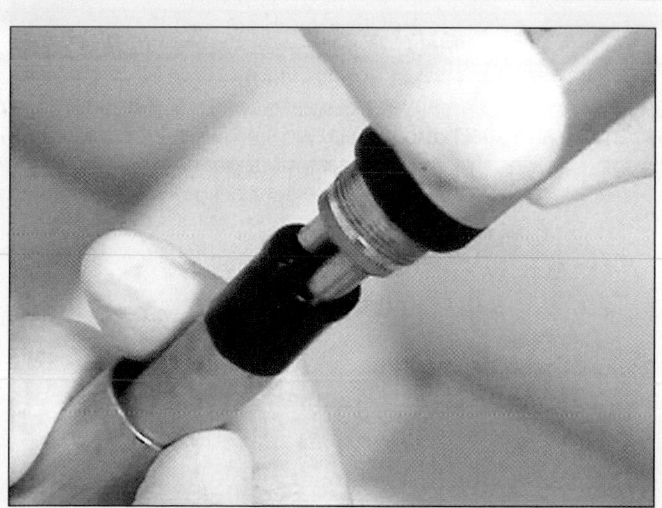

(Continued)

## PROCEDURE 35.1 Identifying and Attaching Dental Handpieces—cont'd

2 Identify and attach the contra-angle attachment onto the straight attachment of the low-speed handpiece, ensuring that the attachment is locked.

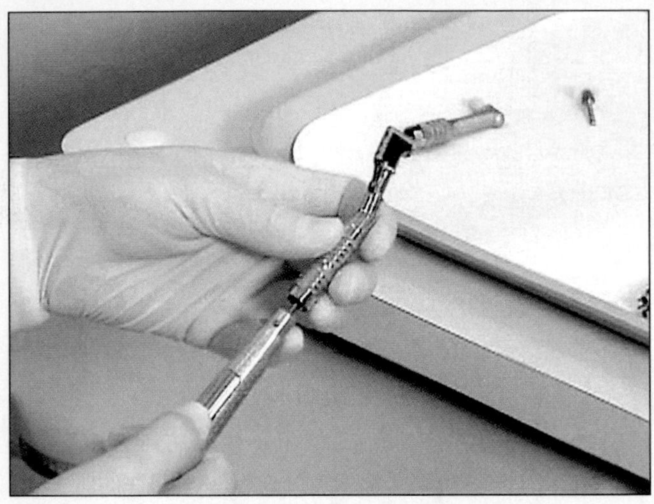

3 Identify and attach the prophylaxis angle attachment onto the straight attachment of the low-speed handpiece, ensuring that the attachment is locked.

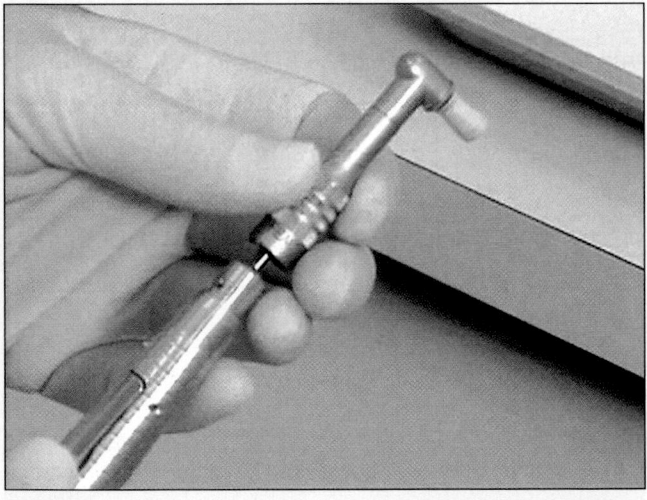

4 Identify and attach the high-speed handpiece to the dental unit, ensuring that the receptors are aligned and that the handpiece fits correctly onto the correct line.

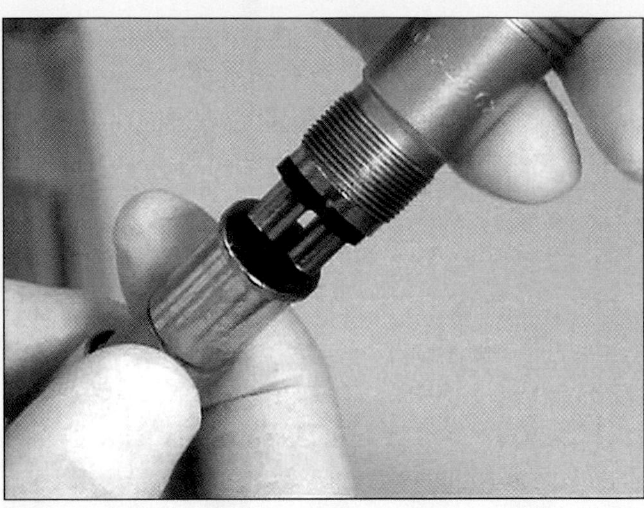

5 Identify and attach the handpiece to the dental unit, ensuring that the receptors are aligned and that the handpiece fits correctly onto the correct line.

PROCEDURE 35.2

# Identifying and Attaching Burs for Rotary Cutting Instruments

## EQUIPMENT AND SUPPLIES

- ✔ Various types of dental rotary instruments, including carborundum, diamond, finishing, abrasive, and laboratory burs
- ✔ Low-speed handpiece
- ✔ High-speed handpiece
- ✔ Contra-angle attachment
- ✔ Mandrel

## PROCEDURAL STEPS

1 Identify specific dental burs, such as carborundum, diamond, finishing, and abrasion burs, by their name and number sequence.

2 Attach latch-type burs to the contra-angle attachment on the low-speed handpiece, ensuring that the bur is locked in place.

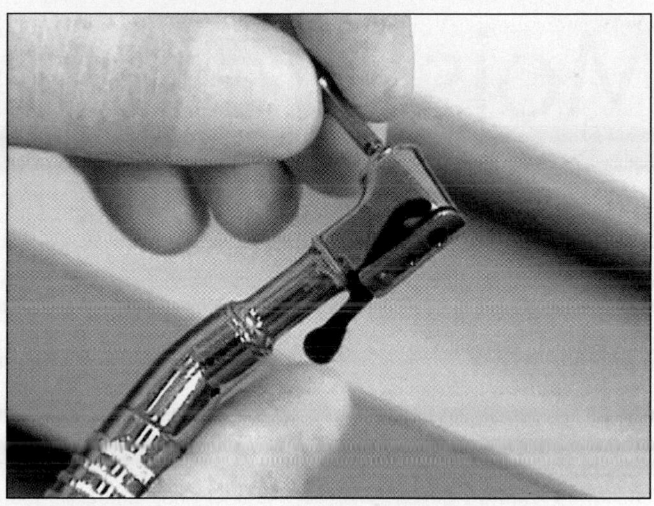

3 Attach the friction-grip bur to the high-speed handpiece, ensuring that the bur is locked in place.

4 Attach abrasive discs to the mandrel correctly by screwing to tighten or by positioning the metal opening onto the mandrel, ensuring that the disc is securely locked.

36

# Moisture Control

## KEY TERMS

**Aspirate (AS-pi-rayt)** To draw back or to draw within.
**Bow** Rounded part of clamp that extends through the dental dam.
**Exposed** Pertaining to selected teeth visible through the dam; *isolated.*
**Invert (in-VURT)** To reverse the position, order, or condition. To turn inside out or upside down.
**Isolated** Pertaining to selected teeth visible through the dam; *exposed.*
**Jaws** Part of a clamp that is shaped into four prongs to help stabilize the clamp on the tooth.
**Malaligned (mal-uh-LINED)** Displaced out of line, especially teeth displaced from normal relation to the line of the dental arch; also called *malposed.*
**Septum (SEP-tum)** Dental dam material located between the holes of the punched dam.
**Stylus (STYE-lus)** Sharp, pointed tool used for cutting.
**Universal** Pertaining to the same clamp that can be placed on the same type of tooth in the opposite quadrant.
**Winged clamp** Type of dental dam clamp that has extensions to help retain the dental dam.

## LEARNING OUTCOMES

*On completion of this chapter, the student will be able to achieve the following objectives:*

1. Pronounce, define, and spell the key terms.
2. Discuss oral evacuation systems, including the following:
   - Describe the two types of oral evacuation systems used in dentistry.
   - Describe the grasp and positioning of the high-volume evacuator tip.
3. Discuss rinsing the oral cavity, including the use of the air-water syringe.
4. List isolation techniques used to decrease moisture during a dental procedure.
5. Describe the dental dam and its role in moisture control, including the following:
   - List the equipment and supplies required for dental dam application.
   - Describe the placement of the dental dam.
   - Explain special applications for the dental dam.

## PERFORMANCE OUTCOMES

*On completion of this chapter, the student will be able to meet competency standards in the following skills:*

- Perform the grasp and positioning of the high-volume evacuator during a procedure.
- Perform limited-area and full-mouth rinses.
- Place cotton rolls for isolation.
- Prepare, place, and remove the dental dam as an expanded function.

## ELECTRONIC RESOURCES

***Additional information related to content in Chapter 36 can be found on the companion Evolve Web site.***

- Practice Quiz
- Tray Setup Drag-and-Drop Exercise: Dental Dam
- Tray Setup Questions
- Videos: Positioning the High-Volume Evacuator During a Procedure; Preparing, Placing, and Removing the Dental Dam

When assisting in a dental procedure, one of the most important responsibilities of the chairside dental assistant is to maintain moisture control and keep a clean oral environment. The assistant maintains the operating field free of excess water, saliva, blood, tooth fragments, and excess dental materials.

This chapter describes several moisture control techniques and their incorporation into the dental procedure.

## Oral Evacuation Systems

The term **oral evacuation** describes the process of removing excess fluid and debris from the mouth. The use of an oral evacuator completes this process before, during, and after a dental procedure. The two types of evacuators most often used in a dental procedure are the **saliva ejector** and the **high-volume evacuator (HVE).**

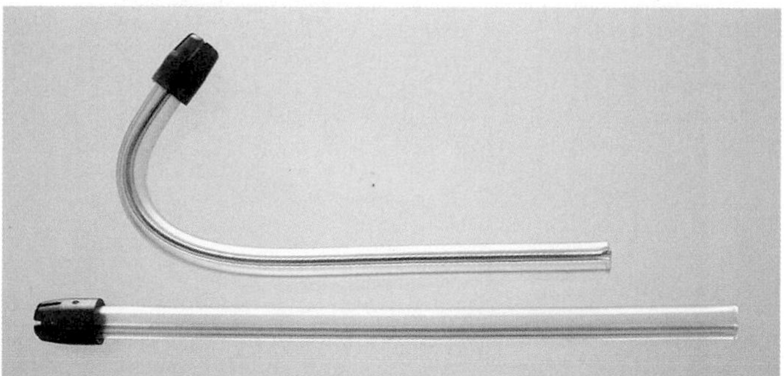

FIG. 36.1 Saliva ejector. *(From Boyd LRB: Dental instruments: a pocket guide, ed 6, St Louis, 2018, Elsevier.)*

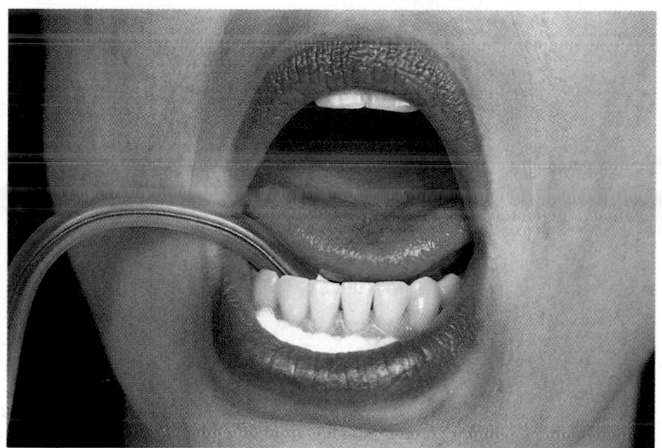

FIG. 36.2 Saliva ejector placed under the tongue for a procedure.

## Saliva Ejector

The saliva ejector is a small, straw-shaped oral evacuator that is used during less-invasive dental procedures (Fig. 36.1). The main function of the saliva ejector is to remove liquids from the mouth; it is not powerful enough to remove solid debris. Indications for using the saliva injector include the following:

- Preventive procedures, such as prophylaxis, placement of sealants, and fluoride treatments
- Control of saliva and moisture accumulation under the dental dam
- Cementation of crown and bridge prostheses
- Orthodontic bonding procedures

The saliva ejector is made of a soft plastic tubing that can be shaped for easy placement in the oral cavity. The saliva ejector can be held (1) throughout the procedure, with the use of repeated sweeps of the mouth to remove fluids; or (2) by positioning the suction tip in the mouth during a procedure.

To place the saliva ejector in a stationary position, bend and form the tubing into the shape of a candy cane (Fig. 36.2). This shape allows the saliva ejector to be positioned under the tongue, where most fluids accumulate. When placing the saliva ejector, insert a cotton roll to act as a buffer, so that it cannot traumatize oral tissues. When positioning the saliva ejector for a procedure, position it on the opposite side from where the dentist is working to reduce the number of items in the operating field.

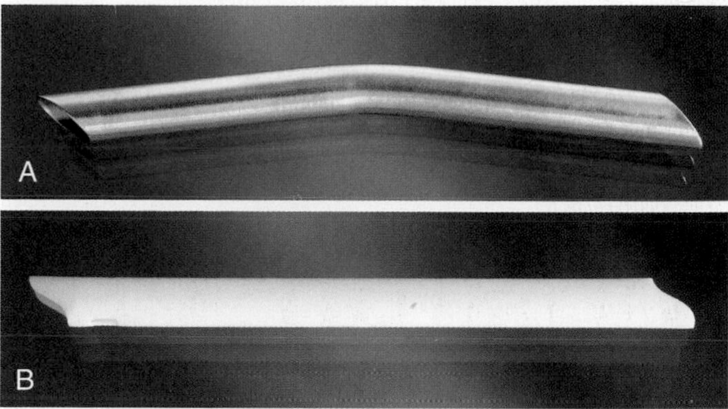


FIG. 36.3 High-volume evacuator (HVE) tips. A, Stainless steel evacuator tip. B, Plastic evacuator tip. *(From Boyd LRB: Dental instruments: a pocket guide, ed 6, St Louis, 2018, Elsevier.)*

## High-Volume Evacuator

The HVE is used to remove saliva, blood, water, and debris during a dental procedure. The HVE system, also known as the **oral evacuator,** works on a vacuum principle similar to that of a household vacuum cleaner. It is able to take up water and debris because of the high volume of air that is moved into the vacuum hose at low pressure to create the strong suction. The HVE has three main purposes:

- To keep the mouth free of saliva, blood, water, and debris
- To retract the tongue and cheek away from the field of operation
- To reduce the bacterial aerosol caused by the high-speed handpiece

### Suction Tips

Oral evacuation tips for the HVE system are designed to accommodate different types of procedures.

**Operative suction tips** are larger in circumference and designed with a straight or slight angle in the middle. Each opening has a beveled (having a surface angle that meets another angle) working end, so that the tip can be positioned parallel to the site for better suction. Most HVE tips are made of a durable plastic and are disposed of after a single use, or stainless steel, which must be sterilized before reuse (Fig. 36.3).

**Surgical suction tips** are smaller in circumference. The size is critical to placement within the surgical site, which typically is more limited in size and visibility. The concern in a surgical procedure is the removal of blood, tissue, and debris, rather than a large amount of water and fluid. Surgical tips are made of stainless steel and are part of the surgical setup (Fig. 36.4). Refer to Chapter 56 for further discussion.

### Grasping the Evacuator

The HVE may be held in the **thumb-to-nose grasp** or the **pen grasp** (Fig. 36.5). Either method provides the dental assistant with control of the tip, which is necessary for patient comfort and safety.

**FIG. 36.4** Stainless steel *(top)* and plastic *(bottom)* surgical evacuation tips. *(From Boyd LRB: Dental instruments: a pocket guide, ed 6, St Louis, 2018, Elsevier.)*

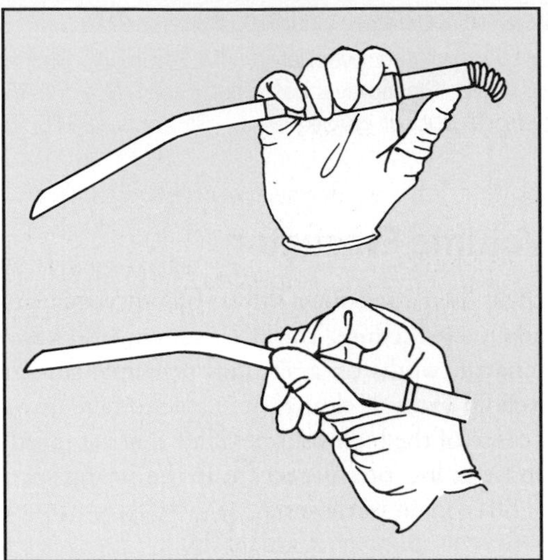

**FIG. 36.5** Grasps used for operating the high-volume evacuator (HVE). *Top,* Thumb-to-nose grasp. *Bottom,* Pen grasp.

## Positioning the Evacuator

Depending on the resistance of the tissue to be retracted and the area being treated, you may wish to alternate between the way of positioning the evacuator tip. When assisting a right-handed dentist, the assistant grasps the evacuator in the right hand. When assisting a left-handed dentist, the assistant grasps the evacuator in the left hand. The hand that is not holding the suction is free to operate the air-water syringe or to participate in the transfer of instruments to the dentist as needed. HVE positions discussed in this chapter are for use with a right-handed dentist.

As a dental assistant, you must understand your role in placing and operating the oral evacuation system. The timing of when suction is used, when the HVE is positioned, and when suction is removed from the mouth is critical to the efficient and effective performance of the procedure. Specific guidelines for positioning the HVE include the following:

- Place the evacuator before the dentist positions the handpiece and the mouth mirror.
- Position the suction tip on the surface of the operative tooth closest to you (Fig. 36.6).
- Position the bevel of the suction tip so that it is parallel to the tooth surface.
- Keep the edge of the suction tip even with or slightly beyond the occlusal surface or the incisal edge (Fig. 36.7).

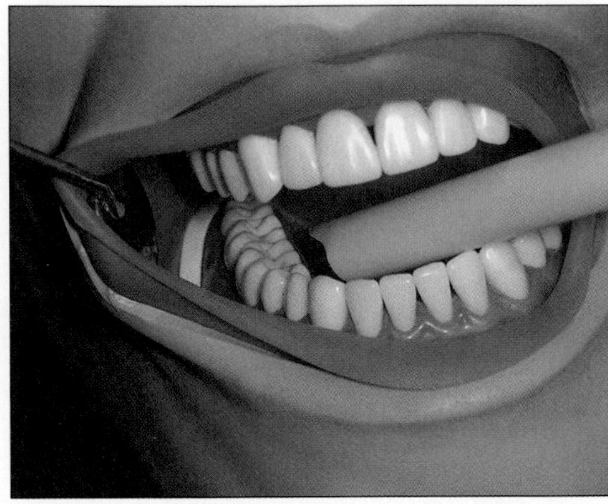

**FIG. 36.6** High-volume evacuator (HVE) tip positioned on a posterior tooth closest to you.

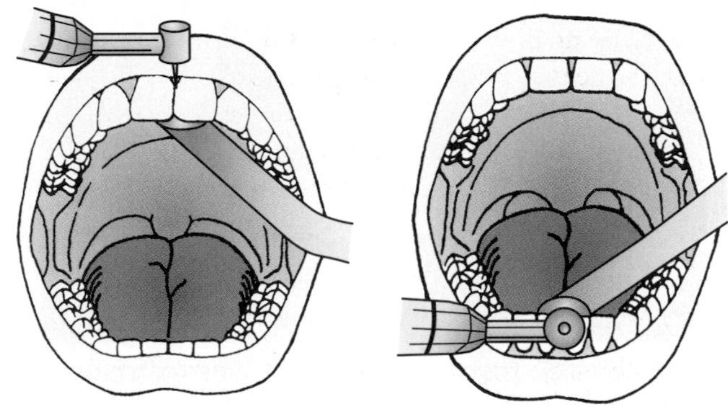

**FIG. 36.7** High-volume evacuator (HVE) tip positioned on anterior tooth opposite of handpiece placement. *(From Robinson D, Bird D: Essentials of dental assisting, ed 6, St Louis, 2017, Elsevier.)*

See Procedure 36.1: Positioning the High-Volume Evacuator During a Procedure.

## Daily Maintenance of the Evacuation System

As with any piece of equipment, the HVE must undergo daily upkeep to maintain proper working order. Specific maintenance guidelines for the evacuation systems and the air-water syringe include the following:

- Follow infection control policies when handling contaminated items.
- Flush the hoses at the end of the day with an antimicrobial solution.
- Check the disposable traps weekly, and replace if needed.
- Open the saliva ejector hoses, and clean or replace the screens as needed.

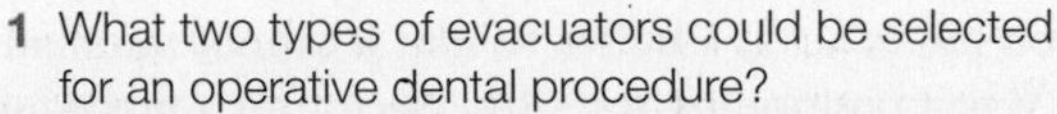

1. What two types of evacuators could be selected for an operative dental procedure?
2. What is the main function of the saliva ejector?
3. What are operative suction tips made from?

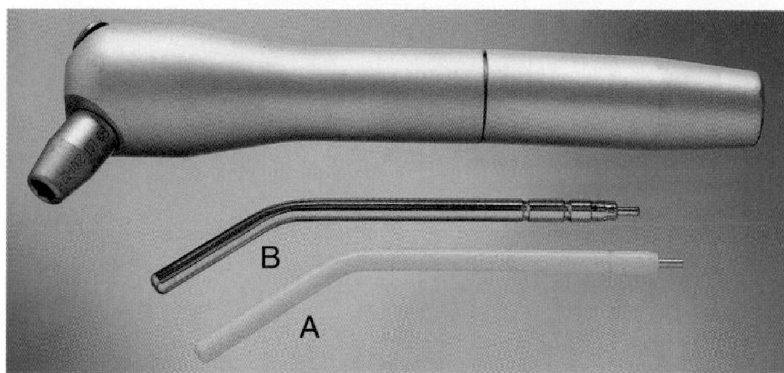


**FIG. 36.8** Air-water syringe with multiple tips. A, Disposable plastic syringe tip for single use. B, Metal syringe tip. *(From Boyd LRB: Dental instruments: a pocket guide, ed 6, St Louis, 2018, Elsevier.)*

## Rinsing the Oral Cavity

Frequent rinsing of the oral cavity maintains a clear operating field for the dentist and keeps the patient comfortable. Rinsing also removes debris from the patient's mouth before dismissal. The two basic types of rinsing procedures used in dentistry are limited-area rinsing and complete mouth rinsing, also referred to as a full-mouth rinse.

### Limited-Area Rinsing

This is performed frequently throughout a procedure as debris accumulates during the preparation and restoration of a tooth. This rinsing is accomplished quickly and efficiently, causing no delay in the procedure. Limited-area rinsing is frequently accomplished when the dentist exits the mouth and pauses for inspection.

### Full-Mouth Rinsing

The full-mouth rinse is used when the patient's entire mouth needs freshening. Complete mouth rinsing may be completed after a long restorative procedure, after dental prophylaxis, or before patient dismissal following any dental procedure.

The saliva ejector can be used as an alternative to the HVE in the complete mouth rinse procedure when the assistant performs this alone.

### Air-Water Syringe

To complete the rinsing process, the air-water syringe is used for convenience and accuracy. As described in Chapter 32, the air-water syringe is connected to the dental unit and provides air, water, or a combination through a small sterile tip. The attached disposable tip can be positioned for the maxillary and mandibular arches by directing the end toward the specific arch (Fig. 36.8). Guidelines for using the air-water syringe include the following:

- Direct the syringe tip toward the tooth that is being treated.
- Keep a close distance between the operative site and the syringe tip. Being too far away from the working site will cause aerosol to be splattered.
- Use the air on the mouth mirror continuously when indirect vision is involved.
- When you hear the handpiece stop, rinse and dry the site.
- When completing a limited-area or full-mouth rinse, move the tip while spraying the area.

See Procedure 36.2: Performing a Mouth Rinse.

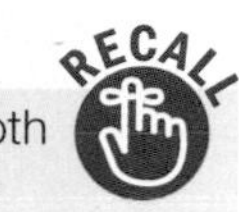


4 The dentist has just completed preparing the tooth for a restorative material. What type of rinsing technique is performed at this time?

## Isolation of Teeth

For optimum results in a dental procedure, a tooth, a quadrant, or even the entire arch must be kept dry and isolated from its normal environment. For ideal conditions during a dental procedure, the following features should characterize the isolation technique:

- Easy to apply
- Protective of soft and hard tissues
- Comfortable for the patient
- Retraction that provides better visualization for the operator
- Prevention of moisture contamination
- Isolation of the area of concern

Various techniques are used to isolate a specific area of the mouth. The three most common isolation methods are (1) cotton roll isolation, (2) dry angles, and (3) the dental dam. The clinical situation will dictate which isolation technique is best suited for the procedure.

### Cotton Roll Isolation

Cotton roll isolation is the use of tightly formed absorbent cotton that is preshaped to be positioned close to the salivary gland ducts to absorb the flow of saliva, and close to the working field to absorb excess water (Fig. 36.9). Cotton roll isolation is the most common type of isolation used for short procedures, such as examinations, application of sealants, cementation of castings, and simple restorations.

Advantages and disadvantages of using cotton rolls include the following:

Advantages
- Easy application.
- No additional equipment is required.
- Cotton rolls are available in a variety of sizes and are flexible for easy adaptability to areas of the mouth.

Disadvantages
- Does not provide complete isolation.
- Does not protect the patient from aspiration.
- If removed improperly, a dry cotton roll may stick to the oral mucosa and cause injury.

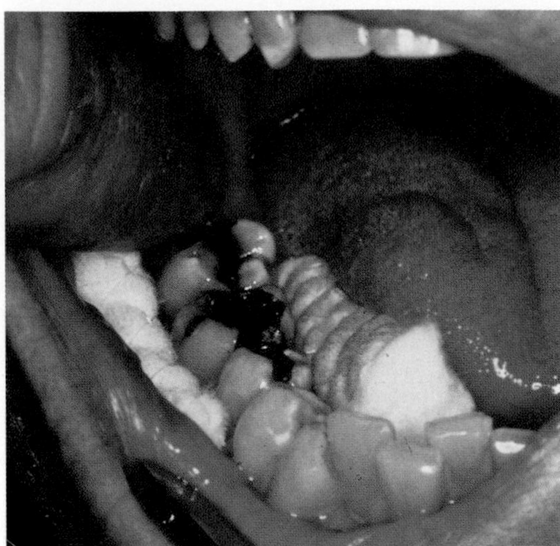

FIG. 36.9 Cotton roll isolation in the mandibular quadrant.

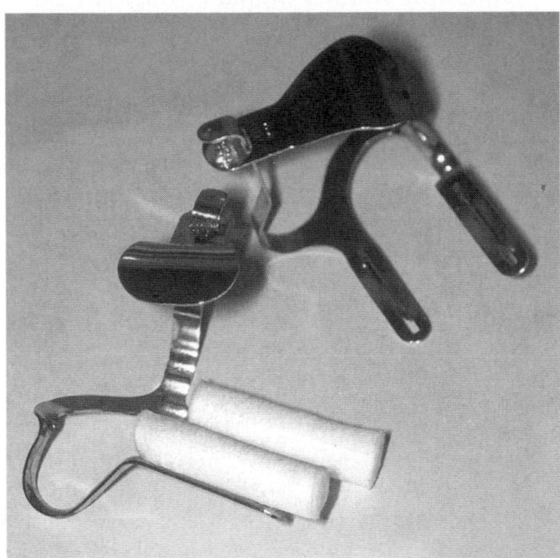

FIG. 36.10 Cotton roll holder.

- Cotton rolls must be replaced frequently because of saturation.
- Limited retraction.

See Procedure 36.3: Placing and Removing Cotton Rolls.

### Cotton Roll Holders

Cotton roll holders are designed to hold multiple cotton rolls in a more secure manner for the mandibular quadrant (Fig. 36.10). Holders are especially important when the operator is working alone, without an extra pair of hands to maintain isolation.

A metal or plastic prong is slid into each cotton roll. The rolls are then seated with one roll positioned on the buccal side and the other on the lingual side. A sliding bar is attached to the base of the holder. After it has been positioned under the chin, the bar is slid upward to secure the cotton roll holder in place.

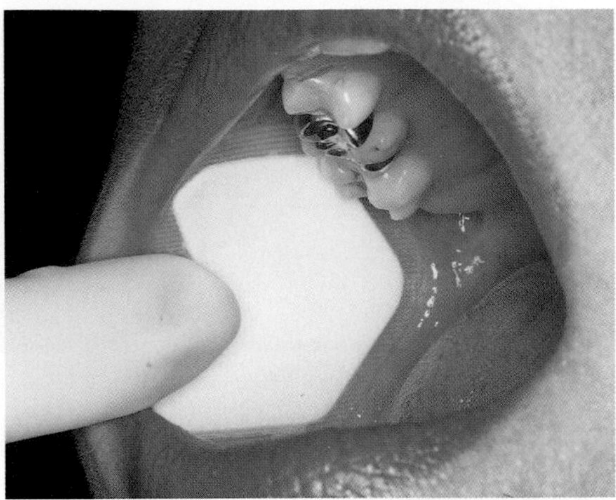

FIG. 36.11 Placement of dry angle in the buccal mucosa.

## Dry-Angle Isolation

An additional isolation technique involves the use of a triangular absorbent pad called the **dry angle.** This pad helps isolate posterior areas in the maxillary and mandibular arches. The pad is placed on the buccal mucosa over the Stensen's duct, which extends from the parotid gland and is located opposite the maxillary second molar (Fig. 36.11). These pads block the flow of saliva and protect the tissues in this area.

Follow the manufacturer's instructions for placement, and, if necessary, replace pads if they become soaked before the procedure has been completed. To remove, use water from the air-water syringe to wet the pad thoroughly before separating it from the tissues.

RECALL

5 Give three types of isolation methods often used in dentistry.
6 What type of isolation is frequently chosen for shorter procedures?
7 Why is it important to wet a cotton roll before removal from the mouth?

## The Dental Dam

The dental dam is a thin, stretchable material that becomes a barrier when it is appropriately applied to selected teeth. When the dam is in place, only selected teeth are visible through the dam. These teeth are described as being **isolated** or **exposed.**

The dental dam is routinely placed after the local anesthetic has been administered. An efficient dental team can place the dam in about 2 minutes. The expanded-functions dental assistant (EFDA) working alone can complete this procedure within 3 to 5 minutes.

Indications for dental dam use include the following:

- Serves as an important infection control barrier in the preparation of teeth
- Safeguards the patient's mouth against contact with debris, dental materials, or other liquids during treatment

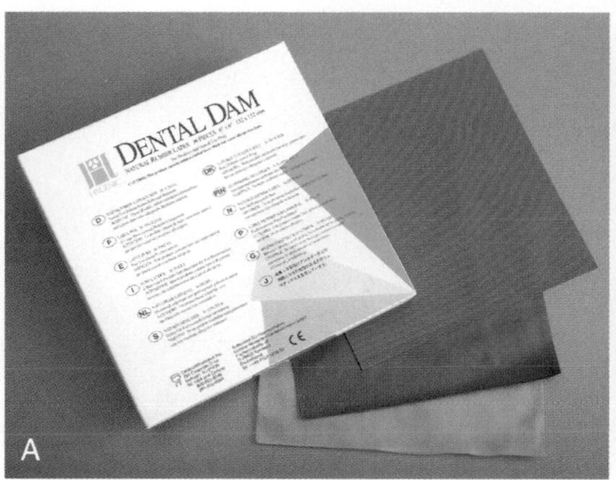


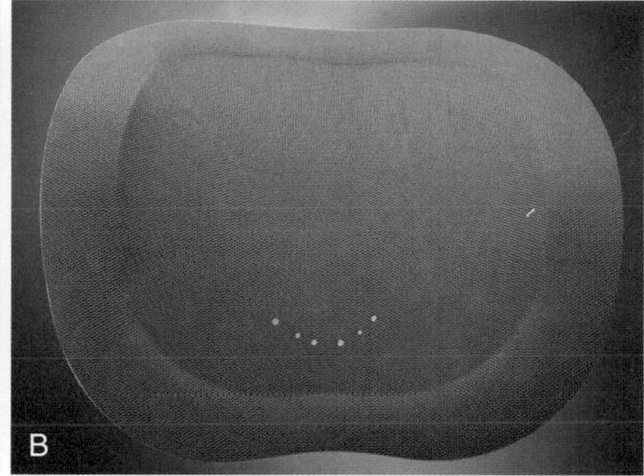


**FIG. 36.12** A, Dental dam material. B, Preframed dental dam. *(From Boyd LRB: Dental instruments: a pocket guide, ed 6, St Louis, 2018, Elsevier.)*

- Protects the patient from accidentally **aspirating** or swallowing debris, such as small fragments of a tooth or scraps of restorative material
- Protects the tooth from contamination by saliva or debris if pulpal exposure accidentally occurs
- Protects the oral cavity from exposure when an infected tooth is opened during endodontic treatment
- Provides the moisture control that is essential for the placement of restorative materials
- Improves access by retracting the lips, tongue, and gingiva from the field of operation
- Provides better visibility because of the contrasting colors of the dam and the tooth
- Increases dental team efficiency by discouraging patient conversation and reducing the time required for treatment

## Dental Dam Equipment

### Dental Dam Material

The dental dam is made from a latex rubber material or a silicone latex-free material (see Chapter 19 for specific information on latex allergies). The type of dental dam selected for each application is based on the operator's choice of size, color, and thickness (Fig. 36.12, *A*).

### Size

The dental dam is available in a continuous roll or in two precut sizes. The 6 × 6–inch size is used for applications on the posterior teeth in the permanent dentition. The 5 × 5–inch size is used for primary dentition or for anterior application on permanent dentition. The dam is also available as one disposable unit that combines the dam material and frame as one (Fig. 36.12, *B*).

### Color

The dental dam is available in a wide range of colors from light to dark, including green, blue, and pastels. Scented and flavored dams also are available. The brighter colors are widely used and have good patient acceptance, but some dentists prefer a darker color because it provides contrast to tooth structure and reduces glare.

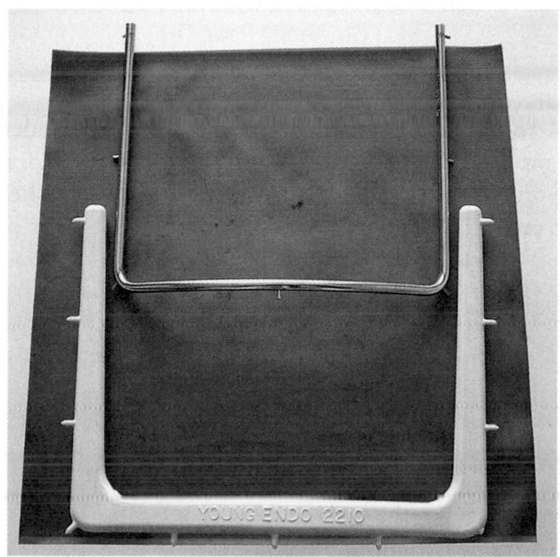


**FIG. 36.13** Dental dam frames. *(From Boyd LRB: Dental instruments: a pocket guide, ed 6, St Louis, 2018, Elsevier.)*

### Thickness

Dam thicknesses or gauges range from thin (light) to medium and heavy. *Thin* is most frequently used for endodontic applications. Because only one tooth is isolated, less stretch is required. *Medium* is widely used in operative procedures because of its ease of handling and ability to isolate selected teeth. *Heavy* is selected when tissue retraction and extra resistance to tearing are important. Examples of this include placement over a crown, fixed bridge, or teeth with tight contacts.

### Dental Dam Frame

A frame is necessary to stabilize and stretch the dam, so it fits tightly around the teeth and is out of the operator's way. Plastic and metal frames are available, and both can be sterilized for reuse (Fig. 36.13).

The **plastic U-shaped frame** is placed *under* the dam (next to the patient's face). Because this frame is *radiolucent* (does not block radiographs), it is not necessary to remove it when radiographs are required during treatment.

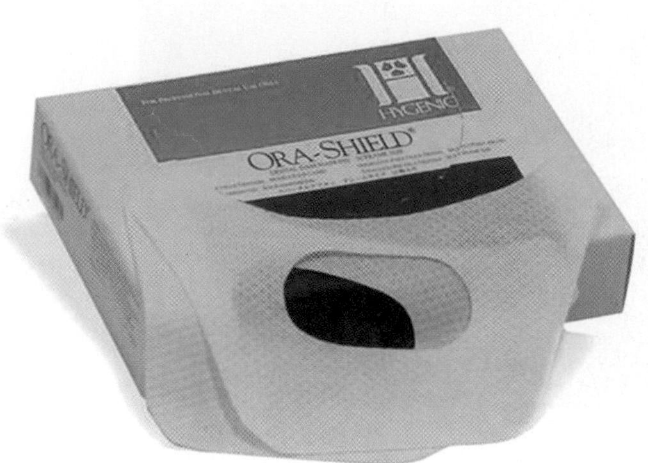


FIG. 36.14 Dental dam napkin. (Courtesy Coltène/Whaledent Inc., Cuyahoga Falls, OH.)

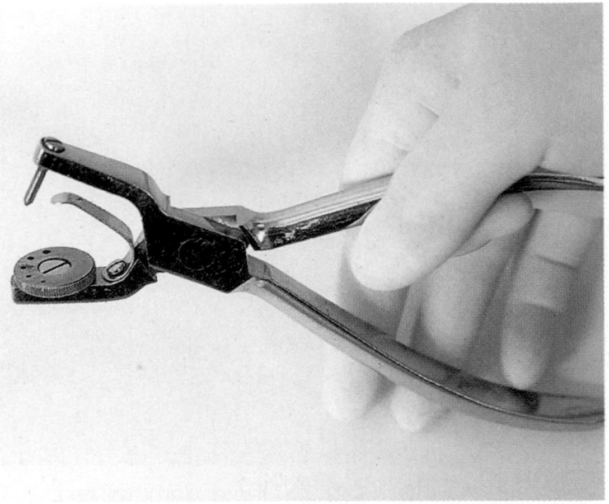

FIG. 36.15 Dental dam punch.

The **Young frame** is a stainless steel U-shaped holder with sharp projections on its outer margin. The Young frame is placed on the *outside* of the dam, and the dam is stretched over the projection of the frame. This approach increases patient comfort by holding the dam away from the patient's face.

The **Ostby frame** is a round plastic frame with sharp projections on its outer margin. It also is placed *outside* the dam, and the dam is stretched over the projections of the frame.

A newer version is the **preframed dam** which includes the dam and frame as one piece and is disposed of after its use.

## Dental Dam Napkin

The disposable dental dam napkin can be used and is placed between the patient's face and the dam. The primary purpose of the napkin is to increase patient comfort by absorbing moisture. The napkin also protects the patient's face from direct contact with the dam, reducing the risk that the patient may develop a latex sensitivity (Fig. 36.14).

## Lubricants

When the dam is placed, two types of lubricants may be selected. One lubricant is placed on the patient's lips to ensure patient comfort. Some operators use zinc oxide ointment for this purpose; others use petroleum jelly.

The second lubricant is *water soluble* and is placed on the *underside* of the dam to help the dam material slide over the teeth and through the interproximal spaces. Petroleum jelly should not be used for this purpose because it interferes with the setting of certain dental materials and breaks down the latex in the dam material.

## Dental Dam Punch

The dental dam punch is used to create holes in the dental dam needed to expose the teeth to be isolated (Fig. 36.15). The working end of the punch has an adjustable **stylus** (cutting tip) that makes the hole as it strikes an opening in the punch plate. The *punch plate* is a rotary platform with five or six holes of different sizes cut into the face of the plate. These holes are approximately 1 mm deep and have sharp edges to accommodate the stylus.

The position of the punch plate is rotated to produce holes of different sizes. When the punch plate is turned, a slight click may be heard as the plate falls into position. This click indicates that the stylus is positioned directly over the hole in the punch plate. The correct position of the stylus is checked by slowly lowering the stylus point over the hole in the punch plate. If the stylus is not placed properly, it may be dulled or broken.

In addition, the holes may not be punched cleanly. If the holes have ragged edges, they may tear easily as the dam is placed over the crown of the tooth. The holes also may irritate the gingiva and may allow leakage of moisture around the tooth.

**SIZE OF HOLES ON THE PUNCH PLATE.** The holes on the punch plate are graduated in size and are numbered from 1 to 5, with 1 being the smallest size. Each size has specific recommended uses. Fig. 36.16 provides recommended uses for each size of hole.

## Dental Dam Stamp and Template

The **dental dam stamp** and inkpad are used to mark the dental dam with predetermined markings for average adult and pediatric arches (Fig. 36.17).

The use of a **dental dam template,** which has holes where the teeth should be marked, provides greater flexibility when one or more teeth in the arch are out of alignment. The template is placed on the dental dam, and a pen is used to mark through the template to indicate the location of the punch holes.

## Dental Dam Forceps

Dental dam forceps are for the placement and removal of the dental dam clamp (Fig. 36.18). The beaks of the forceps fit into holes on the jaws of the clamp (Fig. 36.19).

The handles of the forceps work with a spring action. The beaks of the forceps are turned toward the arch that is being

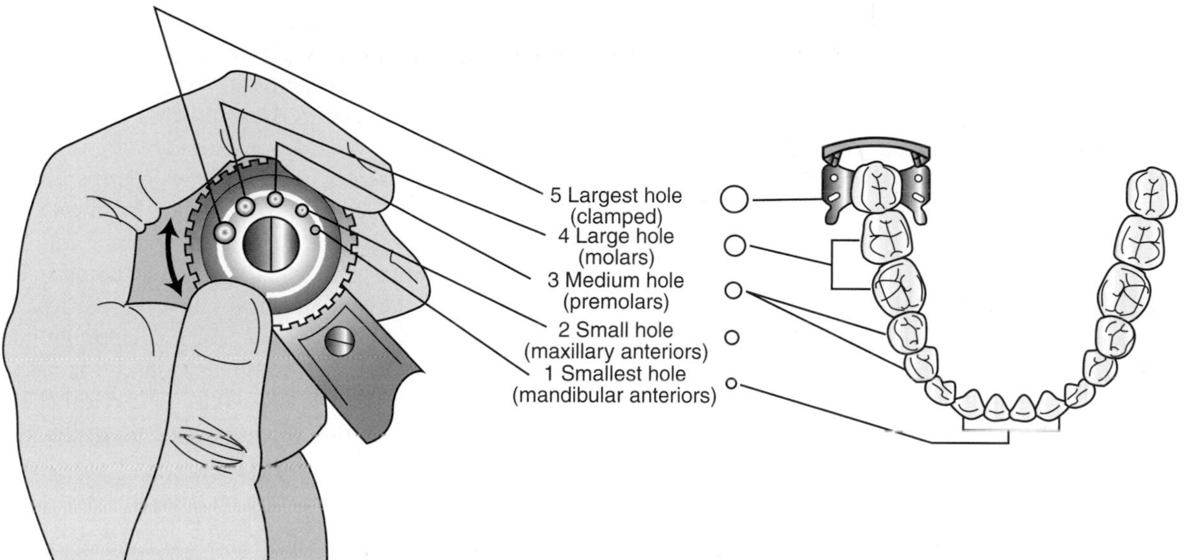


**FIG. 36.16** Sizes of holes for punching the dental dam and coordinating teeth with the sizes of punched holes. *(Adapted from Baum L, Phillips RW, Lund MR: Textbook of operative Dentistry, ed 3, Philadelphia, 1995, Saunders.)*

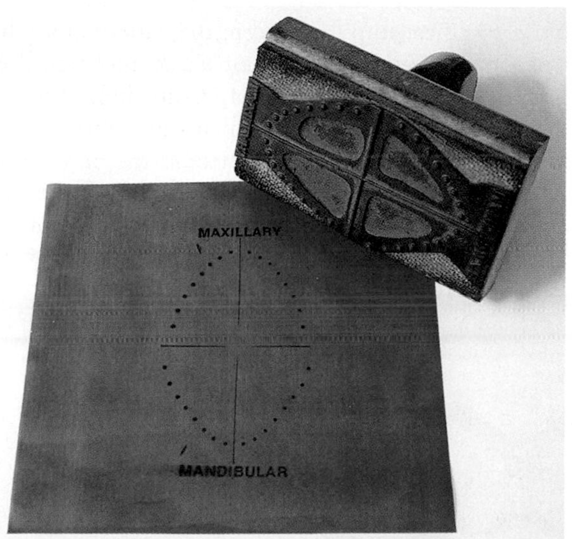


**FIG. 36.17** Dental dam stamp. *(From Boyd LRB: Dental instruments: a pocket guide, ed 6, St Louis, 2010, Elsevier.)*

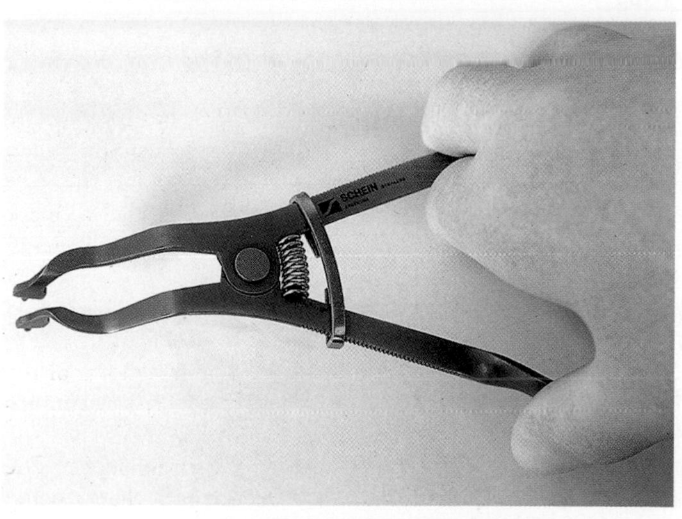


**FIG. 36.18** Dental dam forceps.

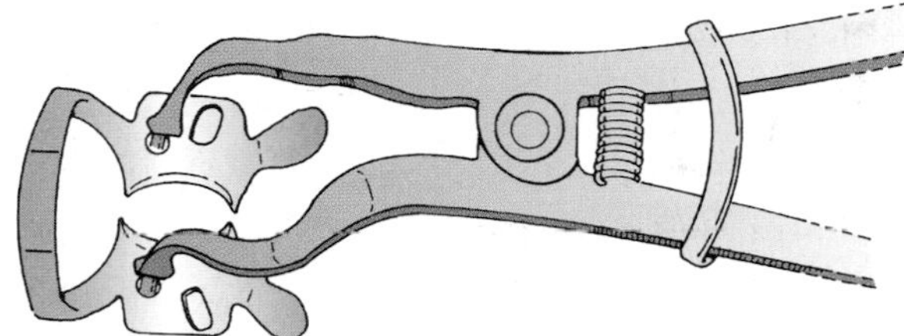

**FIG. 36.19** Positioning the beaks of the dental dam forceps into the clamp properly. *(From Baum L, Phillips RW, Lund MR: Textbook of operative dentistry, ed 3, Philadelphia, 1995, Saunders.)*

treated. A sliding bar keeps the handles of the forceps in a fixed position while the clamp is being held and positioned on the tooth. The handles are squeezed to release the clamp. This permits the operator to place or remove the clamp without having to rotate the forceps to put them into position.

### Dental Dam Clamps

The dental dam clamp is the primary means of anchoring and stabilizing the dental dam. Clamps are made of chrome or nickel-plated steel and are designed to hold the dental dam securely at the end nearest the tooth that is being treated. The opposite end of the dental dam application will also be stabilized, and this is accomplished with the use of either another clamp, a dental dam stabilizing cord, or dental floss or tape. This technique is known as **ligating** the dam.

**PARTS OF THE DENTAL DAM CLAMP.** Parts of the clamp that are important to identify are the bow and the jaws (Fig. 36.20). The **bow** is the rounded portion of the clamp that extends through the dental dam. The clamp is always positioned on the tooth so that the bow is located at the distal aspect.

The **jaws** encircle the tooth and are shaped into four prongs. All four prongs must be firmly seated on the tooth to create the facial-to-lingual balance necessary to stabilize the clamp. A hole is located on each side of the jaw of the clamp. The beaks of the dental dam forceps fit into these holes to allow placement and removal of the clamp.

A **winged clamp** "W" is designed with extra extensions to help retain the dental dam. *Wingless* clamps have numbers/letters that begin with the letter W and do not have extra projections to engage the clamp.

**FITTING THE DENTAL DAM CLAMP.** Dental dam clamps are available in many sizes and designs to accommodate different needs (Fig. 36.21). The jaws of the clamps are designed to fit the *cervical area* of the tooth below the height of contour and at, or slightly below, the cementoenamel junction. The *height of contour* is the widest point on the facial and lingual contours of the tooth.

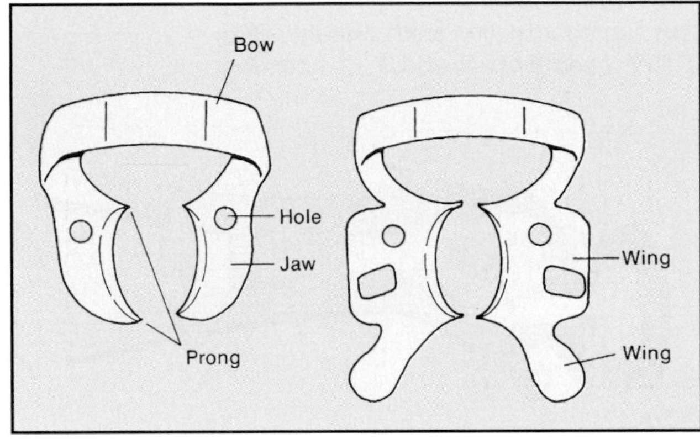


**FIG. 36.20** Parts of the dental dam clamp.

The clamp must be positioned with all four prongs firmly in place on the tooth *before* the clamp forceps are loosened. If the clamp is not placed properly, it may spring off the tooth, possibly injuring the patient, the dentist, or the assistant.

*Posterior dental dam clamps* are used for the maxillary and mandibular posterior teeth. These clamps are **universal**, meaning that the same clamp can be placed on the same type of tooth in the opposite quadrant. Clamps 7 and W7 are universal mandibular molar clamps, and clamps 8 and W8 are universal maxillary molar clamps.

*Anterior dental dam clamps,* such as clamps 9 and W9, are designed to (1) retract the gingiva on the facial surface, (2) improve visibility for the restoration of cervical class V cavities, and (3) permit isolation of an anterior tooth during endodontic treatment.

*Pediatric dental dam clamps* for primary teeth are designed to accommodate the smaller size and shape of the primary teeth or partially erupted permanent teeth. Clamps for primary teeth are available in sizes 00, W00, and 2.

**LIGATURES ON CLAMPS.** Dental floss or dental tape should *always* be attached to the bow of the dental dam clamp as a ligature *before* the clamp is placed in the patient's mouth. *This is an important safety step that must not be omitted.* The ligature makes it possible to retrieve a clamp should it accidentally become dislodged and then inhaled or swallowed by the patient (Fig. 36.22).

The ends of this ligature are always kept out of the patient's mouth on the outside of the dental dam material and within easy reach. During treatment, the ligature may be attached to the dam frame to keep it available yet out of the operator's way.

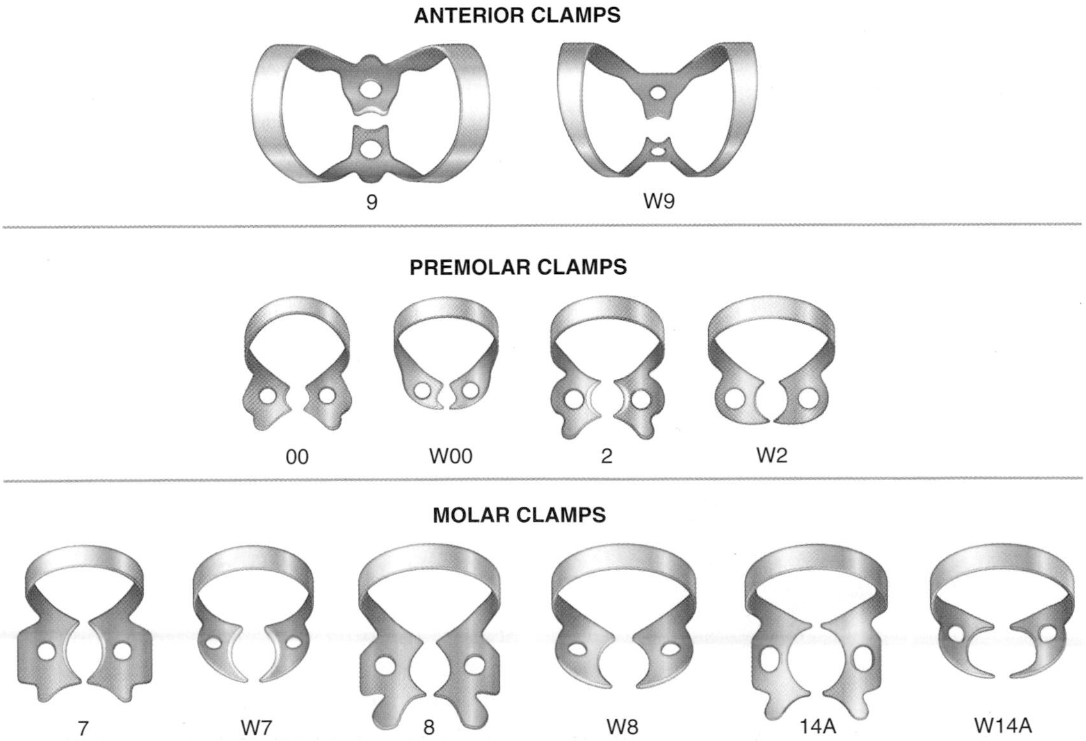

ANTERIOR CLAMPS

9 W9

PREMOLAR CLAMPS

00 W00 2 W2

MOLAR CLAMPS

7 W7 8 W8 14A W14A

**FIG. 36.21** Types of dental dam clamps. (© Elsevier Collection.)

### Dental Dam Stabilizing Cord

The dental dam stabilizing cord, also referred to as a *wedjet,* is a disposable latex cord that provides an alternative to the conventional clamp method of securing the dental dam. The cord is available in three sizes: extra small, small, and large.

During insertion, the cord is stretched so that it becomes narrow and slips easily between the teeth. Once placed and released, the cord resumes its original shape and holds the dam tightly in place. The *size* of the cord selected depends on the amount of contact space available. The *length* of the cord depends on the application.

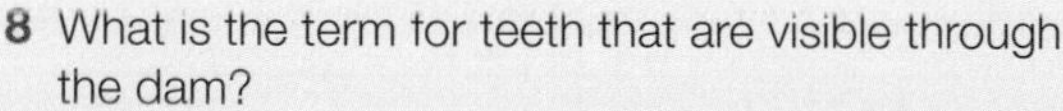
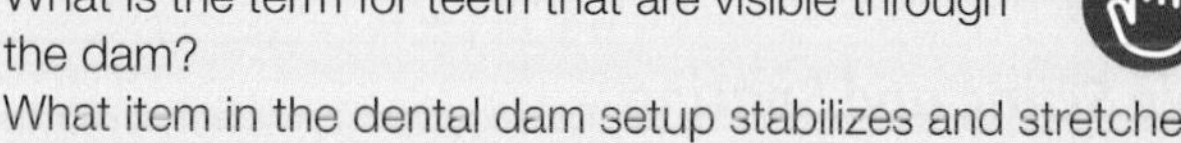

RECALL

**8** What is the term for teeth that are visible through the dam?

**9** What item in the dental dam setup stabilizes and stretches the dam away from the tooth?

**10** If you are unable to slide the dam interproximally, what could be placed on the underside of the dam to help in the application?

## Dental Dam Preparation

Each application of the dam is preplanned to accommodate the dentist's preferences, the tooth or teeth involved, and the procedure to be performed. The following factors must be included in the planning for holes to be punched in the dental dam:

- Maxillary or mandibular arch
- Shape of the arch
- Any irregularities, such as missing teeth, a fixed prosthesis, or malpositioned teeth
- Teeth to be isolated
- Identification of the anchor tooth and location of the key-punch hole
- Size and spacing of the other holes to be punched

The **anchor tooth** holds the dental dam clamp, and the *key-punch hole* covers the anchor tooth.

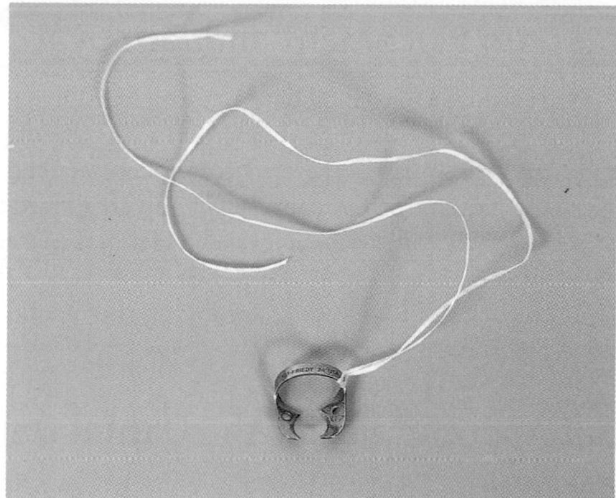

**FIG. 36.22** Ligature placed on the bow of the clamp for protective reasons.

### Maxillary Arch Application

In preparation for maxillary application, the dam material is stamped or marked, and the holes are punched. Because the holes for the maxillary anterior teeth are punched 1 inch down from the upper edge of the dam, it is helpful to stamp or mark the extension in back of the punch plate of the dental dam punch to indicate 1 inch (Fig. 36.23). This mark automatically designates the margin of the dam for these holes. If the patient has a mustache or a very thick upper lip, it is necessary to allow slightly more than a 1-inch margin from the edge.

### Mandibular Arch Application

In preparation for a mandibular application, the dam is stamped or marked, and the holes are punched, leaving a 2-inch margin from the edge (Fig. 36.24). Because of the small size of the mandibular teeth, the holes are punched closer together than for posterior teeth. Extra care should be taken when punching

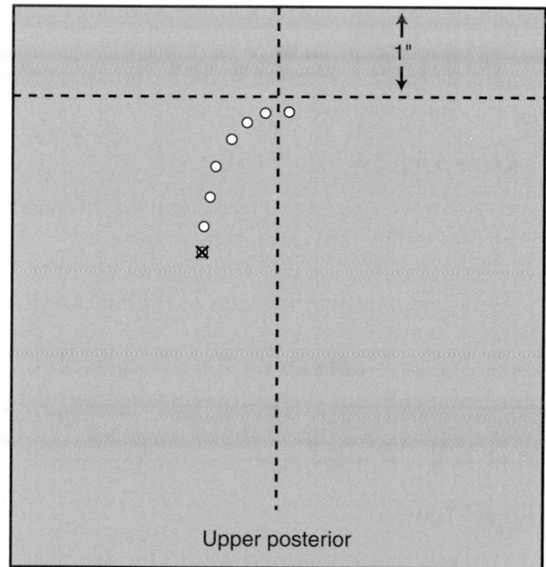


**FIG. 36.23** Punching the dam for a maxillary application.

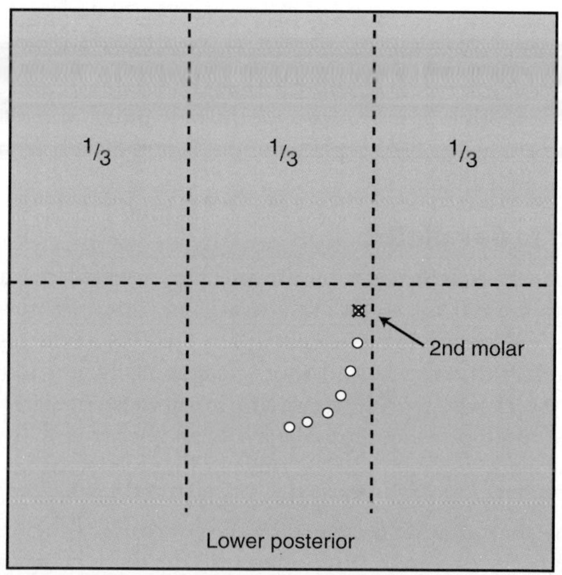


**FIG. 36.24** Punching the dam for a mandibular application.

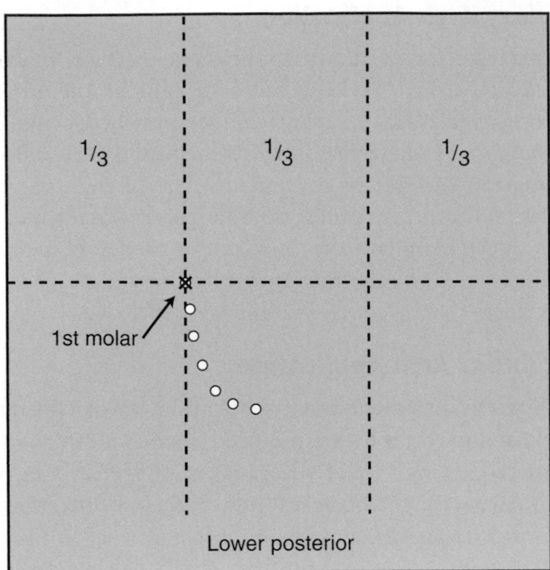


**FIG. 36.25** Punching the dam for a malaligned tooth.

holes for anterior teeth. Use a water-soluble lubricant if crowding or tight contacts are noted in this area.

### Curve of the Arch

It may be necessary to make adjustments to punching the dam to accommodate an extremely narrow or wide arch. Failure to accommodate for this will increase the difficulty of complete isolation, causing inversion of the edges of the holes in the dam.

Bunching and stretching on the lingual aspect of the dental dam occur if the curve of the arch is punched too flat or too wide. *Folding* and stretching of the dam on the facial aspect occurs if the arch is punched too curved or too narrow.

### Malaligned Teeth

If a tooth or teeth are **malaligned** within the dental arch, special consideration of their position is needed *before* the dental dam is punched.

If the tooth is *lingually malposed,* the hole-punch size remains the same, but the hole is placed about 1 mm lingually from the normal arch alignment (Fig. 36.25).

If the tooth is *facially malposed,* the hole-punch size remains the same, but the hole is placed about 1 mm facially from the normal arch alignment.

### Teeth to Be Isolated

*Single-tooth isolation* is typically used for selected restorative procedures and for endodontic treatment. Some dentists isolate only the tooth to be treated; others prefer to have two teeth isolated so that the second tooth acts as an anchor tooth to hold the clamp. During treatment in the posterior area, this second tooth provides greater stability and better visibility.

For *multiple-tooth isolation,* three or four teeth—or for optimum stability, six to eight teeth—are isolated to counteract the pull on the dam that is created by the curvature of the teeth in the arch. At least one tooth posterior to the tooth being treated should be isolated.

When maxillary anterior teeth are to be isolated, maximum stability is achieved by isolating the six anterior teeth (canine to canine).

### Keypunch Hole

As mentioned, the anchor tooth holds the dental dam clamp, and the keypunch hole is punched in the dental dam to cover the anchor tooth. The largest hole (#5) is necessary for the keypunch because it also must accommodate the clamp.

Selection of the anchor tooth and location of the keypunch hole are important considerations in the application of the dental dam. For maximum stability and ease of access, the keypunch hole is placed one or two teeth distal to the tooth that is receiving treatment.

### Hole Sizing and Spacing

The size of each hole selected on the dental dam punch must be appropriate for the tooth to be isolated. A correctly sized hole allows the dam to slip easily over the tooth and fit snugly in the cervical area. This is important to prevent leakage around the dam.

In general, the holes are spaced with 3.0 to 3.5 mm between the edges, not the centers, of the holes. This allows adequate spacing between the holes to create a septum that can slip between the teeth without tearing or injuring the gingiva.

The **septum** is the dental dam material between the holes of the punched dam. During application, this portion of the dam is passed between the contacts.

**TROUBLESHOOTING HOLE SIZING AND SPACING.** If the holes are *too large,* the dam will not fit tightly around the tooth. This may allow saliva to leak through the hole.

If the holes are *too small,* the dam will not slip easily over the tooth. This may cause the dam to stretch or tear and may leave the gingiva exposed.

If the holes are *too close,* the dam may tear or stretch. The stretched holes may leave the gingiva exposed and may cause leakage.

If the holes are *too far apart,* excess material is present between the teeth. This may block the dentist's vision or catch in instrumentation.

## Dental Dam Placement and Removal

Two methods are used for dental dam placement. The main difference between the two is the sequencing in placement of the clamp and the dental dam. The remaining steps are the same In the *one-step method,* the dam and the clamp are placed at the same time. In the *two-step method,* first the clamp is placed and then the dental dam material is stretched over it. See Procedure 36.4: Preparing, Placing, and Removing the Dental Dam (Expanded Function).

## Special Applications for the Dental Dam

### Anterior Teeth

When the dam is applied to the anterior teeth, the isolation and application procedures change. The isolation of anterior

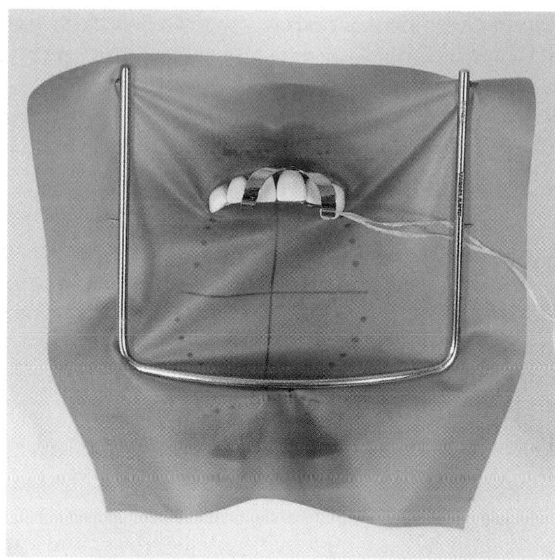

**FIG. 36.26** Maxillary anterior dam application.

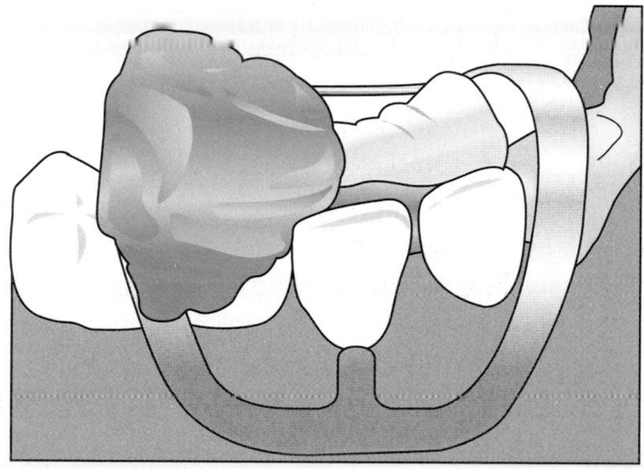

**FIG. 36.27** Compound wax used to stabilize anterior clamp. *(Adapted from Baum L, Phillips RW, Lund MR: Textbook of operative dentistry, ed 3, Philadelphia, 1995, Saunders.)*

teeth occurs typically from canine to canine. When the isolation is complete, a dental dam clamp is not required. The dental dam will remain secure with placement of dental tape or with stretching of a small corner of the dental dam interproximally between the canine and the first premolar on each side.

A cervical or anterior clamp, as seen in Fig. 36.26, may be required if the gingival third of a tooth is to be restored and if the gingival tissue must be retracted for better exposure. The jaws of this type of clamp are positioned lightly on the cementum of the root, just below the carious lesion.

**STABILIZING THE CERVICAL CLAMP.** Occasionally, additional stabilization of the cervical clamp is necessary. Softened stick compound may be used for this purpose (Fig. 36.27). A heat source such as a butane torch or a Bunsen burner is needed; the steps involved in stabilization are as follows:

- Soften the red or green stick compound by holding it over a flame until the tip bends. Then place the tip in hot water for 5 seconds.
- Twist off approximately 1 inch of the tip, and shape it into a cone.
- Very carefully reheat the cone of the compound in the flame. Then place the softened compound under the bow of the clamp (occlusal surface), away from the area to be treated.
- Repeat this procedure for the second bow on the opposite side of the clamp.
- On completion of treatment, remove the compound before you remove the dam and the clamp.

### Fixed Bridge

A fixed bridge is a prosthetic device that is cemented in place to replace one or more adjacent missing teeth. Because the units of the bridge are joined together, it is not possible to place the dental dam septum between each tooth. For this reason, placement of a dental dam on fixed bridgework requires a specialized technique.

When you are punching the dental dam, punch a hole for each fully crowned tooth, but do *not* punch holes for the teeth that are replacing missing teeth. A clamp is placed on the distal aspect of the bridge, and in some situations, a second clamp is placed on the mesial portion. The remainder of the application and the removal are performed as usual.

RECALL

**11** The hole sizes on the dental dam punch range from 1 to 5. Which is the smallest size?

**12** For what purpose would you use an anterior dental dam clamp?

**■ Patient Education** Patients are not aware of the amount of saliva, water, and debris that accumulates in the mouth during a procedure. It is your responsibility to inform and educate patients about the importance of keeping their mouth open, refraining from talking, and remaining still during a procedure. If moisture penetrates an exposed tooth, or if dental material is exposed to moisture, the operative site has been contaminated. The dental team must then repeat certain steps in the procedure, which causes lost time for the office and patient.

Many patients have never had a dental dam placed, or when they did, they found it very confining and uncomfortable. As the EFDA/RDA, your role is to become competent in educating the patient about the importance of the dental dam. As an EFDA/RDA, master the skills involved in placement to provide complete isolation of a tooth or teeth while ensuring comfort for the patient. ■

**■ Legal and Ethical Implications** If your patient begins coughing during a procedure and suddenly swallows a crown, or a bur from the handpiece, you will then understand the importance of using a dental dam. The dental dam provides much more than moisture control for the patient and the dental team. By using the dental dam, you are protecting the health of the patient, as well as the tooth or teeth being treated.

If you are practicing in a state where placement and removal of the dental dam are *expanded functions,* follow all guidelines for proper placement; these include attaching a ligature to the clamp for safe and quick removal. ■

**■ Eye to the Future** Your dental office may take moisture control one step further, by having patients use an oral antiseptic before undergoing any dental treatment. Therapeutic antiseptics are prescribed daily for patients with susceptibility to infection or disease. Phenol, chlorhexidine, and *Sanguinaria* products can be used as a mouthwash before a procedure, reducing bacterial concentration and thus risk of disease for the patient and the dental team. ■

## ■ Critical Thinking

1. You are an EFDA/RDA, and the dentist has requested that you place sealants on teeth #19 and 30. What isolation technique could you use for this procedure, and why?
2. The dentist is preparing tooth #4 for a disto-occlusal amalgam. Where will you place the HVE tip during this procedure?
3. The dentist is halfway through preparing tooth #4 and pulls the handpiece out of the mouth to examine the extent of the remaining decay with the mirror and explorer. What would you do at this moment?
4. You will be assisting today in a composite procedure on tooth #24. How will you punch the dental dam for this procedure?
5. What hole sizes would be punched for the isolation of teeth #18 through #22, with the anchor tooth being #18? ■

PROCEDURE 36.1 

# Positioning the High-Volume Evacuator During a Procedure

### EQUIPMENT AND SUPPLIES

- Sterile high-volume evacuator (HVE) tip
- Plastic barrier cover for HVE handle and hose
- Cotton rolls

### PROCEDURAL STEPS

1 Place the HVE tip in the holder by pushing the end of the tip into the holder through the plastic barrier.
**PURPOSE** Leaves the opposite end exposed and ready for use.

2 If necessary, use the HVE tip or a mouth mirror to gently retract the cheek or tongue.

### Posterior Placement

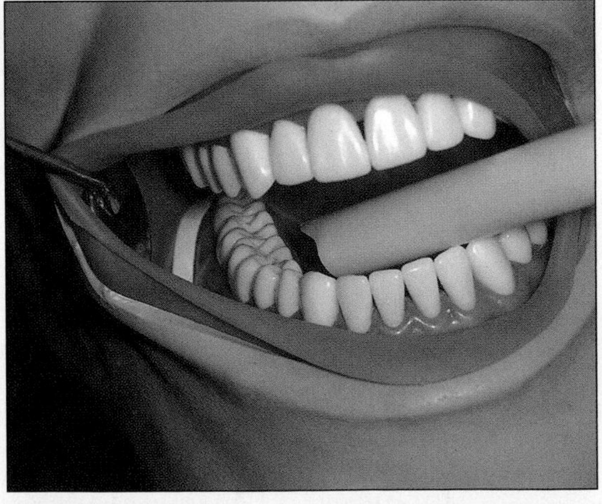

1 For a mandibular site, place a cotton roll under the suction tip.
**PURPOSE** Provides patient comfort, aids in stabilizing tip placement, and prevents injury to the tissues.

2 Place the bevel of the HVE tip as close as possible to the tooth that is being prepared.
**PURPOSE** Suction will draw the water into the tip immediately after it leaves the tooth that is being prepared.

3 Position the bevel of the HVE tip parallel to the buccal or lingual surface of the tooth that is being prepared.

4 Place the upper edge of the HVE tip so that it extends slightly beyond the occlusal surface.
**PURPOSE** Suction will catch the water spray from the handpiece as it leaves the tooth that is being prepared.

### Anterior Placement

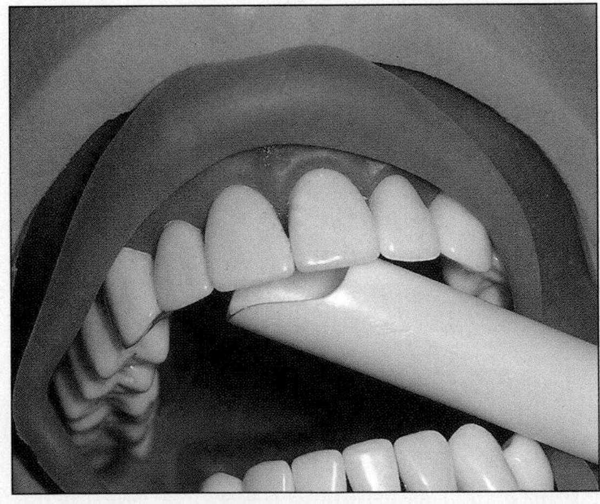

1 When the dentist is preparing the tooth from the *lingual* aspect, position the HVE tip so that it is parallel to the facial surface and extends slightly beyond the incisal edge.

2 When the dentist is preparing the tooth from the *facial* aspect, position the HVE tip so that it is parallel to the lingual surface and extends slightly beyond the incisal edge.

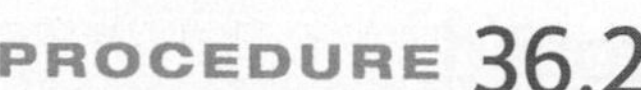

PROCEDURE 36.2

## Performing a Mouth Rinse

### EQUIPMENT AND SUPPLIES

- ✓ High-volume evacuator (HVE) tip
- ✓ Saliva ejector
- ✓ Air-water syringe

### PROCEDURAL STEPS

1 Decide which oral evacuation system would be best for use in the rinsing procedure.

2 Grasp the air-water syringe in your left hand and the HVE or saliva ejector in your right hand.

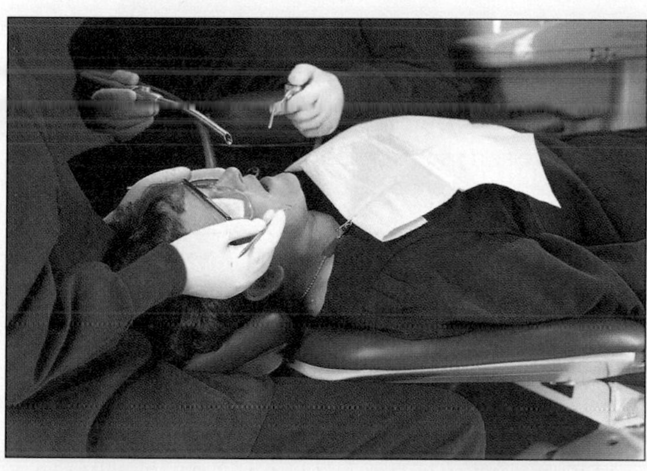

### Limited-Area Mouth Rinse

1 Turn on the suction, and position the tip toward the site for a limited-area rinse.

2 Spray the combination of air and water onto the site to be rinsed.
**PURPOSE** The combination of air and water provides greater force to clean the area thoroughly.

3 Suction all fluid and debris from the area, making sure to remove all fluids.

4 Dry the area by pressing the air button only.

### Full-Mouth Rinse

1 Have the patient turn toward you.
**PURPOSE** Turning the head allows the water to pool on one side, making it easier for you to suction.

2 Turn on the HVE or saliva ejector, and position it in the vestibule of the patient's left side.
**NOTE** Position the tip carefully so that it does not come into contact with soft tissue.

3 With the HVE or saliva ejector tip positioned, direct the air-water syringe from the patient's maxillary right across to the left side, spraying all surfaces.

4 Continue down to the mandibular arch, following the same sequence from right to left.
**PURPOSE** This pattern of rinsing forces the debris to the posterior mouth, where the suction tip is positioned, for easier removal of fluids and debris.

PROCEDURE 36.3

## Placing and Removing Cotton Rolls

### EQUIPMENT AND SUPPLIES

- ✓ Basic setup
- ✓ Cotton rolls
- ✓ Air-water syringe

### PROCEDURAL STEPS

### Maxillary Placement

1 Have the patient turn toward you with the chin raised.
**PURPOSE** Provides better visualization and easier placement of cotton roll.

2 Using the cotton pliers, pick up a cotton roll so that it is positioned evenly with the beaks of the cotton pliers.

3 Transfer the cotton roll to the mouth, and position it securely in the mucobuccal fold closest to the working field.
**NOTE** Once you place the cotton roll with the pliers, you may wish to use your finger to push the cotton roll farther into the mucobuccal fold.

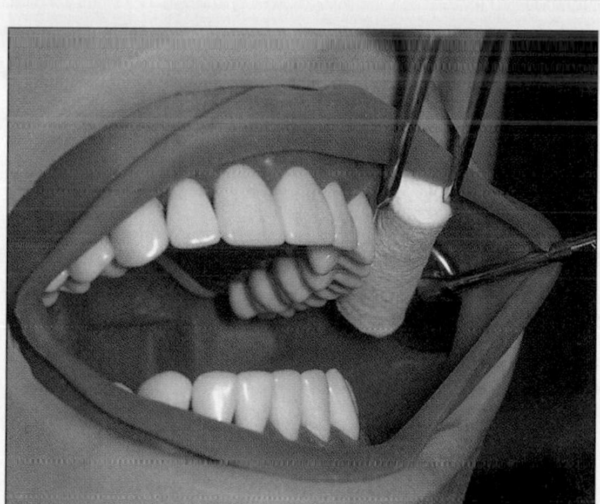

(Continued)

## PROCEDURE 36.3 Placing and Removing Cotton Rolls—cont'd.

4 This placement can be used for any location on the maxillary arch.

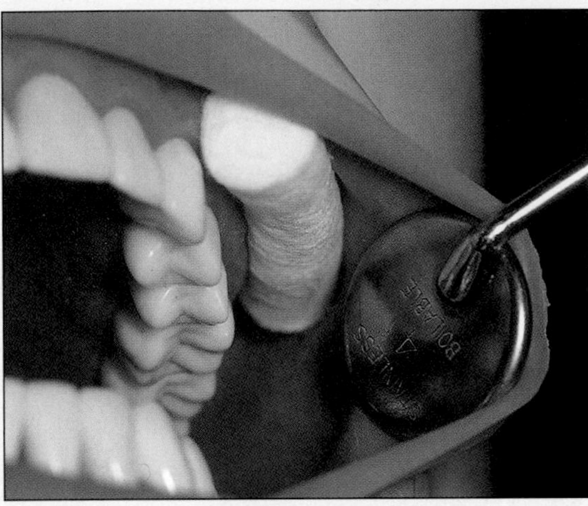

### Mandibular Placement

1 Have the patient turn toward you with the chin lowered.
**PURPOSE** Provides better visualization and facilitates placement of the cotton roll.

2 Using the cotton pliers, pick up a cotton roll so that it is positioned even with the beaks of the pliers.

3 Transfer the cotton roll to the mouth, and position it securely in the mucobuccal fold closest to the working field.

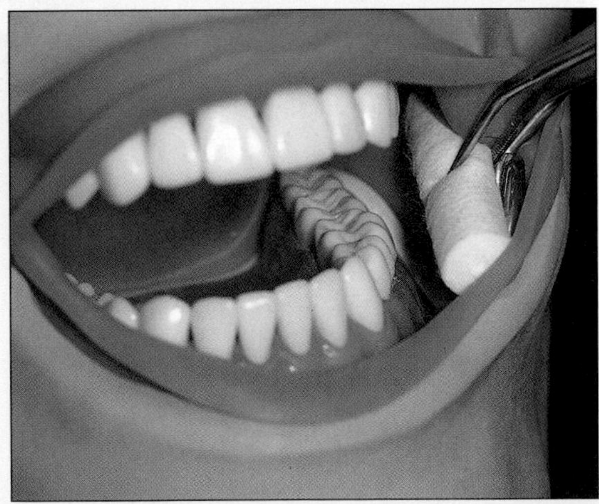

4 Carry the second cotton roll to the mouth, and position it in the floor of the mouth between the working field and the tongue.
**NOTE** Have the patient lift the tongue during placement and then relax, to help secure the cotton roll in position.

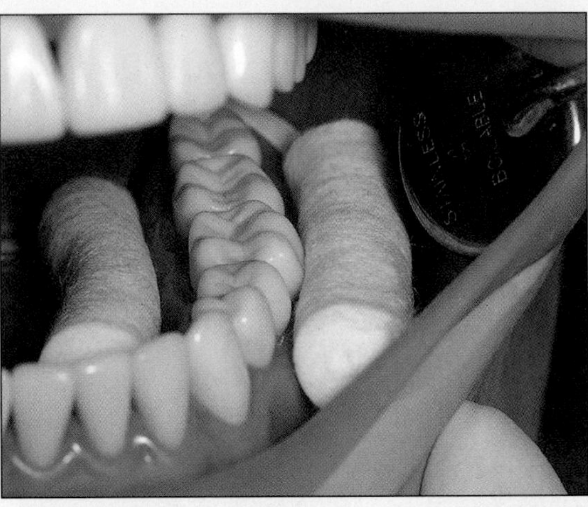

5 If you are placing cotton rolls for the mandibular anterior region, bend the cotton roll before placement for better fit.

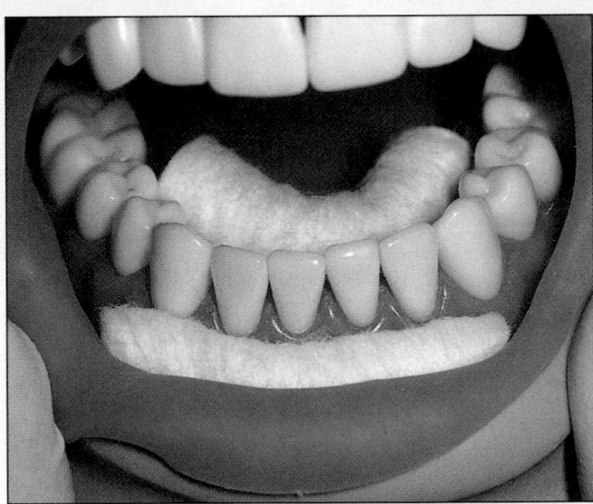

6 If you are using a saliva ejector for the procedure, place it after the cotton roll is in position in the lingual vestibule.

### Cotton Roll Removal

1 At the completion of a procedure, remove the cotton roll before the full-mouth rinse. If the cotton roll is dry, moisten it with water from the air-water syringe.
**PURPOSE** Dry cotton rolls will adhere to the oral mucosal lining, and tissues may be damaged when a dry cotton roll is pulled away from the area.

2 Using cotton pliers, retrieve the contaminated cotton roll from the site.

3 If appropriate for the procedure, perform a limited rinse.

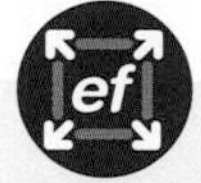

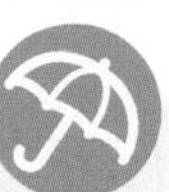

**PROCEDURE 36.4**

# Preparing, Placing, and Removing the Dental Dam (Expanded Function)

**PREREQUISITES FOR THE EXPANDED-FUNCTIONS DENTAL ASSISTANT (EFDA) WHEN PERFORMING THIS FUNCTION**

- ✔ Mirror skills
- ✔ Operator positioning
- ✔ Dental anatomy
- ✔ Instrumentation

**EQUIPMENT AND SUPPLIES**

- ✔ Basic setup
- ✔ Precut 6 × 6–inch dental dam
- ✔ Dental dam stamp and inkpad *or* template and pen
- ✔ Dental dam punch
- ✔ Dental dam clamp or clamps with ligature attached
- ✔ Dental dam clamp forceps
- ✔ Young frame
- ✔ Dental dam napkin
- ✔ Dental tape or waxed floss
- ✔ Cotton rolls
- ✔ Lubricant for patient's lips
- ✔ Lubricant for dam
- ✔ Black spoon
- ✔ Crown and bridge scissors

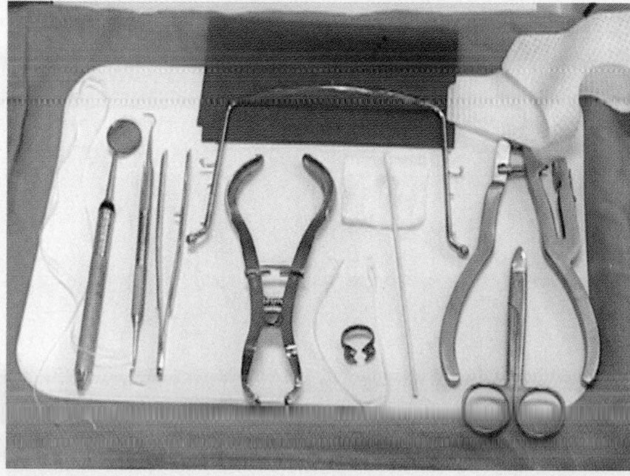

**PROCEDURAL STEPS**

## Patient Preparation

1 Check the patient's record for contraindications, and identify the area to be isolated. Inform the patient of the need to place a dental dam, and explain the steps involved.

2 Assist the dentist in the administration of local anesthetic. The dentist will determine which teeth are to be isolated and will note whether any malposed teeth must be accommodated.

3 Apply lubricating ointment to the patient's lip with a cotton roll or a cotton-tip applicator.

**NOTE** The patient's comfort is a matter of concern throughout placement and removal of the dental dam.

4 Place yourself in the operator's position, and adjust your patient for easier access.

5 Use the mouth mirror and the explorer to examine the site where the dam is to be placed. It should be free of plaque and debris.

**PURPOSE** If the dam is placed in an area with plaque and debris, the dam could push the plaque and debris into the sulcus and irritate the gingival tissues.

**NOTE** If debris or plaque is present, selective coronal polishing is performed on these teeth before the dental dam is applied.

6 Floss all contacts involved in placement of the dental dam.

**PURPOSE** Any tight contacts may tear the dam.

## Punching the Dental Dam

7 Use a template or stamp to mark on the dam the teeth to be isolated.

8 Correctly punch the marked dam according to the teeth to be isolated. Be sure to use the correct size of punch hole for the specific tooth.

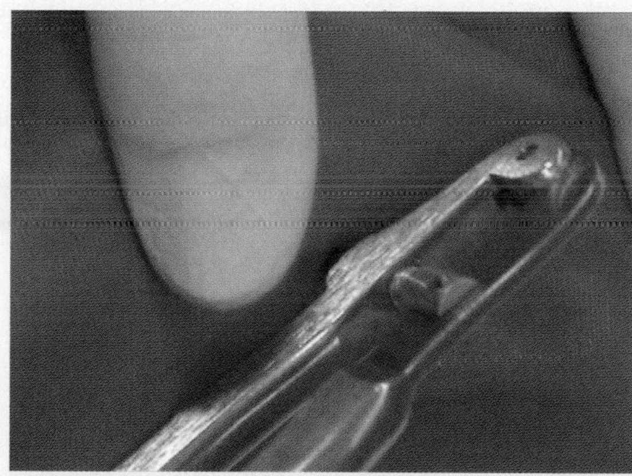

9 If teeth have tight contacts, lightly lubricate the holes on the tooth surface (undersurface) of the dam.

**PURPOSE** This eases placement of the dam over the contact area of the teeth.

## Placing the Clamp and the Frame

10 Select the correct size of clamp.

**NOTE** The W7 clamp has been selected for this procedure.

11 Secure the clamp by tying a ligature of dental tape on the bow of the clamp.

(Continued)

## PROCEDURE 36.4 Preparing, Placing, and Removing the Dental Dam (Expanded Function)–cont'd

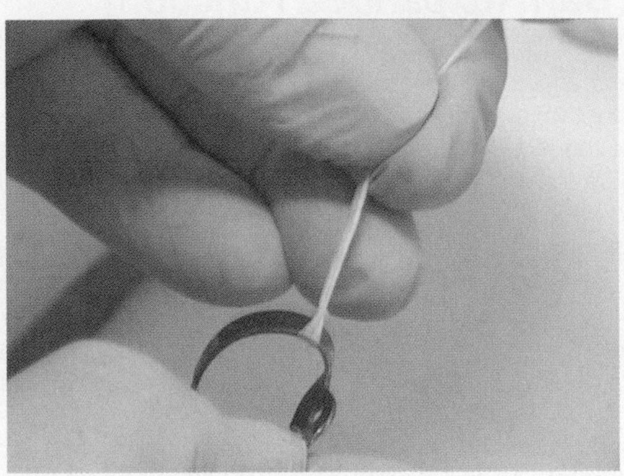

12 Place the beaks of the dental dam forceps into the holes of the clamp. Grasp the handles of the dental dam forceps, and squeeze to open the clamp. Turn upward, and allow the locking bar to slide down to keep the forceps open for placement.

13 Retrieve the dental dam forceps. Position the lingual jaws of the clamp first, then the facial jaws. During placement, keep an index finger on the clamp to prevent the clamp from coming off before it has been stabilized on the tooth. Check the clamp for fit.

**PURPOSE** Lingual jaw placement serves as a fulcrum for placement of the facial jaws.

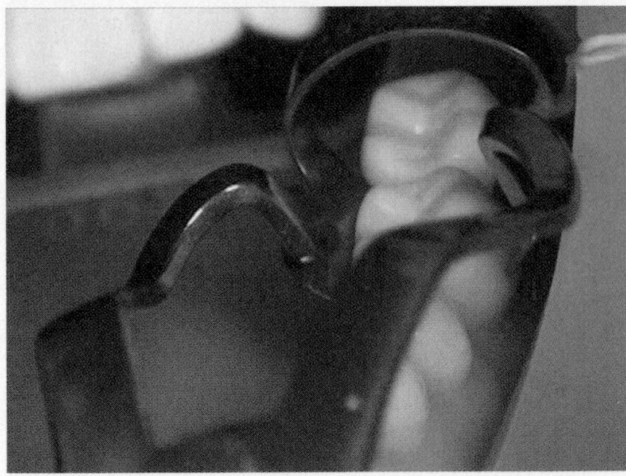

14 Transfer the dental dam to the site; stretch the punched hole for the anchor tooth over the clamp.

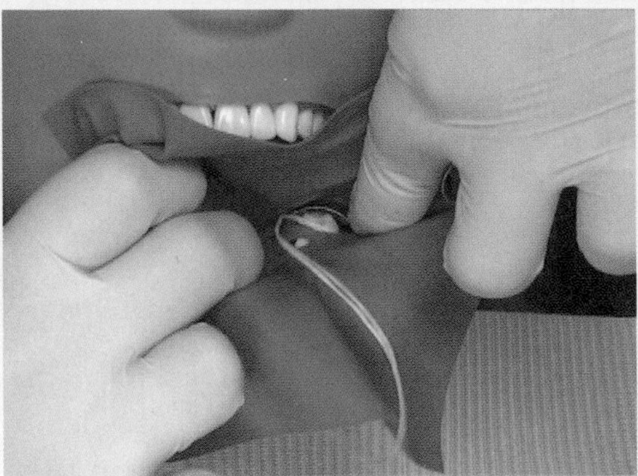

15 Use cotton pliers to retrieve the ligature and pull it through, so that it is exposed and easy to grasp if necessary.

16 Position the frame over the dam, and slightly pull the dam, allowing it to hook onto the projections of the frame.

**PURPOSE** Ensures a smooth and stable fit.

17 Fit the last hole of the dam over the last tooth to be exposed at the opposite end of the anchor tooth.

**PURPOSE** This stabilizes the dam and aids in locating the remaining punch holes for the teeth to be isolated.

18 Using the index fingers of both hands, stretch the dam on the lingual and facial surfaces of the teeth so that the dam slides through each contact area.

19 With a piece of dental tape or waxed floss, floss through the contacts, pushing the dam below the proximal contacts of each tooth to be isolated.

**NOTE** Slide the floss through the contact rather than pulling it back through the contact. This will keep the dam in place.

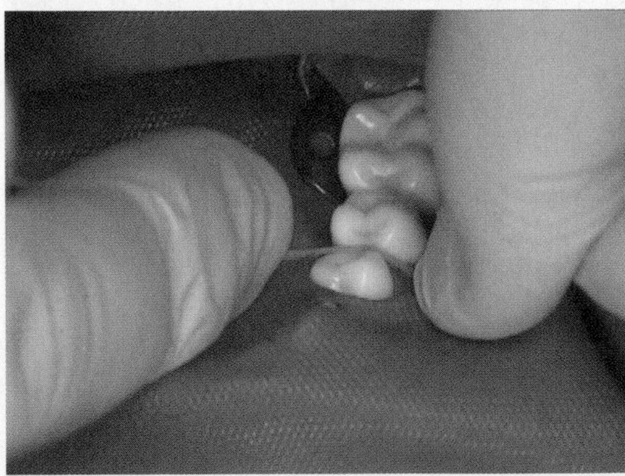

20 If the contacts are extremely tight, use floss or a wooden wedge placed into the interproximal area to separate the teeth slightly.

21 A ligature is placed to stabilize the dam at the *opposite* end of the anchor tooth.

# PROCEDURE 36.4 Preparing, Placing, and Removing the Dental Dam (Expanded Function)–cont'd

## Inverting the Dam

**22** Invert, or reverse, the dam by gently stretching it near the cervix of the tooth.

**PURPOSE** Inverting the dam creates a seal to prevent the leakage of saliva.

**23** Apply air from the air-water syringe to the tooth that is being inverted to help in turning the dam material under.

**PURPOSE** When the tooth surface is dry, the margin of the stretched dam usually inverts into the gingival sulcus as the dam is released.

**24** A black spoon, FP1, or beaver tail burnisher can be used to invert the edges of the dam.

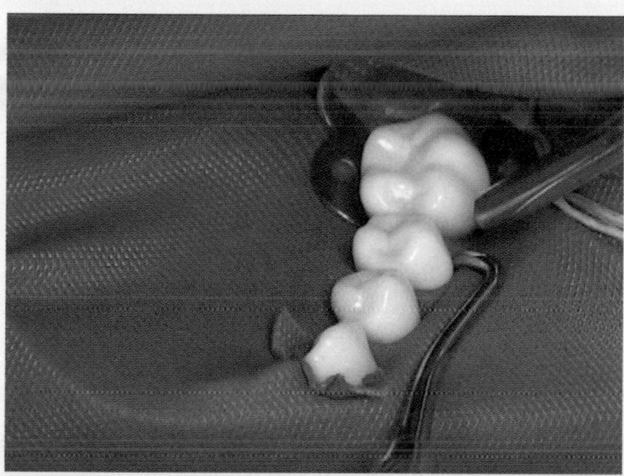

**25** When all punched holes are properly inverted, the dental dam application is complete.

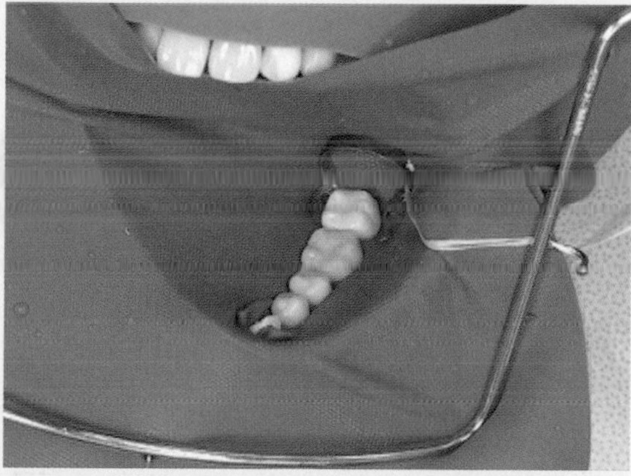

**26** If necessary for patient comfort, a saliva ejector may be placed under the dam. This is positioned on the floor of the patient's mouth on the side *opposite* the area being treated.

**27** If the patient is uncomfortable and has trouble breathing only through the nose, cut a small hole in the palatal area of the dam by pinching a piece of dam with cotton pliers and cutting a small hole near the palatal area.

## Removing the Dam

**28** If a ligature was used to stabilize the dam, remove it first. If a saliva ejector was used, remove it.

**29** Slide your finger under the dam parallel to the arch and pull outward, so you are stretching the holes away from the isolated teeth.

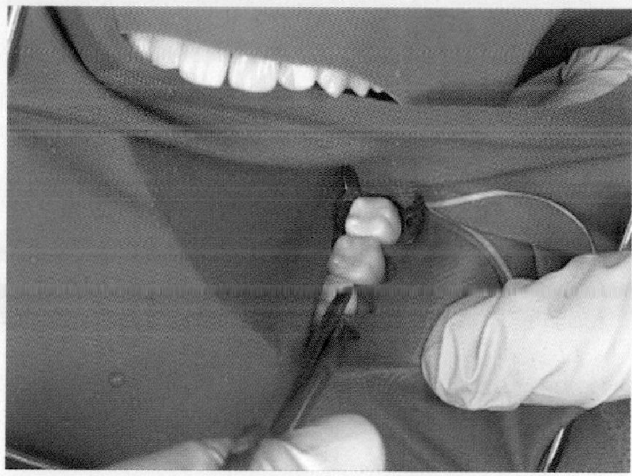

**30** Working from posterior to anterior, use the crown and bridge scissors to cut from hole to hole, creating one long cut.

**31** When all septa are cut, the dam is pulled lingually to free the rubber from the interproximal space.

**32** Using the dental dam forceps, position the beaks in the holes of the clamp, and open the clamp by squeezing the handle. Gently slide the clamp from the tooth.

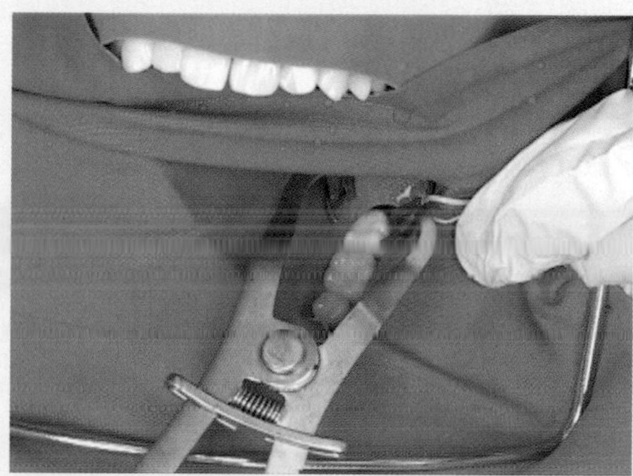

**33** Remove both the dam and the frame at the same time.

**34** Use a tissue or the dam napkin to wipe moisture from the patient's mouth, lips, and chin.

**35** Inspect the dam to ensure that the entire pattern of the torn septa of the dental dam has been removed.

(Continued)

## PROCEDURE 36.4 Preparing, Placing, and Removing the Dental Dam (Expanded Function)–cont'd

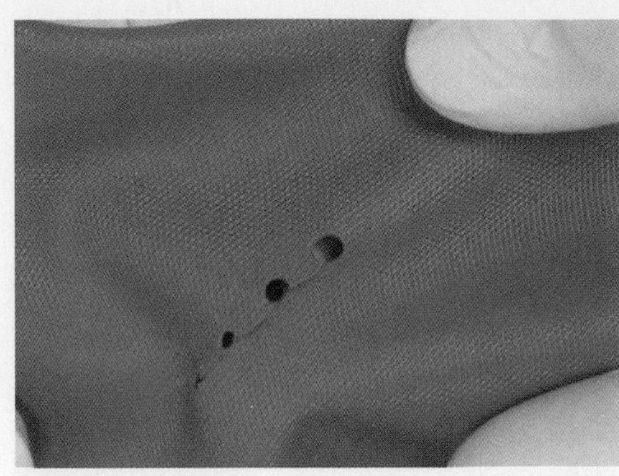

**36** If a fragment of the dental dam is missing, use dental floss to check the corresponding interproximal area of the oral cavity.
**PURPOSE** Fragments of the dental dam left under the free gingiva can cause gingival irritation.

37

# Anesthesia and Pain Control

## KEY TERMS

**Analgesia (an-ul-JEE-zee-uh)** Stage of anesthesia in which the patient is relaxed and conscious.
**Anesthesia (an-es-THE-zhuh)** Temporary loss of feeling or sensation.
**Anesthetic** Medication that produces temporary loss of feeling or sensation.
**Aspirate (AS-pi-rayt)** To draw back or to draw within.
**Diffuse (di-FYOOZ)** To spread from an area of high concentration to one of low concentration.
**Duration (duh-RAY-shun)** Time from induction to complete reversal of anesthesia.
**Gauge** Standard dimension or measurement of the thickness of an injection needle.
**Induction (in-DUK-shun)** Time from injection to effective anesthesia.
**Innervation (in-ur-VAY-shun)** Supply or distribution of nerves to a specific body part.
**Lumen (LOO-men)** The hollow center of the injection needle.
**Oximetry (ok-SIM-uh-tree)** Measurement of oxygen concentration in the blood.
**Permeate (PUR-mee-ayt)** To spread or flow throughout.
**Porous (POR-us)** Describes an object with minute openings that allow the passage of gas or fluid.
**Systemic toxicity (sis-TEM-ik tok-SIS-i-tee)** A harmful reaction to a drug that affects one or more of the body systems.
**Tidal volume** Amount of air inhaled and exhaled with each breath.
**Titrate (TYE-trayt)** To determine the effective dosage of analgesic by increasing the dosage until the desired effect is achieved.
**Vasoconstrictor (vay-zoe-kun-STRIK-tor)** Type of drug that constricts (narrows) blood vessels; used to prolong anesthetic action.

## LEARNING OUTCOMES

*On completion of this chapter, the student will be able to achieve the following objectives:*

1. Define, pronounce, and spell the key terms.
2. Discuss the importance of pain control in dentistry.
3. Describe the composition and application of topical anesthetics.
4. Discuss local anesthesia, including the following:
    - Explain the composition and application of local anesthetic agents.
    - Describe injection techniques used for local anesthesia administration.
    - Describe the setup for local anesthesia.
    - List possible complications and precautions that the dental team should be aware of when administering local anesthesia.
5. List the benefits of electronic anesthesia.
6. Discuss inhalation sedation, including the following:
    - Describe nitrous oxide/oxygen sedation and its use in dentistry.
    - Discuss the importance of reducing the dental team's exposure to nitrous oxide.
7. List the situations where antianxiety drugs may be used.
8. Discuss intravenous sedation and its use in dentistry.
9. Discuss general anesthesia and its use in dentistry, including the four stages of anesthesia.
10. Discuss mind-body medicine.
11. Explain the importance of documenting anesthesia and pain control.

## PERFORMANCE OUTCOMES

*On completion of this chapter, the student will be able to meet competency standards in the following skills:*

- Demonstrate the placement of a topical anesthetic agent.
- Demonstrate the preparation and management of the local anesthetic setup.
- Assist during the administration of local anesthesia.
- Assist in the administration and monitoring of nitrous oxide/oxygen sedation.

## ELECTRONIC RESOURCES

***Additional information related to content in Chapter 37 can be found on the companion Evolve Web site.***

- Practice Quiz
- Tray Setup Drag-and-Drop Exercise: Local Anesthetic Syringe
- Tray Setup Questions
- Videos: Applying a Topical Anesthetic; Assembling the Local Anesthetic Syringe

A wide variety of anxiety and pain control procedures have allowed the dental profession to extend oral healthcare to millions of individuals who would otherwise remain untreated. **Anesthesia** is the term used for temporary loss of feeling or sensation, and **anesthetics** are the drugs that produce the temporary loss of feeling or sensation.

**Anxiety and pain control** is defined as the practice of various psychological, physiologic, and chemical approaches to the prevention and treatment of preoperative, operative, and postoperative anxiety and pain. Methods of pain control used in dentistry to alleviate or reduce anxiety and pain include the following:

- Topical anesthesia
- Local anesthesia
- Inhalation sedation
- Antianxiety agents
- Intravenous sedation
- General anesthesia
- Mind-body medicine

# Topical Anesthesia

The primary purpose of topical anesthesia in dentistry is to provide a numbing effect in a specific area where an injection is to take place. Topical anesthetic agents provide a temporary numbing effect on nerve endings located on the surface of the oral mucosa. The drug makeup in topical anesthetics are concentrated to allow penetration of the mucous membranes and action at the nerve endings.

Topical anesthetic agents' active ingredient is either benzocaine or lidocaine, and these agents are available in the form of ointments, liquids, sprays, and patches, with each form having a slightly different application process (Fig. 37.1). For today's products, a gel type of topical anesthetic should remain on the site of injection for a minimum of 15 to 30 seconds and a maximum of 1 to 2 minutes to have optimum effectiveness.

See Procedure 37.1: Applying a Topical Anesthetic.

Spray topical anesthetic agents are applied to larger surface areas of the oral tissues. These anesthetics are useful when applied at the back of the throat in patients with a strong gag reflex when an impression or intraoral radiographs are to be taken. It should be noted that topical sprays can pose a potential danger if too much is administered. Because topical anesthetics are prepared in a higher concentration, the anesthetic would be absorbed into the bloodstream, possibly causing an overdose reaction to the anesthetic.

The topical patch is a product that when placed provides topical anesthesia within 10 seconds. The patch is used for injections and for alleviation of discomfort from denture sores and oral ulcers (Fig. 37.2).

RECALL

1 Why are topical anesthetics used in dentistry?

# Local Anesthesia

Local anesthetics were first discovered in the mid-1800s and have greatly played an important role in reducing pain and discomfort during dental care. Local anesthetic agents are the most frequently used form of pain control in dentistry. This method of pain control provides a safe, effective, and dependable method of anesthesia of suitable duration for virtually all forms of dental treatment.

## Characteristics of Local Anesthetics

- Nonirritating to the tissues in the area of the injection
- Associated with minimal toxicity (cause the least possible damage to body systems)

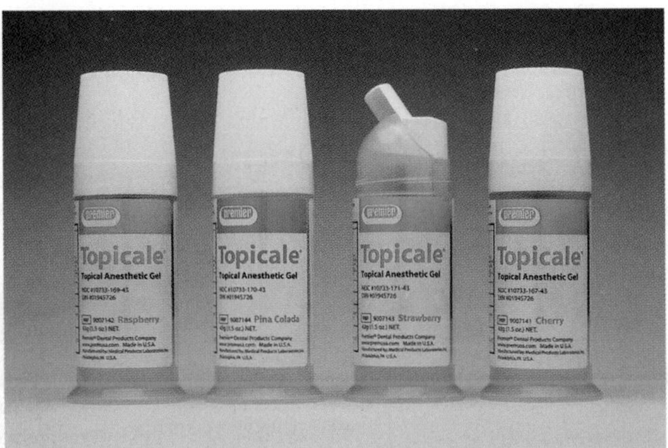


**FIG. 37.1** Topical anesthetic. *(Courtesy Premier Dental Products Company, Plymouth Meeting, PA.)*

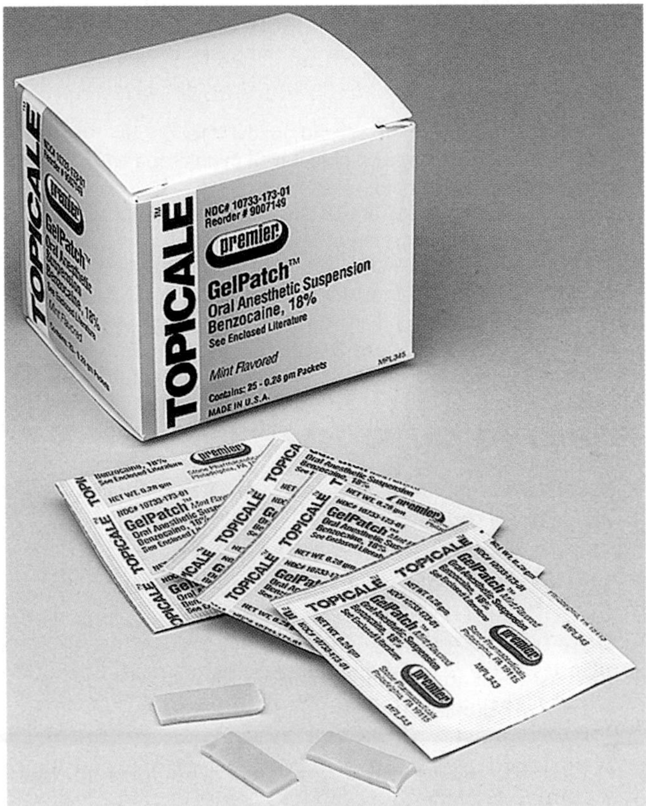


**FIG. 37.2** Topical gel patch. *(Courtesy Premier Dental Products Company, Plymouth Meeting, PA.)*

- Rapid onset (take effect quickly)
- Able to provide profound anesthesia (completely eliminate the sensation of pain during a procedure)
- Sufficient duration (remain effective long enough for the procedure to be completed)
- Completely reversible (leave the tissue in its original state after the patient's recovery from anesthesia)
- Sterile or capable of being sterilized by heat without deterioration

## Method of Action

Local anesthesia is obtained by injecting an anesthetic solution near the nerve where treatment is to take place. The local anesthetic agent temporarily blocks the ability of the nerve membrane to generate an impulse.

After the injection is completed, the anesthetic **diffuses**, or spreads, into the nerve and blocks its normal action, causing the patient to feel numb in the area. For the dentist to obtain complete anesthesia after the injection, the nerve must be sufficiently **permeated** by a concentration of the anesthetic base to inhibit conduction in all fibers. The action of local anesthesia becomes reversed as the bloodstream carries away the solution, causing the patient to lose numbness in the area.

## Chemical Composition of Anesthetics

Local anesthetic solutions for dental use come under two chemical groups: *amides* and *esters*. The amides were first introduced into clinical practice in the 1940s and have maintained the standards by which all other local anesthetics are measured. Ester-type anesthetic solutions are used primarily as topical anesthetics. The difference between the two groups can be seen in how they are metabolized by the body. Amide local anesthetics are metabolized by the liver, and ester local anesthetics are metabolized primarily in the plasma.

Each local anesthetic cartridge contains a combination of the following ingredients:

- **Local anesthetic drug:** The choice depends on the procedure, the health of the patient, and the dentist's preference.
- **Sodium chloride,** which makes the solution isotonic with body tissues
- **Distilled water,** which supplies an added volume of solution

## Time Span of Anesthetics

An important consideration for the dentist when selecting a local anesthetic is the time span of pain control required. **Induction** is the length of time from injection of the anesthetic solution to complete and effective conduction blockage. **Duration** is the length of time from induction until the reversal process is complete. Depending on the type of injection, the type of anesthetic, amount of anesthetic, and location of the injection will determine the duration of the local anesthesia:

- A short-acting local anesthetic agent can last approximately 30 minutes.
- An intermediate-acting local anesthetic agent lasts approximately 60 minutes. Most local anesthetic agents in this group are used for general dental procedures.
- A long-acting local anesthetic agent approximately lasts 90 minutes.

## Vasoconstrictors in Anesthetics

A **vasoconstrictor** is an agent that when combined with the anesthetic slows down the uptake of an anesthetic agent into the bloodstream and increases the duration of action. When a vasoconstrictor is used:

- Blood vessels to the site of administration are constricted.
- Absorption into the cardiovascular system is slowed.
- Local anesthetic toxicity is minimized because the vasoconstrictor lowers the blood level of local anesthetic.
- The effect of the anesthetic agent is prolonged by decreasing blood flow in the immediate area of injection.
- Bleeding at the injected area is decreased, which is especially important for surgical procedures.

Types of vasoconstrictors used with local anesthetic agents include *epinephrine, levonordefrin,* and *Neo-Cobefrin.* A very small quantity of vasoconstrictor is added to the local anesthetic solution in the ratio of vasoconstrictor-to-anesthetic solution of 1:20,000; 1:50,000; 1:100,000; or 1:200,000. With the concentration levels of a vasoconstrictor, the smaller the ratio, the higher the percentage of vasoconstrictor. In most situations, it is desirable to use as high a ratio as possible.

### *Contraindications to Vasoconstrictors*

Because a vasoconstrictor may cause strain on the heart as the local anesthetic solution is absorbed into the body, the use of an anesthetic solution *without a vasoconstrictor* is recommended for patients with a history of heart disease. Such conditions include unstable angina (heart-related chest pain), recent myocardial infarction (heart attack), recent coronary artery bypass surgery, untreated or uncontrolled severe hypertension (high blood pressure), and untreated or uncontrolled congestive heart failure.

The vasoconstrictor action may interact with other drugs the patient is taking. Therefore the dental team must be aware of the patient's current medication intake and always instruct the patient to update and communicate any changes in his or her medical history.

Before you prepare a syringe, always confirm with the dentist as to the type of local anesthetic solution to be given and the desired vasoconstrictor-to-anesthetic solution ratio. See Table 37.1 for the types of routinely used dental anesthetics.

RECALL

2 What is the most frequently selected form of pain control used in dentistry?
3 For local anesthesia to be affective, where does the local anesthetic need to be injected?
4 What is added to a local anesthetic to prolong its effect?

**TABLE 37.1 Commonly Used Dental Anesthetics**

| Formulation | Brand Name | Vasoconstrictor/ Concentration |
|---|---|---|
| Articaine 4% | Septocaine | 1:100,000 or 1:200,000 epinephrine |
| Benzocaine 20% or 15% | | |
| Bupivacaine 0.5% | Marcaine<br>Sensorcaine | 1:200,000 epinephrine |
| Chloprocaine | Nesacaine 2% or 3% | |
| Etidocaine | Duranest | 1:200,000 epinephrine or plain |
| Diphenhydramine | Benadryl | No vasoconstrictor |
| Lidocaine 2% | Daicaine<br>Diocaine<br>L-Caine<br>Nervocaine<br>Xylocaine<br>Lidoject | 1:50,000 and 1:100,000 epinephrine |
| Mepivacaine | Carbocaine 3%<br>Carbocaine 2% | 2% with levonordefrin 1:20,000 |
| Prilocaine 4% | Citanest | 1:200,000 epinephrine |

Modified from Malamed SF: Handbook of local anesthesia, ed 6, St Louis, 2013, Mosby.

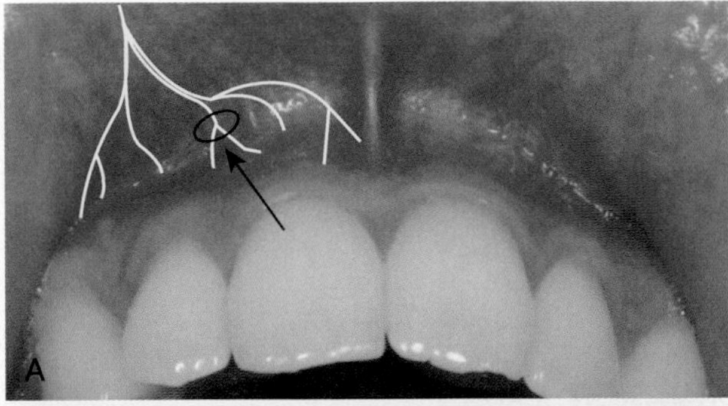


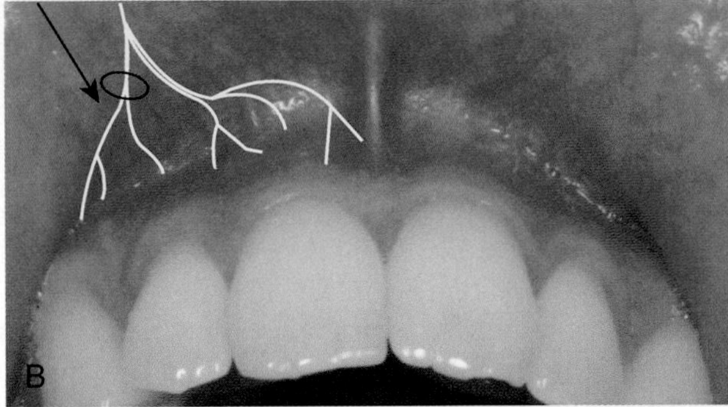


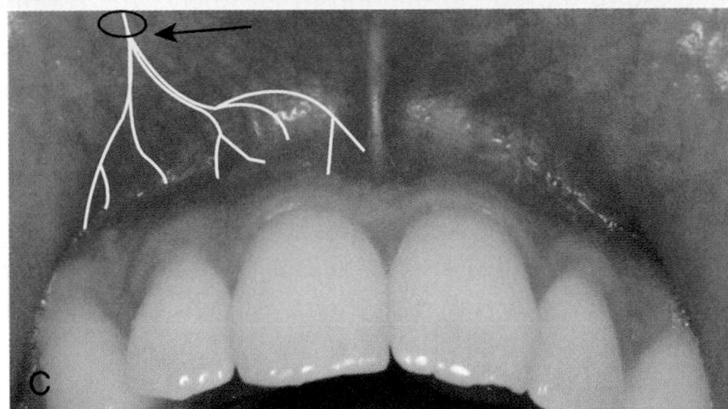


**FIG. 37.3** Maxillary injections. A, Local infiltration. B, Field block. C, Nerve block. *(From Malamed SF: Handbook of local anesthesia, ed 6, St Louis, 2013, Mosby.)*

## Injection Techniques

The location and the **innervation** of the tooth or teeth to be anesthetized will determine where topical anesthetic is placed and the type of injection to be given.

### *Maxillary Anesthesia*

Local anesthesia injection techniques differ from mandibular approaches because of the **porous** nature of alveolar cancellous bone in the maxilla. This type of bone structure allows the anesthetic solution to diffuse through the bone and reach the apices of the teeth in a different manner.

Three major types of local anesthetic injections may be given in the maxillary arch. **Local infiltration** is completed by injecting into a small, isolated area; **field block** refers to the injection of anesthetic near a larger terminal nerve branch. When two or three teeth are being restored, a field block is indicated. **Nerve block** occurs when local anesthetic is deposited close to a main nerve trunk. This type of injection is indicated for quadrant dentistry. Examples of these types of injections are the posterior superior alveolar, the anterior superior alveolar, and the nasopalatine nerve block (Fig. 37.3).

### *Palatal Anesthesia*

Local anesthesia in the palatal area may be necessary for procedures that involve the soft tissues of the palate. Common palatal injections are the **anterior (or greater) palatine nerve block,** which provides anesthesia in the posterior portion of the hard palate, and the **nasopalatine nerve block,** which produces anesthesia in the anterior hard palate (Fig. 37.4).

For many patients, this procedure can be a very painful experience. It is best to advise patients that they may have some discomfort during the injection.

### *Mandibular Anesthesia*

Because of the dense, compact nature of the mandibular bone, anesthetic solution does not diffuse easily through it. Therefore block anesthesia is the type of injection that is frequently required for most mandibular teeth. This solution is injected near a major nerve, and the entire area served by that nerve branch is numbed.

**Inferior alveolar nerve block,** often referred to as **mandibular nerve block,** is obtained by injecting the anesthetic solution near, but not into, the branches of the inferior alveolar nerve close to the mandibular foramen. The nerve and

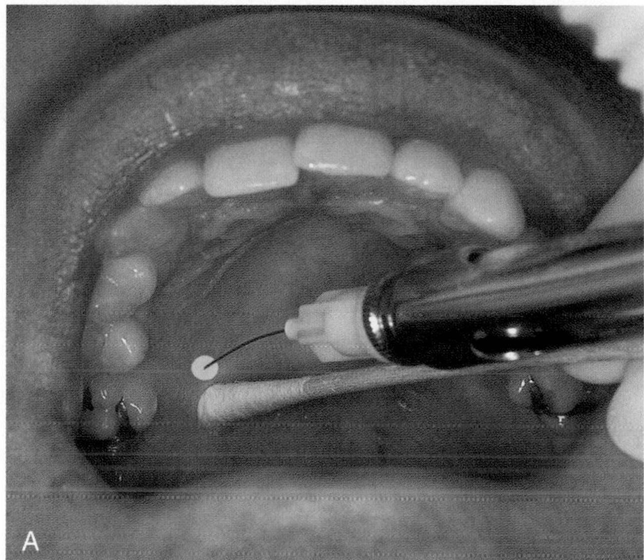


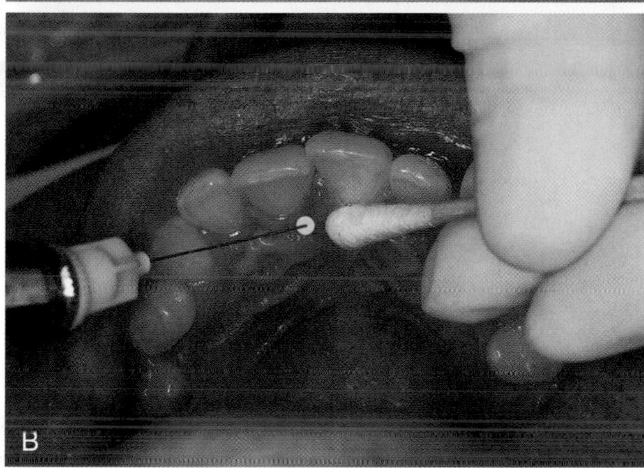


**FIG. 37.4** Palatal injections. A, Greater palatine. B, Nasopalatine nerve block. *(Courtesy of Margaret J. Fehrenbach, RDH, MS.)*

blood supplies are close to each other, and the dentist must be careful not to inject directly into a blood vessel (see later discussion). The patient will experience numbness over half of the lower jaw, including the teeth, tongue, and lip. **Buccal nerve block** provides anesthesia to the buccal soft tissues closest to the mandibular molars; **incisive nerve block** is given only when the mandibular anterior teeth or premolars require anesthesia. The incisive block injection is given at the site of the mental foramen. The branch of this nerve continues within the mandibular canal to the apices of the anterior teeth (Fig. 37.5).

### *Periodontal Ligament Injection*

An alternative infiltration technique involves injection of the anesthetic solution under pressure directly into the periodontal ligament and surrounding tissues. Periodontal ligament injection is generally an *adjunct* (addition) to conventional techniques (Fig. 37.6). This type of injection may be completed with the use of a conventional syringe or a special periodontal ligament injection syringe.

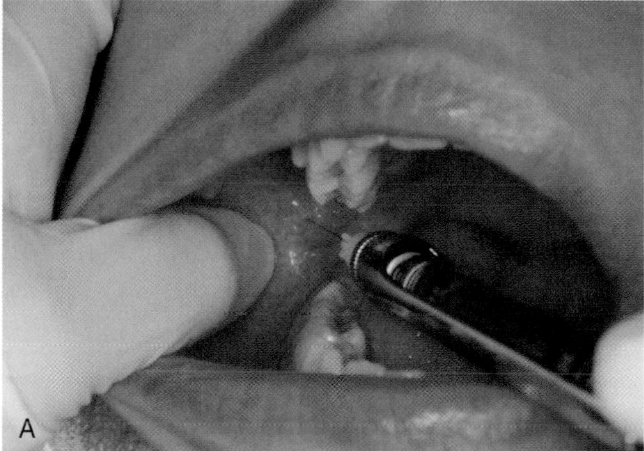


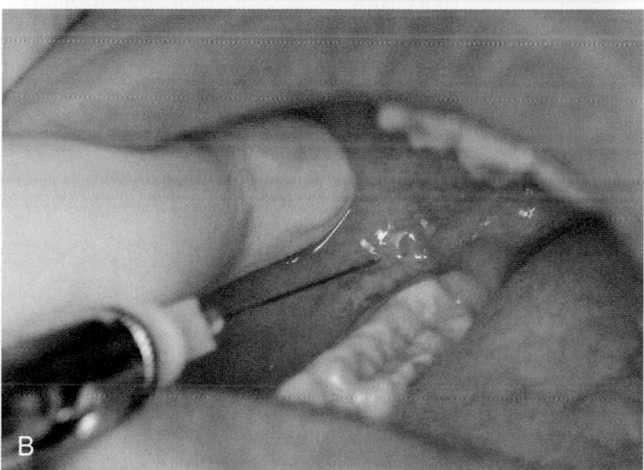


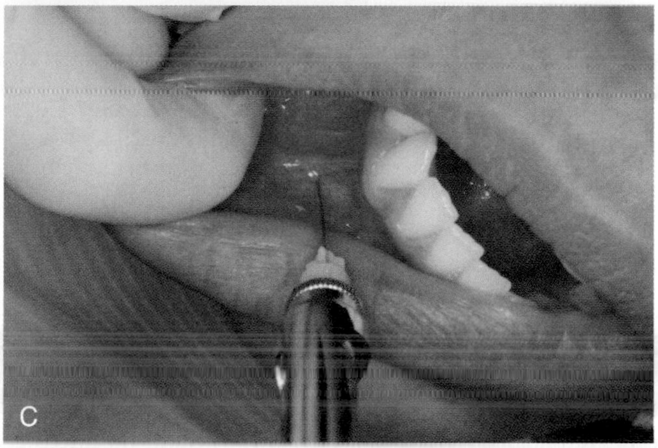


**FIG. 37.5** Mandibular injections. A, Inferior alveolar. B, Buccal nerve block. C, Incisive nerve block. *(From Malamed SF: Handbook of local anesthesia, ed 6, St Louis, 2013, Mosby.)*

## Local Anesthesia Setup

### *Anesthetic Syringe*

Fig. 37.7 provides a diagram of the type of syringe that is used in the administration of local anesthesia. It is made up of the following parts:

- **Thumb ring, finger grip.** These parts allow the dentist to control the syringe firmly and to aspirate effectively with one hand.
- **Harpoon.** The harpoon is a sharp hook that locks into the rubber stopper of the anesthetic cartridge, so the stopper

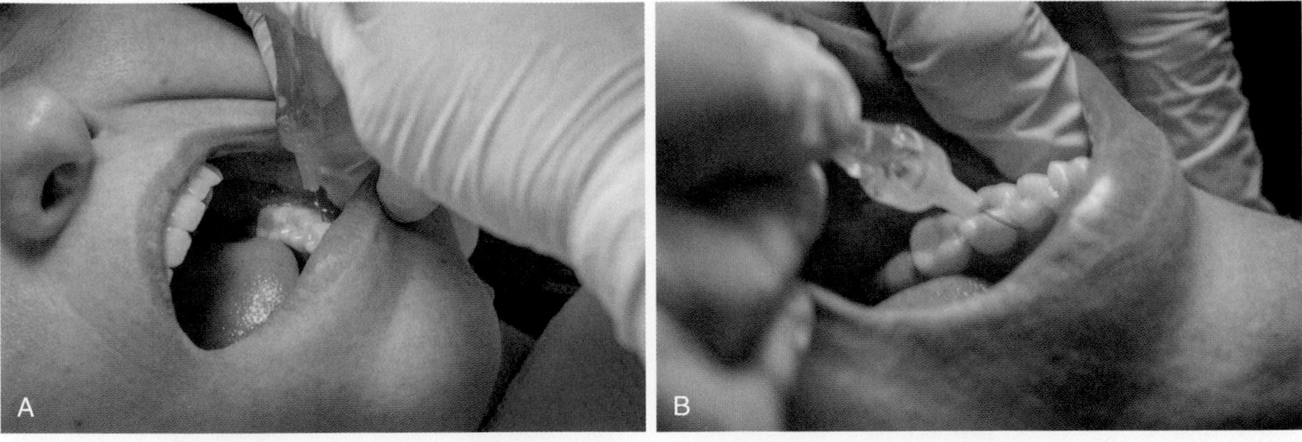

FIG. 37.6 Periodontal ligament injection. *(From Logothetis DD: Local anesthesia for the dental hygienist, ed 2, St Louis, 2017, Elsevier.)*

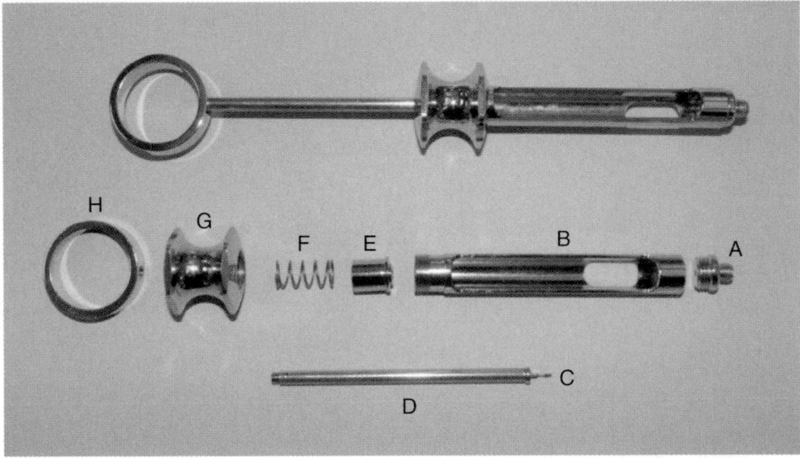


FIG. 37.7 Components of a standard local anesthetic syringe. A, Needle adaptor. B, Syringe barrel. C, Harpoon. D, Piston. E, Guide gearing. F, Spring. G, Finger grip. H, Thumb ring. *(From Logothetis DD: Local anesthesia for the dental hygienist, ed 2, St Louis, 2017, Elsevier.)*

can be retracted by pulling back on the piston rod. This action makes aspiration possible.

- **Piston rod.** This rod pushes the rubber stopper of the anesthetic cartridge and forces the anesthetic solution out through the needle.
- **Barrel of the syringe.** The barrel firmly holds the anesthetic cartridge in place. The cartridge is loaded through the open side of the barrel. A window on the other side allows the dentist to watch for blood during aspiration.
- **Threaded tip (needle adaptor).** The hub of the needle is attached to the syringe on the threaded tip. The cartridge end of the needle passes through the small opening in the center of the threaded tip, puncturing the rubber diaphragm of the anesthetic cartridge.

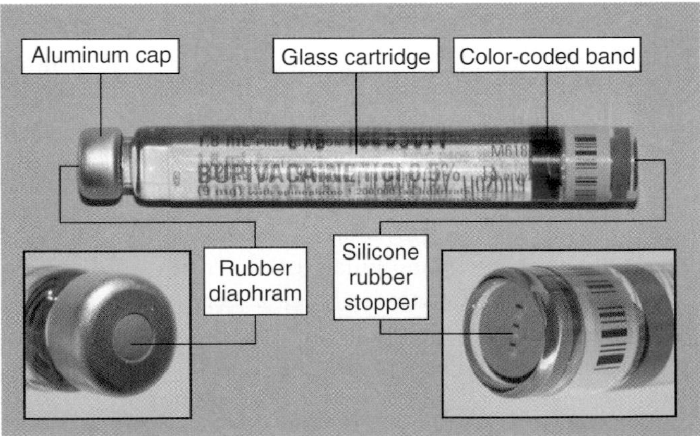


FIG. 37.8 Anesthetic cartridge. *(From Logothetis DD: Local anesthesia for the dental hygienist, ed 2, St Louis, 2017, Elsevier.)*

## Anesthetic Cartridges

Local anesthetic solutions are supplied in glass cartridges. These cartridges have a rubber or silicone stopper at one end and an aluminum cap with a rubber diaphragm at the other end (Fig. 37.8). Cartridges are supplied in "blister packs," which are already sterilized and have been stored in a sealed environment (Fig. 37.9).

**COLOR-CODING OF LOCAL ANESTHETIC CARTRIDGES.** A color-coding system designed by the American Dental Association Council on Scientific Affairs created standardization for all injectable local anesthesia products that chose to participate in this system. This standardization was introduced so that the dental practitioner could easily recognize different

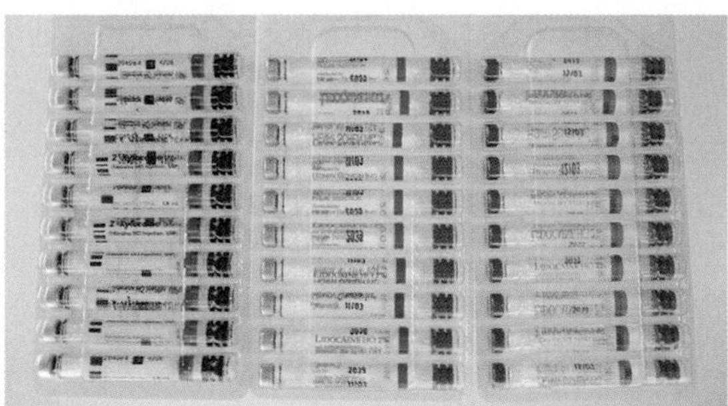

**FIG. 37.9** Local anesthetic cartridges packaged in blister packs. *(From Boyd LRB: Dental instruments: a pocket guide, ed 6, St Louis, 2018, Elsevier.)*

**Local anesthetic cartridge color codes**

Mandated uniform system for local anesthetic cartridges bearing the ADA Seal of Acceptance.*

| PRODUCT | COLOR |
|---|---|
| Lidocaine 2% with epinephrine 1:100,000 | |
| Lidocaine 2% with epinephrine 1:50,000 | |
| Lidocaine 2% plain | |
| Mepivacaine 2% with levonordefrin 1:20,000 | |
| Mepivacaine 3% plain | |
| Prilocaine 4% with epinephrine 1:200,000 | |
| Prilocaine 4% plain | |
| Bupivacaine 0.5% with epinephrine 1:200,000 | |
| Articaine 4% with epinephrine 1:100,000 | |
| Articaine 4% with epinephrine 1:200,000 | |

* This chart originally appeared in ADA News.

**FIG. 37.10** Anesthesia color codes. *(ADA News July 14, 2003; 34(13)12. Copyright © 2003 American Dental Association. All rights reserved. Reproduced with permission.)*

types and concentrations of anesthetic (Fig. 37.10). Each anesthetic cartridge has a band of color that is placed 3 mm from the stopper end, with durable black lettering that follows U.S. Food and Drug Administration (FDA) labeling guidelines.

Learn to identify these color codes, and always take care to select the ratio specified by the dentist. Also, always take the precaution of double-checking the patient's record before you select an anesthetic solution.

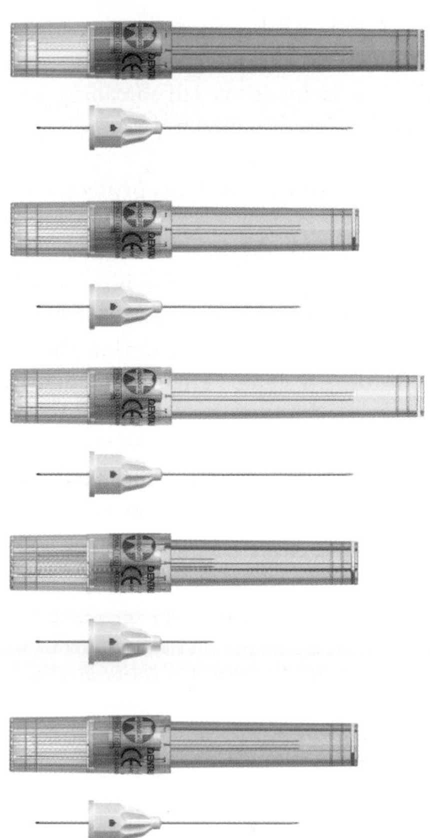

**FIG. 37.11** Outer covering for the needle (top to bottom: 25 gauge long, 27 gauge short, 27 gauge long, 30 gauge x-short, 30 gauge short). *(Courtesy of Septodont, Lancaster, PA.)*

## GUIDELINES FOR HANDLING ANESTHETIC CARTRIDGES

- Cartridges should be stored at room temperature and protected from direct sunlight. Heat and sun may cause the solution to deteriorate and be less effective.
- Never use a cartridge that has been frozen. An *extruded* (pushed out) rubber stopper and a large air bubble are signs that the solution may have been frozen.
- Do not use a cartridge if it is cracked, chipped, or damaged in any way. The glass may shatter under the pressure of injection.
- Never use a solution that is discolored or cloudy or has passed the expiration date shown on the package. The solution may no longer be effective.
- Do not leave the syringe preloaded with the needle attached for an extended period. The metal ions from the needle may be released into the solution, which may cause swelling and edema after injection of the solution.
- Once the needle and syringe have been assembled, the cartridge must be used or discarded.
- Never save a cartridge for reuse.

### *Disposable Needle*

The sterile needle used for injection is protected by a two-part plastic covering (Fig. 37.11). The outer plastic casing consists of two parts that are sealed together to ensure sterility. The needle should not be used if this seal is broken.

The *cartridge end* of the needle is the shorter end of the needle. It fits through the threaded tip of the syringe and punctures the rubber diaphragm or the anesthetic cartridge. The protective plastic cap covers the cartridge end of the needle.

The *needle hub* is made of self-threading plastic or prethreaded metal. It is used to attach the needle to the threaded tip of the syringe.

The *injection end* of the needle is protected by the needle guard and is 1 inch or 1⅝ inches in length. Most often, the 1-inch *short needle* is used for infiltration anesthesia and the 1⅝-inch *long needle* is used for block anesthesia (Fig. 37.12). This end of the needle is *beveled* (angled). Before the injection, the needle is turned so that the beveled angle is toward the bone. This angle enables the dentist to deposit the solution next to the bone without actually contacting the bone.

The **lumen** is the hollow center of the needle through which the anesthetic solution flows. The **gauge** refers to the thickness or size of the needle. Gauges are numbered as follows:

- The *larger* the gauge number, the *thinner* the needle.
- The *smaller* the gauge number, the *thicker* the needle.

Because a longer needle requires more strength, these needles are generally used in a smaller gauge number. The most frequently used gauge numbers are 25, 27, and 30.

See Procedure 37.2: Assembling the Local Anesthetic Syringe.

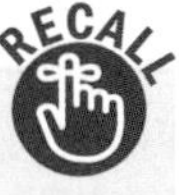


5 What type of injection technique will the dentist most frequently use to anesthetize teeth #2 through #4?

6 How many lengths of needles are used in dentistry, and what are they used for?

## Complications and Precautions

### Injecting into a Blood Vessel

A local anesthetic solution injected directly into a blood vessel can alter the function of vital organs, notably the heart. To be certain that the solution is not being injected into a vessel, the dentist will always **aspirate** before injecting any local anesthetic solution. The dentist inserts the needle into the mucosa and advances it to the desired depth. When the tip of the needle reaches the target area, the dentist slowly pulls back on the thumb ring of the syringe. This creates a negative pressure within the anesthetic cartridge.

If the needle has entered a blood vessel, a thin line of red blood cells will be drawn into the anesthetic cartridge. In this event, the dentist repositions the needle before injecting the solution.

### Infected Areas

Local anesthetic agents are not effective when injected into an area where a tooth or soft tissue is abscessed or infected. Because of an increase in the pH, the acidity in the area of infection increases, which interferes with the anesthetic solution not being able to penetrate the nerves. Injection into an infected area can also carry the risk of the diffusion of infection.

### Toxic Reactions

**LOCALIZED REACTIONS.** The local anesthetic solution is generally tolerated by the oral tissues but the introduction may produce a variety of local tissue changes. In some sensitive individuals, even slight contact with solutions that contain local anesthetic agents can cause *contact dermatitis,* which is an inflammation of the tissues caused by an allergic reaction to the anesthetic solution.

**SYSTEMIC REACTIONS.** Although local anesthetic solutions are remarkably safe in their use, the importance of their **systemic toxicity** cannot be ignored. Most often a systemic toxicity involves the central nervous system or the cardiovascular system. Manifestations of these toxic actions are variable and depend on the following:

- Individual patient physiology
- Local anesthetic solution
- Rate of injection
- Rate of absorption
- Quantity of anesthetic injected
- Other drugs in the patient's system

### Temporary Numbness

Because local anesthesia effectively blocks all pain sensation, the patient must be cautioned against biting the tongue, cheek, or lip when numb. This temporary numbness disappears as the effect of the anesthetic agent wears off.

Because the brain is not receiving normal nerve sensations, the numb area may feel swollen when it is not. The patient may complain that her or his lip feels "fat."

### Paresthesia

Paresthesia is a condition in which numbness lasts after the effects of local anesthetic solutions have worn off. Paresthesia may be caused by the following:

- Use of contaminated anesthetic solution, most often contamination with alcohol or sterilizing solution used to disinfect the anesthetic cartridge before use
- Trauma (injury) to the nerve sheath during the injection or surgery
- Hemorrhage (bleeding) into or around the nerve sheath

Paresthesia may be temporary or permanent. Most paresthesia is resolved in about 8 weeks without treatment. Paresthesia is permanent only if damage to the nerve is severe.

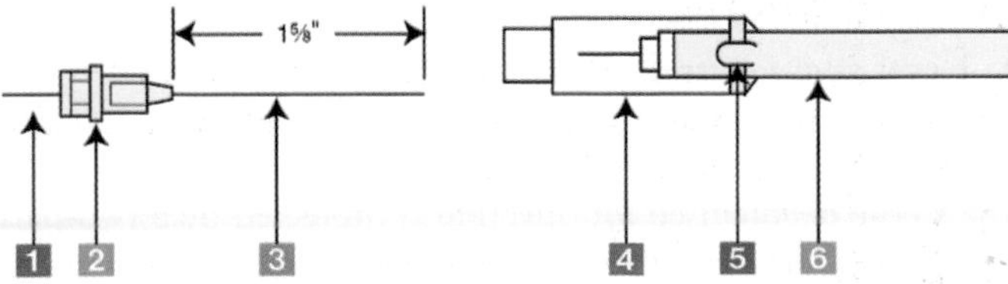


**FIG. 37.12** Sterile needle. *1,* Cartridge end of needle; *2,* needle hub; *3,* injection end of needle; *4,* protective cap; *5,* seal on cap; *6,* needle guard. *(From Boyd LRB: Dental instruments: a pocket guide, ed 6, St Louis, 2018, Elsevier.)*

See Procedure 37.3: Assisting in the Administration of Local Anesthesia.

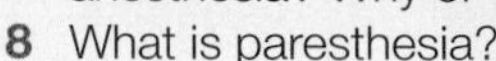

7 Should a patient with an abscess receive local anesthesia? Why or why not?
8 What is paresthesia?

# Electronic Anesthesia

An electronic anesthesia system is an innovative, noninvasive form of anesthesia. The system is designed to block pain electronically with the use of a low current of electricity. Contact pads target a specific electronic waveform directly to the nerve bundle at the root of the tooth (Fig. 37.13).

The patient is seated and is positioned with hand pads placed on the back of each hand. The area of the operative site is determined, isolated, and dried. The third pad, the *intraoral receptor*, is attached to the lingual side 3 to 5 mm from the gingival margin. As instructed, the patient has control in activating the unit and gradually increasing the level of the pain-blocking signal.

This alternative psychological and physiologic approach to local anesthesia benefits the patient for the following reasons:

- No needles
- No postoperative numbness or swelling
- Chemical-free method of anesthesia
- No risk of cross-contamination
- Reduced fear and anxiety in patients
- Patient control over own comfort level

# Inhalation Sedation

Inhalation sedation, also referred to as nitrous oxide/oxygen ($N_2O/O_2$) **analgesia**, may be the safest type of sedation method used in dentistry if used properly. The use of $N_2O$ in dentistry dates back to 1844, when Horace Wells (the first dentist) used these gases on his patients.

$N_2O/O_2$ sedation produces stage I anesthesia/analgesia by using a combination of $N_2O$ and $O_2$ gases. The patient inhales these gases through a nosepiece feeling the effect almost immediately.

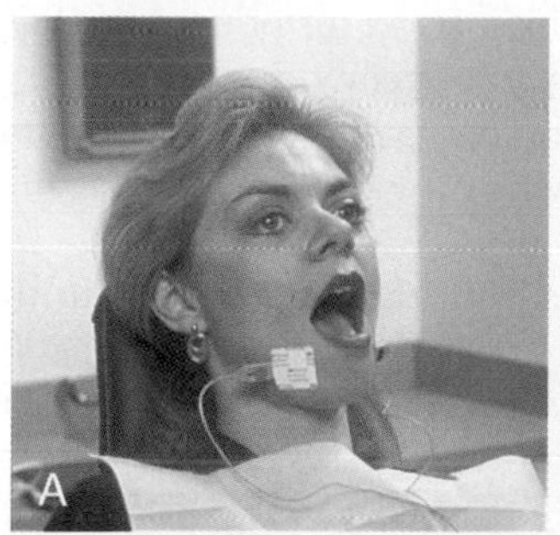


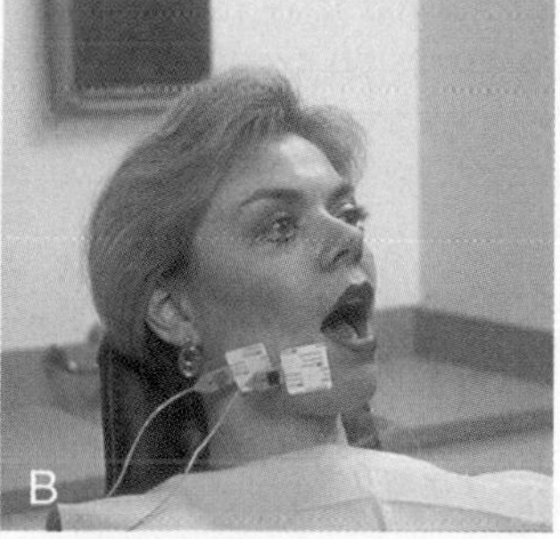


**FIG. 37.13** Electronic anesthesia showing electrode placement for mandibular procedures. A, Anterior and premolar teeth. B, Posterior teeth. *(From Malamed SF: Handbook of local anesthesia, ed 6, St Louis, 2013, Mosby.)*

## Advantages of $N_2O$ Use

- Administration is relatively simple and is easily managed by the dentist.
- Although special training is required for the dentist and the dental assistant, the services of an anesthetist or other special personnel are not necessary.
- This type of sedation has an excellent safety record, and the adverse effects are minimal.
- $N_2O/O_2$ sedation produces a pleasant, relaxing experience for the patient.
- The patient is awake and is able to communicate at all times.
- Recovery is rapid and is complete within a matter of minutes.
- $N_2O/O_2$ sedation may be used with patients of all ages.

## Disadvantages of $N_2O$ Use

- Some patients may experience nausea or vertigo, which can be unpleasant.
- Patients who have behavioral challenges may react in an adverse way and act out those behavior issues.

## Contraindications to $N_2O$ Use

There are certain medical conditions or chronic disorders that make N2O/O2 analgesia a contraindication:

- Pulmonary disorders
- Respiratory infections
- Pregnancy
- Psychiatric disorders
- Immune compromised disorder
- Multiple sclerosis
- Frequent user of marijuana or hallucinogenic drugs
- Middle ear blockage
- Apprehensive patient
- Alcoholic or recovering alcoholic

### *Pregnancy*

No evidence indicates that enough $N_2O$ crosses the placenta to damage the fetus. However, $N_2O/O_2$ analgesia is usually administered to a pregnant patient *only* after the first trimester and *only* with the permission of her obstetrician.

### *Nasal Obstruction*

Any type of nasal obstruction, such as a head cold or allergies, can prevent the patient from breathing in and out normally and not be able to obtain the benefit of $N_2O$.

### *Emphysema and Multiple Sclerosis*

Patients with emphysema or multiple sclerosis may have breathing difficulties while receiving $N_2O/O_2$ sedation. Increased oxygen delivery during administration may lower the stimulus to breathe as often as necessary.

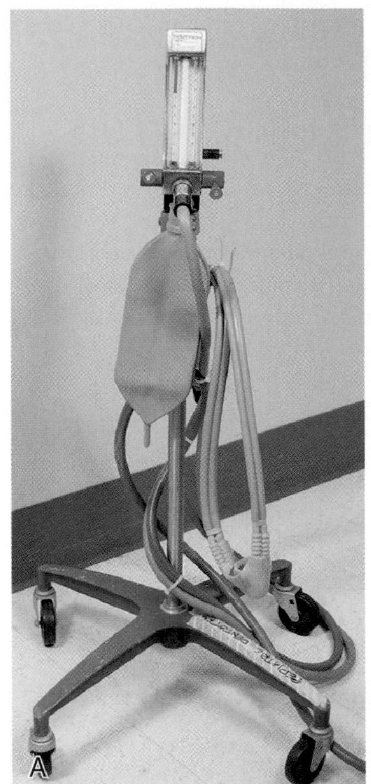

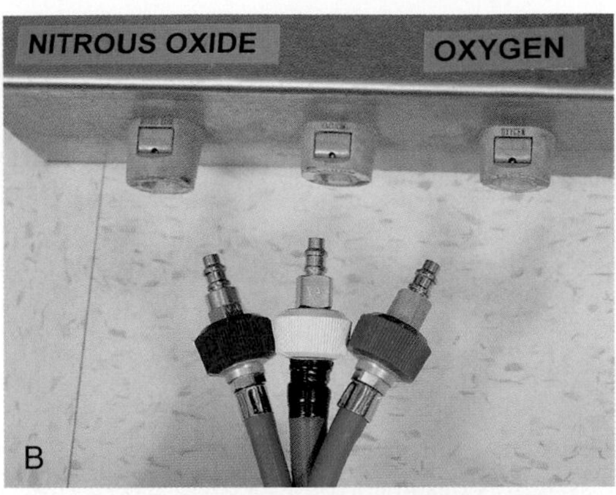


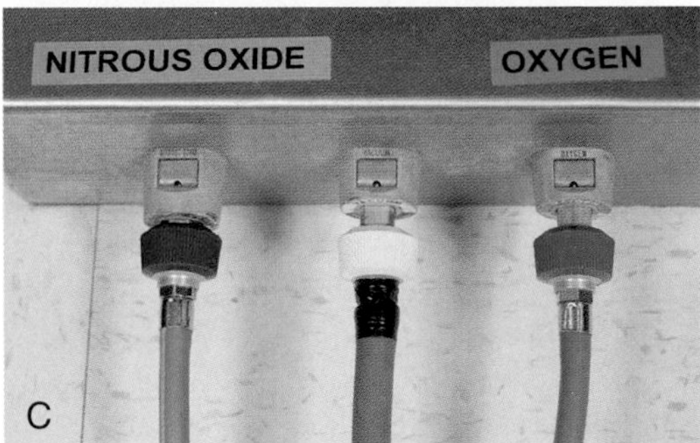


**FIG. 37.14** Portable $N_2O$ system unit. A, Mobile nitrous oxide/oxygen unit. B, Color coded outlets to connect nitrous unit. C, Proper connection for nitrous and oxygen. *(Courtesy Dr. Mark Dellinges and Cory Price.)*

### *Emotional Instability*

The altered perception of reality produced by $N_2O/O_2$ analgesia may intensify a patient's emotional instability, which may provide an undesirable effect.

## Chemical Makeup

$N_2O$, chemical name *dinitrogen monoxide,* is a tasteless, odorless, colorless gas that is compressed into a blue cylinder. This cylinder stores the $N_2O$ liquid/gas combination in equilibrium at 650 to 900 lb per square inch (psi), with only the gas being delivered to the patient.

## Effects of Nitrous Oxide

$N_2O$ is a toxic substance if used improperly. For the clinical dental team, the safest maximum allowable amount of $N_2O$ in the dental environment is 50 parts per million (ppm). $N_2O$ is used only during patient treatment. $N_2O$ is never administered unnecessarily or used for recreational purposes, which could lead to abuse of this substance.

## Equipment

The dental office may be equipped with built-in $N_2O/O_2$ equipment in the treatment area, or an alternative is the use of a portable unit that is moved from room to room as needed (Fig. 37.14).

In most states, ordering of a new supply of these gases involves the dentist's signature and license number. It is also necessary to comply with Occupational Safety and Health Administration (OSHA) and state requirements for safe installation and storage of these supplies.

*$N_2O$ and $O_2$ gas cylinders* are color-coded, green for oxygen and blue for nitrous oxide (Fig. 37.15). Cylinders should be stored in an upright position, away from a heat source, and should be chained to the wall (or portable unit) to prevent them from falling on the valve stem, which could cause them to explode.

*Control valves* are used to control the flow of each gas.

A *flow meter* indicates the rate of flow of the gas. Current flow meters employ a fail-safe mechanism that stops the flow of $N_2O$ whenever the percentage of $O_2$ drops to below 30 percent. This mechanism also prevents the delivery of $N_2O$ in concentrations greater than 70 percent. This feature, introduced in 1976, is standard on every flow meter unit currently manufactured.

The *reservoir bag* is where the two gases are initially combined. The patient inhales, drawing the gases from the bag into the gas hose.

The *gas hose* carries the gases from the reservoir bag to the mask or nosepiece.

*Masks,* also referred to as *nosepieces,* are the nasal inhalers through which the patient breathes the gases. Masks are supplied in varying sizes for adults and children (Fig. 37.16). The masks are made from a rubber type material that can be sterilized or disinfected after each use. The masks are also available in a disposable variety that is discarded after a single use.

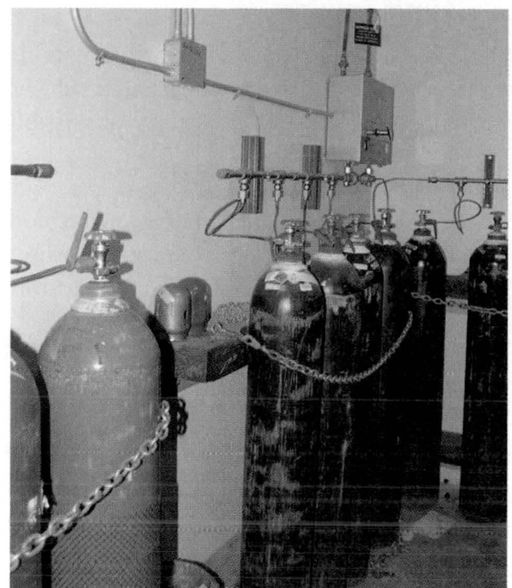

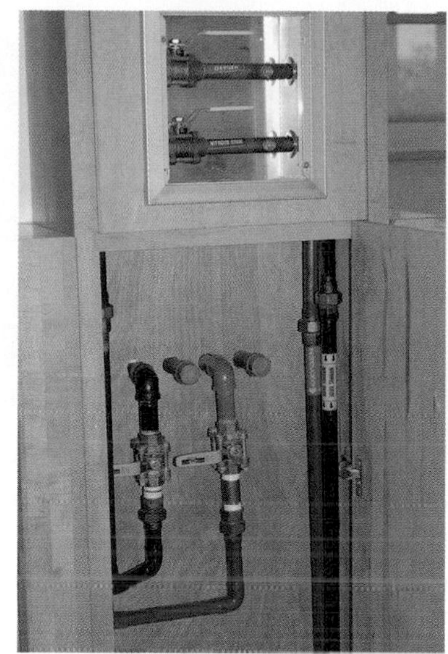

**FIG. 37.15** $N_2O$ and $O_2$ cylinders are stored away from the clinical setting. *(Courtesy Dr. Mark Dellinges and Cory Price.)*

## Patient Assessment and Monitoring

Always review the patient's medical history before administering $N_2O/O_2$ analgesia. Keep in mind that the sedative effects of $N_2O/O_2$ may enhance the effects of other medications directly or indirectly.

The vital signs of blood pressure, pulse, and respiration should be recorded before, during, and after administration of $N_2O/O_2$ analgesia. Preoperative readings provide a baseline against which postoperative readings can be compared. Postoperative readings are used to confirm the patient's recovery or to identify adverse responses.

## Patient Education

Before $N_2O/O_2$ administration begins, the patient should be informed about what to expect. The dentist or the assistant should describe (1) how the gas is administered, (2) proper use of the mask and the importance of nasal breathing, and (3) the sensations of warmth and tingling that the patient will experience. Reassure patients by instructing them that while receiving $N_2O/O_2$, they will remain conscious, aware, and in control of their actions.

## Administration

Under the Dental Practice Act in some states, the dental assistant, following certification, is permitted to aid in monitoring the administration of $N_2O/O_2$ only under the direct supervision of the dentist. To ensure the patient's safety, it is vital for the assistant to understand the process and the assistant's role in its administration.

$N_2O/O_2$ sedation should begin with the administration of 100 percent $O_2$. Start with pure $O_2$ while establishing the patient's **tidal volume**, and then slowly **titrate**, or determine the concentration of, the $N_2O$ until desired results are

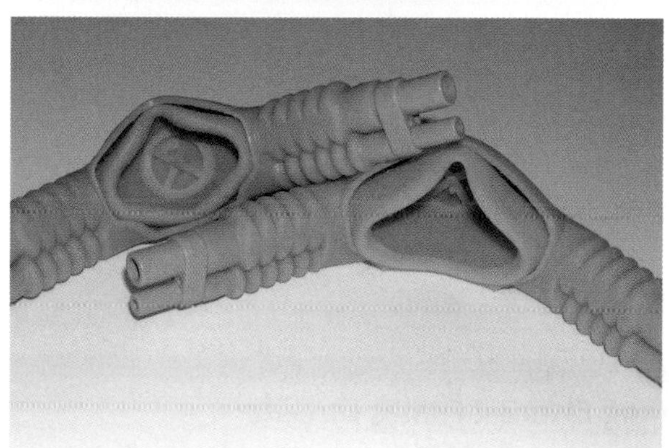

**FIG. 37.16** Nasal masks used for inhalation. *(From Clark M, Brunick A: Handbook of nitrous oxide and oxygen sedation, ed 4, St Louis, 2015, Mosby.)*

achieved. Patients can respond differently to $N_2O$ from one appointment to the next. The dosage at one appointment may seem excessive or insufficient for the patient at a later visit. There is no set dosage regimen, only the goal of **titration** to the patient's needs.

Patients should refrain from talking or mouth breathing. This can expel $N_2O$ into the air that the dental team can inhale and can reduce the concentration of $N_2O$ inhaled by the patient.

The $N_2O/O_2$ analgesia should end with the administration of 100 percent $O_2$ for 3 to 5 minutes. Assess the patient for dizziness, headache, or lethargy, and continue 100 percent $O_2$ if such symptoms exist.

After the patient feels normal, obtain postoperative vital signs and compare them with preoperative recordings. Do not let patients drive themselves home if you believe they pose a risk to themselves or others.

See Procedure 37.4: Assisting in the Administration and Monitoring of Nitrous Oxide/Oxygen Sedation (Expanded Function).

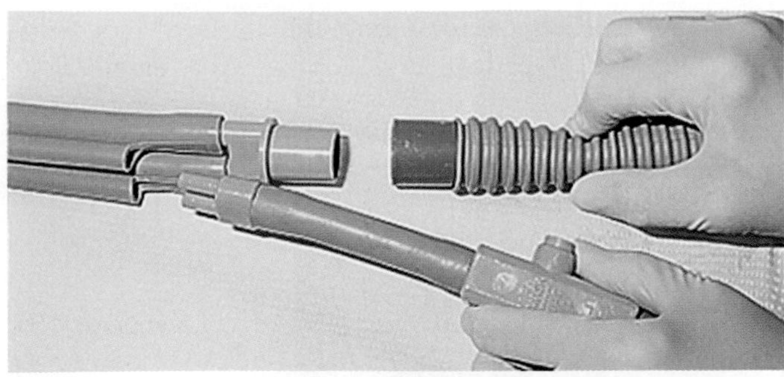

**FIG. 37.17** Scavenger system attached to mask and evacuation unit to redirect unused $N_2O$ gas. *(From Darby ML, Walsh MM: Dental hygiene: theory and practice, ed 4, St Louis, 2015, Saunders.)*

## Safety Work Practices for the Clinical Team

A dental office can safely provide nitrous oxide/oxygen to its patients, but all members of the office staff must adopt general work practices into their daily routine to make it a safe work environment.

### Scavenger System

Every $N_2O/O_2$ system should be equipped with a scavenging system. The use of a scavenger system reduces the $N_2O$ released into the treatment room, which escapes into the atmosphere and is then inhaled. Scavenger systems should have a vacuum flow rate of 45 liters per minute (L/min) and should be incorporated within the nasal mask, or *hood* (Fig. 37.17).

### Venting Exhaust Fumes Outside

Chronic exposure to $N_2O$ for several hours a week have been associated with adverse health effects. To remedy this, exhaust fumes should be vented to the outside. To ensure that this is safe, the exhaust system should not be close to the fresh-air intake vents.

### Testing Pressure Connections

Testing of the pressure connections for leaks of the nitrous system when first turned on and each time a gas cylinder is changed should be done routinely. High-pressure line connections should be tested for leaks quarterly by using a soap solution applied to the lines and connections to test for leaks. You can also purchase a portable infrared spectrophotometer to test these connections.

### Inspection of the equipment

On a daily basis, inspect all of the system components—reservoir bag, tubings, masks, connectors—for wear, cracks, holes, or tears, and replace any damaged pieces.

### Properly Fitting Mask

The mask should be properly fitted to each patient. Check that the reservoir bag does not overinflate or underinflate while the patient is breathing oxygen, before the nitrous is administered.

### Limit Talking

Inform your patients to limit talking during administration of the nitrous and to try to breathe through their nose, and avoid breathing through the mouth if possible.

### Exposure Assessment

Clinical staff, particularly those who work with the nitrous oxide delivery, can be assessed for exposure by wearing dosimetry badges or by placing an infrared spectrophotometer in the room.

RECALL

**9** Who was the first dentist to use $N_2O$ on his patients?
**10** What color code is used for $N_2O$ tanks?
**11** What can be included in making a safe environment when administering $N_2O$?
**12** What is given to the patient before and after $N_2O/O_2$ sedation?

## Antianxiety Agents

Drugs that are administered for the relief of anxiety are called **antianxiety drugs,** or *anxiolytics.* In larger doses, these drugs can produce sleep, sedation, and anesthesia. Antianxiety agents can be administered orally, intravenously, or by inhalation (gases). Before administering any form of these agents, the dentist is required to have specialized training and credentialing.

Sedatives may be prescribed for the following situations:

- Patients are very nervous and apprehensive about an upcoming procedure.
- The procedure itself is a long or difficult procedure.
- A mentally challenged patient is receiving treatment.
- Very young children who are undergoing extensive treatment.

The most common pharmacologic methods for sedation and control of anxiety involve the use of a short-acting benzodiazepine (examples are diazepam and midazolam), either alone or in combination with an opioid analgesic (fentanyl, morphine).

With these types of drugs, the patient will be asked to take the drug orally 30 to 60 minutes before the appointment. Patients must be informed that these drugs induce drowsiness and that they should not drive themselves to the appointment.

## Intravenous Sedation

The process of starting, monitoring, and removing intravenous (IV) sedation is completed only by an individual who is trained and certified in this area. The oral and maxillofacial surgeon and the periodontist are the two dental specialists who most often receive this additional training. Specialty offices often employ a registered nurse to administer and monitor IV sedation procedures. Some states credential the certified dental assistant to monitor and remove IV lines only after completion of a board-approved course.

Before the administration of IV conscious sedation, a physical examination is performed, and a pertinent history and signed consent are obtained. Parental or guardian informed consent is required for children. Baseline vital signs, level of consciousness, and motor function; **oximetry** (blood oxygen concentration) results; and the electrocardiogram (ECG) are completed and recorded (see Chapter 27 for more information on oximetry and ECG). The patient's weight should be recorded for dose determination.

IV conscious sedation results in a minimally depressed level of consciousness. The patient maintains the ability to keep an open airway and respond appropriately to physical or verbal stimulation. Specific antianxiety drugs are administered intravenously (directly into a vein) throughout the procedure at a slower rate, providing deeper stage I analgesia. IV lines are placed in a vein in the forearm or hand. A strong rubber tie, called a tourniquet, is wrapped around the upper arm to enlarge the veins in the lower arm by restricting blood flow through them. The skin over the vein is cleansed with an antiseptic. A small butterfly needle is inserted into the large vein on the top of the hand and is kept in place with tape and the tourniquet is released.

Throughout the surgery, the IV line should be monitored to make sure that there is no inflammation of the vein or pain at the insertion site, or that the needle has become dislodged and is leaking fluid under the skin. IV lines can become clotted or may crack. Frequent monitoring of the IV line helps avoid these problems. Most of these complications require removal of the IV catheter. If these problems occur, alert the surgeon immediately.

During IV conscious sedation, IV access must be maintained continuously. All patients are monitored throughout the procedure, as well as in the recovery phase. Physiologic measurements should be taken and recorded at least every 15 minutes. These measurements include, but are not limited to, level of consciousness, respiratory function, oximetry, blood pressure, heart rate, and cardiac rhythm. Supplemental $O_2$, suction, and a defibrillator must be available immediately and used as needed in case of an emergency situation.

**13** Is the patient conscious during intravenous sedation?

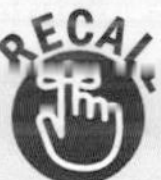


# General Anesthesia

Another method to administer antianxiety agents is through general anesthesia. General anesthesia is a controlled state of unconsciousness characterized by loss of protective reflexes, including the ability to maintain an airway independently and to respond appropriately to physical stimulation or verbal command. This method provides a controlled state of loss of consciousness, or stage III general anesthesia.

General anesthesia is achieved via a combination of gases—$N_2O/O_2$, halothane, or enflurane mixture—and IV agents such as thiopental and methohexital.

General anesthesia is most safely administered in a hospital setting or at outpatient surgical setting with the necessary equipment for administration and management of an emergency. **Anesthesiologists** are physicians who specialize in this form of anesthesia.

## Four Stages of Anesthesia

Specific antianxiety agents or a combination of agents can produce different levels of consciousness and unconsciousness. These levels are called *stages* of anesthesia.

*Stage I:* Analgesia is the stage during which a patient is relaxed and fully conscious. The patient is able to keep the mouth open without assistance and is capable of following directions. The patient experiences a sense of euphoria and a reduction in pain. Vital signs are normal. Depending on the agent, the patient can move into different levels of analgesia.

*Stage II:* Excitement is the stage during which the patient is less aware of immediate surroundings and may start to become unconscious. The patient may become excited and unmanageable. Nausea and vomiting may occur. Excitement is an undesirable stage.

*Stage III:* General anesthesia is the stage of anesthesia that begins when the patient becomes calm after stage II. The patient feels no pain or sensation. The patient soon becomes unconscious. This stage of anesthesia can be achieved only under the guidance of an anesthesiologist in a controlled environment such as a hospital setting.

*Stage IV:* Respiratory failure or cardiac arrest occurs when the lungs and heart slow down or stop functioning. If this stage is not reversed quickly, the patient can die.

## Patient Preparation

The patient must undergo a preoperative physical examination, laboratory tests, or both before the general anesthetic agent is administered. The patient or legal guardian must sign a consent form before anesthesia can be provided and the procedure performed.

## Patient Education

The dentist reviews the procedure, as well as the risks of and probable reactions to the general anesthesia. Most surgical procedures are scheduled in the early morning because patients must not eat or drink 8 to 12 hours before receiving general anesthesia (nothing-by-mouth, or nil per os [NPO], status). The patient must have a driver for transport home after the procedure.

## Patient Recovery

Once the procedure is completed, the patient is monitored closely until normal reflexes return. The patient should respond to name and be able to move the limbs, turn the head, and speak coherently. The patient should not be left alone while regaining consciousness.

14 Is the patient conscious during general anesthesia?
15 In what environment is general anesthesia most often administered?

## Mind-Body Medicine

Mind-body medicine is a method of reducing anxiety and pain through different nonpharmacologic techniques. Patients are instructed to train their mind to focus on their body and not what is unpleasant to them. Some of the most common techniques include the following:

- Distraction, in which the patient is distracted from the surroundings by something pleasant. Examples are listening to music, watching something on an iPad or screen with ear buds, or the use of virtual-reality goggles.
- Relaxation techniques, which can include the following:
  - Guided imagery or imagining a pleasant experience or soothing environment.
  - Deep breathing, which involves deep and slow breathing that floods the body with oxygen and other chemicals that enter the CNS and improve comfort.
  - Biofeedback, which teaches you how to relax and alter your behaviors, thoughts, and feelings of pain and anxiety.
  - Hypnosis can be self-induced or aided to help produce a relaxed state.
  - Acupuncture involves the placement of very thin needles to certain locations on the body. The body responds by releasing certain chemicals that produce an analgesic effect.

## Documentation of Anesthesia and Pain Control

Maintaining accurate records is an essential aspect of pain and anxiety analgesia. Always document the following measures and observations:

- Review of patient's medical history
- Preoperative and postoperative vital signs
- Type of anesthesia used
- Tidal volume if inhalation sedation was provided
- Time anesthesia began and ended
- Peak concentration administered
- Postoperative time (minutes) for patient recovery
- Adverse events or patient complaints

Record this information in the progress notes section of the patient record or on a separate form.

**■ Patient Education** Many patients are hesitant to discuss their fears about dental care because it is either "hearsay" from someone who had a negative experience, or is based on what they think will occur during the dental procedure. It is important for the patient to be aware of the types of pain and anxiety control measures that are available for patients. *Good communication* is the key to your patients being well informed, feeling confident about dental care, and becoming knowledgeable and compliant patients at future appointments. ■

**■ Legal and Ethical Implications** Some degree of risk is always associated with the use of any drug, even when administered by trained individuals. The dentist and the dental team have a responsibility to minimize risk to patients undergoing dental treatment by following these guidelines:

- Use only sedation methods with which they are thoroughly familiar.
- Limit the use of sedation methods to patients who require them.
- Conduct a comprehensive preoperative evaluation of the patient.
- Monitor the patient continuously.
- Document all drugs used in terms of dosage, vital signs, reactions, and recovery.
- Treat high-risk patients in an appropriate setting. ■

**■ Eye to the Future** How about a new field in dentistry called "nanodentistry"? Yes, little dental "nanorobots" could be programmed to crawl or swim through the body to interrupt or alter nerve impulses in individual nerve cells as a means of anesthesia. Researchers in Tokyo are looking into all types of applications in this field. ■

**■ Critical Thinking**

1. You are assisting in a restorative procedure. The dentist will be placing an amalgam in tooth #14. The dentist has indicated that a short-acting anesthetic agent will be used. What is the time frame for a short-acting anesthetic agent?
2. Describe where you will place the topical anesthetic for tooth #14 and what type of injection the dentist will perform for this procedure.
3. The dentist has completed giving anesthesia and transfers the syringe back to you. What is wrong with this scenario, and how do you handle it with the patient in the chair?
4. A 5-year-old child is scheduled to have a tooth restored with a stainless steel crown. The patient record already notes that there is pulpal damage, which means the tooth will require a pulpotomy. The patient is very apprehensive about the visit and what to expect. Describe additional anxiety and pain control measures that the dentist could use in combination with local anesthesia.
5. A patient is scheduled to have her third molars extracted. What type of pain control might the surgeon select to prolong the anesthesia and decrease bleeding around the surgical site?
6. You are scheduled to assist in a procedure that includes the monitoring of $N_2O/O_2$ sedation. You check all the equipment and review the procedure with the patient. You note that the patient seems to have some type of respiratory problem. When you inquire about this, the patient indicates that his allergies have been bothering him. How will this affect the administration of $N_2O$? ■

PROCEDURE 37.1 

# Applying a Topical Anesthetic

## EQUIPMENT AND SUPPLIES

- 2 × 2–inch gauze squares
- Topical anesthetic ointment
- Sterile cotton-tip applicator

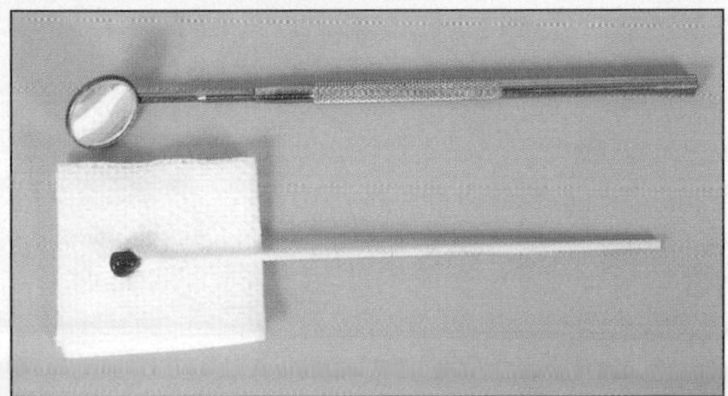

## PROCEDURAL STEPS

### Preparation

1 Place a small amount of topical ointment on the cotton-tip applicator, and then replace the cover of the ointment.

**NOTE** Never insert the same applicator into the ointment after it has been used and contaminated.

2 Explain the procedure to the patient.

**PURPOSE** Patients are more comfortable and less anxious when they are well informed and know what to expect.

3 Identify the injection site, and gently dry the site with gauze squares.

**PURPOSE** Drying the site allows the ointment to penetrate the surface area better and to not become diluted by saliva, which would decrease its effectiveness.

### Placement

4 Place the ointment directly onto the injection site.

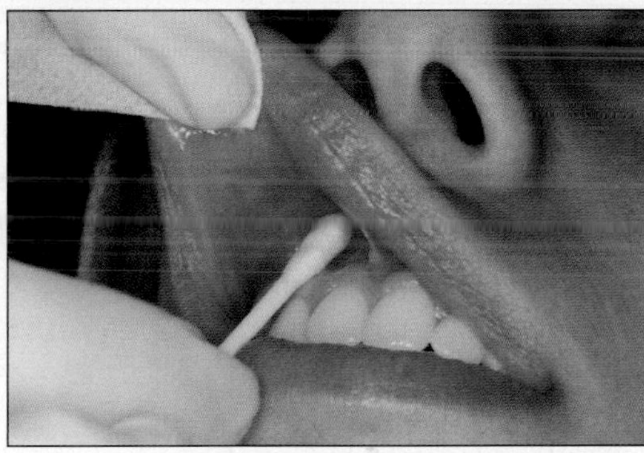

5 Repeat previous steps if multiple injections are to be given.

6 Allow the applicator to remain on the site for 15 to 30 seconds.

7 Remove the applicator just before the dentist gives the injection.

**PURPOSE** The site should not be wet with saliva; this would decrease the effect of the ointment.

PROCEDURE 37.2 

# Assembling the Local Anesthetic Syringe

## EQUIPMENT AND SUPPLIES

- Sterile syringe
- Sealed disposable needle or needles
- Sterile local anesthetic cartridges

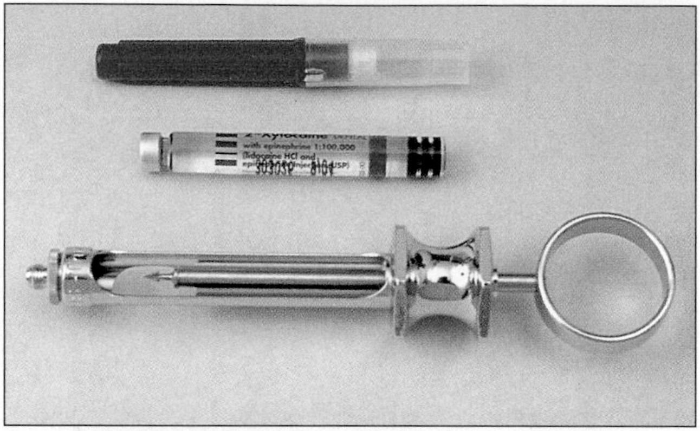

## PROCEDURAL STEPS

### Selecting the Anesthetic

1 The location of the injection will determine the needle length. The dentist determines the type of anesthetic solution to be used.

**PURPOSE** These choices depend on the patient's medical-dental history and the procedure.

2 Organize supplies, and position the items at chairside out of the patient's view.

3 Wash hands before preparing the syringe.

### Loading the Anesthetic Cartridge

4 Hold the syringe in one hand, and use the thumb ring to pull back the plunger.

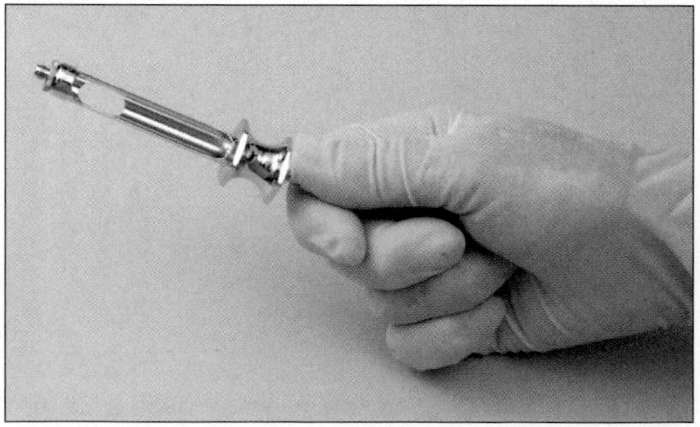

5 With the other hand, load the anesthetic cartridge into the syringe. The stopper end goes in first, toward the plunger.

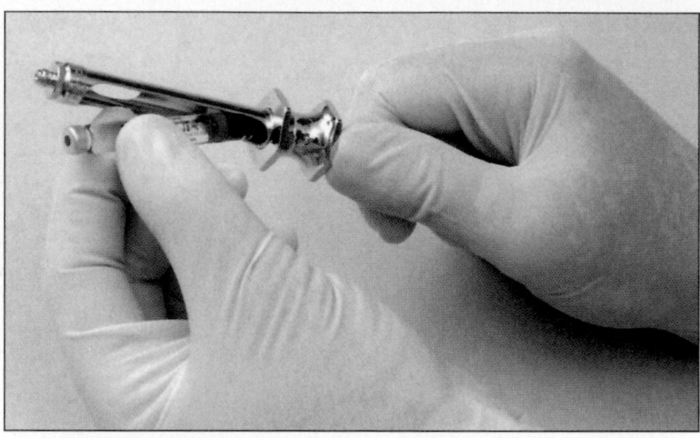

6 Release the thumb ring, and allow the harpoon to engage into the stopper.

7 Use gentle finger pressure to engage the piston forward until the harpoon is engaged into the stopper.

**NOTE** Do *NOT* hit the piston with the palm of your hand in an effort to engage the harpoon. This leads to fracturing of glass cartridges.

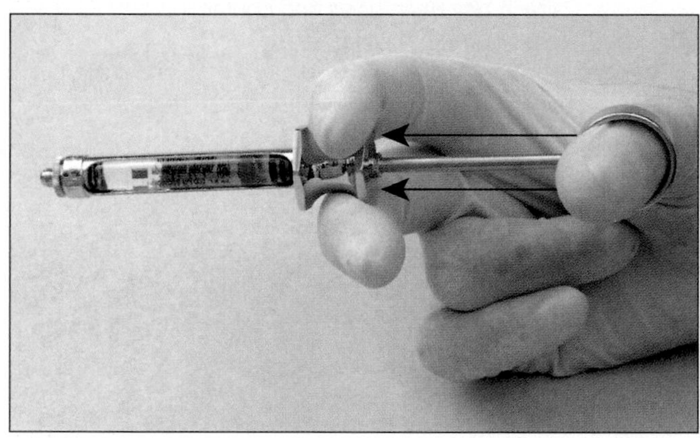

8 To check that the harpoon is securely in place, gently pull back on the plunger.

**PURPOSE** The harpoon must be securely engaged so the dentist can aspirate during the injection.

### Placing the Needle on the Syringe

9 Break the seal on the needle and remove the protective cap from the needle. The protective guard (clear plastic) is removed at this time. The needle guard is not yet removed.

10 Screw the needle into position on the syringe. Take care to position the needle so it is straight and firmly attached.

**PURPOSE** If the needle is not positioned correctly, the anesthetic solution may leak or may not flow properly.

## PROCEDURE 37.2 Assembling the Local Anesthetic Syringe—cont'd

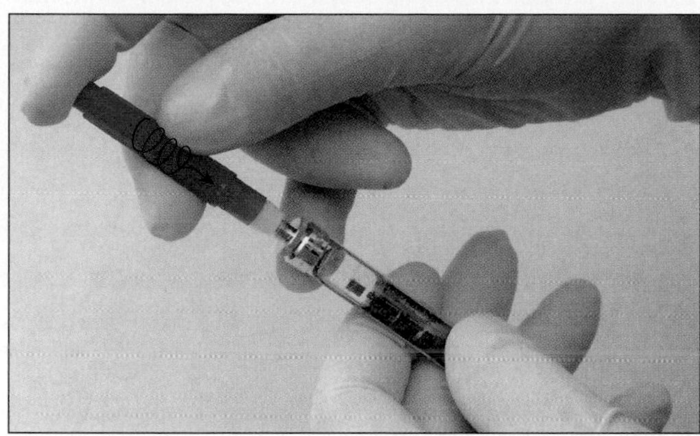

**11** Place the prepared syringe on the tray ready for use and out of the patient's sight.

**NOTE** It has been common teaching for years that the needle should be attached to the syringe before the anesthetic cartridge is placed. Stanley Malamed recommends the sequence stated here because it virtually eliminates the possibility of a broken cartridge or leakage of anesthetic solution during the procedure.

Photos in procedure from Malamed SF: Handbook of local anesthesia, ed 6, St Louis, 2013, Mosby.

## PROCEDURE 37.3

## Assisting in the Administration of Local Anesthesia

### EQUIPMENT AND SUPPLIES

- ✔ Topical anesthetic ointment
- ✔ Sterile cotton-tip applicators
- ✔ Sterile gauze sponges
- ✔ Sterile assembled local anesthetic syringe

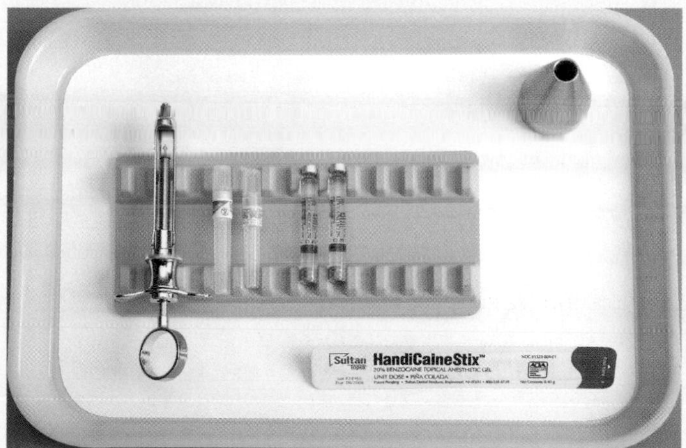


### PROCEDURAL STEPS

**1** Apply topical anesthetic to the appropriate area of injection (see Procedure 37.1).

**2** Loosen the needle guard.

**3** Transfer the syringe to the operator by placing the thumb ring over the dentist's thumb.

**NOTE** This exchange takes place just below the patient's chin and out of the patient's line of vision.

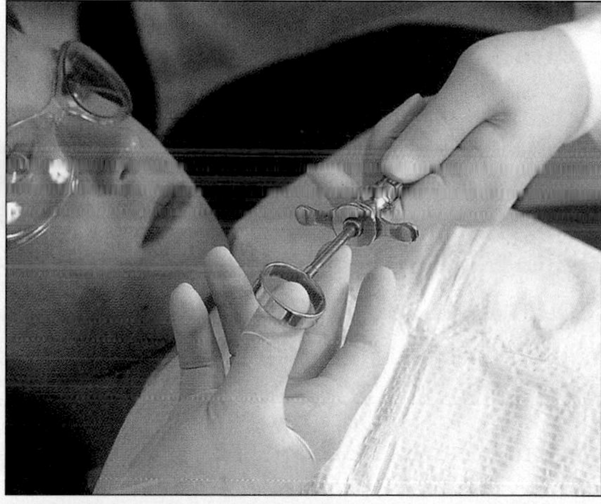

**4** While the dentist is giving the injection, monitor the patient for any adverse effects, and project a calming and relaxed manner.

**5** The dentist will replace the needle guard on the syringe by using a one-handed scoop technique or a recapping device.

**PURPOSE** This prevents the possibility of a needle stick injury.

(Continued)

## PROCEDURE 37.3 Assisting in the Administration of Local Anesthesia–cont'd

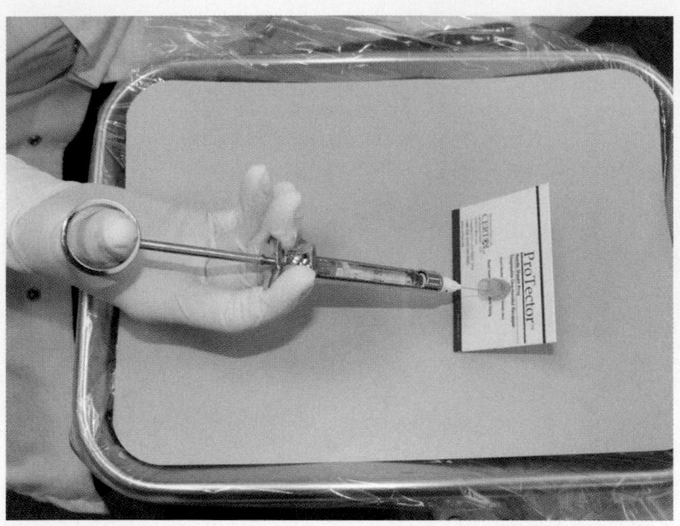


From Logothetis: DD: Local anesthesia for the dental hygienist, ed 2, St Louis, 2017, Elsevier.

6 After the injection is completed, have the patient turn toward you. Rinse the patient's mouth using the air-water syringe and the high-volume evacuator or the saliva ejector.
7 Continue monitoring the patient throughout the procedure for any adverse effects.
8 At the completion of the procedure, instruct the patient about the numbness, and tell the patient not to bite his or her lip or cheek.
9 Before leaving the dental treatment area, remove the used needle with the needle guard still in place, and dispose of it in the sharps container.
10 Remove the anesthetic cartridge and dispose of it with the medical waste. Place the syringe on the tray to be returned to the sterilization center.
11 Document the procedure.

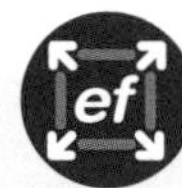

## PROCEDURE 37.4

# Assisting in the Administration and Monitoring of Nitrous Oxide/Oxygen Sedation (Expanded Function)

### PREREQUISITES FOR THE EFDA AND THE RDA

- Background knowledge of $N_2O/O_2$
- Equipment assembly and operation
- Taking and recording of vital signs

### EQUIPMENT AND SUPPLIES

- $N_2O/O_2$ system
- Scavenger-type masks (adult and child sizes)
- Equipment for measuring vital signs

### PROCEDURAL STEPS

1 Seat the patient, update the medical history, and take and record vital signs.
2 Review the use of $N_2O$ with the patient.
**PURPOSE** Informing the patient before administration helps eliminate fear of the unknown.
3 Place the patient in a supine position.

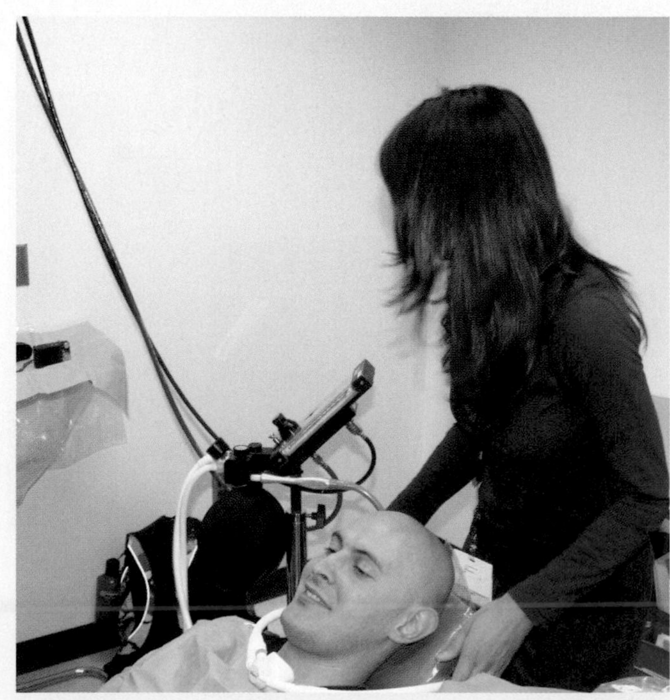

*From Malamed SF: Sedation: a guide to patient management, ed 5, St Louis, 2010, Saunders.*

## PROCEDURE 37.4 Assisting in the Administration and Monitoring of Nitrous Oxide/Oxygen Sedation (Expanded Function)–cont'd

4 Select and place a mask of appropriate size on the tubing.

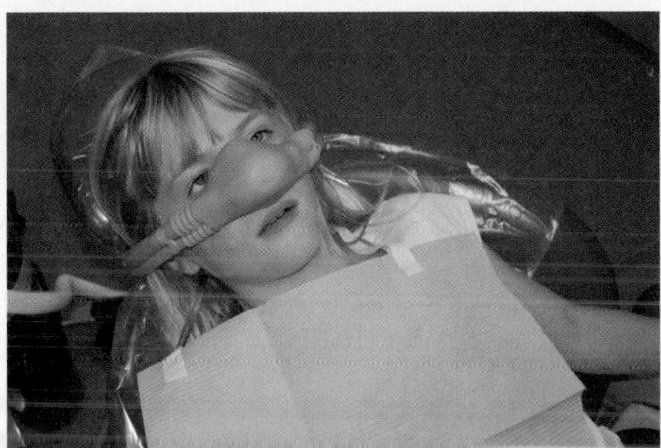

*From Clark MS, Brunick AL: Handbook of nitrous oxide and oxygen sedation, ed 4, St Louis, 2015, Mosby.*

5 Have the patient put on the mask, and adjust the fit.

6 Tighten the tubing once it is comfortable for the patient.

**PURPOSE** To eliminate the need for the patient to hold the mask in place, and to prevent leakage from around the mask.

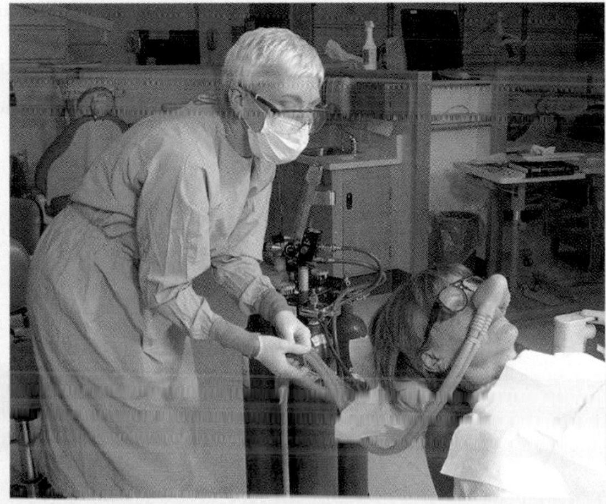

7 If the mask pinches or causes discomfort, place a gauze square under the edge.

### Administration

8 At the dentist's instructions, begin adjusting the flow meter for $O_2$ flow only. The patient is given 100 percent $O_2$ for at least 1 minute.

**PURPOSE** To assist the dentist in determining the patient's tidal volume.

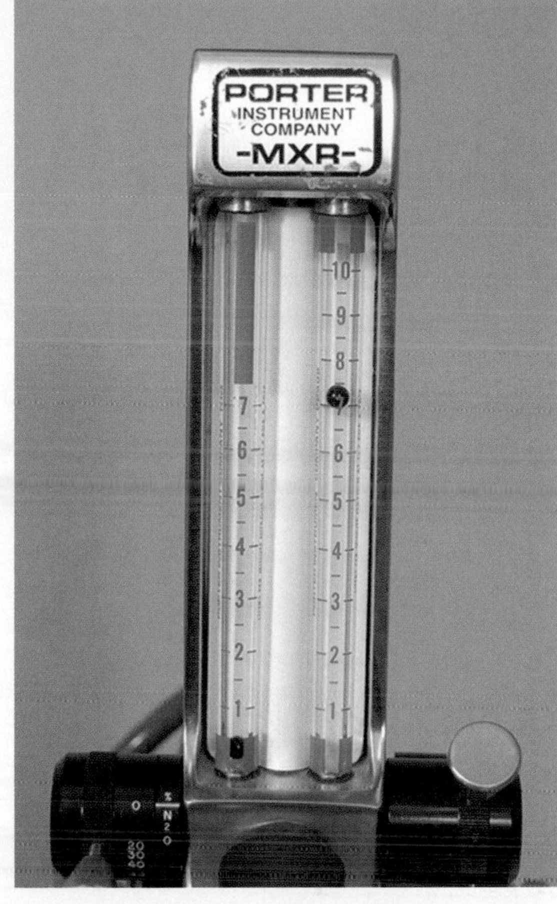


9 At the dentist's direction, adjust $N_2O$ flow in increments of 0.5 to 1 L/min, and reduce $O_2$ flow by a corresponding amount.

**NOTE** Most machines perform this function automat cally.

10 At 1-minute intervals, the previous step is repeated until the dentist determines that the patient has reached the baseline reading.

**PURPOSE** This slow process minimizes the risk of administoring too much $N_2O$

11 Note the patient's baseline level.

12 Monitor the patient closely throughout the procedure.

### Oxygenation

13 Toward the end of the procedure, $N_2O$ is depleted and 100 percent $O_2$ is administered, as directed by the dentist.

**PURPOSE** Oxygenation of patients for a minimum of 5 minutes helps prevent *diffusion* hypoxia, which creates a feeling of light-headedness.

14 After oxygenation is complete, remove the mask. *Slowly* position the patient upright.

**PURPOSE** Bringing the patient upright too quickly may cause postural hypotension (fainting).

15 Record the patient's baseline levels of $N_2O$ and $O_2$ and response during analgesia.

**PURPOSE** This documentation provides a legal record of care and serves as a reference for future care and administration of $N_2O/O_2$ sedation (analgesia).

16 Take and record vital signs.

17 Document the procedure.

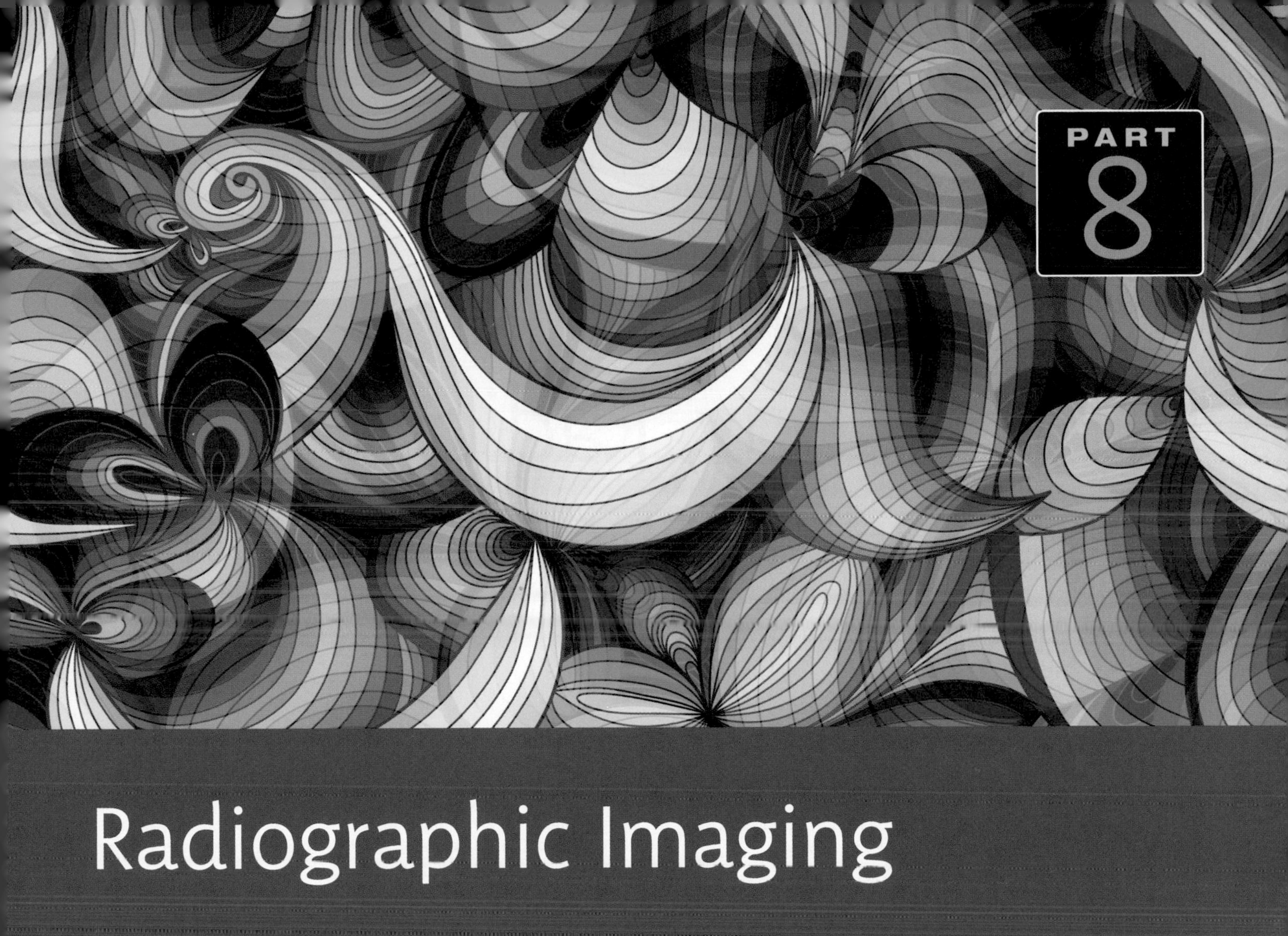


# Radiographic Imaging

Radiographic imaging involves the use of x-radiation to produce dental images that are essential in the practice of dentistry. These images may be produced on conventional x-ray film or by digital technology. Regardless of the technique that is used, a quality diagnostic image is necessary to identify and diagnose conditions that may otherwise go undetected. Your role as a dental assistant is to use x-radiation to produce diagnostic-quality images. You will also be responsible to manage the patient, maintain proper infection control, and *always* follow radiation safety procedures. Producing diagnostic-quality images with minimal exposure to radiation is your professional responsibility.

The chapters in this section will provide you with the information you need to understand radiation and how to use it safely in the dental office. You will learn the basic principles and techniques for film-based and digital imaging.

38

# Foundations of Radiography, Radiographic Equipment, and Radiation Safety

## KEY TERMS

**ALARA concept** Concept of radiation protection that states that all exposures should be kept "*a*s *l*ow *a*s *r*easonably *a*chievable."

**Anode (AN-ode)** The positive electrode in the x-ray tube.

**Atom** The basic unit of matter.

**Bremsstrahlung radiation** "Braking radiation." The sudden deceleration of electrons as they interact with highly positively charged nuclei.

**Cathode (KATH-ode)** The negative electrode in the x-ray tube.

**Central ray** X-rays at the center of the beam.

**Contrast** Differences in degrees of blackness on an image.

**Control panel** The portion of the x-ray unit that contains the master switch, the indicator light, the selector buttons, and the exposure button.

**Density** The overall darkness or blackness of an image.

**Dental radiography (ray-dee-OG-ruh-fee)** The process of recording images of the teeth and adjacent structures by exposure to x-radiation.

**Digital imaging** A filmless method of capturing an image and displaying it by using an image receptor, an electronic signal, and a computer to process and store the image.

**Distortion** Change in the size of an image caused by incorrect vertical angulation.

**Dose (of radiation)** The amount of energy absorbed by tissues.

**Dosimeter** A device used to detect and measure an accumulated dosage of radiation.

**Electron** A negatively charged particle in the atom.

**Energy** The ability to do work.

**Extension arm** Flexible arm that is attached to the x-ray tubehead.

**Genetic (juh-NE-tik) effects** Effects of radiation that are passed on to future generations through genetic cells.

**Image** Film-based or digitally produced recordings of anatomic structures.

**Image receptor** A recording medium for an image, normally film, phosphor storage plate (PSP), or a digital sensor.

**Intensity** The total energy of the x-ray beam.

**Ion (EYE-on)** An electrically charged particle.

**Ionization (eye-uh-ni-ZAY-shun)** Process by which electrons are removed from atoms, causing the harmful effects of radiation in humans.

**Ionizing (EYE-uh-nye-zing) radiation** Radiation that produces ionization, resulting in harmful effects.

**Kilovoltage (KIL-uh-voel-tuj) peak (kVp)** Highest voltage of x-ray tube used during an exposure.

**Latent (LAY-tent) period** Time between exposure to ionizing radiation and appearance of symptoms.

**Lead apron** Device used to protect the reproductive and blood-forming tissues from scatter radiation.

**Magnification** The proportional enlargement of an image.

**Master switch, indicator light, selector buttons, exposure button** Components of control panel.

**Matter** Anything that occupies space and has form or shape.

**Milliampere (mil-ee-AM-peer) (mA)** One one-thousandth (1/1000) of an ampere; a unit of measurement used to describe the intensity of an electrical current.

**Penumbra (puh-NUM-bruh)** The blurred or indistinct area that surrounds an image.

**Personal radiation monitoring badge** A device that measures exposure of personnel to ionizing radiation by measuring the intensity of visible light emitted from a crystal in the detector when heated. The intensity of light emitted is dependent upon the radiation exposure.

**Photon (FOE-ton)** A minute (tiny) bundle of pure energy that has no weight or mass.

**Primary beam** The most penetrating beam produced at the target of the anode.

**Primary radiation** Same as *primary beam.*

**Quality (of x-ray beam)** The mean energy or penetrating ability of the x-ray beam.

**Quantity (of x-ray beam)** The number of x-rays produced in the dental unit; the quantity of x-rays produced is controlled by milliamperage.

**Radiation** Forms of waves of energy emission through space or material.

**Radiograph (RAY-dee-oe-graf)** Image produced on photosensitive film by exposing the film to radiation and then processing it.

**Radiology (ray-dee-OL-uh-jee)** The science or study of radiation as used in medicine.

**Scatter radiation** A form of secondary radiation that occurs when an x-ray beam has been deflected from its path by interaction with matter.

**Secondary radiation** X-radiation that is created when the primary beam interacts with matter.

**Sensor** A solid-state image receptor that contains a silicon chip with an electric circuit.

**Sharpness** A measure of how well an image reproduces the fine details or outline of an object.

**Somatic (soe-MAT-ik) effects** Effects of radiation that cause illness and are responsible for poor health (such as cancer, leukemia, and cataracts) but are not passed on to offspring.

**Thyroid collar** A flexible lead shield that is placed securely around the neck.

**Tubehead** The part of the x-ray unit that contains the x-ray tube, the high-voltage and low-voltage transformers, and insulating oil.

**Tungsten target** A focal spot in the anode.

**X-radiation** High-energy ionizing electromagnetic radiation.

## LEARNING OUTCOMES

*On completion of this chapter, the student will be able to achieve the following objectives:*

1. Pronounce, define, and spell the key terms.
2. Describe uses of dental imaging.
3. Discuss the discovery of x-radiation and the pioneers in the history of dental radiography.
4. Discuss radiation physics, including the following:
   - Explain what happens during ionization.
   - Describe the properties of x-rays.
5. Identify the parts of the dental x-ray machine and the x-ray tube.
6. Explain how x-rays are produced.
7. Identify the types of radiation.
8. Discuss the characteristics of the x-ray beam, including the following:
   - Describe the three characteristics of the x-ray beam.
   - Describe how the kilovoltage affects the quality of the x-ray beam.
   - Describe how the milliamperage affects the quality of the x-ray beam.
   - Describe the difference between contrast and density.
9. Discuss the effects of radiation, including the following:
   - Discuss the biologic effects of radiation exposure on the human body.
   - Identify the critical organs that are sensitive to radiation.
10. Discuss how radiation is measured.
11. Discuss radiation safety, including the following:
    - Describe methods of protecting the patient from excess radiation.
    - Describe measures used to protect the operator from excess radiation.
    - Explain the ALARA concept.

## ELECTRONIC RESOURCES

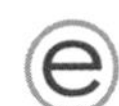

***Additional information related to content in Chapter 38 can be found on the companion Evolve Web site.***

- Canadian Content Corner
- Practice Quiz

The dental assistant must have a thorough knowledge and understanding of the importance and uses of dental imaging. Dental images are a necessary component of a comprehensive dental examination, as well as a part of the dental patient's permanent record. **Note:** The term **image receptor** is used in this text when referring to either a digital imaging sensor or to film because the image is recorded on one or the other, depending on the system being used.

Dental imaging enables the dentist to see conditions that are not visible in the oral cavity and to identify many conditions that might otherwise remain undetected. Many dental diseases and conditions have no clinical signs or symptoms and are typically discovered *only* through the use of dental imaging.

### Uses of Dental Images

- Detect dental caries in the early stages.
- Identify bone loss in the early stages.
- Locate abnormalities in surrounding hard and soft tissues.
- Evaluate growth and development.
- Provide information during dental procedures (such as root canal therapy).
- Document a patient's condition at a specific time.

To understand how dental **images** are produced, the dental assistant must first understand the fundamental concepts of atomic structure and have a working knowledge of ionizing radiation and the components of x-ray equipment. These are discussed later in this chapter.

**Radiation**, which is used to produce all types of dental images, has the ability to cause damage to all types of living tissues. Any exposure to radiation, *no matter how small,* has the potential to cause harmful biologic changes in the operator and the patient. The dental assistant must thoroughly understand the principles of safety when dealing with radiation.

This chapter provides a brief history of **dental radiography** and introduces you to radiation physics and the characteristics of radiation. You will learn the guidelines for radiation safety and methods used to protect the patient and yourself as the operator.

# Discovery of X-Radiation

Wilhelm Conrad Roentgen (RENT-guhn), a Bavarian physicist, discovered the x-ray in 1895 (Fig. 38.1). This monumental discovery revolutionized diagnostic capabilities and changed the practice of medicine and dentistry forever.

Before discovering the x-ray, Roentgen had experimented with the production of cathode rays (streams of electrons). He used a Crookes tube (vacuum tube), an electrical

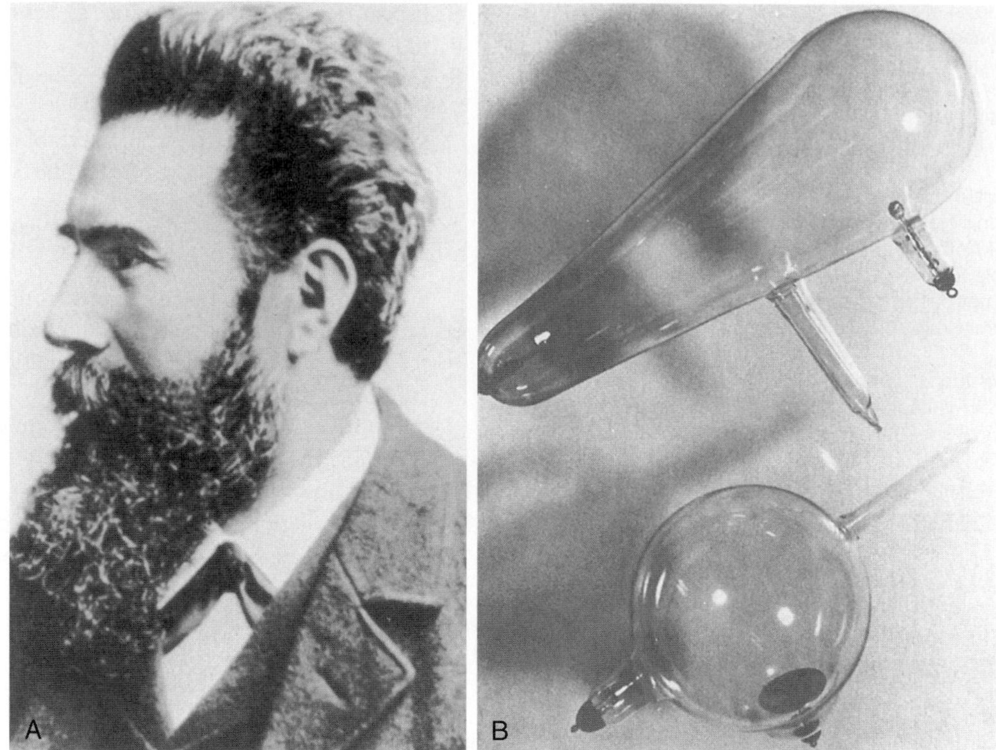


**FIG. 38.1** A, Wilhelm Conrad Roentgen (1845–1923), the discoverer of x-rays. B, A Crookes tube, which Roentgen worked with at the time of his discovery of x-rays in 1895. *(A, From Frommer HH, Stabulus JJ: Radiology for the dental professional, ed 9, St Louis, 2011, Mosby; B, from Goaz PW, White SC: Oral radiology and principles of interpretation, ed 2, St Louis, 1987, Mosby.)*

current, and special screens covered with a material that glowed *(fluoresced)* when exposed to x-rays. While working in a darkened laboratory with a vacuum tube, Roentgen noticed a faint green glow *(fluorescence)* coming from some screens across the room. He realized that something was causing the glow and knew he had discovered a powerful and unknown ray. He named his discovery the *x-ray.* (The symbol *x* is used in mathematics to represent the unknown.)

In the following weeks, Roentgen continued experimenting with the unknown rays. He replaced the fluorescent screens with photographic plates. He demonstrated that shadowed images could be permanently recorded on the photographic plate by placing objects between the tube and the plate. Roentgen placed his wife's hand on a photographic plate and exposed it to the unknown rays for 15 minutes. When he developed the photographic plate, the outline of the bones in her hands could be seen, representing the first radiograph of the human body (Fig. 38.2).

To honor Wilhelm Roentgen for his discovery, for many years x-rays were referred to as *roentgen rays,* **radiology** was referred to as *roentgenology,* and **radiographs** were known as *roentgenographs.* During his lifetime, Roentgen was awarded many honors and distinctions, including in 1901 the first Nobel Prize ever awarded in physics.

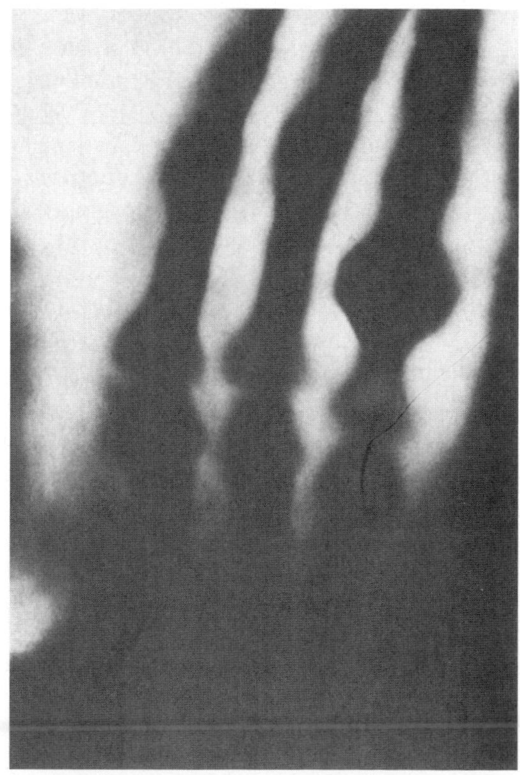

**FIG. 38.2** First radiograph of the human body, showing the hand of Roentgen's wife. *(From Goaz PW, White SC: Oral radiology and principles of interpretation, ed 2, St Louis, 1987, Mosby.)*

TABLE 38.1 Highlights in the History of Dental Radiography

| Year | Event | Individual/Group |
|---|---|---|
| 1895 | Discovery of x-radiation | W. C. Roentgen |
| 1896 | First dental radiograph<br>First U.S. dental radiograph (skull)<br>First U.S. dental radiograph (live patient) | O. Walkhoff<br>W. J. Morton<br>C. E. Kells |
| 1901 | First paper on dangers of x-radiation | W. H. Rollins |
| 1904 | Introduction of bisecting technique | W. A. Price |
| 1913 | First dental text*<br>First prewrapped dental films<br>First x-ray tube | H. R. Raper<br>Eastman Kodak<br>W. D. Coolidge |
| 1920 | First machine-made film packets | Eastman Kodak |
| 1923 | First dental x-ray machine | Victor Radiograph |
| 1925 | Introduction of bitewing technique | H. R. Raper |
| 1933 | Proposal of rotational panoramics concept | |
| 1947 | Introduction of long-cone paralleling technique | F. G. Fitzgerald |
| 1948 | Introduction of panoramic radiography | |
| 1955 | Introduction of D-speed film | |
| 1957 | First variable-kilovoltage dental x-ray machine | General Electric |
| 1978 | Introduction of dental xeroradiography | |
| 1981 | Introduction of E-speed film | |
| 1987 | Introduction of intraoral digital radiography | |
| 1999 | Oral and maxillofacial radiology recognized as a dental specialty | American Dental Association |
| 2001 | Introduction of F-speed intraoral film | Eastman Kodak |
| 2003 | Introduction of cone beam 3-D technology | |

*Modified from Iannucci J, Jansen Howerton L: Dental radiography: principles and practice, ed 4, St Louis, 2012, Saunders.

## Pioneers in Dental Radiography

Although Roentgen discovered the x-ray, others later helped to develop the field of dental radiography (Table 38.1). In fact, many of the early pioneers died from overexposure to x-rays. At the time x-rays were discovered, no one knew about the hidden dangers associated with the use of these penetrating rays.

In 1896 German dentist Otto Walkhoff made the first *dental* radiograph. He placed a glass photographic plate wrapped in black paper and rubber in his mouth and submitted himself to 25 minutes of x-ray exposure. Also in 1896 a New York physician made the first dental radiograph in the United States using a skull.

New Orleans dentist C. Edmund Kells is credited with the first practical use of radiographs in dentistry in 1896. During his many experiments, Dr. Kells exposed his hands to x-rays every day for years. This overexposure to **x-radiation** caused numerous cancers to develop on his hand. His dedication to the development of dental radiography eventually cost Dr. Kells his fingers, later his hand, and then his arm. After enduring much pain and faced with the prospect of becoming a burden to his family, he committed suicide in 1928.

Dr. W. H. Rollins in Boston was a pioneer in the field of radiation safety, and we follow his basic principles to this day.

Dental radiography has progressed from these early discoveries to its current status as an invaluable science. New technology continues to improve dental imaging capabilities.

## History of Dental X-Ray Equipment

William D. Coolidge, an electrical engineer, developed the first hot-cathode x-ray tube, a high vacuum tube that contained a tungsten filament. This was the prototype for modern x-ray tubes.

In 1923 a miniature version of the x-ray tube was placed in the head of an x-ray machine and immersed in oil (Fig. 38.3). This was the precursor for all modern dental x-ray machines. From that time on, the dental x-ray machine changed very little until a variable kilovoltage machine was introduced in 1957. In 1966 a recessed long-beam tubehead was introduced.

# Radiation Physics

All things in the world are composed of energy and matter. **Energy** is defined as the ability to do work. Although energy cannot be created or destroyed, it can change form. **Atoms** are

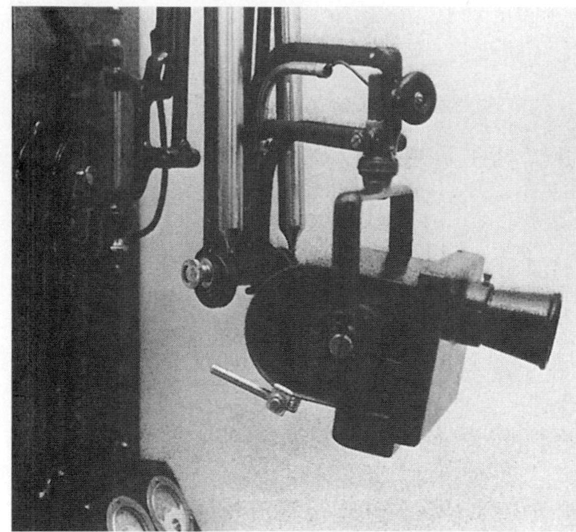

FIG. 38.3 Victor CDX shockproof tube housing (1923). *(From Goaz, White SC: Oral radiography and principles of interpretation, ed 2, St Louis, 1987, Mosby.)*

the basic form of *matter,* and they contain energy. **Matter** is anything that occupies space and has form or shape.

Matter has many forms, including solids, liquids, and gases. Matter is composed of atoms grouped together in specific arrangements called *molecules* (Fig. 38.4). A molecule is the smallest particle of substance that retains the property of the original substance. The fundamental unit of matter for discussion in this chapter is the atom.

## Atomic Structure

The *atom* consists of two parts: a central nucleus and orbiting electrons (see Fig. 38.4). An atom is identified by the composition of its nucleus and the arrangement of its orbiting electrons. The arrangement within the atom is similar to that of the solar system: The atom has a nucleus (sun) at its center, and the electrons (planets) revolve (orbit) around the nucleus. Electrons remain stable in their orbit unless disturbed or moved. X-rays can disturb the orbiting electrons.

### Nucleus

The nucleus, or dense core of the atom, is composed of particles known as *protons* and *neutrons.* Protons carry positive electrical charges, whereas neutrons carry no charge.

Dental x-rays do not affect the tightly bound nucleus of the atom and are changed only in direction, or scattered. Dental x-rays *cannot make atoms radioactive;* that is, patients do not give off x-rays after the x-ray machine stops producing x-rays.

### Electrons

**Electrons** are tiny, negatively charged particles that have very little mass. The orbital path of an electron around the nucleus is called an *electron shell.* Each shell can contain only a specific number of electrons. Electrons are maintained in orbit by electron binding energy, a force similar to gravity.

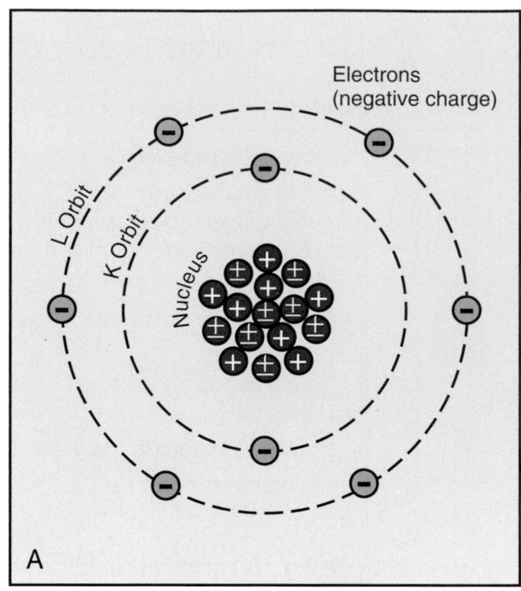


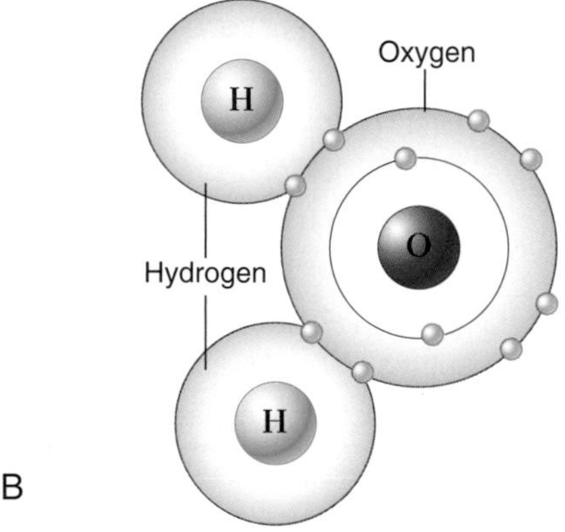


FIG. 38.4 A, Diagrammatic representation of an oxygen atom. B, A molecule of water ($H_2O$) consists of two atoms of hydrogen connected to one atom of oxygen. *(B, From Patton KT, Thibodeau GA: Anatomy and physiology, ed 9, St Louis, 2016 Mosby.)*

### Bremsstrahlung Radiation

**Bremsstrahlung radiation** is produced when an electron passes near the nucleus of an atom. The negatively charged (–) electron is deflected by the positively charged (+) nucleus. Energy lost by deceleration of the electron is emitted in the form of a photon of radiation called *bremsstrahlung* (from the German word for "braking"). Braking radiation is the primary kind of radiation produced in the dental x-ray tubehead (Fig. 38.5).

## Ionization

Electrons remain stable in their orbit around the nucleus until radiograph photons collide with them. A **photon** is a minute (tiny) bundle of pure energy that has no weight or mass.

**Ions** are atoms that gain or lose an electron and become electrically unbalanced. X-rays have enough energy to produce ions because of a process called **ionization**. In this process, electrons are removed from the orbital shells of electrically stable atoms through collisions with x-ray photons (Fig. 38.6).

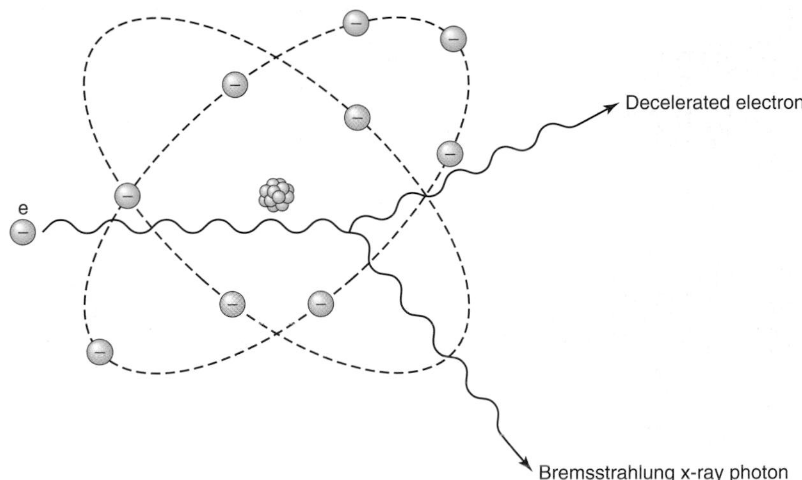


**FIG. 38.5** Bremsstrahlung radiation. This radiation occurs in the target anode material. The incoming electron (from the cathode) slows as it is drawn to the nucleus of the atom. Some of the energy lost in the deceleration is emitted as an x-ray photon with energy equal to that lost by the electron. *(From Miles DA, Van Dis ML, Williamson GF, et al: Radiographic imaging for the dental team, ed 4, St Louis, 2009, Saunders.)*

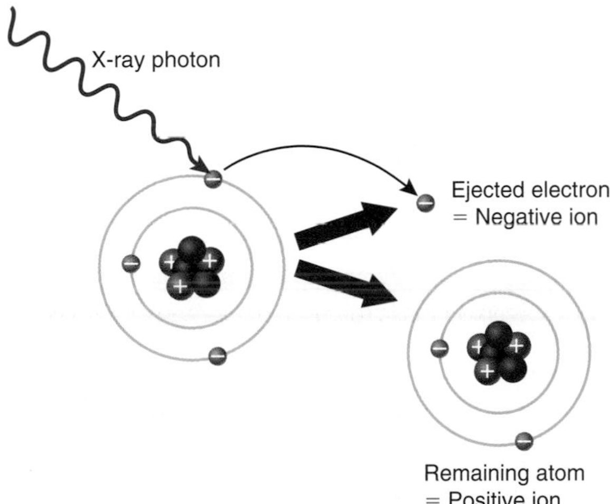


**FIG. 38.6** Ionization occurs when an electron is removed from the orbital shell of the electronically stable atom. *(© Elsevier Collection.)*

## Properties of X-Rays

The dental assistant must be familiar with the unique characteristics of x-rays (Box 38.1). X-rays are a form of energy that can penetrate matter. X-rays belong to a group classified as *electromagnetic radiation* (Fig. 38.7). Visible light, radar, radio, and television waves are also classified as electromagnetic radiation. Electromagnetic radiation is made up of photons that travel through space at the speed of light in a straight line with a wavelike motion.

The *shorter* the wavelength of the x-ray, the *greater* is its energy. Because of their high energy, short wavelengths can penetrate matter more easily than longer wavelengths, making shorter wavelengths especially useful in dentistry (Fig. 38.8).

**BOX 38.1 Characteristics of X-Rays**

- Invisible and undetectable by the senses
- No mass or weight
- No charge
- Travel at speed of light
- Travel in short-wavelength, high-frequency waves
- Travel in straight line and can be deflected or scattered
- Absorbed by matter
- Cause ionization
- Can cause certain substances to fluoresce
- Can produce image on photographic film
- Cause changes in living cells

Modified from Iannucci J, Jansen Howerton L: Dental radiography: principles and techniques, ed 4, St Louis, 2012, Saunders.

1 Who discovered x-rays?
2 Who was the first person to make practical use of x-rays in dentistry?
3 What is ionization?

## The Dental X-Ray Machine

Depending on the age and the manufacturer, dental x-ray machines may vary slightly in size and appearance, but all machines have three primary components: the **tubehead**, an **extension arm**, and the **control panel** (Fig. 38.9).

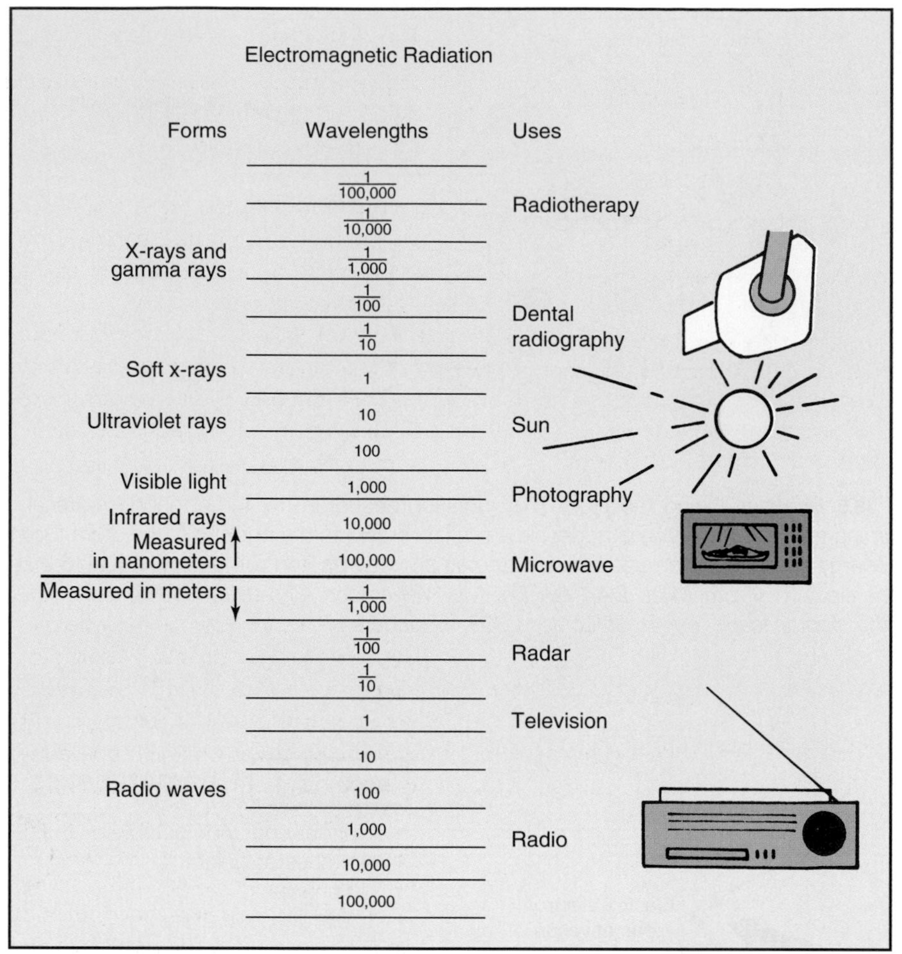


**FIG. 38.7** Electromagnetic spectrum, showing the various wavelengths of radiation typically used.

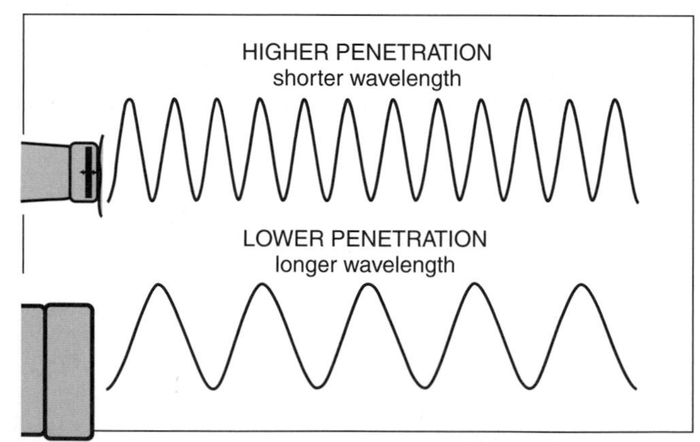


**FIG. 38.8** A wavelength is the distance between the crest (peak) of one wave and the crest of the next. Frequency is the number of wavelengths that pass a given point in a certain amount of time. The shorter the wavelength, the higher the frequency will be, and vice versa. *(From Hagen-Ansert SL: Textbook of diagnostic sonography, ed 7, St Louis, 2012, Mosby.)*

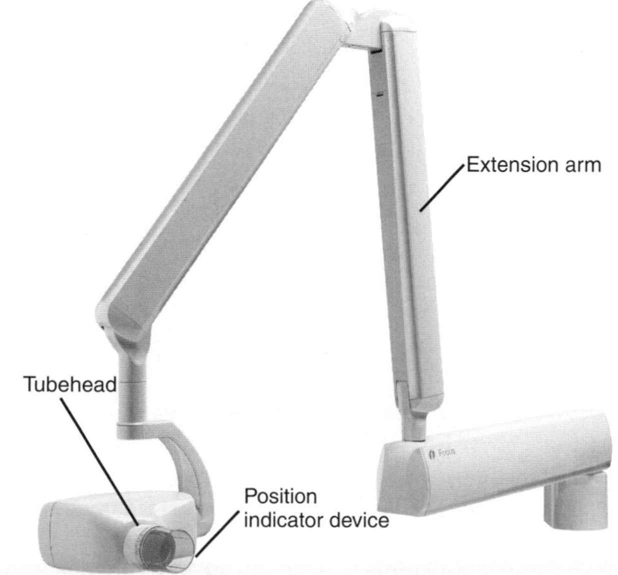


**FIG. 38.9** GX-770 intraoral x-ray machine. *(Courtesy of KaVo Kerr.)*

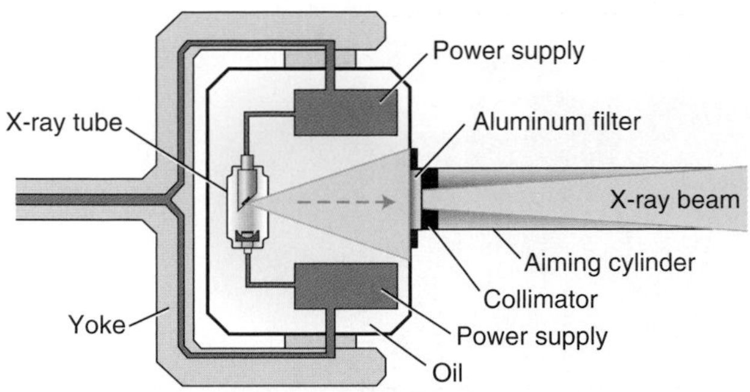


**FIG. 38.10** Tubehead showing a recessed x-ray tube, components of the power supply, and oil that conducts heat away from the x-ray tube. Path of useful x-ray beam (blue) from the anode, through the glass wall of the x-ray tube, oil, and finally an aluminum filter. The size of the beam is restricted by the metal tube housing and collimator. Low-energy photons are removed by the filter. *(From White SC, Pharoah MJ: Oral radiology: principles and interpretation, ed 7, St Louis, 2014, Mosby.)*

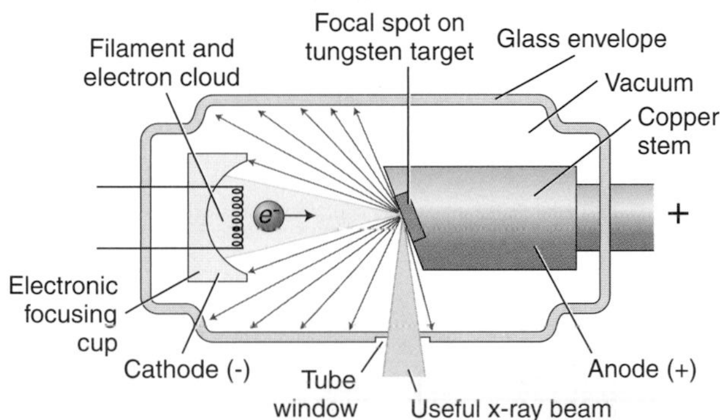


**FIG. 38.11** X-ray tube with the major components labeled. The path of the electron beam is shown in yellow. X-rays produced at the target travel in all directions. The useful x-ray beam is shown in blue. *(From White SC, Pharoah MJ: Oral radiology: principles and interpretation, ed 7, St Louis, 2014, Mosby.)*

## Tubehead

The x-ray tubehead is a tightly sealed, heavy metal housing that contains the radiograph tube. The components of the tubehead are as follows (Fig. 38.10):

- The housing is the metal body that contains the x-ray tube.
- Insulating oil fills the housing and surrounds the x-ray tube. Oil prevents overheating by absorbing the heat created by the production of x-rays.
- The tubehead seal, made of leaded glass or aluminum, keeps the oil in the tubehead and acts as a filter for the x-ray beam.
- The x-ray tube is where x-rays are produced (Fig. 38.11).
- The transformer alters the voltage of incoming electrical current.

The lead collimator is a metal disc with a small opening in the center. It is located inside the position indicator device (PID), in the path of the x-ray beam. The small opening forms the size and shape of the x-ray beam as it leaves the tubehead. The collimator limits the size of the x-ray beam to a circular 2-inch opening at the PID. When the size and shape of the beam are changed to a rectangle only slightly larger than the film, the amount of tissue exposed to radiation can be reduced by more than one half (Fig. 38.12).

The aluminum filter is a 0.5-mm-thick sheet located inside the PID in the path of the x-ray beam that filters out the nonpenetrating, longer-wavelength radiographs.

The PID is the open-ended lead-lined cylinder that extends from the opening of the metal housing.

## X-Ray Tube

The x-ray tube is the heart of the x-ray–generating system. It is made of glass and is about 6 inches long and 1 inch in diameter. Air has been removed from the tube to create a vacuum. This vacuum environment allows electrons to flow with minimum resistance between the electrodes (cathode and anode) (Fig. 38.13).

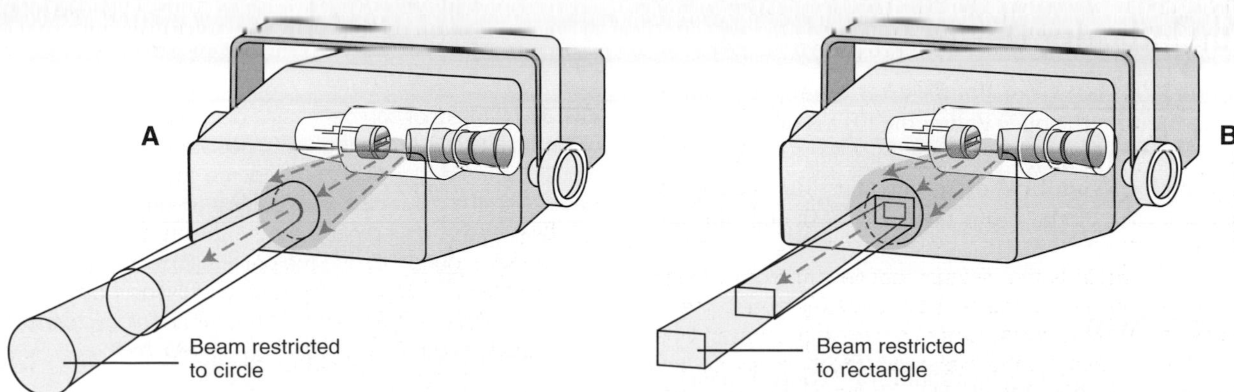


**FIG. 38.12** Collimation of an x-ray beam (blue) is achieved by restricting its useful size. A, Circular collimator. B, Rectangular collimator restricts area of exposure to just larger than the detector size and thereby reduces unnecessary patient exposure. *(From White SC, Pharoah MJ: Oral radiology: principles and interpretation, ed 7, St Louis, 2014, Mosby.)*

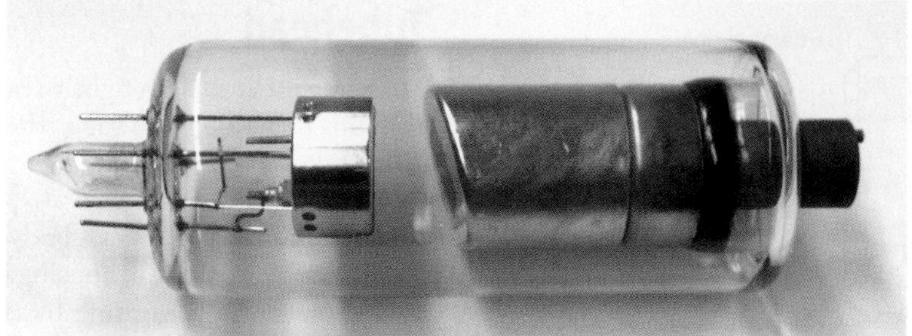

FIG. 38.13 Dental stationary x-ray tube with cathode on left and copper anode on right. *(From White SC, Pharoah MJ: Oral radiology: principles and interpretation, ed 7, St Louis, 2014, Mosby.)*

### Cathode

The **cathode**, or *negative (–) electrode,* consists of a tungsten filament in a focusing cup made of molybdenum. The purpose of the cathode is to supply the electrons necessary to generate x-rays. Electrons are generated in the x-ray tube at the cathode. The hotter the filament becomes, the more electrons are produced.

The *focusing cup* keeps electrons suspended in an electron cloud at the cathode. When the exposure button is pressed, the circuit within the tubehead is completed, and electrons rapidly cross from the cathode to strike the anode.

### Anode

The **anode**, or *positive (+) electrode,* acts as the target for the electrons. It is composed of a **tungsten target** (a small block of tungsten) that is embedded in the larger copper stem. The copper around the target conducts the heat away from the target, thus reducing wear on the target.

The tungsten target serves as a focal spot and converts the bombarding electrons into x-ray photons. The oil absorbs about 99 percent of the x-rays generated by this process, and this energy is given off as heat. The remaining 1 percent exits the tubehead through the port (opening) as a divergent beam toward the patient. The x-rays at the center of this beam are known, collectively, as the **central ray**.

## Position Indicator Device

The lead-lined PID is used to aim the x-ray beam at the film in the patient's mouth. The open end of the PID is placed close to the patient's face during film exposure (Figs. 38.14 and 38.15). The PID may be cylindrical or rectangular. The rectangular PID limits the size of the beam to that of a dental film (see Chapter 39).

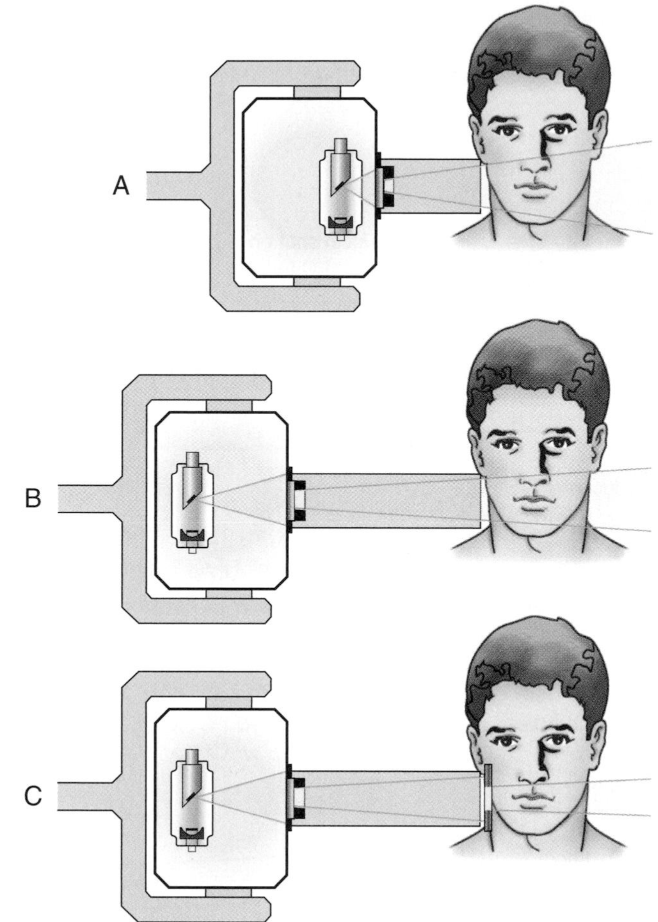


FIG. 38.14 Effect of source-to-skin distance and collimation on the volume of tissue irradiated. A larger volume of irradiated tissue results with the use of a short source-to-skin distance (A) compared with the use of a longer source-to-skin distance (B), which produces a less divergent beam. Using a rectangular collimator between the round PID and the patient (C) results in a smaller, less divergent beam and a smaller volume of tissue irradiated than A or B. *(From White SC, Pharoah MJ: Oral radiology: principles and interpretation, ed 7, St Louis, 2014, Mosby.)*

## Extension Arm

The wire between the tubehead and the control panel is enclosed in the hollow extension arm. The arm also has an important function in positioning the tubehead.

The tubehead is attached to the extension arm by means of a yoke that can be turned 360 degrees horizontally (Fig. 38.16). *Horizontally* means to move in a side-to-side motion. *Vertically* means to move in an up-and-down motion. These movements are necessary to align the tubehead and the film.

The extension arm folds up and can be swiveled from side to side. Never leave the extension arm in an extended position when the machine is not in use, because the weight of

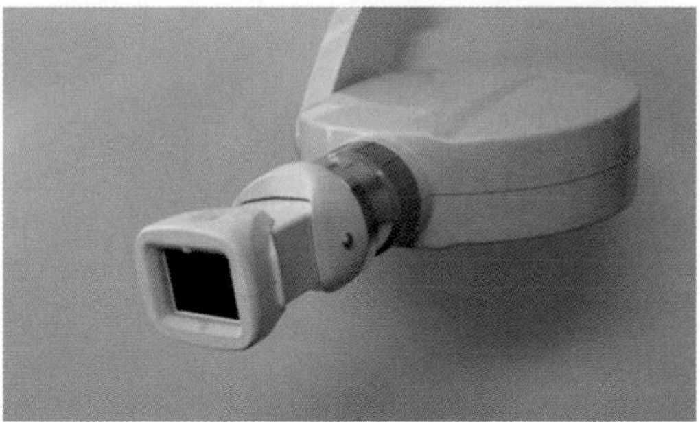

**FIG. 38.15** A rectangular PID mounted on an x-ray machine provides a means to limit the shape of the x-ray beam to just larger than the film or digital sensor. *(Courtesy Margraf Dental Manufacturing, Inc.,* www.margrafdental.com.*)*

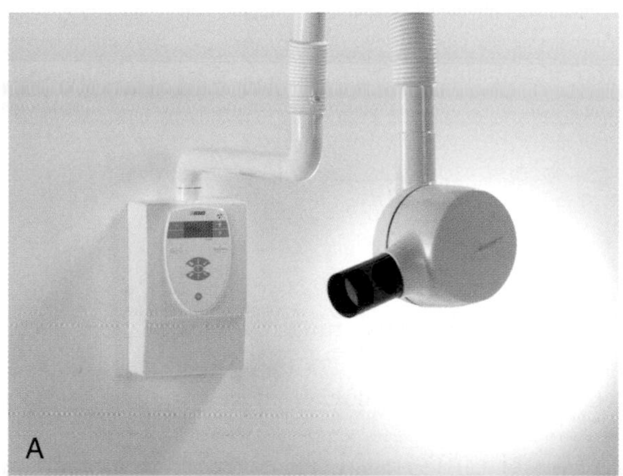


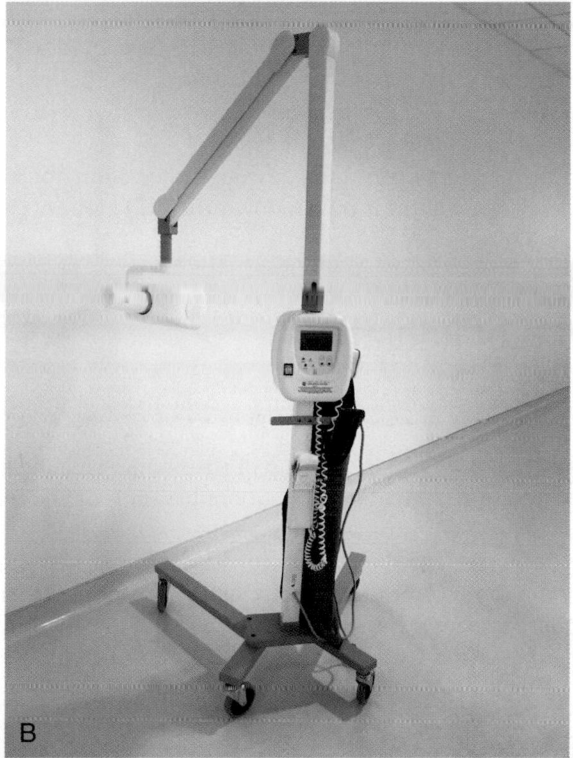


**FIG. 38.16** A, Heliodent intraoral x-ray machine. B, Portable dental x-ray unit. *(A, Courtesy Sirona Dental Inc., Charlotte, NC.)*

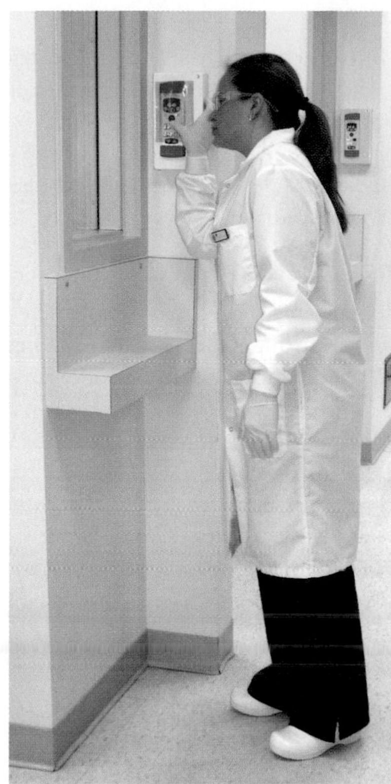

**FIG. 38.17** The operator stands at the control panel located outside the x-ray room.

the tubehead can cause it to become loose. If the tubehead is loose, it can *drift* (slip out of position) after it is positioned for an exposure. This movement can cause a *cone cut* (central ray positioned off the film). If the tubehead drifts, the arm should be repaired immediately. The dental assistant or the patient must *never* hold the tubehead to keep it in place during exposure.

## Control Panel

The control panel is located on a wall outside the x-ray area to prevent radiation exposure to the operator while the film is exposed (Fig. 38.17). The control panel contains the **master switch**, an **indicator light**, **selector buttons**, and an **exposure button**. The selector button is used to select the exposure time, **milliamperage (mA)**, and kilovoltage (kV), thereby regulating the x-ray beam. A single, centrally located control panel may be used to operate several tubeheads located in separate treatment rooms.

### *Master Switch and Indicator Lights*

The master switch is used to turn the machine on and off. An orange indicator light shows when the master switch is on. The x-ray machine may be safely left on all day because it does not produce radiation unless the exposure button is being pushed. The red emission indicator light comes on *only* when the exposure button is being pushed and x-rays are being emitted.

### Exposure Button

The exposure button controls the flow of electricity to generate the x-rays. The timer is electronically controlled to provide precise exposure time, and x-rays are generated *only* while the exposure timer is pressed. The exposure time is measured in fractions of a second, called *impulses* (60 impulses = 1 second; 30 impulses = 0.5 second).

### Milliamperage Selector

The mA of a dental x-ray machine is a measure of the electrical current that passes through the tungsten filament. The milliamperage selector controls the number of electrons produced. Increasing the milliamperage increases the quantity of electrons available for the production of x-rays. This is discussed in greater detail later in this chapter.

### Kilovoltage Selector

The **kilovoltage peak (kVp)** selector is used to control the penetrating power of the x-ray beam. Dental x-ray machines generally operate at 70 or 90 kVp. The effects of kilovoltage settings are discussed later in this chapter.

RECALL

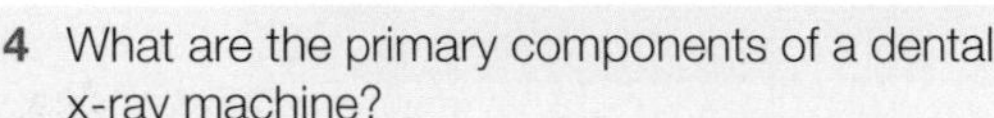

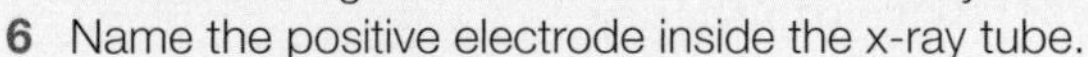

4 What are the primary components of a dental x-ray machine?
5 Name the negative electrode inside the x-ray tube.
6 Name the positive electrode inside the x-ray tube.
7 What does the control panel contain?

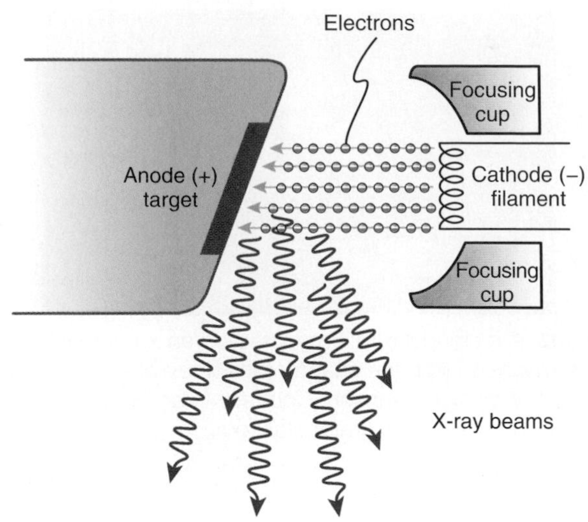


**FIG. 38.18** The production of dental images occurs in the x-ray tube. When the filament circuit is activated, the filament heats up, and thermionic emission occurs. When the exposure button is activated, the electrons are accelerated from the cathode to the anode. Electrons strike the tungsten target, and their kinetic energy is converted to x-rays and heat. *(From Langlais RP, Miller CS: Exercises in oral radiology and interpretation, ed 5, St Louis, 2017, Elsevier.)*

## X-Ray Production

When the x-ray machine is plugged into the wall outlet and the machine is turned on, the electrical current enters the control panel, and the following events occur in an *instant:*

- The current travels from the control panel to the tubehead through electrical wires in the extension arm.
- The current travels through the step-down transformer to the filament of the cathode. The purpose of the step-down transformer is to decrease the voltage from the incoming 110 or 220 volts to 3 to 5 volts.

The filament circuit uses the 3 to 5 volts to heat the tungsten filament in the cathode portion of the x-ray tube. Heating of the filament results in thermionic emission. *Thermionic emission* is the release of electrons from the tungsten filament when the electrical current passes through it and heats it up. The electrons stay in an electron cloud around the tungsten filament within the focusing cup, until the high-voltage circuit is activated by pushing the exposure button.

Then, after the exposure button is engaged, x-rays are produced in an instant in the following way (Fig. 38.18).

- Pushing the exposure button activates the high-voltage circuit. The electrons in the cloud are shot across the x-ray tube to the anode. The molybdenum cup in the cathode directs the electrons to the tungsten target in the anode.
- The electrons speed from the cathode to the anode. When the electrons strike the tungsten target, their energy of motion *(kinetic energy)* creates x-rays and heat. Less than 1 percent of the energy is converted to x-rays, with 99 percent lost as heat.
- The heat is carried away from the copper stem and is absorbed by the insulating oil in the tubehead.
- The x-rays travel through the unleaded glass window of the tube, the tubehead seal, and the aluminum filter. The aluminum filter removes the longer-wavelength x-rays from the beam.
- The x-ray beam then travels through the collimator, where its size is restricted; it travels down the PID and exits at the opening.

## Types of Radiation

X-radiation is described as primary, secondary, or scatter radiation (Fig. 38.19).

**Primary radiation** is made up of the x-rays that come from the target of the x-ray tube. Primary radiation is often referred to as the *useful beam,* or **primary beam**.

**Secondary radiation** refers to x-radiation that is created when the primary beam interacts with matter. For example, secondary radiation is created when the x-rays of the primary beam contact the patient's tissues. Secondary radiation is *less* penetrating than primary radiation. Secondary radiation is *not* useful radiation because it produces fog on the radiograph, damaging the diagnostic quality.

**Scatter radiation** is a form of secondary radiation that occurs when an x-ray beam has been deflected from its path

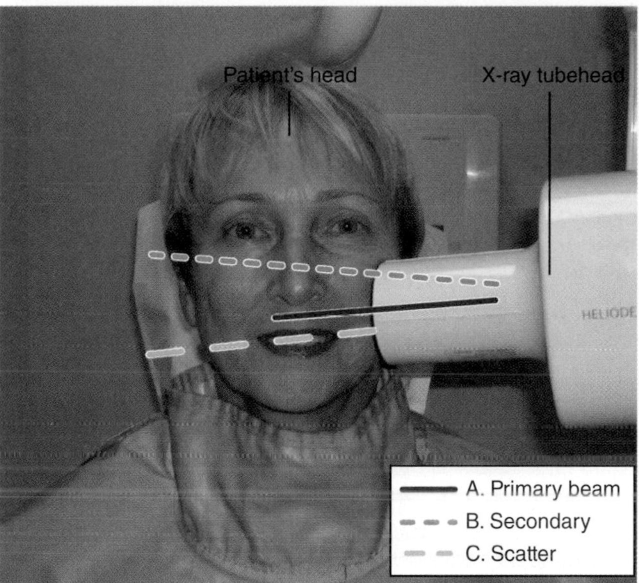


**FIG. 38.19** Types of radiation interaction with the patient: primary, secondary, and scatter.

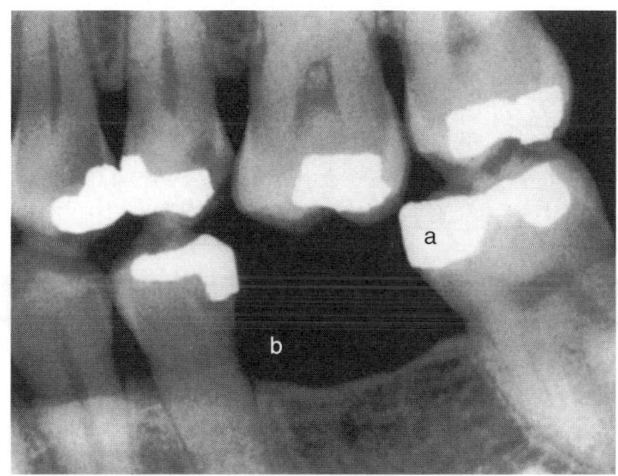


**FIG. 38.20** Bitewing radiograph showing radiopaque (white, *a*) area of amalgam restoration and radiolucent (black, *b*) area of air and cheek tissue.

through interaction with matter. Scatter radiation is deflected in all directions by patient tissues and travels to all parts of the patient's body and to all areas of the dental operatory. Scatter radiation is dangerous to both the patient and the operator.

## Radiolucent and Radiopaque Characteristics

Body structures that radiation can easily pass through appear *radiolucent* (dark) on an image. For example, air spaces, soft tissues, abscesses, tooth decay, and dental pulp appear as radiolucent images (Fig. 38.20).

Body structures that radiation does not easily pass through appear *radiopaque* (white or light gray) on an image. Tooth enamel, dense areas of bone, and metal restorations are examples of radiopaque images.

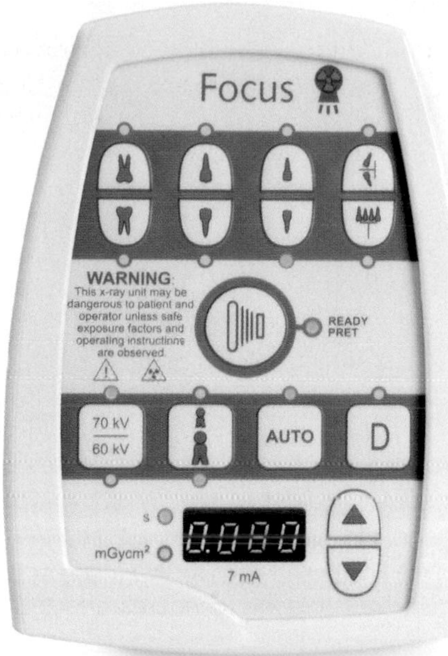


**FIG. 38.21** Kilovoltage peak (kVp) and milliamperage (mA) controls. *(Courtesy Instrumentarium Dental Inc., Milwaukee, WI.)*

RECALL

8 Name the three types of radiation.
9 Describe the difference between radiopaque and radiolucent.
10 Give examples of structures that appear radiolucent on a radiograph.
11 Give examples of structures that appear radiopaque on a radiograph.

# Characteristics of X-Ray Beam

There are three characteristics of the x-ray beam. They are described as the **quality**, **quantity**, and **intensity** of the x-ray beam. These characteristics determine the contrast, density, and image detail—the qualities necessary for a good image. On older x-ray units, the kilovoltage peak, milliamperage, and time could all be changed manually. Modern dental radiographic equipment has predetermined settings for the various areas of the mouth (Fig. 38.21). Even though the modern equipment is easy and convenient to use, the dental assistant should understand how variations in these three characteristics of the x-ray beam influence the quality of the images.

## Quality

In dental radiography, the term *quality* is used to describe the energy or penetrating ability of the x-ray beam. The quality or wavelength and energy of the x-ray beam are controlled by kilovoltage. The use of 85 to 100 kV produces more penetrating dental x-rays with more energy and shorter wavelengths. The use of 65 to 75 kV produces less penetrating dental

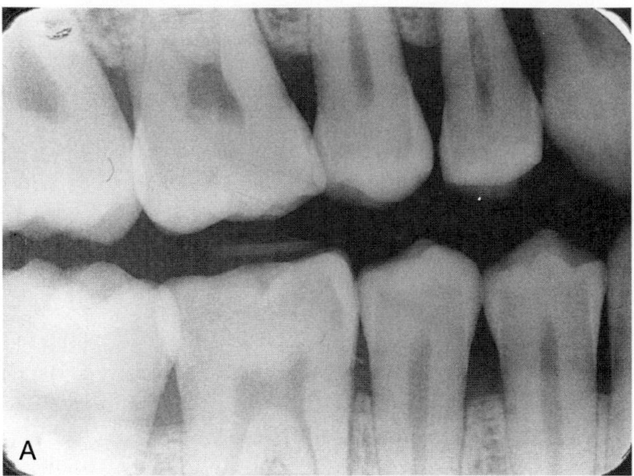


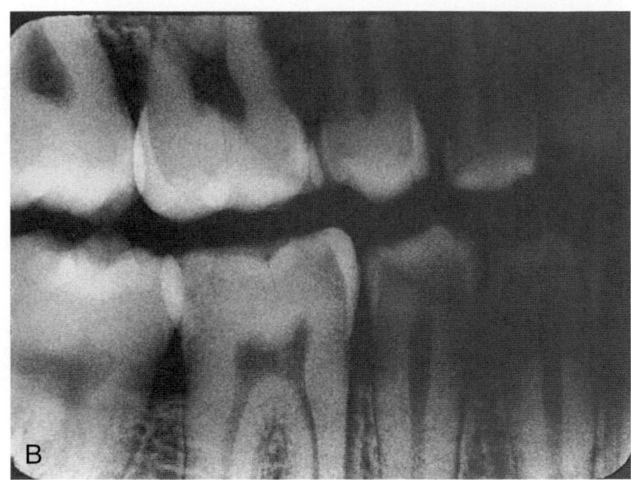


**FIG. 38.22** A, Diagnostic radiograph. B, Increase in kilovoltage results in an image that exhibits increased density; the image appears darker. *(From Iannucci J, Jansen Howerton L: Dental radiography: principles and techniques, ed 5, St Louis, 2017, Elsevier.)*

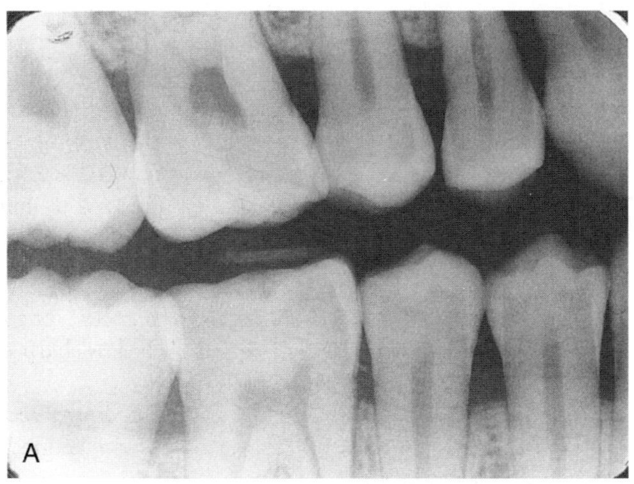


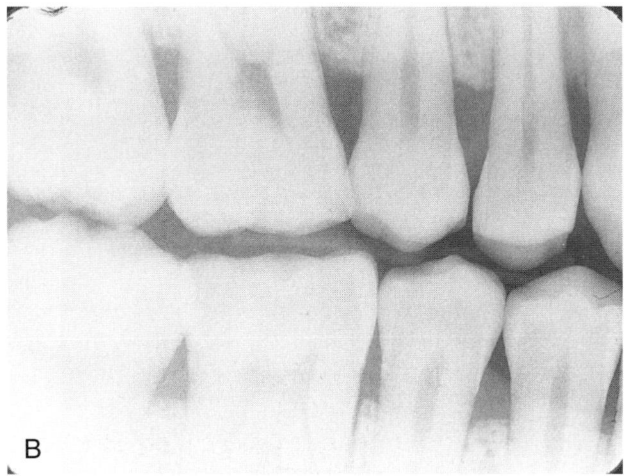


**FIG. 38.23** A, Diagnostic radiograph. B, Decrease in kilovoltage results in an image that exhibits decreased density; the image appears lighter. *(From Iannucci J, Jansen Howerton L: Dental radiography: principles and techniques, ed 5, St Louis, 2017, Elsevier.)*

x-rays with less energy and longer wavelengths. A higher kilovoltage should be used when the area to be examined is dense or thick. **Density** is the overall darkness or blackness of an image. A change in the kP (kilovoltage peak) results in a change in the density of a dental radiograph (Figs. 38.22 and 38.23).

## Quantity

Quantity of the x-ray beam refers to the number of x-rays produced in the dental x-ray unit. The **ampere (A)** is the unit of measurement used to describe the number of electrons, or current flowing through the cathode filament. Because the number of amperes needed to operate a dental x-ray unit is very small, amperage is measured in milliamperes (mA). One milliampere is equal to 1/1000 of an ampere. In dental radiography, the use of 7 to 15 mA is required; a setting above 15 mA is not recommended because it would cause excessive heat production in the x-ray tube.

## Intensity

Intensity is the combination of the number of x-ray photons (quantity) and the energy of each photon (quality). The intensity of the x-ray beam is affected by a number of factors, including the kilovoltage peak, milliamperage, exposure time, and distance (Table 38.2).

## Contrast

The image on a radiograph appears in a range of shades from black to white with multiple shades of gray (Fig. 38.24). This range is referred to as the *gray scale.*

The range of shades of gray to black to white is called **contrast**. The ideal contrast of a film clearly shows the radiopaque white of a metal restoration, the radiolucent black of air, and the many shades of gray between these extremes. *Higher* kilovoltage produces more penetrating radiographs and *lower* radiographic contrast, as follows:

- A 90-kVp setting requires less exposure time and produces an image that has low contrast (more shades of gray).
- A 70-kVp setting requires a slightly longer exposure time and produces an image with high contrast (fewer shades of gray).
- The amount of contrast in a film often reflects the dentist's preference. Some dentists prefer images with more contrast, whereas others prefer low contrast.

## Density

**Density** is the overall blackness or darkness of a film. An image with the correct density enables the dentist to view black areas (air spaces), white areas (enamel, dentin, and bone), and gray areas (soft tissues). The degree of density is controlled by the *milliampere seconds (mAs).*

The mAs control the amount of time given to exposure of the image. If the exposure time is too short, or a low **milliampere (mA)** setting is used, the resulting image will not have the correct overall density or will be light in appearance (see Table 38.2). Other factors that influence the density of an image include the following:

- *Distance from the x-ray tube to the patient.* If the operator lengthens the source-film distance without changing the exposure settings, resulting images will be light or less dense.
- *Developing time and temperature.* If the processing time is too long, the image will appear dark.
- *Body size of the patient.* A patient who is very small or thin requires less radiation than a husky, heavy-boned person.

**TABLE 38.2** Influence of X-Ray Beam Factors on Density and Contrast of Images

| Factor | Effect |
|---|---|
| **Milliamperage (mA)** | |
| ↑ | Increased density |
| ↓ | Decreased density |
| **Kilovoltage Peak (kVp)** | |
| ↑ | Long-scale contrast; low contrast<br>Increased density |
| ↓ | Short-scale contrast; high contrast<br>Decreased density |
| **Time** | |
| ↑ | Increased density |
| ↓ | Decreased density |

## Geometric Characteristics

Three geometric characteristics affect the quality of the image: sharpness, magnification, and distortion.

**Sharpness** refers to how well an image reproduces the fine details or distinct outlines of an object. Sharpness is sometimes referred to as *detail, resolution,* or *definition* as is seen on a high-definition television. The fuzzy or blurred area that surrounds an image is called the **penumbra**. The sharpness of an image is influenced by the following factors:

- *Focal spot size.* A machine with a small focal spot produces a sharper image than a machine with a larger focal spot size.
- *Film composition.* Fast film speeds result in less sharp detail because of the large crystal size.
- *Movement.* Any movement of the patient or image receptor (the film or **sensor**), no matter how slight, will degrade the sharpness of the image.

**Distortion** refers to the disproportionate change in the size of images that is caused by excessive or insufficient vertical angulation. Elongation and foreshortening of images are discussed in Chapter 41.

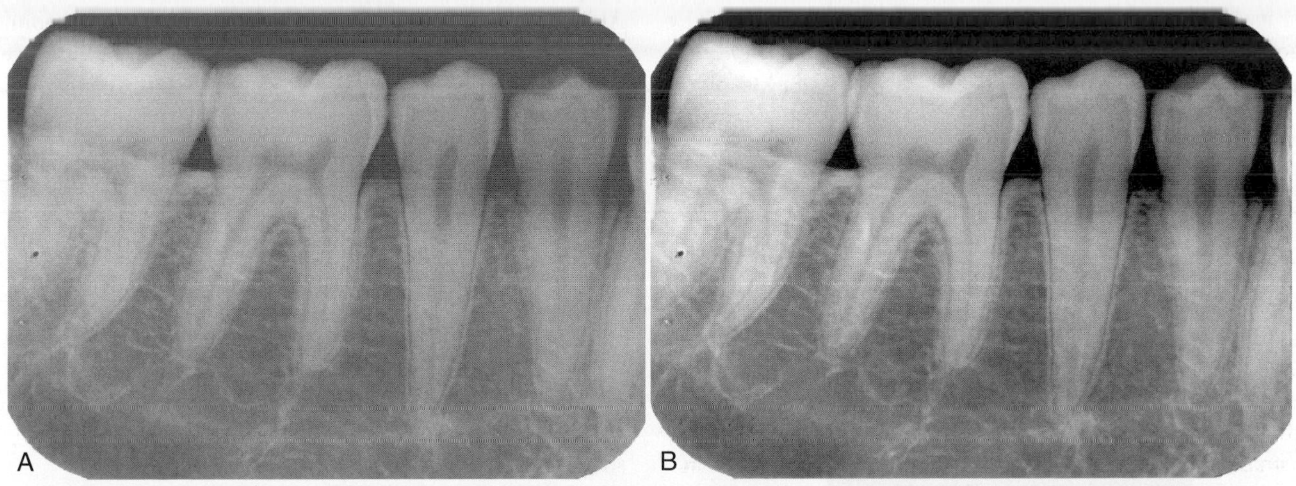


**FIG. 38.24** Radiograph showing low contrast (A) and high contrast (B). *(From White SC, Pharoah MJ: Oral radiology: principles and interpretation, ed 7, St Louis, 2014, Mosby.)*

**Magnification** refers to the proportionate enlargement of a dental image.

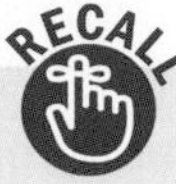


12 What are the three characteristics of the x-ray beam?
13 Which exposure factor controls contrast?
14 What is meant by density on a dental radiograph?

## Radiation Effects

All **ionizing radiation** is harmful and produces biologic changes in living tissues. Although the amount of x-radiation used in dental imaging is small, biologic changes do occur. Thus the dental assistant must know how the harmful effects of radiation occur and how to discuss radiation risks with patients. The entire x-ray area is considered a radiation hazard area, and a radiation hazard area sign must be posted in sight of all personnel and patients (Fig. 38.25).

## Tissue Damage

In dental radiography, not all x-rays pass through the patient and reach the dental film; the patient's tissues absorb some x-rays. When the energy from the x-ray photon is absorbed, chemical changes result in biologic damage.

### Ionization

Ionization results in the harmful effects of x-rays in humans. Ionization can cause disruption of cellular metabolism and permanent damage to living cells and tissues (see earlier discussion). The atoms that lose electrons become positive ions; as such, they are unstable structures capable of interacting with and damaging other atoms, tissues, or chemicals.

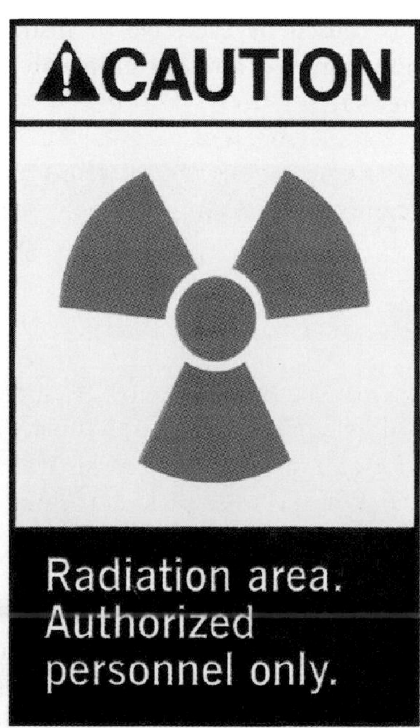


**FIG. 38.25** Sign indicating a radiation hazard area.

## Biologic Effects

Exposure to radiation can bring about changes in body chemicals, cells, tissues, and organs. The effects of radiation may not become evident for many years after the time the x-rays were absorbed. This time lag is called the **latent period.**

### Cumulative Effects

Exposure to radiation has a cumulative effect over a lifetime. This means that when tissues are exposed to x-rays, some damage occurs. Although tissues can repair some damage, the tissues do not return to their original state. The cumulative effect of radiation exposure can be compared with the cumulative effect from repeated exposure over the years to the rays of the sun (Table 38.3).

### Acute and Chronic Radiation Exposure

*Acute radiation exposure* occurs when a large **dose** of radiation is absorbed in a short period, such as in a nuclear accident. *Chronic radiation exposure* occurs when small amounts of radiation are absorbed repeatedly over a long period. The effects of chronic radiation exposure may not be observed until years after the original exposure.

### Genetic and Somatic Effects

Table 38.4 compares the relative radiation sensitivity (high to low) of cells and tissues. Note that the skin, eye, and oral mucosa, all of which might be affected by dental imaging, have a "fairly high" sensitivity to radiation.

X-rays affect both genetic and somatic cells. *Genetic* cells are the reproductive cells (sperm and ova). Damage to genetic cells *is* passed on to succeeding generations. These changes from **genetic effects** are referred to as *genetic mutations.*

All other cells in the body belong to the group of *somatic* tissues (*somatic* refers to the body). X-rays can damage somatic tissue, but damage from **somatic effects** is *not* passed on to future generations (Fig. 38.26).

## Critical Organs

Although the risk associated with dental x-rays is minimal, some tissues and organs are exposed to more radiation when

**TABLE 38.3** Disorders of Critical Organs Resulting from Cumulative Radiation Exposure

| Critical Organ | Disorder |
|---|---|
| Lens of the eye | Cataracts |
| Bone marrow | Leukemia |
| Salivary gland | Cancer |
| Thyroid gland | Cancer |
| Skin | Cancer |
| Gonads | Genetic abnormalities |

**TABLE 38.4** Relative Radiation Sensitivity of Cells and Tissues

| Radiation Sensitivity | Cell/Tissue |
|---|---|
| High | Small lymphocyte<br>Bone marrow<br>Reproductive cells |
| Fairly high | Skin<br>Lens of eye<br>Oral mucosa |
| Medium | Connective tissue<br>Small blood vessels<br>Developing bone and cartilage |
| Fairly low | Mature bone and cartilage<br>Salivary gland<br>Thyroid gland<br>Kidney<br>Liver |
| Low | Muscle tissue<br>Nerve tissue |

Modified from Miles DA, Van Dis ML, Williamson GF, et al: Radiographic imaging for the dental team, ed 4, St Louis, 2009, Saunders.

dental images are exposed. The following organs are more sensitive to radiation and thus are called *critical organs:*

- *Skin.* Because it is exposed during dental imaging procedures, skin is considered a critical organ. The effects of radiation on skin can be seen as reddening, or erythema, similar to sunburn. This effect requires moderate to high doses of radiation, which are not used in normal dental radiography.
- *Thyroid gland.* If a thyroid collar were not used, the radiation dose to the thyroid gland could be significant. In adults, thyroid tissue is considered fairly resistant to radiation, but the thyroid gland in children is radiation sensitive.
- *Lens of the eye.* High doses of radiation to the lens of the eye can cause cataracts (a cloudiness of the lens). However, many experts no longer consider the lens of the eye a critical organ in dental imaging because of the low dose. Using the paralleling technique further reduces exposure to the eye (see Chapter 40).
- *Bone marrow.* Significant radiation-induced changes in bone marrow can result in leukemia. Bone marrow sites are active in the mandible and skull, and this should be a consideration in dental imaging.

RECALL

15 What is the name of the process that results in the harmful effects of x-rays?
16 What is the name of the time period between x-ray exposure and the appearance of symptoms?
17 What is meant by genetic effects of radiation?

# Radiation Measurement

Radiation can be measured in a manner similar to time, distance, and weight. Just as distance can be measured in

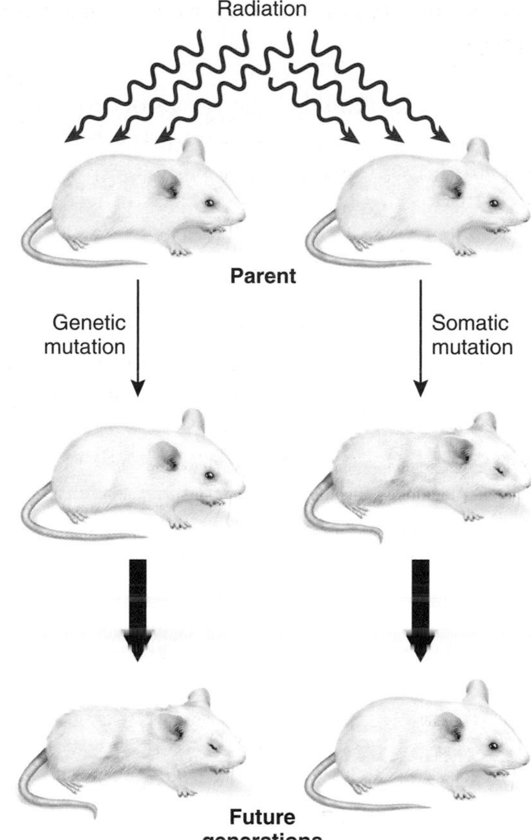


**FIG. 38.26** Comparison of somatic and genetic effects of radiation. *(© Elsevier Collection.)*

miles or kilometers and time can be measured in hours or minutes, two sets of systems are used to define the ways in which radiation is measured. The older system is referred to as the *traditional system,* or *standard system.* The newer system is the metric equivalent known as the *Système Internationale (SI).*

The traditional units of radiation measurement include (1) the *roentgen* (R), (2) the *radiation **a**bsorbed **d**ose* (rad), and (3) the *roentgen equivalent in [hu]man* (rem). SI units include (1) *coulombs* per kilogram (C/kg), (2) the *gray* (Gy), and (3) the *sievert* (Sv). Both systems are presented in Table 38.5.

# Maximum Permissible Dose

The maximum permissible dose (MPD) is defined by the National Council on Radiation Protection and Measurements (NCRP) as the maximum dose equivalent that a body is permitted to receive in a specified period of time. The MPD is the dose of radiation that the body can endure with little or no injury.

The NCRP published recommendations specifying dose limits for exposure to ionizing radiation. The most recent report in 2003 states that the current MPD for persons occupationally exposed to radiation is 5000 millirem (mrem), or 5.0 rems/year (0.05 Sv/year). For non–occupationally exposed persons, the current MPD is 0.1 rem/year (0.001 Sv/year).

Dental personnel should strive for an occupational dose of *zero* by adhering to strict radiation protection practices. Zero exposure is not difficult to achieve when radiation safety precautions are taken. Dental personnel should not exceed the *maximum accumulated lifetime dose,* calculated as follows:

$$(N-18)\times 5\text{ rems/year or }(N-18)\times 5\text{ Sv/year}$$

In this formula, $N$ is the operator's age.

RECALL

**18** Name the two systems of radiation measurement.
**19** What is the maximum permissible dose of radiation for occupationally exposed persons?

### Dentist's Responsibilities for Dental Imaging

- Prescribe only images that are required for diagnostic purposes.
- Ensure that all radiographic equipment is maintained in safe working condition.
- Ensure that appropriate shielding protects staff and patients from the effects of radiation.
- Require that all personnel who obtain images be properly trained, credentialed, and appropriately supervised while exposing images.
- Use only techniques that will produce diagnostic-quality images with minimal radiation exposure to the patient and operator.
- Follow the state, province, or territory's radiographic licensing requirements, rules, and regulations.
- Participate in obtaining informed consent from patient and family.
- Review the patient's record to determine when images were last taken.

## Radiation Safety

We are exposed to radiation every day of our lives. *Background radiation* comes from natural sources such as radioactive materials in the ground and cosmic radiation from space (Table 38.6).

Exposure from medical or dental sources is an additional radiation risk. Because of concerns, patients frequently say, "I've heard x-rays are bad for me. Do you really have to take them?" The dental assistant should anticipate this patient reaction and should be prepared to explain to the patient the risks and diagnostic benefits of dental imaging techniques.

When dental images are prescribed and properly taken, the benefit of disease detection far outweighs the risk for biologic damage associated with receiving small doses of radiation (Table 38.7). However, when images must be retaken because of poor operator technique, the patient is exposed to unnecessary additional radiation.

The decision to expose new radiographic images must be based on how recently previous film images were obtained and the clinical need for additional images. Dental images should never be taken on a "routine basis."

## Protective Devices

Other measures that provide further patient protection include the use of properly operating radiographic equipment. The x-ray tubehead must be equipped with appropriate aluminum filters, lead collimators, and PIDs. Equipment should be checked on a regular basis by state or federal regulating agencies. Faulty or malfunctioning equipment should be repaired immediately.

### *Aluminum Filtration*

The purpose of the aluminum filter is to remove the low-energy, long-wavelength, least-penetrating x-rays from the beam. These x-rays are harmful to the patient and are not useful in producing a diagnostic-quality image.

X-ray machines operating at 70 kVp or greater must have aluminum filtration of 2.5 mm. This is a federal requirement.

### *Collimator*

The collimator, used to restrict the size and shape of the x-ray beam to reduce patient exposure, may have a round or a rectangular opening. A rectangular collimator restricts the beam to an area slightly larger than size 2 intraoral film and significantly reduces patient exposure.

**TABLE 38.5** Units of Radiation Measurement

| Quantity | SI Units | Traditional Units | Conversion |
|---|---|---|---|
| Exposure | Coulombs per kilogram (C/kg) | Roentgen (R) | 1 C/kg = 3380 R |
| Dose | Gray (Gy) | Rad | 1 Gy = 100 rad |
| Dose equivalence | Sievert (Sv) | Rem | 1 Sv = 100 rem |

From Miles DA, Van Dis ML, Williamson GF, et al: Radiographic imaging for the dental team, ed 4, St Louis, 2009, Saunders.

### Position Indicator Device

The PID, which is used to direct the x-ray beam, has a round or rectangular shape and is available in two lengths: *short* (8-inch) and *long* (16-inch). PIDs used in dentistry are usually 8, 12, or 16 inches long. The length selected is determined by the imaging technique that is being used. However, a long (12- to 16-inch) PID is more effective than a short (8-inch) PID in reducing exposure to the patient because it causes less *divergence* (spreading out) of the beam (Fig. 38.27).

## Patient Protection

With the use of proper radiation protection measures, the amount of x-radiation to the patient can be minimized. Patient protection begins with understanding and practicing general guidelines for obtaining dental images in pediatric, adolescent, and adult patients.

**TABLE 38.6 Radiation Sources and Whole Body Exposure**

| Source | Exposure: Millirems/Year | Exposure: Sieverts/Year |
|---|---|---|
| Radon | 200.00 | 0.002 |
| Cosmic | 27.00 | 0.00027 |
| Terrestrial | 28.00 | 0.00028 |
| Internal | 39.00 | 0.00039 |
| Medical/dental | 53.00 | 0.00053 |
| Consumer products | 9.00 | 0.00009 |
| Other | | |
| Occupational | <1.00 | <0.00001 |
| Nuclear fuel cycle | <1.00 | <0.00001 |
| Fallout | <1.00 | <0.00001 |

Modified from Iannucci J, Jansen Howerton L: Dental radiography: principles and techniques, ed 4, St Louis, 2012, Saunders.

### Lead Apron and Thyroid Collar

A lead apron and a thyroid collar must be used on *all* patients for *all* exposures (Fig. 38.28). This rule applies to all patients regardless of age or gender or the number of images being exposed.

The **lead apron** should cover the patient from the neck and extend over the lap area to protect the reproductive and blood-forming tissues from scatter radiation. Many states mandate the use of a lead apron.

The **thyroid collar** is a flexible lead shield that is placed securely around the patient's neck to protect the thyroid gland from scatter radiation. The collar may be a separate shield or part of the lead apron. The lead protects the highly sensitive thyroid gland from scatter radiation. A low rate of exposure to dental x-rays has *not* been shown to cause thyroid disease, but the use of collars further minimizes the patient's exposure to x-radiation.

Lead aprons and thyroid collars must *not be folded* when stored. Folding eventually cracks the lead and allows radiation leakage. Instead, the lead apron and thyroid collar should be hung up or laid over a rounded bar.

### Fast-Speed Film

When conventional film-based exposures are used, the film speed refers to the amount of radiation required to obtain the image. The faster the film speed, the less radiation exposure to the patient occurs.

The size of the silver bromide crystals on the film is the main factor in determining the film speed: the larger the crystals, the faster the film.

Fast-speed film is a very effective method of reducing a patient's exposure to x-radiation. Fast film is available for both intraoral and extraoral radiography (see Chapter 39).

### Image Receptor–Holding Devices

The use of an image receptor–holding device keeps the patient's hands and fingers from being exposed to x-radiation (Fig. 38.29). These devices also hold the image receptor in a stable position and assist the operator in properly positioning the PID. Individual types of holding devices are discussed in Chapter 39.

**TABLE 38.7 Examples of Selection Criteria for Prescribing Radiographs**

| Type of Patient | Child (Mixed Dentition) | Adult |
|---|---|---|
| New patient | Individualized examination consisting of panoramic examination with posterior bitewings *or* posterior bitewings with selected periapical views | Individualized examination consisting of posterior bitewings and selected periapicals; a full mouth survey is appropriate when patient presents with clinical evidence of generalized dental disease or a history of extensive dental treatment |
| Recall patient with no clinical caries and low risk factors for caries | Posterior bitewing examination at 12- to 24-month intervals | Posterior bitewing examination at 24- to 36-month intervals |
| Recall patient with clinical caries or high risk factors for caries | Posterior bitewing examination at 6-month intervals until no carious lesions are evident | Posterior bitewing examination at 12- to 18-month intervals |

From Miles DA, Van Dis ML, Williamson GF, et al: Radiographic imaging for the dental team, ed 4, St Louis, 2009, Saunders.

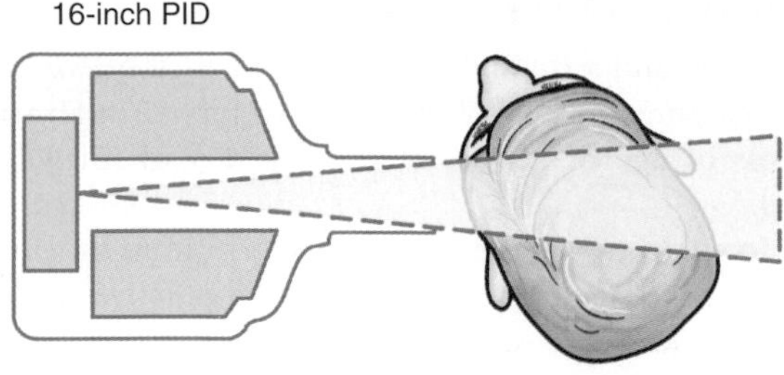


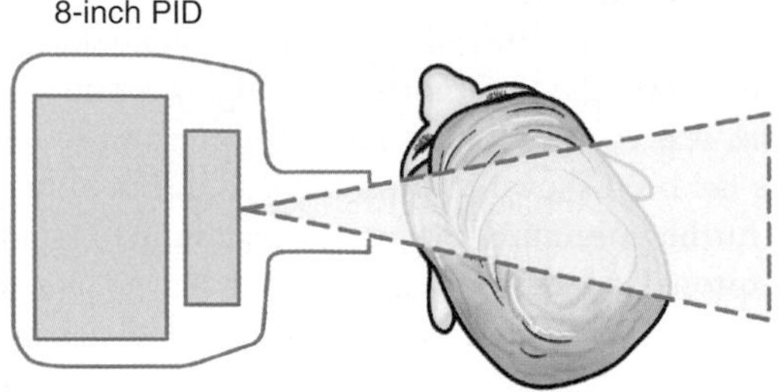


**FIG. 38.27** The longer (16-inch) position indicator device (PID) is preferred to the short (8-inch) PID because it produces less divergence of the x-ray beam. *(Modified from Frommer H, Stabulas-Savage J: Radiology for the dental professional, ed 9, St Louis, 2011, Mosby.)*

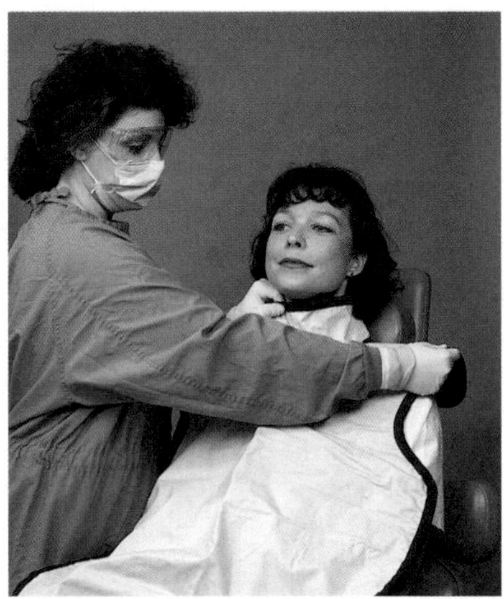

**FIG. 38.28** The lead apron and the thyroid collar must be large enough to cover the seated patient from the neck to above the knees.

### *Exposure Factor*

Using the proper exposure factors also limits the amount of x-radiation exposure to the patient. Adjusting the selectors for kVp, mA, and time controls the exposure factors. A setting of 70 to 90 kVp keeps patient exposure to a minimum. On some dental units, the kVp and mA settings are preset by the manufacturer and cannot be adjusted.

### *Proper Technique*

Using the correct technique is necessary for ensuring the diagnostic quality of images and reducing the amount of exposure to a patient. Images that are nondiagnostic must be retaken; this results in additional radiation exposure to the patient. Retakes are the major cause of unnecessary radiation to patients and must be avoided.

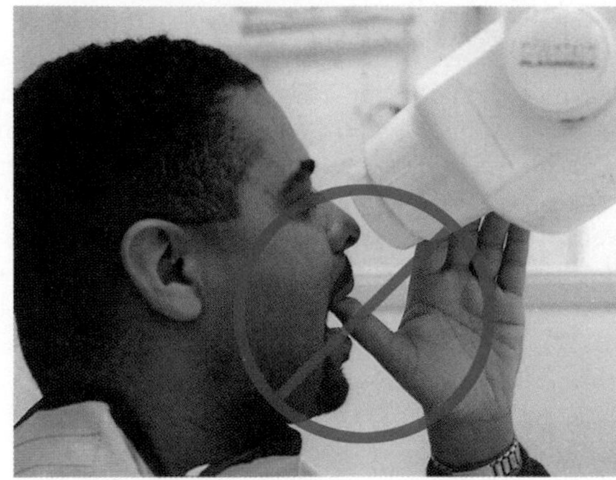

**FIG. 38.29** The patient's fingers are unnecessarily exposed to radiation when film/sensor holders are not used.

## Pregnancy

The manual *Guidelines for Prescribing Dental Radiographs,* issued by the American Dental Association (ADA) and the U.S. Food and Drug Administration (FDA), states that dental radiographic procedures "do not need to be altered because of pregnancy." When a lead apron is used during dental imaging procedures, the amount of radiation received in the pelvic region is nearly zero. The embryo or fetus receives no detectable exposure with the use of a lead apron.

Although scientific evidence indicates that dental x-ray procedures can be performed during pregnancy, many dentists and pregnant patients prefer to postpone such x-ray procedures because of the patient's concern.

RECALL

**20** What is the purpose of the collimator?
**21** What is the purpose of the aluminum filter?
**22** What precautions should be taken when one is handling the lead apron?
**23** What is the most effective measure in reducing a patient's exposure to radiation?

## Operator Protection and Monitoring

The dental assistant must use proper operator protection measures to avoid occupational exposure to radiation, including primary radiation, leakage radiation, and scatter radiation. The assistant must carefully follow the safety guidelines and use radiation monitoring devices.

A dental assistant who fails to follow the rules of radiation protection may suffer the results of chronic radiation exposure. By following these rules, dental personnel can keep their radiation exposure to zero (Fig. 38.30).

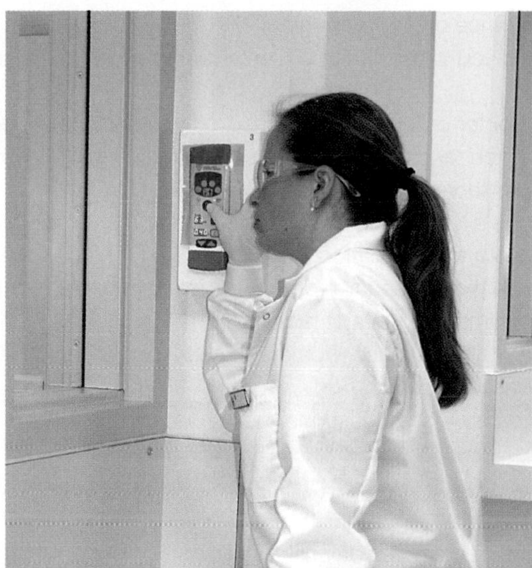

FIG. 38.30 For safety, the dental assistant must stand out of the path of the primary beam.

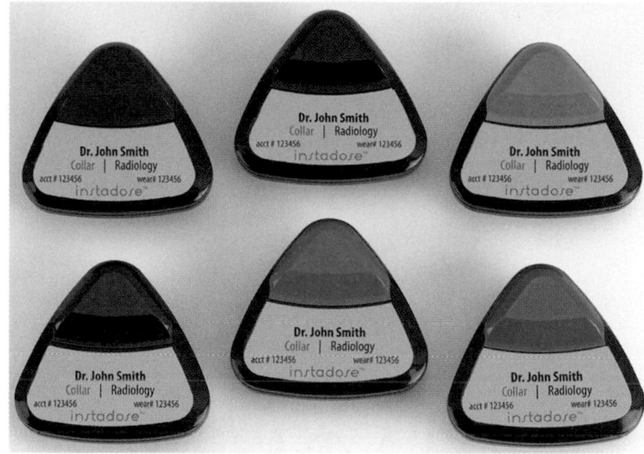


FIG. 38.31 A direct ion storage (DIS) dosimeter constructed with non-volatile analog memory cells is surrounded by gas filled ion chambers. It measures the ionizing radiation exposure dose incident by calculating the amount of proportional change in the voltage across the memory cells. *(Courtesy Mirion Technologies, Dosimetry Service Division, Irvine, CA [www.mirion.com].)*

### *Radiation Monitoring*

Radiation monitoring can be used to protect the operator by identifying occupational exposure to radiation. Both equipment and dental personnel can be monitored. Three types of monitoring devices are used to determine the amount of radiation exposure to personnel: (1) film badge, (2) pocket dosimeter (pen style), and (3) thermoluminescent device (TLD).

A **dosimeter** is used to measure the amount of occupational exposure to ionizing radiation. A commonly used type of measurement tool is the **dosimeter personal radiation monitoring badge**. The badge measures the intensity of visible light emitted from a crystal in the detector when heated. The intensity of light emitted is dependent upon the radiation exposure. The dosimeter badge is commonly labeled with the wearer's name, identification number, and the location on the body where to attach the badge for best radiation exposure reading (Fig. 38.31).

The dosimeter badge should be worn at all times while the employee is at work. At the end of the radiation exposure monitoring period, usually every 3 to 4 weeks, the badge is returned to the monitoring service company for reporting. The company processes the badge and prepares a dose read report that is returned to the dental office. The dose read report contains the radiation exposure results for the radiation exposure monitoring period, as well as accumulated quarterly, yearly, and sometimes lifetime exposures of the individual.

There are also personal radiation monitoring badges that do not require the dental office to collect and return employee badges, but instead offer the opportunity for the wearer to get their exposure feedback with on-demand dose reads and programmable automatic dose reads using a mobile device or a cloud-based relay station at their location.

Dosimeter badges should not be worn outside the office or in any way or body location different than what the badge manufacturer recommends. Personal radiation monitoring badges must be removed when the wearer is having medical or dental x-ray films taken because the badges are only intended to measure occupational exposure.

#### Rules of Radiation Protection

- Never stand in the direct line of the primary beam.
- Always stand behind a lead barrier or a proper thickness of drywall. If a lead barrier is not available, stand at right angles to the beam.
- Never stand closer than 6 feet from the x-ray unit during an exposure, unless you are behind a barrier.

## Equipment Monitoring

Dental x-ray machines must be monitored for *leakage* radiation, or any radiation (except for the primary beam) that is emitted from the tubehead. If an x-ray tubehead has a faulty seal, leakage radiation results. Dental x-ray equipment can be monitored through a device available from the manufacturer or the state health department.

## Pediatric Patients

If the patient is a child who is unable to cooperate, the patient may be seated on the parent's lap in the dental chair (Fig. 38.32). Both parent and child are covered with the lead apron, and the parent holds the film in place.

Having the parent hold the film or sensor is acceptable because this is a single exposure for the parent. If the assistant were to hold the film in this manner, he or she would have repeated exposures and would suffer the cumulative effects of radiation.

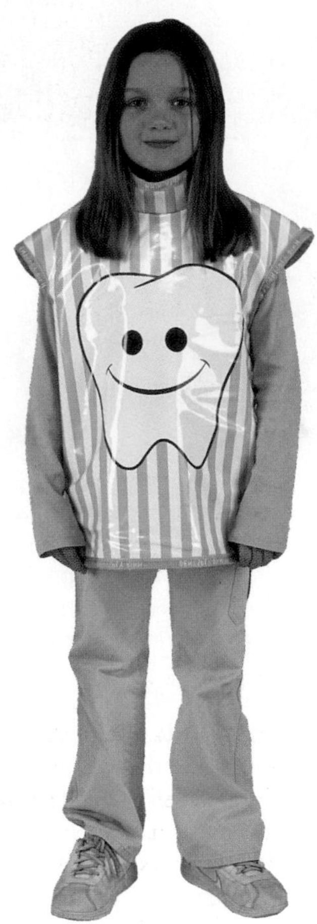

**FIG. 38.32** Leaded apron with thyroid collar. Children are more sensitive to radiation than adults, and so the use of leaded aprons with thyroid collars is especially important for this population. *(Courtesy Densply Rinn:* http://rinncorp.com/.*)*

## ALARA Concept

The **ALARA concept** states that all exposure to radiation must be kept to a minimum, or "*as low as reasonably achievable*." Every possible method of reducing exposure to radiation should be used to minimize risk.

The radiation protection measures detailed in this chapter should be used to minimize patient, operator, and staff exposure, thus keeping radiation exposure "ALARA."

■ **Patient Education** Patients often have questions and concerns about radiation. As a dental assistant, you must be prepared to answer their questions and educate them about the importance of dental imaging. The following examples are comments you can make to patients during informal discussions:

- "The doctor orders images based on your individual needs."
- "Our office takes every step possible to protect you from unnecessary radiation."
- "We use a lead apron and a thyroid collar to protect your body from stray radiation."
- "We use high-speed film or **digital imaging** that requires only minimal amounts of radiation."
- "We use film or sensor holders so that your fingers are not exposed to radiation."
- "Do you have any questions before we begin?" ■

■ **Legal and Ethical Implications** Although the risks of radiation exposure involved in dental imaging are not significantly greater than other everyday risks in life, it is important that dental professionals do everything possible to protect patients from unnecessary exposure to x-radiation.

Every patient's dental condition is different, and consequently, every patient should be evaluated for dental images on an individual basis. Radiographic examinations should not be based on a standard number of images, and images should not be taken at predetermined times. For example, the dentist who prescribes a set number of images (such as four bitewing views) at a set interval (such as every 6 months) for every patient is not considering the individual needs of the individual patient. ■

■ **Eye to the Future** Dental manufacturers are continually striving to develop products that will minimize exposure to radiation. For conventional film-based imaging, F-speed film has cut previous exposure times in half, and digital imaging systems use even less radiation. In addition, dental x-ray machines now being manufactured are operating at lower settings.

Other imaging machines that do not require the use of radiation are currently used in medicine and in the future will be available for dentistry as well. ■

■ **Critical Thinking**

As a dental assistant, how would you answer the following patient questions regarding dental x-rays?

1. "Are dental x-rays really necessary?"
2. "Should I have x-rays every 6 months?"
3. "Why do you use a lead apron?"
4. "Should x-rays be taken during pregnancy?"
5. "Why do you leave the room when x-rays are taken?"
6. "Are dental x-rays safe?" ■

39

# Digital Imaging, Dental Film, and Processing Radiographs

## KEY TERMS

**Automatic processor** Machine that automates all film processing steps.
**Beam alignment device** Assists in the positioning of the position indicator device (PID).
**Bitewing** Image view that shows the crowns of both arches on one film.
**Calcium tungstate** Common type of phosphor.
**Cassette** Contains extraoral films during exposure.
**Cephalometric film** Shows the bony and soft tissue areas of the facial profile.
**Charge-coupled device (CCD)** A solid-state image sensor used in intraoral digital imaging.
**Digital image** Electronic signals captured by sensors and displayed on computer monitors.
**Digitize** Scanning of traditional film-based radiographs into a digital image.
**Duplicating film** Film designed for use in film duplicating machines.
**Emulsion (ee-MUL-shun)** A coating on the x-ray film that contains energy-sensitive crystals.
**Extraoral film** Film designed for use in cassettes.
**Film speed** The sensitivity of the emulsion on the film to radiation.
**Intensifying screen** The part inside an extraoral cassette that converts x-ray energy into visible light, which in turn exposes screen film.
**Intraoral film** Film designed for placement in the patient's mouth.
**Label side** Colored side of the film that faces the tongue.
**Latent image** The invisible image on the x-ray film after exposure but before processing.
**Occlusal** Radiographic view that shows large areas of the maxilla or mandible.
**Panoramic film** Used in cassettes to provide a wide view of both the upper and lower jaws.
**Periapical (per-ee-AP-i-kul)** Radiographic view that shows the crown, root tip, and surrounding structures.
**Phosphor storage plate (PSP)** Reusable film-sized plates coated with phosphor as the image receptor.
**Positioning instruments** Intraoral devices used to position and hold the film, sensor, or PSP.
**Processing** A series of steps that change exposed film into a radiograph. Steps include developing, rinsing, fixing, washing, and drying.
**Radiograph (RAY-dee-oe-graf)** Image produced on photosensitive film by exposing the film to radiation and then processing it.
**Teledentistry** Process of using electronic transfer of images and other information for consultation and/or insurance purposes in dentistry.
**Tube side** Solid white side of the film packet that faces the x-ray tube.

## LEARNING OUTCOMES

*On completion of this chapter, the student will be able to achieve the following objectives:*

1. Pronounce, define, and spell the key terms.
2. Describe the purposes and uses of digital radiography.
3. Explain the fundamental systems of digital radiography, including the following:
   - List and describe the equipment necessary for digital radiography.
   - Identify the types of dental image receptors.
   - Describe the purpose for scanning and clearing phosphor plates.
   - Describe the process for digitizing radiographs using a scanner.
   - List and describe the advantages and disadvantages of digital radiography.
   - Describe the changes to the image that a digital imaging software can make.
4. Do the following regarding x-ray film and film processing:
   - Identify correct terminology used in conventional film based techniques.
   - Describe common types of beam alignment devices.
5. Discuss dental film, including the following:
   - Explain why it is important to know the film speed.
   - Name the five basic sizes of intraoral dental film.
   - Describe the contents of an extraoral x-ray film packet.
   - Explain the purpose of an intensifying screen.
   - Name two types of extraoral films.
   - Describe the process for duplicating radiographs.
   - Explain how dental film should be stored.
6. Discuss film processing, including the following:
   - Describe the features and necessary requirements of a darkroom.
   - Identify the component parts of an automatic film processor.
   - Describe common time and temperature errors during film processing.

- Describe chemical contamination errors during film processing.
- Describe film handling errors that can occur during film processing.
- Describe some common lighting errors during film processing.

## PERFORMANCE OUTCOMES

*On completion of this chapter, the student will be able to meet competency standards in the following skills:*

- Duplicate a set of dental radiographs.
- Process dental x-ray films with the use of a manual tank.
- Successfully process dental films using a daylight loader.

## ELECTRONIC RESOURCES

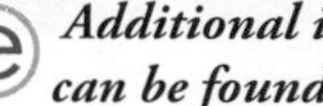

***Additional information related to content in Chapter 39 can be found on the companion Evolve Web site.***

- Canadian Content Corner
- Practice Quiz
- Videos: Duplicating Radiographs; Manual Processing of Dental Radiographs; Automatic Processing of Dental Radiographs; Digital Imaging (Setting Up the System; Maxillary Canine Exposure; Maxillary Molar Exposure; Bitewing Exposure)

In this chapter, you will learn the advantages and basic concepts of digital radiography, including scanning and digitizing dental images. You will learn the various types and uses of intraoral and extraoral images. Using conventional x-ray film, you will learn how to use manual and automatic processing techniques and how to duplicate films. You will also learn how to recognize common errors in film processing and how to prevent them from occurring.

# Digital Radiography

Digital radiography has revolutionized dentistry (Fig. 39.1). Digital imaging eliminates chemical processing and hazardous wastes from chemicals and lead foil. Images can be electronically transferred to other healthcare providers without loss of the original image quality. A significant advantage is that it requires less radiation than film, thus reducing radiation to the patient. Finally, digital imaging allows enhancements, measurements, and corrections that are not available with film (Fig. 39.2). Digital systems also have disadvantages compared with film. The initial cost is relatively high, and the sensors can be damaged if handled improperly and are costly to replace.

When digital radiography is discussed, the term **digital images** is used instead of **radiographs**, x-rays, or films. The digital images are not radiographs but electronic signals that are captured by sensors and displayed on a computer monitor almost instantaneously. These images can be emailed to insurance companies and other dentists for consultations. If desired, hard copies of these images can be printed on image-quality paper.

Although digital imaging systems are high tech, a conventional x-ray machine is still needed to expose the image, and the position of the image receptor (sensor or phosphor storage plate [PSP]) in the mouth is identical to positioning with film. In addition, strict infection control measures must be used because the sensors and PSPs are reused time and again. U.S. Food and Drug Administration (FDA)–cleared disposable, fluid-impervious barriers must be used on digital image sensors and phosphor plates. Digital image receptors are *not* able to tolerate heat sterilization.

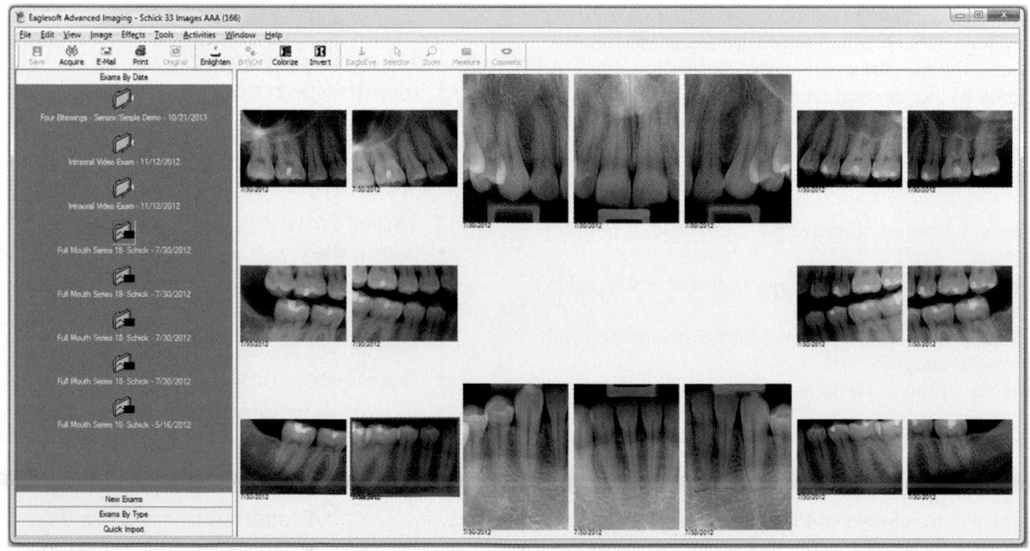


**FIG. 39.1** Computer monitor illustrating a variety of images, including panoramic and cephalometric images. *(Courtesy Sirona Dental, Inc., Long Island City, NY.)*

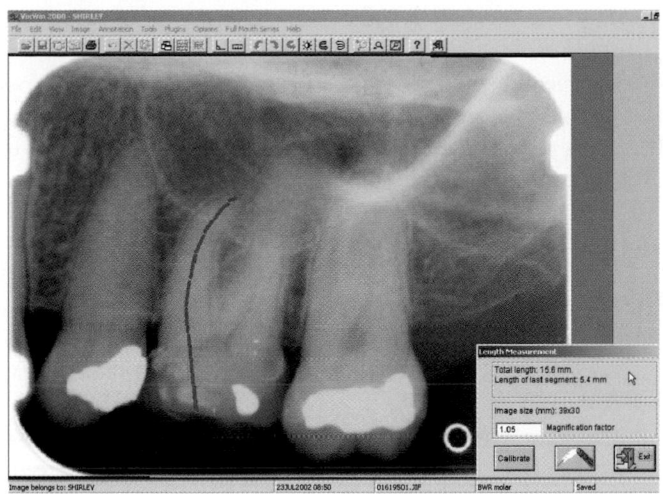


**FIG. 39.2** Example of a measurement tool to determine the length of the crown and mesiobuccal root of the first molar. *(From White SC, Pharoah MJ: Oral radiology: principles and interpretation, ed 7, St Louis, 2014, Mosby.)*

Step-by-step procedures for the use of digital radiography systems vary by manufacturer. It is *critical* to refer to the manufacturer's instruction booklet for information concerning operation of the system, equipment preparation, patient preparation, and exposure factors. Only general guidelines on sensor preparation and placement are discussed here. The videos that accompany the text show placement for a maxillary canine exposure, maxillary molar exposure, and bitewing exposure.

# Types of Digital Imaging Systems

There are two basic systems used to acquire a digital image: **direct imaging** and **indirect imaging.**

## Direct Digital Imaging

In direct imaging, a solid-state sensor is the image receptor. It contains an x-ray–sensitive silicon chip with an electronic circuit embedded in the silicon (Fig. 39.3). The sensor, available

**TrueComfort™ Design** 1

To maximize both patient comfort and ease of use, DEXIS has enhanced its own great sensor housing design by refining the curvatures, redesigning the cable exit, upgrading the materials, and giving it a slimmer profile.

Four beveled corners and a smooth, rounded casing ensure there are no sharp edges against the palate or soft tissue. The smaller, angled dome makes precise placement in posterior regions easy.

**Integrated Electronics** 2

A smart design places the electronics on the sensor's back to maximize the active imaging area. The on-board electronics provide the USB functionality, allowing direct connection to the computer.

**ScatterGuard™** 3

A protective shield affixed to the interior wall of the rear housing protects the patient by preventing X-ray back scattering.

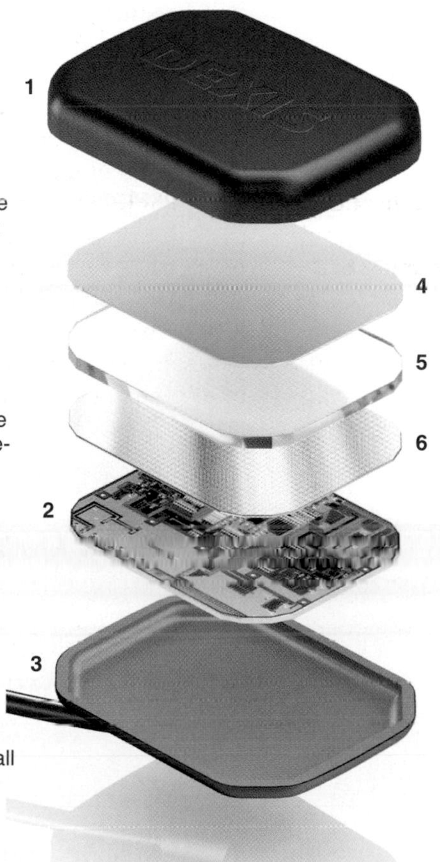


**PureImage™ Technology**

The ability to see subtleties in x-ray images is crucial to diagnosis, collaboration, and patient communication. Through a combination of advanced hardware and software technologies, the DEXIS Platinum sensor is able to deliver clinically meaningful images that are extremely clear and highly detailed.

A premium quality **Caesium Iodide scintillator** 4 converts the x-ray beam into visible light and guides it through its micro-columnar structures.

**Fiber optics** 5 then transmit the light precisely to the CMOS sensor surface. This efficient design allows for a high signal-to-noise ratio, resulting in clean images with virtually no visual noise.

Our **high-resolution CMOS sensor** 6 features an exclusive architecture that maximizes active area at the pixel level to bring out the smallest details.

**FIG. 39.3** Dexis platinum sensor. *1,* Sensor housing. *2,* Integrated electronics to maximize the imaging area. *3,* Scatter guard to prevent x-ray backscatter. *4,* The x-ray beam is converted into visible light. *5,* Fiber optics transmit light to the sensor for clear images. *6,* High-resolution sensor brings out the smallest details. *(Courtesy of KaVo Kerr.)*

in a variety of sizes, is positioned in the patient's mouth instead of film (Fig. 39.4).

The sensor, or **charge-coupled device (CCD)**, is the most commonly used digital receptor (Fig. 39.5). The technology is used in a variety of other imaging devices, such as telescopes, fax machines, personal data assistants (PDAs), video cameras, and even some panoramic machines and other extraoral imaging systems such as cone beam volumetric imaging (see Chapter 42).

Like telephones, some CCDs are wireless, and other types have a cable connected directly from the sensor to the computer. The wireless type of sensor uses radio frequency transmission to instantly transmit the image to the computer via radio waves.

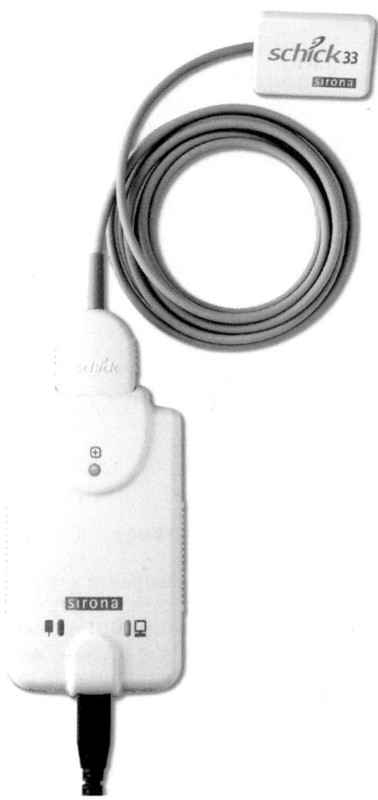


**FIG. 39.4** Cable-type sensor. *(Courtesy Dentsply Sirona, Charlotte, NC.)*

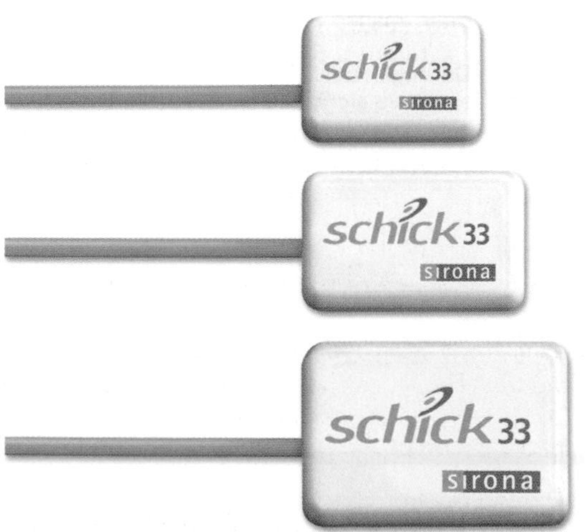


**FIG. 39.5** Various sizes of digital sensors. *(Courtesy Sirona Dental, Inc., Long Island City, NY.)*

## Indirect Digital Imaging

### *Phosphor Storage Imaging*

In **phosphor storage plate (PSP)** imaging systems the image receptor is a thin, flexible plate, the size of a conventional x-ray film that has been coated with phosphor crystals (Fig. 39.6). The phosphor layer is able to store the energy of the x-ray photons for some time. The PSP is placed in a barrier envelope to be ready for use on a patient. Following exposure, scanning is required to "read" the information stored on the plate by using a laser beam to release the energy from the plate and convert it into a digital image (Fig. 39.7). The latent image will remain on the phosphor plate before the scanning phase for minutes to hours, depending on the environment in which the plates are stored. They should not be exposed to bright light or warmth because this will release the energy before it is read by the scanner. After the plates are scanned, they are exposed to bright light that erases all remaining energy, and the plates are ready to be used again.

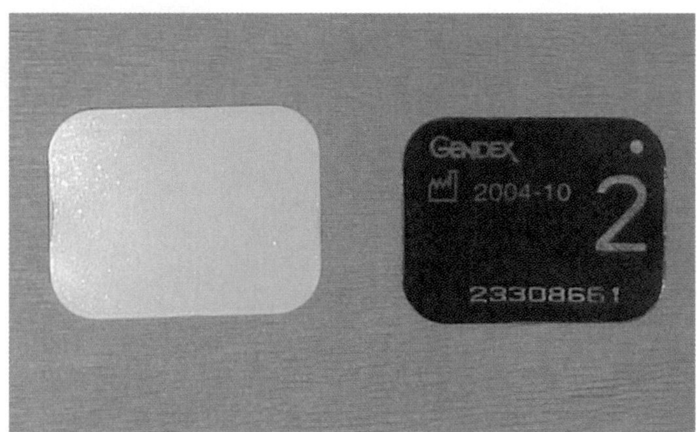


**FIG. 39.6** Front and back sides of phosphor plate.

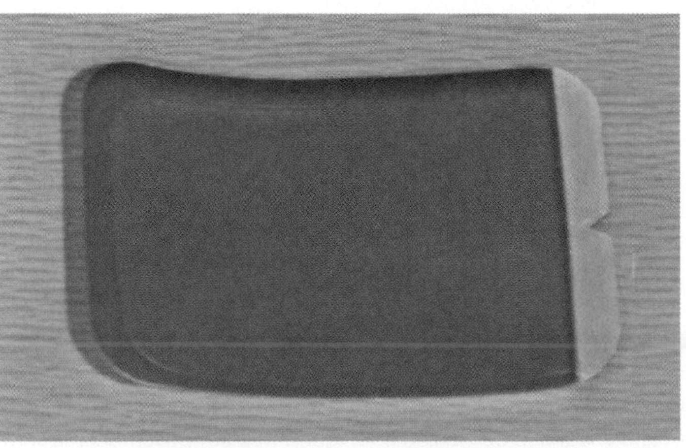

**FIG. 39.7** Barrier envelope for phosphor plate.

For infection control, the imaging plate is inserted into a specially designed barrier envelope. The barrier envelope is sealed by removing the adhesive strip and pressing the envelope closed. The imaging plate is protected and then can be used intraorally. The imaging plate is positioned in the patient's mouth using the same positioning techniques as are used with conventional dental x-ray film. After exposure, the imaging plate is carefully removed from the barrier envelope and then is placed in a scanner that uses a laser to display the image on the computer.

The imaging plates cannot be autoclaved, and extreme care must be taken when handling to avoid scratches or dust.

## Digitizing Images

Film-based radiographs may be digitized for viewing on a computer in much the same way as any other document. Desktop scanners capture and **digitize** the light signal of whatever is placed inside them (Fig. 39.8). This process is similar to placing a film on a duplicator lightbox (discussed later in this chapter). This type of indirect digital imaging is slightly less detailed than direct digital imaging because the resultant image is similar to a "copy" of the image versus the "original" (Fig. 39.9).

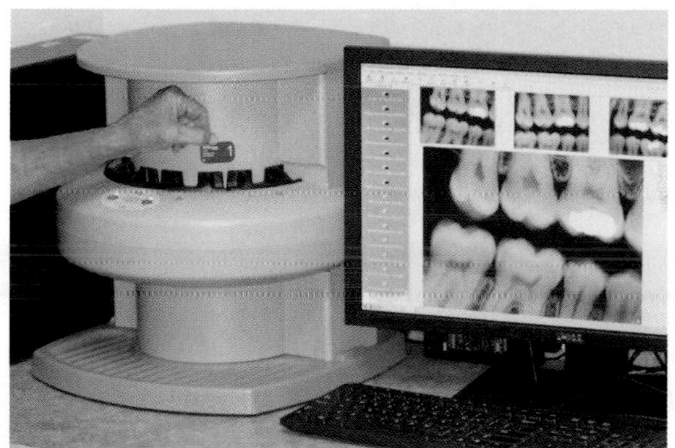

**FIG. 39.8** Laser scanner for reusable plates (PSP). *(From Darby ML, Walsh M: Dental hygiene: theory and practice, ed 4, St Louis, 2015, Saunders.)*

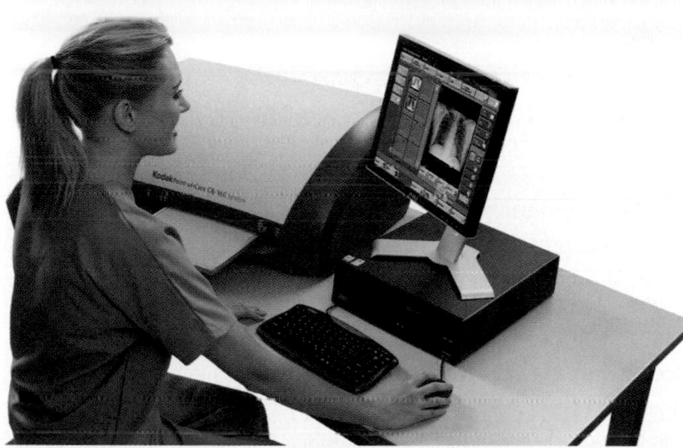

**FIG. 39.9** The desktop scanner scans the radiographs and digitizes the images to be viewed on a computer. *(Courtesy Carestream Health, Rochester, NY.)*

## Digital Imaging Software Programs

Most computer software programs that are used in digital imaging are capable of performing electronic image enhancement. This means that the operator can change the following image variables together or separately (Fig. 39.10 and Box 39.1):

- Contrast
- Brightness
- Image size (zoom)
- Sharpness
- Inversion (white to black and black to white)
- Pseudocolor alteration

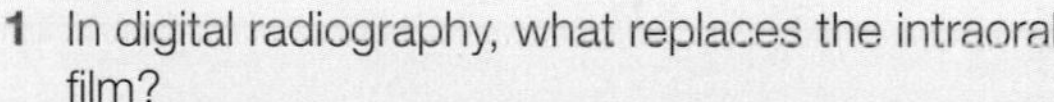

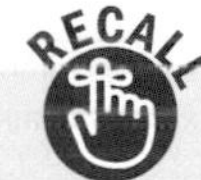


1 In digital radiography, what replaces the intraoral film?
2 What are the two fundamental techniques for intraoral digital radiography?
3 Which of the digital techniques requires scanning of image receptors?

# X-Ray Film and Film Processing

Although many dental practices are transitioning to digital techniques, a significant number of private dental practices are still using conventional film-based techniques. The dental assistant must thoroughly understand the procedures and techniques necessary to process films into high-quality diagnostic dental images. It is also important to use the correct terminology. *Film* is the correct term to use *before* it has been processed. The *film* is in the packet; the *film* is placed in the bite-block; the *film* is exposed and processed. *After* the film has been processed, it becomes an image or radiograph.

## Positioning Instruments

**Positioning instruments** (dental film and sensor holders) are used to position and hold dental x-ray films or the digital sensor in the patient's mouth. The use of a positioner keeps the patient's fingers from being exposed to x-radiation. Positioners also assist the operator in properly placing the film or sensor and the position indicator device (PID). When a rectangular PID is used, a film holder is absolutely necessary to avoid *cone cuts,* or clear areas of the film that are not exposed to radiation (see Chapter 38).

Various types of intraoral positioning instruments are currently available. The sensor holders used in digital radiography are almost identical to the x-ray film holders used in conventional techniques. The primary difference is seen in the size and shape of the holder.

Double-ended instruments used for the bisecting technique hold the film or phosphor plate between two serrated plastic grips that can be locked into place (Fig. 39.11).

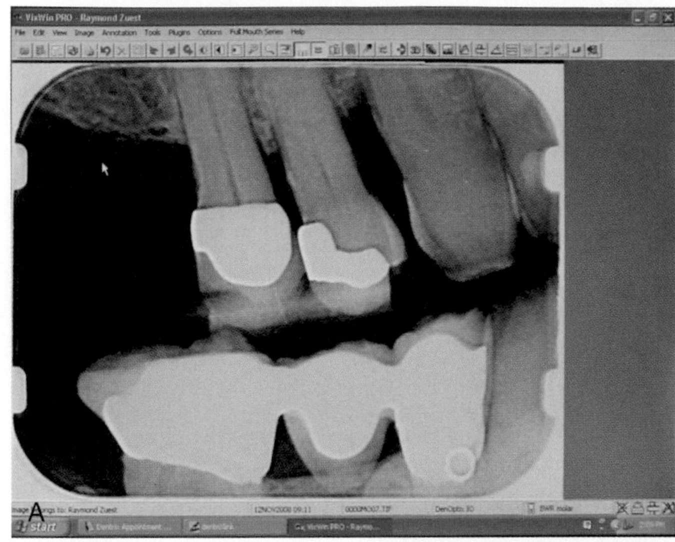


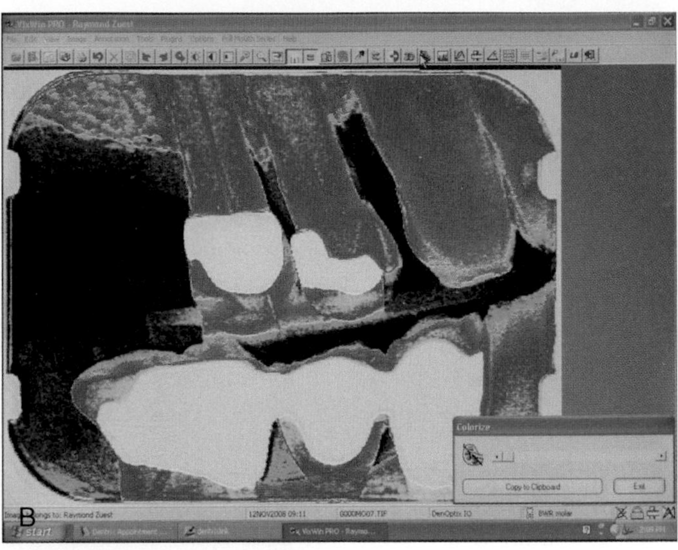


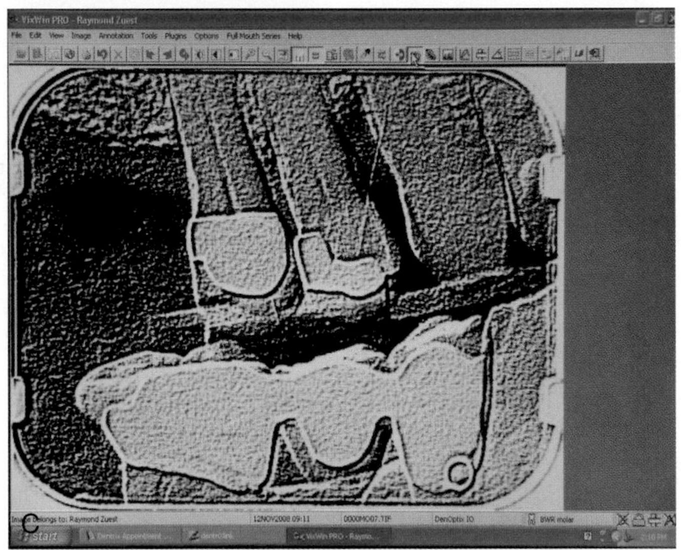


**FIG. 39.10** Examples of how images can be manipulated with the software program. A, Changed contrast. B, Pseudocolor alteration. C, Inversion of image.

## BOX 39.1 Advantages and Disadvantages of Digital Radiography

### Advantages

#### Immediate Viewing of Images

In conventional radiography, reading the image is delayed because the film must be processed. Being able to immediately view the image is a significant clinical advantage

*Note:* Only charge-coupled devices (CCDs) provide immediate viewing. Phosphorous plate digital technology requires that the irradiated sensor be placed in a processing device to scan it and put the information into a computer, so that the image can be viewed.

#### Less Radiation

Digital radiography requires *much less x-radiation* than conventional film-based radiography because the sensor is *more sensitive* to x-rays than is conventional film. Exposure times for digital radiography are 70 to 80 percent less than those required for radiography with conventional film. With less radiation, the absorbed dose to the patient is significantly lower.

#### No Chemicals

It is not necessary to maintain, change, and dispose of processing chemicals. The need for a darkroom is eliminated, and gone are the stains and odors from the developing and fixing solutions.

#### Ability to Enhance Images

Digital radiography allows the dentist to change the contrast (to lighter or darker), enlarge images, place color enhancements, and so forth. It also allows for immediate and effective patient education.

#### Communication with Other Dentists

Digital radiography provides the ability to send images to other practitioners in a matter of minutes. This can be useful when consulting with another practitioner, especially when the patient is still in the chair. Email is the method most commonly used to send images.

**BOX 39.1** Advantages and Disadvantages of Digital Radiography—cont'd

**No More Lost Films**

Occasionally, a film is lost from a patient's chart and cannot be replaced. With adequate backup procedures, stored digital images will not be lost.

**Remote Consultation Capability**

Digital images can be sent electronically by email or other electronic means. This is very useful for consultation or for insurance purposes. This process has been termed teledentistry.

**Disadvantages**

**Cost**

At the present time, the cost of purchasing a digital radiography setup can be substantial depending on the configuration. When considering the cost, one should carefully consider the advantages and disadvantages of digital radiography.

**Converting Previous Records to Digital**

Previous patient radiographs must be digitized (scanned) into digital records. To do this at one time for all the patient records in the practice can be very costly. It is best to do this gradually as patients come in for recall appointments. Spreading the labor costs over many months is more manageable.

**Learning the Computer Software**

As with all computer programs, users need time to become comfortable with the software. Software programs vary, depending on the manufacturer.

**Thickness and Rigidity of Sensors**

CCD sensors vary in thickness depending on the manufacturer. Care must be taken during placement to avoid discomfort to the patient. Phosphor storage plates (PSPs) are the thinnest, but they do not offer the advantage of immediate viewing of the image.

A sensor is used in place of intraoral dental film. When the x-ray beam strikes the sensor, an electronic charge is produced on the surface of the sensor. This electronic signal is digitized, or converted into "digital" form. The digital sensor in turn transmits this information to the computer. Software in the computer is used to store the image electronically.

**Infection Control**

The sensor or phosphor plate must be carefully covered with a barrier because it cannot be heat sterilized. Care must be taken when removing the barrier to avoid contamination of the sensor under the barrier. Follow the manufacturer's recommendations regarding surface disinfection of the sensor. At this time, sensors and PSPs cannot withstand heat sterilization.

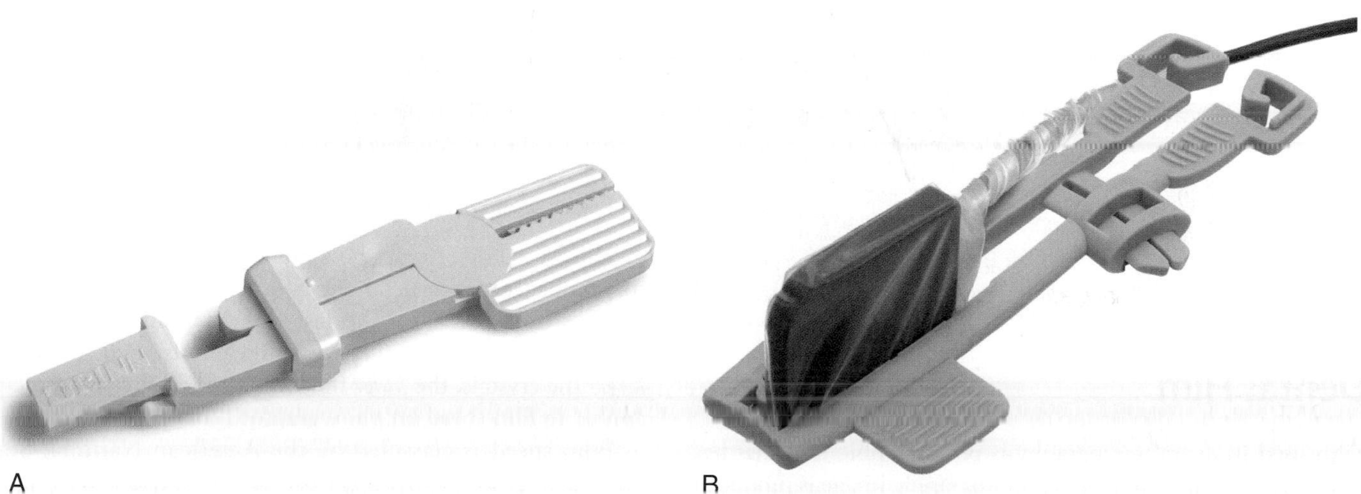


**FIG. 39.11** A, Snap-a-Ray Xtra Film and phosphor plate holder for the bisecting technique. B, Eezee-Grip Digital Sensor Holder for the bisecting technique. *(Courtesy Dentsply Rinn, Elgin, IL.)*

A basic style of film holder is the disposable polystyrene (Styrofoam) bite-block with a backing plate and a slot for film retention (Fig. 39.12). Other devices include the EndoRay (Dentsply International, York, PA) (Fig. 39.13), which is used for images with endodontic instruments in the canal.

## Beam Alignment Devices

Devices used to align the beam are available from several manufacturers for both film-based and digital techniques. The **beam alignment device** assists in positioning of the PID in relation to the tooth and film or sensor. Rinn XCP instruments (Dentsply Rinn, Elgin, IL) use color-coded plastic bite-blocks, plastic aiming rings, and metal indicator arms for film-based techniques, and Rinn XCP-DS are examples of instruments used for holding digital sensors. *Note:* Several manufacturers produce digital sensors, and the size and shape of sensors vary slightly. You must be sure that you use a digital sensor holder designed to fit the specific brand of sensor you are using (Fig. 39.14).

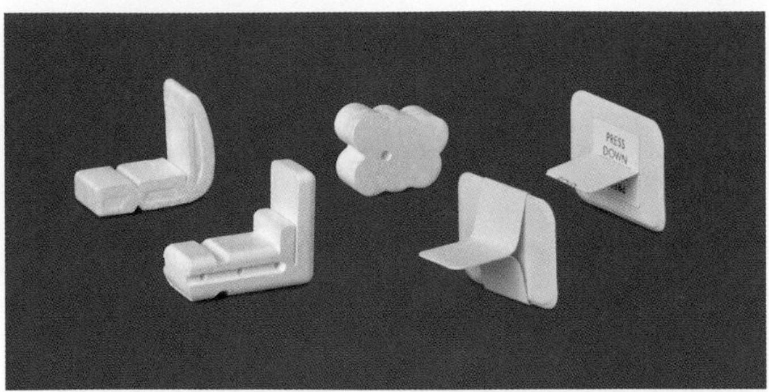


**FIG. 39.12** Plastic- and Styrofoam-type disposable bite-block film holders. *(Courtesy Dentsply Rinn, Elgin, IL.)*

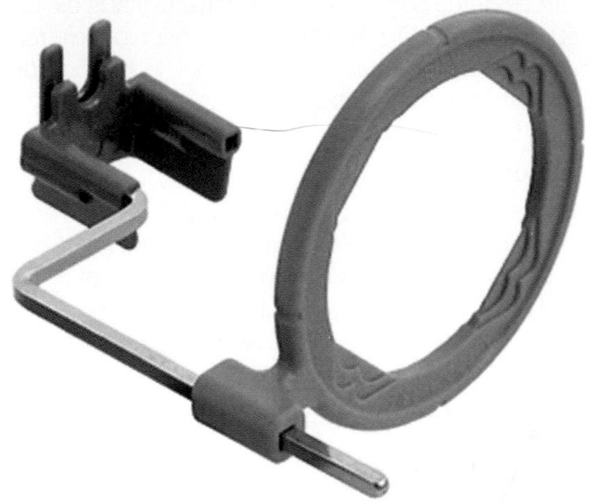

**FIG. 39.13** The EndoRay is designed to be used for images of teeth with endodontic instruments in them. *(Courtesy Dentsply Rinn, Elgin, IL.)*

RECALL

4 How does the use of positioning instruments protect the patient from unnecessary radiation?
5 What is the primary difference between a film holder and a digital sensor holder?
6 What is the purpose of a beam alignment device?

# Dental Film

Film used in dental radiography is photographic film that has been adapted for dental use. A photographic image is produced on dental x-ray film when it is exposed to x-rays that have passed through teeth and adjacent tissues. The concept is similar to an image that is recorded on photographic film after it has been exposed to light through the shutter and lens of a camera.

The dental assistant must understand the composition of x-ray film and latent image formation. The assistant also must be familiar with the types of film used in dental radiography, as well as methods of film storage and protection.

## Film Composition

**Intraoral film** consists of a semiflexible acetate film base that is coated on both sides with an **emulsion** of silver bromide, silver halide, and silver iodide that is sensitive to radiation. Beginning with the film base, the following layers make up a dental x-ray film (Fig. 39.15):

- The film base is made of clear cellulose acetate.
- The thin adhesive layer attaches the emulsion to the film base.
- The gelatin suspends the emulsion of microscopic silver crystals over the film base. During film processing, the gelatin absorbs the processing solutions and allows the chemicals to react with the silver halide crystals.
- The silver halide crystals absorb radiation during x-ray exposure and store energy emitted from the radiation (Fig. 39.16).
- The protective layer is a thin transparent coating that protects the emulsion surface.

## Latent Image

When radiation interacts with the silver halide crystals in the film emulsion, the image on the film is produced. This image is not visible before processing and is called the **latent image**.

An example of another type of latent image is *fingerprints*. If you touch an item, you leave your fingerprints even though you cannot see them on the object. When the item is treated, however, your fingerprints become visible.

## Film Speed

**Film speed** refers to the amount of radiation that is required to produce a radiograph of standard density (darkness). Film speed is determined by the following:

- Size of the silver halide crystals
- Thickness of the emulsion
- Presence of special radiosensitive dyes

Film speed determines how much exposure time is required to produce the image on the film. For example, a fast film requires less radiation. The fast film responds more quickly because the silver halide crystals in the emulsion are larger; the *larger* the crystals, the *faster* the film speed. This same principle applies to film speed on photographic film.

Film speed is classified by the American National Standards Institute (ANSI) with use of the letters A through F. Only D, E, and F speeds are used in intraoral dental radiography. *F-speed,* the newest and fastest film currently available, reduces radiation exposure to the patient by 20 to 60 percent compared with E-speed and D-speed film, respectively (Fig. 39.17).

The film speed is clearly indicated on the label side of the intraoral film packet, as well as on the outside of the film box or container.

## Types of Film

The three types of x-ray film used in dental radiography are intraoral film, extraoral film, and duplicating film.

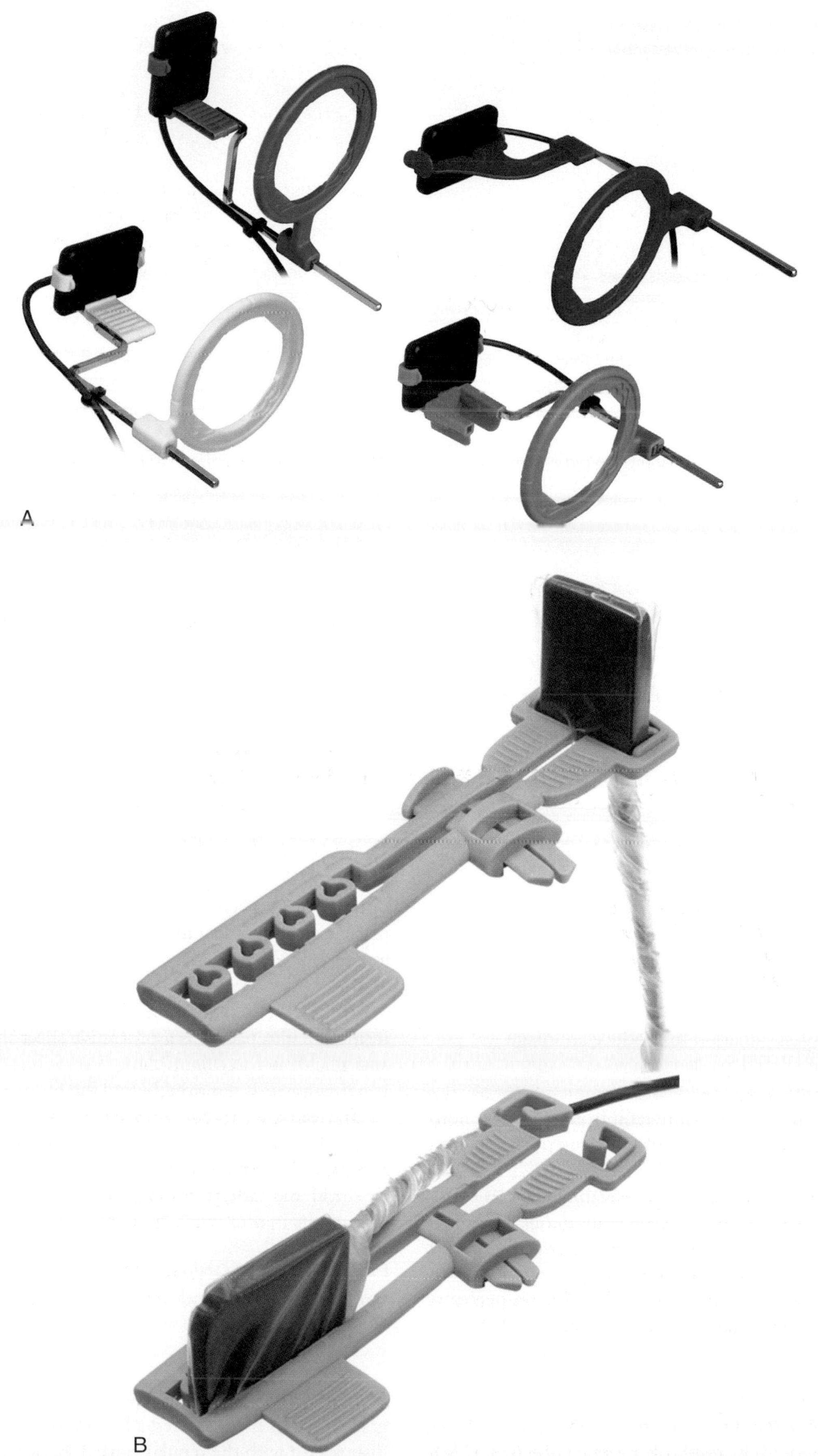

**FIG. 39.14** A, Rinn sensor holders suitable for Gendex, VisualiX, USB/GX, Cygnus, and Visiodent systems. B, Digital sensor holding device. *(Courtesy Dentsply Rinn, Elgin, IL.)*

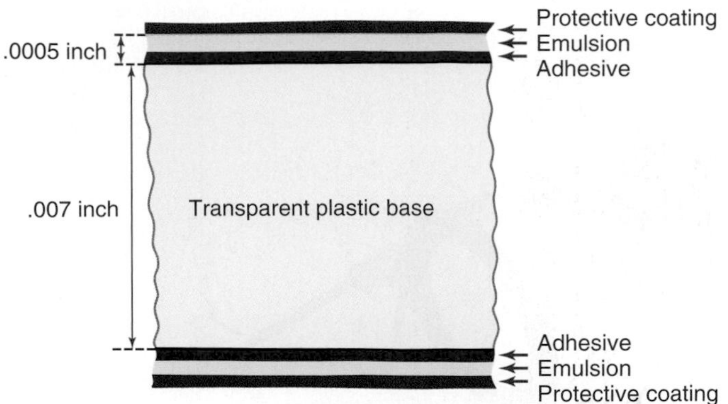


**FIG. 39.15** Cross-sectional diagram of film base and emulsion. *(From Frommer H, Stabulas-Savage JJ: Radiology for the dental professional, ed 9, St Louis, 2011, Mosby.)*

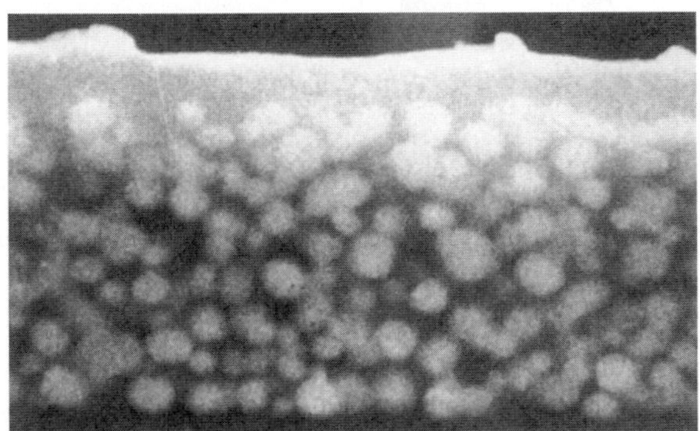

**FIG. 39.16** Scanning electron micrograph of unprocessed emulsion of pre-2006 Kodak Ultra-Speed dental film (5000× magnification). Note white-appearing, unexposed silver bromide grains. *(Courtesy Carestream Health, Inc., Rochester, NY.)*

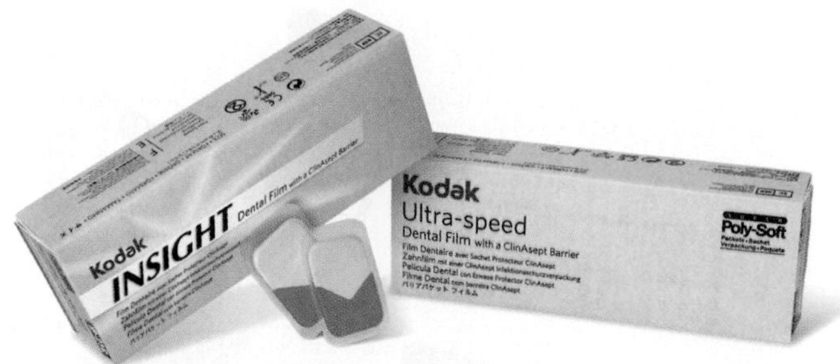


**FIG. 39.17** Insight is the F-speed film available from Kodak. *(Courtesy Carestream Health, Inc., Rochester, NY.)*

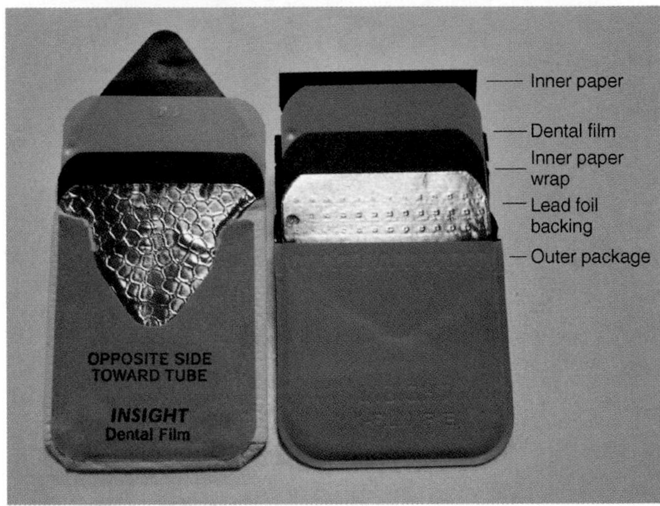


**FIG. 39.18** Contents of a moisture-proof dental film packet. *(Courtesy Carestream Dental, a division of Carestream Health, Inc.)*

## Intraoral Film

An intraoral film is placed *inside* the mouth (*intra*orally) during x-ray exposure. Intraoral radiographs are used to examine the teeth and supporting structures. Intraoral x-ray film has emulsion on *both sides* of the film instead of only on one side because it requires less radiation to produce an image.

### Film Packet

Film is sealed in a film packet to protect it from light and moisture. The terms *film packet* and *film* often are used interchangeably (Fig. 39.18).

Intraoral film packets are typically available in boxes of 25, 100, or 150 films. The film packet may contain one film (one-film packet) or two films (two-film packet). A two-film packet (also referred to as a *double film packet*) produces two identical radiographs with the same amount of radiation necessary to produce a single radiograph. The two-film packet is used when duplicate radiographs are necessary, such as for insurance claims and referrals to a specialist.

**PACKET INFORMATION.** Boxes of film are labeled with (1) type of film, (2) film speed, (3) number of films per individual packet, (4) total number of films in the box, and (5) film expiration date.

On one corner of the film packet is a small raised bump known as the *identification dot.* This bump or dot is used to differentiate the left side from the right side when the film is placed. The dot is also important when one is mounting radiographs (see Chapter 41).

**WRAPPER AND LEAD SHEET.** The black paper film wrapper inside the film packet is a protective sheet that covers the film and shields it from light. Always make certain that the black paper wrapper is removed before the film is processed.

The lead foil sheet is a single piece of foil that is included in the film packet behind the film and wrapped in black protective paper. The thin lead foil sheet is positioned *behind* the film to shield the film from back-scattered (secondary) radiation that results in film fog (Fig. 39.19).

**PACKAGE POSITIONING.** If the film packet is inadvertently positioned in the mouth backward and then is exposed, a *herringbone* pattern will be visible on the radiograph. This pattern is caused by the embossed pattern on the lead foil (Fig. 39.20).

**PACKAGE DISPOSAL.** In many states, the lead foil from radiograph packets is considered a hazardous waste and must not be disposed of with the regular trash. Check with the department of environmental health in your state, province, or territory.

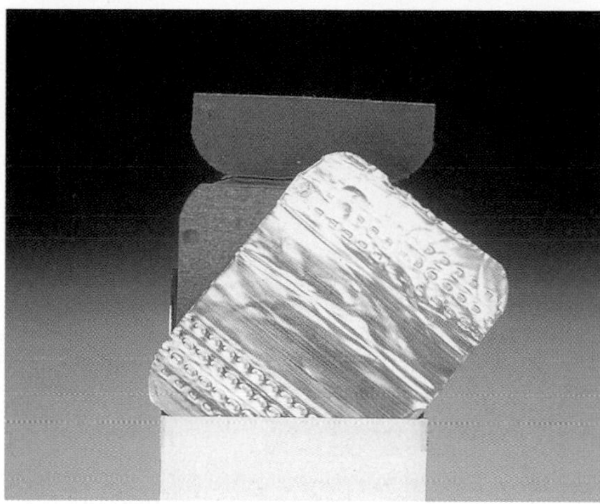

FIG. 39.19 The lead foil insert in this package has a raised diamond pattern across both ends.

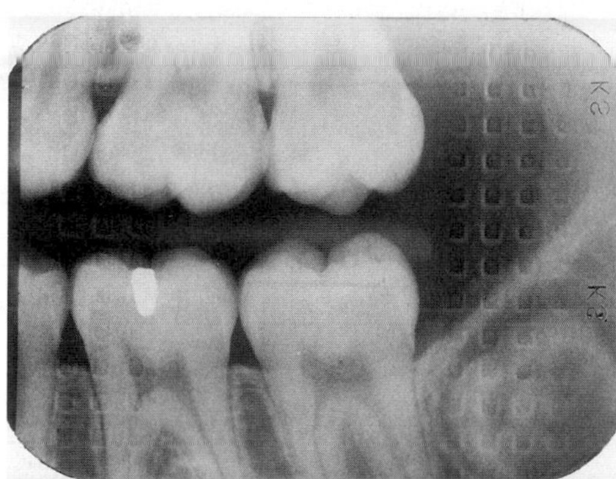

FIG. 39.20 A radiograph that was positioned backward in the mouth will have a herringbone pattern on it. *(From Langlais RP, Miller CS: Exercises in oral radiology and interpretation, ed 5, St Louis, 2017, Elsevier.)*

Recycling programs are available for the lead foil from radiograph packets.

### Outer Packet

The outer packet wrapping is a soft vinyl or paper wrapper that seals the film packet, protective black paper, and lead foil sheet. The outer wrapper protects the film from exposure to light and saliva.

**TUBE SIDE.** The **tube side** is solid white and has the raised bump on one corner. When placed in the mouth, the white side (tube side) of the film faces toward the teeth and tubehead, and the raised dot points toward the incisal/**occlusal** surface.

**LABEL SIDE.** The **label side** of the film packet has a flap that is used to open the film packet before processing. The label side is the color-coded side that is used to identify films. Color codes are used to distinguish between one-film and two-film packets and between film speeds. When placed in the mouth, the color-coded side of the packet faces toward the tongue.

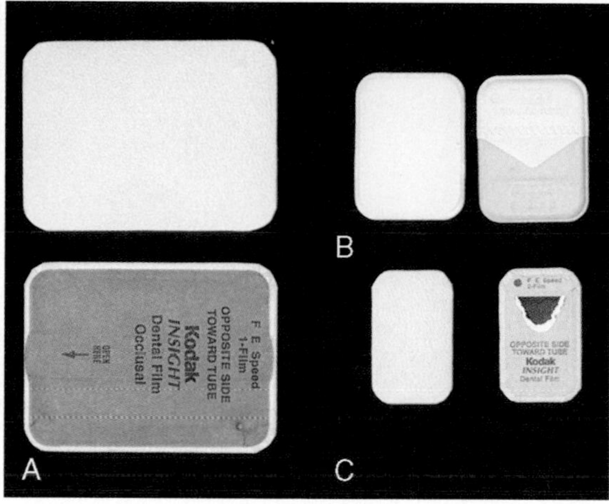


FIG. 39.21 The white side of the film packet faces the tube. A, Size #4 occlusal film. B, Size #2 film. C, Size #1 film.

### Film Sizes

Intraoral film packets come in five basic sizes (Fig. 39.21), as follows:

- Child size (#0): children younger than 3 years
- Narrow anterior (#1): anterior views on adults and children
- Adult size (#2)
- Preformed **bitewing** (#3): infrequently used
- Occlusal (#4)

Full-mouth radiographic surveys for adults usually involve film sizes #1 and #2. For adult bitewing examinations, #2 film is generally used.

RECALL

7 What are the five components of intraoral film?
8 What is a latent image?
9 How can you tell which side of the film is placed toward the tube?
10 What number film is used for adult radiographs?
11 What size film is used for occlusal radiographs?

## Extraoral Film

An **extraoral film** is placed *outside* the mouth (*extra*orally) during x-ray exposure. Extraoral films are used to examine large areas of the head or jaws.

Common extraoral films include panoramic and cephalometric films. A **panoramic film** shows a panoramic (wide) view of the upper and lower jaws on a single radiograph (Fig. 39.22). A **cephalometric film** shows the bony and soft tissue areas of the facial profile (Fig. 39.23).

### Film Packaging

Extraoral radiography uses a film-screen system, which means that the film is used with intensifying screens, as is discussed later.

Extraoral film is supplied in boxes of 50 or 100 films. Extraoral film used in dental radiography is available in 5 × 7–inch and 8 × 10–inch sizes. Boxes of extraoral film are labeled with

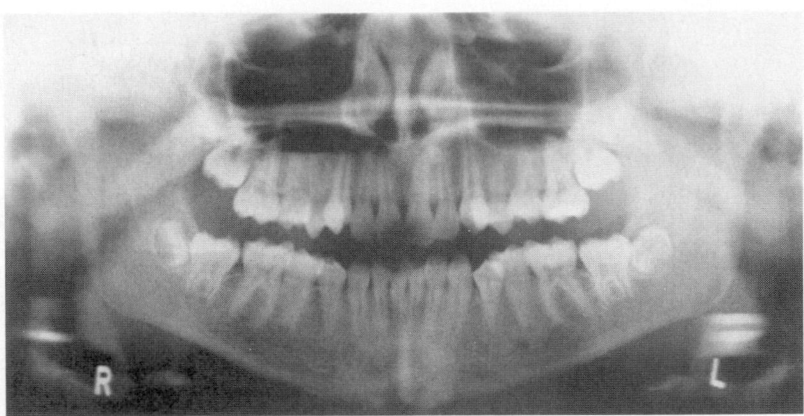


FIG. 39.22 Panoramic x-ray film. *(Courtesy Carestream Health, Inc., Rochester, NY.)*

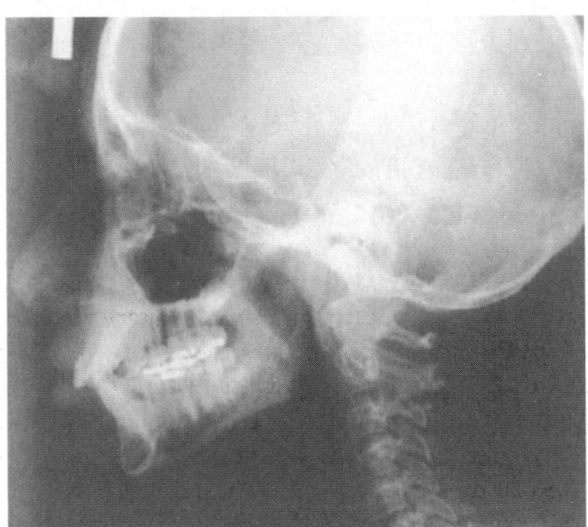

FIG. 39.23 Cephalometric radiograph. *(Courtesy Carestream Health, Inc., Rochester, NY.)*

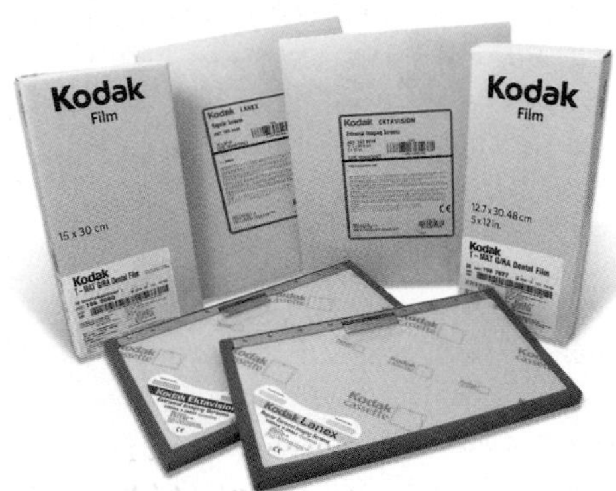


FIG. 39.24 Boxes of extraoral x-ray film. *(Courtesy Carestream Health, Inc., Rochester, NY.)*

(1) type of film, (2) film size, (3) total number of films enclosed, and (4) film expiration date.

Extraoral film is not supplied in film packets. This film is stacked in the box much in the way a deck of cards would be. *Important note:* Extraoral film boxes must be opened in the darkroom and the film then placed into a film cassette. The film in the box is not protected with paper wrappers as is intraoral film. If the box is opened where light is present, all the film in the box will be exposed and ruined (Fig. 39.24).

## Film Cassette

A **cassette** is a plastic or metal case that is used to hold the film and protect it from exposure to light. The cassette also holds the film in tight contact with the intensifying screen. Cassettes are available in rigid and flexible styles (Fig. 39.25).

Extraoral film does not have a raised dot on it. Therefore, to distinguish the patient's left from right, as on intraoral films, the front of the cassettes must be marked with the letter *L* (left side) or *R* (right side). After exposure, the letter will be superimposed on the radiograph. The front side of the cassette is typically constructed of plastic to permit passage of the x-ray beam, whereas the back side is made of metal to reduce scatter radiation. *The front side of the cassette must always face the patient during exposure.*

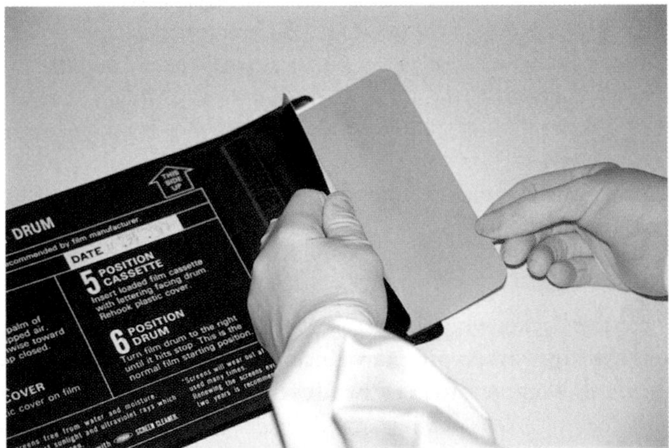


FIG. 39.25 The dental assistant removes a film from a flexible film cassette.

## Intensifying Screen

An intensifying screen is mounted on the front and back of the inside surfaces of a rigid-type film cassette (Fig. 39.26). The flexible-type film cassette uses removable intensifying screens.

An **intensifying screen**, as the name implies, is a device that intensifies or increases the effect of radiation and thus decreases the amount of exposure time needed. The intensifying screen is coated with a material called *phosphor,* which gives off light when struck by x-radiation. *This is the same material*

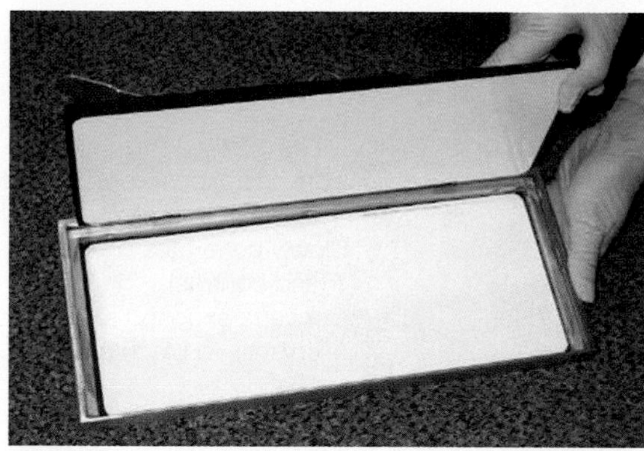

**FIG. 39.26** Rigid-type film cassette with an intensifying screen.

*that is used to coat the plates in the phosphor intraoral digital imaging system.* The film inside the cassette is sandwiched between the intensifying screens and is affected by the light from the phosphor *and* the x-radiation. The intensified beam results in a slight loss of image detail, however, because the light produces a *halo* effect at the edge of the image field.

Intensifying screens vary in their speed and exposure requirements, similar to the D, E, and F speeds of intraoral film. The speed of the screen depends on the type of phosphor and the size of the crystal; the larger the crystal, the faster the screen, but the poorer the definition. One type of screen uses a common type of phosphor called **calcium tungstate**, which produces a *blue light.*

The other types of phosphors are called rare earth elements; they produce a *green light.* Rare earth element screens are 4 times more efficient in converting x-ray energy into light than are calcium tungstate screens; therefore, they are faster and require less exposure time. Be certain to use the appropriate film for the type of intensifying screen that is in use.

When film is placed in and removed from the cassette, care must be taken not to scratch the intensifying screen. If an intensifying screen is badly scratched and the phosphor is removed, a white streak will appear on any films taken with this cassette.

### Film Types

The two types of film that may be used in extraoral radiography are screen film and nonscreen film.

Screen film is sensitive to the light emitted from the intensifying screen; this means that the film is more sensitive to light emitted by the phosphor in the intensifying screen than it is to radiation. The use of screen-type film and intensifying screens *reduces* the amount of radiation to the patient. The two types of screen film used in extraoral radiography are as follows:

- *Green-sensitive* film is used with cassettes that have rare earth intensifying screens.
- *Blue-sensitive* film is used with cassettes that have calcium tungstate intensifying screens.

Nonscreen film is an extraoral film that does *not* require the use of intensifying screens for exposure. A nonscreen extraoral film is exposed directly to x-rays; the emulsion is sensitive to direct x-ray exposure rather than to fluorescent light. A nonscreen extraoral film requires more exposure time than does a screen film and is *not* recommended for use in dental radiography.

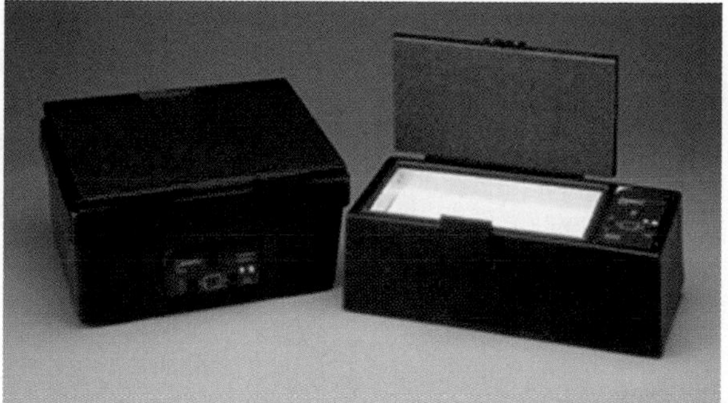

**FIG. 39.27** Examples of film duplicators. *(Courtesy Dentsply Rinn Corporation, Elgin, IL.)*

RECALL

12 What are the two types of extraoral film cassettes?
13 What is an intensifying screen?
14 How does extraoral film react differently from intraoral film?

## Duplicating Film

Duplication of radiographs may be necessary when one is referring patients to specialists, for insurance claims or legal purposes, or when patients change dentists and request that copies of their records be sent to the new dentist. Film duplication creates an identical copy of an intraoral or extraoral radiograph. Special duplicating film and a duplicating machine are needed to duplicate radiographs (Fig. 39.27). See Procedure 39.1: Duplicating Dental Radiographs.

**Duplicating film** is used only in a darkroom setting and is *never* exposed to x-rays. Duplicating film is sensitive to light and has emulsion on one side only. The emulsion side of the film appears dull, whereas the side without emulsion appears shiny. Duplicating film is available in all **periapical** sizes, as well as in 5 × 12–inch and 8 × 10–inch sheets.

The duplicating machine produces white light to expose the film. Because the film is light sensitive, the duplication process is performed in the darkroom with the safelight.

## Film Storage

All dental films should be stored according to the manufacturer's instructions; this involves providing protection from light, heat, moisture, chemicals, and scatter radiation. Optimum temperature for film storage ranges from 50° F to 70° F, and relative humidity levels range from 30 to 50 percent.

To avoid exposure to secondary or scatter radiation, film should not be kept in the treatment room or near the radiograph unit.

The box of x-ray film is marked with an expiration date. If expired film is accidentally used, the radiographs produced may be fogged and may not be of diagnostic quality. This effect is also known as *age fog.*

Always check the expiration date on the box when new film is purchased. If the expiration date on the box indicates that the film soon will be out of date, you should immediately return the box to the dental supplier. Always rotate the supply of film by using the oldest packages first.

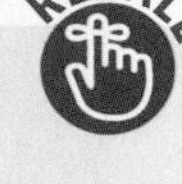


15 When might it be necessary to duplicate x-rays?
16 What precautions should be taken when storing x-ray film?
17 How can you find the expiration date of a package?

# Film Processing

**Processing** is a series of steps that change the latent image on the exposed film into a radiograph by producing a visible image on the film. Proper processing is just as important as the exposure technique is in producing diagnostic-quality radiographs. Radiographs that are nondiagnostic because of poor processing techniques must be retaken, resulting in unnecessary exposure of the patient to additional radiation.

In many practices, intraoral films are processed in an automatic processor. In some dental offices, however, it is still necessary to know how to process the film manually. Whichever method of processing is used, the steps are the same. Both manual and automatic methods are discussed in this chapter.

## Five Steps in Processing

Developing is the first step in processing film. A chemical solution called *developer* is used. The purpose of the developer is to chemically reduce the exposed silver halide crystals into black metallic silver. The developer solution softens the film emulsion during this process (Table 39.1).

- Rinsing the film is necessary to remove the developer from the film, so the development process stops.
- Fixing uses an acidic solution to remove the unexposed silver halide crystals from the film emulsion. The fixer also hardens the film emulsion during this process.
- Films that are not properly fixed will fade and turn brown in a short time. Leaving films in the fixer for a long period (such as over a weekend) can remove the image from the film (Table 39.2).
- Washing follows fixation. A water bath is used to wash the film.
- Drying the film is the final step in film processing.

## Processing Solutions

Film processing solutions are available in three forms: powder, ready-to-use liquid, and liquid concentrate.

The powder and liquid concentrate forms must be mixed with distilled water. The liquid concentrate is the most widely used form and is the preference of many dental offices; it is easy to mix and occupies little storage space (Fig. 39.28). Always follow the manufacturer's recommendations for preparing solutions.

**TABLE 39.1 Developer Composition**

| Ingredient | Chemical | Function |
|---|---|---|
| Developing agent | Hydroquinone | Converts exposed silver halide crystals to black metallic silver<br>Slowly generates black tones and contrast |
| | Elon | Converts exposed silver halide crystals to black metallic silver<br>Quickly generates gray tones |
| Preservative | Sodium sulfite | Prevents rapid oxidation of developing agents |
| Accelerator | Sodium carbonate | Activates developer agents<br>Provides necessary alkaline environment for agents<br>Softens gelatin of film emulsion |
| Restrainer | Potassium bromide | Prevents developer from developing unexposed silver halide crystals |

From Iannucci J, Jansen Howerton L: Dental radiography: principles and techniques, ed 4, St Louis, 2012, Saunders.

**TABLE 39.2 Fixer Composition**

| Ingredient | Chemical | Function |
|---|---|---|
| Fixing agent | Sodium thiosulfate, ammonium thiosulfate | Removes all unexposed, undeveloped silver halide crystals from emulsion |
| Preservative | Sodium sulfite | Prevents deterioration of fixing agent |
| Hardening agent | Potassium alum | Shrinks and hardens gelatin in emulsion |
| Acidifier | Acetic acid, sulfuric acid | Neutralizes alkaline developer and stops further development |

From Iannucci J, Jansen Howerton L: Dental radiography: principles and techniques, ed 4, St Louis, 2012, Saunders.

Fresh chemicals produce the best radiographs. To maintain freshness, film processing solutions must be replenished daily and changed every 3 to 4 weeks. More frequent changing of solutions may be necessary when large numbers of films are processed. "Normal" use is defined as 30 intraoral films per day.

18 What are the five steps in processing dental radiographs?
19 Which is the most widely used form of processing solution?
20 How often should processing solutions be replenished?

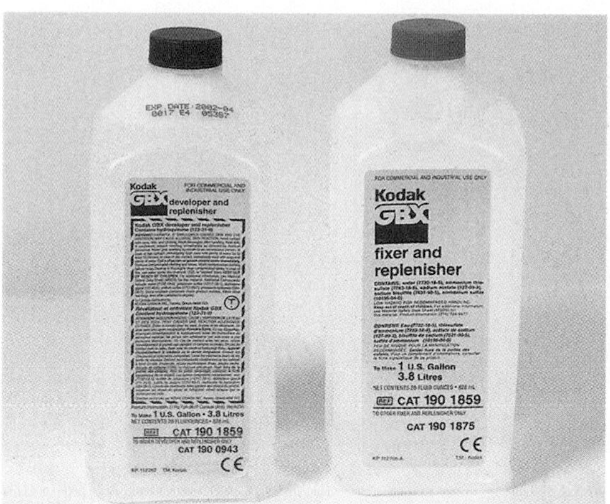


**FIG. 39.28** Concentrated solutions of film developer and fixer. *(Courtesy Carestream Health, Inc., Rochester, NY.)*

## The Darkroom

A well-organized darkroom facilitates the processing of dental x-ray films. The ideal darkroom is the result of careful planning. The darkroom should (1) have adequate working space, proper lighting, and good ventilation; (2) be kept clean at all times; and (3) be equipped with the necessary devices and supplies.

### Requirements for a Film Processing Darkroom

- Infection control items (gloves, disinfectant, spray, paper towels)
- Container with a biohazard label for contaminated film packets or barriers (see Chapter 23)
- Recycling container for lead foil pieces, which should not be thrown in the trash
- "Light-tight" room with no cracks around doors or corners that would allow light leaks
- Processing tanks for the developer and fixer solutions and a circulating water bath
- Running water supply with mixing valves to adjust the temperature
- Both a safelight and a source of white (normal) light
- Accurate timer
- Accurate floating thermometer to indicate the temperature of the solutions
- Stirring rod or paddle to mix the chemicals and equalize the temperature of the solutions
- Safe storage space for chemicals
- Film hangers
- A film-drying rack and a film dryer

### *Lighting*

The darkroom must be completely dark. The term *light-tight* is often used to describe the darkroom. To be light-tight, no light leaks can be present.

Any white light that "leaks" into the darkroom, such as from around the door, is termed a *light leak.* When you are in the darkroom with the light turned off, no white light should be seen. If you see *any* light leaks around the door, such as through a vent or a keyhole, this must be corrected with weather stripping or black tape. X-ray film is *extremely* sensitive to visible white light. Any leaks of white light can cause film fog. A fogged film appears dull gray, lacks contrast, and is nondiagnostic.

Two types of lighting are essential in a darkroom: room lighting and "safelighting."

**ROOM LIGHTING.** The darkroom must have an overhead white light that provides adequate lighting when one is performing tasks such as cleaning, restocking materials, and mixing chemicals.

**SAFELIGHTING.** A *safelight* is a low-intensity light in the red-orange spectrum. Safelighting provides enough illumination in the darkroom to process films safely without exposing or damaging the film.

A safe distance must be maintained between the light and the working area. Also, exposure to the safelight must be kept as short as possible by working quickly. Unwrapped films that are left too close to the safelight or that are exposed to the safelight for longer than 2 to 3 minutes appear fogged. A safelight must be placed at least 4 feet away from the film and working area (Fig. 39.29).

Of the many types of safelights available, some are made only for intraoral films, others only for extraoral films, and some for both intraoral and extraoral films. A good universal safelight filter for *both* extraoral screen films and intraoral films is the GBX-2 safelight filter by Kodak (Carestream Health, Rochester, NY). Recommendations for specific safelights and filters are provided on the film package.

### *Processing Tanks*

Manual processing is a method that is used to develop, rinse, fix, and wash dental radiograph films (Table 39.3). The essential piece of equipment required for manual processing is a processing tank. The processing tank is divided into compartments to hold the developer solution, water bath, and fixer solution. A processing tank has two insert tanks and one master tank (Fig. 39.30).

The temperature of the circulating water in the master tank controls the temperatures of the developer and fixer solutions. The water temperature is controlled through a mixing valve, which functions similarly to those found in bathroom showers. The optimum temperature for the water bath is 68° F (20° C).

RECALL

21 What is a safelight?
22 What is the minimum distance between the safelight and the working area?
23 What is the optimum temperature for the water in the manual processing tanks?

## Automatic Processor

Automatic film processing is a fast and simple method that is used to process dental radiograph films (Fig. 39.31). Other

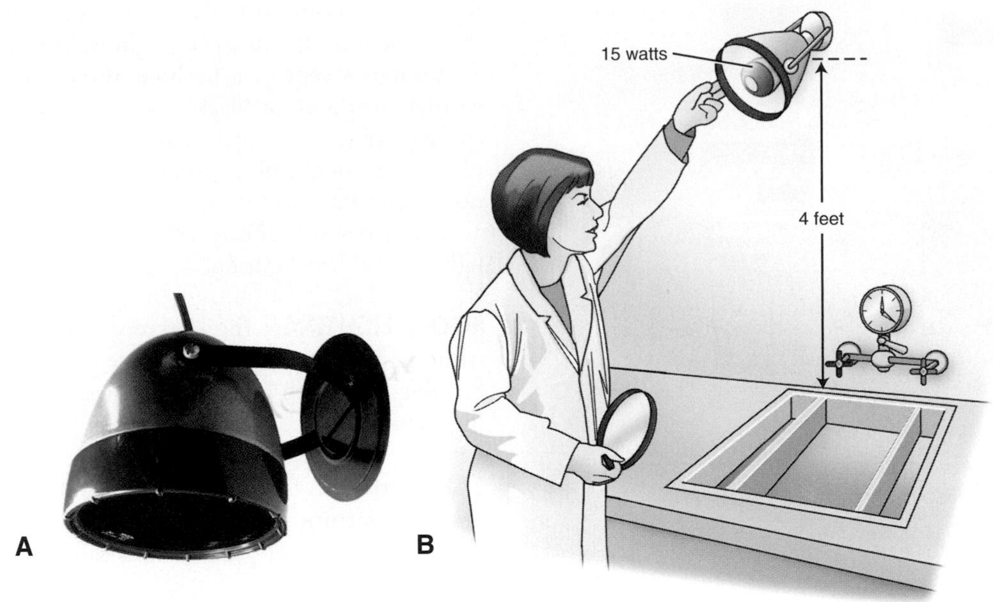


**FIG. 39.29** A, A safelight may be mounted on the wall or ceiling in the darkroom and should be at least 4 feet from the work surface. B, The safelight uses a GBX-2 filter and 15-watt bulb. *(From White SC, Pharoah MJ: Oral radiology: principles and interpretation, ed 7, St Louis, 2014, Mosby.)*

**TABLE 39.3** Processing Temperatures and Times

| Solution Temperature, ° F (° C) | Time in Processing Step (Minutes) | | | |
|---|---|---|---|---|
| | **Developer** | **Rinse** | **Fixer** | **Wash** |
| 65 (18.5) | 6 | ½ | 10–12 | 20 |
| 68 (20.0) | 5 | ½ | 10 | 20 |
| 70 (21.0) | | ½ | 9–10 | 20 |
| 72 (22.0) | 4 | ½ | 8–9 | 20 |
| 75 (24.0) | 3 | ½ | 6–7 | 20 |
| 80 (26.5) | | ½ | 5–6 | 20 |

Modified from Iannucci J, Jansen Howerton L: Dental radiography: principles and techniques, ed 4, St Louis, 2012, Saunders.

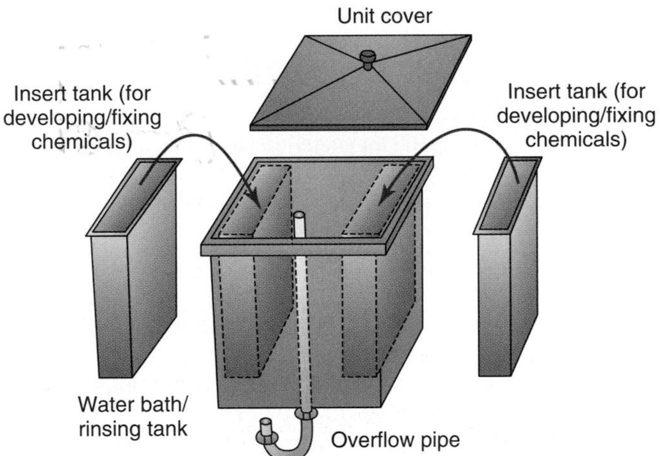


**FIG. 39.30** Processing tanks show developing and fixing tank inserts in bath of running water. *(From Iannucci J, Jansen Howerton L: Dental radiography: principles and techniques, ed 4, St Louis, 2012, Saunders.)*

than opening the film packet, the **automatic processor** automates all film processing steps.

Advantages of automatic film processing include the following:

- Less processing time is required.
- Time and temperatures are automatically controlled.
- Less equipment is used.
- Less space is required.

Automatic film processing requires only 4 to 6 minutes to develop, fix, wash, and dry a film, whereas manual processing and drying techniques require approximately 1 hour. In addition, the automatic processor maintains the correct temperature of the solutions and adjusts the processing time. Provided that the automatic processor is maintained properly, the chance of error during film processing is reduced.

Many dental offices with automatic processors maintain manual processing equipment as a standby or backup for when the automatic processor malfunctions. See Procedure 39.2: Processing Dental Films Manually and Procedure 39.3: Processing Dental Films in an Automatic Film Processor.

## Components

Automatic processors use a roller transport system to move the unwrapped dental x-ray film through the developer, fixer,

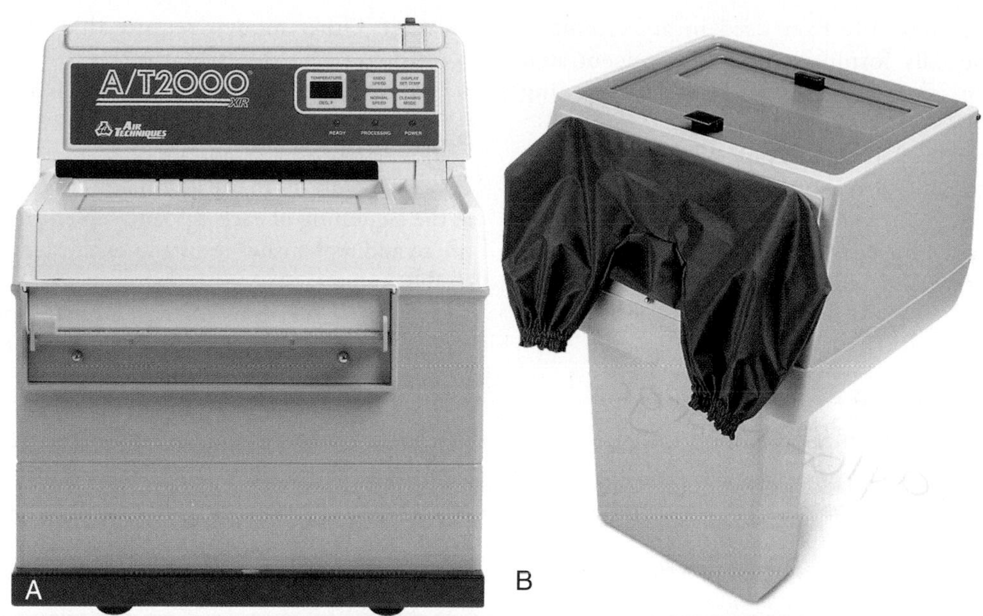


**FIG. 39.31** A, A typical automatic film processor used in the dental office. B, A daylight loader, which may be attached to the top of an automatic processor. *(Courtesy Air Techniques, Inc., Melville, NY.)*

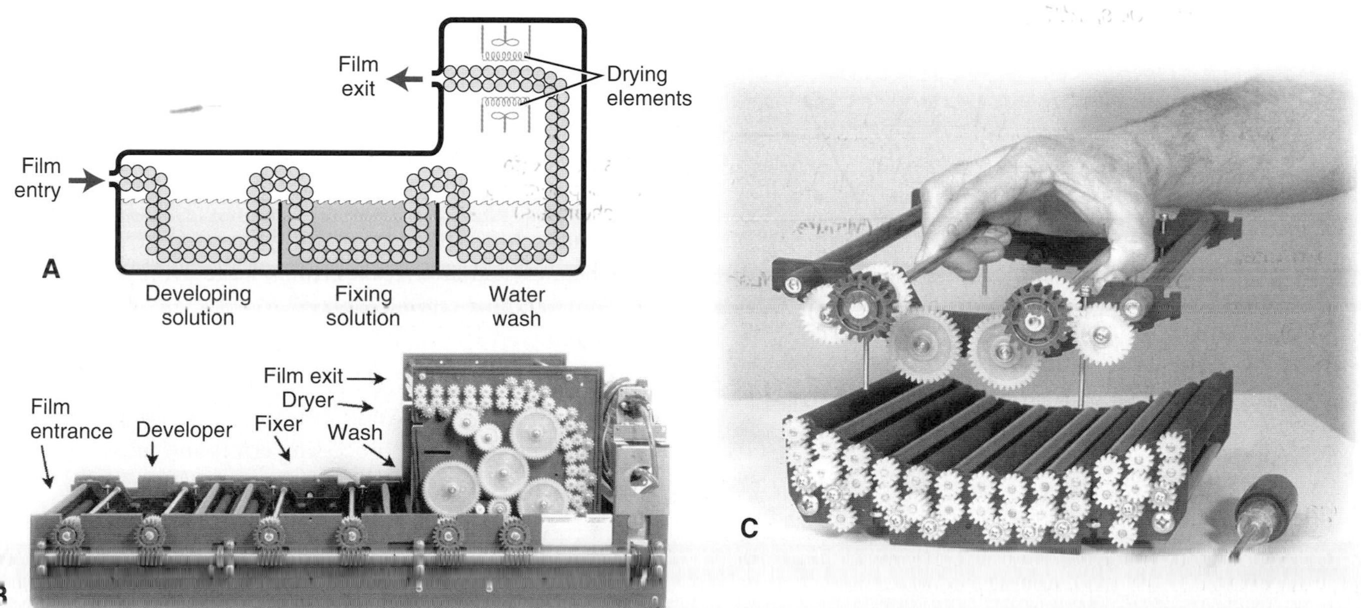


**FIG. 39.32** Component parts of the automatic processor. A, Automatic film processors typically consist of a roller assembly that transports the film through the developing, fixing, washing and drying solutions. B, Assembly of the film transport mechanism. C, One roller assembly. *(A, From White SC, Pharoah MJ: Oral radiology: principles and interpretation, ed 7, St Louis, 2014, Mosby. B and C, Courtesy AFP Manufacturing, Peachtree City, GA.)*

water, and drying compartments. Each component has its own special function (Fig. 39.32), as follows:

- The processor housing covers all the component parts of the automatic processor.
- The film feed slot is where the unwrapped films are inserted into the automatic processor.
- The roller film transporter is a system of rollers that rapidly moves the film through the developer, fixer, water, and drying compartments. The rollers are turned by motor-driven gears or belts.
- The developer compartment holds the developer solution. The developer used in an automatic processor is a specially formulated solution that is designed to react at temperatures between 80° F and 95° F. Because of the high temperatures, development occurs rapidly.
- The fixer compartment holds the fixer solution. The film is transported directly from the developer into the fixer

without a rinsing step. The fixer used in an automatic processor is a specially formulated, highly concentrated chemical solution that contains additional hardening agents.

- *Note:* The chemicals used in manual processing should never be used in an automatic processor.
- The water compartment holds circulating water. Water is used to wash the films after fixation. Some units have a plumbed water system that provides continuous fresh water. Other models require that the water be changed manually.
- The drying chamber holds heated air and dries the wet film.

### Processing Solutions

Levels of solutions in the automatic processor must be checked at the beginning of each day and replenished as necessary. Failure to add replenisher results in exhausted solutions and poor-quality radiographs.

Processing solutions in the automatic processor should be replaced every 2 to 6 weeks, depending on the number of films processed and the replenishment schedule. Follow the manufacturer's recommendations carefully. Some units have pumps that add replenisher solutions automatically to maintain proper solution concentrations and levels. Other models require the operator to replenish the solutions (Box 39.2).

**BOX 39.2 Preventing Problems in Automatic Processors**

- Keep the cover open slightly, particularly over the motor, when the processor is *not in use.* Accumulated fumes will fog films if not vented, and the moisture around the motor will cause premature rusting and breakdown. Be sure to replace the cover tightly before processing films.
- Lubricate the moving parts as indicated in the owner's manual.
- Check the temperature of the solutions regularly. A few degrees' difference in the developer temperature will change the density of the films.
- Check each day to see that the rollers are locked in the proper position to prevent loss of films.
- *Replenish the chemicals* as described previously.
- Feed the films slowly into the machine and keep them straight. If they turn sideways even slightly, they may merge and stick together.
- Count 10 to 15 seconds after feeding each film into the processor before inserting another film.
- Alternate slots or sides when possible.
- Check to be sure that the black paper has been completely removed and double-pack films have been separated; place only the films into the processor.
- Do *not* put wet films into the processor, as they will contaminate the rollers.

From Miles DA et al: Radiographic imaging for the dental team, ed 4, St Louis, 2009, Saunders.

RECALL

**24** What is the major advantage of automatic film processing?

**25** How often should the levels of solution in the automatic processor be checked?

**26** Are manual processing solutions and automatic processing solutions interchangeable?

## Processing Errors

Processing errors may result in nondiagnostic radiographs. Films must be free from processing errors to be of diagnostic quality. Poor-quality radiographs may result from the following:

- Time and temperature errors (Table 39.4)
- Chemical contamination errors (Table 39.5)
- Film handling errors (Table 39.6)
- Lighting errors (Table 39.7)

Many processing errors can be attributed to one or more errors. The dental assistant must be able to recognize the appearance of common processing errors and must know what actions are needed to prevent a recurrence (Fig. 39.33).

**TABLE 39.4 Time and Temperature Errors and Solutions for Manual Processing**

| Example | Appearance | Error | Solution |
|---|---|---|---|
| Underdeveloped film | Light | Inadequate development time<br>Developer solution too cool<br>Inaccurate timer or thermometer<br>Depleted or contaminated developer solution | Check development time.<br>Check developer temperature.<br>Replace faulty timer or thermometer.<br>Replenish developer with fresh solution as needed. |
| Overdeveloped film | Dark | Excessive developing time<br>Developer solution too hot<br>Inaccurate timer or thermometer<br>Concentrated developer solution | Check development time.<br>Check developer temperature.<br>Replace faulty timer or thermometer.<br>Replenish developer with fresh solution as needed. |
| Reticulation of emulsion | Cracked | Sudden temperature change between developer and water bath | Check temperature of solutions and water bath. Avoid extreme temperature changes. |

Modified from Iannucci J, Jansen Howerton L: Dental radiography: principles and techniques, ed 4, St Louis, 2012, Saunders.

TABLE 39.5 Chemical Contamination Errors and Solutions for Manual Processing

| Example | Appearance | Error | Solution |
|---|---|---|---|
| Developer spots | Dark or black spots | Developer contacts film before processing | Use clean work area in darkroom. |
| Fixer spots | White or light spots | Fixer contacts film before processing | Use clean work area in darkroom. |
| Yellow-brown stains | Yellowish brown color | Exhausted developer or fixer<br>Insufficient fixation time<br>Insufficient rinsing | Replenish chemicals with fresh solutions as needed.<br>Ensure adequate fixation time.<br>Rinse for at least 20 minutes. |

Modified from Iannucci J, Jansen Howerton L: Dental radiography: principles and techniques, ed 4, St Louis, 2012, Saunders.

TABLE 39.6 Film Handling Errors and Solutions for Manual Processing

| Example | Appearance | Error | Solution |
|---|---|---|---|
| Developer cutoff | Straight white border | Undeveloped part of film from low level of developer | Check developer level before processing; add solution if needed. |
| Fixer cutoff | Straight black border | Unfixed part of film from low level of fixer | Check fixer level before processing; add solution if needed. |
| Overlapped films | White or dark areas | Two films in contact during processing | Separate films to prevent contact during processing. |
| Air bubbles | White spots | Air trapped on film surface after film placed in solution | Gently agitate film racks after placing in processing solutions. |
| Fingernail artifact | Black crescent-shaped marks | Film emulsion damaged by operator's fingernail during rough handling | Gently handle films only by the edges. |
| Fingerprint artifact | Black fingerprint | Film touched by fingers contaminated with fluoride or developer | Wash and dry films thoroughly before processing. |
| Static electricity | Thin, black, branching lines | Occurs when film pack is opened quickly<br>Occurs when film pack is opened before operator touches conductive object | Open film packs slowly.<br>Touch a conductive object before unwrapping film. |
| Scratched film | White lines | Soft emulsion removed from film by sharp object | Use care when handling films and film racks. |

Modified from Iannucci J, Jansen Howerton L: Dental radiography: principles and techniques, ed 4, St Louis, 2012, Saunders.

TABLE 39.7 Lighting Errors and Solutions

| Example | Appearance | Error | Solution |
|---|---|---|---|
| Light leak | Black (exposed area) | Accidental exposure of film to white light | Examine film packs for defects before using.<br>Never wrap films in presence of white light. |
| Fogged film | Gray; lack of detail and contrast | Improper "safelighting"<br>Light leaks in darkroom or autoprocessor<br>Outdated (expired) films<br>Improper film storage<br>Contaminated solutions<br>Solution too hot | Check filter and bulb wattage of safelight.<br>Check darkroom and autoprocessor for light leaks.<br>Check expiration date on the box of film.<br>Store films in cool, dry area.<br>Avoid contamination by covering tanks after each use.<br>Check temperature of developer. |

Modified from Iannucci J, Jansen Howerton L: Dental radiography: principles and techniques, ed 4, St Louis, 2012, Saunders.

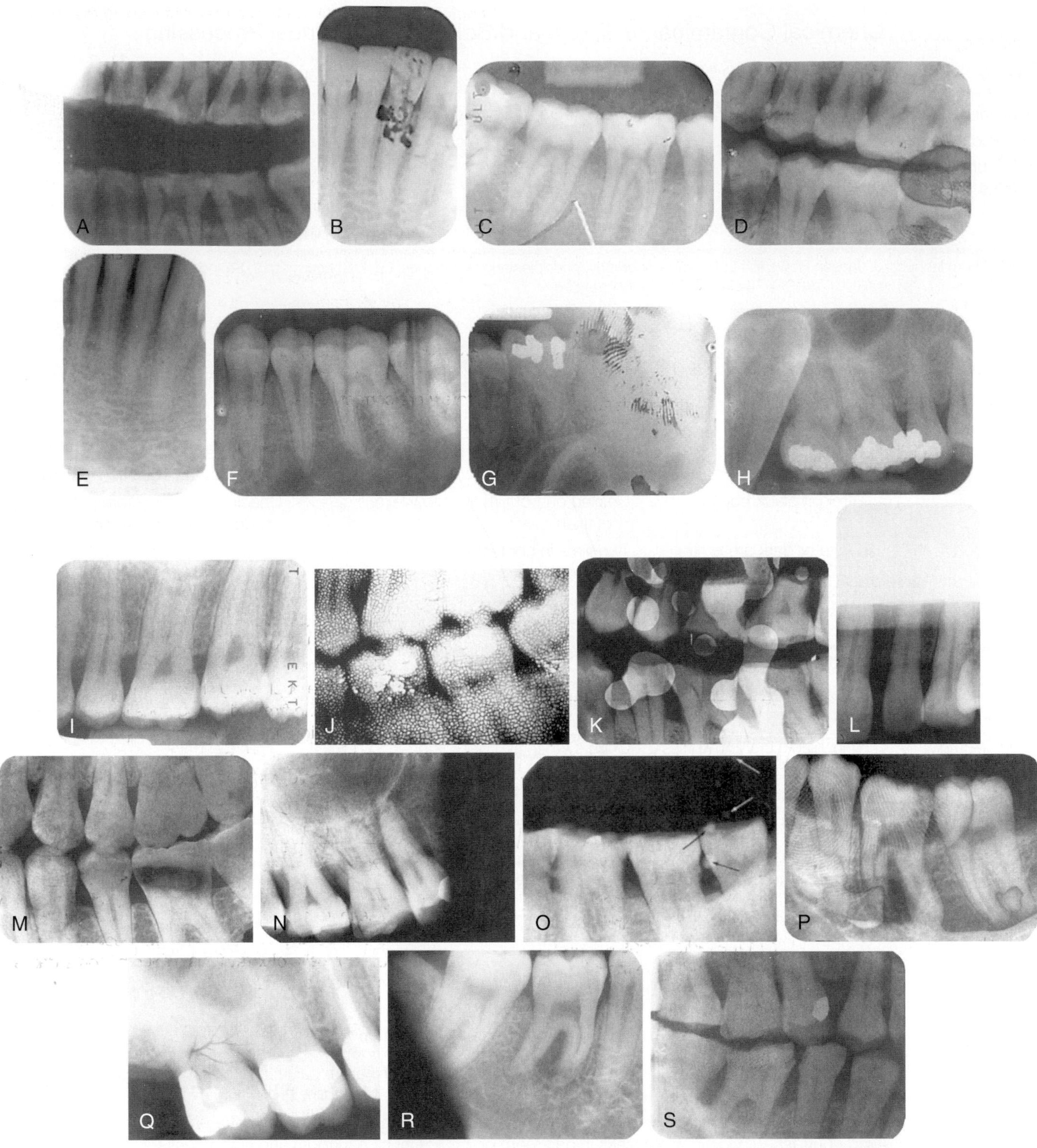


**FIG. 39.33** Radiograph processing errors. A, Overdevelopment. B, Developer splash. C, Scratched film. D, Water spots. E, Solution too low. F, Roller marks. G, Fingerprints. H, Overlapped films. I, Underdeveloped. J, Reticulation. K, Fixer spots. L, Developer cutoff. M, Number of errors. N, Fixer cutoff. O, Air bubbles. P, Black fingerprint. Q, Static electricity. R, Exposure to light. S, Fogged film. *(From Iannucci J, Jansen Howerton L: Dental radiography: principles and techniques, ed 5, St Louis, 2017, Elsevier.)*

**■ Legal and Ethical Implications** Dental images are a critical component of the patient's permanent record. The diagnostic quality of a digital image or a properly processed radiograph must never be compromised. It may be considered malpractice for a dentist to provide treatment using images that are inadequate for proper diagnosis.

When films with processing errors make it necessary to retake the film, the patient is exposed to unnecessary additional radiation. ■

**■ Eye to the Future** Digital imaging has distinct advantages over film. One of the primary advantages of digital imaging is that it eliminates the need for x-ray film, processing solutions, running water, and a darkroom. It is also better for the environment by eliminating disposal of hazardous chemicals. The digital imaging techniques of the future will even further reduce the amount of radiation exposure to the patient. Imaging techniques of the future may not involve the use of radiation at all. ■

## ■ Critical Thinking

1. Jason Marks is a 2-year-old patient in your office, and you are going to take bitewing radiographs on him. What size film do you think you will need?
2. Your dental office has recently transitioned to digital radiography. Mr. Huang, who has not been in the office for almost 3 years, begins to ask you questions about the safety of digital imaging and wants to know why you are using sensors instead of film. How would you respond?
3. Nancy is a new dental assistant in your office, and she just finished manually processing some dental radiographs. When you look at the films, you notice that they are very light. You exposed the films, so you are certain that the exposure factors were correct. What could have gone wrong? ■

PROCEDURE 39.1 

## Duplicating Dental Radiographs

### GOAL

To duplicate a set of dental radiographs.

### EQUIPMENT AND SUPPLIES

- ✔ Darkroom environment
- ✔ Duplicating film
- ✔ Duplicating machine
- ✔ Radiograph label
- ✔ Pen

### PROCEDURAL STEPS

1. Turn on the safelight and turn off the white light.
2. Place the radiographs on the duplicator machine glass.
3. Open the box of duplicating film and remove one film.
4. Place the duplicating film on top of the radiographs with the emulsion side against the radiographs, and close the lid.
5. Turn on the light in the duplicating machine for the manufacturer's recommended time.

   **PURPOSE** The light passes through the radiographs and strikes the duplicating film.
6. Remove the duplicating film and radiographs from the machine.
7. Process the duplicating film as you would other film, using manual or automatic techniques.
8. Return the original radiographs to the patient's file.
9. Document the duplication in the patient's record.

| Date | Procedure | Operator |
|---|---|---|
| 8/15/17 | Duplicated FMX and mailed to Delta Dental Insurance | PJL |

**NOTE** The longer the duplicating film is exposed to light, the lighter the duplicate films will become. This is the opposite of x-ray films, which become darker when exposed to light.

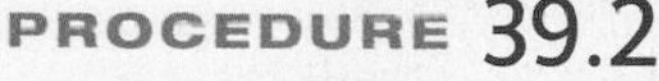 

## Processing Dental Films Manually

### GOAL

To process dental films using a manual tank.

### EQUIPMENT AND SUPPLIES

- ✔ Fully equipped darkroom
- ✔ Surface barriers or disinfecting solution for counters
- ✔ Exposed films
- ✔ Film rack
- ✔ Timer
- ✔ Pencil
- ✔ Film dryer (optional)

### PROCEDURAL STEPS

#### Preparation

1. Follow all the infection control steps discussed in Chapter 40.
2. Stir the solutions with the corresponding paddle.

**(Continued)**

## PROCEDURE 39.2 Processing Dental Films Manually—cont'd

**PURPOSE** The chemicals are heavy and tend to settle to the bottom of the tank. Do not interchange mixing paddles, or cross-contamination will occur.

3 Check the temperature of the developer solution and refer to the processing chart to determine the times (see Table 39.3).

**PURPOSE** The temperature of the solution determines the processing time.

4 Label the film rack with the patient's name and date of exposure.

5 Turn on the safelight; then turn off the white light.

6 Wash hands and put on gloves.

7 Open the film packets and allow the films to drop onto the clean paper towel. Take care not to touch the films.

**PURPOSE** The films have not been contaminated. Films that have been touched become contaminated and may remain contaminated even after processing.

### Processing

8 Attach each film to the film rack so the films are parallel and are not touching each other.

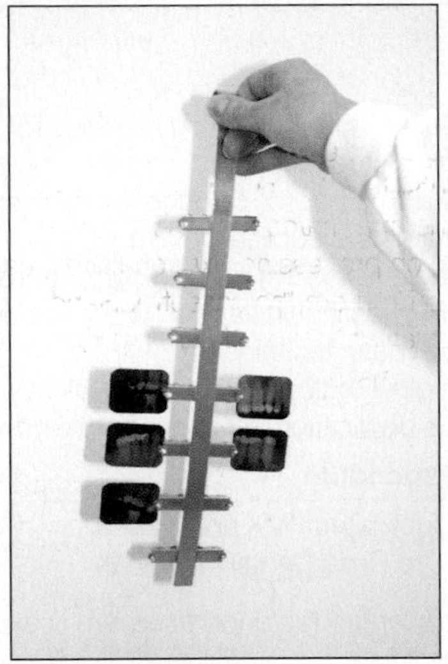

9 As you immerse the film rack in the developer solution, agitate (jiggle) the rack slightly.

**PURPOSE** Agitating the film rack prevents air bubbles from forming on the film.

10 Start the timer. The timer is set according to the recommendations stated on the processing chart (e.g., 5 minutes if the solution is 68° F [20° C]).

11 When the timer goes off, remove the rack of films and rinse it in the circulating water in the center tank for 20 to 30 seconds. Let the excess water drip off the films.

**PURPOSE** Water dripping from the racks into the fixer will dilute it.

12 Insert the rack of films into the fixer tank, and set the timer for 10 minutes.

**PURPOSE** For permanent fixation, the film is kept in the fixer for a minimum of 10 minutes. However, films may be removed from the fixing solution after 3 minutes for viewing; this is a wet reading. The films must be returned to the fixer to complete the process.

13 Return the rack of films to the center tank of circulating water for at least 20 minutes.

**PURPOSE** Incomplete washing will cause the films to eventually turn brown.

14 Remove the rack of films from the water and place it in the film dryer. If a film dryer is not available, it is recommended to hang the films to air-dry.

**PURPOSE** Films may be air-dried at room temperature in a dust-free area or placed in a heated drying cabinet. Films must be completely dried before they can be handled for mounting and viewing.

15 When the radiographs (films) are completely dry, remove them from the rack, and mount and label (see Chapter 41).

PROCEDURE 39.3 

# Processing Dental Films in an Automatic Film Processor

## EQUIPMENT AND SUPPLIES

- Automatic x-ray processor with daylight loader
- Exposed dental films
- Chemical disinfection spray
- Two disposable cups or containers for lead foil and film packets
- Paper towel

## PROCEDURAL STEPS

**1** At the beginning of the day, turn on the machine and allow the chemicals to warm up according to the manufacturer's recommendations.

**PURPOSE** The heating unit must warm the chemicals to the correct temperature so the films will be of diagnostic quality.

**2** Follow the infection control steps discussed in Chapter 40.

**PURPOSE** The film packets are contaminated because they have been in the patient's mouth.

**3** Wash and dry hands.

**4** Open the lid on the daylight loader and place a paper towel over the bottom. Then place two disposable cups on the towel.

**PURPOSE** The paper towel will act as a surface barrier on the bottom of the daylight loader. One disposable cup is for the lead foil in the film packet; the other is for use in disposing of the paper towel, film packets, and gloves.

**5** Put on gloves and slide gloved hands through the sleeves of the daylight loader.

**6** Remove the film from its packet, and check to be sure that the black paper has not stuck to the film. If the black paper is left on the film, or if double film packets have not been separated, the films will be ruined and the automatic processor could jam.

**7** Feed the film into the machine.

**PURPOSE** Open the film packets and feed films in one at a time to avoid having films overlap during loading.

**8** While the film is feeding into the machine, remove the lead foil from the packet and place it into one of the disposable cups. Then drop the empty packet onto the paper towel.

**9** Keep the films straight as they are fed slowly into the machine. Allow at least 10 seconds between insertion of each film into the processor and insertion of the next film. Place films in alternate film slots when possible.

**10** After the last film is inserted into the machine, carefully remove gloves and drop them into the center of the paper towel. Touching only the corners and underside of the paper towel, wrap the paper towel over the contaminated film packets and gloves. Place the wrapped paper towel into the second cup.

**PURPOSE** Handling the paper towel only by the corners and underside will help eliminate cross-contamination during film processing procedures.

**11** Remove the cup that contains the lead foil and take it to the recycling container.

**12** Remove the processed radiographs from the film recovery slot on the outside of the automatic processor. Allow 4 to 6 minutes for the automated process to be completed.

**NOTE** When processing extraoral films, carefully remove the film from the cassette. Handle all films by the edges only, to avoid fingerprints and scratches on the films.

40

# Legal Issues, Quality Assurance, and Infection Prevention

## KEY TERMS

**Artifact** A blemish or unintended radiographic image that is not present in the actual structure.

**Confidentiality** Never revealing any personal information about the patient.

**Disclosure** Process of informing the patient about a procedure, for example, the procedure for taking x-rays.

**Image receptor** Recording medium for an image—a digital sensor, a phosphor storage plate (PSP), or conventional dental x-ray film.

**Informed consent** Permission granted by a patient after being informed about the risks, benefits, and alternatives of a procedure.

**Liability** Accountability or legal responsibility.

**Malpractice** Professional negligence.

**Negligence** The failure to provide a proper or reasonable level of care.

**Phosphor storage plates (PSPs)** Reusable film-sized flexible plates coated with phosphor as the image receptor.

**Positioning devices** Intraoral devices used to position and hold the film, sensor, or PSP.

**Quality assurance (QA)** A plan to ensure that the dental office produces consistent, high-quality images with a minimum of exposure to patients and personnel.

**Quality control tests** Specific tests used to ensure quality in dental x-ray equipment, supplies, and film processing.

**Risk management** Policies and procedures that will reduce the chance that a malpractice lawsuit will be brought against the dentist. Key areas of risk management include *patient informed consent, patient records, confidentiality, liability issues,* and *patient education.*

**Standard of care** Level of knowledge, skill, and care comparable with that of other dentists who are treating similar patients under similar conditions.

**Stepwedge** Device constructed of layered aluminum steps to demonstrate film densities and contrasts.

**View box** An illuminated boxlike device used to view radiographs.

## LEARNING OUTCOMES

*On completion of this chapter, the student will be able to achieve the following objectives:*

1 Pronounce, define, and spell the key terms.
2 Discuss the three major categories of legal considerations, including the following:
   - Describe the types of laws that affect the practice of dental radiography.
   - Describe the Consumer-Patient Radiation Health and Safety Act.
   - Describe the components of informed consent with regard to dental imaging.
   - Identify the individual who legally "owns" the dental images.
3 Discuss quality assurance in the dental office, including the following:
   - Name the annual tests recommended for x-ray equipment.
   - Describe quality control tests for processing solutions, including the use of a reference radiograph and stepwedge radiograph.
   - Describe the components of a quality assurance program.
4 Discuss infection control, including the following:
   - Implement the Centers for Disease Control and Prevention (CDC) guidelines for infection control in dental radiology.
   - Explain the infection control requirements for preparing a radiography operatory.
   - Describe the infection control protocol when making exposures using conventional dental x-ray film.
   - Describe the infection control protocol when making exposures using phosphate storage plates.
   - Describe the infection control protocol when making exposures using digital sensors.
   - Describe procedures during and after x-ray exposure.
   - Describe procedures during x-ray film processing.

## PERFORMANCE OUTCOMES

*On completion of this chapter, the student will be able to meet competency standards in the following skills:*

- Perform infection control practices required for all dental imaging techniques.
- Practice infection control measures when in the darkroom.
- Practice infection control measures when using the daylight loader in processing dental films.
- Scan images from phosphor plates.

## ELECTRONIC RESOURCES

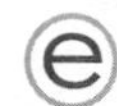
***Additional information related to content in Chapter 40 can be found on the companion Evolve Web site.***

- Practice Quiz
- Video: Preparing Operatory/Equipment to Take Radiographs
- Canadian Content Corner

Dental radiography is an important part of patient care, including the diagnosis of dental disease and treatment planning. When dental radiographs are either not properly exposed or used, there is the possibility of a claim of negligent care. As a dental assistant, it is your responsibility to understand the laws that apply to you when you are exposing dental images.

Federal and state regulations control the use of dental x-ray equipment. Individual state requirements also determine the educational qualifications of dental personnel who expose dental radiographs.

To ensure the highest quality dental images and the least risk for radiation exposure to patients and personnel, a *quality assurance program* is necessary. **Quality assurance (QA)** means regular testing to detect equipment malfunctions, monitoring techniques, and scheduled maintenance. Regular testing of equipment also helps to ensure compliance with state and federal regulations.

Regardless of whether film-based or digital techniques are used, the potential is always present for cross-contamination of equipment and environmental surfaces if good infection control procedures are not practiced.

In this chapter, you will learn the details and the step-by-step infection control procedures that are required in the various techniques of dental radiography. Refer to Part 4 of this text for a detailed discussion of disinfection, sterilization, and other general infection control measures.

# Legal Considerations

Three major categories of legal considerations regarding the use of images in dentistry have been identified: (1) federal and state *regulations* regarding x-ray equipment and its use, (2) *licensure* for individuals who expose dental images, and (3) **risk management** to reduce the chances of a patient taking legal action.

## Federal and State Regulations

The use of dental x-ray equipment is regulated by *federal* and *state* regulations. All dental x-ray machines manufactured or sold in the United States after 1974 must meet federal regulations. These include safety specifications for minimum filtration and accuracy of the milliamperage, time, and kilovoltage settings.

All x-ray equipment is also subject to state, county, or city radiation health codes. These codes may include regulations pertaining to barriers, film speeds, position of the operator, and image processing. Many states require that x-ray machines must be registered and charge a fee for this registration. In addition, most states have laws that require inspection of dental x-ray equipment on a regular basis, such as every 5 years. Be certain that you understand the requirements in your state.

## Licensure Requirements

The Consumer-Patient Radiation Health and Safety Act is a federal law that requires that all persons who use x-rays to take dental radiographs must be properly trained and certified. It is then up to the individual state to establish its own policies.

Thus requirements for certification in radiography for dental assistants vary from state to state. Some states require Dental Assisting National Board (DANB) certification, and other states may require an additional examination. Because each state deals with dental radiography differently, it is your responsibility to become informed about the specific requirements in your particular state.

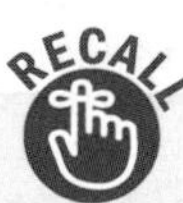


1 What federal act requires persons who take radiographs to be trained and certified?

## Risk Management

Risk management involves following policies and procedures that will reduce the chance that a **malpractice** lawsuit will be brought against the dentist. Key areas of risk management include patient informed consent, patient records, **confidentiality**, **liability** issues, and patient education, as discussed in the following sections.

In today's society, people tend to file more malpractice lawsuits than in the past. Thus the dental assistant should always practice risk management. For example, the assistant must be careful not to make casual negative comments about the radiograph equipment or its operation. Statements made without thinking, such as "The timer must be off," "This thing never works right," or "The solutions are weak," are unnecessary and can make the patient feel uncomfortable. Remember, statements made by anyone at the time of an alleged negligent act are admissible as evidence in court (see Chapter 5).

## Informed Consent

It is the dentist's responsibility to discuss with the patient the need for dental images and treatment procedures, but the dental assistant may participate in the process of obtaining **informed consent**. Patients must give their informed consent for dental images, in addition to other procedures. Before patients can give informed consent, they must be provided with the following information in *terms the patient can understand:*

- Risks and benefits of radiographic procedures
- Person who will be exposing the radiographs
- Number and type of radiographs that will be taken
- Consequences of not having the radiographs
- Alternative diagnostic aids that may provide the same information as dental radiographs

The process of informing the patient about the nature and purpose of dental radiographs is termed **disclosure**. After disclosure, the patient may give informed consent or may refuse the radiographs. If the dentist has *not* obtained informed consent from a patient before exposure of dental radiographs, a patient may legally claim malpractice or **negligence**.

## Liability

Under state laws, the supervising dentist is legally responsible, or *liable,* for the actions of dental auxiliary personnel. Known as the *respondeat superior* doctrine, this means that the employer is responsible for the actions of the employee.

Even though dental assistants work under the supervision of a licensed dentist, they still can be held legally liable for their *own* actions. Most often, the dentist is the only person sued for negligence or malpractice, but in some cases the dentist and the dental assistant have been sued for the actions of the dental assistant. You must be aware of the laws in your state, province, or territory, and practice accordingly.

## Patient Records

Whether conventional film or digital images are obtained, they are a part of the patient's dental record and must be regarded as a legal document. The dental record must accurately reflect all aspects of patient care (see Chapter 26). Documentation of all radiographs must include the following information:

- Informed consent
- Number and type of radiographs
- Rationale for requiring radiographs
- Diagnostic interpretation

It is important to document the exposure of dental radiographs. The number of exposures and the quality of the radiographs may be important issues in a malpractice suit. If poor-quality radiographs are used in court, this reflects poorly on the dentist.

### *Ownership of Dental Radiographs*

Legally, dental radiographs are the property of the dentist, even though the patient or the patient's insurance company paid for them, because dental radiographs are a part of the patient's *dental records.*

However, patients have a right to reasonable access to their records. When patients transfer to another dentist, it is reasonable for them to have a copy of their records, including dental radiographs, forwarded to the new dentist. Patients may request a copy of their radiographs; this request should be written and signed by the patient. The dentist should be informed of the patient's request, and an entry should be made in the chart stating when and to whom duplicate radiographs or digital images were sent. A reasonable fee may be charged. *Never* give or send the original radiographs to a patient. If a lawsuit should occur, no defense is possible without the dental radiographs.

Dental radiographs and other dental records should be retained indefinitely. Statutes of limitation may vary, and the question of when to destroy or discard a patient record may not always have a simple answer. Patient records and computer data must be stored carefully so they do not become damaged or lost. Computer files should always be backed up both within the dental office and at an off-site storage facility. It is critical that a protocol and labeling system is used to ensure that computer records are not accidentally overwritten.

## Digital Files Security

An advantage of digital files is that they can be sent over computer networks. Before doing so, you must check with local, state, and federal regulations about patient confidentiality. It may be necessary to encrypt the files or use virtual private networks (VPNs) rather than sending files over the public Internet.

## Patient Refusal

On occasion, patients may refuse to have dental radiographs. This refusal presents a difficult situation because the dentist must decide whether an accurate diagnosis can be made without radiographs, and whether treatment should be provided. In most cases, a lack of radiographs compromises the patient's diagnosis and treatment. The use of dental radiographs is now the accepted **standard of care**.

Every effort should be made to educate the patient about the importance of dental radiographs. No document can be signed that totally releases the dentist from liability for treating a patient without taking dental radiographs. Even if the patient suggests signing a release or waiver that would release the dentist from liability, such a document would be considered invalid if an injury were to result. Legally, a patient cannot consent to negligent care. It should be stated in the patient's record if a patient refuses recommended radiographs. The dentist then must make the decision as to whether to proceed without dental radiographs.

## Patient Education

As a dental assistant, you should understand and be sensitive to the patient's concern and fears about exposure to radiation during radiographs. The patient often feels more comfortable

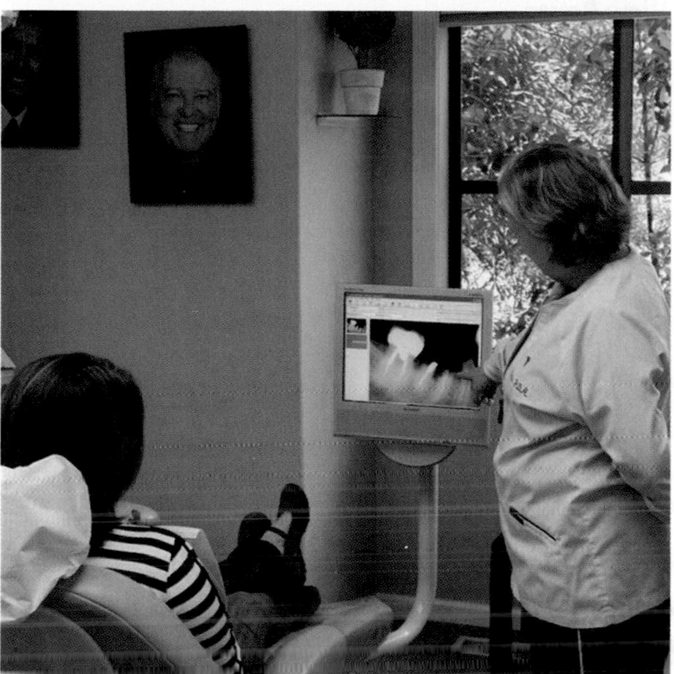

**FIG. 40.1** The dental assistant explains the importance of radiographs and answers the patient's questions regarding the safety of dental x-rays.

confiding these fears to the dental assistant rather than to the dentist.

The dental assistant can explain to the patient the importance of dental radiographs in detecting disease and planning treatment (Fig. 40.1). The dental assistant can inform patients of the federal and state laws enacted for their protection. In addition, you can give patients educational materials on the subject (e.g., American Dental Association pamphlets, such as Dental Radiograph Examinations, Your Dentist's Advice, and The Benefits of Radiograph Examinations, or the U.S. Food and Drug Administration's Radiographs: Get the Picture on Protection). These educational materials also can be placed in the reception room. Furthermore, the dental assistant can remind patients that the dose from four bitewing images is about the same as a single day's worth of natural background radiation.

RECALL

2 What type of consent is necessary before a patient is exposed for dental images?
3 Under state laws, who is allowed to prescribe dental images?
4 Who is the legal owner of a patient's dental images?

# Quality Assurance in the Dental Office

QA is a way of ensuring that everything possible is being done to produce high-quality diagnostic images. QA includes *quality control tests* that monitor dental x-ray equipment, supplies, and image processing. It also involves *quality administration procedures* that include keeping schedules of maintenance and record-keeping logs.

The benefits of a QA program far outweigh the associated time, effort, and costs. Fewer retakes mean time and cost savings for both patients and operators.

## Quality Control Tests

**Quality control tests** are specific tests that are used to monitor dental x-ray equipment, supplies, and film processing. The American Academy of Dental Radiology recommends a number of annual tests for dental x-ray machines. These tests are designed to identify minor malfunctions, including (1) variations in radiation output, (2) inadequate collimation, (3) tubehead drifting, (4) errors in timing, and (5) inaccurate kilovoltage and milliamperage readings.

### Types of Quality Control Tests

*Dental film:* Test each new box for freshness.
*Dental x-ray machine:* Calibrate equipment regularly.
*Cassettes and phosphor storage plates (PSPs):* Clean and examine for scratches.
*Safelighting:* Check for light-tightness in darkroom.
*Automatic processor:* Follow manufacturer's recommendations carefully regarding maintenance.
*Manual processor:* Replenish daily and change every 3 to 4 weeks.

### *Dental X-Ray Machines*

Regulations require that dental x-ray machines must be inspected periodically. Some state and local regulatory agencies provide inspections of dental x-ray equipment without charge as part of their registration and licensing procedures. Dental x-ray machines also must be *calibrated,* or adjusted for accuracy, at regular intervals. A qualified technician must check the x-ray machine performance and calibrate the dental x-ray equipment. For risk management purposes, it is important to keep a record of the calibration service.

The dentist, the dental assistant, or the manufacturer's service representative can perform annual tests for dental x-ray machines. These tests are easy to perform and require only basic test materials and test logs to record the results. You can obtain a free pamphlet called *Quality Control Tests for Dentistry* from Eastman Kodak (Rochester, NY). This easy-to-follow pamphlet describes step-by-step procedures for performing each of these tests.

### X-Ray Machine Quality Control Steps

1. Test output of x-rays.
2. Test size of focal spot.
3. Test tubehead for stability.
4. Test timer for accuracy.
5. Test milliamperage.
6. Test kilovoltage.

### Dental X-Ray Film

You should check each box of film while opening it. Even though the film may not be expired, the box may have been improperly stored before it reached your office. Follow these easy steps to test the film for freshness:

1. In the darkroom, unwrap one unexposed film from the newly opened box.
2. Process the film with the use of fresh chemicals.
3. Check the results.
4. If the processed film appears clean with a slight blue tint, the film is fresh and has been properly stored and handled. This film is safe for use.
5. If the processed film appears fogged, the film has been improperly stored or exposed to radiation. This film must not be used.

### Phosphor Storage Plates

Reusable **phosphor storage plates (PSPs)** are used with digital radiography instead of a rigid sensor. The PSP must be handled with care to avoid scratching the surface. Scratched surfaces will result in artifacts on the image (see Chapter 39).

### Screens and Cassettes

Intensifying screens inside the extraoral cassette should be periodically checked for dirt and scratches. Screens should be cleaned monthly with a commercially available cleaner. After cleaning, an antistatic solution should be applied to the screen to prevent static electricity that may affect film quality. Screens that appear visibly scratched should be replaced.

Cassettes should be checked for worn closures, light leaks, and warping, which may result in fogged and blurred radiographs; damaged cassettes must be repaired or replaced. Follow these easy steps to test the cassette for adequate film-screen contact:

1. In the darkroom, insert one film between the screens in the cassette.
2. Place a wire mesh test object on top of the loaded cassette.
3. Using a 40-inch target-film distance, direct the central ray perpendicular to the cassette.
4. Expose the film with the use of 10 mA, 70 kVp, and 15 impulses.
5. Process the exposed film.
6. View the film on a view box in a dimly lit room at a distance of 6 feet.
7. Check the results.
8. If the wire mesh image seen on the film exhibits uniform density, good film-screen contact has taken place. The cassette and the screen are safe to use.
9. If the wire mesh image seen on the film exhibits varying densities, poor film-screen contact has taken place. Areas of poor film-screen contact appear darker than good-contact areas. If the film-screen contact is poor, the cassette should be repaired or replaced.

RECALL

5 What is meant by quality assurance?
6 What are quality control tests?
7 When should you check a box of film for freshness?
8 Should you use a film cassette that has scratches?

### View Boxes

A properly functioning **view box** is necessary for the interpretation of conventional radiographs (Fig. 40.2). The view box contains fluorescent bulbs that emit light through an opaque plastic or Plexiglas front. The view box should emit a uniform and subdued light when functioning properly.

The view box should be periodically checked for dirt and discoloration of the Plexiglas surface. The surface of the view box should be wiped clean daily. Permanently discolored Plexiglas or blackened fluorescent bulbs must be replaced.

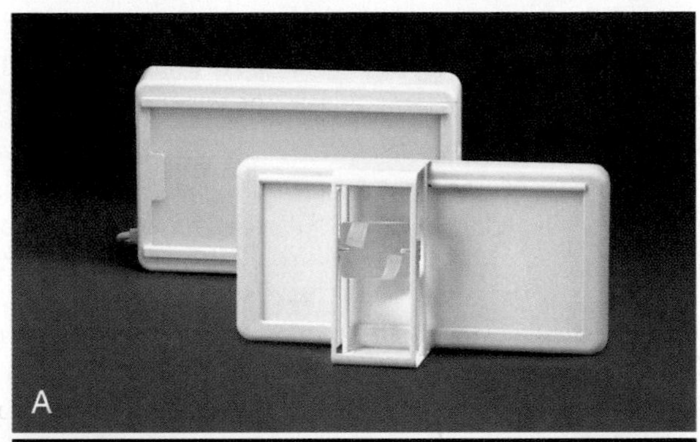

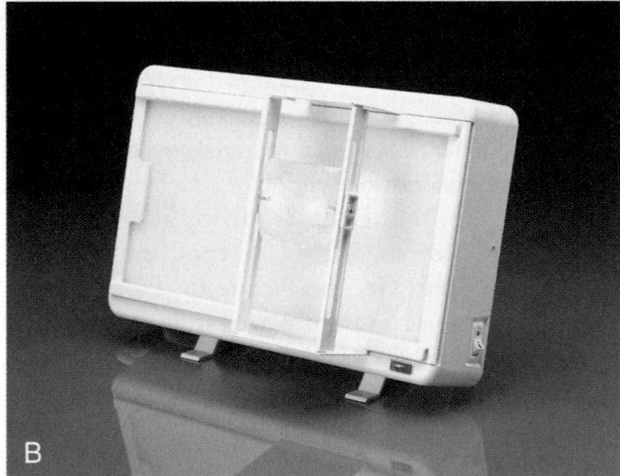

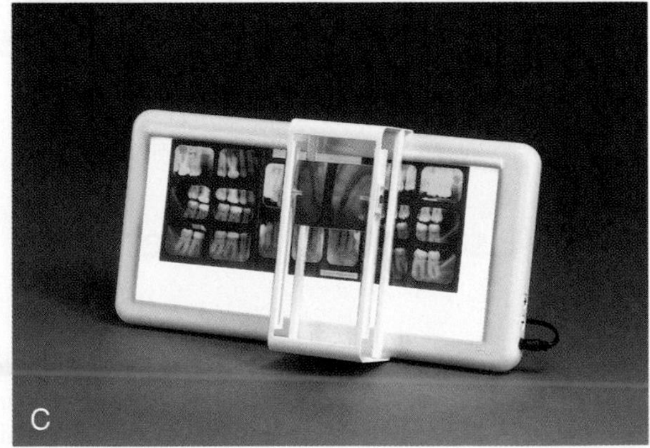

**FIG. 40.2** Examples of view boxes in sizes. *(Courtesy Densply Rinn, Elgin, IL.)*

### Darkroom Lighting

Check the darkroom for light leaks every 6 months. Follow these easy steps to test the darkroom for light leaks:

1. While standing in the darkroom, turn off all the lights, including the safelight.
2. Once your eyes become accustomed to the darkness, look around the room for any signs of white light. Check around the door, the seams on the walls and ceilings, the vent area, and the keyhole for light leaks.
3. Check the results.
4. If the darkroom has no visible light leaks, the room is safe for processing films.
5. If light leaks are present, they must be corrected with weather stripping or black electrical tape before film processing is continued.

**SAFELIGHT TEST.** The "light-tightness" of the darkroom must be confirmed before you can test the effectiveness of the safelight. Follow these easy steps to use the *coin test* to check the safelight:

1. Turn off all the lights in the darkroom, including the safelight.
2. Unwrap one unexposed film. Place the film on a flat surface at least 4 feet away from the safelight. Place a coin on top of the film (Fig. 40.3, *A*).
3. Turn on the safelight. Allow the film and the coin to be exposed to the safelight for 3 to 4 minutes.
4. Remove the coin and process the film as usual.

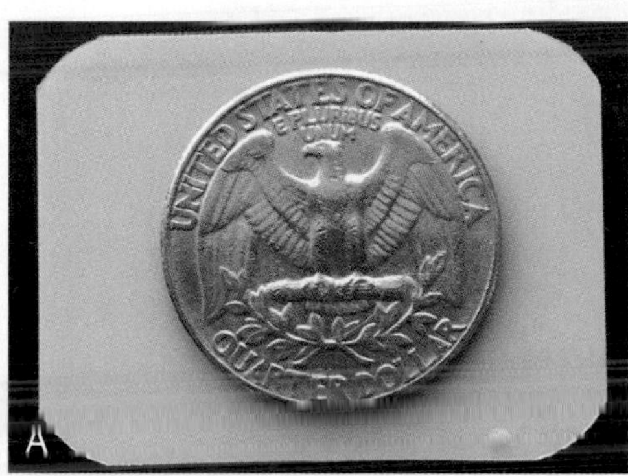

**FIG. 40.3** A, Unexposed film with coin on it. B, Radiograph showing outline of coin.

5. Check the results.
6. If no image is visible on the film, the safelight is functioning, and it is safe to process other films.
7. If the image of the coin and a fogged background appear on the processed film, the safelight is not safe to use with that type of film (Fig. 40.3, *B*). Safelighting problems must be corrected before film processing is continued.

### Film Processing

Perform quality control procedures routinely because film processing is one of the most critical aspects of a quality control program and must be monitored on a daily basis.

**MANUAL PROCESSING.** With the manual system, the thermometer and the timer must be checked for accuracy. The temperature and levels of the water bath, developer, and fixer solutions also must be checked. Always strictly follow the processing time and temperature recommendations of the solution manufacturer.

**AUTOMATIC PROCESSING.** With automatic equipment, you must check the water circulation system, the solution levels, the replenishment system, and temperatures. Always follow the manufacturer's procedure and maintenance directions carefully. Each day, you should process two test films in the automatic processor. Follow these steps to verify the functioning of the automatic processor:

1. Unwrap two unexposed films; expose one to light.
2. Process both films in the automatic processor.
3. Check the results.
4. If the unexposed film appears clear and dry, and if the film exposed to light appears black and dry, the automatic processor is functioning properly.
5. If the unexposed film does not appear clear and dry, or if the exposed film does not appear completely black and dry, the automatic processor must be checked. Corrections must be made before patient films are processed.

**PROCESSING SOLUTIONS.** The processing solutions are the most critical component in the quality control of film processing. As discussed in Chapter 39, you must replenish the processing solutions daily and change them every 3 to 4 weeks, as recommended by the manufacturer.

As an alternative to using the calendar to determine the freshness of solutions, quality control tests can be used to monitor the strength of the developer and fixer solutions. You should check the processing solutions each day *before* any patient films are processed.

**DEVELOPER STRENGTH.** As the developer loses strength, the time-temperature chart is no longer accurate. An easy way to check the strength of the developer solution is to compare film densities against a standard. This can be done with the use of a reference radiograph or a stepwedge radiograph.

**REFERENCE RADIOGRAPH.** A reference radiograph is processed under ideal conditions and then is used to compare the film densities of radiographs that are processed daily. Use the following steps to create a reference radiograph:

1. Expose fresh film, using correct exposure factors.
2. Process the film using fresh chemicals at the recommended time and temperature.
3. View the reference radiograph and the daily radiographs side by side on a view box.
4. Check the results.
5. If the densities seen on the reference radiograph match the densities seen on the daily radiographs, the developer solution strength is adequate. You may process patient films.
6. If the densities seen on the daily radiograph appear *lighter* than those seen on the reference film, the developer solution is either weak or cold.
7. If the densities seen on the daily radiograph appear *darker* than those seen on the reference radiograph, the developer solution is either too concentrated or too warm.
8. Weakened or concentrated developer solution must be replaced. If the developer solution is too warm or too cold, the temperature must be adjusted before patient films are processed.

**STEPWEDGE RADIOGRAPH.** A **stepwedge** is a device that is constructed of layered aluminum steps. When a stepwedge is placed on top of a film and then is exposed to radiographs, the different steps absorb varying amounts of radiation. When the film is processed, different densities are seen on the dental radiograph as a result of the stepwedge.

Use the following steps to create stepwedge radiographs:

1. Use a total of 20 fresh films (one for each workday in the month). Place an aluminum stepwedge on top of one film.
2. Expose the film. Then expose the remaining films using the same exposure factors.
3. Using fresh chemicals, process only *one* of the exposed films. This processed radiograph will exhibit different densities as a result of the stepwedge, and it becomes the *standard stepwedge radiograph.*
4. Store the remaining 19 exposed films in a cool dry area protected from x-radiation.
5. Each day, after the chemicals have been replenished, process one of the exposed stepwedge films.
6. Compare the *standard stepwedge radiograph* and the daily radiograph side by side on a view box. Compare the densities seen on the daily radiograph with the densities seen on the standard radiograph (Fig. 40.4).
7. Check the results.
8. Use the middle density seen on the standard stepwedge radiograph for comparison. If the density seen on the standard radiograph matches the density seen on the daily radiograph, the developer solution strength is adequate for processing patient films.
9. If the density on the daily radiograph differs from that on the standard stepwedge radiograph by more than two steps, the developer solution is depleted and must be changed before patient films are processed.

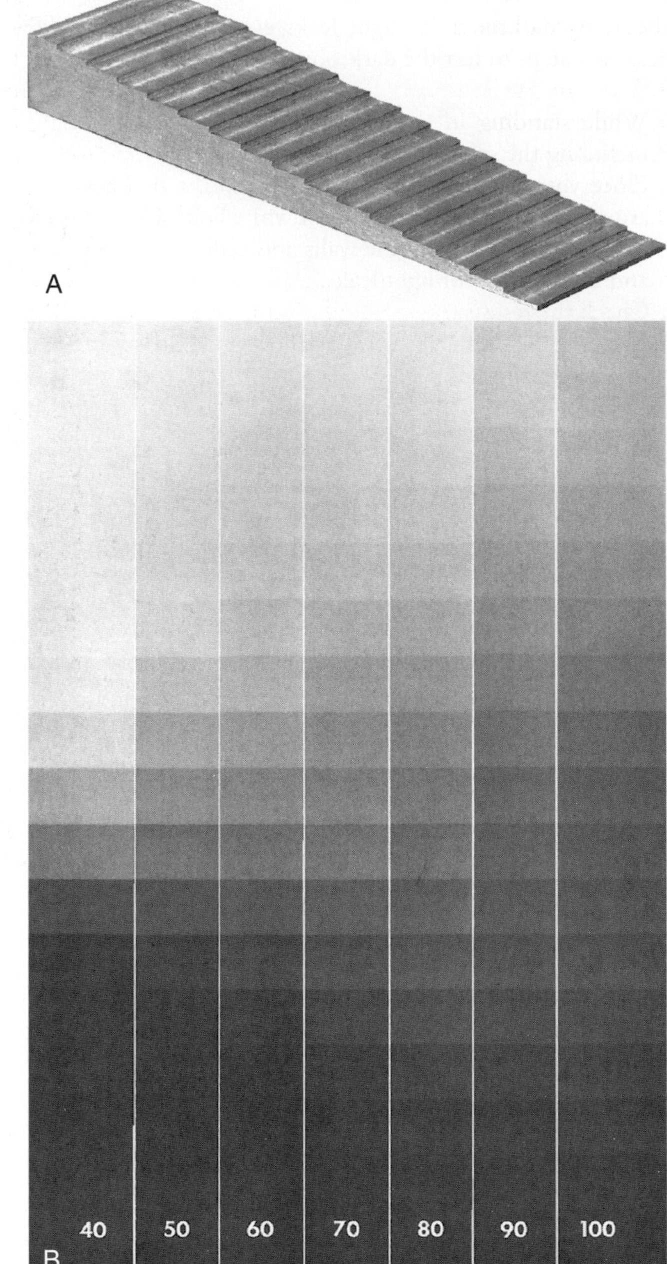

**FIG. 40.4** A, Aluminum stepwedge. B, Seven radiographs of a stepwedge made at 50 to 100 kVp shown side by side. Note the radiographs taken at 40 kVp have a high contrast (short contrast scale) and those taken at 100 kVp show many shades of gray (long-contrast scale). *(A, From White SC, Pharoah MJ: Oral radiology: principles and interpretation, ed 7, St Louis, 2014, Mosby. B, Courtesy Carestream Dental, a division of Carestream Health, Inc.)*

**FIXER STRENGTH.** When the fixer solution loses its strength, the film takes a longer time to "clear," or become transparent, in unexposed areas. When the fixer is at full strength, a film should clear within 2 minutes. Follow these steps to monitor the strength of the fixer:

1. Unwrap one unexposed film and immediately place it in the fixer solution.
2. Check the film for clearing. Note the amount of time the film takes to clear.
3. If the film clears in 2 minutes, the fixer strength is adequate.
4. If the film is not completely clear in 3 to 4 minutes, the fixer is depleted. The fixer solution must be replaced before patient films are processed.

RECALL

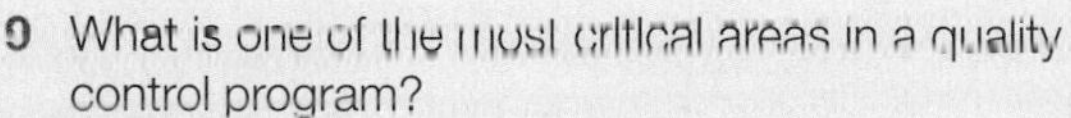

9 What is one of the most critical areas in a quality control program?

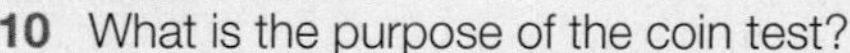

10 What is the purpose of the coin test?
11 How often should processing solutions be replenished?
12 Why are the reference radiograph and the stepwedge used?
13 How can you tell when the fixer loses its strength?

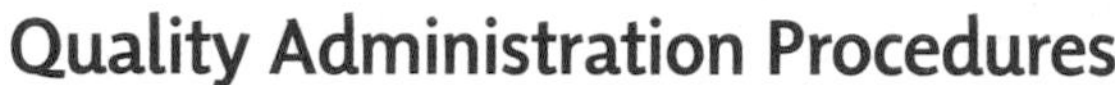

## Quality Administration Procedures

Quality administration deals with the management of the QA program in the dental office. Although the dental assistant may be responsible for performing quality control tests, the dentist is ultimately responsible for overall QA.

### Administrative Quality Control Steps

1. Develop and maintain a written description of the quality assurance plan.
2. Assign specific duties to staff members, and ensure that each individual is thoroughly trained to perform those assigned duties.
3. Maintain records of monitoring and maintenance.
4. Review the plan periodically and revise it as necessary.

### Description

A detailed, *written description* of the QA plan should be available to all staff members. Each staff member involved in the QA program must understand the quality standards, as well as the importance of maintaining quality control of imaging procedures.

### Monitoring

A *written* monitoring schedule should be posted in the office. This schedule should describe all quality control tests and the frequency of testing for all dental imaging equipment, supplies, and film processing.

### Maintenance

A *record-keeping log* of all quality control tests should be maintained and should include the specific test performed, the date the test was performed, and test results. A *processing solutions log* that lists the dates of solution replacement/replenishment and processor or tank cleaning should be kept as well (Fig. 40.5).

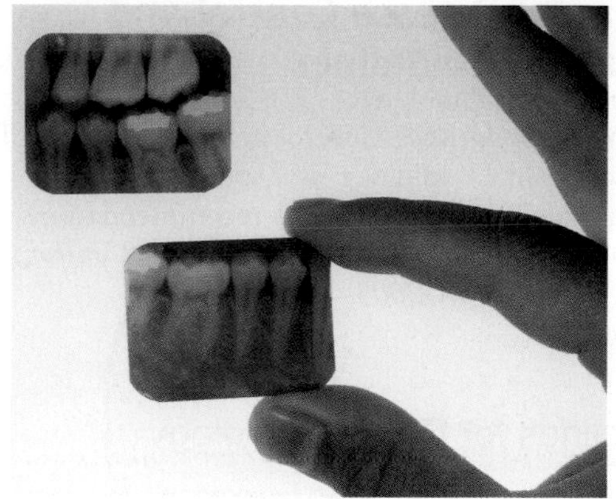

**FIG. 40.5** Radiographs should be checked daily against a reference film. As processing solutions become exhausted, the daily images become lighter and lose contrast. *(From White SC, Pharoah MJ: Oral radiology: principles and interpretation, ed 7, St Louis, 2014, Mosby.)*

### Evaluation

A *written plan* for periodic evaluation and revision of the existing QA program also should be included in the quality administration plan.

### Training

*In-service* training should be provided to all staff members so they can upgrade and improve their imaging exposure techniques and processing procedures.

RECALL

14 What is the purpose of a quality administration program?
15 Which staff members have to be aware of the quality administration program?

## Infection Control

Dental radiography presents unique infection control problems because of the potential for cross-contamination of equipment and environmental surfaces with blood and saliva. Think of the many opportunities for cross-contamination in the procedure: You place the **image receptor** (film, PSP, or sensor) into the mouth, move to the exposure controls outside the operatory, and then return to remove or reposition the image receptor from the mouth. Opportunities for cross-contamination occur in the darkroom or when PSPs are scanned, and with use of the computer and mouse. Direct digital imaging systems can reduce the potential for cross-contamination of surfaces caused by contaminated film packets or PSP wrappers and holders. However, digital sensors and PSPs require careful placement and removal of barriers to avoid contamination.

## Centers for Disease Control and Prevention Guidelines

The Centers for Disease Control and Prevention (CDC) has recognized dental radiology as a potential source of cross-contamination and has provided recommendations for dental radiology in the *Guidelines for Infection Control in Dental Health-Care Settings—2003.*

### Guidelines for Dental Radiology 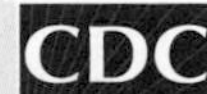

- Wear gloves when exposing radiographs and handling contaminated film packets. Use other personal protective equipment (PPE) (e.g., protective eyewear, mask, gown) as appropriate if spattering of blood or other body fluids is likely.
- Use heat-tolerant or disposable intraoral devices whenever possible (e.g., film-holding and positioning devices). Clean and heat-sterilize heat-tolerant devices between patients.
- Transport and handle exposed film in an aseptic manner to prevent contamination of the developing equipment.
- The following apply for digital radiography sensors:
  - Use FDA-cleared barriers.
  - Clean and heat-sterilize, or high-level–disinfect, between patients, barrier-protected semicritical items. If an item cannot tolerate these procedures, then, at a minimum, protect with an FDA-cleared barrier, and clean and disinfect with an EPA-registered hospital disinfectant with intermediate-level (i.e., tuberculocidal claim) activity, between patients. Consult the manufacturer for methods of disinfection and sterilization of digital radiography sensors and for protection of associated computer hardware.

*EPA,* Environmental Protection Agency; *FDA,* U.S. Food and Drug Administration.

Adapted from Centers for Disease Control and Prevention: Guidelines for infection control in dental health-care settings—2003, Atlanta, GA, 2003, U.S. Department of Health and Human Services.

## The Radiography Operatory

The radiography operatory and the darkroom are not usually associated with spatter of blood or saliva. Transmission of infectious diseases is still possible, however, because x-ray equipment, operatory surfaces, **positioning devices**, and image receptors are contaminated.

Your first step in preparation of the operatory is to identify the surfaces to be protected with barriers or disinfected with a high-level surface disinfectant. In general, surfaces that cannot be easily cleaned and disinfected should be protected by *barriers,* usually plastic or foil. Surface barriers are preferred on electrical switches because of the possibility that the cleaner and disinfectant may cause an electrical short (Fig. 40.6).

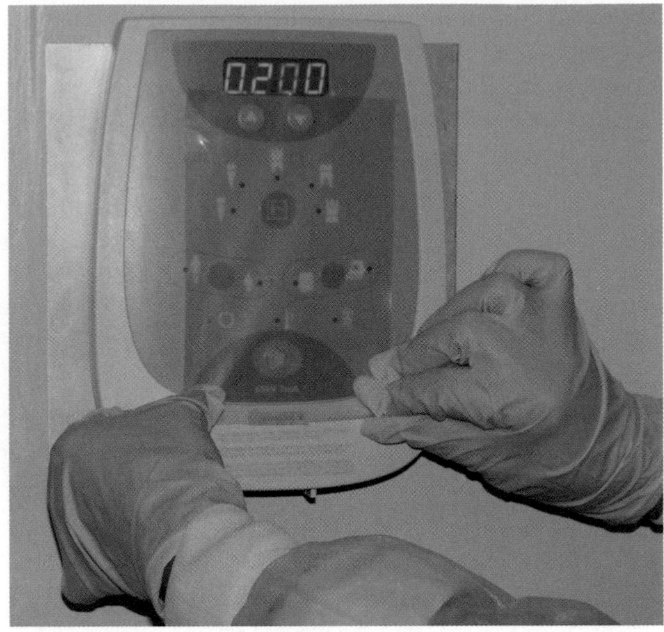


**FIG. 40.6** The exposure control should be covered with a clean barrier and changed after every patient. *(From White SC, Pharoah MJ: Oral radiology: principles and interpretation, ed 7, St Louis, 2014, Mosby.)*

### Checklist for Infection Control in Dental Radiography

**Before Exposure**

**Treatment Area (Covered or Disinfected)**

- X-ray machine
- Dental chair
- Work area
- Lead apron
- Computer keyboard/mouse

**Equipment and Supplies (Prepared Before Seating Patient)**

- Image receptor (film, sensor, or phosphor storage plate [PSP])
- Positioning devices
- Cotton rolls
- Paper towel
- Disposable container

**Patient Preparation (Performed Before Putting on Gloves)**

1. Adjust chair.
2. Adjust headrest.
3. Place lead apron.
4. Remove personal objects.

**Operator Preparation (Completed Before Exposure)**

1. Wash hands.
2. Put on gloves.
3. Assemble positioning devices.

**During Exposure**
Film/PSP Handling
1. Dry exposed film or PSP with paper towel.
2. Place dried film in disposable container or transfer box.

Positioning Devices
1. Transfer positioner from work area to mouth.
2. Transfer positioner from mouth back to work area.
*Note:* Never place a positioner on uncovered countertop.

**After Exposure**
Before Glove Removal
1. Dispose of all contaminated items.
2. Place positioning devices in designated area for contaminated equipment.

After Glove Removal
1. Wash hands.
2. Remove lead apron.

Modified from Iannucci J, Jansen Howerton L: Dental radiography: principles and techniques, ed 4, St Louis, 2012, Saunders.

## Surfaces Likely to Be Contaminated During X-Ray Procedures

- X-ray tubehead and position indicator device (PID)
- X-ray control panel
- Exposure button
- Lead apron
- Dental chair controls
- Operatory counter surfaces
- Darkroom equipment
- Sleeves on automatic processors/scanners
- Computer, monitor, and mouse

### X-Ray Machine

The tubehead, position indicator device (PID), control panel, and exposure button must be covered or carefully disinfected (Fig. 40.7, *A*)

### Dental Chair

The back and arms of the chair, the headrest, and the headrest adjustment controls must be covered or disinfected. Once the radiography operatory is set up, you can set up the image receptors and holders (Fig. 40.7, *B*).

### Lead Apron

The lead apron should be considered contaminated and wiped with a disinfectant after each use (Fig. 40.8).

### Work Area

The work area where the films, PSPs, or sensors and positioners are placed during exposure should be disinfected. Then a barrier, such as a paper sheet, paper towels, or plastic cover, should be placed.

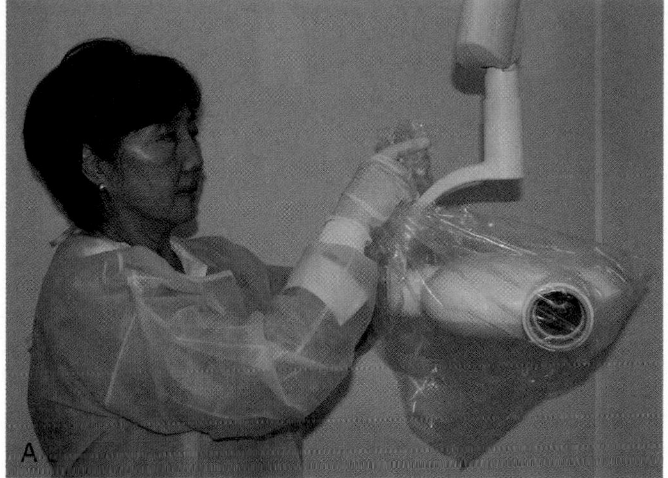

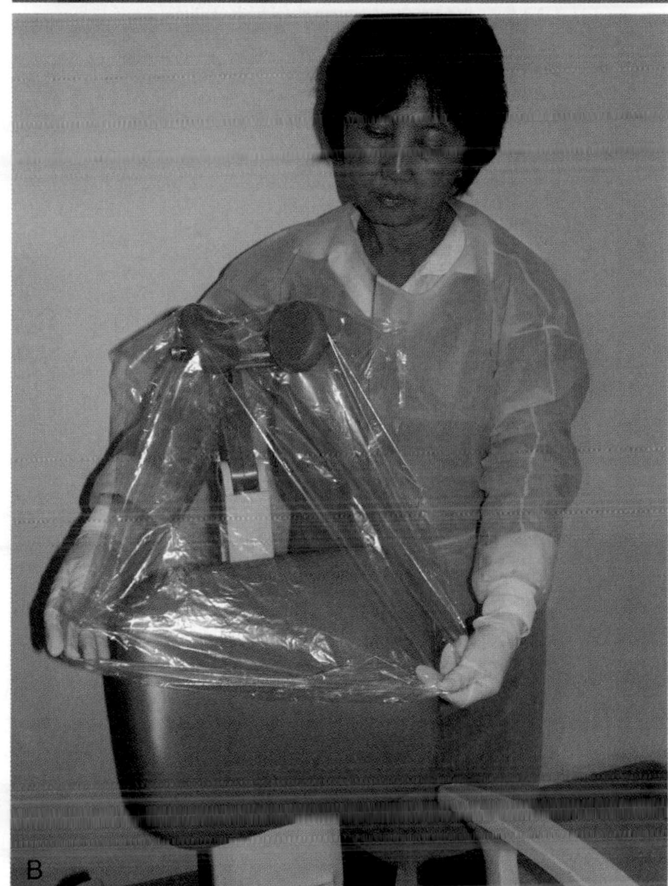

**FIG. 40.7** A, A plastic bag is slipped over the x-ray tube head, pulled tight and secured. B, A new plastic bag is placed over the chair and headrest for each patient. *(From White SC, Pharoah MJ: Oral radiology: principles and interpretation, ed 7, St Louis, 2014, Mosby.)*

Once the procedure is completed, discard the barriers. If counter surfaces are not protected by barriers, or if the barriers have become torn or damaged, they should be cleaned and disinfected.

## Equipment and Supplies

Before beginning the procedure, gather all necessary supplies to decrease the chance of cross-contamination. For example,

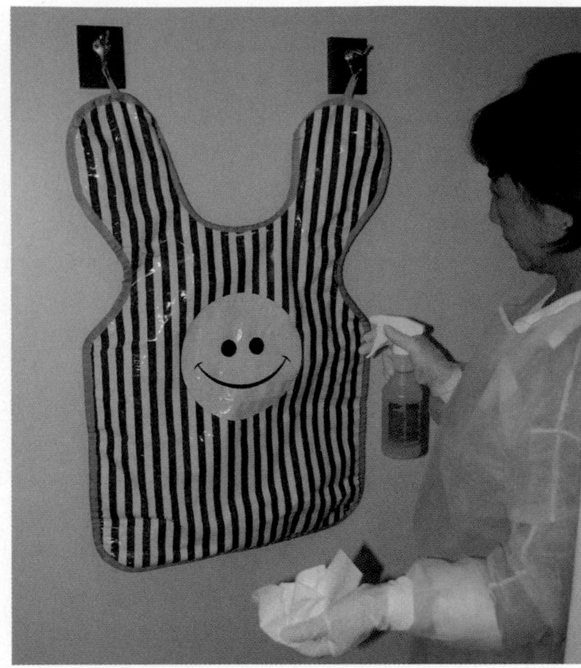

FIG. 40.8 Hanging apron is sprayed with disinfectant and then dried. *(From White SC, Pharoah MJ: Oral radiology: principles and interpretation, ed 7, St Louis, 2014, Mosby.)*

think about the types of film or sensor positioning devices, barrier sleeves, cotton rolls, bitewing tabs, and so forth, that you may need.

*Note:* If you need additional supplies during the procedure, use overgloves (food handler's gloves) or ask for assistance.

### Film and Phosphor Storage Plates

Dispense the film or PSPs from a central area in a disposable container, such as a paper cup.

**FILM.** Once films are removed from the mouth, they are obviously contaminated and should be handled only with gloved hands. One technique that is used to minimize contamination is to place a clear-plastic barrier envelope over the film packet. Some commercially available films are enclosed in a clear-plastic barrier packet (Fig. 40.9). Barrier-protected film packets are exposed and are brought to the processing area. The barriers are contaminated, and one must remove them carefully without touching the inner packet, so the packet can be handled with bare hands. When films are not protected by barrier envelopes, you will need to use a technique to open the film packet without contaminating the film (Fig. 40.10).

**PSPs.** PSPs are reusable and *must* be placed in a sealed barrier packet before exposure (Fig. 40.11). Caution must be used to prevent cross-contamination when the plate is removed from the barrier packet.

### Digital Sensors

Intraoral digital sensors come into contact with mucous membranes and ideally should be cleaned and heat-sterilized

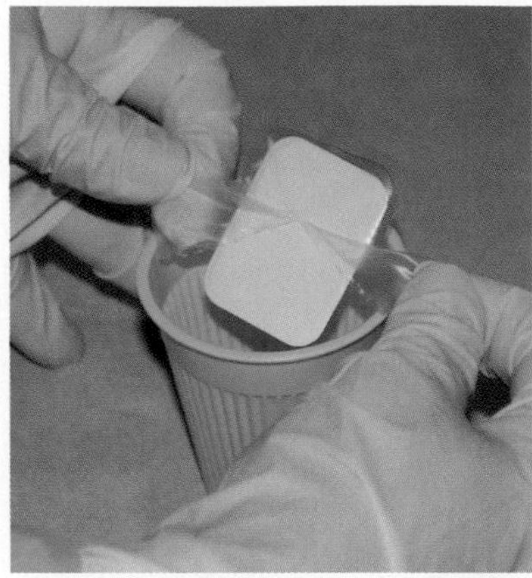

FIG. 40.9 Dental film with a plastic barrier to protect the film from saliva. During opening, the plastic is removed and the clean film is allowed to drop into a container. *(From White SC, Pharoah MJ: Oral radiology: principles and interpretation, ed 7, St Louis, 2014, Mosby.)*

or high-level disinfected between patients. At this time, however, sensors *cannot* withstand heat sterilization or immersion in a high-level disinfectant. Until this technology changes, the CDC recommends at a minimum using an FDA-cleared plastic barrier (Fig. 40.12). The barrier is placed over the sensor and part of the attached cable (unless a wireless sensor is used).

### Image Receptor Positioning Instruments

Image receptor positioning instruments that are placed in the patient's mouth are *semicritical items* that should be sterilized before reuse. The alternative is to use disposable positioners and discard them after a single use (Fig. 40.13).

Sterilized positioning instruments should remain packaged until the patient is seated and can view the opening of the package. Patients appreciate knowing that proper infection control procedures are in place throughout the office.

RECALL

16 What unique infection control problems occur in dental imaging?
17 What surfaces must be covered with barriers?
18 What personal protective equipment should the operator wear while exposing radiographs?
19 When should the packages that contain positioning instruments be opened?

## Procedures During and After X-Ray Exposure

### Operator Preparation

Always wear gloves and protective clothing while exposing images and handling contaminated items (Fig. 40.14). You should also wear a mask and eyewear if there is a likelihood that blood or other body fluids may spatter. Masks also are indicated if you or the patient has a cough or a cold.

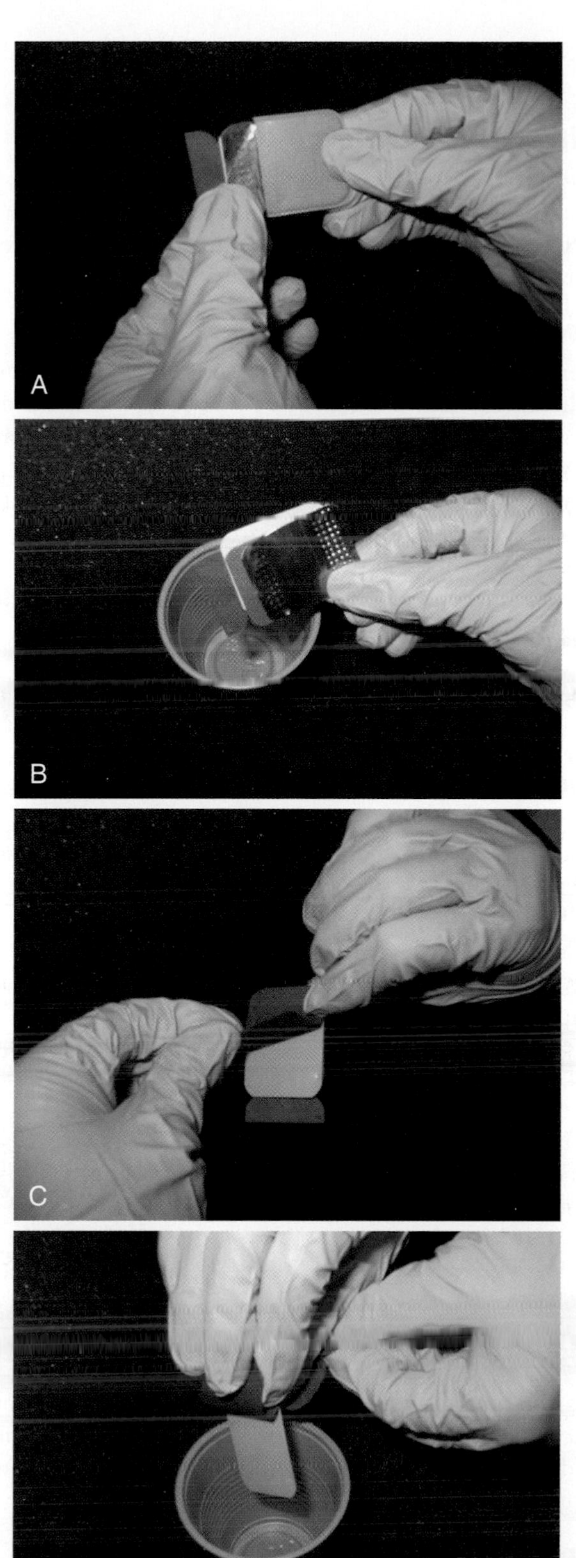


**FIG. 40.10** Steps to open a size 2 film packet without contaminating the film. A, Method for removing films from packet and not touching them with contaminated gloves. Open tab, and slide lead foil and black interleaf paper from wrapping. B, Rotate contaminated film packet away from black paper and foil and discard. C, Peel back paper wrapping away from film. D, Allow film to fall into a clean cup. *(From Iannucci J, Jansen Howerton L: Dental radiography: principles and techniques, ed 5, St Louis, 2017, Elsevier.)*

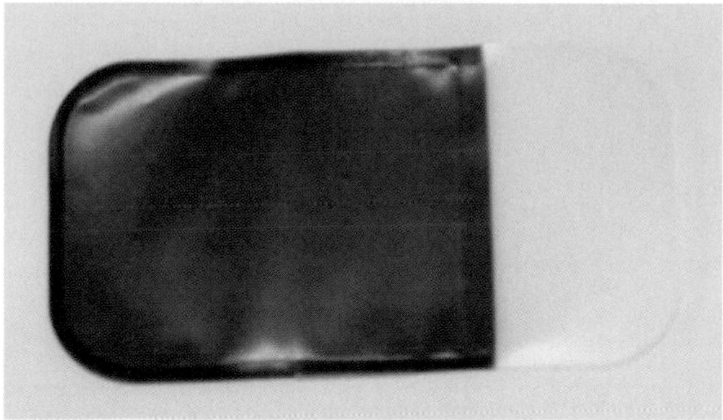

**FIG. 40.11** Protective packet barrier over phosphor storage plate (PSP).

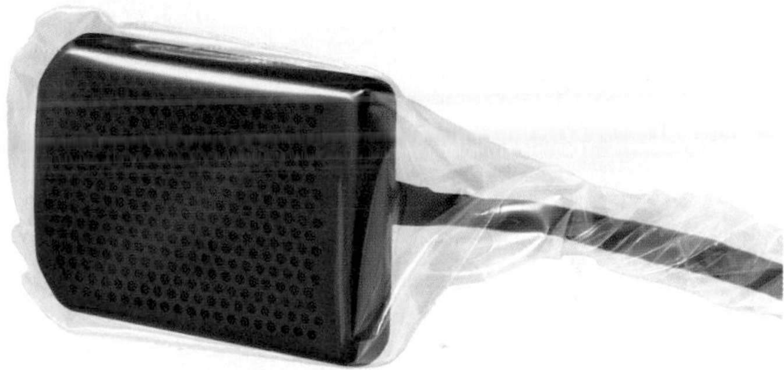

**FIG. 40.12** FDA-cleared sensor and cable barriers. *(Courtesy Dentsply Rinn, Elgin, IL.)*

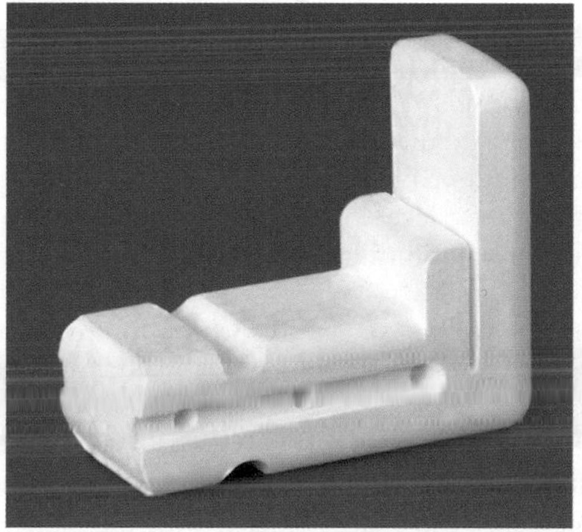

**FIG. 40.13** Disposable film positioner. *(Courtesy Dentsply Rinn, Elgin, IL.)*

After putting on gloves, be careful not to touch any surfaces that are not covered. The best approach is to develop a sequence in which you touch as few surfaces as possible. See Procedure 40.1: Practicing Infection Control During Film Exposure.

## Drying of Exposed Film or PSP

The contaminated film or PSP packet is a major source of cross-contamination during dental imaging procedures. When you remove the film packet or PSP from the patient's mouth, it is

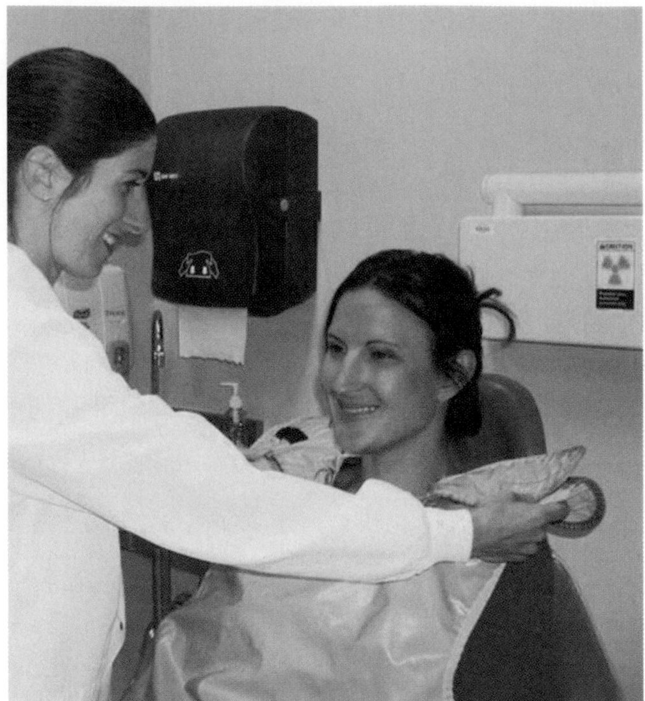

FIG. 40.14 After placing the lead apron and assembling materials, the dental assistant will put on her PPE.

coated with saliva (or occasionally, contaminated with blood). For this reason, you must *always* wear gloves while handling contaminated packets or PSPs. After you remove each exposed receptor from the patient's mouth, wipe saliva off using a dry 2 × 2–inch gauze sponge or a paper towel. Do *not* attempt to sterilize the film or the PSP packet or sensor. Heat sterilization will destroy them.

Some dental film manufacturers permit light spraying of contaminated film packets with a disinfectant spray. However, immersion of the packet in a disinfecting solution can result in seeping of the solution into the emulsion and damage to the image.

It is always the best policy to check with the manufacturer regarding infection control protocol.

### Collection of Contaminated Films and PSPs

Once the film or PSP envelope has been dried, place it into a disposable paper cup that is labeled with the patient's name. If the PSPs are not going to be scanned immediately, while gloved, carefully remove the PSPs from the sealed envelope, open the barrier envelopes, and place the PSPs into a black transfer box. If the PSPs are going to be scanned immediately, there is no need to store the PSPs in the transfer box. The black transfer box is used to protect the PSP from excessive light before scanning. The paper cup can be used to transport films to the darkroom and PSPs to the scanner. Be careful not to touch the outside surface of the paper cup or transfer box with gloved hands.

To prevent film fog caused by radiation, never place the paper cup or transfer box in a room where additional films are being exposed.

PSPs or film should *never* be placed in the operator's laboratory coat or uniform pocket.

### Positioning Instruments

During exposure, always take the positioning instruments from the covered work area to the patient's mouth and then back to the covered area. Never place contaminated film holders on an uncovered surface.

### Disposal of Contaminated Items

When you finish all exposures, all contaminated items must be discarded, and any uncovered surfaces must be disinfected. Handle contaminated items in the same manner that you handle contaminated dental instruments. You must always wear gloves while disposing of contaminated items, including disposable surface coverings, packets, barriers, and so forth. All covered surfaces should be uncovered carefully; be sure not to touch the actual surfaces with gloved hands.

While still wearing gloves, remove the contaminated positioning instrument from the treatment area and place it in the area designated for contaminated instruments.

### Handwashing

After all contaminated items have been removed and disposed of, remove your gloves and wash your hands.

### Surface Disinfection

While wearing protective eyewear and chemical-resistant utility gloves, clean and disinfect any uncovered areas in the radiography operatory that were contaminated during exposure. Use a hospital-grade disinfectant that is registered and approved by the Environmental Protection Agency (EPA).

20 What precautions should be taken when one is handling contaminated film or PSPs?

21 What type of gloves should be worn while one is disinfecting the radiography operatory?

## Procedures During X-Ray Film Processing

After the films have been exposed, specific infection control procedures must be followed during transport of the films to the darkroom, during film handling, and during automatic and manual film processing.

### Transporting Film

You should never touch the disposable container with your gloved hands. Only after your gloves have been removed, your hands washed and dried, the patient dismissed, and the area cleaned and disinfected should you carry the container with contaminated films to the darkroom.

Procedures 40.2, 40.3, 40.4, and 40.5 review infection control steps to be followed when processing films in the darkroom, when using daylight film loaders, when using digital sensors, and when using PSPs.

## Infection Control Steps in Dental Imaging

**Treatment Area**

1. Place barriers or disinfect the x-ray machine, dental chair, work area, computer, mouse, and lead apron.
2. Before seating the patient, gather positioning devices, cotton rolls, paper towels, and disposable cup.

**Preparation of Patient and Operator**

1. Before gloving, seat the patient, and adjust the chair and headrest. Ask the patient to remove objects from the face and mouth. Place the lead apron.
2. Wash hands, put on gloves, and assemble positioning devices.

**Exposure of Image**

1. After each exposure, dry image receptor.
2. Never place a positioner on uncovered surfaces.

**After Exposure of Images**

1. Before removing gloves, dispose of contaminated items (such as cotton rolls).
2. Place positioner device in area for contaminated instruments.
3. Remove gloves, wash hands, and remove the lead apron.

RECALL

**22** What precautions must be taken when films are transported to the darkroom?

**■ Legal and Ethical Implications** Dental malpractice results when the dental practitioner is negligent in the delivery of dental care. Because dental radiographs are an essential part of diagnosis and treatment planning, negligence may result from radiographic-related action or inaction of the dental practitioner. For example, a patient of Dr. Daniels refused x-rays, and Dr. Daniels decided to treat the patient anyway. Later, the patient developed an abscess, resulting from undetected caries under a filling. Dr. Daniels could be held liable in this case because she should not have treated the patient without radiographs. Treating a patient without the diagnostic aid of radiographic examination may result in significant harm to the patient. Harm for which the dentist could be held liable may include stress, embarrassment, loss of income, and expenses incurred in seeking additional treatment. ■

**■ Eye to the Future** The Internet has changed the way information is communicated. Patients are exposed to increasing amounts and sources of information, and many patients have heard or read about the harmful effects of radiation. Media coverage often highlights the dangers of radiation and casts doubt on the benefits of dental imaging. Such reports are misleading and often are poorly researched. Many times, these reports cause patients to avoid or refuse images out of a fear of exposure to x-radiation.

As new information becomes available and as communications improve, the dental assistant must continue to educate patients now and in the future about the importance, benefits, and relative safety of dental imaging techniques. ■

## ■ Critical Thinking

1. You are the person in your office assigned the responsibility of replenishing and maintaining the processing solutions. What tasks will you have to perform, and how often will you need to do them?
2. You are using a stepwedge film to evaluate the quality of the developer solution. You note that the middle density on the daily film is much lighter than the middle density on the stepwedge film. What is the problem, and how do you solve it?
3. Mrs. Johnstone, a patient in your office, stops by one morning and asks to pick up her radiographs because she is moving to another city. Kathy, the receptionist, explains to Mrs. Johnstone that her films need to be duplicated, which will take some time. Mrs. Johnstone becomes angry and wants her films immediately, saying, "Those films belong to me. I paid for them, and I want them." What should Kathy tell Mrs. Johnstone? ■

PROCEDURE 40.1

# Practicing Infection Control During Film Exposure

## GOAL

To perform all infection control practices during film exposure.

## EQUIPMENT AND SUPPLIES

- Barriers for the operatory
- Paper towels
- Dental film (sizes as necessary)
- Packaged positioning device
- Film barriers *(optional)*
- Lead apron with thyroid collar
- Disposable container for exposed films (labeled with patient's name)
- Surface cleaner/disinfectant

## PROCEDURAL STEPS

1. Wash and dry hands.
2. Place surface barriers on equipment and work area.

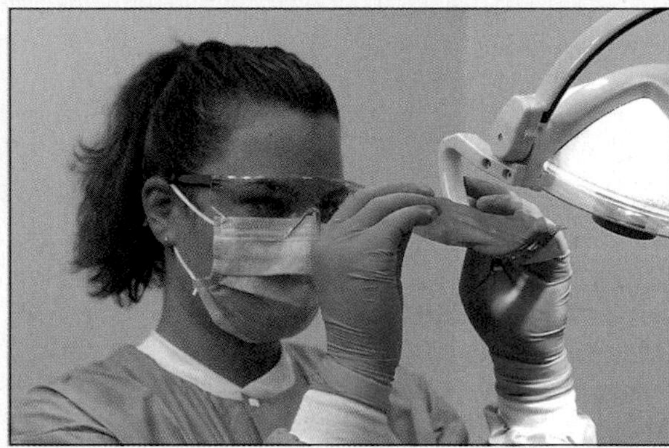

3. Set out the packaged positioning device, film, labeled container for exposed film, paper towel, and other miscellaneous items you might need.

   **PURPOSE** Once gloved, you should not have to leave the operatory area for additional materials.

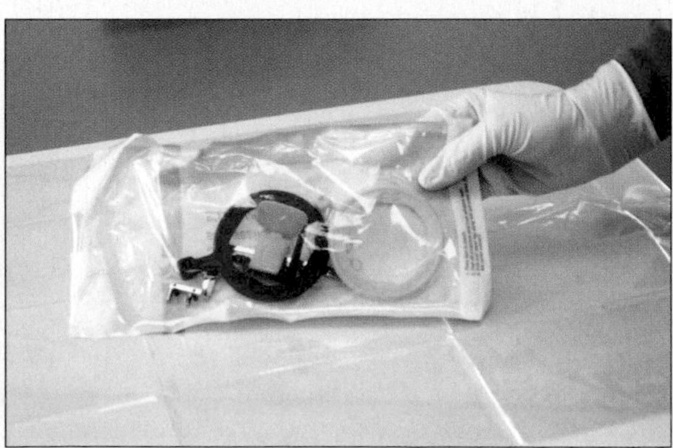

4. Seat the patient and place the lead apron.
5. Wash and dry hands and don gloves.
6. After each exposure, wipe excess saliva from the film using a paper towel.
7. Place each exposed film into the container, being careful not to touch the external surface.

   **PURPOSE** Your contaminated gloves will contaminate the outer surface of the container.

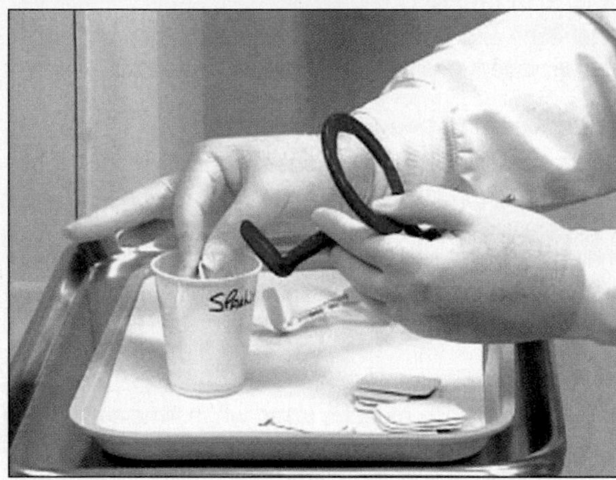

8. After the exposures are complete, remove the lead apron and dismiss the patient.
9. While still gloved, remove barriers, taking care not to touch the surfaces underneath.

   **PURPOSE** You must wear gloves while removing barriers, because they are contaminated. If you touch a surface underneath the barrier while you are removing it, that surface will become contaminated and then must be disinfected.
10. Dispose of barriers and paper towels.
11. Place the positioning device on a tray to be returned to the instrument processing area.
12. Wash and dry hands.
13. Take exposed films to the processing area.

PROCEDURE 40.2

# Practicing Infection Control in the Darkroom

## GOAL

To practice infection control measures when in the darkroom.

## EQUIPMENT AND SUPPLIES

- ✓ Paper towels
- ✓ Clean gloves
- ✓ Clean paper cup
- ✓ Container for lead foil

## PROCEDURAL STEPS

1 Place a paper towel and a clean cup on the counter near the processor.

**PURPOSE** The paper towel provides a barrier for the work surface, and the cup is used to discard the opened film packets.

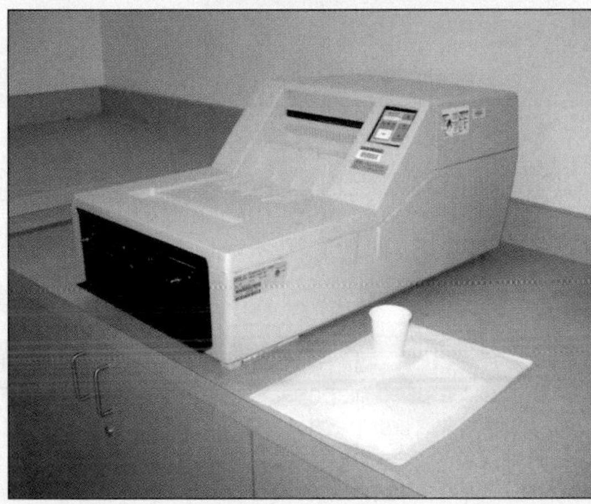

2 Wash hands and put on a new pair of gloves, preferably the type that does not contain powder.

**PURPOSE** Powder remaining on the hand can cause artifacts on the exposed film.

3 Turn on the safety light, then turn off the white light. Open the film packets and allow each exposed film to drop onto the paper towel. Be careful that the unwrapped films do not come in contact with the gloves.

**PURPOSE** The film must remain free from contamination.

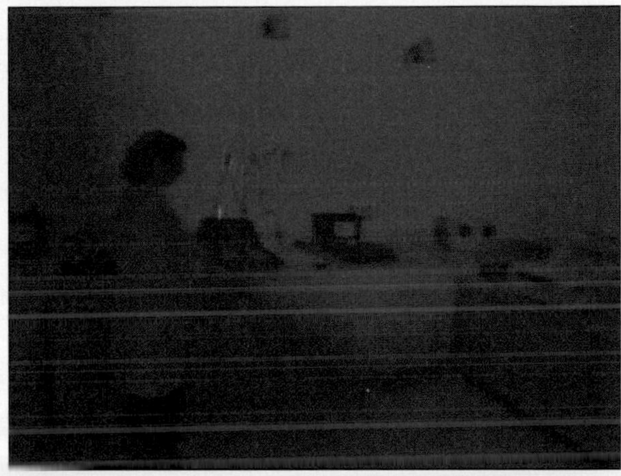

4 Remove the lead foil from the packet and place into the foil recycling container

**PURPOSE** Lead foil is considered an environmental hazard and should not be discarded with the general waste.

5 Place the empty film packets into the clean cup.

6 Discard the cup. Remove your gloves by turning them inside out; then discard them.

7 Place the films into the processor or on developing racks with bare hands.

**NOTE** If you used films with plastic barriers, you would have already removed the protective barrier in the operatory with gloved hands. You would then open the packets with your bare hands and feed the films into the processor.

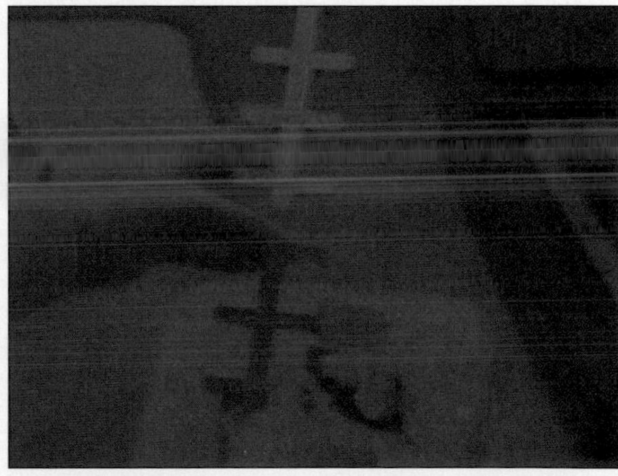

PROCEDURE 40.3

# Practicing Infection Control with Use of Daylight Loader

## GOAL

To practice infection control measures when using the daylight loader in processing dental films.

## EQUIPMENT AND SUPPLIES

- ✔ Paper towels
- ✔ Clean gloves
- ✔ Clean cup
- ✔ Container for lead foil

## PROCEDURAL STEPS

1 Wash and dry your hands; then place a paper towel or a piece of plastic as a barrier to cover the bottom of the daylight loader.

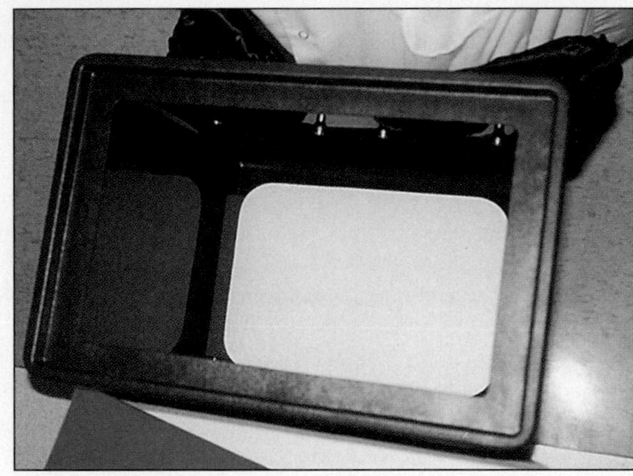

2 Place the following into the bottom of the daylight loader: the cup containing the contaminated film, a clean pair of gloves, and a second empty paper cup. Then close the top.

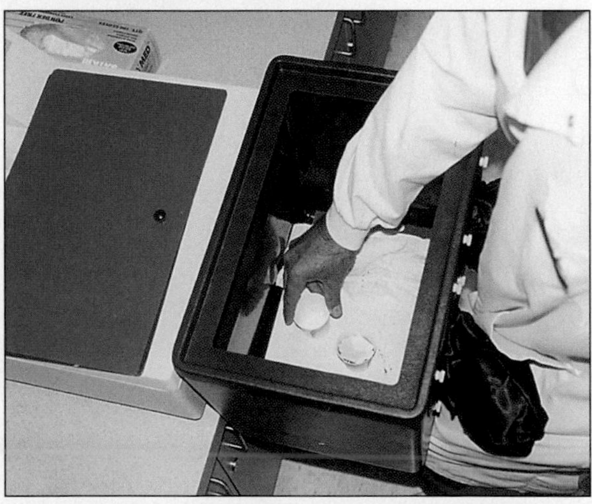

3 Put your clean hands through the sleeves of the daylight loader; then put on the gloves.

**PURPOSE** Clean hands prevent contamination of the sleeves. Contaminated gloves should never be placed through the sleeves of the daylight loader.

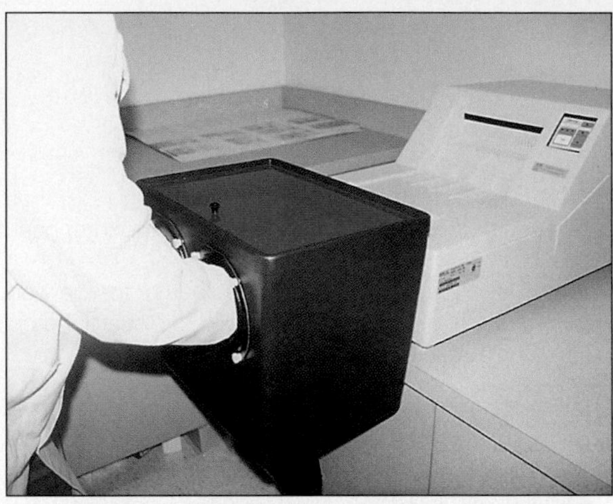

4 Open the packets and allow the films to drop onto the clean barrier.

**PURPOSE** The clean barrier keeps dust or powder from the film.

5 Place the contaminated packets into the second cup, and place the lead foil into the foil container.

**PURPOSE** The cup confines the contaminated film packets and makes disposal easier.

6 After you open the last packet, remove your gloves by turning them inside out. Insert the films into the developing slots.

**PURPOSE** The film remains uncontaminated, which eliminates the question of whether organisms can survive in the solutions.

## PROCEDURE 40.3 Practicing Infection Control with Use of Daylight Loader–cont'd

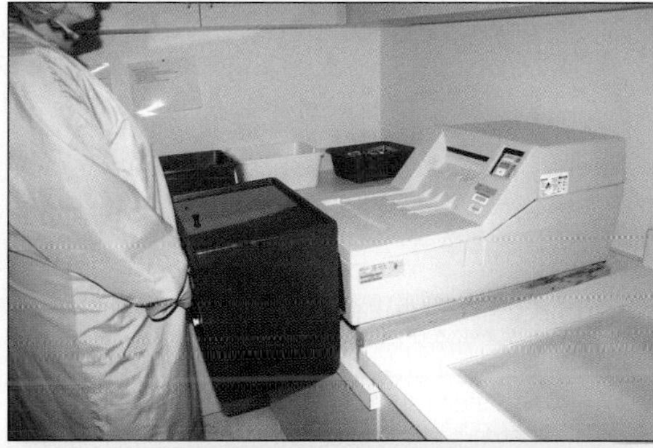

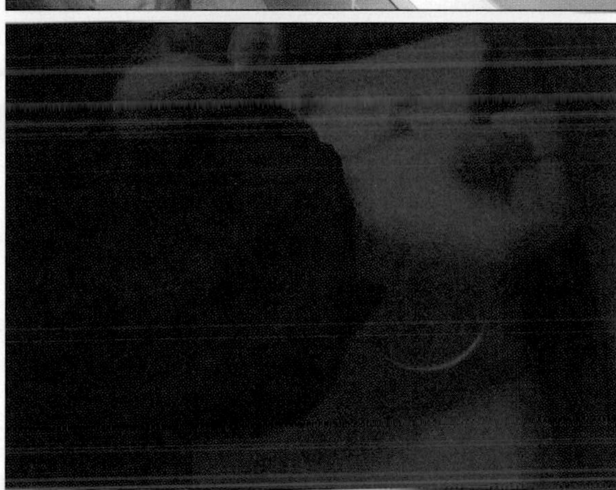

7 After you insert the last film, pull your ungloved hands through the sleeves.
8 Open the top of the loader; then carefully pull the ends of the barrier over the paper cup and used gloves and discard.
**NOTE** Be careful not to touch the contaminated parts of the barrier with your bare hands.

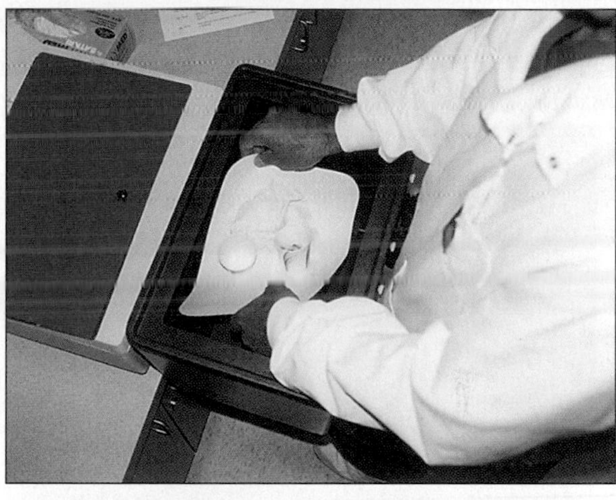

9 Wash your hands.
10 Label a film mount, paper cup, or envelope with the patient's name. Use these to collect the processed films.

## PROCEDURE 40.4

# Practicing Infection Control with Digital Sensors

### GOAL

To perform all infection control practices using digital sensor exposure.

### EQUIPMENT AND SUPPLIES

- Barriers for the operatory, including the sensor, computer keyboard, and mouse
- Paper towels or gauze squares
- Digital sensor (sizes as necessary)
- Packaged positioning device
- Wraps or cushions for sensor *(optional)*
- Sensor and cable barriers
- Lead apron with thyroid collar
- Surface cleaner/disinfectant

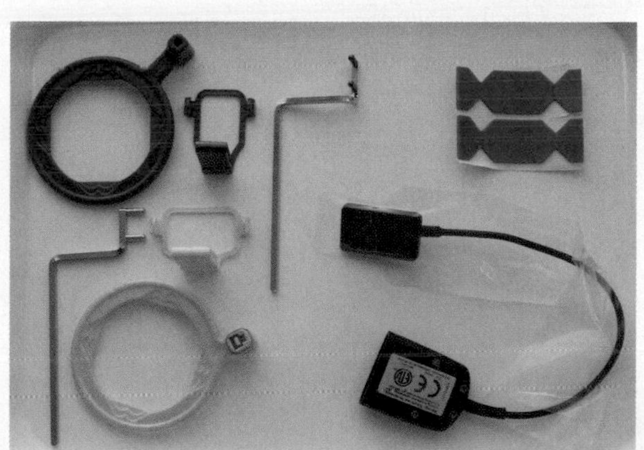

**(Continued)**

# PROCEDURE 40.4 Practicing Infection Control with Digital Sensors—cont'd

**PROCEDURAL STEPS**

**1** Wash and dry hands.

**2** Place surface barriers on equipment, computer keyboard and mouse, and work area.

**3** Set out the packaged positioning device, barriers for the sensor and cable, a paper towel or gauze squares, and miscellaneous items you might choose.

**PURPOSE** Once gloved, you should not have to leave the operatory area for additional materials.

**4** Secure the barrier around the digital sensor.

**PURPOSE** Sensors are reused on patients and cannot be heat-sterilized. Therefore it is essential to protect them with FDA-cleared barriers.

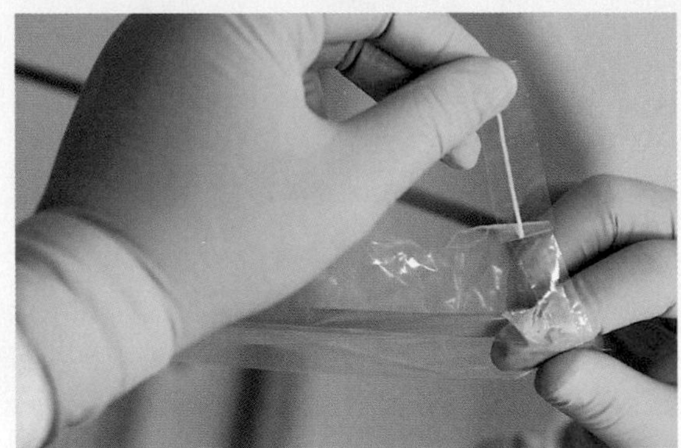

*(© 2017 Crosstex International, Inc.)*

**5** Seat the patient and place the lead apron.

**6** Wash and dry hands and don gloves.

**7** After all exposures are complete, remove the lead apron and dismiss the patient.

**NOTE** To remove the lead apron and still maintain aseptic technique, you can wear overgloves to remove the apron, or you can take off your gloves and remove the apron barehanded.

**8** Put on utility gloves and remove barriers from the x-ray equipment, taking care not to touch the surfaces underneath.

**PURPOSE** Chemical-resistant utility gloves are necessary when performing surface disinfection. If you touch a surface underneath the barrier while you are removing it, that surface will become contaminated and then must be disinfected.

**9** Dispose of barriers and paper towels.

**10** Place the positioning device on a tray to be returned to the instrument processing area.

**11** Disinfect the lead apron and any surfaces that may have become contaminated during the removal of surface barriers.

**12** Carefully disinfect the sensor according to the manufacturer's recommendations.

**PURPOSE** Sensors are very expensive and can be damaged if improperly handled. Several leading brands of digital sensors are available. Cleaning and disinfecting protocol may vary according to the individual manufacturer.

**13** Wash and dry hands.

# PROCEDURE 40.5

## Practicing Infection Control with Phosphor Storage Plates (PSPs)

**GOAL**

To perform all infection control practices when using phosphor storage plates.

**EQUIPMENT AND SUPPLIES**

- Barriers for the operatory
- Barriers for the computer and mouse
- Paper towels or gauze
- Cotton rolls
- PSP (sizes as necessary)
- Barrier PSP envelopes
- Packaged positioning device
- Lead apron with thyroid collar
- Black transfer box
- Paper cup
- Image scanner
- Surface cleaner/disinfectant

**PROCEDURAL STEPS**

**1** Turn on the computer.

**2** Log on to link the patient's images to his or her chart.

**3** Choose the image layout you wish to use.

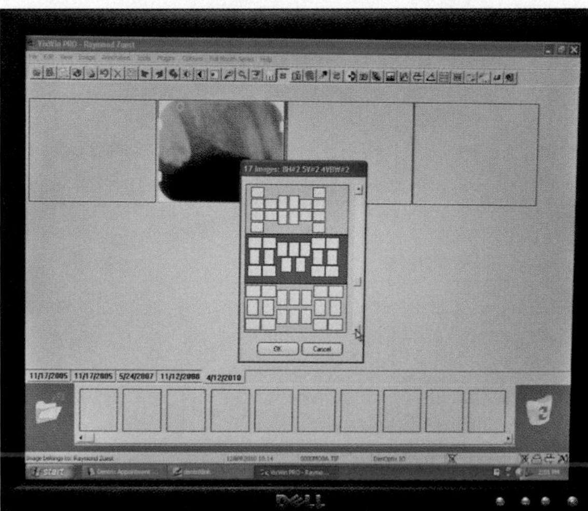

**4** Wash and dry hands.

**5** Place surface barriers on equipment and work area.

# PROCEDURE 40.5 Practicing Infection Control with Phosphor Storage Plates (PSPs)–cont'd

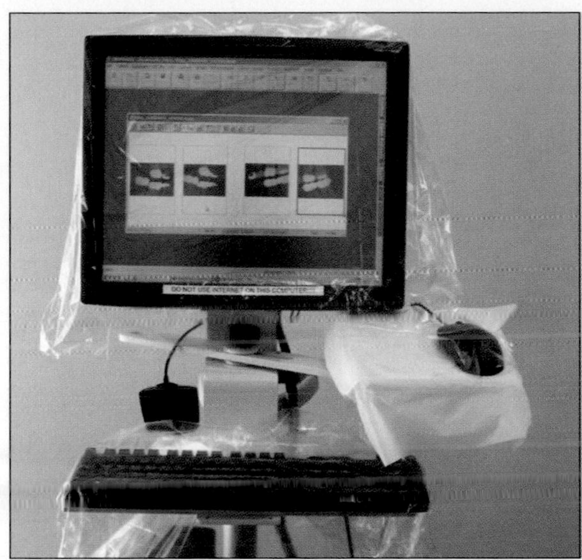

6 Slide the phosphor plates into barrier envelopes. Seal barrier by removing the protective strip, and gently press to seal the edge.

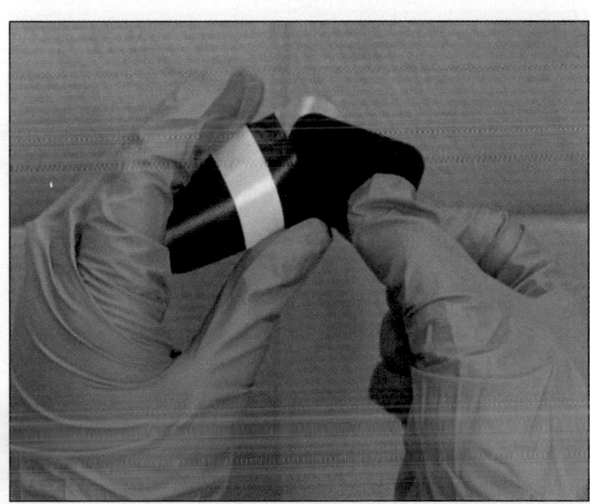

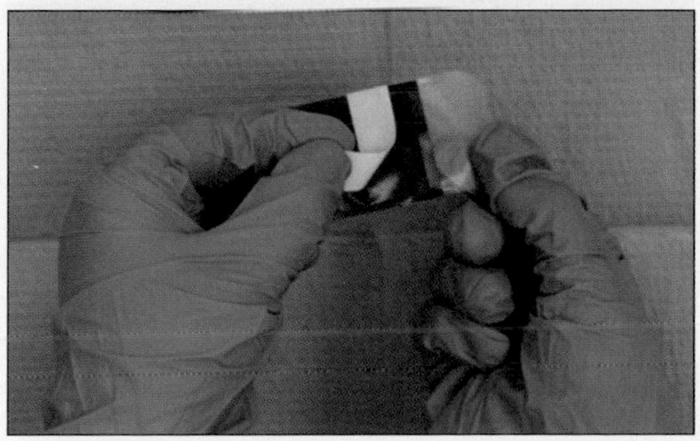

7 Set out the packaged positioning device, paper cup, transfer box, paper towel, and other miscellaneous items you might need.

**PURPOSE** Once gloved, you should not have to leave the operatory area for additional materials.

## Exposures

8 Seat the patient and place the lead apron.

9 Wash and dry hands and don gloves.

10 Place the PSP into the film holder for each exposure.

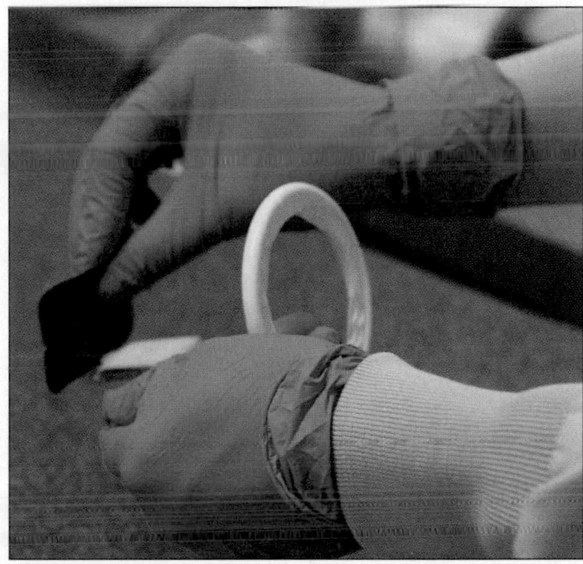

11 After each exposure, wipe excess saliva from the PSP envelope using a paper towel.

12 Place each exposed PSP into the paper cup labeled with the patient's name or directly into the black transfer box.

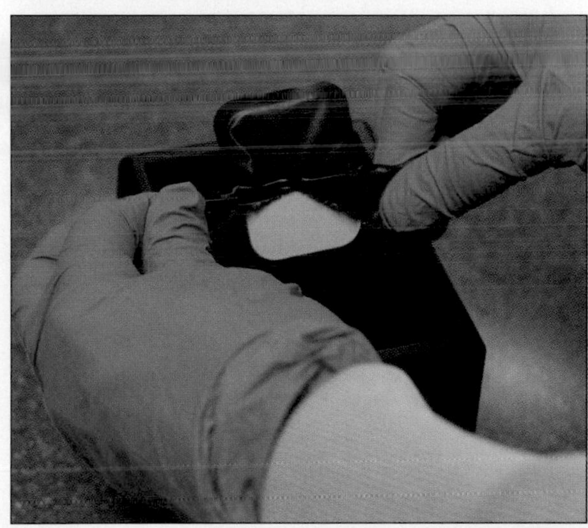

(Continued)

## PROCEDURE 40.5 Practicing Infection Control with Phosphor Storage Plates (PSPs)–cont'd

**13** After the exposures are complete, remove the lead apron and dismiss the patient.

**14** While still gloved, remove barriers, taking care not to touch the surfaces underneath.

**PURPOSE** You must wear gloves while removing barriers, because they are contaminated. If you touch a surface underneath the barrier while you are removing it, that surface will become contaminated and then must be disinfected.

**15** Dispose of barriers and paper towels. Place the used positioning device on a tray to be returned to the instrument processing area.

### Preparing PSPs for Scanning

**NOTE** If scanning is done immediately following exposure, it is not necessary to use the black transfer box step, and the PSPs can be scanned immediately. The black transfer box is necessary because the PSPs should not be exposed very long to bright light or warmth because this will release the energy before it is read by the scanner.

**16** While gloved, remove each PSP from the paper cup and carefully open the sealed envelope and allow the PSP to drop into the black transfer box. Use care not to touch the outside of the transfer box to avoid contamination.

**PURPOSE** Gloves must be worn because the PSP envelopes are contaminated.

**17** Dispose of contaminated envelopes.

**18** Remove gloves and wash and dry hands.

### Scanning the PSP

**19** Scanning machines vary greatly depending on the manufacturer, so reading the specific instructions for the specific machine being used is critical.

**NOTE** The PSP plates are no longer contaminated and are carefully handled with clean bare hands. The plates are easily scratched or damaged.

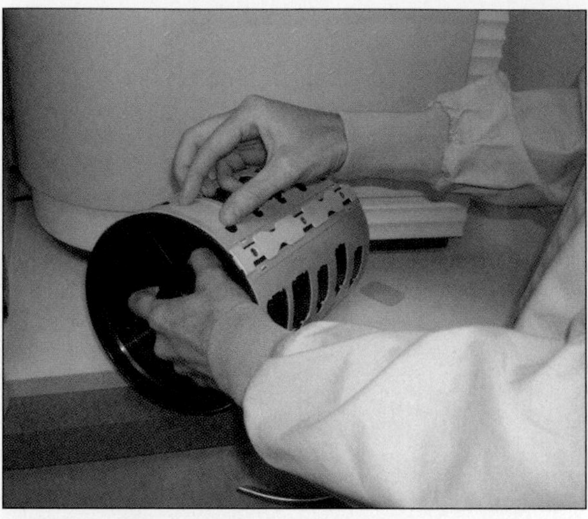

**20** Insert the PSP into the scanner according to the manufacturer's instructions.

**PURPOSE** The scanning machine will convert the fluorescent "signal" into a digital image that will appear on the monitor.

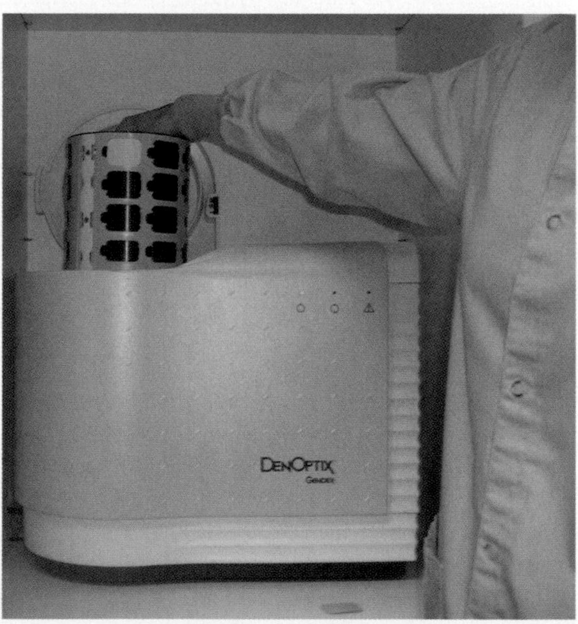


**21** When the imaging is complete, log off the system.

**22** Document the procedure in the patient's record.

41

# Intraoral Imaging

## KEY TERMS

**Angulation** Alignment of central ray of x-ray beam in horizontal and vertical planes.

**Bisecting (bisection of the angle) technique** Intraoral technique of exposing dental images.

**Bitewing** Type of image used for interproximal examination.

**Central ray** X-ray at center of beam.

**Contact area** Area of the mesial or distal surfaces of a tooth that touches an adjacent tooth in the same arch.

**Crestal bone** Coronal portion of alveolar bone found between the teeth.

**Developmental disability** Impairment of mental or physical functioning that usually occurs before adulthood and lasts indefinitely.

**Diagnostic quality** Referring to images with the proper structures and necessary density, contrast, definition, and detail for diagnostic purposes.

**Interproximal** Between two adjacent surfaces.

**Intersecting** Cutting across or through.

**Long axis of the tooth** Imaginary line dividing the tooth longitudinally (vertically) into two equal halves.

**Occlusal technique** Used to examine large areas of the upper or lower jaw.

**Parallel** Moving or lying in the same plane, always separated by the same distance.

**Paralleling technique** Intraoral technique of exposing periapical and bitewing images.

**Perpendicular** Intersecting at or forming a right angle.

**Physical disability** Impairment in certain function(s) of the body, such as vision, hearing, or mobility.

**Positioning instrument** Intraoral device used to position and hold the film, sensor, or PSP.

**Right angle** Angle of 90 degrees formed by two lines perpendicular to each other.

## LEARNING OUTCOMES

*On completion of this chapter, the student will be able to achieve the following objectives:*

1. Pronounce, define, and spell the key terms.
2. Explain the reasons that the number of images in an FMX might vary.
3. Name the two primary types of projections used in an intraoral technique.
4. Discuss the paralleling technique, including the following:
   - State the five basic rules of the paralleling technique.
   - Describe how to prepare a patient for dental imaging.
   - Explain why an image receptor* holder is necessary with the paralleling technique.
   - Describe the sequence of exposure for anterior and posterior teeth.
5. Discuss the bisecting technique, including the following:
   - Identify the types of image receptor holders that can be used with the bisecting technique.
   - Describe the result of incorrect horizontal angulation.
   - Describe the result of incorrect vertical angulation.
   - Identify the image receptor size used in the bisecting technique.
6. Discuss the bitewing technique, including the following:
   - Explain the basic rules for the bitewing technique.
   - Name the recommended vertical angulation for all bitewing exposures.
7. Explain the technique for exposing occlusal radiographs.
8. Describe techniques for managing patients with special medical needs.
9. Describe techniques for managing patients with special dental needs, including a hypersensitive gag reflex.
10. Describe the appearance of the most common dental image technique errors.
11. Explain the two methods of mounting dental radiographs.

* *Note:* The term "image receptor" refers to either a conventional dental film, PSP, or digital sensor.

## PERFORMANCE OUTCOMES

*On completion of this chapter, the student will be able to meet competency standards in the following skills:*

- Describe how to prepare a patient for dental imaging.
- Assemble the XCP instruments.
- Using the paralleling technique, expose a full series of images using both dental film and sensors.
- Using the bisection angle technique, expose a full-mouth series of images using both dental film and digital sensors.
- Using both dental film and sensors, expose a series of bitewing images.
- Using dental film, expose a maxillary and a mandibular occlusal radiograph.
- Mount and label a full series of dental radiographs.

## ELECTRONIC RESOURCES

***Additional information related to content in Chapter 41 can be found on the companion Evolve Web site.***

- Canadian Content Corner
- Practice Quiz
- Videos: Positioning the Patient for Dental Imaging; Assembling XCP Instruments; Mounting Dental Radiographs; Paralleling Technique; Bisecting Technique; Bitewing Technique; Occlusal Technique

It is possible for every dental assistant to be successful in producing quality dental images that are free from distortion, have the correct density and contrast, and can be used for the detection of dental disease. You can create such images by carefully following the steps in image receptor *placement, exposure,* and *processing* (Fig. 41.1).

Your patients will come in a variety of sizes, physical and mental abilities, types of dentitions, and personalities. Often, you will take x-rays on patients with special needs. For example, you will explain x-rays to a 6-year-old patient differently than you will to an adult. Your technique will vary depending on whether you are using digital sensors, phosphor storage plates (PSPs), or conventional dental film. In addition, you will have to modify your technique if your patient has a palate that is very flat and narrow, or your patient has a sensitive gag reflex. This chapter provides guidelines about various situations you are likely to encounter in your career.

Even the most skilled operators can make errors; the ability to recognize errors and to know the steps to take to prevent their recurrence is most important. This chapter explains common technique errors and how to prevent them. In addition, you will learn to recognize and use normal anatomic landmarks in mounting radiographs.

## Full-Mouth Survey

No dental examination can be complete without dental images, and, in almost all cases, the full-mouth survey is the preferred technique.

An intraoral *full-mouth survey (FMX)* contains both *periapical* and *bitewing* images. The bitewing image shows the upper and lower teeth in occlusion. Only the crowns and a small portion of the root are seen. This view is used for detecting **interproximal** decay, early periodontal disease, recurrent decay under restorations, and the fit of metallic fillings or crowns (Fig. 41.2). The periapical image shows the entire tooth from occlusal surface or incisal edge to about 2 to 3 mm beyond the apex to show the periapical bone. This view is used to diagnose pathologic conditions of the tooth, root, and bone, as well as tooth formation and eruption (Fig. 41.3). Periapicals are essential in endodontics and in oral surgical procedures.

For the average adult, a full-mouth series consists of 18 to 20 images—generally, 14 periapical views and 4 to 6 bitewing views. The number may vary, however, depending on the dentist's preference and the number of teeth present. For example, for the patient without teeth, 14 periapical views are enough to cover the edentulous arches; bitewings are not necessary. For the patient with a full dentition, the number of periapical views varies depending on whether the paralleling or the bisecting technique is used.

The *anterior* area is the region in which the number of images varies. Variables include the size of the sensor, if you are using digital, and the technique used (Fig. 41.4, *A*). When using dental film and the bisecting technique, three anterior views are taken on each arch (maxillary and mandibular) with size #2 film. For the paralleling technique, three or four size #1 films would be used on each arch (Fig. 41.4, *B*).

## Intraoral Imaging Techniques

Whether using conventional film, digital sensors, or PSPs, two basic techniques can be used to obtain periapical images: the paralleling technique and the **bisecting (bisection of the angle) technique**. The American Academy of Oral and Maxillofacial Radiology and the American Dental Education Association (ADEA) recommend use of the **paralleling technique** because it provides the most accurate image with the least amount of radiation exposure to the patient. In some situations, however, such as a small mouth, a shallow palate, or tori, the operator may need to use the bisecting technique. This chapter provides step-by-step procedures on how to produce diagnostic-quality images with both techniques (Fig. 41.5).

RECALL

1 What is the difference between a bitewing and a periapical image?
2 What are the two techniques for obtaining periapical images?

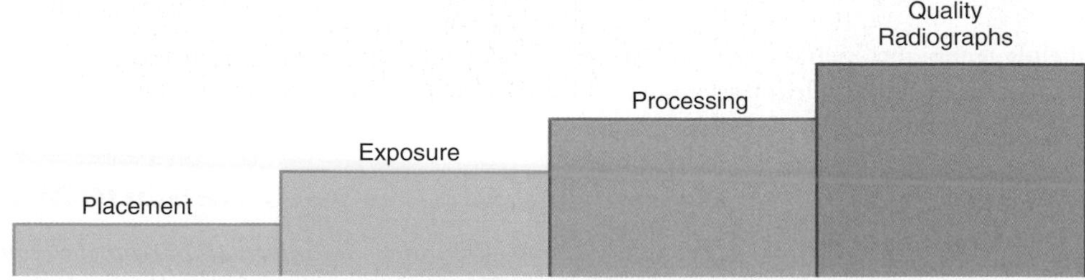


**FIG. 41.1** Steps to quality dental images. *(© Elsevier Collection.)*

## Paralleling Technique

The paralleling technique is also known as the *extension-cone paralleling (XCP), right-angle,* or *long-cone* technique. To use the paralleling technique competently, you must understand the terminology, including **parallel** (Fig. 41.6), **intersecting**, **perpendicular**, **right angle**, **long axis of the tooth** (Fig. 41.7), and **central ray**, in addition to the five basic rules.

### Five Basic Rules

The following basic rules *must* be followed when the paralleling technique is used:

1. Image receptor *placement.* The image receptor must be placed in the mouth, so that it will cover the correct teeth to be examined.
2. Image receptor *position.* The image receptor must be positioned parallel to the long axis of the tooth. The image receptor, in the appropriate holder (**positioning instrument**), must be placed away from the teeth and toward the middle of the mouth (Fig. 41.8).
3. *Vertical angulation.* The central ray of the x-ray beam must be directed perpendicular (at a right angle) to the image receptor and the long axis of the tooth.
4. *Horizontal angulation.* The central ray of the x-ray beam must be directed through the **contact areas** between the teeth (Fig. 41.9).
5. *Central ray.* The x-ray beam must be centered on the image receptor to ensure that all areas are exposed. Failure to center the x-ray beam results in a partial image, or *cone cut* (Fig. 41.10).

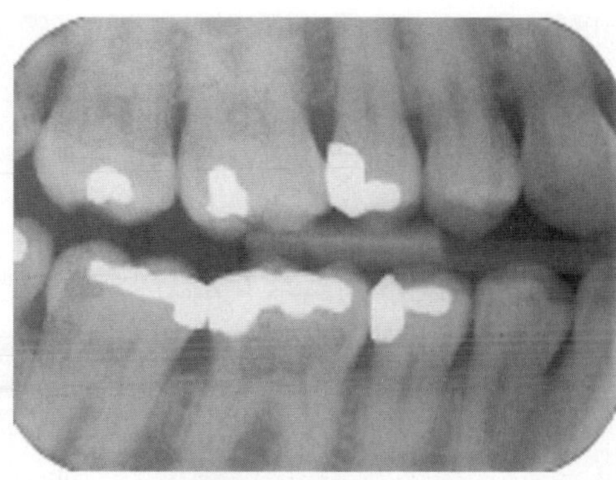

**FIG. 41.2** Bitewing radiograph. Note that only the crowns and the alveolar ridge are visible, but not the entire root.

## Patient Preparation

The patient who is having dental images taken should be seated after the room has been prepared and infection control procedures completed. See Procedure 41.1: Preparing the Patient for Dental Imaging.

## Exposure Sequence for Image Receptor Placement

You should plan an exposure sequence, or a definite order, for periapical image receptor placement when you are exposing images. When working with dental film without a planned exposure sequence, you are more likely to omit an area or to expose the same area twice. This does not occur as easily when using direct digital imaging because the image most recently exposed appears on the computer screen.

### *Anterior Exposure Sequence*

When exposing periapical views with the paralleling technique, *always* start with the anterior teeth (canines and incisors) for the following reasons:

- The size of the anterior image receptor (#1) is small and is easier for patients to tolerate.

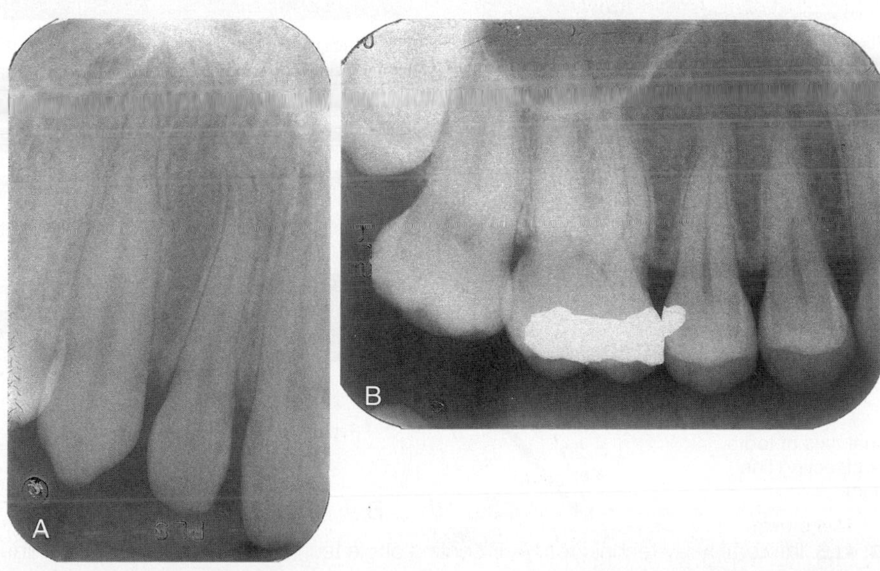


**FIG. 41.3** A, Anterior periapical. B, Posterior periapical. Note that the entire tooth and surrounding bone are visible on the radiograph.

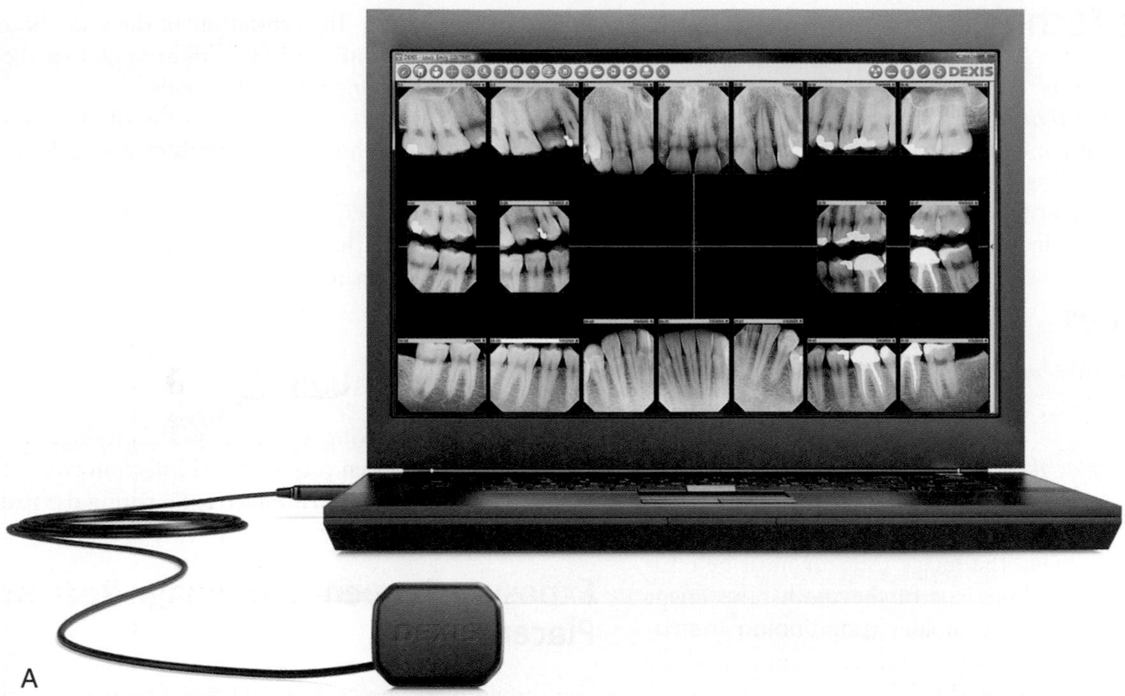


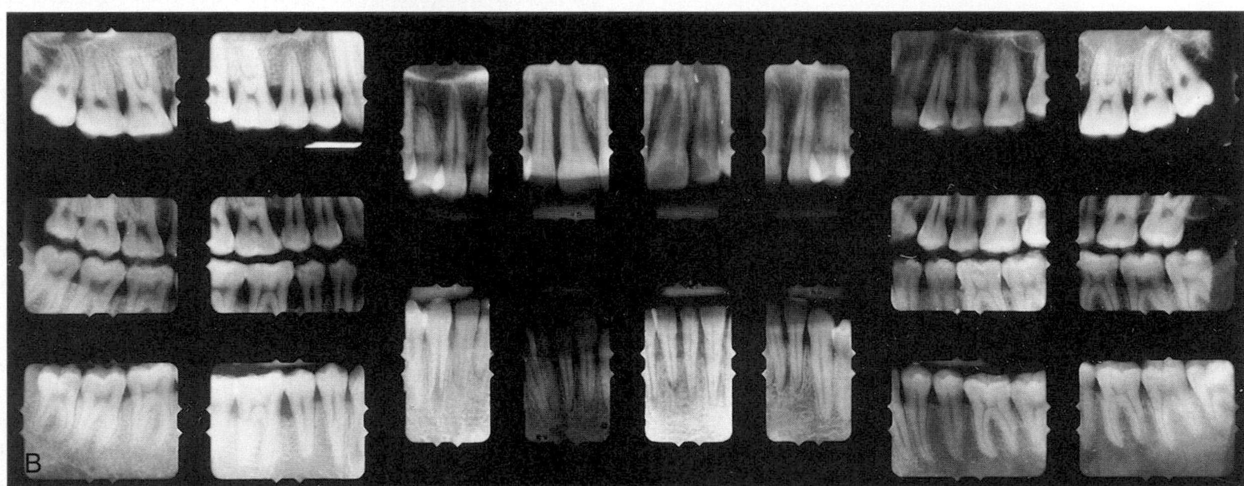


**FIG. 41.4** A, Full-mouth survey using digital sensor. B, Mounted full-mouth series with eight anterior films using the paralleling technique. *(A, Courtesy of KaVo Kerr.)*

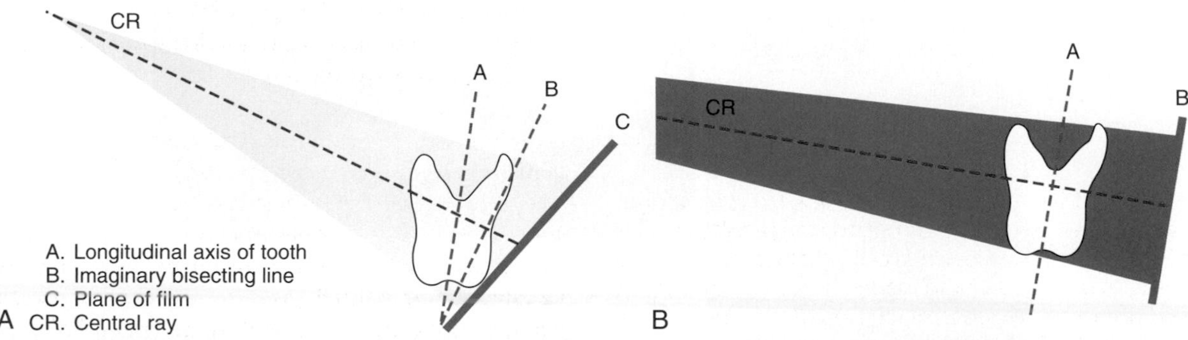


**FIG. 41.5** Intraoral x-ray techniques. A, Bisecting angle technique. B, Paralleling technique.

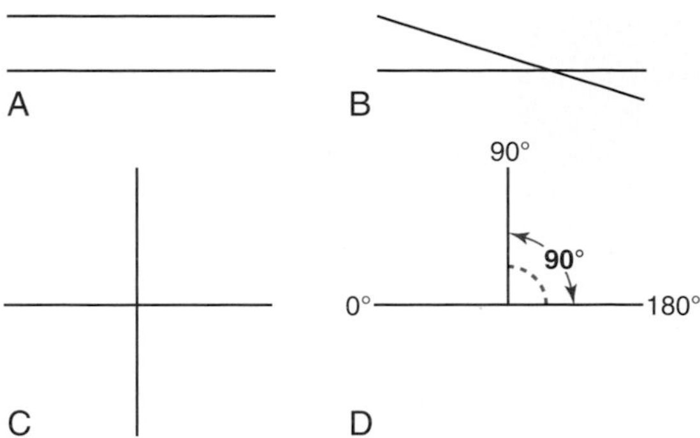


**FIG. 41.6** A, Parallel lines are always separated by the same distance and do not intersect. B, Intersecting lines cross one another. C, Perpendicular lines intersect one another to form right angles. D, Right angle measures 90 degrees and is formed by two perpendicular lines. *(From Iannucci J, Jansen Howerton L: Dental radiography: principles and techniques, ed 5, St Louis, 2017, Elsevier.)*

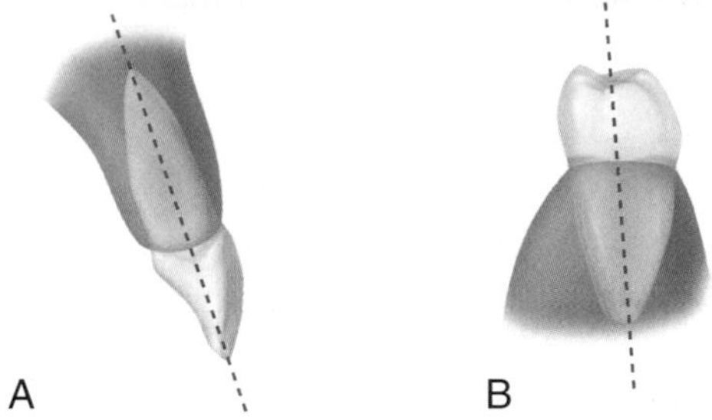


**FIG. 41.7** A, Long axis of maxillary incisor divides the tooth into two equal halves. B, Long axis of mandibular premolar divides the tooth into two equal halves. *(From Iannucci J, Jansen Howerton L: Dental radiography: principles and techniques, ed 5, St Louis, 2017, Elsevier.)*

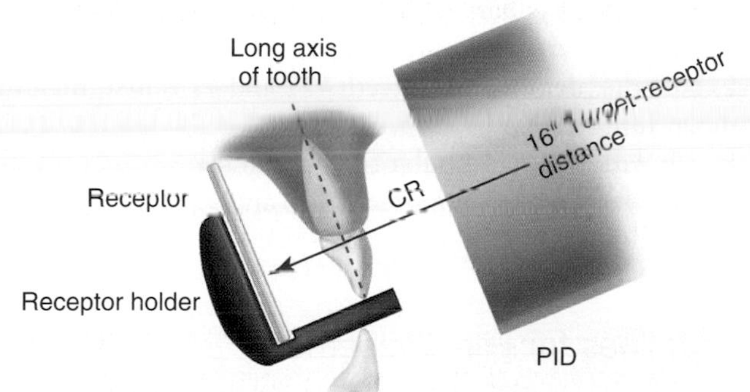


**FIG. 41.8** Position of the film sensor, teeth, position indicator device (PID), and central ray of the x-ray beam in the paralleling technique. The film sensor and the long axis of the tooth are parallel. The central ray (CR) is perpendicular to the tooth and the film sensor. An increased distance (16 inches) is required. *(From Iannucci J, Jansen Howerton L: Dental radiography: principles and techniques, ed 5, St Louis, 2017, Elsevier.)*

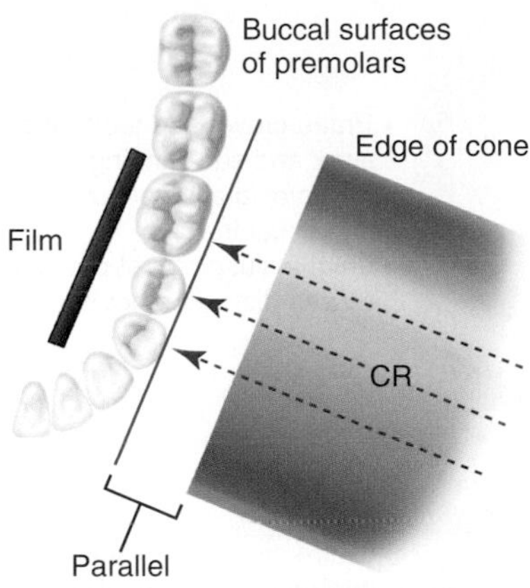


**FIG. 41.9** In this diagram, x-rays pass through the contact areas of the premolars because the central ray is directed through the contacts and perpendicular to the film. If the central ray (CR) is not directed through the contacts, overlap of the premolar contacts occurs. *(From Iannucci J, Jansen Howerton L: Dental radiography: principles and techniques, ed 4, St Louis, 2012, Saunders.)*

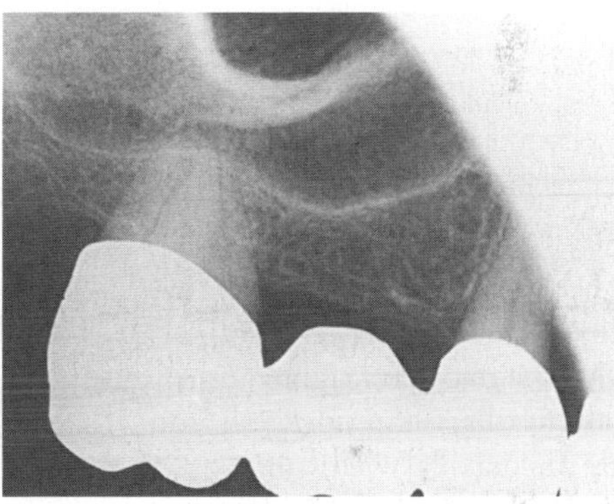

**FIG. 41.10** This radiograph demonstrates a cone cut, that is, a clear unexposed area on the film. The position indicator device was positioned too far distally, so the anterior portion of the film received no exposure. *(From Frommer HH, Stabulus JJ: Radiology for the dental professional, ed 9, St Louis, 2011, Mosby.)*

- Patients more easily adapt to the anterior image receptor holder.
- Patients are less likely to gag with anterior image receptor placement. Once the gag reflex is stimulated, the patient may gag on subsequent views that would normally be tolerated (see later discussion).

When using a size #1 film/sensor, a total of seven or eight anterior placements are used in the paralleling technique: four maxillary exposures and three mandibular exposures (Fig. 41.11). Some operators will choose to expose four maxillary and four mandibular anterior views. If size #2 film/sensor is used instead, six anterior placements are needed: three maxillary and three mandibular exposures. The authors recommend the use of #1 film/sensor for the anteriors.

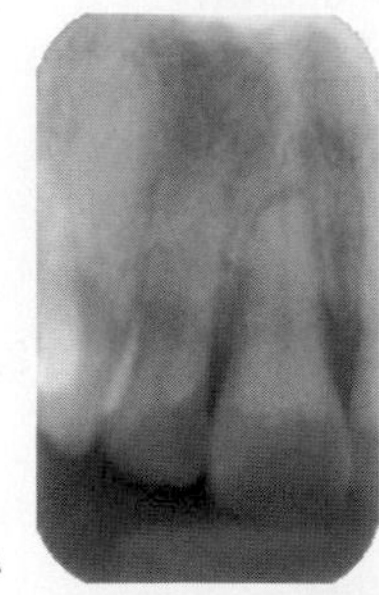

A

- Entire crown and tooth of canine, including apex and surrounding structures.
- Interproximal alveolar bone and mesial contact of canine.
- Lingual cusp of first premolar usually obscures distal contact of canine.

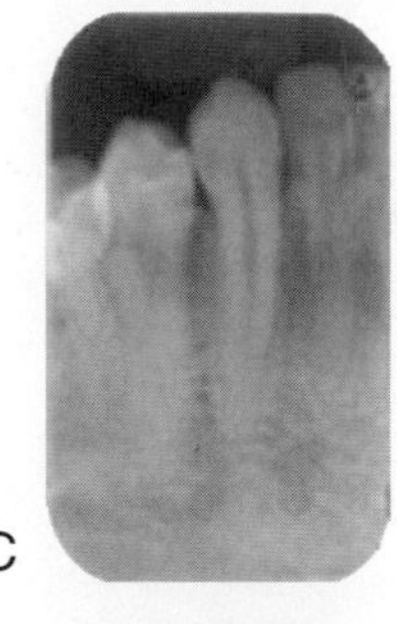

C

- Entire crown and root of canine, including apex and surrounding structures.
- Interproximal alveolar bone and mesial and distal contacts.

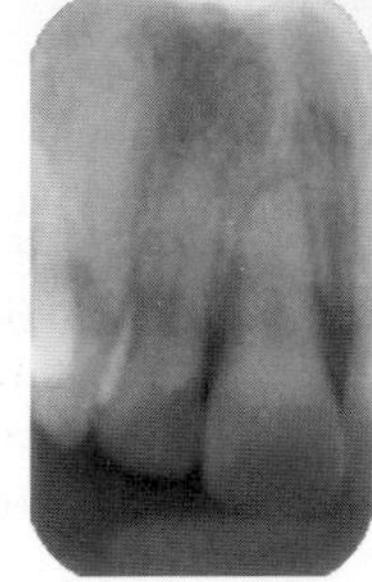

B

- Entire crown and roots of one lateral and one central incisor, including apices of teeth and surrounding structures.
- Interproximal alveolar bone between central and lateral contact areas, mesial and distal contact areas, and surrounding regions of bone.
- Mesial contacts of adjacent central incisor and adjacent canine.

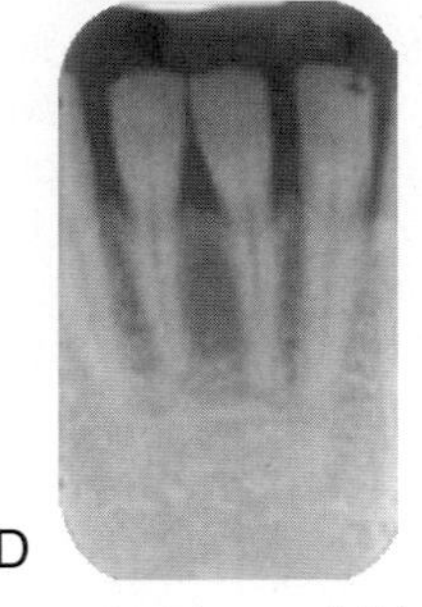

D

- Entire crown and roots of four mandibular incisors, including apices of teeth and surrounding structures.
- Contacts between central incisors and between central and lateral incisors.
- In most cases, not necessary to see distal contacts of lateral incisors.

**FIG. 41.11** Anterior periapical film placement shows structures visible on the radiograph. A, Maxillary canine exposure. B, Maxillary incisor exposure. C, Mandibular canine exposure. D, Mandibular incisor exposure. *(From Iannucci J, Jansen Howerton L: Dental radiography: principles and techniques, ed 5, St Louis, 2017, Elsevier.)*

The recommended anterior exposure sequence for the Rinn XCP instruments (Dentsply Rinn, Elgin, IL) is as follows:

1. Assemble the anterior XCP instrument. See Procedure 41.2: Assembling the XCP (Extension-Cone Paralleling) Instruments.
2. Begin with the maxillary right canine (tooth #6).
3. Expose all maxillary anterior teeth from *right* to *left*.
4. End with the maxillary left canine (tooth #11).
5. Move to the mandibular arch.
6. Begin with the mandibular left canine (tooth #22).
7. Expose all mandibular anterior teeth from *left* to *right*.
8. Finish with the mandibular right canine (tooth #27).

No wasted movement or shifting of the position indicator device (PID) occurs when you work from right to left in the maxillary arch, and then from left to right in the mandibular arch. You may find an exposure sequence that works better for you. The most important thing is to always use the same sequence. This allows you to keep track of the last exposure if you are interrupted. See Procedure 41.3: Producing Full-Mouth Radiographic Survey Using Paralleling Technique.

### Posterior Exposure Sequence

After you have completed the anterior teeth, begin the posterior teeth. *Always* begin with the premolar view before the molar view, for the following reasons:

- Premolar image receptor placement is easier for the patient to tolerate than molar placement.
- Premolar exposure is less likely to bring on the gag reflex.
- With the paralleling technique, eight posterior image receptor placements are used: four maxillary exposures and four mandibular exposures (Fig. 41.12).

The recommended posterior exposure sequence for the XCP instruments is as follows:

1. Begin with the maxillary right quadrant.
2. Assemble the posterior XCP instrument for this area. See Procedure 41.2.
3. Expose the premolar view (teeth #4 and #5) first, then the molar view (teeth #1, #2, and #3).
4. Without reassembling the XCP instrument, move to the mandibular left quadrant.
5. Expose the premolar view (teeth #20 and #21) first, then the molar view (teeth #17, #18, and #19).
6. Move to the maxillary left quadrant and reassemble the posterior XCP instrument for this area.
7. Expose the premolar film (teeth #12 and #13) first, then the molar film (teeth #14, #15, and #16).
8. Finish with the mandibular right quadrant.
9. Expose the premolar film (teeth #28 and #29) first, then the molar film (teeth #30, #31, and #32).

#### Guidelines for Film Placement

- The white side of the film always faces the teeth.
- Anterior films are always placed vertically.
- Posterior films are always placed horizontally.
- The identification dot on the film is always placed in the slot of the film holder (dot in the slot).
- The film holder is always positioned away from the teeth and toward the middle of the mouth.
- The film is always centered over the areas to be examined.
- The film is always placed parallel to the long axis of the teeth.

A

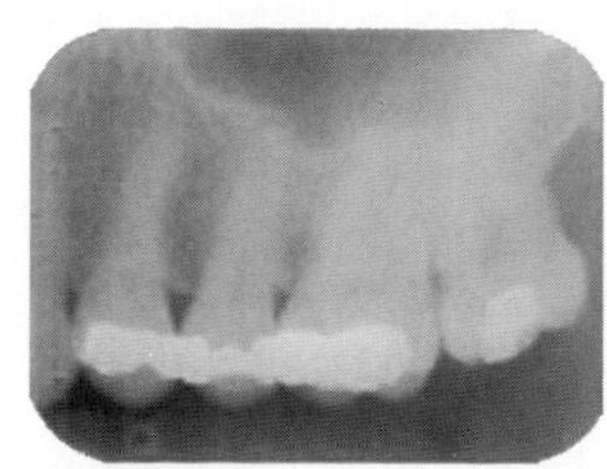

- All crowns and roots of first and second premolars and first molar, including apices, alveolar crests, contact areas, and surrounding bone

B

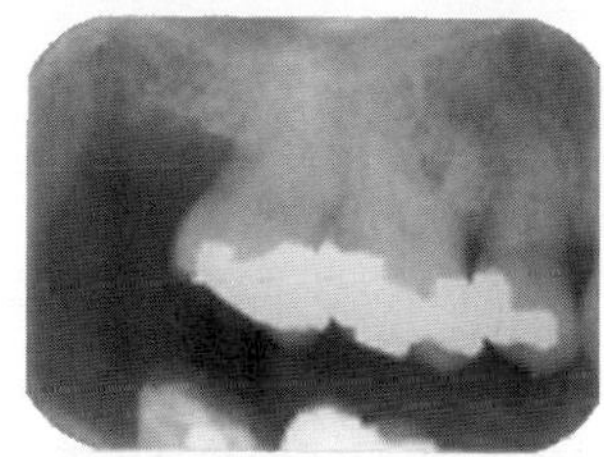

- All crowns and roots of first, second, and third molars, including apices, alveolar crests, contact areas, surrounding bone, and tuberosity region

C

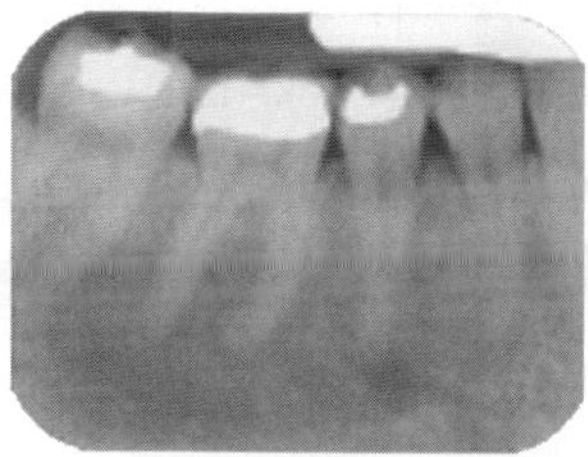

- All crowns and roots of first and second premolars and first molar, including apices and surrounding bone
- Distal contact of mandibular canine

D

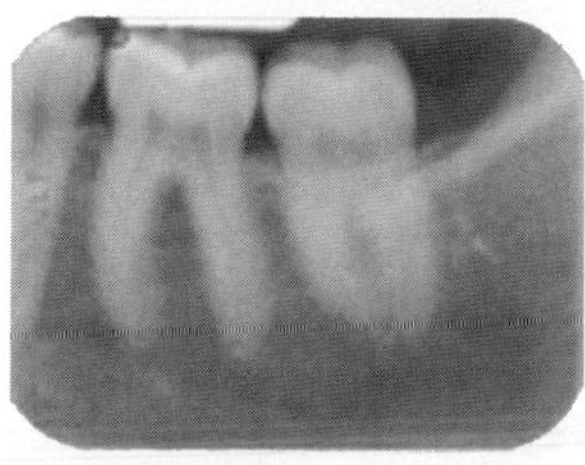

- All crowns and roots of first, second, and third molars, including apices and surrounding bone

**FIG. 41.12** Posterior periapical film placement showing structures visible on the radiograph. A, Maxillary premolar exposure. B, Maxillary molar exposure. C, Mandibular premolar exposure. D, Mandibular molar exposure. *(From Iannucci J, Jansen Howerton L: Dental radiography: principles and techniques, ed 5, St Louis, 2017, Elsevier.)*

### Guidelines for Sensor Placement

- Use the paralleling technique and a sensor positioning device.
- Place the sensor parallel to the teeth, but not necessarily against the tooth.
- For maxillary views, place the sensor at the midline of the palate.
- For mandibular views, place the sensor more toward the tongue.
- For mandibular molar views, make sure the bite-block is fully inside the patient's mouth.
- If the patient has difficulty closing, have the patient stabilize the arm of the holder with his or her finger.
- Make sure the position indicator device (PID) is parallel to the arm of the holder and is directed at the center of the aiming ring.
- Use a cotton roll as a cushion between the sensor and tori.
- For especially sensitive patients, foam cushions are made specifically for use with sensors. These can make placement much more comfortable.

Adapted from Schick by Sirona, *Sensor Placement Tutorial.*

### *Film Placement*

There are specific teeth and structures that must be clearly visible on each image for every projection (see Figs. 41.11 and 41.12).

RECALL

3 Why is an exposure sequence important?
4 When exposing images, in which area of the mouth should you begin?
5 Which projection should be the first for posterior exposures?

## Bisecting Technique

Another method of exposing periapical views is the bisecting technique, also known as the *bisecting-angle, bisection of the angle,* or *short-cone* technique. Although the bisecting technique was first used with a short cone, this technique can be used with a short or a long PID, and with any type of image receptor.

The American Academy of Oral and Maxillofacial Radiology recommends the paralleling technique as the technique of choice for periapical images. Therefore the bisecting technique should be used only as an alternative method in special circumstances, when it is not possible to use the paralleling technique. Such special circumstances include patients with very small mouths, children, and patients with low or flat palatal vaults.

The bisection of the angle technique is based on the geometric principle of equally dividing a triangle. In contrast to the paralleling technique, in which you move the image receptor away from the teeth to make the film and the teeth parallel, the bisecting technique places the film *directly against* the teeth to be exposed. Thus the film and the teeth are not parallel, but are at an angle.

With the bisecting technique, the angle formed by the long axes of the teeth and the image receptor is bisected into two equal parts, and the x-ray beam is directed perpendicular to the bisecting line (Fig. 41.13).

The major disadvantage of this technique is that the image is dimensionally distorted.

## Image Receptor Holders

When the bisecting technique is being used, you may see some operators asking the patient to hold the film with his or her fingers to stabilize the film in the mouth. This practice is *not* recommended. Holding the film exposes the patient's hand and finger to unnecessary radiation.

Available types of image receptor holders for the bisecting technique include the following:

- The bisecting-angle instrument (BAI; Dentsply Rinn) includes plastic bite-blocks, plastic aiming rings, and metal indicator arms.
- The Stabe bite-block (Dentsply Rinn) is a disposable bite-block that can be used with the paralleling technique or the bisecting technique. With the bisecting technique, the scored front section is removed, and the image receptor is placed *as close as possible* to the teeth.

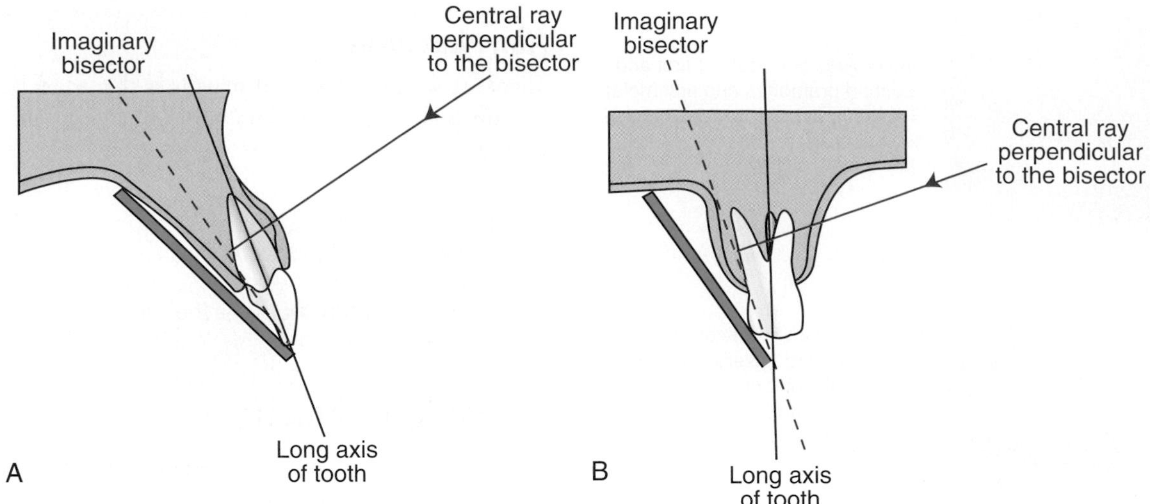


**FIG. 41.13** A, A diagram of an anterior tooth with the central ray perpendicular to the "imaginary" bisector of the angle between the long axis of the tooth and the film plane. B, A posterior tooth using the bisecting angle concept. *(From Miles DA, Van Dis ML, Williamson GF, et al: Radiographic imaging for the dental team, ed 4, St Louis, 2009, Saunders.)*

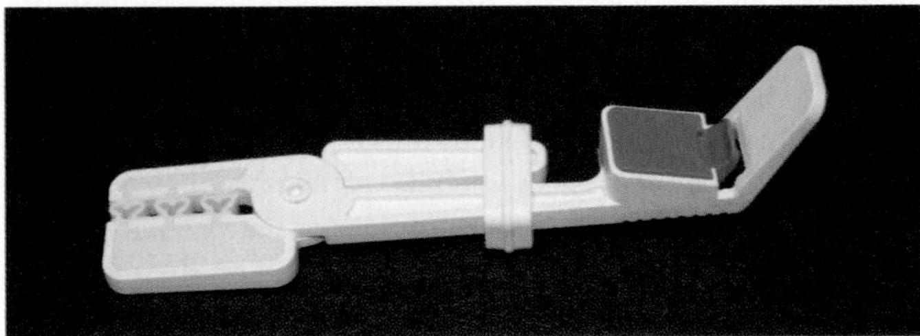

**FIG. 41.14** EeZee-Grip (Dentsply Rinn) sensor holder for both anterior and posterior digital images.

- The EeZee-Grip holder (Dentsply Rinn) is a sensor-holding device that is used in the bisecting technique (Fig. 41.14).

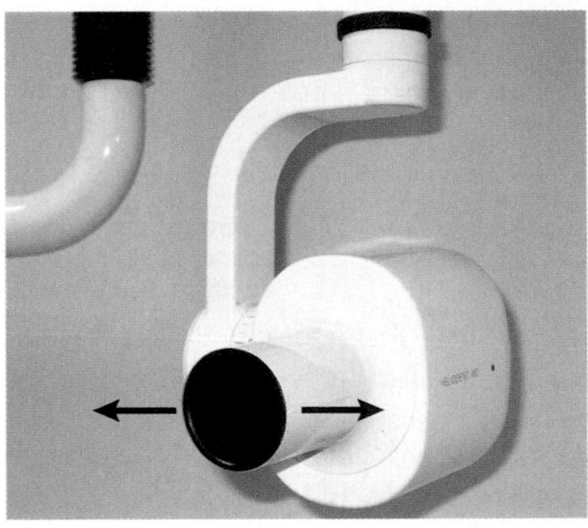

**FIG. 41.15** The arrows indicate movement in a horizontal direction.

## Angulation of Position Indicator Device

In the bisecting technique, the angulation of the PID is *critical.* **Angulation** is the term that is used to describe the alignment of the central ray of the x-ray beam in the horizontal and vertical planes. Angulation can be changed by moving the PID in a horizontal or a vertical direction. BAI instruments with aiming rings dictate the proper PID angulation. However, when the finger-holding method or the EeZee-Grip method is used, the operator must determine both the horizontal and the vertical angulation.

### Horizontal Angulation

Horizontal angulation refers to the positioning of the tubehead and the direction of the central ray in a horizontal, or side-to-side, plane. Horizontal angulation *remains the same* whether you are using the paralleling or the bisecting technique (Fig. 41.15).

**CORRECT HORIZONTAL ANGULATION.** With correct horizontal angulation, the central ray is directed perpendicular to the curvature of the arch and through the contact areas of the teeth (Fig. 41.16).

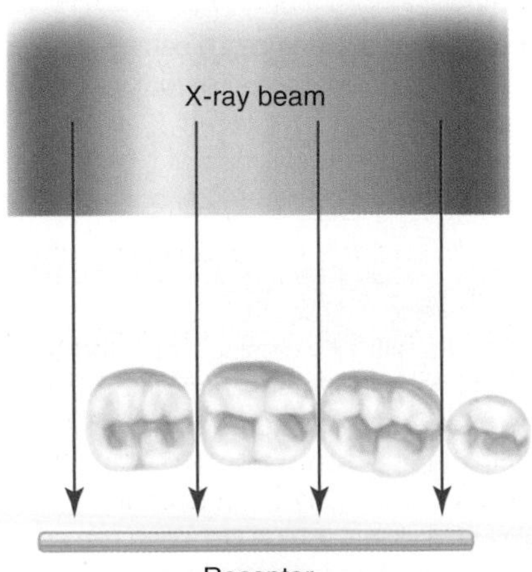


**FIG. 41.16** Correct horizontal angulation. *(From Iannucci J, Jansen Howerton L: Dental radiography: principles and techniques, ed 5, St Louis, 2017, Elsevier.)*

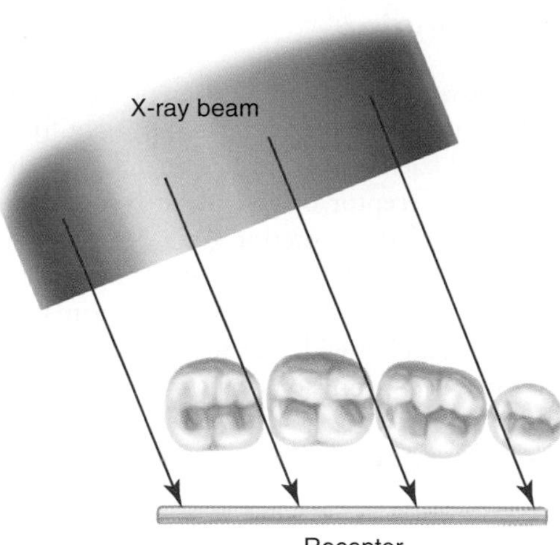


**FIG. 41.17** Incorrect horizontal angulation. *(From Iannucci J, Jansen Howerton L: Dental radiography: principles and techniques, ed 5, St Louis, 2017, Elsevier.)*

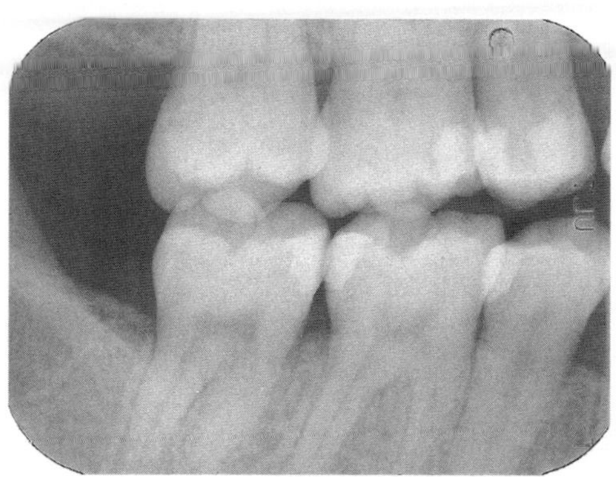

**FIG. 41.18** Overlapped contact areas.

**INCORRECT HORIZONTAL ANGULATION.** Incorrect horizontal angulation results in overlapped (unopened) contact areas (Fig. 41.17). A film with overlapped contact areas cannot be used to examine the interproximal areas of the teeth (Fig. 41.18).

## *Vertical Angulation*

Vertical angulation refers to the positioning of the PID in a vertical, or up-and-down, plane (Fig. 41.19). Angulation is measured in degrees according to the markings on the outside of the tubehead. Vertical angulation differs according to the x-ray technique that is being used, as follows:

- With the paralleling technique, the vertical angulation of the central ray is directed perpendicular to the image receptor and the long axis of the tooth.
- With the bisecting technique, the vertical angulation is determined by the imaginary bisector; the *central ray is directed perpendicular to the imaginary bisector.*
- With the bitewing technique, the vertical angulation is predetermined; the central ray is directed at +10 degrees to the occlusal plane (see later discussion).

**CORRECT VERTICAL ANGULATION.** Correct vertical angulation results in a radiographic image that is the same length as the tooth (Table 41.1).

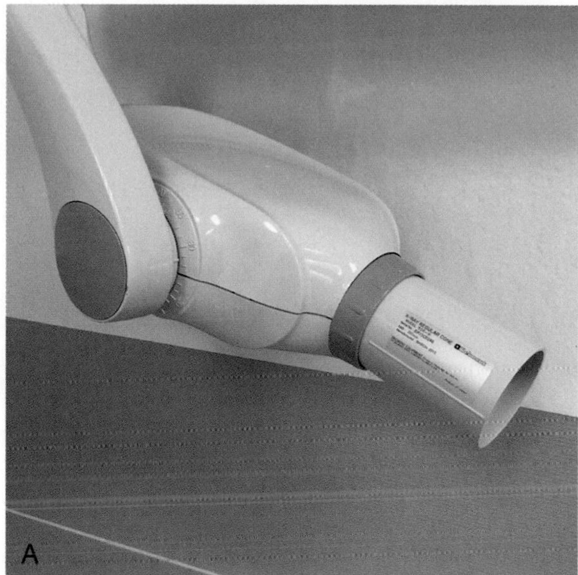


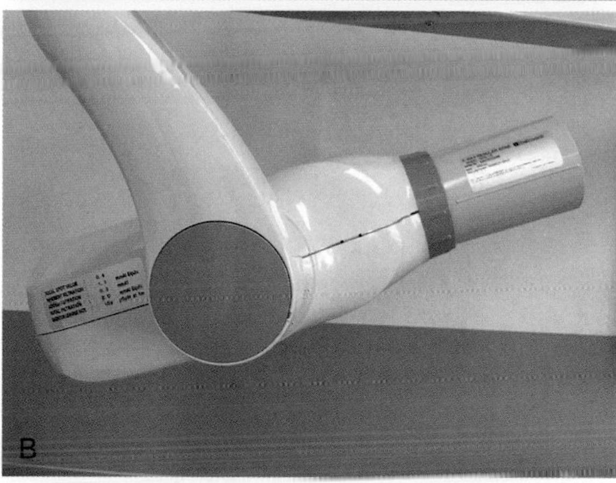


**FIG. 41.19** A, Positive vertical angulation. B, Negative vertical angulation. (Courtesy of Dr. Kamran Azmoudeh, Santa Rosa, CA.)

**TABLE 41.1** Recommended Vertical Angulation Ranges for Bisecting Technique

| Dentition | Maxillary, Degrees | Mandibular, Degrees |
|---|---|---|
| Canines | +45 to +55 | −20 to −30 |
| Incisors | +40 to +50 | −15 to −25 |
| Premolars | +30 to +40 | −10 to −15 |
| Molars | +20 to +30 | −5–0 |

From Iannucci J, Jansen Howerton L: Dental radiography: principles and techniques, ed 4, St Louis, 2012, Saunders.

**INCORRECT VERTICAL ANGULATION.** Incorrect vertical angulation results in an image that is not the same length as the tooth that is being x-rayed. The image appears longer or shorter. *Elongated* or *foreshortened images* are not diagnostic.

To better understand this concept, think of the sun and your own shadow. When the sun (central beam) is high in the sky, your shadow is shorter than you are. When the sun (central ray) is low in the sky, your shadow is longer than you actually are.

**FORESHORTENED IMAGES.** On a foreshortened image, the teeth appear too short. Foreshortening of images results from *excessive* vertical angulation (Fig. 41.20).

**ELONGATED IMAGES.** On elongated images, the teeth appear too long. Elongation of images is caused by *insufficient* (not enough) vertical angulation, or vertical angulation that is too "flat" (Fig. 41.21).

## Image Receptor Size and Placement

In the bisecting technique, the image receptor is placed close to the crowns of the teeth to be x-rayed and extends at an angle into the palate or the floor of the mouth. The image receptor should extend beyond the incisal or occlusal aspect of the teeth by about 1/8 inch. Image receptor holders for the bisection of the angle technique, including some with alignment indicators, are available commercially.

## Patient Positioning

The patient's midsagittal plane should be perpendicular to the floor. This means that the patient's head is upright for maxillary films and is tipped back slightly for the mandibular arch.

A size #2 image receptor is used in both the anterior (in a vertical position) and the posterior (in a horizontal position) regions. Only three views are needed in the maxillary anterior region because all four maxillary incisors can be imaged on a #2 film or sensor if the arch is wide. If the arch is narrow, it may be necessary to use four #1 films or sensors.

## Beam Alignment

The x-ray beam is directed to pass between the contacts of the teeth that are being x-rayed in the horizontal dimension, just as it is in the paralleling technique. The vertical angle, however, must be directed at 90 degrees to the imaginary bisecting line. Too much

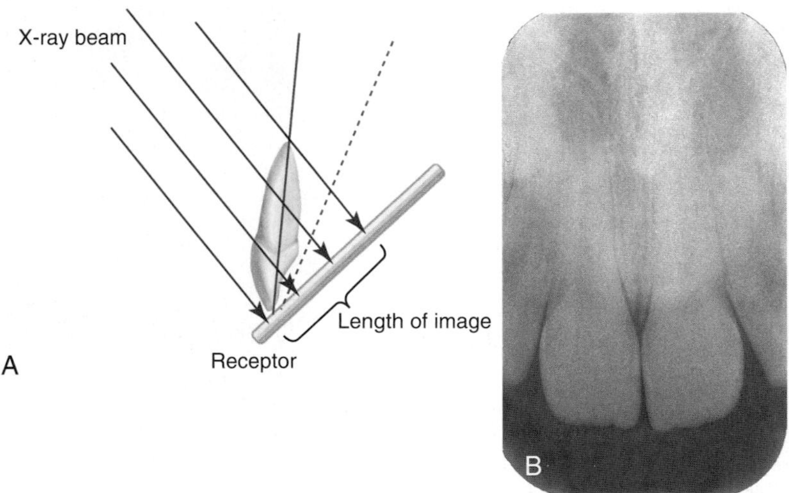


**FIG. 41.20** A, If the vertical angulation is too steep, the image on the film is shorter than the actual tooth. B, Foreshortened image. *(A, From Iannucci J, Jansen Howerton L: Dental radiography: principles and techniques, ed 5, St Louis, 2017, Elsevier.)*

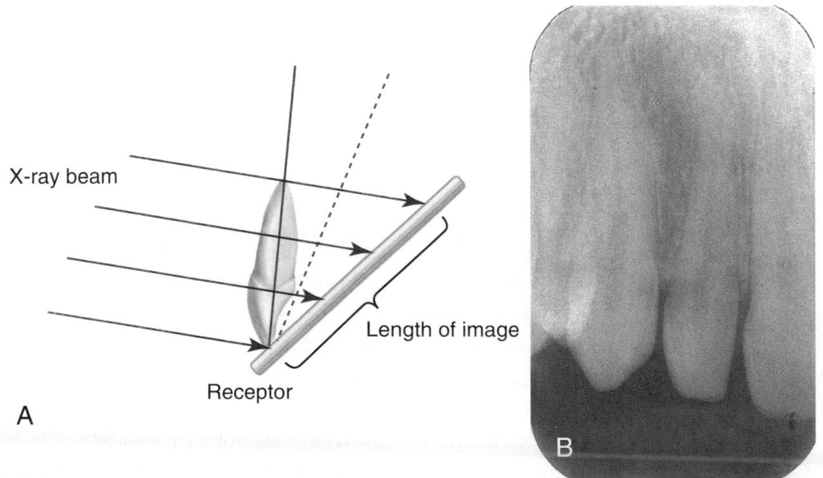


**FIG. 41.21** A, If the vertical angulation is too flat, the image on the film is longer than the actual tooth. B, Elongated image. *(A, From Iannucci J, Jansen Howerton L: Dental radiography: principles and techniques, ed 5, St Louis, 2017, Elsevier.)*

vertical angulation produces images that are too *short* (foreshortened; see Fig. 41.20), and too little vertical angulation results in images that are too *long* (elongated; see Fig. 41.21). The beam must be centered to avoid cone cutting. See Procedure 41.4: Producing Full-Mouth Radiographic Survey Using Bisecting Technique.

RECALL

6 Why is it not recommended to have the patient hold the film or sensor during exposure?
7 What type of film or sensor holders can be used in the bisecting technique?
8 What error occurs when the horizontal angulation is incorrect?
9 What two errors occur when the vertical angulation is incorrect?
10 In the bisecting technique, how is the film or sensor placed in relation to the teeth?

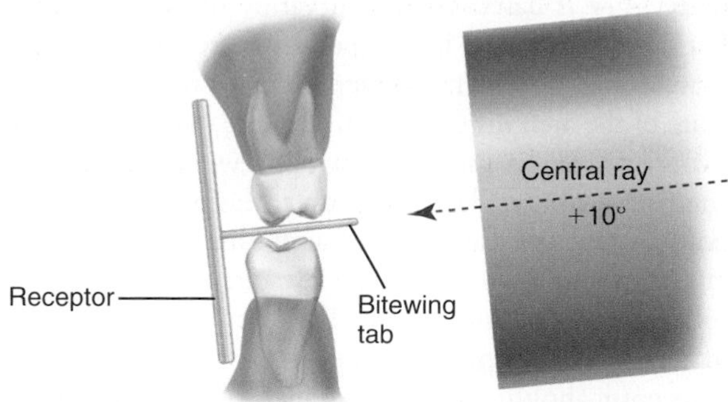


**FIG. 41.22** Positions of the receptor, bitewing tab, and central ray in the bitewing technique. The receptor is parallel to the crowns in the maxillary and mandibular teeth. The central ray is directed slightly downward (+10 degrees of vertical angulation). *(From Iannucci J, Jansen Howerton L: Dental radiography: principles and techniques, ed 5, St Louis, 2017, Elsevier.)*

## Bitewing Technique

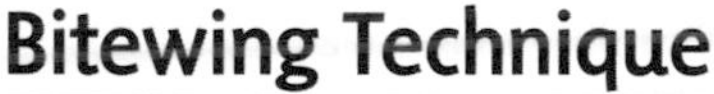

A **bitewing** view shows the crowns and interproximal areas of the maxillary and mandibular teeth and the areas of **crestal bone** on a single image. Bitewing views are used to detect interproximal caries (tooth decay) and are particularly useful in detecting early carious lesions that are not clinically evident. Bitewing views are also useful in examining crestal bone levels between the teeth.

The basic principles of the bitewing technique are as follows:

- The image receptor is placed in the mouth parallel to the crowns of both the upper and lower teeth.
- The image receptor is stabilized when the patient bites on the bitewing tab or the bitewing film holder.
- The central ray of the x-ray beam is directed through the contacts of the teeth, using +10 degrees of vertical angulation (Fig. 41.22).

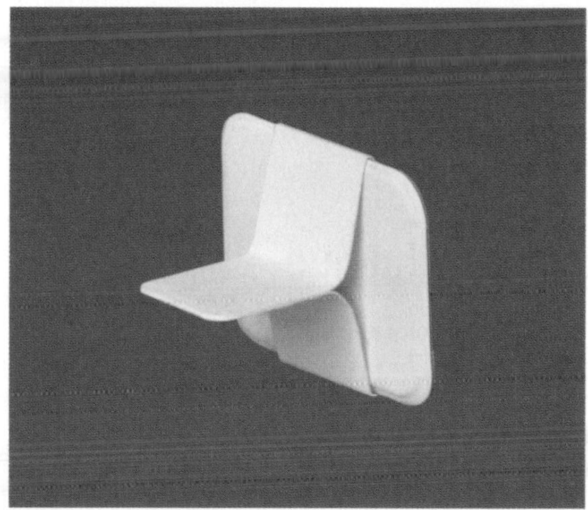

**FIG. 41.23** Bitewing tab and film holder. *(Courtesy Dentsply Rinn, Elgin, IL.)*

## Image Receptor Holder and Bitewing Tab

In the bitewing technique, a holding device or a bitewing tab is used to stabilize the image receptor (Fig. 41.23). When using a Rinn type of image receptor, red is the universal color for bitewing holders.

## Angulation of Position Indicator Device

The angulation of the PID is critical in the bitewing technique. The image receptor–holding instruments and aiming rings provide the proper angulation. When a bitewing tab is used, however, the operator must determine both the horizontal and the vertical angulation. Even a slight error will result in an image that is not diagnostic (Fig. 41.24).

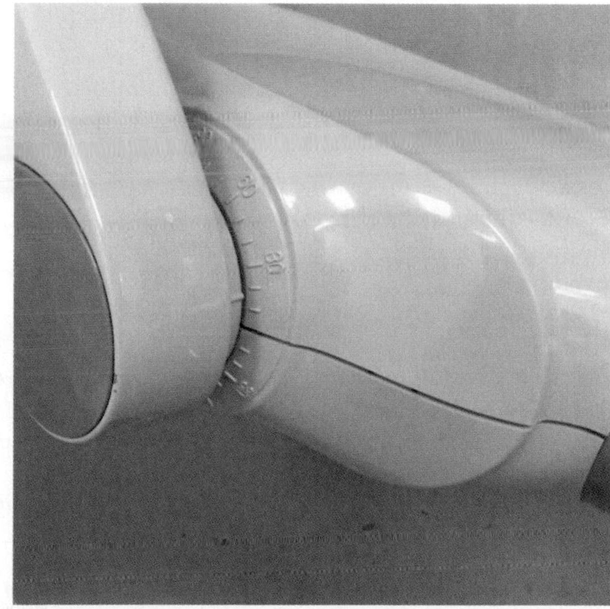

**FIG. 41.24** Vertical angulation is measured in degrees on the outside of the tubehead. (Courtesy of Dr. Kamran Azmoudeh, Santa Rosa, CA.)

## Exposure for Image Receptor Placement

Bitewing images are always parallel views regardless of the technique used for the periapical images. The number of bitewing views necessary is based on the curvature of the arch and the number of teeth present in the posterior areas. The curvature of the arch often differs in the premolar and molar areas. If the curvature of the arch differs, it is impossible to open *all* the posterior contact areas on a single bitewing view. Consequently, two bitewing views are usually exposed on each side of the arch.

Because the curvature of the arch differs in most adult patients, a total of four bitewing views are exposed: one right premolar, one right molar, one left premolar, and one left molar. The image receptor is positioned (with a bite tab or an image receptor–holding device) parallel to the crowns of both upper and lower teeth, and the central ray is directed perpendicular to the image receptor.

The *premolar* bitewing image should include the distal half of the crowns of the canines, both premolars, and often the first molars on both maxillary and mandibular arches. The *molar* view should be centered over the second molars. See Procedure 41.5: Producing Four-View Radiographic Survey Using Bitewing Technique.

**11** What is the purpose of bitewing images?
**12** What horizontal angulation should be used for bitewing images?

## Occlusal Technique

The **occlusal technique** is used to examine large areas of the upper or lower jaw. The occlusal technique is so named because the patient bites or "occludes" the entire film. In adults, size #4 intraoral film is used, but #2 film is used in children. The occlusal technique is used when large areas of the maxilla or mandible must be radiographed. See Procedure 41.6: Producing Maxillary and Mandibular Radiographs Using Occlusal Technique.

Occlusal radiographs can be used for the following purposes:

- Locate retained roots of extracted teeth.
- Locate supernumerary (extra) unerupted or impacted teeth.
- Locate salivary stones in the duct of the submandibular gland.
- Locate fractures of the maxilla and mandible.
- Examine the area of a cleft palate.
- Measure changes in the size and shape of the maxilla or mandible.

The basic principles of the occlusal technique follow:

- The film is positioned with the white side facing the arch that is being exposed.
- The film is placed in the mouth between the occlusal surfaces of the maxillary and mandibular teeth.
- The film is stabilized when the patient gently closes on the surface of the film.

**13** What size film is used for adults in the occlusal technique?
**14** When are occlusal radiographs indicated?

### Guidelines for Dental Treatment of Patients with Disabilities

- Do not ask personal questions about the patient's disability.
- Do offer assistance, for example, to push a wheelchair or direct a person who is blind. Often, a blind patient may prefer to hold your arm rather than having you hold the patient's arm.
- Do talk directly to the person with a disability. It is rude to talk to the caregiver instead of the patient. For example, instead of asking the caregiver, "Can Mrs. Jones get out of her wheelchair?" speak directly to Mrs. Jones.

## Patients with Special Medical Needs

Radiographic examination techniques often must be modified to accommodate patients with special needs. You must be prepared to alter your radiographic technique to meet the specific needs of the individual patient.

A person with a **physical disability** may have problems with vision, hearing, or mobility. You must make every effort to meet the individual needs of such patients. In many cases, a family member or a caregiver accompanies the person with a physical disability to the dental office. You can ask this person to assist you with communicating or with the physical needs of the patient. You should be aware of common disabilities and the modifications necessary to assist patients who have such problems.

### Vision Impairment

If your patient is blind or visually impaired, you must communicate using clear verbal explanations. You must keep your patient informed of what you are doing and explain each procedure *before* performing it. You must *never* gesture to another person in the presence of a person who is blind. Blind persons are sensitive to this form of communication and perceive that you are "talking behind their backs."

### Hearing Impairment

If your patient is deaf or hearing impaired, you have several options. You may ask a caregiver to act as an interpreter, use gestures, or use written instructions. If the patient can read lips, you will need to remove your mask, face the patient, and speak clearly and slowly.

### Mobility Impairment

If your patient is in a wheelchair and does not have use of the lower limbs, you may need to expose the necessary radiographs with the patient seated in the wheelchair (Fig. 41.25).

If your patient does not have use of the upper limbs, and a holder cannot be used to stabilize the image receptor in the mouth, you may ask the patient's caregiver to assist with holding the image receptor. This person must wear a lead apron and a thyroid collar during exposure of the images. In this case give the caregiver specific instructions on how to hold the image receptor or the patient.

Remember, regardless of the situation, you must *never* hold an image receptor for a patient during an exposure.

## Developmental Disabilities

A **developmental disability** is a substantial impairment of mental or physical functioning that occurs before adulthood and lasts indefinitely. Examples of developmental disabilities include autism, cerebral palsy, epilepsy, and mental impairment. You must make every effort to meet the individual needs of the patient with a developmental disability.

A person with a developmental disability may have problems with *coordination* or *comprehension* of instructions. As a result, you may have difficulties in obtaining intraoral images. If coordination or comprehension is a problem, mild sedation may be useful.

It is important that you recognize situations in which the patient *cannot tolerate* intraoral exposures. Intraoral images should *not* be attempted in these patients; such exposure results only in nondiagnostic images and needless radiation exposure of the patient. In patients who cannot tolerate intraoral exposures, extraoral images such as lateral jaw and panoramic x-rays may be used.

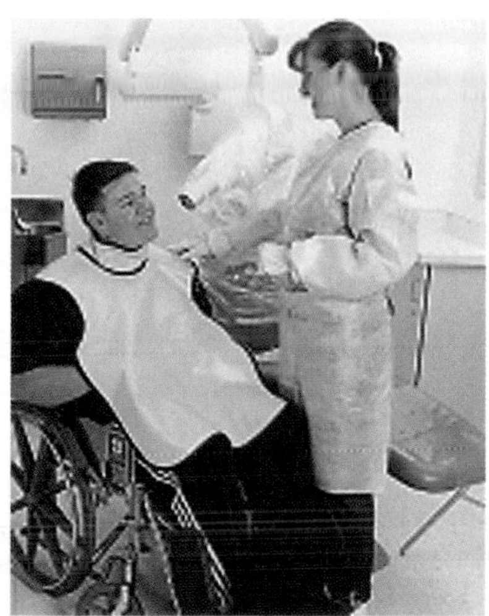
FIG. 41.25 X-rays can be taken with a patient sitting in his or her wheelchair.

RECALL

**15** What physical disabilities may affect dental patients?
**16** Under what circumstance would you hold a film sensor for a patient?

# Patients with Special Dental Needs

Dental images are indicated for a variety of patient needs. Often, you may need to modify the basic x-ray techniques to accommodate patients with special dental needs, including edentulous, pediatric, and endodontic patients.

## Edentulous Patient

*Edentulous* means "without teeth." Dental images on edentulous patients may be required for the following reasons:

- Detect retained root tips, impacted teeth, and lesions (cysts, tumors).
- Identify objects embedded in bone.
- Observe the quantity and health of the bone.

Radiographic examination of an edentulous patient may include a panoramic image (see Chapter 42), periapical images, or a combination of occlusal and periapical views (Fig. 41.26).

Radiographic images must be taken in all areas of the arches, whether or not teeth are present. For edentulous patients, the bisecting or the paralleling technique may be used. Because no teeth are present, the distortion inherent in the bisecting technique does not interfere with diagnostic intrabony conditions.

For *partially edentulous* patients, image receptor–holding instruments can be used by placing a cotton roll on the

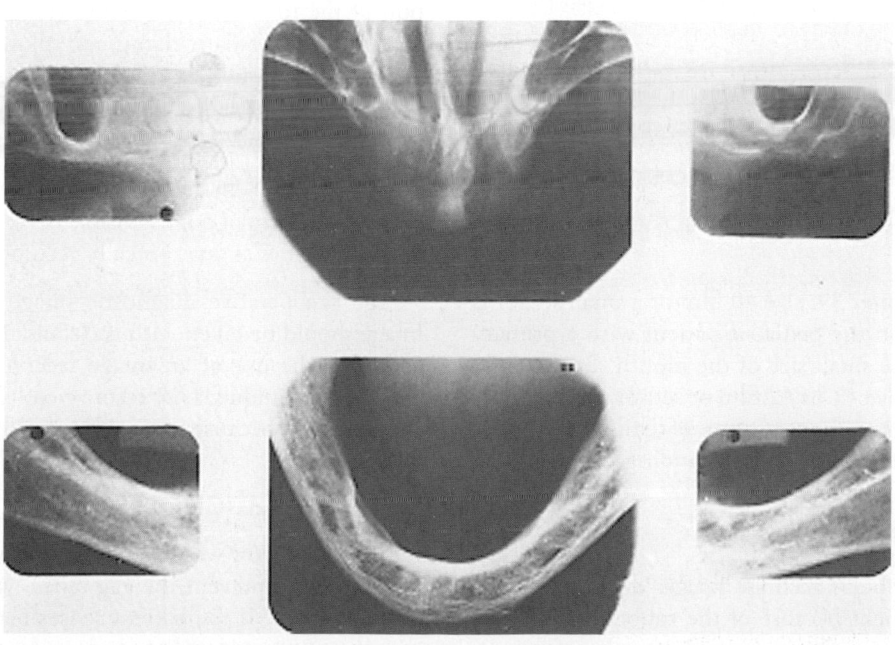
FIG. 41.26 Mixed occlusal-periapical edentulous survey.

bite-block where the crowns of the missing teeth would have been, and then following standard exposure procedures.

## Pediatric Patient

In children, images are useful for (1) detecting conditions of the teeth and bones, (2) showing changes related to caries and trauma, and (3) evaluating growth and development (see Chapter 57).

You must explain the x-ray procedures you are about to perform in terms that the child can easily understand. For example, you can refer to the tubehead as a "camera," the lead apron as a "coat," and the image as a "picture."

Exposure factors (milliamperage, kilovoltage, exposure time) must be reduced because of the smaller size of the pediatric patient. The shorter exposure time will reduce the effect of blurring if the child should move. All exposure factors should be set according to the recommendations of the equipment and film manufacturers (Fig. 41.27).

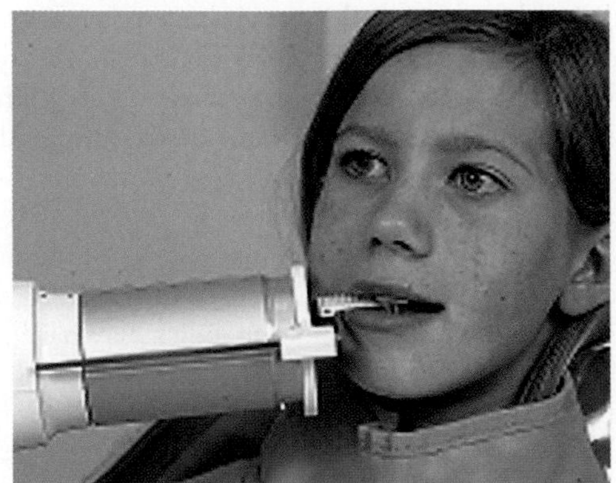

**FIG. 41.27** Extension-cone paralleling (XCP) instruments can be used for the pediatric patient. Exposure time is reduced because of the size of the patient. Follow the recommendations of the manufacturer.

### Guidelines for Dental Radiography of Pediatric Patients

- *Show and tell.* Most children are curious. The "show and tell" approach best prepares the child for the x-ray procedure.
- *Be self-assured.* Most children will respond well to the authority of a self-assured and capable operator. Be patient with the child.
- *Reassure the child.* Most children are afraid of the unknown. A frightened child is not a cooperative patient, so you must reassure the child that everything will be safe.
- *Demonstrate actions.* Show children exactly what you want them to do. For example, if you want them to open wide or move their tongue, demonstrate this action first, and then ask them to do the same thing.
- *Request assistance.* If the child cannot sit still or hold the image receptor in the mouth, you can ask the accompanying adult to help. The adult can hold the image receptor or the child during the x-ray exposure. Be sure that the adult and the child are wearing lead aprons and thyroid collars.
- *Postpone imaging (if indicated).* If a child is particularly frightened or uncooperative and the procedure is not an emergency, it is often better to postpone the x-rays rather than force the child to undergo the procedure. It may be better to try again on the second or third visit to the office, rather than instilling fear of the dental office in the child.

As described in Chapter 39, size #0 film or a small sensor is recommended for use in the pediatric patient with a primary dentition because of the small size of the mouth. In the child with mixed dentition, size #1 or #2 film or sensor may be used.

Always remember that management of children requires you to be confident, patient, and understanding.

## Endodontic Patient

It often is difficult to obtain accurate images during *endodontic* ("root canal") treatment because of the rubber dam clamp, endodontic instruments, or filling material extending from the tooth. The EndoRay image receptor holder (Dentsply Rinn) can be used to aid in positioning the image receptor during this portion of the root canal procedure (Fig. 41.28). This holder fits around a rubber dam clamp and allows space for endodontic instruments and filling materials to protrude from the tooth.

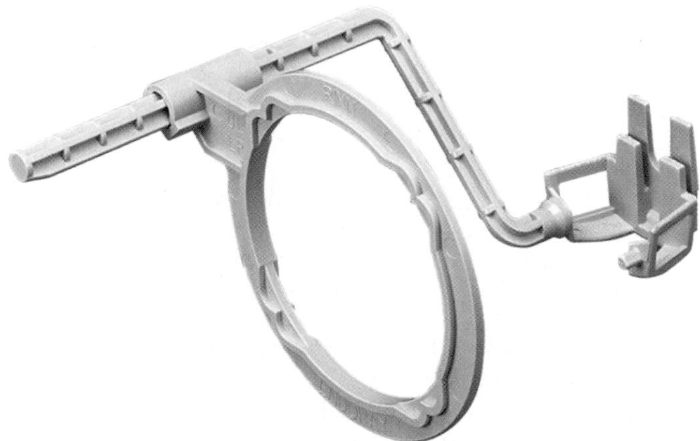

**FIG. 41.28** The EndoRay II film holder is designed for use during endodontic procedures when x-rays must be taken while instruments are in the canal. *(Courtesy Dentsply Rinn, Elgin, IL.)*

A diagnostic-quality endodontic image must have the following qualities:

- The tooth is centered on the image.
- At least 5 mm of bone is visible beyond the apex of the tooth.
- The image is as anatomically accurate as possible.

The preoperative diagnostic image and the postoperative image should be taken with the standard paralleling technique and with the use of an image receptor–holding device. The bisecting technique is *not* recommended for preoperative diagnostic images because of the inherent dimensional distortion.

## Gagging Patient

On occasion, you will have a patient with a *hypersensitive gag reflex.* To help prevent the gag reflex, you must convey a confident attitude. If the patient senses nervousness, a *psychogenic stimulus* may result and cause the gag reflex.

In addition, be patient, tolerant, and understanding. Explain the procedure, and then compliment the patient as each exposure is completed. As the patient becomes more confident with the procedure, the patient is less likely to gag.

## Guidelines to Reduce Gag Reflex in Dental Patients

- *Never* ask a patient about the gag reflex. The power of suggestion can trigger it.
- *Reassure the patient.* If the patient begins to gag, remove the image receptor quickly. Reassure the patient that such a response is not unusual. Patients may feel embarrassed. Remain calm and in control.
- *Suggest breathing techniques.* Instruct the patient to "breathe deeply" through the nose during image receptor placement and exposure. For the gag reflex to take place, respiration must cease; therefore, if the patient is breathing, the gag reflex cannot occur.
- *Distract the patient.* You can instruct the patient to do one of the following during image receptor placement and exposure: (a) Bite as hard as possible on the holder, or (b) raise a leg or arm in the air. These actions help to divert the patient's attention and lessen the likelihood that the gag reflex will be elicited.
- *Reduce tactile stimuli.* You can try one of the following techniques before placing and making the exposure: (a) Give the patient a cup of ice water to drink, or (b) place a small amount of ordinary table salt on the tip of the tongue. These techniques help to "confuse" the sensory nerve endings and lessen the likelihood that the gag reflex will be stimulated.
- *Consider use of topical anesthetic.* In the patient with a severe gag reflex, a topical anesthetic may be used. A spray or gel may be used to numb the areas that elicit the gag reflex. You should instruct the patient to exhale while the anesthetic is sprayed on the soft palate and posterior tongue.

*Note:* Caution must be used to ensure that the patient does not inhale the spray, because inflammation of the lungs may occur.

- The topical anesthetic spray takes effect after 1 minute and lasts for approximately 20 minutes.

*Note:* Topical anesthetic sprays should *not* be used in patients who are allergic to benzocaine. Not all states allow dental assistants to place topical anesthetic. Check the regulations in your state, province, or territory before you apply topical anesthetics.

### Exposure Sequencing

As was discussed earlier, exposure sequencing plays an important role in preventing the gag reflex. Anterior images are easier for the patient to tolerate and are less likely to elicit the gag reflex. With posterior image receptor placements, you should always expose the premolar film before the molar view.

The maxillary molar image receptor placement is the one most likely to cause the gag reflex. For the patient with a hypersensitive gag reflex, you should expose the maxillary molars last.

### Image Receptor Placement

**AVOID THE PALATE.** When you position image receptors in the maxillary posterior, do not slide them along the palate. This elicits the gag reflex. Instead, position the image receptor lingual to the teeth, and then firmly bring it into contact with the palatal tissues in a single motion.

**DEMONSTRATE IMAGE RECEPTOR PLACEMENT.** In the areas that are most likely to elicit the gag reflex, rub a finger along the tissues near the intended area of image receptor placement while telling the patient, "This is where the image receptor will be positioned." Then quickly position the image receptor. This technique demonstrates where the image receptor will be placed and desensitizes the tissues in the area.

### Extreme Cases

At times, you may encounter a patient with an *uncontrollable* gag reflex. In such patients, intraoral images are impossible to obtain, and you must use extraoral images such as panoramic or lateral jaw views.

RECALL

**17** For partially edentulous patients, how can you modify the technique for using a bite block?
**18** When exposing images on a pediatric patient, how can you best describe the tubehead for the patient?
**19** What changes must be made in exposure factors when one is exposing dental images on a pediatric patient?
**20** What size of film is recommended for a pediatric patient with all primary dentition?
**21** Why is the exposure sequence especially important when one is taking x-rays on a patient with a severe gag reflex?

# Dental Imaging Technique Errors

The purpose of dental images is to benefit the patient. However, only images of **diagnostic quality** benefit the patient. Diagnostic-quality images are those that have been properly *placed, exposed,* and *processed;* errors in any of these three areas may result in nondiagnostic images. Nondiagnostic images must be retaken, which results in additional exposure of the patient to ionizing radiation.

You must be able to recognize image errors, identify their causes, and know what steps are necessary to prevent them from happening again (Fig. 41.29).

# Mounting Dental Radiographs

## Recognizing Anatomic Landmarks

To mount dental radiographs correctly, the dental assistant must be able to recognize the normal anatomic landmarks on intraoral radiographs (Fig. 41.30).

Processed radiographs are arranged in anatomic order in holders, called *mounts,* to make it easier for the dentist to view the films. The mount must always be labeled with the patient's name and the date that the radiographs were exposed. The dentist's name and address should also be on the mount. When using a digital system, the computer program automatically "mounts" the images on the computer monitor.

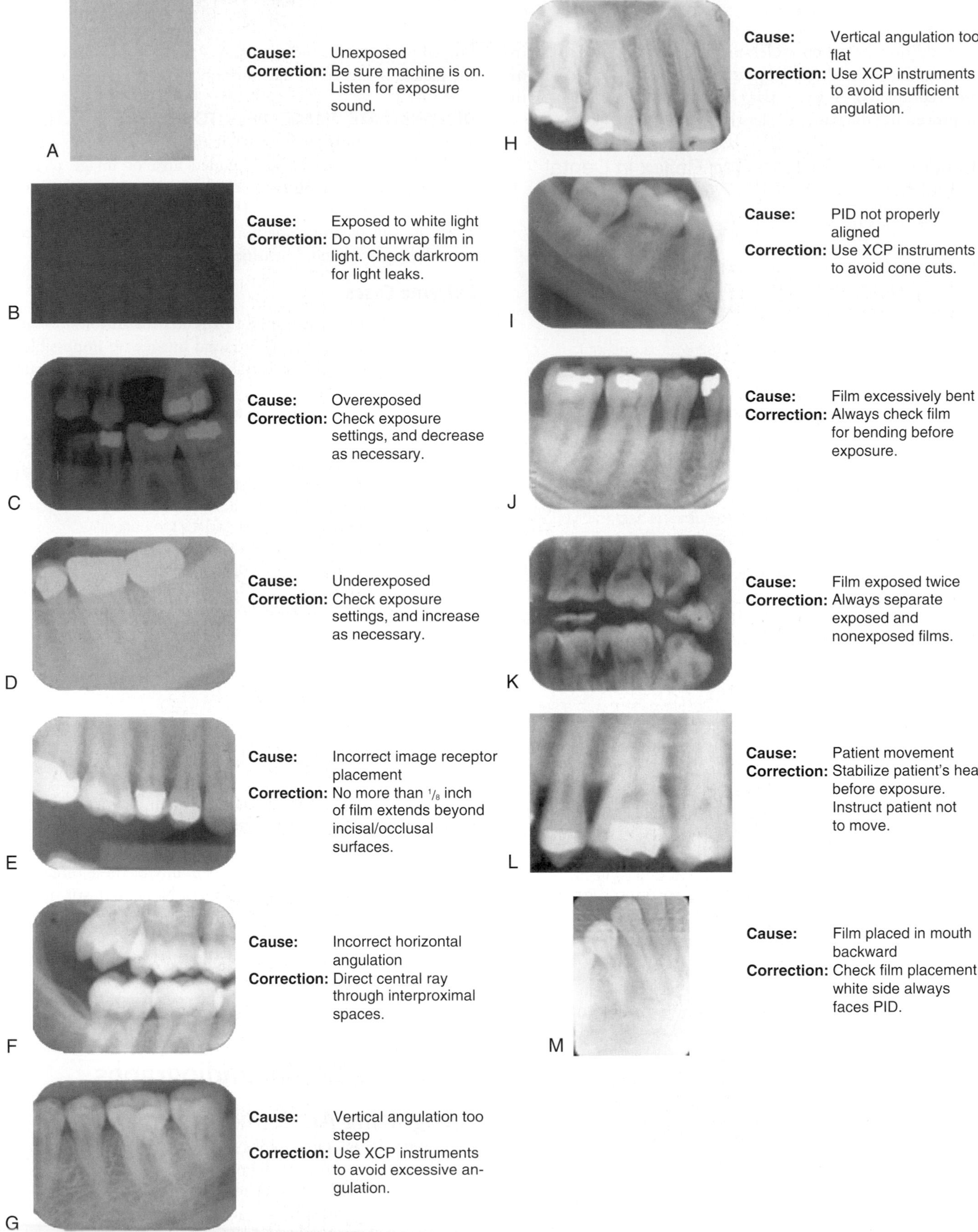


**FIG. 41.29** Radiographic exposure errors. A, Clear. B, Black. C, Dark. D, Light. E, No apices. F, Overlapped contacts. G, Foreshortened image. H, Elongated image. I, Cone cut. J, Distorted image with dark lines on corners. K, Double image. L, Blurred image. M, Light image with herringbone pattern. *XCP,* Extension-cone paralleling; *PID,* position indicator device. *(Radiographs from Iannucci J, Jansen Howerton L: Dental radiography: principles and techniques, ed 5, St Louis, 2017, Elsevier.)*

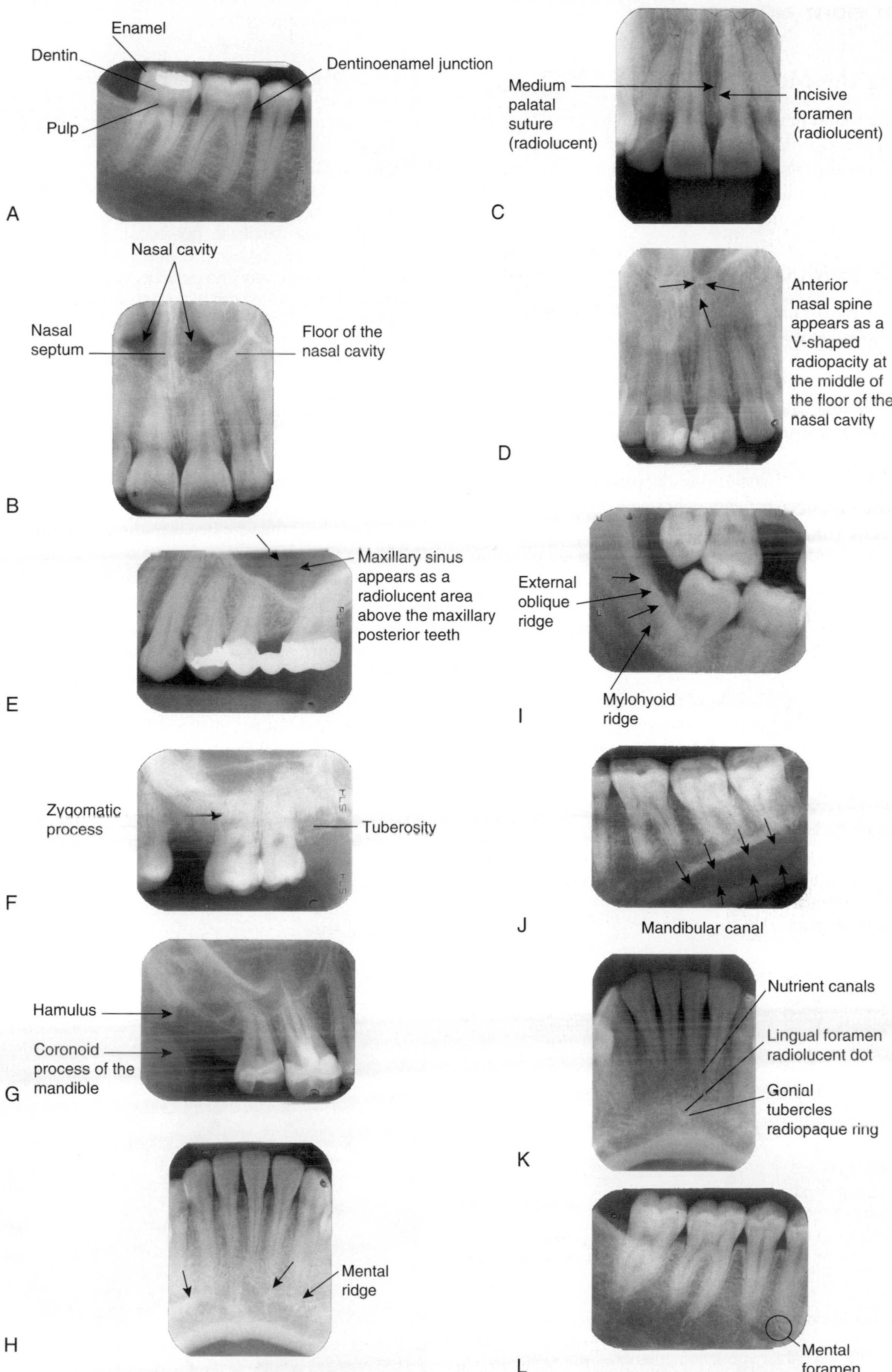


**FIG. 41.30** Radiographic landmarks of normal anatomy. A, Structures of the tooth. B through D, Maxillary structures. Radiographic landmarks of normal anatomy. E through G, Maxillary structures. H through L, Mandibular structures.

## Selecting the Mount

Mounts are available in many sizes, with different numbers and sizes of *windows* (openings) to accommodate the number and sizes of views in the patient's radiographic survey. The mounts most often used for radiographic surveys are available in black, gray, and clear plastic.

## Methods of Mounting

Two methods can be used when mounting radiographs. Both methods rely on identification of the raised *(embossed)* dot on the film.

In the first method, the *labial mounting method,* films are placed in the mount with the raised dots facing up *(convex).* The American Dental Association (ADA) recommends this method of mounting radiographs. Radiographs are viewed as if the viewer is looking directly at the patient; thus the patient's left side is on the viewer's right, and the patient's right side is on the viewer's left (Fig. 41.31). See Procedure 41.7: Mounting Dental Radiographs.

In the second mounting method, radiographs are placed in the mount with the raised dots facing down *(concave).* With this method, radiographs are viewed as if the viewer is inside the patient's mouth and looking out; that is, the patient's left side is on the viewer's left, and the patient's right side is on the viewer's right.

*Note:* It is critical to know how the dentist prefers to have radiographs mounted. Mistakes in mounting radiographs have resulted in errors in treatment of the dental patient.

### Guidelines for Mounting Radiographs

- Handle films only by the edges.
- Learn the normal anatomy of the maxilla and the mandible.
- Label and date the film mount *before* mounting the films. Include the patient's full name, the date of exposure, and the dentist's name.
- Mount films immediately after processing.
- Use clean, dry hands.
- Use the order of the teeth to distinguish the right side from the left.
- Use a definite order for mounting films. For example, start with maxillary anterior periapical films, proceed to mandibular anterior periapical and bitewing views, and finish with maxillary and mandibular posterior periapical views.
- Mount bitewing radiographs with the curve of Spee (occlusal plane between the maxillary and mandibular teeth) directed *upward* toward the distal. The result resembles a smile.

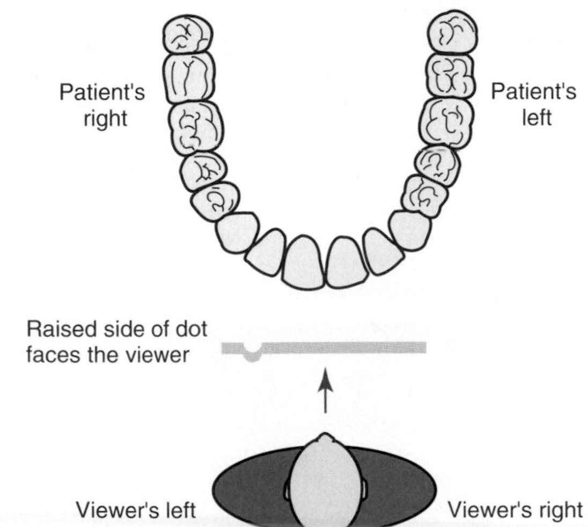


**FIG. 41.31** With the labial mounting method, radiographs are viewed as if the dental radiographer were looking directly at the patient. *(From Iannucci J, Jansen Howerton L: Dental radiography: principles and techniques, ed 5, St Louis, 2017, Elsevier.)*

## Portable Imaging

There are a variety of situations that make it difficult or impossible for a patient to come to the dental office. The U.S. Food and Drug Administration has approved a portable battery-powered machine that can be taken directly to the patient (Fig. 41.32).

With a portable handheld x-ray generator and digital imaging, it is possible to take the x-ray machine to a patient in a nursing home, hospital, or in remote areas.

For operator safety it has internal shielding materials to reduce leakage exposure and a shield on the aiming cylinder to minimize backscatter from the patient. These units are approved for use in many states, but not in all.

RECALL

22 What is the definition of a diagnostic-quality image?
23 When mounting radiographs, what is the ADA's recommendation concerning placement of the raised dot?
24 Why is it important for the dental assistant to recognize anatomic landmarks?
25 Why is it important to avoid retakes?

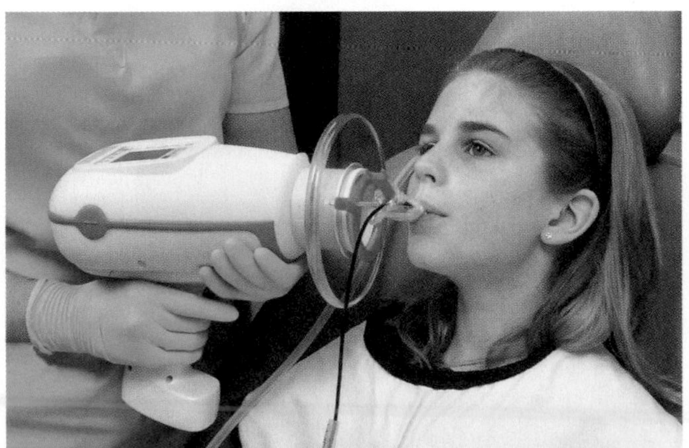

**FIG. 41.32** Handheld x-ray machine useful for patients in nontraditional dental settings. *(Courtesy Aribex, Inc., Orem, UT.)*

**Legal and Ethical Implications** Public awareness of the harmful effects of x-radiation has caused dental patients to question the value and necessity of having dental x-rays. The dental assistant should be prepared to explain to the patient the amount of risk that is associated with dental imaging. A patient should never be exposed to x-rays unless he or she understands the need for the dental images and has given consent.

To avoid retakes and unnecessary radiation to the patient, the dental assistant must be competent in performing various imaging techniques. ■

**Eye to the Future** The focus of dental imaging in the future will be on the continued development of methods and machines to further reduce the amount of radiation to the patient and enhance the quality of the images. Digital imaging and conventional F-speed film are excellent steps in this direction.

Dental professionals must recognize the need for lifelong learning to remain current with technological advances in dental imaging. ■

## Critical Thinking

1. Mr. Li Trung is a 65-year-old patient in your office who needs a full-mouth survey. You notice that Mr. Trung has a very small mouth and a very shallow palate. What technique would you use? Why?
2. Mrs. Jackson has brought her 14-year-old son Jamal into your office for an examination. During the examination, the dentist explains to Mrs. Jackson that Jamal's maxillary canine teeth have not erupted into the mouth and may be impacted in the palate. What type of intraoral image will the dentist most likely request? Why?
3. You are using a digital x-ray system, and as the image of the left premolar bitewing appears on the monitor, you notice that the premolars are overlapped. You realize you must do an immediate retake to obtain a diagnostic image. What caused this error, and what must you do to correct it on the retake? ■

PROCEDURE 41.1 

# Preparing the Patient for Dental Imaging

### GOAL

To follow the basic steps in preparing a patient for intraoral x-ray procedures.

### EQUIPMENT AND SUPPLIES

- ✓ Lead apron with thyroid collar
- ✓ Plastic container for prosthetic devices
- ✓ Tissue to remove lipstick

### PROCEDURAL STEPS

1 Update the medical history. Explain the x-ray procedure to the patient. Ask whether the patient has any questions.

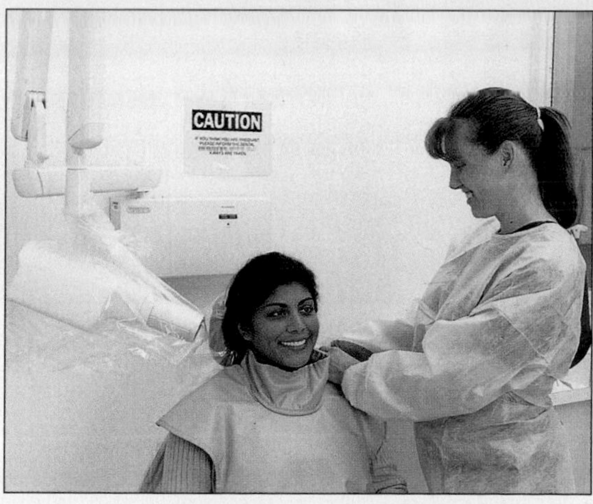


2 Ask the patient to remove all objects from the mouth, including dentures, retainers, chewing gum, and any pierced tongue or pierced lip objects. Place any objects into a plastic container.

**PURPOSE** Objects in the mouth can cause artifacts on the radiograph.

3 Make sure the exposure settings on the x-ray machine are correct.

4 Adjust the chair so that the patient is positioned upright. The level of the chair must be adjusted to a comfortable working height for the operator.

5 Adjust the headrest to support and position the patient's head. The patient's head must be positioned so that the upper arch is parallel to the floor and the midsagittal (midline) plane is perpendicular to the floor.

6 Place and secure the lead apron with the thyroid collar on the patient.

PROCEDURE 41.2 

# Assembling the Extension-Cone Paralleling (XCP) Instruments

## GOAL

To assemble the Rinn XCP instruments (Dentsply Rinn, Elgin, IL) for all areas of the mouth in preparation for radiographic surveys.

## EQUIPMENT AND SUPPLIES

- Sterilized Rinn XCP instruments (film or brand-specific sensor holders)

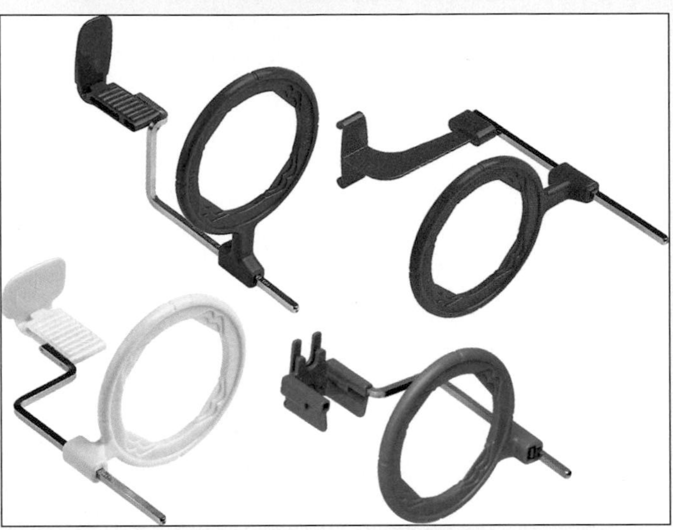

Extension-cone paralleling (XCP) instruments for film. *(Courtesy Dentsply Rinn, Elgin, IL.)*

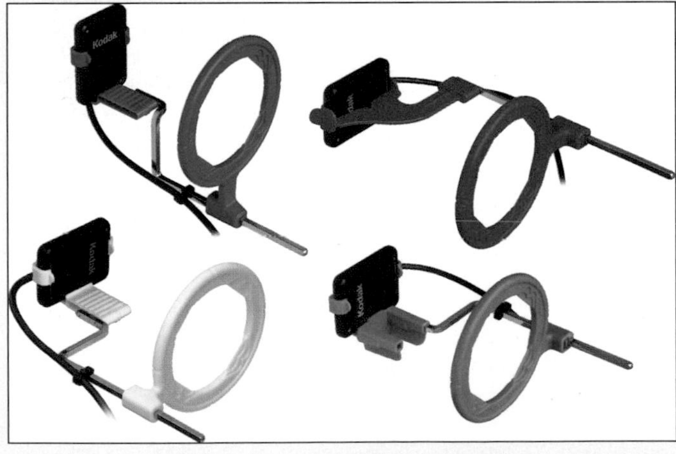

Extension-cone paralleling (XCP-DS) instruments for digital sensors. *(Courtesy Dentsply Rinn, Elgin, IL.)*

**NOTE** Depending on the manufacturer, digital sensors vary in size and thickness. Some brands are available in two or three sizes, and some are available in only one size. Sensor holders are available for each brand of digital system. Phosphor plates can be used with film-type holders.

## PROCEDURAL STEPS

### Anterior Assembly

1 Lay out the blue parts for the anterior XCP instrument.

**PURPOSE** Blue is the universal color for anterior film sensor–holding instruments.

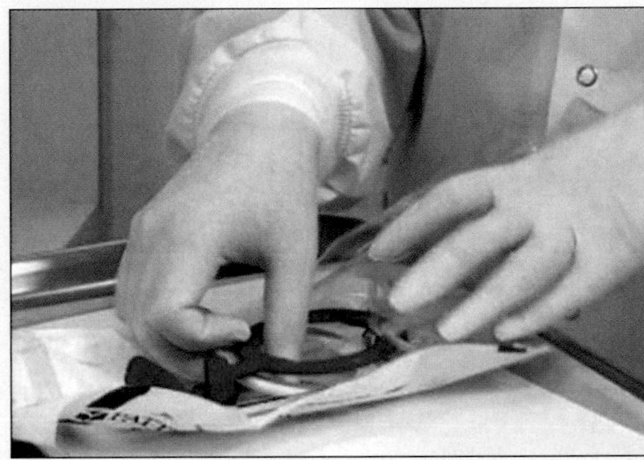

2 Assemble the anterior XCP instrument by inserting the two prongs of the blue anterior indicator arm into the openings in the blue anterior bite-block.

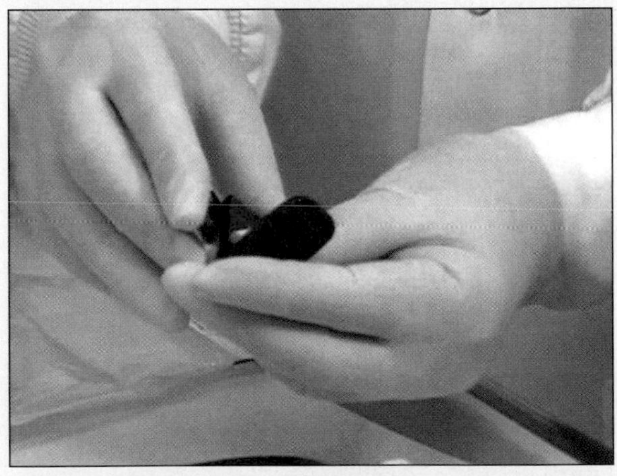

3 Insert the anterior indicator arm into the opening on the blue anterior aiming ring.

## PROCEDURE 41.2 Assembling the Extension-Cone Paralleling (XCP) Instruments–cont'd

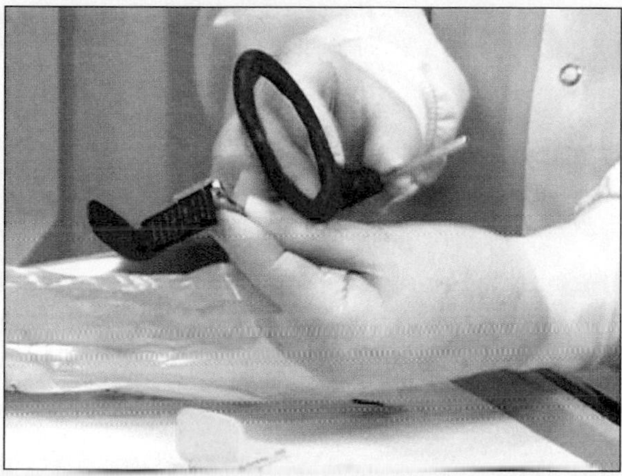

4 For films, flex the plastic backing of the blue bite-block to open the film slot for easy insertion of the anterior film packet. For sensors, slide the sensor into position.

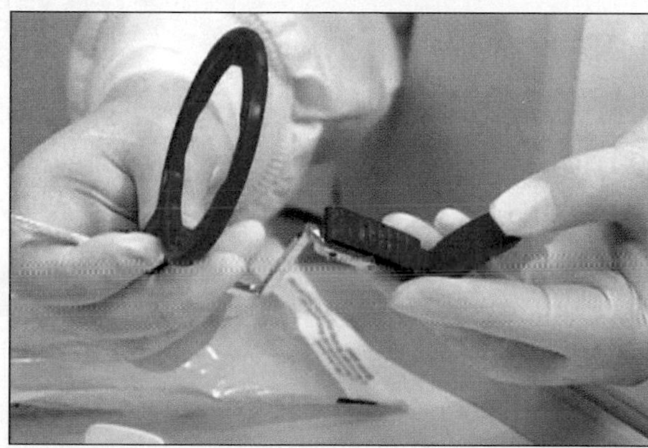

5 The blue anterior XCP instrument is correctly assembled when the film sensor is seen centered in the middle of the aiming ring.

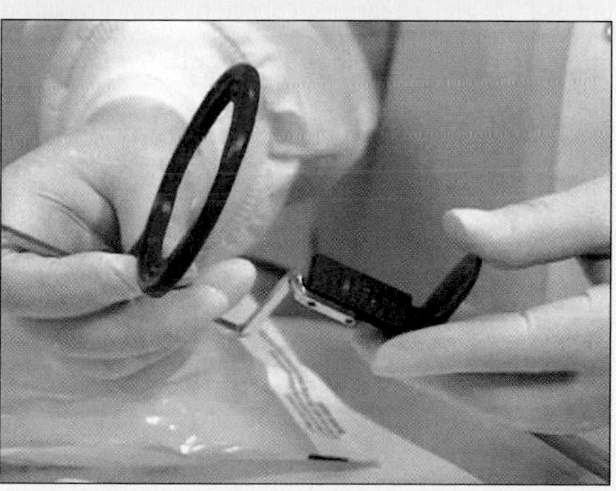

### Posterior Assembly

1 Lay out the yellow parts for the posterior XCP instrument.
**PURPOSE** Yellow is the universal color for posterior film sensor–holding instruments.

2 Assemble the yellow posterior XCP instrument by inserting the two prongs of the yellow posterior indicator arm into the openings in the yellow posterior bite-block, as shown.

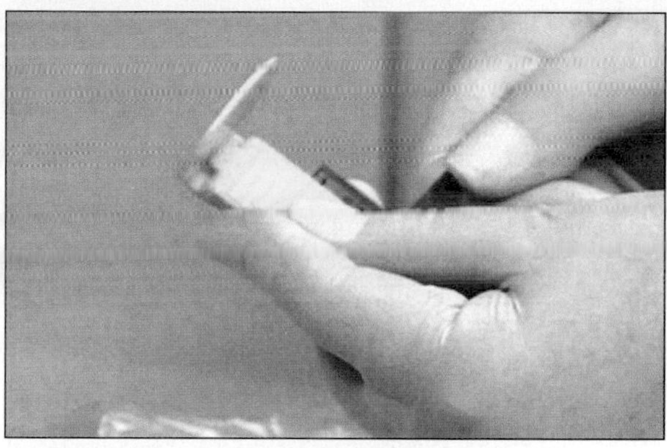

3 Insert the yellow posterior indicator arm into the opening on the yellow posterior aiming ring, as shown.

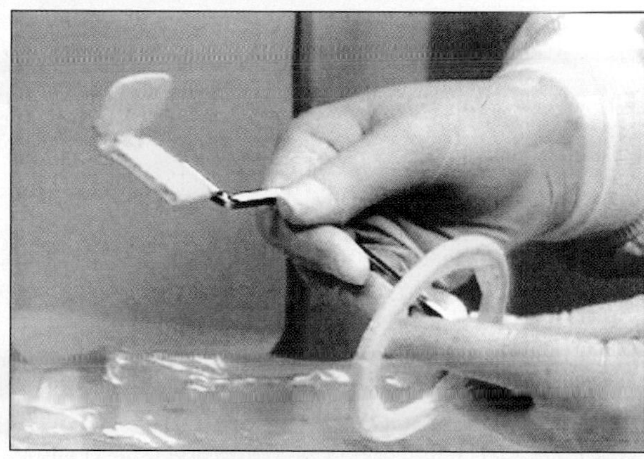

4 For film, flex the plastic backing of the yellow bite-block to open the film slot for easy insertion of the posterior film packet. For sensors, slide the sensor into position on the holder.

(Continued)

## PROCEDURE 41.2 Assembling the Extension-Cone Paralleling (XCP) Instruments–cont'd

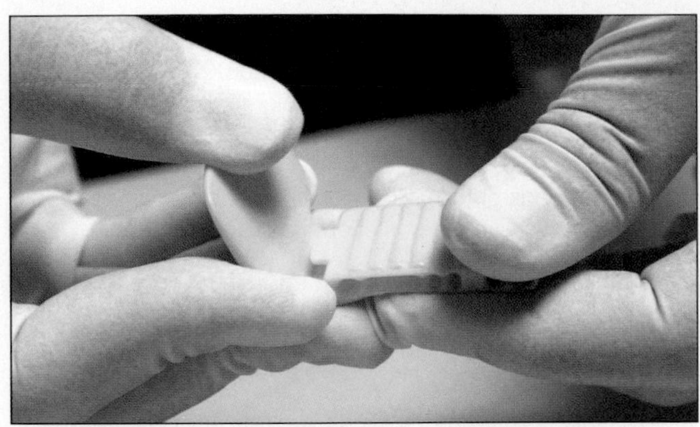

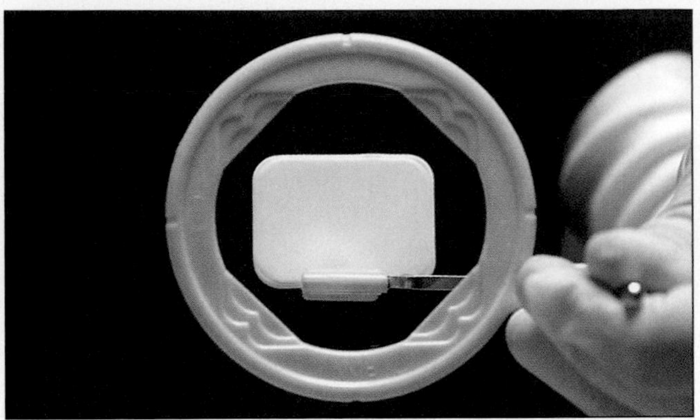

5 The posterior XCP instrument is correctly assembled when the film sensor is seen centered in the middle of the aiming ring.

## PROCEDURE 41.3 

# Producing Full-Mouth Radiographic Survey Using Paralleling Technique

### GOAL

To follow the proper steps to produce a full-mouth survey using the paralleling technique with conventional dental film or digital technology.

### EQUIPMENT AND SUPPLIES

- ✓ Appropriate number and size of image receptors (radiographic films, sensors, or phosphor storage plates [PSPs] in barrier envelopes).
- ✓ Appropriate infection control materials (paper cup, barriers, paper towel, and impervious surface cover)
- ✓ Lead apron and thyroid collar
- ✓ Sterile packaged extension-cone paralleling (XCP) instruments
- ✓ Cotton rolls
- ✓ Patient chart

### PROCEDURAL STEPS

#### Preparation Before Seating Patient

1 Prepare the operatory with all infection control barriers.

**PURPOSE** Any object that is touched and was not covered with a barrier must be disinfected after the patient is dismissed.

2 Determine the number and type of images to be exposed through a review of the patient's chart, directions from the dentist, or both.

3 For films or PSPs, label a paper cup with the patient's name and the date. Place it outside the room where the x-ray machine will be used.

**PURPOSE** This is the transfer cup for storing and moving exposed films or PSPs.

4 Turn on the x-ray machine and check the basic settings (kilovoltage, milliamperage, exposure time).

5 Wash and dry your hands.

6 Dispense the desired number of films or PSPs, and store them outside the room where the x-ray machine is being used.

**PURPOSE** To prevent fogging caused by scatter radiation.

#### Additional Preparation Requirements for Digital Technologies

1 Turn on the computer and the monitor.

2 Place barriers on the keyboard, mouse, sensors, and cables.

3 Log on to link the patient's chart.

**NOTE** This step will vary depending on the software program being used.

4 Choose the layout you will use for the images.

**PURPOSE** The layout will appear on the screen. This is the digital equivalent of mounting radiographs.

## PROCEDURE 41.3 Producing Full-Mouth Radiographic Survey Using Paralleling Technique–cont'd

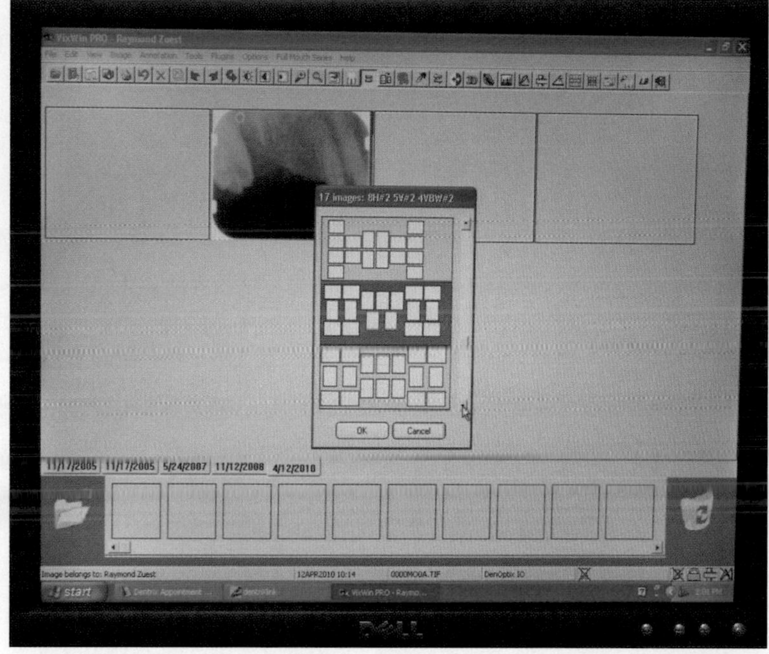

### Positioning Patient

1 Seat the patient comfortably in the dental chair, with the back in an upright position and the head supported.

2 Ask the patient to remove eyeglasses and bulky earrings.

**PURPOSE** These objects may cause radiopaque images to be superimposed over the dental images.

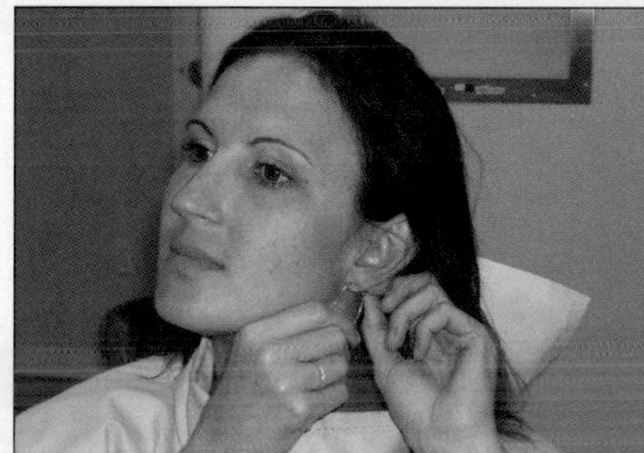

3 Ask the patient to remove prosthotic appliances or objects from the mouth.

**NOTE** Always wear gloves when handling a prosthetic appliance.

4 Position the patient so that the occlusal plane of the jaw being x-rayed is parallel to the floor when the mouth is open.

5 Drape the patient with a lead apron and a thyroid collar.

6 Wash and dry hands, and put on clean examination gloves.

7 Open the package, and assemble the sterile film sensor–holding instruments.

**PURPOSE** Allowing the patient to observe you washing your hands, putting on clean gloves, and opening the sterile package of instruments assures the patient that appropriate infection control measures are being taken.

**NOTE** When using dental film, the white side of the film always faces the tube. When using PSPs, follow the specific manufacturer's instructions to determine which side faces the tube.

### Maxillary Canine Exposure

1 Insert the #1 image receptors vertically into the anterior biteblock.

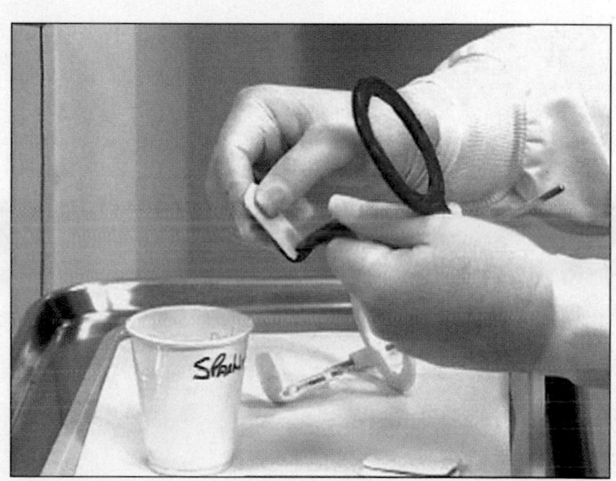

2 Position the image receptors with the canine and the first premolar centered. Position image receptors as far posterior as possible.

3 With the film-holding instrument and image receptors in place, instruct the patient to close the mouth slowly but firmly.

4 Position the localizing ring and the position indicator device (PID); then press the exposure button.

**(Continued)**

## PROCEDURE 41.3 Producing Full-Mouth Radiographic Survey Using Paralleling Technique–cont'd

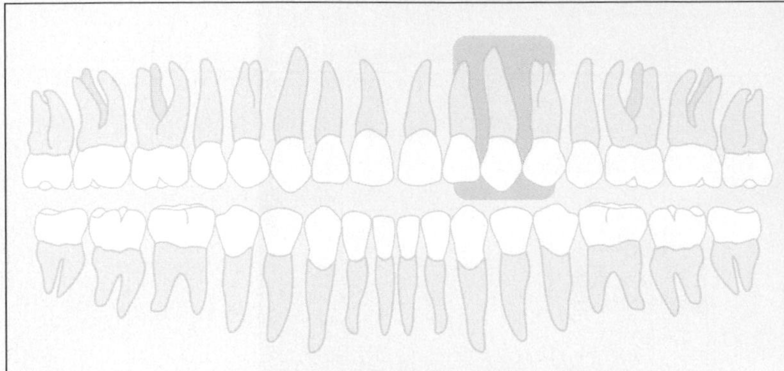

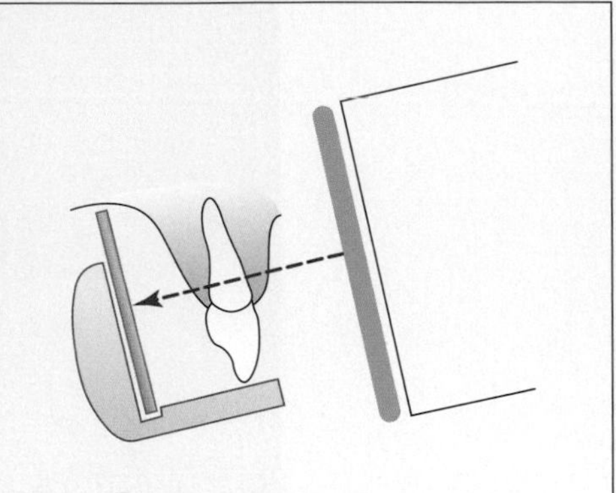

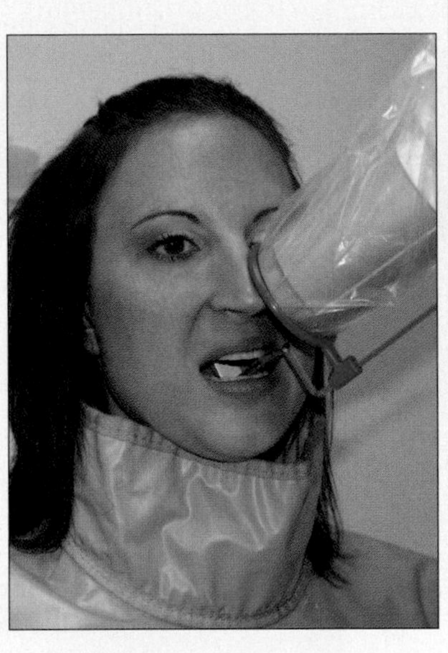

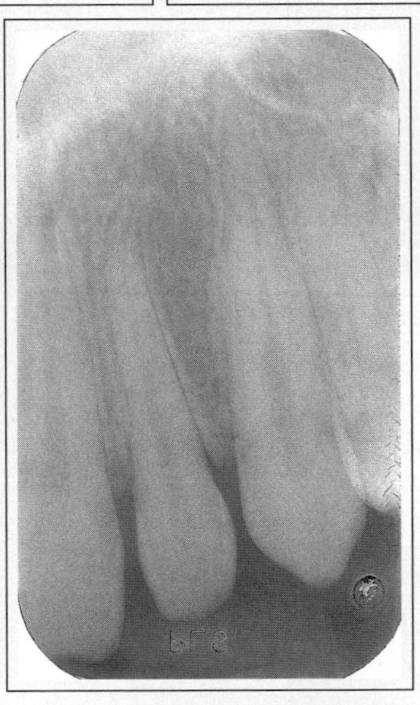

**NOTE** The image of the lingual cusp of the first premolar is usually superimposed on the distal surface of the canine because of the curvature of the maxillary arch. This contact area must be "opened" on the view of the premolar region.

### Maxillary Central/Lateral Incisor Exposure

1 Insert the #1 image receptor vertically into the anterior block.
2 Center the image receptor between the central and lateral incisors. Position the film sensor as posterior in the mouth as possible.
3 With the instrument in place, instruct the patient to close the mouth slowly but firmly.
4 Position the localizing ring and the PID; then push the exposure button.

# PROCEDURE 41.3 Producing Full-Mouth Radiographic Survey Using Paralleling Technique—cont'd

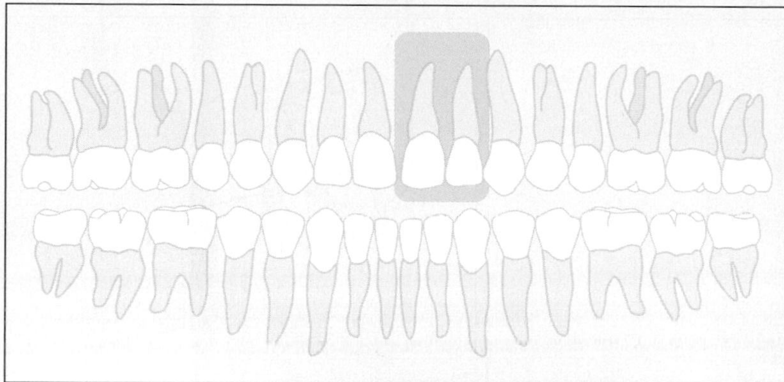

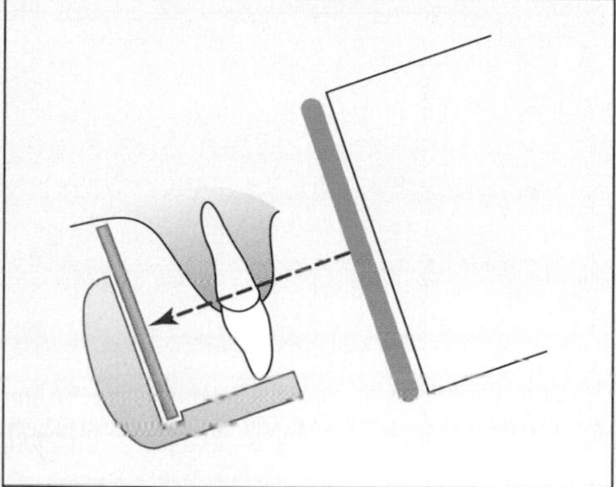

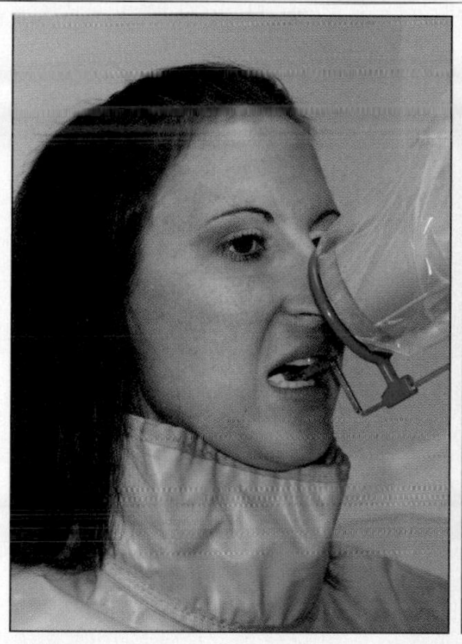

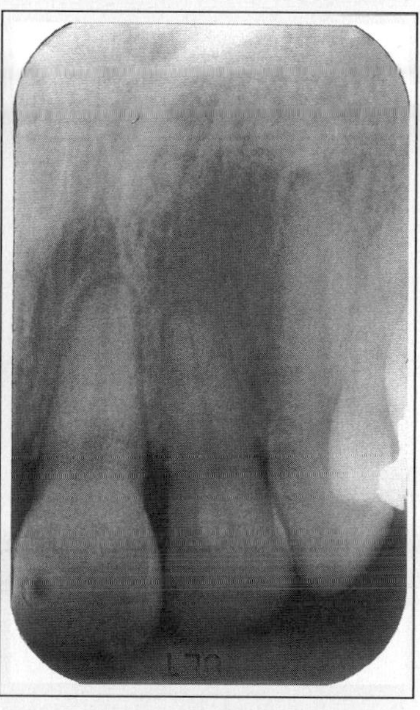

## Mandibular Canine Exposure

1 Insert the #1 image receptor vertically into the anterior bite-block.

2 Center the image receptor on the canine. Position the film sensor as far in the lingual direction as the patient's anatomy will allow.

**NOTE** A cotton roll may be placed between the maxillary teeth and the bite-block to prevent rocking of the bite-block on the canine tip and to increase patient comfort.

3 With the instrument and image receptors in place, instruct the patient to close the mouth slowly but firmly.

4 Position the localizing ring and the PID; then press the exposure button.

(Continued)

## PROCEDURE 41.3 Producing Full-Mouth Radiographic Survey Using Paralleling Technique—cont'd

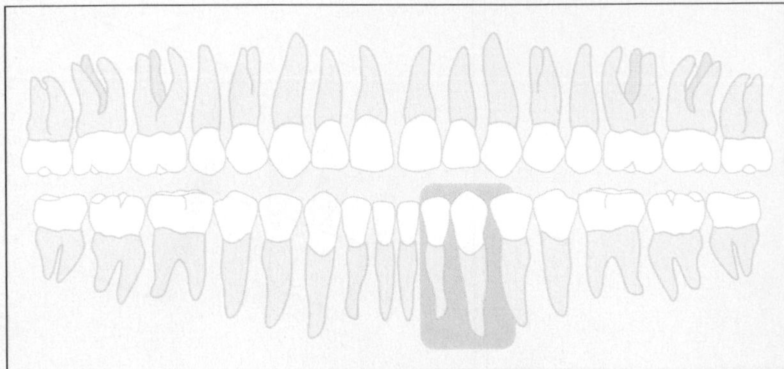

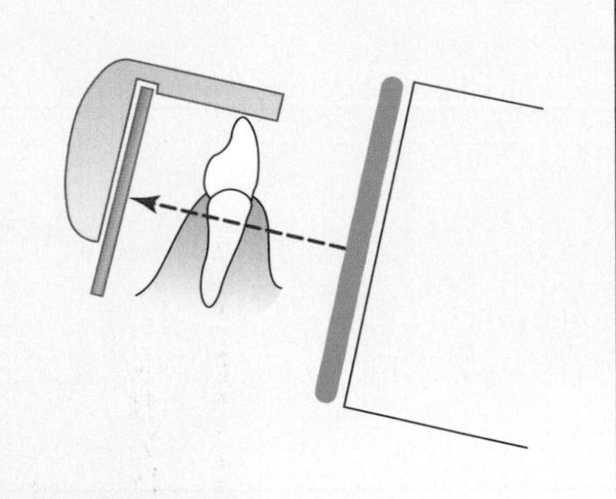

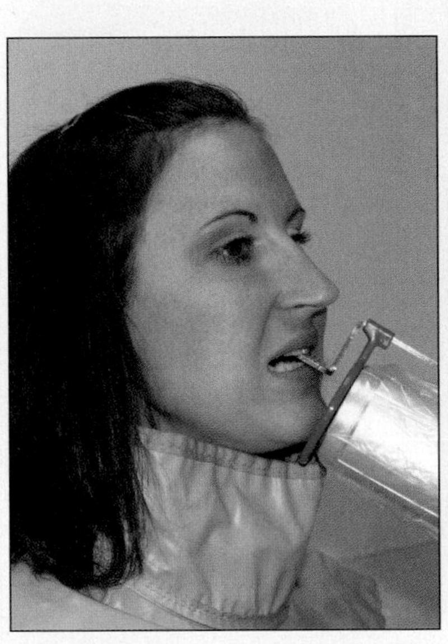

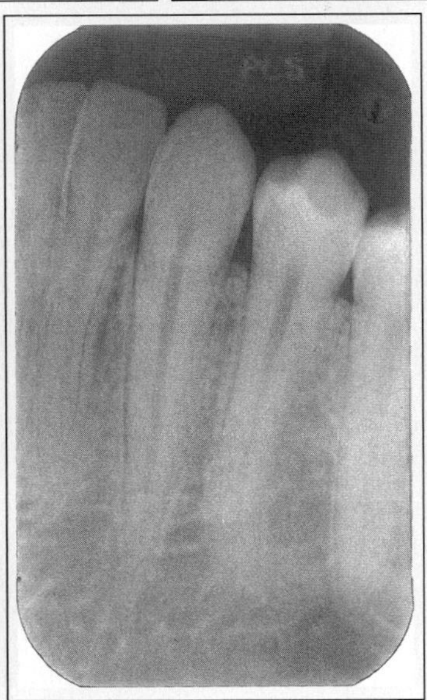

### Mandibular Incisor Exposure

1 Insert the #1 image receptor vertically into the anterior bite-block.
2 Center the image receptor between the central incisors. Position the image receptor as far in the lingual direction as the patient's anatomy will allow.
3 With the instrument and image receptor in place, instruct the patient to close the mouth slowly but firmly.
4 Slide the localizing ring down the indicator rod to the patient's skin surface.
5 Position the localizing ring and the PID; then press the exposure button.

## PROCEDURE 41.3 Producing Full-Mouth Radiographic Survey Using Paralleling Technique–cont'd

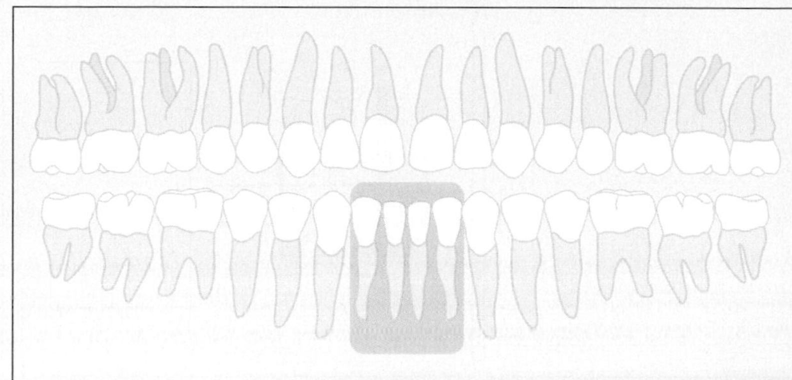

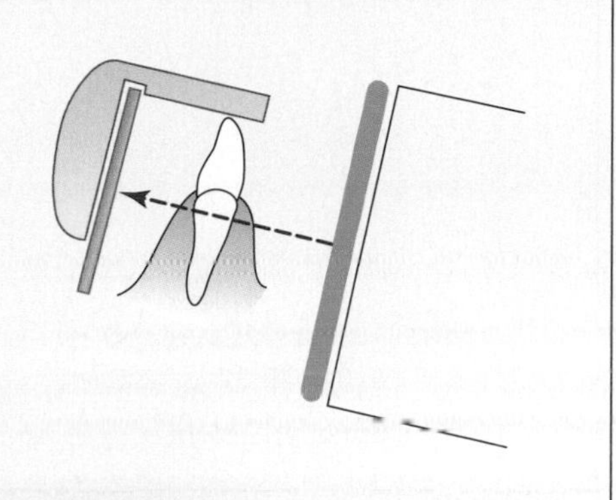

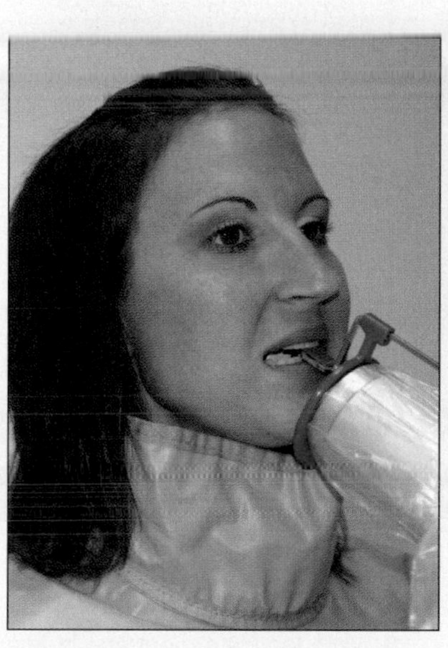

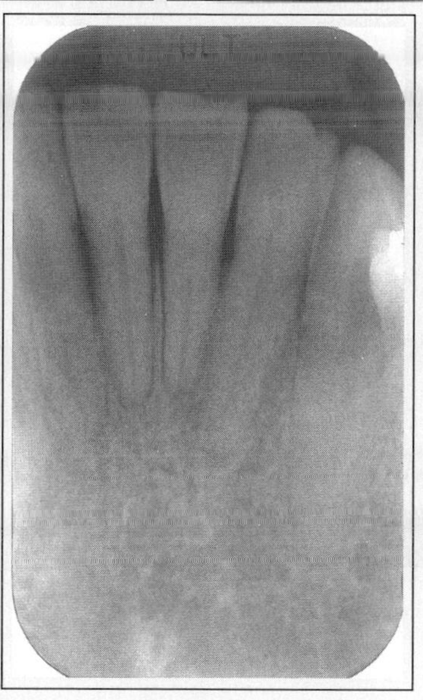

### Maxillary Premolar Exposure

1 Insert the image receptor horizontally into the posterior bite-block, pushing the image receptor all the way into the slot.
2 Center the image receptor on the second premolar. Position the film sensor in the midpalatal area.
3 With the instrument and image receptor in place, instruct the patient to close the mouth slowly but firmly.
4 Position the localizing ring and the PID; then push the exposure button.

(Continued)

## PROCEDURE 41.3 Producing Full-Mouth Radiographic Survey Using Paralleling Technique—cont'd

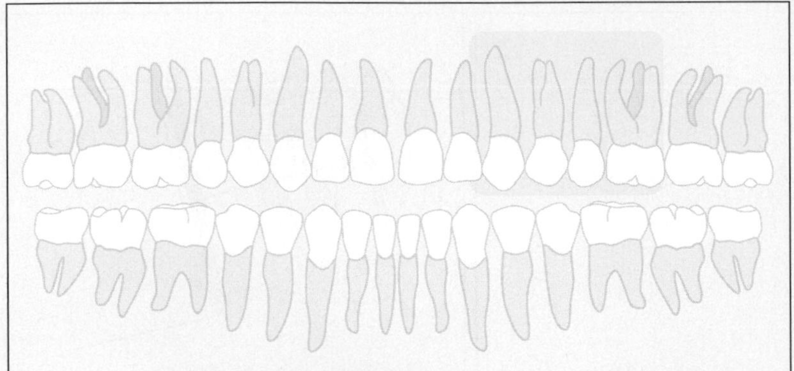

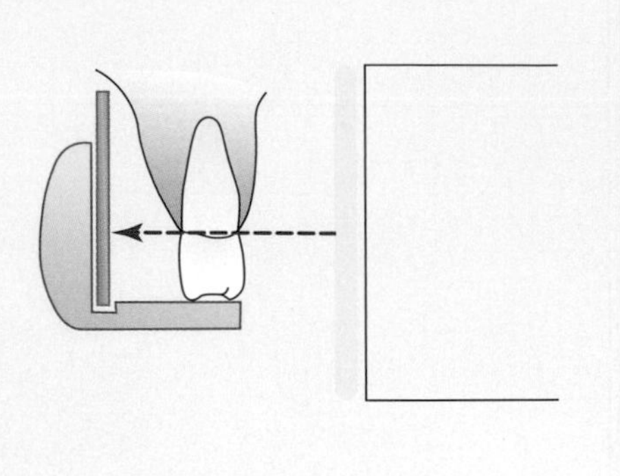

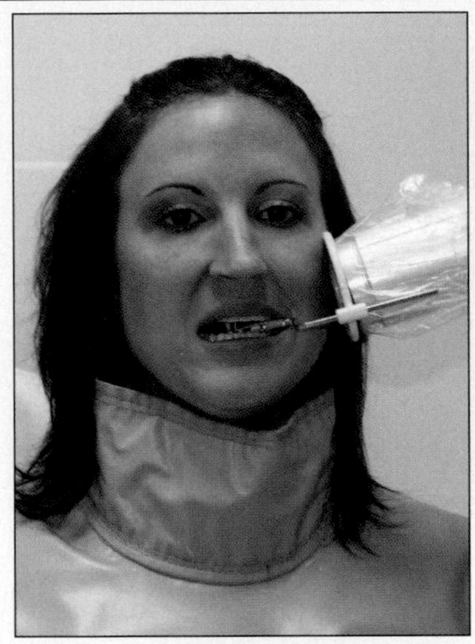

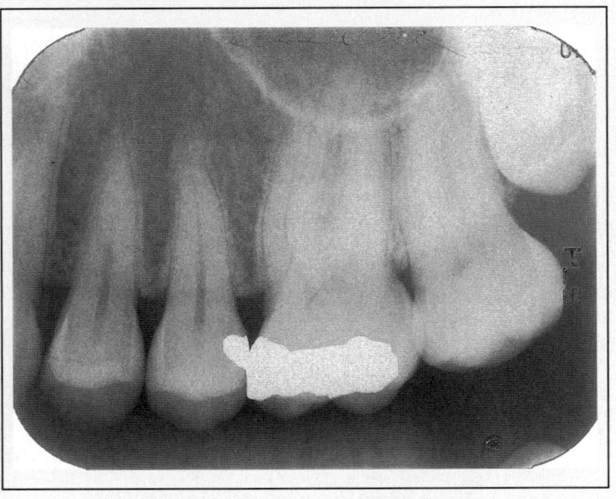

### Maxillary Molar Exposure

1. Insert the image receptor horizontally into the posterior bite-block.
2. Center the image receptor on the second molar. Position the film in the midpalatal area.
3. With the instrument and image receptor in place, instruct the patient to close the mouth slowly but firmly.
4. Position the localizing ring and the PID; then push the exposure button.

## PROCEDURE 41.3 Producing Full-Mouth Radiographic Survey Using Paralleling Technique–cont'd

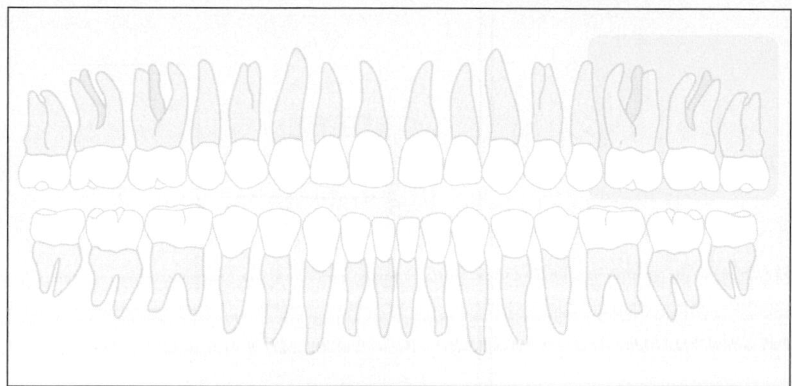

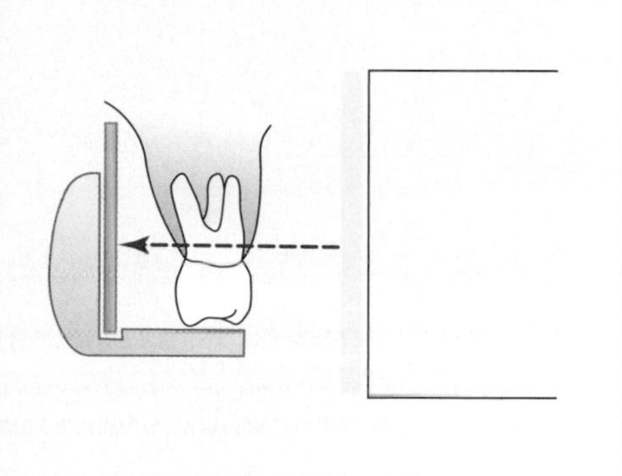

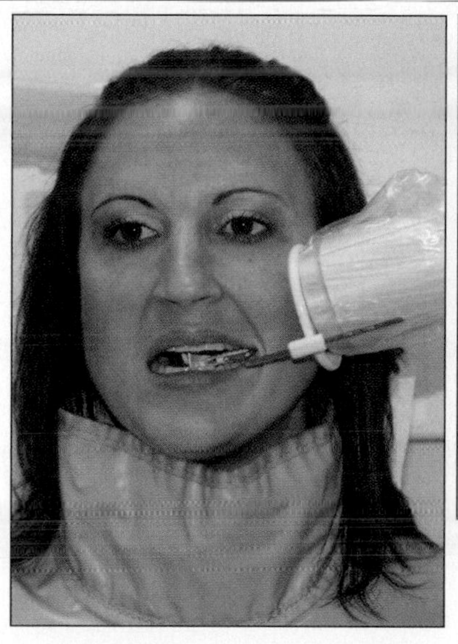

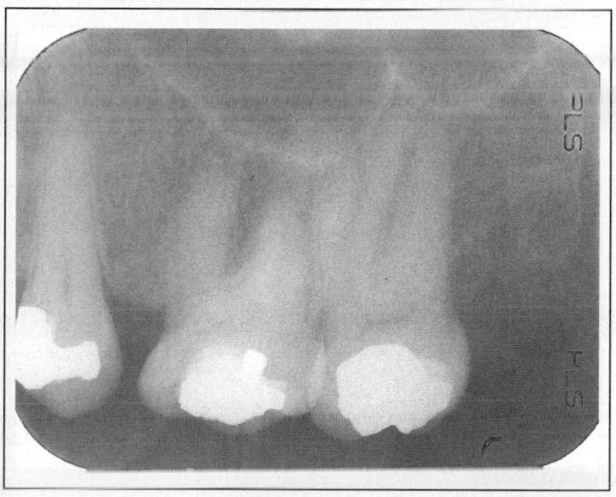

### Mandibular Premolar Exposure

1 Insert the #2 image receptor horizontally into the posterior bite-block.
2 Center the image receptor on the contact point between the second premolar and the first molar. Position the image receptor as far lingual as the patient's anatomy will allow.
3 With the instrument and image receptor in place, instruct the patient to close the mouth slowly but firmly.
4 Slide the localizing ring down the indicator rod to the patient's skin surface.
5 Position the localizing ring and the PID; then push the exposure button.

(Continued)

# PROCEDURE 41.3 Producing Full-Mouth Radiographic Survey Using Paralleling Technique—cont'd

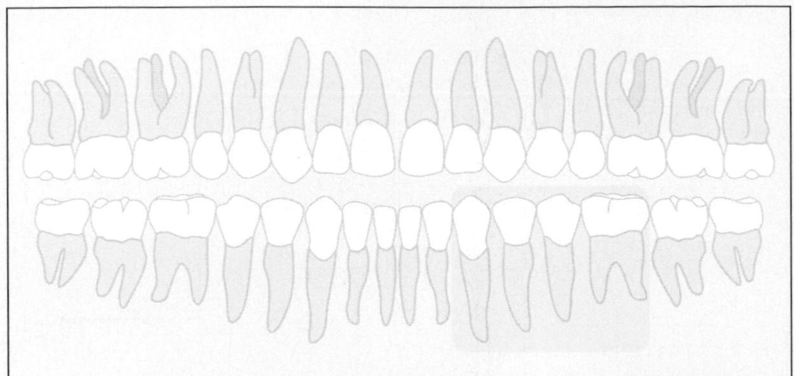

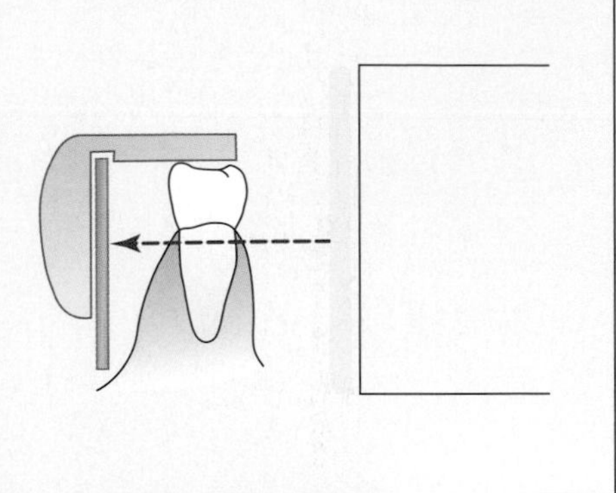

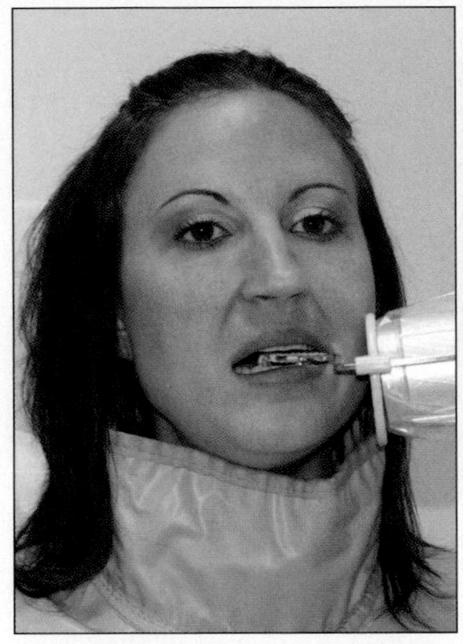

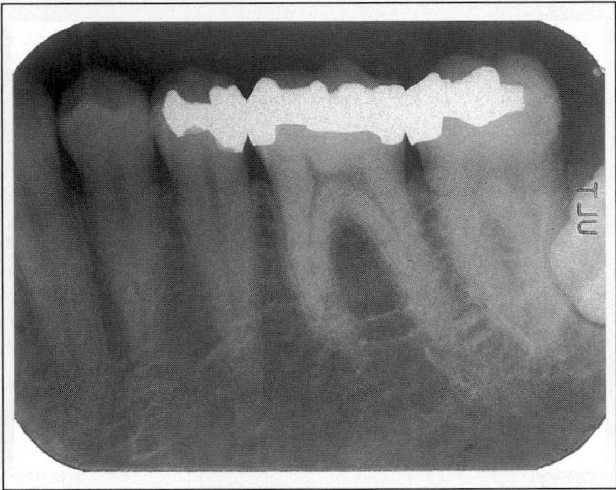

### Mandibular Molar Exposure

1 Insert the #2 image receptor horizontally into the posterior bite-block.
2 Center the image receptor on the second molar. Position the film sensor as far lingual as the tongue will allow.
   **NOTE** This position will result in placement of the image receptor closer to the teeth than for the premolar and anterior views.
3 With the instrument and image receptor in place, instruct the patient to close the mouth slowly but firmly.
4 Slide the localizing ring down the indicator rod to the patient's skin surface.
5 Position the localizing ring and the PID; then press the exposure button.

## PROCEDURE 41.3 Producing Full-Mouth Radiographic Survey Using Paralleling Technique–cont'd

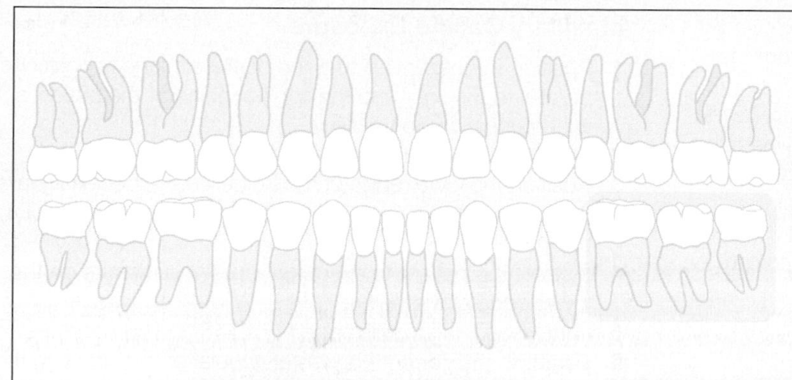

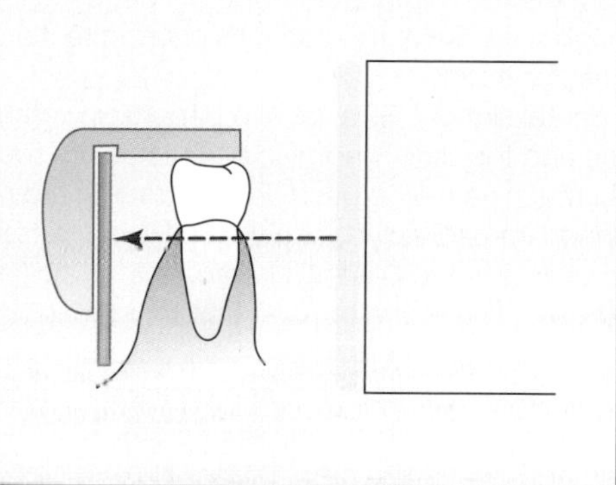

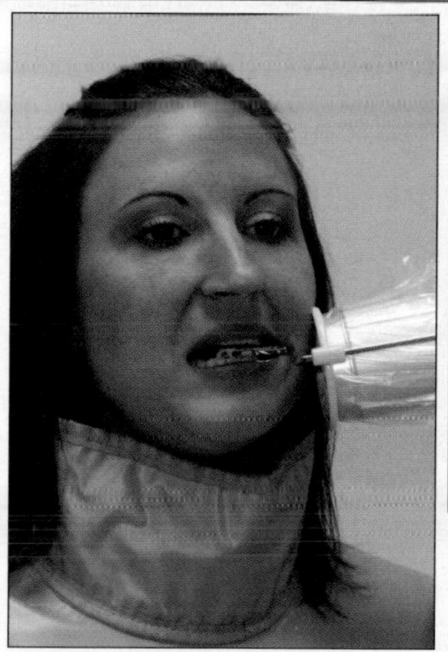

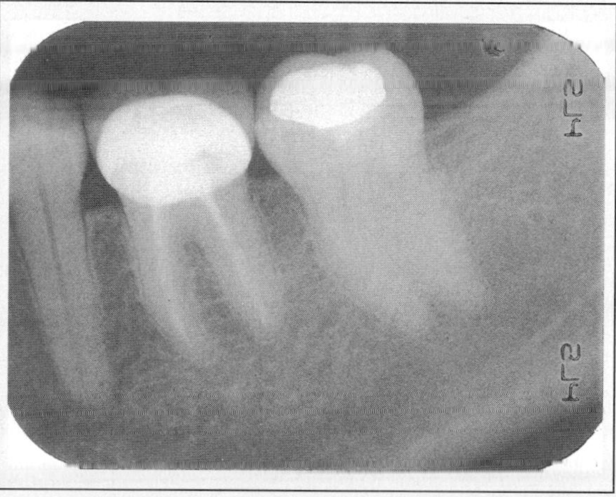

### Documentation

1 Document the procedure.

## PROCEDURE 41.4

# Producing Full-Mouth Radiographic Survey Using Bisecting Technique

### GOAL

To produce a full-mouth series of images using the bisecting technique.

### EQUIPMENT AND SUPPLIES

- Appropriate number and size of x-ray film, sensors, or phosphor storage plates (PSPs)
- Appropriate infection control materials (paper cup, barriers, paper towel, and impervious surface cover)
- Lead apron and thyroid collar
- Sterile packaged EeZee-Grip instruments (film or sensor type) or bite-block
- Cotton rolls
- Patient chart

### PROCEDURAL STEPS

#### Preparation Before Seating Patient

1 Prepare the operatory with all infection control barriers.

**PURPOSE** Any object that is touched and was not covered with a barrier must be disinfected after the patient is dismissed.

(Continued)

## PROCEDURE 41.4 Producing Full-Mouth Radiographic Survey Using Bisecting Technique—cont'd

2 Determine the number and type of images to be exposed through a review of the patient's chart, directions from the dentist, or both.
3 For dental film or PSPs, label a paper cup with the patient's name and the date, and place it outside the room where the x-ray machine will be used. For PSPs that are not going to be scanned immediately, place the PSPs in the transfer box that is labeled with the patient's name.
   **PURPOSE** This is the transfer cup for storing and moving exposed films.
4 Turn on the x-ray machine, and check the basic settings (kilovoltage, milliamperage, exposure time).
5 Wash and dry hands.
6 Dispense the desired number of films or PSPs, and store them outside the room where the x-ray machine is being used.
   **PURPOSE** This prevents fogging caused by scatter radiation.

### Maxillary Canine Exposure

1 Position the patient so that the occlusal plane is positioned parallel to the floor and the sagittal plane of the patient's face is perpendicular to the floor.
2 Center the image receptor on the canine.
3 Position the lower edge of the holder to the occlusal plane so that it extends about 1/8 inch below the incisal edge of the canine.
4 Instruct the patient to exert light but firm pressure on the lower edge of the holder.
5 Vertical angulation will range from +45 to +55 degrees.
6 Establish the correct horizontal angulation by directing the central ray between the contacts of the canine and the first premolar.
7 Center the PID over the image receptor to avoid cone cutting.
8 Press the exposure button.

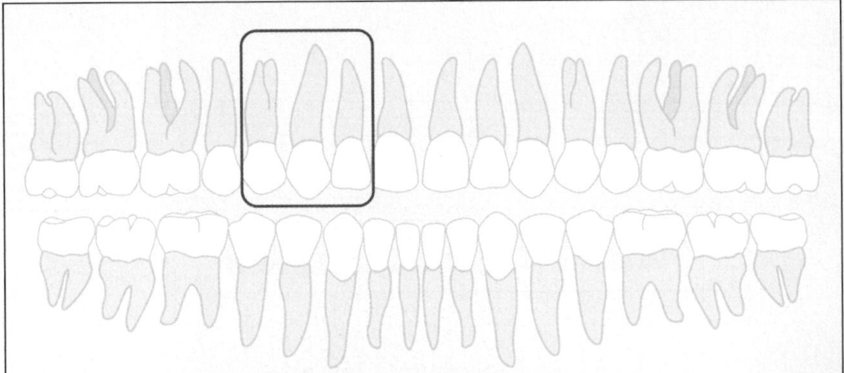

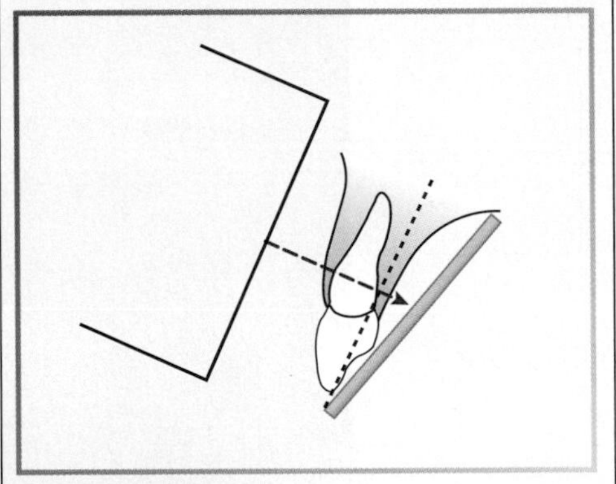

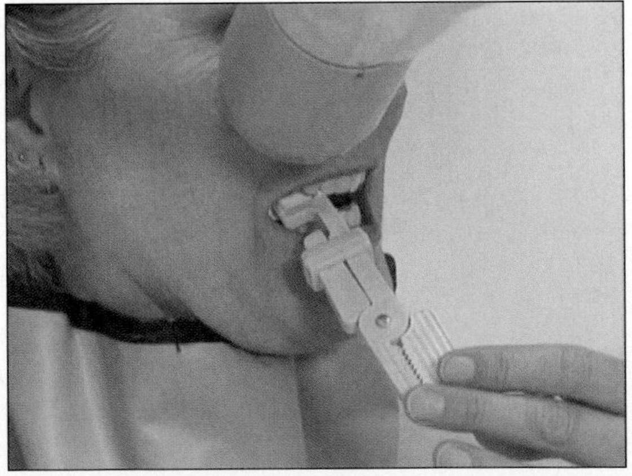

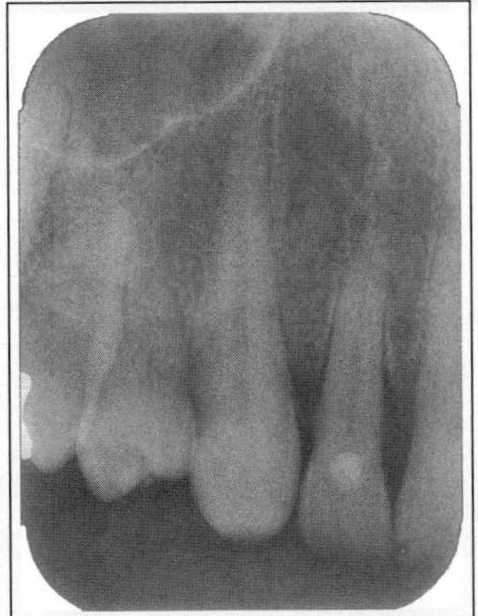

# PROCEDURE 41.4 Producing Full-Mouth Radiographic Survey Using Bisecting Technique–cont'd

**Maxillary Incisor Exposure**

1. Position the patient so that the occlusal plane is parallel to the floor and the sagittal plane of the patient's face is perpendicular to the floor.
2. Place the image receptor vertically into the holder.
3. Position the edge of the image receptor on the incisal edge of the incisors. Position the image receptor as close as possible to the lingual surface of the incisors.
4. Instruct the patient to bite lightly on the edge of the image receptor.
5. Vertical angulation will range from +40 to +50 degrees.
6. Establish the correct horizontal angulation by directing the central ray between the contacts of the central incisors.
7. Center the PID over the image receptor to avoid cone cutting.
8. Press the exposure button.

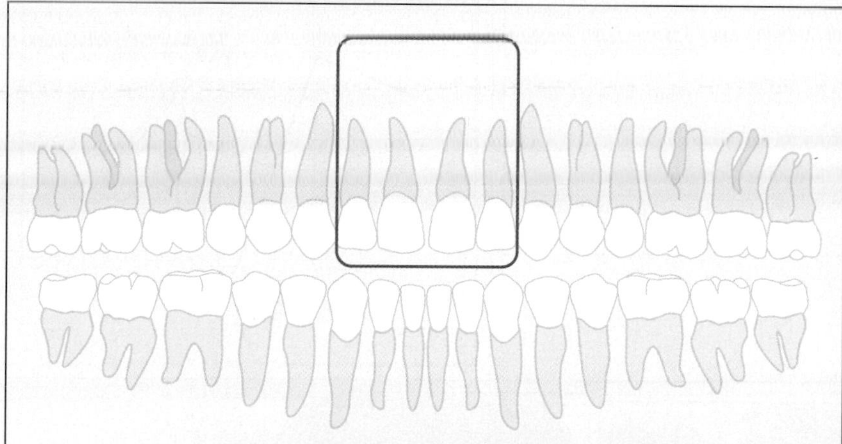

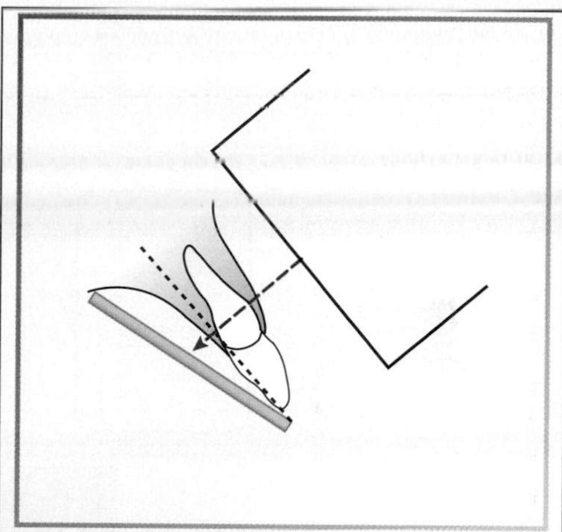

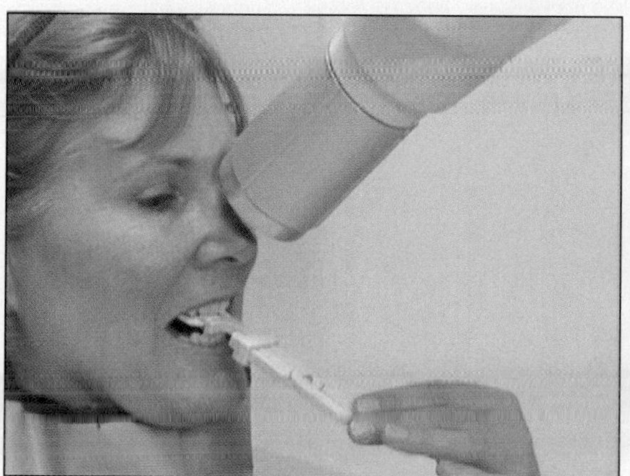

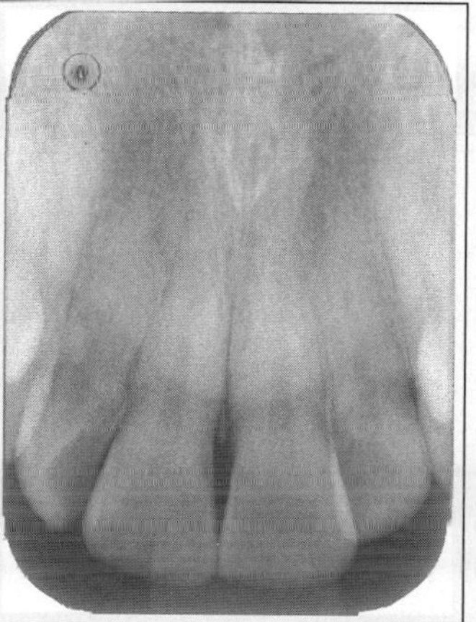

(Continued)

# PROCEDURE 41.4 Producing Full-Mouth Radiographic Survey Using Bisecting Technique–cont'd

## Mandibular Canine Exposure

1. Position the patient so that when the mouth is open, the maxillary occlusal plane is parallel to the floor and the sagittal plane of the patient's face is perpendicular to the floor.
2. Place the image receptor vertically into the film holder.
3. Position the edge of the image receptor on the incisal edge of the canine.
4. Instruct the patient to bite lightly but firmly on the edge of the image receptor.
5. Vertical angulation will range from −20 to −30 degrees.
6. Establish the correct horizontal angulation by directing the central ray between the contacts of the canine and the first premolar.
7. Center the PID over the image receptor to avoid cone cutting.
8. Press the exposure button.

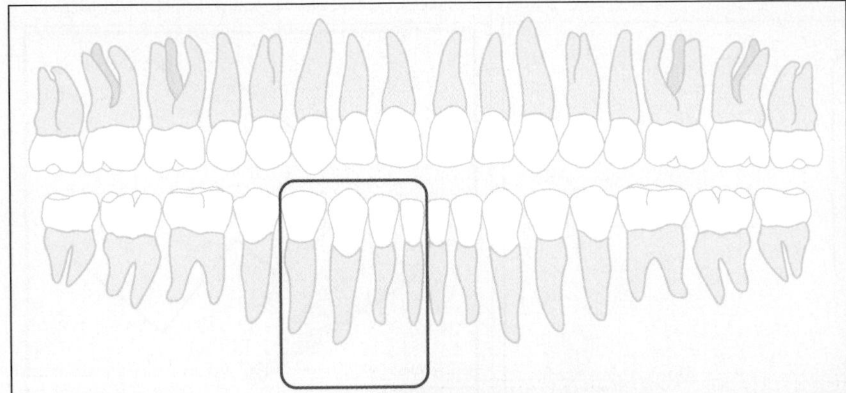

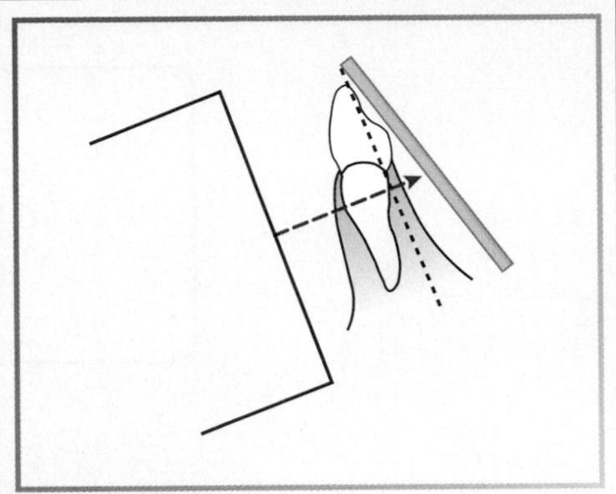

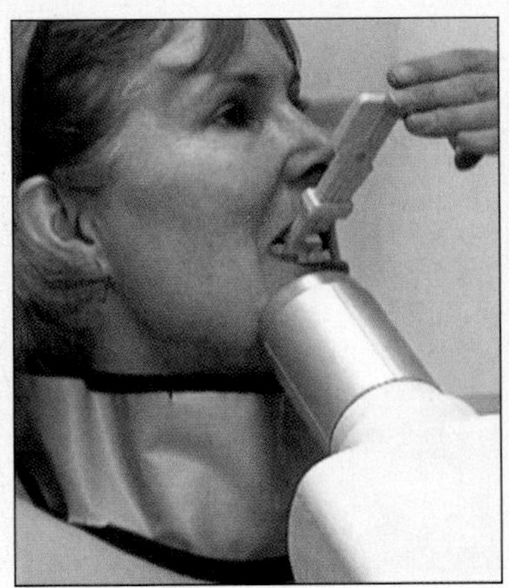

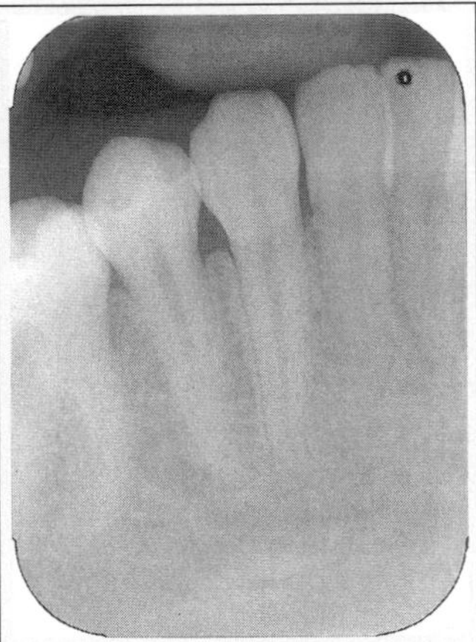

## PROCEDURE 41.4 Producing Full-Mouth Radiographic Survey Using Bisecting Technique—cont'd

### Mandibular Incisor Exposure

1 Position the patient so that when the mouth is open, the mandibular occlusal plane is parallel to the floor and the sagittal plane of the patient's face is perpendicular to the floor.
2 Place the image receptor vertically into the film holder.
3 Center the image receptor on the contact between the two central incisors and against the lingual surfaces of the incisors.
4 Instruct the patient to bite lightly but firmly on the edge of the image receptor.
5 Vertical angulation will range from −15 to −25 degrees.
6 Establish the correct horizontal angulation by directing the central ray between the contacts of the central incisors.
7 Center the PID over the image receptor to avoid cone cutting.
8 Press the exposure button.

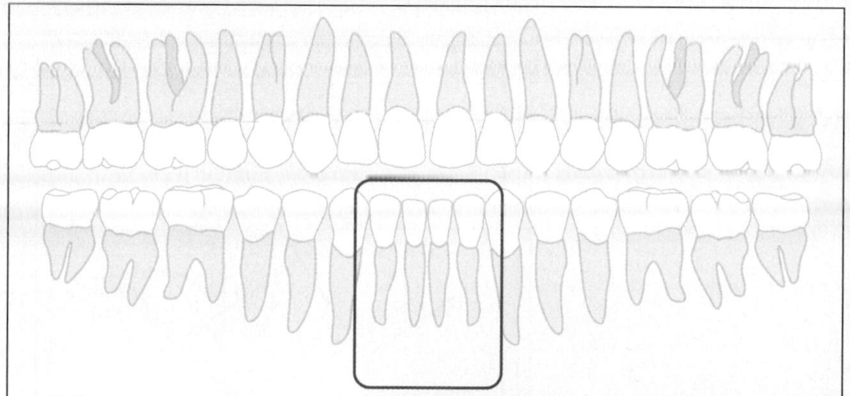

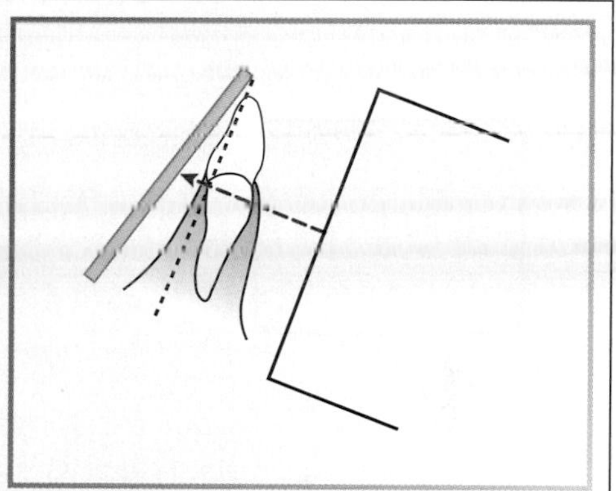

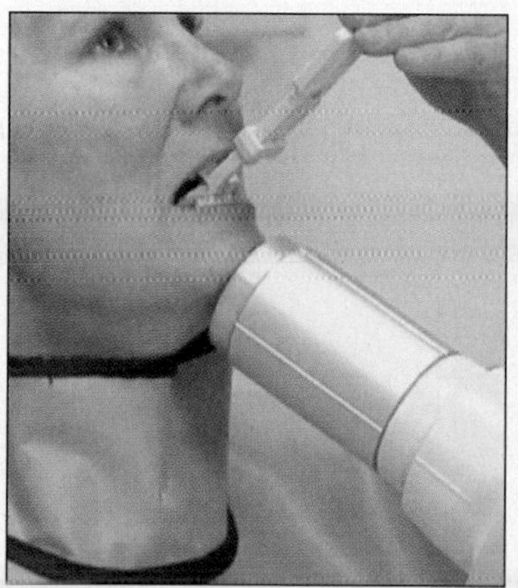

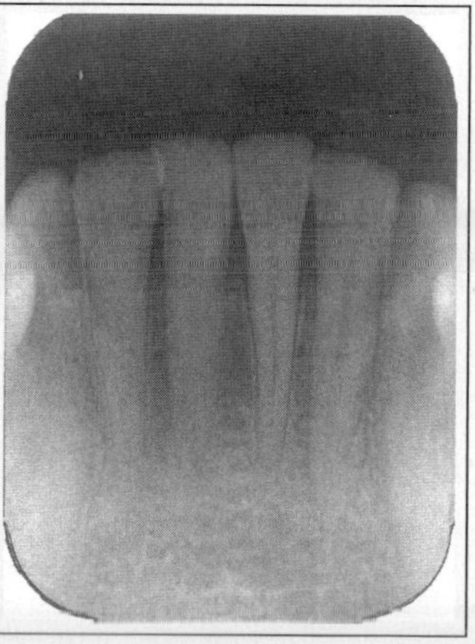

(Continued)

# PROCEDURE 41.4 Producing Full-Mouth Radiographic Survey Using Bisecting Technique—cont'd

### Maxillary Premolar Exposure

1. Position the patient so that when the mouth is open, the maxillary occlusal plane is parallel to the floor and the sagittal plane of the patient's face is perpendicular to the floor.
2. Place the image receptor horizontally into the holder.
3. Center the image receptor on the second premolar against the lingual surfaces of the teeth. Avoid shaping the film packet or PSP to the arch.
4. The central ray is directed at the most anterior part of the cheekbone. Vertical angulation will range from +30 to +40 degrees.
5. Establish the correct horizontal angulation by directing the central ray between the contacts of the premolars.
6. Center the PID over the image receptor to avoid cone cutting.
7. Press the exposure button.

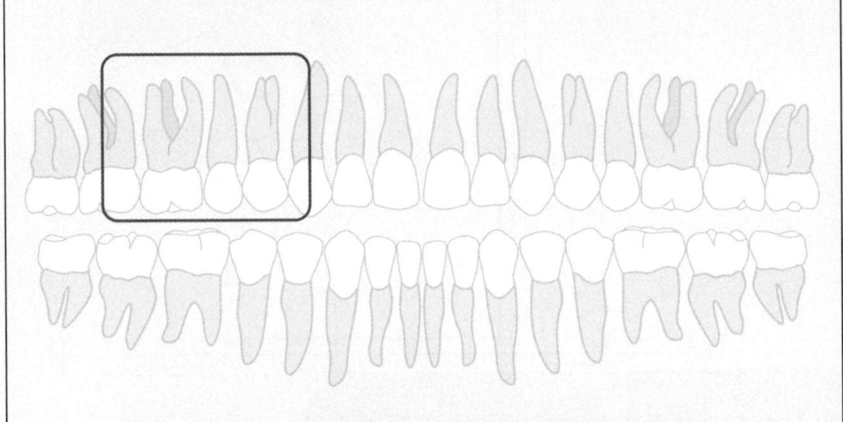

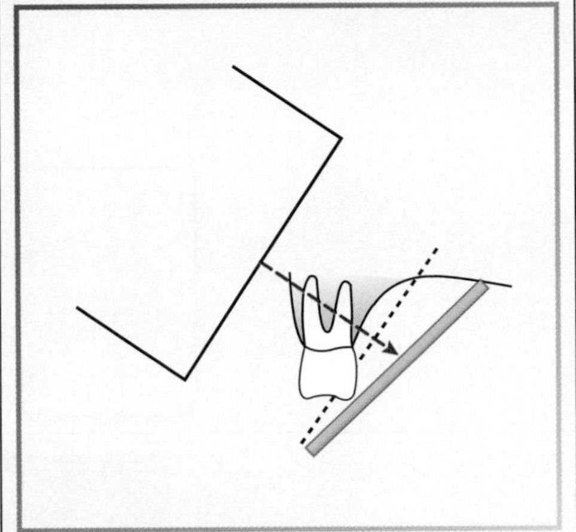

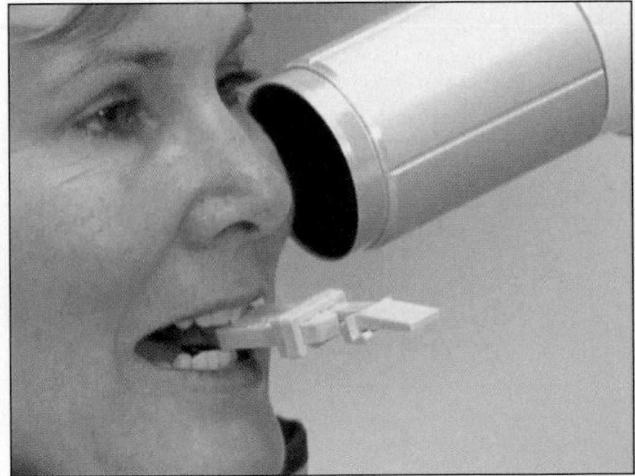

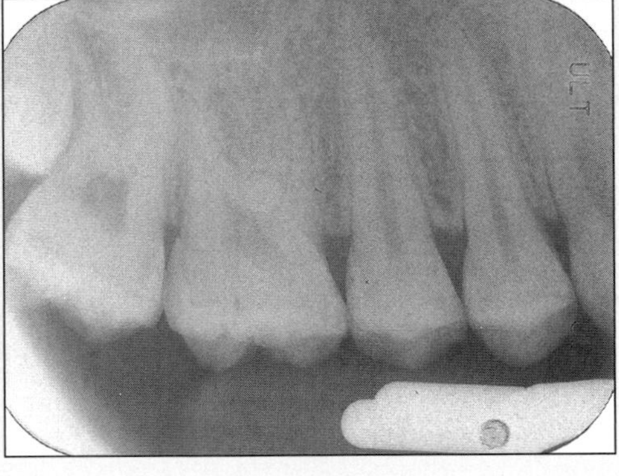

# PROCEDURE 41.4 Producing Full-Mouth Radiographic Survey Using Bisecting Technique–cont'd

### Maxillary Molar Exposure

1 Position the patient so that when the mouth is open, the maxillary occlusal plane is parallel to the floor and the sagittal plane of the patient's face is perpendicular to the floor.
2 Place the image receptor horizontally into the holder.
3 Center the image receptor on the second molar, and place it against the lingual surfaces of the teeth.
4 The central ray is directed through the zygomatic arch at the center of the image receptor. The distal edge of the PID should not be distal to the outer corner of the eye. Vertical angulation will range from 20 to 30 degrees.
5 Establish the correct horizontal angulation by directing the central ray between the contacts of the molars.
6 Center the PID over the image receptor to avoid cone cutting.
7 Press the exposure button.

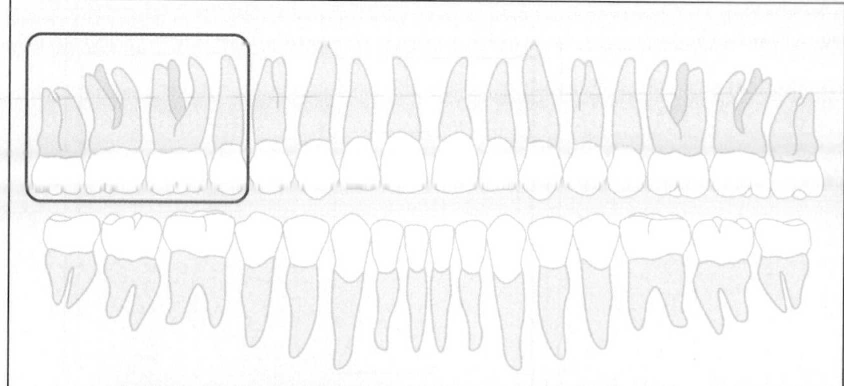

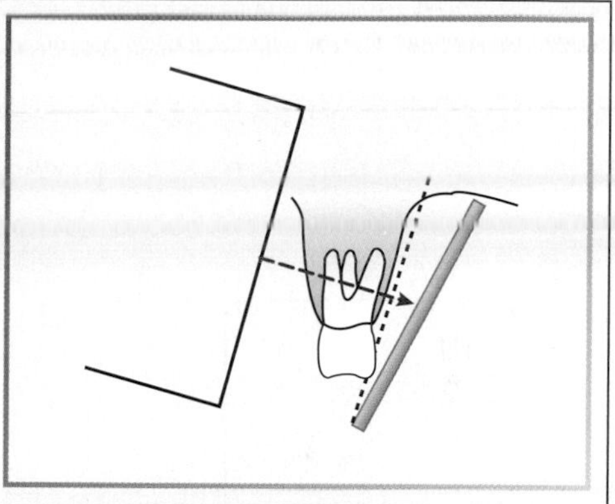

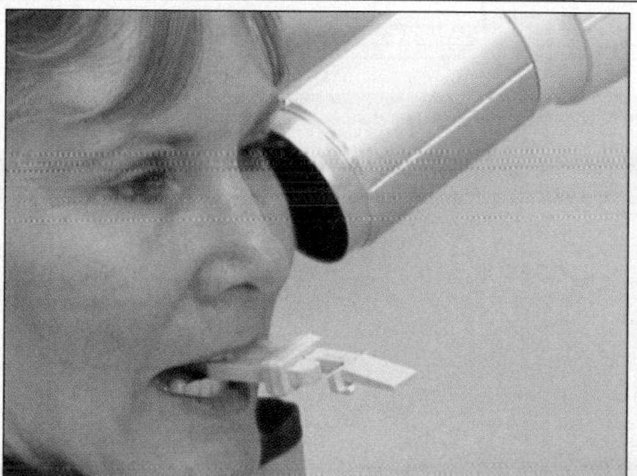

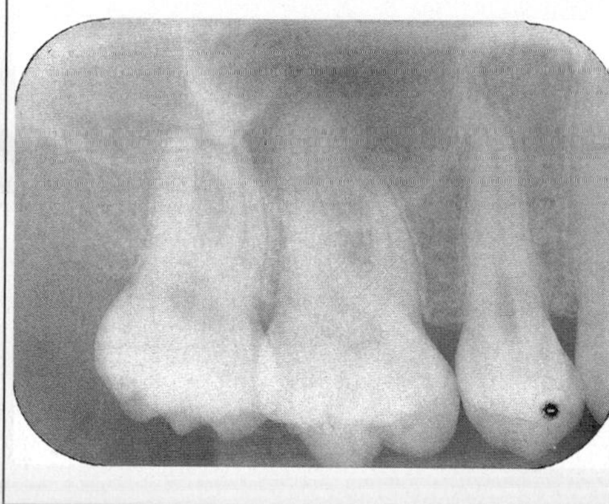

(Continued)

# PROCEDURE 41.4 Producing Full-Mouth Radiographic Survey Using Bisecting Technique—cont'd

### Mandibular Premolar Exposure

1 Position the patient so that when the mouth is open, the mandibular occlusal plane is parallel to the floor and the sagittal plane of the patient's face is perpendicular to the floor.
2 Place the image receptor horizontally into the holder.
3 Center the image receptor on the second premolar; the front edge of the image receptor should be aligned with the mesial aspect of the canine. Position the image receptor against the lingual surfaces of the teeth.
4 Instruct the patient to bite gently but firmly on the holder.
5 The central ray is directed at the mental foramen, aimed at the center of the image receptor. Vertical angulation will range from −10 to −15 degrees.
6 Establish the correct horizontal angulation by directing the central ray between the contacts of the premolars.
7 Center the PID over the image receptor to avoid cone cutting.
8 Press the exposure button.

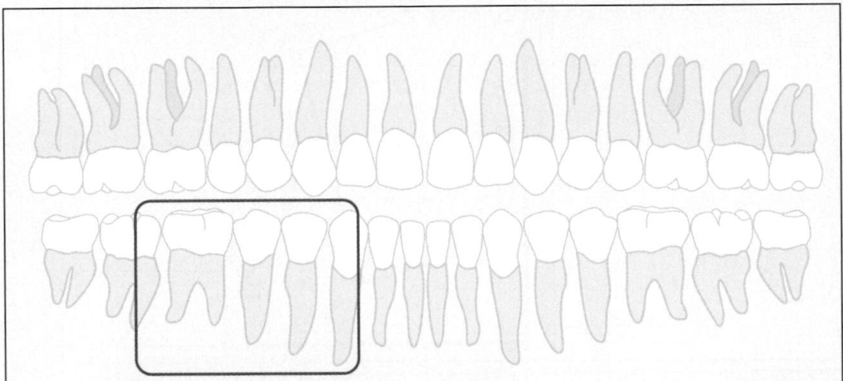

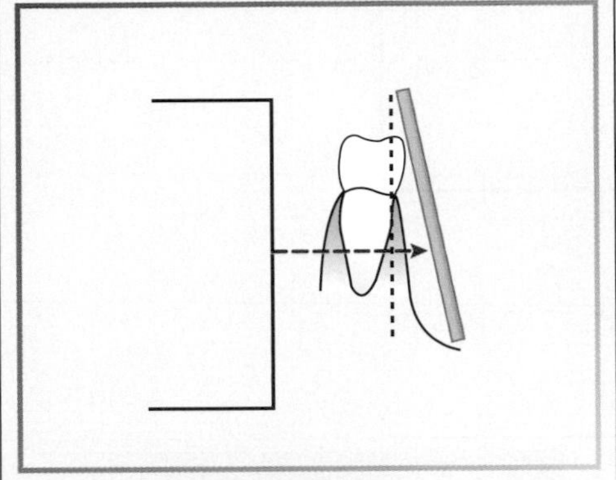

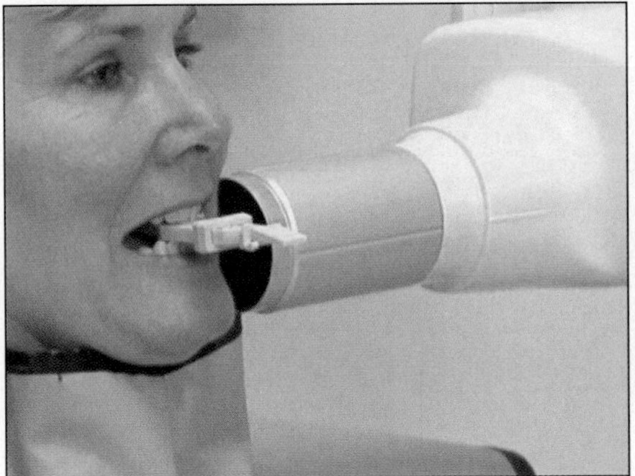

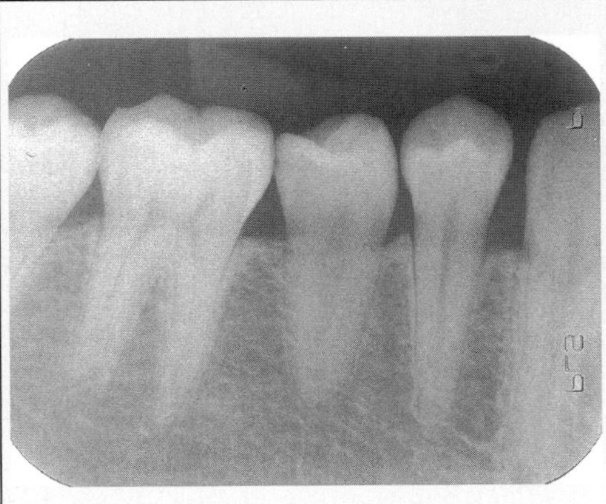

# PROCEDURE 41.4 Producing Full-Mouth Radiographic Survey Using Bisecting Technique–cont'd

## Mandibular Molar Exposure

1 Position the patient so that when the mouth is open, the mandibular occlusal plane is parallel to the floor and the sagittal plane of the patient's face is perpendicular to the floor.
2 Place the image receptor horizontally into the holder.
3 Center the holder and image receptor on the second molar; the front edge of the image receptor should be aligned with the midline of the second premolar.
**NOTE** Because of the anatomy of the area, the image receptor is almost parallel to the long axis of the tooth; therefore most molars radiographed with the bisecting technique actually produce parallel views.
4 Instruct the patient to close gently but firmly on the holder.
**NOTE** You may have to ask the patient to raise the chin so that the occlusal surfaces are parallel to the floor.
5 The central ray is directed at the roots of the molars. Vertical angulation will range from −5 to 0 degrees.
6 Establish the correct horizontal angulation by directing the central ray between the contacts of the molars.
7 Center the PID over the image receptor to avoid cone cutting.
8 Press the exposure button.

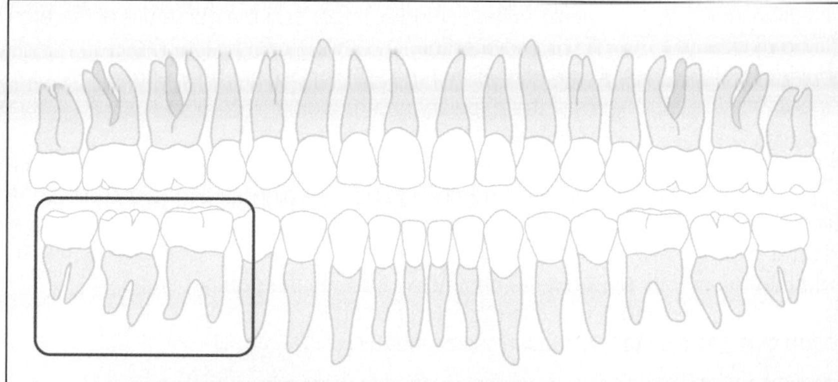

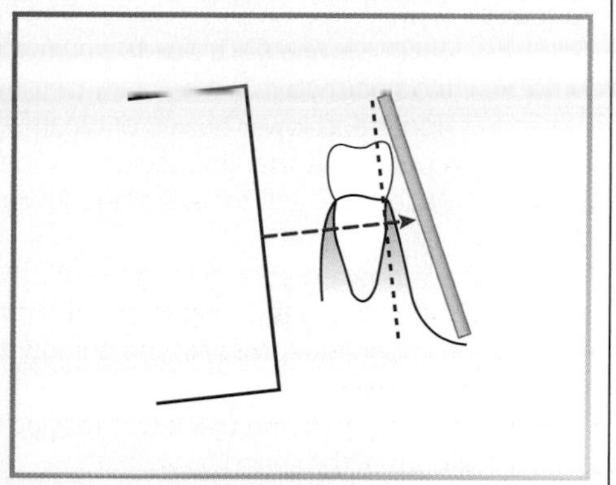

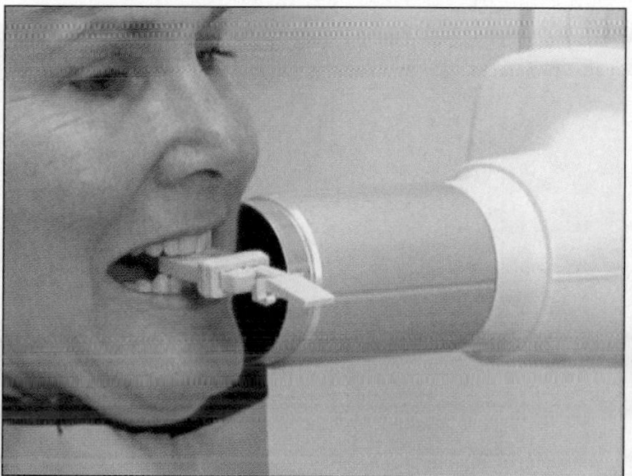

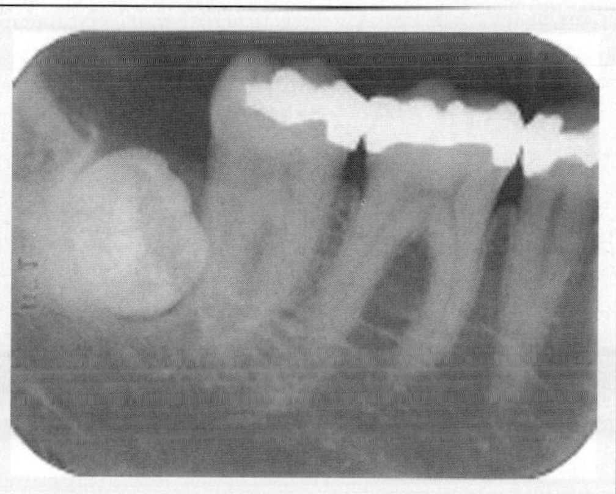

## Documentation

1 Document the procedure.

PROCEDURE 41.5 

# Producing Four-View Radiographic Survey Using Bitewing Technique

## GOAL

To produce a four-view series of images using the bitewing technique.

## EQUIPMENT AND SUPPLIES

- Four size #2 films, phosphor storage plates (PSPs), or sensor
- Paper cup or transfer box
- Lead apron and thyroid collar
- Bitewing tab or film sensor–holding device

## PROCEDURAL STEPS

### Premolar Bitewing Exposure

1 Set vertical angulation at +10 degrees.
**PURPOSE** A positive angulation means that the position indicating device (PID) points downward. This places the beam so that it is nearly perpendicular to both upper and lower halves of the image receptor.

2 Position the patient so that the occlusal plane is parallel to the floor. If necessary, ask the patient to lower or raise the chin.

3 Position the image receptor in the patient's mouth by placing the lower half between the tongue and the mandibular teeth. Position the image receptor with the anterior border at the middle of the canine.

4 Hold the image receptor in place by pressing the tab over the occlusal aspect of the mandibular teeth.
**PURPOSE** To prevent the image receptor from slipping out of position.

5 Ask the patient to close the mouth slowly. Take care not to allow the patient to close on the fingertip of your glove.

6 Do not pull the image receptor too tightly against the lower teeth as the patient closes the mouth.
**PURPOSE** This can cause the image receptor to push against the lingual aspect of the maxillary alveolar ridge and can force the image receptor down into the floor of the mouth.

7 Stand in front of the patient to set the horizontal angulation. To better visualize the curvature of the arch, place your index finger along the premolar area. Align the open end of the PID parallel with your index finger and the curvature of the arch in the premolar area.

8 Make certain that the PID is positioned far enough forward to cover the maxillary and mandibular canines to avoid a cone cut.
**PURPOSE** To check for a cone cut, stand directly behind the tubehead and look along the side of the PID. No portion of the image receptor should be covered by the PID.

9 Direct the central ray through the contact areas.

10 Press the exposure button.

11 Document the procedure.

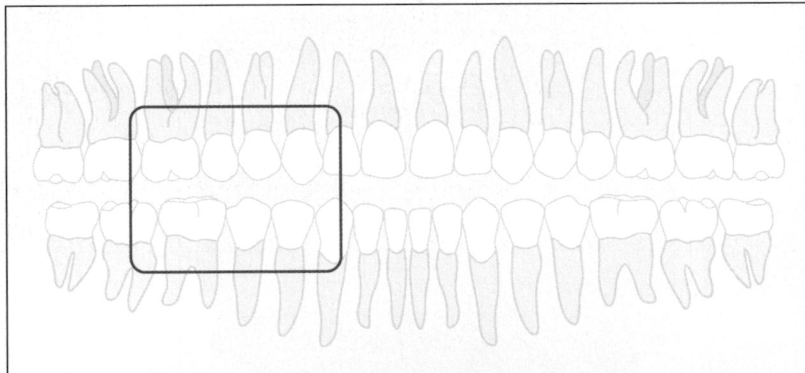

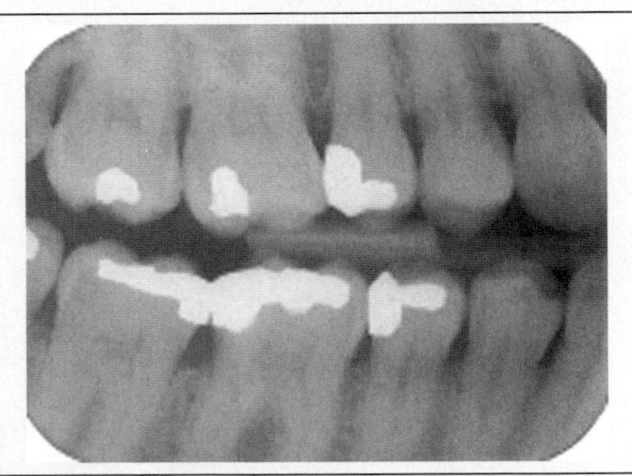

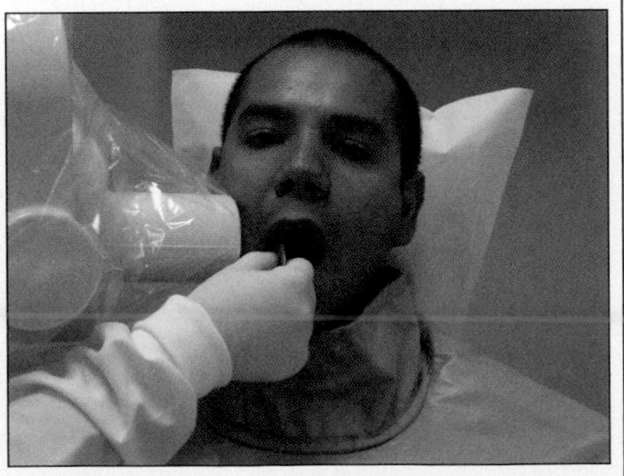

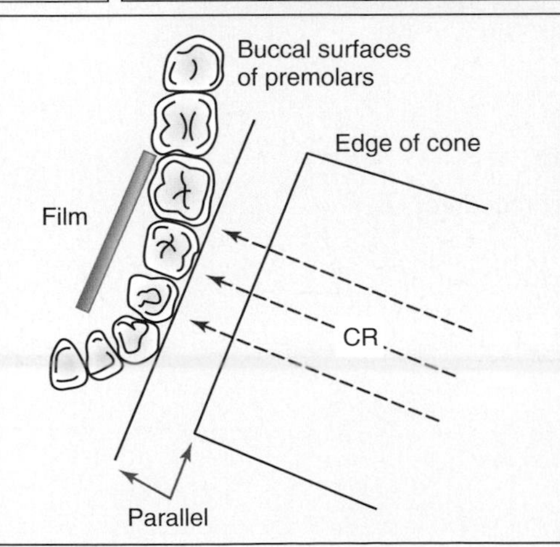

## PROCEDURE 41.5 Producing Four-View Radiographic Survey Using Bitewing Technique—cont'd

### Molar Bitewing Exposure

1 Set vertical angulation at +10 degrees.

**PURPOSE** A positive angulation means that the PID points downward. This places the beam so that it is nearly perpendicular to both upper and lower halves of the image receptor.

2 Position the patient so that the occlusal plane is parallel with the floor. If necessary, ask the patient to lower or raise the chin.

3 Position the image receptor in the patient's mouth by placing the lower half between the tongue and the mandibular teeth. Center the image receptor on the second molar; the front edge of the image receptor should be aligned with the middle of the mandibular second premolar.

4 Hold the image receptor in place by pressing the tab over the occlusal aspect of the mandibular tooth.

**PURPOSE** To prevent the image receptor from slipping out of position.

5 Ask the patient to close the mouth slowly. Take care not to allow the patient to close on the fingertip of your glove.

6 Do not pull the image receptor too tightly against the lower teeth as the patient closes the mouth.

**PURPOSE** This can cause the image receptor to push against the lingual aspect of the maxillary alveolar ridge and can force the image receptor down into the floor of the mouth.

7 Stand in front of the patient to set the horizontal angulation. To better visualize the curvature of the arch, place your index finger along the premolar area. Align the open end of the PID parallel with your index finger and the curvature of the arch in the molar area.

**PURPOSE** Different image receptor placement and horizontal angulations are needed to open the proximal contact areas.

8 Make certain that the PID is positioned far enough forward to cover the maxillary and the mandibular canines to avoid a cone cut.

**PURPOSE** To check for a cone cut, stand directly behind the tubehead and look along the side of the PID. No portion of the image receptor should be visible; the image receptor should be covered by the PID.

9 Direct the central ray through the contact areas.

10 Press the exposure button.

11 Document the procedure.

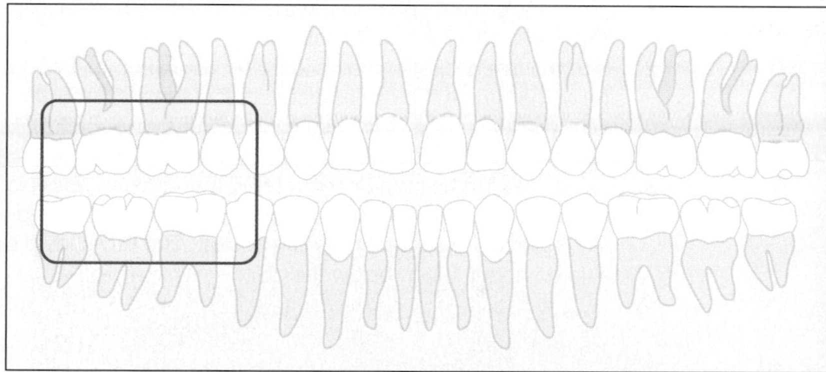

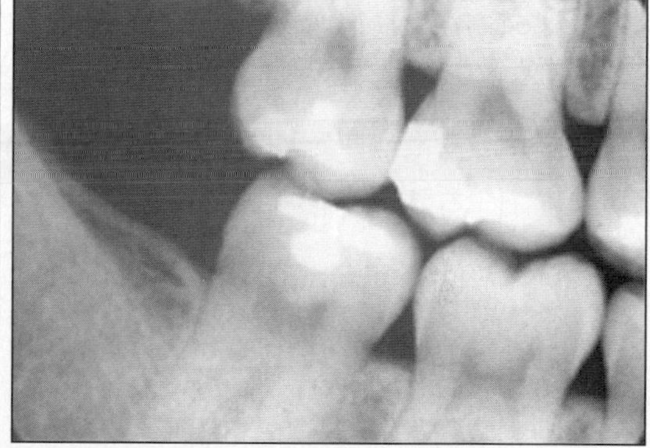

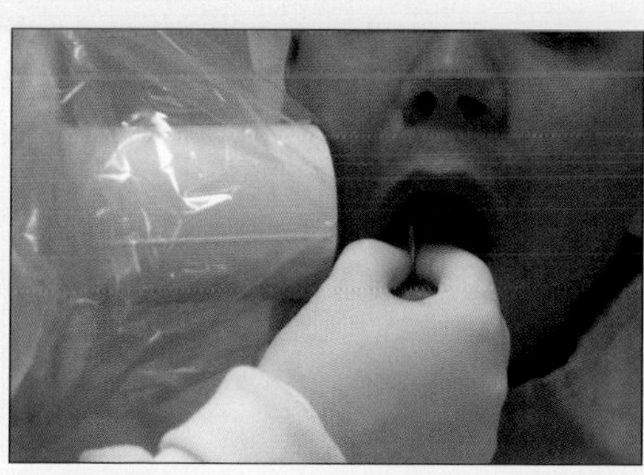

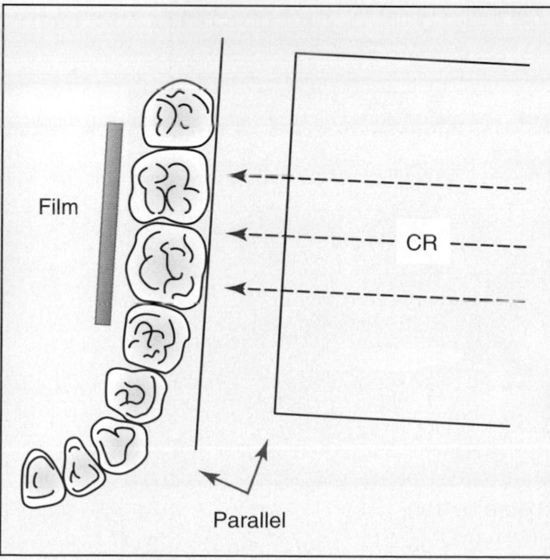

PROCEDURE 41.6 

# Producing Maxillary and Mandibular Radiographs Using Occlusal Technique

## GOAL

To follow the steps of the occlusal technique in producing diagnostic-quality maxillary and mandibular x-ray films.

## EQUIPMENT AND SUPPLIES

- Two #4 films
- Paper cup
- Lead apron and thyroid collar

## PROCEDURAL STEPS

### Maxillary Occlusal Technique

1 Ask the patient to remove prosthetic appliances or objects from the mouth.
2 Place the lead apron and thyroid collar.
3 Position the patient's head so the film plane is parallel to the floor and the midsagittal plane is perpendicular to the floor.
4 Place the film packet in the patient's mouth with the white side of the film on the occlusal surfaces of the maxillary teeth. The long edge of the film is placed in a side-to-side direction.
5 Place the film as far posterior as possible.
6 Position the PID so that the central ray is directed at +65 degrees through the center of the film. The top edge of the PID is placed between the eyebrows on the bridge of the nose.

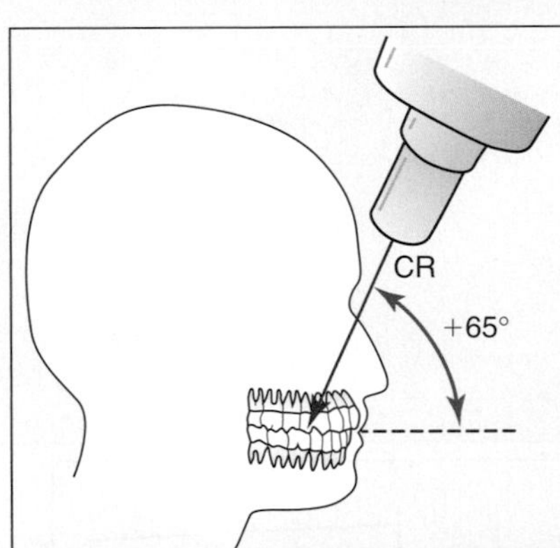


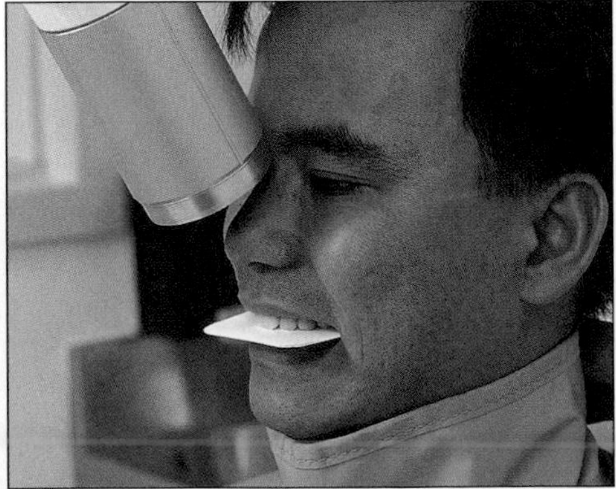

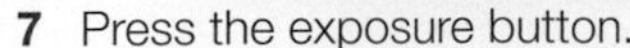

7 Press the exposure button.

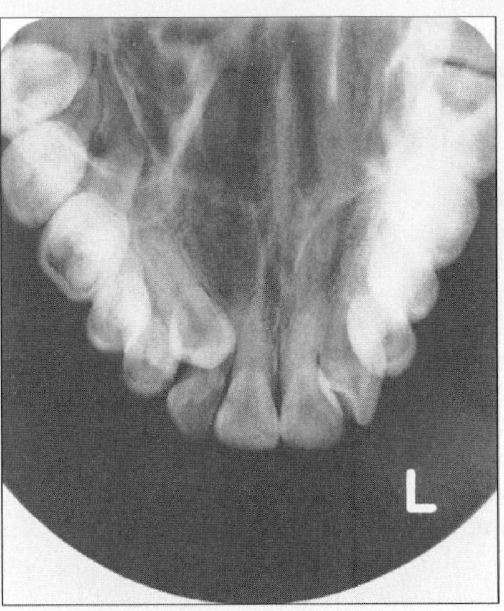


8 Document the procedure.

### Mandibular Occlusal Technique

1 Recline the patient and position the head with the midsagittal plane perpendicular to the floor.
2 Place the film packet in the patient's mouth with the white side of the film on the occlusal surfaces of the mandibular teeth. The long edge of the film is placed in a side-to-side direction.
3 Position the film as far posterior on the mandible as possible.
4 Position the PID so that the central ray is directed at a 90-degree angle to the center of the film packet. The PID should be centered about 1 inch below the chin.

## PROCEDURE 41.6 Producing Maxillary and Mandibular Radiographs Using Occlusal Technique–cont'd

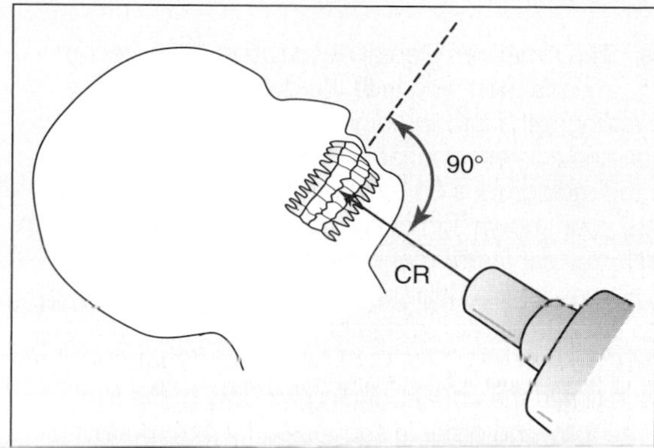


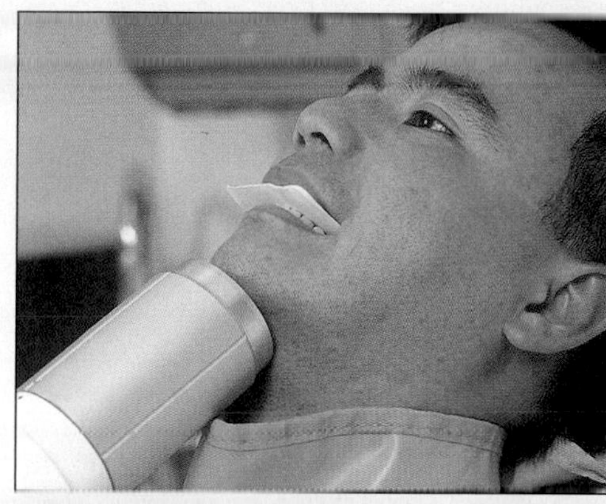

**5** Press the exposure button.

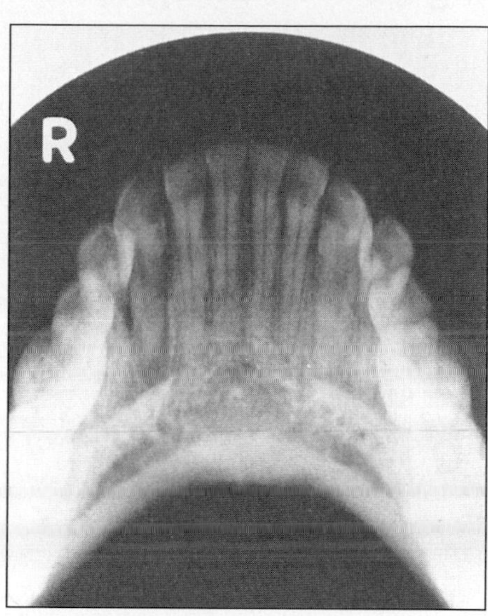


**6** Document the procedure.

PROCEDURE 41.7 

# Mounting Dental Radiographs

## GOAL

To mount a full-mouth series of dental radiographs.

## EQUIPMENT AND SUPPLIES

- ✔ Appropriate size of film mount
- ✔ Pencil
- ✔ View box
- ✔ Paper towel
- ✔ Processing for full-mouth series of radiographs

## PROCEDURAL STEPS

1 Place a clean paper towel over the work surface in front of the view box.
**PURPOSE** To keep the films clean.

2 Turn on the view box.

3 Label and date the film mount.

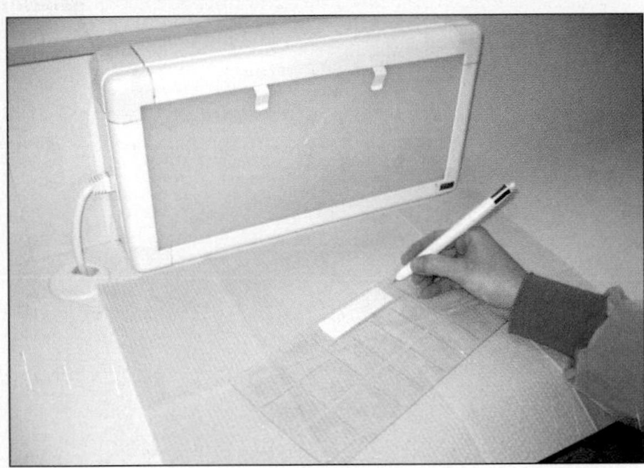

4 Wash and dry your hands.
**PURPOSE** To prevent finger marks on the radiographs.

5 Identify the embossed dot on each radiograph; place the film on the work surface with the dot facing up.
**PURPOSE** The American Dental Association (ADA) recommends mounting with the dot up.

6 Sort the radiographs into three groups: bitewing, anterior periapical, and posterior periapical views.

7 Arrange the radiographs on the work surface in anatomic order. Use your knowledge of normal anatomic landmarks to distinguish maxillary from mandibular radiographs.

8 Arrange all maxillary radiographs with the roots pointing upward and all mandibular radiographs with the roots pointing downward.

9 Place each film in the corresponding window of the film mount. The following order is suggested for film mounting:
   a Maxillary anterior periapical films
   b Mandibular anterior periapical films
   c Bitewing films
   d Maxillary posterior periapical films
   e Mandibular posterior periapical films

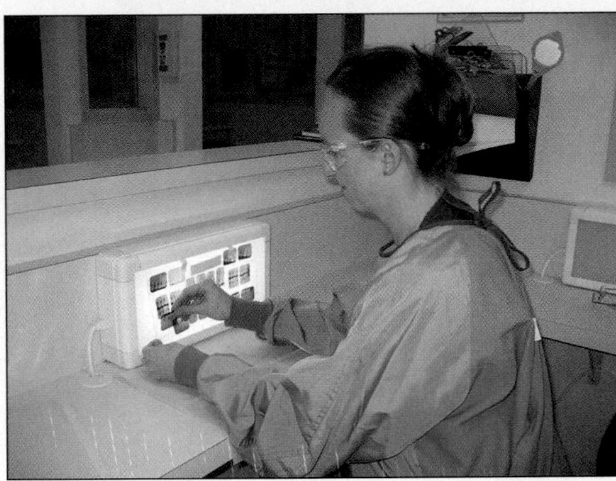

10 Check the mounted radiographs to ensure that (a) the dots are all oriented properly, (b) the films are arranged properly in anatomic order, and (c) the films are secure in the mount.

42

# Extraoral Imaging

## KEY TERMS

**Cephalostat** Special device that allows the operator to easily position both film and patient.

**Computed tomography (toe-MOG-ruh-fee) (CT)** Radiographic technique that produces images or "slices" of one layer or section of the specific areas. Also referred to as computed axial tomography (CAT scan).

**Cone beam computed tomography (CBCT)** A three-dimensional digital imaging method that uses a cone-shaped beam of radiation that rotates around the patient.

**Digital panoramic units** A filmless method of recording a panoramic image and displaying it by using an electronic sensor and a computer to process and store the image.

**Exposure controls** Feature that allows the operator to adjust the milliamperage and kilovoltage settings.

**Extraoral images** Images taken when large areas of the skull or jaw must be examined.

**Extraoral imaging** An image of the teeth and bones made by placing the film or cassette against the face or the head and projecting the x-rays from the opposite side.

**Field of view** The area that can be shown when performing imaging procedures.

**Focal trough (trof)** Imaginary three-dimensional horseshoe-shaped zone used to focus panoramic radiographs.

**Frankfort plane** Imaginary plane that passes through the top of the ear canal and the bottom of the eye socket.

**Midsagittal plane** Imaginary line that divides the patient's face into right and left sides.

**Temporomandibular (tem-puh-roe-man-DIB-yoo-lur) joint (TMJ)** Joint on each side of the head that allows movement of the mandible.

**Three-dimensional digital imaging** An image that demonstrates the anatomy in three dimensions.

## LEARNING OUTCOMES

*On completion of this chapter, the student will be able to achieve the following objectives:*

1. Pronounce, define, and spell the key terms.
2. Discuss panoramic imaging, including the following:
   - Describe the purpose and uses of panoramic imaging.
   - Describe the equipment used in panoramic imaging.
   - Describe the steps for patient preparation and positioning in panoramic imaging.
   - Describe the errors that may occur during patient preparation and positioning during panoramic imaging.
3. Discuss three-dimensional imaging, including the following:
   - Explain the difference between a CT scan and cone beam computed tomography (CBCT).
   - Describe the uses of three-dimensional imaging.
   - Discuss the advantages and disadvantages of CBCT.
4. Identify the specific purpose of each type of the extraoral film projections.

## PERFORMANCE OUTCOMES

*On completion of this chapter, the student will be able to meet competency standards in the following skills:*

- Prepare the equipment necessary for a panoramic image.
- Prepare a patient for a panoramic x-ray.
- Position the patient for a panoramic procedure.

## ELECTRONIC RESOURCES

***Additional information related to content in Chapter 42 can be found on the companion Evolve Web site.***

- Practice Quiz
- Video: Preparing Equipment and Positioning the Patient for Panoramic Imaging
- Canadian Content Corner

**Extraoral images** are useful when large areas of the skull or jaw must be examined, or when patients are unable to open their mouths for image receptor placement. (*Extraoral* means "outside the mouth.") Extraoral images are very useful for evaluating large areas but have never been recommended for detection of subtle changes, such as dental caries or early periodontal changes. The reason for this is that traditional film-based extraoral radiographs do not show details as well as intraoral films. This is changing with the introduction of full-featured **digital panoramic units** and special software programs. Almost all digital extraoral images have better resolution than film-based images.

This chapter focuses on panoramic imaging and a recent technology called cone beam computed tomography (CBCT), and also discusses various other **extraoral imaging** techniques and their advantages and disadvantages.

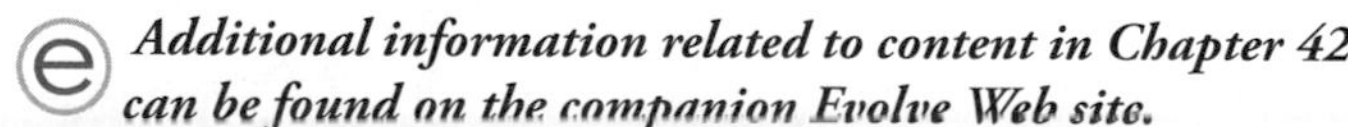
1 When are extraoral radiographs needed?

# Panoramic Imaging

Panoramic imaging allows the dentist to view the entire dentition and related structures on a single image (Fig. 42.1). Small intraoral images cannot adequately show the temporomandibular joint, the maxillary sinuses, or broad areas of the jaws. Panoramic images are used to locate impacted teeth, to detect lesions in the jaw, and to observe eruption patterns.

When extraoral images are taken with radiographic film, the details are not as clear as intraoral images. However, digital extraoral imaging systems have better resolution than the film-based systems. Before digital panoramic units became available, panoramic images were not recommended for diagnosing dental caries, periodontal disease, or lesions because of the overlapping of posterior contact areas. Bitewing images had to be used to supplement the panoramic image (Fig. 42.2). This situation has changed with the introduction of new full-featured digital panoramic units with specialized software. Panoramic digital images produced with this technology can show small interproximal carious lesions. They can "open up" contacts in the premolar areas that traditional film-based panoramic machines showed as being overlapped (Fig. 42.3). As with all imaging techniques, panoramic imaging has advantages and disadvantages (Table 42.1).

## Types of Panoramic Units

Two types of panoramic machines are in use today: *film-based imaging* and *direct digital imaging.* The main difference between direct digital panoramic imaging and film-based panoramic imaging is the image receptor. Digital units use a sensor array rather than film, and the image is produced immediately on the computer monitor rather than on film after processing (Fig. 42.4).

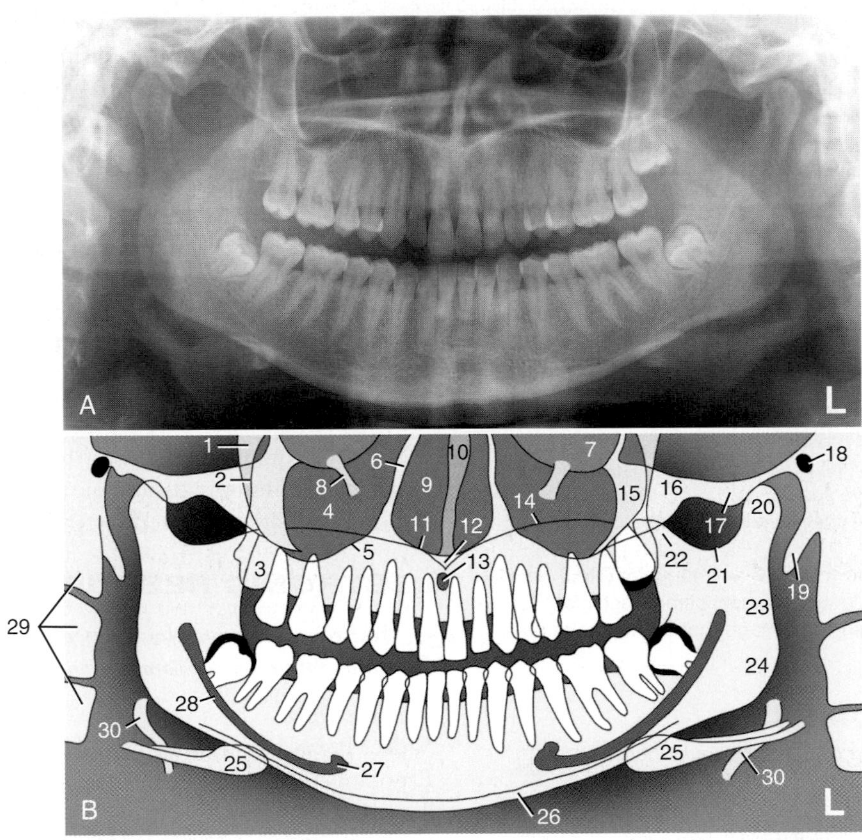


1. Pterygomaxillary fissure
2. Posterior border of maxilla
3. Maxillary tuberosity
4. Maxillary sinus
5. Floor of the maxillary sinus
6. Medial border of maxillary sinus/ lateral border of the nasal cavity
7. Floor of the orbit
8. Infraorbital canal
9. Nasal cavity
10. Nasal septum
11. Floor of the nasal cavity
12. Anterior nasal spine
13. Incisive foramen
14. Hard palate/floor of the nasal cavity
15. Zygomatic process of the maxilla
16. Zygomatic arch
17. Articular eminence
18. External auditory meatus
19. Styloid process
20. Mandibular condyle
21. Sigmoid notch
22. Coronoid process
23. Posterior border of ramus
24. Angle of mandible
25. Hyoid bone
26. Inferior border of mandible
27. Mental foramen
28. Mandibular canal
29. Cervical vertebrae
30. Epiglottis

**FIG. 42.1** A, Panoramic image of an adult patient. B, This diagram outlines some of the structures that can be visualized on a panoramic image. *(From White SC, Pharoah MJ: Oral radiology: principles and interpretation, ed 7, St Louis, 2014, Mosby.)*

## Basic Concepts

In panoramic imaging, the image receptor and the tubehead rotate around the patient, producing a series of individual images. When these images are combined on a single film, an overall view of the maxilla and mandible is created (Fig. 42.5).

## Focal Trough

The **focal trough**, also known as the *image layer,* is a three-dimensional (3D) horseshoe-shaped zone (Fig. 42.6). When the patient's jaws are positioned within this zone, the resulting radiograph is reasonably clear and well defined. If the jaws are positioned outside of this zone, images on the radiograph appear blurred or indistinct. Imagine this trough as an area of ideal focus.

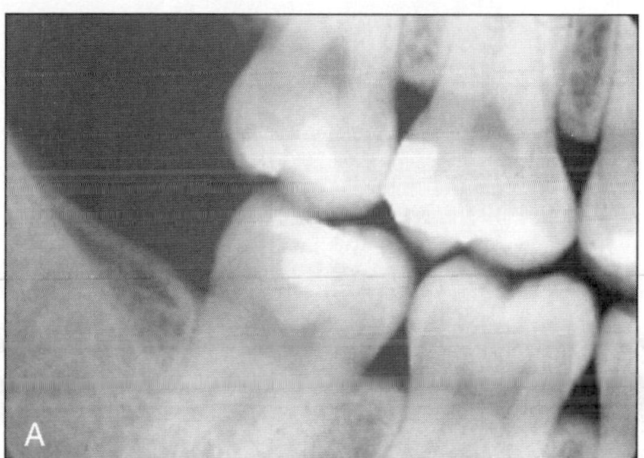


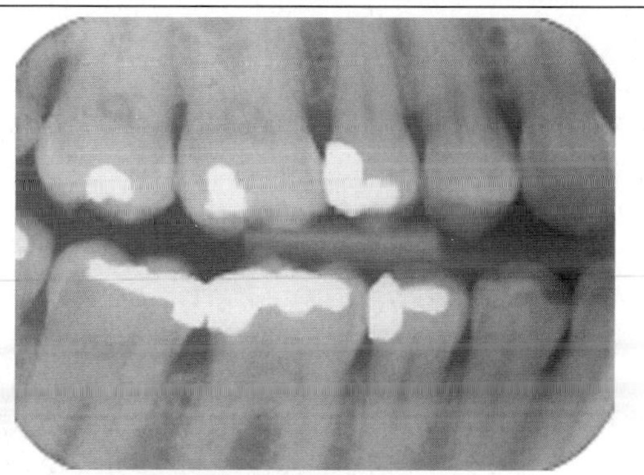

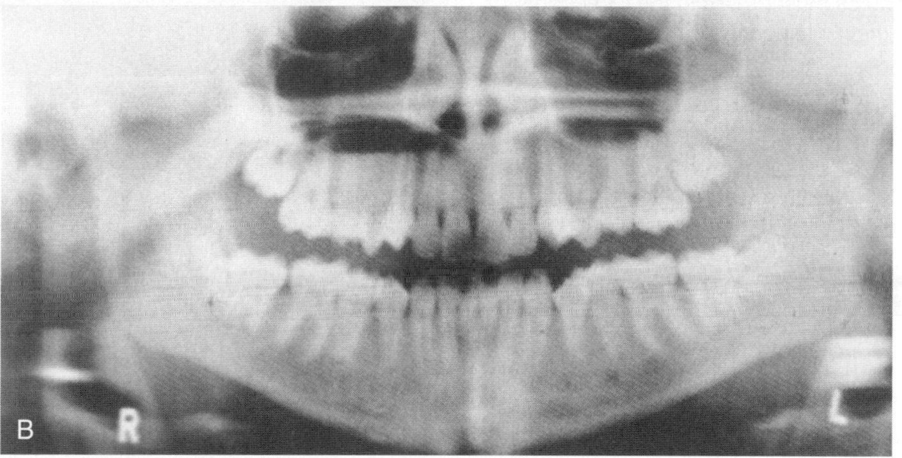


**FIG. 42.2** A, Open contacts on a bitewing film. B, The posterior contacts are closed on this panoramic film. (B, *From Iannucci J, Jansen Howerton L: Dental radiography: principles and techniques, ed 4, St Louis, 2012, Saunders.)*

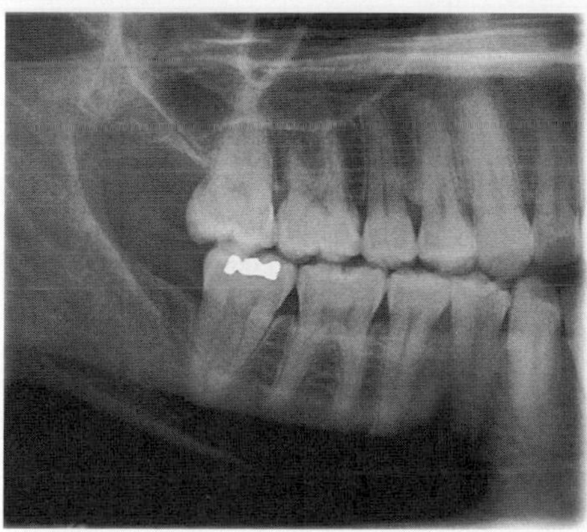

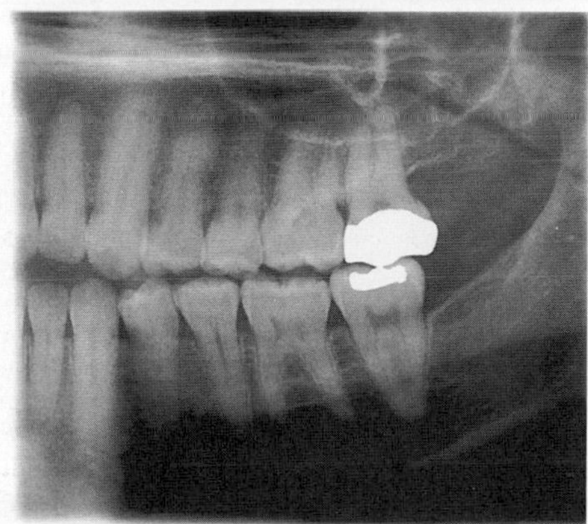

**FIG. 42.3** A specialized program in the digital software allows this type of "panoramic bitewing." Note that the interproximal contacts are opened. This set of bitewings also displays the posterior region of all posterior teeth.

**TABLE 42.1 Advantages and Disadvantages of Panoramic Imaging**

| | |
|---|---|
| **Advantages** | |
| Field size | The entire maxilla and mandible can be seen on one panoramic image. |
| Ease of use | Learning how to expose a panoramic image is relatively quick and easy. |
| Patient acceptance | Most patients prefer the panoramic image because they do not have to hold uncomfortable film in their mouths. |
| Less radiation exposure | The patient receives less radiation exposure compared with the full-mouth survey. |
| **Disadvantages** | |
| Image sharpness | On older film-based panoramic units, the images seen are not as sharp as those seen on an intraoral film. This is changing because of the development of digital full-featured panoramic units. These units can open contacts and detect small carious lesions. |
| Focal trough limitations | Structures must be within the focal trough, or they will appear out of focus. |
| Distortion | If proper positioning and technique are not used, there will always be some overlapping of the teeth and distortion of the images. |
| Cost of equipment | Compared with the cost of an intraoral radiograph unit, a panoramic unit is more expensive. |

The size and shape of the focal trough vary with the manufacturer of the panoramic unit. Panoramic x-ray units are designed to accommodate the average size jaw. The quality of the resulting radiograph depends on how the patient's jaws are positioned within the trough and how closely the patient's jaws conform to the focal trough, which is designed for the average jaw.

Each manufacturer provides specific instructions about patient positioning to ensure that the teeth are positioned within the focal trough. When the jaws are outside this area, the resulting images are distorted. Proper positioning errors are important and are discussed later in this chapter.

## Equipment

Film-based panoramic radiography requires the use of a panoramic x-ray unit, screen-type film, intensifying screens, and cassettes (see Chapter 39).

A number of different panoramic x-ray units are on the market today. Although each manufacturer's panoramic unit is slightly different, all machines have similar components. The main components of the panoramic unit include the panoramic x-ray tubehead, the head positioner, and exposure controls (Fig. 42.7).

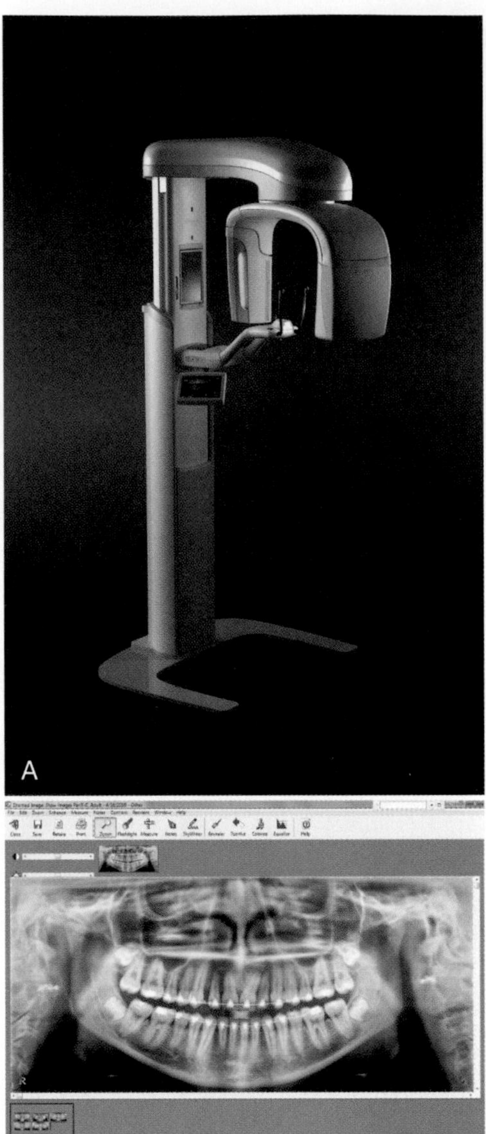


**FIG. 42.4** A, Panoramic machine used with digital imaging. B, An example of a panoramic digital image. *(A, Courtesy Midmark. B, Courtesy Schick Technologies, Long Island City, NY.)*

### Tubehead

The components of a panoramic x-ray tubehead are similar to an intraoral tubehead in that it has a filament that produces electrons and a target that produces radiographs. The *collimator* used in the panoramic x-ray machine is a lead plate with an opening shaped like a narrow vertical slit.

Different from the intraoral tubehead, the vertical angulation of the panoramic tubehead is not adjustable. In addition, the tubehead of the panoramic unit always rotates *behind* the patient's head as the film rotates in front of the patient.

### Head Positioner

Each panoramic unit includes a head positioner that is used to align the patient's teeth as accurately as possible. Each head positioner consists of a chin rest, a notched bite-block,

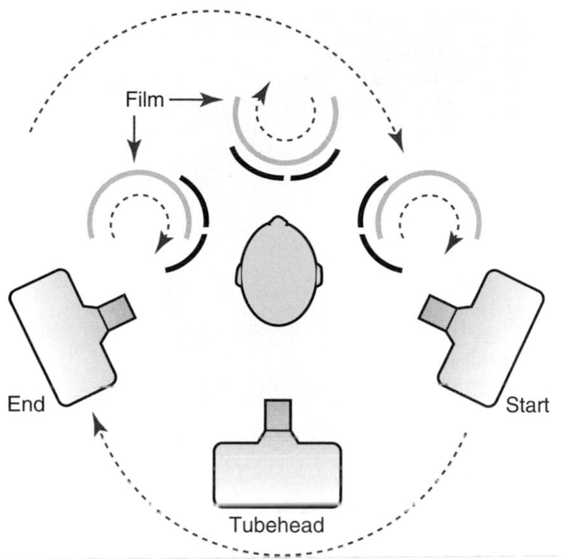


FIG. 42.5 The film and x-ray tubehead move around the patient in opposite directions in panoramic radiography. *(Courtesy Dr. Robert M. Jaynes, Columbus, OH.)*

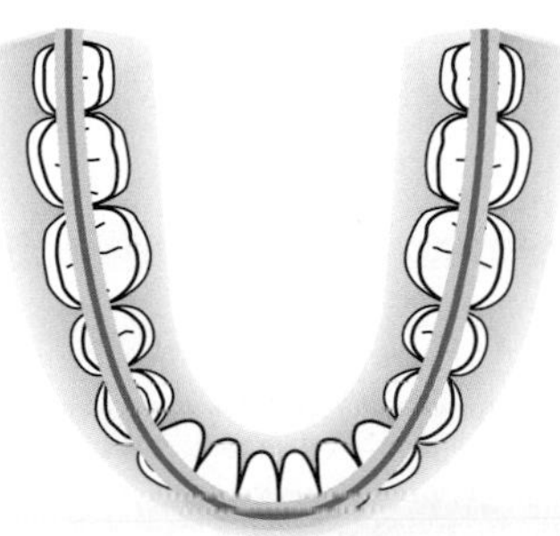

FIG. 42.6 Schematic representation of the focal trough, or image layer, of a panoramic machine. Structures in the middle of the layer (darkest area) will be sharply depicted; those toward the periphery will be less sharply depicted. All structures outside the layer will be blurred and magnified. *(From Miles DA, Van Dis ML, Williamson GF, et al: Radiographic imaging for the dental team, ed 4, St Louis, 2009, Saunders.)*

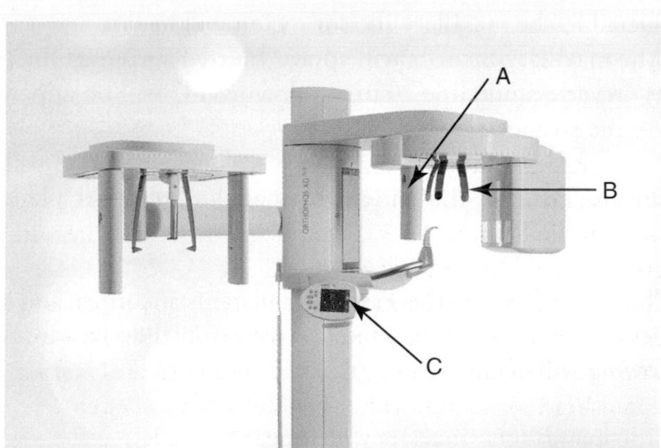


FIG. 42.7 Exposure controls on the Orthophos XG can be used to adjust exposure factors. The main components of the machine are A, x-ray tubehead; B, head positioner; C, exposure controls. *(Courtesy Sirona USA, Charlotte, NC.)*

a forehead rest, and lateral head supports or guides. Each panoramic unit is unique, and the operator must follow the manufacturer's instructions to position the patient correctly in the focal trough.

### Exposure Controls

**Exposure controls** allow the milliamperage and kilovoltage settings to be adjusted to accommodate patients of different sizes. However, *the exposure time cannot be changed.*

Step-by-step procedures for the exposure of a panoramic image include equipment preparation (Procedure 42.1), patient preparation (Procedure 42.2), and patient positioning (Procedure 42.3).

### Film and Intensifying Screens

Film-based panoramic imaging uses a type of extraoral screen film that is held in a film cassette. This type of film is sensitive to the light emitted from intensifying screens in the film-holding cassette. Refer to Chapter 39 for a review of extraoral films and cassettes.

## Common Errors

To produce a diagnostic panoramic image while minimizing patient exposure, you must avoid mistakes. To do this, you must be able to recognize the following common patient preparation and positioning errors and understand what you can do to prevent such errors from occurring.

### Patient Preparation Errors

**GHOST IMAGES.** If all metallic or radiodense objects, including eyeglasses, earrings, necklaces, piercing jewelry, removable partial dentures, orthodontic retainers, and hearing aids, are not removed from the patient before exposure of a panoramic film, a "ghost" image results. A ghost image looks similar to the real object except that it appears on the opposite side of the film.

For example, if an earring was on the patient's left side, the ghost image on the radiograph would appear on the right side and slightly higher than the real object. In addition, the ghost image of the earring would appear blurred and larger (Fig. 42.8).

**Solution.** The patient must be instructed to remove all objects from the head and neck region before being positioned for a panoramic radiograph.

**LEAD APRON ARTIFACT.** If the lead apron is incorrectly placed, or if a lead apron with a thyroid collar is used during exposure of panoramic films, a radiopaque cone-shaped artifact results that interferes with the diagnostic information (Fig. 42.9).

**Solution.** Use a lead apron *without* a thyroid collar, and place the lead apron low around the neck of the patient so that it does not block the x-ray beam. Follow the recommendations of the manufacturer of the panoramic unit regarding the specific style of apron that should be used.

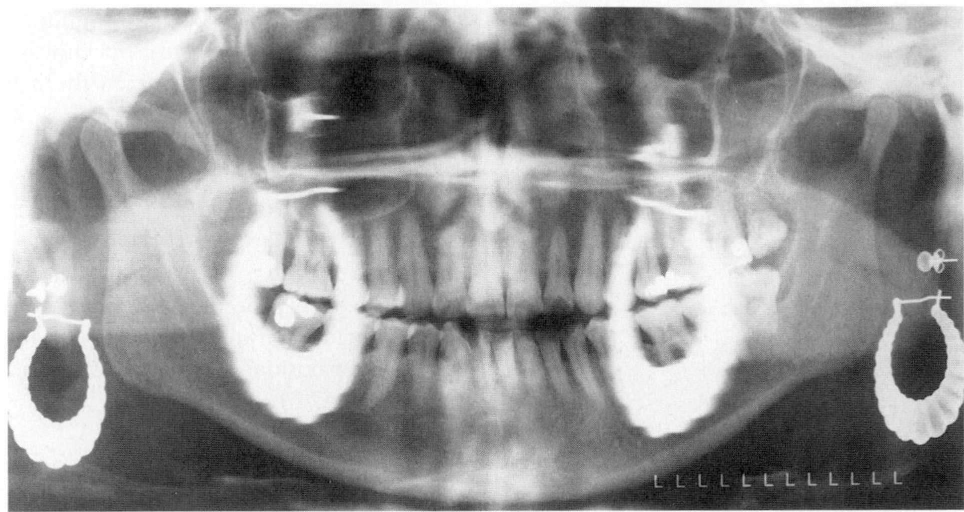

**FIG. 42.8** Hoop earrings and "ghost" images. The ghost image of the earring appears on the opposite side of the image and is enlarged and laterally distorted. *(From Langlais RP, Miller CS: Exercises in oral radiology and interpretation, ed 5, St Louis, 2017, Elsevier.)*

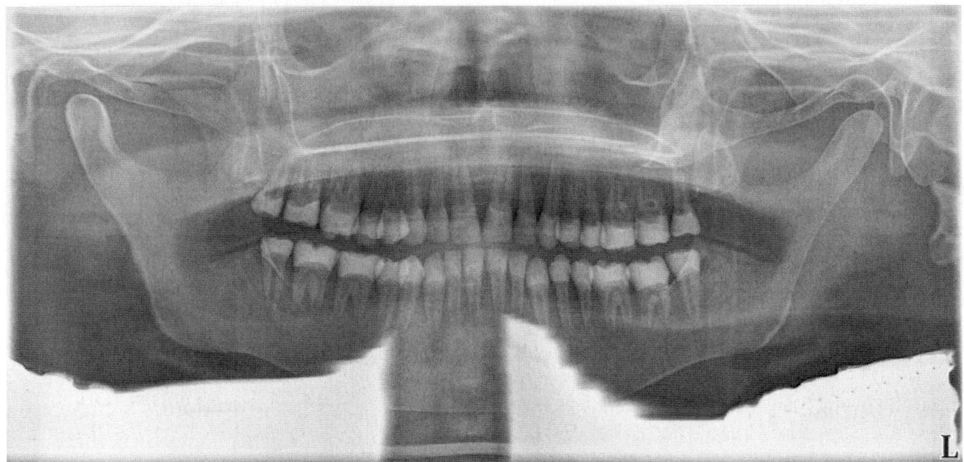

**FIG. 42.9** On a panoramic image, a thyroid collar artifact appears as a bilateral radiopaque artifact obscuring the mandible. *(From Iannucci J, Jansen Howerton L: Dental radiography: principles and techniques, ed 5, St Louis, 2017, Elsevier.)*

## Patient Positioning Errors

**LIPS AND TONGUE.** The patient's lips must be closed on the bite-block during exposure of a panoramic film. If they are not, the result is a dark radiolucent shadow that obscures the anterior teeth. Also, the tongue must be in contact with the palate during exposure of a panoramic film. If it is not, the result is a dark radiolucent shadow that obscures the apices of the maxillary teeth (Fig. 42.10).

***Solution.*** The patient must be instructed to close the lips around the bite-block. The patient must also be instructed to swallow and then raise the tongue up to the palate during exposure of the film.

**CHIN TOO HIGH (POSITIONING OF FRANKFORT PLANE).** If the **Frankfort plane** is incorrect and the patient's chin is positioned too high or is tipped upward, the following problems will occur:

- The hard palate and the floor of the nasal cavity will appear superimposed over the roots of the maxillary teeth.
- Detail in the maxillary incisor region will be lost.
- The maxillary incisors will appear blurred and magnified.
- A "reverse smile line" (curved downward) will be apparent on the radiograph (Fig. 42.11).

***Solution.*** Position the patient so that the Frankfort plane is parallel to the floor.

**CHIN TOO LOW.** If the Frankfort plane is incorrect and the patient's chin is positioned too low or is tipped downward, the following will occur:

- The mandibular incisors will appear blurred.
- Detail in the anterior apical regions will be lost.
- The condyles will not be visible.
- An "exaggerated smile line" (curved upward) will be apparent on the radiograph (Fig. 42.12).

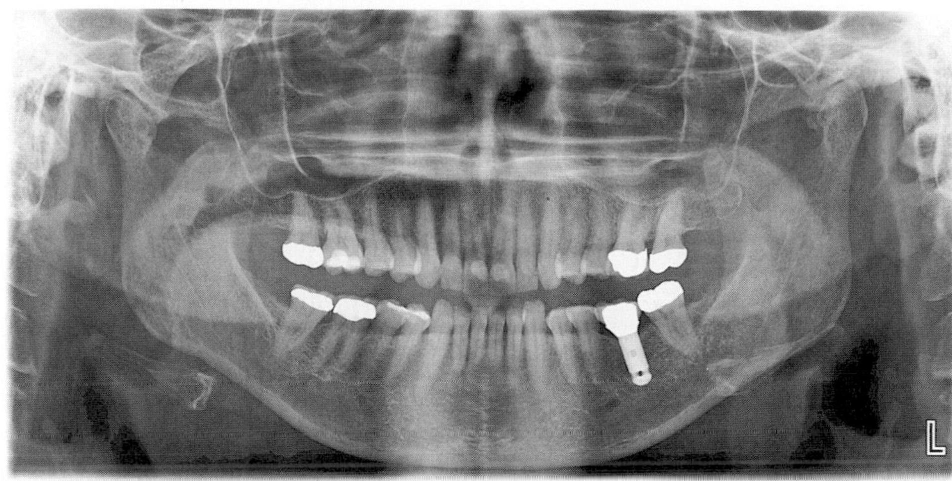


**FIG. 42.10** A radiolucent shadow will be superimposed over the apices of the maxillary teeth if the patient does not keep the tongue against the palate throughout the entire exposure. *(From Langlais RP, Miller CS: Exercises in oral radiology and interpretation, ed 5, St Louis, 2017, Elsevier.)*

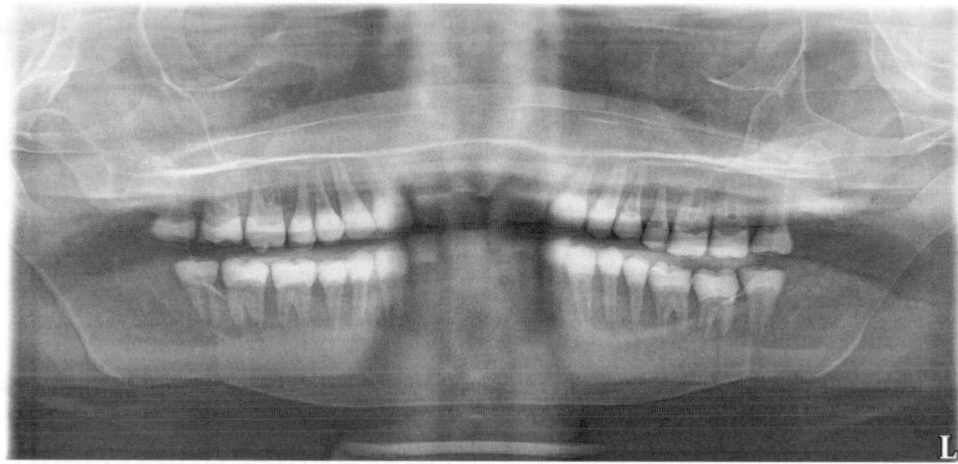


**FIG. 42.11** A "reverse smile line" is seen on a panoramic image when the patient's chin is tipped up. The condyles do not appear on the image. *(From Iannucci J, Jansen Howerton L: Dental radiography: principles and techniques, ed 5, St Louis, 2017, Elsevier.)*

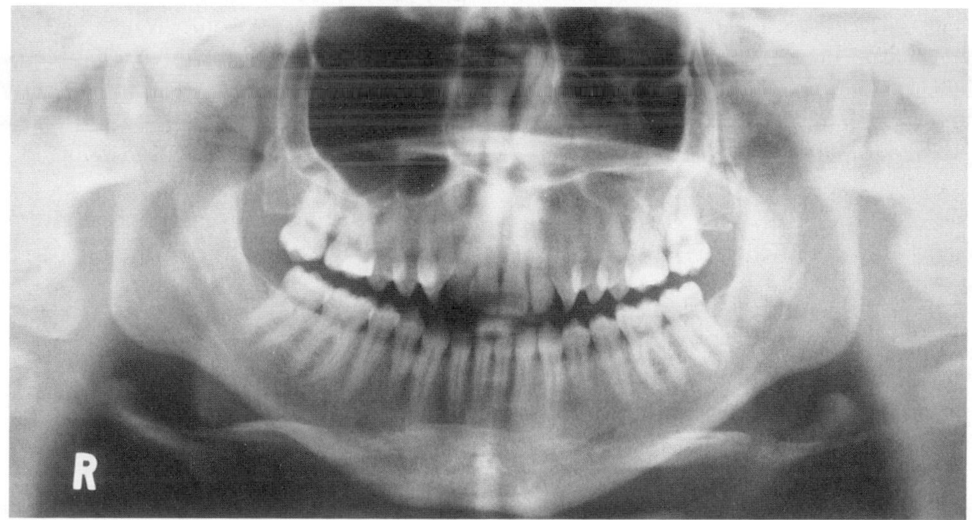


**FIG. 42.12** An "exaggerated smile line" is seen on a panoramic image when the patient's chin is tipped down. The anterior body of the mandible is widened vertically. *(From Langlais RP, Miller CS: Exercises in oral radiology and interpretation, ed 5, St Louis, 2017, Elsevier.)*

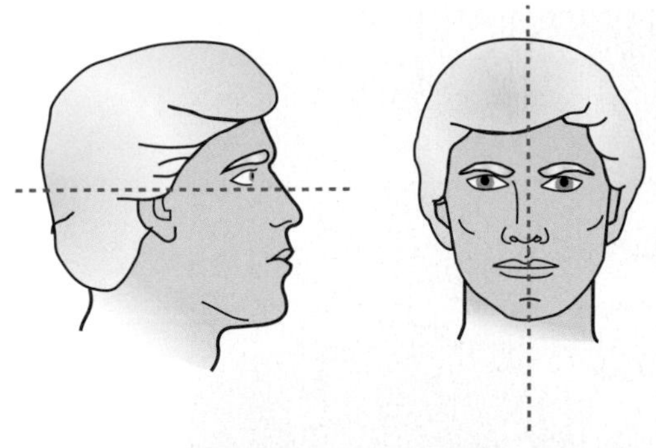


**FIG. 42.13** Frankfort and midsagittal planes. The Frankfort plane passes through the floor of the orbit and the external auditory meatus. The midsagittal plane divides the face in half into right and left sides. *(From Olson SS: Dental radiography laboratory manual, Philadelphia, 1995, Saunders.)*

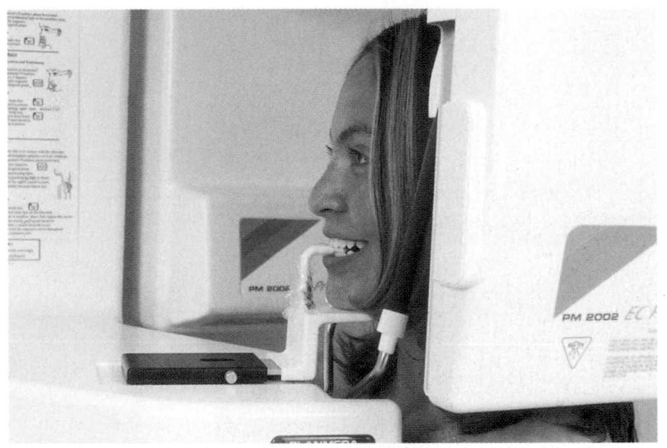

**FIG. 42.14** Patient is biting too far back on the bite stick.

***Solution.*** Position the patient so that the Frankfort plane is parallel to the floor (Fig. 42.13).

**POSTERIOR TO FOCAL TROUGH.** If the patient's anterior teeth are positioned too far back on the bite-block, or posterior to the focal trough (Fig. 42.14), the anterior teeth appear "fat" and out of focus on the radiograph (Fig. 42.15).

***Solution.*** Position the patient so that the anterior teeth are placed in an end-to-end position in the groove on the bite-block.

**ANTERIOR TO FOCAL TROUGH.** If the patient's anterior teeth are not positioned in the groove on the bite-block and are too far forward, or anterior to the focal trough, the teeth appear "skinny" and out of focus (Fig. 42.16).

***Solution.*** Position the patient so that the anterior teeth are placed in an end-to-end position in the groove on the bite-block.

**SPINE NOT STRAIGHT.** If the patient is not standing or sitting with a straight spine, the cervical spine appears as a radiopacity in the center of the film and obscures diagnostic information (Fig. 42.17).

***Solution.*** The patient must be instructed to stand or sit "as tall as possible" with a straight back.

### Tips for Success When Exposing Panoramic Images

- Use a plastic barrier on the bite-block.
- Use the manufacturer's recommendations for exposure factors.
- Explain the procedure to the patient.
- Place the proper type of lead apron.
- Ask the patient to remove all radiolucent objects.
- Ask the patient to sit or stand as straight as possible.
- Ask the patient to place the anterior teeth in the groove on the bite-block.
- Position the patient with the midsagittal plane perpendicular to the floor.
- Position the patient with the Frankfort plane parallel to the floor.
- Ask the patient to close the lips on the bite-block and to swallow and place the tongue against the roof of the mouth.
- Ask the patient to remain still during the exposure.

2 What type of image might have been needed to supplement a panoramic image taken with radiographic film? Why?
3 What is a focal trough?

## Three-Dimensional Digital Imaging

To better understand cone beam technology (CBCT), you should first understand what regular **computed tomography (CT)** is. CT imaging, also referred to as a computed axial tomography (CAT) scan, produces a *two-dimensional (2D) image.* It involves the use of x-ray equipment that rotates around the head, and it is combined with a digital computer to obtain images (slices) of specific areas of the body. CT images are digital and need no film; however, x-radiation is used as the energy source. CT images have long been used in medicine because CT has the ability to provide clear images of bone, muscle, and blood vessels. In dentistry it has been used primarily for diagnosing lesions and planning implant cases.

### Cone Beam Computed Tomography

All of the radiographic images discussed until this point have been 2D images. A new technology termed **cone beam computed tomography (CBCT)** now allows the viewing of the head and neck in *three dimensions.* CBCT is so named because it uses a cone-shaped x-ray beam to acquire 3D information. **Three-dimensional digital imaging** in dentistry

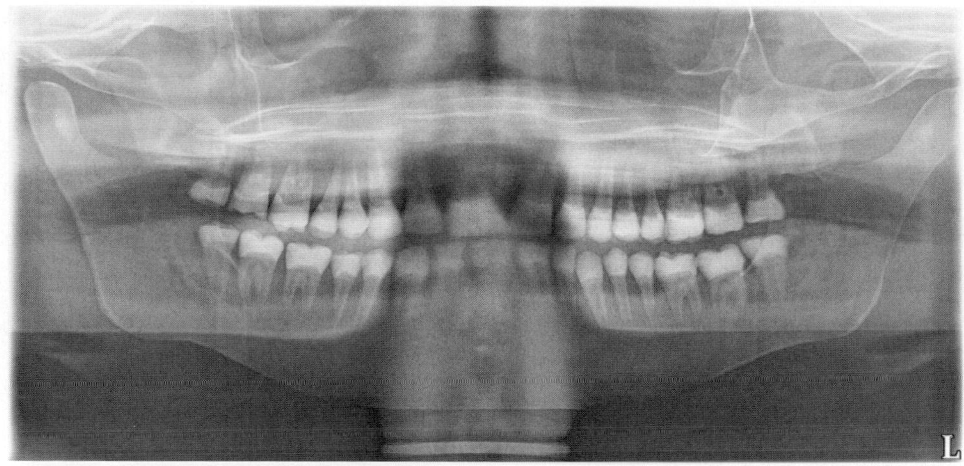


**FIG. 42.15** Anterior teeth appear widened and blurred on the panoramic image when the patient's teeth are positioned too far back on the bite-block. *(From Iannucci J, Jansen Howerton L: Dental radiography: principles and techniques, ed 5, St Louis, 2017, Elsevier.)*

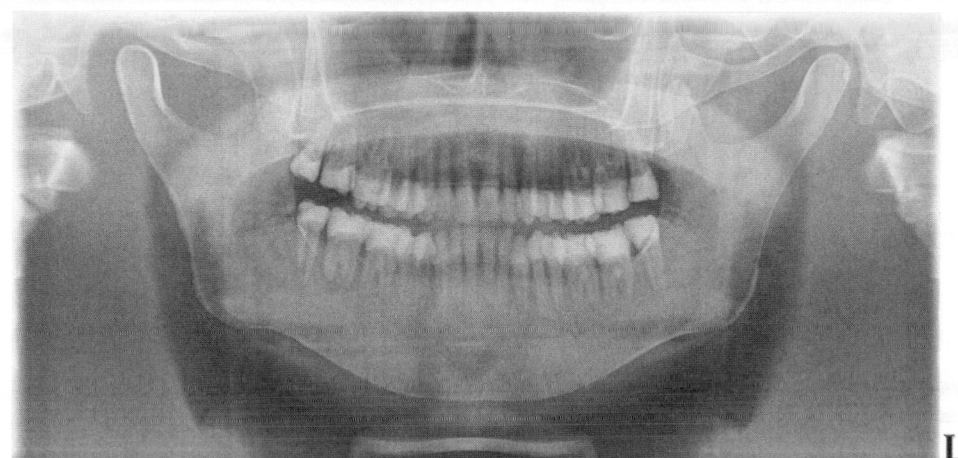


**FIG. 42.16** Anterior teeth appear narrowed and blurred on the panoramic image when the patient's teeth are positioned too far forward on the bite-block. *(From Iannucci J, Jansen Howerton L: Dental radiography: principles and techniques, ed 5, St Louis, 2017, Elsevier.)*

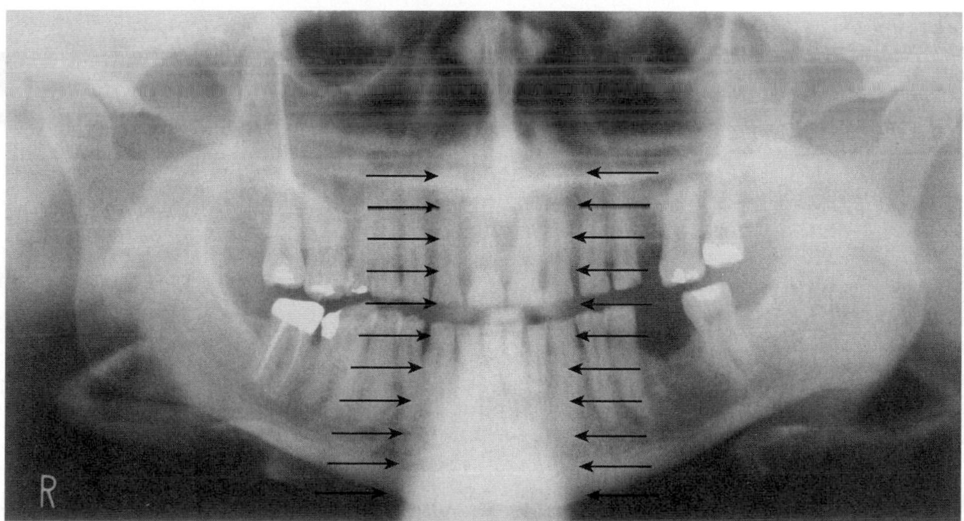


**FIG. 42.17** If the patient is not standing erect, superimposition of the cervical spine *(arrows)* may be seen at the center of the panoramic image. *(From Langlais RP, Miller CS: Exercises in oral radiology and interpretation, ed 5, St Louis, 2017, Elsevier.)*

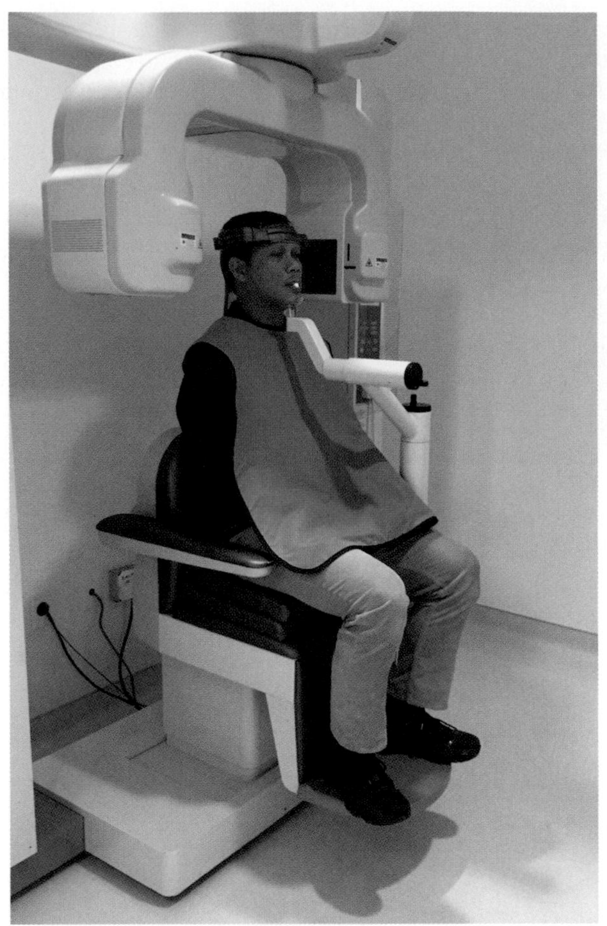

**FIG. 42.18** Next-generation i-CAT dental imaging system. Cone beam computed tomography (CBCT) machines have a small footprint and are equivalent to a digital Panorex. The patient is comfortably seated within the machine and does not feel claustrophobic.

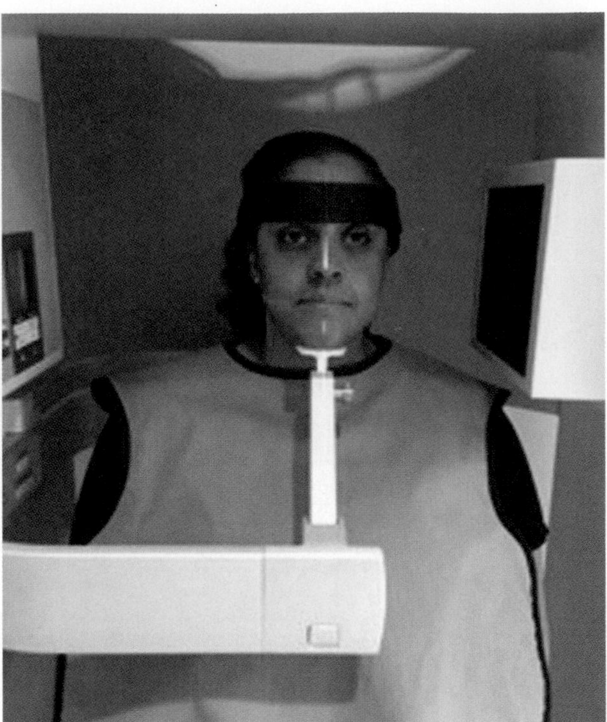

**FIG. 42.19** Lighting assists the operator in properly adjusting the machine.

has become very important because of the detailed information it provides.

### How CBCT Works

During a cone beam CT examination, the arm rotates around the patient's head in a complete 360-degree rotation. While doing this, it takes anywhere from 200 to 600 2D images that the software collects, and then digitally combines them to form a 3D image that can provide the dentist or oral surgeon with valuable information. The floor space required for a CBCT scanner is about the same as that required for a panoramic unit. Compared with traditional CT procedures, cone beam imaging involves a lower radiation dose to the patient. Studies have determined the dose given for a typical CBCT scan to be comparable with the dose given for three or four full-mouth series of intraoral radiographs. Scan times vary between 7 and 30 seconds. The short exposure time decreases the chances for motion artifacts to occur. Motion artifacts occur when a patient moves during the radiographic procedure. This type of artifact may occur with both 2D and 3D imaging. To minimize movement, CBCT machines are equipped with devices to stabilize the head and the neck of the patient, and the patient also should be given oral instructions to remain still during exposure (Figs. 42.18 and 42.19).

When using conventional imaging techniques, periapical and bite-wing images focus on specific teeth. When using CBCT, however, the area of interest is termed the **field of view**. Manufacturers of 3D imaging use a variety of sizes to accommodate the appropriate field of view for diagnostic purposes.

Unlike conventional 2D imaging, this amazing technology provides 3D views of the mouth, face, and jaw from any direction (Fig. 42.20). The manufacturers of these units can provide software programs that make it possible to see all anatomic structures clearly, including soft tissue. Some programs even overlay the patient's facial image onto the radiographic image (Fig. 42.21).

The digital images can be easily adjusted, manipulated, and colorized on the computer (Fig. 42.22). Because the images are digitized, they can be easily sent over the Internet, allowing for collaboration and consultation on cases.

## Advantages of Three-Dimensional Views

Panoramic images are 2D and therefore cannot provide any information about buccal or lingual width or locations, nor can they distinguish between types of soft tissues. CBCT has greatly enhanced the diagnostic abilities of the dentist by providing 3D information that is vital for the exact placement

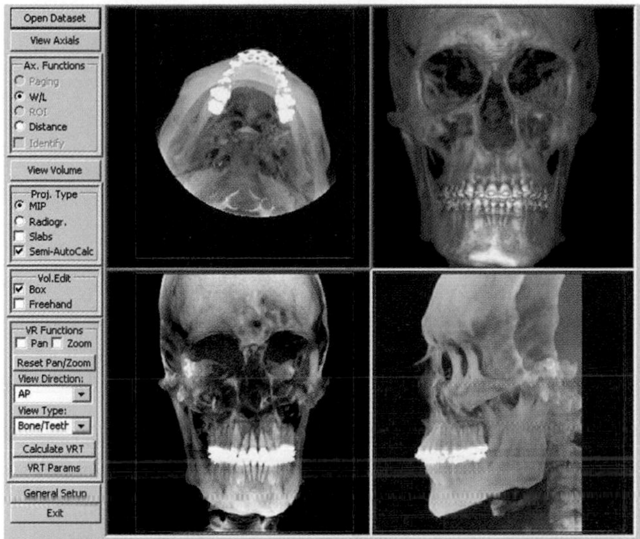


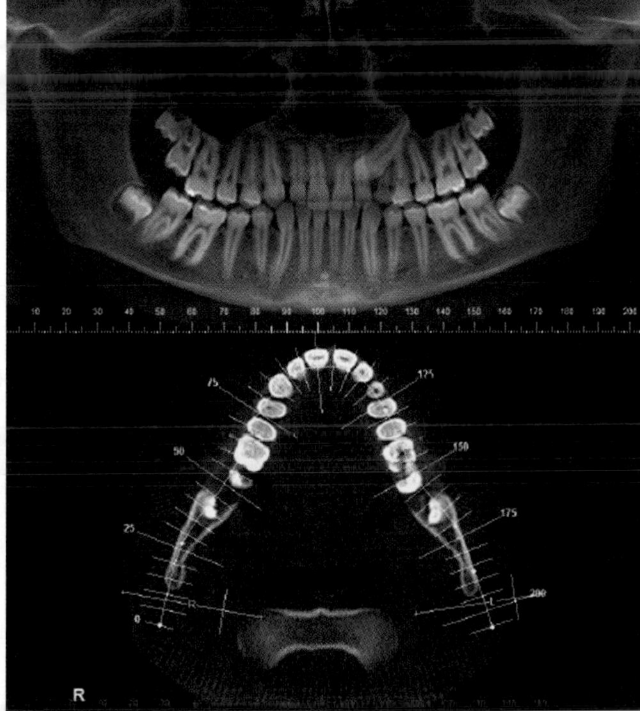


FIG 42.20 A sample of the types of views offered by software modules. Most have settings to customize contrast and to select only the area of interest. *(Courtesy of KaVo Kerr.)*

of implants, the buccal/lingual position of impacted teeth that are to be removed, and determination of the exact location of the mandibular nerve before surgery is performed (Fig. 42.23).

## Common Uses of Cone Beam Computed Tomography

CBCT is revolutionizing the practice of dentistry. Some of the common uses of 3D imaging include the following: implant placement (Fig. 42.24), extraction or exposure of impacted teeth, endodontic assessment, evaluation of temporomandibular joint (TMJ) disorders, orthodontic evaluation, and pathology evaluation.

More dentists and especially dental specialists (periodontists, orthodontists, oral maxillofacial surgeons, and general dentists who are doing implants) are investing in CBCT units for their offices (Fig. 42.25). Dentists without a CBCT unit in their own office may refer a patient needing a 3D image to a colleague who does have a CBCT unit to have the images taken.

It is not difficult to learn to use the CBCT hardware, but time for training is necessary. The training is very similar to that needed to take panoramic images. Additional training is required for the dentist to learn to interpret the images because they are presented in a 3D view, or as tomographic slices.

Three-dimensional digital imaging has become increasingly important in dentistry and is quickly becoming the desired technology because of the accurate information it provides.

### Uses for CBCT

- Surgical planning for impacted teeth
- Diagnosing temporomandibular joint (TMJ) disorder
- Accurate placement of dental implants
- Evaluation of the jaw, sinuses, nerve canals, and nasal cavity
- Detecting, measuring, and treating tumors of the jaw
- Determining bone structure and tooth orientation
- Locating the origin of pain or pathology
- Cephalometric analysis for orthodontics
- Reconstructive surgery

### Advantages and Disadvantages of CBCT

**Advantages**

- Lower radiation dose
- Brief scanning time
- Anatomically accurate images
- Ability to save and easily transport images

**Disadvantages**

- Patient movement causes artifacts
- Size of field of view
- Cost of equipment and need to learn a new computer language
- Training in interpretation of image data

RECALL

4 Why is a CBCT image better than a periapical image?
5 Why are CBCT images better than a panoramic image?

## Specialized Extraoral Imaging

### Equipment

As with intraoral images, extraoral images may be obtained using film-based or digital systems. A standard intraoral x-ray machine may be used for a variety of extraoral

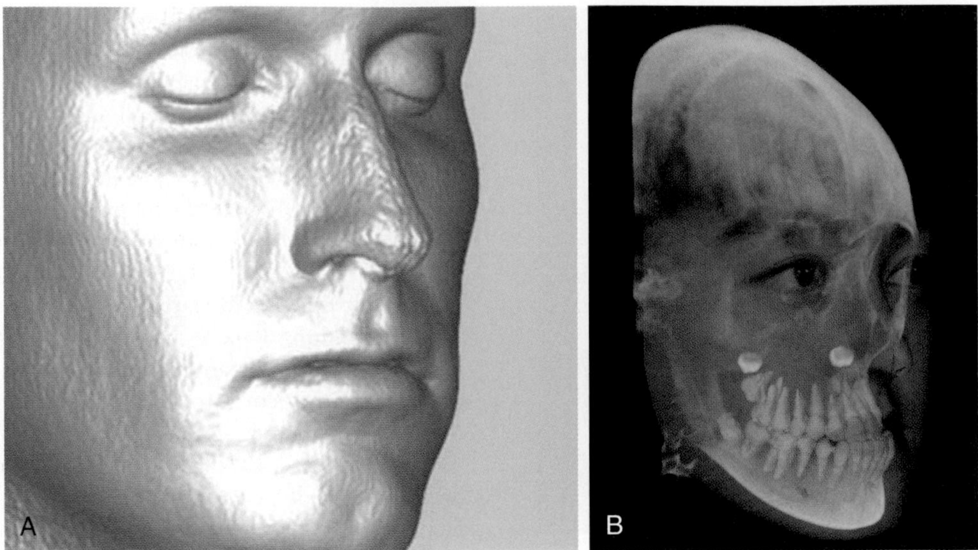


**FIG. 42.21** A, Soft-tissue anatomy captured using cone beam computed tomography (CBCT) technology (i-CATVision software). B, Skeletal anatomy captured from CBCT data and superimposed on a digital photograph (InVivo Dental 3-D Imaging Software). This allows the practitioner to see how dental and skeletal changes will alter facial soft tissue. *(A, Courtesy of KaVo Kerr. B, Courtesy Anatomage, San Jose, CA.)*

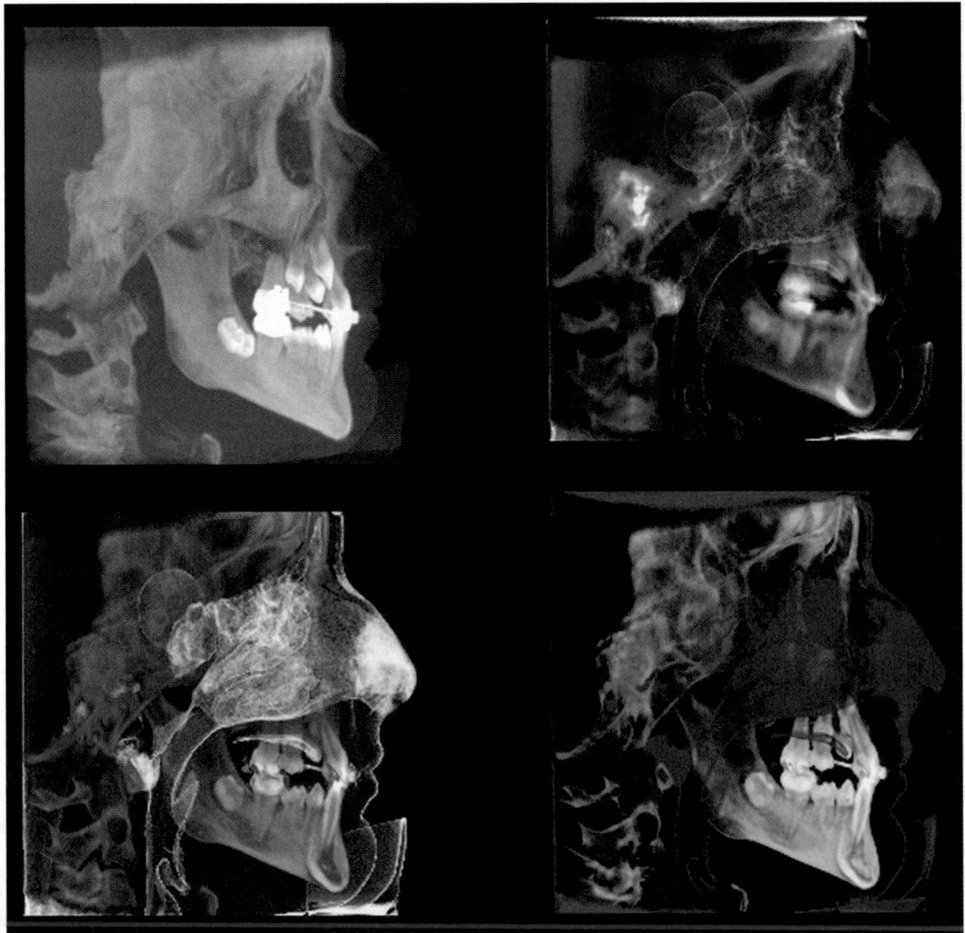

**FIG. 42.22** Digital images allow for custom coloring of soft tissues to assess airway anatomy and sinus morphology (InVivo Dental 3-D Imaging Software). They provide information on the entire maxillofacial region. *(Courtesy Anatomage, San Jose, CA.)*

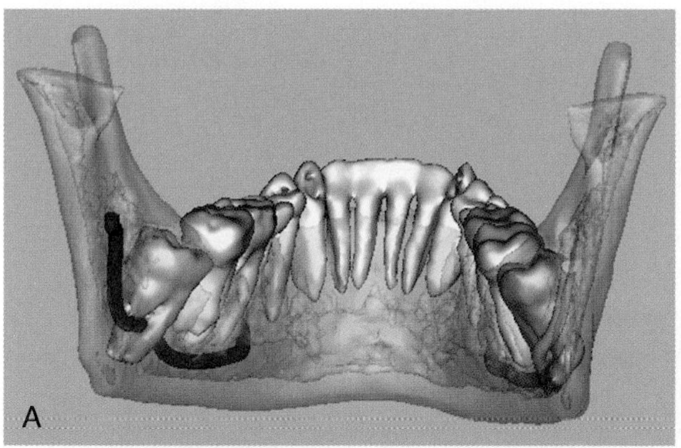


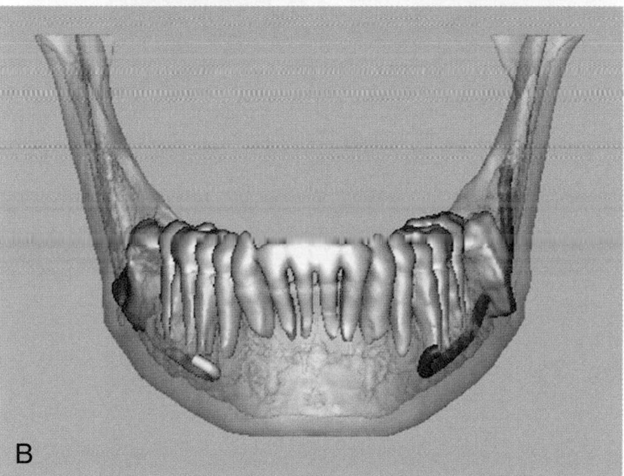


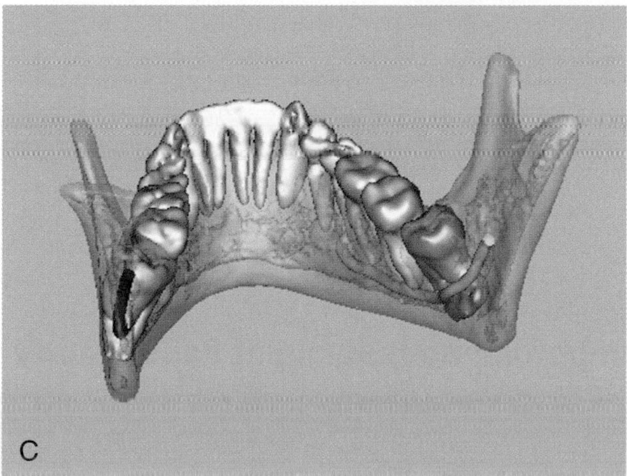


**FIG. 42.23** A, Impacted mandibular third molars (tooth #17 in green; tooth #32 in pink). Note the roots of #17 surrounding the mandibular canal. B, Teeth #17 and #32 positioned facial to the mandibular canal. C, Transparent mandible showing full view of the location of the mandibular. *(Courtesy Carolina OMF Imaging, Dr. Bruce Howerton, Jr., Raleigh, NC.)*

projections, including transcranial and lateral jaw. Special head positioning and beam alignment devices are attached to the intraoral x-ray machine for use in positioning the patient's head. Some panoramic x-ray units also may be fitted with special devices known as *cephalostats.* The **cephalostat** includes a film holder and a head positioner; these allow the operator to easily position both the film and the patient (Fig. 42.26).

### Film and Intensifying Screens

Most extraoral exposures use screen film placed in a cassette that has an intensifying screen. An occlusal film (size #4) may be used for some extraoral radiographs, such as lateral jaw or transcranial projections. An occlusal film is a *nonscreen film* that does not require a cassette; however, it requires more radiation than is needed with a screen film (see Chapter 39).

### Grid

A grid is a device that is used to reduce the amount of *scatter radiation* that reaches an extraoral film during exposure (Fig. 42.27). As is discussed in Chapter 39, scatter radiation causes film fog and reduces film contrast. A grid decreases film fog and increases the contrast of the radiographic image.

A grid is composed of a series of thin lead strips embedded in plastic that permits passage of the x-ray beam. The grid is placed between the patient's head and the film. During exposure, the grid permits passage of the beam between the lead strips. When certain x-rays interact with the patient's tissues, scatter radiation is produced, which is then directed at the grid and film at an angle. As a result, scatter radiation is absorbed by the lead strips and does not reach the surface of the film to cause film fog.

Despite the benefits of grid use, exposure time must be increased to compensate for the lead strips found in the grid. Therefore a grid should be used only when improved image quality and high contrast are necessary to minimize radiation to the patient.

## Procedures

Step-by-step procedures for the exposure of an extraoral film involve the same equipment preparation, patient preparation, and patient positioning as for panoramic radiographs (see Procedures 42.1 to 42.3). Before an extraoral film is exposed, infection control procedures must be completed (see Chapter 40). If an extraoral x-ray unit with a cephalostat is used, the ear rods must be wiped with a disinfectant between patients.

## Skull Radiography

Skull radiography is used most often in oral surgery and orthodontics. Although some skull films can be exposed with a standard intraoral radiograph machine, most require the use of an extraoral unit and cephalostat.

Skull radiographs may be difficult to interpret because of the numerous anatomic structures that exist in this area. Often, these structures appear superimposed over one another. In many cases, multiple exposures may be

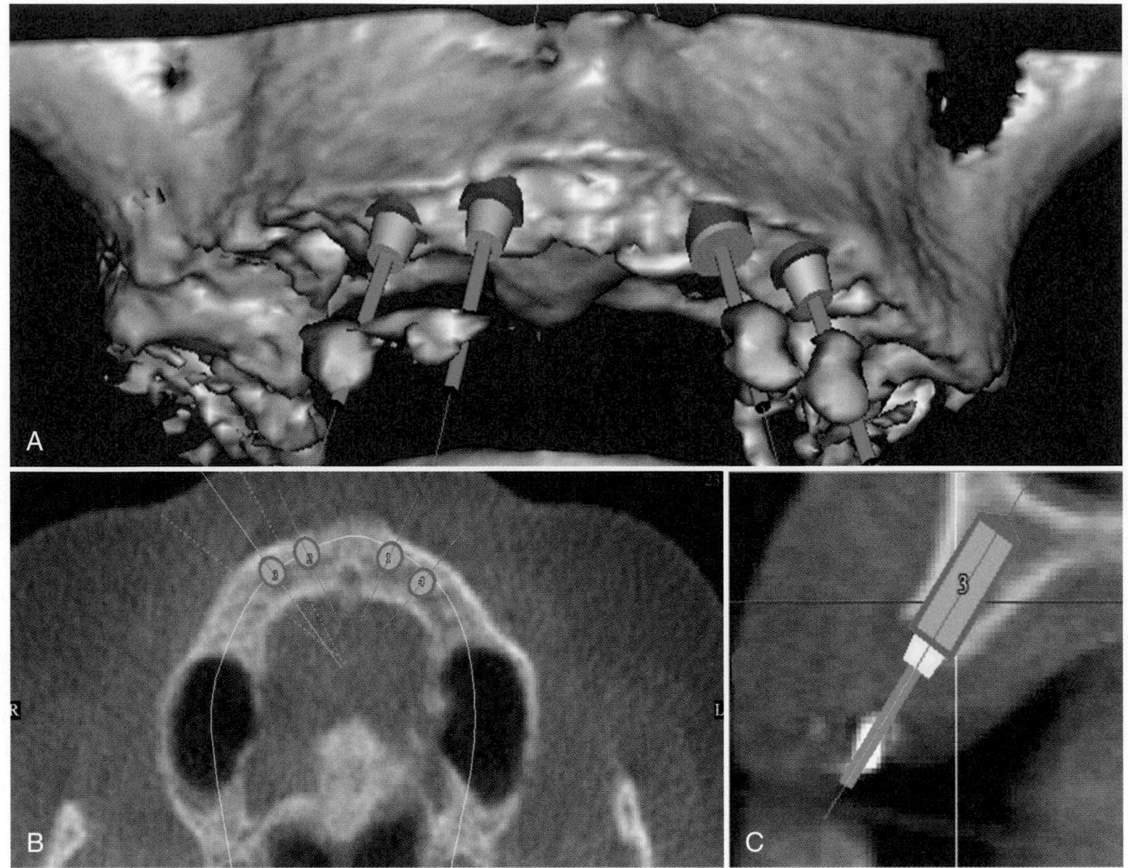


**FIG. 42.24** Visual simulation for implant placement. A, A totally edentulous maxilla showing alignment of four virtual implant fixtures. B, Anterior-posterior spread of the position of the implants. C, Cross-sectional image of the right maxillary canine shows the buccopalatal emergence profile (green line) and position (implant in light pink). *(From White SC, Pharoah MJ: Oral radiology: principles and interpretation, ed 7, St Louis, 2014, Mosby. Images created with Virtual Implant Placement (VIP), Biohorizons IPH, Inc. Birmingham, AL.)*

necessary to obtain a clear view of the area in question. The most common skull radiographs used in dentistry include the following:

- Lateral cephalometric projection
- Posteroanterior projection
- Temporomandibular joint projection

### Lateral Cephalometric Projection

The lateral cephalometric projection is used to evaluate facial growth and development, trauma, disease, and developmental abnormalities. This projection shows the bones of the face and skull, as well as the soft tissue profile (Fig. 42.28).

### Posteroanterior Projection

The posteroanterior projection is used to evaluate facial growth and development, trauma, disease, and developmental abnormalities. This projection shows the frontal and ethmoid sinuses, the orbits, and the nasal cavities (Fig. 42.29).

## Temporomandibular Joint Radiography

The **temporomandibular joint (TMJ)** is the *jaw joint.* This area can be very difficult to examine radiographically because of the multiple adjacent bony structures.

Radiography *cannot* be used to examine the articular disc and other soft tissues of the TMJ. Instead, special imaging techniques such as arthrography and CBCT must be used. Radiographic projections of the TMJ, however, can be used to show the bone and the relationship of the jaw joint. For example, changes in bone can be seen on transcranial TMJ radiographs (Fig. 42.30).

6 What is the name of the device that may be added to a panoramic unit to allow the operator to easily position the film and patient?
7 What is the purpose of a grid?
8 What type of imaging is best for soft tissues of the TMJ?

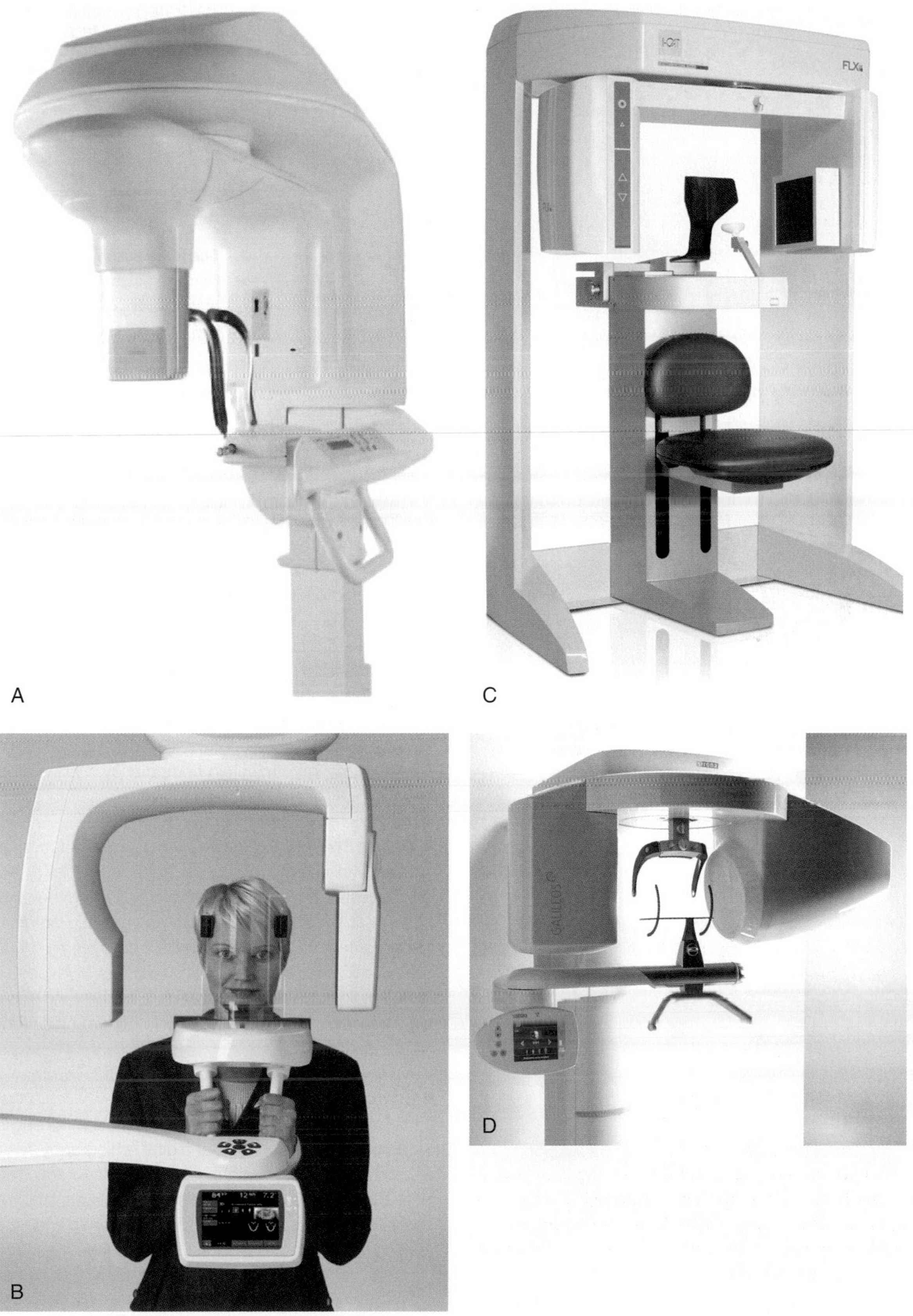


**FIG. 42.25** Examples of cone beam computed tomography machines. A, CS 9000D 3D Extraoral Imaging System. B, Planmeca Promax 3D. C, i-CAT FLX Cone Beam 3D system. D, Comfort 3D Imaging System. E, NewTom VGi. *(A, Courtesy Carestream Health, Inc., Rochester, NY.* B, *Courtesy Planmeca USA, Inc., Roselle, IL.* C, *Imaging Sciences International, Inc., Hatfield, PA.* D, *Courtesy Sirona Dental Systems, Charlotte, NC.* E, *Courtesy NewTom, Verona, Italy.)*

E

FIG. 42.25, Cont'd

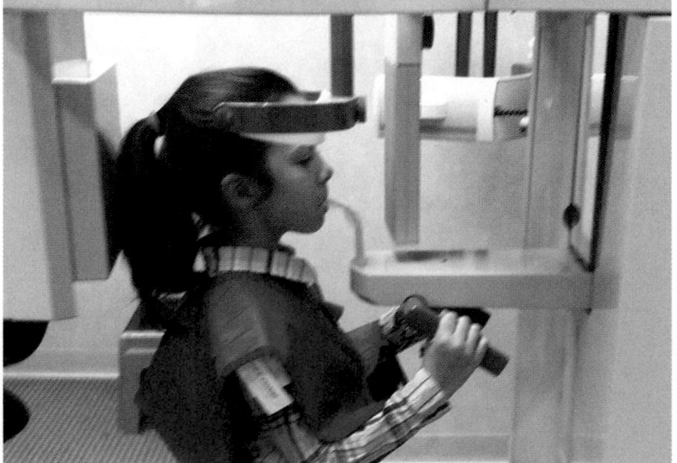

FIG. 42.26 Panoramic images being taken on a patient. Note the head positioner in place.

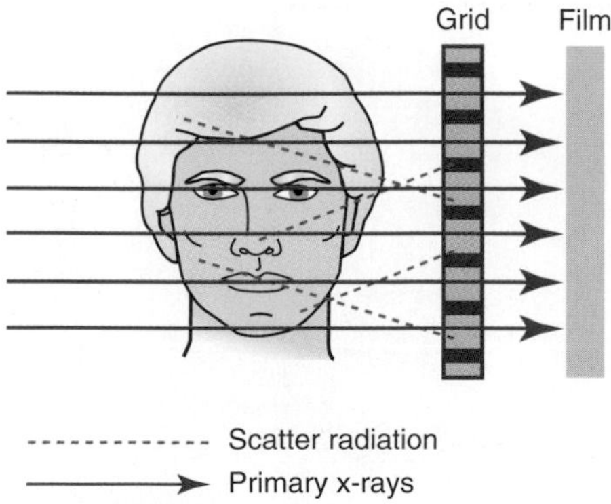


**FIG. 42.27** A grid decreases the amount of scatter radiation that reaches the extraoral film. *(Courtesy Dr. Robert M. Jaynes, Columbus, OH.)*

**■ Legal and Ethical Implications** It is the dentist who is ultimately responsible for the diagnostic quality of all dental radiographs exposed in his or her office, regardless of who exposes and processes the film. In the majority of dental offices, the dental assistant is most often the person who actually exposes and processes the film. The dentist relies on the dental assistant to be competent in both exposure and processing techniques. If the dental assistant produces a nondiagnostic image, the radiograph must be retaken. If there is an error in processing, the radiograph must be retaken. Whatever the reason, *all* retakes cause unnecessary exposure to x-radiation for the patient. It is the dental assistant's ethical responsibility to continually strive to maintain competency in all types of dental imaging. ■

**■ Eye to the Future** In the not too distant future, patients who are well informed will understand the benefits of CBCT and will request to have one taken before allowing their dentist to perform an extraction or to place an implant. Parents will come to expect that a CBCT for their children is an important part of orthodontic treatment. There is little doubt by experts involved in dental radiography, dental implant placement, orthodontics, and legal issues that CBCT will, one day, become the standard of care in dentistry. ■

## ■ Critical Thinking

1. You have just begun a new job in a beautiful and modern dental office that has total digital radiography. Mr. McKenzie is a new patient scheduled for a panoramic radiograph and a dental examination. In your previous job, you always took bitewings in addition to a panoramic image for patients who were going to have a dental examination. Your new employer told you that bitewings would not be necessary. Why do you think bitewing images would not be necessary in this case?

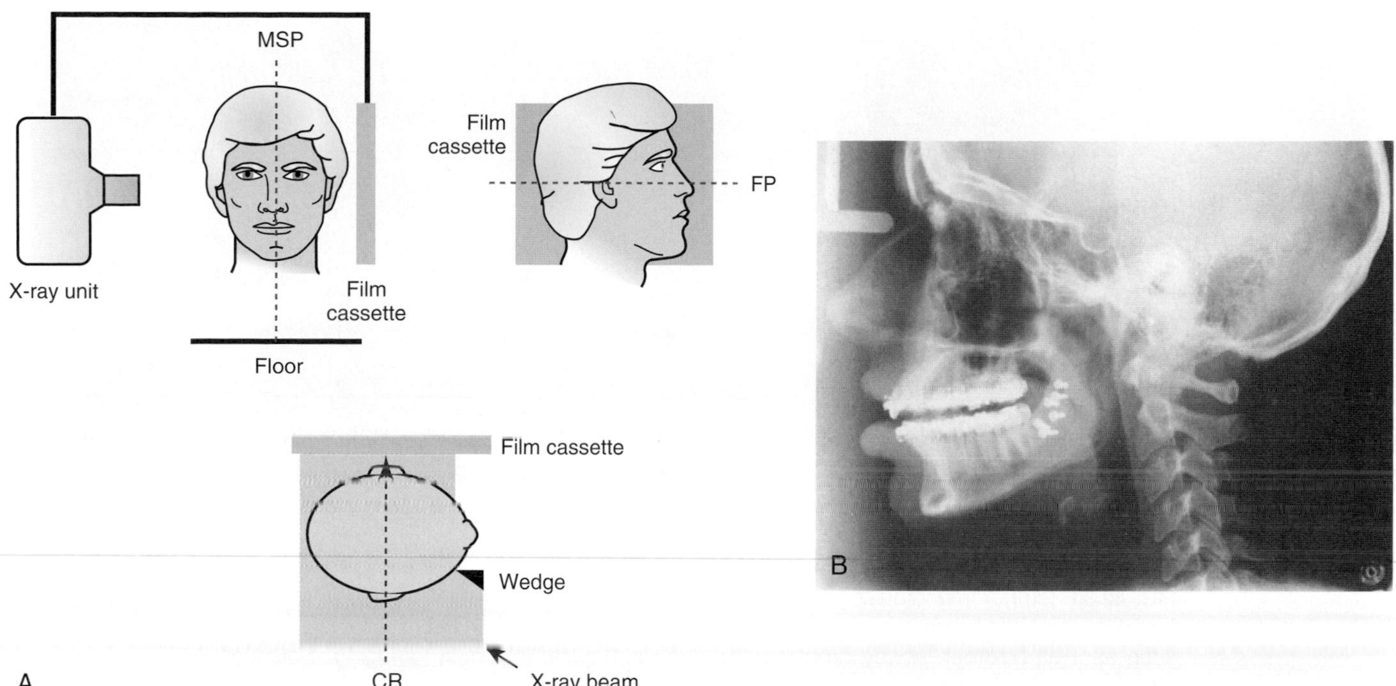


**FIG. 42.28** A, For the lateral cephalometric projection, proper patient and film positioning is shown as viewed from the front, side, and top of the patient. *CR,* Central ray; *FP,* Frankfort plane; *MSP,* midsagittal projection. B, Lateral cephalometric radiograph. *(Courtesy Dr. Robert M. Jaynes, Columbus, OH.)*

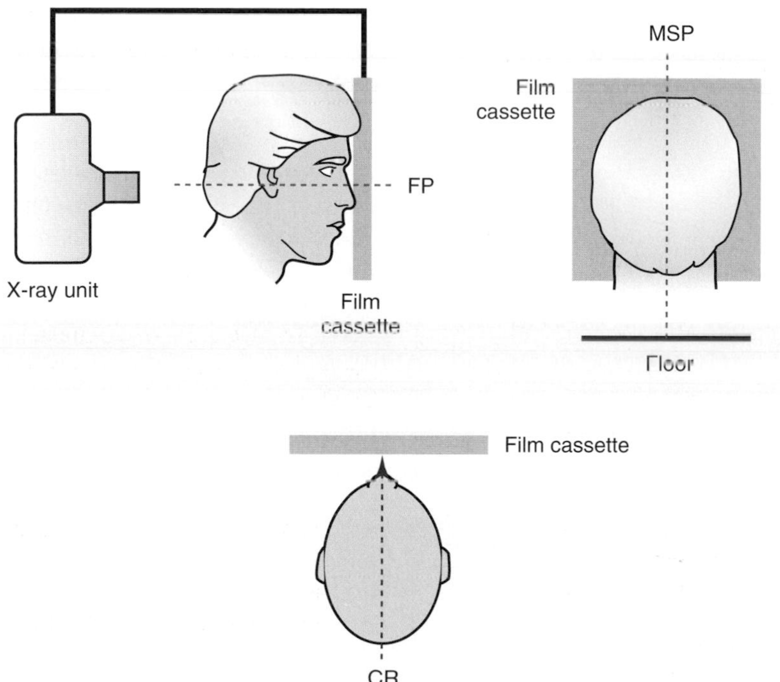


**FIG. 42.29** For the posteroanterior skull projection, proper patient and film positioning is shown as viewed from the side, back, and top of the patient. *CR,* Central ray; *FP,* Frankfort plane; *MSP,* midsagittal projection. *(Courtesy Dr. Robert M. Jaynes, Columbus, OH.)*

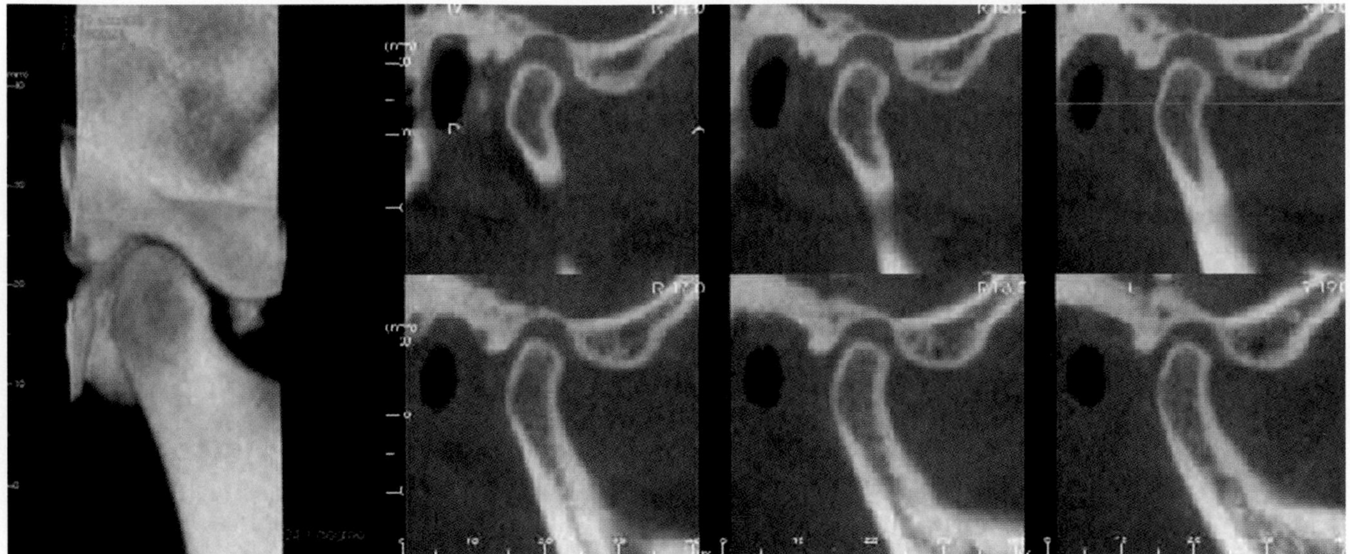

**FIG. 42.30** Temporomandibular joint (TMJ) pathology viewed from three dimensions. Cone beam imaging can be used in diagnosing a variety of conditions within the maxillofacial region, such as TMJ disorder, airway problems, tumors, and cysts. *(Courtesy Imaging Sciences International Inc., Hatfield, PA.)*

2. After processing Mr. McKenzie's panoramic film, you notice that the anterior teeth appear very wide and distorted. What could have been the problem?
3. A good friend is going to have two dental implants placed, and her dentist recommended a CBCT first. Your friend told you that she has never heard of this procedure and asks you for your opinion whether or not she should agree with the dentist and have a CBCT before having the implants placed. How would you answer your friend's question? ■

PROCEDURE 42.1

## Preparing Equipment for Panoramic Imaging

**GOAL**

To prepare the equipment necessary for a panoramic procedure.

**EQUIPMENT AND SUPPLIES FOR FILM-BASED UNITS**

- ✔ Extraoral film
- ✔ Cassette
- ✔ Infection control barriers

**PROCEDURAL STEPS**

1 Load the panoramic cassette in the darkroom under safelight conditions. Handle the film only by its edges to avoid fingerprints.
**PURPOSE** The panoramic film is sensitive to light, and the remainder of the film in the box will be ruined if it is exposed to light.

2 Place all infection control barriers and containers.

3 Cover the bite-block with a disposable plastic barrier. If the bite-block is not covered, it must be sterilized before it is used on the next patient.
**PURPOSE** The bite-block is considered a semicritical item that must be disposable or sterilized.

4 Cover or disinfect (or both) any part of the machine that comes in contact with the patient.
**PURPOSE** Parts of the machine that touch the patient but are not used intraorally are considered noncritical items and must be disinfected with a high-level disinfectant.

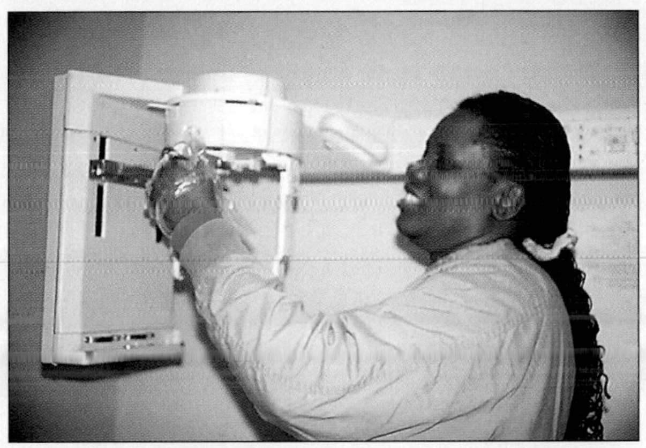

5 Set the exposure factors (kilovoltage, milliamperage) according to the manufacturer's recommendations.

6 Adjust the machine to accommodate the height of the patient; align all movable parts properly.

7 Load the cassette into the carrier of the panoramic unit.

PROCEDURE 42.2

## Preparing the Patient for Panoramic Imaging

**GOAL**

To prepare a patient for a panoramic image.

**EQUIPMENT AND SUPPLIES**

- ✔ Double-sided lead apron (or style recommended by the manufacturer)
- ✔ Plastic container

**PROCEDURAL STEPS**

1 Explain the procedure to the patient. Give the patient the opportunity to ask questions.
**PURPOSE** The patient has the right to be informed and must give consent to the procedure.

2 Ask the patient to remove all objects from the head and neck area; this includes eyeglasses, earrings, lip-piercing and tongue-piercing objects, necklaces, napkin chains, hearing aids, hairpins, and complete and partial dentures. Place objects in a container.
**PURPOSE** If not removed, these objects will appear on the image and could superimpose on diagnostic information.

3 Place a double-sided (for protecting the front and back of the patient) lead apron on the patient, or use the style of lead apron recommended by the manufacturer.
**NOTE** The apron should not cover the back of the patient's neck.
**NOTE** A thyroid collar is not recommended for all panoramic units because it blocks part of the beam and obscures important anatomic structures. Refer to the manufacturer's instructions for the unit you use.

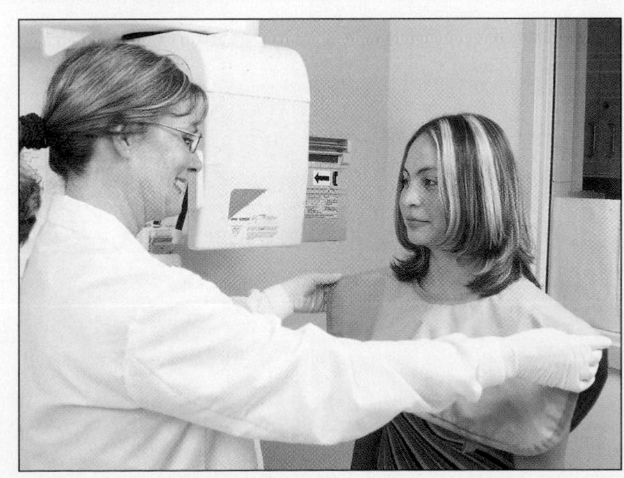

PROCEDURE 42.3 

# Positioning the Patient for Panoramic Imaging

## GOAL

To position the patient for a panoramic procedure.

## PROCEDURAL STEPS

1 Instruct the patient to sit or stand "as tall as possible" with the back straight and erect.

**PURPOSE** The spinal column is very dense; if the spine is not straight, a white shadow appears over the middle of the image and obscures diagnostic information.

2 Instruct the patient to bite on the plastic bite-block and then slide the upper and lower teeth into the notch (groove) on the end of the bite-block.

**PURPOSE** The groove aligns the teeth in the focal trough.

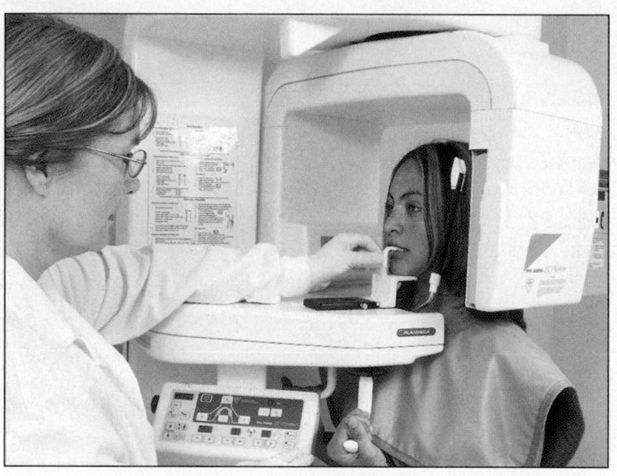

3 Position the midsagittal plane perpendicular to the floor.

**PURPOSE** If the patient's head is tipped or tilted to one side, a distorted image will result.

4 Position the Frankfort plane (the imaginary plane that passes through the top of the ear canal and the bottom of the eye socket) parallel with the floor.

**PURPOSE** The occlusal plane will be positioned at the correct angle.

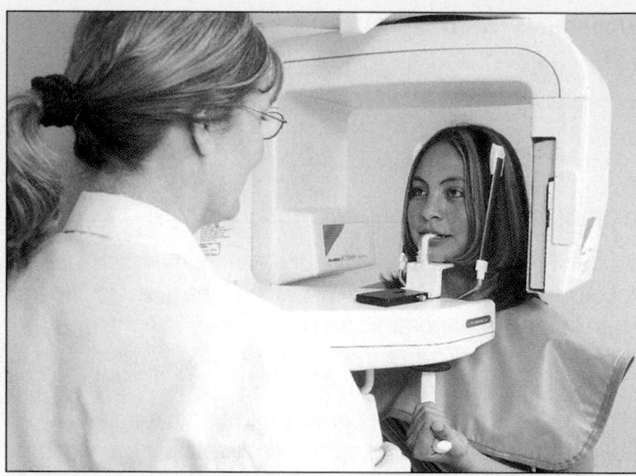

5 Instruct the patient to position the tongue on the roof of the mouth and then to close the lips around the bite-block.

**PURPOSE** If the tongue is not placed on the roof of the mouth, a radiolucent shadow will be superimposed over the apices of the maxillary teeth.

6 After the patient has been positioned, instruct him or her to remain still while the machine rotates during exposure.

**PURPOSE** Any movement of the patient will result in a blurred image.

7 Expose the film and proceed with film processing as described in Chapter 39.

8 Document the procedure.

| Date | Procedure | Operator |
|---|---|---|
| 8/15/17 | Exposed panoramic image | PJL |

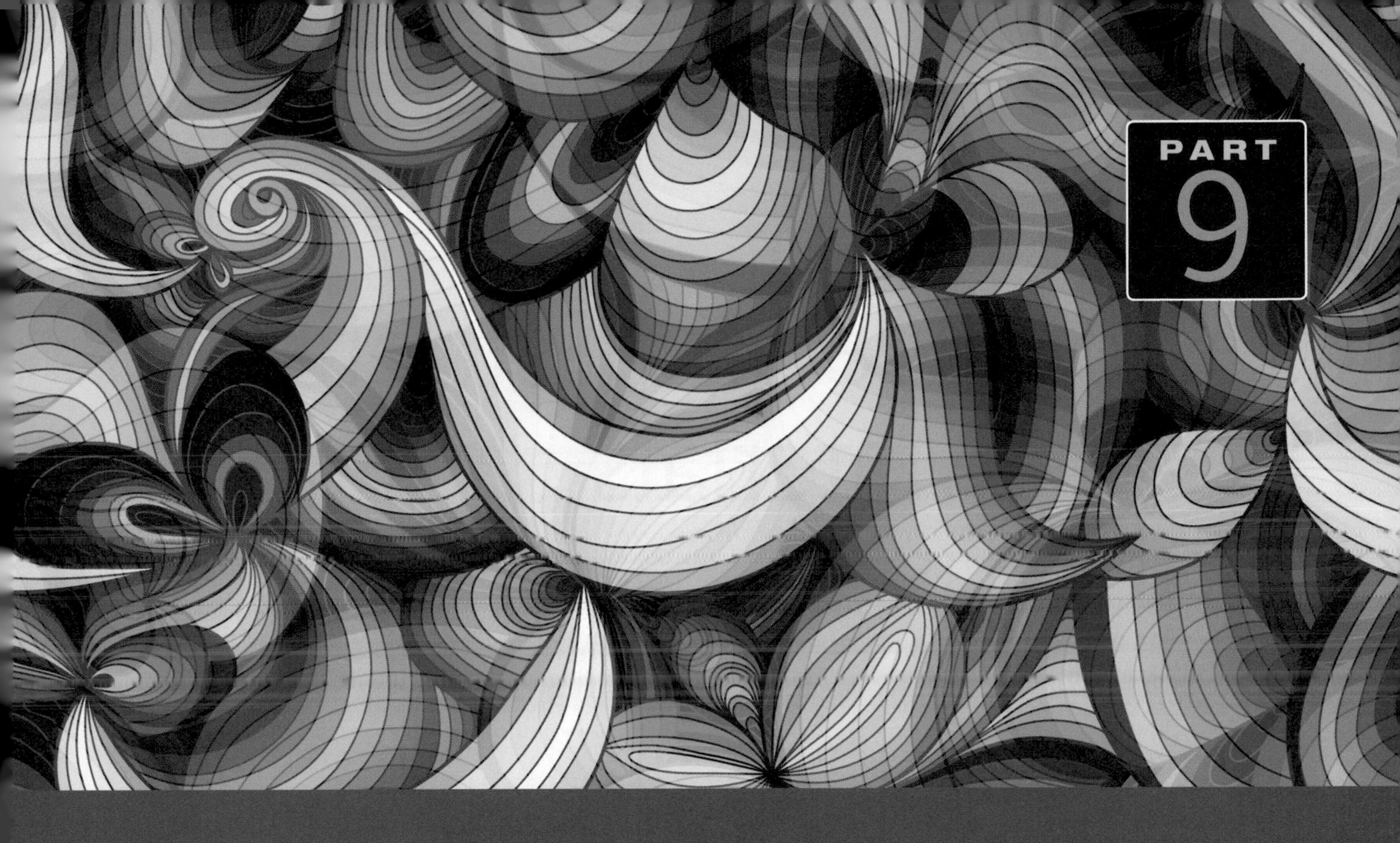


# Dental Materials

The clinical use of dental materials is an essential component of most dental procedures. The role of the dental assistant in the preparation and application of a dental material is an integral part of this process.

The chapters in this section will provide you with the level of background knowledge and skill necessary to become competent with the dental materials used today in the clinical setting. The presentation of dental materials in the following chapters will guide and advance your skill level for working in the general and specialized areas of dentistry.

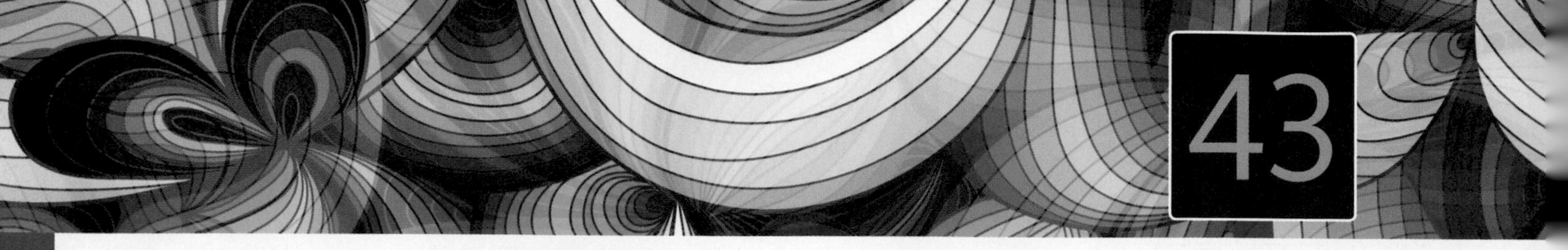


# Restorative and Esthetic Dental Materials

## KEY TERMS

**Adhere** To stick or glue two items together.
**Alloy** A mixture of two or more metals that are dissolved with each other when in the liquid state.
**Amalgam (uh-MAL-gum)** An alloy, with one of the constituents being mercury.
**Auto-cured** Hardened or set by a chemical reaction of two materials.
**Ceramic** Hard, brittle, heat- and corrosive-resistant material such as clay.
**Coupling agent** Agent that strengthens resin by bonding filler to the resin matrix.
**Cured** Preserved or finished by a chemical or physical process.
**Dual-cured** A composite resin material that has both light-cure and auto-cure properties.
**Esthetic (aesthetic) (es-THET-ik)** Artistically pleasing and beautiful appearance.
**Filler** Inorganic material that adds strength and other characteristics to composite resins.
**Force** Any push or pull on an object.
**Galvanic (gal-VA-nik)** An electrical current that takes place when two different or dissimilar metals come together.
**Gold** A soft, yellow, corrosive-resistant metal that is used in the making of indirect restorations.
**Irregular** Not straight, uniform, or symmetric.
**Malleability (mal-ee-uh-BIL-uh-tee)** The ability of a material to withstand permanent deformation under compressive stress without sustaining permanent damage.
**Matrix (MAY-triks)** Foundation that binds a substance together; continuous phases (organic polymer) in which particles of filler are dispersed in composite resin.
**Microleakage (mye-kroe-LEE-kuj)** Microscopic space located at the interface of the tooth structure and the sealant or restoration.
**Palladium (puh-LAY-dee-um)** Soft, steel-white, tarnish-resistant metal that occurs naturally with platinum.
**Percolation (PER-ko-LAY-shun)** The process of a liquid substance passing through a porous substance.
**Pestle (PES-ul, PES-tul)** An object that is moved vertically to pound or pulverize a material.
**Platinum (PLAT-i-num)** Silver-white noble metal that does not corrode in air.
**Porcelain (POR-se-lun)** Hard, white, translucent ceramic material fabricated by firing and then glazing it to match the tooth color.
**Restorative (re-STOR-uh-tiv)** To restore or bring back to its natural appearance.
**Retention (ree-TEN-shun)** The act of holding something by means of an adhesive or mechanical locking, or both.
**Spherical (SFEER-i-kul)** Round.
**Strain** Distortion or change produced as a result of stress.
**Stress** Internal reaction or resistance to an externally applied force.
**Tarnish (TAR-nish)** A discoloration.
**Viscosity (vis-KOS-i-tee)** Physical property of fluids responsible for resistance to flow.
**Wetting** Covering or soaking something with a liquid.

## LEARNING OUTCOMES

*On completion of this chapter, the student will be able to achieve the following objectives:*

1. Pronounce, define, and spell the key terms.
2. Discuss how a dental material is evaluated before it is marketed to the profession.
3. Discuss the properties of dental materials, including the following:
   - List the properties of dental materials and ways that they affect their application.
   - Describe the factors that affect how dental materials are manufactured for the oral cavity.
4. Discuss direct restorative and esthetic materials, including the following:
   - Describe the properties of amalgam and its application in restoring teeth.
   - Describe the properties of composite resin materials and their application in restoring teeth.
   - Describe the properties of glass ionomers and their application in restoring teeth.
5. Describe the properties of temporary restorative materials and their application in restoring teeth.
6. Discuss the use of tooth-whitening products.
7. Discuss indirect restorative materials, including the following:
   - Discuss the differences between direct and indirect restorative materials.
   - Describe the properties of gold alloys and their application in restoring teeth.
   - Describe the properties of porcelain and its application in restoring teeth.

## PERFORMANCE OUTCOMES

*On completion of this chapter, the student will be able to achieve competency standards in the following skills:*

- Mix and transfer amalgam.
- Prepare composite resin material.
- Mix intermediate restorative material.
- Prepare acrylic resin for provisional coverage.

## ELECTRONIC RESOURCES

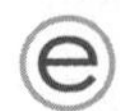

***Additional information related to content in Chapter 43 can be found on the companion Evolve Web site.***

- Practice Quiz
- Video: Mixing and Transferring Amalgam

Dental materials fulfill an important role in the way dentistry is delivered today. Selection of the appropriate dental material(s) for a procedure will depend on several variables: the extent of decay; the type of defect in the tooth; the condition of the entire mouth; the location of the restoration; and cost factors.

The restorative and esthetic dental materials used most commonly in dentistry today include the following:

- Amalgam
- Composite resin
- Glass ionomer
- Temporary restorative materials
- Tooth-whitening products
- Gold alloy
- Ceramic castings

**Restorative** is a term in dentistry that describes the ability to remove decay or disease and bring back the proper function of a tooth. **Esthetic** (sometimes spelled **aesthetic**) is a term that refers to recreating the tooth or teeth with an artistically pleasing appearance.

The types of dental materials introduced in this chapter are restorative and esthetic materials most often used by the general dentist. An understanding of these dental materials will provide you with the knowledge necessary to recognize the types of procedures practiced by the general dentist.

As a clinical dental assistant, it is essential that you learn the general characteristics of each type of dental material, the selection criteria, and ways to prepare the restorative and esthetic materials for a procedure. It will be your responsibility to assemble the setup for each material while being attentive to the manufacturer's recommended proportions and mixing techniques.

# Standardization of Dental Materials

When a new dental material is developed, the product undergoes a strict evaluation and assessment before it is marketed to the profession. The Council on Dental Materials, Instruments, and Equipment was formed as a subcommittee by the American Dental Association (ADA) in combination with federal organizations to ensure that standards and strict specifications are followed by dental material manufacturing companies when new dental materials are developed (Fig. 43.1).

# Criteria for a New Dental Material

- It must *not* be poisonous or harmful to the body.
- It must *not* be harmful or irritating to the tissues of the oral cavity.
- It must help protect the tooth and tissues of the oral cavity.
- It must resemble the natural dentition as closely as possible so as to be esthetically pleasing.
- It must be easily formed and placed in the mouth to restore the mouth's natural contour.
- It must conform and function despite limited access, wet conditions, and poor visibility.

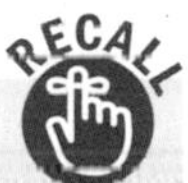


1 Which professional organization evaluates a new dental material?

# Properties of Dental Materials

The types of dental materials used to restore teeth must respond to and withstand specific factors associated with oral conditions. The following characteristics enhance the ability of dental materials to withstand the oral environment and allow for easy application.

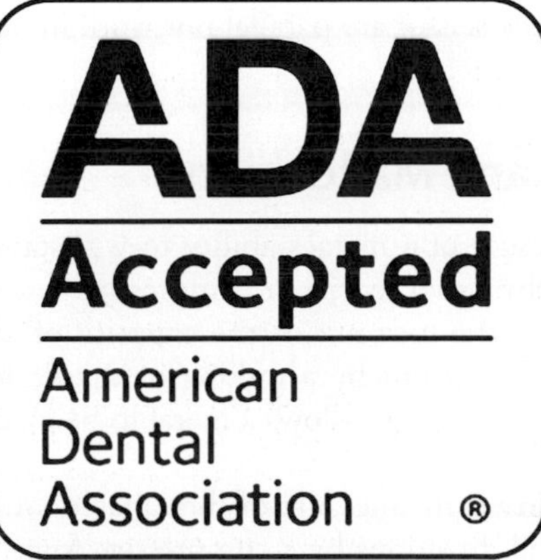


**FIG. 43.1** ADA Council on Dental Materials seal. The seal is viewed on consumer products.

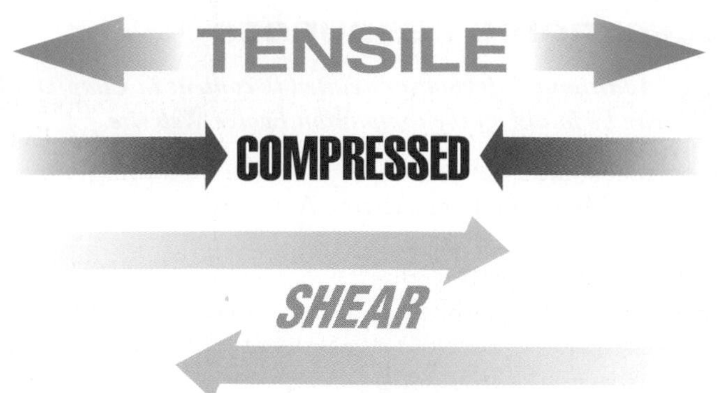


FIG. 43.2 Types of stress and strain: tensile, compressed, and shear. *(© Elsevier Collection.)*

## Mechanical Properties

The average biting and chewing **force** that takes place in the posterior area of the mouth of people with natural teeth is approximately 170 pounds (77 kg). This averages out to 28,000 pounds of pressure per square inch (psi) on a single cusp of a molar tooth. Dental materials used in restoring posterior teeth must have sufficient strength to withstand such force.

A force is any push or pull on matter, which produces a stress and a strain. **Stress** is the internal resistance or force that can cause distortion. **Strain** is the *change* or deformation of a material as the result of stress. Stress and strain are applicable to both liquids and solids. Stress and strain go together; you cannot have one without the other.

### *Types of Stress and Strain*

- **Tensile stress and strain pulls** and stretches the material. Think about tug-of-war as an example (Fig. 43.2, *A*).
- **Compressive stress and strain** results from two forces directed toward each other. An example would be chewing (Fig. 43.2, *B*).
- **Shear stress and strain** occurs from the two forces of material parallel to each other sliding in opposite directions. Think about cutting a piece of paper with scissors. The blades of the scissor are parallel but work in opposite directions (Fig. 43.2, *C*).

## Ductility and Malleability

This is a measure of a metal's ability to withstand permanent deformation by either tensile or compressive forces.

Ductility is the measure of the capacity of a metal to be stretched or drawn out by a pulling or tensile force without fracturing. This property allows a metal to be made into a thin wire.

**Malleability** is the measure of the capacity of a metal to be extended in all directions by a compressive force, such as rolling or hammering. This property allows a metal to be shaped into a thin sheet or plate.

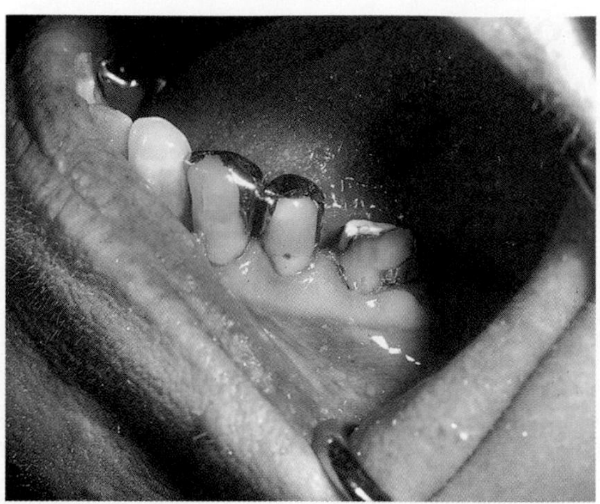

FIG. 43.3 A galvanic action can occur when different types of metals touch each other.

## Thermal Change

When a person drinks hot coffee and then immediately eats ice cream, the temperature in the mouth can change from 150° F to 100° F (66° C–38° C) within seconds. These thermal changes are of major concern for two reasons: (1) contraction and expansion, and (2) the need to protect the pulp from thermal shock from extreme differences in temperature.

### *Contraction and Expansion*

When temperature changes occur, each type of dental material will contract or expand at its own rate. It is essential that the tooth structure and the restorative material have, as nearly as possible, the same rate of contraction and expansion. Significant changes in the degree of contraction and expansion can cause a dental material to pull away from the tooth, which can result in **microleakage**, or a faulty restoration. This microscopic separation of material and tooth can allow oral fluids, debris, and microorganisms to enter between the restoration and the wall of a cavity preparation. The term for this process is **percolation**.

## Electrical Properties

An electrical current (also referred to as **galvanic** action or shock) can take place in the oral cavity when two different or dissimilar metals are present (Fig. 43.3). Conditions that can create these electrical currents include the following:

- Saliva contains salt, which makes it a good conductor of electricity.
- Two metallic components of different composition (two different types of metals in the restorations or a metal object such as a fork placed in the mouth) can act as the battery.

## Corrosive Properties

**Corrosion** is the reaction that occurs within a metal when it is exposed to corrosive factors such as temperature, humidity,

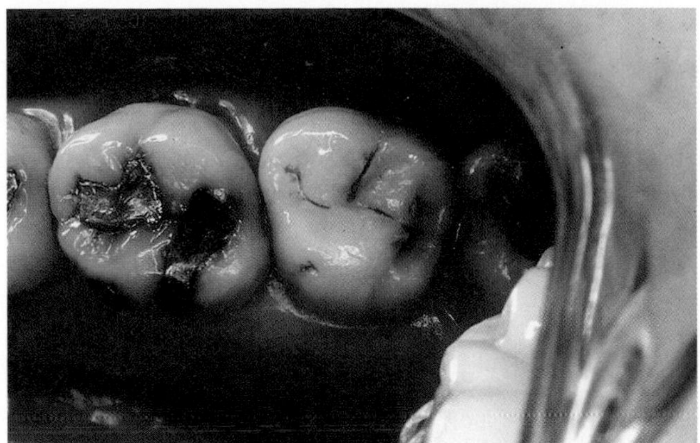

FIG. 43.4 Corrosion can occur on certain metals.

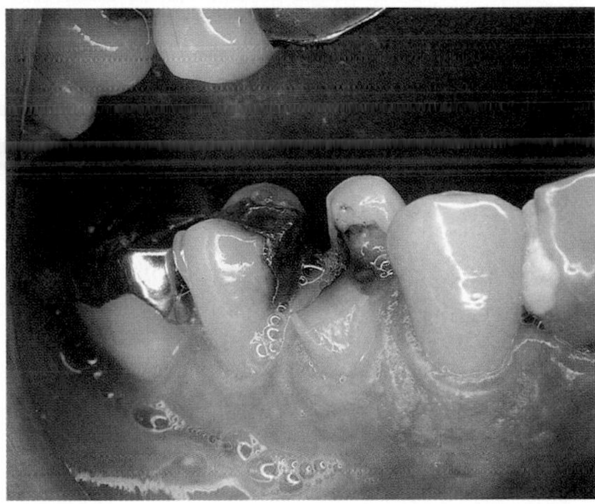

FIG. 43.5 Dental materials must withstand the solubility of saliva in the oral cavity.

and saline. Certain foods contain metallic forms that cause corrosion of a dental material. The surface discoloration that we see in older amalgam restorations in the mouth is referred to as **tarnish** (Fig. 43.4). Most corrosion, however, involves surface discoloration and can be removed easily with the use of polishing agents.

## Hardness

This is a measure of the resistance of a metal to indentation, scratching, or abrasion. It is an indication of strength and wear-ability.

## Solubility

**Solubility** is the degree to which a substance will dissolve in a given amount of another substance. For example, sand has *low* solubility because it does not dissolve easily; sugar has *high* solubility because it does dissolve easily. The solubility of a dental material placed in the mouth is a matter of concern (Fig. 43.5). A material that dissolves easily in the oral environment is of limited use because it will wash away and leave the tooth structure exposed.

## Application Properties

For a dental material to have specific mechanical properties, steps must occur in the application of the dental material. Techniques used in the application help create the following effects.

### Flow

When decay is removed from a diseased tooth, and healthy tooth structure remains and is prepared to receive a permanent filling material, the dental material must be pliable enough to be adapted in the preparation. Dental materials are designed to have a certain amount of flow for placement; this allows the material to fill in the preparation of the tooth.

### Adhesion

**Adhesion** is the ability of two unlike materials to **adhere** to each other. Adhesion between a dental material and the tooth structure is a major concern. Without proper adhesion, microleakage can occur, and the restoration could come out. Characteristics of dental materials that can affect the adhesion process are wetting, viscosity, surface characteristics, and film thickness.

**Wetting** is the ability of a liquid to flow over the surface and come into contact with the small irregularities that may be present. For example, water has *high* wetting ability because it flows easily.

**Viscosity** is the property of a liquid that causes it *not* to flow easily. A liquid with high viscosity, such as maple syrup, does not flow easily and is not effective in wetting a surface.

The surface characteristics that are important in wetting are the chemical nature of the tooth surface and how the dental material flows on that surface. An example of this is how rain on your windshield runs, but when a chemical is added to the windshield to help repel the rain, the rain beads up.

For adhesion to take place and remain permanent, the cement must have a thin film thickness of 25 microns or less to join the tooth and restoration. It is important to remember that the thinner the film thickness, the stronger the adhesive junction.

### Retention

**Retention** is the ability to hold two things firmly together when they will not adhere to each other naturally. For example, amalgam (silver fillings) and cast metals will not naturally adhere directly to tooth structure. Retention is an extremely important concept in dentistry because dental restorations, casting, and appliances must be held in place with the use of materials and retention methods.

Because amalgam and tooth structure do not adhere to each other, a traditional cavity preparation must include a retention form within the tooth structure. The dentist will use a bur or a hand (manual) cutting instrument to produce this retention form (creating a crevice in the tooth that the material can lock into). Even though retention holds the material in place, it does not completely seal the two structures together. Microleakage can still occur between the material and the tooth if an additional material such as a bonding material is not placed to create a seal.

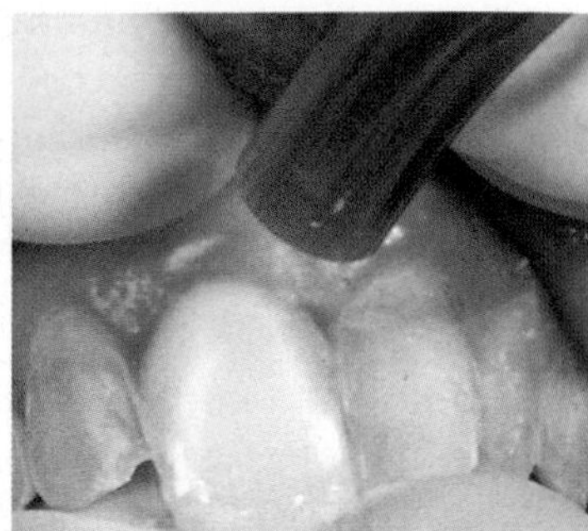

FIG. 43.6 Light-curing of a composite resin.

### Curing

**Curing** is a setting process of a dental material that is initiated by a chemical reaction or by light in a blue wave spectrum. Curing of most dental materials is the process of placing a paste-type material into the tooth preparation for adaptation. After the material is in place, it is then **cured** to harden.

An **auto-cured** or self-cured material hardens as the result of a chemical reaction of the materials when mixed together. The curing action proceeds from start to finish by itself. Because of urgency, the material must be mixed and placed within working and setting times for that material.

A **light-cured** material does not harden until it has been exposed to a curing light (Fig. 43.6). This allows a more flexible working time.

With a **dual-cured** material, some curing takes place as the material is mixed. However, the final cure does not occur until the material has been exposed to a curing light.

RECALL

2 What type of reaction does a dental material undergo when distortion occurs?
3 What happens to a dental material when it is exposed to hot and cold?
4 What is a source of galvanic action?
5 What are the four properties that must be considered in the application of a dental material?
6 How does an auto-cured material harden or set up?

# Direct Restorative and Esthetic Materials

Direct restorative and esthetic materials are applied to a tooth or teeth while the material is pliable and can still be adapted, carved, and finished. Materials selected for these types of restorative and esthetic procedures are amalgam, composite resins, glass ionomers, temporary restorative materials, and tooth-whitening products.

## Amalgam

For longer than 150 years, billions of dental amalgam fillings have been used to restore decayed teeth. **Amalgam** is the technical name for "silver fillings" (Fig. 43.7). Actually, amalgam consists of several different metals, with silver being the predominant metal. These metals are in powder form and are mixed with mercury to form a soft, pliable mixture. When placed into a prepared tooth, condensed, carved, and allowed to harden, the mixture becomes a permanent amalgam restoration.

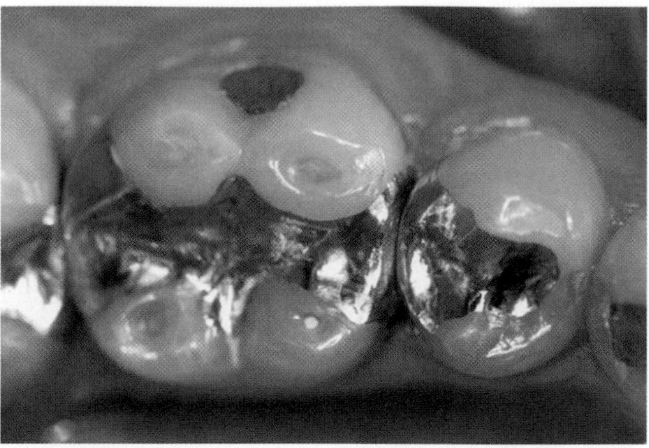

FIG. 43.7 Example of class II amalgam restoration. *(From Heymann HO, Swift EJ, Ritter AV: Sturdevant's art and science of operative dentistry, ed 6, St Louis, 2013, Mosby.)*

Dental amalgam is a safe, affordable, and durable material used predominantly to restore premolars and molars.

### Indications for Using Dental Amalgam

- Primary and permanent teeth
- Stress-bearing areas of the mouth
- Small to medium-sized cavities in the posterior teeth
- Severe destruction of tooth structure
- As a foundation for cast-metal, metal-ceramic, and ceramic restorations
- When a patient's commitment to personal oral hygiene is poor
- When moisture control is problematic
- When cost is an overriding patient concern

### Contraindications to the Use of Dental Amalgam

- When esthetics is particularly important, such as in the anterior teeth or in facial surfaces that can be viewed
- With patients who have a history of allergy to mercury or other amalgam components
- When a large restoration is needed and the cost of other restorative materials is not a significant factor in the treatment decision

### Composition of Dental Amalgam

Dental amalgam is the end result of mixing approximately equal parts of mercury (43 to 54 percent) and an amalgam **alloy** powder (46 to 57 percent) (Fig. 43.8). The alloy powder is a combination of metals. Amalgam alloy powder is composed of the following metals:

- **Silver,** which gives it its strength
- **Tin,** for its workability and strength

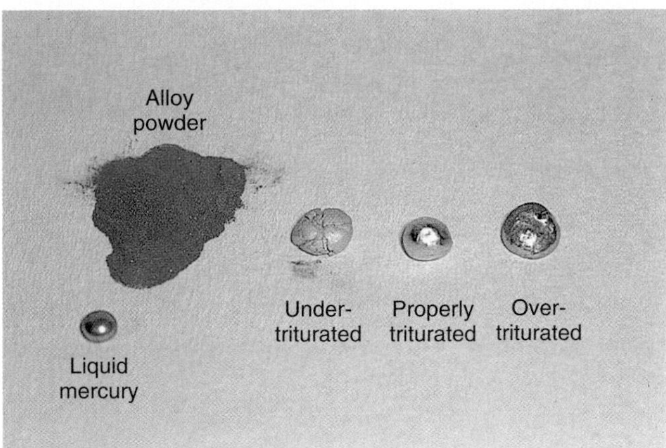


**FIG. 43.8** The mercury and alloy powder are in their purest form before trituration. *(From Hatrick CD, Eakle WS: Dental materials: clinical applications for dental assistants and dental hygienists, ed 3, St Louis, 2016, Elsevier.)*

- **Copper,** for its strength and corrosion resistance
- **Zinc,** to suppress oxidation

The main differences in the composition and classification of dental amalgam alloy powders are based on (1) alloy particle shape and size, (2) copper content, and (3) zinc content.

## High-Copper Alloys

**High-copper alloys,** frequently used in dentistry, are named this because they contain a higher percentage of copper than previous alloys. High-copper alloys are classified according to their particle shape: **spherical** (round particles) or **irregular** (rough, lathe-cut particles) (Fig. 43.9). These particle shapes influence the trituration and working characteristics (condensing and carving) of the resulting amalgam mixture.

A high-copper alloy is made up of 40 to 70 percent silver, 8 to 28 percent copper, and 15 to 30 percent tin. The percentages are expressed as percentages of the composition by weight. Table 43.1 describes the composition and classification of dental amalgam alloy powders.

## Mercury-to-Alloy Ratios

The appropriate mercury-to-alloy ratio is very important. The ratio must contain just enough mercury to make the mix workable without containing an excessive amount of mercury. A 1:1 mercury-to-alloy ratio, also known as the **Eames technique,** is widely used. This ratio is one portion of mercury to one portion of alloy by weight.

## Nonmercury Alloys

A nonmercury alloy called Galloy, composed of gallium, indium, and tin, was approved by the American Dental Association (ADA), but has not been researched for its potential because of the advancement of composite resins.

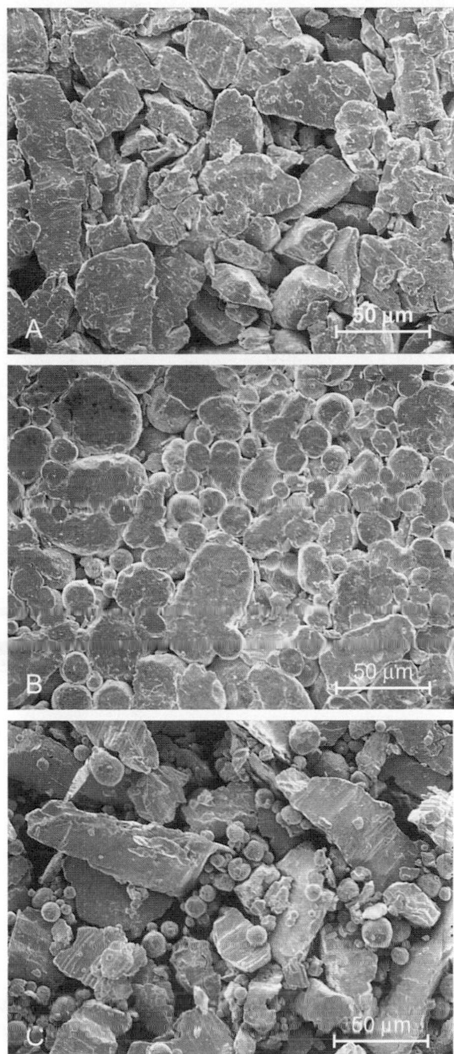


**FIG. 43.9** Microscopic view of alloy powder particles. A, Irregular. B, Spherical. C, Mixed. *(Courtesy of S.C. Bayne, School of Dentistry, University of Michigan, Ann Arbor, MI.)*

## Controversial Issues in Mercury

Mercury in dental amalgam has been under controversy for many years. The controversy has evolved in the following two directions: (1) potential harm to patients from the mercury within the amalgams placed in their teeth, and (2) the toxicity level of mercury vapors affecting dental personnel exposed over a long period.

When mercury is combined with other materials in dental amalgam, its chemical nature changes so that it is essentially harmless. The amount released in the mouth under the pressure of chewing and grinding is extremely small and presents no cause for alarm. In fact, this amount is less than what patients are routinely exposed to in food, air, and water. The ADA and the National Institute of Health–Nations Administration have agreed that there is no basis for claims that amalgam is a significant health hazard; they firmly support the use of dental amalgams for the permanent restoration of

TABLE 43.1 Composition and Classification of Dental Amalgam Alloy Powders

| Amalgam Alloys | Classification | Particle Type | AG (Silver) | SN (Tin) | CU (Copper) | ZN (Zinc) | HG (Mercury) | Other |
|---|---|---|---|---|---|---|---|---|
| New True Dentalloy | Low copper | Lathe-cut | 70.8 | 25.8 | 2.4 | 1 | 0 | |
| Micro II | Low copper | Lathe-cut | 70.1 | 21 | 8.6 | .3 | 0 | |
| Dispersity | High copper | Mixed | 69.5 | 17.7 | 11.9 | .9 | 0 | |
| Tytin | High copper | Spherical | 59.2 | 27.8 | 13 | 0 | 0 | |
| Sybraloy | High copper | Spherical | 41.5 | 30.2 | 28.3 | 0 | 0 | |
| Cupralloy | High copper | Mixed | 62.2 | 15.1 | 22.7 | 0 | 0 | |
| Aristalloy CR | High copper | Spherical | 58.7 | 28.4 | 12.9 | 0 | 0 | |
| Indiloy | High copper | Lathe-cut | 60.5 | 24 | 12.1 | 0 | 0 | 3.4 In |
| Valiant | High copper | Lathe-cut | 49.5 | 30 | 20 | 0 | 0 | .5 Pd |
| Valiant PhD | High copper | Mixed | 52.7 | 29.7 | 17.4 | 0 | 0 | .5 Pd |

From Heymann HO, Swift EJ, Ritter AV: Sturdevant's art and science of operative dentistry, ed 6, St Louis, 2013, Mosby; data from Osborne JW, Gale EN, Chew CL: Clinical performance and physical properties of 12 amalgam alloys, J Dent Res 57:983–988, 1978, and Vrijhoef MMA et al: Dental amalgam, Chicago, 1980, Quintessence.

teeth. It is believed that amalgam is the best dental material that can be used in posterior restorations.

The health risk for dental personnel is greater than that for a patient (Fig. 43.10). With the use of precapsulated amalgam, the risk has definitely decreased, but care must still be maintained to avoid hazards in the routine use of amalgam. Careful amalgam handling procedures must be followed. The dentist and the assistant who are exposed to mercury vapors daily should be aware of their toxic effects. An increase in exposure can result in tremors, kidney dysfunction, depression, and central nervous system disorders (Box 43.1).

## The Application of Dental Amalgam

**PREPARATION.** Amalgam is supplied by the manufacturer in sealed single-use capsules with the proper ratio of alloy powder in one side of the capsule and mercury in the other side, separated by a thin membrane. This ensures an accurate ratio and reduces the possibility of exposure to any of the materials. Immediately after use, the capsule is reassembled and is discarded with nonregulated waste.

Capsules are available in 600 mg of alloy, which is the appropriate amount of material for a small or single-surface restoration, or 800 mg of alloy, which is used for a larger restoration (Fig. 43.11). If more than this amount of amalgam is required, additional capsules are placed within the setup and triturated as needed.

**TRITURATION.** Also known as **amalgamation, trituration** is the process by which mercury and alloy powders are mixed together to form the mass of amalgam needed to restore the tooth. The preloaded capsule of amalgam alloy and mercury contains a **pestle**, which aids in the mixing process.

Before the capsule is placed into the amalgamator, many types of capsules require the use of an activator, which breaks the separating membrane (Fig. 43.12). The activated capsule is placed into the amalgamator, and the cover is closed to prevent mercury vapors from escaping during trituration.

The amalgamator is set to operate for the length of time specified in the manufacturer's directions (Table 43.2). In a proper mix, the mass of amalgam is free of dry alloy particles and holds together as a single unit. The mix is placed from the capsule into an amalgam well; the pestle is removed, and the mix is loaded into the amalgam carrier.

Amalgam should appear soft, pliable, and easily shaped when first triturated. At this stage, amalgam is transferred to the dentist in the amalgam carrier to be placed and condensed into the prepared tooth. Once it hardens, amalgam forms a very strong restoration that can withstand the mechanical properties mentioned.

See Procedure 43.1: Mixing and Transferring Dental Amalgam.

**CONDENSATION.** The amalgam is carried to the tooth by the amalgam carrier and is placed in increments into the prepared tooth, and each increment is condensed immediately with the use of an amalgam condenser. The purpose of condensation is to pack the amalgam tightly into all areas of the prepared cavity and to aid in removing any excess mercury from the amalgam mix (Fig. 43.13).

**CARVING AND FINISHING.** With the use of hand carving instruments, the dentist is able to carve back the amalgam material to the tooth's normal anatomy, which was removed during cavity preparation (Fig. 43.14). A burnisher is used to smooth the amalgam, making sure that no irregularities are present in the restoration. Once most of the carving has been completed, the patient is instructed to bite down lightly on articulating paper. This allows the dentist to check how the new restoration occludes with the opposing tooth, and then final carvings can be made.

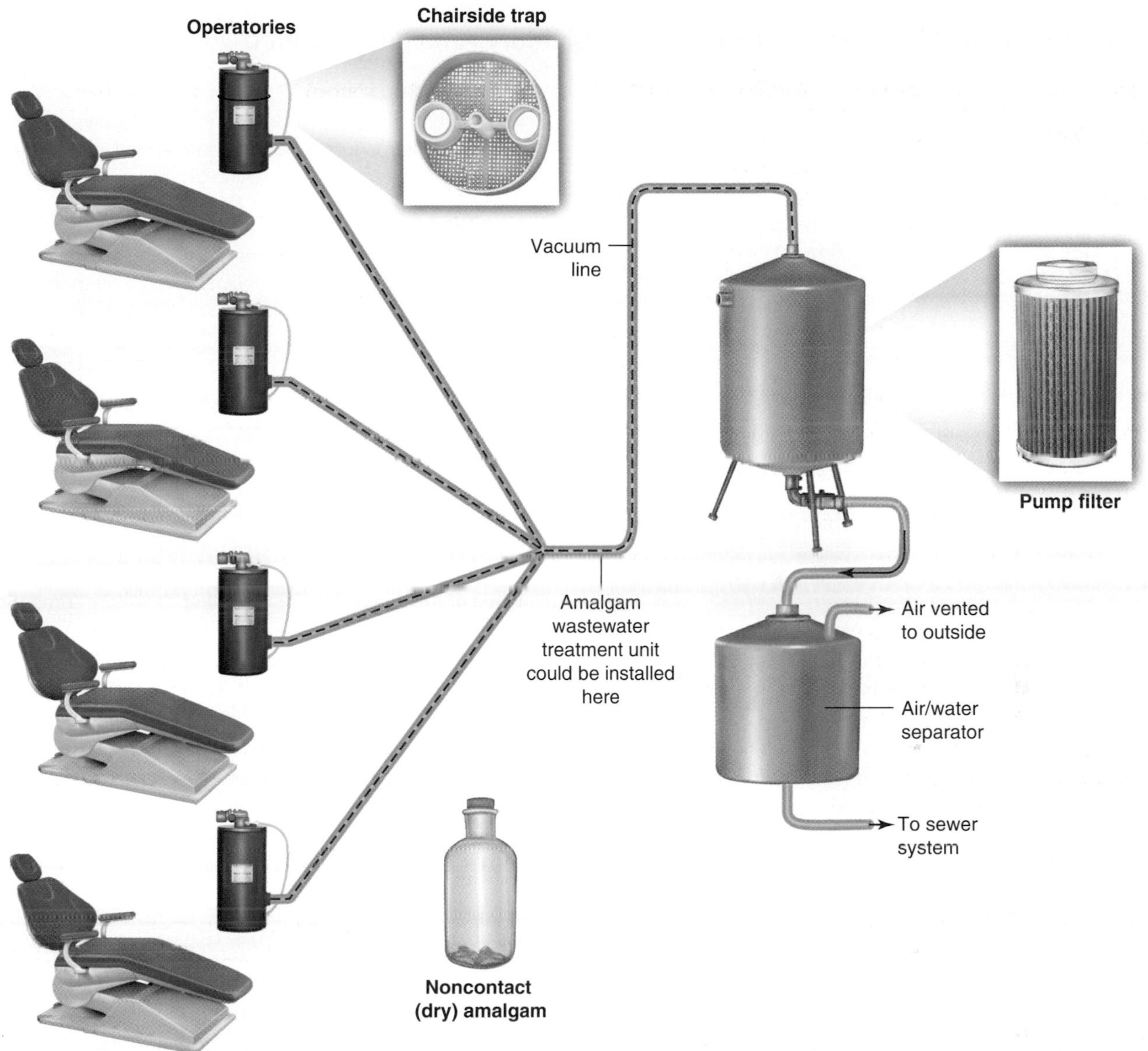


**FIG. 43.10** Management practices for mercury amalgam. *(© Elsevier Collection.)*

**BOX 43.1 Best Management Practices for Mercury Amalgam**

**Noncontact (Scrap) Amalgam**

- Place noncontact, scrap amalgam in a wide-mouthed, airtight container that is marked "Noncontact Amalgam Waste for Recycling."
- Make sure the container lid is well sealed.
- When the container is full, send it to a recycler.

**Amalgam Capsules**

- Stock amalgam capsules in a variety of sizes.
- After mixing amalgam, place the empty capsules in a wide-mouthed, airtight container that is marked "Amalgam Capsule Waste for Recycling."
- Capsules that cannot be emptied should likewise be placed in a wide-mouthed, airtight container that is marked "Amalgam Capsule Waste for Recycling."
- Make sure the container lid is well sealed.
- When the container is full, send it to a recycler.

**Disposable Chairside Traps**

- Open the chairside unit to expose the trap.
- Remove the trap and place it directly into a wide-mouthed, airtight container that is marked "Contact Amalgam Waste for Recycling."
- Make sure the container lid is well sealed.
- When the container is full, send it to a recycler.
- Traps from dental units dedicated strictly to hygiene may be placed in with the regular garbage.

**Reusable Chairside Traps**

- Open the chairside unit to expose the trap.
- Remove the trap and empty the contents into a wide-mouthed, airtight container that is marked "Contact Amalgam Waste for Recycling."
- Make sure the container lid is well sealed.
- When the container is full, send it to a recycler.

*Continued*

**BOX 43.1 Best Management Practices for Mercury Amalgam—cont'd**

- Replace the trap into the chairside unit. (Do *not* rinse the trap under running water as this could introduce dental amalgam into the waste stream.)

**Vacuum Pump Filters**

- Change the filter according to the manufacturer's recommended schedule. *Note:* The following instructions assume that your recycler will accept whole filters; some recyclers require different handling of this material, so check with your recycler first.
- Remove the filter.
- Put the lid on the filter and place the sealed container in the box in which it was originally shipped. When the box is full, the filters should be recycled.

**Amalgam Separators**

- Select an amalgam separator that complies with ISO 11143.
- Follow the manufacturer's recommendations for maintenance and recycling procedures.

**Line Cleaners**

- Use nonbleach, nonchlorine–containing line cleaners, which will minimize amalgam dissolution, such as those listed in the Additional Resources section of this document.

From Best Management Practices for Amalgam Waste, American Dental Association, October 2007. Accessed at www.ada.org May 9, 2013.

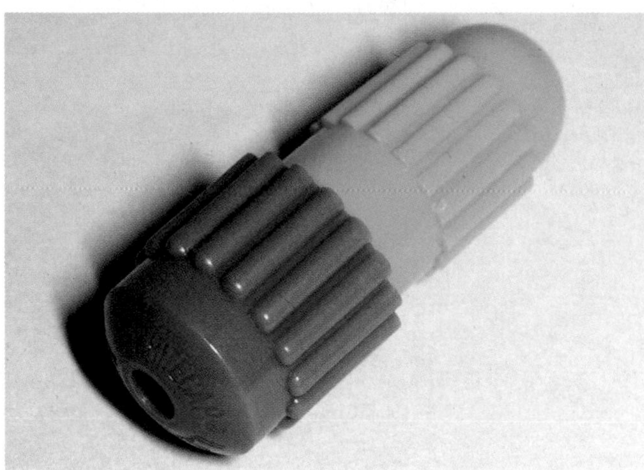

**FIG. 43.11** Precapsulated amalgam.

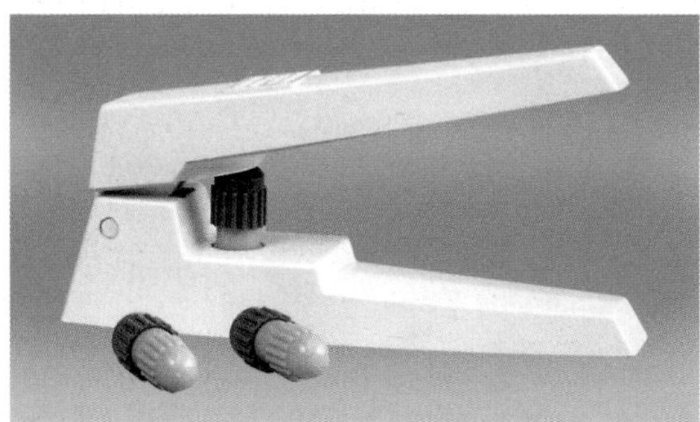

**FIG. 43.12** Activator used to break the separating membrane in the capsule.

**RECALL**

7 What metals make up the alloy powder in amalgam?
8 Would dental amalgam be placed in anterior or posterior teeth?
9 What does copper provide to an amalgam restoration?
10 Where do you dispose of amalgam scraps?
11 How is the amalgam triturated?
12 How long would you triturate Sybraloy?

**TABLE 43.2 Amalgamation Time**

| Types of Amalgam | Setting | Time (Seconds) |
|---|---|---|
| Dispersalloy | M-2 | 13 |
| Tylin | M-2 | 4–5 |
| Sybraloy | M-2 | 13 |
| Spheralloy | M-2 | 15 |
| Valiant | M-2 | 13 |
| Valiant PhD | M-2 | 15 |
| Velvalloy | M-2 | 20 |

## Composite Resins

Composite resins have become the most widely accepted and utilized material of choice by dentists and patients (Fig. 43.15). Composite resins are now being placed throughout the mouth; in anterior teeth because of their esthetic qualities, but with new advances in their makeup, they are being placed in posterior teeth as well.

Composite resins were not as strong as amalgams or gold alloy restorations, but they are now being designed to meet the needs of a specific area of a tooth or mouth. This tooth-colored material is versatile, with many indications.

### *Indications for Using Composite Resins*

- Restoration of class I, II, III, IV, and V restorations
- Restoration of surface defects such as hypocalcification, attrition, abrasion, and congenital abnormalities
- Closure of diastema
- Esthetic recontouring of teeth such as peg laterals

### *Contraindications for Using Composite Resins*

- When esthetics is not an important factor
- With patients who do not have daily proper oral hygiene habits, especially in the posterior area
- When the cost of the restorative materials is a significant factor in the treatment decision

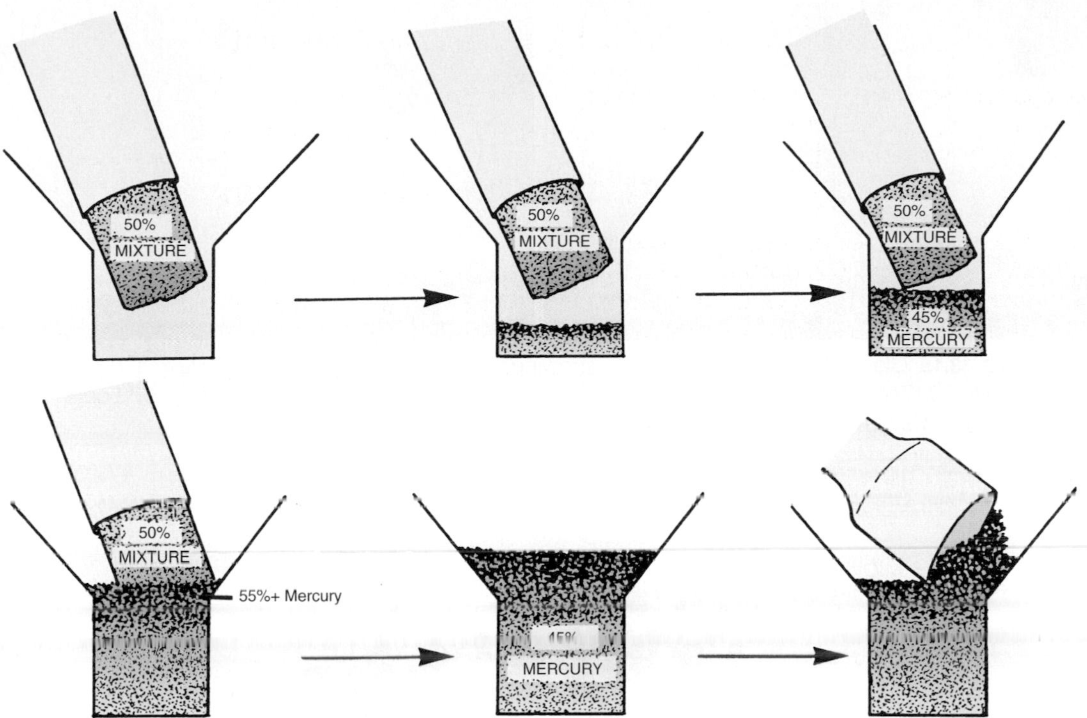


FIG. 43.13 Increments of amalgam placed. *(From Baum L, Phillips RW, Lund MR: Textbook of operative dentistry, ed 3, Philadelphia, 1995, Saunders.)*

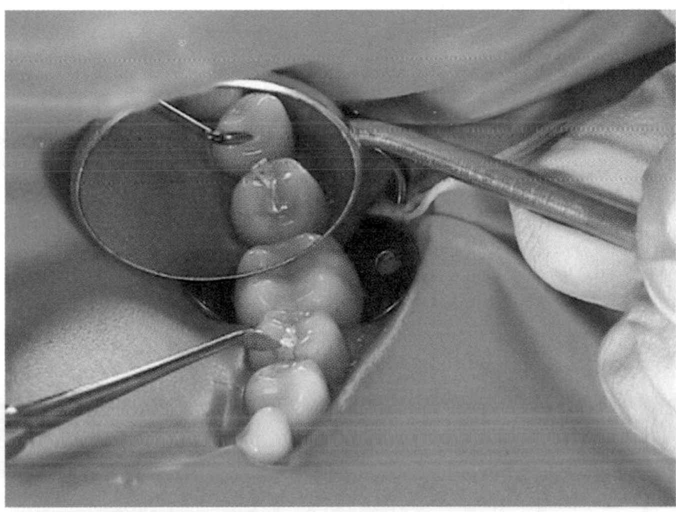

FIG. 43.14 Carving an amalgam restoration.

## Composition of Composite Resins

The composition of composite resins is a chemical mix, which includes (1) an organic resin **matrix**, (2) inorganic **fillers**, (3) a **coupling agent**, and (4) tooth-colored pigments.

**RESIN MATRIX.** The resin matrix component of composite is a fluid-like material called *dimethacrylate,* which is also referred to as *BIS-GMA.* This fluid, which is the monomer, is used to make synthetic resins. BIS-GMA is the foundation of resins. By itself, it is not strong enough to be used as a restorative dental material. The addition of fillers and coupling agents provides the strength needed for the material to withstand the forces of mastication. Additional additives included in this process are the initiator, the accelerator, the retarder, and the ultraviolet (UV) light stabilizers.

**FILLER.** Inorganic fillers used in composite resins include **quartz** (a hard rock-forming mineral), glass, **silica** (white or colorless crystalline compound) particles, and colorants. These fillers add the strength and other characteristics that are needed in a restorative material. The ability of these materials to reflect light facilitates the creation of an esthetically pleasing restoration. The amount of filler, the particle size, and the types of fillers used are important factors in determining the strength and wear resistant characteristics of the material (Fig. 43.16). These factors also influence the polished finish of the restoration. Composites are classified by particle size as *megafill, macrofill, midifill, minifill, microfill,* and *nanofill.* Composites that have a combination or mixed range of particle sizes are referred to as **hybrids** (Fig. 43.17).

**Macrofilled composites,** also known as *conventional or traditional composites,* were used primarily in the 1960s and 1970s. This type of composite contained the largest of filler particles, providing the greatest strength, but its use resulted in a duller, rougher surface. Macrofilled composites are self-cured and were used in areas where greater strength was required to resist fracture.

**Microfilled composites** came about in the 1980s; the main difference noted with this type of composite resin was that it contained inorganic fillers that were much smaller than those in a macrofilled composite. Microfilled composite

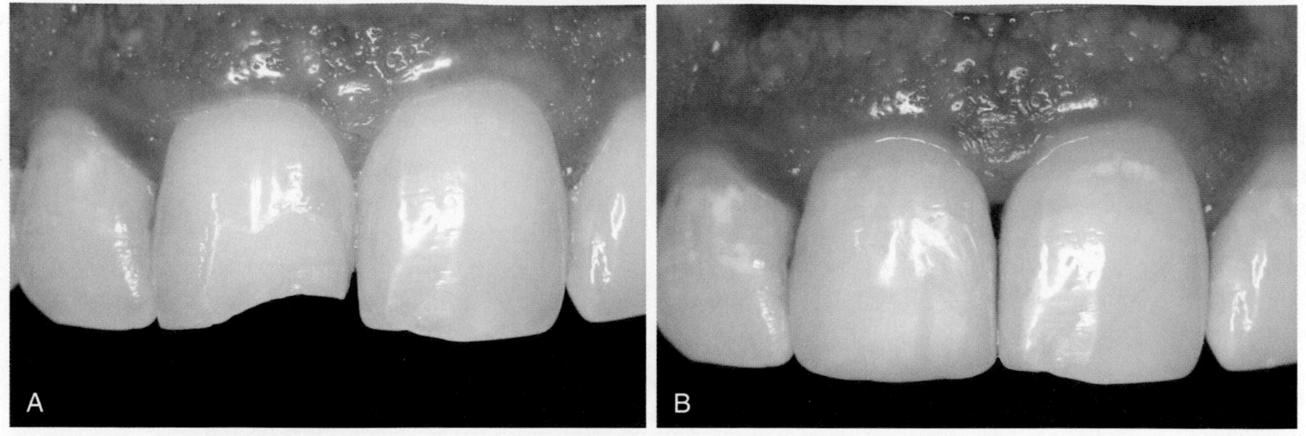


**FIG. 43.15** Class IV composite restoration showing before (A) and after (B). *(From Heymann HO, Swift EJ, Ritter AV: Sturdevant's art and science of operative dentistry, ed 6, St Louis, 2013, Mosby.)*

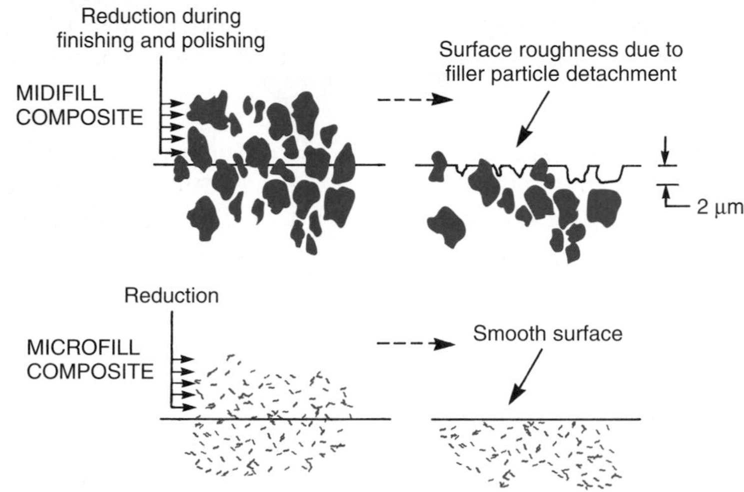


**FIG. 43.16** Effect of particle size on surface finish of composite. *(Courtesy of S.C. Bayne, School of Dentistry, University of Michigan, Ann Arbor, MI.)*

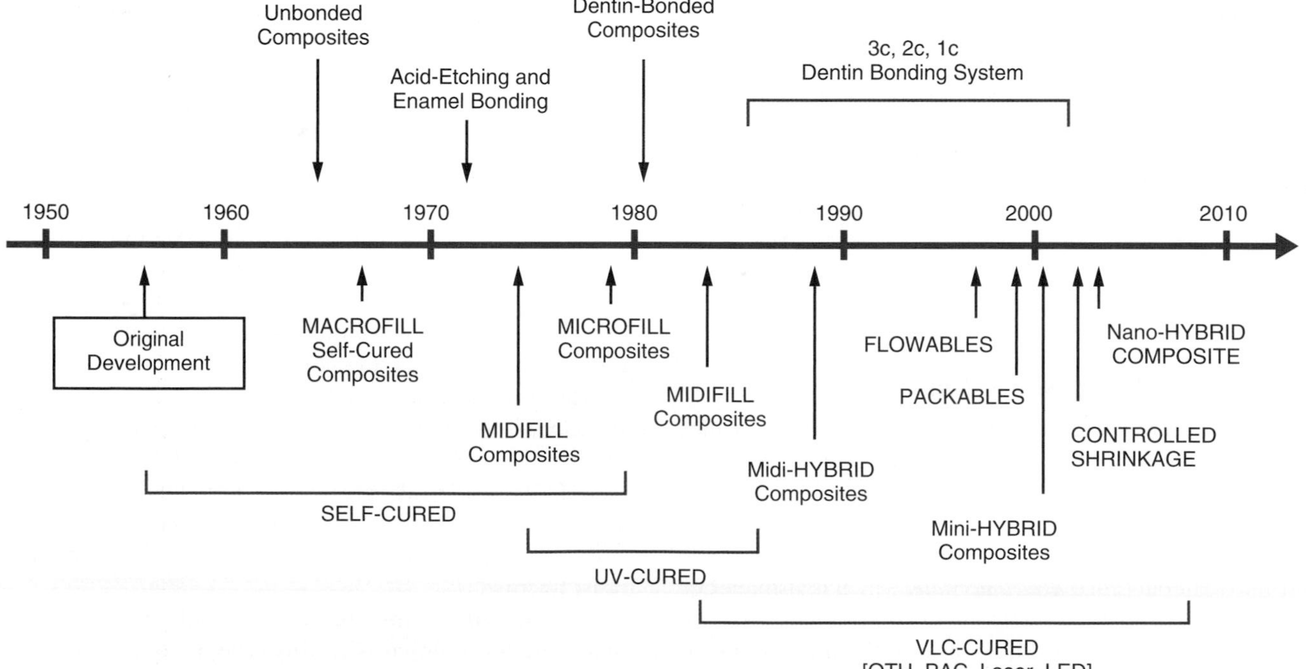


**FIG. 43.17** Summary of the historical evolution of dental composites, curing methods, and accompanying bonding systems. *(Courtesy of S.C. Bayne, School of Dentistry, University of Michigan, Ann Arbor, MI.)*

resins are light-cured and are capable of producing a highly polished finished restoration; they were used primarily in anterior restorations, for which smoothness and esthetics were of primary concern.

**Hybrid composites** are used most often today. They contain a mixed range of particle sizes. Hybrid composites are cured with a visible light–curing method and can be polished smoother than macrofilled composites, yet they have greater strength than is seen with microfilled composites. Hybrid composites also have high wear resistance and excellent shading characteristics.

**Flowable composites** are supplied as a hybrid or nanofilled composite with enough filler included to make the material wear resistant. *Flow* is the key term in describing this type of composite. The material is designed to flow more easily into the more conservative preparation. An example would be a class V noncarious lesion caused by toothbrush abrasion. Flowable composites are provided in a syringe-like device that permits precise placement of the material in the cavity preparation.

**Sealant composites** resemble flowable composites but have the viscosity to allow the material to flow into the pits and fissures of the tooth surface. No preparation with the handpiece or hand instruments is needed for placement, but the tooth surface is etched to prepare for application of the material.

**COUPLING AGENT.** The coupling agent is important because it strengthens the resin by chemically bonding the filler to the resin matrix. To achieve this, filler particles are coated with an organosilane compound. The *silane* portion of the molecule bonds with the quartz, glass, and silica filler particles. The *organic* portion bonds with the resin matrix, thus bonding the filler to the matrix.

**PIGMENTS.** For a composite material to match a tooth color, coloring must be added. Most often, the coloring comes from an inorganic substance.

### Commercial Examples of Composite Resins

| Classification | Brand |
|---|---|
| Microfilled | Durafill, Renamel, Matrixx, Epic, Heliomolar, Ivoclar, Vivadent, Virtuoso, Sculptable |
| Hybrids | Herculite, Prodigy, Spectrum, Charisma, |
| Microhybrid | Filtek, Synergy, Gradia, Point 4, Renamel, Tetric, Venus |
| Nanofilled | Premise, Aelite Esthetic Enamel, Clearfill Majesty, Artiste |

## Application of Composites

Important differences in the application or technique of an amalgam restoration versus a composite restoration include the following:

- The cavity preparation for a composite resin is designed to hold the resin material by means of a bonding system rather than by retention added into the preparation.
- Some dental materials cannot be used with composite resins.
- The matrix system will vary with composite resins.
- Placement of composite resin may be accomplished in increments if it is a large restoration; light-curing is performed before additional increments are added.

**SHADE SELECTION.** Color matching is one of the most critical aspects when working with composite resins. If the correct shade is not selected, this will be apparent to the patient after the restoration is in place. A shade guide is always used when determining the correct shade for application (Fig. 43.18).

The composite kit may include its own shade guide; most manufacturers cross-reference their shades with those of the

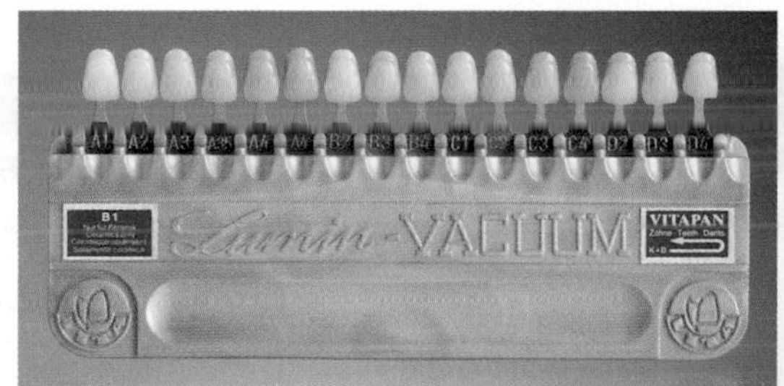


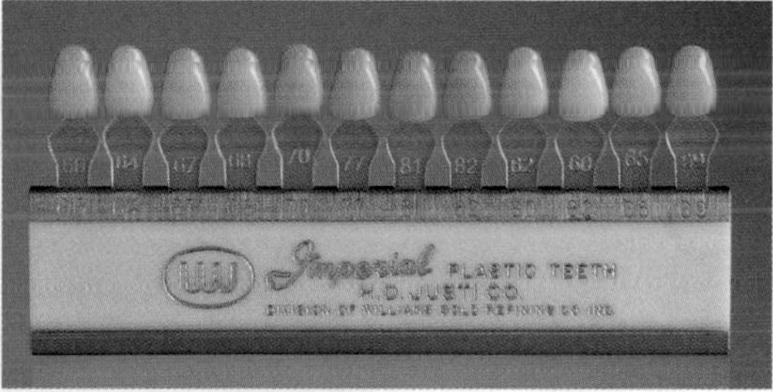


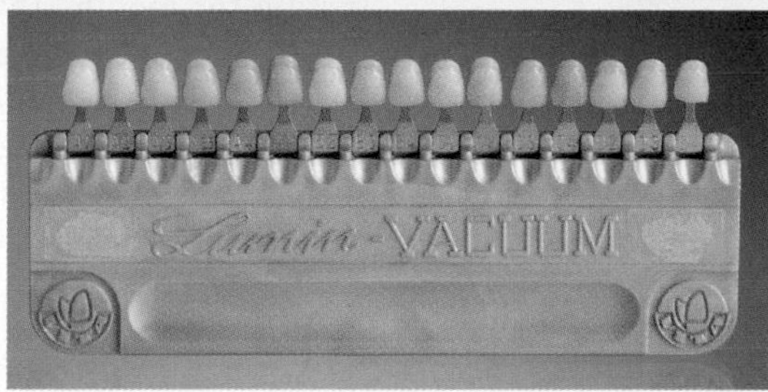


**FIG. 43.18** Use of a shade guide for color matching. *(From Boyd LRB: Dental instruments: a pocket guide, ed 6, St Louis, 2018, Elsevier.)*

VITA Shade Guide, which is a universally adopted shade guide.

### *Tips When Choosing a Shade*

- Determine tooth shades if possible in daylight or with standardized daylight lamps and not under normal ambient lighting.
- The entire surroundings should be kept free from bright colors. If necessary, ask the patient to remove lipstick and to cover brightly colored clothing.
- Make your choice quickly; always accept the first decision because the eyes begin to tire after approximately 5 to 7 seconds.

**APPLICATION.** Light-cured composite resins are supplied in a single-paste, lightproof syringe. These resins do not require mixing and are used directly from the syringe with the addition of a syringe tip. The paste contains both the photo initiator and the amine activator and will not polymerize until it is exposed to the curing light. The material is supplied in a kit that includes varying shades of the composite resin, along with an etching and bonding system that works specifically for the application process of that material (Fig. 43.19).

Traditional composite resin material was to be placed incrementally in layers and cured before placing another increment. With the advancement in makeup of composites, bulk-filling for posterior composites through a syringe tip allows for precise application and a reduction in time.

### *Polymerization*

Polymerization is the process by which resin material is changed from a pliable state (in which it can be molded or shaped) into a hardened restoration. Polymerization occurs through autocuring or light-curing.

The **light-curing process** uses either a high-intensity blue light source, which is a combination of tungsten and a halogen, or an LED curing light. The exact curing time depends on the following:

- Composite manufacturer's instructions (most often, 20–60 seconds)
- Thickness and size of the restoration (when larger quantities of the material are being placed)
- Shade of the restorative material used (the darker the shade, the longer the required curing time)

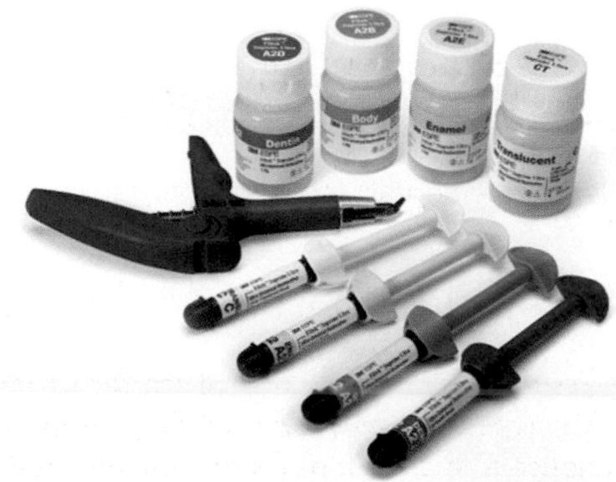


**FIG. 43.19** Composite resin kit. *(Courtesy 3M ESPE, St Paul, MN.)*

### *Finishing and Polishing*

The finishing and polishing of composite resins are much different from the completion steps in an amalgam procedure. Because composite materials go from a soft pliable state to being completely hardened by polymerization, the dentist is not able to carve or make adjustments with hand instruments. Finishing burs and abrasive materials are used to contour and polish a finished composite resin.

**STEPS IN FINISHING A COMPOSITE RESIN.**

- Reduction of the material is completed by the use of a white stone or a finishing diamond.
- Fine finishing is performed with carbide finishing burs, then with diamond burs.
- Polishing the resin begins with medium discs and finishes with superfine discs.
- Finishing strips assist in polishing of the interproximal surfaces.
- Polishing paste applied to a rubber cup completes the step.

See Procedure 43.2: Preparing Composite Resin Materials.

RECALL

13 What is the common term used for dimethacrylate?
14 Which filler type of composite resin is recommended because of its versatility?
15 When composite resins are light-cured, what factors might contribute to the need for a longer curing time for the material?
16 What item is used to determine the color of composite for a procedure?
17 What is the final step in finishing a composite resin?

## Glass Ionomers

Glass ionomers represent one of the most versatile dental materials available. This material has been shown to have an excellent biocompatibility within the oral environment. The adaptability of the glass ionomer by altering the chemical properties allows the material to be used for different purposes within the mouth. This chapter discusses glass ionomers used in the restorative sense such as for restorations core buildups and as sealants. Chapters 44 and 45 introduce glass ionomers used as liners, bonding agents, and cements.

Because glass ionomers have the ability to adhere chemically (not mechanically) to teeth, the need to prepare the tooth structure is not as extensive as the preparation for an amalgam or composite resin. The most unique feature of glass ionomers is the release of *fluoride* after the final setting. This provides the added advantage of inhibiting decay.

This type of material is especially desirable for the following applications:

- *Primary teeth:* Because of the fluoride release and minimal cavity preparation requirement, glass ionomers are the material of choice for the restoration of carious primary teeth.
- *Final restorations in nonstressed areas such as class V and root surfaces:* This material is widely used to restore lost tooth structure such as occurs as a consequence of decay or cervical abrasion.
- *Sealants:* The material is mixed to a more fluid consistency to allow flow into the depths of the pits and fissures of the posterior teeth.
- *Core material for buildups:* Some dentists favor glass ionomers over amalgam because of ease of placement, adhesion, fluoride release, and thermal qualities.
- Provisional (longer-term temporary) restorations

In the term *glass ionomer,* the word *glass* actually refers to a combination of glass, ceramic particles, and a glassy matrix. From this special glass combination, the material derives its translucency and prolonged fluoride release. *Ionomer* refers to ion–cross-linked polymers, such as acrylic acid, tartaric acid, and maleic acid (common materials found in most dental cements). The type of polymer and its molecular weight ensure excellent adhesion and resistance to acid erosion.

### Resin Modified

Over the past several years, glass ionomer materials have improved in terms of physical properties and esthetic qualities through the addition of resin. Resin gives the material better strength, greater wear resistance, and an improved esthetic quality. The resin component also allows the material to be light-cured, auto-cured, or both.

### Metal Reinforcement

The blend of spherical silver-tin alloy with glass ionomer produces a strong, abrasion-resistant dental material. The glass component provides a desirable balance between working and setting times, together with sustained fluoride release. The particles are a polymer of **acrylic acid,** which provides toughness and resistance to acid erosion. The level of metal addition also provides an optimal level of radiopacity. This product is extremely versatile in its clinical application for core buildups; for repair of fractured cusps and amalgam fillings in class I, II, and V cavities; as a base; and as an abutment for overdentures.

### Fabrication and Application

When supplied as a powder and a liquid for cement, glass ionomers are manually mixed together on a treated paper pad, with the powder incorporated into the liquid in several increments (Fig. 43.20). The material must be completely mixed in less than 45 seconds.

For restorative purposes, glass ionomers are supplied in light-protected tubes, cartridges, tubs, or premeasured capsules (Fig. 43.21). The material can be either manipulated with a spatula and placed in the applicator, or triturated and then placed in the applicator and applied to the tooth and light-cured.

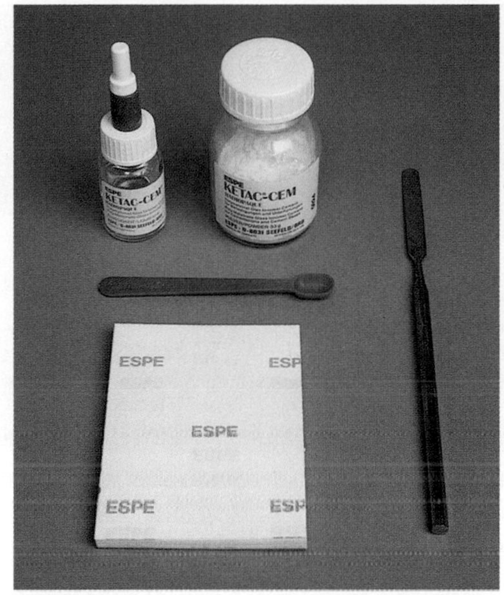


**FIG. 43.20** Setup for mixing glass ionomer liquid and powder.

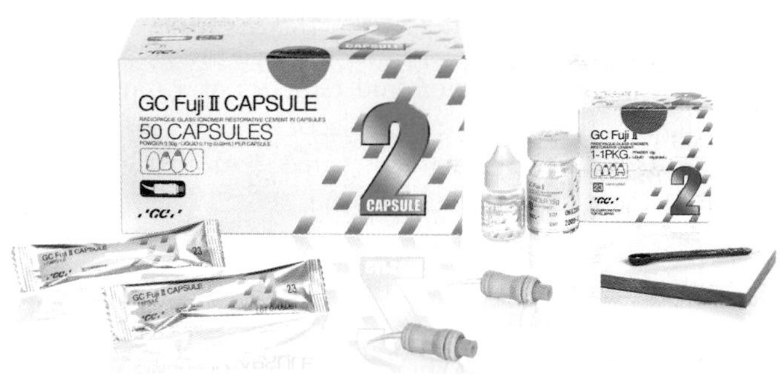


**FIG. 43.21** Glass ionomers are supplied in capsules, cartridges, and individual powder and liquid bottles. *(Courtesy GC America Inc., Alsip, IL.)*

### Cautions for Placing Glass Ionomers

- Avoid water contamination/contact with the material.
- Be aware that when the material's glossy appearance has disappeared, the setting stages have begun.
- Protect the matrix band from the material; the material will adhere to the metal band.

RECALL

18 What are some of the most common uses of glass ionomer materials?

19 What could contaminate the setting of glass ionomers?

## Temporary Restorative Materials

Temporary restorative materials are utilized for various dental situations. The type of material selected for a temporary restoration is designed to maintain or restore function and keep the

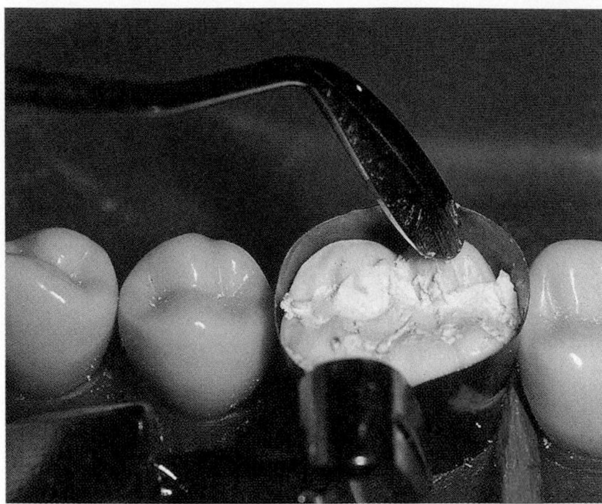

**FIG. 43.22** Placement of intermediate restorative material (IRM) into a molar.

patient comfortable for a limited time. Temporary restorative materials are used for the following reasons:

- To reduce the sensitivity and discomfort of a tooth to determine its diagnosis
- To maintain the function and esthetics of a tooth until a permanent restoration can be placed
- To protect the margins of a prepared tooth that will receive a permanent casting at a later time
- To prevent shifting of adjacent or opposing teeth caused by an open space

The type of temporary restorative material selected depends on the location and amount of the tooth structure that needs to be restored. If a tooth has lost a filling or has a small pit within the enamel, an intermediate restorative material would be selected. If a cusp is gone, or if the dentist has prepared the tooth for a cast restoration involving the gingival margin, a provisional coverage material would be selected.

## Intermediate Restorative Materials

An intermediate restoration is frequently recommended by the dentist as a short-term restoration. The material most often selected for this procedure is the **intermediate restorative material,** or **IRM** (Fig. 43.22). IRM is a reinforced zinc oxide–eugenol composition. The **eugenol** has a sedative effect on the pulp, and fillers are added to improve the strength and durability of the material.

Common uses of IRM include the following:

- Restoration of primary teeth (when permanent teeth are 2 years or less from eruption)
- Restorative emergencies
- Caries management programs
- Placement as a base

IRM is supplied as a powder and a liquid, which are mixed manually on a treated paper pad, or as premeasured capsules that are activated and then triturated.

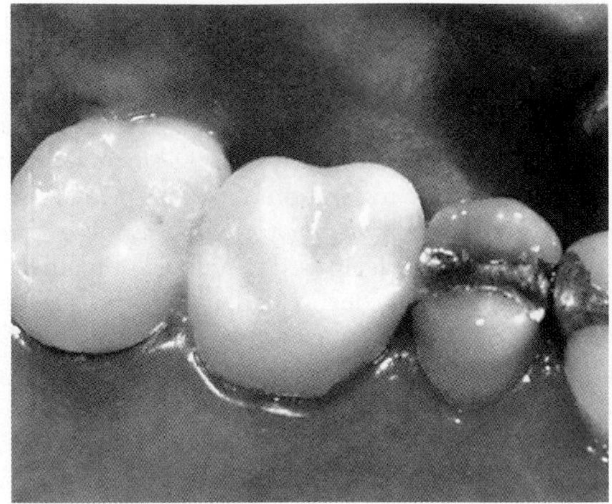

**FIG. 43.23** Example of provisional coverage material.

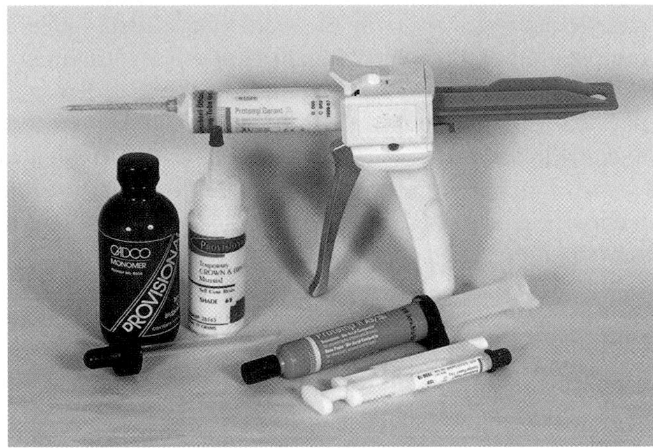


**FIG. 43.24** Acrylic resin is supplied as liquid/powder, tubes, and automix cartridges. *(From Hatrick CD, Eakle WS: Dental materials: clinical applications for dental assistants and dental hygienists, ed 3, St Louis, 2016, Elsevier.)*

Because an intermediate restoration is not considered permanent, this procedure can be performed as an expanded function of the dental assistant in most states. Chapter 48 provides the skill process for this advanced function.

See Procedure 43.3: Mixing Intermediate Restorative Materials.

## Provisional Restorative Materials

A provisional restorative material is designed to cover the major portion, if not the entire clinical portion, of a tooth or several teeth for a longer period. Because of this, these materials must withstand biting forces and the daily wear and tear of oral conditions (Fig. 43.23).

Acrylic resins are supplied in several applications: as a liquid/powder, in premeasured tubes, and in automix cartridges. An auto-cured acrylic (methylmethacrylate) or light-cured composite resin (different properties from composite restorative material) is selected (Fig. 43.24). The material is placed in an alginate impression or a vacuum-formed tray and is seated over the prepared tooth and allowed to cure. The occlusion is adjusted, and the temporary is polished and cemented in place with temporary cement.

Because a provisional restoration is not considered permanent, this procedure can be performed by the expanded-function dental assistant. Chapter 51 provides the skill process for this expanded function.

See Procedure 43.4: Preparing Acrylic Resin for the Fabrication of Provisional Coverage.

RECALL

20 What does the abbreviation IRM stand for?
21 How could IRM be utilized in a pediatric practice?
22 What material would you use to prepare for provisional coverage?
23 How many drops of monomer per tooth are recommended when acrylic resin is mixed for a provisional restoration?

## Tooth-Whitening Materials

Tooth whitening, also referred to as *bleaching,* is one of the most popular and cost-effective ways of restoring the esthetic appearance of teeth. Whitening products can be found in many everyday items such as toothpaste, fluoride, mouth rinses, and even chewing gum.

### Composition of Whitening Materials

Most tooth-whitening products are made from a peroxide-based ingredient. Peroxide-based solutions are supplied in different concentrations. Peroxide-based whitening products work deep within the enamel to remove staining and discoloration that have come from years of accumulated stain and aging. Teeth become discolored and stained for many reasons, most commonly aging; consumption of staining substances such as coffee, tea, colas, and tobacco; trauma; use of tetracycline (antibiotic); excessive fluoride; nerve degeneration; and aging of restorations.

When the peroxide-based product contacts the teeth, it allows oxygen to enter the enamel and dentin, thereby whitening the colored substances. The structure of the tooth is not altered; the tooth is simply made lighter and whiter (Fig. 43.25).

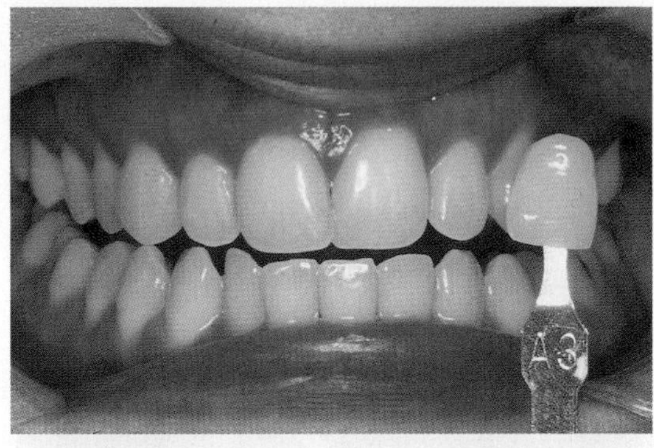


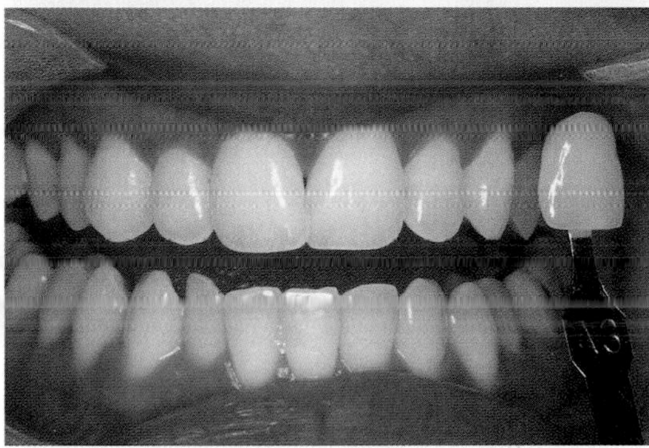

**FIG. 43.25** Before and after the use of a whitening product.

### Methods of Tooth Whitening

Patients can choose from two distinct options when wanting to whiten their teeth: "in office" or "at home." Most in-office bleaching procedures use a bleaching agent that is carbamide peroxide, which breaks down in the mouth to form hydrogen peroxide. The bleaching gel typically contains between 10 percent and 30 percent carbamide peroxide (15 percent is recommended), which is roughly equivalent to a 3 percent to 10 percent hydrogen peroxide concentration.

A newer choice for in-office whitening is power or light-accelerated bleaching, also referred to as laser bleaching. This technique uses light energy to speed the process of bleaching. Different types of energy can be used in this procedure, with the most common being the halogen light. A power bleaching treatment typically involves isolation of soft tissue with a resin-based, light-curable barrier; application of a professional dental-grade hydrogen peroxide whitening gel (25 to 38 percent hydrogen peroxide); and exposure to the light source for 6 to 15 minutes. Most power teeth-whitening treatments can be done in approximately 30 minutes to 1 hour, in a single visit.

Teeth whitening at home can be accomplished by using high-concentration carbamide peroxide; this can be more cost-effective than the in-office procedure. Whitening is performed by applying a concentration of an oxidizing agent to the teeth using thin plastic trays or strips for a short period of time; this produces results in a few days to a week. The application ideally should be well fitted to retain the bleaching gel, ensuring even and full tooth exposure to the gel. Typically, the material will stay on the teeth for about 15 to 20 minutes. Trays or strips are then removed, and the procedure is repeated over several days.

See Chapter 48 for specific procedures with whitening products.

## Indirect Restorative Materials

An indirect restoration is one that is fabricated outside the mouth by a dental laboratory technician. These restorations, also referred to as **castings,** involve a sequence of procedures that include preparing the tooth, taking a final impression, waxing a pattern, investing the pattern, casting the restoration, finishing and polishing the casting, and cementing the restoration in place.

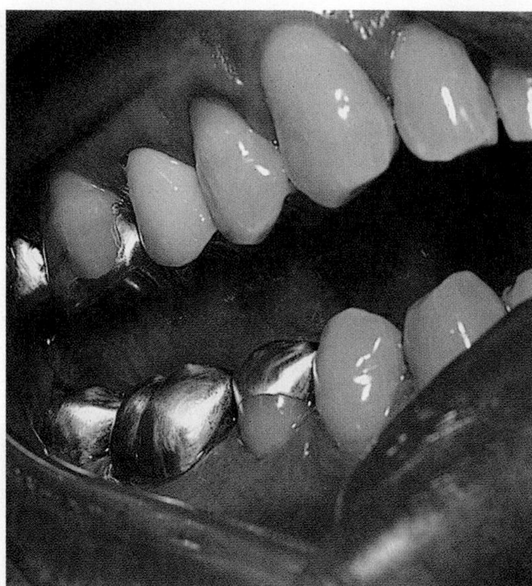

**FIG. 43.26** Gold crown. *(Courtesy Dr. David Graham, San Francisco, CA.)*

Indirect restorative materials include gold alloys and ceramic materials. The finished castings of these materials are bonded or cemented into place.

## Gold–Noble Metal Alloys

Gold in its purest form has the ability to resist tarnish and etching when exposed to harsh conditions in the mouth, but it is much too soft for use in cast dental restorations. However, gold can be combined with other metals to form an alloy; this material provides the characteristics and hardness required of an indirect restoration (Fig. 43.26). One way of describing the alloys used in indirect restorations is to discuss their noble and base metal content.

**Noble metals** used for cast restorations consist of **gold** (Au), **palladium** (Pd), and **platinum** (Pt). All other metals in the alloys that are not classified as noble metals are considered to be base metals. A *base metal* is a metal of relatively low value that has inferior properties such as lack of resistance to corrosion and tarnish. Iron, tin, and zinc are examples of base metals.

Gold alloys are described according to their hardness, malleability, and adaptability. With the use of this descriptive system, the four types of gold alloys are as follows:

- Soft, **type I alloys** have 83 percent noble metals and are used for casting inlays, which are subject to slight stress during mastication.
- Medium, **type II alloys** have 78 percent noble metals and can be used for almost all types of cast inlays and posterior bridge abutments.
- Hard, **type III alloys** have 77 percent noble metals and are acceptable for inlays, full crowns, three-quarter crowns, and anterior or posterior bridge abutments.
- Extra hard, **type IV alloys** have 75 percent noble metals and are also referred to as partial denture alloys; they are designed for crowns, bridges, and cast-removable partial dentures.

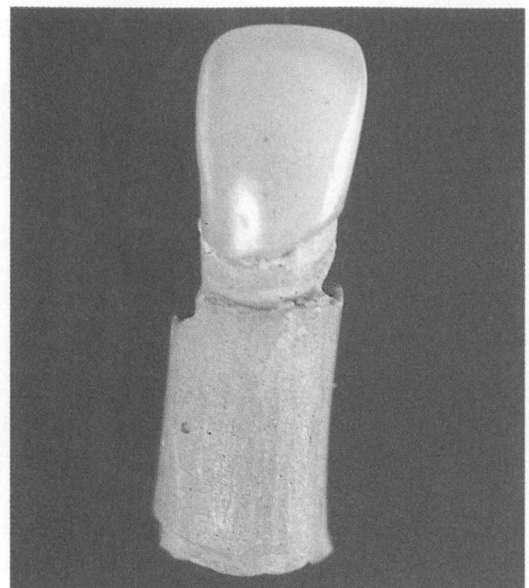

**FIG. 43.27** Porcelain crown.

## Ceramic Castings

**Ceramic** is a type of material that is similar to that used in the dishes or pottery in your home. Ceramics are **compounds,** which are combinations of metallic and nonmetallic elements. As with dishes and pottery, ceramic castings are made of a claylike material with a **glaze** that has metallic components to make it durable and able to withstand temperature change. A ceramic material can be adhered to a metal casting, creating the "best of both worlds" in strength and esthetics. Combinations of ceramic-metal restorations include the following:

- Porcelain fused to metal (PFM)
- Porcelain bonded to metal (PBM)
- Ceramico-metal (C/M)
- Porcelain-metal (P/M)

## Porcelain

The type of ceramic most often used in dentistry is **porcelain**. This type of ceramic combines strength, translucency, and the ability to match natural tooth color (Fig. 43.27). Because laboratory fabrication techniques incorporate heat and pressure, these restorations are stronger than *direct* restorations, such as composite resins, which are created in the mouth. The ceramic porcelain is fused to a metal backing shell; then it is glazed and fired to produce a highly smooth surface that is extremely hard and similar to enamel.

Porcelain material is chosen for the following reasons:

- The shading of colors matches tooth color well.
- Porcelain improves the esthetic appearance of anterior teeth.
- The material has the strength of metal.
- Porcelain is a good insulator.
- The material has a low coefficient of thermal expansion.

24 What are the three noble metals used in dentistry?
25 What type of restoration is made in the dental laboratory?

**■ Patient Education** Most patients are concerned not only with the appearance of their teeth, but also with the safety and quality of the dental materials that are being placed in their mouth. When scheduling patients for a temporary or a permanent restoration, be sure to inform them of their needs and to explain why the dentist has made the decision to use a specific dental material for the procedure. Use of visual aids that allow the patient to view different restorations can greatly alleviate the patient's fear of the unknown. ■

**■ Legal and Ethical Implications** As with any procedure, it is important to indicate in the patient's record what material was used during the restoration. If a patient has any negative medical reaction to a specific material or develops a problem associated with the restoration that requires attention, the dentist will have a record of what might be causing the problem. This also provides the patient with a sense of assurance that the dentist is following through to provide complete treatment. ■

**■ Eye to the Future** In the near future, the new term for restoration may be *regeneration.* This may sound like something from *Star Trek,* but decayed or missing teeth soon will be regrown, either in the mouth or in the laboratory. A group of scientists are currently working on a cavity treatment that will stimulate the growth of dentin. This new treatment eventually will be applied to the cavity before it is filled, thus helping the tooth to heal itself. ■

## ■ Critical Thinking

1. An emergency patient is being seen today because of a lost "filling" (M-O on # 5). The dentist examines the tooth and requests that a radiograph be taken and to schedule the patient for a new restoration. The dentist asks you to place a temporary restoration until the patient can return for a scheduled appointment. Which temporary dental material would most likely be used to replace the lost filling?
2. A patient has discussed her concern over the large quantity of amalgam fillings in her mouth; she fears that the mercury may be harming her health. She has scheduled an appointment to discuss this with the dentist. If you were the dentist, how would you respond to this patient?
3. With regard to direct restorative dental materials, which dental material would you say is the most versatile and widely used, and why?
4. Tooth whitening has become one of the most often requested procedure by patients. Why is this procedure so popular with patients, and why is it best to have the dentist involved in the process?
5. What is the difference between composite resins and ceramics? ■

PROCEDURE 43.1

# Mixing and Transferring Dental Amalgam

### EQUIPMENT AND SUPPLIES

- ✓ Amalgam capsule
- ✓ Capsule activator
- ✓ Amalgamator
- ✓ Amalgam well or cloth
- ✓ Amalgam carrier

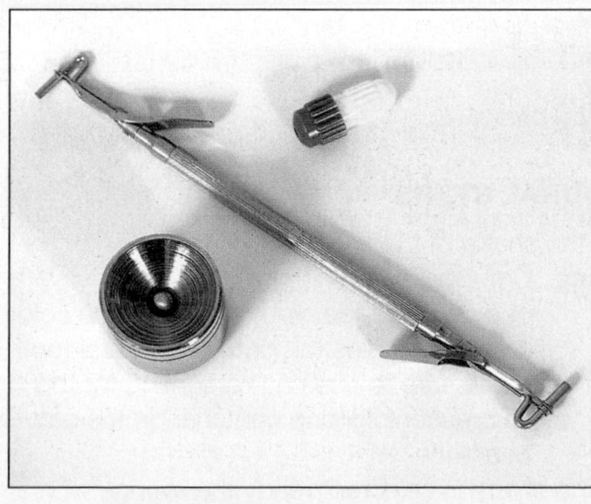

### PROCEDURAL STEPS

1 Activate the amalgam capsule using the activator, if required for the particular type of amalgam.
**PURPOSE** This breaks the separating membrane to allow the mercury and alloy powders to mix.

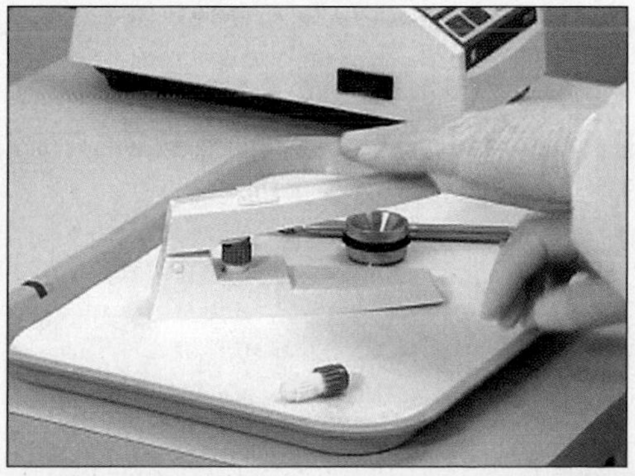

2 Place the capsule into the amalgamator.

**(Continued)**

## PROCEDURE 43.1 Mixing and Transferring Dental Amalgam—cont'd

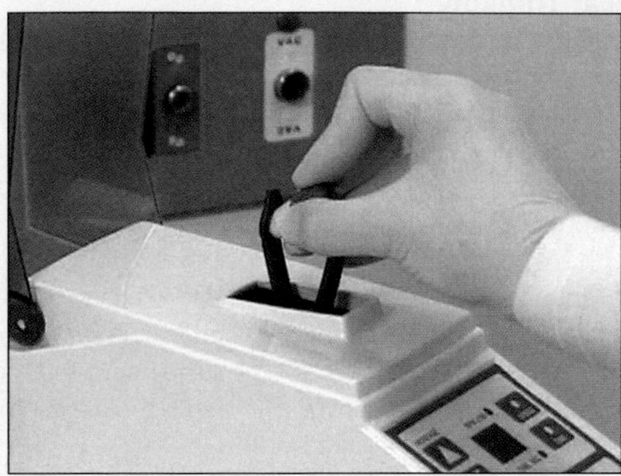

3 Adjust the settings on the amalgamator according to the type of amalgam.
4 Close the cover on the amalgamator and begin trituration.
5 Remove the capsule, twist it open, and dispense amalgam in the well or amalgam cloth.

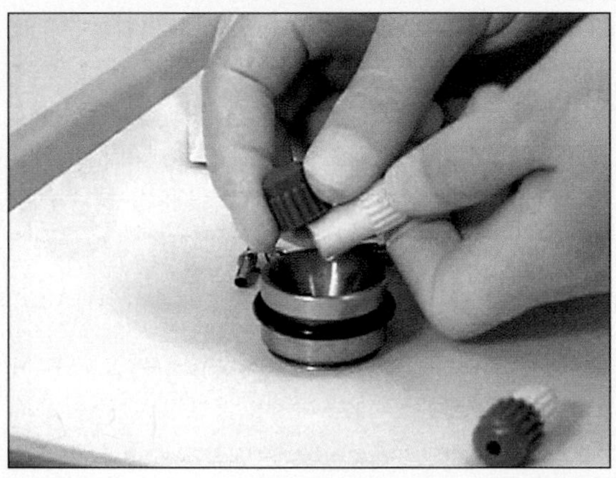

6 Fill the small end of the carrier first; then transfer the carrier, making sure the end of the carrier is directed toward the preparation.

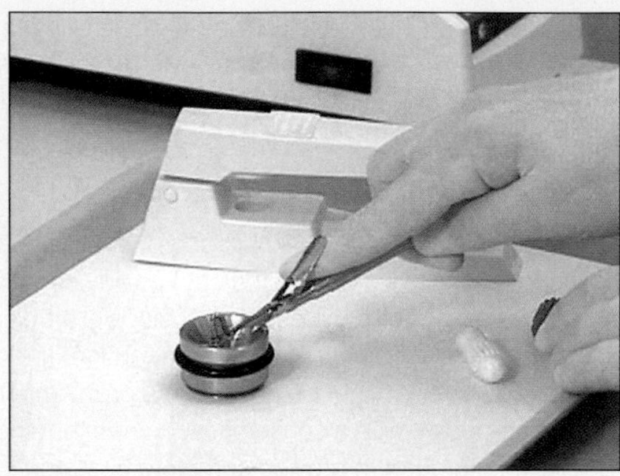

7 Transfer the carrier to the operator with the small end facing toward the tooth to be filled.

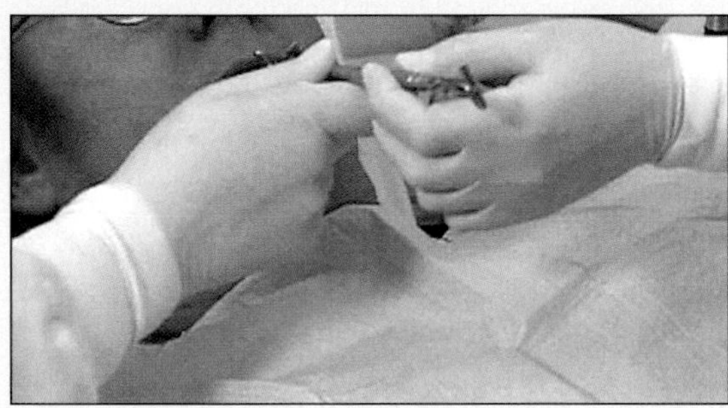

8 Continue this process until the preparation is overfilled.

## PROCEDURE 43.2

# Preparing Composite Resin Materials

### EQUIPMENT AND SUPPLIES

- ✓ Shade guide
- ✓ Composite resin material
- ✓ Syringe tip
- ✓ Composite instrument
- ✓ 2 × 2–inch alcohol gauze pads
- ✓ Curing light

### PROCEDURAL STEPS

1 Select the shade of the tooth.

**PURPOSE** Composites come in varying shades; with the use of a shade guide, you can select the color that most resembles the patient's natural tooth color.

**NOTE** Make sure to use natural lighting for this decision. Fluorescent lighting can change the natural appearance.

2 Once the shade is selected, ready the syringe with a new tip for application.

## PROCEDURE 43.2 Preparing Composite Resin Materials–cont'd

**NOTE** If using a paste, express a very small amount on a paper pad or well.

3 Transfer the composite instrument and material to the transfer zone for the dentist.

4 The dentist may ask that the liquid bonding resin or alcohol gauze be available during placement of material increments.
**PURPOSE** These will aid in the flow of the material.

5 Have the curing light readied during placement of the material. It is best when the material can be light-cured as increments are placed.
**PURPOSE** This completes the final setting of the material.

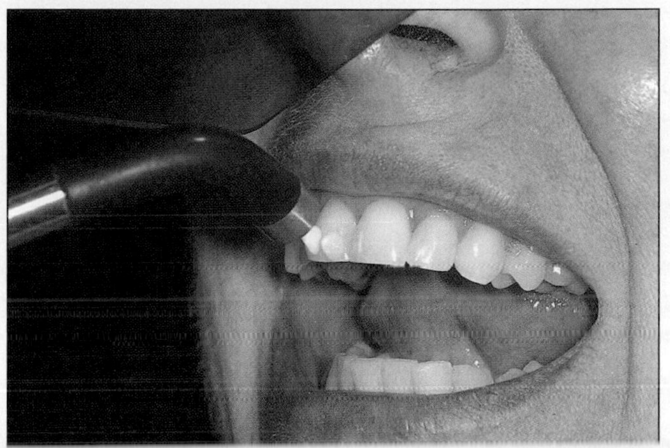

## PROCEDURE 43.3

# Mixing Intermediate Restorative Materials

### EQUIPMENT AND SUPPLIES

- ✔ Treated paper pad
- ✔ Spatula (flexible stainless steel)
- ✔ Intermediate restorative material (IRM) powder and dispenser
- ✔ IRM liquid and dropper
- ✔ 2 × 2–inch alcohol gauze

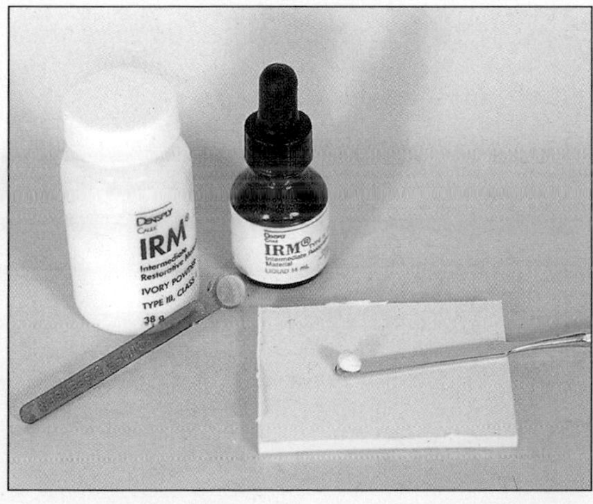


### PROCEDURAL STEPS

1 Shake the powder before dispensing; then measure the powder onto the mixing pad.
**PURPOSE** When the powder is fluffed, it will not be as packed, thus creating a drier mix.

2 Make a well in half the powder; then dispense the liquid into the mix. Recap the containers.
**NOTE** IRM is dispensed in equal ratios, meaning 1 scoop of powder to 1 drop of liquid.

3 Incorporate the remaining powder into the mixture in two or three increments, and mix thoroughly with the spatula. The mix will be quite stiff at this stage.

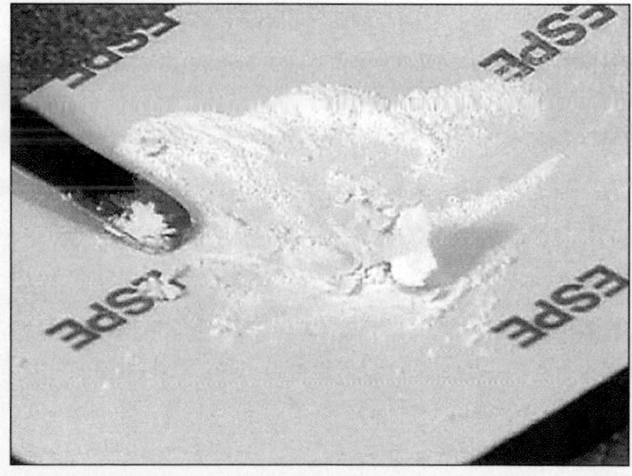


4 Wipe the mix back and forth on the mixing pad for 5 to 10 seconds. The resulting mix should be smooth and adaptable. The mix must be completed within 1 minute.

5 Clean and disinfect the equipment immediately.

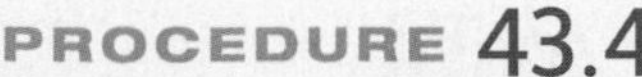

PROCEDURE 43.4

# Preparing Acrylic Resin for the Fabrication of Provisional Coverage

## EQUIPMENT AND SUPPLIES

- ✓ Self-curing acrylic resin (liquid and powder)
- ✓ Dropper
- ✓ Spatula (small metal)
- ✓ Dappen dish or disposable dish available with material

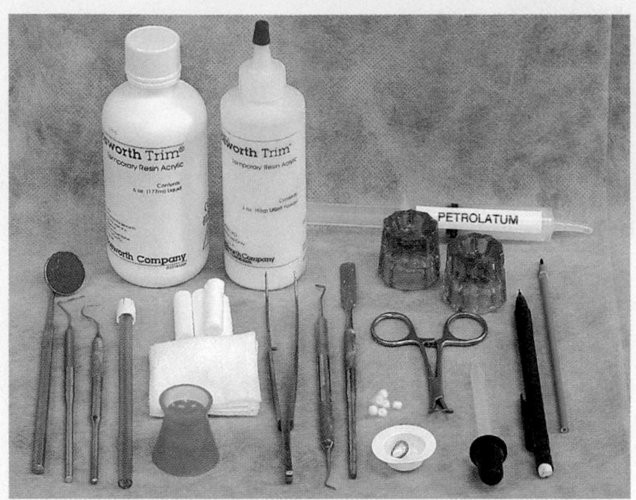


Rosenstiel SF, Land MF, Fujimoto J: Contemporary fixed prosthodontics, ed 5, St Louis, 2016, Elsevier.

## PROCEDURAL STEPS

1 Using the dropper provided, dispense liquid monomer into the mixing container. The recommended amount is 10 drops of liquid per tooth.

**NOTE** Cover the monomer container immediately. This material is volatile.

2 Quickly dispense the selected shade of self-curing powder (polymer) into the liquid until the liquid is overfilled. Quickly turn over the dish onto a paper towel, removing excess powder that was not absorbed by the liquid.

3 Use a small spatula to blend the powder and liquid into a homogeneous mix.

4 Allow the material to sit untouched until the mix loses some of its shine and changes to a doughlike state.

5 The material is ready to be placed in the impression or tray.

44

# Dental Liners, Bases, and Bonding Systems

## KEY TERMS

**Desiccate (DES-i-kayt)** To remove all moisture from an item, or to dry out.
**Etchant (ECH-unt)** Chemical agent used to prepare a tooth surface for a dental material.
**Etching (ECH-ing)** Process of cutting into a surface with the use of an acid product.
**Eugenol (YOO-je-nol)** Colorless liquid made from clove oil and used for its soothing qualities.
**Hybrid (HYE-brid)** Material that produces a similar outcome to its natural counterpart.
**Insulating** Preventing the passage of heat or electricity.
**Micromechanical (mye-kroe-me-KAN-i-kul)** Means by which a material and a structure lock onto one another through minute cuttings.
**Obliterating (oe-BLIT-uh-rayt-ing)** Removing something completely.
**Polymerize (pah-LIM-uh-rize)** To subject a material to the bonding process of two or more monomers.
**Sedative (SED-uh-tiv)** Having a soothing effect.
**Smear layer** Very thin layer of debris on newly prepared dentin.
**Thermal (THUR-mul)** Relating to heat.

## LEARNING OUTCOMES

*On completion of this chapter, the student will be able to achieve the following objectives:*

1. Pronounce, define, and spell the key terms.
2. Discuss how preparation of a tooth is determined.
3. Discuss how the sensitivity of a tooth determines what type of dental material is selected for a procedure.
4. Discuss how and why cavity liners are used in restoring tooth structure.
5. Discuss how and why cavity sealers, including varnish, are used in restoring tooth structure.
6. Discuss how and why desensitizers are used in restoring tooth structure.
7. Discuss how and why dental bases are used in restoring tooth structure.
8. Describe the etching process of a tooth and its importance in the bonding of tooth and material.
9. Describe the bonding systems and how they provide better adherence of dental materials to the tooth structure.

## PERFORMANCE OUTCOMES

*On completion of this chapter, the student will be able to achieve competency standards in the following skills:*

- Apply calcium hydroxide to a prepared tooth surface.
- Apply dental varnish to a prepared tooth surface.
- Apply a desensitizer to a prepared tooth surface.
- Mix and place three types of base on a prepared tooth surface.
- Apply etchant material.
- Apply a bonding system to the prepared tooth structure.

## ELECTRONIC RESOURCES

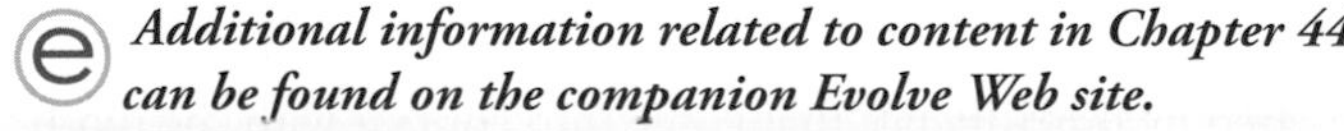

***Additional information related to content in Chapter 44 can be found on the companion Evolve Web site.***

- Practice Quiz
- Videos: Mixing and Applying Calcium Hydroxide; Mixing and Applying Zinc Oxide–Eugenol Cement as a Base; Mixing Polycarboxylate Cement as a Base

A variety of supplemental dental materials are often incorporated into a restorative and esthetic procedure for the health and well-being of the tooth being restored. This chapter describes these materials and guides you in the use of liners, bases, varnishes, desensitizers, and etching and bonding materials that provide added protection for the pulp and surrounding tooth structures in the final restoration process.

When a dentist begins to prepare a tooth, he or she is never 100 percent certain as to the extent of the disease present in the tooth's structure until the tooth has been accessed by a rotary or hand (manual) cutting instrument. If decay has extended into the dentin or has moved close to the pulp, a moderately deep or deep preparation is required. When this happens, the tooth will require additional materials to be placed, such as a liner, base, varnish, desensitizer, bonding agent, or a combination of the five, before the permanent restoration is placed.

Table 44.1 summarizes the use of supplemental materials discussed in this chapter and presents the order in which they would be placed for specific procedures.

## Prepared Tooth Structures

If you look at existing restorations in your mouth, you will see a specific outline or design of the restoration. These cavity designs are used for the sole purpose of creating strength within the tooth; this determines how well the tooth will hold the restoration in place and withstand the normal chewing and biting forces. The more natural tooth structure that the dentist leaves, the easier it is to hold the restorative material in place. If the tooth structure is weak or has little foundation, the dentist will rely on dental materials for their retaining properties.

## Pulpal Responses

As was mentioned in earlier chapters, if decay has progressed from the enamel and into the dentin, a patient may have greater sensitivity and discomfort even after the placement of a permanent restoration. The patient may experience sensitivity immediately, a month after placement, or even several months after placement. For the dentist to be proactive, he or she must decide at this point what supplemental materials will be placed to provide healing and protection against a pulpal response.

### Types of Pulpal Stimuli

Because the pulp is living tissue with nerves and blood vessels, a tooth can respond to different stimuli occurring in the mouth.

- **Physical stimuli** result from **thermal** changes such as hot and cold, air used for drying a tooth, or electrical energy created by other metals that come into contact with the tooth.
- **Mechanical stimuli** can include the vibration from a handpiece when the tooth is being prepared. It can also be associated with traumatic occlusion, which occurs when a person's "bite" does not occlude properly, and added pressure is placed on a specific area of the tooth. Also, if the person grinds his or her teeth, this can create a response to stimuli.
- **Chemical stimuli** can occur as a result of acidic materials reaching pulpal tissues, such as saliva reaching an exposed pulp or by means of microleakage.
- **Biologic stimuli** can also be the result of bacteria from saliva coming into contact with pulpal tissues, or if carious tissue was not completely removed during the preparation of the tooth.

## Cavity Liners

A cavity liner does exactly what its name implies: It is a thin layer of a flowable material placed in the most excavated area of the dentin layer for a therapeutic effect. This thin barrier between the tooth and final restorative material protects the pulpal tissue from irritation caused by physical, mechanical, chemical, and biologic elements. The dentist will determine which lining agent to use based on the health and condition of the tooth being restored.

### Calcium Hydroxide

Calcium hydroxide is one of the most frequently selected types of cavity liner because of its unique characteristics. Examples include Dycal, VLC Dycal, and Life. Some of its unique characteristics include the following:

- It protects the pulp from chemical irritation through its sealing abilities.
- It stimulates the production of reparative or secondary dentin.
- It is used for pulp capping of pulpal exposures and near exposure.
- It is compatible with all types of restorative materials.

**TABLE 44.1** Supplemental Dental Materials and Application in Order of Use

| Type of Restorative Material | Shallow Preparation | Moderately Deep Restoration | Deep Restoration |
|---|---|---|---|
| Amalgam | Desensitizer<br>Etching/bonding system | Base<br>Varnish or desensitizer<br>Etching/bonding system | Liner<br>Base<br>Varnish or desensitizer<br>Etching/bonding system |
| Composite resin | Etching/bonding system | Etching/bonding system | Liner<br>Etching/bonding system |
| Gold inlays/onlays | | Base | Liner<br>Base |
| Ceramic | Bonding system | Bonding system | Liner<br>Bonding system |

## Glass Ionomer

Resin-modified glass ionomer liners are indicated to form a strong bond to dentin, sealing the restoration to reduce microleakage and helping to reduce post-operative sensitivity. Examples include Vitrebond, Ketac bond, and Fuji Lining.

## Application

Liners are supplied either as a two-paste system (base and catalyst) or as a light-cured material. The material is prepared and placed with the use of a Dycal applicator. The liner is placed in the deepest *dentin* surface of the preparation. It is important to note that this material is not to be placed on enamel or in retentive grooves of the preparation.

The expanded functions dental assistant (EFDA), or registered dental assistant (RDA), can place dental liners if this function is legal in the state or provinces in which the assistant is practicing. Because of variations in cavity preparations, you must be certain of where the liner is to be placed. Knowledge of pulpal anatomy and knowledge of how a cavity preparation appears will assist you in your placement (Fig. 44.1).

See Procedure 44.1: Applying Calcium Hydroxide (Expanded Function).

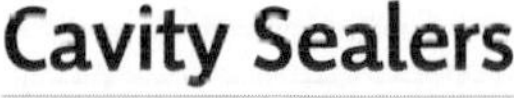


1 What is the function of a dental liner?
2 Within the cavity preparation, where is a liner placed?
3 What are the unique qualities of calcium hydroxide?

# Cavity Sealers

If you are familiar with refinishing furniture, you will understand the significance of using a sealer to protect the wood from its environment. A cavity sealer works in the same way for the restoration of a tooth; it is applied in a thin film that provides a protective layer within the prepared cavity.

## Varnish

Dental varnish is a type of sealer that consists of one or more natural resins dissolved in an organic solvent. Varnish is placed within the entire preparation. Examples include Copalite, Plastodent, and Barrier. Application of a varnish accomplishes the following:

- Seals dentinal tubules (Fig. 44.2)
- Reduces microleakage around a restoration
- Acts as a barrier to protect the tooth from highly acidic base or cements such as zinc phosphate

### *Fluoride Varnish*

Fluoride varnish was developed and utilized in Europe and Canada for many years for caries prevention and was approved in the early 1990s for placement in the United States for this purpose, as well as for use as a highly effective cavity varnish and desensitizer (Fig. 44.3). Fluoride varnish has a higher fluoride concentration than any other fluoride marketed, being 5% or 22,600 ppm fluoride. The main advantage of this type of varnish is its versatility in use. This gel-like substance is designed to release fluoride on enamel, root structure, and dentin structure. Specific indications for the use of fluoride varnish are as follows:

- Professional topical fluoride application
- Treatment of hypersensitive cervical areas
- Orthodontic patients
- Cavity varnish
- Dentin sealant

See Chapter 13 for the procedure for a preventive application of fluoride varnish.

### *Application*

Varnish is applied with a small disposable applicator. It is important to note that the varnish is placed *after* the liner is applied (Fig. 44.4).

Because dental varnish interferes with the bonding and setting reaction of composite resins and glass ionomer restorations, the use of varnish is contraindicated with these materials.

The EFDA (RDA) can place dental varnish if the function is legal where the assistant is practicing.

See Procedure 44.2: Applying Dental Varnish (Expanded Function).

# Desensitizer

A desensitizer is a type of sealer used to protect the tooth from hypersensitivity. A desensitizer is an agent that would be used in place of a varnish. This works like a varnish, but the difference is the makeup of the product. GLUMA, Barrier, and Protect are examples of this type of material utilized for sealing dentin tubules with hydroxyethyl methacrylate (HEMA) and glutaraldehyde. This material is ideal for use under *all* direct and indirect restorations because no surface layer of the preparation has to be prepared.

## Application

Because of the makeup and the toxic element in desensitizers, it is very important that this material is used sparingly and should not come into contact with soft tissue.

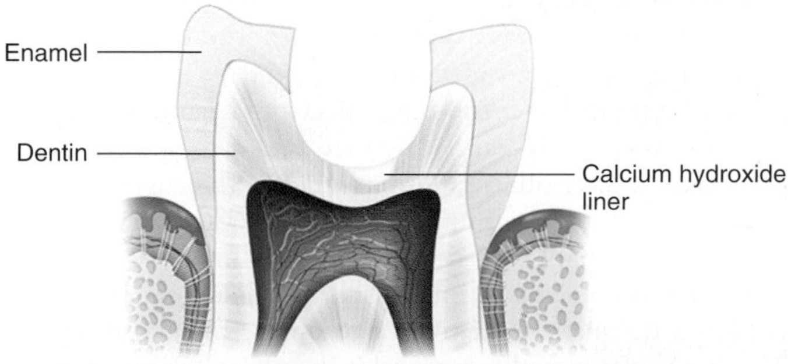


**FIG. 44.1** Placement of a liner. *(© Elsevier Collection.)*

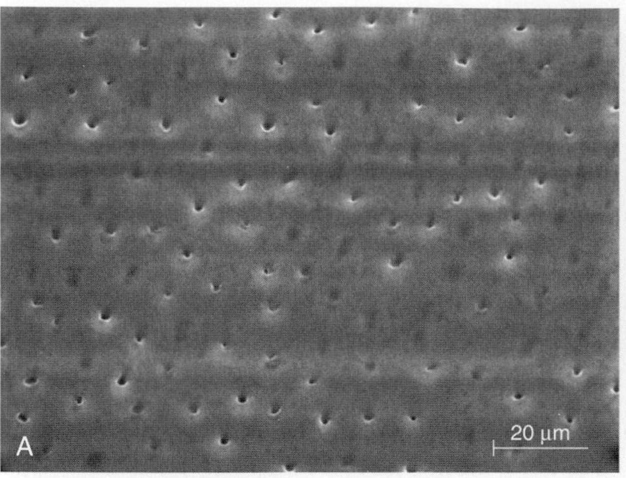


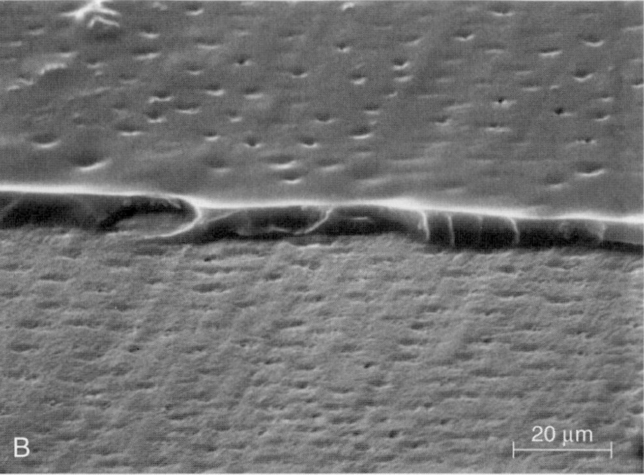


**FIG. 44.2** Microscopic view of dentin structure with exposed dentinal tubules. A, Showing one layer of varnish. B, Two layers of varnish sealing the dentinal tubules. *(Courtesy of S.C. Bayne, School of Dentistry, University of Michigan, Ann Arbor, MI.)*

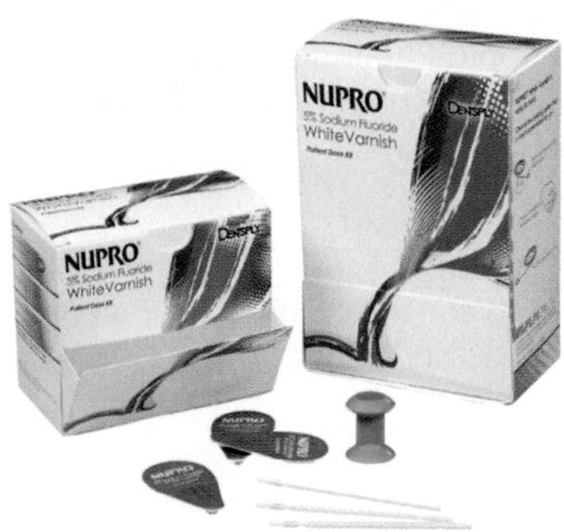


**FIG. 44.3** An example of a fluoride varnish product. *(Courtesy DENTSPLY Professional, York, PA.)*

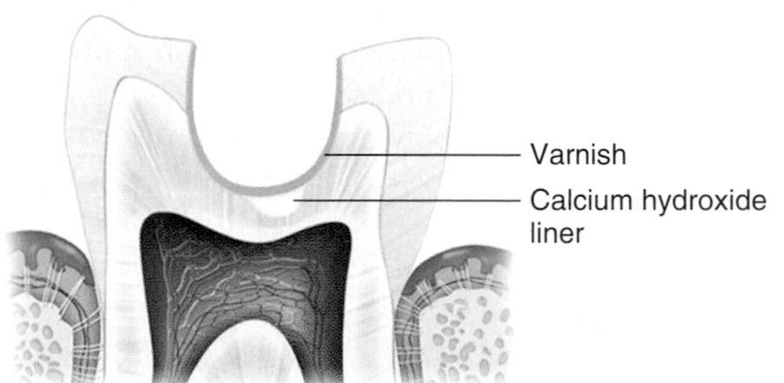


**FIG. 44.4** Location for placement of cavity varnish. *(© Elsevier Collection.)*

The EFDA (RDA) can place desensitizers if the function is legal where the assistant is practicing.

See Procedure 44.3: Applying a Desensitizer (Expanded Function).

RECALL

4 What is the main ingredient in varnish?
5 Can varnish be placed under all restorative materials? If not, with which materials is it contraindicated?
6 What toxic element is in a desensitizer?
7 What does a desensitizer do?

## Dental Bases

When a tooth preparation becomes moderately deep to deep, the preparation will require an additional layer or base to be placed before the permanent restorative material.

A base is designed to provide pulpal defense in the following three ways:

- **Protective bases** are placed when it is necessary to protect the pulp before the restoration is placed. Without this protection, postoperative sensitivity and damage to the pulp may occur.
- **Insulating bases** are placed in a deep cavity preparation to protect the tooth from thermal shock. (**Thermal shock** occurs when sudden temperature changes occur within the tooth.)
- **Sedative bases** help soothe a pulp that has been damaged by decay or has been irritated during the process of removing the decay.

## Types of Materials Used

Different types of cement products are used to form these specialized bases under permanent restorations. Dental cements have a versatile quality to be used as a base or a cement based on the mixing technique. See Chapter 45 for cement use.

**Zinc oxide–eugenol (ZOE)** can be selected for use as an **insulating** base and as a **sedative** base. The unique quality of this material is the eugenol in the liquid. With its oil from cloves, **eugenol** has a soothing effect on a painful, irritated pulp. However, ZOE cannot be used under composite resins, glass ionomers, or other resin restorations. The eugenol in the liquid will affect the setting process of the resin materials.

**Zinc phosphate** cement is an excellent material to use as a base because of its thermal insulation qualities. The material has a thermal conductivity rate similar to that of dentin. The disadvantage to this material is the phosphoric acid liquid component, which can be irritating to the pulp. Because of this, it is necessary to place a cavity liner before the zinc phosphate insulating base.

**Polycarboxylate** cements are selected as a base for their protective and insulating qualities. Polycarboxylate is nonirritating to the pulp and can be placed under all types of direct and indirect restorations.

**Glass ionomer** cement can also be utilized as a base. It is characterized by its excellent adhesion to enamel and dentin. Glass ionomer liner/base combines light-cure convenience with true glass ionomer fluoride release and bond strength.

### Examples of Commercial Cement Bases

**Zinc Oxide–Eugenol**

- IRM
- ZOE
- ZOE 2200

**Zinc Phosphate**

- Dropsin
- Fleck's Extraordinary
- HyBond SP
- Modern Tenacin
- Zinc Cement Improved

**Polycarboxylate**

- Carboxylon
- Chemit
- Durelon
- Durelon Fast Set
- Hybond
- PC Cement
- Polybond
- Poly-F Plus
- Tylok

**Glass Ionomer**

- ASPA
- Chembond
- Dentin Cement LC
- Fuji Lining LC
- Ketac-Bond
- Vitrebond
- Zionomer

**Resin-Modified Glass Ionomer**

- Fuji Duet
- Vitremer Cement

## Application

For a base application, the material is mixed into a putty-like consistency and condensed into the cavity preparation to provide a buffer or layer between the pulp and the restoration. The entire pulpal floor is covered with a base to a thickness of 1 to 2 mm (Fig. 44.5). The EFDA (RDA) can place a base if the function is legal in the state in which the assistant is practicing.

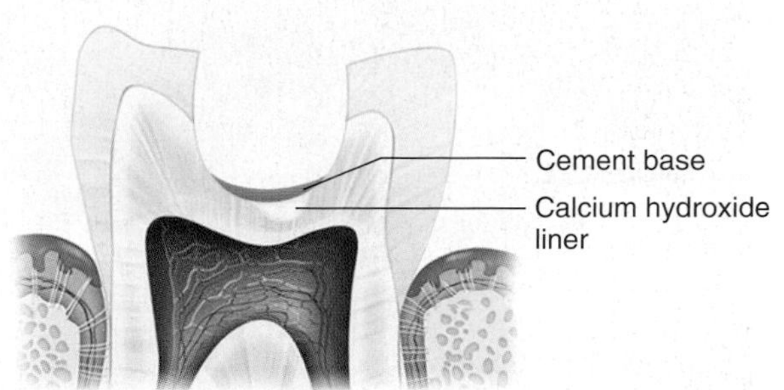


**FIG. 44.5** Location for placement of a base. *(© Elsevier Collection.)*

See Procedure 44.4: Mixing and Placing Zinc Oxide–Eugenol Cement as a Base (Expanded Function), Procedure 44.5: Mixing and Placing Zinc Phosphate Cement as a Base (Expanded Function), and Procedure 44.6: Mixing and Placing Polycarboxylate Cement as a Base (Expanded Function).

RECALL

8 What does an insulating base provide for the restoration of a tooth?
9 What base material contains eugenol? What effect does eugenol have on the pulp?
10 Where is a base applied in the preparation?
11 What dental instrument is used to adapt a base into the cavity preparation?

## Dental Etchant

In tooth preparation when using a bonding material, the tooth surface (enamel or dentin, or both) will need to be etched with an acidic **tooth conditioner.** In many ways, an etched surface of a tooth resembles etched glass. If you run your hand over frosted glass, you can feel that its surface has a texture. This is because at a microscopic level, the surface of the glass is very rough. You also know that etched glass has a frosted appearance. The surface of an etched tooth resembles this effect. When you rinse and dry an etched surface, it will have the same distinctive "frosted" appearance.

The preparation of a tooth surface is critical for both enamel and dentin surfaces of a cavity preparation to form a better chemical bond between the tooth and the permanent restorative material. The use of a bur or by applying a **phosphoric acid** solution to the dentin removes the **smear layer** in preparation for adhesion of a composite resin or sealant material to the tooth surface (Fig. 44.6).

## Application

The **etchant** material is supplied as a liquid or a gel, with gel being packaged in a syringe-type applicator (Fig. 44.7). Syringe dispensing through pre-bent dispenser needles provides precise placement of the material where it is needed in and around the preparation. The allotted time for placement will depend on the procedure. Fifteen to twenty seconds is the most common recommended time from the manufacturers of etchants.

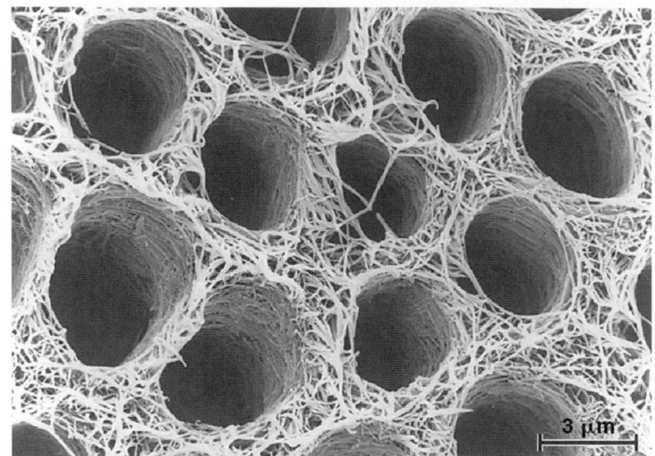


FIG. 44.6 Microscopic view of dentin after etching. *(From Heymann HO, Swift EJ, Ritter AV: Sturdevant's art and science of operative dentistry, ed 6, St Louis, 2013, Mosby.)*

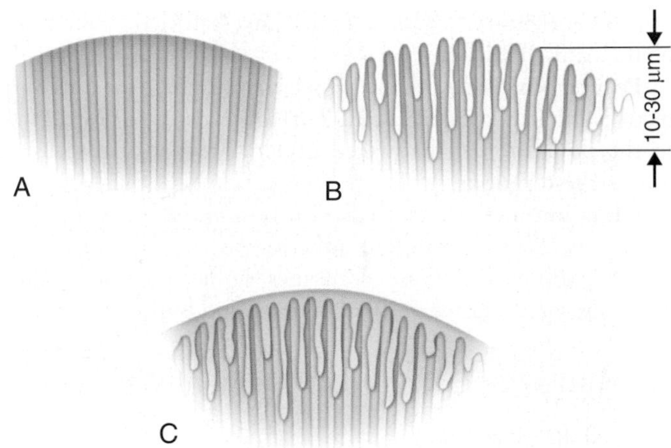


FIG. 44.8 Process of bonding. A, Enamel rods unetched. B, Enamel rods etched. C, Bonding agent mechanically bonding to tooth. *(© Elsevier Collection.)*

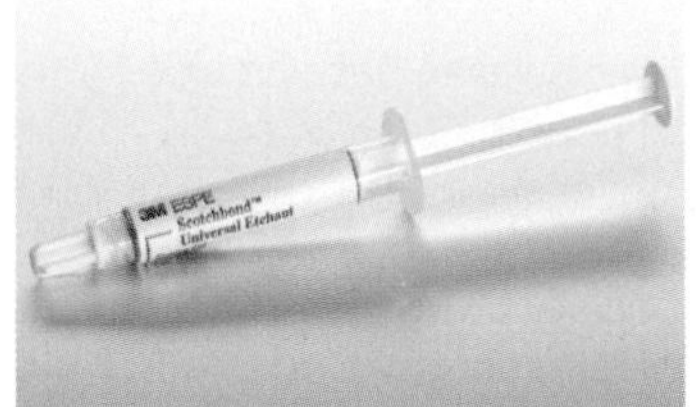

FIG. 44.7 Example of etchant material. *(Courtesy 3M ESPE, St Paul, MN.)*

An understanding of the application process is important for the dental assistant. The EFDA (RDA) can apply the etchant and place the bonding material if the function is legal in the state in which the assistant is practicing.

See Procedure 44.7: Applying an Etchant Material (Expanded Function).

# Dental Bonding

Many of the retention problems associated with dental materials have been remedied by the addition of a bonding material. Dental bonding, also referred to as **dental adhesion,** is the process of attaining a solid and/or liquid contact of one material with another at a single margin. Retaining properties of bonding systems have been improved by the creation of **micromechanical** retention between the tooth structure and the restoration. With the use of bonding materials, it is now possible to bond restorative materials to enamel and dentin.

## Enamel Bonding

Examples of enamel bonding include the placement of *sealants,* the bonding of orthodontic *brackets,* and the use of resin-bonded *bridges.* Most of these are attached directly to the intact enamel surface. For resin-bonded *veneers,* a thin layer of enamel is removed with the use of rotary instruments before the **etching** and bonding process is begun.

When sealant, resin cement, or restorative material is placed on an etched surface, the bonding material flows in and around the enamel tags (Fig. 44.8). The material hardens in this location to form a strong mechanical bond with the enamel.

## Dentin Bonding

Different from enamel, dentin consists of a range of organic substances, and the bonding of restorative dental materials can be difficult. A major factor in the success of bonding a material to dentin is the removal of the smear layer, which is a very thin layer (5–10 microns) of debris composed of fluids and tooth components that remain on the dentin after cavity preparation has been completed (Fig. 44.9).

The smear layer, which has been described as "nature's bandage," protects the tooth by **obliterating** the openings of the dentinal tubules. However, before dentin bonding is performed, the smear layer must be removed through the application of an etchant, which allows the dentin tubules to become opened, for the bonding material to flow into. As part of the bonding process, the tubules are sealed with the bonding material, and protection is restored to the tooth. Also, different from the enamel bonding, a slight amount of moisture must be maintained on the dentin so as not to **desiccate**, or "dry out," the tooth. If dentin is completely dried, the tooth structure could be harmed.

## Application

Bonding applications are available as self-curing, dual-cured, and light-cured systems. Some systems use a single application, whereas others require mixing of two liquids. Each bonding system is different, and the material from one system is not interchangeable with that from another. It is essential that the manufacturer's instructions be followed exactly with each product.

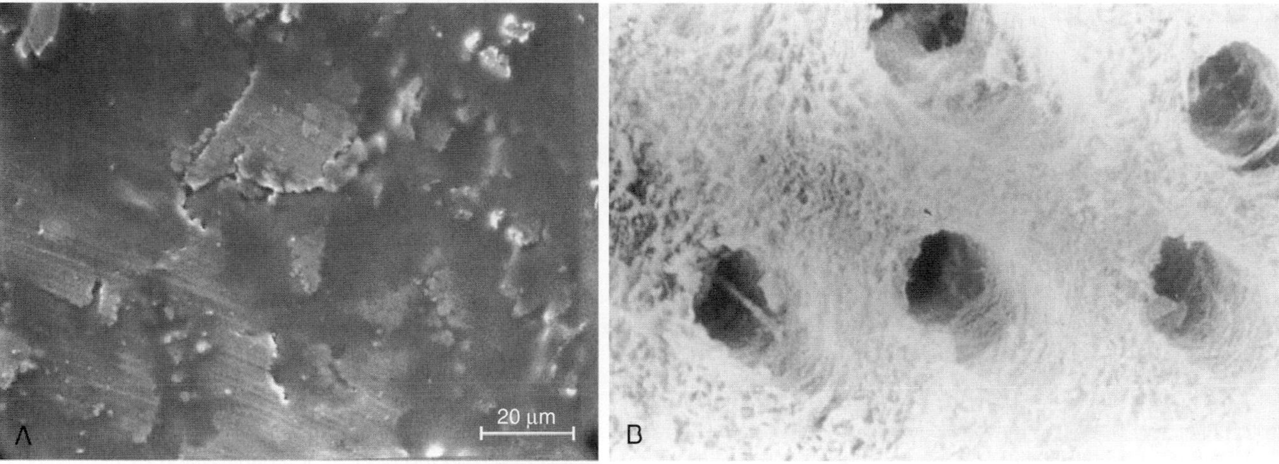


FIG. 44.9 Microscopic view in various stages of etching. A, Unetched dentin with smear layer. B, Overetched dentin. *(A, Courtesy of S.C. Bayne, School of Dentistry, University of Michigan, Ann Arbor, MI; B, Courtesy of K. Bruggers, School of Dentistry, University of North Carolina, Chapel Hill, NC.)*

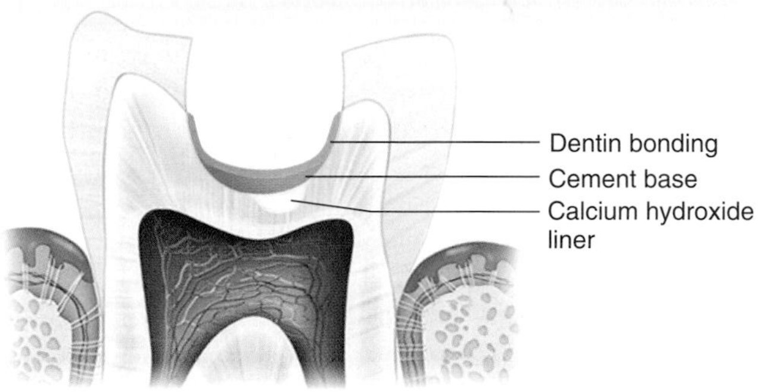


FIG. 44.10 Location for placement of dentin bonding. *(© Elsevier Collection.)*

The following general description outlines what occurs in the bonding system: The tooth surface receives the etchant material, which removes the smear layer; then the bonding component is allowed to flow into these small defects and into the partially opened tubules. Once this material is placed, it will be allowed (1) to harden and act as a **hybrid layer**, or (2) to remain in a liquid state while the restoration is being placed, to bond together the tooth and the dental material (Fig. 44.10).

## Guidelines for Clinical Application of Bonding Products

- Perform the steps in the bonding process precisely.
- Avoid expiration, contamination, and thickening of liquids.
- Remove any plaque or debris before beginning the bonding process.
- Avoid overdrying the dentin; these products work best on a slightly moist tooth structure.
- Note that too much bonding material is better than too little; multiple layers work best.
- Ensure that the bonding solution covers all surfaces.
- Avoid any contamination with saliva, blood, or debris, which will require the entire procedure to be redone.
- Allow as much time as possible for the bond to mature before completing the restoration and removing the cotton rolls or dental dam.

See Procedure 44.8: Applying a Bonding System (Expanded Function).

RECALL

12 What is the purpose of a dental bonding material?
13 What is an example of enamel bonding?
14 What must be removed from the tooth structure for bonding material to adhere to dentin?
15 Which material is applied first—the bonding or etchant material?

**■ Patient Education** A patient comes to you with concern over the sensitivity and discomfort he is experiencing in a specific tooth. You must be able to discuss and interpret these sensations with the patient. You also must be able to distinguish these problems for the dentist.

A patient may experience many types of sensitivities from a dental procedure. You have to become the "detective" in this process and ask the following specific questions about the type of discomfort the patient is experiencing:

- How long has this been bothering you?
- Is there a certain time of day that it seems to bother you the most?
- Does hot or cold beverages bother you?
- When you bite down, does it bother you?
- Does air that you breathe into your mouth bother you?

By understanding the materials discussed in this chapter, you will have a better knowledge of how dental liners, bases, and bonding systems work to eliminate the discomfort and sensitivity that a patient may experience from a tooth restoration. ■

**■ Legal and Ethical Implications** If the dentist and the dental team do not treat a patient's sensitivity or discomfort from a dental procedure as a serious concern, a problem—and perhaps even a legal issue—could arise. Follow through with a patient who is experiencing discomfort; bring the patient into the office and complete any diagnostic evaluations needed to determine the source of the problem. Too often, dental professionals say to patients, "It is common to experience discomfort or sensitivity from a procedure." With the materials and techniques currently available, patients should be pain-free after their dental experience. ■

**■ Eye to the Future** One area of dentistry that is ever-changing is the application of supplemental dental materials. It is difficult to believe that these products are even easier to mix and use today than they were just a few years ago. Companies are now providing materials in easy-to-use packets, syringes, capsules, and applicators; soon the whole process of restorative materials and supplemental materials will be supplied as a single application. This approach will save an enormous amount of time for the dental team and will reduce the steps required to complete the restorative procedure. ■

## ■ Critical Thinking

1. You are assisting in a class II composite restorative procedure on tooth #12. The preparation is moderately deep and has extended into the dentin. The dentist indicates to set out additional materials for the procedure. What base material would be contraindicated for this procedure?
2. Three types of base materials are discussed in this chapter. You are assisting in a procedure that requires a base that is nonirritating and provides protection and insulation. Which of the three would most likely be selected?
3. You are assisting in a four-surface amalgam procedure on tooth #30. The preparation becomes very deep. Describe the supplemental materials that would be set out for this procedure, and give the order in which they would be placed.
4. Describe how the design of a preparation relates to the types of supplemental materials used in restorative dentistry.
5. Are any of the procedures in this chapter considered an "expanded function" for dental assistants in your state? If so, what additional techniques do you find are important for you as the operator? ■

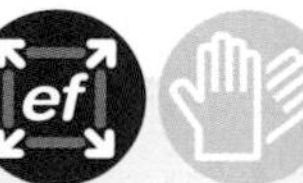

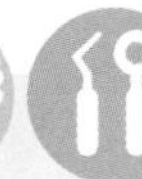
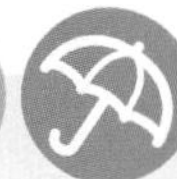

**PROCEDURE 44.1** 

# Applying Calcium Hydroxide (Expanded Function)

### PREREQUISITES FOR PERFORMING THIS PROCEDURE

- ✔ Appropriate operator positioning
- ✔ Knowledge of cavity classifications and oral anatomy
- ✔ Knowledge of application technique
- ✔ Appropriate intraoral instrumentation
- ✔ Mirror skills

### EQUIPMENT AND SUPPLIES

- ✔ Small paper mixing pad
- ✔ Small spatula
- ✔ Calcium hydroxide applicator
- ✔ Calcium hydroxide base and catalyst paste (from the same manufacturer)
- ✔ 2 × 2–inch gauze pads

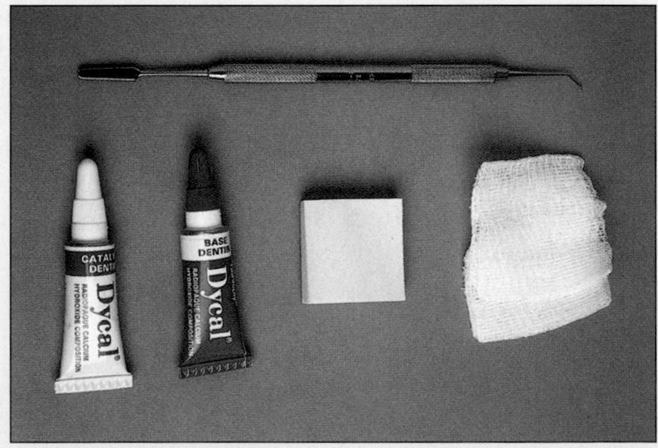


### PROCEDURAL STEPS

1. Position yourself as the operator.
2. Using the mirror and the explorer, examine the cavity outline of the preparation, and determine where the material is to be placed. This should be discussed with the dentist.
3. Rinse and dry the preparation, and isolate with cotton rolls or dental dam.

## PROCEDURE 44.1 Applying Calcium Hydroxide (Expanded Function)—cont'd

4 Dispense small, equal amounts of the catalyst and base paste onto the paper mixing pad.
**PURPOSE** The area to be covered will be 0.5 to 1 mm, depending on the size of the cavity preparation.

5 Using a circular motion, quickly mix (10–15 seconds) the material over a small area of the paper pad with the spatula.

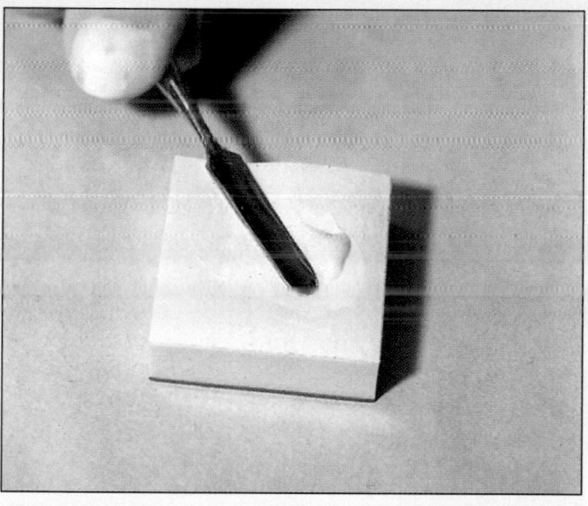

6 Use gauze to clean the spatula.

7 With the tip of the applicator, pick up a small amount of the material, and apply a thin layer at the deepest area of the preparation.

8 Use an explorer to remove any material from the enamel before drying.

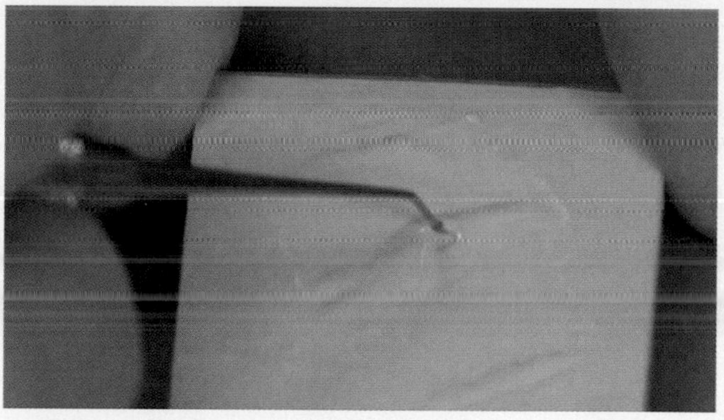

9 Have the dentist evaluate your skills.

10 Document the procedure.

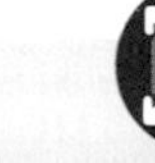

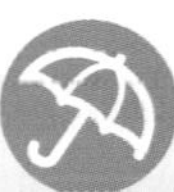

## PROCEDURE 44.2

# Applying Dental Varnish (Expanded Function)

### PREREQUISITES FOR PERFORMING THIS PROCEDURE

- ✔ Appropriate operator positioning
- ✔ Knowledge of cavity classifications and oral anatomy
- ✔ Knowledge of application technique
- ✔ Appropriate intraoral instrumentation
- ✔ Mirror skills

### EQUIPMENT AND SUPPLIES

- ✔ Mirror and explorer
- ✔ Microbrush applicators (2)
- ✔ Dental varnish

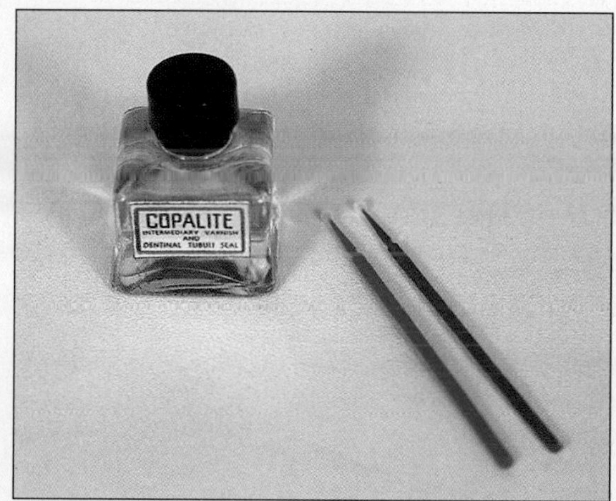


### PROCEDURAL STEPS

1 Position yourself as the operator.

2 Using the mirror and the explorer, examine the cavity outline of the preparation, and determine where the material is to be placed.

*(Continued)*

## PROCEDURE 44.2 Applying Dental Varnish (Expanded Function)—cont'd

3 Rinse and dry the preparation, and isolate with cotton rolls or dental dam.
4 Retrieve a new applicator.
5 Open the bottle of varnish, and place the tip of the applicator into the liquid.
6 Replace the cap on the bottle immediately.
**PURPOSE** When varnish is exposed to air, evaporation causes this liquid to thicken. If it becomes too thick, a thinning agent must be added.
7 Place a thin coating of the varnish on the walls, floor, and margin of the cavity preparation. Allow to air-dry.

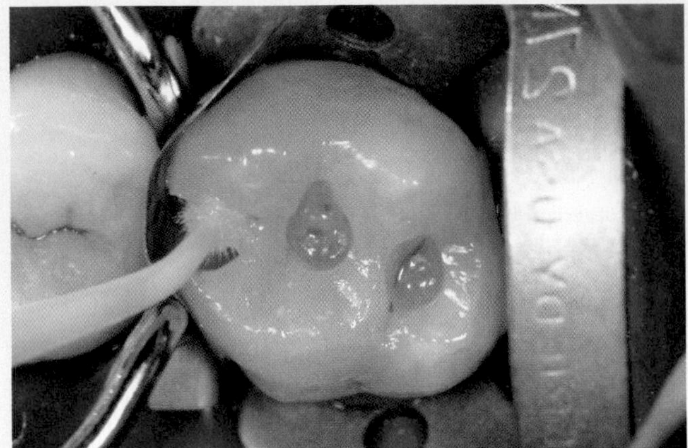

*From Heymann HO, Swift EJ, Ritter AV: Sturdevant's art and science or operative dentistry, ed 6, St Louis, 2013, Mosby.*

8 Apply a second coat; repeat steps 3 through 6.
9 Have the dentist evaluate your skills.
10 Document the procedure.

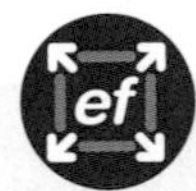

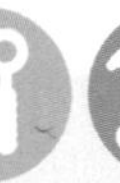
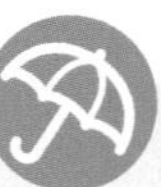

## PROCEDURE 44.3

# Applying a Desensitizer (Expanded Function)

### PREREQUISITES FOR PERFORMING THIS PROCEDURE

- Appropriate operator positioning
- Knowledge of cavity classifications and oral anatomy
- Knowledge of application technique
- Appropriate intraoral instrumentation
- Mirror skills

### EQUIPMENT AND SUPPLIES

- Basic setup
- Desensitizer material
- Microbrush applicator
- Air-water syringe
- Oral evacuation system

### PROCEDURAL STEPS

1 Position yourself as the operator.
2 Using the mirror and the explorer, examine the cavity outline of the preparation, and determine where the material is to be placed.
3 Provided that the tooth and the tissues are not sensitive, rinse the area with water, but avoid overdrying.
4 With the applicator, apply the desensitizer over all areas of the dentin.
**PURPOSE** To assist with delivery of the solution to all affected dentinal tubules.

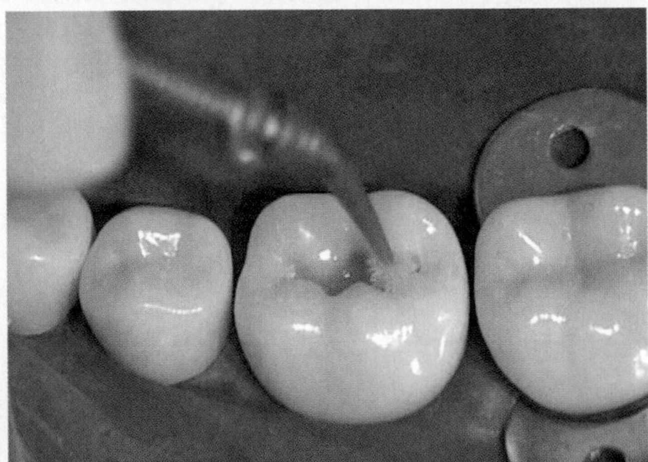

*Courtesy Aldridge D. Wilder, DDS.*

5 Wait 30 seconds; then dry thoroughly *(do not rinse).*
6 Repeat application if sensitivity has been a problem with the patient.
7 Have the dentist evaluate your skills.
8 Document the procedure.

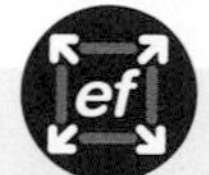

**PROCEDURE 44.4**

# Mixing and Placing Zinc Oxide–Eugenol Cement as a Base (Expanded Function)

## PREREQUISITES FOR PERFORMING THIS PROCEDURE

- ✔ Appropriate operator positioning
- ✔ Knowledge of cavity classifications and oral anatomy
- ✔ Knowledge of application technique
- ✔ Appropriate intraoral instrumentation
- ✔ Mirror skills

## EQUIPMENT AND SUPPLIES

- ✔ Basic setup
- ✔ Treated paper pad
- ✔ Spatula (flexible stainless steel)
- ✔ Zinc oxide powder and dispenser
- ✔ Eugenol liquid and dropper
- ✔ Plastic instrument (for placement)
- ✔ Amalgam condenser (for condensation)
- ✔ 2 × 2–inch gauze pads

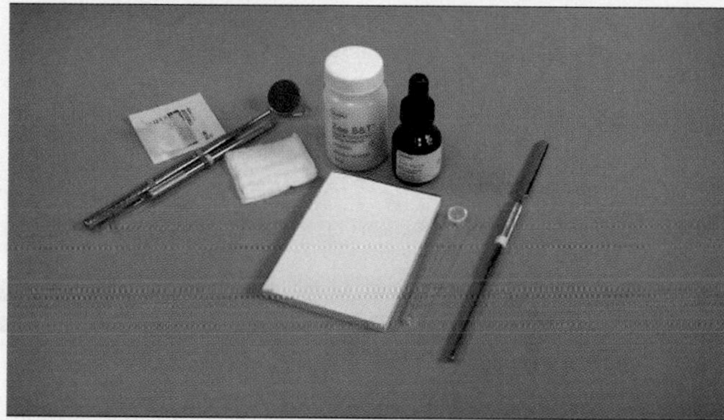

## PROCEDURAL STEPS

1. Position yourself as the operator.
2. Using the mirror and the explorer, examine the cavity outline of the preparation, and determine where the material is to be placed.
3. Rinse and dry the preparation, and isolate with cotton rolls or dental dam.
4. Measure the powder onto the mixing pad. Replace the cap immediately.
5. Dispense the liquid near the powder on the mixing pad. Replace the cap immediately.

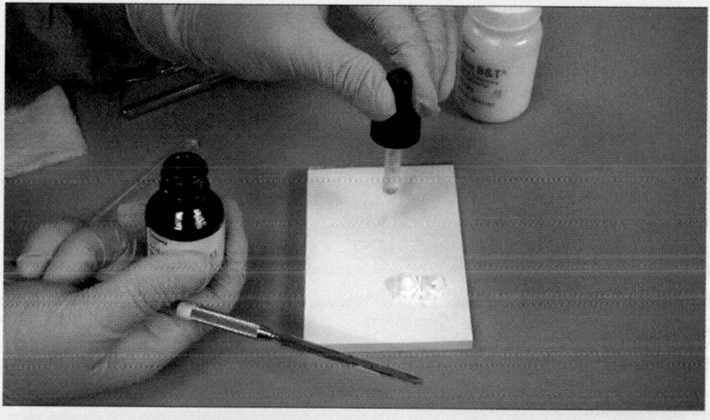

6. Incorporate half the powder into the liquid; mix with the spatula for 20 to 30 seconds.
7. Incorporate the remaining portion into the mixture. Continue mixing for an additional 20 to 30 seconds. The material should be thick and putty-like.
8. Pick up half the material with your spatula, and roll it into a small ball. Do this with the other portion as well.

   **PURPOSE** To make the material easier to place into the cavity preparation.
9. Pick up the material by placing the condenser into the material; then carry it to the preparation.
10. Use a light tapping stroke to adapt the material into place.

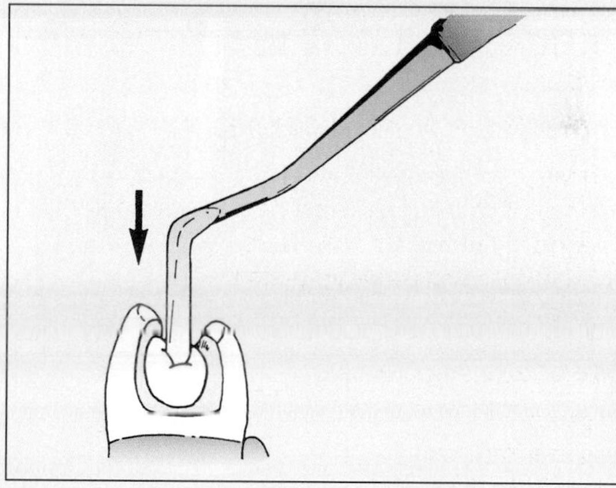

*From Baum L, Phillips RW, Lund MR: Textbook of operative dentistry, ed 3 Philadelphia, 1995, Saunders.*

11. Ensure that the entire pulpal floor is covered with the base.
12. Have the dentist evaluate your skills.
13. Document the procedure.

PROCEDURE 44.5

# Mixing and Placing Zinc Phosphate Cement as a Base (Expanded Function)

## PREREQUISITES FOR PERFORMING THIS PROCEDURE

- Appropriate operator positioning
- Knowledge of cavity classifications and oral anatomy
- Knowledge of application technique
- Appropriate intraoral instrumentation
- Mirror skills

## EQUIPMENT AND SUPPLIES

- Basic setup
- Glass slab (cool)
- Spatula (flexible stainless steel)
- Zinc phosphate powder and dispenser
- Zinc phosphate liquid and dropper
- Plastic instrument (for placement)
- Amalgam condenser (for condensation)
- 2 × 2–inch gauze pads

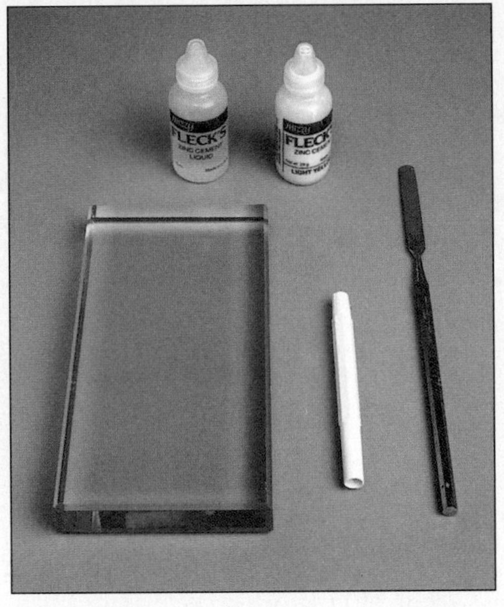


## PROCEDURAL STEPS

1. Position yourself as the operator.
2. Using the mirror and the explorer, examine the cavity outline of the preparation, and determine where the material is to be placed.
3. Rinse and dry the preparation, and isolate with cotton rolls or dental dam.
4. Dispense the powder and the liquid onto the slab. Use the powder-to-liquid ratio recommended to produce a thick, putty-like mix.

   **NOTE** This requires more powder in proportion to the amount of liquid used.
5. Mix to the desired consistency.
6. Form the completed mix into a small ball.
7. Pick up the material by placing the condenser into the material; then carry it to the preparation.
8. Using a light tapping stroke, adapt the material into place.
9. Ensure that the entire pulpal floor is covered with the base.
10. Have excess powder available for use when the material is condensed into the tooth.

    **PURPOSE** This powder will prevent the instrument from sticking to the material.
11. Have the dentist evaluate your skills.
12. Document the procedure.

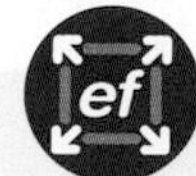

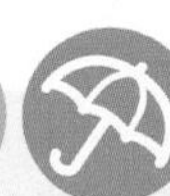

PROCEDURE 44.6 

# Mixing and Placing Polycarboxylate Cement as a Base (Expanded Function)

## PREREQUISITES FOR PERFORMING THIS PROCEDURE

- ✔ Appropriate operator positioning
- ✔ Knowledge of cavity classifications and oral anatomy
- ✔ Knowledge of application technique
- ✔ Appropriate intraoral instrumentation
- ✔ Mirror skills

## EQUIPMENT AND SUPPLIES

- ✔ Basic setup
- ✔ Treated paper pad
- ✔ Spatula (flexible stainless steel)
- ✔ Polycarboxylate powder and dispenser
- ✔ Polycarboxylate liquid (in squeeze bottle or calibrated syringe)
- ✔ Plastic instrument (for placement)
- ✔ Amalgam condenser (for condensation)
- ✔ 2 × 2–inch gauze pads

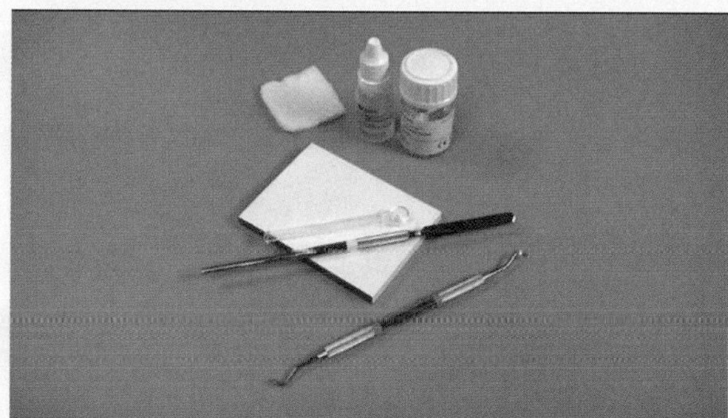

## PROCEDURAL STEPS

1 Position yourself as the operator.
2 Using the mirror and the explorer, examine the cavity outline of the preparation, and determine where the material is to be placed.
3 Rinse and dry the preparation, and isolate with cotton rolls or dental dam.
4 Dispense the powder and liquid onto the pad.

**NOTE** When used for a base, the liquid portion is decreased to make a thicker consistency.

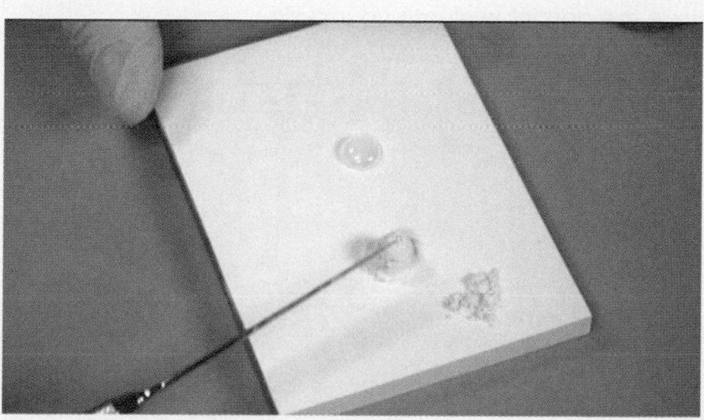

5 Incorporate all the powder into the liquid, with total mixing time not to exceed 45 seconds.
6 Form the completed mix into a small ball.

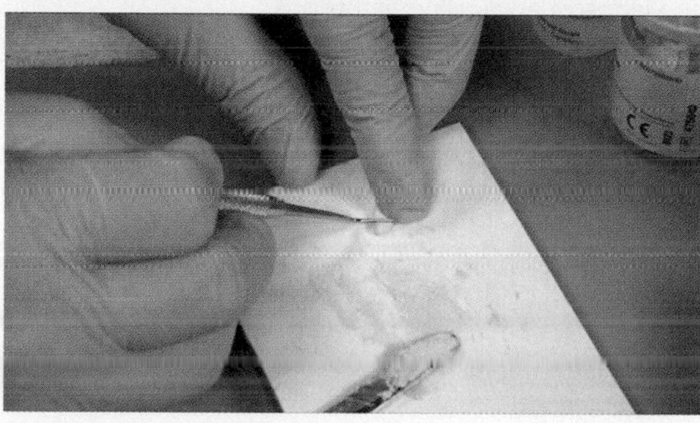

7 Pick up the material by placing the condenser into the material; then carry it to the preparation.
8 Using a light tapping stroke, adapt the material into place.

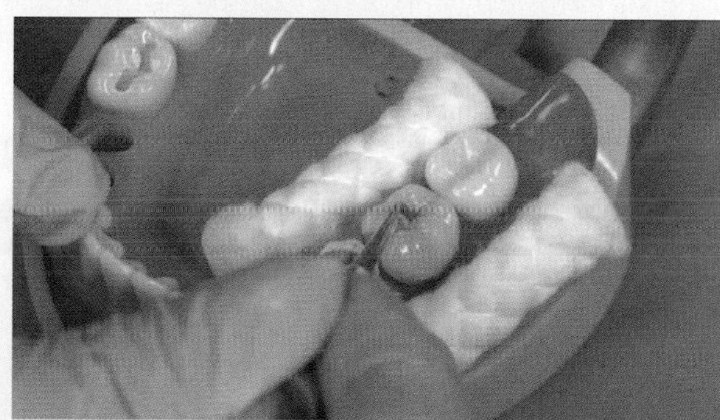

9 Ensure that the entire pulpal floor is covered with the base.
10 Clean and disinfect the equipment immediately.

**NOTE** This cement must set for approximately 5 minutes before placement of the permanent restoration.

11 Have the dentist evaluate your skills.
12 Document the procedure.

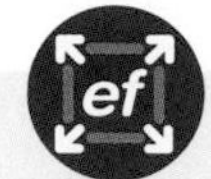    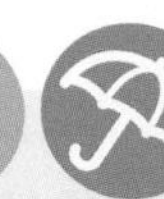 

PROCEDURE 44.7

# Applying an Etchant Material (Expanded Function)

## PREREQUISITES FOR PERFORMING THIS PROCEDURE

- ✔ Appropriate operator positioning
- ✔ Knowledge of cavity classifications and oral anatomy
- ✔ Knowledge of application technique
- ✔ Appropriate intraoral instrumentation
- ✔ Mirror skills

## EQUIPMENT AND SUPPLIES

- ✔ Basic setup
- ✔ Cotton rolls/dental dam for isolation
- ✔ Applicator (cotton pellets for liquid etchant and syringe tip for gel)
- ✔ Etchant material
- ✔ High-velocity evacuator
- ✔ Air-water syringe
- ✔ Timer

## PROCEDURAL STEPS

1 Position yourself as the operator.

2 Using the mirror and the explorer, examine the cavity outline of the preparation, and determine where the material is to be placed.

3 The prepared tooth must be isolated from contamination. A dental dam or cotton rolls are placed before the etching process begins.

**PURPOSE** Saliva must not contaminate the preparation.

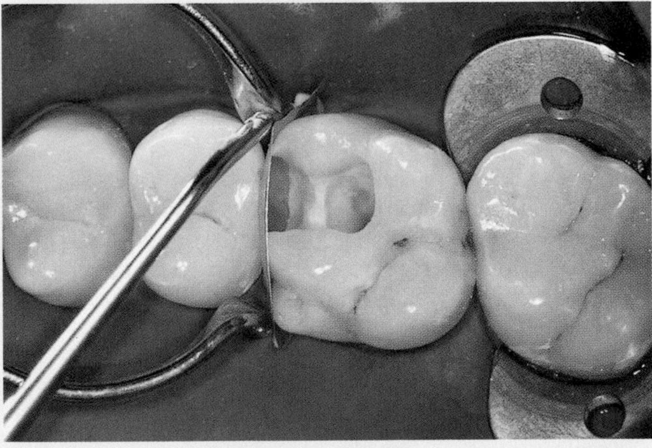

4 The surface of the tooth structure must be clean and free of any debris, plaque, or calculus before etching is begun.

**PURPOSE** Debris on the surface may interfere with the etching process.

5 After cleaning, the surface is carefully dried but is not desiccated.

**PURPOSE** Too much drying of the tooth structure will harm the tooth.

6 The etchant is selected. Most manufacturers supply a gel etchant in a syringe that can be applied to enamel or dentin.

**PURPOSE** The gel allows the etchant to be carefully placed *only* where it is needed.

7 The tooth structure is etched for the length of time recommended by the manufacturer; this usually ranges from 15 to 30 seconds.

**PURPOSE** The exact time depends on the material and the use. For example, etching time for placing sealants is not the same as etching time for bonding orthodontic brackets.

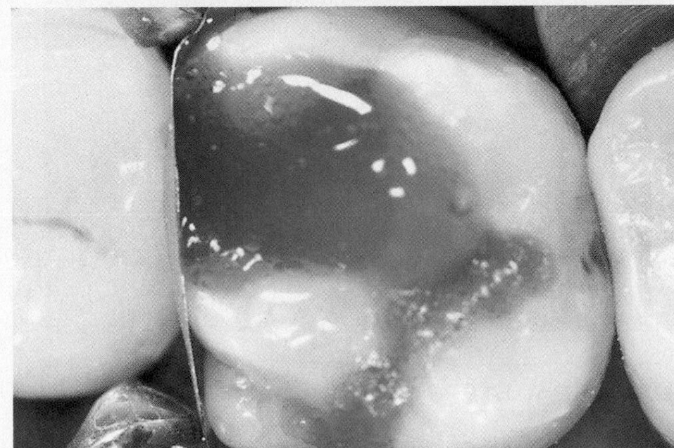

8 After etching, the surface is thoroughly rinsed and dried for 15 to 30 seconds.

9 An etched surface has a frosty-white appearance. If the surface does not have this appearance or has been contaminated with moisture, it is necessary to repeat the etching process.

10 Have the dentist evaluate your skills.

11 Document the procedure.

Photos in this procedure courtesy Dr. William Libenberg.

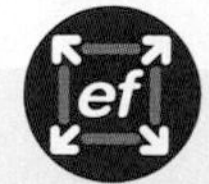

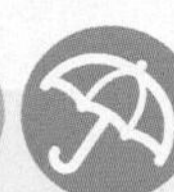

**PROCEDURE 44.8**

# Applying a Bonding System (Expanded Function)

## PREREQUISITES FOR PERFORMING THIS PROCEDURE

- ✔ Appropriate operator positioning
- ✔ Knowledge of cavity classifications and oral anatomy
- ✔ Knowledge of application technique
- ✔ Appropriate intraoral instrumentation
- ✔ Mirror skills

## EQUIPMENT AND SUPPLIES

- ✔ Bonding agent
- ✔ Applicator device or brush
- ✔ Air-water syringe
- ✔ Oral evacuation system
- ✔ 2 × 2–inch gauze pads

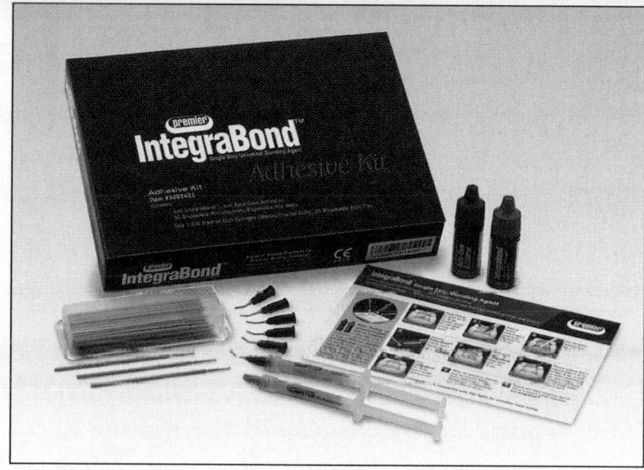


## PROCEDURAL STEPS

1. Position yourself as the operator.
2. Using the mirror and the explorer, examine the cavity outline of the preparation, and determine where the material is to be placed.
3. The cavity preparation and the enamel margins should be etched according to the manufacturer's directions.
4. If a metal matrix band is used, the band is prepared with cavity varnish or wax before placement around the tooth.

**PURPOSE** This prevents the bonding resin and the amalgam from adhering to the surface (see Chapter 49 for the application of a matrix).

**CAUTION** No varnish should come in contact with the tooth because this would interfere with the bonding effects of the resin primers.

5. The dual-cured adhesive resin is placed in the entire cavity preparation and is lightly air-thinned. The resin should appear unset or partially set.

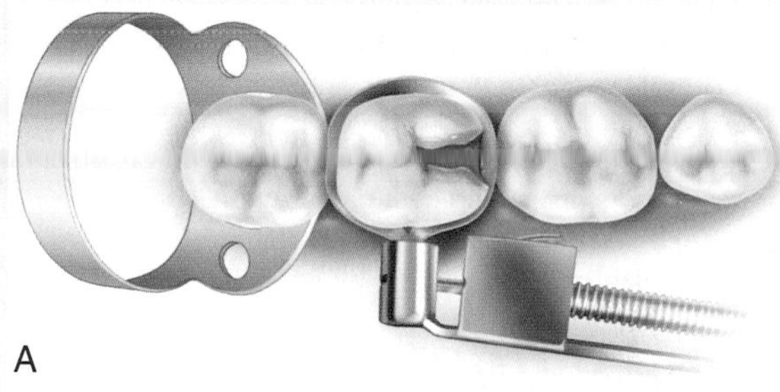


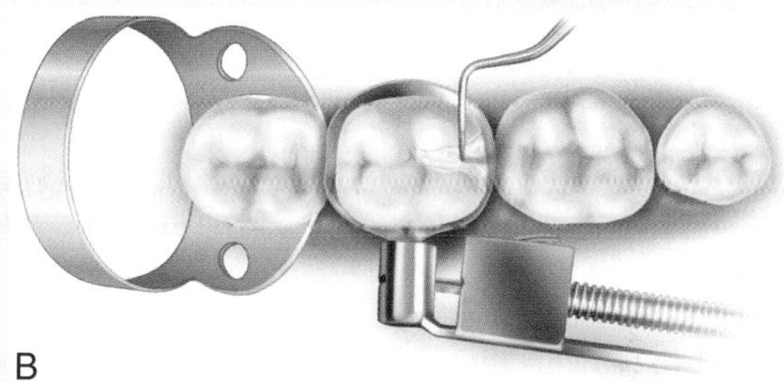


*© Elsevier Collection.*

6. The restorative material is mixed and then is readied for placement into the cavity preparation.

**PURPOSE** To integrate the restorative material and bonding material at the preparation walls before the resin has time to polymerize (set).

7. Have the dentist evaluate your skills.
8. Document the procedure.

45

# Dental Cements

## KEY TERMS

**Dissipate (DI-suh-payt)** To cause something to scatter, or become dispersed, and gradually disappear.
**Exothermic (ek-so-THUR-mik)** Characterized by the release of heat from a chemical reaction.
**Luting (LOO-ting) agent** Cement-type substance used to seal a surface.
**Provisional** Referring to temporary coverage made for crown or bridge preparations and worn during cast preparation.
**Retard (ree-TAHRD)** To slow down a process.
**Spatulate (SPACH-uh-layt)** To mix using a spatula-type instrument.

## LEARNING OUTCOMES

*On completion of this chapter, the student will be able to achieve the following objectives:*

1. Pronounce, define, and spell the key terms.
2. Discuss the classification of dental cements, including the following:
   - Describe the three types of luting cements.
   - Differentiate between permanent and temporary cements.
3. Discuss the variables that influence final cementation.
4. List the five cements discussed in this chapter and identify their similarities and differences.
5. Discuss the steps in cement removal.

## PERFORMANCE OUTCOMES

*On completion of this chapter, the student will be able to achieve competency standards in the following skills:*

- Mix and prepare glass ionomer for permanent cementation.
- Mix and prepare composite resin for permanent cementation.
- Mix and prepare two-paste zinc oxide–eugenol (Tempbond) for temporary cementation.
- Mix and prepare zinc oxide–eugenol for permanent cementation.
- Mix and prepare polycarboxylate for permanent cementation.
- Mix and prepare zinc phosphate cement for permanent cementation.
- Remove cement from permanent and temporary permanent cementations.

## ELECTRONIC RESOURCES

***Additional information related to content in Chapter 45 can be found on the companion Evolve Web site.***

- Practice Quiz
- Videos: Mixing Glass Ionomer for Permanent Cement; Mixing Zinc Oxide–Eugenol for Temporary Cementation; Mixing Zinc Oxide–Eugenol for Permanent Cementation; Mixing Polycarboxylate as a Permanent Cement; Mixing Zinc Phosphate for Permanent Cementation; Removing Cement

Dental cements are a category of dental materials that are versatile in their use. Dental cements are routinely used as a permanent adhesive material when working with indirect restorations. Additional uses are as a base for protection of the pulp, as a temporary cement, and to retain restorations or appliances in a fixed position within the mouth. In addition, certain cements are used for specialized purposes in prosthodontic, endodontic, orthodontic, periodontics, and surgical fields of dentistry.

## Classification of Dental Cement

The American Dental Association (ADA) and the International Standards Organization (ISO) have classified dental cements into three types according to their properties and their intended use in dentistry:

- **Type I cements** are classified as a **luting agent**. This type of cement is designed to act as an adhesive to hold an indirect restoration to the tooth structure, or to adhere brackets to the tooth surface during orthodontic treatment. This group includes permanent and temporary cements.

- **Type II cements** involve materials that can be used as a restorative material, such as intermediate restorative material (see Chapter 43), and dental sealants (see Chapter 59).
- **Type III cements** include the liners and bases that are placed within the cavity preparation. These were discussed in Chapter 44.

## Permanent Cements

Permanent cements are luting agents that are used for the long-term cementation of cast restorations such as inlays, crowns, bridges, laminate veneers, and orthodontic fixed appliances. As discussed in Chapter 43, permanent indirect restorations, such as those produced from gold and ceramic, are designed and cast by a dental laboratory technician. Once prepared in the laboratory, cast restorations are delivered to the dentist for the cementation appointment.

Because these types of restorations are seated on a prepared tooth structure, the hollow, shell-like structure of the indirect restoration requires that a luting agent should have qualities that do not interfere with a proper fit (Fig. 45.1).

## Temporary Cements

Temporary cementation of an indirect restoration may be completed if the dentist needs to remove the indirect restoration at a later date; if the tooth is sensitive or is exhibiting other symptoms that might require removal of the cast restoration; or when temporary cementation of provisional coverage is required while the patient waits until the laboratory technician completes the cast restoration. **Provisional** coverage is a temporary coverage that is placed on a tooth to protect the tooth until the permanent restoration is ready to be cemented (see Chapter 51).

# Variables Affecting Final Cementation

A number of factors can influence actual cementation with a luting cement. Cementing errors can be the result of improper mixing technique, time, humidity, or incorrect temperature of the glass slab.

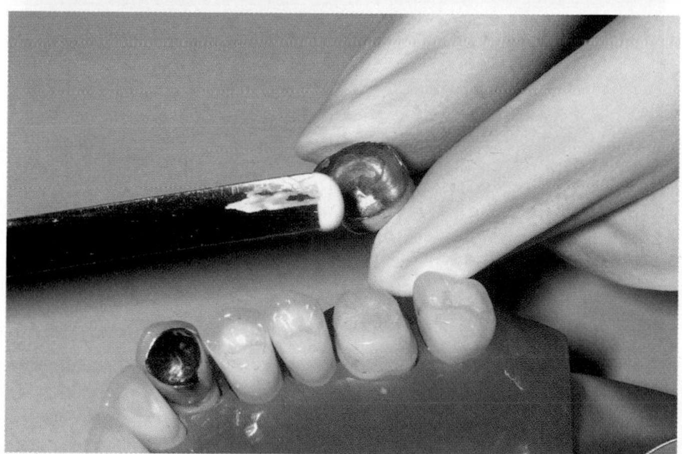

FIG. 45.1 Casting ready to be cemented.

## Mixing Time

One of the first and foremost rules in the preparation of a cement material is to follow the manufacturer's directions regarding a material's exact mixing time, working time, and delivery time. Any delay between completion of the mix and seating of the cast restoration will result in the initial setting process, which could cause the casting not to seat properly.

Regardless of the type of dental cement used, basic guidelines must be followed.

### *Guidelines for Mixing Dental Cements*

- Before mixing, read and carefully follow the manufacturer's directions for the type of cement being mixed.
- Determine the use of the cement (restorative, liner, base, cement); then measure out the powder and liquid according to the manufacturer's instructions.
- Place the powder toward one end of the glass slab or paper pad and the liquid toward the opposite end (the space between allows room for mixing).
- Divide the powder into increments. Each manufacturer uses a slightly different system for sectioning the powder. Some manufacturers divide the powder into equal parts, whereas others divide the powder into progressively smaller increments. When increment sizes vary, use the smaller increments first.
- Incorporate each powder increment into the liquid; then mix thoroughly. The mixing time per increment will vary according to the type of material and its use.

### *Automix System*

Many types of cements today are supplied in a cartridge where they are automatically mixed as they are expressed onto the pad or directly onto the tooth surface you are working on. The advantages of using an automix system are that it provides an exact measurement of material, easy mix and application, and easy cleanup.

## Humidity

If the clinical area is warm, or if it is a humid day, premature exposure of the cement to these environmental conditions can create loss of water from the liquid or addition of moisture to the powder. Always dispense the powder first, *then* the liquid, to minimize the loss of water from evaporation. Wait until it is time to mix the material before placing it on the pad. Do not set it out at the beginning of the procedure.

## Powder-to-Liquid Ratio

Incorporating too much or too little powder will alter the consistency of the cement. Be sure to fluff the powder in the bottle before dispensing the powder in the measuring scoop. Always hold the bottle or vial upright to ensure drops of consistent size when dispensing the liquid (Fig. 45.2).

### Temperature

Specific types of cement will have a chemical reaction during the setting stage. An example of this is seen when the material zinc phosphate generates heat; this is referred to as an **exothermic** reaction. In such cases, it is beneficial to cool a glass slab in the refrigerator before mixing the cement. If the glass slab is kept in the refrigerator, make sure to thoroughly wipe the slab dry before dispensing the material, so as not to incorporate any moisture condensation into the material.

RECALL

1 What is another name used for permanent cement?
2 When is a temporary cement used instead of a permanent cement?
3 What variable affects the addition or loss of water in a dental cement?

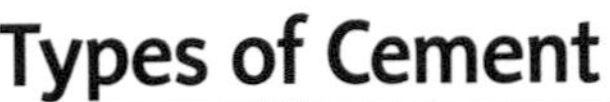

## Types of Cement

The cements described in this chapter are designed to be versatile in their properties, uses, and mixing techniques. Many of the cements that were traditionally used for routine cementation through the 1990s have been replaced by newer makeup and mixing techniques. The selection of cement for a specific procedure requires knowledge of the chemical and physical properties of each particular cement type for the specific restorative process to be performed.

### Glass Ionomer Cement

Glass ionomer cement is one of the most versatile types of cement used in dentistry. Glass ionomer cements are a hybrid of silicate and polycarboxylate cements. This type of cement adheres to enamel, dentin, and metallic materials. Glass ionomer cements are supplied in special formulations according to their use:

- **Type I** is a luting cement used for the cementation of indirect restorations.
- **Type II** is designed for restoring areas of erosion in Class V.
- **Type III** is used for liners and bases.
- **Type IV** is used for pit and fissure sealants.
- **Type V** is used in the cementation of orthodontic bands and brackets.
- **Type VI** is used for the core buildup of a restoration.

Glass ionomer's popularity in use is because of its advantages:

- The powder is an acid-soluble calcium. The slow release of fluoride from this powder aids in inhibiting recurrent decay.
- The cement causes less trauma or shock to the pulp than is caused by many other types of cement.
- The cement has low solubility in the mouth.
- The cement adheres to a slightly moist tooth surface.
- The cement has a very thin film thickness, which is excellent for ease of seating a casting.
- Glass ionomer cements can be formulated for use as a dentin substitute or base material.

#### Chemical Makeup of Glass Ionomer Cement

- *Liquid:* polyacrylic acid copolymer and water
- *Powder:* Silica, alumina, aluminum fluoride, calcium fluoride, sodium fluoride, aluminum phosphate

#### Application

Glass ionomers are available in self-curing or light-cured formulas. The cements are supplied in bottles of powder and liquid, which can be mixed manually on a paper pad or a cool, dry glass slab. Use of the glass slab increases the working time of the cement. Glass ionomer material is also supplied in premeasured capsules, which are triturated and expressed through a dispenser (Fig. 45.3). These capsules have the advantages of

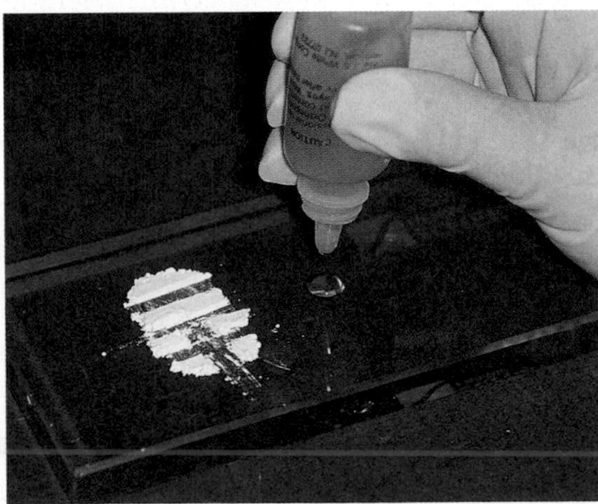

FIG. 45.2 Hold the bottle upright when dispensing the liquid of a cement.

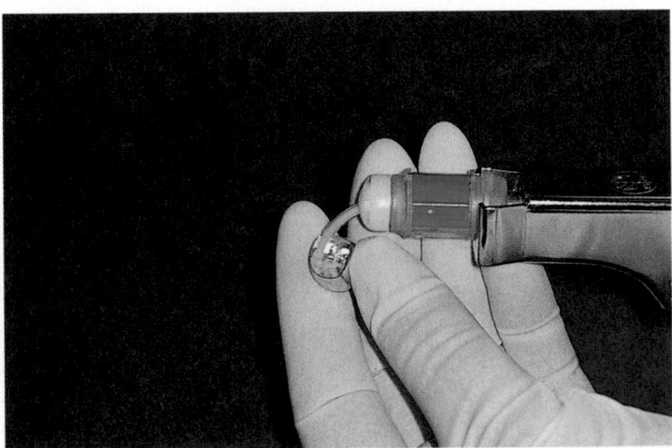

FIG. 45.3 Premeasured capsules of glass ionomer permanent cement. *(From Hatrick CD, Eakle WS: Dental materials: clinical applications for dental assistants and dental hygienists, ed 3, St Louis, 2016, Elsevier.)*

(1) being more convenient to use, (2) requiring less mixing time, and (3) producing consistent mixes because of the controlled powder-to-liquid ratio.

See Procedure 45.1: Mixing Glass Ionomer for Permanent Cementation.

## Examples of Commercial Glass Ionomer Cement

- Aspa
- Ionomer
- Fuji
- Ketac-Cem
- Vitrebond
- Biobond
- Aquacem
- Rely X
- Dyract
- Permacen

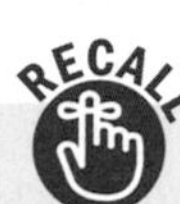


4 Can a glass ionomer cement be used as a restorative material?

5 What ingredient in the powder of glass ionomer cement helps inhibit recurrent decay?

## Composite Resin Cement

A newer classification of cement material is the **composite resin cement,** which has been designed especially for the following indications:

- Ceramic or porcelain inlays, onlays, crowns, and bridges
- Ceramic veneers
- Orthodontic bands
- Direct bonding of orthodontic brackets
- Metal-based crowns and bridges

### *Chemical Makeup of Composite Resin Cement*

Composite resin cements have physical properties comparable with those of composite resins, including thin film thickness and virtual insolubility in the mouth. An important aspect of the selection of composite resin cements is that the tooth must be free of all plaque and debris and must be prepared by etching or by treating the tooth surface with a bonding system before cementation.

### *Application*

Composite resin cements are supplied (1) as a powder and liquid mix, (2) in a syringe-type applicator as a base and catalyst, and (3) in a versatile light-cured/dual-cured system (Fig. 45.4). Recommended portions of either application are dispensed onto a paper pad and mixed rapidly with a spatula. See Procedure 45.2: Mixing Composite Resin for Permanent Cementation.

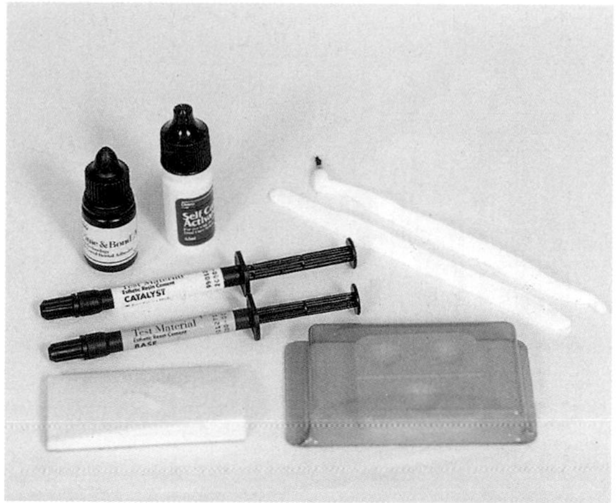

**FIG. 45.4** Examples of composite resin cements supplied in variable systems.

## Commercial Resin Cements

- Comspan
- Panavia
- Enforce
- Opal Luting
- Compolute
- Nexus

RECALL

6 Can resin cements be used under metal castings?

7 In the composite resin cementation procedure, what step is important to complete on the tooth surface before cementation of the material?

## Zinc Oxide–Eugenol Cement

Zinc oxide–eugenol (ZOE) cement is one of the most versatile cements available. As you learned in Chapter 44, ZOE can be used as a base because the eugenol in ZOE is nonirritating to the pulp. Eugenol actually has a soothing effect on pulp and is often used in procedures when postoperative sensitivity may be a concern.

**ZOE type I** lacks strength and long-term durability. For this reason, type I is used for temporary cementation or provisional coverage. ZOE type I (Temp-Bond is the brand name) is supplied as a two-paste system for temporary cement (Fig. 45.5). Temp-Bond is now supplied with and without eugenol. These pastes are dispensed in equal lengths on a paper pad and are mixed according to the manufacturer's directions.

**ZOE type II** includes added reinforcing agents. For this reason, type II is used for permanent cementation of cast restorations or appliances (Fig. 45.6).

### *Chemical Makeup of Zinc Oxide–Eugenol Cement*

- *Liquid:* eugenol, water, acetic acid, zinc acetate, and calcium chloride
- *Powder:* zinc oxide, magnesium oxide, and silica

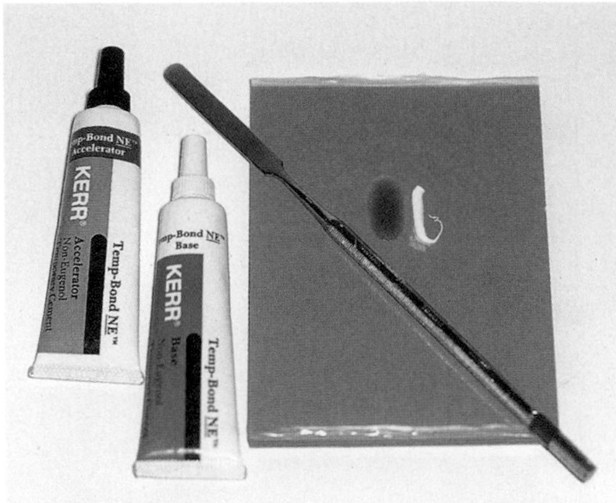


FIG. 45.5 Temp-Bond NE, a type I temporary cement.

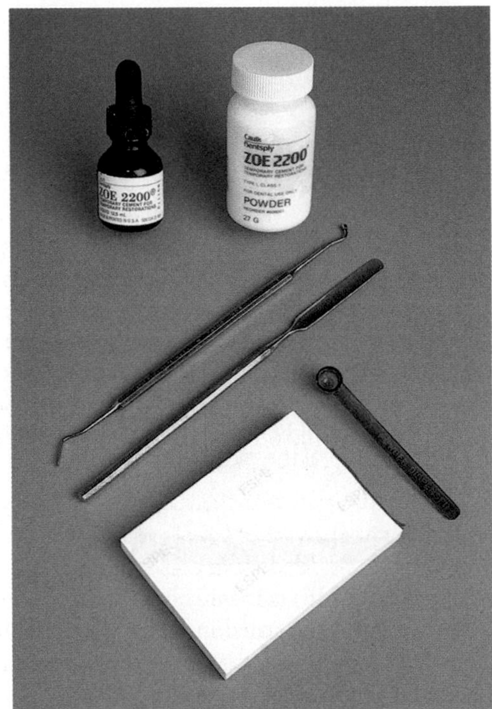


FIG. 45.6 ZOE type II cement for permanent cementation.

ZOE has a pH level close to 7.0, which makes it less acidic than most other cements. ZOE is one of the least irritating of all dental cements. The eugenol can have a strong odor, which may be offensive to some patients.

### Application

Because eugenol is an oil-based liquid, ZOE is mixed on an oil-resistant paper pad that will not absorb any of the liquid. Take care when using a eugenol product because of its irritating qualities to the oral mucosa. Try not to allow the liquid to come into direct contact with tissue.

When a slower set is required, a glass slab can be used. The thickness of the mix is determined by the powder-to-liquid ratio, as recommended by the manufacturer. For use as a luting agent, a thinner mix is necessary. The normal mixing time ranges from 30 to 60 seconds. The normal setting time in the mouth ranges from 3 to 5 minutes.

See Procedure 45.3: Mixing Zinc Oxide–Eugenol for Temporary Cementation and Procedure 45.4: Mixing Zinc Oxide–Eugenol for Permanent Cementation.

#### Examples of Commercial ZOE Cement

- ZOE 2200
- Zogenol
- TempBond
- Fynal

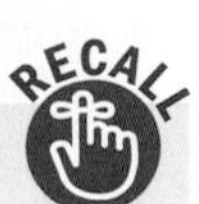

8 What type of ZOE is used for permanent cementation?
9 On what mixing surface is ZOE mixed?
10 How is Temp-Bond supplied?

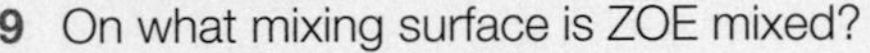
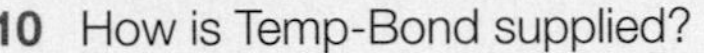

## Polycarboxylate Cement

Polycarboxylate cement, which was developed in the 1960s, was one of the first cements scientifically designed to provide an adhesive bond to tooth structure. This cement has changed from its original chemical makeup over the past few years. The original acid polymer was polyacrylic acid; now the cement contains two or more monomers, so it is technically referred to as a polyalkenoate cement. This cement generally has been used as permanent cement for cast restorations, stainless steel crowns, and orthodontic bands. Polycarboxylate also maintains its versatility as a nonirritating base under composite and amalgam restorations and as an intermediate restoration.

### Chemical Makeup of Polycarboxylate Cement

- *Liquid:* polyacrylic acid, itaconic acid, maleic acid, tartaric acid, and water
- *Powder:* zinc oxide, magnesium oxide, aluminum oxide, and other reinforcing fillers

When properly mixed, polycarboxylate cement is similar to zinc phosphate cement in terms of solubility and tensile strength. The pH increases rapidly as the material sets, and after 24 hours the cement is similar to zinc phosphate cement. Polycarboxylate cement is less irritating to the pulp than is zinc phosphate cement, and the pulpal reaction is similar to that of ZOE cement.

### Application

Polycarboxylate cement is available in powder and liquid forms. The liquid can be measured by using the plastic squeeze bottle or the calibrated syringe-type liquid dispenser supplied by the manufacturer (Fig. 45.7). The liquid is syrup-like in consistency and has a limited shelf life because it will thicken as the water evaporates. Before actual mixing, read and follow the manufacturer's instructions. The material is recommended to be mixed on a nonabsorbent paper pad. If it is necessary to increase the working time, however, a cool, dry glass slab can be used.

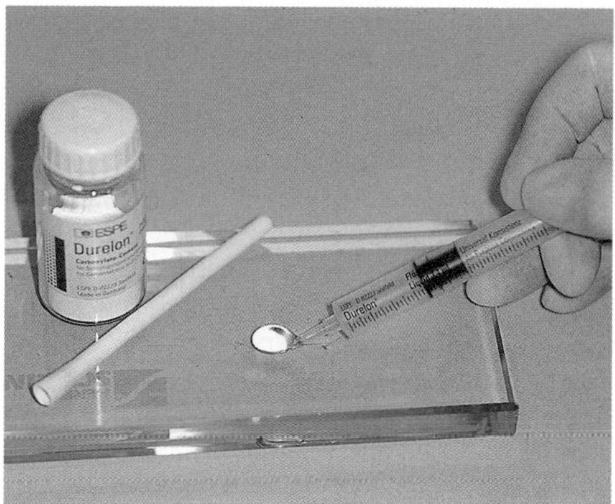


FIG. 45.7 Powder and calibrated syringe of polycarboxylate cement.

See Procedure 45.5: Mixing Polycarboxylate for Permanent Cementation.

### Examples of Commercial Polycarboxylate Cement

- Tylok
- Durelon
- Chemit
- Carboxylon
- Poly F

RECALL

11 In what two forms is the polycarboxylate cement liquid supplied?
12 How should polycarboxylate cement appear after the mixing process?

## Zinc Phosphate Cement

Zinc phosphate, one of the oldest dental cements in use, is classified as two types.

**Type I (fine-grain)** zinc phosphate cement is used for the permanent cementation of cast restorations such as crowns, inlays, onlays, and bridges. This material creates a very thin film layer, which is necessary for accurate cementation of castings (Fig. 45.8).

**Type II (medium-grain)** zinc phosphate cement is recommended for use as an insulating base for deep cavity preparations (see Chapter 44).

### Chemical Makeup of Zinc Phosphate Cement

- *Liquid:* 50 percent phosphoric acid in water, buffered with aluminum phosphate and zinc salts to control the pH
- *Powder:* 90 percent zinc oxide and 10 percent magnesium oxide

When using zinc phosphate, the phosphoric acid is an ingredient that can be irritating to the pulp. Because of the irritating factors, a liner, sealer, or desensitizer should be placed first to reduce sensitivity to the phosphoric acid.

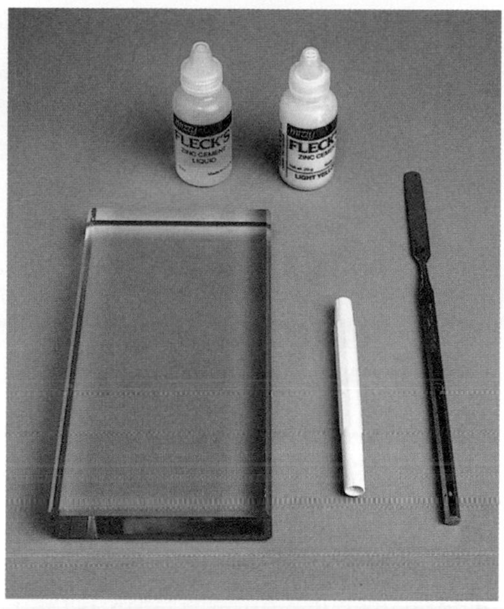


FIG. 45.8 Zinc phosphate type I cement for permanent cementation.

### Application

During the mixing and setting process, zinc phosphate cement undergoes an exothermic reaction giving off heat. To **dissipate** this heat before cementation on a prepared tooth, the cement is **spatulated** over a wide area of a cool, dry, thick glass slab. The temperature of the glass slab is an important variable in the mixing time for zinc phosphate cement. The ideal slab temperature should be 68° F. This temperature allows a longer working time and permits a maximum amount of powder to be incorporated into the liquid without making the mix too thick.

The powder is divided into increments that vary in size, with each increment spatulated slowly and thoroughly before the next increment is added. It is critical that the powder be added to the liquid in very small increments. This method dissipates the heat of the chemical action and **retards** the setting of the cement. See Procedure 45.6: Mixing Zinc Phosphate for Permanent Cementation.

### Examples of Commercial Zinc Phosphate Cement

- Modern Tenacin
- Fleck's Extraordinary
- Smith's Zinc Cement
- Lang-C B
- Elite

13 What is the main component in the liquid form of zinc phosphate cement?
14 How do you dissipate the heat from zinc phosphate during the mixing process?
15 What size of powder increment is first brought into the liquid of zinc phosphate during mixing?
16 Do you “fill” or “line” a crown with a permanent cement?

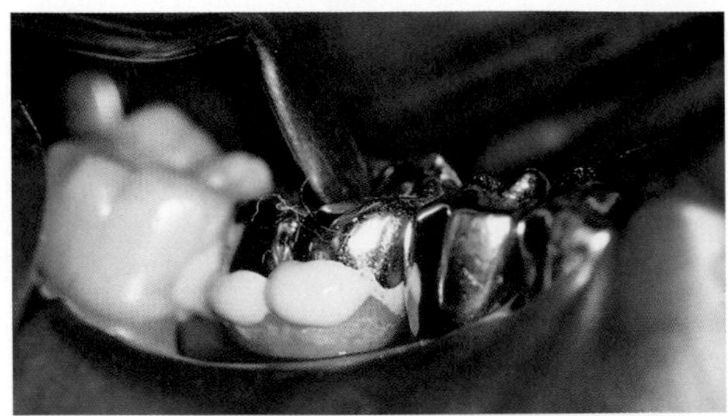

**FIG. 45.9** Excess cement must be removed after the setting process.

## Cement Removal

When the dentist has completed the cementation procedure for an indirect restoration, the patient is instructed to bite down for a few minutes on a cotton roll for the initial setting process. The material selected will determine the correct time at which to remove excess cement from around the margins, interproximal spaces, and adjacent areas covered with excess cement (Fig. 45.9). If excess cement is not removed from in and around the gingival margin and sulcus of a tooth, the cement can irritate the area and cause inflammation and discomfort.

Cement removal may be an *expanded function* for dental assistants in the state or province in which you are practicing. Therefore it is important that you understand your role as an operator with the knowledge of (1) instruments used in the procedure (explorer, mouth mirror, scaler), (2) proper use of a fulcrum, and (3) use of dental floss in and around the embrasure areas.

See Procedure 45.7: Removing Cement from Permanent or Temporary Cementation (Expanded Function).

**■ Patient Education** Cementation of an indirect restoration can be a stressful and demanding process for the dentist and dental assistant if the procedural steps do not go smoothly. Patients must express how the indirect restoration feels to their "bite," as well as the overall feeling within their mouth. When preparing cement for the cementation, remind your patients the importance of keeping their mouth open and not getting the area wet. Explain how the material will react during the setting phase.

Your role in preparing the cement must be exact in the mixing and delivery steps, so that the restoration is seated properly. Explain to the patient that a cement requires 24 hours to complete its final setting. Advise the patient to take care when chewing sticky or hard foods on the side of the restoration during this period. ■

**■ Legal and Ethical Implications** When an indirect restoration has been cemented with a permanent cement, the tooth is considered completed. This means that the dentist has done everything possible to treat this tooth. Is this correct?

No, the above statement is not correct. Many other treatments could have been provided to the patient, such as extraction, root canal therapy, or implants. Just because the tooth has undergone a final restoration procedure does not mean that the tooth will not need future work. The patient needs to understand that when a restoration, crown, or bridge is placed, the tooth may still require further treatment, and if this occurs, the dentist has not provided inadequate care to the patient. ■

**■ Eye to the Future** The future of dental cements and adhesives will include biogenetic research into human tissue made from dentin and enamel stem cells. These materials will be designed to be so similar to actual tooth structure that when they are applied to an indirect restoration, the tooth and the restoration will become one over time. ■

**■ Critical Thinking**

1. You are mixing a permanent cement and notice halfway through the mixing process that the material is setting faster than it should. What factors may be associated with the setting of the mix?
2. You are a clinical assistant in an orthodontic office. What types of cementation procedures would be used in this specialty? What three types of cements listed in this chapter typically could be used in an orthodontic practice?
3. What is the difference between preparing ZOE for permanent cementation and for temporary cementation?
4. You are preparing to mix a dental cement for the permanent cementation of a bridge. You note that after you have incorporated half the powder into the liquid, the cement is starting to thicken. Should you (a) stop mixing and use the material at this point, (b) keep incorporating all of the powder, or (c) start over? Why did you select your answer?
5. One cement presented in this chapter requires procedural steps before cementing an indirect restoration that are different from the steps required for the other materials discussed. Which material has this unique characteristic, and why are these initial steps taken for this cement? ■

# PROCEDURE 45.1 

## Mixing Glass Ionomer for Permanent Cementation

### EQUIPMENT AND SUPPLIES

- Paper mixing pad
- Spatula (flexible stainless steel)
- Glass ionomer powder and dispenser
- Glass ionomer liquid and dropper
- 2 × 2–inch gauze pads

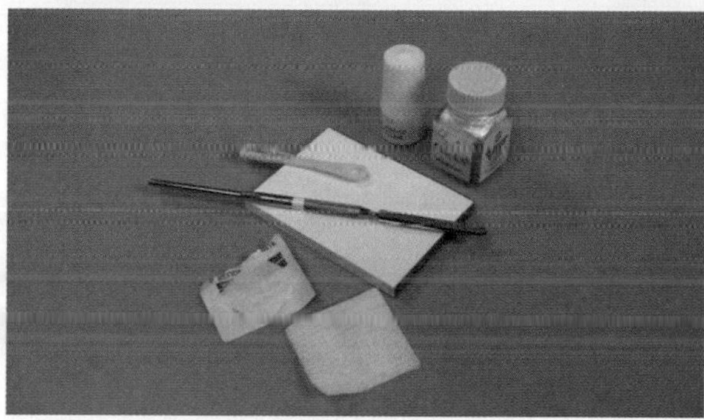

### PROCEDURAL STEPS

1 Dispense the manufacturer's recommended proportion of the liquid on one half of the paper pad.

2 Dispense the manufacturer's recommended proportion of the powder on the other half of the pad; this is usually divided into two or three increments.

3 Incorporate the powder into the liquid, following the recommended mixing time. The material should have a glossy appearance.

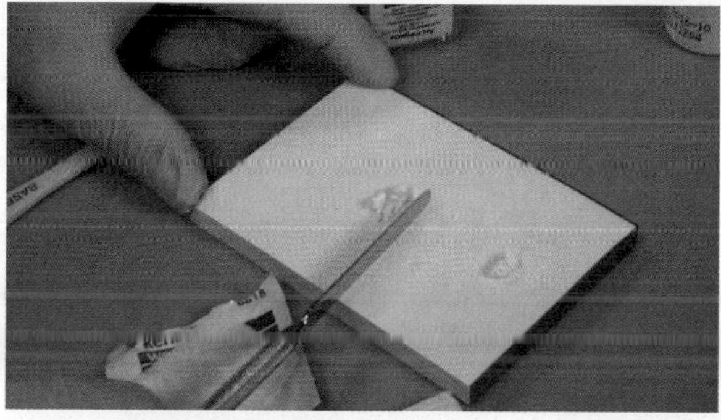

4 Clean and disinfect the equipment immediately.

# PROCEDURE 45.2

## Mixing Composite Resin for Permanent Cementation

### EQUIPMENT AND SUPPLIES

- Basic setup
- Etching system
- Cotton pellets
- Applicators
- Bonding system
- Resin cement (supplied in powder/liquid or syringe type)
- Mixing pad
- Spatula
- 2 × 2–inch gauze pads

### PROCEDURAL STEPS

1 Apply etchant to enamel and dentin for 15 seconds; then rinse. Blot excess water with a moist cotton pellet, leaving the tooth moist.

**PURPOSE** During this procedure, you do not want the tooth completely dry.

2 Apply a bond adhesive to enamel and dentin; then dry gently. Avoid excess adhesive on all prepared surfaces.

3 Light-cure each surface for 10 seconds.

4 Apply primer to etched porcelain or roughened metal surfaces. Dry for 5 seconds.

5 Dispense a 1:1 ratio onto a mixing pad; then mix for 10 seconds. Apply a thin layer of cement to the bonding surface of the restoration.

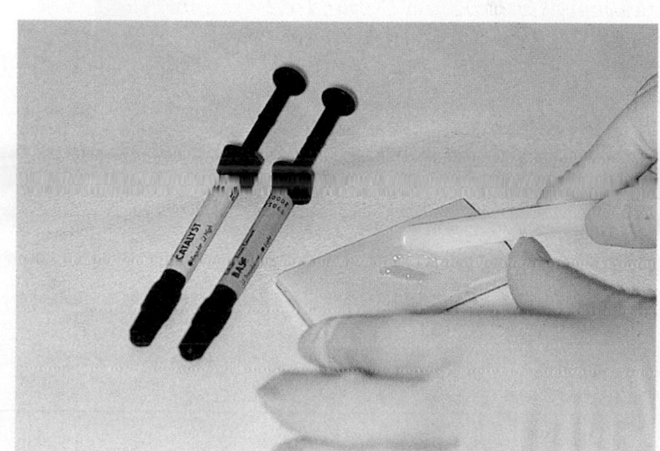


*From Hatrick CD, Eakle WS: Dental materials: clinical applications for dental assistants and dental hygienists, ed 3, St Louis, 2016, Elsevier.*

6 Once the crown is seated, margins may be light-cured for 40 seconds or allowed to self-cure for 10 minutes from the start of the mixing.

**NOTE** For porcelain and precured composite crowns, margins must be light-cured for 40 seconds.

PROCEDURE 45.3 

# Mixing Zinc Oxide–Eugenol for Temporary Cementation

## EQUIPMENT AND SUPPLIES

- Treated paper pad
- Spatula (flexible stainless steel)
- ZOE catalyst paste
- ZOE accelerator paste
- 2 × 2–inch gauze pads

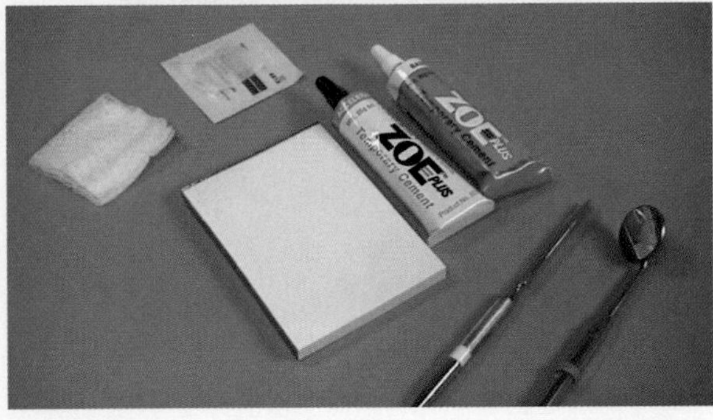


## PROCEDURAL STEPS

1 Measure the pastes onto the mixing pad at equal lengths, approximately ½ inch per unit of restoration.
2 Replace the caps immediately.
3 Incorporate the two pastes together.

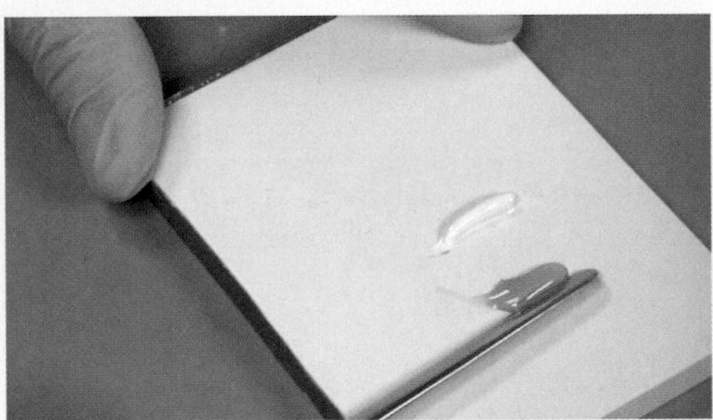

4 Mix while wiping the material over an area of the mixing pad.
5 The material should be smooth and creamy and prepared within 20 to 30 seconds.

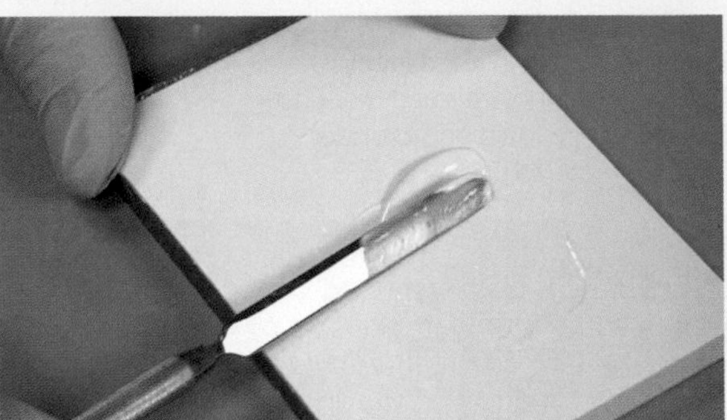

6 Immediately fill the temporary coverage with the cement.
**PURPOSE** Because the material has weaker properties than are seen in the permanent cement, fill the provisional rather than line it.
7 Clean and disinfect the equipment immediately.

## PROCEDURE 45.4

# Mixing Zinc Oxide–Eugenol for Permanent Cementation

### EQUIPMENT AND SUPPLIES

- Treated paper pad or glass slab
- Spatula (flexible stainless steel)
- Zinc oxide powder and dispenser
- Eugenol liquid and dropper
- 2 × 2–inch gauze pads

### PROCEDURAL STEPS

1. Measure the powder and place it onto the mixing pad. Replace the cap on the powder immediately.
2. Dispense the liquid near the powder on the mixing pad. Replace the cap on the liquid container immediately.

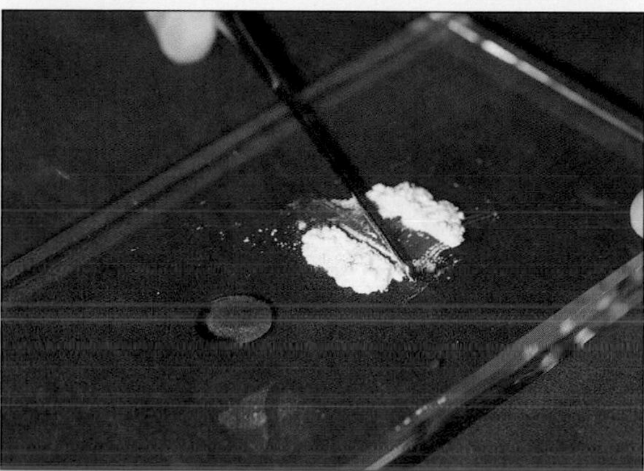

*From Hatrick CD, Eakle WS: Dental materials: clinical applications for dental assistants and dental hygienists, ed 3, St Louis, 2016, Elsevier.*

3. Incorporate the powder into the liquid all at once; spatulate for 30 seconds.
4. Initially, the mix is putty-like, but with additional mixing for 30 seconds, it will become more fluid for loading into a casting.
5. Clean and disinfect the equipment immediately.

## PROCEDURE 45.5 

# Mixing Polycarboxylate for Permanent Cementation

### EQUIPMENT AND SUPPLIES

- Treated paper pad or glass slab
- Spatula (flexible stainless steel)
- Polycarboxylate powder and dispenser
- Polycarboxylate liquid (in plastic squeeze bottle or calibrated syringe)
- 2 × 2–inch gauze pads

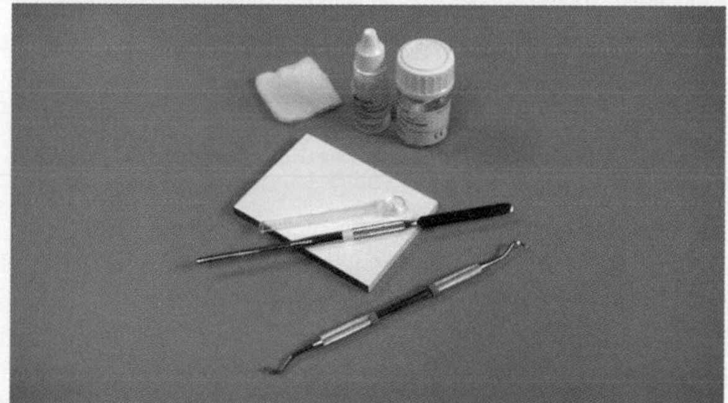

### PROCEDURAL STEPS

1. Gently shake the powder to fluff the ingredients. Measure the powder onto the mixing pad and immediately recap the container.
2. Dispense the liquid; then recap the container.
3. Use the flat side of the spatula to incorporate all the powder quickly into the liquid at one time. The mix must be completed within 30 seconds.
4. A correct mix should be somewhat thick and should have a shiny, glossy surface.

   **NOTE** If the material has lost its glossiness or exhibits a stringy "weblike" consistency, it has begun the setting process and should not be used.

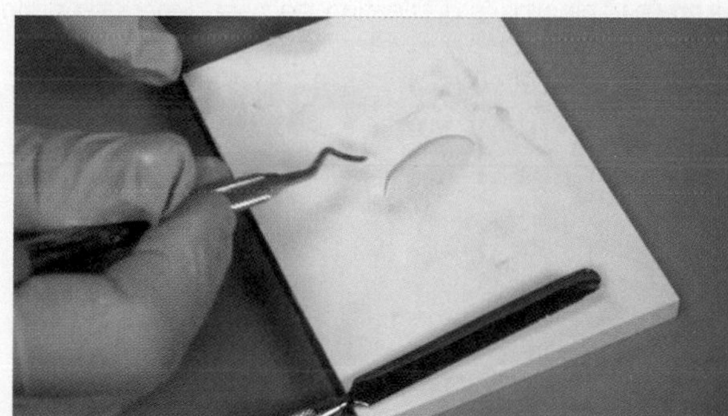

5. Clean and disinfect the equipment immediately.

PROCEDURE 45.6 

# Mixing Zinc Phosphate for Permanent Cementation

## EQUIPMENT AND SUPPLIES

- Glass slab (cool)
- Spatula (flexible stainless steel)
- Zinc phosphate powder and dispenser
- Zinc phosphate liquid and dropper
- 2 × 2–inch gauze pads

## PROCEDURAL STEPS

### Preparing the Mix

1 Dispense the powder toward one end of the slab and the liquid toward the opposite end.

2 Recap the containers.
**PURPOSE** These materials can be affected by prolonged exposure to the humidity.

3 Divide the powder into small increments as directed by the manufacturer.

4 Incorporate each powder increment into the liquid.
**NOTE** When increment sizes vary, smaller increments are used first. Mixing time per increment also varies; the time is approximately 15 to 20 seconds.

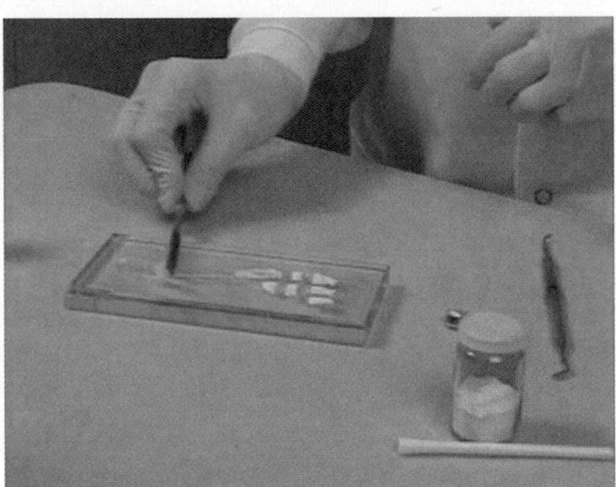

5 Spatulate the mix thoroughly, using broad strokes or a figure-8 movement over a large area of the slab.
**PURPOSE** This aids in dissipating the heat generated during mixing.

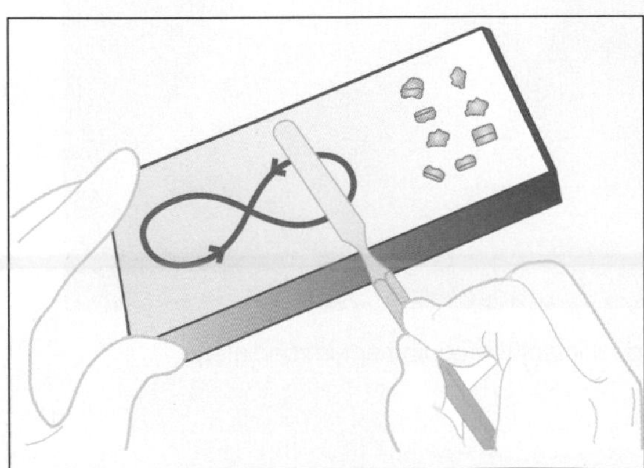

6 Test material for appropriate cementation consistency. The cement should string up and break about 1 inch from the slab. Total mixing time is approximately 1 to 2 minutes.

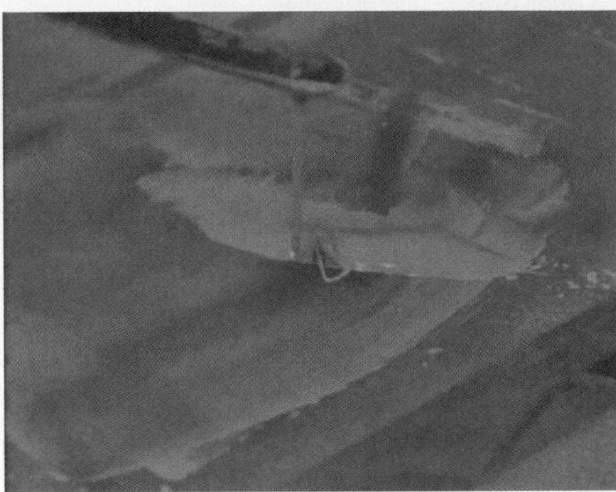

### Placing Cement in the Casting

7 In addition to preparing and mixing the material, the assistant will have the important responsibility of placing the cement in the casting.

8 Hold the casting with the inner portion facing upward.

9 Retrieve the cement onto the spatula. Scrape the edge of the spatula along the margin to cause the cement to flow from the spatula into the casting.

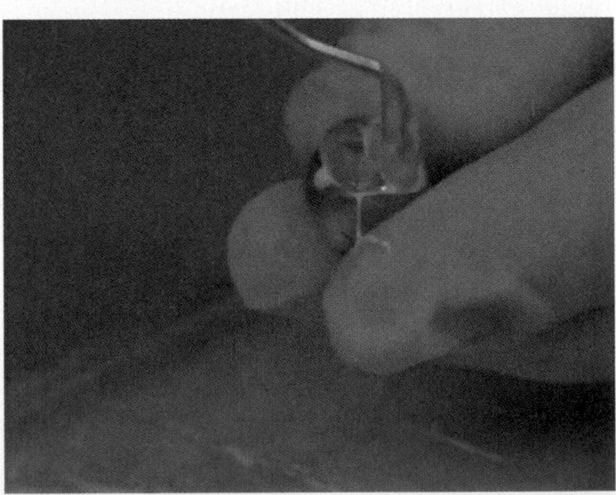

10 Place the tip of the spatula or a black spoon into the bulk of the cement; move the material so that it covers all internal walls with a thin lining of cement.

11 Turn the casting over in your palm and transfer it to the dentist.
**PURPOSE** By having the outer portion of the casting facing up, the dentist can rotate it safely to attain a better grasp for seating it.

12 Transfer a cotton roll so that the patient can bite down on it to help seat the crown and displace the excess cement.

13 Clean and disinfect the equipment immediately.

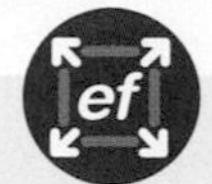

PROCEDURE 45.7

# Removing Cement from Permanent or Temporary Cementation (Expanded Function)

## PREREQUISITES FOR PERFORMING THIS PROCEDURE

- ✔ Operator positioning
- ✔ Identifying cavity classifications and oral anatomy
- ✔ Fulcrum application
- ✔ Intraoral instrumentation
- ✔ Mirror skills

## EQUIPMENT AND SUPPLIES

- ✔ Basic setup
- ✔ Spoon excavator
- ✔ Dental floss
- ✔ 2 × 2–inch gauze

## PROCEDURAL STEPS

1 After the cement has completed its initial setting, remove the cotton rolls from the area.

2 Using your explorer, examine the material to ensure the proper set.

3 With a firm fulcrum, take the edge of the explorer and carefully move the instrument in a horizontal direction, pulling the excess material away from the tooth.

**PURPOSE** Pulling the material down away from the casting will stretch or weaken the material directly under the margins.

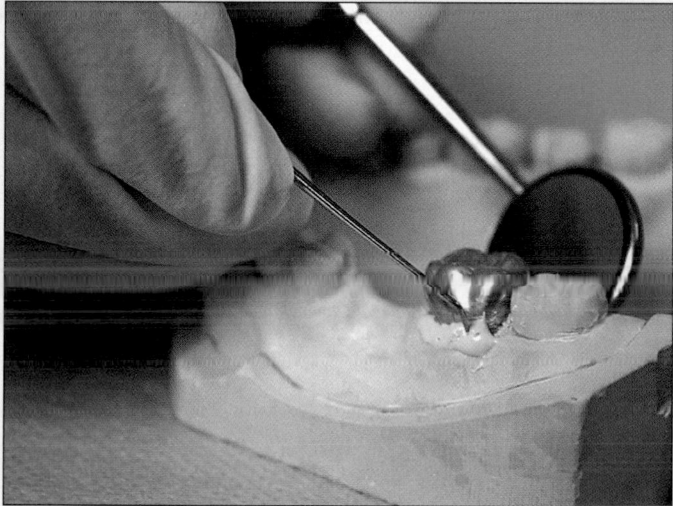

4 With the tip of the instrument at the gingival edge of the crown, use overlapping strokes to remove the bulk of the cement.

5 Follow along the margin to remove small pieces that are still adhering to the surface.

6 Tie a knot in the middle of the dental floss, and pass it through the contact on both sides to remove excess cement from the interproximal area.

**PURPOSE** The knot adds extra mass for removing the cement from this space.

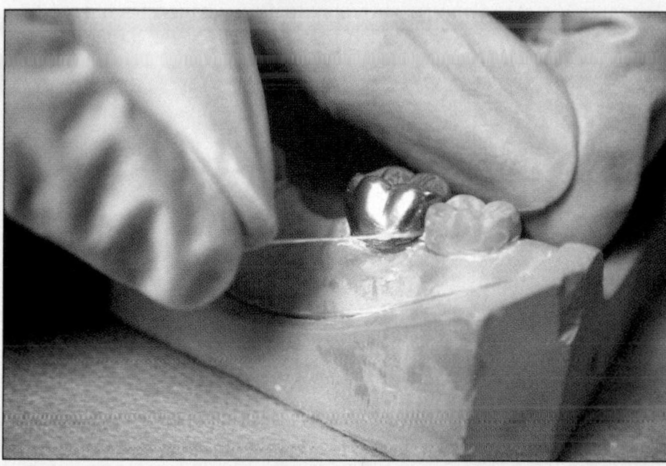

7 After the excess cement has been removed, thoroughly rinse and dry the area for evaluation of the procedure.

46

# Impression Materials

## KEY TERMS

**Agar (AG-ahr)** Gelatin-type material derived from seaweed.

**Alginate (AL-ji-nayt)** Irreversible hydrocolloid material used for taking preliminary impressions.

**Base** Foundation or the basic ingredient of a material.

**Border molding** Process of using finger pressure to contour a closer adaptation of the margins of an impression while still in the mouth.

**Catalyst (KAT-uh-list)** Substance that modifies or increases the rate of a chemical reaction.

**Centric (SEN-trik)** Having an object centered, such as maxillary teeth centered over mandibular teeth in correct relation.

**Colloid (KOL-oid)** A suspension of particles in a dispersion medium such as water. Its two phases are sol and gel.

**Elastomeric (ee-las-tuh-MER-ik)** Material having elastic properties from rubber.

**Hydro-** Prefix meaning "water."

**Hysteresis** A change in temperature that causes the reversible hydrocolloid material to transform from one physical state to another.

**Imbibition (im-bi-BI-shun)** Absorption of water, causing an object to swell.

**Occlusal (o-KLOO-sul; o-KLOO-zul) registration** Reproduction of a patient's bite with the use of wax or elastomeric material.

**Syneresis (si-ner-E-sus)** Loss of water, causing something to shrink.

**Tempering (TEM-pur-ing)** Bringing a material to a desired consistency.

**Viscous, Viscosity (vis-KOS-i-tee)** Physical property of a fluid related to resistance to flow.

## LEARNING OUTCOMES

*On completion of this chapter, the student will be able to achieve the following objectives:*

1 Pronounce, define, and spell the key terms.
2 Give the three types of impressions taken in a dental office.
3 Describe the types of impression trays and their characteristics of use.
4 Discuss hydrocolloid impression materials and their uses, mixing techniques, and application.
5 Discuss elastomeric impression materials and their uses, mixing techniques, and application.
6 Explain the importance of an occlusal registration and describe its use in a procedure.

## PERFORMANCE OUTCOMES

*On completion of this chapter, the student will be able to achieve competency standards in the following skills:*

- Mix alginate impression material at competency level.
- Take a maxillary and a mandibular preliminary impression at competency level.
- Mix a paste final impression material.
- Prepare an automix impression material.
- Take a wax bite registration.
- Prepare and assist in a closed bite registration procedure with polysiloxane material and zinc oxide–eugenol material.

## ELECTRONIC RESOURCES

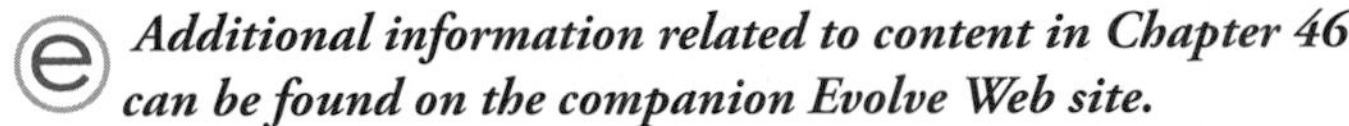

***Additional information related to content in Chapter 46 can be found on the companion Evolve Web site.***

- Practice Quiz
- Video: Mixing Alginate and Taking Preliminary Impressions

There are a range of dental procedures in which impression materials are used to take an impression of the teeth and surrounding oral tissues. Impressions are a **negative** reproduction of those structures, and the model created from the impression is the **positive** reproduction of the structures. The type of impression material selected for a procedure will depend on how the impression will be utilized.

As a clinical assistant, you will be responsible for knowing what type of impression tray to prepare, what material to set out, and the proper mixing sequence to use for the procedure. Your role is to assist in taking the final impression, or, as an expanded-functions dental assistant (EFDA) or registered dental assistant (RDA), in the actual taking of the impression.

## Classification of Impressions

The three classifications of impressions applied in dental procedures consist of **preliminary, final,** and **occlusal,** which can also be referred to as **(bite) registration.** The type of dental material selected by the dentist for these types of impressions will depend on what will be fabricated from the impression. This chapter describes the two types of hydrocolloid and

**elastomeric** impression materials, as well as the bite registration materials regularly used for dental procedures.

### Preliminary Impressions

Preliminary impressions are taken by the dentist or by the EFDA/RDA and are used to create a reproduction of the teeth and surrounding tissues. A preliminary impression is used for the following procedures:

- Diagnostic models/casts
- Custom trays
- Provisional coverage
- Orthodontic appliances
- Pretreatment and posttreatment records

### Final Impressions

Final impressions are to be taken by the dentist and are used to produce the most accurate reproduction of the teeth and the surrounding tissue. A final impression provides the dentist and the dental laboratory technician with essential information needed for the creation of indirect restorations, partial or full dentures, and implants.

### Bite Registrations

Bite or occlusal registrations are taken by the dentist or the EFDA/RDA to produce a reproduction of the occlusal relationship of the maxillary and mandibular teeth when the mouth is occluded. This provides the dentist and the laboratory technician with an accurate registration of the patient's **centric** relationship between the maxillary and mandibular arches.

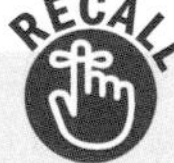


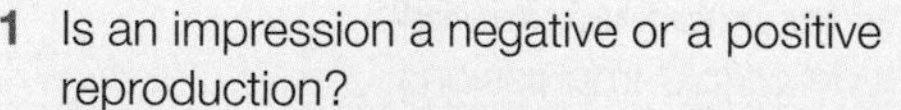

1 Is an impression a negative or a positive reproduction?
2 Of the three classifications of impressions, which can the EFDA legally take?
3 Which of the three classifications of impressions is used for occlusal relationships?

## Impression Trays

Impression trays are used to hold the impression material within the mouth. These trays must be sufficiently rigid to (1) carry the impression material into the oral cavity, (2) hold the material close to the teeth, (3) avoid breaking during removal, and (4) prevent warping the completed impression.

Impression trays are of two basic types: stock trays and custom trays.

### Stock Trays

Stock trays are manufactured in several ways and are available in a range of sizes and styles. Fig. 46.1 illustrates the different types of stock trays that are used most often during a dental procedure.

#### Characteristics

Impression trays are supplied in one of the following ways (Fig. 46.2):

- **Quadrant trays,** which cover half of an arch
- **Section trays,** which are used to cover the anterior portion of the arch
- **Full-arch trays,** which cover the entire arch

An impression tray is also characterized by whether the surface of the tray is perforated or smooth. When a **perforated** surface tray is used, the impression material oozes through the holes of the tray, creating a mechanical lock to hold the material in place. When a **smooth** surface tray is used, there is no mechanical lock, so the interior of the tray is painted or sprayed with an adhesive to hold the impression material securely in the tray.

#### Sizing of Tray

Impression trays are selected for size by trying the tray in the patient's mouth before taking the impression. The correct size of tray accomplishes the following:

- Is comfortable for the patient
- Extends slightly beyond the facial surfaces of the teeth
- Extends approximately 2 to 3 mm beyond the third molar, retromolar, or tuberosity area of the arch
- Is sufficiently deep to allow 2 to 3 mm of material between the tray and the incisal or occlusal edges of the teeth

#### Adaptation

If necessary, the depth or length of the tray can be extended by adding utility wax to the border of the tray. This addition might be necessary if the tray does not completely cover the posterior teeth (Fig. 46.3). For a patient with an unusually high palate, softened utility wax can be added to the palate area of the impression tray.

### Custom Trays

A custom tray is constructed to fit the mouth of a specific patient. The dental assistant or the laboratory technician constructs the custom tray in the laboratory from a diagnostic model made from a preliminary impression of the arch *before* the dentist has prepared the teeth. Chapter 47 describes the construction of a custom tray by using acrylic resin, light-cured resin, or a thermoplastic resin technique.

### Tray Adhesives

Tray adhesive helps ensure that an impression remains firmly attached to the tray on removal from the mouth so as not to cause deformity. It is important that an adhesive be dry before the impression material is loaded into the tray. If the adhesive has not had time to dry, the impression will pull away from

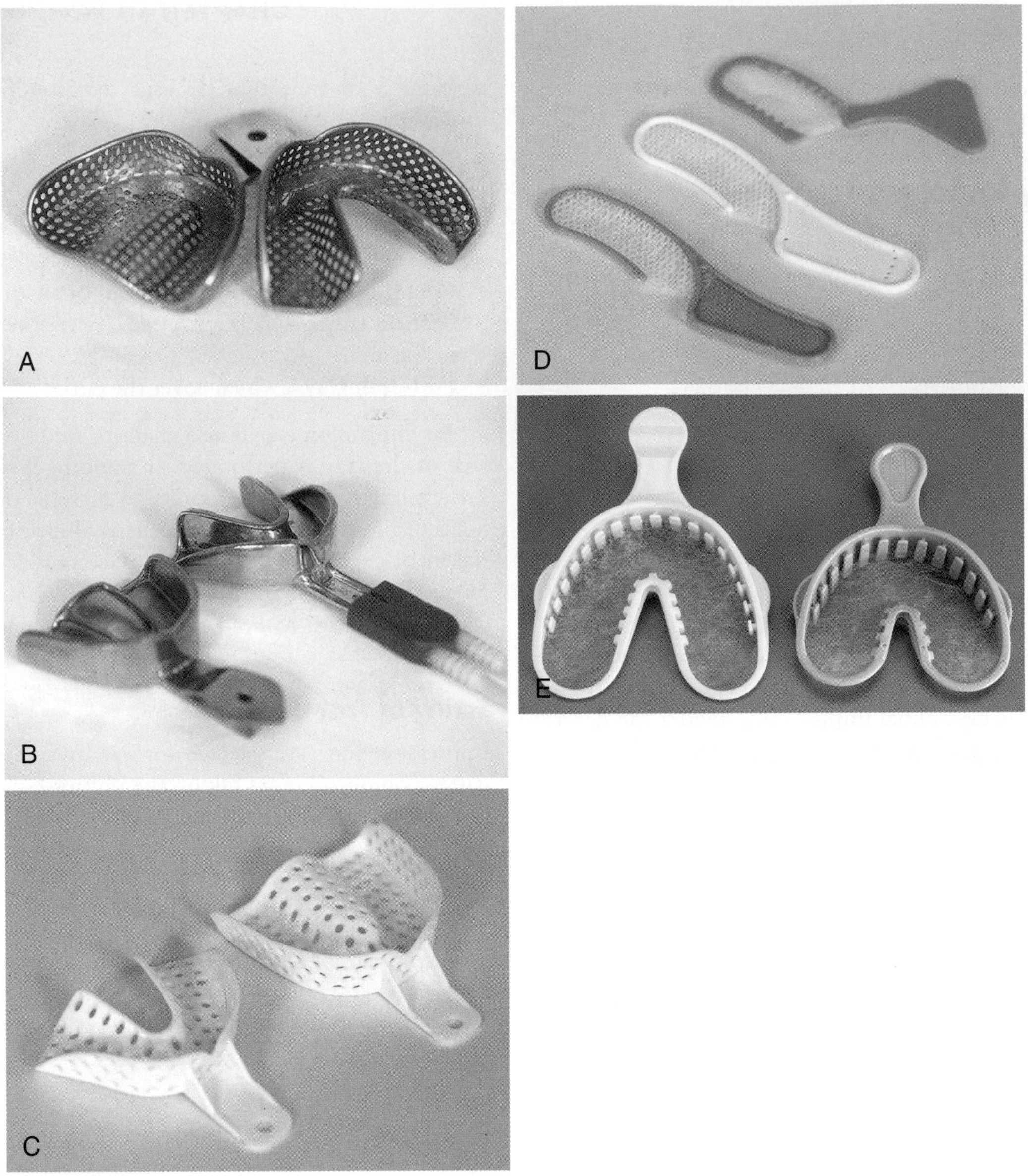

**FIG. 46.1** Types of stock trays. A, Metal perforated tray used most often for preliminary impressions. B, Metal water coolant tray used most often with reversible hydrocolloid impressions. C, Plastic perforated tray used for preliminary and final impressions. D, Bite tray used for final impressions and bite registrations. E, Triple tray designed to eliminate steps by taking final impressions and bite registration at the same time. *(E, From Boyd LRB: Dental instruments: a pocket guide, ed 6, St Louis, 2018, Elsevier.)*

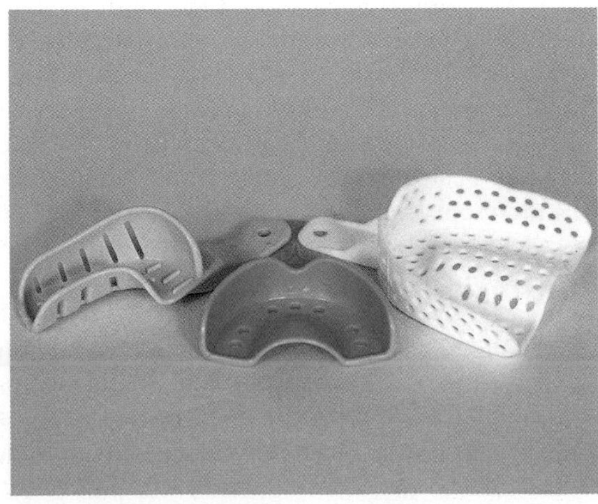

**FIG. 46.2** Examples of a quadrant, sectional, and full-arch impression trays.

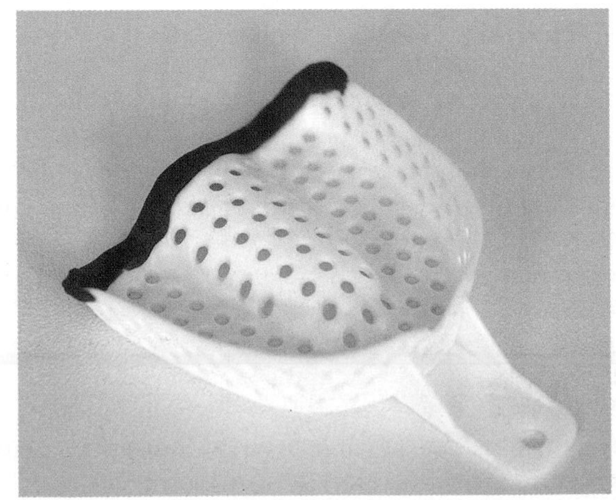

**FIG. 46.3** Extending impression tray with utility wax.

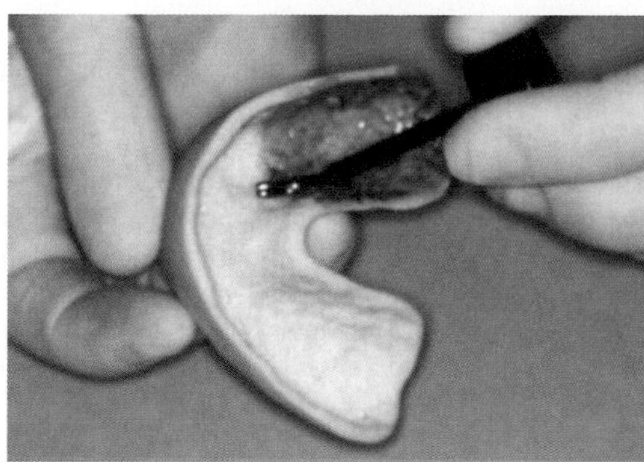

**FIG. 46.4** Impression tray with adhesive applied. *(From Rosenstiel SF, Land MF, Fujimoto J: Contemporary fixed prosthodontics, ed 5, St Louis, 2016, Elsevier.)*

the tray, causing deformity in the impression. Paint or spray the tray with the adhesive at least 15 minutes before use (Fig. 46.4). Specific adhesives used with specific impression materials are as follows:

- **VPS adhesives** (blue)—used with polyvinyl siloxane (polysiloxane) and polyether impression materials
- **Rubber base adhesives** (brown)—used with rubber base impression materials
- **Silicone adhesives** (orange-pink)—used with silicone impression materials

RECALL

4 Which type of impression tray covers half the arch?
5 Which type of tray allows impression material to lock on mechanically?
6 Which type of tray is designed to fit a specific patient?
7 What is used to extend the length of a tray?

# Hydrocolloid Materials

Hydrocolloid (**hydro-** meaning water and **colloid** meaning a gelatinous substance) is a material used to obtain preliminary and final impressions. Depending on the type of hydrocolloid, the physical change from **sol (solution)** to **gel (solid)** can be **irreversible** (changed by chemical factors) or **reversible** (changed by thermal factors).

## Irreversible Hydrocolloid: Alginate

Hydrocolloid impression materials that cannot return to the sol state after they become a gel are termed **irreversible hydrocolloids.** The change in this physical state results from a chemical change in the material. Cake mix is an example of an irreversible change. When water is added to the powder in a cake mix, a chemical reaction occurs. It is impossible to remove the water and return the mixture to powder.

**Alginate** is an irreversible hydrocolloid that is most widely used for preliminary impressions.

### Composition and Chemistry

The main components of alginate include the following:

- **Potassium alginate,** derived from seaweed, is used as a thickening agent. This ingredient is used in some ice creams for the same reason.
- **Calcium sulfate** reacts with the potassium alginate to form the gel.
- **Trisodium phosphate** is added to slow down the reaction time for mixing.
- **Diatomaceous earth** is a filler that adds bulk to the material.
- **Zinc oxide** adds bulk to the material.
- **Potassium titanium fluoride** prevents interference with the setting and surface strength of the product used when making the model.

### Physical Phases

Hydrocolloid impression materials have two physical phases. First, in the *sol* (solution) phase, the material is in a liquid or semiliquid form. Second, in the *gel* (solid) phase, the material is semisolid, similar to a dessert pudding. The gel strength of hydrocolloid is not as great as that of elastomeric impression materials. The hydrocolloids have difficulty withstanding tensile stress *(tearing)* and elastic strain *(stretching).*

### Strength

It is important for alginate to be sufficiently strong to resist tearing when the impression is removed from the patient's mouth. The strength of the material will continue to increase even after it appears to be set. Because of this setting process, leaving the impression in the mouth for the full length of time recommended by the manufacturer is important toward achieving maximum strength.

### Dimensional Change

Because so much of the alginate material is made from water, a slight change in the surroundings can distort the impression and cause **dimensional** change. Alginate impression materials must be "poured up" within 1 hour of taking the impression—a requirement dictated by the environment.

If an alginate impression is stored in water or in a saturated paper towel, the alginate acts like a sponge and will actually absorb the additional water and expand. This condition is called **imbibition**.

If an alginate impression remains in the open air, moisture will evaporate from the material, causing the impression to shrink and distort. This condition is called **syneresis.**

Storage of the disinfected impression in a plastic biohazard bag covered with a slightly moistened towel will provide an atmosphere close to 100 percent relative humidity, which causes the least amount of distortion.

### Packaging and Storage

Alginate can be purchased in a variety of packaging. Containers the size of a coffee can are the most common form of packaging. Premeasured, individual packages are more expensive than other types of packaging, but they save time by eliminating the need for measurement of the powder (Fig. 46.5). The material is also supplied with flavoring and changes color when set. Alginate can deteriorate very quickly if exposed to elevated temperatures and moisture, causing the material to not set or to set too rapidly. The shelf life of alginate is approximately 1 year.

### Types of Setting

Alginate is available in two settings: **normal set** and **fast set.** The types of alginate refer to the working time and the setting time. Normal-set alginate has a working time of 2 minutes and a setting time of up to 4½ minutes after mixing. Fast-set alginate has a working time of 1¼ minutes and a setting time of 1 to 2 minutes.

**Working time** is the time allowed for mixing the alginate, loading the tray, and positioning the tray in the patient's mouth.

**Setting time** is the time required for the chemical action to be completed, after which the impression is ready to be removed from the patient's mouth.

There is no difference in the makeup of the completed impression between the two setting types of alginates. The decision as to which type to use is based on time-related factors, such as the following:

- Difficulty in seating the impression tray (normal set allows more time for insertion and placement of the tray)
- Whether or not the operator is working alone (normal set allows the operator more time to mix the alginate, load the impression tray, and seat the tray in the mouth)
- Patients with a severe gag reflex (fast set allows the tray to be removed from the mouth much sooner)

### Altering Setting Time

Room temperature water (21° C/70° F) is best to use when mixing alginate. If additional time is needed for the procedure, using cooler water will increase or lengthen the setting time. Warmer water will decrease or shorten the setting time of the procedure.

### Water-to-Powder Ratio

It is important to accurately measure the alginate powder and the water to be mixed. To help ensure accuracy, the manufacturer supplies a plastic scoop for dispensing the bulk powder and a plastic cylinder for measuring the water (Fig. 46.6). The water-to-powder ratio for mixing alginate is clearly marked on these measures. The mixture is equal in ratio: one scoop of powder to one "measure" of water.

- An adult **mandibular impression** generally requires two scoops of powder and two measures of water.
- An adult **maxillary impression** generally requires three scoops of powder and three measures of water.

### Mixing Techniques

The most common mixing technique used for alginate materials is manual spatulation with a rubber bowl and beavertail wide spatula. An additional technique is the use of an alginator, which is a rubber flexible bowl attached to an electrical component with a low or high speed (Fig. 46.7).

See Procedure 46.1: Mixing Alginate Impression Material.

### Taking an Alginate Impression

It is important for the EFDA/RDA to gain competence in mixing the alginate, loading the tray, and keeping the patient comfortable while taking the impression.

### Explain Procedure to Patient

Before an impression is taken, the procedure is explained to the patient to ensure his or her comfort. The patient is instructed on the following:

- The material will feel cool to the teeth, there is no unpleasant taste, and the material will set quickly.
- To not talk, but to use a hand signal to communicate any discomfort.

If a patient has a strong gag reflex, this is one procedure that can easily trigger the patient to gag. To reduce the chance

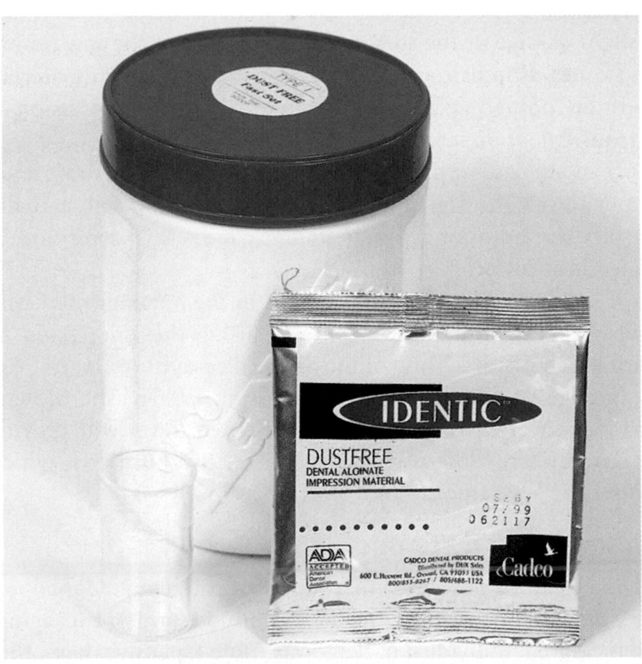

FIG. 46.5 Packaging of alginate.

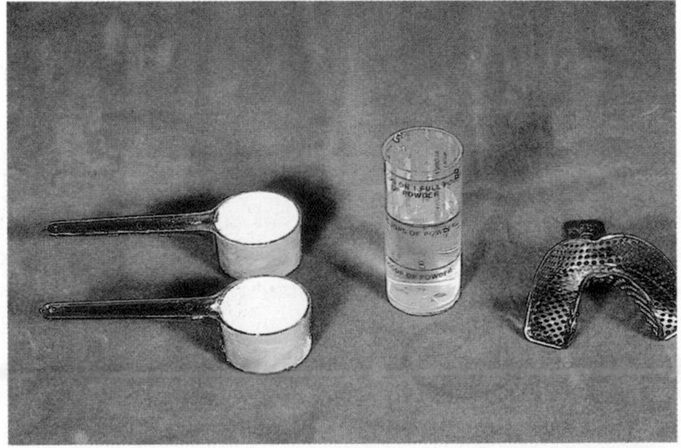
FIG. 46.6 A plastic scoop and a plastic cylinder are supplied with alginate.

of triggering a gag reflex while the impression is seated in the mouth you can use the following suggestions:

- **Breathe through the nose**—instruct the patient to focus on breathing deeply through his or her nose. Explain that this will help the patient relax and be more comfortable.
- **Drooling**—can be embarrassing, causing the patient to try to swallow. Have a saliva ejector to remove saliva from the mouth and a paper towel to wipe the patient's mouth.
- **Distraction**—by having a stress ball to squeeze, a video on the screen, or something that will focus the patient's mind away from the dental procedure—will help the time go by.
- **Talk to your patient**—by continually talking to your patient (as long as you are not asking questions) the distraction can help reduce the chance of gagging.
- **Sit upright with the head tilted forward**—the impression material will ooze forward, rather than toward the patient's throat.

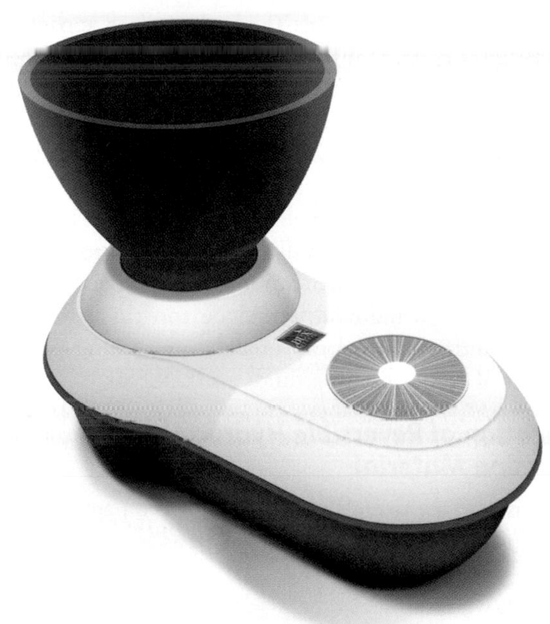

FIG. 46.7 Example of an alginator. *(Courtesy DUX Dental, Oxnard, CA.)*

- **Administer nitrous oxide**—for severe gaggers, nitrous oxide has a significant effect on reducing the gag reflex.

## Evaluating Alginate Impression

An acceptable alginate impression must meet specific criteria (Fig. 46.8):

- The impression tray should be centered over the central and lateral incisors.
- There is a complete "peripheral roll," which includes all the *vestibular* areas.
- The tray is not *overseated* (pushed down too far), which would result in exposure of areas of the impression tray.
- The impression is free from tears or voids *(holes).*
- Sharp anatomic detail of all teeth and soft tissues is provided.
- The *retromolar* area, lingual frenum, tongue space, and mylohyoid ridge are reproduced in the *mandibular* impression.
- The *hard palate* and tuberosities are recorded in the maxillary impression.

See Procedure 46.2: Taking a Mandibular Preliminary Impression (Expanded Function) and Procedure 46.3: Taking a Maxillary Preliminary Impression (Expanded Function).

## Impressions of Edentulous Arches

Taking an alginate impression of an edentulous arch differs from taking other alginate impressions in two ways: (1) The height of the teeth is missing, and (2) it is important to include more extensive tissue details. An edentulous tray is used to take this impression. This tray is not as deep as other trays used for alginate impressions. In addition, attaching sticky wax or similar material to the edges will modify the borders of the tray. This modification allows **border molding**, also known as **muscle trimming,** to achieve closer adaptation of the edges of the impression of the tissues in the mucobuccal fold.

Border molding is performed after the impression tray is in place. The dentist uses the fingers to gently massage the area of the face over these borders. This action shapes the wax-covered edges of the tray so that these edges more closely approximate the tissues.

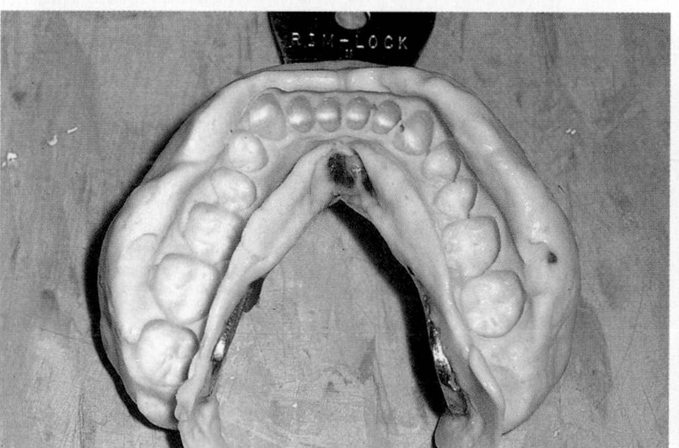



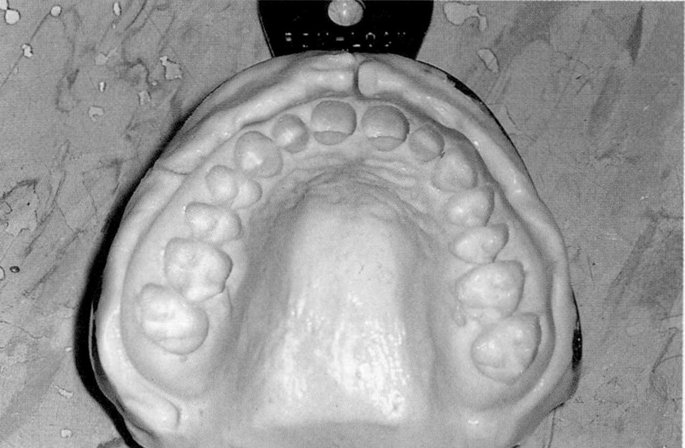

FIG. 46.8 How a centered mandibular and maxillary impression will appear.

RECALL

8 What is the most widely used irreversible hydrocolloid for preliminary impressions?
9 What is the organic substance within hydrocolloid materials?
10 Why would you select a fast-set alginate over a normal-set alginate?
11 What is the water-to-powder ratio for taking a maxillary impression?
12 What does the prefix "hydro-" mean?
13 Do you mix irreversible hydrocolloid on a paper pad or in a mixing bowl?

## Reversible Hydrocolloid

Hydrocolloid impression materials that change physical states from a sol to a gel and then back to a sol are called **reversible hydrocolloids.** A change in temperature causes the reversible hydrocolloid material to transform from one physical state to another.

Ice cream is a good example of a reversible hydrocolloid. When ice cream is frozen, it is in the gel state. **Hysteresis** is a term used to describe the change in temperature that causes the reversible hydrocolloid material to transform from one physical state to another. An example of this change is when ice cream is left at room temperature, the ice cream melts and turns into a *sol* (solution) state. When returned to the freezer, the ice cream again becomes a *gel* (solid) state.

Reversible hydrocolloid material is approximately 85 percent water and 13 percent **agar**. As in alginate, agar is an organic substance derived from seaweed. Additional chemical modifiers are added to enhance the handling characteristics.

For the reversible hydrocolloid to change from one consistency to another, a specialized conditioning bath is used. The following three compartments maintain water at three different temperatures (Fig. 46.9):

- The first bath is for **liquefying** the semisolid material. Immersing the tube of material in a special water bath called a *hydrocolloid conditioner* at 212° F (100° C) liquefies the material. After liquefying, the preset thermostat automatically cools the temperature to 150° F (65.5° C).
- The second bath becomes a *storage* bath that cools the material, readying it for the impression. At this temperature, the tubes are waiting for use.
- A third temperature in a separate bath is kept at 110° F (44° C) for **tempering** the material after it has been placed in the tray.

### Tray Material

Reversible hydrocolloid material is packaged in plastic tubes. Each tube holds enough material to fill a full-arch, water-cooled tray (Fig. 46.10).

The material needs enough viscosity to keep it from flowing out of the tray when dispensed at 150° F (65.5° C). An impression tray is filled and then immersed in the 110° F (43.3° C) bath for a few minutes to further increase viscosity and reduce the temperature to a comfortable level for the patient.

### Syringe Material

A conventional hydrocolloid is dispensed directly onto the prepared and surrounding teeth. It is less **viscous** (has a lower **viscosity**) than tray material. The hydrocolloid is packaged in plastic or glass cartridges that fit a syringe, or it comes in preloaded syringes or preformed sticks that refill special hydrocolloid inlay syringes.

The syringe material is liquefied by placing it in the same 150° F (65.5° C) storage bath as the tray material. Because it requires easy flow, the syringe material is never tempered at 110° F (43.3° C). As the small stream flows through the dispensing needle, it cools to a comfortable temperature. If tempered, the syringe material would be too thick for accurate placement and would gel too quickly, preventing proper displacement of contaminating fluids and bubbles.

### Application of Reversible Hydrocolloid Impression Material

The dentist and the dental assistant must coordinate the following steps to ensure that the impression will be as accurate as possible:

- A stock water-cooled tray is selected, making sure that the tray does not impinge on any of the teeth or soft tissues.

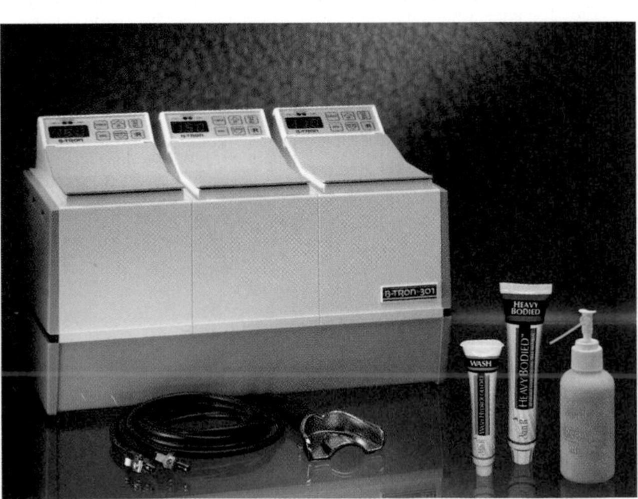


**FIG. 46.9** Conditioning bath for reversible hydrocolloid.

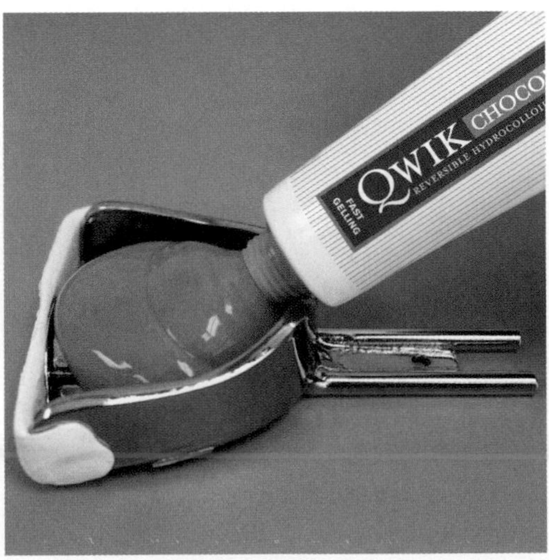


**FIG. 46.10** Filling tray with heavy body material from the storage bath. *(Courtesy Dux Dental, Oxnard, CA.)*

- Plastic stops are placed in the tray to help keep the tray from sticking to the teeth.
- Tubing is connected to the tray and to the water outlet for drainage.
- The material is liquefied and is moved to the storage bath (second bath).
- The light-bodied material is placed in the syringe; the heavy-bodied material is placed in the tray and is moved to the tempering bath (third bath).
- The light-bodied material is expressed around the prepared tooth, and the dentist seats the tray.

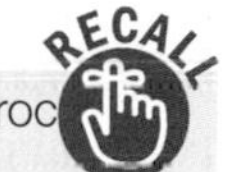


**14** Before an impression is taken with reversible hydroc
where is the material kept?

# Elastomeric Materials

Elastomeric impression materials are used when an accurate impression is essential (Fig. 46.11). The term **elastomeric** indicates "having elastic or rubber-like qualities." This rubber-like quality makes it possible to remove the impression after it has set, without creating any distortion or tearing.

## Characteristics

Elastomeric impression materials are self-curing and supplied as a **base** and a **catalyst**. The base is supplied as a paste in either a tube, a cartridge with syringe tip, or as putty in a jar. The catalyst, also known as the **accelerator,** is packaged as a paste in a tube, in a cartridge, or as a liquid in a bottle with a dropper top.

These materials are supplied with the appropriate base and catalyst in the same package, and should always be used together and not with other types of materials. If the base from one box is mixed with the catalyst from another, the material may not set properly or may lack important characteristics.

## Forms of Materials

Elastomeric impression materials generally are supplied in three forms: light-bodied, regular, and heavy-bodied.

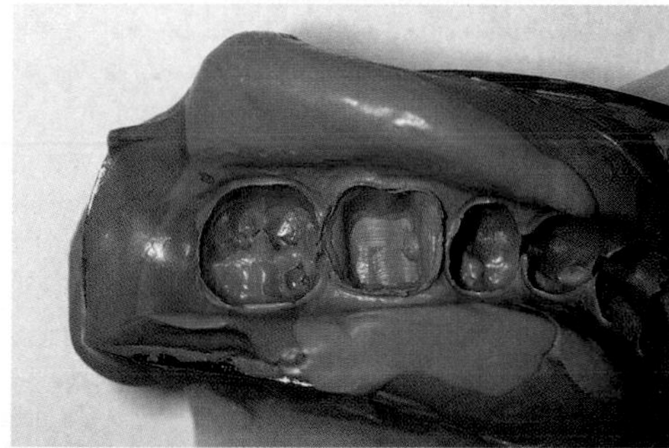

**FIG. 46.11** Example of a final impression. *(From Hatrick CD, Eakle WS: Dental materials: clinical applications for dental assistants and dental hygienists, ed 3, St Louis, 2016, Elsevier.)*

### Light-Bodied Material

**Light-bodied** material, also referred to as **syringe-type or wash-type** material, is used because of its ability to flow into and around the details of the prepared tooth. A special syringe, or **extruder,** is used to apply light-bodied material immediately around the prepared teeth.

### Regular and Heavy-Bodied Materials

**Regular** and **heavy-bodied** materials, also referred to as **tray-type** materials, are much thicker than light-bodied impression materials and are used to fill the tray. Their stiffness helps force the light-bodied material into close contact with prepared teeth and surrounding tissues to ensure a more accurate impression and details of a preparation.

### Basic Impression Technique

- The material selected depends on the dentist's preference and the type of impression required for the procedure.
- The dentist prepares the tooth (or teeth) for the impression.
- Gingival retraction cord is placed in the sulcus in preparation of the light body material (see Chapter 50).
- The light-bodied material is prepared, loaded into the syringe, and transferred to the dentist.
- The dentist removes the retraction cord while placing the light-bodied material into the sulcus, around and over the prepared teeth, and onto the surrounding tissues.
- The heavy-bodied material is prepared, loaded into the tray, and transferred to the dentist.
- When the impression material has reached final set, the impression is removed and is inspected for accuracy.
- The impression is disinfected, placed in a biohazard bag, labeled, and readied for the laboratory technician.

## Curing Stages and Types

The curing reaction *(polymerization),* as the elastomeric material changes from a paste into a rubber-like material, begins as soon as the base and the catalyst are brought together. The change occurs in a three-stage process: initial set, final set, and final cure.

1. **Initial set** results in stiffening of the paste without the appearance of elastic properties. The material may be *manipulated* only during this first stage. The mix must be completed within the limited working time specified by the manufacturer.
2. **Final set** begins with the appearance of elasticity and proceeds through a gradual change to a solid, rubbery mass. The material must be in place in the mouth before the elastic properties of the final set begin to develop.
3. **Final cure** occurs within 1 to 24 hours. Only slight dimensional change is noted in the details of the impression during this time.

## Mixing of Materials

Many different mixing techniques are available for use with impression materials. The most common sequence, however, involves preparing the light-bodied material *first,* then the heavy-bodied material.

### Paste System

When working with an elastomeric material in a paste system, *timing* is the most important reason for having the equipment and material prepared and ready to mix when the dentist signals the go-ahead. Make sure that you have enough material placed out for the type of tray you are using. See Procedure 46.4: Mixing a Two-Paste Final Impression Material.

### Automix System

Automix systems are designed by manufacturers to complete the mixing process for the procedure. The unique automix system provides a homogeneous mix with the appropriate amount of material without waste. The extruder is used to automatically mix and dispense elastomeric impression materials. The unit can be used with any viscosity (light-bodied, medium, or heavy-bodied material) and is operated with a trigger-like handle. The extruder is loaded with dual cartridges that consist of a tube of catalyst and a tube of base material. See Procedure 46.5: Preparing an Automix Final Impression Material.

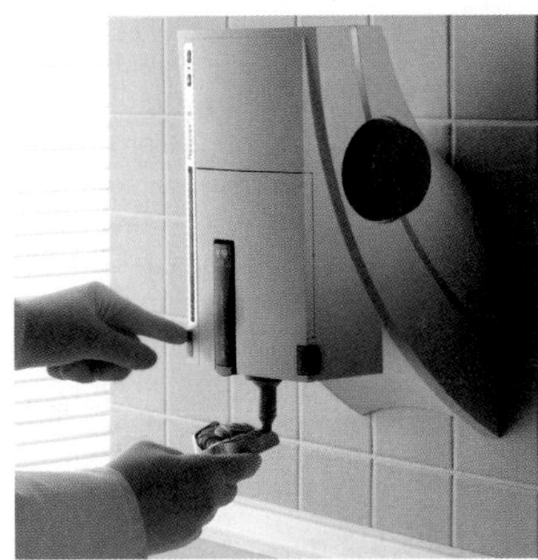

**FIG. 46.12** Mixing unit for final impression material. *(Copyright © 3M 2017. All rights reserved.)*

### Mixing Unit System

In a dental office in which a lot of impressions are taken, a table-top or wall-mounted mixing unit may save time (Fig. 46.12). Several factors make this process easier:

- *Controlled dispensing*—No excess material remains on the mixing pad.
- *Infection control*—Less time is spent cleaning and disinfecting guns and cartridges.
- *Versatility*—A variety of impression materials can be mixed and dispensed from this unit.

### Putty System

Putty impression material provides all the benefits of true putty, including a higher viscosity than seen with heavy-bodied materials. Because the material is kneaded in the palms, putty is already warm when it is seated in the mouth; it helps warm up the syringe material, actually accelerating setting time without reducing the intraoral working time.

## Types of Elastomeric Materials

The four types of elastomeric impression materials most often used in dental practice are *polysulfide, polyether, silicone,* and *polysiloxane* (polyvinyl siloxane) (Table 46.1). Although the materials have some common aspects, each material has slightly different properties and characteristics. Of particular concern when using these materials are dimensional stability and permanent deformation:

- **Dimensional stability** is the ability of the material to keep its shape after it has been removed from the mouth.
- **Deformation** is the ability of the material to resist permanent change caused by stresses during removal from the mouth.

**TABLE 46.1** Properties of Final Impressions Materials

| Type | Characteristics | Working Ability |
|---|---|---|
| **Polysulfide** | A paste material supplied in two tubes. A strong odor and taste are associated with the material. The stiffness and stability of the material are poor. | A harder material to mix. It has a longer mixing time of 60 seconds and a longer setting time of 10–20 minutes. |
| **Polyether** | A paste material supplied in tubes or cartridges that has an acceptable odor and taste. The stiffness and stability of the material are very good. | An easy material to mix, with a short mixing time of 30–45 seconds and a fast setting time of 6–7 minutes. |
| **Condensation silicone** | Material supplied as a paste and a liquid. It has an acceptable odor and taste. The stiffness and stability are average. | A fairly easy material to mix, with an average mixing time of 30–60 seconds and an average setting time of 6–10 minutes. |
| **Addition silicone** | A paste material supplied as a two-paste system, as a putty material, or in cartridges. This material has an acceptable odor and taste. The stiffness and stability are excellent. | An easy material to mix, with a short mixing time of 30–45 seconds and an average setting time of 6–8 minutes. |

From Robinson DS, Bird DL: Essentials of dental assisting, ed 5, St Louis, 2013, Saunders.

- **Permanent deformation** means that the material was changed and will not regain its previous shape.

### Polysulfide

Polysulfide, also referred to as **rubber base,** has been used in dentistry as a final impression material for many years (Fig. 46.13). Polysulfide impression materials are available in light-bodied, regular, and heavy-bodied forms.

The material is supplied as a two-paste system: the base and the catalyst. Disadvantages of rubber base material are its strong odor and the fact that it can easily stain clothing.

Polysulfide material has a relatively long working and setting time. Its stiffness is low, which allows this material to maintain some flexibility on removal from the mouth and separation from the cast.

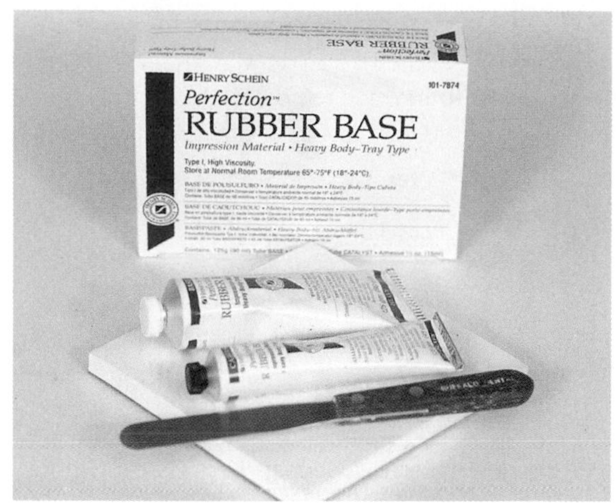


**FIG. 46.13** Polysulfide material.

#### Chemical Makeup and Mixing Guidelines for Polysulfide Impression Material

**Chemical Makeup**

- Base: mercaptan polysulfide
- Cross-linking agent: sulfur or lead peroxide
- Catalyst: copper hydroxide, zinc peroxide, or organic hydroperoxide
- Filler: zinc sulfate, lithopone, or calcium sulfate dihydrate

**Guidelines for Using Material**

- Dispense pastes at the top of the mixing pad.
- Mix pastes with the tip of the spatula to incorporate the material first.
- Transfer material to a fresh surface of the pad.
- Refer to the excess mixed material on the pad to monitor setting time.
- Water, saliva, and blood affect polysulfide material.
- Impressions should be removed quickly after setting; do not rock the tray.
- Adhesive to the tray must be thin and dry before impression material is added.
- Wait 20 to 30 minutes before pouring the impression for stress relaxation to occur in the material.
- Some research shows that the sulfur in the powder of latex gloves can affect the setting properties of the impression material.

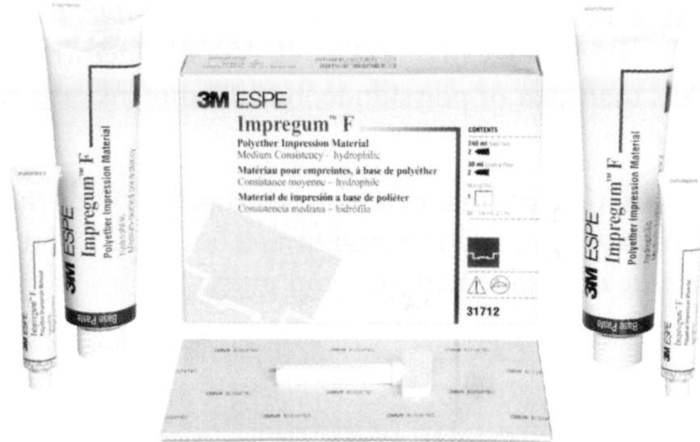


**FIG. 46.14** Impregum F polyether impression material. *(Copyright © 3M 2017. All rights reserved.)*

### Polyether

Polyether impression material provides better mechanical properties than polysulfide and less dimensional change than silicone (Fig. 46.14). Because the set material is quite stiff, a third component called a *thinner* (or body modifier) is included. The thinner is added to the mix to reduce the thickness of the mix and improve the finished impression.

Polyether material is supplied as a two-paste system (the base and the catalyst) and as cartridges. The tubes are *not* the same size; however, when equal lengths are dispensed, the correct amount of each material is delivered.

#### Chemical Makeup and Mixing Guidelines for Polyether Impression Material

**Chemical Makeup**

- Base: polyether
- Cross-linking agent: sulfate
- Catalyst: glycol-based plasticizers
- Filler: silica

**Guidelines for Using Material**

- Excellent impression accuracy and dimensional stability are necessary.
- Material is very stiff, which makes it difficult to remove without rocking.
- When removing the impression, break the seal and rock slightly to prevent tearing.
- Water, saliva, and blood affect the setting process of polyether material.
- Added moisture will increase the impression's marginal discrepancy.
- Increased water absorption occurs if a thinning agent is used.
- Impressions can be dispensed from an automated extruder and mixer.

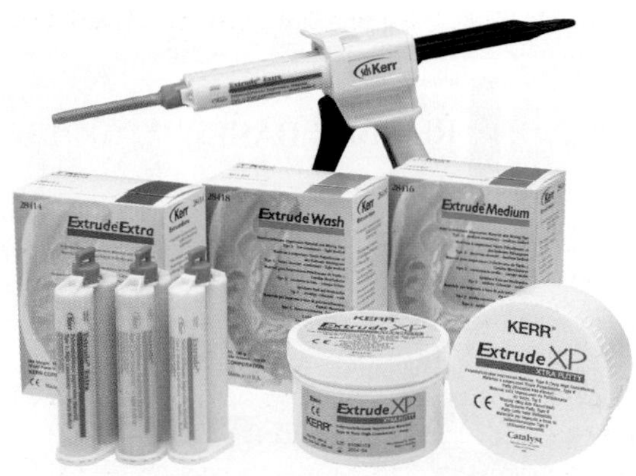


FIG. 46.15 Silicone material. *(Courtesy Kerr Corp., Orange, CA.)*

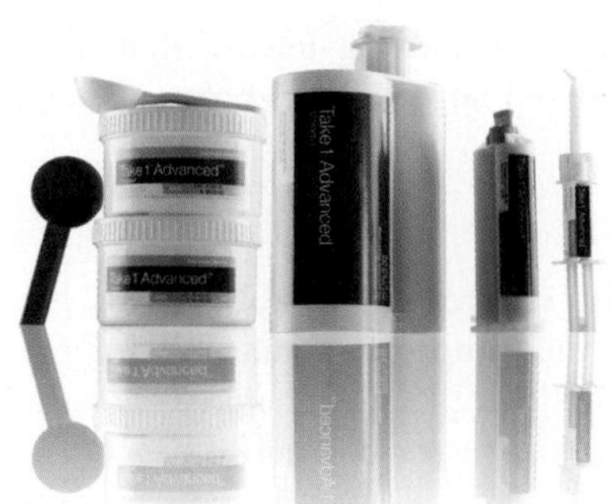


FIG. 46.16 Polysiloxane (polyvinyl siloxane) material. *(Courtesy Kerr Corp., Orange, CA.)*

### *Silicone*

Condensation silicone is a material that is odor-free, nonstaining, and relatively easy to mix (Fig. 46.15). The deformation is much less than that of polysulfide, but the dimensional stability is superior.

Condensation silicone materials are supplied with the base as a paste in a tube, and the catalyst as a liquid in a bottle or a smaller tube of paste, cartridges, and putty.

#### Chemical Makeup and Mixing Guidelines for Silicone Impression Material

**Chemical Makeup**

- Base: polydimethyl siloxane
- Cross-linking agent: alkyl orthosilicate or organo hydrogen siloxane
- Catalyst: organo tin compounds
- Filler: silica

**Guidelines for Using Material**

- The material has a limited shelf life.
- The tray requires a special tray adhesive.
- No syneresis or imbibition occurs, but silicone material does respond with shrinkage over time.
- The material is more flexible, so the chance of distortion during removal is greater.
- Wait 20 to 30 minutes before pouring models for stress relaxation to occur.

### *Polysiloxane*

Polysiloxane (polyvinyl siloxane) materials have high dimensional stability and low tear resistance, making them easy to handle when taking final impressions (Fig. 46.16). The material has no taste or odor, which makes it acceptable to patients.

Polysiloxane impression material is available in light-bodied, regular, and heavy-bodied forms. It is supplied in cartridges and in putty consistencies for single-impression or double-impression techniques.

#### Chemical Makeup and Mixing Guidelines for Polysiloxane Impression Material

**Chemical Makeup**

- Base: silica-based polymers
- Catalyst: chloroplatinic acid
- Filler: silica

**Guidelines for Using Material**

- For dimensional stability, polysiloxane is the best impression material.
- Pouring of the model can be delayed up to 7 to 10 days.
- Stiffness of the material makes removal of the tray difficult.
- Material is dispensed with the use of an automixer and mixing tips.

**15** Is an elastomeric material used for preliminary impressions or final impressions?
**16** In which three ways are elastomeric materials supplied?
**17** What technique is used to place light-bodied material around a prepared tooth?
**18** What impression material will the dentist first apply to a prepared tooth—the heavy-bodied or the light-bodied form?
**19** What system completes the mixing of a final impression material for you?
**20** What is another term for polysulfide?

## Occlusal (Bite) Registration

In addition to having an accurate impression of the prepared teeth, the dentist and the laboratory technician will require a registration of the normal **centric** relationship of the maxillary and mandibular arches (Fig. 46.17). This relationship is recorded as the **occlusal registration**, which is most often referred to as the bite registration. There are several techniques that can be used to obtain the bite registration.

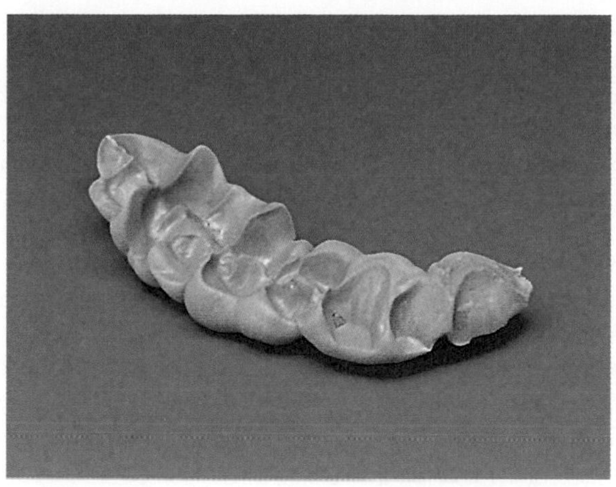

FIG. 46.17 Example of a bite registration using ZOE. *(Copyright © 3M 2017. All rights reserved.)*

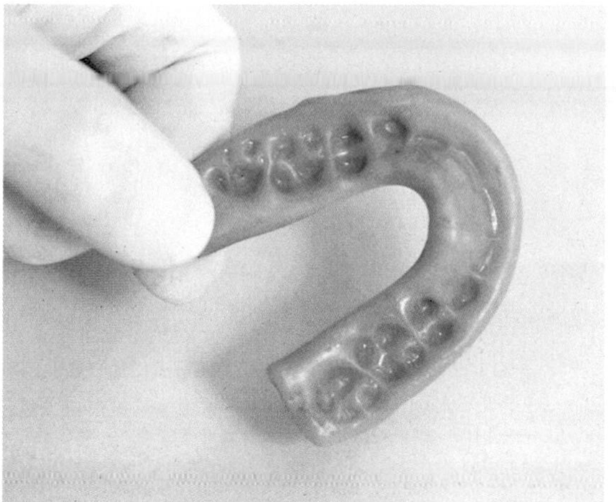

FIG. 46.18 Wax bite registration. *(Copyright © 3M 2017. All rights reserved.)*

## Wax Bite Registration

A wax bite registration is used to show the occlusal relationship of the maxillary and mandibular teeth (Fig. 46.18). It is particularly useful when the diagnostic casts are trimmed. The easiest technique employs a softened baseplate wax.

See Procedure 46.6: Taking a Wax Bite Registration (Expanded Function).

## Polysiloxane Bite Registration Paste

One of the most popular materials used for bite registrations is polysiloxane. The material is supplied as a paste system and in cartridges. Polysiloxane provides the following benefits for the dentist and the laboratory technician:

- The material is fast-setting.
- The paste has no resistance to biting forces.
- The paste has no odor or taste for the patient.
- Polysiloxane material gains dimensional stability over time.
- The material is convenient to use.

See Procedure 46.7: Mixing Polysiloxane Material for a Bite Registration.

## Zinc Oxide–Eugenol Bite Registration Paste

When a more durable material is needed for a bite registration, a zinc oxide–eugenol (ZOE) material may be selected. ZOE paste has little to no resistance to bite closure and is a fast-setting material. The material is supplied in a paste system, which is dispensed onto a paper pad, mixed, and placed onto a gauze tray for the patient to bite into.

See Procedure 46.8: Mixing Zinc Oxide–Eugenol Bite Registration Material.

RECALL

**21** Which type of bite registration material is most popular?

**22** What type of tray is used when ZOE bite registration paste is applied?

**23** Do you cool or warm the wax before placing the tray in the patient's mouth for a bite registration?

**■ Patient Education** As you complete this chapter you should have a clearer understanding of the importance and versatility of impressions in dentistry. It is common to hear patients express anxiety or discomfort when having an impression taken. Patients tend to lose their sense of control when a tray with impression material is placed in their mouth. Also, this procedure can be uncomfortable if patients are not used to breathing through their nose or if they have an oversensitive gag reflex.

Be prepared to explain the impression procedure to your patient. When your confidence and skills are evident, the patient will have a much easier time allowing the dental team to complete this important procedure. ■

**■ Legal and Ethical Implications** The EFDA/RDA is allowed to take preliminary impressions because these impressions are used for procedures that will not permanently alter a patient's dentition. Final impressions, though, are used solely for the making of indirect restorations, partials, dentures, and implants. These types of procedures do alter a patient's dentition and are the full responsibility of the dentist. Always check with your state board regarding your legal qualifications in taking preliminary impressions. ■

**■ Eye to the Future** With advances in biomechanics and computer technology, impression materials soon will be a thing of the past. The use of computers in dentistry is allowing dentists to construct indirect restorations, partial dentures, and implants completely in the dental laboratory within the office. Time and effort instead will be spent on enhancing and increasing patient care, and waiting time for construction of the restoration will be virtually eliminated. ■

**■ Critical Thinking**

1. You are taking a preliminary impression on an 8-year-old girl. While seating the mandibular tray, the child grabs the handle

of the tray and states, "I do not want that in my mouth." You need to take this impression for diagnostic models. Describe techniques you can use with this child to obtain the impression.

2. You have finally convinced your 8-year-old patient to have impressions taken. When seating the maxillary tray, however, she starts to gag. Describe some concepts or techniques you could use to make this procedure a positive experience for the patient.
3. You are assisting in taking a final impression of a patient's mandibular arch, using an automix material. After transferring the syringe material to the dentist, you ready the heavy-bodied material for the tray. While you are preparing the tray, the cartridge runs out of material before the tray is completely filled. What could have prevented this? What should you do now?
4. Your dentist has a habit of "getting behind" with patients. You have worked with this dentist for 12 years, and you know exactly what steps are taken for every procedure. Because he is behind schedule, the dentist asks you to go ahead and take the final impression while he sees the next patient. He notes that by the time you get the tray in, he will be in the room to take the impression out. Do you feel confident in following through? What do you think about this request by the dentist?
5. When you assist the dentist in taking a final impression, you must always obtain a bite registration as well. Explain why the dental laboratory technician needs a reproduction of the opposing arch for designing an indirect restoration. ■

PROCEDURE 46.1 

## Mixing Alginate Impression Material

### EQUIPMENT AND SUPPLIES

- ✓ Alginate
- ✓ Powder measure
- ✓ Water measure
- ✓ Medium-sized rubber bowl
- ✓ Beavertail-shaped wide-blade spatula

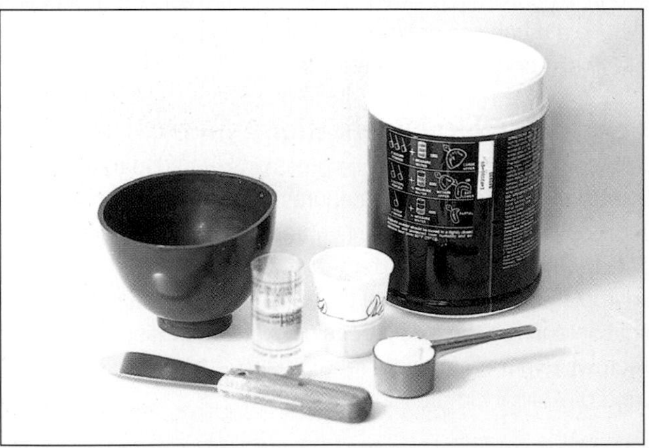

### PROCEDURAL STEPS

1 Place the appropriate amount of water into the bowl.

2 Shake the can of alginate to "fluff" the contents. After fluffing, carefully lift off the lid to prevent the particles from flying into the air.

**PURPOSE** Alginate is fluffed because the material tends to settle and pack down in the can, which can make the measurement inaccurate. When preweighed packages are used, fluffing is not necessary.

3 Sift the needed amount of powder into the water and use the spatula to mix with a stirring action to wet the powder until all has been moistened.

**PURPOSE** *Mixing order is important:* Adding the powder to the water ensures that the powder particles are wet evenly. If mixed in reverse (the water is added to the powder), the chemical reaction will start early with some particles setting faster than others.

4 Firmly spread the alginate between the spatula and the side of the rubber bowl.

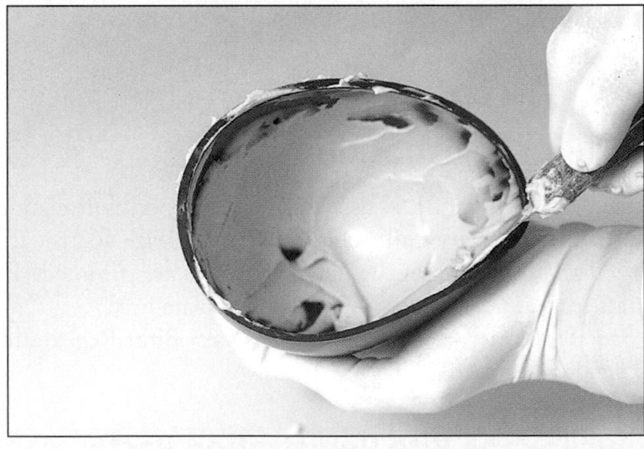

5 Mix with the spatula for the appropriate length of time. The mixture should appear smooth and creamy.

**PURPOSE** Inadequate mixing of alginate causes the mix to contain air bubbles and a grainy texture, which may produce an unsatisfactory impression.

6 Wipe the alginate mix into one mass on the inside edge of the bowl.

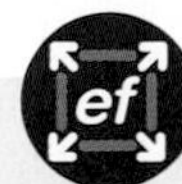

**PROCEDURE 46.2**

# Taking a Mandibular Preliminary Impression (Expanded Function)

## PREREQUISITES FOR PERFORMING THIS PROCEDURE

- ✔ Operator positioning
- ✔ Intraoral instrumentation

## EQUIPMENT AND SUPPLIES

- ✔ Alginate powder
- ✔ Alginate measure scoop (provided by the manufacturer)
- ✔ Water measure (provided by the manufacturer)
- ✔ Room temperature water
- ✔ Rubber bowl
- ✔ Wide-blade spatula
- ✔ Sterile impression trays
- ✔ Tray adhesive (used on nonperforated trays)
- ✔ Utility wax (if tray must be extended)
- ✔ Saliva ejector
- ✔ Precaution (biohazard) bag

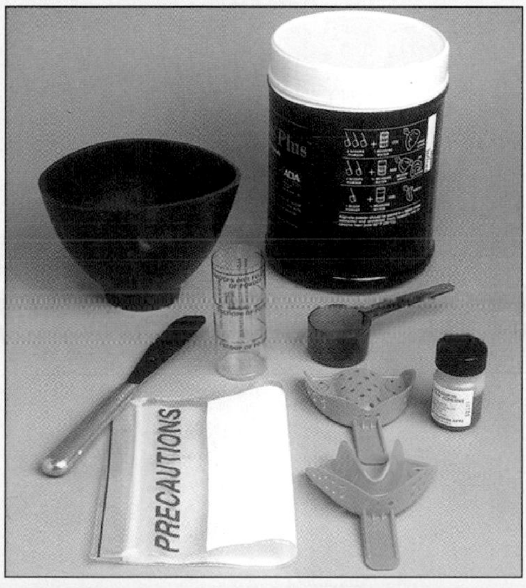


## PROCEDURAL STEPS

### Preparation

1. Gather all necessary supplies.
2. Seat and prepare the patient.
3. Explain the procedure to the patient.
4. Select and prepare the mandibular impression tray.
5. Take two measures of room temperature water with two scoops of alginate. Mix the material as specified in Procedure 46.1.

### Loading the Mandibular Impression Tray

6. Gather half the alginate in the bowl onto the spatula, then wipe alginate into one side of the tray from the lingual side. Quickly press the material down to the base of the tray.
   **PURPOSE** To remove any air bubbles trapped in the tray.

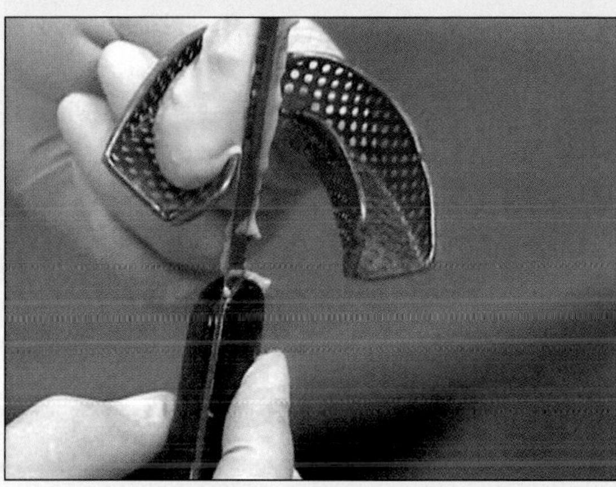

7. Gather the remaining half of the alginate in the bowl onto the spatula; then load the other side of the tray in the same way.
8. Smooth the surface of the alginate by wiping a moistened finger along the surface.

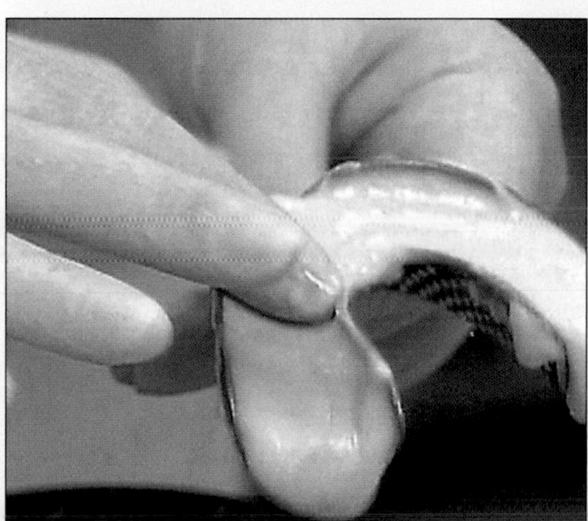

### Seating the Mandibular Impression Tray

9. Place additional material over the occlusal surfaces of the mandibular teeth.
   **PURPOSE** To place extra material in the fissures and interproximal surfaces to create less discrepancy in the anatomy of the impression.
10. Retract the patient's cheek with your index finger.
11. Turn the tray slightly sideways when placing it into the mouth.
12. Center the tray over the teeth.
13. Press down the posterior border of the tray first.
    **PURPOSE** To form a seal.

(Continued)

## PROCEDURE 46.2 Taking a Mandibular Preliminary Impression (Expanded Function)—cont'd

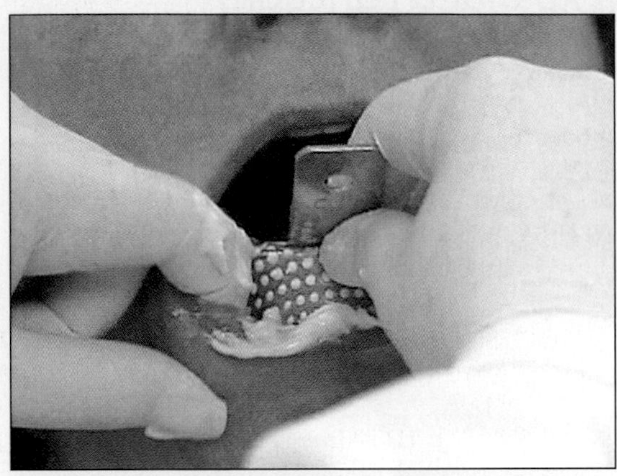

14 Push down the anterior portion of the tray and ask the patient to lift the tongue to the roof of the mouth and then relax it.

**PURPOSE** To allow the alginate to form an impression of the lingual aspect of the alveolar process.

15 Instruct the patient to breathe normally while the tray is in place.

16 Observe the alginate around the tray to determine when the material has set.

**NOTE** When set, the material should not register a dent when pressed with a finger.

### Removing the Mandibular Impression

17 First, place your fingers on the top of the impression tray.

**PURPOSE** To protect the maxillary teeth from damage during removal of the mandibular tray.

18 Gently break the seal between the impression and the peripheral tissues by moving the inside of the patient's cheeks or lips with your finger.

19 Grasping the handle of the tray with your thumb and index finger, use a firm lifting motion to break the seal.

20 Snap up the tray and impression from the dentition.

21 Have the patient rinse with water to remove any excess alginate material.

22 Evaluate the impression for accuracy.

23 Rinse, disinfect, wrap in a slightly moistened towel, and place the impression in the appropriate precaution bag.

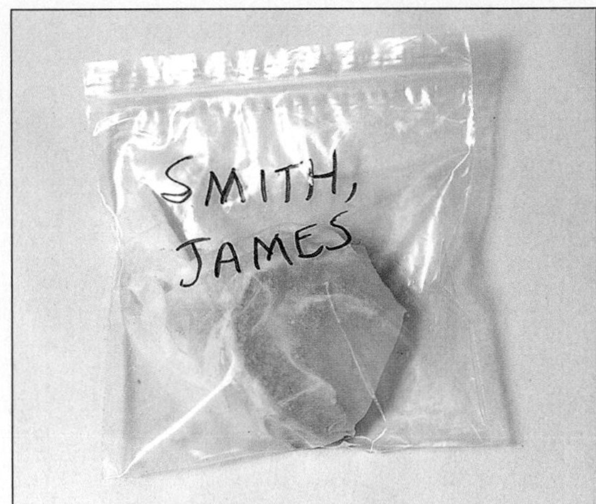


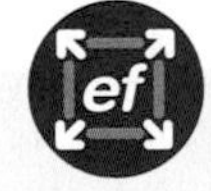

## PROCEDURE 46.3

# Taking a Maxillary Preliminary Impression (Expanded Function)

### PREREQUISITES FOR PERFORMING THIS PROCEDURE

- ✔ Operator positioning
- ✔ Intraoral instrumentation

### EQUIPMENT AND SUPPLIES

- ✔ Maxillary tray

Other equipment and supplies are the same as for a mandibular impression (see Procedure 46.2). If the same bowl and spatula are being reused, make certain they are clean and dry before beginning the next mix. For a maxillary impression, 3 measures of water are mixed with 3 scoops of powder.

### PROCEDURAL STEPS

#### Preparation

The preparation of the material is the same as in Procedure 46.2.

#### Loading the Maxillary Impression Tray

1 Load the maxillary tray in one large increment, using a wiping motion to fill the tray from the posterior end.

**PURPOSE** To help prevent the formation of air bubbles in the material.

## PROCEDURE 46.3 Taking a Maxillary Preliminary Impression (Expanded Function)—cont'd

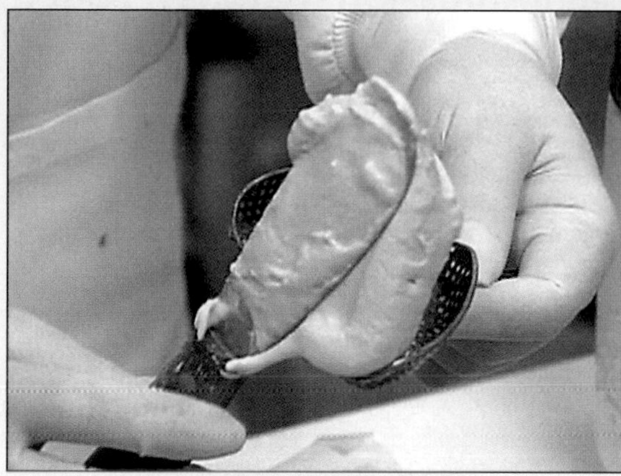

2 Place the bulk of the material toward the anterior palatal area of the tray.

**PURPOSE** To prevent the alginate from flowing beyond the tray and into the throat during tray placement.

3 Moisten fingertips with tap water and smooth the surface of the alginate.

### Seating the Maxillary Impression Tray

4 Use your index finger to retract the patient's cheek.

5 Turn the tray slightly sideways to position the tray in the mouth.

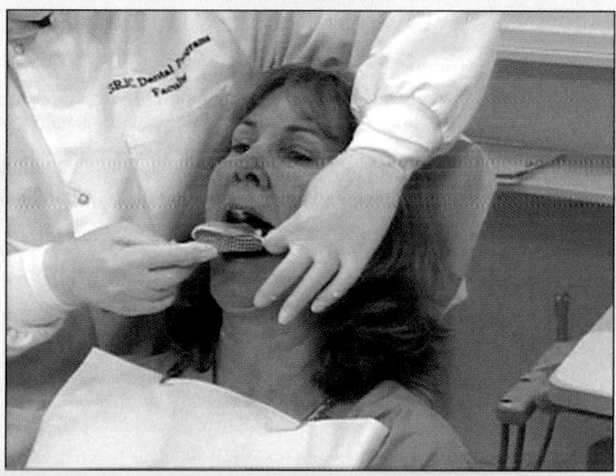

6 Center the tray over the patient's teeth.

7 Seat the posterior border (back) of the tray up against the posterior border of the hard palate to form a seal.

**PURPOSE** To prevent excess material from going toward the back of the mouth.

8 Direct the anterior portion of the tray upward over the teeth.

9 Gently lift the patient's lips out of the way as the tray is seated.

**PURPOSE** This retraction allows the material to flow into the vestibular areas.

10 Check the posterior border of the tray to ensure that no material is flowing into the patient's throat. If necessary, wipe excess material away with a cotton-tip applicator.

**PURPOSE** This technique helps prevent triggering of the gag reflex when the material touches the soft palate area.

11 Hold the tray firmly in place while the alginate sets.

### Removing the Maxillary Impression

12 To avoid injury to the impression and the patient's teeth, place a finger along the lateral borders of the tray to push down and break the palatal seal.

13 Use a straight, downward snapping motion to remove the tray from the teeth.

14 Instruct the patient to rinse with water to remove any excess alginate impression material.

### Caring for Alginate Impressions

15 Gently rinse the impressions under cold tap water to remove any blood or saliva.

**PURPOSE** Bioburden will interfere with the setting of gypsum products.

16 Spray the impression with an approved disinfectant.

17 If the impression must be stored before pouring, wrap it in a damp paper towel and store the impression in a covered container or a plastic bag labeled with the patient's name.

### Before Dismissing the Patient

18 Examine the patient's mouth for any remaining fragments of alginate and remove them using an explorer and dental floss.

19 Use a moist facial tissue to remove any alginate from the patient's face and lips.

## PROCEDURE 46.4

## Mixing a Two-Paste Final Impression Material

### EQUIPMENT AND SUPPLIES

- Stock or custom tray with appropriate adhesive
- Large, stiff, tapered spatulas (2)
- Large paper pads (2)
- Light-bodied base and catalyst
- Heavy-bodied base and catalyst
- Impression syringe with sterile tip
- 2 × 2–inch gauze pads

### PROCEDURAL STEPS

### Preparing Light-Bodied Syringe Material

1 Dispense approximately to 2 inches of equal lengths of the base and catalyst of the light-bodied material onto the top third of the pad, making sure that the materials are not too close to each other.

**PURPOSE** Some paste materials tend to start spreading on the pad, and it is important to prevent a premature reaction.

**(Continued)**

## PROCEDURE 46.4 Mixing a Two-Paste Final Impression Material—cont'd

2 Wipe the tube openings clean with gauze; recap immediately.
**PURPOSE** Cleaning the top of the tube and the threads prevents the cap from becoming messy and sticking.

3 Using the spatula, pick up the catalyst mixing it into the base; then mix in a swirling direction for approximately 5 seconds.

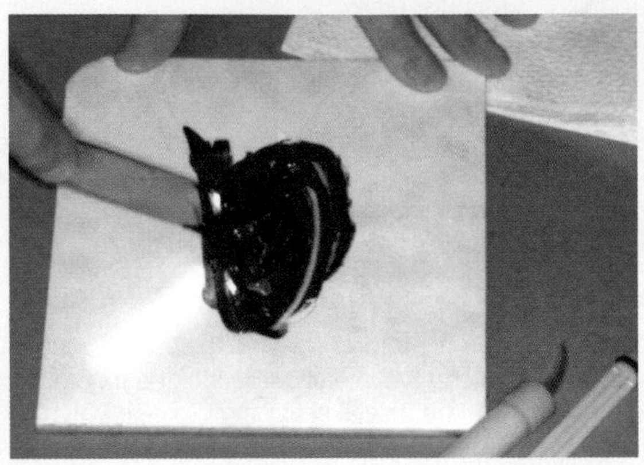

4 Gather the material onto the flat portion of the spatula. Place it on a clean area of the pad, preferably the center.
**PURPOSE** By beginning the mix on a clean area of the pad, you will obtain a more homogeneous mix.

5 Spatulate smoothly, wiping back and forth and trying to use only one side of the spatula during the mixing process.
**PURPOSE** Material is lost when both sides of the blade are used.

6 To obtain a more homogeneous mix, pick the material up by the spatula blade and wipe it onto the pad.
**PURPOSE** To pull the material from the bottom to the top of the mix.

7 Gather the material together and take your syringe tube and begin "cookie cutting" the material into the syringe. Insert the plunger and express a small amount of the material to make sure it is in working order.

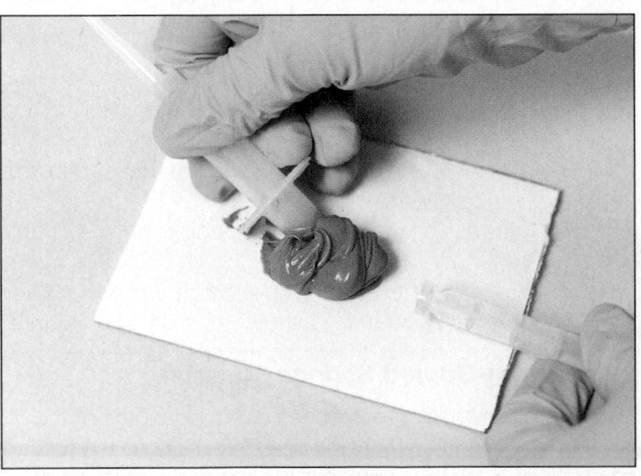

8 Transfer the syringe to the dentist, making sure the tip of the syringe is directed toward the tooth.

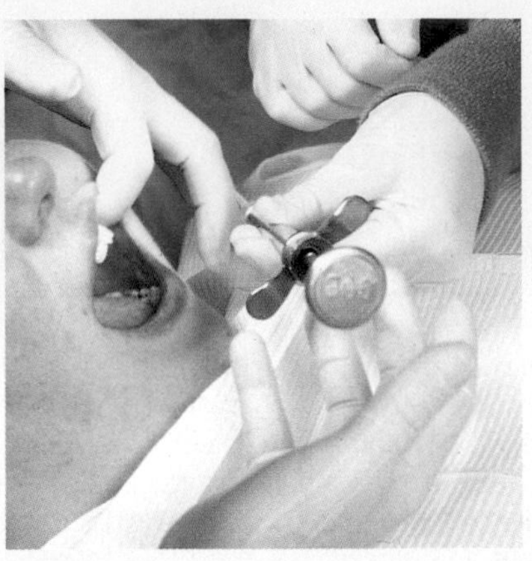

### Preparing Heavy-Bodied Tray Material

1 Dispense approximately 3 to 4 inches of equal lengths of the base and the catalyst of the heavy-bodied material on the top third of the pad for a quadrant tray.
**NOTE** The amount of material placed depends on whether you are using a quadrant tray or a full-arch tray.

2 Place the tip of the spatula blade into the catalyst and base; then mix in a swirling direction for approximately 5 seconds.

3 Gather the material onto the flat portion of the spatula and place it on a clean area of the pad, preferably the center.
**PURPOSE** Starting the mix on a clean area of the pad results in a more homogeneous mix.

4 Spatulate smoothly, wiping back and forth and trying to use only one side of the spatula during the mixing process.
**PURPOSE** Material is lost when both sides of the blade are used.

5 To get a more homogeneous mix, pick the material up by the spatula blade and wipe it on the pad.
**PURPOSE** To pull the material from the bottom to the top of the mix.

6 Gather the bulk of the material with the spatula and load it into the tray. The best way to do this without incorporating air is to use the flat side of the spatula and follow around the outside rim of the tray, while "wiping" the material into the tray.

7 Using the tip of the spatula, spread the material evenly from one end of the tray to the other without picking up the material.
**PURPOSE** When you pull the material in an upward direction, you are incorporating air into the mixture.

8 Retrieve the syringe from the dentist and transfer the tray, making sure the dentist is able to grasp the handle of the tray properly.

Photo for Step 3 of preparing light-bodied syringe material from Rosenstiel SF, Land MF, Fujimoto J: Contemporary fixed prosthodontics, ed 5, St Louis, 2016, Elsevier.

PROCEDURE 46.5

# Preparing an Automix Final Impression Material

## EQUIPMENT AND SUPPLIES

- Stock or custom tray with appropriate adhesive
- Extruder units (2)
- Extruder mixing tips (2)
- Light-bodied mixing tip
- Cartridge of light-bodied material
- Cartridge of heavy-bodied material
- 2 × 2–inch gauze pads

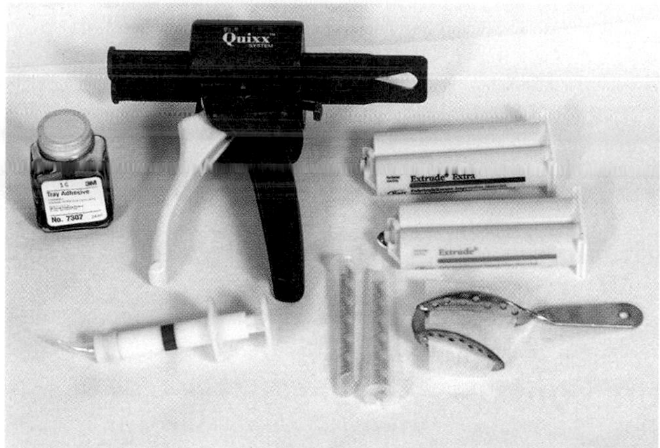


*From Hatrick CD, Eakle WS: Dental materials: clinical applications for dental assistants and dental hygienists, ed 3, St Louis, 2016, Elsevier.*

## PROCEDURAL STEPS

1 Load the extruder with dual cartridges of the base and the catalyst of light-bodied material.

2 Remove the caps from the tubes and extrude (force or push out) a small amount of unmixed material onto the gauze pad.

**PURPOSE** To ensure that no air bubbles are in the mix and to remove any hardened material that might remain.

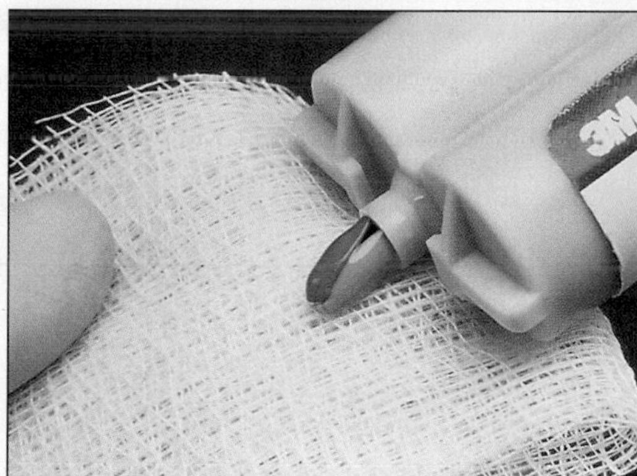




3 Attach a mixing tip on the extruder, along with a syringe tip for light-bodied application by the dentist.

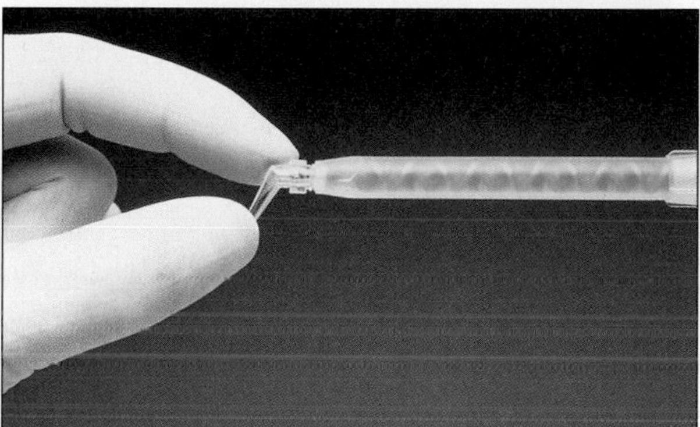



4 When the dentist signals readiness, begin squeezing the trigger until the material has reached the tip.

5 Transfer the extruder to the dentist, making sure that the tip is directed toward the area of the impression.

6 The dentist places the light-bodied material over and around the prepared teeth and onto the surrounding tissues.

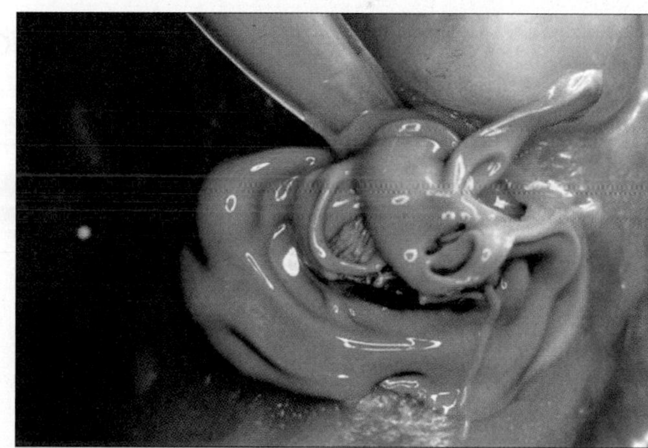

7 Place the heavy-bodied cartridges into the extruder, making sure to express a small amount (same as with the light-bodied material). Attach the mixing tip to the cartridge.

8 At the dentist's "okay," begin squeezing the trigger, thus mixing the heavy-bodied material.

9 Load the impression tray with heavy-bodied material, making sure not to trap air within the material.

**NOTE** Begin expressing the material at one end of the tray and follow through to the other end without taking the tip out of the material.

10 Transfer the tray, making sure the dentist is able to grasp the handle of the tray.

11 When the impression materials have reached final set, the impression is removed and inspected for accuracy by the dentist.

**(Continued)**

## PROCEDURE 46.5 Preparing an Automix Final Impression Material–cont'd

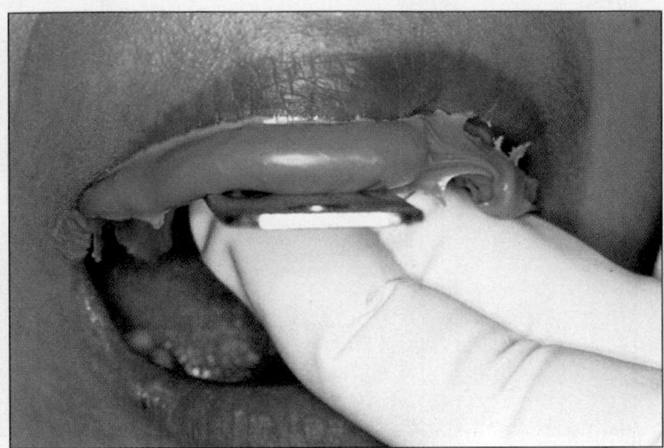



12 The impression is disinfected, placed in a precaution bag, labeled with the patient's name, and taken to the laboratory.

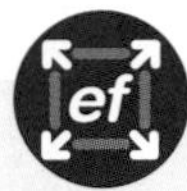

## PROCEDURE 46.6

# Taking a Wax Bite Registration (Expanded Function)

### PREREQUISITES FOR PERFORMING THIS PROCEDURE

- ✔ Operator positioning
- ✔ Identification of cavity classifications and oral anatomy
- ✔ Intraoral instrumentation

### EQUIPMENT AND SUPPLIES

- ✔ Baseplate wax
- ✔ Laboratory knife
- ✔ Heat source (warm water, Bunsen burner, or torch)

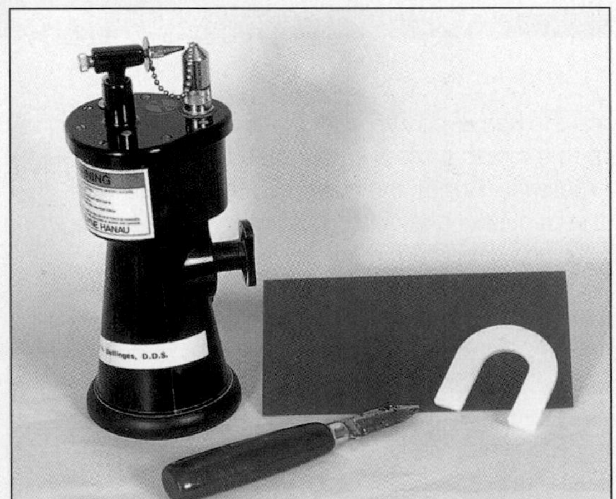

### PROCEDURAL STEPS

1 Explain the procedure to the patient. Reassure the patient that the wax placed will be warm, not hot.

2 Have the patient practice opening and closing the mouth normally.

**PURPOSE** To ensure that the correct position will be recorded in the wax. When the wax is in place, the patient may close the teeth together instead of biting directly into the wax, resulting in an inaccurate bite registration.

3 Place the wax over the biting surfaces of the teeth and check the length. If the wax extends so far beyond the last tooth that the patient is uncomfortable, remove the wax from the patient's mouth. Use the laboratory knife to shorten the length of the wax.

4 Use a heat source to soften the wax.

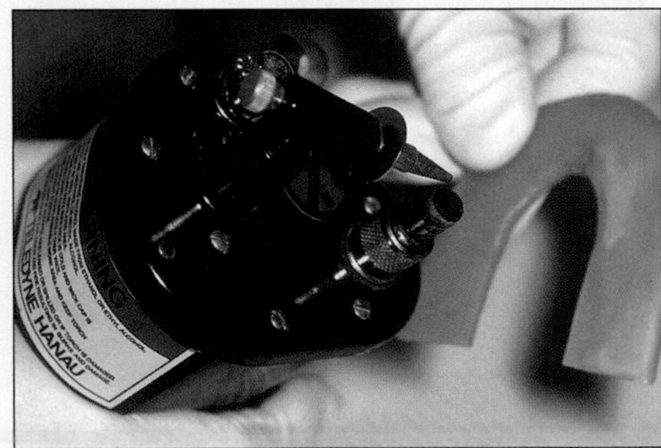

5 Place the softened wax against the biting surfaces of the teeth.

6 Instruct the patient to bite gently and naturally into the wax.

# PROCEDURE 46.6 Taking a Wax Bite Registration (Expanded Function)—cont'd

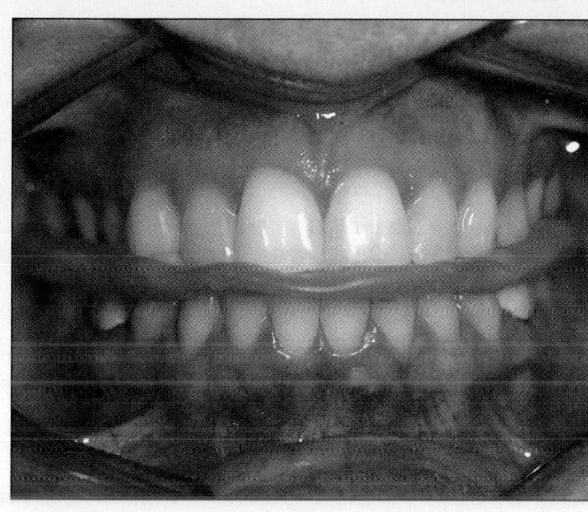

7 Allow the wax to cool.

**NOTE** The wax will cool quickly and may be removed from the mouth in 1 to 2 minutes.

8 Remove the wax bite registration carefully to avoid distortion.

9 Write the patient's name on a piece of paper and keep it with the wax bite registration.

10 Store the wax bite registration with the impressions or casts until it is needed during trimming of the casts.

# PROCEDURE 46.7

## Mixing Polysiloxane Material for a Bite Registration

### EQUIPMENT AND SUPPLIES

- ✓ Extruder unit
- ✓ Cartridge of bite registration material (base and catalyst)
- ✓ Mixing tip
- ✓ Tray

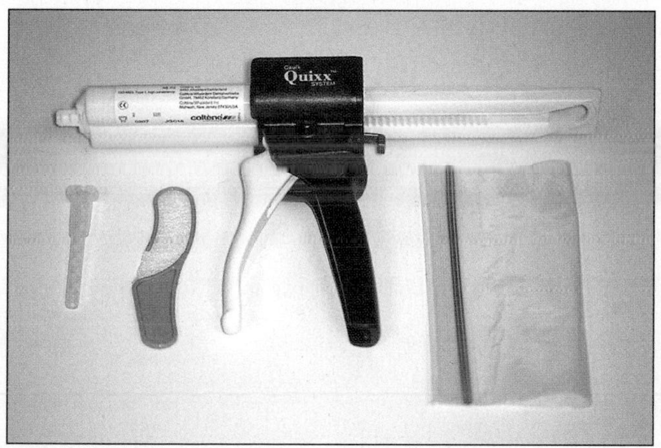


### PROCEDURAL STEPS

1 Mix the material and dispense it with an extruder.

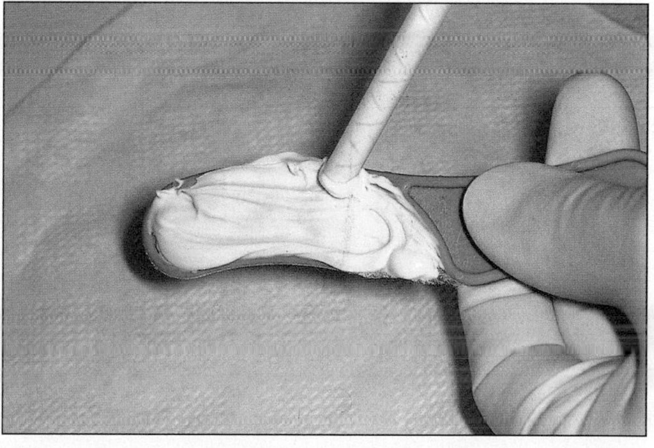

2 Extrude the material directly onto the tray, making sure to fill both sides of the tray.

3 Instruct the patient to close in proper occlusion.

4 After the material has set (about 1 minute), remove the impression and check it for accuracy.

5 Rinse, disinfect, and dry the impression; then send it to the laboratory with the written prescription and with other impressions.

Photos in this procedure from Hatrick CD, Eakle WS, Bird WF: Dental materials: clinical applications for dental assistants and dental hygienists, ed 3, St Louis, 2016, Saunders.

PROCEDURE 46.8

# Mixing Zinc Oxide–Eugenol Bite Registration Material

## EQUIPMENT AND SUPPLIES

- ✔ ZOE bite registration material (base and catalyst)
- ✔ Mixing pad
- ✔ Heavy spatula
- ✔ Bite tray
- ✔ 2 × 2–inch gauze pads

## PROCEDURAL STEPS

1. Dispense 1 to 2 inches of base and catalyst paste onto the pad.
2. Mix the material thoroughly for 45 seconds.
3. Gather half the material on the spatula; then wipe the material onto one side of the gauze tray. Gather the remaining half and wipe onto the other side of the tray.

   **PURPOSE** It is important to have material on both sides of the tray to ensure that you have the patient's bite from the maxillary and mandibular arches.
4. Place the tray in the patient's mouth over the desired areas and have the patient bite down. The material should set within 1 minute.
5. Have the patient open the mouth; then remove the tray.
6. Rinse, dry, and disinfect the bite registration. Send it to the laboratory with the written prescription and with other impressions.

47

# Laboratory Materials and Procedures

## KEY TERMS

**Anatomic (an-uh-TOM-ik) portion** The structural portion of a dental model created from the alginate impression.

**Articulator (ar-TIK-yoo-lay-tur)** Dental laboratory device that simulates mandibular and temporomandibular joint movement when models of the dental arches are attached to it.

**Crystallization (kris-tul-i-ZAY-shun)** Chemical process in which crystals form a structure.

**Die** An accurate replica of the prepared portion of a tooth used in the laboratory during the fabrication of a cast restoration.

**Dihydrate (dye-HYE-drayt)** Related to gypsum products and indicating two parts of water to one part of calcium sulfate.

**Dimensionally (di-MEN-shun-uh-lee) stable** Resistant to changes in width, height, and length.

**Face bow** Portion of articulator used to measure the upper teeth compared with the temporomandibular joint.

**Gypsum (JIP-sum)** Mineral used in the formation of plaster of Paris and stone.

**Hemihydrate (hem-ee-HYE-drayt)** Removal of water to become one-half part water to one part of calcium sulfate, forming the powder product of gypsum.

**Homogenous (hoe-MOJ-uh-nus), homogeneous (hoe-moe-JEE-nee-us)** Having a uniform quality and consistency throughout.

**Lathe (layth)** Machine used for cutting or polishing dental appliances.

**Model** Replica of the maxillary and mandibular arches made from an impression.

**Monomer (MON-oe-mur)** A molecule that, when combined with other molecules, forms a polymer.

**Polymer (POL-i-mur)** Compound of many molecules.

**Slurry (SLUR-ee)** Mixture of gypsum and water used in the finishing of models.

**Volatile (VOL-uh-til)** Substance that can evaporate easily and is very explosive.

## LEARNING OUTCOMES

*On completion of this chapter, the student will be able to achieve the following objectives:*

1. Pronounce, define, and spell the key terms.
2. Discuss the safety precautions that should be taken in the dental laboratory.
3. List the types of equipment found in a dental laboratory and describe their uses.
4. Discuss dental models, including the following:
   - Explain the role of dental models in dentistry.
   - Discuss gypsum products and their role in the making of dental models.
   - Name the three methods of pouring dental models.
5. List the three types of custom impression trays and describe their use in dentistry.
6. Identify the types of dental waxes and describe their use in dentistry.

## PERFORMANCE OUTCOMES

*On completion of this chapter, the student will be able to achieve competency standards in the following skills:*

- Take a face-bow registration.
- Mix dental plaster.
- Pour a set of dental models using the inverted-pour method.
- Trim and finish a set of dental models.
- Construct an acrylic resin custom tray.
- Construct a light-cured custom tray.
- Construct a vacuum-formed custom tray.

## ELECTRONIC RESOURCES

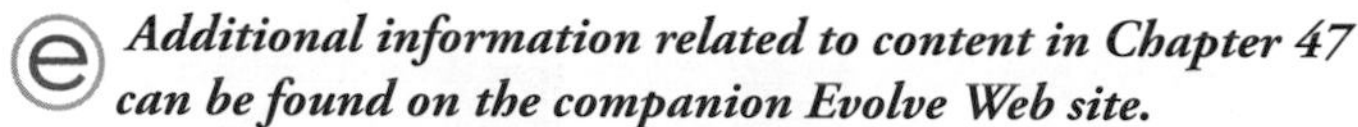

***Additional information related to content in Chapter 47 can be found on the companion Evolve Web site.***

- Practice Quiz
- Videos: Constructing a Vacuum-Formed Tray; Pouring Models Using the Inverted-Pour Method

The dental laboratory is a separate area of the dental office (away from the patient treatment area) where the dentist and the clinical staff complete the following procedures:

- Pour up preliminary impressions
- Trim and finish diagnostic models
- Prepare custom trays
- Polish provisional, partial or full dentures, and indirect restorations

Specialty practices, such as fixed and removable prosthodontics, orthodontics, and pediatrics, will have a more extensive laboratory because of higher demands of laboratory work to be completed. By having laboratory equipment available within a dental practice, the dentist and dental assistant are able to handle case work without having to send it out to a private dental laboratory, which keeps overhead costs to a minimum. If a case cannot be handled in the laboratory, it will be sent to a commercial dental laboratory (Fig. 47.1).

# Safety in the Dental Laboratory

When working in the laboratory, you must make safety your first concern. It is essential to follow safety precautions and infection control procedures. Remember, items brought into the laboratory from the treatment room area are contaminated, and exposure control is just as important here as when you are with the patient.

## Laboratory Rules

- No eating, drinking, or smoking is permitted.
- Keep all cosmetics away from the area.
- Wear personal protective equipment (PPE) when working in the laboratory.
- Keep hair pulled back.
- Report all accidents to the dentist immediately.
- Follow the manufacturer's instructions for equipment operation.
- Clean the work area before and after every procedure.

## Physical Safety

When working around electrical equipment or items that produce high heat, you must become familiar with the location of the fire extinguisher and with fire escape routes. Keep all equipment in good working order, and always follow the manufacturer's directions when handling equipment.

## Chemical Safety

Dental materials in the laboratory area may include corrosive, toxic, or carcinogenic substances. Take care when handling and using these materials, and take special precautions to avoid coming in direct contact with chemicals that could be inhaled, absorbed, or ingested. (See Chapter 23 on exposure to and protection from hazardous chemicals.)

## Biohazards

Biohazards are associated with the treatment area and the sterilization center. However, impressions and other items brought into the laboratory can harbor blood and saliva that can be infectious. The laboratory area and contaminated items must be disinfected before and after each use when biohazards are a concern.

RECALL

1. Where would the dental laboratory be located in a dental office?
2. What specialty practices might have a more extensive laboratory setup?
3. What would be an example of a contaminated item that would be brought into the dental laboratory?

# Dental Laboratory Equipment

The dental laboratory is equipped with a countertop and cabinets to provide adequate work areas and safe storage for supplies and equipment used in the laboratory (Fig. 47.2).

Wall-mounted bins are used to store bulk supplies of plaster, stone, and investment materials. These bins protect materials from moisture contamination and make it easy to remove gypsum products as needed. After the material has been retrieved, the cover should immediately be placed back on the bin.

Work pans are open plastic containers with identification labels used to hold the laboratory work in progress for an individual patient. Pans may be color-coded to indicate the type of procedure to be performed.

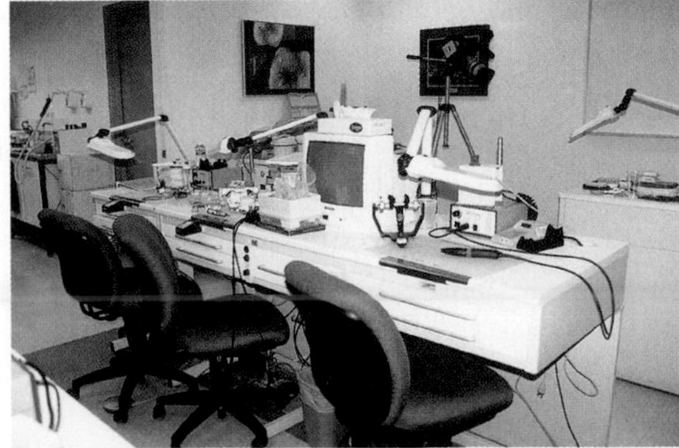

**FIG. 47.1** Commercial dental laboratory.

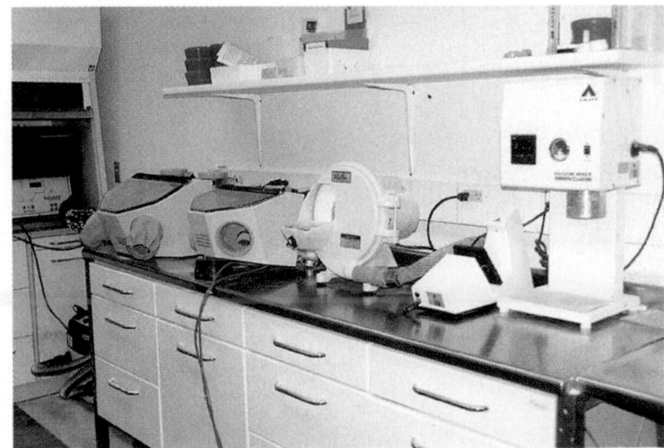

**FIG. 47.2** Dental laboratory within a dental office.

## Heat Sources

A heat source is required in the laboratory to heat wax or other materials. A **propane** or **butane** torch is used for this purpose. If a gas line has been installed in the laboratory, rubber hosing will be attached to a **Bunsen burner** and then to the gas outlet. Remember to turn the handle completely *on* or completely *off.* Otherwise, gas can escape, thereby creating a dangerous environment.

## Model Trimmer

The model trimmer is a machine used to trim stone or plaster models (Fig. 47.3). The model trimmer has an abrasive grinding wheel used to grind away excess plaster or stone. This wheel works more effectively if it is kept clean, which prevents stone or plaster from building up. Models are placed on the work surface and are held in place by firm pressure with the hands or with a holding device that can be attached.

To control the dust level from the cast and to facilitate cutting, a gentle stream of water continuously runs on the wheel when in use. Used water drains directly into a sink equipped with a plaster trap that catches the grindings and prevents the drain from clogging.

## Vacuum Former

A vacuum former is a small electrical appliance used to construct custom trays for bleaching, mouth guards, and positioners for orthodontics (Fig. 47.4). The upper part of the unit is a heating element that warms and softens a sheet of thermoplastic resin. The work surface has holes that allow the vacuum to pull and shape the warmed plastic around the model.

## Vibrator

A vibrator is used to remove air from the mix of plaster or stone and to aid in the flow of material when a diagnostic model is poured up (Fig. 47.5). The vibrator has a flat working surface that vibrates the bowl or tray. To help keep the vibrator clean, a disposable cover can be placed on the work surface before it is used. After use, this cover is discarded.

## Laboratory Handpiece

A low-speed laboratory handpiece is used for many tasks, such as trimming custom impression trays, adjusting dentures, and polishing provisional and indirect restorations. The laboratory handpiece and burs are discussed further in Chapter 35.

## Sandblaster

A sandblaster is a handheld unit that sprays sand at a high rate of speed, creating an etching or pitting on a surface area of metals, porcelain, or acrylic (Fig. 47.6). These elevations in the surface area create added retention through surface roughening. Sandblasting is suitable for the repair of crowns, dentures, and appliances, as well as for the cementation of crowns, bridges, and inlays.

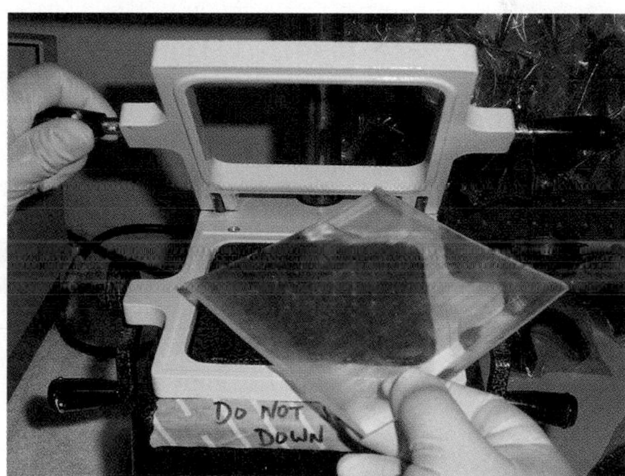


**FIG. 47.4** Vacuum former. *(Courtesy Gwen Essex, UCSF School of Dentistry.)*

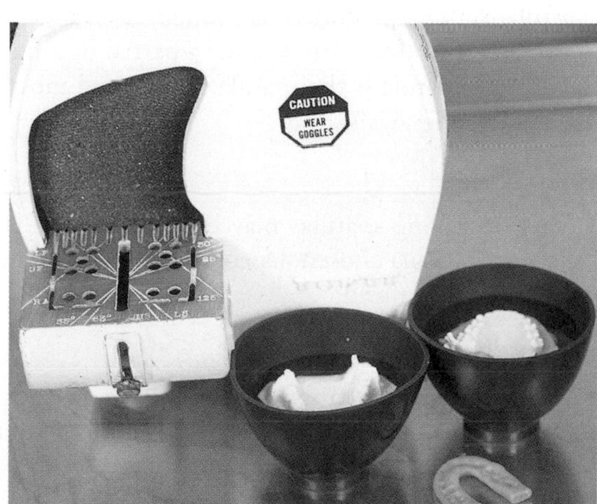


**FIG. 47.3** Model trimmer.

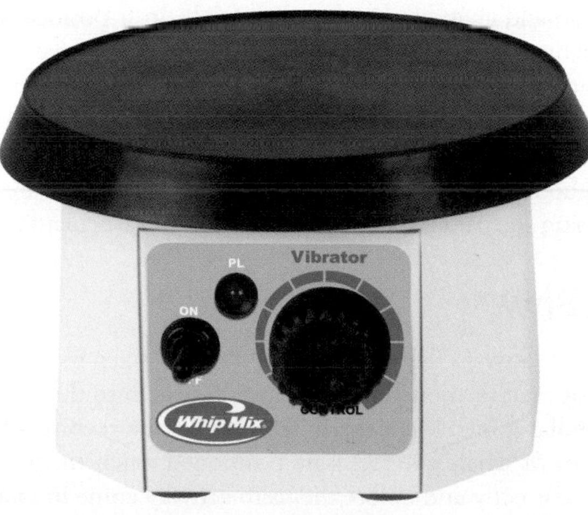


**FIG. 47.5** Vibrator. *(Courtesy Whip Mix Corp., Louisville, KY.)*

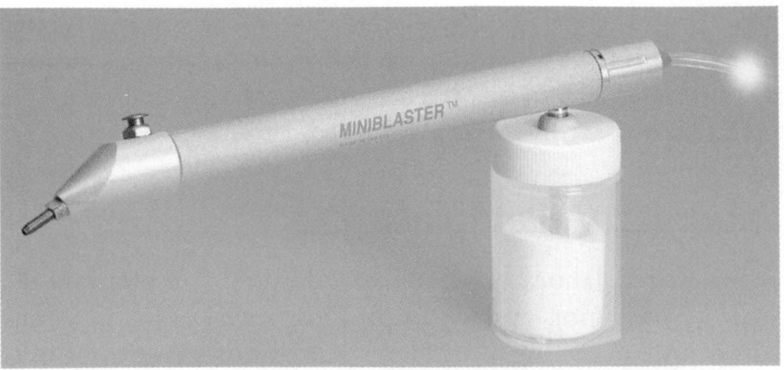


FIG. 47.6 Sandblaster. *(Courtesy Johnson-Promident, Valley Cottage, NY.)*

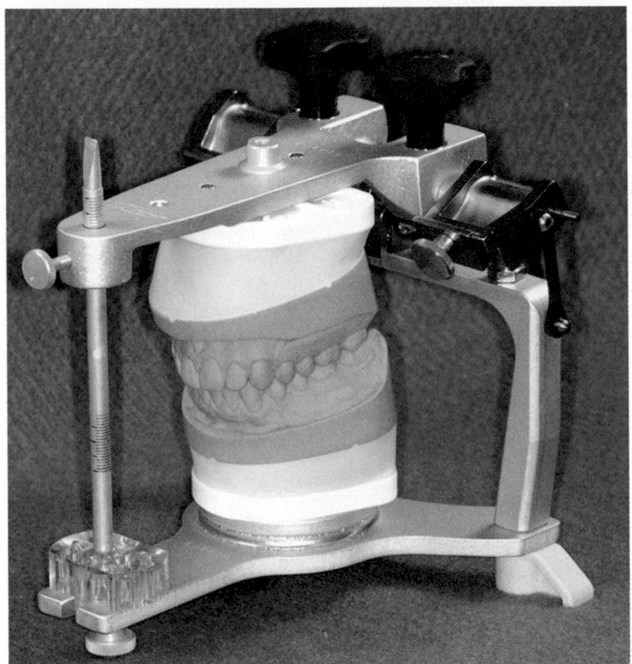

FIG. 47.7 Articulator. *(Courtesy Whip Mix Corp., Louisville, KY.)*

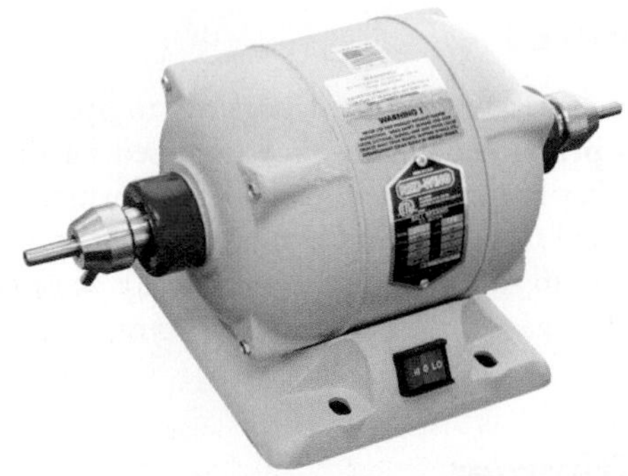

FIG. 47.8 Dental lathe. *(Courtesy Handler Red Wing Int'l., Westfield, NJ.)*

## Articulator

An **articulator** is a mechanical device used in dentistry to hold maxillary and mandibular dental **models** in a position to aid in reproduction of the mandible in relation to the maxilla. The articulator allows the dentist and the dental laboratory technician to fabricate removable prosthodontic appliances (dentures), fixed prosthodontic restorations (crowns, bridges, inlays, and onlays), and orthodontic appliances (Fig. 47.7). Special records are taken to position the dental models accurately on the articulator.

## Face Bow

The **face bow** is the first step the dentist takes to determine the positional relationship of the maxillary arch to the temporomandibular joints. The **centric relation** or **bite record** is a measurement of where the teeth are positioned when the joints are aligned correctly and before the teeth actually come in contact.

In some states, it is legal for the expanded-function dental assistant (EFDA)/registered dental assistant (RDA) to perform the technique for taking a face-bow registration.

See Procedure 47.1: Taking a Face-Bow Registration (Expanded Function).

## Dental Lathe

The dental **lathe** is used to polish or trim custom trays, provisionals, dentures, and indirect restorations. The lathe is designed with a protective plastic see-through shield that is brought down over the work area. The lathe has revolving threaded extensions from each end of the motor. Attachments such as an abrasive grinding wheel or a rag wheel are placed on these extensions. After each use, these attachments must be sterilized before reuse (Fig. 47.8).

**Pumice** and other polishing agents are used during polishing. A protective pan behind and under the wheel is used to hold the pumice and catch the spatter.

## Specialized Spatulas and Bowls

A few specialized instruments are used frequently in the dental laboratory. As with any instruments, these must be sterilized and stored properly after each use.

### Wax Spatulas

A wax spatula is a double-ended instrument used in waxing a pattern, or when working with wax for a partial or a full denture. The #7 wax spatula is the spatula that is used most often in the laboratory (Fig. 47.9).

### Mixing Spatulas

Several types of mixing spatulas may be found in the laboratory. The type of spatula chosen depends on the strength of the dental material being mixed.

### Rubber Bowls

Rubber bowls are used for mixing of alginate in the treatment area and for mixing of stone or plaster in the laboratory setting. Make sure to have an adequate supply of rubber bowls in the office (Fig. 47.10).

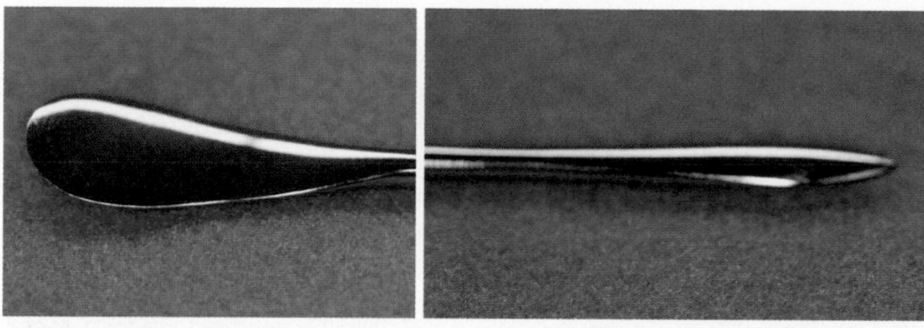

**FIG. 47.9** Number 7 Wax spatula. *(From Rosenstiel SF, Land MF, Fujimoto J: Contemporary fixed prosthodontics, ed 5, St Louis, 2016, Elsevier.)*

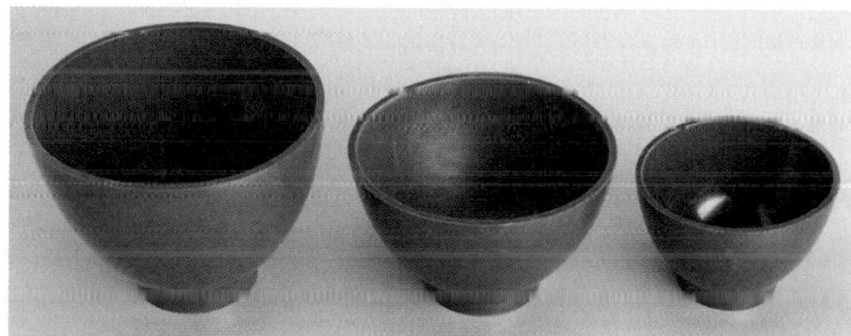

**FIG. 47.10** Different sizes of rubber flexible bowls. *(From Boyd LB: Dental instruments: a pocket guide, ed 6, St Louis, 2018, Elsevier.)*

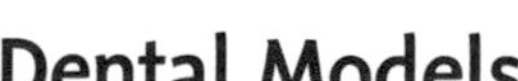


4 What piece of equipment is used to grind away plaster or stone?
5 What piece of equipment does the dentist use to determine centric relation on a diagnostic model?
6 What is the most common wax spatula size used in the laboratory?

## Dental Models

Dental models, also referred to as **study casts,** are a three-dimensional reproduction of the teeth and surrounding soft tissues of the patient's maxillary and mandibular arches (Fig. 47.11). A model is created by using an alginate impression. The alginate impression is taken to the laboratory and then is poured into a gypsum product to create the completed model.

Because these models show a three-dimensional view of conditions, they are a valuable diagnostic tool. The dentist can use these models to analyze the patient's mouth from viewpoints that are impossible to evaluate from the clinical examination. Dental models are used for the following procedures in dentistry:

- Diagnosis for planning a fixed or removable prosthetic device
- Diagnosis of orthodontic treatment
- Visual presentation of dental treatment
- Production of custom trays
- Creation of orthodontic appliances
- Making of provisional coverage
- Making of mouth guards

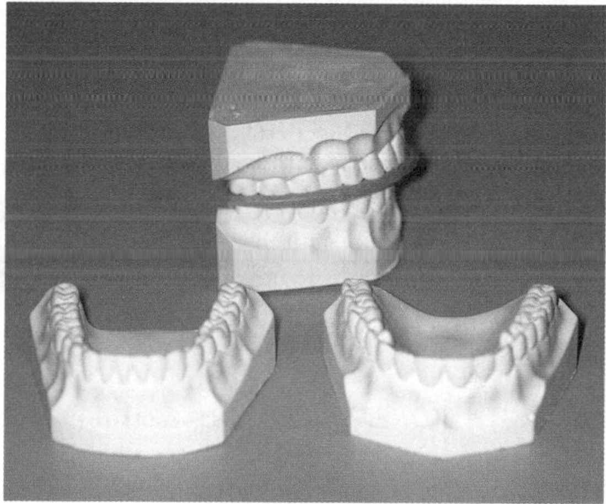

**FIG. 47.11** Dental models.

## Gypsum Products

**Gypsum** products are used extensively in dentistry to make dental models. Many characteristics and properties affect the use of gypsum.

### Chemical Properties

Gypsum is a mineral mined from the earth. In its unrefined state, gypsum is the **dihydrate** form of calcium sulfate, which means it consists of 2 parts water to every 1 part calcium sulfate. When gypsum is heated during the manufacturing process, the water is removed, and the gypsum is converted into a powdered **hemihydrate**, which consists of ½ part water to 1 part calcium sulfate.

### Setting Reactions

When you mix gypsum powder with water, the hemihydrate crystals dissolve in the water to form clusters known as the **nuclei of crystallization.** These nuclei are so close together that as the gypsum crystals expand during the setting process, they intermesh and become entangled with each other. As more intermeshing of crystals occurs, the strength, rigidity, and hardness of the final product is increased.

### Forms

Three forms of gypsum products are used in pouring up study models: *model plaster, dental stone,* and *high-strength stone.* All three of these forms consist of hemihydrate crystals. The only differences between the three are seen in the size, shape, and porosity of the hemihydrate crystals. Differences between the hemihydrate crystals determine the characteristics and water-to-powder ratios for each type of gypsum product.

**DENTAL PLASTER.** Also commonly referred to as **plaster of Paris,** model plaster is white and used primarily for pouring up preliminary impressions to make diagnostic models for a case presentation, or in the use of orthodontics. The crystals in plaster are irregularly shaped and very porous, similar in appearance to a sponge. Because of the porous and irregular crystals, model plaster requires the greatest quantity of water for mixing, which produces the weakest of the three forms of study model.

**DENTAL STONE.** Dental stone is a form of gypsum that is typically yellow in color and is used when a more durable diagnostic cast is required, or when a working model is needed for the fabrication of a fixed or removal prosthetics, retainer, and custom tray. The crystals in dental stone are more uniform in shape and less porous than those in plaster. The result is a study model that is much stronger and denser than one made from plaster.

**HIGH-STRENGTH STONE.** Also known as **densite** or **improved dental stone,** high-strength stone has a strength, hardness, and dimensional accuracy that make it ideal for use by the dental laboratory technician in creating a **die** for use in the fabrication of a wax pattern with the production of crowns, bridges, and indirect restorations. The crystals in high-strength stone are smooth and very dense and require the least amount of water for mixing.

### *Powder-to-Water Ratio*

The powder-to-water ratio has a significant effect on the setting time and strength of the gypsum product. Each gypsum material has an optimal ratio as specified by the manufacturer. These ratios should be observed carefully because deviations can change the consistency of the material and the properties of the set cast.

Recommended powder-to-water ratios for gypsum products are as follows:

| | | |
|---|---|---|
| Dental plaster (100 g) | to | 45–50 ml water |
| Dental stone (100 g) | to | 30–32 ml water |
| High-strength stone (100 g) | to | 19–24 ml water |

When **too little** water is used, the mix will be dry, which will provide a shorter working time. If additional water is added to thin the mixture, the **crystallization** (setting) process will be disturbed, and the model will not have the desired strength.

When **too much** water is used, the mix will be thin and runny and will take longer to set; this creates a model that is considerably weaker. If additional powder is added after the stirring has begun, continued stirring will break up the crystals that have begun to form. The result is a cast that is weak and brittle.

Measurements of the powder and water in each mix must be exact. The water is measured by volume with a measuring device such as a large syringe or a milliliter-graduated cylinder. The powder is measured by weight with the use of a scale. Remember to adjust the scale for this weight *before* the powder is weighed. If a scale is not available, the powder may be measured by volume.

See Procedure 47.2: Mixing Dental Plaster.

RECALL

7 What is another term for a dental model?
8 What dental materials are used to make dental models?
9 What are the three forms of gypsum?
10 What is the water-to-powder (g/ml) ratio of plaster?
11 When mixing gypsum materials, do you add the "powder to the water" or the "water to the powder"?
12 In what are gypsum materials mixed?

## Pouring Dental Models

A model consists of two parts: the **anatomic portion**, which is created from the alginate impression, and the **art portion,** which forms the base of the cast (Fig. 47.12). Three different pouring methods can be used to create the base or art portion of the cast (Fig. 47.13).

### *Double-Pour Method*

The anatomic portion of the cast is poured first. Then a second mix of plaster or stone is used to prepare the art portion. A free-form base may be created by hand, or a commercial rubber mold can be used.

### *Box-and-Pour Method*

The impression is surrounded with a "box" made from boxing wax. The completed box should extend at least 1 inch above the palatal area of the maxillary impression and 1 inch above the tongue area of the mandibular impression.

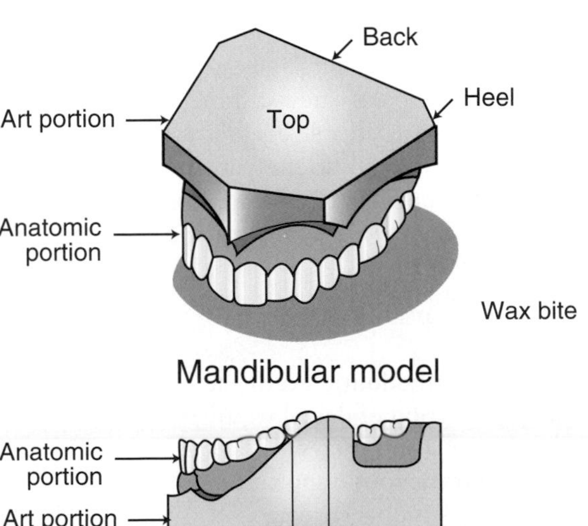


**FIG. 47.12** Anatomic and art portions of a dental model.

### Inverted-Pour Method

The inverted-pour approach consists of mixing one large mixture of plaster or stone and pouring up the impression first, and then placing a base of material on a tile or counter to invert the impression in a single step. This is the most common way of "pouring up" an impression.

See Procedure 47.3: Pouring Dental Models Using the Inverted-Pour Method.

RECALL

13 What are the two parts of a dental model?
14 When pouring an impression, where in the maxillary impression do you begin to place the gypsum material?
15 How long should you wait before you separate the model from the impression?

## Trimming and Finishing Dental Models

When models are to be used for a case presentation or as part of the patient's permanent record, they must have a professional appearance. This is accomplished by trimming the models to a **geometric standard.** The wax bite registration is used to articulate casts during the trimming process.

### Anatomic and Art Portions

The anatomic portion of the dental model includes the teeth, oral mucosa, and muscle attachments. This portion makes up two thirds of the overall trimmed cast. The art portion of the model forms the base and should make up one third of the overall trimmed cast.

### Polishing Plaster Models

Many dental offices use the dental model for presentation of the diagnosis and treatment plan. It is important for the model to have a professional-quality appearance.

To create a more polished look for a plaster model, soak the model in a soapy solution for 24 hours, allow to dry, and then polish with a soft cloth. An alternative to this solution is a commercial model gloss spray that can be used for the same purpose.

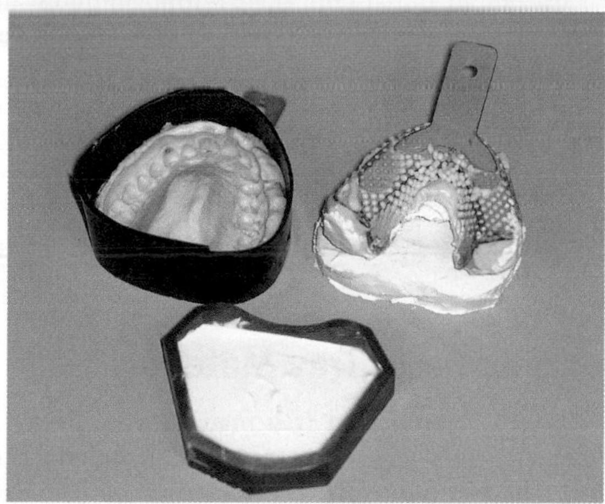

FIG. 47.13 Examples of pouring methods. *Upper left,* boxed; *upper right,* inverted; *lower middle,* double-pour.

See Procedure 47.4: Trimming and Finishing Dental Models.

### Overview of Pouring, Trimming, and Finishing Study Casts

**Pouring Impressions**

1. Remove excess water from impression using air syringe.
2. Mix either stone or plaster.
3. Add material to impression slowly, using the vibrator to remove air bubble from the mix.
4. Place filled impression onto base.
5. Allow stone to set a minimum of 45 minutes before separating cast from impression.

**Pretrim Check**

1. Review cast for air bubble and remove as needed.
2. Trim any excess plaster that could interfere with occluding the maxillary cast to the mandibular cast.
3. Soak models in water to prepare for trimming.

**Trimming Maxillary Cast**

1. Trim base of cast to be parallel with occlusal plane.
2. Trim heel to be perpendicular with midpalatal raphe.
3. Trim sides of maxillary cast.
4. Trim anterior cuts from canine to midline.
5. Trim posterior angles.

**Trimming Mandibular Cast**

1. Place wax bite, and occlude the cast together.
2. Trim mandibular heel to the maxillary heel.
3. Trim mandibular base parallel with maxillary base.
4. Trim sides of mandibular cast to be flush with maxillary base.
5. Trim distal angles flush with maxillary base.
6. Trim anterior portion of mandibular cast from canine to canine.

**Finishing Casts**

1. Fill any voids with a slurry mixture of plaster/stone and water.
2. Remove any gypsum beads.
3. Smooth and provide model gloss if using as a case presentation.

RECALL

16 Which of the two models (maxillary or mandibular) do you begin measuring and trimming first?
17 What area on the maxillary and mandibular model is trimmed differently?
18 What should be placed between the maxillary and mandibular cast when trimming them together?

## Custom Impression Trays

As was discussed in Chapter 46, custom impression trays are made specifically for an individual patient. Custom trays are created in the dental laboratory within the office, or a dental laboratory technician can prepare these before the patient returns for his or her appointment.

## Criteria for Creating Custom Impression Trays

- Tray must be sufficiently rigid to hold and support materials needed during tray placement and removal.
- Tray must fit and adapt well to the arch and must maintain patient comfort without *impinging* (pressing uncomfortably) on surrounding tissues.
- Tray must provide accurate adaptation to an edentulous or a partially edentulous arch.
- Tray must maintain an even distribution of 3 to 4 mm of impression material between itself and the teeth.
- The completed maxillary tray must cover the teeth and hard palate and extend slightly beyond the gingival margin (but not into the mucobuccal fold).
- The completed mandibular tray must cover the teeth and extend beyond the gingival margin (but not into the mucobuccal fold).
- The primary materials that can be used to construct custom trays are **self-curing acrylic resin, light-cured resin,** and **thermoplastic material.** Regardless of the material used in construction of the tray, a diagnostic model must be prepared first, in accordance with specific guidelines.

## Guidelines and Terminology for Creating a Custom Impression Tray

- **Undercuts:** The first step in cast preparation is to fill all undercuts with wax or other molding material. Air bubbles in the cast, the shape of the arch and ridge, carious lesions, fractured teeth, and deep interproximal spaces and malposed teeth may cause undercuts.
- **Outlining the tray:** The margins of the cast where the finished tray will be seated are outlined in pencil. The outline, which designates the area to be covered by the tray, extends over the attached gingiva to the mucogingival junction and 2 to 3 mm beyond the last tooth in the quadrant.
- **Spacer:** A spacer is placed on the cast to create room in the tray for the impression material. Baseplate wax, a folded moist paper towel, or a commercial nonstick molding material may be used for this purpose. To create the spacer, cut a length of baseplate wax, warm it, and place it on the cast over the area of the tray. A warmed plastic instrument is used to *lute* the wax to the cast.
- **Spacer stops:** Spacer stops are placed to prevent the tray from seating too deeply onto the arch or quadrant. Spacer stops also allow for an adequate quantity of impression material around the preparations. Spacer stops are triangular or round holes that are cut out of the spacer with a laboratory knife or wax spatula. These cutouts will form bumps on the tissue side of the tray. (The *tissue side* is the inner surface of the completed tray.) An *edentulous tray* requires a minimum of four stops: one each on the crest of the alveolar ridge in the area of the first or second molar. Additional stops may be placed on the crest of the ridge in the area of each canine. A tray used to take an impression of prepared natural teeth, as for a crown or a bridge, has the stops placed near, but not on, the prepared teeth.
- **Separating medium:** The prepared cast, spacer, and immediate surrounding area are painted with a separating medium, so that the completed tray can be separated readily from the cast.
- **Handle:** A handle adapted to the tray will allow easier placement into and removal from the patient's mouth. The handle is *always* placed at the anterior of the tray, as near the midline as possible, facing outward and parallel to the occlusal surfaces of the teeth. The handle is formed from a piece of scrap acrylic that was cut away from the tray. The end of the handle and the area where it will be attached to the tray are moistened with tray resin liquid.
- **Spacer removal:** After the tray has been formed, it is necessary to remove the spacer and clean the tissue side of the tray. A small, stiff brush, such as a toothbrush, is used to remove most of the wax at this time. The remainder of the spacer is removed and the interior of the tray is cleaned after the tray reaches its final set.
- **Finishing:** It is *not* necessary to remove rough areas on the *tissue* side of the tray; this surface will be covered with impression material. If the outer edges of the tray are rough, however, it is necessary to smooth them so they do not injure the tissues of the patient's mouth. A laboratory knife can be used to smooth minor rough areas. An acrylic bur in a straight slow-speed handpiece can be used to remove major rough areas. An alternative is to use the laboratory lathe to smooth the edges. The tray is given a final rinse and is disinfected according to the manufacturer's instructions.

## Acrylic Resin Tray Materials

Self-curing acrylic resin provides a strong and easily adaptable material that can be used to create a custom tray. The major disadvantage of this material involves the hazards of working with the liquid monomer, which is highly **volatile**. The vapor is highly flammable, is hazardous if inhaled in large concentrations, and may be irritating to the skin. This material must be handled with great care.

When a self-curing resin is used, polymerization begins when the **monomer** and the **polymer** are mixed together. The material reaches an initial cure stage within minutes; during this time, it hardens and gives off heat, but still can be shaped. The material has reached final set when (1) it can no longer be shaped, and (2) the heat has diminished. The tray material is not **dimensionally stable** for 24 hours. Because of this the custom tray should be fabricated 24 hours before the patient is scheduled.

See Procedure 47.5: Constructing an Acrylic Resin Custom Tray.

## Light-Cured Resin Tray Materials

This premixed, prefabricated tray material is a visible light-cured material that does *not* contain methylmethacrylate monomer (the hazardous material associated with the acrylic resin material). Light-cured resin has very low shrinkage, which provides excellent adaptation of the cast. This tray material is prepared for any impression situation, including dentulous, edentulous, and partially edentulous impressions.

With light-cured resins, a curing light acts as the catalyst to bring about polymerization, which allows the material to remain workable until it has been exposed to the light again. Once exposed, the resin polymerizes and hardens very quickly.

See Procedure 47.6: Creating a Light-Cured Custom Tray.

## Vacuum-Formed Thermoplastic Resin

The vacuum former uses heat and a vacuum to conform a sheet of thermoplastic resin to a diagnostic model. The vacuum former is a versatile machine. The major differences in this technique, compared with acrylic resin and light-cured resin applications, are the model preparation and the weight and type of plastic used.

- When constructing an **impression tray,** you will use a rigid, heavy-gauge plastic that requires a spacer and a handle.
- When constructing **provisional coverage,** you will use a lighter-gauge plastic that does not require a spacer or a handle.
- When constructing a **vital bleaching tray,** you will use a lighter-gauge plastic that does not require a spacer or a handle.
- When constructing a **mouth guard,** you will use a heavier-gauge, flexible plastic that does not require a spacer but does require an attachment for the strap.

See Procedure 47.7: Constructing a Vacuum-Formed Custom Tray.

RECALL

19 Of the three types of custom trays discussed, which technique uses a more hazardous material in the fabrication of the tray?
20 Which type of custom tray is made for a vital bleaching procedure?
21 Name two ways that acrylic resin can harden.
22 Which type of material is used for a vacuum-formed custom tray?
23 What is the purpose of a spacer?
24 How are undercuts corrected on a model when a custom tray is prepared?

## Dental Waxes

Dental waxes have a specific purpose in clinical and laboratory procedures. Each wax is derived from a specific by-product. They are derived from either *natural* products, animal by-products, or *synthetic* products that are made to have certain qualities that cannot be attained from natural sources.

- **Paraffin**—derived from mineral
- **Ceresin**—derived from mineral
- **Beeswax**—derived from animal
- **Candelilla**—derived from plant
- **Carnauba**—derived from plant
- **Gum Dammar**—derived from plant
- **Rosin**—derived from plant

## Classification of Waxes

Dental waxes are categorized into three general classifications: *pattern waxes, processing waxes,* and *impression waxes.*

### Pattern Waxes

Pattern wax is a specific type of wax used in the construction of metal castings, and also for the base in the fabrication of dentures. The three types of waxes in this classification are inlay wax, casting wax, and baseplate wax.

**INLAY WAX.** Inlay wax is a hard, brittle wax made from paraffin wax, carnauba wax, resin, and beeswax (Fig. 47.14). The dental laboratory technician uses this wax to create a pattern of the indirect restoration on a model.

Inlay waxes are classified according to how they flow (hardness), as follows:

- *Type A* is a hard wax used for direct wax patterns in the mouth.
- *Type B* is a medium inlay wax used for indirect wax patterns on dies (Fig. 47.15).
- *Type C* is a soft inlay wax used for indirect waxing techniques in the dental laboratory.

**CASTING WAX.** Casting wax is similar to inlay wax, consisting of paraffin, ceresin, beeswax, and resins. Casting waxes are used for single-tooth indirect restorations and fixed bridges and for casting metal portions of a partial denture. This wax is supplied in sheets of various thicknesses.

**BASEPLATE WAX.** Baseplate wax is supplied in sheets and is made from paraffin or ceresin with beeswax and carnauba wax (Fig. 47.16). It is hard and brittle at room temperature. Baseplate wax is used to record the occlusal rims for the initial arch form, for setting denture teeth, and for denture wax-up.

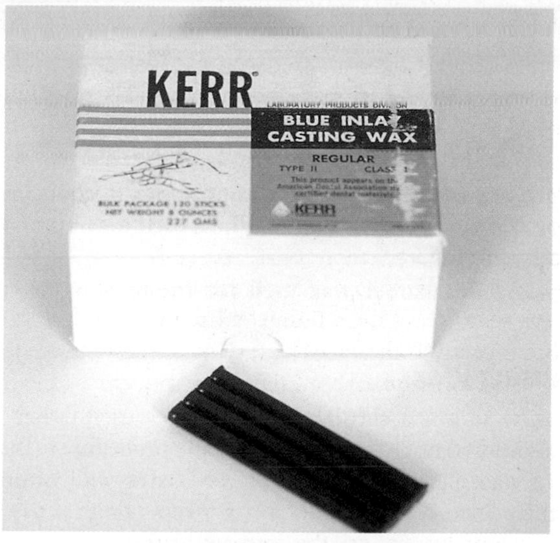


**FIG. 47.14** Inlay casting wax.

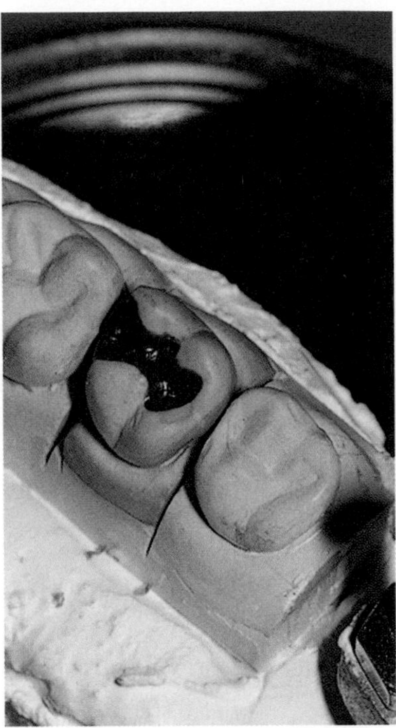

FIG. 47.15 Use of inlay wax on the die. *(From Heymann HO, Swift EJ Jr, Ritter AV: Sturdevant's art and science of operative dentistry, ed 6, St Louis, 2013, Mosby.)*

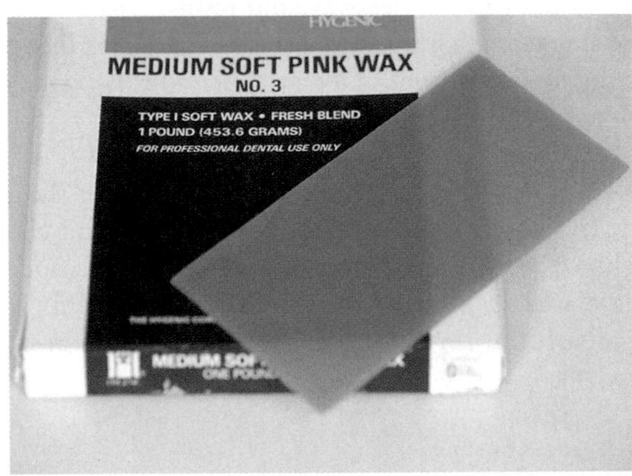


FIG. 47.16 Baseplate wax.

The American Dental Association (ADA) classifies baseplate wax as the following three types:

- *Type I* is a softer wax used for impressions in cool climates.
- *Type II* is a wax of medium hardness used for impressions in moderate climates.
- *Type III* is a harder wax used for impressions in tropical climates.

### *Processing Wax*

Processing wax is a classification of waxes used either in the clinical or laboratory setting for multiple procedures. The three types of waxes in this classification are boxing wax, utility wax, and sticky wax.

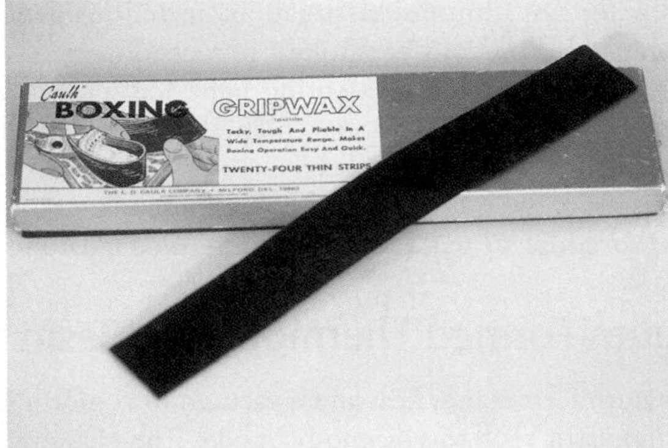


FIG. 47.17 Boxing wax.

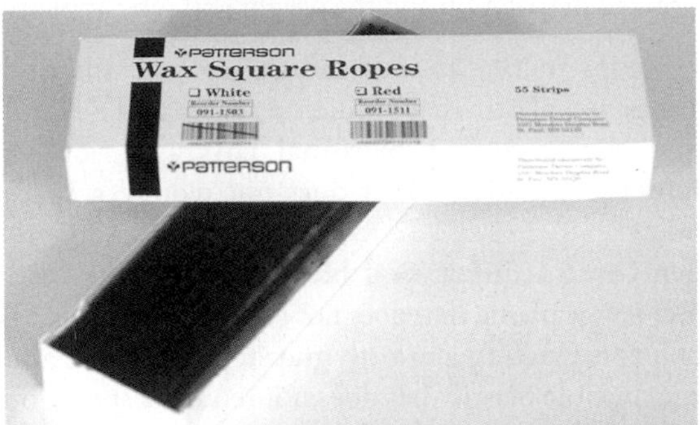


FIG. 47.18 Utility wax.

**BOXING WAX.** Boxing wax is a soft, pliable wax with a smooth, shiny appearance. It is supplied in long, narrow strips measuring 1 to 1 1/2 inches wide by 12 to 18 inches long (Fig. 47.17).

Boxing wax is often used to form a wall or box around a preliminary impression when it is poured up, producing a cleaner model, without the need to trim as much material.

**UTILITY WAX.** Utility wax is a soft, pliable wax with a slightly tacky consistency. This type of wax is supplied in different forms depending on its use. It can be purchased in strips, sticks, or rope form (Fig. 47.18). Utility wax is made of beeswax, petrolatum, and other soft waxes. Uses of utility wax include extending the borders of an impression tray and covering brackets in orthodontic treatment when they are irritating the cheek or lips.

**STICKY WAX.** Sticky wax is a very brittle wax. Its main ingredients are beeswax and resin. This type of wax is supplied in sticks or blocks. Sticky wax is best used in the laboratory in fabrication of castings. When heated, it becomes very tacky and is useful in the casting procedure, creating a wax pattern, or joining acrylic resin together.

### *Impression Waxes*

Impression waxes are a classification of waxes used to take impressions within the oral cavity. The two types within this classification are corrective impression wax and bite registration wax.

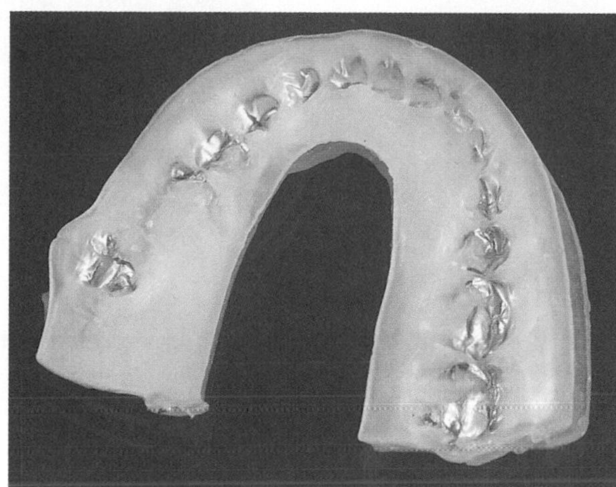

FIG. 47.19 Bite registration wax.

**CORRECTIVE IMPRESSION WAX.** Corrective impression wax is commonly used in the procedure of taking edentulous impressions. This type of wax flows easily at the temperature of the oral cavity, making it useful with other impression materials.

**BITE REGISTRATION WAX.** Bite registration waxes are soft and very similar to casting waxes. After the wax is softened under warm water, the patient is instructed to bite down, so the wax forms an imprint of the teeth.

*Bite wafers* are another example of bite registration wax (Fig. 47.19). This wax is preformed in a horseshoe shape with a thin sheet of aluminum foil between layers.

RECALL

**25** What type of wax could be used to form a wall around a preliminary impression when pouring it up?

**26** To extend an impression tray, what type of wax would you use?

**27** What type of wax would you use to obtain a patient's bite impression?

**28** What is the most common wax used to create a pattern for an indirect restoration?

**■ Patient Education** Dental models is one of the most useful tools in explaining and educating patients about their own mouth. The dentist will use these models when presenting a treatment plan for fixed and removable prosthodontics, pediatrics, orthodontics, surgical procedures, and implants.

Because of their importance, your role in pouring, trimming, and polishing diagnostic models will benefit the patient greatly. Remember that your expertise in this procedure represents your skills as well as the dentist's expertise. ■

**■ Legal and Ethical Implications** As a clinical dental assistant, you may find that your artistic and creative abilities promote interest in a hands-on role with laboratory procedures. The more responsibility you acquire in the laboratory setting, the more aware you must be of the legal limitations in your state, province, or territory regarding what procedures a dental assistant can perform. ■

**■ Eye to the Future** As dentistry becomes more sophisticated, dentists will seek more highly skilled dental assistants for the performance of laboratory procedures to provide optimum treatment for their patients. Dental schools are teaching fewer laboratory skills to dental students, which in turn makes dentists more dependent on the skills and knowledge of the dental assistant and the dental laboratory technician. As a dental assistant, it will be important for you to take an active role in continuing your education and skills with procedures and materials used in the dental laboratory setting. ■

## ■ Critical Thinking

1. You are preparing a preliminary impression to be poured with plaster. How would you ready the impression before pouring it up?
2. You have measured the water and weighed the plaster correctly for a maxillary impression and base. A few seconds after you begin mixing, you note that the mix is very dry. You know you measured correctly. Offer reasons why this happened.
3. It has been approximately a half hour since you poured up the maxillary impression and base. As you remove the impression from the model, two anterior teeth break off. Discuss possible reasons why this happened.
4. In your own words, describe the trimming process of the maxillary and mandibular model.
5. The dentist has asked you to prepare a vital bleaching tray. What types of procedures are involved in making a bleaching tray? ■

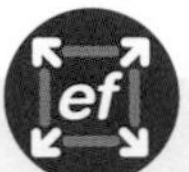

PROCEDURE 47.1

# Taking a Face-Bow Registration (Expanded Function)

## EQUIPMENT AND SUPPLIES

- ✔ Face bow
- ✔ Adhesive or compound bite tabs
- ✔ Warm water if needed to soften the compound bite tabs

## PROCEDURAL STEPS

1 Attach the vertical indicator rod to the analyzer bow.

2 Attach a disposable index tray or a bite-fork to the analyzer bow.

3 Prepare the bite-fork with a disposable index tray or with compound bite tabs.

**NOTE** If using compound bite tabs, they will need to be softened in warm water before placement.

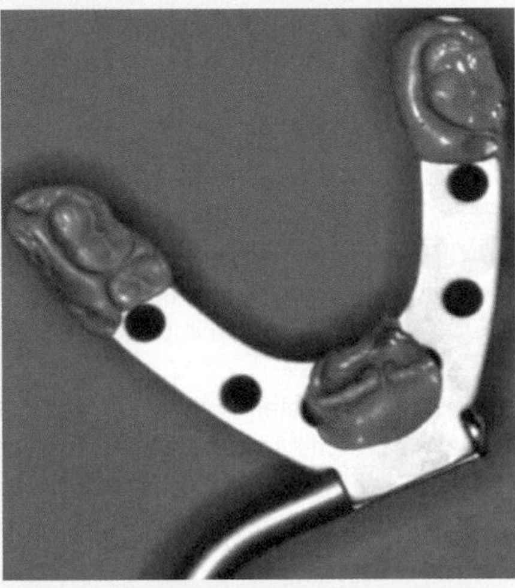

4 When positioning the bite-fork in the mouth, make sure the patient bites slowly.

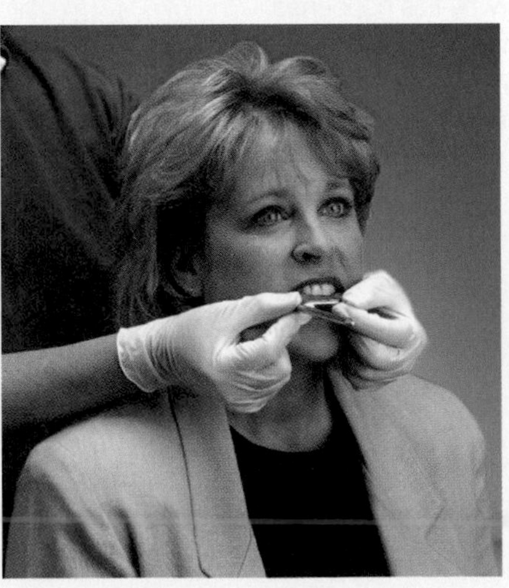

5 Align the vertical indicator rod with the patient's facial midline. This registers the dental midline of the teeth to the frontal plane.

6 While making sure the patient maintains incisal contact with the bite-fork, position the analyzer bow until the lateral wings are level.

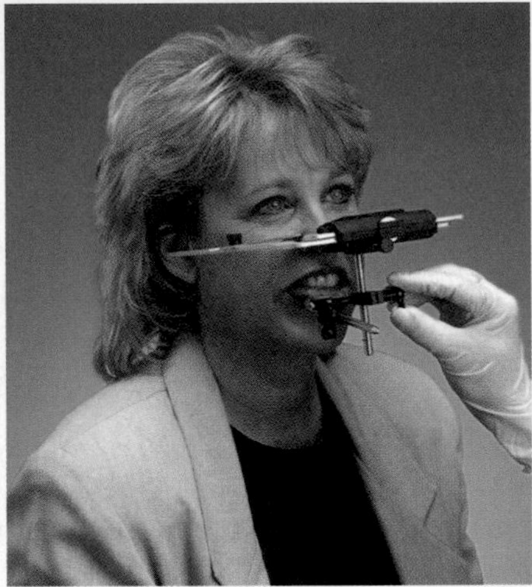

**NOTE** It is best to complete this while standing directly in front of the patient.

7 Remove tray or bite-fork from the bow; this becomes the permanent bite-fork registration record that will be used by the dentist or dental laboratory technician in mounting the study cast.

8 Document the procedure.

Photos in this procedure are courtesy Whip Mix Corporation, Louisville, KY.

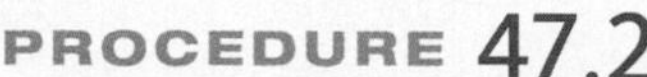

PROCEDURE 47.2

# Mixing Dental Plaster

## EQUIPMENT AND SUPPLIES

- ✓ Flexible rubber mixing bowl (clean and dry)
- ✓ Metal spatula (stiff blade with a rounded end)
- ✓ Scale
- ✓ Plaster (100 g)
- ✓ Water-measuring device
- ✓ Room temperature water (70° F)
- ✓ Vibrator with a disposable cover

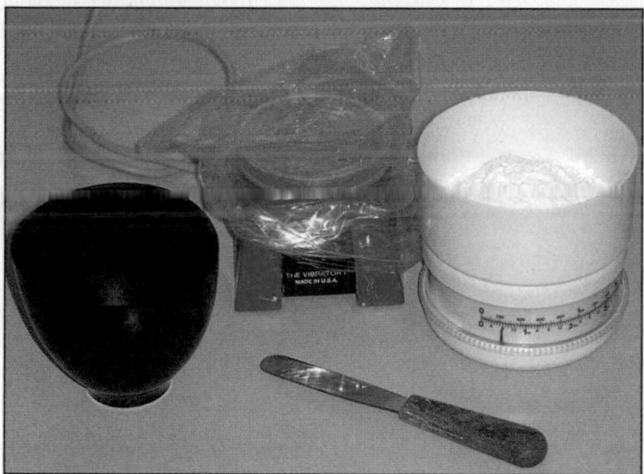

## PROCEDURAL STEPS

1. Measure 45 ml of room temperature water into a clean rubber mixing bowl.
2. Place the paper towel on the scale, and make necessary adjustments.
3. Weigh out 100 g of dental plaster.
4. Add the powder to the water in steady increments. Allow the powder to settle into the water for about 30 seconds.

   **PURPOSE** This helps prevent trapping air bubbles.
5. Use the spatula to incorporate the powder slowly into the water. A smooth and creamy mix should be achieved in about 20 seconds.

   **PURPOSE** This helps prevent spilling the powder.

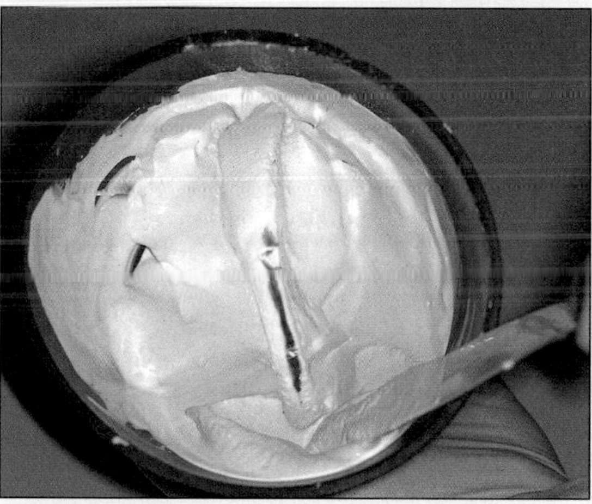

6. Turn the vibrator on at low or medium speed, and place the rubber bowl with the plaster mix on the vibrator platform.

   **PURPOSE** The vibration forces the air bubbles to rise to the surface, which reduces the air in the mix and creates a strong mix.
7. Lightly press and rotate the bowl on the vibrator.
8. Complete mixing and vibration of the plaster for no longer than 2 minutes.

PROCEDURE 47.3 

# Pouring Dental Models Using the Inverted-Pour Method

## EQUIPMENT AND SUPPLIES

- ✓ Maxillary and mandibular impressions
- ✓ Glass slab or tile
- ✓ Laboratory spatula
- ✓ Laboratory knife and cutters
- ✓ 150 g of plaster (additional plaster is needed for the base)
- ✓ 60 ml of water (additional water is needed for the base)
- ✓ Flexible rubber bowl
- ✓ Vibrator

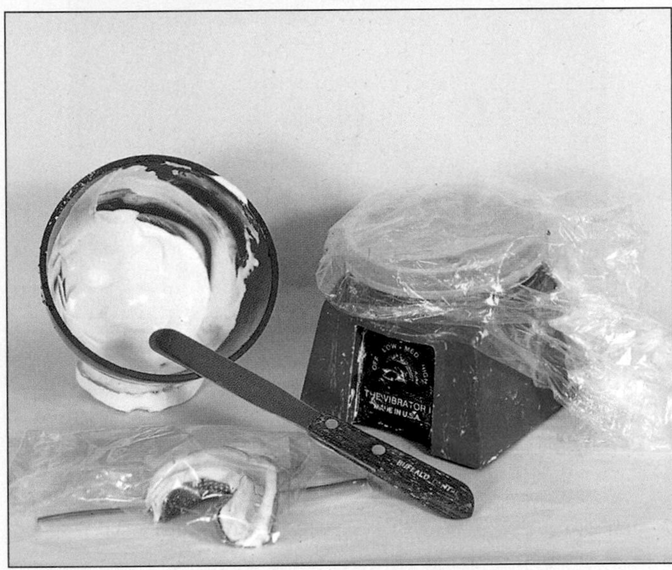

## PROCEDURAL STEPS

### Preparing the Impression

1 Use a gentle stream of air to remove excess moisture from the impression. Be careful not to dry out the impression too much.

**PURPOSE** Overdrying can cause distortion of the material.

2 Use the laboratory knife or laboratory cutters to remove any excess impression material that may interfere with pouring of the model.

### Pouring the Mandibular Model and Base

1 Mix the plaster; then set the vibrator at low to medium speed.

**NOTE** A separate mix will be mixed for the maxillary impression.

2 Hold the impression tray by the handle, and place the edge of the base of the handle on the vibrator.

3 Dip the spatula into the plaster mix, picking up a small increment (about 1 teaspoon).

4 Place this small increment into the impression near the most posterior tooth. Guide the material as it flows lingually.

**PURPOSE** The flowing action pushes out the air ahead of it and eliminates air bubbles.

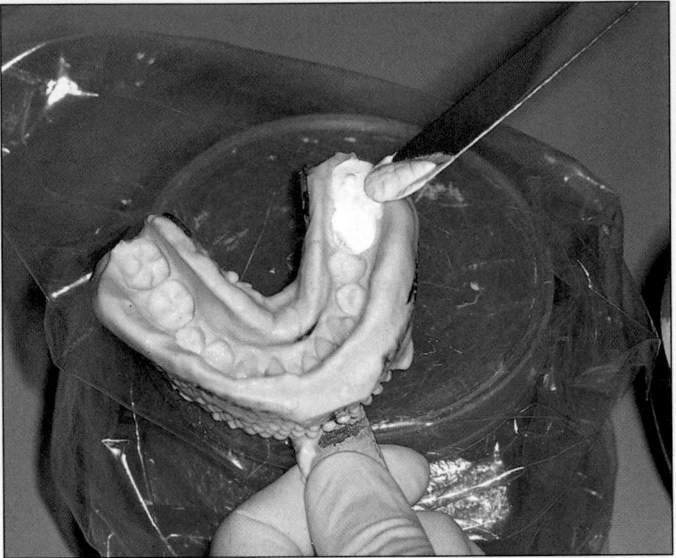

5 Continue to place small increments in the same area as the first increment and allow the plaster to flow toward the anterior teeth.

6 Turn the tray on its side to provide the continuous flow of material forward into each tooth impression.

7 Once all of the teeth in the impression are covered, begin to add larger increments until the entire impression is filled.

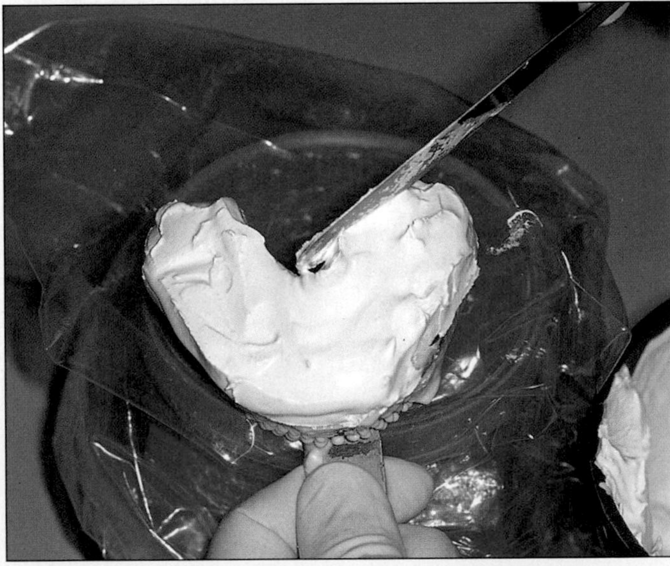

8 Place the additional material onto a glass slab (or tile); shape the base to approximately 2 × 2 inches × 1 inch thick.

**NOTE** Commercial rubber molds are available for making bases. These molds provide symmetry to the cast and reduce the need for trimming.

## PROCEDURE 47.3 Pouring Dental Models Using the Inverted-Pour Method–cont'd

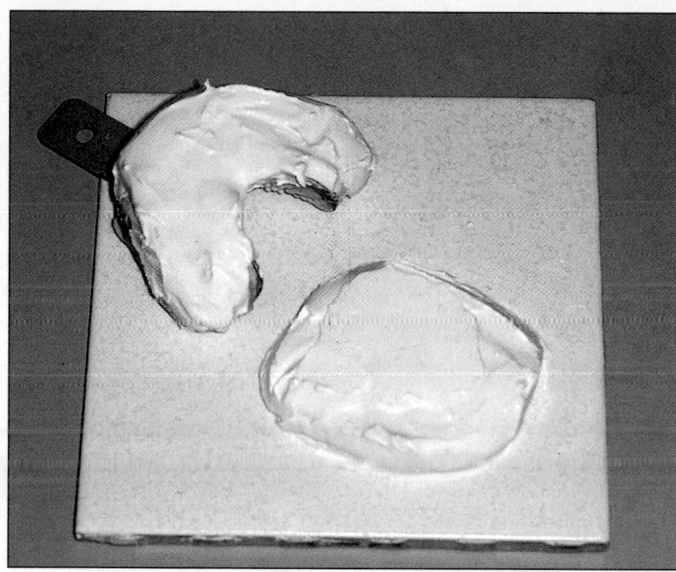

9 Invert the impression onto the new mix. Do not push the impression into the base.

**PURPOSE** When the poured impression is inverted onto the new mix, the fresh material tends to flow excessively. This can result in a base that is too large and too thin.

10 While holding the tray steady, use a spatula to smooth the plaster base mix up onto the margins of the initial pour. Be careful not to cover the impression tray with material, or you will have difficulty removing the cast from the impression.

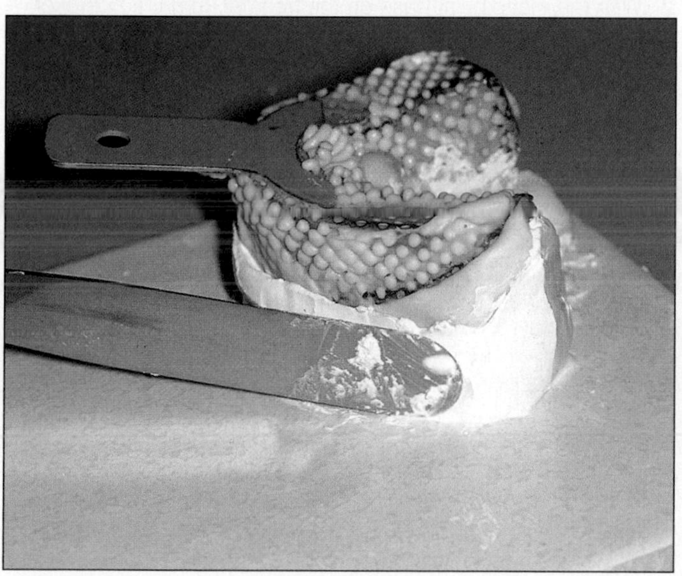

### Pouring the Maxillary Cast

1 Repeat steps 3 through 5 above, using clean equipment for the fresh mix of stone.

2 Place the small increment of plaster in the posterior area of the impression. Guide the material as it flows down into the impression of the most posterior tooth.

3 Continue to place small increments in the same area as the first increment, and allow the plaster to flow toward the anterior teeth.

4 Rotate the tray on its side to provide continuous flow of material into each tooth impression.

5 Once all the teeth in the impression are covered, begin to add larger increments until the entire impression is filled.

6 Place the mix onto a glass slab (or tile), and shape the base to approximately 2 × 2 inches × 1 inch thick.

7 Invert the impression onto the new mix. Do not push the impression into the base.

**PURPOSE** When the poured impression is inverted onto the new mix, the fresh material tends to flow excessively. This can result in a base that is too large and too thin.

8 While holding the tray steady, use a spatula to smooth the stone base mix up onto the margins of the initial pour. Be careful not to cover the impression tray with plaster, or you will have difficulty removing the cast from the impression.

9 Place the impression tray on the base so that the handle and the occlusal plane of the teeth on the cast are parallel to the surface of the glass slab (or tile).

**PURPOSE** To help form a base with uniform thickness.

### Separating the Cast from the Impression

1 Wait 45 to 60 minutes after the base has been poured before separating the impression from the model.

**PURPOSE** The material needs to complete its initial setting stage, or the model will become distorted.

2 Use the laboratory knife to gently separate the margins of the tray.

3 Apply firm, straight, upward pressure on the handle of the tray to remove the impression.

4 If the tray does not separate easily, check to see where the tray is still attached to the impression. Again, use the laboratory knife to free the tray from the model.

5 Pull the tray handle straight up from the model.

**NOTE** Never wiggle the impression tray from side to side while it is on the cast. This can cause the teeth on the cast to fracture.

6 The models are ready for trimming and polishing.

PROCEDURE 47.4

# Trimming and Finishing Dental Models

## EQUIPMENT AND SUPPLIES

- Poured stone maxillary and mandibular dental model
- Wax bite registration
- Pencil
- Ruler
- Laboratory knife
- Model trimmer

## PROCEDURAL STEPS

### Preparing the Model

1 Soak the art portion of the model in a bowl of water for at least 5 minutes.

**PURPOSE** To make the trimming much easier.

### Trimming the Maxillary Model

1 Place the maxillary model on a flat countertop with the teeth setting on the table.
2 Using a ruler, measure up 1 1/4 inches from the counter, and draw a line around the model using your pencil.

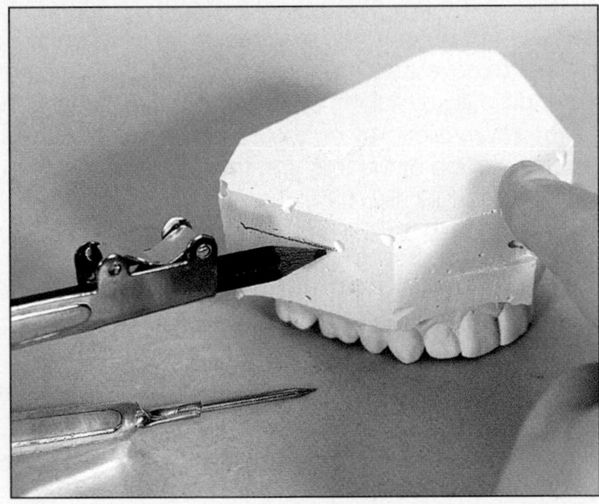

3 Turn on the trimmer, hold the model firmly against the trimmer, and trim the bottom of the base to the line that you drew.
4 Draw a line 1 inch behind the maxillary tuberosities. With the base flat on the trimmer, trim excess plaster in the posterior area of the model to the marked line.
5 To trim the sides of the model, draw a line through the center of the occlusal ridges on one side of the model. Measure out 1 inch from this line, and draw a line parallel to the previous line drawn.

**NOTE** If you need to measure out beyond 1 inch so the mucobuccal fold is not trimmed away, do so.

6 Repeat these measurements on the other side of the model.
7 Trim the sides of the cast to the lines drawn.

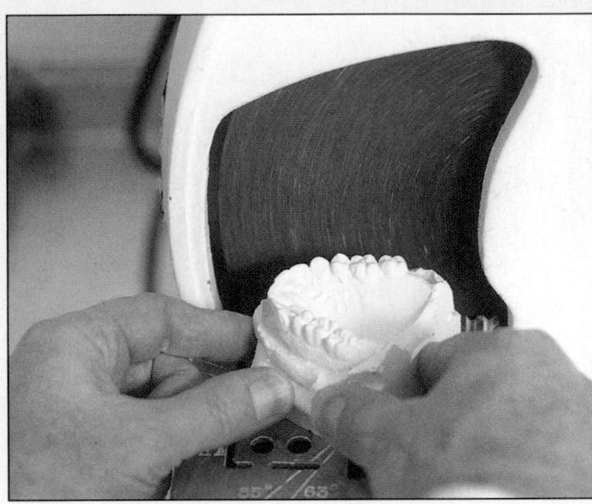

8 Draw a line behind the tuberosity perpendicular to the opposite canine, and trim to that line. This completes the maxillary heel cuts.
9 The final cut is made by drawing a line from the canine to the midline at an angle. Complete this on both sides, and trim to the line.

### Trimming the Mandibular Model

1 Occlude the mandibular model with the maxillary model, using the wax bite.
2 With the mandibular base on the trimmer, trim the posterior portion of the mandibular model until it is even with the maxillary model.
3 Place the models upside down (maxillary base on the table), measure up 3 inches from the surface, and mark a line around the base of the mandibular model.
4 Trim mandibular model base to the line drawn.
5 With models in occlusion with the wax bite, place the mandibular model on the trimmer, and trim the lateral cuts to match the maxillary lateral cuts.
6 Trim the back and heel cuts to match the maxillary heel cuts.

## PROCEDURE 47.4 Trimming and Finishing Dental Models—cont'd

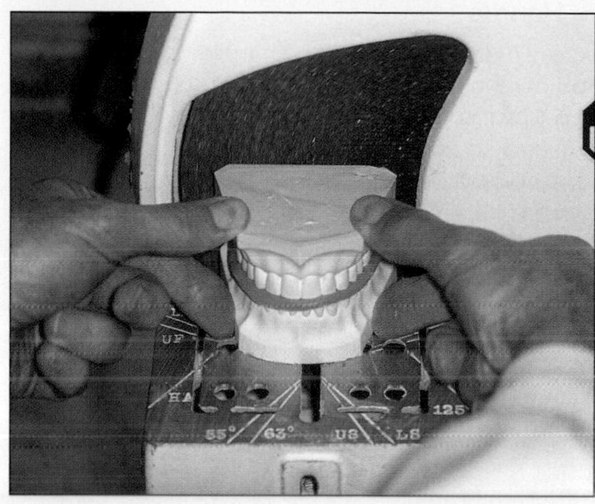

7 Check that the mandibular anterior cut is rounded from the mandibular right canine to the mandibular left canine.
8 The models now are ready to be finished.

### Finishing the Model

1 Mix a **slurry** of gypsum, and fill in any voids.
2 Using a laboratory knife, remove any extra gypsum that occurs as beads on the occlusion or model.

## PROCEDURE 47.5

# Constructing an Acrylic Resin Custom Tray

### EQUIPMENT AND SUPPLIES

- Diagnostic model
- Pencil
- Tray resin (monomer and polymer)
- Measures for liquid and powder
- Baseplate wax
- Separating medium with brush
- Heat source
- Laboratory knife
- Laboratory spatula
- Tongue blade
- Wax spatula #7
- Glass jar with lid or smooth surface paper cup
- Petroleum jelly

### PROCEDURAL STEPS

### Preparing the Model

1 Fill the undercuts on the diagnostic model.
2 Outline the tray in pencil.
3 Place the baseplate wax spacer, trim it, and lute the wax to the cast.

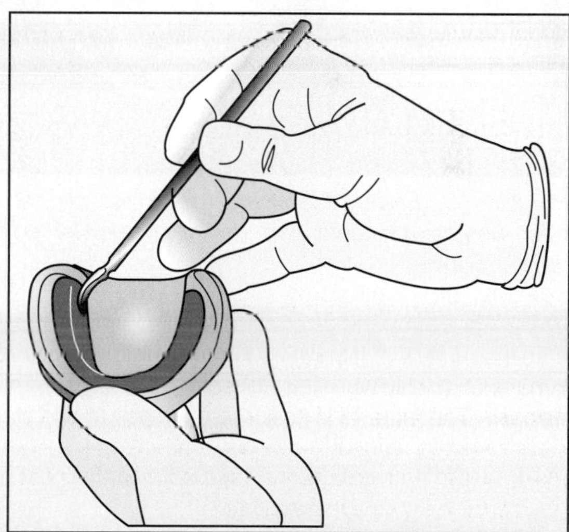

4 Cut the appropriate stops in the spacer.
5 Paint the spacer and surrounding area with separating medium.

### Mixing the Acrylic Resin

6 Use the manufacturer's measuring devices to measure the powder into the mixing container. Then add an equal part of liquid, and recap the container immediately.
**PURPOSE** The fumes are toxic.

(Continued)

## PROCEDURE 47.5 Constructing an Acrylic Resin Custom Tray—cont'd

7 Use tongue blade to mix the powder and liquid. A **homogeneous** mix should be obtained within 30 seconds. The mix will be thin and sticky.

8 Set mix aside for 2 to 3 minutes to allow polymerization. If the manufacturer specifies a covered container, place the cover during this time.

### Forming the Tray

9 When the mix has reached a "doughy" stage, remove it from the container with the spatula.

10 Lubricate the palms of your hands with petroleum jelly, and knead the resin to form a flat patty that is approximately the size of the wax spacer.

**NOTE** Some materials will react with latex gloves and will not set properly. Make sure to read the manufacturer's instructions when working with any material.

11 Place the material on the cast to cover the wax spacer. Adapt it to extend 1 to 1.5 mm beyond the edges of the wax spacer.

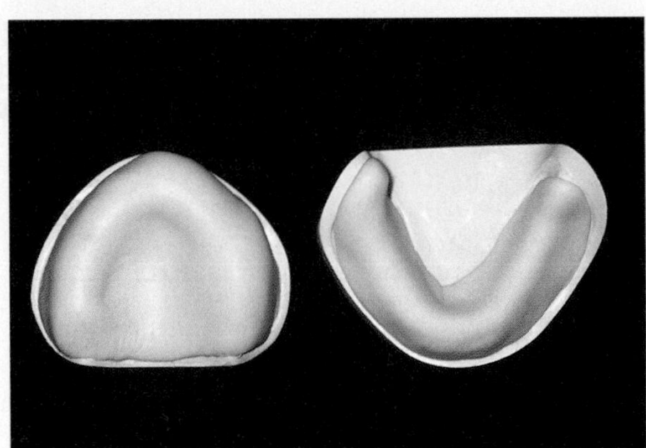

*From Hatrick CD, Eakle WS: Dental materials: clinical applications for dental assistants and dental hygienists, ed 3, St Louis, 2016, Elsevier.*

12 Use an instrument or laboratory knife to trim away excess tray material quickly while it is still soft.

**PURPOSE** The material is easier to cut away at this stage.

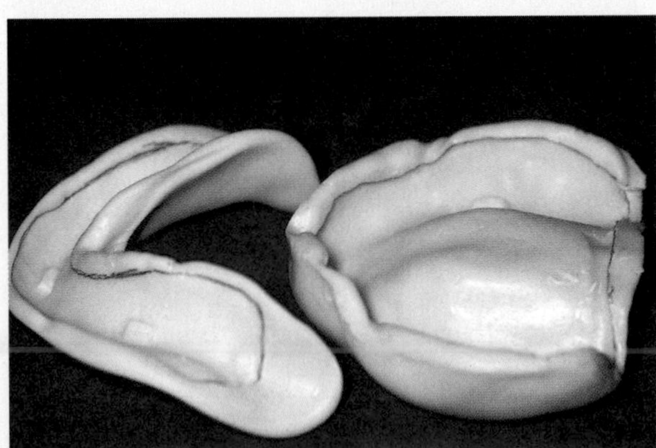

*Hatrick CD, Eakle WS: Dental materials: clinical applications for dental assistants and dental hygienists, ed 3, St Louis, 2016, Elsevier.*

### Creating the Handle

13 Use the excess material to shape the handle.

14 Place a drop of monomer on the handle and on the tray, where they will join.

15 Attach the handle so that it extends out of the mouth and is parallel to the occlusal surfaces of the teeth.

16 Hold the handle in place until it is firm.

### Finishing the Tray

17 After the initial set (7 to 10 minutes), remove most of the spacer, and return the tray to the cast.

18 Clean the wax completely from the inside of the tray after the tray resin has reached final cure.

19 Finish the edges; then clean and disinfect the tray.

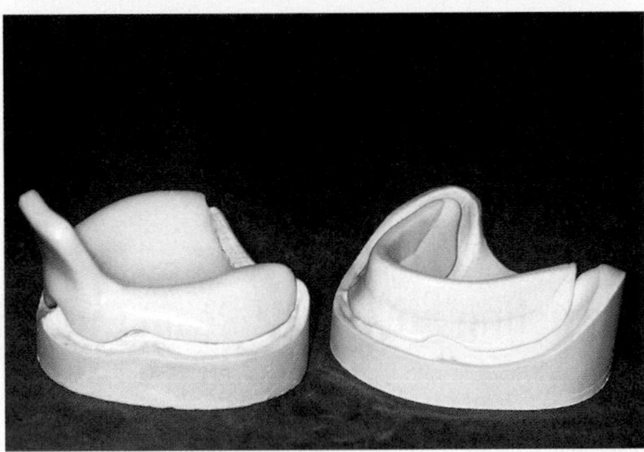

*Hatrick CD, Eakle WS: Dental materials: clinical applications for dental assistants and dental hygienists, ed 3, St Louis, 2016, Elsevier.*

PROCEDURE 47.6

# Creating a Light-Cured Custom Tray

## EQUIPMENT AND SUPPLIES

- Diagnostic model
- Pencil
- Prefabricated tray material
- Baseplate wax
- Separating medium with brush
- Scalpel or laboratory knife
- Curing light system
- Barrier coating

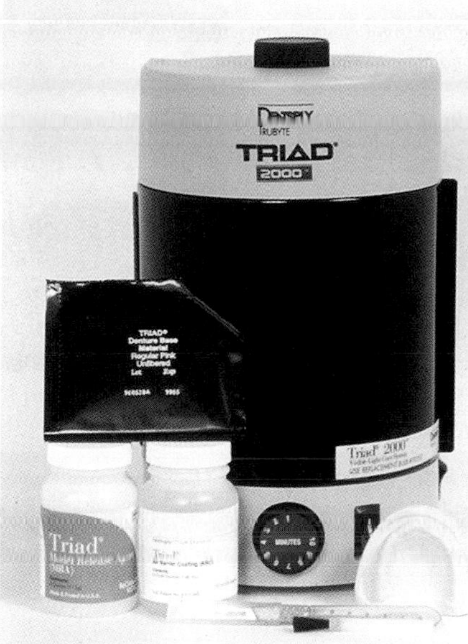


## PROCEDURAL STEPS

1 A model is completed before tray construction.

2 Use a pencil to outline the vestibular area and the posterior tray border on the stone model.

3 Paint separating medium on the model before placing the material.

**NOTE** The material is supplied in uniform precut sheets and is stored in a dark container to prevent premature curing.

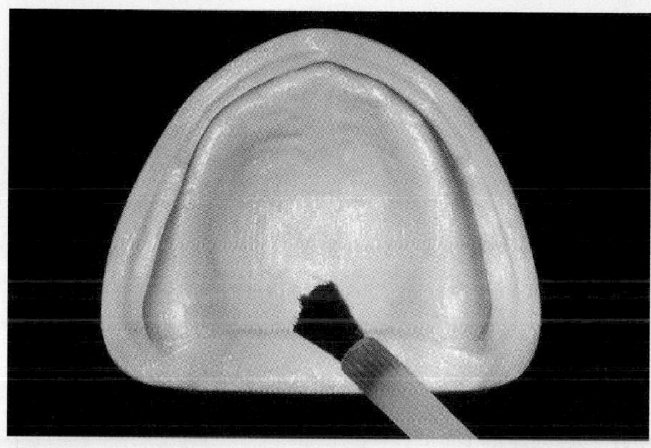

4 Adapt precut sections of the custom tray material for use on the maxillary model with full palatal coverage and on the mandibular model without full palatal coverage.

5 Mold the sheet of tray material to conform to the study model, using your thumb and forefinger with minimal pressure.

**NOTE** Be sure to push material through the "occlusal stop" areas of the tray so that acrylic will be in contact with the occlusal surfaces.

6 Trim away excess tray material with a laboratory knife.

**NOTE** If desired, the excess material can be used to form a handle on the tray.

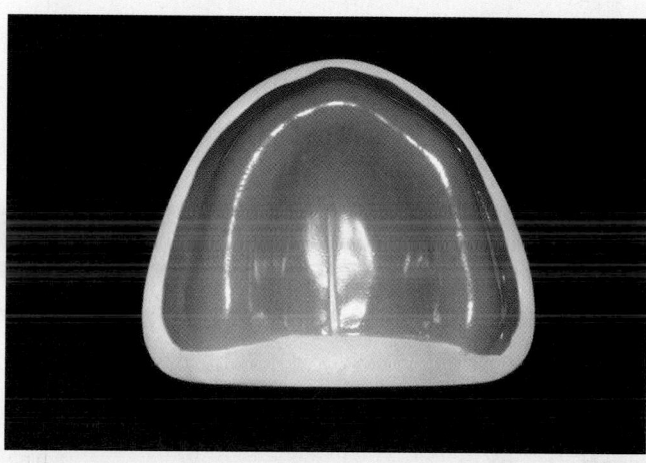

7 Place the model and the tray in a light-curing unit. Cure the tray for 2 minutes.

(Continued)

## PROCEDURE 47.6 Creating a Light-Cured Custom Tray—cont'd

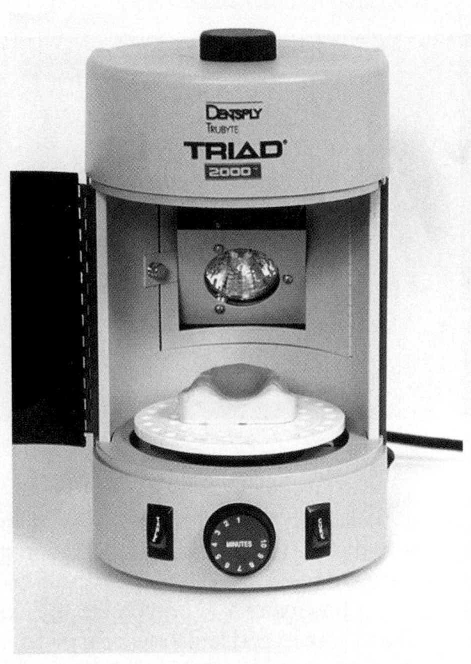


8 After curing, place the model and the tray in cool water to solidify the wax spacer and facilitate separation of the tray from the model.
9 Use the acrylic extruded through the holes in the spacer to create occlusal stops on the inside of the tray.
10 Remove the wax spacer from the tray using a #7 wax spatula.
11 Place the tray in hot water to remove any remnants of wax from the inside.
12 Trim the borders of the tray using an acrylic laboratory bur.

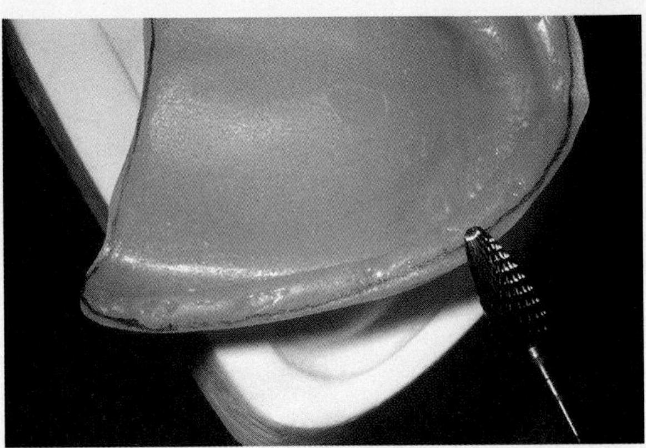

13 A thin acrylic bur can be used to perforate the custom tray if needed.

**NOTE** Perforations and tray adhesives ensure a solid lock of the impression material to the custom tray.

14 Using a laboratory acrylic bur, trim the borders of the edentulous tray to 2 mm short of the vestibule to allow for border molding material.

Photos from Hatrick CD, Eakle WS, Bird WF: Dental materials: clinical applications for dental assistants and dental hygienists, ed 3, St Louis, 2016, Saunders.

PROCEDURE 47.7 

# Constructing a Vacuum-Formed Custom Tray

## EQUIPMENT AND SUPPLIES

- Diagnostic model
- Thermoplastic resin material
- Crown and bridge scissors
- Vacuum former

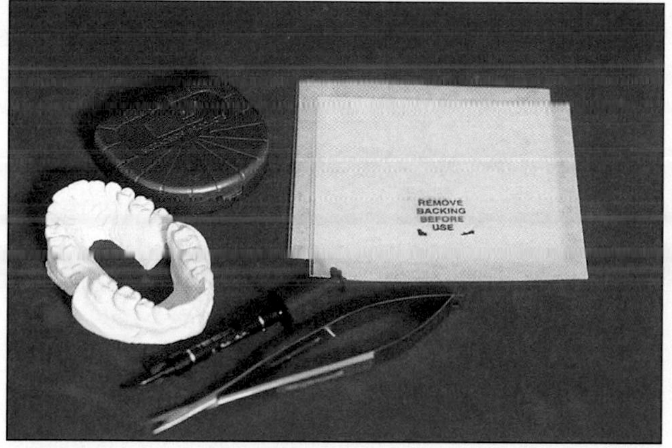


## PROCEDURAL STEPS

1 Trim the model so that it extends 3 to 4 mm past the gingival border.

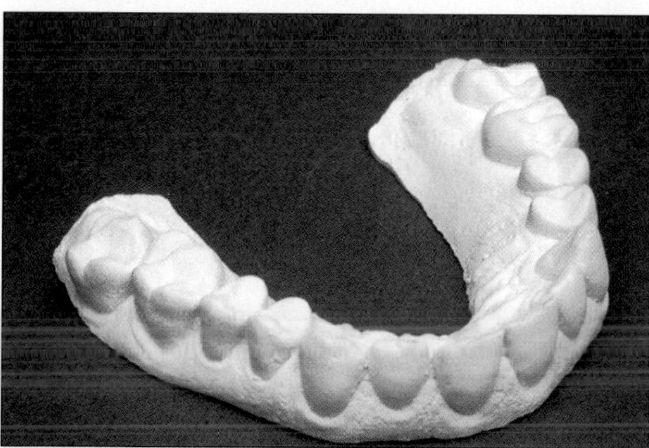

2 To extend the tray from the teeth for the purpose of holding bleaching solution, place a spacer material on the facial surfaces of the teeth on the model.

**NOTE** Some materials will require the tray to be light-cured.

3 Using a vacuum former, heat a tray sheet until it sags to 1 inch.

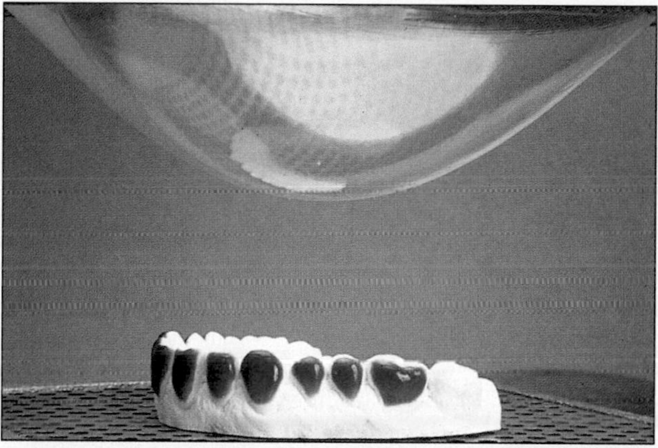

4 Lower the sheet over the model, and turn on the vacuum for 10 seconds.

5 Remove the sheet after allowing it to cool completely.

6 Using your scissors, cut the excess material from the tray.

7 Use small, sharp scissors to trim the tray approximately 0.5 mm away from the gingival margin.

**PURPOSE** You want to avoid having the tray irritate the patient's gingiva.

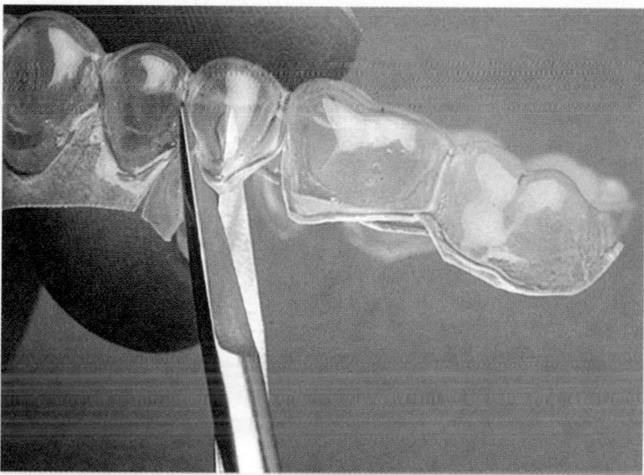

8 Place the tray onto the original model, and check gingival extensions.

9 If necessary, apply a thin coat of petroleum jelly to the facial surface. Using a low flame, gently heat and readapt the margins on the model so that the entire tooth is covered, taking care to avoid overlapping onto the gingiva.

10 After readapting all the margins, retrim excess material. If any areas appear to be too short, or if accidental perforation occurs, simply reheat the tray and stretch the material by pushing it in the desired direction.

11 Leave the tray on the model until the delivery appointment, at which time it should be washed in cold, soapy water and then cold-sterilized.

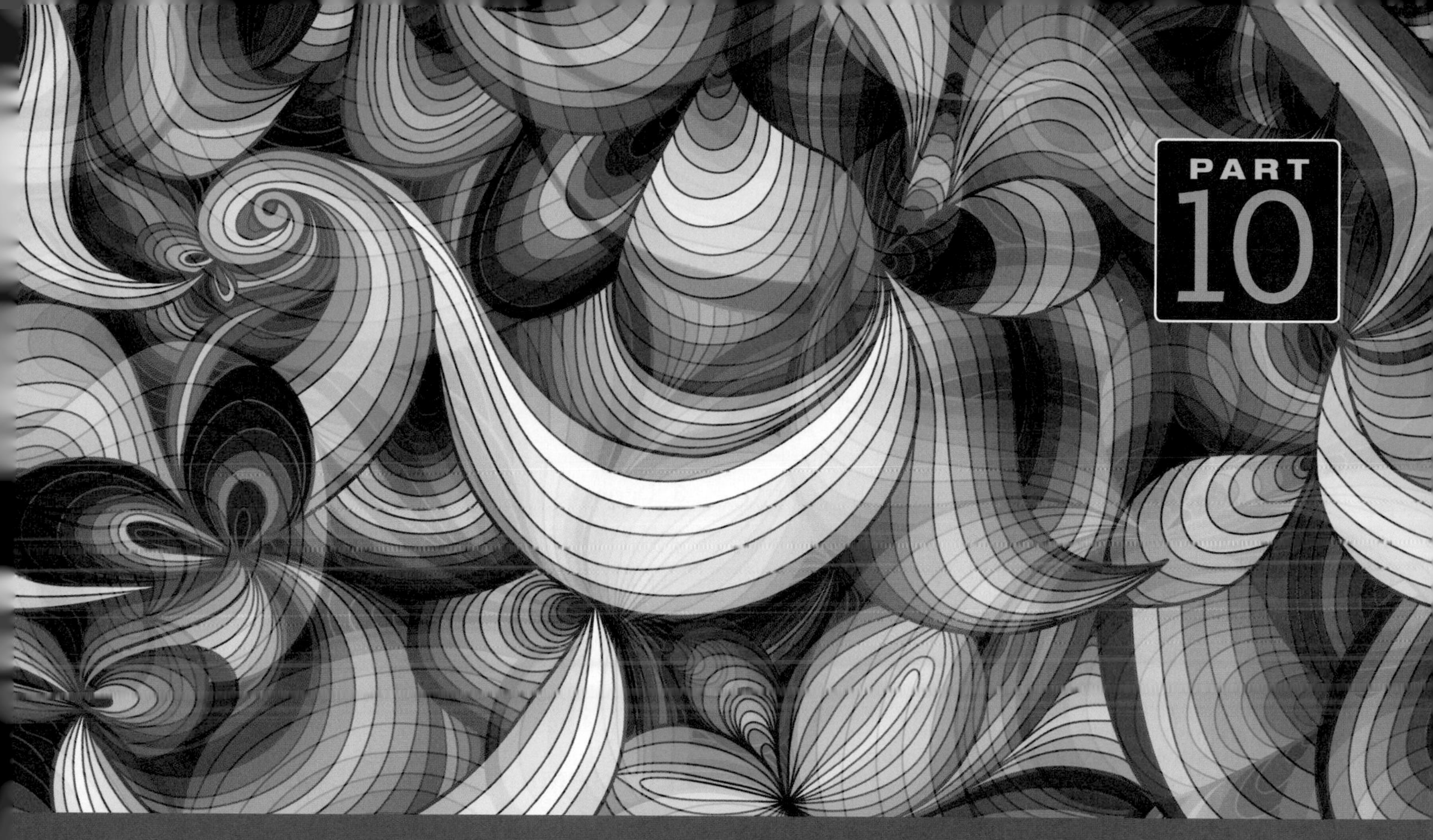


# Assisting in Comprehensive Dental Care

Practicing as a clinical dental assistant is one of the most challenging and rewarding professions in dentistry. The diversity of clinical responsibilities is unlimited in both general and specialized settings.

The chapters in this section are intended to provide a level of knowledge and skill that will prepare you for clinical dentistry. As you progress and demonstrate competency in the general and specialized areas of dentistry, you will be better prepared for graduation, the Dental Assisting National Board, and a career in dental assisting.

48

# General Dentistry

## KEY TERMS

**Axial (AK-see-ul) wall** Internal surface of a cavity preparation positioned in the same vertical direction as the pulp within the tooth.
**Cavity** Pitted area in a tooth caused by decay.
**Cavity preparation** Process of decay removal and tooth design in preparation for restoring a tooth.
**Cavity wall** Internal surface of a cavity preparation.
**Convenience form** Cavity preparation step that allows the dentist easier access when restoring a tooth.
**Diastema (dye-uh-STEE-muh)** A space between two teeth.
**Esthetic (es-THET-ik) dentistry** Type of dentistry that improves the appearance of teeth by camouflaging defects and whitening teeth.
**Line angle** Junction of two walls in a cavity preparation.
**Operative dentistry** Term commonly used to describe restorative and esthetic dentistry.
**Outline form** Design and initial depth of sound tooth structure used by the dentist when restoring a tooth.
**Pulpal (PUL-pul) wall** Surface of the cavity preparation perpendicular to the pulp of a tooth.
**Resistance (ree-ZIS-tuns) form** Shape and placement of cavity walls in preparation for tooth restoration.
**Restoration (res-tuh-RAY-shun)** Use of a dental material to restore a tooth or teeth to a functional permanent unit.
**Restorative (re-STOR-uh-tiv) dentistry** Type of dentistry that restores teeth by removing decay and restoring defects.
**Retention (ree-TEN-shun) form** Shaping of the cavity walls to aid in retaining the restoration.
**Retention (retentive) pin** Basis of a stronger system used to retain and support a tooth restoration.
**Veneer (vuh-NEER)** Thin layer of composite resin or porcelain bonded or cemented to a prepared facial surface.

## LEARNING OUTCOMES

*On completion of this chapter, the student will be able to achieve the following objectives:*

1. Define, spell, and pronounce the key terms.
2. Describe the process and principles of cavity preparation.
3. Discuss the differences in assisting with the different classes of permanent restorations.
4. Discuss why retention pins would be selected for a complex restorative procedure.
5. Describe the need for placement of an intermediate restoration.
6. Describe the procedure of applying composite veneers.
7. Describe tooth-whitening procedures and explain the role of the dental assistant.

## PERFORMANCE OUTCOMES

*On completion of this chapter, the student will be able to achieve competency standards in the following skills:*

- Prepare the setup and assist in a class I restoration.
- Prepare the setup and assist in a class II restoration.
- Prepare the setup and assist in a class III restoration.
- Prepare the setup and assist in a class IV restoration.
- Prepare the setup and assist in a class V restoration.
- Prepare the setup and place and carve an intermediate restoration (expanded function).
- Assist in the placement of a veneer.

## ELECTRONIC RESOURCES

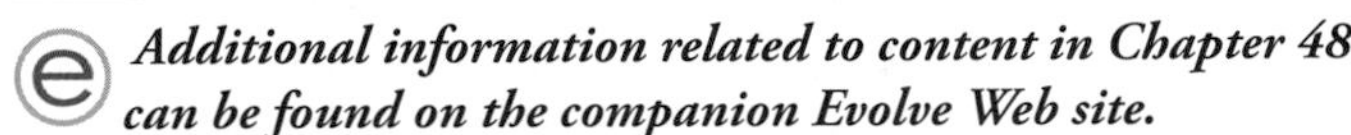
***Additional information related to content in Chapter 48 can be found on the companion Evolve Web site.***

- Practice Quiz
- Tray Setup Drag-and-Drop Exercises: Amalgam Restoration; Composite Procedures (Class III and IV; Class I, II, and V); Bleaching
- Tray Setup Questions
- Videos: Assisting in a Class II Amalgam Restoration; Placing an Intermediate Restoration

General dentistry, also referred to as **operative dentistry**, is the primary focus of the general dentist. This chapter presents the background knowledge and introduces the skills required for the clinical dental assistant of procedures such as amalgam restorations, composite resin restorations, intermediate restorations, resin veneers, and tooth-whitening procedures.

General dentistry can be thought of as *restorative dentistry* and *esthetic dentistry.* In either area, the dentist ensures that the tooth structure is healthy and sound before restoring it to its proper function or improving the appearance.

**Restorative dentistry** is indicated when a tooth is to be restored to its original form and shape through the use of direct and indirect restorative materials. Specific conditions that determine the need for restorative dentistry include the following:

- Initial or recurring decay (**cavity**)
- Replacement of a failed restoration

- Abrasion or wearing away of tooth structure
- Erosion of tooth structure

**Esthetic dentistry** is devoted to improving the appearance of teeth by repairing imperfections with direct and indirect restorative materials, or by using whitening techniques. Specific conditions that result in the need for esthetic treatment include the following:

- Discoloration caused by extrinsic or intrinsic staining
- Anomalies caused by developmental disturbances
- Abnormal spacing between teeth
- Trauma

## Restoration Process

To restore a tooth to its normal function or improve an esthetic appearance, the dentist will master a clinical technique that follows specific steps to complete the process of restorative dentistry. Each time a dentist prepares a tooth for a permanent **restoration**, the dentist has the understanding about the direction of the enamel rods, the thickness of the enamel, the body of the dentin, the size and position of the pulp, and the contours in the crown of the tooth as it relates to the gingival tissues.

G. V. Black's principle of cavity preparation is still used today as the basic steps in the process of designing a cavity preparation. **Cavity preparation** is the process of removing diseased tooth structure while leaving healthy tooth structure for the tooth to maintain a restoration.

The dentist follows these steps in a precise order so that ideal results are achieved.

### Initial Preparation

Cavity preparation first involves the initial design and extension of the preparation's external walls to a limited depth. The factors listed below are intended to help the dentist gain access to the decay or defect and reach sound tooth structure. The objectives for initial cavity preparation are as follows:

- **Outline form**—The dentist decides on the design and initial depth of sound tooth structure (Fig. 48.1).
- **Resistance form**—The dentist determines the primary shape and placement of the cavity walls (Fig. 48.2).
- **Retention form**—The dentist knows where to place retention in the preparation to help in securing the restoration in place (Fig. 48.3).
- **Convenience form**—The dentist has accessibility in preparing and restoring the tooth (Fig. 48.4).

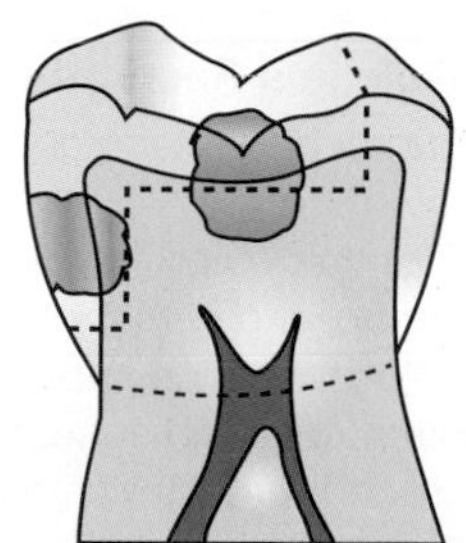

**FIG. 48.1** Outline form of a cavity preparation.

## Terminology

Throughout the restorative process, there is specific terminology that describes the anatomic structures as they relate to cavity preparation. These terms are especially helpful for the expanded-functions dental assistant (EFDA)/registered dental assistant (RDA) in the application of dental materials and intermediate restorations. An understanding of the terminology of a cavity preparation will help to know which dental instruments, dental accessories, and dental materials to have ready at the appropriate times throughout a procedure. See Box 48.1 for tooth preparation terms.

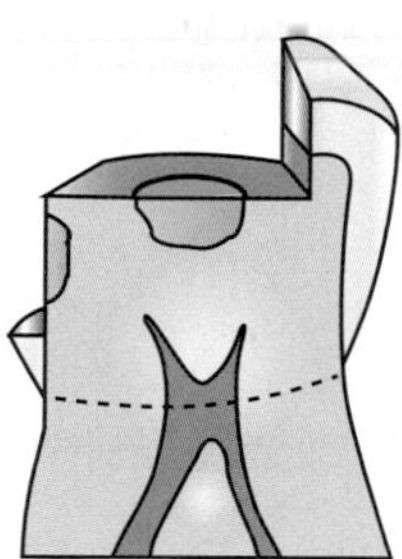

**FIG. 48.2** Resistance form of a cavity preparation.

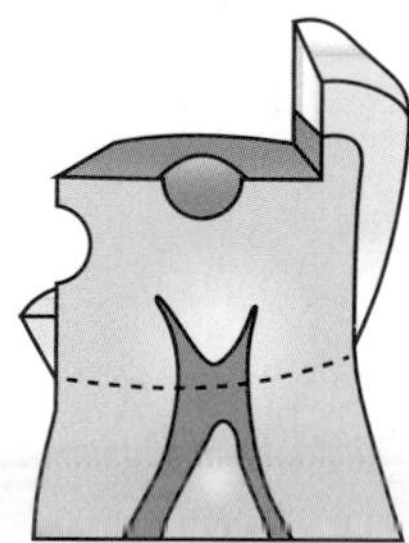

**FIG. 48.3** Retention form placed in the cavity preparation.

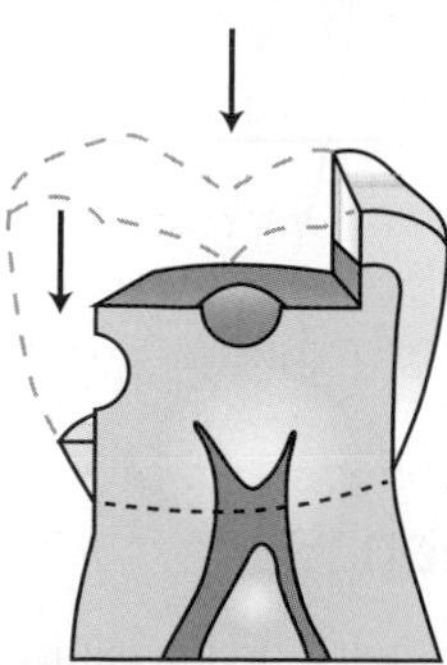

**FIG. 48.4** Convenience form used for easy access to tooth decay.

### BOX 48.1 Terminology Related to Cavity Preparation

**Tooth Preparation Walls**

Cavity wall: Internal surface of the tooth prepared for the restoration.

Internal wall: Cavity wall/surface that does not extend to the external tooth surface.

External wall: Surface of the tooth preparation that extends to the external tooth surface; named according to the tooth surface involved: distal, mesial, facial, lingual, or gingival.

Axial wall: Internal wall/surface of the prepared tooth that runs parallel to the long axis of the tooth.

Pulpal wall: Internal wall/surface of a prepared tooth that is perpendicular to the long axis of the tooth; also known as the *pulpal floor*.

Enamel wall: Portion of a prepared external wall that consists of enamel.

Dentinal wall: Portion of a prepared external wall that consists of dentin.

**Tooth Preparation Angles**

Line angle: Angle formed by the junction of two walls/surfaces in a cavity preparation (similar to the angle formed when two walls of a room meet to form a corner). To identify a line angle, the names of the two involved walls/surfaces are combined. For example, the angle formed by the *mesial* and *lingual* walls is called the *mesiolingual line angle;* the suffix *-al* of mesial is dropped and the letter *o* is added. The two terms are then combined to form the term *mesiolingual.* It is important not to confuse the names of these angles with the names used to describe the surfaces involved in the restoration itself.

Point angle: Junction of three walls/surfaces that are coming from a different orientation.

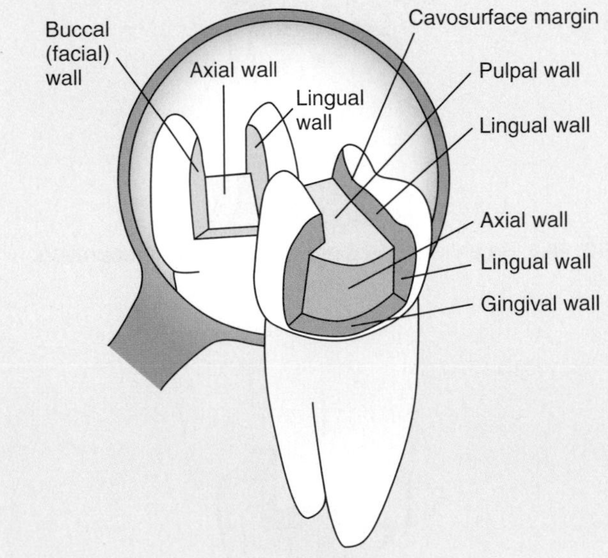


## Final Preparation

Following the initial cavity preparation, the dentist will continue the procedure with the final cavity preparation. This includes:

- Removing any remaining enamel within the preparation, diseased dentin, or old restorative material (or a combination)
- Inserting additional resistance and retention notches, grooves, and coves to provide strength in maintenance of the restoration
- Placing dental materials, which can include lining agents, bases, and desensitizing for protective purpose, or bonding agents, for pulpal protection and better retention

**RECALL**

1 What is restorative and esthetic dentistry often referred to as?
2 What is a common term used to describe decay?
3 Which step in the initial preparation allows the dentist to determine the shape and placement of the cavity walls?
4 Which wall of a cavity preparation is perpendicular to the long axis of the tooth?

## Permanent Restorations

A permanent restoration can range from a small class I restoration to an extensive class II multisurface foundation and continue with classes III, IV, and V. With the exception of steps added to the process by using supplementary accessories and dental materials, a restorative procedure will follow a standardized format.

### Standardized Plan for a Restorative Procedure

- Communicate with the patient about the procedure and about what to expect during treatment.
- Position the patient correctly for the dentist and the type of procedure (see Chapter 33).
- The dentist will evaluate the tooth to be restored (see Chapter 28).
- The dentist will administer local anesthesia (see Chapter 37).
- Prepare the type of moisture control to be used for the procedure (cotton roll, dry angles, dental dam; see Chapter 36).
- The dentist will prepare the tooth for the restoration (this includes the use of dental hand instruments and dental handpieces with rotary instruments; see Chapters 34 and 35).
- The dentist will determine the types of dental materials to be used (see Chapters 43 and 44).
- Apply the dental materials. Burnish, carve, or finish the dental material.
- Check the occlusion of the restoration.
- Finish and polish the restoration.

**Dental Assistant's Role in a Restorative Procedure**

- Be familiar with the procedure, and anticipate the dentist's needs.
- Prepare the setup for the restorative procedure.
- Provide moisture control and better visualization for the dentist by using high-velocity suction and an air-water syringe.
- Transfer dental instruments and accessories.
- Provide a proper mix and transfer of dental materials.
- Perform any required legal expanded functions.
- Maintain patient comfort throughout the procedure.
- Maintain appropriate infection control precautions.

## Class I Restorations

The class I cavity, or *lesion,* is a one-surface lesion involving the pits and fissures of a tooth. Because of this anatomic feature, plaque and debris tend to accumulate within these areas, making it difficult for a patient to keep the area clean. Therefore the pits and fissures are highly susceptible to decay. Class I decay involves the following areas of concern:

- Occlusal pits and fissures of premolars and molars (Fig. 48.5, *A*)
- Buccal pits and fissures of mandibular molars (Fig. 48.5, *B*)
- Lingual pits and fissures of maxillary molars (Fig. 48.5, *C*)
- Lingual pits of maxillary incisors, most frequently near the cingulum (Fig. 48.5, *D*)

### Tooth Preparation

The occlusal or lingual class I cavity preparation is a simple preparation for the dentist. The outline of the cavity preparation involves the pit, the groove, or a fissure that is decayed. The dentist will use a bur to open the enamel, taking care not to create any sharp angles or corners within the preparation. This preparation should be smooth throughout the internal structure (Fig. 48.6).

The location and size of the restoration will determine the type of permanent restorative material to be used.

### Special Considerations

With any type of restoration that involves the occlusal or incisal surface, the dentist must evaluate the patient's occlusion after replacing tooth structure. An easy way for the dentist to review how the tooth occludes with an opposing tooth is to mark the occlusion with **articulating paper** after the restorative process.

See Procedure 48.1: Assisting in a Class I Restoration.

## Class II Restorations

The class II lesion is an extension of the class I cavity into the proximal surfaces of the premolars and molars. The proximal surfaces of a tooth can be more difficult to keep decay free, especially if a patient is not disciplined with a routine flossing regimen. Class II decay involves the following areas:

- Two-surface restoration of a posterior tooth (Fig. 48.7, *A*)
- Three-surface restoration of a posterior tooth (Fig. 48.7, *B*)
- Multisurface restoration (four or more surfaces) of a posterior tooth (Fig. 48.7, *C*)

### Tooth Preparation

Because of the difficulty involved in reaching the proximal surfaces with a handpiece or a hand instrument, the dentist will involve the occlusal surface in the preparation and restoration of the tooth. A class II restoration can be termed **conservative,** where it involves two surfaces of a tooth, or **comprehensive,** where it involves four or more surfaces and the removal of a cusp. The decay may extend from the enamel into the dentin, which would require the placement of additional retention in the cavity preparation with the

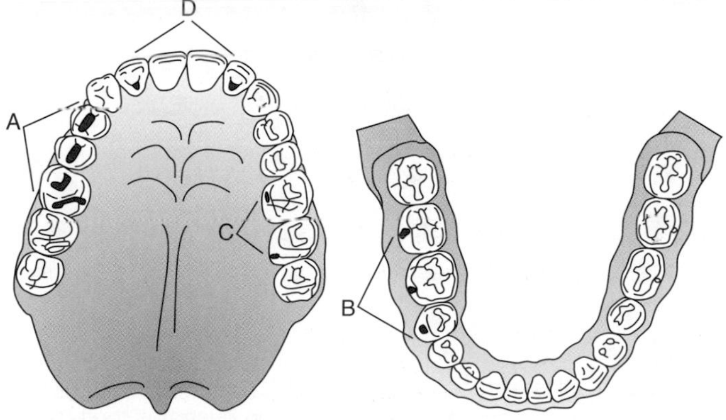


FIG. 48.5 Class I restorations. A, Occlusal pits and fissures of premolar/molar. B, Buccal pits and fissures of mandibular molars. C, Lingual pits and fissures of maxillary molars. D, Lingual pits of maxillary incisors.

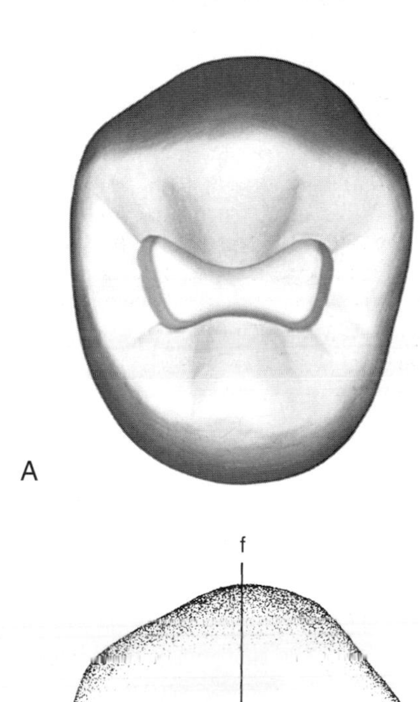


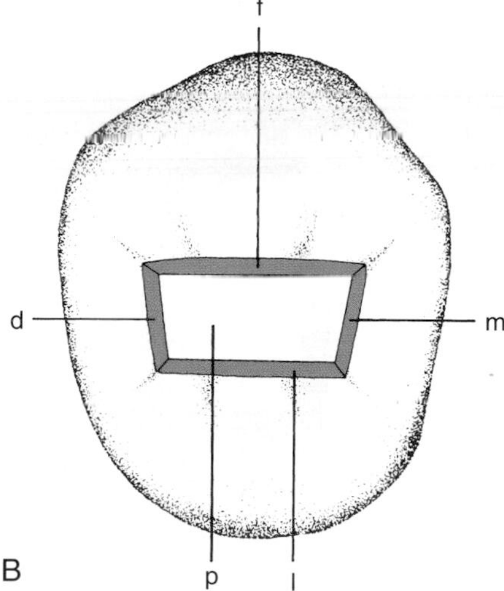


FIG. 48.6 A, Typical class I tooth preparation for amalgam on maxillary premolar. B, Schematic representation illustrates tooth preparation walls: facial *(f)*, mesial *(m)*, distal *(d)*, pulpal floor *(p)*, and lingual *(l)*. *(From Roberson TM, Heymann HO, Swift EJ: Sturdevant's art and science of operative dentistry, ed 5, St Louis, 2006, Mosby.)*

use of rotary instruments and the use of bonding materials (Fig. 48.8).

Either amalgam or composite resin can be selected as a direct restorative material for a class II restoration.

### *Special Considerations*

The outline of a class II preparation involves the removal of one or both of the proximal surfaces. Because the mesial or distal (or both) walls of the tooth are missing, little to no support is available to hold the material in place. A **matrix system** is required for this procedure. See Chapter 49 on the description and placement of a posterior matrix.

See Procedure 48.2: Assisting in a Class II Restoration.

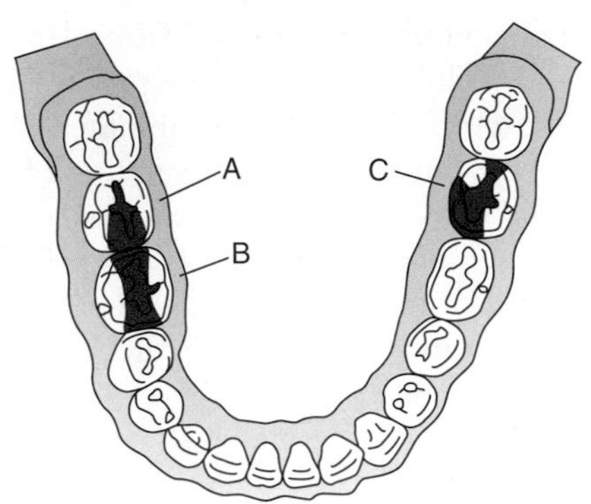


**FIG. 48.7** Class II restorations. A, Two-surface restoration. B, Three-surface restoration. C, Multisurface restoration.

## Class III and IV Restorations

A class III lesion affects the interproximal surfaces (mesial or distal) of incisors and canines (Fig. 48.9). A class IV lesion involves a larger surface area (mesial or distal), which includes the incisal edge and the interproximal surfaces of incisors and canines (Fig. 48.10).

### *Tooth Preparation*

The anatomy of anterior teeth is such that the dentist is able to access the interproximal surface without affecting other surfaces of the tooth. If possible, the dentist will enter the tooth from the lingual surface to reduce the size of the restoration from the facial aspect. If the decay has progressed subgingival, special precautions are used to keep the area isolated and dry during the restorative process.

Because incisors and canines are visible, esthetics is a concern. The dentist will select a **composite resin** when restoring the class III or IV preparation (Fig. 48.11). It is important to pay special attention to the shade selection

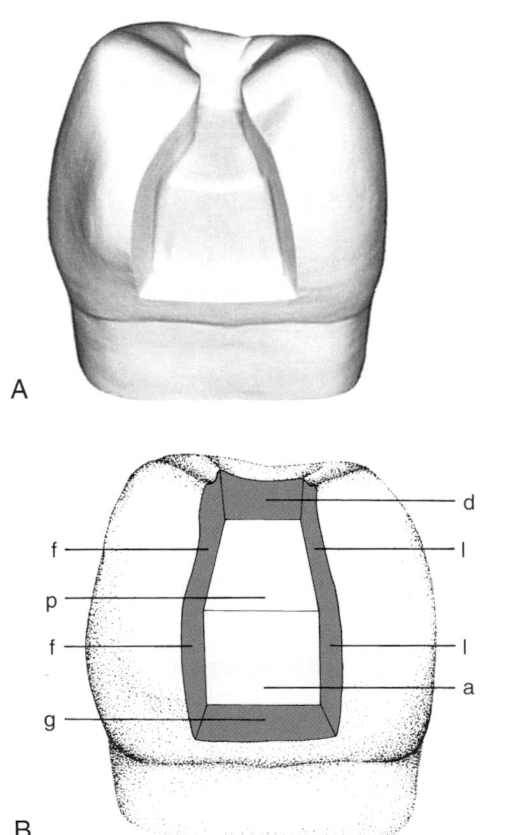


**FIG. 48.8** A, Typical class II MO conventional tooth preparation for amalgam on a maxillary molar. B, Schematic representation illustrates tooth preparation walls: molar *(a)*, facial *(f)* of proximal and incisal portions, gingival *(g)*, and lingual *(l)* of proximal and incisal portions. *(From Roberson TM, Heymann HO, Swift EJ: Sturdevant's art and science of operative dentistry, ed 5, St Louis, 2006, Mosby.)*

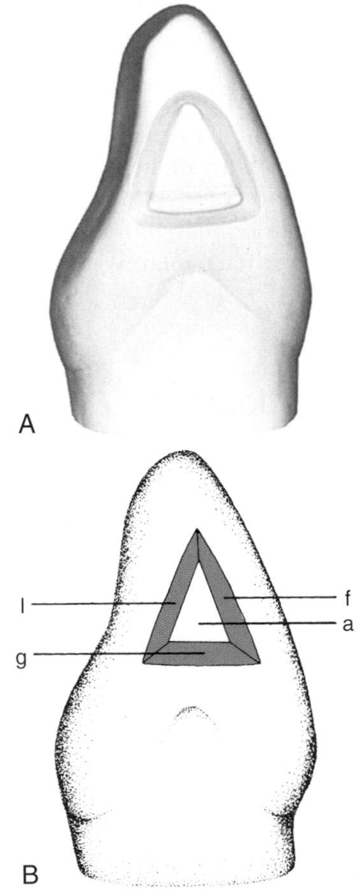


**FIG. 48.9** A, Class III conventional tooth preparation on maxillary central incisor. B, Schematic representation illustrates tooth preparation walls: axial *(a)*, facial *(f)* of proximal and incisal portions, gingival *(g)*, and lingual *(l)* of proximal and incisal portions. *(From Roberson TM, Heymann HO, Swift EJ: Sturdevant's art and science of operative dentistry, ed 5, St Louis, 2006, Mosby.)*

of the composite resin material. Use natural lighting, and involve the patient in the selection of the shade of the material.

### Special Considerations

It is advisable to use a dental dam during the preparation and restoration of class III and IV lesions. This type of isolation provides better retraction of gingival tissue and maintains a drier environment when applying dental materials.

The dentist will pay close attention to the contouring of a class III or IV restoration, making sure to reproduce the correct contours and contacts. To help in the contouring process, a **Mylar matrix system** is used in the restoration process. See Chapter 49 on the description and placement of an anterior matrix.

See Procedure 48.3: Assisting in a Class III or IV Restoration.

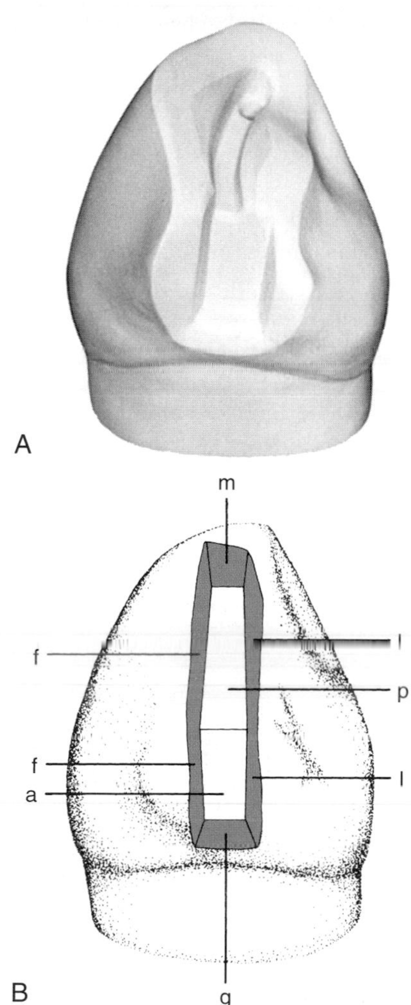


**FIG. 48.10** A, Class IV conventional tooth preparation of maxillary canine. B, Schematic representation illustrates tooth preparation walls: axial *(a)*, facial *(f)* of proximal and incisal portions, gingival *(g)*, lingual *(l)* of proximal and incisal portions, and mesial *(m)*. *(From Roberson TM, Heymann HO, Swift EJ: Sturdevant's art and science of operative dentistry, ed 5, St Louis, 2006, Mosby.)*

## Class V Restorations

The class V restoration is classified as a **smooth surface restoration.** These decayed lesions occur on the gingival third of the facial or lingual surface of any tooth (Fig. 48.12). In the older population, class V lesions also tend to progress near the cementoenamel junction, and possibly onto the root of the tooth.

### Tooth Preparation

As with class I restorations, the class V lesion is prepared by having a smooth outline with no angles. The location of a class V lesion determines the type of material selected. The dentist would prefer to use a composite resin material for esthetic purposes, but the moisture control factor in this area may prohibit its use.

### Special Considerations

One of the most important considerations for the dentist when restoring this area of the tooth is the proximity of the gingiva to the lesion. It is important to be able to retract the gingiva away from the lesion during the preparation and restoration stages and keep the area as clean and dry as possible. The application of the dental dam provides this added gingival retraction. A cervical clamp is used in this procedure to move the dam subgingivally. If a dental dam is not placed, the dentist may select the placement of a gingival retraction cord for better visibility and for reduction in moisture and hemorrhage from that area.

See Procedure 48.4: Assisting in a Class V Restoration.

RECALL

5 Where in the mouth would you find a class I restoration?
6 How many surfaces can be involved in a class II restoration?
7 Would a class II restoration be located in the anterior or posterior teeth?
8 What restorative material would you set up for a class IV procedure?
9 What type of moisture control is recommended for class III and IV restorations?
10 What population has a higher incidence of class V lesions that progress onto the root of the tooth?

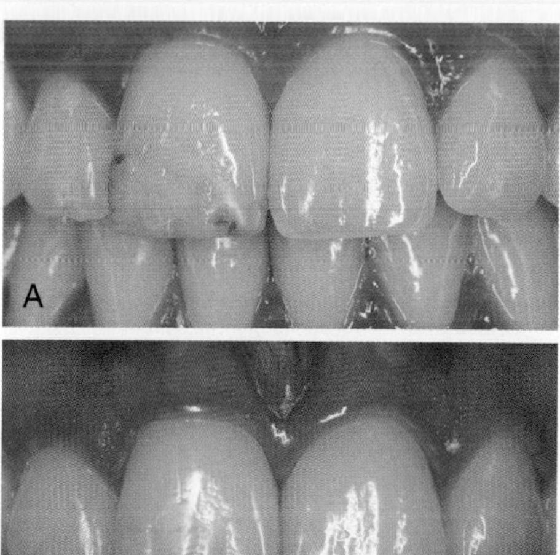


**FIG. 48.11** Class IV composite restoration with decay affecting the distal-incisal surfaces. *(Courtesy of Dr. Didier Dietschi.)*

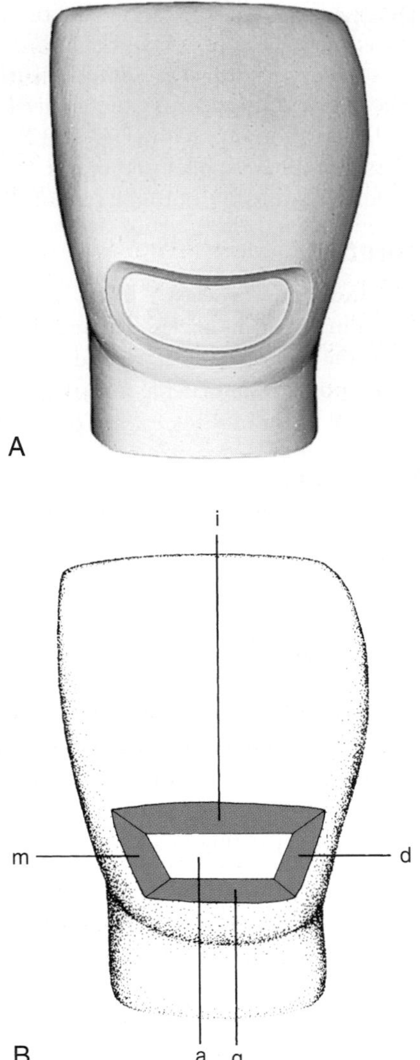


**FIG. 48.12** A, Class V conventional tooth preparation of maxillary canine. B, Schematic representation illustrates tooth preparation walls: axial *(a)*, facial *(f)*, distal *(d)*, gingival *(g)*, incisal *(i)*, and mesial *(m)*. *(From Roberson TM, Heymann HO, Swift EJ: Sturdevant's art and science of operative dentistry, ed 5, St Louis, 2006, Mosby.)*

# Complex Restorations

There are situations, during tooth preparation, when the loss of tooth structure will become greater than what is remaining of the natural tooth. In these cases, the dentist will decide whether to (1) move ahead and restore the tooth with a direct restoration, or (2) change the treatment plan and advise the patient that an indirect restoration such as an onlay or crown would be more suitable. If the dentist and the patient agree to move ahead with a direct restoration, additional techniques can be used to help retain or hold the restoration in place.

## Retention Pins

When decay has extended beyond a specific classification, it may be necessary for the dentist to use a stronger system to retain and support the restoration other than retentive grooves or bonding materials. **Retention (retentive) pins** can provide this additional means. For example, a pin may be required when tooth decay has extended into the distolingual cusp, undermining the enamel and dentin. In general, when retention is required, one pin is placed for each missing cusp (Fig. 48.13).

Pins are available in several diameters (widths) and styles. The retention pin has deep threads that grip the dentin when screwed into the tooth structure. The other end of the pin grips the restorative material. Because all pins are very small and are easily misplaced or dropped, it is essential that the dental dam be in place during the process of preparing and placing the pins.

# Intermediate Restorations

An intermediate restoration is a temporary restoration that can be placed in any tooth or surface for a short period of time. The use of this type of restoration is a preliminary step toward providing a patient with a permanent restoration. The dentist would recommend placement of an intermediate restoration for three primary reasons: (1) to wait and determine the health of a tooth, (2) while waiting to receive a permanent restoration, or (3) for financial reasons.

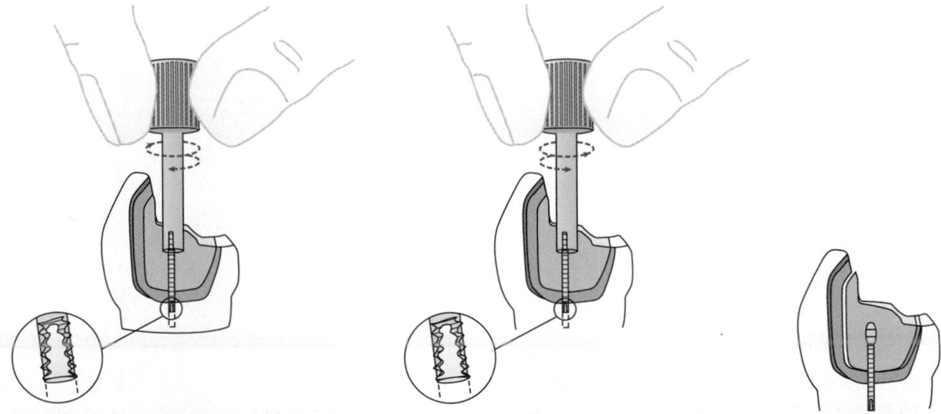

**FIG. 48.13** Retention (retentive) pins placed in tooth structure for retaining and supporting a restoration.

Chapter 43 discusses the types of dental materials commonly used when a temporary restoration is required. Intermediate restorative material (IRM) is the type of material most commonly used for this procedure when tooth structure is replaced.

Because this is a short-term rather than a permanent restoration, many states, provinces, and territories have approved this procedure as an **expanded function** for the certified dental assistant.

See Procedure 48.5: Placing and Carving an Intermediate Restoration.

**11** What are three reasons why an intermediate restoration would be placed rather than a permanent restoration?
**12** Is the placement of an intermediate restoration an expanded function of the dental assistant?

## Veneers

A **veneer** is a thin layer of tooth-colored material that is applied to the facial surface of a prepared tooth. A veneer may be placed on one or more anterior teeth for an esthetic purpose. Veneers are used to improve the appearance of teeth that are slightly abraded, eroded, discolored with intrinsic stains, or darkened following endodontic treatment (Fig. 48.14). Veneers can also improve the alignment of teeth or close a **diastema** (Fig. 48.15).

There are two distinctive techniques used in the placement of veneers. The **direct technique** uses a composite resin to create a veneer that is bonded directly to the prepared facial tooth surface. The **indirect technique,** which is a more complex procedure, is a porcelain veneer that is prepared by the dental laboratory technician and cemented to the prepared facial tooth surface. See Chapter 50 for the indirect technique.

Regardless of the type of veneer that is applied, the patient is advised of the following instructions:

- Veneers have a limited life span and must be watched for any wear, chipping, or discoloration that may occur and require replacement.
- Good oral hygiene is important to keep the surfaces and margins free of plaque and food debris.
- Biting on hard substances such as ice and hard candy can fracture the veneer.

See Procedure 48.6: Assisting in the Placement of a Direct Veneer.

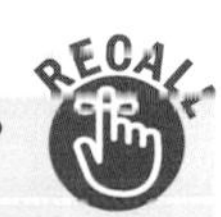


**13** What tooth surface most often receives a veneer?
**14** What is the difference between a direct and an indirect veneer?

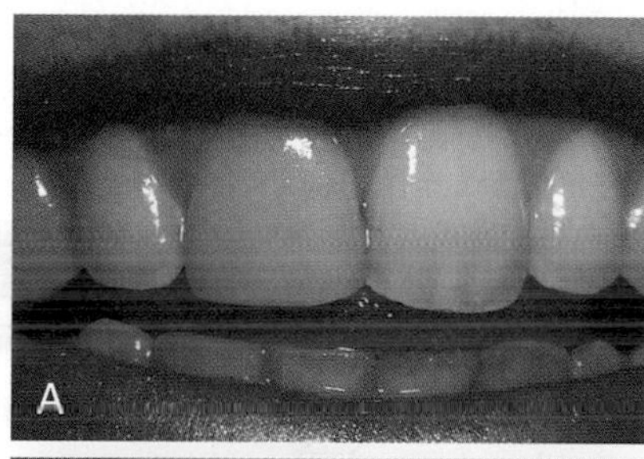


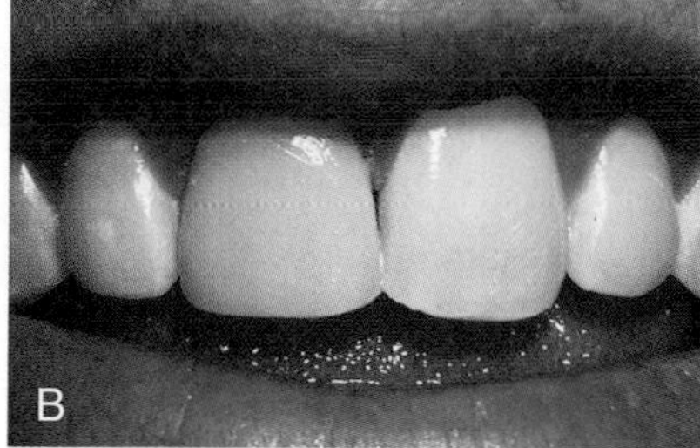


**FIG. 48.14** Veneers placed on tooth #8 and tooth #9 to reduce discoloration and cover stain. A, Before placement. B, After placement. *(From Heymann HO, Swift EJ, Ritter AV: Sturdevant's art and science of operative dentistry, ed 6, St Louis, 2013, Mosby.)*

## Tooth Whitening

Tooth whitening, also referred to as **vital bleaching,** is a noninvasive method of lightening stained or discolored teeth. There are three primary indications for prescribing a tooth-whitening procedure:

1. Extrinsic stains, which are stains that appear on the surface of the teeth as a result of exposure to coffee, tea, red wine, certain foods, or tobacco products (Fig. 48.16)
2. Aged teeth; as a person ages and with routine wear and tear the enamel wears down, teeth become more transparent, and the yellow color of dentin begins to show through
3. Intrinsic stains, such as trauma, aging, exposure to tetracycline during tooth formation, and/or the ingestion of fluoride causing fluorosis (Fig. 48.17)

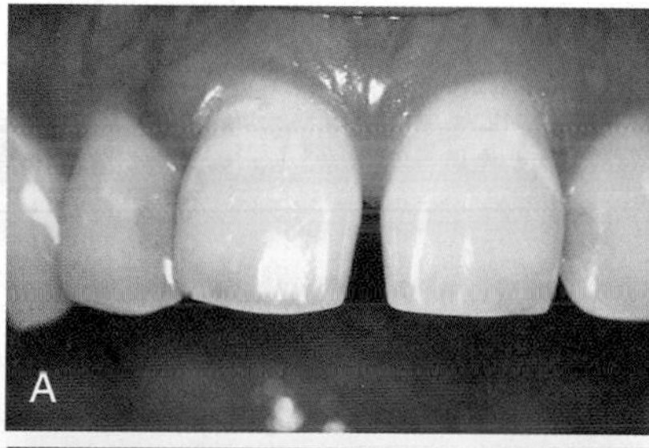


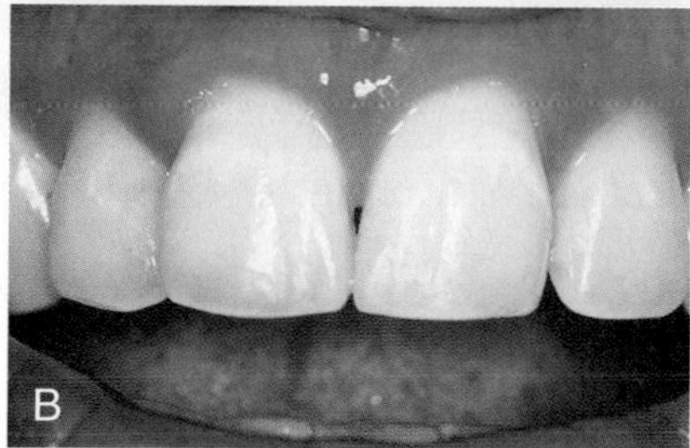


**FIG. 48.15** Veneers placed to close diastema. *(From Heymann HO, Swift EJ, Ritter AV: Sturdevant's art and science of operative dentistry, ed 6, St Louis, 2013, Mosby.)*

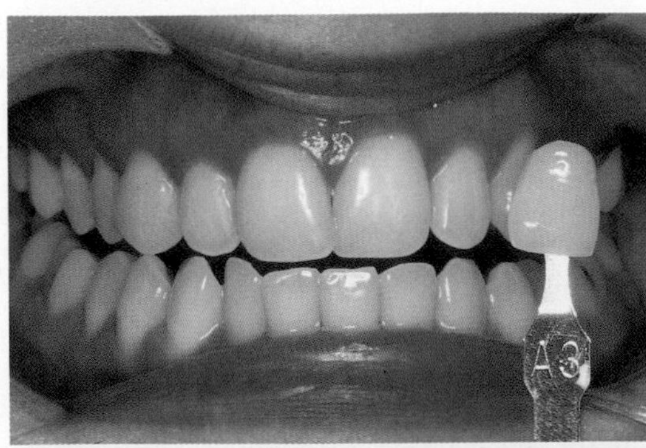


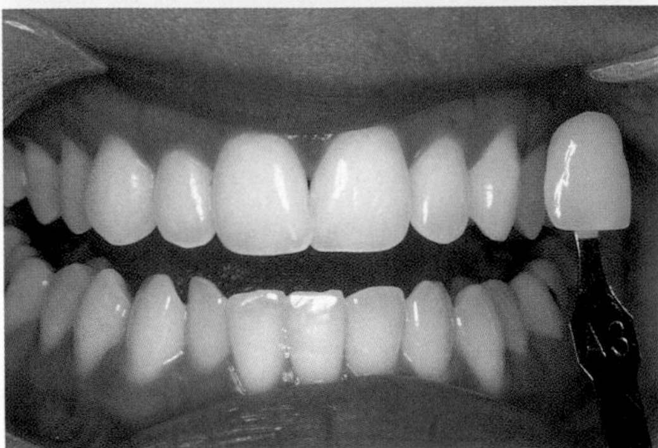


**FIG. 48.16** Before and after photos of tooth whitening used for extrinsic stains.

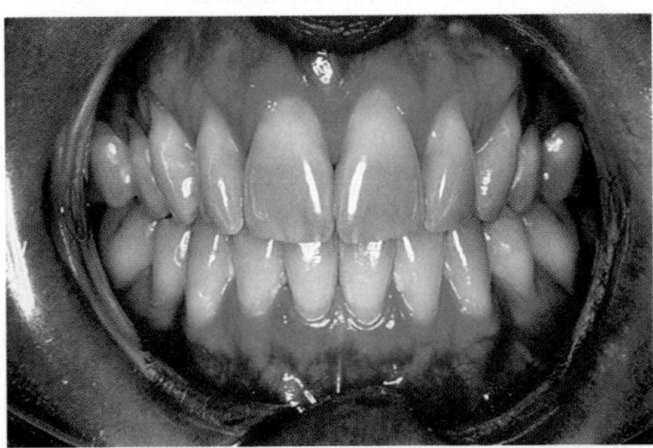

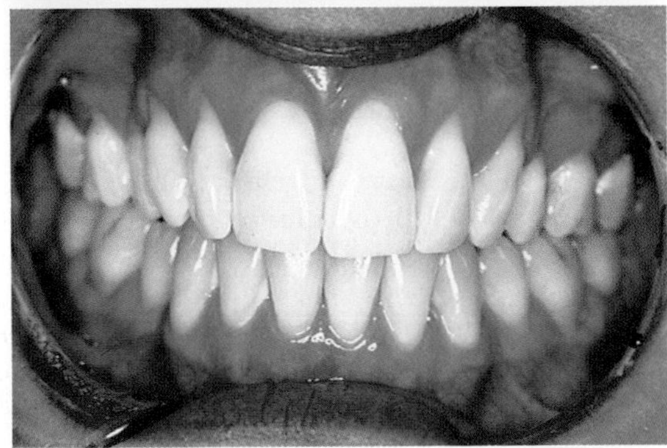

**FIG. 48.17** Before and after photos of tooth whitening used for intrinsic stains. *(From Heymann HO, Swift EJ, Ritter AV: Sturdevant's art and science of operative dentistry, ed 6, St Louis, 2013, Mosby.)*

Chapter 58 provides an in-depth background in different types of stains.

Tooth whitening is often requested by the patient and has become a routine procedure that includes both in-office options and professionally supervised at-home options. The patient must be made aware that the results are not guaranteed and are not permanent. Most whitening systems last for 3 to 5 years.

Not everyone can be recommended a tooth-whitening procedure. Teeth that have existing resin-colored restorations, veneers, or fixed restorations fabricated with porcelain cannot be whitened from hydrogen or carbamide peroxide. The materials will not whiten past the color they were originally made from.

Chapter 43 describes the composition of whitening products.

## Treatment Options

There are three major teeth-whitening options available today. All three rely on a different concentration of peroxide and varying application times. The main ingredient in tooth-whitening products is hydrogen or carbamide peroxide, which is what actually whitens the enamel. The concentration or strength of the gel can range from 10 percent for over-the-counter products, to 16 percent in the at-home whitening procedure, to 22 percent with the in-office procedure.

### *In-Office Treatment*

Professionally applied tooth whitening can be accomplished by the dentist in as little as 1 hour. The patient will see results, with the teeth becoming as much as five shades lighter. This appointment requires the dental team to follow specific criteria in the application:

- Complete isolation of the teeth involved (includes use of the dental dam or a light-reflective resin barrier)
- Whitening agent at a higher concentration applied to the facial surfaces of teeth
- Light or laser source used to enhance the application

### *At-Home Treatment*

The decision to use a whitening product at home under the care of a dentist is another option for a patient who wants this procedure. The patient will see results within a couple of weeks and can anticipate up to six shades lighter from this process. The patient must follow specific criteria for application:

- Having a custom-fitted tray made in the dental office to hold the peroxide-based gel (Fig. 48.18)
- Having a supply of peroxide-based gel available for application for the suggested length of time (Fig. 48.19)

Usage regimens vary. Some products are used twice a day for 2 weeks, and others are intended for overnight use for 1 to 2 weeks.

### *Over-the-Counter Options*

A variety of over-the-counter tooth-whitening products are available today. Most of the products that are manufactured by the larger oral health companies are safe, reliable, and effective. However, these products will not achieve the dramatic changes that may be made with dentist-supervised products. The three types of over-the-counter tooth-whitening systems

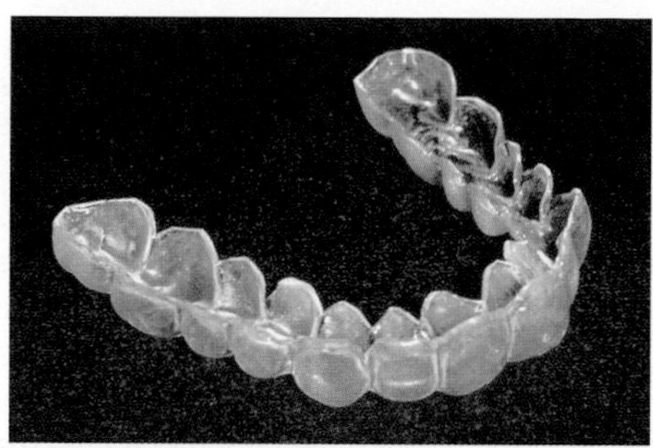

**FIG. 48.18** Custom-fitted tray for bleaching procedure.

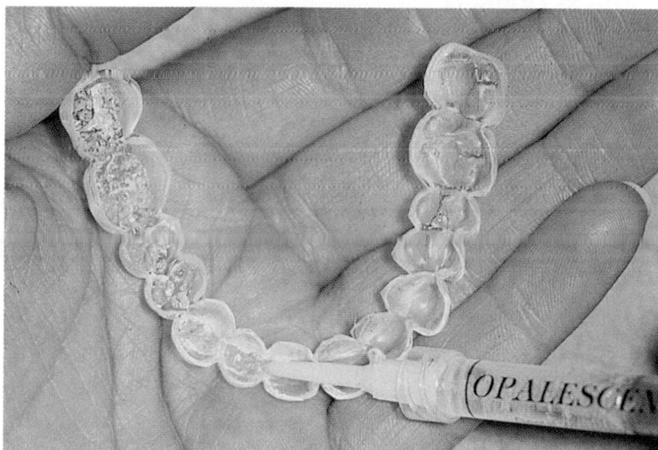


**FIG. 48.19** Loading peroxide gel into custom-fitted tray. *(Courtesy Ultradent, South Jordan, UT.)*

that are most commonly used are brush-on whitening, whitening strips, and trays with bleaching gels.

**BRUSH-ON WHITENING.** Brush-on whitening gel can be purchased at most drugstores. The gel contains peroxide that, after it has been painted on the facial surfaces of the teeth, will whiten surface stains through an oxidation process. It is important to explain to your patients that they should expect a minimum amount of whitening from this technique. Other tooth-whitening methods are much more effective. For this type of whitening, the brush-on gel must remain on the teeth for a specified time, but saliva flow inhibits the effectiveness of this method. If they are not used properly, brush-on whiteners can cause blotches on the teeth.

**WHITENING STRIPS.** These thin, flexible strips are coated with an adhesive hydrogen peroxide whitening gel. The patient peels off the backing like a bandage and then presses the strip to the facial anterior teeth, ensuring that the upper edge of the strip is at the gingival margin. The remaining portion of the strip is folded onto the lingual surface. New advanced bleaching components have been added to the strips and stronger adhesive qualities are available, making this choice of whitening technique very popular, with visible results in 7 to 10 days.

**TRAYS WITH BLEACHING GELS.** Teeth-whitening kits have become very popular because the process is affordable, the patient receives good results, and the results are long lasting with minimal adverse effects. Teeth-whitening gel trays are very similar to what a patient would receive in the dental office, except that the bleaching process is completed at home. The type of kit most commonly used involves a tray that is molded to the mouth by boiling it in water; the tray is allowed to cool slightly, and then it is placed in the mouth until it molds to the teeth. Once the tray is completely cooled, it is filled with peroxide gel and placed in the mouth for the prescribed time, which is typically around 30 minutes.

## Dental Assistant's Role in Tooth Whitening

The role of the dental assistant in the tooth-whitening process involves the following functions and procedural steps:

- Assist in recording the medical and dental history.
- Make the shade selection.
- Take intraoral photographs before and after the whitening procedure.
- Take and pour up the preliminary impression for the custom tray.
- Fabricate and trim the tray.
- Provide preoperative instructions on use of the material.
- Assist in weekly or biweekly clinic visits.

## Patient Instructions for Tooth Whitening

Patient instructions for the gel tooth-whitening procedure include the following:

- Brush and floss before tray placement.
- Place gel in tray in equal limited amounts; less material is better than more.
- Seat the tray.
- Do not eat or drink when wearing the tray.
- Wear the tray for the recommended time.
- Discontinue using the tray if adverse effects occur.
- Discuss adverse effects or other problems with the dentist.

## Abuse of Whitening Products

With at-home and over-the-counter whitening products, the patient may have a greater potential for abuse. A patient will abuse a whitening product by not following directions or by overusing it to achieve whiter teeth. Most adverse effects are temporary, but on rare occasions, irreversible tooth damage can occur.

## Adverse Effects of Tooth Whitening

### *Sensitivity*

Bleaching procedures can create a short-term increase in sensitivity to temperature, pressure, and touch. Individuals at greatest risk for sensitivity are those with gum recession, minute cracks in their teeth, or microleakage resulting from a faulty restoration. Sensitivity can be immediate, may last a day or two, and in some cases can persist up to a month. A sensitive toothpaste can be recommended to the patient to relieve the sensitivity.

### Tissue Irritation

Gingival tissue may be exposed to excess gel because of improper fitting of the tray, allowing the material to ooze onto the gingiva. Advise the patient not to overfill the tray with material, and remind the patient to remove any excess when seating the tray.

RECALL

**15** What are the three primary indications for tooth whitening?
**16** What is used to hold whitening gel to the teeth?
**17** What is the main ingredient of whitening strip products?
**18** What adverse effects may a patient experience during tooth whitening?

**■ Patient Education** The treatment and procedures discussed in this chapter involve the process of restoring teeth to their normal function and performing procedures for esthetic purposes. Looking fit and healthy with an attractive smile is important in today's society regardless of age. Educating your patients about the way their smile can be improved is a service that helps them feel better about themselves. ■

**■ Legal and Ethical Implications** An important reason why a patient continues to seek care at a dental practice is because of the type of dental work that is performed. It is the dental team's responsibility and obligation to update their knowledge of procedures and materials on a continuing base.

If it is legal in your state to perform expanded functions such as placement of liners and bonding agents, matrices, and intermediate restorations, ensure that you are trained in the new materials and techniques being used for restorative procedures. Remember that you are putting your patient, yourself, and your dentist at liability by performing these procedures if you have not prepared and become certified in the application process. ■

**■ Eye to the Future** The future of restorative dentistry seems unlimited with the new materials being designed today. More dental products will become available as over-the-counter products for in-home use by the consumer. The dentist then will focus on more complex procedures that require the expertise of the dental assistant and the use of dental equipment. ■

## ■ Critical Thinking

1. The schedule indicates that your next patient is noted for a class II on tooth #4. Are there any additional items that you would set out for the procedure that would not be included for a class III on tooth #9?
2. Ms. Campbell will be coming in today to have a distal restoration replaced on tooth #10. Why would a patient have a restoration replaced?
3. A new patient indicates on his dental history form that he is unhappy with the appearance and color of his teeth. During initial examination and further discussion about his habits, you find out he is a coffee drinker. What procedures could be recommended to the patient to lighten the stains and color of his teeth?
4. You are assisting in a complex restoration (MODF) on tooth #30. During the final carving of the amalgam, a portion of the amalgam breaks off the distofacial cusp. What should the dentist consider to create a better retention between the amalgam and the tooth for such a large restoration?
5. Dr. Stewart is in the next operatory, finishing a surgery that is taking longer than expected. She asks you to finish etching, place primer, and begin adding increments of composite to the small class I pit. What are you legally permitted to do in this procedure? ■

PROCEDURE 48.1

# Assisting in a Class I Restoration

## EQUIPMENT AND SUPPLIES

- ✓ Restorative tray (basic setup, hand cutting instruments, composite placement instrument, amalgam carrier, condensers, burnishers, carvers, articulating paper holder)
- ✓ Local anesthetic setup
- ✓ Dental dam setup
- ✓ High-volume oral evacuator (HVE) tip
- ✓ Saliva ejector
- ✓ High-speed and low-speed handpieces
- ✓ Burs, assorted (dentist's choice)
- ✓ Cotton pellets, cotton rolls, 2 × 2–inch gauze
- ✓ Dental liners, base, sealers, bonding agents
- ✓ Permanent restorative material (composite or amalgam)
- ✓ Dental floss

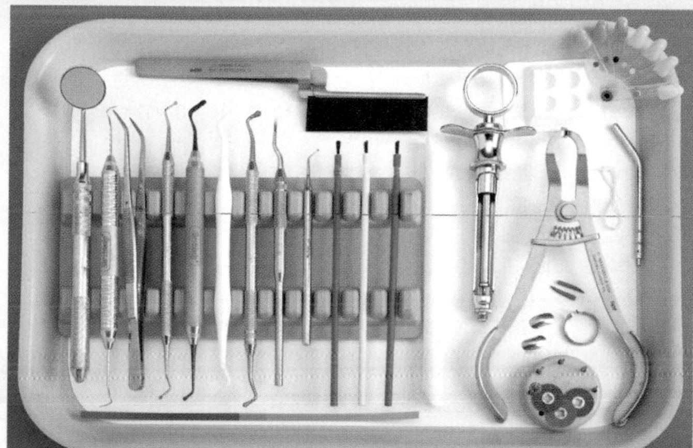

*From Boyd LB: Dental instruments: a pocket guide, ed 6, St Louis, 2018, Elsevier.*

## PROCEDURAL STEPS

### Preparing the Tooth

1 Transfer the mouth mirror and explorer to the dentist.

**PURPOSE** The dentist will examine the tooth to be prepared.

2 Assist in administration of topical and local anesthetic agents.

3 Place and secure cotton rolls or dental dam.

### Preparing the Cavity

4 Transfer the mirror and the high-speed handpiece with a cutting bur to the dentist.

5 During cavity preparation, use the HVE and the air-water syringe, adjust the light, and retract the patient's cheek as necessary to maintain a clear field for the dentist.

**PURPOSE** With efficient placement and use of the HVE and the air-water syringe, the operating field will remain clean and clear for the dentist, and this will provide comfort for the patient.

6 Transfer the explorer, excavators, and hand cutting instruments as needed throughout the cavity preparation.

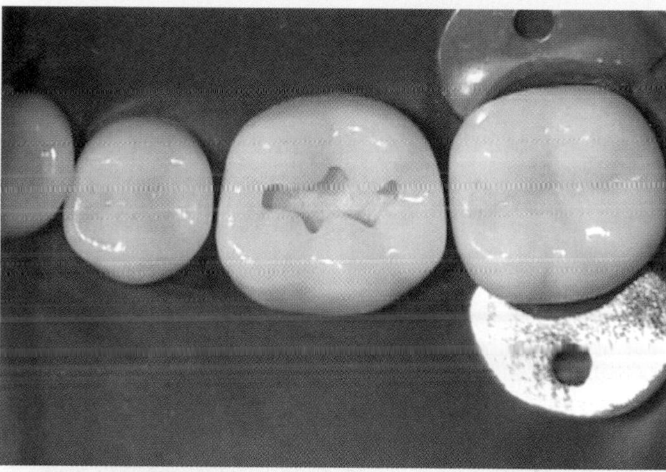

*From Heymann HO, Swift EJ, Ritter AV: Sturdevant's art and science of operative dentistry, ed 6, St Louis, 2013, Mosby.*

### Placing Dental Materials

7 Rinse and dry the preparation for the dentist to evaluate.

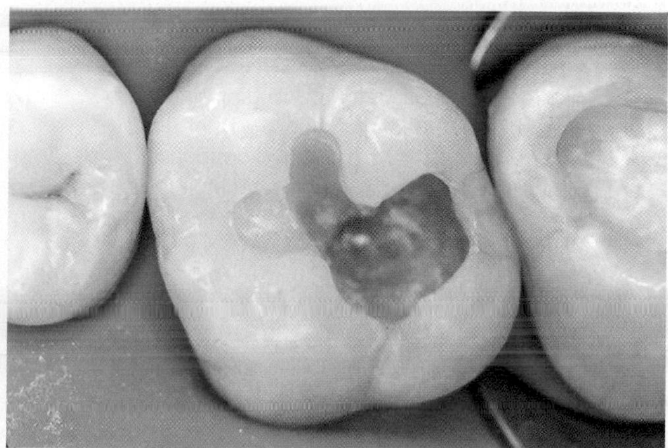

*From Heymann HO, Swift EJ, Ritter AV: Sturdevant's art and science of operative dentistry, ed 6, St Louis, 2013, Mosby.*

8 If a base, liner, or sealer is required, mix and transfer or apply the materials in the proper sequence.

(Continued)

## PROCEDURE 48.1 Assisting in a Class I Restoration–cont'd

9 After the tooth is etched and primed, prepare and transfer or apply the bonding material before the permanent material is readied.

10 If using amalgam, activate the capsule, place in the amalgamator, close the cover, and mix according to the recommended time.

11 If using composite, place a small amount of a universal color material on a paper pad, protecting it from transient light, and ready the material for placement.

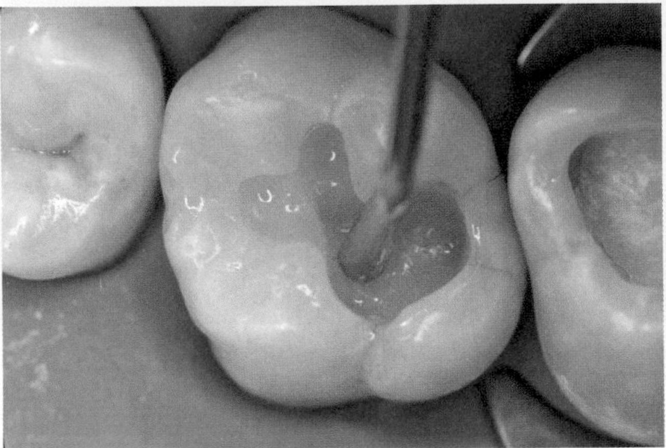

*From Heymann HO, Swift EJ, Ritter AV: Sturdevant's art and science of operative dentistry, ed 6, St Louis, 2013, Mosby.*

### Placing Permanent Material

12 With amalgam, fill the smaller end of the amalgam carrier and transfer the carrier to the dentist for placement, with the condenser in the transfer position ready for use.

13 Assist as the process of placing and condensing the amalgam is repeated until the preparation is slightly overfilled.

14 When the preparation is slightly overfilled, exchange the condenser for the burnisher so that the dentist can burnish the surface and margins of the restoration.

**PURPOSE** This strengthens the finished restoration by burnishing the excess mercury to the surface.

15 With composite, carry the material to the transfer zone with the composite placement instrument. The dentist will apply the material to the preparation in increments, following each placement with the curing light.

**NOTE** The depth of the restoration will determine how often the curing light is used.

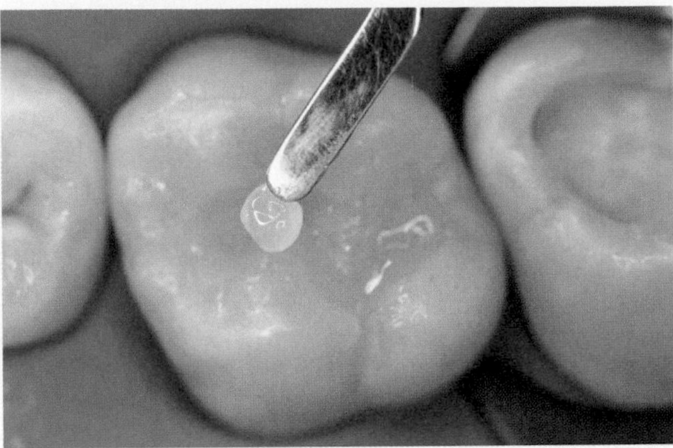

*From Heymann HO, Swift EJ, Ritter AV: Sturdevant's art and science of operative dentistry, ed 6, St Louis, 2013, Mosby.*

### Final Carving or Finishing

16 For amalgam, transfer the carvers until the carving is complete.

17 For composite, transfer the high-speed handpiece with finishing burs.

18 Keep the tip of the HVE close to the restoration during the carving and finishing process.

**PURPOSE** To remove all particles as soon as possible. This step is especially important when a dental dam is not used.

### Occlusal Adjustment

19 Remove the cotton rolls or the dental dam, and rinse and dry the area.

20 Position the articulating paper within the quadrant, and instruct the patient to "tap" his or her teeth together very gently, and then to move his or her bite from side to side.

**NOTE** Heavy blue marks will appear on any high spots on the new restoration. The patient is cautioned to not bite too hard, or the restoration may fracture.

21 Assist with transfers as necessary while the dentist uses a carver or a finishing bur to remove any remaining high spots.

**NOTE** This step is repeated as often as necessary to bring the new restoration into proper occlusion.

22 Transfer a moistened cotton pellet or cotton roll to gently clean the surface of the restoration.

**PURPOSE** To remove any remaining small surface irregularities.

## PROCEDURE 48.1 Assisting in a Class I Restoration–cont'd

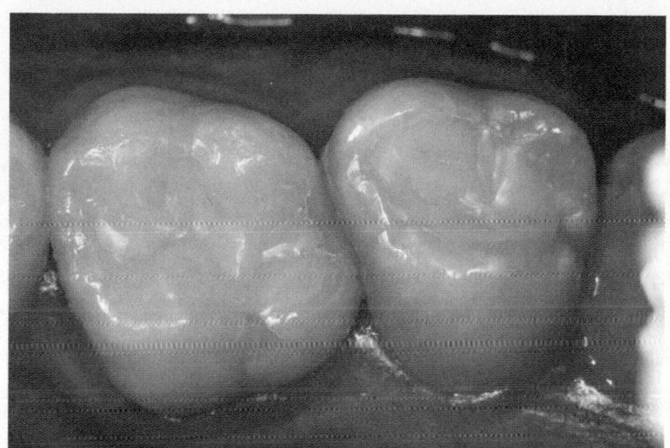

*From Heymann HO, Swift EJ, Ritter AV: Sturdevant's art and science of operative dentistry, ed 6, St Louis, 2013, Mosby.*

### Postoperative Instructions

**23** Caution the patient not to chew on a new amalgam restoration for a few hours.

**PURPOSE** Amalgam takes several hours to reach its maximum strength, and biting or chewing on that side could cause the restoration to fracture.

### Documentation

**24** Document the procedure.

| Date | Tooth | Surface | Charting Notes |
|---|---|---|---|
| 7/20/17 | 3 | O | 1 cartridge Xylocaine w/o epi, dam application, glass ionomer base, Filltec. Procedure well tolerated by patient. Return for 6 mo recall. |

T. Clark, CDA/L, Stewart, DDS

  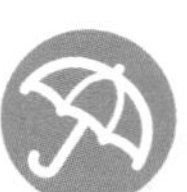 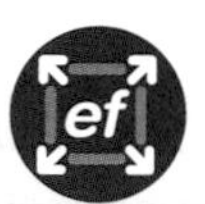

## PROCEDURE 48.2 

# Assisting in a Class II Amalgam Restoration

### EQUIPMENT AND SUPPLIES

- Restorative tray (basic setup, hand cutting instruments, composite placement instrument, amalgam carrier, condensers, burnishers, carvers, articulating paper holder)
- Local anesthetic setup
- Dental dam setup
- High-volume oral evacuator (HVE) tip
- Saliva ejector
- High-speed and low-speed handpieces
- Burs, assorted (dentist's choice)
- Matrix setup
- Dental liners, base, sealers, bonding agents
- Premeasured amalgam capsules
- Dental floss
- Articulating paper
- Cotton pellets, cotton rolls, 2 × 2–inch gauze
- Dental floss

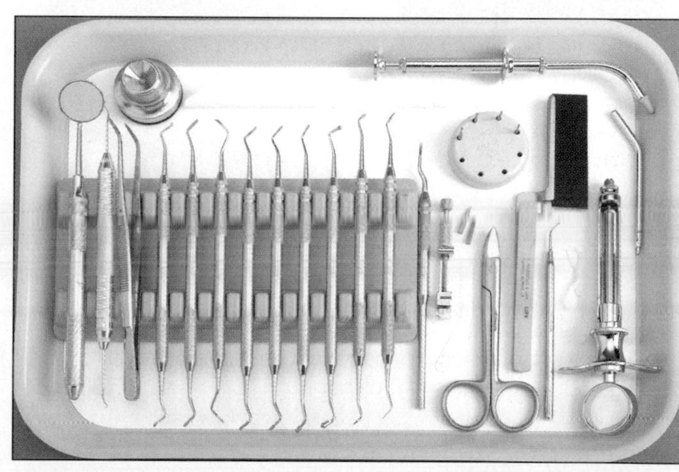

*From Boyd LB: Dental instruments: a pocket guide, ed 6, St Louis, 2018, Elsevier.*

### PROCEDURAL STEPS

### Preparing the Tooth

**1** Transfer the mouth mirror and explorer to the dentist

**PURPOSE** The dentist examines the tooth to be prepared.

(Continued)

## PROCEDURE 48.2 Assisting in a Class II Amalgam Restoration—cont'd

2 Assist in administration of the local anesthetic agent.
3 Place and secure moisture control techniques (cotton roll, dental dam).

### Preparing the Cavity

4 Transfer the mirror and the high-speed handpiece with cutting bur to the dentist.
5 During cavity preparation, use the HVE and the air-water syringe, adjust the light, and retract the patient's cheek as necessary to maintain a clear field for the dentist.

**PURPOSE** With efficient placement and use of the HVE and the air-water syringe, the operating field will remain clean and clear for the dentist, and this will provide comfort to the patient.

6 Transfer the explorer, excavators, and hand cutting instruments as needed throughout the cavity preparation.

### Placing the Base and Cavity Liner (Expanded Function)

7 After examination, rinse and dry the preparation. Mix and place any necessary cavity liners or bases.

### Placing the Matrix Band and Wedge (Expanded Function)

8 Assist or place the preassembled universal (Tofflemire) retainer and matrix.

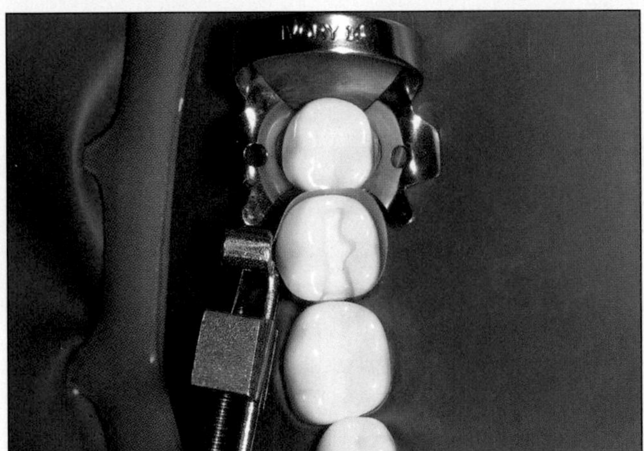

9 Assist or place the wedge or wedges in the proximal box using cotton pliers or #110 pliers.

### Placing the Bonding Agent (Expanded Function)

10 After the tooth has been etched and primed, assist the dentist in preparing and placing the bonding material.

### Mixing the Amalgam

11 Activate the capsule, place in the amalgamator, close the cover, and set the timer for the time recommended by the manufacturer.
12 At the signal from the dentist, start the amalgamator.
13 Open the capsule, and remove the pestle with cotton pliers. Drop the amalgam into the amalgam well.
14 Reassemble and discard the capsule.

**PURPOSE** To prevent mercury vapor from escaping into the air.

### Placing and Condensing the Amalgam

15 Fill the smaller end of the amalgam carrier, and transfer the carrier to the dentist.
16 Assist when necessary as the dentist exchanges the carrier for a condenser and begins condensing the first increments of amalgam with the smaller end of the condenser.

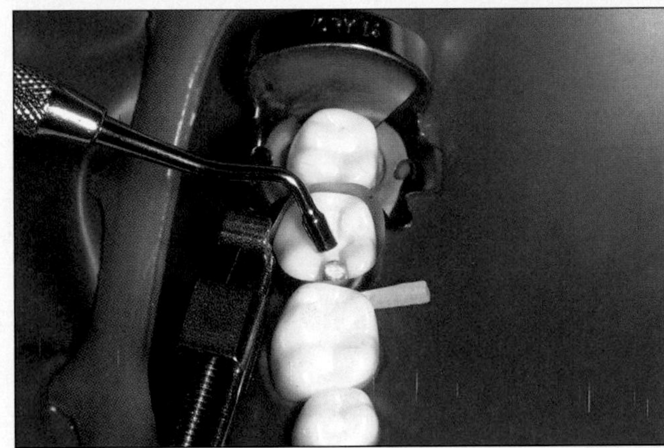

17 Assist as the process of placing and condensing the amalgam is repeated until the cavity has been slightly overfilled.
18 When the cavity preparation is slightly overfilled, exchange the condenser for the burnisher, so that the dentist can burnish the surface and margins of the restoration.

**PURPOSE** This strengthens the filled restoration by burnishing the excess mercury to the surface.

## PROCEDURE 48.2 Assisting in a Class II Amalgam Restoration–cont'd

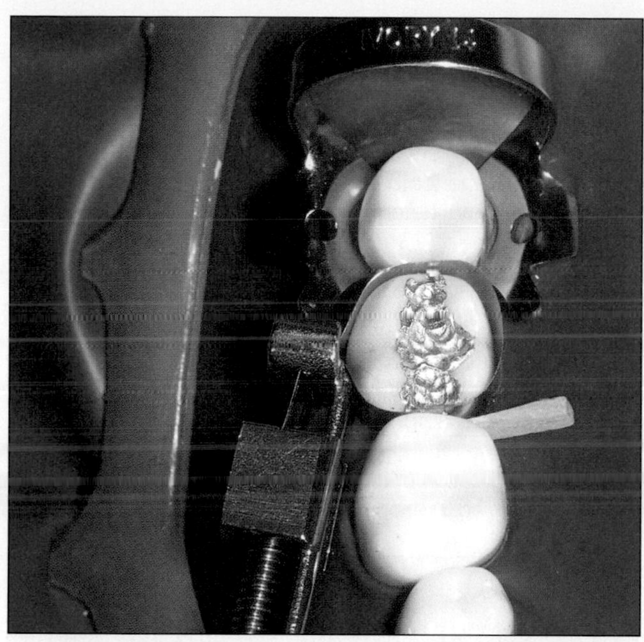

### Initial Carving

19 Assist while the dentist uses an explorer and a discoid/cleoid carver to remove excess amalgam from the occlusal surface, from between the matrix band, and at the marginal ridge of the tooth.

**PURPOSE** This prevents the restoration from fracturing during removal of the matrix band.

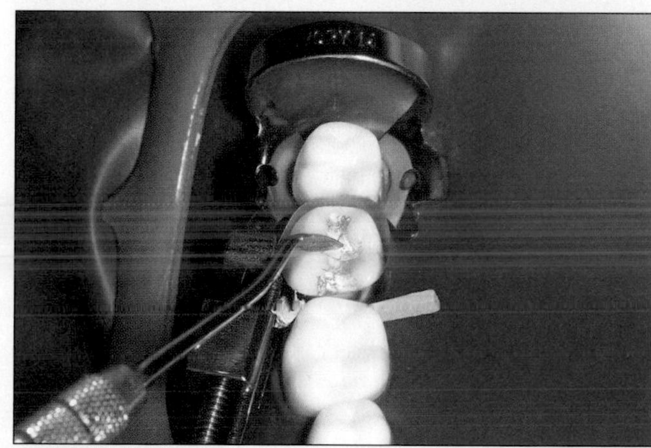

20 Assist in removing the Tofflemire retainer, matrix band, and wedge.

### Final Carving

21 Transfer the amalgam carvers until the carving is complete.

22 Keep the tip of the HVE close to the restoration during the carving process.

**PURPOSE** To remove all amalgam particles as soon as possible.

**NOTE** This step is especially important when a dental dam is not used.

### Occlusal Adjustment

23 Remove moisture control materials (cotton rolls, dental dam).

24 Position the articulating paper within the quadrant, and instruct the patient to "tap" his or her teeth together very gently, and then to move his or her bite from side to side.

**NOTE** Heavy blue marks will appear on any high spots on the new restoration. The patient is cautioned to not bite too hard, or the restoration may fracture.

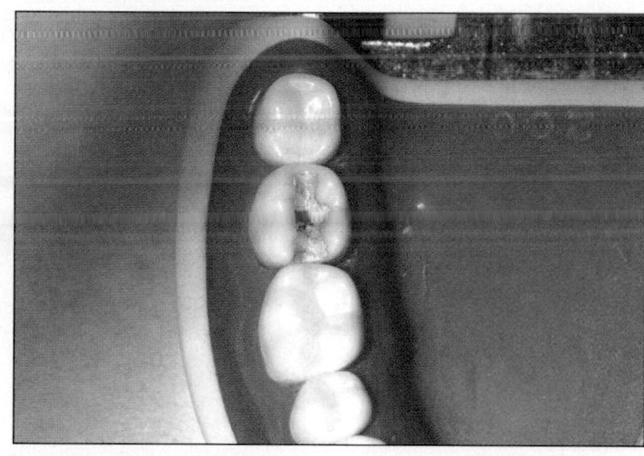

25 Assist with transfers as the dentist uses an amalgam carver to remove any remaining high spots.

**NOTE** This step is repeated as often as necessary to bring the new restoration into proper occlusion.

26 Transfer a moist cotton pellet in cotton pliers to gently rub the surface of the amalgam.

**PURPOSE** To remove any remaining small surface irregularities.

### Postoperative Instructions

27 Caution the patient not to chew on a new amalgam restoration for a few hours.

**PURPOSE** Amalgam takes several hours to reach its maximum strength, and biting or chewing on that side could cause the restoration to fracture.

### Documentation

28 Document the procedure.

| Date | Tooth | Surface | Charting Notes |
|---|---|---|---|
| 7/20/17 | 3 | MO | 1 cartridge Xylocaine w/o epi, dam isolation, dycal/etch/bond. 2 capsules of Sybralloy. Procedure well tolerated by patient. Return for 6 mo recall.<br>T. Clark, CDA/L, Stewart, DDS |

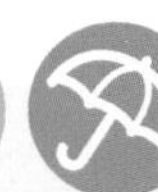

PROCEDURE 48.3

# Assisting in a Class III or IV Restoration

## EQUIPMENT AND SUPPLIES

- Restorative tray (basic setup, hand cutting instruments, composite placement instrument, amalgam carrier, condensers, burnishers, carvers, articulating paper holder)
- Composite shade guide
- Local anesthetic setup
- Dental dam setup
- HVE tip
- Saliva ejector
- High-speed and low-speed handpieces
- Burs, assorted (dentist's choice)
- Mylar matrix setup
- Dental liners, base, sealers, bonding agents
- Composite material
- Curing light with protective shield
- Finishing burs and diamonds
- Dental floss
- Articulating paper
- Cotton pellets, cotton rolls, 2 × 2–inch gauze
- Dental floss
- Abrasive strips
- Articulating paper
- Polishing kit (disc and mandrel)
- Polishing paste

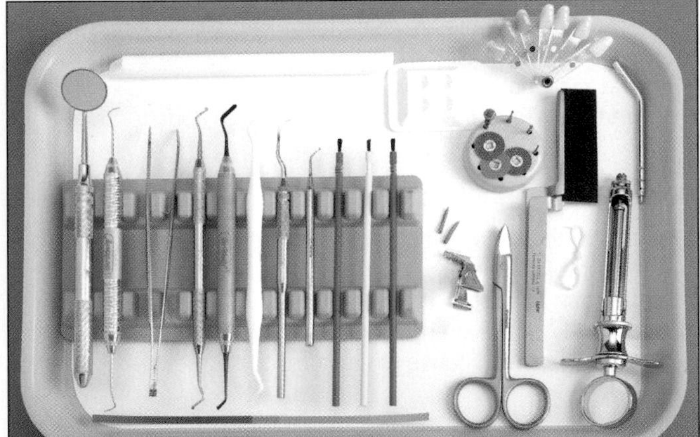

*From Boyd LB: Dental instruments: a pocket guide, ed 6, St Louis, 2018, Elsevier.*

## PROCEDURAL STEPS

### Preparing the Tooth

1 Transfer the mouth mirror and explorer to the dentist.
**PURPOSE** The dentist examines the tooth to be prepared.

2 Assist in administration of the local anesthetic.

3 Assist in selection of the shade of the composite material.

4 Place and secure moisture control techniques (cotton roll, dental dam).

### Preparing the Cavity

5 Transfer the high-speed handpiece and hand cutting instruments so the dentist can remove decayed tooth structure. Use the HVE to maintain a clear operating field.

6 Rinse and dry the tooth throughout the procedure. If indicated, the dentist will determine whether a cavity liner should be placed.

### Etching, Bonding, and Composite Placement

7 After the tooth has been prepared, the dentist will have you etch, rinse, and dry according to the manufacturer's instructions.

8 Place the matrix strip. If indicated, a wedge should also be placed.

9 Assist in application of the primer and bonding resin, which are light-cured in accordance with the manufacturer's instructions.

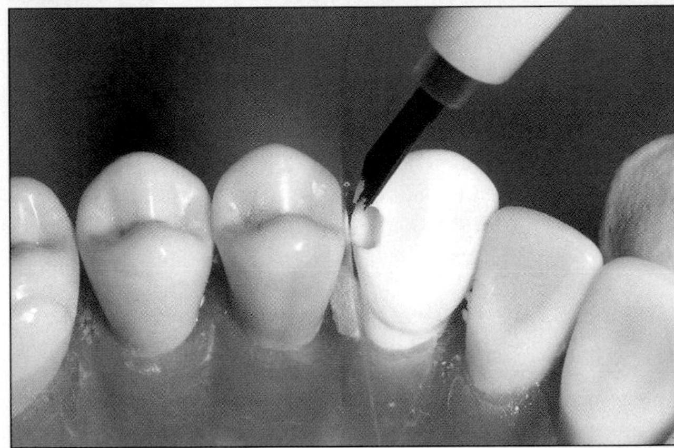

10 Dispense the composite material on a paper pad, or insert the capsule into the composite syringe, and transfer it along with the composite instrument to be placed into the preparation.

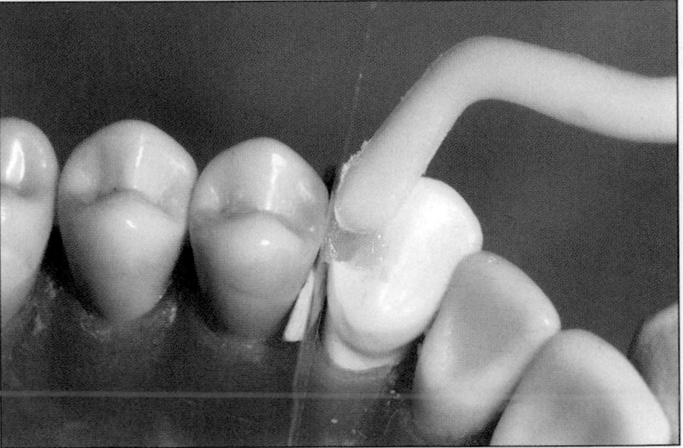

## PROCEDURE 48.3 Assisting in a Class III or IV Restoration–cont'd

**11** Assist as the matrix is pulled and held tightly around the tooth while the composite material is light-cured from the lingual and facial surfaces.

### Finishing the Restoration

**12** Assist in removal of the matrix strip and wedge.
**13** Assist with transfers as the dentist uses finishing burs or diamonds in the high-speed handpiece to contour the restoration.
**14** If indicated, transfer finishing strips to smooth the interproximal surface.
**15** Remove the moisture control technique, and use articulating paper to check the occlusion. Adjustments are made as necessary.
**16** Assist while the dentist uses polishing discs, points, and cups in the low-speed handpiece to polish the restoration

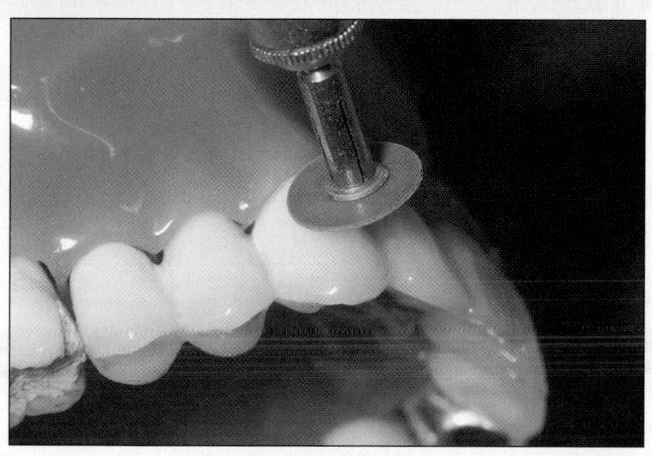

### Documentation

**17** Document the procedure.

| Date | Tooth | Surface | Charting Notes |
|---|---|---|---|
| 7/20/14 | 8 | MI | 1 cartridge Xylocaine w/o epi, dam isolation, etching/bonding/Silux, shade YL. Procedure well tolerated by patient. Return for 6 mo recall.<br>T. Clark, CDA/L, Stewart, DDS |

PROCEDURE 48.4

# Assisting in a Class V Restoration

## EQUIPMENT AND SUPPLIES

- ✓ Restorative tray (basic setup, hand cutting instruments, composite placement instrument, amalgam carrier, condensers, burnishers, carvers, articulating paper holder)
- ✓ Local anesthetic setup
- ✓ Dental dam setup (cervical clamp)
- ✓ Retraction cord and packer
- ✓ HVE tip
- ✓ Saliva ejector
- ✓ High-speed and low-speed handpieces
- ✓ Burs, assorted (dentist's choice)
- ✓ Cotton pellets, cotton rolls, 2 × 2–inch gauze
- ✓ Dental liners, base, sealers, bonding agents
- ✓ Permanent restorative material (composite or amalgam)
- ✓ Dental floss

## PROCEDURAL STEPS

### Preparing the Tooth

1 Transfer the mouth mirror and explorer to the dentist.
**PURPOSE** The dentist examines the tooth to be prepared.

2 Assist in administration of topical and local anesthetic agents.

3 Place and secure cotton rolls or dental dam.

### Preparing the Cavity

4 Transfer the mirror and the assembled high-speed handpiece with a cutting bur to the dentist.

5 During cavity preparation, use the HVE and the air-water syringe, adjust the light, and retract the patient's cheek as necessary to maintain a clear field for the dentist.
**PURPOSE** With efficient placement and use of the HVE and the air-water syringe, the dentist will maintain a clear operating field while ensuring the comfort of the patient.

6 Transfer the explorer, excavators, and hand (manual) cutting instruments as needed throughout the cavity preparation.

### Placing Dental Materials

7 Rinse and dry the preparation for evaluation. If a base, liner, or sealer is required, mix and transfer these materials in proper sequence.

8 After the tooth has been etched and primed, prepare and transfer the bonding material to the dentist before inserting the permanent material.

9 If using amalgam, activate the capsule, place it in the amalgamator, close the cover, and mix according to the recommended time.

10 If using composite, place a small amount of universal color material on a paper pad, and cover it from the light.

### Placing Permanent Material

11 With amalgam, fill the smaller end of the amalgam carrier and transfer the carrier to the dentist for placement, with the condenser in the transfer position ready for use.

12 Assist the dentist as the process of placing and condensing the amalgam is repeated until the preparation is slightly overfilled.

13 When the preparation is slightly overfilled, exchange the condenser for the burnisher, so the dentist can burnish the surface and margins of the restoration.
**PURPOSE** To strengthen the finished restoration by burnishing the excess mercury to the surface.

14 If using composite, carry the material to the transfer zone with the composite placement instrument. The dentist adds the material to the preparation in increments, curing after each placement with the curing light.
**NOTE** The depth of the restoration will determine how often the curing light is used.

### Final Carving or Finishing

15 For amalgam, transfer the carvers until the carving is complete.

16 For composite, transfer the high-speed handpiece with finishing burs.

17 Keep the tip of the HVE close to the restoration during the carving and finishing process.
**PURPOSE** To remove all particles as soon as possible.
**NOTE** This step is especially important when a dental dam is not used.

### Documentation

18 Document the procedure.

| Date | Tooth | Surface | Charting Notes |
|---|---|---|---|
| 7/20/17 | 11 | F | 1 cartridge Xylocaine w/o epi, dental dam isolation, etching/bonding/Silux, shade Y. Procedure well tolerated by patient. Return for 6 mo recall.<br>T. Clark, CDA/L, Stewart, DDS |

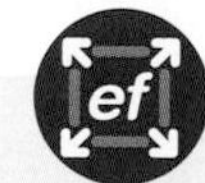

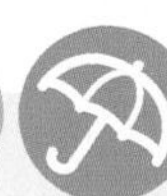

PROCEDURE 48.5

# Placing and Carving an Intermediate Restoration (Expanded Function)

### PREREQUISITES FOR PERFORMING THIS PROCEDURE

- ✔ Mirror skills
- ✔ Operator positioning
- ✔ Dental anatomy
- ✔ Instrumentation

### EQUIPMENT AND SUPPLIES

- ✔ Basic setup
- ✔ Tofflemire matrix retainer (for class II)
- ✔ Matrix band system (for classes II, III, and IV)
- ✔ Wedge (for classes II, III, and IV)
- ✔ Intermediate restoration material (IRM) setup (material, treated pad, spatula)
- ✔ Plastic instrument
- ✔ Condenser
- ✔ Discoid/cleoid carvers
- ✔ Hollenback carver
- ✔ Cotton pellet
- ✔ Articulating paper

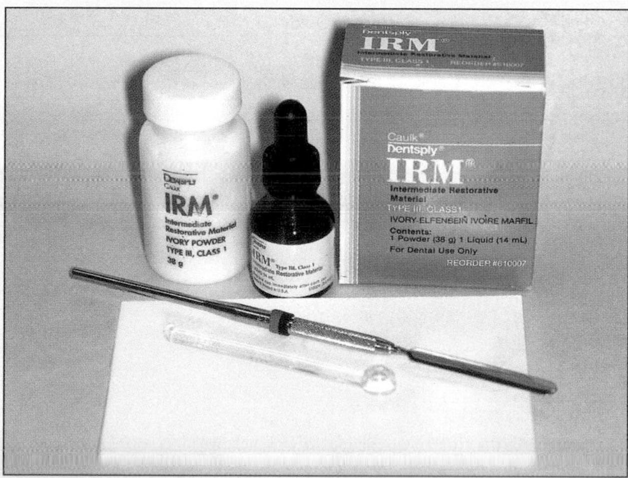


### PROCEDURAL STEPS

1 Clean, dry, and isolate the site with cotton rolls or a dental dam.

2 Examine the tooth and preparation, making sure to keep a mental note of the outline of the preparation.

**PURPOSE** When you begin carving, you need to know how far to carve back to the tooth structure.

3 If the preparation includes a proximal wall, you will need to place the appropriate matrix and wedge for the preparation. (See Chapter 49 for matrix selection and application.)

4 Mix the IRM to the appropriate consistency.

5 Using your plastic instrument (FP-1), take increments of the material to the preparation. If an interproximal box is present, begin filling this area first.

**PURPOSE** This area is more difficult to see, and material must be packed against the tooth for proper contour.

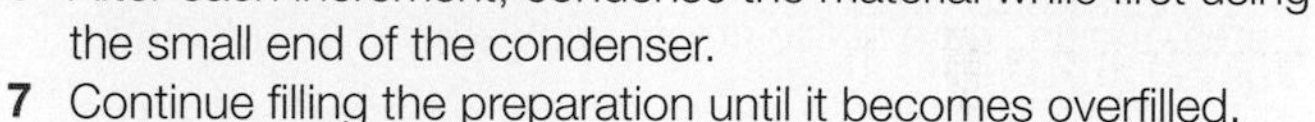

6 After each increment, condense the material while first using the small end of the condenser.

7 Continue filling the preparation until it becomes overfilled.

**PURPOSE** You want enough material to be able to carve back to the tooth structure.

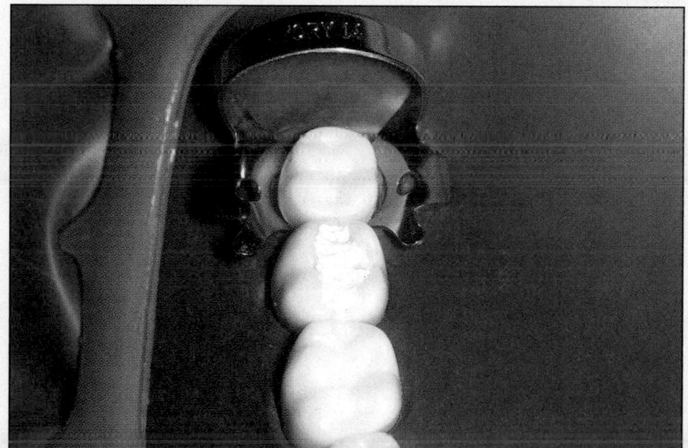

### Carving Stage

8 If a matrix system was used, use an explorer to run around the matrix band to remove any excess material from the marginal ridge and the proximal box. Remove the matrix at this time, leaving the wedge in place.

9 Remove any excess material from the occlusal surface, using the discoid/cleoid carver.

**PURPOSE** To keep the interproximal space open for easier carving.

10 Complete the final carving of the occlusal surface with the discoid/cleoid carver, making sure to carve back to the normal anatomy of the tooth.

**NOTE** Look at the same tooth on the opposite side of the arch for anatomic landmarks.

(Continued)

## PROCEDURE 48.5 Placing and Carving an Intermediate Restoration (Expanded Function)—cont'd

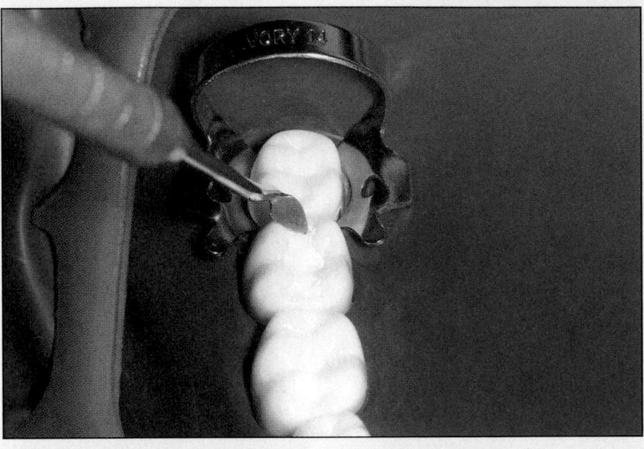

**11** If an interproximal surface was involved, use the Hollenback carver to remove any excess material from the interproximal area, making sure not to create an overhang or indentation in the material.
**12** Once all carving has been completed, remove the wedge.
**13** To check the occlusion, instruct the patient to bite down gently on articulating paper.
**14** After the final carving, take a wet cotton pellet and wipe over the restoration.
**15** Inform the patient that this restoration is "short term," and instruct him or her to not chew sticky foods on that side.

### Documentation

**16** Document the procedure.

| Date | Tooth | Surface | Charting notes |
|---|---|---|---|
| 7/20/17 | 3 | OL | Filling came out while chewing ice, cotton roll isolation, IRM placed. Reschedule pt for a permanent 2 surface composite |
| | | | T. Clark, CDA/L, Stewart, DDS |

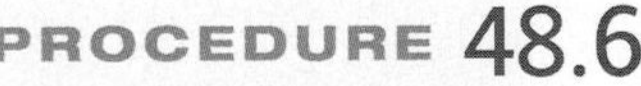

## PROCEDURE 48.6

# Assisting in the Placement of a Direct Veneer

### EQUIPMENT AND SUPPLIES

- Restorative tray (basic setup, hand [manual] cutting instruments, composite placement instrument, articulating paper holder)
- Composite shade guide
- Local anesthetic setup (if needed)
- Dental dam setup
- HVE tip
- Saliva ejector
- High-speed and low-speed handpieces
- Burs, assorted (dentist's choice)
- Mylar matrix setup
- Dental liners, base, sealers, bonding agents
- Composite material
- Curing light with protective shield
- Finishing burs and diamonds
- Dental floss
- Articulating paper
- Cotton pellets, cotton rolls, 2 × 2–inch gauze
- Abrasive strips
- Polishing kit (disc and mandrel)
- Polishing paste

### PROCEDURAL STEPS

**1** A local anesthetic agent may not be required for this procedure.

**PURPOSE** Because only a small amount of tooth structure is removed, the procedure should not be uncomfortable for the patient.

**2** The shade is selected.
**3** Application of cotton rolls or the dental dam is completed.
**4** The tooth is measured to determine the appropriate crown form size. If necessary, the form is trimmed to fit the gingival contour.

## PROCEDURE 48.6 Assisting in the Placement of a Direct Veneer–cont'd

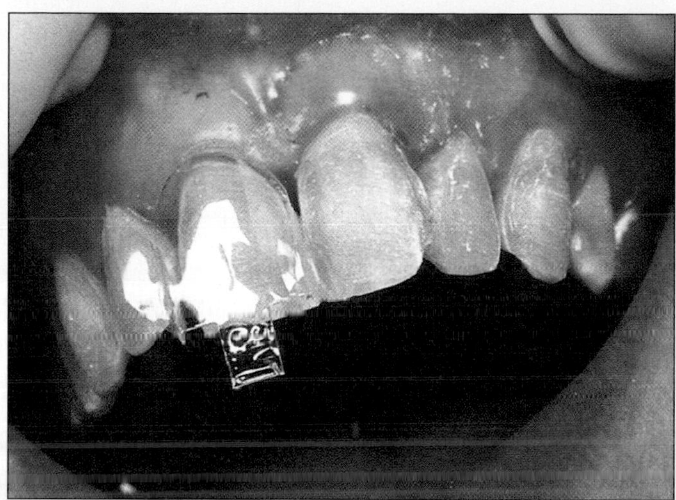

5 The required amount of enamel is removed with the use of diamond burs.

6 Before materials are placed, celluloid matrix strips are placed interproximally.

**PURPOSE** This will prevent the etchant, bonding, and resin materials from affecting adjacent teeth.

7 The tooth is etched, rinsed, and dried, and bonding material is applied.

8 If the veneers are being placed to cover dark stains, an opaque material may be placed to block out the stains.

9 The composite is placed on the inner surface of the crown form. The form is placed on the tooth with the matrix strips between the teeth. With one hand, the form is slowly pushed into place. With the other hand, the interproximal strips are pinched together at the lingual side of the tooth.

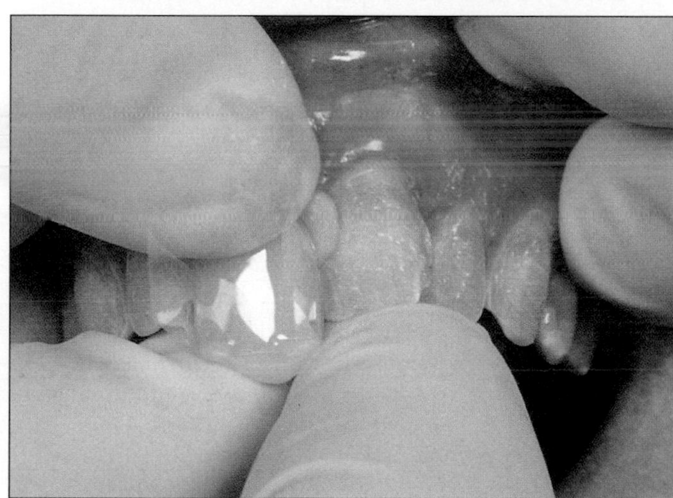

10 An explorer is used to trim away excess composite material that has extruded beyond the crown form.

11 With the crown form properly positioned, the material is light-cured for the length of time recommended by the manufacturer. When curing is complete, remove and discard the form.

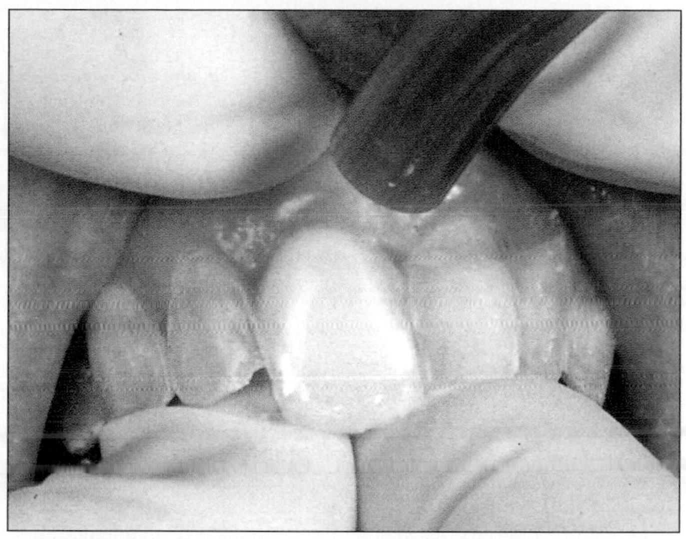

12 The dentist will use a series of sandpaper discs (coarse to fine) to adjust the tooth to the proper length. Finishing burs are used to trim and smooth the veneer.

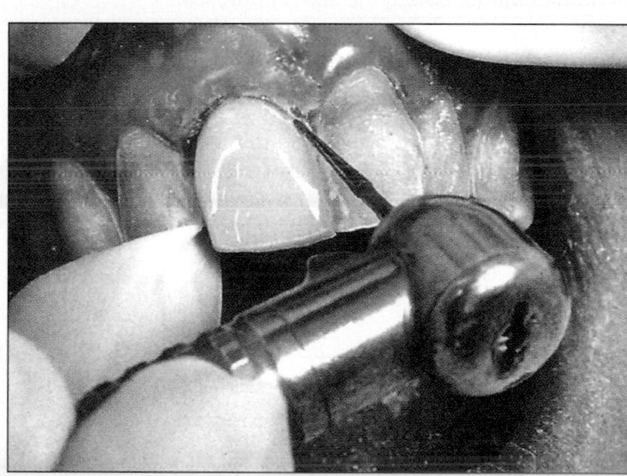

13 Assist as needed as these steps are repeated for each tooth that is to receive a veneer.

### Documentation

14 Document the procedure.

| Date | Tooth | Surface | Charting Notes |
|---|---|---|---|
| 7/20/17 | 8, 9 | F | Veneer—dental dam isolation, etching/bonding/Silux shade YL. Procedure well tolerated by patient. Return for 6 mo recall. |
| | | | T. Clark, CDA/L, Stewart, DDS |

49

# Matrix Systems for Restorative Dentistry

## KEY TERMS

**AutoMatrix (aw-toe-MAY-triks)** Matrix system designed to establish a temporary interproximal wall for the restoration of a tooth surface without the use of a retainer.

**Celluloid (SEL-yoo-loid) strip** Clear plastic strip used to provide a temporary interproximal wall for the restoration of an anterior tooth surface.

**Cupping** Form created by a concave tooth surface that has not been contoured properly.

**Matrix (MAY-triks)** Foundation that binds or holds the dental material and tooth together during the setting process.

**Mylar (MYE-lahr)** Brand name for clear plastic strip used to provide a temporary wall for restoration of an anterior tooth.

**Overhang** Excess restorative material that extends beyond the cavity margin.

**Universal retainer** Dental device used to hold a matrix band in place during restoration of a class II cavity.

**Wedge** Wooden or plastic triangular device placed in the embrasure to provide the contour needed when a class II lesion is restored.

## LEARNING OUTCOMES

*On completion of this chapter, the student will be able to achieve the following objectives:*

1. Pronounce, define, and spell the key terms.
2. Describe the use of a matrix system in class II, III, and IV restorations.
3. Describe the types of matrices used for posterior restorations, including the purpose and use of a wedge.
4. Describe the types of matrices used for anterior restorations.
5. Discuss alternative methods for matrix systems used in restorative dentistry.

## PERFORMANCE OUTCOMES

*On completion of this chapter, the student will be able to achieve competency standards in the following skills:*

- Assemble a matrix band and universal retainer.
- Place and remove a matrix band and wedge for a class II restoration.
- Place and remove a matrix band and wedge for a class III restoration.

## ELECTRONIC RESOURCES

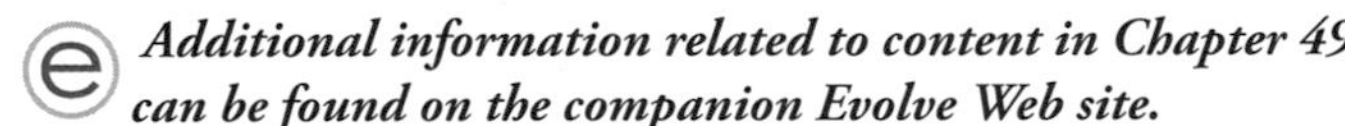
***Additional information related to content in Chapter 49 can be found on the companion Evolve Web site.***

- Practice Quiz
- Videos: Assembling a Matrix Band and Universal Retainer; Placing a Matrix Band and Wedge for a Class II Restoration

When a tooth is prepared for a class II, III, or IV restoration, at least one interproximal wall of the tooth has been removed (Fig. 49.1). A **matrix** system is designed to create a temporary interproximal wall for the amalgam, composite resin, or intermediate restorative material to be placed against during the restorative procedure. (The plural term for *matrix* is **matrices.**) Besides acting as a temporary wall, the matrix system has specific characteristics:

- To stablize and hold material during the placement and curing stage of the dental material
- To restore interproximal anatomic contours
- To restore the correct interproximal contact with the adjacent tooth
- To create a smooth external surface for the restorative material to be packed against

Placement and removal of the matrix system may be a legal expanded function in the state in which you are practicing. Pay special attention to the type of tooth preparation, the type of matrix system to be prepared and placed, and the techniques of placement and removal.

## Posterior Matrix Systems

The matrix system commonly used today for the class II restoration is the universal retainer and matrix band. To avoid unnecessary delays in a procedure, the assistant will have the retainer and band assembled at the beginning of the procedure.

## Universal Retainer

The **universal retainer**, also referred to as the **Tofflemire retainer,** is a mechanical device that holds the matrix band snugly in position. This type of retainer is most commonly positioned from the *buccal* surface of the tooth that is being restored.

If the dentist is restoring a premolar or molar tooth, and the interproximal wall extends onto the buccal surface, there is a contra-angle retainer that has been designed with a slight bend in the body to accommodate positioning from the lingual surface.

### Components of a Universal Retainer

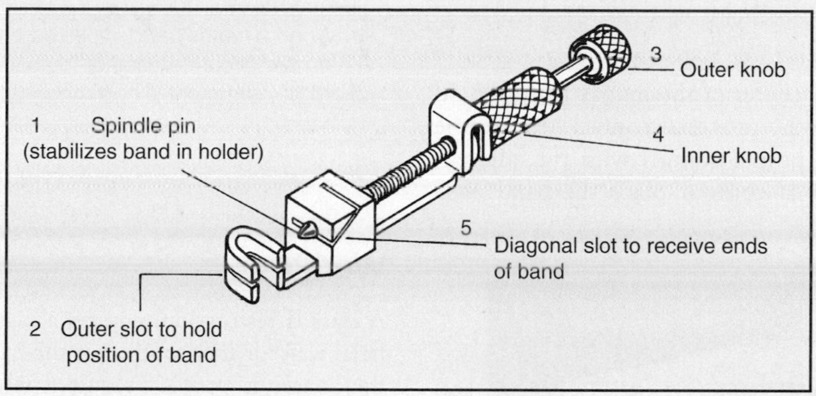


1. **Spindle:** Internal screwlike pin that fits into the diagonal slot to hold the ends of the matrix band. When the retainer is assembled, the spindle point must be clear of the slot while the band is slid into the slot, and then tightened.
2. **Outer guide slots:** Also known as guide channels; these are located at the end of the retainer and serve as channels to guide the loop of the matrix band. The channel selected is determined according to the quadrant that is being treated.
3. **Outer knob:** Used to tighten or loosen the spindle within the diagonal slot; this holds the matrix band securely in the retainer. To tighten the spindle, turn the outer knob away from you. To loosen the spindle, turn the outer knob toward you. Be careful not to turn it too far, or the diagonal slot vise will fall off the spindle. If this happens, insert the end of the spindle into the diagonal slot vise, and turn the outer knob away from you.
4. **Inner knob:** Used to increase or decrease the size of the matrix band loop. The size of the loop formed by the band depends on the tooth to be restored. When the band is placed over the tooth, the size of the loop circumference should be larger than the tooth, and the band should be tightened after placement.
5. **Diagonal slot:** Slot within the boxlike structure used to position the ends of the matrix band into the vise; the retainer is always positioned in the mouth with this slot facing *toward the gingiva.*

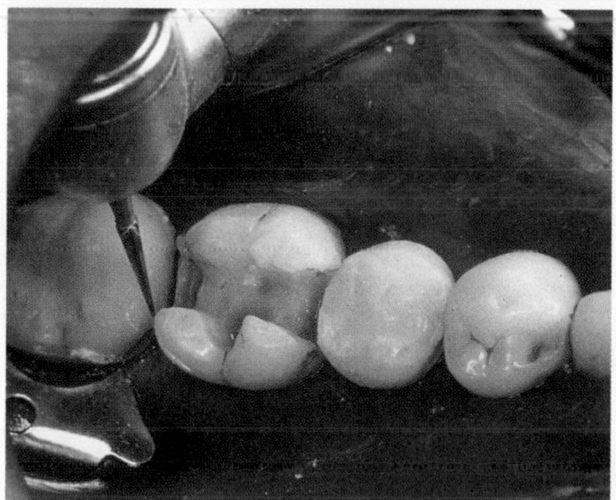

**FIG. 49.1** Tooth preparation with mesial and distal proximal walls missing. *(Courtesy Garrison Dental Solutions, Spring Lake, MI.)*

## Matrix Band

The matrix band is a thin flexible stainless steel material. This type of band is commonly used for the placement of amalgam because of its thinness and ability to be contoured and adapted to the preparation.

There are two designs of the matrix band; the **universal band** and the **extension band** (Fig. 49.2). The *universal band* is selected for the class II preparation when the proximal "box" is prepared to a minimum depth and width and the cusps are intact (Fig. 49.3). The *extension band* would be selected for a class II preparation with a more extensive preparation and requires gingival extensions to compensate for the loss of a cusp (Fig. 49.4). The universal band would not be selected because it would not have the additional height for the occlusal surface of the tooth as required.

The matrix band is designed in such a way that when the ends of the band are brought together, the band forms a circle. One side of the **circumference** (perimeter or outside edge) of the circle will be smaller than the other opening side, resembling a cone effect. The circumference guides you in how the band is placed on the tooth:

- The *smaller circumference* of the band is the *gingival edge* and is always positioned toward the gingiva.
- The *larger circumference* of the band is the *occlusal edge* and is always positioned on the tooth facing the occlusal part of the tooth.

### Contouring

In preparation for use, the center of the matrix band should be **contoured** (shaped) in the proximal contact area, so the final restoration will have proper contact with the adjacent tooth. To provide additional contour place the band on a paper pad. Using a *burnisher* or an end of the mirror handle, rub against the inner surface of the band until the ends begin to curl (Fig. 49.5).

See Procedure 49.1: Assembling a Matrix Band and Universal Retainer.

RECALL

1 Which cavity classifications use a posterior matrix system?
2 What is the plural of matrix?
3 What is used to hold a posterior matrix band in position intraorally?
4 When a matrix band is placed on the tooth, where is the smaller circumference of the band placed?
5 What instrument is commonly used to contour the matrix band?

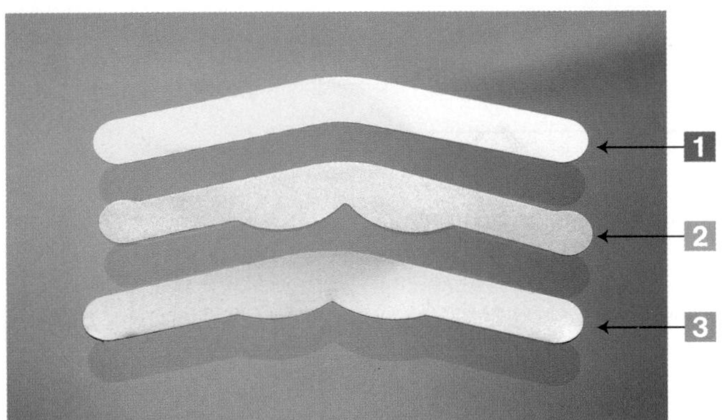


**FIG. 49.2** Three designs of the matrix band: *1*, universal band; *2 and 3*, extension bands. *(From Boyd LRB: Dental instruments: a pocket guide, ed 6, St Louis, 2018, Elsevier.)*

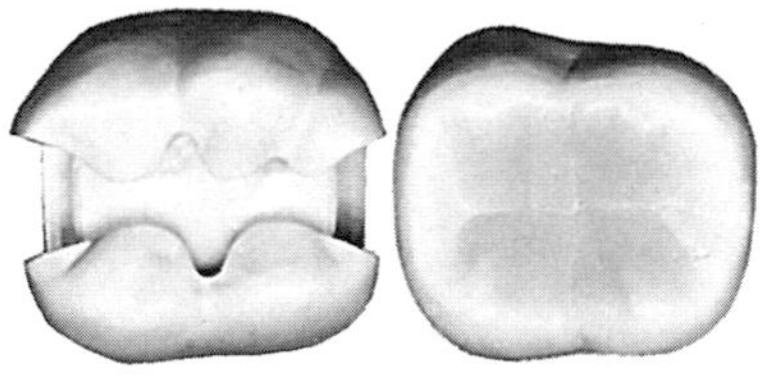

**FIG. 49.3** Ideal class II with minimal extension. *(From Heymann HO, Swift EJ, Ritter AV: Sturdevant's art and science of operative dentistry, ed 6, St Louis, 2013, Mosby.)*

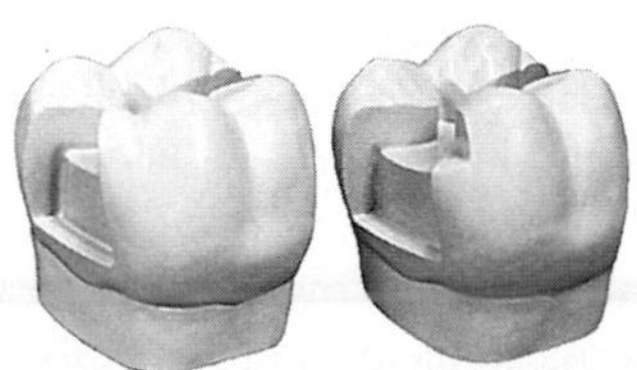

**FIG. 49.4** Extended preparation with distal cusp removed. *(From Heymann HO, Swift EJ, Ritter AV: Sturdevant's art and science of operative dentistry, ed 6, St Louis, 2013, Mosby.)*

## Wedges

A class II restoration requires a matrix band to act as an artificial wall for that tooth, but the band alone does not provide the anatomic contour required interproximally. A **wedge** is inserted into the lingual embrasure to hold the matrix band firmly against the gingival margin of the preparation (Fig. 49.6). This added pressure pushes the matrix band against the

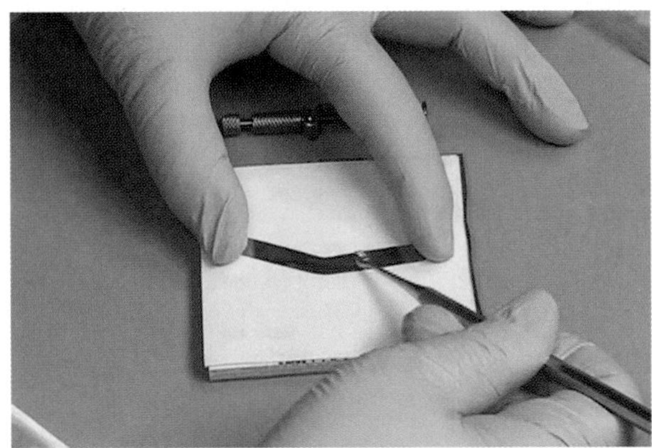

**FIG. 49.5** Contouring the interproximal surface of the band.

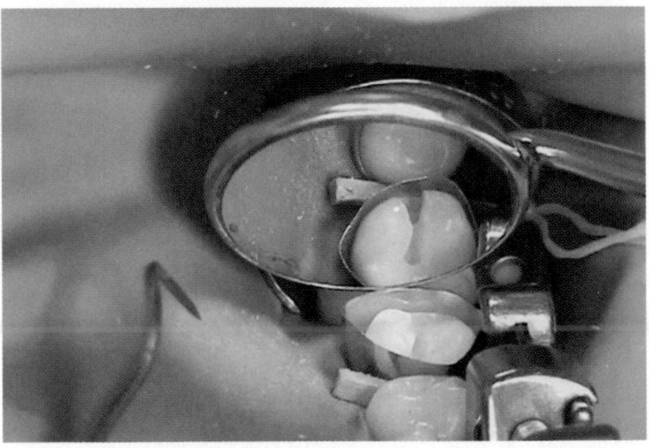

**FIG. 49.6** Wedge correctly positioned interproximally.

proximal surface of the tooth, allowing the contour of the finished restoration to match that of the natural tooth structure it replaces.

Wedges are made in various sizes, forms (triangular or round), and materials (wood and plastic). The most commonly used type of wedge is the triangular or round wooden wedge (Fig. 49.7). When a wedge is selected, the following should be considered:

- The wedge must be wide enough that pressure is applied to the apical and gingival walls of the preparation.
- The wedge presses the band against the tooth and causes a slight separation of the teeth.
- The wedge is slightly wider than the distance between the cervical portions of adjacent teeth.

The instrument used for inserting the wedge is the #110 (Howe) pliers. The design of the plier allows the operator to have the proper grasp and pressure to position the wedge firmly into the embrasure. For posterior restorations, the wedge is most commonly positioned from the lingual side.

The key criterion to consider when placing a wedge is to create a seamless transition where the tooth and the restoration meet. Improper wedge and band placement can result in an **overhang** or in **cupping** of the final material (Fig. 49.8, *A* and *B*). If a restoration is not contoured properly it can result in an overhang; if the restoration is indented because of improper contouring, it can result in cupping. Either result can create a noticeable condition for the patient, because it can cause the following:

- Trap food, which could result in possible recurrence of decay
- Make it difficult to floss

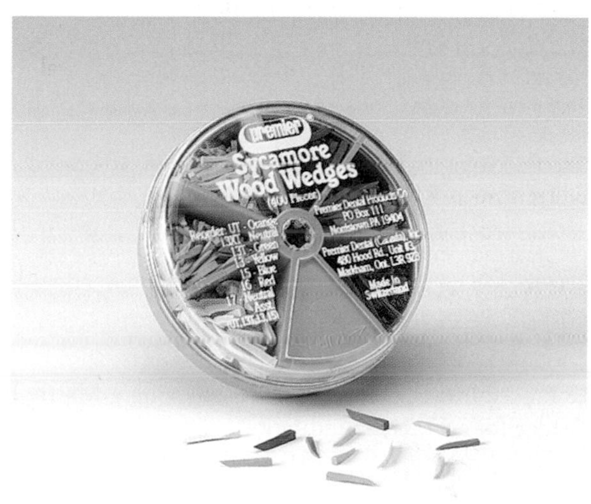


**FIG. 49.7** Assortment of precontoured wedges. *(Courtesy Premier Dental Products Company, Plymouth Meeting, PA.)*

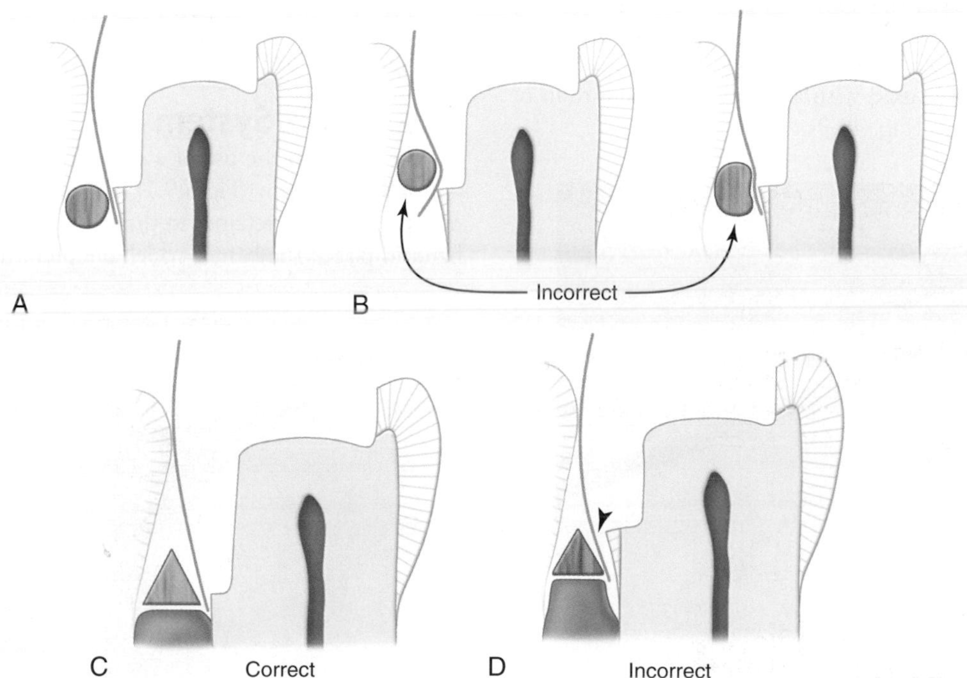


**FIG. 49.8** A and B, The diagrams show the correct and incorrect position when using a round toothpick wedge. C and D, The diagrams show the correct and incorrect position when using a triangular wedge. *(From Heymann HO, Swift EJ, Ritter AV: Sturdevant's art and science of operative dentistry, ed 6, St Louis, 2013, Mosby.)*

- Contribute to inflamed gingival tissue and periodontal disease
- Cause long-term bone loss

### Criteria for Placing the Posterior Matrix Retainer and Band

- Prepare the matrix band and retainer before the procedure.
- Determine the number and type of wedges.
- The diagonal slotted surface of the retainer is positioned toward the gingiva.
- The retainer is positioned from the buccal surface of the tooth.
- The handle of the retainer extends out from the oral cavity at the corner of the lips.
- The seated band extends approximately 1 mm below the gingival margin of the preparation.
- The seated band extends no farther than 2 mm above the occlusal surface of the tooth.

See Procedure 49.2: Placing and Removing a Matrix Band and Wedge for a Class II Restoration.

**6** What additional item is used in the matrix system to reestablish proper contact with an adjacent tooth?
**7** What can result from improper wedge placement?

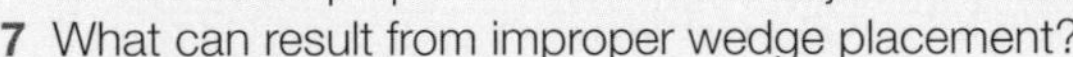

## Anterior Matrix Systems

A different type of matrix system is used for anterior teeth because of the types of dental materials used and the unique design in how the tooth is restored. A clear plastic matrix is a type of matrix system used with anterior composite resin or glass ionomer materials (Fig. 49.9).

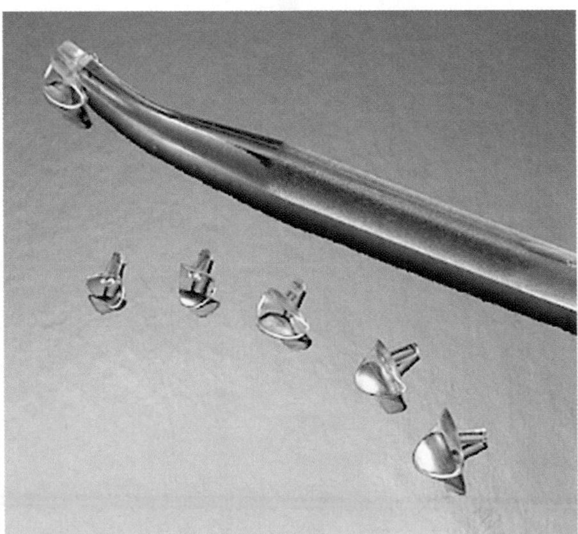

**FIG. 49.9** A clear matrix system. *(Courtesy Premier Dental Products, Plymouth Meeting, PA.)*

The clear plastic matrix, also referred to as the **celluloid** strip or **Mylar** strip, is used for a class III or IV restoration when the proximal wall of an anterior tooth is missing. No retainer is needed to hold the matrix in place, making this system an easier application. The plastic matrix and wedge serve the following three purposes during the restoration process:

1. The matrix is placed between the teeth before etching and priming of the tooth to *protect adjacent teeth* from these materials.
2. After placement of the composite material, the matrix is pulled tightly around the tooth to *help in reconstructing* its natural contour.
3. The clear plastic allows the curing light to penetrate the material, thereby *completing the curing process.*

Because anterior teeth have a slight curvature of their interproximal surfaces, contouring the matrix before placement helps keep it in place. To contour a plastic matrix strip, pull the matrix lengthwise over the rounded end of the cotton pliers or mirror handle (Fig. 49.10). Lingual surfaces hold the matrix in place while the material is adapted to the preparation. When the restorative material has reached its final set, the matrix is removed for the finishing and polishing stages.

See Procedure 49.3: Placing a Matrix for a Class III or Class IV Restoration.

**8** What is another term for a clear plastic matrix?

## Alternative Matrix Systems

### AutoMatrix System

An alternative to the use of a universal retainer and band is the **AutoMatrix** system (Fig. 49.11). This system has an advantage over the universal retainer in that no retainer is used to hold the band in place. The bands, which are preformed into a circle, are

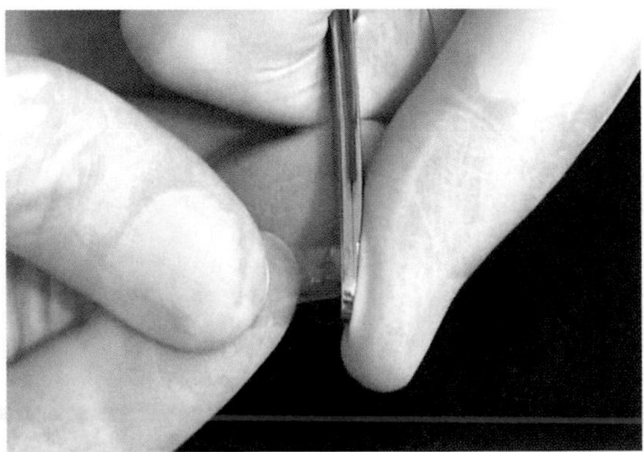

**FIG. 49.10** Contouring a plastic matrix band. *(Courtesy Aldridge D. Wilder, DDS.)*

available in assorted sizes in both metal and plastic. Each band has a coil-like autolock loop. The tightening wrench is inserted into the coil and is turned clockwise to tighten the band. No additional retainer is necessary, and wedges are placed as indicated.

When the procedure is finished, the tightening wrench is inserted into the coil and is turned counterclockwise to loosen the band. The removing pliers are used to cut the band. The band is removed and discarded in the sharps container. The wedge(s) is then removed. The tightening wrench and the removing pliers are sterilized or disinfected in accordance with the manufacturer's instructions.

## Sectional Matrices

Posterior composite restorations require a different type of matrix system than is used with the universal band and retainer. Examples of these types of matrices are Palodent, Triodent, and Composi-Tight. With a thin polished sectional matrix bands (small, oval stainless steel matrix available in a variety of sizes) and a tension ring, this system is able to produce tight anatomic contacts for composite resin materials (Fig. 49.12).

The thin, contoured *matrix band* is positioned first interproximally, and then the *wedge* is firmly placed to close the cervical margin. The prongs of the *tension ring* are placed between the band and the wedge, thereby creating a solid closure of the cavity preparation.

## Matrix Systems for Primary Teeth

Because of the shape and size of primary molars, the universal retainer and the matrix band do not fit. The T-band and the spot-welded band are two types of matrix systems designed to provide the correct width and depth needed for proper restoration of primary molars.

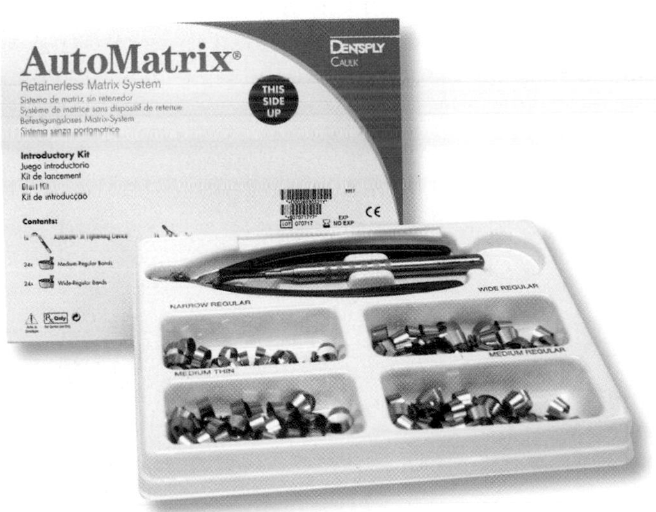


FIG. 49.11 AutoMatrix system. *(Courtesy Dentsply Sirona Restorative.)*

### T-Band

The T-band is a copper band in the shape of a T (Fig. 49.13). When formed, the top portion of the T allows the straight portion to adjust and fit the circumference of the primary molar. Preparing the T-band matrix involves the following steps:

1. Bend the wings of the T-band to form a U-shaped trough.
2. Slip the free end of the band loosely through the U formation.
3. Close the wings, and pull the free end to make a small loop of the band.
4. Holding the free end toward the facial surface, place the band loop on the tooth to be prepared.

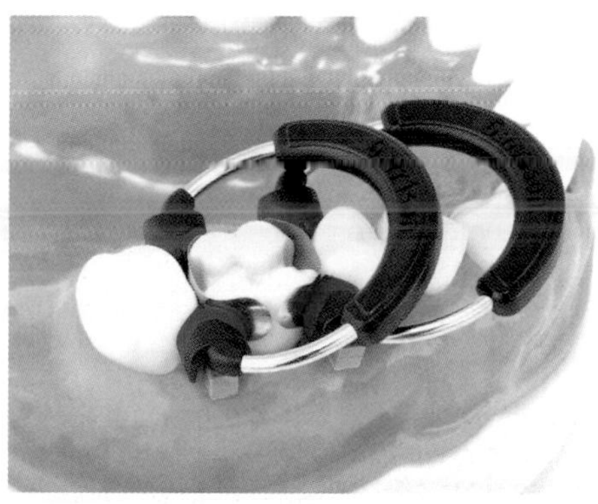

FIG. 49.12 Sectional matrix system. A variety of sizes and shapes accommodate composite and amalgam restorative materials. *(Courtesy Garrison Dental Solutions, Spring Lake, MI.)*

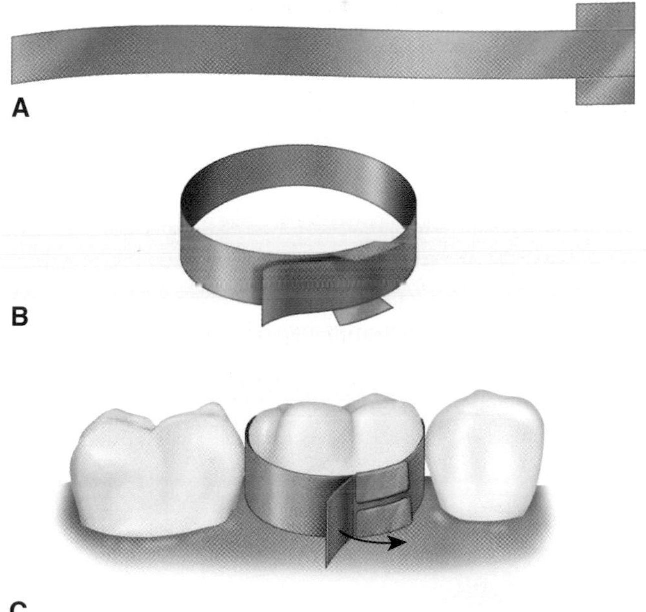


FIG. 49.13 Copper T-band used for primary molars. A, T-band. B, T-band prepared for placement. C, Position the T-band around the tooth and tighten the band by folding the flaps. *(© Elsevier Collection.)*

## *Spot-Welded Band*

The spot-welded band is form-fitted around the tooth with the use of #110 pliers. The band is then removed and placed in the smaller form of a welder that fuses the metal to make a custom band.

Preparing a spot-welded matrix band involves the following steps:

1. Measure to 1 inch of stainless steel matrix material.
2. Fit the matrix material around the prepared tooth.
3. Adapt the band with #110 pliers, ensuring that the ends of the matrix material are at the facial surface for visibility and control.
4. While holding the ends tightly, remove the band in an occlusal direction.
5. Place the band on the plate of the spot welder.
6. Spot-weld the matrix at three positions.

RECALL

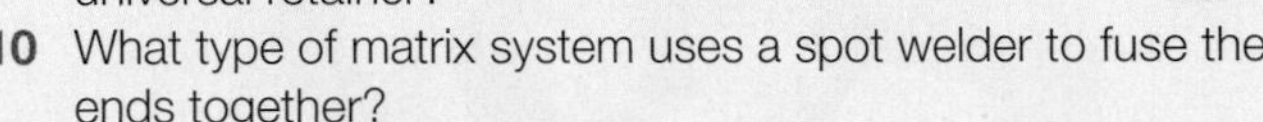

9 What matrix system is an alternative to the universal retainer?

10 What type of matrix system uses a spot welder to fuse the ends together?

11 What is another term for a thin polished matrix band used for posterior composites?

■ **Patient Education** Many instruments and supplies are used throughout a dental procedure in the restoration of a tooth. The patient may never have seen the matrix system. When assisting in a procedure that introduces a piece of dental equipment, such as the universal retainer or the AutoMatrix system, educate the patient on how it is used. This type of ongoing discussion will promote confidence in your patients, which will enhance their dental visit. ■

■ **Legal and Ethical Implications** The placement of a matrix system may be a legal expanded function in the state where you practice. If so, it is essential that you receive training in the proper placement of matrix bands and the insertion of a wedge.

Do not let your dentist take for granted that you have placed a band or wedge correctly. Every time you complete this procedure, request that the dentist critique your work and offer advice about the application. This exchange improves communication in the office and makes you a more valuable member of the dental team. ■

■ **Eye to the Future** The newer composite resin materials that are being placed for posterior restorations require a different type of matrix system. The matrix is thinner and provides more accurate contact with the adjacent tooth or teeth. Always consult with a sales representative regarding what accessories are required for the types of restorative materials that are selected to be placed. ■

## ■ Critical Thinking

1. You are assisting in the restoration of a mesial-occlusal-distal (MOD) amalgam on tooth #13. How many wedges should be set out for this procedure? Where is a wedge(s) positioned for proper contour? From what direction do you position the wedge(s)?
2. You are to prepare the universal retainer and matrix band for tooth #29. When assembling the band into the retainer with the diagonal slot facing you, in which direction should the band go—right, straight, or left?
3. Before you assemble the matrix band and retainer or place the Mylar strip interproximally, what needs to be done to the band to enhance its contouring abilities?
4. The dentist has overfilled tooth #13 and has completed the initial carving and is ready to start the final carving of the occlusal and interproximal surfaces. Describe the sequence involved in removal of the matrix band, retainer, and wedge. ■

PROCEDURE 49.1

# Assembling a Matrix Band and Universal Retainer

## EQUIPMENT AND SUPPLIES

- ✓ Basic setup
- ✓ Universal retainer
- ✓ Matrix band
- ✓ Ball burnisher
- ✓ Paper pad

## PROCEDURAL STEPS

1 Rinse and dry the preparation.

2 Examine the outline of the cavity preparation using a mirror and explorer.

3 Determine the design of the matrix band to be used for the procedure.

**PURPOSE** The band is selected according to the type of tooth and the depth of the cavity preparation.

4 Place the middle of the band on the paper pad, and burnish this area with a burnisher.

**PURPOSE** This creates a thin, slightly contoured area, where the contact will be located.

5 Hold the retainer with the diagonal slot facing you, and turn the outer knob counterclockwise until the end of the spindle is visible and away from the diagonal slot in the vise.

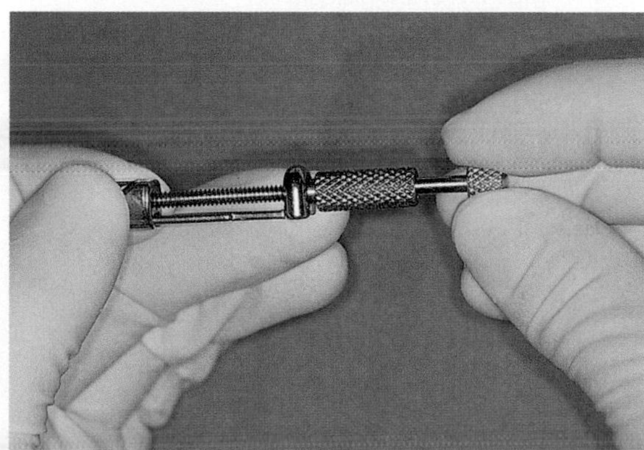

6 Turn the inner knob until the vise moves next to the guide slots.

**PURPOSE** The retainer is ready to receive the matrix band.

7 Bring together the ends of the band to identify the occlusal and gingival aspects of the matrix band. The occlusal edge has the larger circumference. The gingival edge has the smaller circumference.

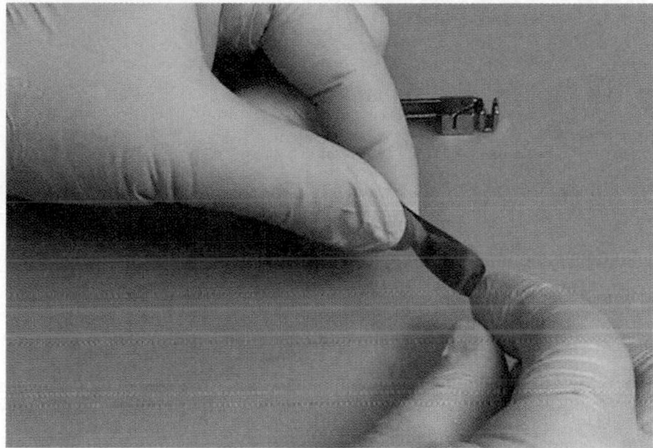

8 With the diagonal slot of the retainer facing toward you, slide the joined ends of the band, *occlusal edge first (wider circumference),* into the diagonal slot on the vise.

9 Guide the band into the correct guide slots.

**PURPOSE** The position of the band loop in the guide slots depends on whether the tooth being restored is maxillary, mandibular, right, or left.

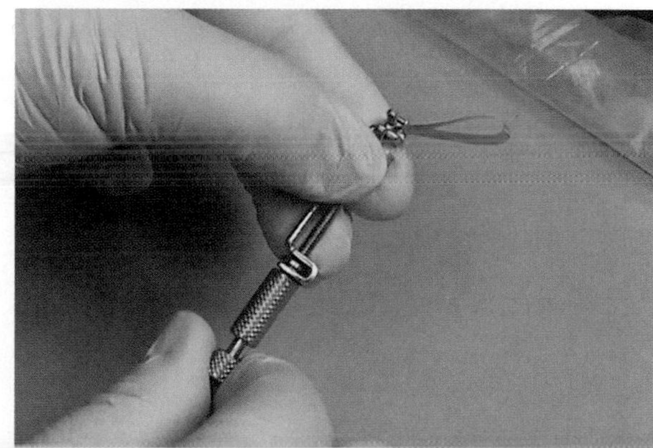

10 Tighten the outer knob on the retainer to secure the band.

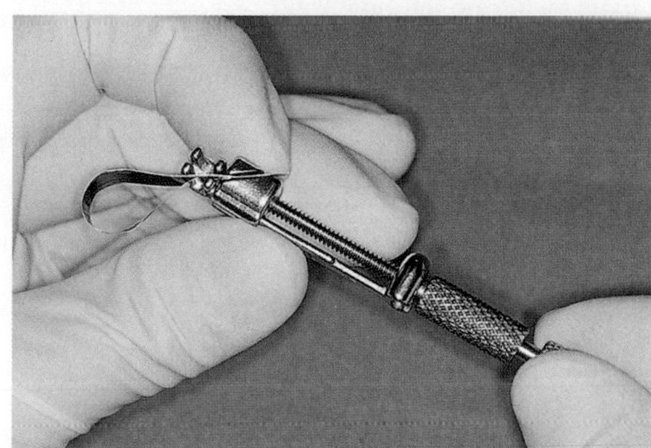

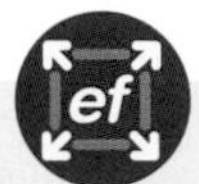

PROCEDURE 49.2 

# Placing and Removing a Matrix Band and Wedge for a Class II Restoration (Expanded Function)

## PREREQUISITES FOR PERFORMING THIS PROCEDURE

- ✔ Mirror skills
- ✔ Operator positioning
- ✔ Dental anatomy
- ✔ Instrumentation

## EQUIPMENT AND SUPPLIES

- ✔ Basic setup
- ✔ Prepared matrix band and retainer
- ✔ Wedge for each proximal space involved
- ✔ #110 pliers

## PROCEDURAL STEPS

### Preparing the Band Size

**1** If necessary, use the handle end of the mouth mirror to open the loop of the band.

**PURPOSE** The band can become flattened or bent during placement in the retainer and may not slide easily onto the tooth preparation.

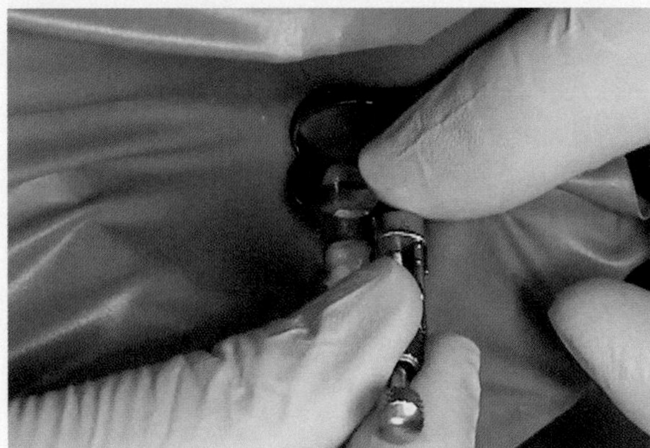

**2** If necessary, adjust the size (diameter) of the loop to fit over the tooth by turning the *inner knob.*

### Placing Matrix Band and Universal Retainer

**3** Position and seat the loop of the band over the occlusal surface, with the retainer parallel to the buccal surface of the tooth. Ensure that the band remains beyond the occlusal edge by approximately 1.0 to 1.5 mm.

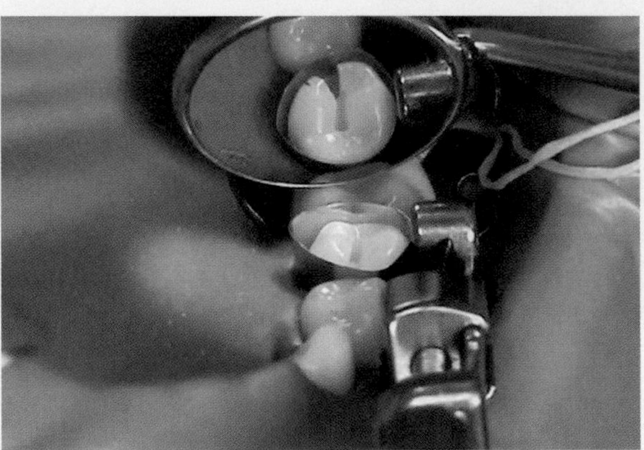

**4** Hold the band securely in place by applying finger pressure over its occlusal surface. Slowly turn the inner knob clockwise to tighten the band around the tooth.

**5** Use the explorer to examine the adaptation of the band.

**PURPOSE** Gingival tissue or dental dam material can become trapped between the band and the proximal box of the cavity preparation.

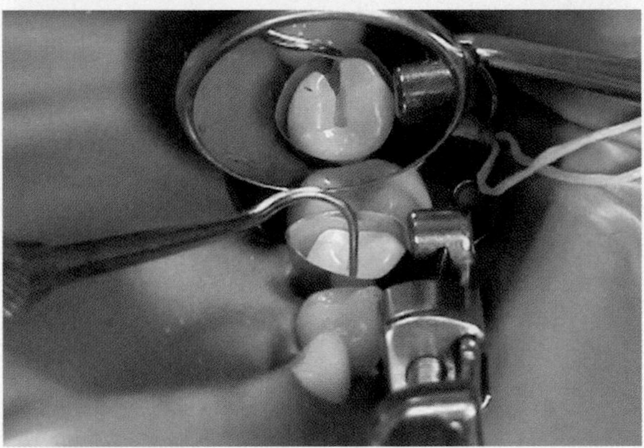

**6** Use a burnisher to contour the band at the contact area, creating a slightly concave area.

### Placing the Wedge

**7** Select the proper wedge size and shape.

**PURPOSE** The size of the embrasure will determine the size and shape of the wedge for complete closure of the band and cavity preparation.

**8** Place the wedge in the pliers so that the flat, wider side of the wedge is toward the gingiva.

**9** Insert the wedge into the lingual embrasure next to the preparation and the band.

**NOTE** If both proximal surfaces (mesial and distal) are being restored, a wedge is inserted for each open contact.

# PROCEDURE 49.2 Placing and Removing a Matrix Band and Wedge for a Class II Restoration (Expanded Function)–cont'd

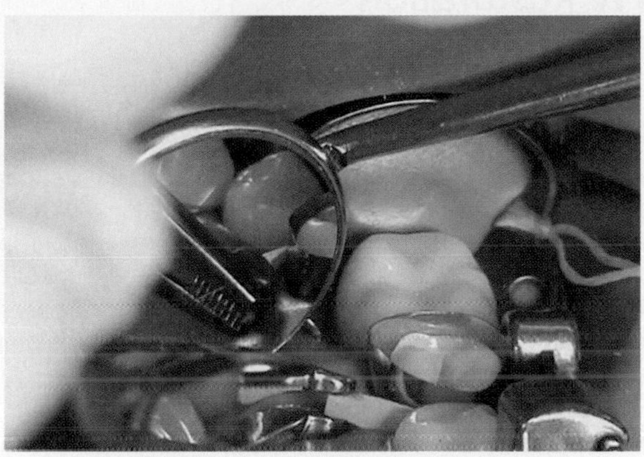

10 Check the proximal contact to ensure that the seal at the gingival margin of the preparation is closed.

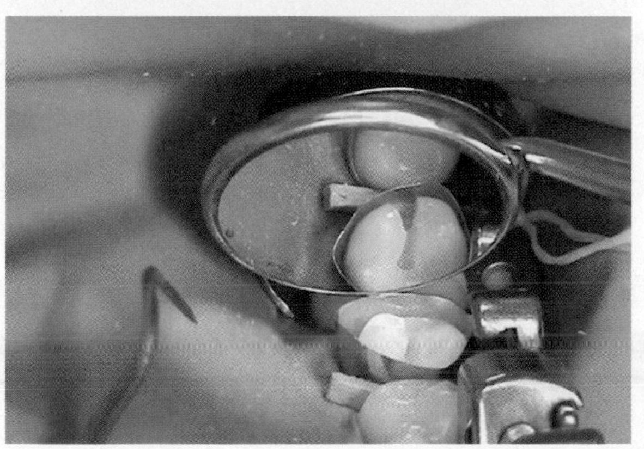

## Removing Universal Retainer, Matrix Band, and Wedge

11 After the dentist completes the initial carving of the restorative material, loosen the retainer from the band by placing a finger over the occlusal surface and slowly turning the *outer knob* of the retainer.

12 Carefully slide the retainer toward the occlusal surface, while leaving the band around the tooth.

13 Gently lift the matrix band in an occlusal direction, using a seesaw motion.

**PURPOSE** To avoid fracturing the newly placed material.

14 Discard the matrix band into the sharps container.

15 Using #110 pliers, grasp the base of the wedge to remove it from the lingual embrasure.

**PURPOSE** The wedge remains in place to help prevent fracture of the restoration when the matrix band is removed.

16 The restoration is now ready for the final carving steps.

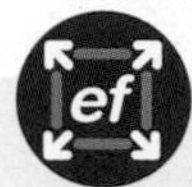

PROCEDURE 49.3

# Placing a Plastic Matrix for a Class III or Class IV Restoration (Expanded Function)

## PREREQUISITES FOR PERFORMING THIS PROCEDURE

- ✔ Mirror skills
- ✔ Operator positioning
- ✔ Dental anatomy
- ✔ Instrumentation

## EQUIPMENT AND SUPPLIES

- ✔ Basic setup
- ✔ Clear matrix strip
- ✔ Wedges
- ✔ #110 pliers

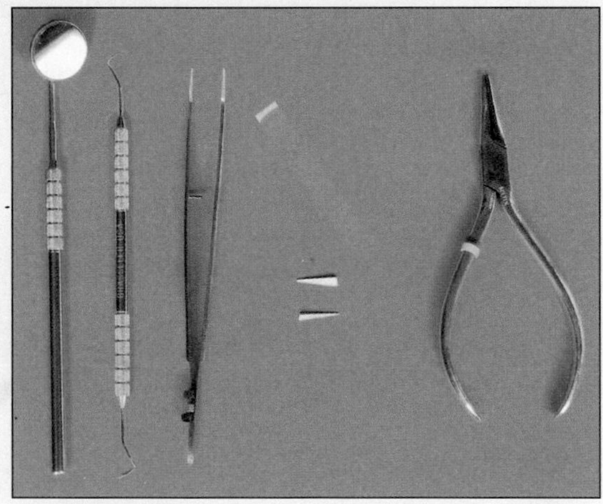

## PROCEDURAL STEPS

1. Examine the contour of the tooth and preparation site, paying special attention to the outline of the preparation.
2. Contour the matrix strip.
3. Slide the matrix interproximally, ensuring that the gingival edge of the matrix extends beyond the preparation.

   **PURPOSE** If the matrix does not completely cover the preparation, the cavity preparation could be filled incorrectly.

   **NOTE** If a matrix is placed during the etching process, make sure a new matrix is used for placement of the composite resin material.

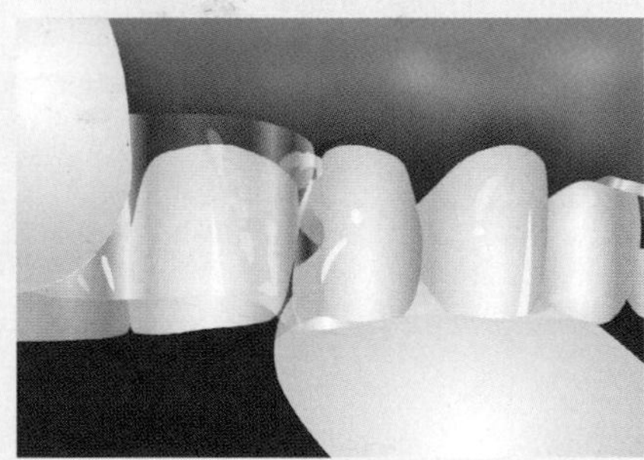

4. Using your thumb and forefinger, pull the band over the prepared tooth on the facial and lingual surfaces.
5. Using pliers, position the wedge within the gingival embrasure.

   **NOTE** The wedge can be positioned from the facial or the lingual side for anterior restorations.
6. After the preparation has been filled and light-cured, the matrix is removed.

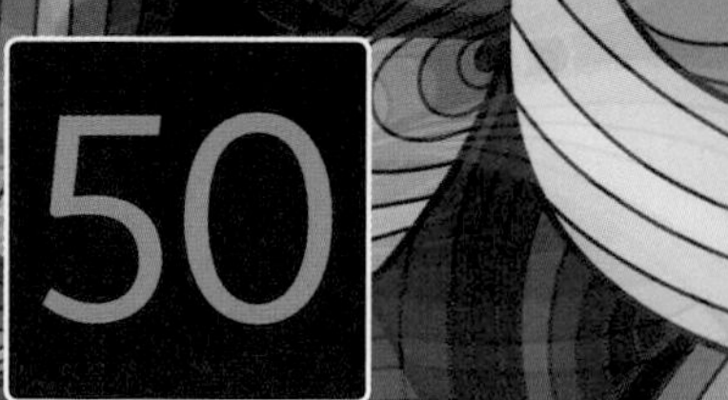

# Fixed Prosthodontics

## KEY TERMS

**Abutment (uh-BUT-munt)** A tooth, root, or implant used for support and retention of a fixed or removable prosthesis.

**Articulator (ar-TIK-yoo-lay-tur)** Dental laboratory device that simulates mandibular and temporomandibular joint movement when models of the dental arches are attached to it.

**Bevel (BEV-ul)** Enamel margin of a tooth preparation.

**Cast post** Metal post placed into the root canal of an endodontically treated tooth to improve the retention of a cast restoration.

**Chamfer (CHAM-fur)** Tapered finish line of the margin at the cervical area of a tooth preparation.

**Core** Portion of a post that extends above the tooth structure.

**Die** An accurate replica of the prepared portion of a tooth used in the laboratory during fabrication of a cast restoration.

**Fixed bridge** Dental prosthesis with artificial teeth fixed in place and supported by attachment to natural teeth.

**Full crown** Cast restoration that covers the entire anatomic crown of the tooth.

**Gingival retraction (jin-JI-vul ree-TRAK-shun)** Means of displacing gingival tissue away from the tooth.

**Hypertrophied (hye-PUR-troe-feed)** Referring to overgrown oral tissues.

**Infuser (in-FYOO-zur)** Syringe that applies hemostatic solution to the gingival retraction cord.

**Inlay (IN-lay)** Cast restoration designed to replace a conservative class II cavity.

**Investment material** Special gypsum product able to withstand extreme heat.

**Master cast** Cast created from a final impression used to construct baseplate, bite rims, wax setups, and finished prosthesis.

**Onlay (ON-lay)** Cast restoration designed to replace a class II cavity that includes the occlusal, one or more cusp, and proximal surfaces of posterior teeth.

**Opaquer (oe-PAY-kur)** Resin material placed under a porcelain restoration to mask tooth discoloration.

**Pontic (PON-tik)** Artificial tooth that replaces a missing natural tooth.

**Porcelain-fused-to-metal (PFM) crown** Indirect restoration in which a thin porcelain material is fused to the facial portion of a gold crown.

**Prosthesis (pros-THEE-sis)** Fabricated replacement for a missing tooth.

**Resin-bonded bridge** Fixed dental prosthesis with wings that are bonded to the lingual surfaces of adjacent teeth; also known as *Maryland bridge.*

**Shade guide** Accessory dental item that contains different shades of teeth used to match the color of a patient's teeth.

**Shoulder** Margins of a tooth preparation for a cast restoration.

**Three-quarter crown** Cast restoration that covers the anatomic crown of a tooth, except for the facial or buccal portion.

**Unit** Each component of the fixed bridge.

**Veneer (vuh-NEER)** Thin layer of composite resin or porcelain bonded or cemented to a prepared facial surface.

## LEARNING OUTCOMES

*On completion of this chapter, the student will be able to achieve the following objectives:*

1. Pronounce, define, and spell the key terms.
2. List indications for and contraindications to a fixed prosthesis.
3. Discuss indirect restorations, including the following:
   - Describe the differences among inlays, onlays, veneer crowns, and full crowns.
   - Describe the uses of porcelain for fixed prosthodontics.
   - Identify the components of a fixed bridge.
4. Identify the role of the laboratory technician and the steps for a diagnostic workup.
5. Explain a crown procedure, including the following:
   - Describe the preparation and placement of a cast restoration.
   - Discuss the uses of core buildups, pins, and posts in crown retention.
   - Describe the use of retraction cord before taking a final impression.
   - Describe the function of provisional coverage for a crown or fixed bridge.
6. Explain a bridge procedure, including the home care instructions for a permanent fixed prosthesis.
7. Describe the steps when using a CAD/CAM system.

## PERFORMANCE OUTCOMES

*On completion of this chapter, the student will be able to achieve competency standards in the following skills:*

- Demonstrate the placement and removal of gingival retraction cord.
- Assist in a crown and bridge preparation.
- Assist in the delivery and cementation procedure of a cast restoration.
- Assist in a CAD/CAM procedure.

## ELECTRONIC RESOURCES

***Additional information related to content in Chapter 50 can be found on the companion Evolve Web site.***

- Practice Quiz
- Video: Placing and Removing a Retraction Cord

Fixed prosthodontics, also referred to as **crown and bridge,** is the specialized area of dentistry involved in replacing missing teeth with either a gold, porcelain, or ceramic fixed **prosthesis** (adjective, *prosthetic*). *Fixed* is an important key to remember with this specialty, meaning that the restoration is permanently cemented into place and cannot be removed by the patient. This chapter reviews the preparation, construction, and placement of indirect restorations, which include inlays, onlays, veneers, single crowns, and bridges.

A **prosthodontist** is the dentist who is committed to the restoration and replacement of teeth by focusing on fixed or removable prosthodontics. This specialty requires an additional 3 years of training in a university- or hospital-based program, leading to a certificate or master of science degree. The program provides education and training for clinicians, researchers, and teachers in prosthodontics.

# Plan of Care

A patient's dental condition is thoroughly evaluated before prosthodontic treatment is initiated. It is necessary to obtain detailed medical and dental histories, a thorough intraoral examination, diagnostic models, and a current series of full-mouth radiographic images. The dentist will then develop a restorative treatment plan that is suited to the needs of the patient.

## Considerations for Prescribing Fixed Prosthodontics

**Indications**

- One or two adjacent teeth are missing in the same arch.
- Supportive tissues are healthy.
- Suitable abutment teeth are present.
- Patient is in good health and wants to have the prosthesis placed.
- Patient has the skills and motivation to maintain good oral hygiene.

**Contraindications**

- Necessary supportive tissues are diseased or missing.
- Suitable abutment teeth are not present.
- Patient is in poor health or is not motivated to have the prosthesis placed.
- Patient has poor oral hygiene habits.
- Patient cannot afford the treatment.

1 What is a common term used to describe the specialty of fixed prosthodontics?
2 If a patient has poor dental hygiene habits, is fixed prosthodontics indicated?

# Indirect Restorations

Indirect restorations, also known as **cast restorations,** are created in a commercial dental laboratory by a dental laboratory technician, or with the use of the computer-aided design/computer-aided manufacturing (CAD/CAM) system.

An indirect restoration is permanent; once received from the laboratory, the finished cast is in its final state and ready to be bonded or cemented into place. The tooth structure that will hold the inlay, onlay, crown, or bridge must be prepared, so that it allows the casting to be seated into place with only minor adjustments required by the dentist.

## Inlays and Onlays

Inlays and onlays are cast restorations designed to fit snugly *within* the preparation of a tooth. An **inlay** resembles a class II restoration and covers a portion of the occlusal and proximal surface (Fig. 50.1). An **onlay** resembles a multisurface restoration and covers the proximal surfaces and most of the entire occlusal surface (Fig. 50.2).

An inlay or onlay can be made from gold, porcelain, or resin materials. The difference is in the appearance of the finished restoration. The dentist will discuss with the patient which is the best type of material to use. If esthetics is not a concern, gold is a good option. Porcelain inlays and onlays offer the best esthetics and are often used in the "smile line" areas. Resin materials may be the best option for people who grind their teeth and/or those with a misaligned bite.

## Veneers

A **veneer** is a thin shell of tooth-colored material. Two types of veneer restorations are available. The direct veneer, which was discussed in Chapter 48, is created directly in the patient's mouth with the use of composite resin material. An **indirect veneer** is fabricated in the dental laboratory from an impression taken of the prepared tooth, or using the CAD/CAM system.

### *Porcelain Veneers*

Porcelain veneers are treatment planned for a patient to improve the esthetics of anterior teeth that are affected by abrasion, erosion, discoloration caused by intrinsic stains, and anomalies such as **enamel hyperplasia** (Fig. 50.3).

An important task in the construction and placement of an indirect veneer involves matching the tooth color. Because of the material's translucence, the color of the finished veneer is affected by the shade of the underlying tooth structure and by the color of the luting agent. The dentist will take these factors into account when selecting the shade. A specific device has been designed for determining a shade for porcelain and ceramic materials; it is called the *spectrophotometer* (Fig. 50.4). This device scans all surfaces involved in the restoration process of the tooth and eliminates the shadows and varying light sources to reveal the most realistic shade.

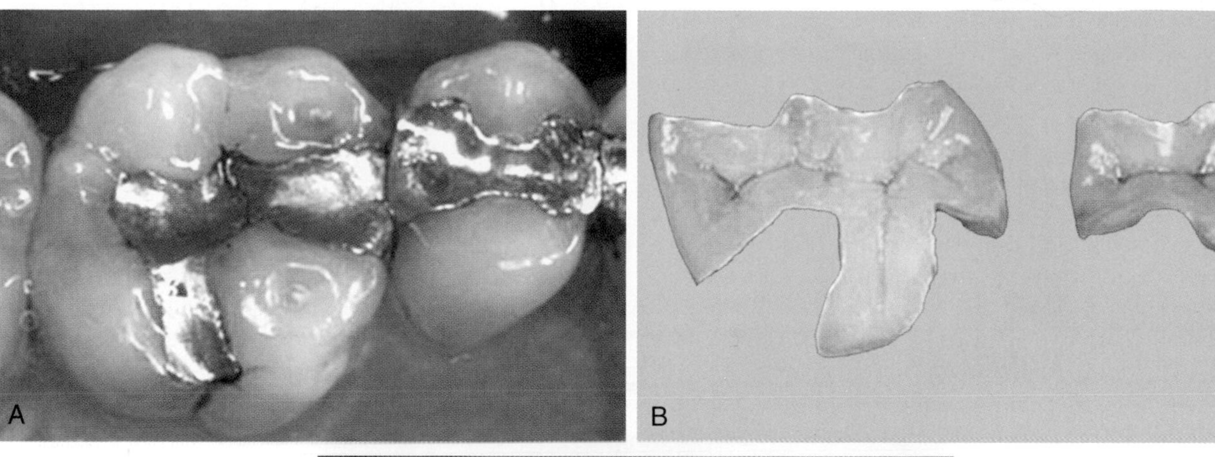


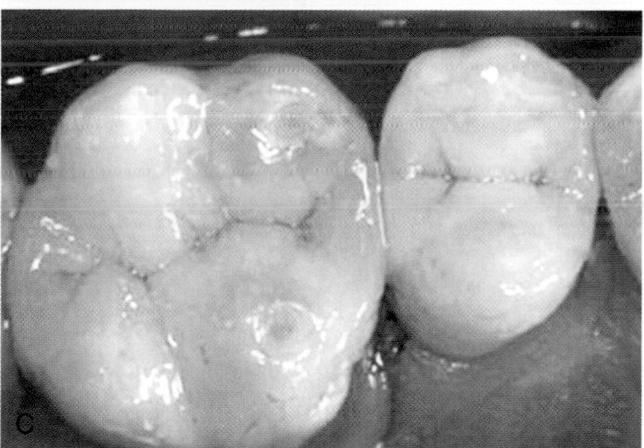


**FIG. 50.1** Inlay cast restoration replacing amalgam restorations. A, Class II amalgam. B, Class II porcelain inlay replacing the amalgam. C, Final placement of porcelain inlay. *(From Freedman G: Contemporary esthetic dentistry, St Louis, 2012, Mosby.)*

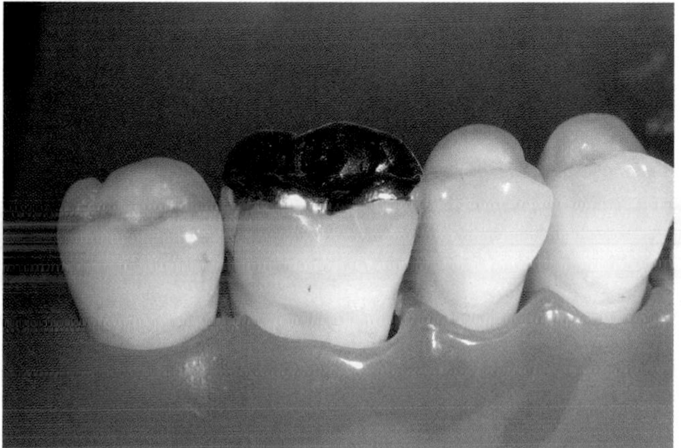

**FIG. 50.2** Onlay cast restoration fabricated from gold. *(From Robinson DS, Bird DL: Essentials of dental assisting, ed 6, St Louis, 2017, Elsevier.)*

In preparing for the final impression, the dentist will use specialized burs and discs to prepare the facial surface of the tooth as conservatively as possible. After the preparation has been completed, gingival retraction is placed and a final impression is taken. Provisional coverage may be needed based on the amount of tooth surface that is removed.

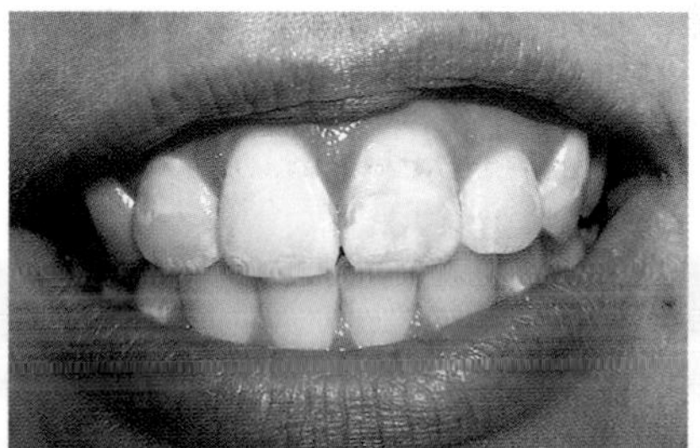

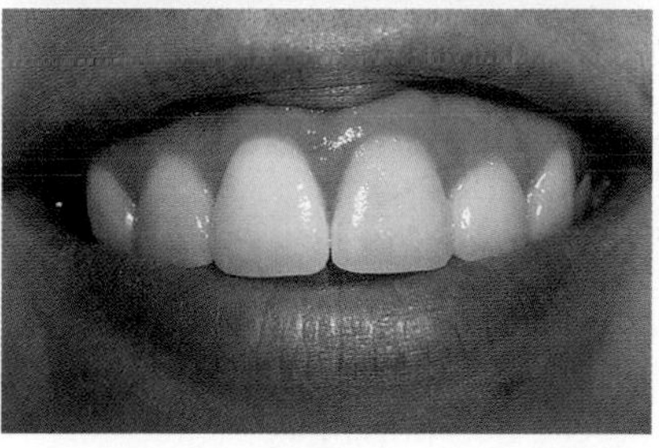

**FIG. 50.3** Porcelain veneers placed to cover hypocalcification defects. *(From Heymann HO, Swift EJ Jr, Ritter AV: Sturdevant's art and science of operative dentistry, ed 6, St Louis, 2013, Mosby.)*

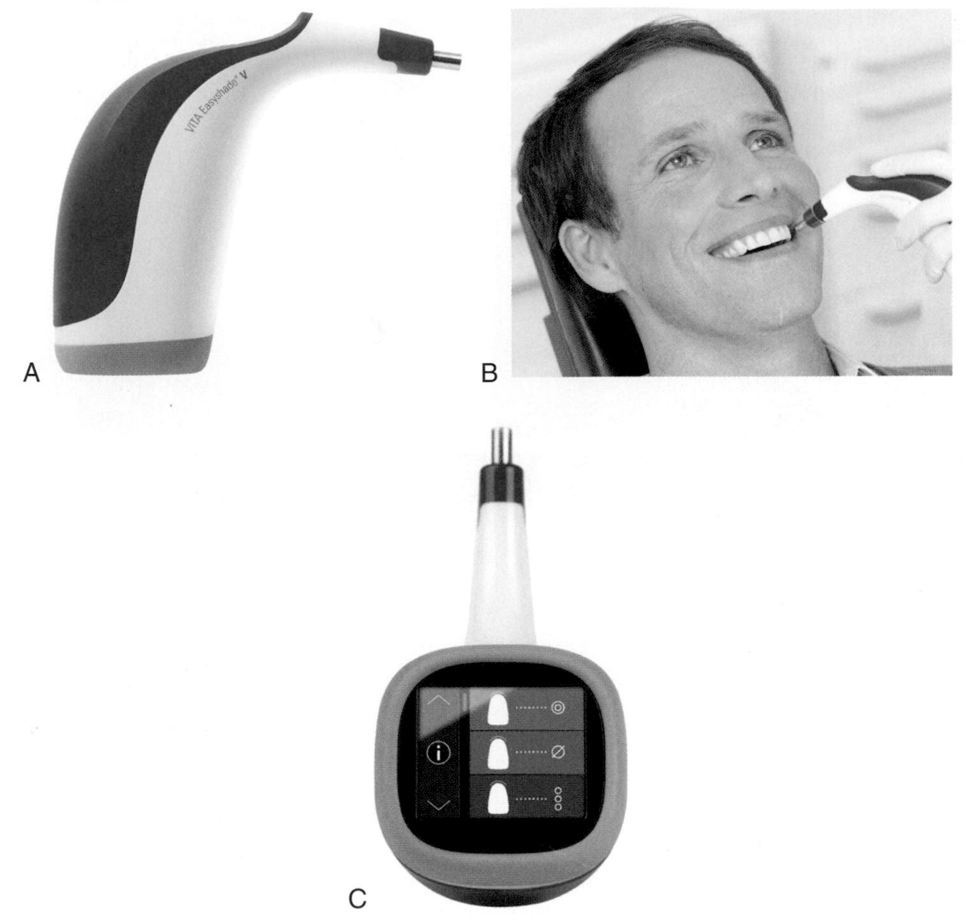


**FIG. 50.4** VITA Easyshade V device. A, VITA Easyshade V device. B, Placement of the device. C, Reading of the shade. *(Courtesy VITA North America, Yorba Linda, CA.)*

At the cementation visit, the dentist will try the veneers for fit and color match. Before cementation, an **opaquer** may be placed on the tooth surface to block out underlying color and structural defects. The cement is selected in a shade to enhance the color match as well. After etching and bonding, the veneers are then cemented into place. Any excess cement is removed, and final adjustments are made.

## Crowns

A **full crown** completely covers the anatomic portion of an individual tooth (Fig. 50.5). The decision to place a full crown is made when a tooth is decayed or fractured and cannot be reconstructed with a conservative restoration. If a tooth is severely broken down, additional retention may be required with the use of retention pins or a post and core (see discussion later in this chapter).

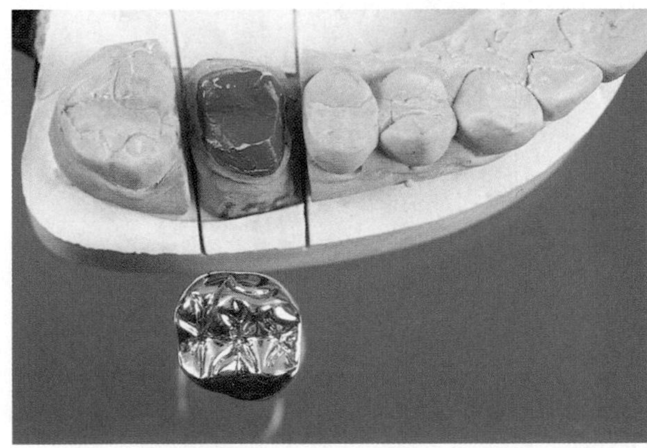

**FIG. 50.5** Posterior gold crown.

The **three-quarter crown** differs from the full crown in that it does not cover the entire anatomic portion of the tooth. Instead, the tooth is prepared so that the facial or buccal surface of the tooth is unchanged. When the crown is placed, the natural enamel on the facial surface is visible, and the crown covers the prepared portion.

A **porcelain-fused-to-metal (PFM) crown** has a metal layer with an outer surface of a thin layer of porcelain. This

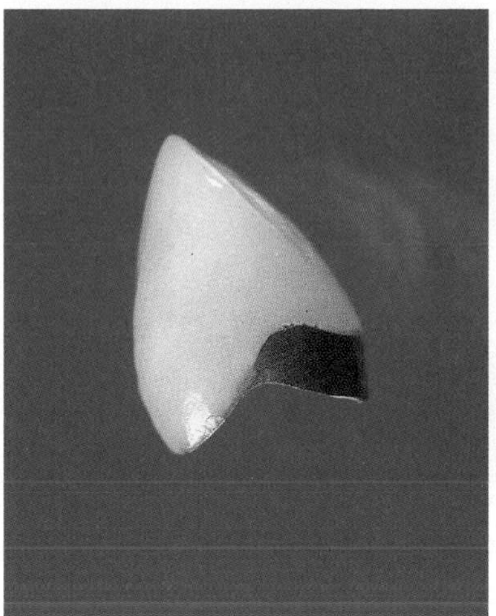

**FIG. 50.6** Anterior porcelain-fused-to-metal (PFM) crown.

type of casting has the strength of a metal crown and the esthetic appeal of a natural tooth color (Fig. 50.6).

A **porcelain jacket crown** is a porcelain ceramic crown which is used to protect the entire surface of a tooth. These restorations are used on anterior teeth and are esthetically pleasing but lack the strength of a PFM crown.

## Fixed Bridge

A **fixed bridge** is a type of prosthesis that is prescribed when one tooth or multiple teeth are missing within the same quadrant (Fig. 50.7). A fixed bridge consists of a series of units joined together for greater strength (Fig. 50.8). The bridge is cemented into place and cannot be removed by the patient. With proper oral hygiene habits, a fixed bridge will provide many years of excellent service.

### Components of a Fixed Bridge

**UNIT.** A bridge is described by the number of **units** (teeth) involved. For example, a bridge that replaces one missing tooth with its adjacent teeth holding the bridge in place would be referred to as a *three-unit bridge* because it consists of three parts (two abutments and a pontic).

**PONTIC.** A **pontic** is the artificial tooth, or the part of the fixed bridge, that replaces the missing natural tooth. When a bridge replaces more than one tooth, a pontic is used for each tooth that is being replaced.

**ABUTMENT.** An **abutment** is the natural tooth that serves as the support for the replacement tooth or teeth in a fixed bridge. There is *at least* one abutment at each end of the bridge. When a longer bridge is constructed to replace several teeth, two abutment teeth may be present at either end. The abutment tooth is commonly restored with an onlay or a cast crown. Because the completed bridge is placed into the mouth as a single piece, the abutment teeth must be in alignment to allow the bridge to slide into place without adding excessive width or length.

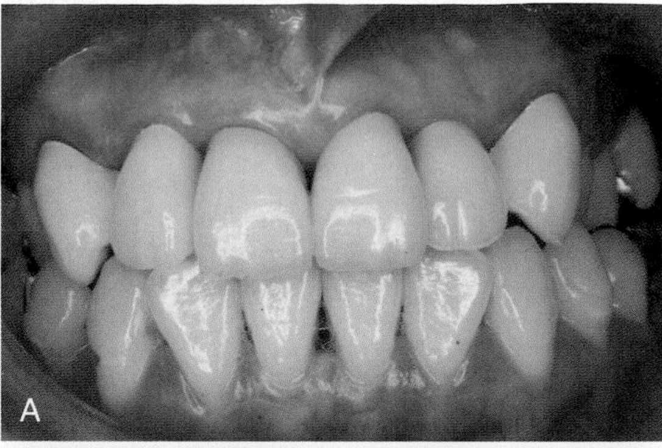



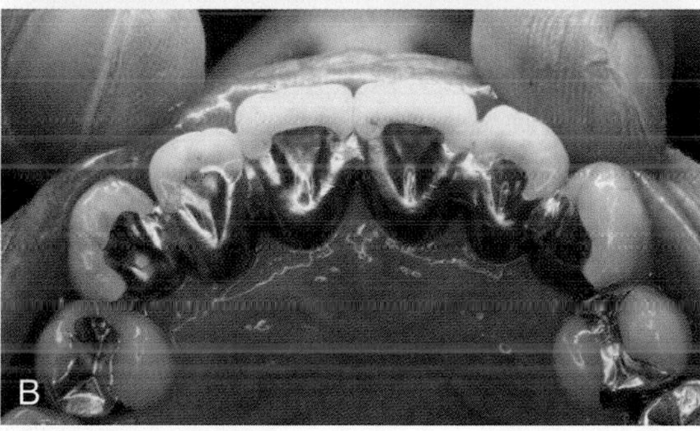



**FIG. 50.7** Six-unit porcelain-fused-to-metal (PFM) anterior fixed bridge. A, Final placement of a 6-unit fixed bridge. B, Lingual position of the bridge. *(From Rosenstiel SF, Land MF, Fuijimoto J: Contemporary fixed prosthodontics, ed 5, St Louis, 2016, Elsevier.)*

### Resin-Bonded Bridge

A **resin-bonded bridge**, also known as a *Maryland bridge*, consists of a pontic (replaces the missing tooth) with winglike extensions from the mesial and distal sides (Fig. 50.9). Bonding of these extensions to the lingual surfaces of the adjacent teeth supports the pontic.

In selected situations, such as the replacement of a single missing anterior tooth or the replacement of congenitally missing lateral incisors, a bonded bridge is an alternative to a traditional bridge. The dentist will decide whether the patient is a candidate for this type of bridge, or is better suited for an implant (see Chapter 53).

The lingual surfaces of the adjacent teeth require limited preparation to accommodate the bridge supports. Some bonded bridges have very thin metal mesh extensions. Others have cast or PFM extensions that require more extensive tooth preparation, so the natural contours of the abutment tooth are maintained when the completed bridge is bonded into place.

RECALL

3 What type of indirect restoration is placed to improve the appearance of the facial surfaces of teeth?
4 What part of the tooth is covered by a full crown?
5 What is the difference between an onlay and a three-quarter crown?

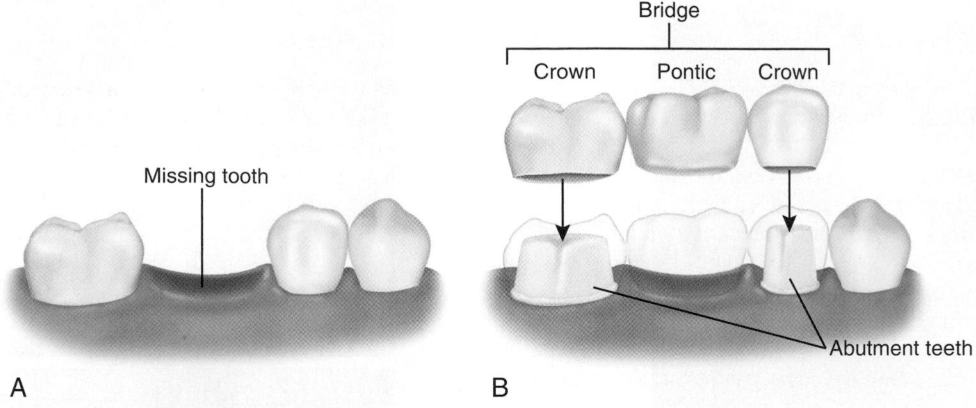


FIG. 50.8 Components of a fixed bridge. (© Elsevier Collection.)

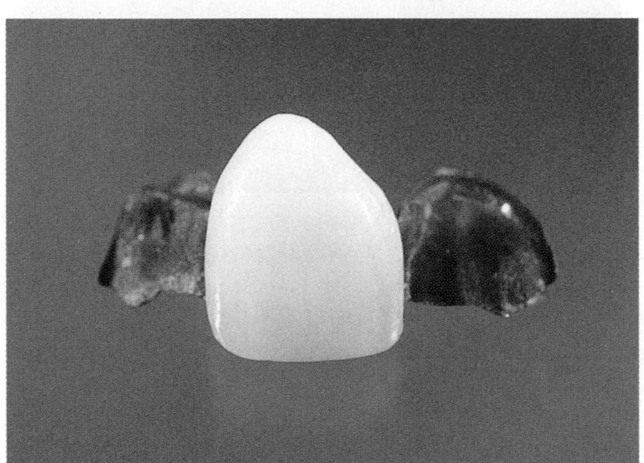

FIG. 50.9 Resin-bonded bridge.

# Role of the Dental Laboratory Technician

A cast restoration is precise and must fit the prepared tooth exactly. The dental laboratory technician carefully fabricates a casting that meets the specific requirements stated on the laboratory prescription (Box 50.1).

## Laboratory Prescription

The laboratory technician can fabricate a casting only on the basis of a written prescription from the dentist (Fig. 50.10). The prescription should be detailed and precise in its description of the restoration or restorations to be fabricated. A copy of the prescription, also known as a *work order* or *requisition,* is included with the case, and a copy is retained with the patient records.

A laboratory prescription contains the following information:

- Dentist's name, license number, address, phone number, and signature
- Identification of the patient (name or case number)
- Type of prosthesis requested
- Types of alloys or other materials to be used
- Exact shade of restoration
- Anatomic characterization, if required
- Date on which the case is expected back at the dental practice

## Laboratory Working Days

The laboratory requires a specific number of working days to complete the cast. This must be taken into consideration when the patient's return appointment is scheduled. Before the patient's next appointment, the assistant must determine whether the case has been completed and returned to the practice. If the case has not been returned or completed, it may be necessary to reschedule the patient's appointment.

RECALL

6 How does a dentist convey to a dental laboratory technician the type of crown or bridge that should be made?
7 What is the term for an exact replica of a tooth prepared by a laboratory technician?
8 What material does a laboratory technician use to create the pattern for a casting?

# Overview of a Crown Procedure

The placement of a cast restoration typically requires two visits. The first appointment includes shade selection, preliminary impression, bite registration, preparation of the tooth, final impression, and fabrication and placement of provisional coverage. The second appointment involves the try-in, cementation, and finishing of the crown or bridge.

## Shade Selection

If the crown is going to be fabricated from porcelain or ceramic, matching the shade of the natural teeth is important and must be completed before the tooth is prepared. A **shade guide**,

**BOX 50.1 Laboratory Steps in Creating an Indirect Restoration**

1. The laboratory receives a prescription, a final impression, and a bite registration for construction of an indirect restoration.
2. The final impression is poured to create the **master casts**. In the master casts, the prepared teeth are poured as dies. A **die** is an exact replica of the prepared portion of a tooth. The die is constructed so it can be taken into and out of the master cast.
3. Occlusal registration is used to position casts properly on an **articulator** to simulate the patient's normal occlusion.
4. A wax pattern is created for casting from the die of the prepared tooth.

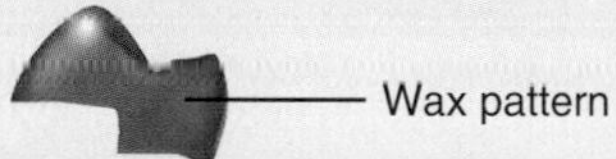


5. The completed wax pattern is removed from the die, and a wax or plastic *sprue* is attached. In the casting process, the sprue forms a channel that allows the molten metal to flow into the mold.

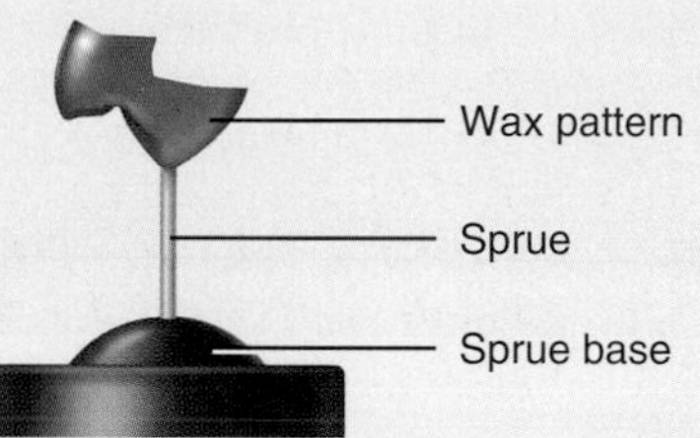


6. The completed pattern and sprue are placed in a casting ring and are *invested (encased)* in **investment material.**

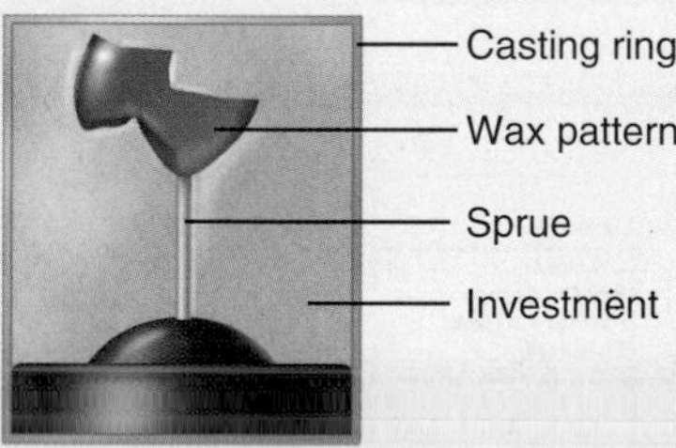


7. The casting ring is placed in a "burnout" oven. During the burnout process, the wax of the pattern and sprue is lost (burned away), and a negative pattern of casting remains in the investment material.

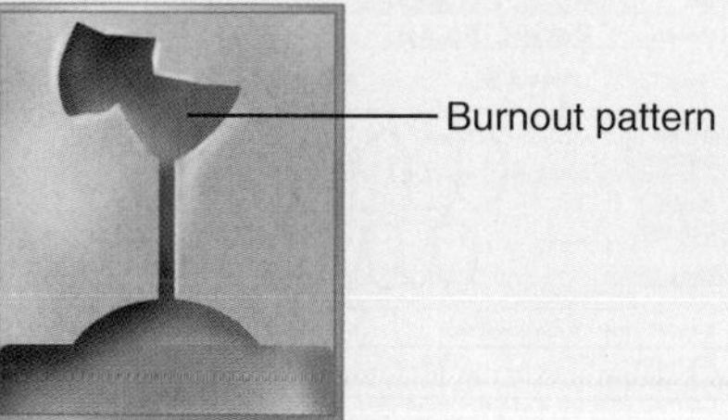


8. The metal alloy is heated until it melts; then, centrifugal force is used to cause the molten metal to flow through the sprue opening and into the pattern. This creates the casting.

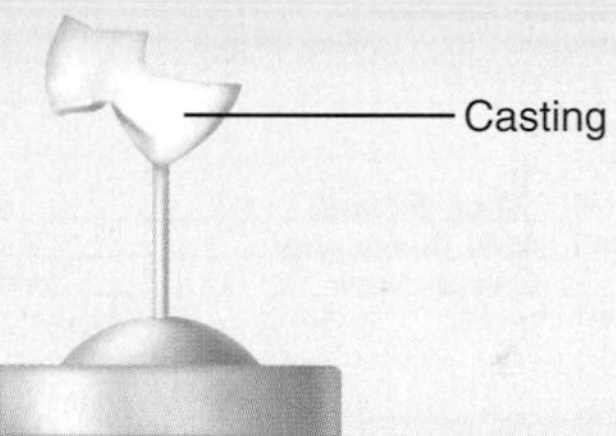


9. The cooled casting ring is placed in water to aid in removal of the investment material, and the casting remains.
10. The *sprue button* (created when molten metal fills the sprue opening) is removed, and the casting is polished and completed.
11. To achieve a truly natural look on restorations, the dentist may instruct the laboratory technician to add characterization to the finished surface. These fine lines and small areas of slight discoloration resemble the stains or cracks that are present on the natural tooth.



which contains samples of all available shades, is used to match the natural tooth color (Fig. 50.11). Most dentists prefer to make the shade selection while waiting for the local anesthetic agent to take effect.

The color sample is moistened and is held close to the tooth to be restored. Because teeth are normally wet, this moisture helps achieve a more accurate match. To determine the shade, the match is selected in a natural light. Many dentists will have a patient move to a window when selecting the shade. The shade selected is identified by number from the shade guide and is noted on the patient record and laboratory prescription.

The shade guide is a semicritical item that cannot withstand the heat of sterilization. After use, it is disinfected with the use of a high-level Environmental Protection Agency (EPA)–registered disinfectant.

## Tooth Preparation

During preparation, the dentist reduces the height and contour of the tooth with rotary instruments (specifically carbide burs) so that the casting will have the necessary strength but the overall size of the restored tooth will not be increased (Fig. 50.12). The prepared tooth is designed so the cast restoration

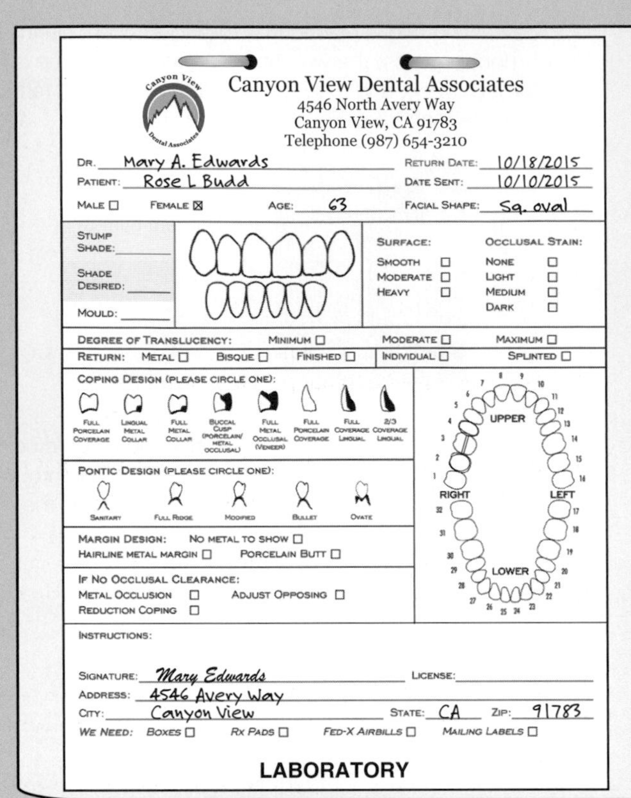

Canyon View Dental Associates
4546 North Avery Way
Canyon View, CA 91783
Telephone (987) 654-3210

Dr. Mary A. Edwards Return Date: 10/18/2015
Patient: Rose L Budd Date Sent: 10/10/2015
Male ☐ Female ☒ Age: 63 Facial Shape: Sq. oval

Stump Shade: ____
Shade Desired: ____
Mould: ____

Surface: Smooth ☐ Moderate ☐ Heavy ☐
Occlusal Stain: None ☐ Light ☐ Medium ☐ Dark ☐

Degree of Translucency: Minimum ☐ Moderate ☐ Maximum ☐
Return: Metal ☐ Bisque ☐ Finished ☐ Individual ☐ Splinted ☐

Coping Design (please circle one):
Full Porcelain Coverage; Lingual Metal Collar; Full Metal Collar; Buccal Cusp (Porcelain/Metal Occlusal); Full Metal Occlusal (Veneer); Full Porcelain Coverage; Full Coverage Lingual; 2/3 Coverage Lingual

Pontic Design (please circle one):
Sanitary; Full Ridge; Modified; Bullet; Ovate

Margin Design: No metal to show ☐
Hairline metal margin ☐ Porcelain butt ☐

If No Occlusal Clearance:
Metal occlusion ☐ Adjust opposing ☐
Reduction coping ☐

Upper Right Left Lower

Instructions:

Signature: Mary Edwards License: ____
Address: 4546 Avery Way
City: Canyon View State: CA Zip: 91783
We Need: Boxes ☐ Rx Pads ☐ Fed-X Airbills ☐ Mailing Labels ☐

**LABORATORY**

**Laboratory Forms**

Laboratory forms are used to communicate instructions to dental laboratory staff in the fabrication of a dental prosthesis. This form or prescription is required in most states to prevent the illegal practice of dentistry. The form contains specific information that communicates to the laboratory what needs to be done.

*Paper:* It is important to keep a copy of this form in the patient's chart for reference. The laboratory prescription includes the patient's name or identification number, along with date, instructions, signature, and license number of the prescribing dentist.

*Electronic:* As with some of the other forms, information required to be entered into the laboratory prescription may be pulled from other parts of the patient or provider files, easing the work of the dental healthcare team.

(Dentrix screen shot courtesy Henry Schein Practice Solutions, American Fork, UT.)

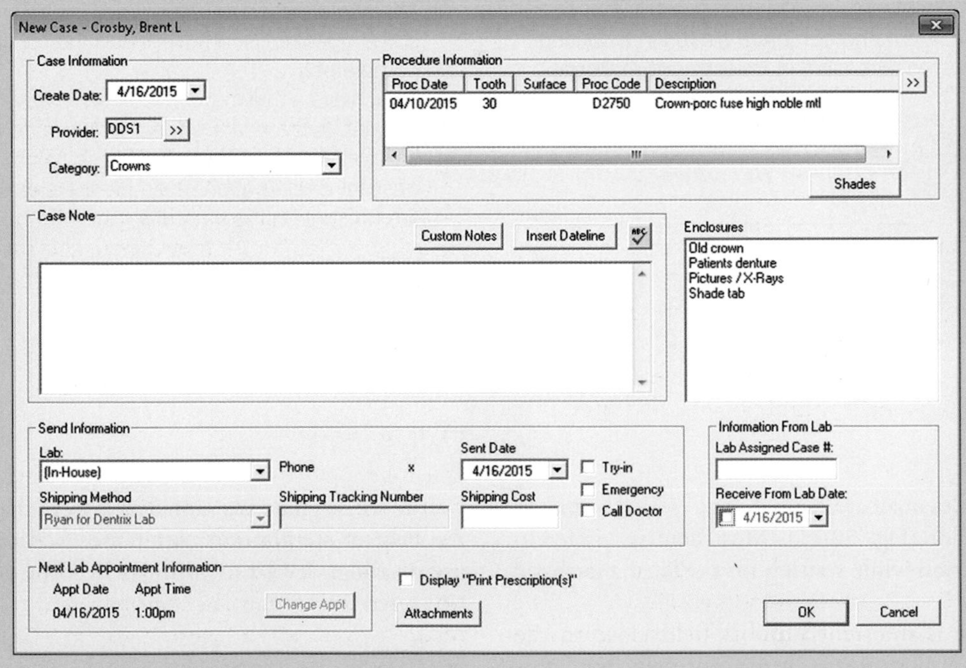


**FIG. 50.10** Laboratory prescription. *(From Gaylor LJ: The administrative dental assistant, ed 4, St Louis, 2017, Elsevier. Dentrix screen shot courtesy Henry Schein Practice Solutions, American Fork, UT.)*

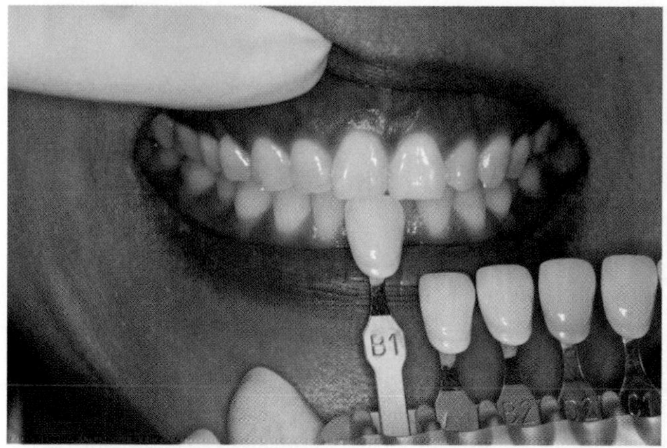


**FIG. 50.11** Shade guide, used to match the exact color of tooth. *(From Freedman G: Contemporary esthetic dentistry, St Louis, 2012, Mosby.)*

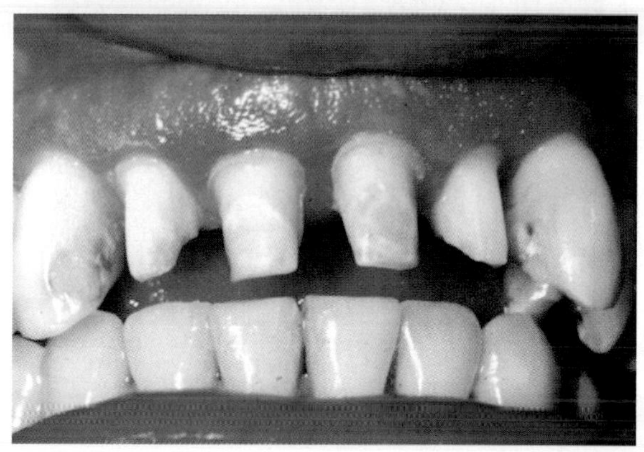

**FIG. 50.12** Prepared tooth structure showing height and contour. *(From Rosenstiel SF, Land MF, Fuijimoto J: Contemporary fixed prosthodontics, ed 5, St Louis, 2016, Elsevier.)*

can slide into place and will be able to withstand the forces of occlusion.

The gingival margins of the preparation are designed to provide a smooth, strong junction of the edges *(margins)* of the casting with the surface of the tooth. These margins are known by several terms, which include **bevel**, **chamfer**, and **shoulder**.

## Retention Aids for Crowns

When the coronal portion of a tooth is extensively decayed or fractured, or has been treated endodontically, it may be necessary to provide additional support for the crown to sit on.

### Core Buildup

If a tooth is vital, a **core** buildup is used. This supports the cast crown and provides a larger area of surface retention for cementation of the crown. If an amalgam restoration is already

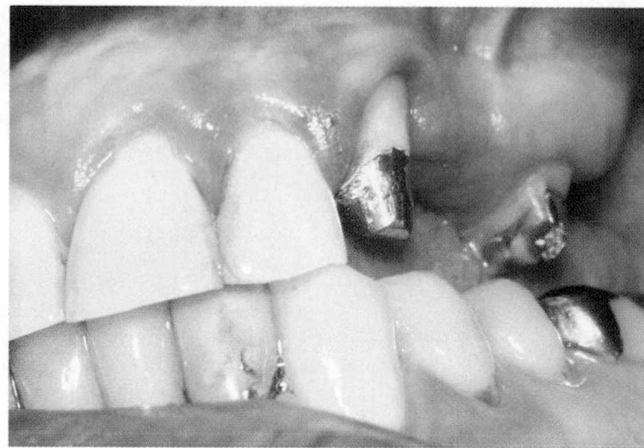

**FIG. 50.13** An existing amalgam restoration is prepared for the core buildup designed to support the crown.

in place, the restoration can be shaped and prepared (similarly to natural tooth structure) as the core (Fig. 50.13). If a restoration is not in place, a self-curing or light-cured composite material or reinforced glass ionomer cement is used for the buildup. The core buildup process is completed through the following steps:

1. The core material is prepared.
2. The material is placed in an anatomic crown form and is placed on the tooth.
3. After the initial set of material, the crown form is cut away. Initial set time will vary depending on the material.
4. After the final set (approximately 10 minutes), the material is reduced with the use of rotary instruments to serve as the foundation of the crown preparation.

### Retention Pins

Pin retention may be necessary to add strength to the core buildup for the crown. The type of crown and the location of the pulp determine the exact location of the pinholes and placement of the pins. When pins are used, they are placed before the core buildup and then are incorporated into the buildup material.

The steps in the preparation and placement of these pins are very similar to those in the placement of pins in an amalgam restoration as discussed in Chapter 48.

### Post and Core

If a tooth is nonvital and has been treated endodontically, a post is fabricated and cemented into the pulpal canal. *Prefabricated posts* are made of titanium and titanium alloys. If it fits accurately, a preformed post may be used. In some cases, a **cast post** is necessary instead of a prefabricated post. A cast post is made from an acrylic pattern and is fabricated by the dental laboratory technician.

To provide strength and stability to the post and crown, the post is placed deeply into the canal. A portion of the post extends out of the canal to the height of the core buildup. After the post has been cemented into place, a core buildup is placed to support the crown.

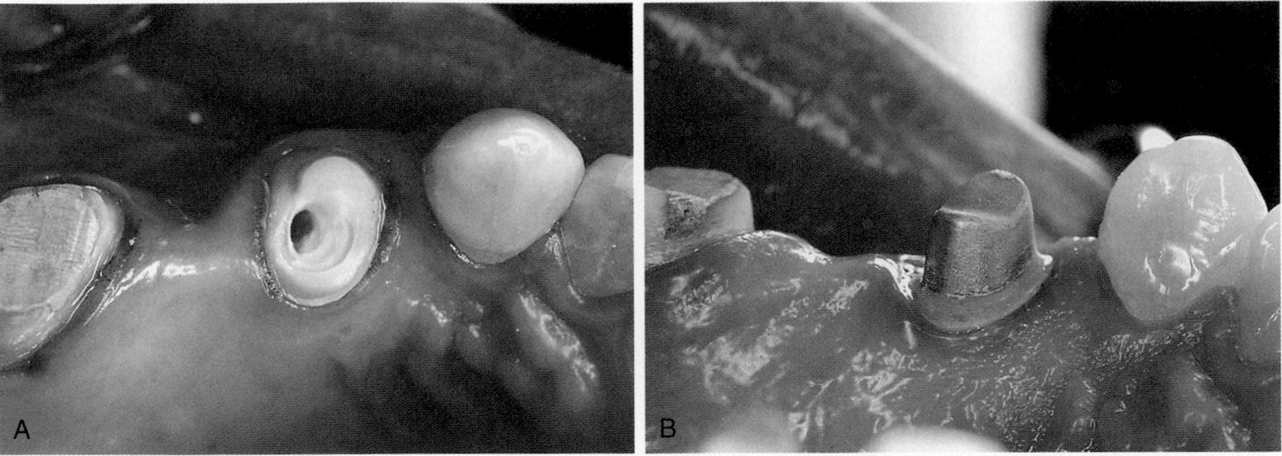

**FIG. 50.14** Tooth #5 was restored using a cast post and core. A, Prepared tooth. B, Cemented cast post and core. *(From Johnson W: Color atlas of endodontics, St Louis, 2002, Saunders.)*

Enlarging the treated pulp canal creates a *post channel,* which is the opening into which the post will be cemented. *Keyway slots* hold the post steady in the canal and are created in the adjacent dentin. After the opening has been prepared, a preformed post is selected and fitted. A *Lentulo spiral,* an endodontic instrument, is used to place the cement into the post channel. Once cementation of the post is complete, the dentist may proceed with the core buildup and tooth preparation (Fig. 50.14).

## Gingival Retraction and Tissue Management

Taking a final impression is a component of the procedure when fabricating a crown or a bridge. The impression should capture the whole tooth preparation as well as some uncut tooth structure past the gingival margin in an apical direction. Obtaining this detail is possible through the use of **gingival retraction**. Gingival retraction temporarily displaces the gingival tissue and widens the sulcus so that the impression material can flow around all parts of the preparation.

Gingival retraction takes place *after* the preparation is complete and *just before* the final impression is taken. Chemical retraction with the use of retraction cord is the most common method. In special situations, however, surgical or mechanical retraction may be required.

### Gingival Retraction Cord

Gingival retraction cords are available as untwisted *(plain),* twisted, or braided. *Untwisted* cords must be twisted just before placement. *Twisted* and *braided* cords do not require additional twisting. Cords are available in various degrees of thickness, and the dentist will decide which thickness is needed (Fig. 50.15).

*Chemical retraction* involves placing gingival retraction cord, also known as *packing cord,* into the sulcus surrounding the tooth. The packing of cord into the sulcus pushes the tissue away from the tooth. The chemical agent within the cord causes the tissues to *contract* (shrink), which temporarily widens the sulcus.

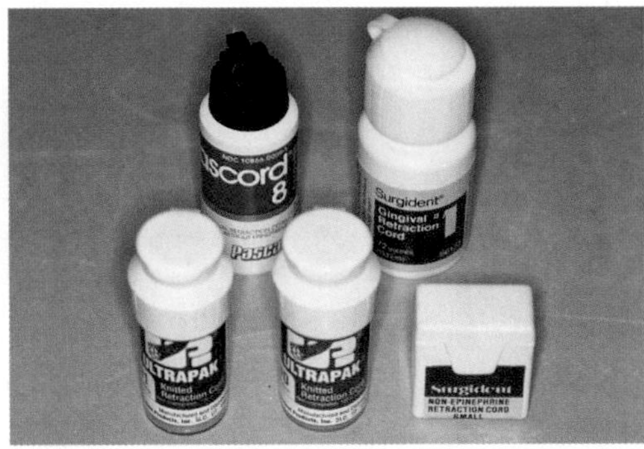

**FIG. 50.15** Types of retraction cords. *(From Rosenstiel SF, Land MF, Fuijimoto J: Contemporary fixed prosthodontics, ed 5, St Louis, 2016, Elsevier.)*

*Nonimpregnated* retraction cord does not contain a chemical agent and retracts the tissues only by force. *Impregnated* retraction cord contains a buffered solution of 10 percent aluminum chloride that helps in controlling bleeding and the desired temporary shrinkage of the tissues.

Cords impregnated with a vasoconstrictor are contraindicated for patients with cardiovascular disease. For this reason, the patient's updated medical history is reviewed *before* the impregnated forms of retraction is used. If the use of epinephrine is contraindicated, a cord impregnated with aluminum chloride may be used instead. *Aluminum chloride* is a mineral astringent that does not produce undesirable cardiovascular effects.

A *hemostatic* solution may be used to control bleeding in the area. The solution can be dispensed into a *dappen dish* and applied by lightly dabbing the area where bleeding is occurring with a cotton pellet moistened with the solution. Alternatively, the solution can be dispensed with an **infuser** syringe with tips. Any solution that is dispensed but is not used must be discarded.

### Retraction Cord Packing

Retraction cord is placed with the use of a blunt cord-packing instrument. This instrument has a straight handle with a broad,

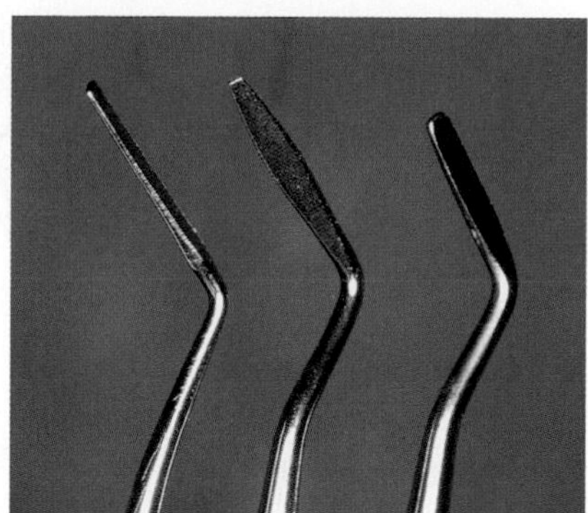

**FIG. 50.16** Gingival retraction cord instrument. *(From Rosenstiel SF, Land MF, Fujimoto J: Contemporary fixed prosthodontics, ed 5, St Louis, 2016, Elsevier.)*

rounded *(blunt)* working end that is used to place the retraction cord gently within the sulcus (Fig. 50.16). Some operators use a plastic instrument with a blunted tip for this purpose. The objective is to place the retraction cord *without* damaging the surrounding gingival tissues.

The retraction cord is removed just prior to the final impression material is seated. Often, the operator removes the cord while the assistant prepares the syringe-type impression material.

See Procedure 50.1: Placing and Removing Gingival Retraction Cord.

### Surgical Retraction

Surgical retraction may be necessary if **hypertrophied** gingival tissue interferes with preparation and placement of a fixed restoration. This excess tissue can be removed electrosurgically or with a surgical knife. *Electrosurgery,* the most common method, is performed with a special electrical tip that quickly cauterizes away excess tissue and controls bleeding. When using a surgical knife, the operator will incise the excess gingiva and remove it from the area. If bleeding occurs, pressure or hemostatic material must be applied to control bleeding.

### Mechanical Retraction

If other retraction methods are not suitable, the dentist may use mechanical retraction to move the tissue away from the tooth. A provisional crown, one that extends into the sulcus, is placed and worn by the patient for several days. It is removed just before the impression is taken.

The use of mechanical retraction requires an extra patient visit to take the final impression. At the end of that visit, normal provisional coverage is placed.

## Final Impression and Bite Registration

The final impression, also referred to as the **master impression,** for an indirect restoration must be accurate and detailed. If the impression is defective, the casting can also be defective. *Elastomeric materials* are generally used to create these extremely accurate impressions. The dentist will select the impression material to be used according to the impression qualities needed. It also will be necessary at this time to obtain a bite registration and an opposing-arch registration. Chapter 46 describes the mixing and taking of final impressions and bite registrations.

## Provisional Coverage

Provisional coverage is a protective temporary tooth covering that is placed after a tooth has been prepared and the final impression obtained. Chapter 51 reviews the types of provisional coverage that are available and explains the role of the expanded-functions dental assistant (EFDA)/registered dental assistant (RDA) in the fabrication.

The four specific rationales of provisional coverage are as follows:

1. To reduce sensitivity and discomfort of the prepared tooth
2. To maintain the function and esthetics of the prepared tooth
3. To protect the margins of the preparation
4. To prevent shifting of adjacent or opposing teeth

Generally, a provisional crown or bridge should maintain or restore function and keep the patient comfortable during the period from tooth preparation to final cementation, usually ranging from several days to a few weeks. Occasionally, patients are required to wear provisional coverage for a longer period to accommodate a more complex treatment plan.

See Procedure 50.2: Assisting in a Crown and Bridge Preparation.

## Delivery Appointment

Before a permanent restoration is placed, the provisional coverage must be removed. A large spoon excavator, scaler, or Backhaus towel forceps may be used for this purpose. The provisional coverage should be placed aside in case it is needed again should a problem arise with the casting. The tooth preparation is examined, carefully cleaned, and dried.

When the casting has been fitted and is acceptable, the dentist cements it with permanent cement. Great care must be taken during this step because once a cast restoration has been permanently cemented, it is almost impossible to remove it without damaging the casting, the tooth, or both. In contrast, if the casting is not cemented properly, the margins may leak, decay may be recurrent, or the crown could come off the preparation.

The cement selected for *luting* is the dentist's choice. Proper mixing of this cement in accordance with the manufacturer's instructions and placement of cement only on the interior surface of the crown are critical steps for the dental assistant. (See Chapter 45 regarding the mixing of certain cements.)

## Provisional Placement of a Permanent Casting

Once a cast restoration has been permanently cemented, it could be difficult to remove without causing damage to the casting. In special situations, where the patient is experiencing sensitivity, the dentist may choose to cement the casting initially with temporary cement, such as that used for provisional coverage. This provisional placement makes it possible to remove the casting without damage if a problem occurs with the tooth. If no problems are noted, the crown is cemented into place with permanent cement within a few weeks.

See Procedure 50.3: Assisting in the Delivery and Cementation of a Cast Restoration.

RECALL

9 How many appointments are commonly required for a crown procedure?
10 What does the dentist use to reduce the height and contour of a tooth for a casting?
11 If a tooth is nonvital, what is fabricated and placed into the pulp for better retention of a crown?
12 What is placed on the tray to displace gingival tissue during a crown and bridge preparation?
13 What type of agent is applied to control bleeding?
14 What term is used for overgrown tissue?
15 What types of impressions are taken during the crown preparation procedure?
16 What is placed on a prepared tooth while the laboratory is making a crown or bridge?
17 Who in the dental office is allowed to cement a crown or bridge permanently?

# Overview of a Bridge Procedure

Preparation for a fixed bridge can be completed in two appointments: preparation and "try-in"/cementation.

## Preparation Appointment

The first visit for a bridge is similar to the first visit for a crown, except it involves the preparation of two or more teeth, which requires a longer appointment. Depending on the case, the abutment teeth are prepared to receive a full crown or an onlay.

After the preparations are complete, the final impressions, occlusal registration, and opposing-arch impression must be taken. A custom provisional or temporary bridge then is placed. The provisional is prepared with the same technique used for coverage of an individual tooth. Refer to Chapter 51 for a more detailed description of the fabrication of a provisional.

## Try-In and Cementation Appointment

Prior to the patient's appointment, the assistant will ensure that the laboratory has returned the finished bridge. The patient will receive a local anesthetic agent if necessary, and the provisional coverage is carefully removed, cleaned, and placed aside for possible reuse if the bridge must be resent to the laboratory.

The casting is tried in and is checked carefully to determine the accuracy of fit. If the casting does not fit properly, final impressions may need to be retaken, and the bridge is returned to the laboratory for adjustments.

If the casting fits, adjustments are made as necessary, and the bridge is cemented into place.

## Patient Instructions

- Good home care is essential to the maintenance of a fixed prosthesis.
- The fixed prosthesis and supporting tissues must be brushed carefully each day.
- The other teeth are flossed as usual.
- A bridge threader is used to thread dental floss under the pontic and down into the sulcus at both abutments of the bridge (see Chapter 15).

RECALL

18 How many appointments are normally required for a three-unit fixed bridge?
19 What accessory is used to help in flossing a bridge?
20 What would be the next step for a dentist if a bridge does not fit properly?

# Computer-Assisted Restorations

CAD/CAM is the acronym for *C*omputer-*A*ided *D*esign/*C*omputer-*A*ided *M*anufacturing (Fig. 50.17). Dentists and dental laboratory technicians use CAD/CAM technology to design the anatomic features, size, and shape of a tooth restoration on a computer. Today, CAD/CAM technology is used for the fabrication of veneers, inlays, onlays, crowns, and bridges. Specific advantages of this technology include the following: one-visit procedure, no impressions, no provisional, reduced tooth sensitivity, and no laboratory costs.

To summarize the procedure, the tooth or teeth are prepared for the type of indirect restoration to be received (Fig. 50.18). The dentist pays special attention to the gingival margins and the outline of the preparation, making sure the area is completely dry and the surrounding tissues are retracted, and that hemorrhage is under control. The tooth is sprayed with a reflective powder and a digital camera is used to scan the area, creating an optical impression (Fig. 50.19). This process projects a three-dimensional (3D) image of the preparation and surrounding structures onto a computer monitor; this allows the dentist to use the CAD portion of the system to design the restoration. The dentist reviews the gingival margins and outline of the restoration, and once the design has been approved, the computer directs a micromilling device (CAM portion of the system) to mill the restoration from ceramic blocks that come in different sizes and shades (Fig. 50.20). Once completed, the indirect restoration is ready for try-in, contouring, cementation, and polishing.

See Procedure 50.4: Assisting in a CAD/CAM Procedure.

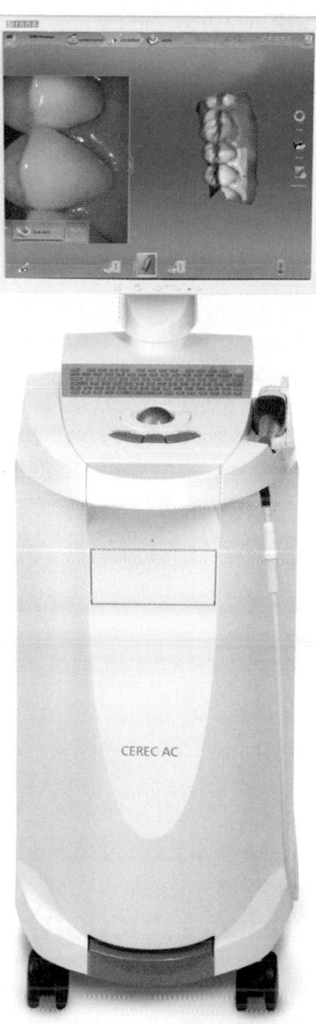


**FIG. 50.17** CEREC CAD/CAM device. *(Courtesy Sirona Dental Inc., Charlotte, NC.)*

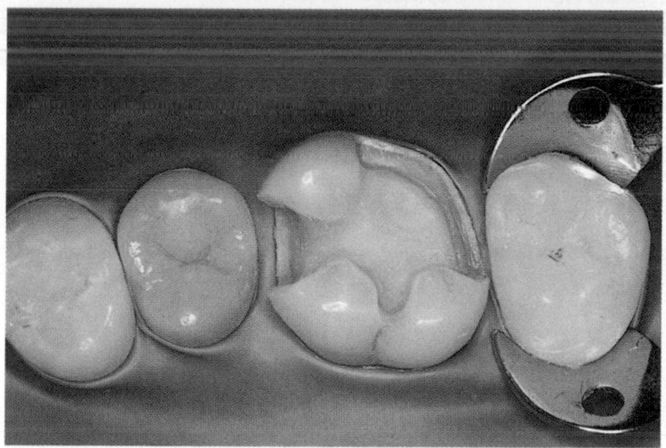

**FIG. 50.18** Molar prepared and readied for the scanning portion of the procedure. *(From Heymann HO, Swift EJ Jr, Ritter AV: Sturdevant's art and science of operative dentistry, ed 6, St Louis, 2013, Mosby.)*

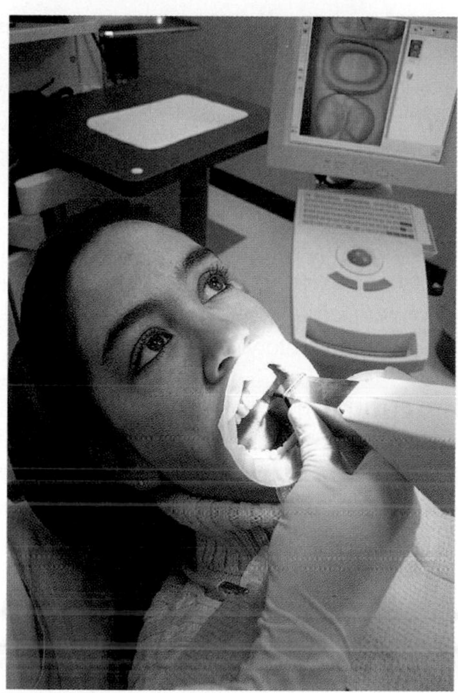

**FIG. 50.19** Optical impression being generated. *(From Freedman G: Contemporary esthetic dentistry, St Louis, 2012, Mosby.)*

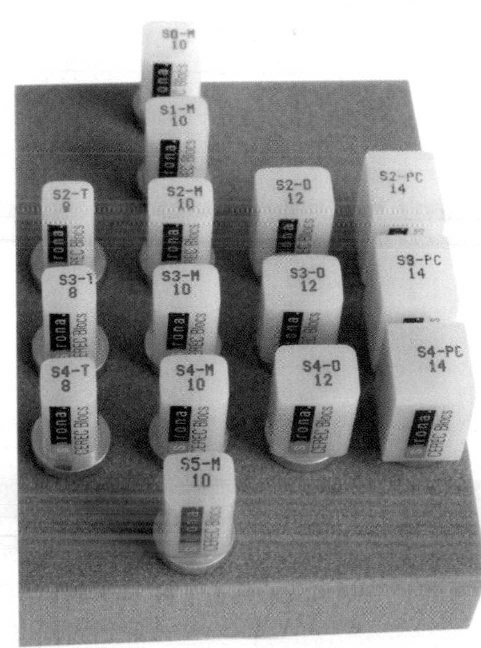


**FIG. 50.20** A series of ceramic blocks in varying sizes and shades used to prepare the indirect restoration. *(Courtesy Sirona Dental Systems, LLC, Charlotte, NC.)*

■ **Patient Education** Your patients are unaware of the amount of time and precision that goes into the preparation, design, and fabrication of a crown or bridge. The delivery of a cast restoration to a patient truly involves a team, including the dentist, dental assistant, business manager, and dental laboratory technician.

Fixed prosthodontics is a tremendous investment for your patients. Acknowledge and educate your patients as they make positive decisions toward their oral health. ■

**■ Legal and Ethical Implications** With many dental professionals involved in the making of a cast restoration, communication is crucial in providing the best care for your patient. As an EFDA, your involvement is important. You may be asked to take preliminary impressions, place the gingival retraction cord, fabricate and temporarily cement the provisional coverage, and assist in the series of appointments.

Remember always to review the patient record before providing treatment. Communicate with the dentist and the dental laboratory technician, and practice only functions that are legal in your state, province, or territory. ■

**■ Eye to the Future** The dental laboratory technician will take on a more important role in the future of dentistry. Until recently, dentists received extensive training in the preparation of laboratory cases. Dental school curricula are ever changing and are becoming more comprehensive in dental techniques, thus eliminating a lot of the hands-on laboratory work. It will eventually become common for certain dental specialties to hire a dental laboratory technician for office patient casework. ■

## ■ Critical Thinking

1. Mrs. Cooper is scheduled today for the preparation of a four-unit bridge to replace teeth #12 and #13. How many abutments and how many pontics will make up this case?
2. When the gingival retraction cord is placed on tooth #20, from which surface of the tooth will the ends of the cord originate? From there, in which direction will you continue to pack the string?
3. The dentist has seated a finished crown and has made all final adjustments. After mixing and loading the crown with cement, the dentist seats the crown and notices that the crown is not seating completely. What do you think happened?
4. Your patient has been given a diagnosis of tetracycline stains. How can this drug affect a person's teeth? What type of procedure could the dentist recommend to this patient to cover and mask this anomaly?
5. A close friend of your family comes to you for advice about whether to spend "a lot of money" for a bridge, or just have the teeth extracted and "get a partial denture." What would be your response? ■

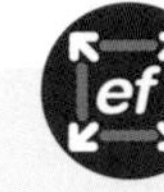

PROCEDURE 50.1 

# Placing and Removing Gingival Retraction Cord (Expanded Function)

### PREREQUISITES FOR PERFORMING THIS PROCEDURE

- ✔ Mirror skills
- ✔ Operator positioning
- ✔ Dental anatomy
- ✔ Instrumentation
- ✔ Fulcrum

### EQUIPMENT AND SUPPLIES

- ✔ Basic setup
- ✔ Cotton rolls
- ✔ Cord-packing instrument
- ✔ Gingival retraction cord
- ✔ Dappen dish
- ✔ Scissors

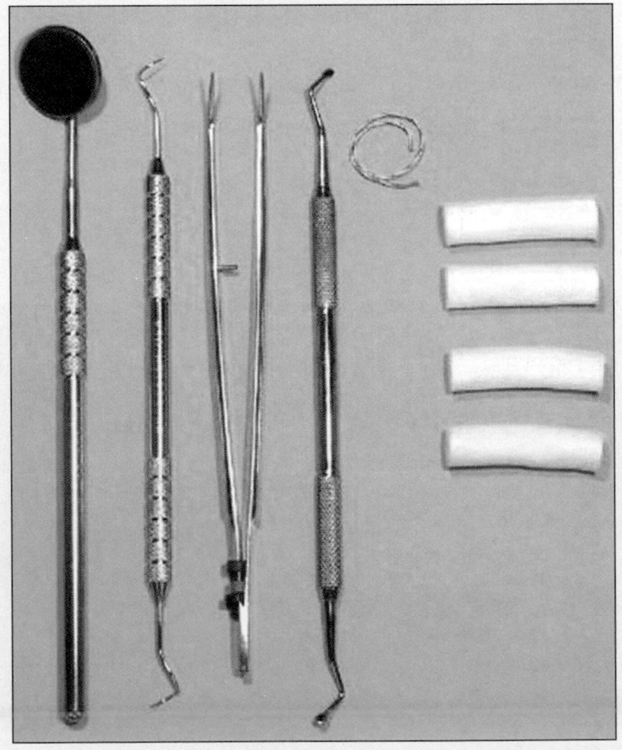

# PROCEDURE 50.1 Placing and Removing Gingival Retraction Cord (Expanded Function)–cont'd

## PROCEDURAL STEPS

### Preparation

1 Rinse and gently dry the prepared tooth; isolate the quadrant with cotton rolls.

**PURPOSE** Dry tissue makes it easier to see the details of the gingival tissue and place the retraction cord.

2 Cut a piece of retraction cord 1 to 1 ½ inches in length, depending on the size and type of tooth under preparation.

**NOTE** The length is determined by the circumference of the prepared tooth and the placement technique to be used.

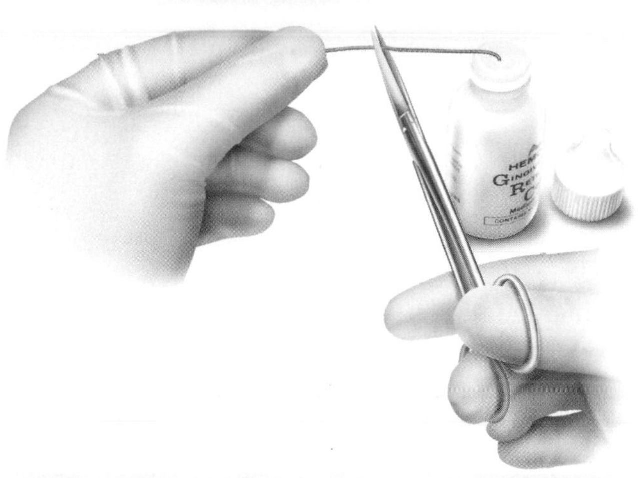

3 Use cotton pliers to form a loose loop of the cord.

**PURPOSE** This makes the cord easy to slip over the tooth, but the loop is not tied or knotted.

### Placement

4 Make a loop in the retraction cord, slip it over the tooth, and position the loop in the sulcus around the prepared tooth.

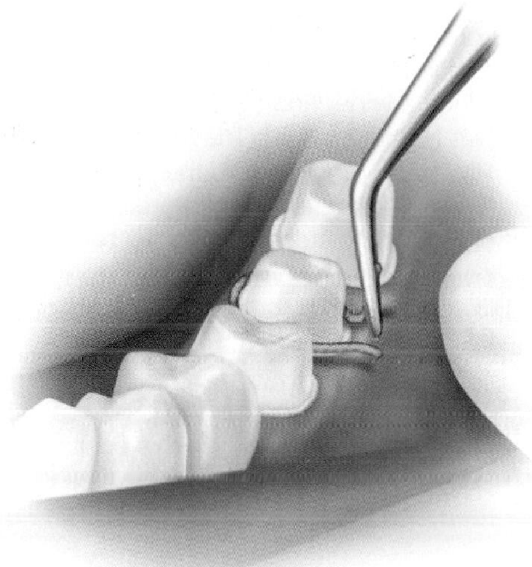

5 Using the cord-packing instrument and working in a *clockwise* direction, pack the cord gently into the sulcus surrounding the prepared tooth, so that the ends are on the facial aspect.

**PURPOSE** The ends in this position are easier to reach for removal of the cord.

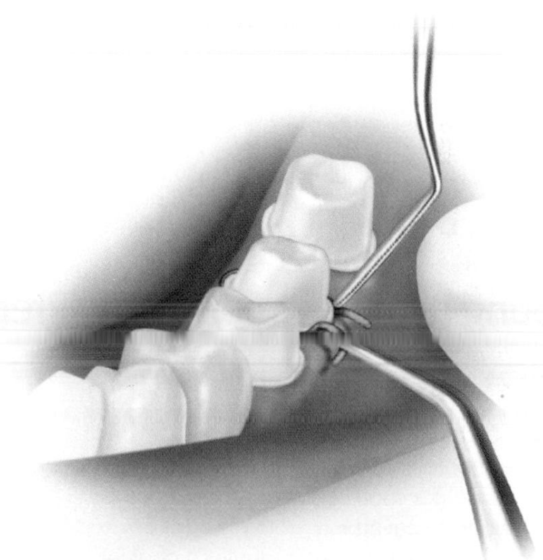

6 Pack the cord into the sulcus by gently rocking the instrument slightly backward as the instrument is moved forward to the next loose section of retraction cord. Repeat this action until the length of cord is packed in place.

7 Overlap the cord where it meets the first end of the cord. The ends may be tucked into the sulcus on the facial aspect.

**(Continued)**

## PROCEDURE 50.1 Placing and Removing Gingival Retraction Cord (Expanded Function)–cont'd

**NOTE** An alternative is to leave a short length of the cord sticking out of the sulcus. This makes it easier to grasp and quickly remove the cord.

**OPTIONAL** When a wider and deeper sulcus is required, two retraction cords may be placed with one on top of the other. *Before* the impression material is taken, remove the top cord. *After* the impression is completed, remove the second retraction cord.

8 The cord should be left in place for a maximum of 5 to 7 minutes. Instruct the patient to remain still to keep the area dry.

**PURPOSE** This time allows the cord to push tissue away from the tooth and stay in this position.

**NOTE** The exact time depends on the type of chemical retraction used.

### Removal

9 Grasp the end of the retraction cord with cotton pliers, and remove it in a *counterclockwise* direction (the reverse of the method used in packing).

10 Remove the retraction cord just before the impression material is placed.

**NOTE** Usually the operator removes the cord while the assistant prepares the syringe-type impression material.

11 Gently dry the area, and apply fresh cotton rolls.

**NOTE** The impression is taken immediately.

### Documentation

12 Document the procedure.

## PROCEDURE 50.2

# Assisting in a Crown or Bridge Preparation

### EQUIPMENT AND SUPPLIES

- ✓ Local anesthetic agent setup
- ✓ Alginate impression setup
- ✓ Shade guide (for tooth-colored restoration)
- ✓ Large spoon excavator
- ✓ Additional hand instruments (dentist's choice)
- ✓ Burs, diamond stones, and discs (dentist's choice)
- ✓ Gingival retraction setup
- ✓ Cotton rolls and gauze sponges
- ✓ High-volume oral evacuator (HVE) tip
- ✓ At this visit, setups are also required for the following:
  - Elastomeric impressions, which may include a custom tray
  - Occlusal (bite) registration
  - Provisional coverage fabrication, adjustment, and cementation supplies

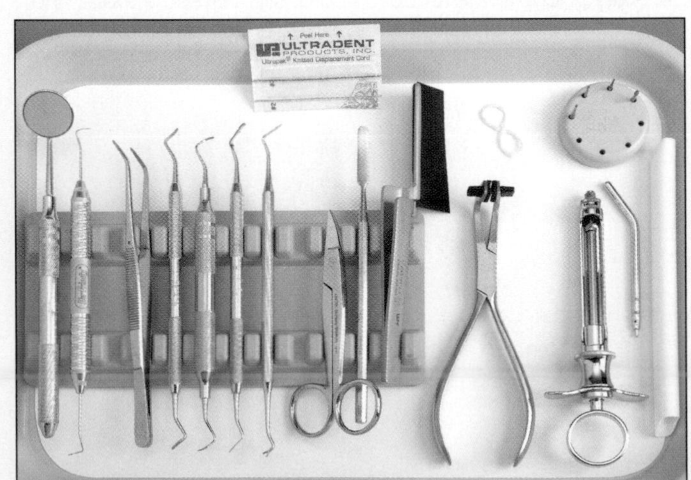


*From Boyd LRB: Dental instruments: a pocket guide, ed 6, St Louis, 2018, Elsevier.*

# PROCEDURE 50.2 Assisting in a Crown or Bridge Preparation—cont'd

## PROCEDURAL STEPS

### Preliminary Steps

1 Assist in administration of the local anesthetic agent.

2 If an alginate impression is needed to fabricate the provisional coverage, the impression is obtained at this time. In addition, an alginate impression of the opposing arch is taken (see Chapter 46).

3 If a silicone two-step impression method is used, the first impression is obtained at this time.

4 If this procedure involves a tooth-colored restoration, the shade is selected at this time.

### Tooth Preparation

5 Throughout the preparation, maintain a clear operating field by using the HVE to retract the lips and tongue and to remove water and debris.

6 The dentist uses diamond stones in the high-speed handpiece to remove all decay or fractured portions of the tooth.

**PURPOSE** Diamond stones are used during crown preparation because they can rapidly remove tooth structure.

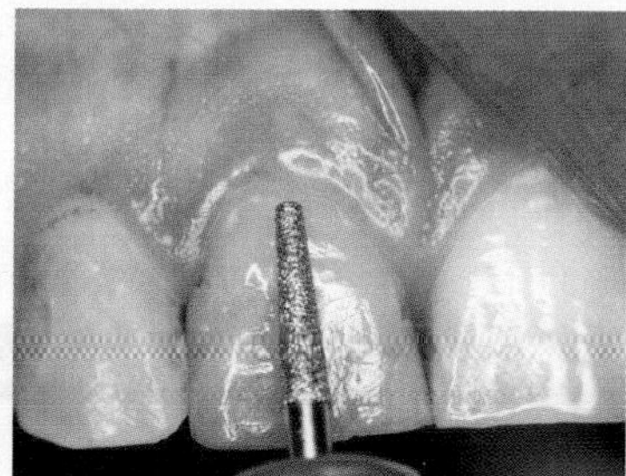

*From Rosenstiel SF, Land MF, Fuijimoto J: Contemporary fixed prosthodontics, ed 5, St Louis, 2016, Elsevier.*

7 Assist in bur changes as necessary while the dentist reduces tooth bulk and completes the preparation using burs of different shapes.

8 When the preparation is complete, the gingival retraction cord is placed.

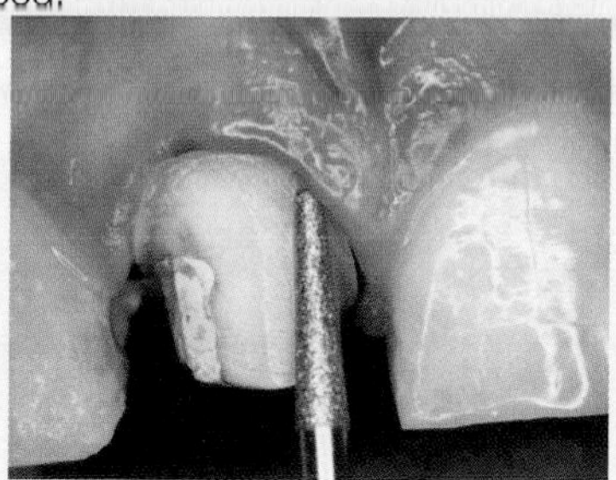

*From Rosenstiel SF, Land MF, Fuijimoto J: Contemporary fixed prosthodontics, ed 5, St Louis, 2016, Elsevier.*

9 Assist in readying the final impression material.

10 Before transferring the light-bodied material, transfer cotton pliers for the dentist to remove the gingival retraction cord.

**NOTE** The dentist may want to rinse and dry the sulcus before applying the light-bodied material.

11 While the dentist is applying the light-bodied material, ready the tray with heavy-bodied material.

12 Have the air-water syringe available for the dentist to "blow" air around the preparation.

**PURPOSE** This procedure thins out the material, allowing it to flow better within the sulcus and around the margins.

13 Retrieve the light-bodied material syringe from the dentist and transfer the tray, ensuring that the dentist can grasp the handle and insert the tray properly.

14 After the recommended time has passed for the material to set, the dentist will remove the tray.

15 The occlusal registration is obtained.

16 Provisional coverage is fabricated and is temporarily cemented to protect the prepared teeth (see Chapter 51).

17 The patient is scheduled for a cementation appointment and then is dismissed.

**NOTE** Ensure that the laboratory has sufficient time to fabricate the crown before scheduling the patient for another appointment.

18 After the dentist writes the laboratory prescription, prepare the case and send it to the laboratory.

### Documentation

19 Document the procedure.

| Date | Tooth | Surface | Charting Notes |
|---|---|---|---|
| 8/15/17 | 4 | PFM | Crown prep, 2 cartridges Xylocaine w/epi, final impression, temporary made and cemented with temp bond, Shade C2 for porcelain. Pt tolerated procedure well. Reschedule in 2 weeks for cementation. |
| | | | T. Clark, CDA/L Stewart, DDS |

PROCEDURE 50.3

# Assisting in the Delivery and Cementation of a Cast Restoration

## EQUIPMENT AND SUPPLIES

- Local anesthetic agent setup (if needed)
- Cast restoration
- Backhaus towel forceps (to remove provisional coverage)
- Large spoon excavator
- Cavity varnish/sealer and applicator *(optional)*
- Bonding supplies (dentist's choice)
- Cementation supplies (dentist's choice)
- Cotton rolls
- Saliva ejector *(optional)*
- Bite stick
- Articulating paper and holder
- Polishing points and stones (dentist's choice)
- Scaler (to remove excess cement)
- Dental floss

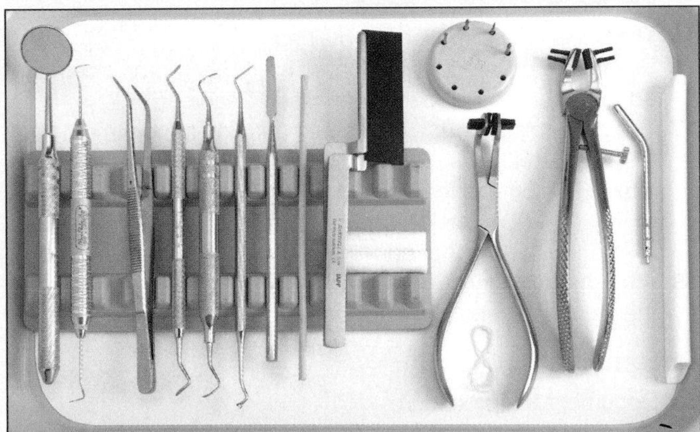

*From Boyd LRB: Dental instruments: a pocket guide, ed 6, St Louis, 2018, Elsevier.*

## PROCEDURAL STEPS

1 Transfer the cast restoration to the dentist to try on for fit. Transfer mirror and explorer.

2 When the dentist signals, mix the prepared cement.

3 Quickly apply the mixed cement in the internal surface of the casting, and transfer the prepared crown to the dentist.

4 The dentist places the crown on the prepared tooth, presses it into place, and then asks the patient to bite down on a wooden bite stick or Burlew wheel to seat the restoration completely.

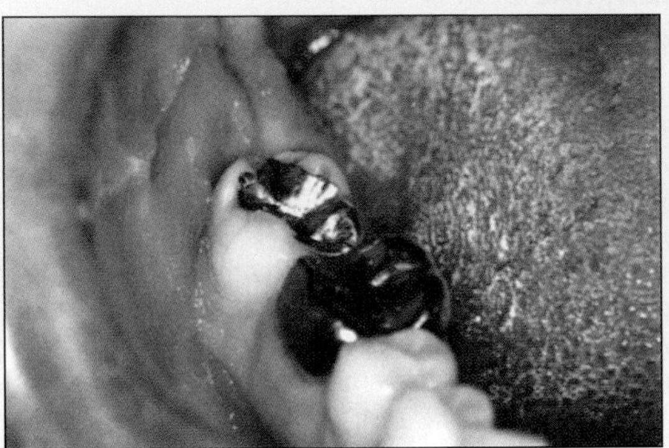

5 Instruct the patient to continue this biting pressure until the cement reaches the initial set, approximately 8 to 10 minutes.

**OPTIONAL** Once the casting is firmly seated, a saliva ejector may be placed in the floor of the patient's mouth.

6 After the cement has set, remove the cotton rolls.

7 An explorer is used to carefully remove excess cement from the crowns of the teeth.

**NOTE** This step is done very carefully so as not to scratch the newly placed crown or injure the gingiva.

8 A firm fulcrum is necessary for the hand that is holding the instrument.

**PURPOSE** The fulcrum prevents the instrument from slipping and consequently injuring the gingiva.

9 The tip of the instrument is placed at the gingival edge of the cement, and overlapping vertical strokes are used to remove the bulk of the cement.

10 Slight lateral pressure is applied (toward the tooth surface) to remove the remaining cement.

11 Dental floss with tied knots is passed between the teeth to remove excess cement from the interproximal areas.

**PURPOSE** The knots provide added bulk in removing the cement.

12 After the excess cement has been removed, the dentist may polish by using polishing points in the low-speed handpiece.

## Documentation

13 Document the procedure.

| Date | Tooth | Surface | Charting Notes |
|---|---|---|---|
| 9/03/17 | 4 | — | Crown delivered, cemented with glass ionomer. Patient pleased with crown's fitting and appearance. |
| | | | T. Clark, CDA/L. Stewart, DDS |

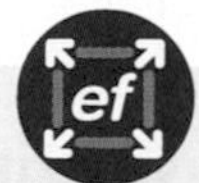

**PROCEDURE 50.4** 

# Assisting in a CAD/CAM Procedure (Expanded Function)

## EQUIPMENT AND SUPPLIES

- ✔ Local anesthetic agent setup
- ✔ Ceramic shade guide
- ✔ Hand instruments (dentist's choice)
- ✔ Burs, diamond stones, and discs (dentist's choice)
- ✔ Gingival retraction setup
- ✔ Cotton rolls, dry angle, or dental dam (operator's preference)
- ✔ High-volume oral evacuator (HVE) tip
- ✔ Optispray
- ✔ Etching material
- ✔ Cementation material

## PROCEDURAL STEPS

### Preliminary Steps

1 The shade of the ceramic is selected.

2 The patient is anesthetized for the specific area.

3 Cotton rolls, Dri-Angle, or dental dam is placed to control moisture.

### Tooth Preparation

4 The tooth and surrounding teeth are powdered with the Optispray to obtain prephotos of the occlusal registration before tooth structure or restorative material is removed.

**PURPOSE** This provides the computer software an occlusal or bite relationship from which to work.

5 All caries and any existing restorations are removed with the use of carbide and diamond burs, along with hand (manual) cutting instruments.

**NOTE** Care is taken by the operator not to produce any voids or undercuts in the cavity preparation to prevent the restoration from locking on during fitting.

6 Once the preparation is completed, the tooth is rinsed, dried, and isolated.

7 Gingival retraction is placed if needed.

8 The preparation and surrounding soft tissue are coated with Optispray for the taking of an optical impression.

**PURPOSE** The coating creates a reflective environment for the camera to pick up details of the preparation.

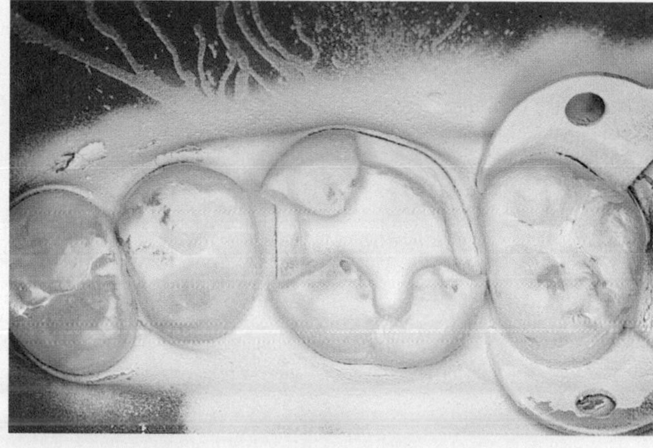

9 A digital impression is taken using the system camera.

**NOTE** Several images are taken to obtain views of the preparation and surrounding tissues.

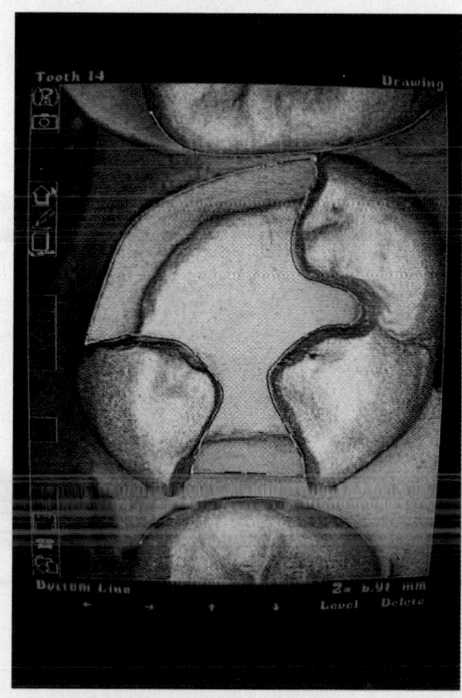


10 Using the images taken, the outline of the new restoration is drawn on the screen. A toggle switch is available to view all sides of the restoration to examine the margins.

11 The contacts and anatomy are viewed, and any needed changes are made on the screen.

12 The computer is instructed to mill the restoration from the ceramic block.

(Continued)

## PROCEDURE 50.4 Assisting in a CAD/CAM Procedure (Expanded Function)—cont'd

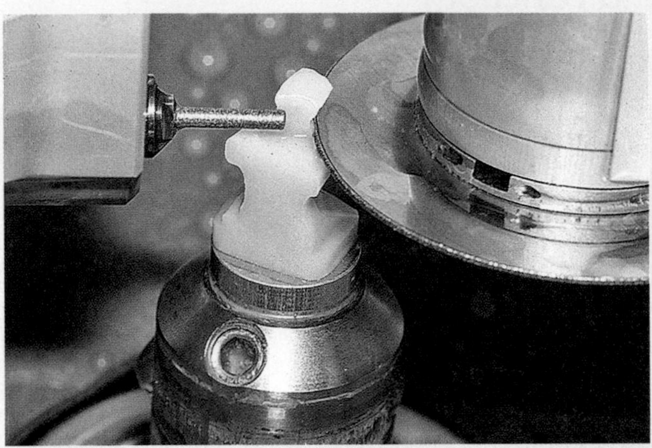

**13** The onlay is tried in and adjusted for fit using discs.

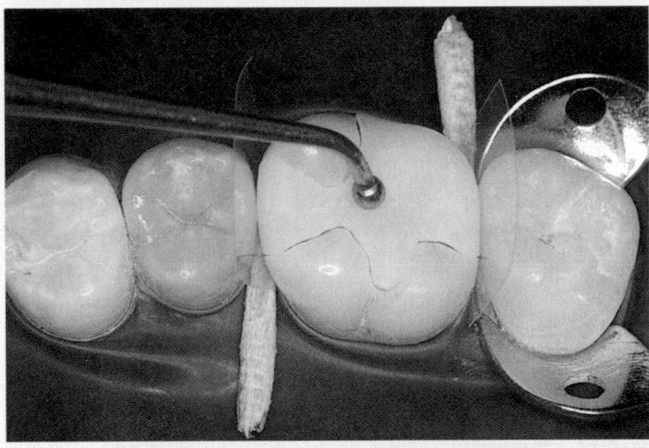

**14** The tooth preparation is etched, rinsed, and dried, and a bonding agent is applied.

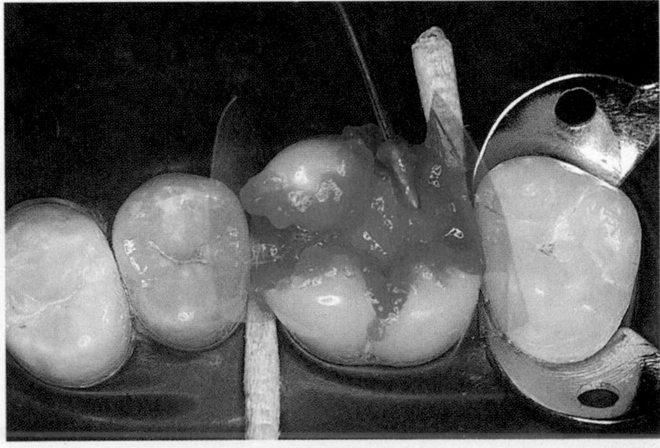

**15** The cement is readied and placed as a thin film on the restoration.

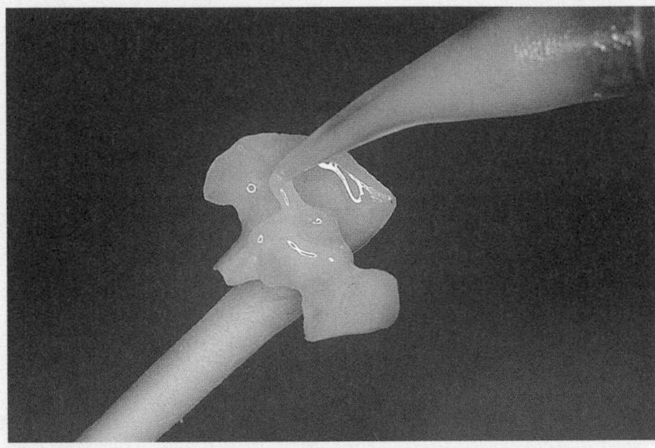

**16** The restoration is cemented, with the occlusal bite and contacts checked for accuracy.

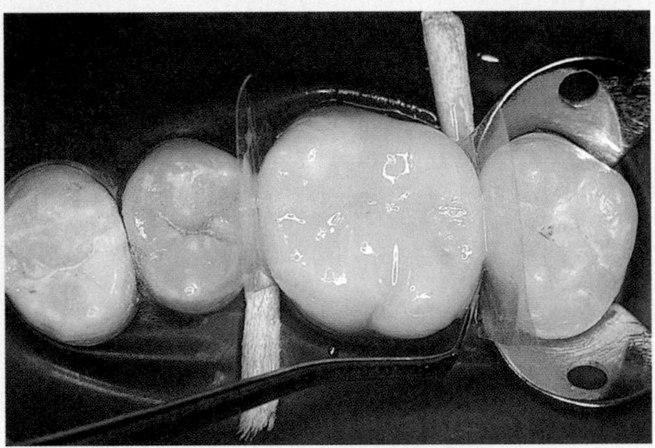

### Documentation

**17** Document the procedure.

| Date | Tooth | Surface | Charting Notes |
|---|---|---|---|
| 8/15/17 | 14 | MODF | CAD/CAM Onlay, 2 cartridges Xylocaine w/epi, Shade C2, Optical impression obtained, Tooth etched and bonded, and cemented with resin cement. Pt tolerated procedure well. |
| | | | T. Clark, CDA/L. Stewart, DDS |

All photos in this procedure from Heymann HO, Swift EJ, Ritter AV: Sturdevant's art and science of operative dentistry, ed 6, St Louis, 2013, Mosby.

51

# Provisional Coverage

## KEY TERMS

**Custom provisional** A temporary custom-made coverage that resembles the tooth being restored.

**Polycarbonate (pol-ee-KAHR-buh-nayt) crown** Provisional crown made from a hard plastic tooth-colored material used for anterior teeth.

**Polymer crown** Provisional coverage designed in a shell-like form.

**Preformed** Referring to provisional coverage that is already shaped as needed.

**Provisional** Referring to temporary coverage made for crown or bridge preparations and worn during cast preparation.

**Stainless steel crown** Thin aluminum crown made from a medium-hard material for good durability.

## LEARNING OUTCOMES

*On completion of this chapter, the student will be able to achieve the following objectives:*

1. Pronounce, define, and spell the key terms.
2. Discuss provisional coverage, including the following:
   - Describe the categories of provisional coverage.
   - Describe the indications for provisional coverage for a crown or fixed-bridge preparation.
3. Discuss the criteria for provisional coverage and cementation, including the dental assistant's role in making a provisional crown or bridge and troubleshooting.
4. Identify home care instructions for provisional coverage.
5. Explain the process of removing a provisional crown or bridge.

## PERFORMANCE OUTCOMES

*On completion of this chapter, the student will be able to achieve competency standards in the following skills:*

- Fabricate and cement a custom acrylic provisional crown.
- Fabricate and cement a custom acrylic provisional bridge.
- Fabricate and cement a preformed polymer crown.

## ELECTRONIC RESOURCES

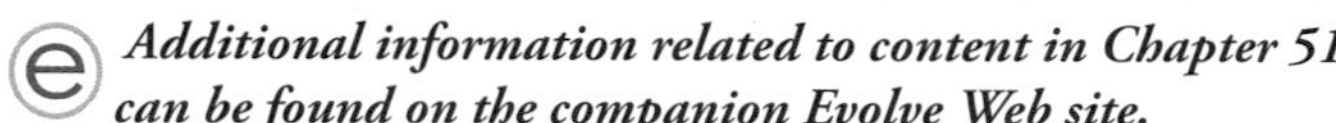
***Additional information related to content in Chapter 51 can be found on the companion Evolve Web site.***

- Practice Quiz
- Tray Setup Drag-and-Drop Exercises: Crown and Bridge Preparation/Cementation
- Tray Setup Questions
- Video: Fabricating a Custom Acrylic Provisional Crown

Provisional coverage is a **temporary** crown or bridge that is temporarily cemented to a tooth that protects the prepared tooth or teeth that will receive an inlay, onlay, single crown, or abutment teeth for a fixed bridge. The patient will wear the provisional coverage for a period of time while the dental laboratory technician is preparing the fixed prosthesis, which will be permanently cemented at a later scheduled appointment.

A **provisional** crown or bridge restores and maintains function to that area of the mouth and keeps the patient comfortable during the period from tooth preparation to final cementation. In most cases, this period can range from 2 weeks to 1 month. There are specific procedures when a patient is required to wear the provisional for a longer period to accommodate a more complex treatment plan. This may include implants or periodontal therapy.

There is an importance to the health of the area of the oral cavity where a tooth or teeth have been prepared for a fixed prosthetic. Indications for provisional coverage include the following:

- Protect pulp from sensitivity
- Maintain periodontal health
- Provide occlusal stability
- Maintain tooth position within the arch
- Protect the margins and preparation from fracture
- Be color compatible with adjacent teeth

## Categories of Provisional Coverage

There are two categories of provisional coverage: a custom provisional or a prefabricated provisional. The dentist will determine the type of coverage that best fits the individual's case and oral condition. The construction and temporary cementation of provisional coverage may be an expanded function in the state, province, or territory where you practice. If this is the case, this procedure may be delegated to you as a major role in your clinical position.

## Custom Provisional

A **custom provisional** represents the type of temporary coverage used for crown and bridge preparations. The procedure for making this type of provisional can be more time-consuming, but it can provide the best-fitting and most natural-looking restoration. This custom technique can be used for posterior or anterior crowns or bridges (Fig. 51.1).

## Prefabricated Crowns

A prefabricated type of provisional coverage can be used for posterior and anterior preparations. These shell-like crowns are available for single-unit teeth. The crown is supplied in several types of materials, depending on the location of the provisional (Fig. 51.2).

**Polycarbonate crowns** have a natural appearance compared with the other preformed provisionals. The crown is made from a polycarbonate material and is customized in varying sizes for incisor, canine, and premolar teeth.

There is a molar design crown made from polymer shell that can be filled with a composite resin material and finished with a laboratory bur.

**Cellulose acetate** is a thin clear shell available in all tooth types. The shell is used as a carrier of the provisional material. After polymerization of the material, the shell is removed and any contouring and finishing is completed with a laboratory bur.

**Aluminum and tin crowns** are thin aluminum crowns designed as either a cylinder shell or anatomic shell for posterior teeth. When using these, care must be taken when contouring the gingival margin because of their thinness.

**Stainless steel crowns** are commonly used for the restoration of primary posterior teeth in cases in which strength is essential and a match with tooth color is not a primary concern. These crowns are trimmed, adapted with contouring pliers, and cemented with a high-strength cement. See Chapter 57 for the complete procedure.

**Laboratory fabricated** provisionals are used less frequently. When several teeth have been prepared, or when a multiunit bridge is being created, a laboratory can complete the provisional prosthesis. A preliminary impression and cast of the teeth are prepared and sent to the laboratory well in advance of the preparation appointment. When the laboratory approach is used, it is important to confirm the provisional coverage has been returned from the laboratory and is ready for use.

RECALL

1 What term is used instead of "temporary" covering for a crown or bridge?
2 How long would a patient normally wear provisional coverage?
3 Why is it possible for the fabrication and cementation of provisional coverage to be an expanded function?
4 What type of provisional coverage provides the most natural-looking appearance?
5 What types of provisional coverage could be used for anterior teeth?
6 When would a stainless steel crown be commonly selected as a provisional?

## Criteria for Provisional Fabrication

Each type of provisional prosthesis follows its own unique fabrication method; you will find that your dentist will prefer a specific type of procedure that works best for that practice. This approach will become the method of choice for patients in the office.

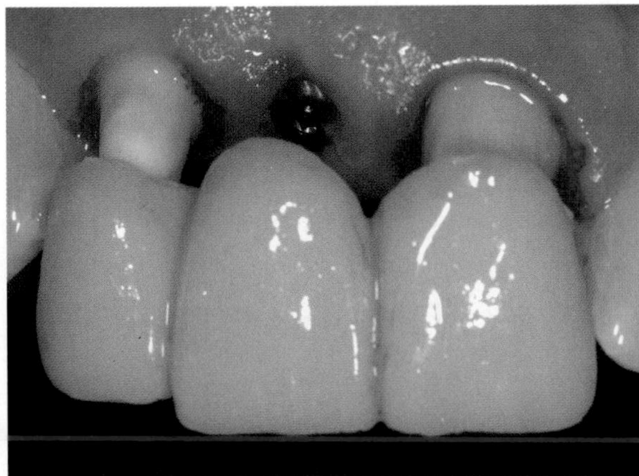

**FIG. 51.1** Custom provisional coverage. *(From Babbush CA, et al: Dental implants: The art and science, ed 2, St Louis, 2011, Saunders. [Surgery by Dr. Javier Suarez Lopez. Prosthetics by Dr. Jose Manuel Martinez].)*

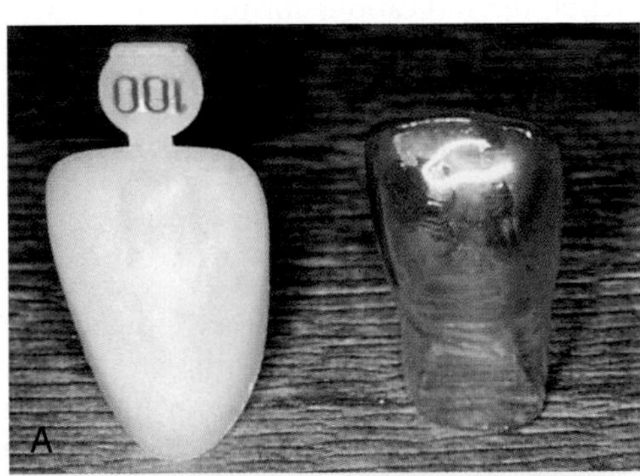


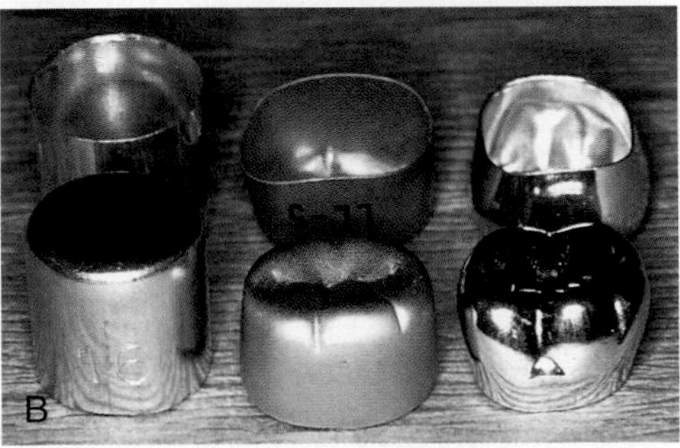


**FIG. 51.2** Types of prefabricated provisional coverage. A, Example of a polycarbonate crown and cellulose crown. B, Examples of aluminum, tin, and stainless steel crowns. *(From Rosenstiel SF, Land MF, Fuijimoto J: Contemporary fixed prosthodontics, ed 5, St Louis, 2016, Elsevier.)*

Regardless of the method used, the following specific criteria must be followed for each fabricated provisional crown or bridge (Fig. 51.3):

- The provisional coverage is esthetically acceptable.
- The contours of the provisional coverage are similar to those of the natural tooth, with adequate interproximal contacts and appropriate alignment within the arch.
- The cervical margin of the provisional coverage is smooth and fits snugly, with no more than 0.5 mm of space between the crown margin and the finish line of the preparation.
- The provisional coverage does not extend below the margin of the preparation.
- The occlusal surface of the provisional coverage is aligned with the occlusal plane of the adjacent teeth.

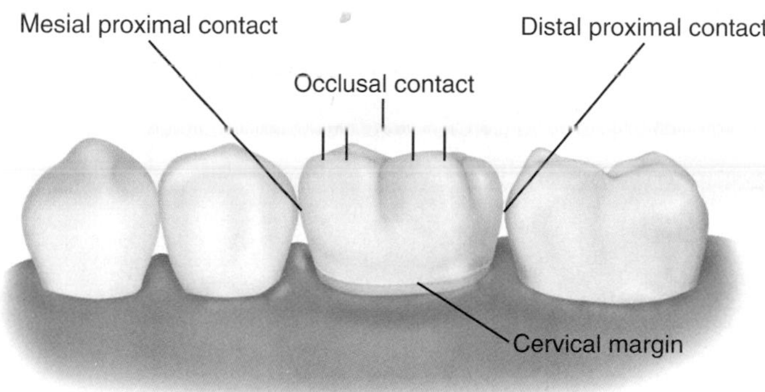


**FIG. 51.3** The provisional should resemble the natural tooth in its appearance, contour, contact, and occlusion. *(© Elsevier Collection.)*

*Alternative:* To avoid any trauma to the prepared tooth, the dentist may decide to intentionally take the crown out of occlusion by making the occlusal surface slightly lower than the adjacent teeth.

- When temporarily cemented, the provisional coverage remains stable, stays in place, and is comfortable for the patient.
- The provisional coverage can be readily removed without damage to the tooth or adjacent tissues.

## Custom Provisional Method

In the making of a custom provisional crown or bridge, the provisional tray or mold has been prepared for use before the dentist prepares the teeth for the final impression.

The common types of molds used for holding the provisional material are as follows (Fig. 51.4):

- Alginate impression
- Baseplate wax impression
- Vacuum-formed tray
- Silicone putty impression

## Custom Provisional Materials

The materials listed can be divided based on their makeup, supply, and setting properties (Fig. 51.5).

### *Powder/Liquid Materials*

These materials set in a 5- to 6-minute period. It is advisable to add the powder to the liquid when mixing to decrease air entrapment

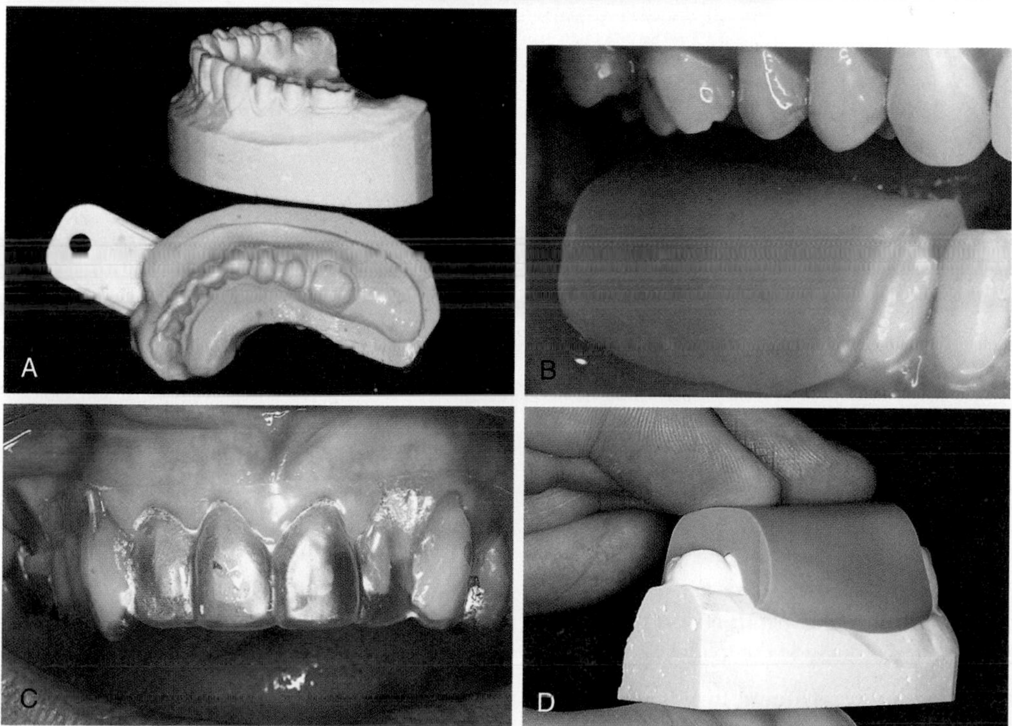


**FIG. 51.4** Types of molds used for holding the provisional material. A, Alginate impression. B, Baseplate wax. C, Vacuum-formed acetate tray. D, Silicone putty impression. *(From Rosenstiel SF, Land MF, Fujimoto J: Contemporary fixed prosthodontics, ed 5, St Louis, 2016, Elsevier.)*

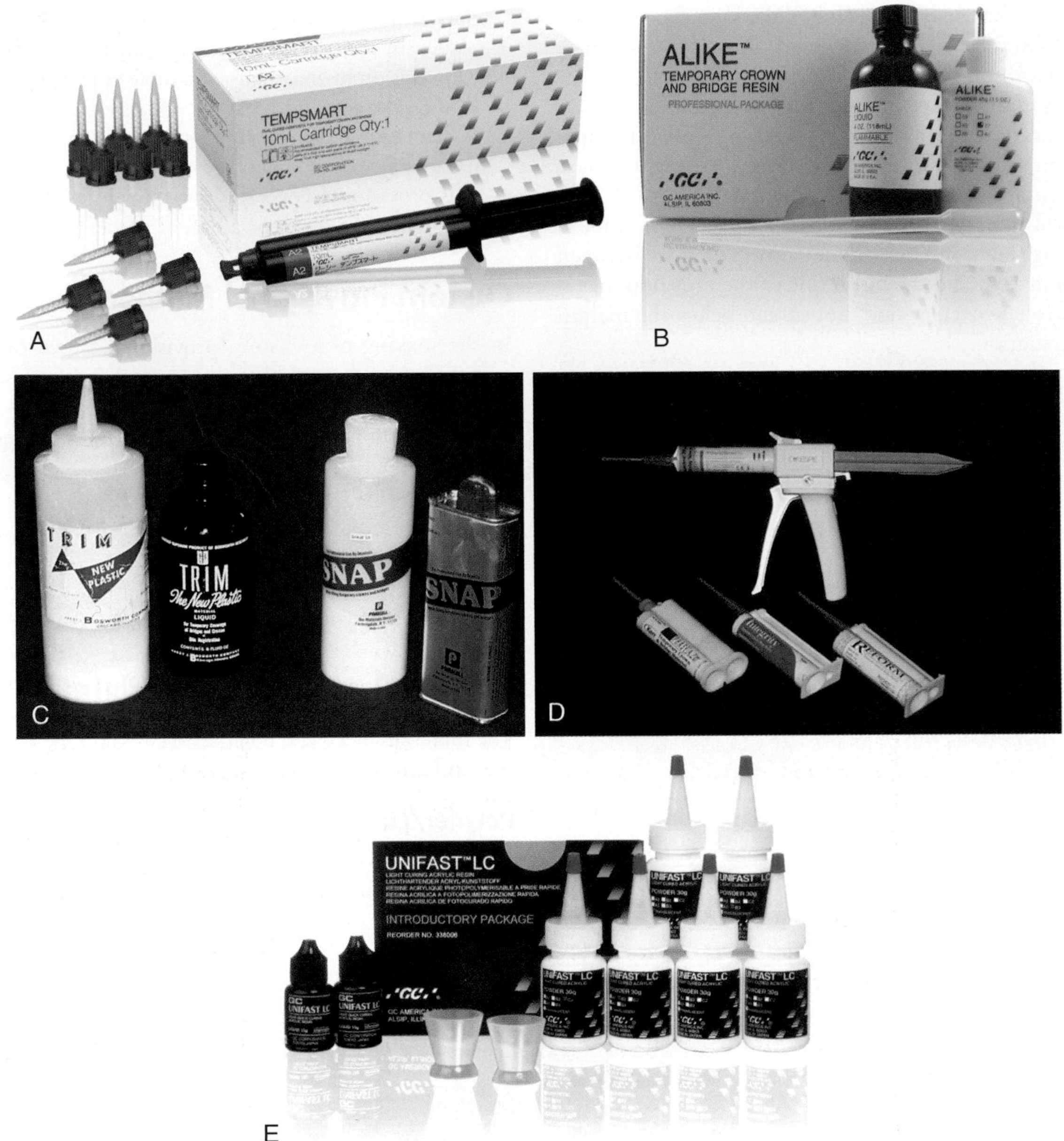


**FIG. 51.5** Different forms of acrylic and composite provisional materials. *A, B, and E, Courtesy GC America Inc., Alsip, IL. C and D, From Rosenstiel SF, Land MF, Fuijimoto J: Contemporary fixed prosthodontics, ed 5, St Louis, 2016, Elsevier.*

in the mixed material. When adding the powder, it should be sprinkled over the liquid and not poured into the mixing dish. It is recommended that minimal mixing be performed, as overmixing introduces air into the mixture leading to voids and a weaker final set material. See Chapter 43 for an in-depth review on preparation. Examples of these materials include the following:

- Methyl methacrylate is a powder/liquid formulation and is self-curing. Examples include Jet, Provisional, and Duralay.
- Ethyl methacrylate resin is a powder/liquid formulation and is self-curing. Examples include Trim and Snap.

## Paste/Paste Materials

This material is dispensed from preloaded syringes or cartridges and mixed through an automix tip. By having a consistent mixture, you will have less air incorporated into the final product. This material is kinder to the underlying pulpal tissue because of little exothermic reaction. Example of these materials include the following:

- Bisacrylic composites. Protemp is an example.
- Bis GMA acrylic provisional resin. TempSpan is an example.

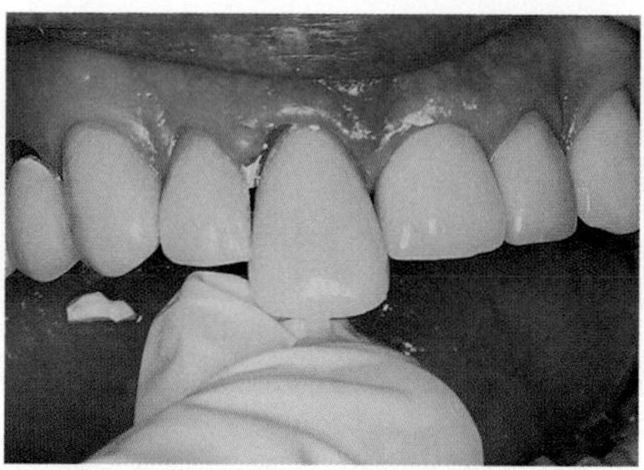

FIG. 51.6 Polycarbonate provisional crown. *(From Rosenstiel SF, Land MF, Fujimoto J: Contemporary fixed prosthodontics, ed 5, St Louis, 2016, Elsevier.)*

### *Light-Polymerized Materials*

Another type of provisional material is self- and light-cured composite provisional materials that have a glass filler content, with a working time of 45 seconds and setting time of 2 to 3 minutes, and complete cure time of 6 to 7 minutes. This type of material makes it an ideal choice for a multiunit temporary bridge. An example of this is LuxaFlow.

See Procedure 51.1: Fabrication and Cementing a Custom Acrylic Provisional Crown and Procedure 51.2: Fabricating and Cementing a Custom Acrylic Provisional Bridge.

## Preformed Crown Method

With the **preformed** technique, you will use fabricated provisional shell-like crowns, sized specifically for each tooth. These shells are made from a polymer or polycarbonate material and are designed with anatomic features of natural teeth. The presence of the shell reduces procedural steps by not requiring a preliminary impression or fabrication of a thermoplastic tray.

The preformed **polymer crown** resin used in this technique is a *hybrid composite* resin-monomer mixture that has a setting time of 90 seconds. The resin and shell then become a single bonded unit, providing the patient with strength and optimal margins for the time required by provisional coverage.

Tooth-colored preformed polycarbonate crowns are used on anterior teeth in cases in which appearance is important (Fig. 51.6). These crowns are available in a variety of sizes, shapes, and shades and have an *identification tab* on the incisal edge that indicates location of placement. This tab is removed once the crown has been selected. This type of crown has the stability and appearance to remain on the tooth preparation as the temporary, but it can also be used as the mold for the acrylic resin when a custom temporary is fabricated. A preformed crown is a semicritical item; if tried in the mouth and *not* selected for use, it must be sterilized before reuse.

See Procedure 51.3: Fabricating and Cementing a Preformed Provisional Crown.

RECALL

7 What step should be completed before tooth preparation when making a custom provisional?
8 What type of tray or mold is used to fabricate a custom provisional?
9 After the acrylic resin is mixed, how would you place it for the prepared tooth?
10 Does a polycarbonate crown remain on a prepared tooth, or is it just a mold for the provisional coverage?

## Criteria for Cementation of a Provisional Crown

The temporary cement selected should provide adequate strength to retain the temporary restoration for function; however, the retention developed by the provisional cement should be weak enough to allow for removal of the provisional restoration without causing damage or alteration to the prepared tooth in preparation of the cementation of the final restoration.

**Zinc oxide–eugenol (ZOE) temporary luting cements** are commonly used because of their sedative effect on sensitive teeth. Research has shown that eugenol is able to penetrate and diffuse throughout the dentin and can affect the bond strength. This material presents an excellent antibacterial effect.

**Polycarboxylate temporary luting cements** are designed to replace eugenol with various types of carboxylic acids that do not interfere with definitive cementation. They are compatible with resin provisional materials and with permanent resin cements and show greater retention compared with ZOE cements but have no sedative effect on the pulp.

**Resin temporary luting cements** present high strength, excellent retention, better esthetics, and easy cleanup. However, these temporary cements have a higher incidence of microleakage, discoloration, and odor associated with their use.

### Questions to Think About When Selecting a Temporary Cement

- How long is the provisional to remain in place? The temporary cement should be able to restore the marginal integrity and resist oral fluids. The temporary cement should maintain the proper seal at the margins for the duration of the temporary restoration. A cement suitable for a 1- or 2-week cementation will not be suitable for a longer period of time such as is required after periodontal surgery.
- How retentive is the preparation? Crown preparations or onlay preparations that have less retention will require a more retentive temporary cement. Preparations that have good retentive features can receive a weaker cement.
- Is an esthetic aspect important? In some cases, on anterior teeth, the temporary cement could discolor the provisional restoration if the provisional is thin. Thin preparations such as veneers may allow show-through of the temporary cement. In such a situation, a clear cement should be used to avoid discoloration.

## Troubleshooting When Fabricating a Provisional

Problems can arise when fabricating provisional restorations:

**Occlusal errors or voids**

*Problem:* When an impression has not been fully reseated after being filled with the provisional material, this can often cause occlusal errors or voids.

*Solution:* Trim away any interproximal tags with scissors before filling, and reseat the impression. When using syringe material, keep the syringe tip in the material to prevent the incorporation of air, which can cause bubbles in the mix.

**Locking on a provisional restoration**

*Problem:* Provisional restorations can become "locked on" to the preparation if material flows into the undercuts formed by the proximal surfaces of adjacent teeth.

*Solution:* While the provisional material is still soft and adaptable, remove the material from the gingival embrasure space with a Hollenback instrument. After removal, any excess flash should be trimmed with a pair of scissors; then the crown should be reseated a number of times to ensure that it does not lock into place when set.

**Marginal discrepancies**

*Problem:* Most distortion of the margins occurs when the provisional crown is first removed from the preparation.

*Solution:* If a marginal discrepancy occurs with a provisional resin crown, the simplest solution is to reline it with more material and then reseat it for setting. To help the seating of the provisional, do not fill the whole crown with resin, but confine the reline material to the inner aspect of the crown margin.

**Removal of provisional**

*Problem:* Once a provisional has been temporarily cemented, you want to be able to remove it easily.

*Solution:* To make removal easier, temporary cement should be applied around the inner aspect of the margin. Equal lengths of base and catalyst with a small amount of modifier or petroleum jelly can be used to weaken the cement for easy removal.

## Home Care Instructions

For the patient with provisional coverage who is waiting for delivery of a crown or bridge, the following instructions must be provided before he or she leaves the office, both verbally and in writing:

- Bite and chew carefully on the side with provisional coverage, and avoid sticky foods.
- When flossing, do not "pop" the floss into and out of the contact. Once the floss is placed below the contact, pull the floss through the contact to the lingual or the facial side.

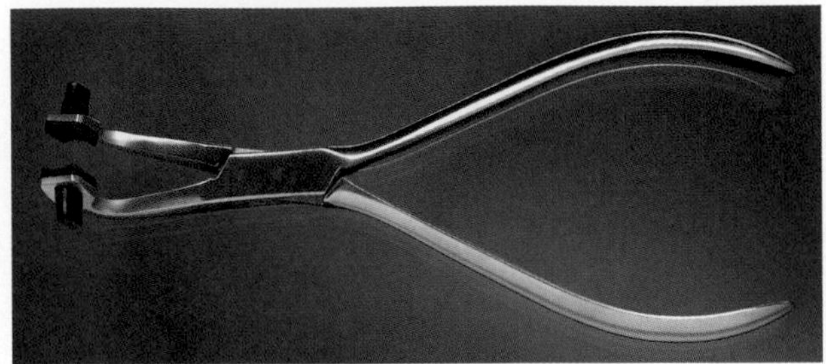

**FIG. 51.7** Provisional crown–removing forceps. *(From Boyd LRB: Dental instruments: a pocket guide, ed 6, St Louis, 2018, Elsevier.)*

- If the provisional coverage is loose or lost, contact the office immediately to have it re-cemented or replaced.

## Removal of the Provisional Crown or Bridge

It is essential that a provisional crown or bridge remain cemented while the fixed prosthesis is being prepared and delivered to the dental office. When the patient returns for the final cementation of a fixed crown or bridge, the provisional should be cautiously removed without causing any fracture or harm, just in case it needs to be re-cemented if the final prostheses must be sent back to the laboratory for adjustments and remake.

Finger pressure or provisional crown–removing forceps can be used to remove the restoration without risking damage to the margins (Fig. 51.7).

■ **Patient Education** Your patient has been informed that he or she will be wearing a "temporary" crown for the next few weeks. More than likely, your patient does not realize the importance of this coverage. If provisional coverage is not appropriately constructed to protect the margins, or if the prosthesis comes off and the dental office is not notified, the patient's crown preparation can be adversely affected. The crown may not fit properly, or the dentist may need to make adjustments to the preparation or restart the procedure.

Be sure to inform and educate your patient about the importance of provisional coverage and appropriate home care. ■

■ **Legal and Ethical Implications** The expanded-functions dental assistant (EFDA)/registered dental assistant (RDA) can play a major role in the fabrication and temporary cementation of a provisional crown or bridge. It is the dentist's and your responsibility to remain current with the new provisional materials and techniques that are available. Remember that this procedure may be an *expanded function,* and it may be legal for you to practice this only if your state permits. Check and keep current with your state's rulings and regulations. ■

■ **Eye to the Future** As mentioned in Chapter 50, the dental laboratory technician will become increasingly involved in the dental practice setting. Many dental offices will have a complete laboratory setup with a dental laboratory technician on staff. By having the technician on hand, and with the availability of new indirect materials, provisional coverage will not be needed. The dentist will be able to prepare the tooth structure while the technician is preparing the crown or bridge. ■

## ■ Critical Thinking

1. A patient is being seen today for a crown preparation on tooth #29/45. Because of the location of the crown, what type of provisional coverage could be recommended?
2. The dentist has anesthetized the patient and started the preparation for a crown on tooth #29. During the course of preparation, you realize that you have not obtained a preliminary impression. What steps could you take with regard to making a provisional crown at this point?
3. After trying the provisional crown on the prepared tooth, you notice the margins are too short. What is your plan of action in adjusting the provisional so that it will fit properly?
4. The dentist asks you to make provisional crowns for teeth #8 and #9. Your choice of coverage is the polycarbonate crown. Because the teeth involved are the maxillary centrals, what are your concerns regarding these provisional crowns?
5. What two temporary cements are most commonly used for provisional coverage? ■

**PROCEDURE 51.1**

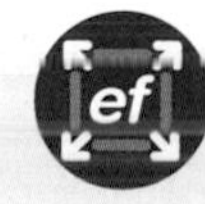


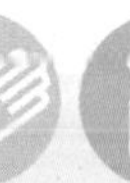

# Fabricating and Cementing a Custom Acrylic Provisional Crown (Expanded Function)

### PREREQUISITES FOR PERFORMING THIS PROCEDURE

- ✔ Operator positioning
- ✔ Differentiation between cavity classifications and oral anatomy
- ✔ Knowledge of application technique
- ✔ Intraoral instrumentation
- ✔ Extraoral use of low-speed handpiece
- ✔ Mirror skills
- ✔ Fulcrum placement

### EQUIPMENT AND SUPPLIES

- ✔ Basic setup
- ✔ Spoon excavator
- ✔ Alginate impression (obtained before preparation of the teeth)
- ✔ Separating medium
- ✔ Cotton rolls
- ✔ Self-curing acrylic resin (liquid and powder)
- ✔ Spatula (small, cement type)
- ✔ Mixing container/dappen dish
- ✔ Scissors
- ✔ Surgical knife (optional)
- ✔ Burnisher ("beaver tail" or ball)
- ✔ Straight handpiece and mandrel
- ✔ Finishing diamond, discs, or burs
- ✔ Polishing discs or burs
- ✔ Articulating paper
- ✔ Pumice paste
- ✔ Lathe and sterile white rag wheel
- ✔ Provisional cementation setup

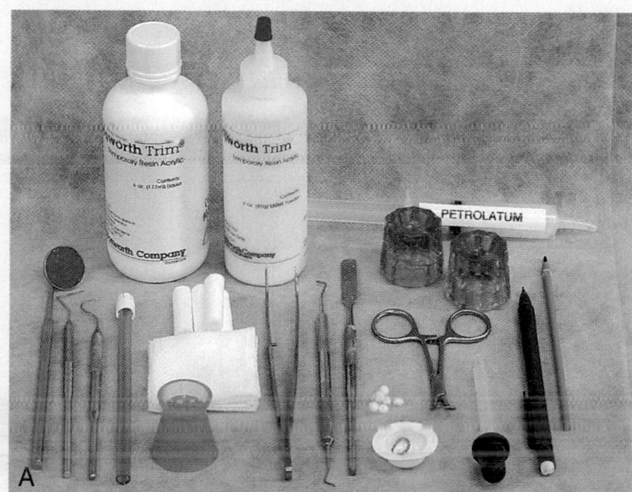


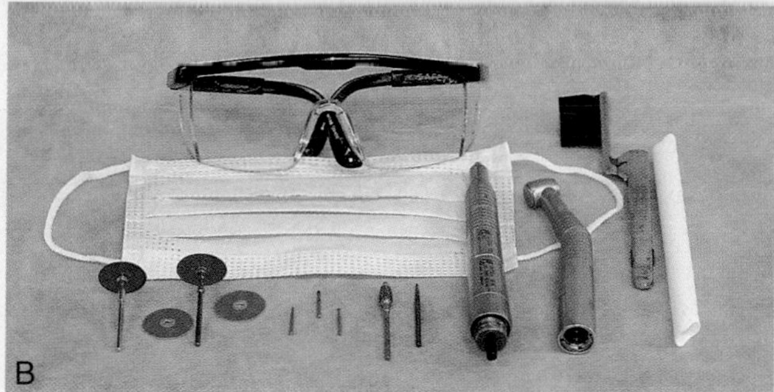


*From Rosenstiel SF, Land MF, Fujimoto J: Contemporary fixed prosthodontics, ed 5, St Louis, 2016, Elsevier.*

**(Continued)**

## PROCEDURE 51.1 Fabricating and Cementing a Custom Acrylic Provisional Crown (Expanded Function)–cont'd

### PROCEDURAL STEPS

1 Obtain an alginate impression of the arch before the teeth are prepared.
**PURPOSE** You want the provisional coverage to be a replica of the tooth before the dentist prepares it.

2 Check the impression to be sure it is free of debris and tears in the area selected for construction of the provisional crown or bridge covering.

3 Disinfect the impression and keep moist until needed.
**PURPOSE** If allowed to dry, the impression will be distorted, and the provisional coverage will not fit.

4 Isolate the prepared tooth with cotton rolls to maintain moisture control.

5 Lightly apply petroleum jelly or a liquid medium to the prepared tooth to facilitate separation of the acrylic dough from the preparations.

6 If using the liquid/powder acrylic material, place the liquid monomer in the glass dappen dish; 10 drops of liquid per unit is recommended. Quickly dispense the selected shade of self-curing powder (polymer) into the monomer until the powder is saturated.
**IMPORTANT** Cover the monomer container immediately; this material is volatile.
**NOTE** If using the syringe-type acrylic material, skip to step 9.

7 Use a small spatula to blend the powder and liquid to a homogeneous mix.

8 Set the mixed material aside for 1 to 2 minutes until the resin reaches a doughy, less glossy stage.
**IMPORTANT** Do not let the resin cure beyond this point.

9 Unwrap the alginate impression, and gently dry the area of the teeth to receive provisional coverage.

10 Remove the resin from the mixing container with a small spatula, and immediately place it within the area of the prepared teeth.
**OPTIONAL** Express the acrylic resin from a syringe directly into the impression.

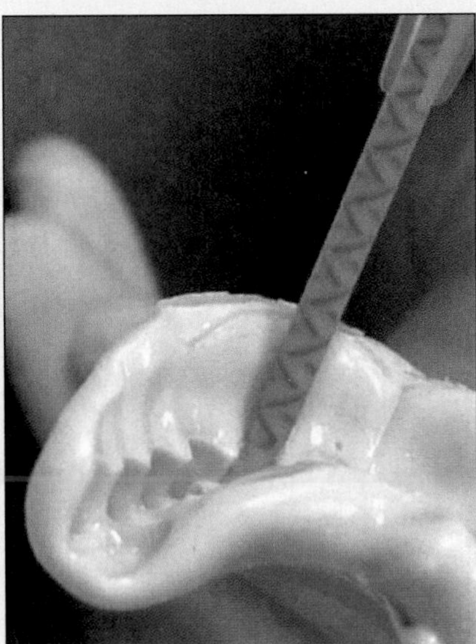

11 Place the acrylic-loaded impression back into the patient's mouth on the prepared tooth or teeth.

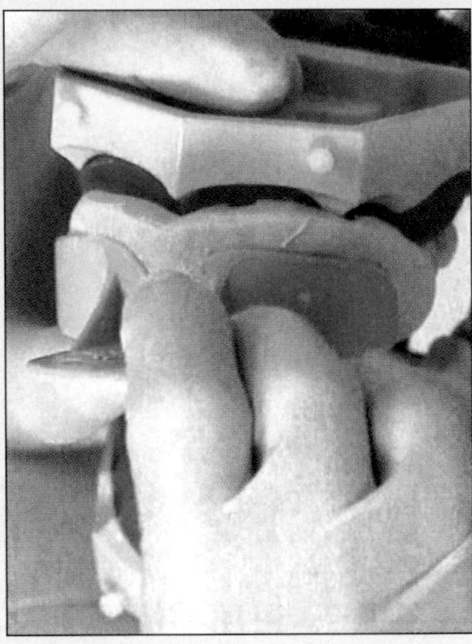

12 Allow the material to reach an initial set, after approximately 3 minutes, and remove the tray from the patient's mouth.

13 Carefully remove the provisional coverage from the alginate impression, and place it onto the patient's teeth.
**PURPOSE** To avoid excess shrinkage during the final curing stage.

14 Mark the marginal border and contact points of the provisional coverage with a pencil to provide better visualization of the markings.

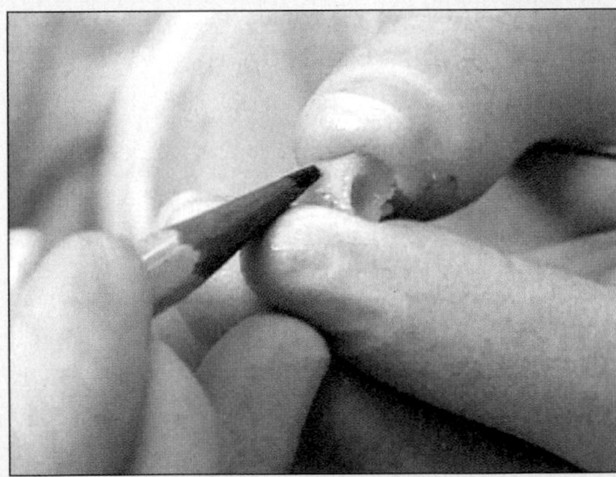

15 Trim the acrylic resin to within 1 mm of the gingival shoulder of the prepared tooth with an acrylic bur or stone.
**NOTE** Any trimming completed by the EFDA/RDA must be completed outside the mouth with the low-speed handpiece and acrylic burs.

16 Check the occlusion, accuracy, and completeness of the provisional coverage, and adjust as necessary. Remove the provisional coverage from the prepared tooth, and complete the trimming with an acrylic bur.

## PROCEDURE 51.1 Fabricating and Cementing a Custom Acrylic Provisional Crown (Expanded Function)–cont'd

17 Remove the provisional coverage and take it to the laboratory, where it is polished with a sterile white rag wheel and pumice on the laboratory lathe.

**CAUTION** Safety goggles must be worn throughout the trimming and polishing procedure. In addition, be aware that the rag wheel could remove a large bulk of acrylic or could overheat and cause distortion of the provisional coverage.

18 Temporarily cement the provisional coverage with provisional cement, such as zinc oxide–eugenol (TempBond) or intermediate restorative material.

19 Check the occlusion with articulating paper. If any reduction is required, the dentist will use an acrylic-trimming bur.

20 Document the procedure.

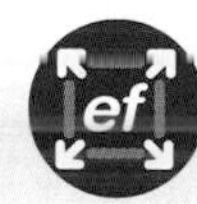

## PROCEDURE 51.2

## Fabricating and Cementing a Custom Acrylic Provisional Bridge (Expanded Function)

### PREREQUISITES FOR PERFORMING THIS PROCEDURE

- ✔ Operator positioning
- ✔ Differentiation between cavity classifications and oral anatomy
- ✔ Knowledge of application technique
- ✔ Intraoral instrumentation
- ✔ Extraoral use of low-speed handpiece
- ✔ Mirror skills
- ✔ Fulcrum placement

### EQUIPMENT AND SUPPLIES

- ✔ Basic setup
- ✔ Spoon excavator
- ✔ Thermoplastic tray
- ✔ Cotton rolls
- ✔ Autocure acrylic resin (syringe type)
- ✔ Spatula (small, cement type)
- ✔ Scissors
- ✔ Surgical knife (optional)
- ✔ Burnisher ("beaver tail" or ball)
- ✔ Straight handpiece and mandrel
- ✔ Finishing diamond, discs, or burs
- ✔ Polishing discs or burs
- ✔ Articulating paper
- ✔ Pumice paste
- ✔ Lathe and sterile white rag wheel
- ✔ Provisional cementation setup

### PROCEDURAL STEPS

1 The thermoplastic tray is prepared before the scheduled appointment and before the teeth are prepared.

**PURPOSE** The provisional coverage should be a replica of the teeth before the dentist prepares them.

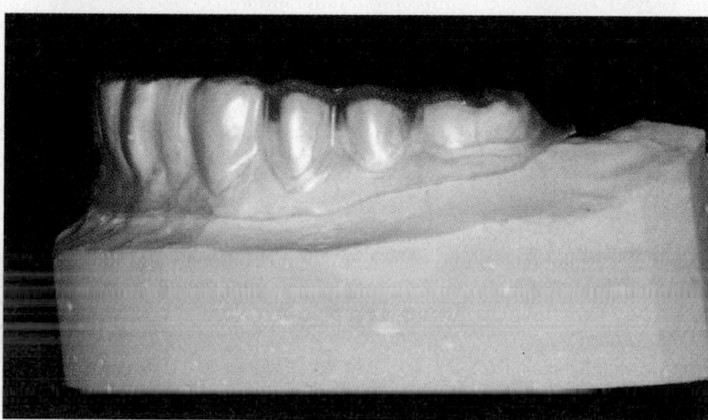

*From Rosenstiel SF, Land MF, Fujimoto J: Contemporary fixed prosthodontics, ed 5, St Louis, 2016, Elsevier.*

2 Isolate the prepared teeth to maintain moisture control.

3 Lightly apply petroleum jelly or a liquid medium to the prepared teeth to facilitate separation of the acrylic dough from the preparations.

(Continued)

## PROCEDURE 51.2 Fabricating and Cementing a Custom Acrylic Provisional Bridge (Expanded Function)–cont'd

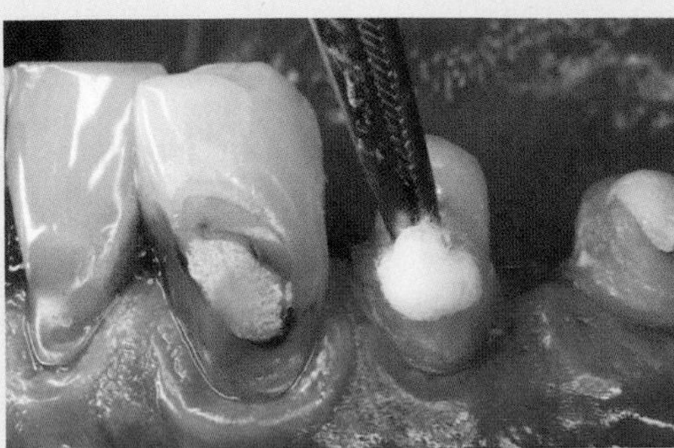

*From Rosenstiel SF, Land MF, Fuijimoto J: Contemporary fixed prosthodontics, ed 5, St Louis, 2016, Elsevier.*

4 Prepare the provisional material cartridge for application.
5 Express the acrylic resin from a cartridge directly into the tray.
6 Place the acrylic-loaded tray back into the prepared teeth.
7 Allow the material to reach an initial set, which takes approximately 3 minutes, and remove the tray from the patient's mouth.
8 Carefully remove the provisional coverage from the tray, and replace it onto the patient's teeth.
   **PURPOSE** To avoid excess shrinkage during the final curing stage.

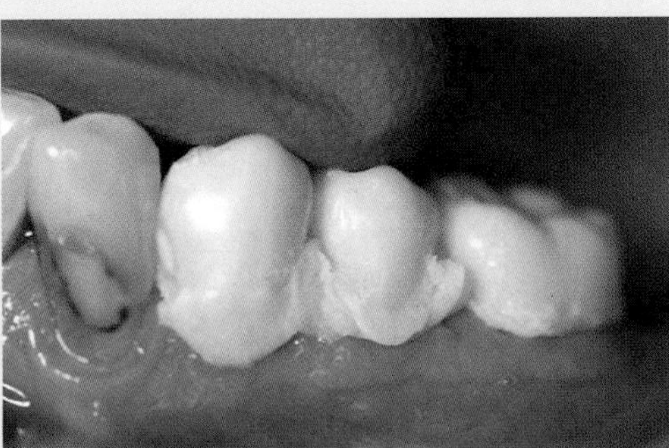

*From Rosenstiel SF, Land MF, Fuijimoto J: Contemporary fixed prosthodontics, ed 5, St Louis, 2016, Elsevier.*

9 After final set, remove the provisional and mark the marginal border and contact points of the provisional coverage with a pencil to provide better visualization of the markings.
10 Trim the acrylic resin to within 1 mm of the gingival shoulder of the prepared tooth with an acrylic bur or stone.
   **NOTE** Any trimming completed by the EFDA must be completed outside the mouth with use of the low-speed handpiece and acrylic burs.

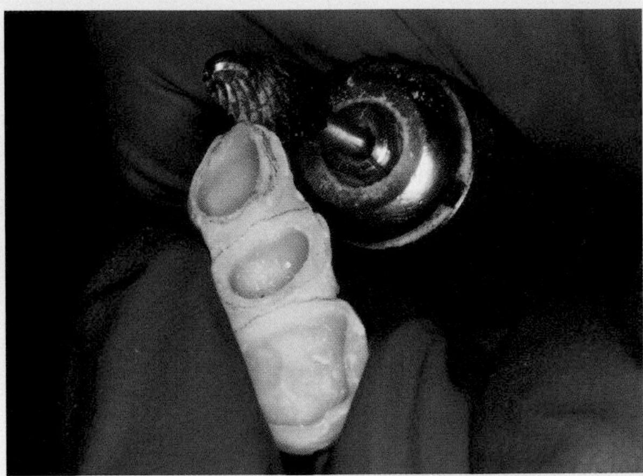

*From Rosenstiel SF, Land MF, Fuijimoto J: Contemporary fixed prosthodontics, ed 5, St Louis, 2016, Elsevier.*

11 Check the occlusion, accuracy, and completeness of the provisional coverage, and adjust as necessary. Remove the provisional coverage from the prepared teeth, and complete the trimming with an acrylic bur.
12 Remove the provisional coverage and take it to the laboratory, where it is polished with a sterile white rag wheel and pumice on the laboratory lathe.
   **CAUTION** Safety eyewear must be worn throughout the trimming and polishing procedure. In addition, be aware that the rag wheel could remove a large bulk of acrylic or could overheat and cause distortion of the provisional coverage.
13 Temporarily cement the provisional coverage with provisional cement, such as zinc oxide–eugenol (TempBond) or intermediate restorative material.
14 Check the occlusion with articulating paper. If any reduction is required, the dentist will use an acrylic-trimming bur.
15 Document the procedure.

PROCEDURE 51.3

# Fabricating and Cementing a Preformed Provisional Crown (Expanded Function)

## PREREQUISITES FOR PERFORMING THIS PROCEDURE

- ✔ Operator positioning
- ✔ Differentiation between cavity classifications and oral anatomy
- ✔ Knowledge of application technique
- ✔ Intraoral instrumentation
- ✔ Extraoral use of low-speed handpiece
- ✔ Mirror skills
- ✔ Fulcrum placement

## EQUIPMENT AND SUPPLIES

- ✔ Basic setup
- ✔ Shell or bridge unit
- ✔ Composite resin mixture
- ✔ Dappen dish
- ✔ Laboratory spatula
- ✔ Crown and bridge scissors
- ✔ Low-speed handpiece
- ✔ Articulating paper and holder
- ✔ Acrylic burs
- ✔ Rubber wheels
- ✔ Temporary cement setup

## PROCEDURAL STEPS

1 With the dentist, examine the prepared tooth for size and shape.

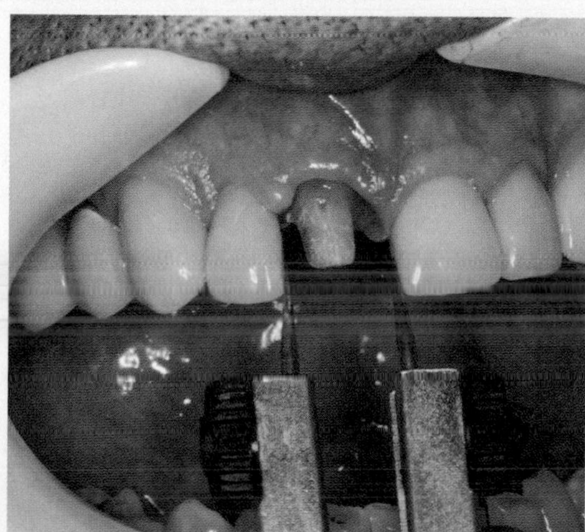

*From Rosenstiel SF, Land MF, Fuijimoto J: Contemporary fixed prosthodontics, ed 5, St Louis, 2016, Elsevier.*

2 Select the preformed crown unit that best suits the area of the mouth.

3 Try on the crown for size and shape, and make any needed adjustments with a slow-speed handpiece outside of the mouth.

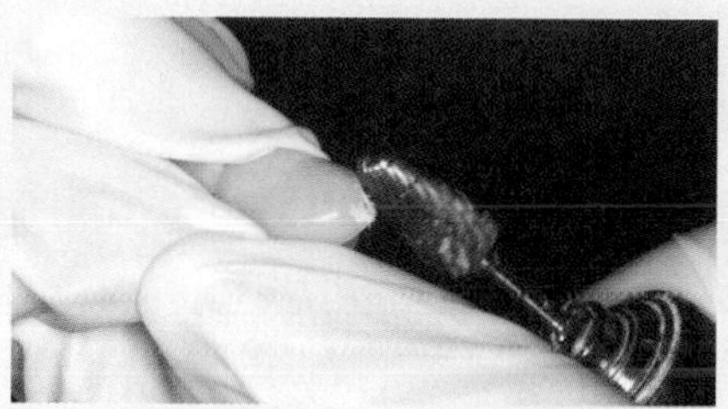

*From Rosenstiel SF, Land MF, Fuijimoto J: Contemporary fixed prosthodontics, ed 5, St Louis, 2016, Elsevier.*

4 Mix the resin as directed and fill the shell, making sure not to trap any air bubbles in the material.

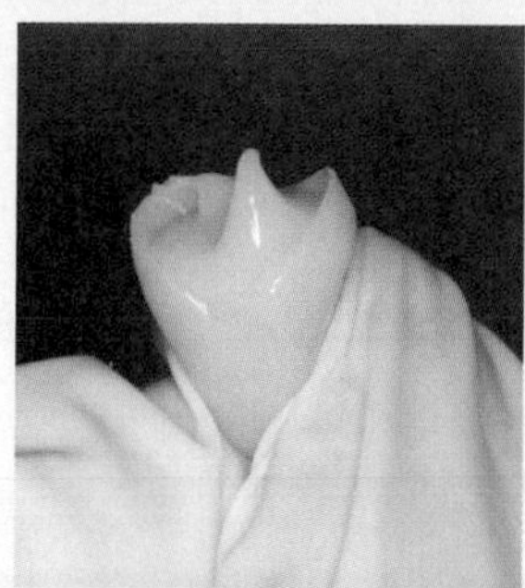

*From Rosenstiel SF, Land MF, Fuijimoto J: Contemporary fixed prosthodontics, ed 5, St Louis, 2016, Elsevier.*

5 Seat the shell over the tooth or teeth, and ask the patient to bite down.

**NOTE** You will notice excess resin flowing from the shell into the margins and contacts.

6 Use your fingers to apply pressure to the buccal and lingual areas of the crown.

7 Remove excess resin from the margins after 20 to 30 seconds.

8 Lift the crown on and off the tooth until the resin has hardened. The time required for setting of this material is approximately 90 seconds.

**PURPOSE** To prevent the crown from locking onto the tooth.

9 Mark the patient's occlusion with articulating paper and with a pencil around the margins and contact points, and then adjust using acrylic burs, discs, and rubber wheels.

(Continued)

## PROCEDURE 51.3 Fabricating and Cementing a Preformed Provisional Crown (Expanded Function)–cont'd

**10** Finish the crown or bridge.
**11** Cement with temporary cement.

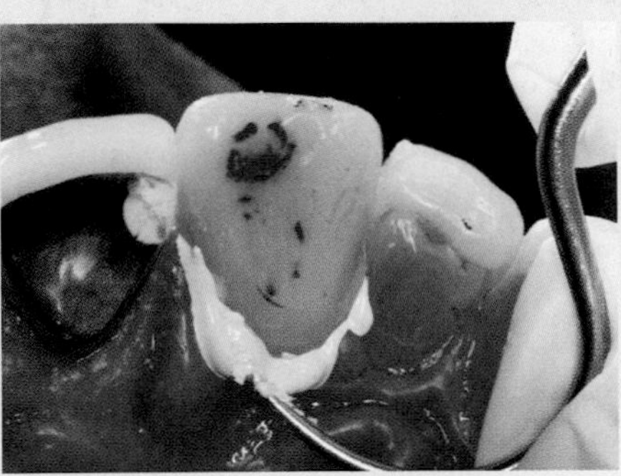

*From Rosenstiel SF, Land MF, Fuijimoto J: Contemporary fixed prosthodontics, ed 5, St Louis, 2016, Elsevier.*

**12** Document the procedure.

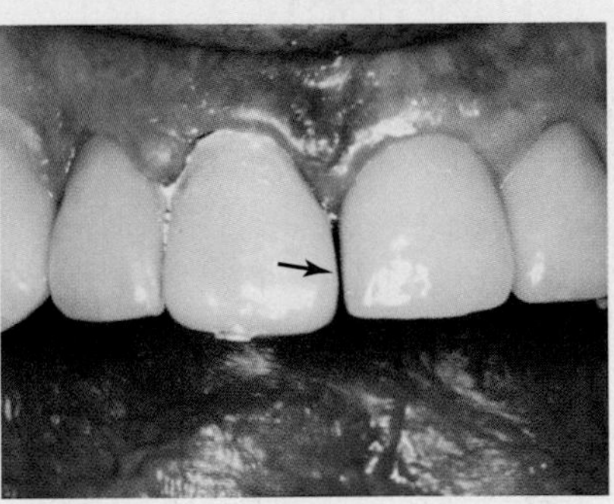

*From Rosenstiel SF, Land MF, Fuijimoto J: Contemporary fixed prosthodontics, ed 5, St Louis, 2016, Elsevier.*

52

# Removable Prosthodontics

## KEY TERMS

**Alveoplasty (al-VEE-uh-plas-tee)** The surgical shaping and smoothing of the margins of the tooth socket after extraction of the tooth, generally in preparation for the placement of a prosthesis.

**Baseplate** A temporary resin form representing the base of a denture used to help establish jaw relationships and the arrangement of teeth.

**Border molding** Process of using fingers to contour a closer adaptation of the margins of an impression while it is still in the mouth.

**Centric (SEN-trik) relation** Having the jaws in a position that produces a centrally related occlusion.

**Connector** Piece of metal that joins the various parts of a partial denture; also called *bar.*

**Coping (KOEP-ing)** Thin metal covering or cap placed over a prepared tooth.

**Edentulous (ee-DEN-tyoo-lus)** To be without teeth.

**Festooning (fes-TOO-ning)** The process of carving the base material of a denture or denture pattern to simulate the contours of the natural tissues.

**Flange (flanj)** Parts of a full or partial denture that extend from the teeth to the border of the denture.

**Framework** Metal skeleton of a removable partial denture.

**Full denture (DEN-chur)** Prosthesis that replaces all of the teeth in one arch.

**Immediate denture** Temporary denture placed after the extraction of anterior teeth.

**Lateral excursion (ek-SKUR-zhun)** Sliding the position of the mandible to the left or right of the centric position.

**Mastication (mas-ti-KAY-shun)** Chewing.

**Occlusal (o-KLOO-sul) rim** Rim built on the baseplate to register vertical dimension and occlusal relationship of the mandibular and maxillary arches.

**Overdenture** Full denture supported by two or more remaining natural teeth.

**Partial denture** Removable prosthesis that replaces teeth within the same arch.

**Post dam** Seal in back of a full denture that holds it in place; also called *posterior palatal seal.*

**Pressure points** Specific areas in the mouth where a removable prosthesis may rub or apply more pressure.

**Protrusion (proe-TROO-zhun)** Position of the mandible placed forward as related to the maxilla.

**Rebasing (ree-BAY-sing)** Procedure to replace the entire denture base material on an existing prosthesis.

**Relining (ree-LYE-ning)** Procedure to resurface the tissue side of a partial or full denture so that it fits more accurately.

**Resorption (ree-SORP-shun)** The body's processes of eliminating existing bone or hard tissue structure.

**Rest** Metal projection on or near the retainer of a partial denture.

**Retainer (ree-TAY-nur)** Device used to hold attachments and abutments of a removable prosthesis in place.

**Retrusion (ree-TROO-zhun)** Position of the mandible posterior from the centric position as related to the maxilla.

**Template (TEM-plut)** Clear plastic tray to represent the alveolus as it should appear after teeth have been extracted.

**Tuberosity (too-buh-ROS-i-tee)** Rounded bony protrusion behind the last molar in the maxilla.

## LEARNING OUTCOMES

*On completion of this chapter, the student will be able to achieve the following objectives:*

1. Pronounce, define, and spell the key terms.
2. Differentiate between a removable partial and a full denture.
3. Identify factors that influence the choice for removable partial and full dentures.
4. Discuss removable partial dentures, including the following:
   - List the components of a partial denture.
   - Describe the appointment sequence needed for the proper construction of a removable partial denture.
   - Identify home care instructions for removable partial dentures.
5. Discuss removable full (complete) dentures, including the following:
   - List the components of a full denture.
   - Describe the appointment sequence needed for the proper construction of a full denture.
   - Identify home care instructions for removable full dentures.
   - Explain what to expect the first month of having a denture.
6. Discuss the construction, surgical template, and placement of an immediate denture.
7. Discuss the process of constructing overdentures.
8. Discuss the process of denture adjustment and relining.
9. Discuss denture repair and duplication.

## PERFORMANCE OUTCOMES

*On completion of this chapter, the student will be able to achieve competency standards in the following skills:*

- Assist in the delivery of a partial denture.
- Assist in the try-in of the wax setup for a full denture.
- Assist in the delivery of a full denture.
- Assist in the repair of a denture.

## ELECTRONIC RESOURCES

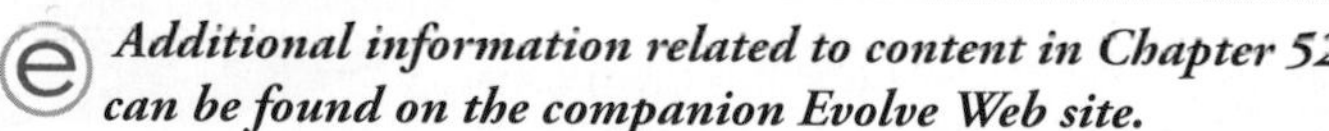


- Practice Quiz

Removable prosthodontics is the dental specialty in which missing teeth are replaced with a prosthesis that the patient can place in and take out of the mouth freely. Two major types of removable prosthetics are as follows:

- **Removable partial denture,** also referred to as a *partial,* replaces one or more teeth in the same arch (Fig. 52.1).
- **Removable full denture,** also referred to as a *denture,* replaces all the teeth in one arch (Fig. 52.2).

## Factors Influencing the Choice of a Removable Prosthesis

The dentist will advise patients who are considering a removable prosthesis that it will never function as well as their natural dentition that is being replaced, regardless of how well it is constructed and fits. The dentist will assess the following extraoral and intraoral factors before recommending this treatment plan for a patient.

### Extraoral Factors

Although extraoral factors are usually beyond the control of the dentist, they should not be ignored when discussing this option with a patient. These factors include the patient's physical and mental health, motivation, age, occupation, and dietary habits, as well as social and economic factors.

#### Physical Health

Certain chronic medical conditions, such as diabetes, can affect how oral tissues tolerate the pressure of a removable prosthesis. Also, the patient who has poor health may be unable to cope during the fabrication of a new prosthesis or unable to adapt to wearing it.

#### Mental Health

Individuals with poor mental health may become agitated or concerned about having a denture in their mouth. Patients with severe mental disability or mental decline may not be able to keep the appliance in place or maintain adequate oral hygiene.

#### Patient Motivation

Occasionally, patients' major motive for having their teeth extracted and replaced with a prosthesis is for **esthetic** reasons, that is, only to improve their appearance. The dentist should explore all acceptable alternative treatment options before giving serious consideration to the request.

#### Age

A prosthesis for a young person must be designed to allow for growth and accommodate for new teeth as they erupt. If the

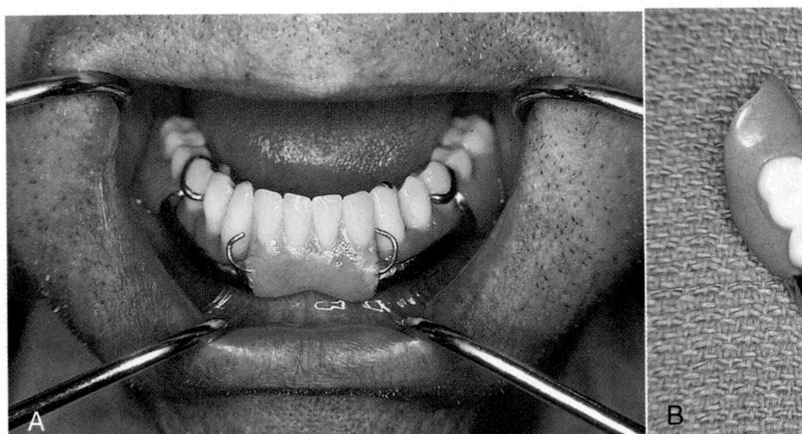


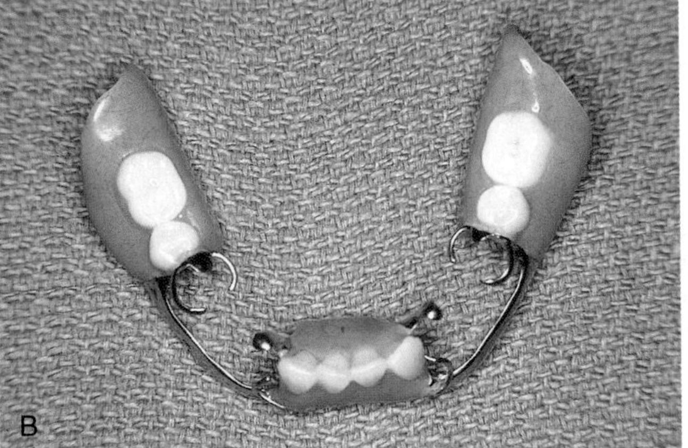


**FIG. 52.1** Partial denture. A, Partial in place. B, Partial outside of the mouth. *(From Carr AB, Brown DT: McCracken's removable partial prosthodontics, ed 13, St Louis, 2016, Elsevier.)*

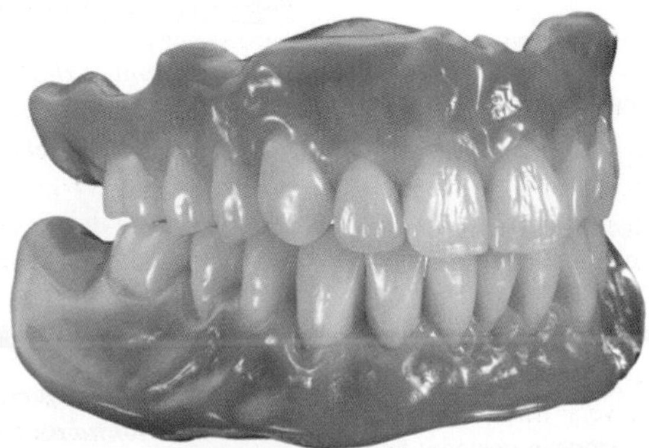

**FIG. 52.2** Full denture. *(Courtesy Ivoclar Vivadent Inc., Amherst, NY.)*

patient is very active or plays contact sports, the strength of the appliance is also an important factor.

A different challenge is found in the attitude of an older patient who associates the loss of teeth with aging and has an unrealistic desire to retain teeth that are structurally unsound.

### Dietary Habits

Healthy oral tissue is an important aspect of removable prosthodontic success. Patients with poor nutritional habits may have poor tissue response to the prosthesis, which can affect the overall tolerance for and comfort of the prosthesis.

### Social and Economic Factors

How important is it to the patient to replace lost teeth? Patients' attitudes about their oral health and appearance will help them decide whether dentures are important.

The ability to pay for the treatment is a major economic factor. There are "denture clinics" or "mail order clinics," which cater specifically to the lower economic population by providing a quick, low-cost method of obtaining a denture.

### Occupation

Patients whose daily activities involve "meeting the public" are concerned about the possible change in their appearance during or after the transition to partial or full dentures. Appointments for surgery and the delivery of the prosthesis should be scheduled without serious disruption to the patient's social and occupational activities.

## Intraoral Factors

The condition of the tissues in the patient's mouth is a key factor in determining whether a removable partial or a complete denture should be recommended.

### Musculature

Facial muscles contribute to retention and functional control of the prosthesis. Strong muscle attachments with good muscle tone are important. On the contrary, a large or very active tongue may cause difficulty in retention and wearing of the prosthesis. A patient with a nervous or physical facial habit may have difficulty retaining and adjusting to a prosthesis.

### Salivary Flow

The presence of something foreign, such as a prosthesis, in the oral cavity may stimulate an excessive flow of saliva. This response usually diminishes and is controlled as the patient becomes accustomed to wearing the prosthesis. However, the prosthesis may make saliva control more difficult to deal with in patients with paralysis of the facial muscles caused by a stroke.

In contrast, a patient with a lack of saliva may find it very difficult to wear a prosthesis and may be very uncomfortable. Physical conditions, medications, or radiation treatment may be the cause of inadequate salivary flow.

### Residual Alveolar Ridge

Successful wearing of a removable prosthesis depends mainly on the support provided by the alveolar ridge. If it is at normal height and is evenly contoured, the alveolar ridge should provide good support, allowing for an even distribution for the stress of **mastication**. If the alveolar ridge has **resorbed** anywhere within the ridge, this can result in a sore spot for the patient. **Resorption** occurs when the alveolar ridge has resorbed, causing an uneven distribution of pressure on the prosthesis, which keeps it from fitting properly.

In some cases, it is necessary for the surgeon to perform an **alveoplasty** to recontour the alveolar ridge surgically to minimize such problems (see Chapter 56). It is a normal ongoing process for the alveolar ridge to continue to decrease in size and shape after teeth are lost. A well-fitted prosthesis minimizes these changes; a poorly fitting prosthesis accelerates the process. Because of these changes, it is important that the patient return periodically for an oral examination and for reevaluation in the fit of the prosthesis.

### Oral Mucosa

When the mucosa that covers the residual ridge is altered by the patient's physical condition, the prosthesis may cause friction and irritation and be difficult for the patient to wear. Likewise, a poorly fitting prosthesis may cause irritation and sore spots, known as **pressure points**, on the oral mucosa. Patients should be seen promptly so the dentist can relieve these sore spots.

### Oral Habits

Oral habits such as clenching or grinding can cause extreme stress on the ridges and remaining teeth, which must be taken into account when selecting a removable prosthesis. Mouth breathing may affect the patient's ability to hold the appliance in place.

### Tori

Tori is a benign overgrowth of bone in a specific area. Mandibular or maxillary tori, when present, can affect the patient's ability to wear a prosthesis in that arch (see Chapter 17). Depending on the type of prosthesis, it may be necessary to have the tori surgically removed before fabrication of the appliance is begun.

RECALL

1 What type of removable prosthesis replaces one or more teeth?
2 How does a person's occupation affect the choice of a removable prosthesis?
3 How will the addition of a prosthesis affect the flow of saliva?
4 Why is it important that the alveolar ridge be evenly contoured for a removable prosthesis?
5 What oral habits can affect the choice of a removable prosthesis?

## Removable Partial Denture

A removable partial denture receives its support and retention from the underlying tissues and remaining teeth that serve as abutments. This type of prosthesis is designed to distribute the forces of mastication between the abutments and the supporting tissues.

### Considerations for Prescribing a Removable Partial Denture

**Indications for a Removable Partial Denture**

- To replace several teeth in the same quadrant or in both quadrants of the same arch
- To serve as a temporary replacement for missing teeth in a child (as necessary, a new appliance is constructed to compensate for the child's growth)
- To avoid additional reduction in tooth structure on primary or permanent dentition of children and adolescents
- To replace missing teeth for a patient who cannot tolerate longer appointments and the extensive preparation required for placement of a fixed bridge or implants
- To allow the patient to maintain good oral hygiene
- To serve as a splint to support periodontally involved teeth

**Contraindications to a Removable Partial Denture**

- A lack of suitable teeth in the arch to support, stabilize, and retain the removable prosthesis
- Rampant caries or severe periodontal conditions that threaten the remaining teeth in the arch
- Lack of patient acceptance for esthetic reasons
- Chronic poor oral hygiene

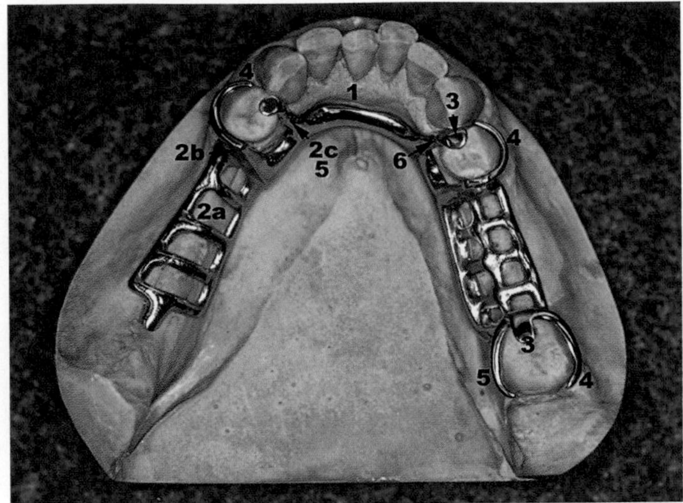


FIG. 52.3 Framework for mandibular removable partial denture with the following components: 1, lingual bar major connector; 2a, minor connector by which the resin denture base will be attached; 2b, minor connector, proximal plate, which is part of clasp assembly; 2c, minor connector used to connect rests to major connectors; 3, occlusal rests; 4, direct retainer arm, which is part of the total clasp assembly; 5, stabilizing or reciprocal components of clasp assembly (includes minor connectors); and 6, an indirect retainer consisting of a minor connector and an occlusal rest. *(From Carr AB, Brown DT: McCracken's removable partial prosthodontics, ed 13, St Louis, 2016, Mosby.)*

## Components of a Partial Denture

The basic components of a removable partial denture are the framework, connectors, denture base, retainers, rests, and artificial teeth (Fig. 52.3).

### Framework

The **framework** is the cast metal skeleton that provides support for the remaining components of the prosthesis. The dental laboratory technician constructs this meshlike portion of the partial denture and then covers the framework with acrylic resin to mirror the appearance of gingiva.

### Connectors

The **connectors**, or *bars,* join together the various parts of the partial denture. The **major connector** is the piece of rigid metal that joins the right-and-left-quadrant framework of the partial denture. This connector also helps provide support for the remaining teeth, so the stress is evenly distributed. A maxillary partial denture will have a **palatal connector,** and the mandibular partial denture will have a **lingual connector.**

A **stress breaker** is a metal device built into a partial denture design to protect the abutment teeth from excessive occlusal loads and stress during mastication. A stress breaker is advised for abutment teeth that have limited support in the alveolar ridge.

The **minor connector** links the major connector to the base and other areas, such as rests and clasps.

### Retainer

A **retainer**, also known as a **clasp,** is the portion of the framework that directly supports and provides stability to the partial denture by partially encircling or resting on an abutment tooth.

The *I-bar retainer,* or *I-bar clasp,* approaches the tooth in a straight line from the apical direction and extends upward against the tooth (Fig. 52.4, *A*). A *circumferential retainer,* or *C-clasp,* originates at the occlusal surface of the tooth and extends downward, so that it partially encircles the tooth (Fig. 52.4, *B*).

### Rest

A **rest** is a metal projection designed to control the seating of a prosthesis as it is positioned in the mouth. Rests prevent the partial denture from moving in a gingival direction, which would place abnormal stress and wear on the abutment tooth. The rest also aids in distributing the retention load of the partial denture to several teeth, not just to a single tooth. It also prevents passage of food between the abutment tooth and the retainer.

Rests are designed to lay within a prepared recess on the occlusal or lingual surface of a tooth. If a cast restoration is in place on the abutment tooth, the rest is positioned to protect the tooth

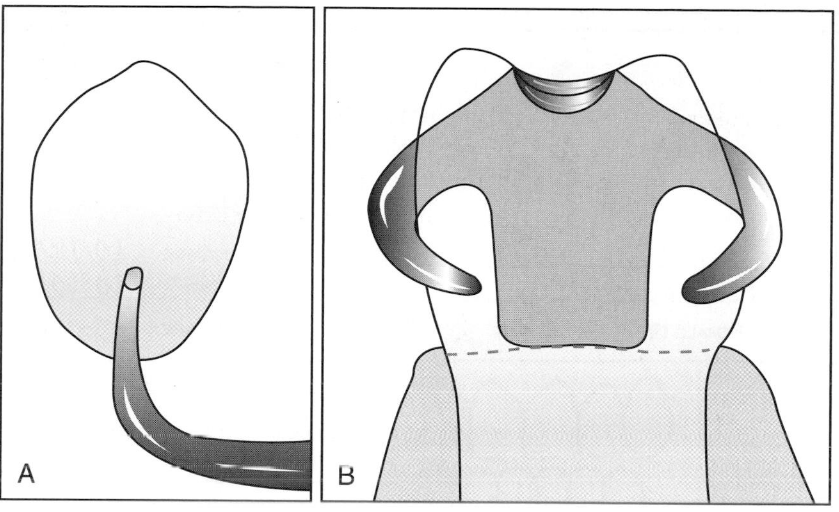


**FIG. 52.4** Different types of clasps. A, I-bar clasp. B, C-clasp.

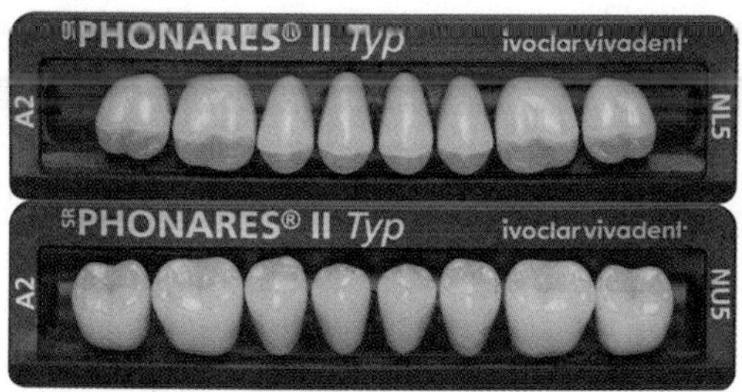


**FIG. 52.5** Artificial teeth. *(Courtesy Ivoclar Vivadent Inc., Amherst, NY.)*

structure against wear. Although the rest fits into the casting, it is not attached to it. Two common types of rests are available:

- The *occlusal rest,* which is used on the occlusal surface of the tooth. This placement minimizes trauma to the tooth by transmitting stress along the long axis of the tooth.
- The *lingual rest* is placed on the cingulum of the lingual surface of the tooth, where support is good but visibility is lacking.

### Artificial Teeth

Artificial teeth can be constructed from acrylic or porcelain (Fig. 52.5). **Acrylic teeth** are selected more often because they do not produce a clicking sound during chewing; however, acrylic teeth tend to wear faster and are more susceptible to staining. **Porcelain teeth** are more susceptible to fracture and tend to cause abrasion of the opposing natural teeth. Placement of acrylic teeth with natural or porcelain teeth in the opposing arch often is a satisfactory compromise.

## Appointment Sequencing for a Partial Denture

The patient who is considering a partial denture should be educated about the sequencing of and commitment to the process of delivering a partial denture. A patient can expect multiple dental appointments before the prosthesis is delivered.

### Appointment One: Records

This appointment involves the preliminary steps taken to gather the diagnostic tools that the dental team and laboratory technician will need to proceed:

- Updated health and dental *history.*
- *Prophylaxis* completed by the dental hygienist.
- *Preliminary impressions* and casts are poured up in stone, for the fabrication of the custom trays either within the office or sent to the dental laboratory.
- *Radiographs. Periapical* radiographs are prescribed for the evaluation of decay, periodontal problems, and other disease that cannot be seen visually. A *panoramic* (Panorex) radiograph may be prescribed to evaluate the alveolar ridge and any additional structures.
- *Photographs* are important to have intraoral and extraoral photographs for the case presentation and for presentation of final results.

### Appointment Two: Preparation

This appointment is the preparation appointment.

- *Selecting the shade and mold of the teeth.* When choosing the tooth shade and mold, the dentist considers the patient's age and body size, length of the lip, and space to be occupied by the artificial tooth or teeth. The goal is to match as closely as possible the color, size, and shape of the patient's natural teeth. When the selection has been made, the mold and shade of the artificial teeth are written on the patient's chart.
- *Preparation of the teeth.* The type of rest selected determines the preparation of the abutment teeth. This preparation may involve one of the following:
  - Slight modification of the tooth structure
  - Modification of an amalgam restorations, if present
  - Placement of a cast metal restoration with a recessed area to receive the rest or precision attachment
- *Taking the final impression.* Because this must be an exact impression, an *elastomeric* material is used. A custom tray may

Canyon View Dental Associates
Canyon View Dental Associates
4546 North Avery Way
Canyon View, CA 91783
Telephone (987) 654-3210

DR. Mary A. Edwards RETURN DATE: 10/18/2015
PATIENT: Rose L Budd DATE SENT: 10/10/2015
MALE ☐ FEMALE ☒ AGE: 63 FACIAL SHAPE: Sq. oval

STUMP SHADE: ______
SHADE DESIRED: ______
MOULD: ______

SURFACE: SMOOTH ☐ MODERATE ☐ HEAVY ☐
OCCLUSAL STAIN: NONE ☐ LIGHT ☐ MEDIUM ☐ DARK ☐

DEGREE OF TRANSLUCENCY: MINIMUM ☐ MODERATE ☐ MAXIMUM ☐
RETURN: METAL ☐ BISQUE ☐ FINISHED ☐ INDIVIDUAL ☐ SPLINTED ☐

COPING DESIGN (PLEASE CIRCLE ONE):
FULL PORCELAIN COVERAGE · LINGUAL METAL COLLAR · FULL METAL COLLAR · BUCCAL CUSP (PORCELAIN/METAL OCCLUSAL) · FULL METAL OCCLUSAL (VENEER) · FULL PORCELAIN COVERAGE · FULL COVERAGE LINGUAL · 2/3 COVERAGE LINGUAL

PONTIC DESIGN (PLEASE CIRCLE ONE):
SANITARY · FULL RIDGE · MODIFIED · BULLET · OVATE

MARGIN DESIGN: NO METAL TO SHOW ☐
HAIRLINE METAL MARGIN ☐ PORCELAIN BUTT ☐

IF NO OCCLUSAL CLEARANCE:
METAL OCCLUSION ☐ ADJUST OPPOSING ☐
REDUCTION COPING ☐

UPPER 1 2 3 4 5 6 7 8 9 10 11 12 13 14 15 16
RIGHT LEFT
LOWER 32 31 30 29 28 27 26 25 24 23 22 21 20 19 18 17

INSTRUCTIONS:

SIGNATURE: Mary Edwards LICENSE: ______
ADDRESS: 4546 Avery Way
CITY: Canyon View STATE: CA ZIP: 91783
WE NEED: BOXES ☐ RX PADS ☐ FED-X AIRBILLS ☐ MAILING LABELS ☐

**LABORATORY**

**FIG. 52.6** Laboratory prescription. *(From Gaylor LJ: The administrative dental assistant, ed 4, St Louis, 2017, Elsevier.)*

be selected for taking the final impression to give the laboratory technician a better form for the surrounding structures.

- *Taking the bite and occlusal registration.* Jaw registration must be recorded to determine the relationship between the maxillary and mandibular arches.
- *Preparing the laboratory prescription.* Before the case is sent to the laboratory, the dentist prepares a written prescription that includes all details regarding construction of the prosthesis (Fig. 52.6). The dentist must sign this prescription, and a copy is retained in the practice records.

### Appointment Three: Try-in

An appointment is scheduled for the initial try-in of the prosthesis. At this point, the appliance consists of the cast framework and the artificial teeth set in wax.

The dentist evaluates the fit, comfort, and function of the appliance. The shade, mold, and arrangement of the teeth are reviewed to ensure that the appearance is acceptable to the patient. If necessary, the dentist may alter the alignment of the teeth in the wax.

When the appliance is acceptable, another bite registration may be required to reflect any changes made during the try-in. Any changes in partial denture design are noted on the laboratory prescription. The *wax-up* is disinfected and is returned to the dental laboratory along with the prescription.

### Appointment Four: Delivery

A 20- to 30-minute appointment is usually adequate for delivery of the partial denture. On the day before the appointment, verify that the case has been returned from the laboratory.

See Procedure 52.1: Assisting in the Delivery of a Partial Denture.

### Appointment Five: Postdelivery Check

The patient is scheduled for an appointment to return within a few days after delivery of the partial denture. A 10- to 20-minute appointment is adequate for this postdelivery visit. The dentist will remove the partial denture and check the mucosa for pressure areas and sore spots. If necessary, minor adjustments are made.

When the dentist and the patient are satisfied that the prosthesis is functioning correctly, the patient is given a recall appointment for several months later. It is important that the patient return for the recall visits so the dentist can evaluate the fit, changes in mucosa, function of the prosthesis, and effectiveness of the patient's oral hygiene.

As time passes, changes in the alveolar ridge and surrounding tissues may make it necessary to *reline* the partial denture (see later in the chapter for discussion).

## Home Care Instructions

Patients with a removable partial must be instructed to maintain good oral hygiene; the importance of this cannot be overemphasized. Patients should be provided home care instructions verbally in the office and written instructions that can be used at home to reinforce education after the patient has left the office.

- Store the prosthesis in water or in a moist, airtight container when not wearing it.
- After eating, remove the partial denture from the mouth, and brush or rinse the retainers, rests, and complete partial prosthesis.
- Carefully brush and floss the abutment teeth and the remaining natural teeth to keep them free of food debris and plaque.
- Do not adjust the partial denture. The patient should contact the dentist if he or she has any difficulties.

RECALL

6 What is the term for the metal skeleton on a partial denture?
7 What is the term for the retainer on a partial denture?
8 What component of a partial denture controls the way it is seated in the mouth?
9 What impression material is typically used when one is taking a final impression for a partial denture?
10 In what are the artificial teeth set during the try-in appointment?

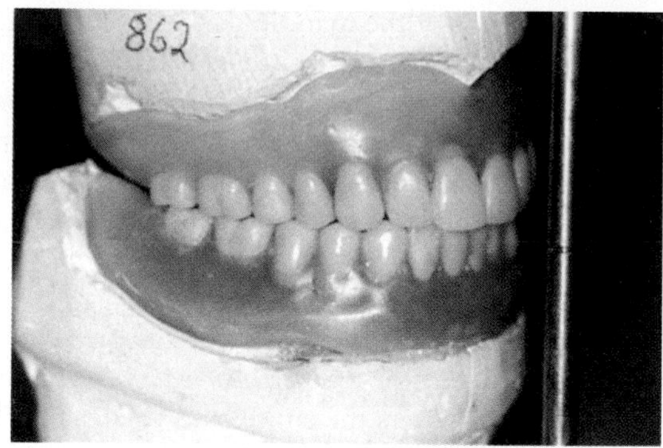


**FIG. 52.7** Components of a full denture: base, flange, post dam, and artificial teeth.

## Full (Complete) Denture

Full dentures are designed to restore the function and esthetics of the natural dentition when all of the natural teeth are missing. A complete denture receives all its support and retention from the underlying tissues, alveolar ridges, hard and soft palate, and surrounding oral mucosa.

### Considerations for Prescribing a Full Denture

**Major indications for a full denture include the following:**

- The patient is totally **edentulous**.
- The remaining teeth cannot be saved.
- The remaining teeth cannot support a removable partial denture, and no acceptable alternatives are available.
- The patient refuses alternative treatment recommendations.

**Contraindications to a full denture include the following:**

- Another acceptable alternative is available.
- Physical or mental illness affects the patient's ability to cooperate during fabrication of the denture and to accept or wear the denture.
- The patient is hypersensitive to the denture materials (a hypoallergenic denture material may be indicated).
- The patient is not interested in replacing missing teeth.

## Components of a Full Denture

The basic components of a denture include the base, flange, post dam, and artificial teeth (Fig. 52.7).

### Base

The base is designed to fit over the residual alveolar ridge and surrounding gingival area. The base is commonly made from denture *acrylic.* To provide additional strength, however, it may be reinforced with a metal mesh embedded in the acrylic.

### Flange

The **flange** is the part of the base that extends over the attached mucosa from the cervical margin of the teeth to the border of the denture. The flange of the mandibular denture base extends over the residual ridge and attached mucosa, down to the *oblique ridge* and *mylohyoid ridge,* and over the *genial tubercles* and *retromolar pads.* The flange of the maxillary denture base extends beyond the residual ridge and over the attached mucosa to the tuberosities and the junction of the hard and soft palates.

### Post Dam

Retention of a maxillary denture depends on the suction seal known as the **post dam**, or the *posterior palatal seal.* The base of a maxillary denture covers the entire hard palate, and the seal is formed at the junction of the tissues and the posterior border of the denture. The post dam extends across the entire posterior portion of the denture from one buccal space across the back of the palate behind the maxillary **tuberosity** (rounded area on the outer surface of the maxillary bones) to the opposite buccal space.

Retention for a mandibular denture depends on the support of the remaining alveolar ridge and the suction achieved between the prosthesis and the tissues covering the ridge. Achieving good retention of a mandibular denture can be difficult. A mandibular denture lacks the broad suction area found in a maxillary denture, and the constant action of the tongue can dislodge it. For these reasons, retained teeth or implants are desirable to help hold the appliance in place.

### Artificial Teeth

Denture teeth are fabricated from acrylic or porcelain and are designed to be retained in the acrylic base of the denture. Third molars are not included in dentures because space is needed in the posterior region to allow the patient to close, chew, swallow, and speak normally. A full denture will have 14 teeth per arch; each arch acts as a single unit, whereas a natural tooth functions as an individual unit.

## Appointment Sequencing for a Full Denture

The patient who is considering a complete denture must be educated about the sequencing and commitment to the process of delivering a denture. It is common for a patient to have six dental appointments for delivery of a denture.

### Appointment One: Records

This appointment involves the preliminary steps involved in gathering the diagnostic tools that the dental team and dental laboratory technician will require to proceed with the removable prosthodontic procedure:

- Updated health and dental *history.*
- *Preliminary impressions.* An alginate impression of an edentulous arch differs from other alginate impressions in two ways: (1) The height of the teeth is missing, and (2) more extensive tissue details are needed. An *edentulous tray* will be used to take this impression. This tray is not as deep, but if the tray requires modification to accommodate space and depth in the mucobuccal fold, a rope wax may be added to the borders of the tray.

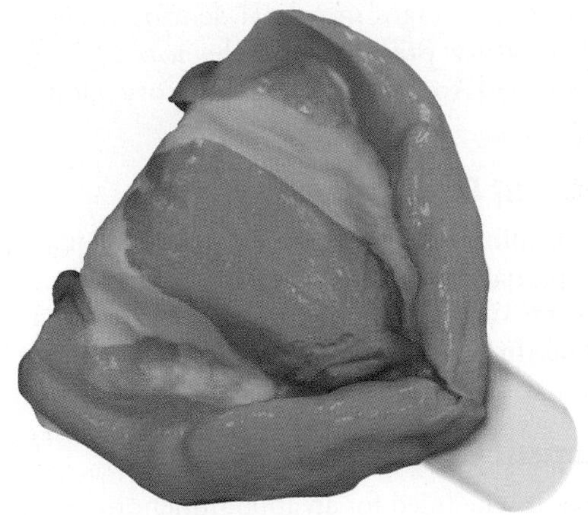

**FIG. 52.8** Final impression for a full denture. *(Courtesy Ivoclar Vivadent Inc., Amherst, NY.)*

- Tray modification allows **border molding**, also known as *muscle trimming,* to achieve closer adaptation of the edges of the impression to the tissues in the mucobuccal fold. Border molding is performed after the impression tray is in place. The dentist will use his or her fingers to gently massage the facial area over these borders. This action shapes the tray's wax-covered edges, so that they more closely resemble the tissues.
- *Radiographs.* A *panoramic* radiograph may be prescribed for the dentist to evaluate the underlying bone structure and observe any disease that may not be visible.
- *Photographs.* It is important to have intraoral and extraoral photographs for the case presentation and final results.

### Appointment Two: Final Impression

The dental laboratory technician requires a final impression to create the base of a denture. Before the impression is taken, a custom tray is fabricated. Because of the shape of the edentulous arch, custom trays are required for the final impression. Custom trays are constructed from the diagnostic casts and are prepared before the patient's appointment for the final impression (see Chapter 47). The edges of the custom tray for an edentulous arch are modified with beading wax to allow border molding. The edges of the tray should extend to 2 mm *short* of the mucobuccal fold.

Because accuracy is essential, an *elastomeric* impression material is selected for the final impression for creation of the baseplates and **occlusal rims** (Fig. 52.8).

#### Essentials of a Final Impression for Dentures

- The impression material should be free of bubbles and should be distributed evenly over the tray and its margins, so that landmarks of the dental arches are accurately reproduced.
- The maxillary impression should include the *hamular notches,* post dam, tuberosities, and *frenum attachments.*
- The mandibular impression should include the retromolar pads; oblique ridge; outline of the mylohyoid ridge; genial tubercles; and lingual, labial, and buccal frenula.

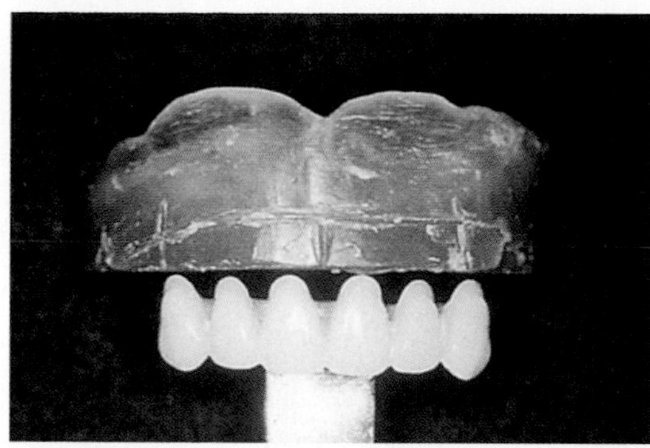

FIG. 52.9 Recording made from the baseplate–occlusal rim assembly: vertical dimensions, occlusal relationship, smile line, and canine eminence.

The **baseplate**, which is constructed on the master casts, is made of a semirigid material such as shellac and self-curing or heat-cured resins. If necessary for added stability, acrylic baseplates may be reinforced with wires or mesh metal sheets embedded in the material at processing.

The occlusal rims are built of wax on the alveolar crest of the baseplate and are sufficiently high and wide to occupy the space of the missing dentition.

### Appointment Three: Try-in of Baseplate and Occlusal Rim

The baseplate–occlusal rim assembly is returned to the dental office on an articulator, a dental laboratory device that simulates movement of the mandible and the temporomandibular joint. Before it is tried in the patient's mouth, the baseplate–occlusal rim is removed from the articulator, disinfected, and rinsed. On the occlusal rims, the dentist records the following:

- *Vertical dimension:* space occupied by the height of the teeth in normal occlusion
- *Occlusal relationship:* centric, protrusive, retrusive, and lateral excursions
- *Smile line:* line representing the area of the teeth that is visible when the patient is smiling
- *Canine eminence:* vertical line that indicates the locations of the canines

**ARTIFICIAL TEETH.** At this appointment, the mold, shade, and material of the artificial teeth to be placed in the denture are selected (Fig. 52.9). These factors are determined in the same way as for the teeth of a partial denture.

When placing the teeth in the denture, the laboratory technician is able to modify the arrangement as requested to produce a more natural appearance for the patient, for example, by lightly overlapping the mesial incisal margin of the maxillary lateral incisor over the distal margin of the central incisor. In addition, the technician may set (position) the teeth to expose less or more of the cervical area of the teeth to emulate the natural setting of the teeth according to the patient's age. Less cervical area is shown in a younger patient; more area is visible in an older patient to simulate gingival recession.

**OCCLUSAL REGISTRATION.** During construction of a complete denture, the laboratory technician must have an accurate and extensive record of the patient's occlusion. The technician uses this information to articulate the casts, so the completed prosthesis will replicate these normal motions.

The measurements most frequently used are the patient's bite registered in the following positions:

- **Centric relation**, with the jaws closed, relaxed, and comfortably positioned
- **Protrusion**, with the mandible placed as far forward as possible from the centric position
- **Retrusion**, with the mandible placed as far posterior as possible from the centric position
- **Lateral excursion**, which involves sliding the mandible to the left or right of the centric position

These exaggerated motions simulate the actual movements of the mandible as it functions during the acts of mastication, biting, yawning, and speaking. Various measuring devices are used to obtain these measurements.

**FUNCTIONALLY GENERATED PATH TECHNIQUE.** The functionally generated path technique uses the patient's ability to create his or her own occlusal relationship by tracing in wax the movements of the mandible on the maxilla. Establishment of a functionally generated path involves the following steps:

1. Place the baseplates and occlusal rims for the new prosthesis in the patient's mouth.
2. Prepare a double thickness of specially formulated baseplate wax in a horseshoe shape, and lay it over the occlusal surface of the mandibular teeth.
3. Instruct the patient to close firmly into the wax and simulate the act of chewing as accurately as possible.
4. Remove the wax bite in approximately 20 to 30 seconds.
5. In the treatment room, rinse and disinfect the wax bite and place in a precaution bag.
6. In the laboratory, pour the wax bite in stone immediately after the patient's dismissal.

### Appointment Four: Try-In

The wax setup consists of the baseplate with the artificial teeth set in wax that resembles gingival tissue. The shaping of the wax to simulate normal tissue contours, grooves, and eminences is known as **festooning**. The teeth are articulated according to the bite registration of the patient's occlusion, as established on the articulator through a functional arch tracing.

The complete denture try-in, which has been fabricated in wax by the laboratory technician on an articulator, is returned to the dental office before the patient's appointment. The wax setup is removed from the articulator and is disinfected before it is tried in the patient's mouth (Fig. 52.10).

See Procedure 52.2: Assisting in a Wax Denture Try-in.

Patients may require more than one wax try-in appointment to achieve the esthetics they are seeking. It is important for the

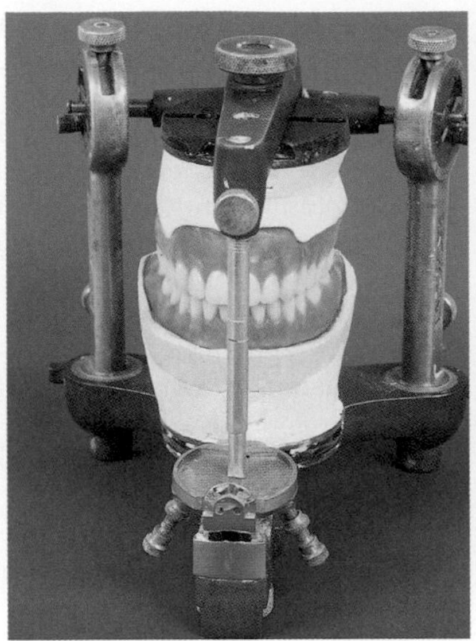
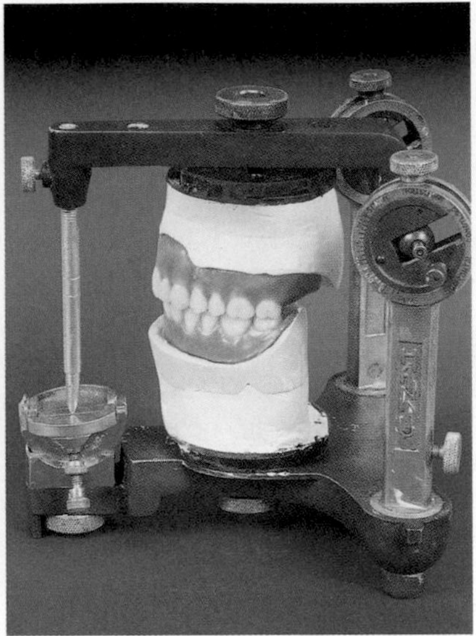

FIG. 52.10 Wax setup within the articulated cast.

dentist, laboratory technician, and patient to work together to achieve the patient's acceptance and satisfaction.

### Appointment Five: Delivery

The completed dentures are delivered to the dental office in a sealed, moist container. The dentures must be disinfected before they are placed in the patient's mouth.

See Procedure 52.3: Assisting in the Delivery of a Full Denture.

### Appointment Six: Postdelivery

The patient is scheduled to return 2 to 3 days after delivery of the full denture. A 10- to 20-minute appointment is usually adequate for this postdelivery visit.

The dentist removes the denture and checks the mucosa for pressure areas and sore spots. If necessary, minor adjustments are made to the denture. Patients usually need more than one adjustment appointment after the delivery of a complete denture. When the patient and the dentist are satisfied that the prosthesis is functioning properly, the patient is given a recall appointment for several months later.

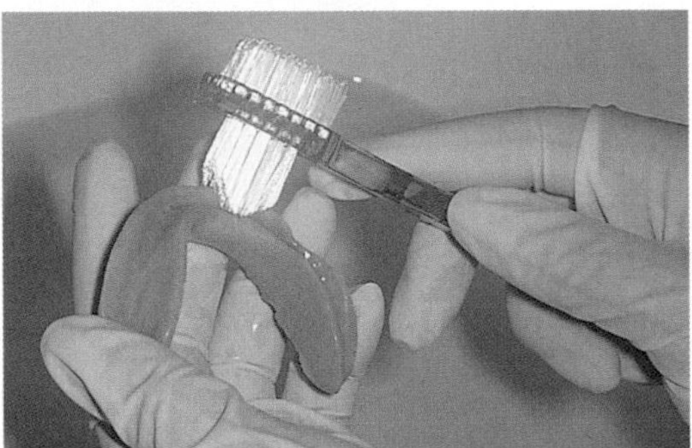
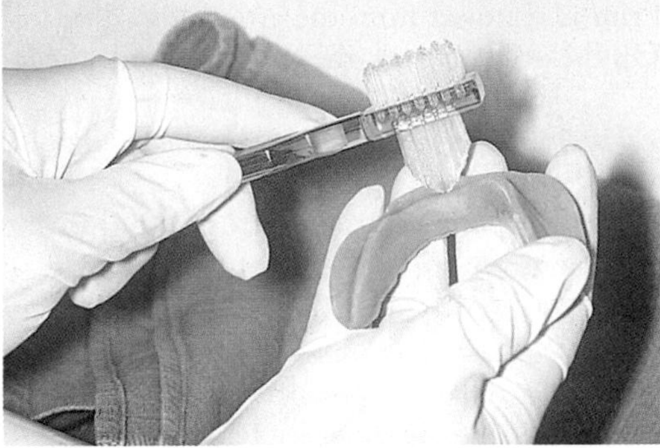

FIG. 52.11 Denture and denture brush. *(From Daniel SJ, Harfst SA, Wilder R: Mosby's dental hygiene: concepts, cases, and competencies, ed 2, St Louis, 2008, Mosby.)*

## Home Care Instructions

As with partial dentures, the patient should be given home care instructions in writing to reinforce the verbal instructions:

- With the denture removed, thoroughly rinse the oral tissues at least once daily.
- On removal, thoroughly clean all surfaces of the denture; a special denture brush may be used. Avoid harsh abrasives such as toothpaste (Fig. 52.11).
- During cleaning, carefully hold the denture over a sink half-filled with cool water.
- Do not soak the denture in hot water or a strong solution such as undiluted bleach, because these liquids will damage the denture.
- When not in the mouth, store dentures in a moist, airtight container to prevent drying and warping. If the prosthesis is not stored in a safe container, it may be accidentally knocked to the floor, stepped on, or broken.
- Do not wear the denture at night.

## What To Expect the First Month

**Day 1**—Your "adjusting to dentures" journey is just beginning; even for experienced denture wearers, new dentures can be a challenge. Many first-time denture wearers say that eating soft foods that are gentle on your gums/teeth makes this new experience easier.

**Days 2 to 14**—Your mouth is adjusting to the new dentures; you will likely experience increased salivation. You might also experience sore spots in your mouth from the dentures. Rinsing your mouth with warm salt water may help. If soreness persists, return to your dentist for an adjustment. Expect a longer denture adjustment and healing time if you recently had teeth extracted or are a full-plate wearer.

**Days 15 to 29**—You are still learning to talk and eat all over again. You also are adjusting to the foreign-object feeling in your mouth. The saliva flow and sore spots have lessened. This is the best time to start using an adhesive to improve the fit and feel of your dentures. Be careful not to use too much, and follow the usage instructions! The more you wear your dentures, the more quickly you will adjust.

**Day 30**—You've made it through 1 month with dentures! Reward yourself with your favorite food. Remember to visit your prosthodontist on a regular basis to have your dentures checked. It is usually recommended that you get new dentures in 5 to 10 years.

RECALL

**11** What is the suction seal created between the denture and the mouth?
**12** How many teeth are included in a full set of dentures?
**13** What technique does the dentist use to modify the borders of an impression?
**14** What is a smile line?
**15** What are the four jaw positions that the dentist measures when articulating a denture?

## Immediate Dentures

An **immediate denture** is a prosthesis that is placed immediately after the extraction of a patient's remaining anterior teeth. During the healing process, this type of denture serves as a compress and bandage to protect the surgical area. Although an immediate denture may be placed in either arch, placement of a *maxillary* immediate denture is more common because it restores function and spares the patient the embarrassment of being without teeth.

Before agreeing to receive an immediate denture, the patient must be aware that normal healing and resorption can change in the alveolar ridge. Because of these changes, the denture placed immediately after surgery must be replaced or relined in 3 to 6 months.

### Construction

When a patient's posterior teeth have been extracted and healing is complete, but before the anterior teeth are extracted, the try-in of the wax setup includes only the posterior teeth. These teeth are aligned in the occlusal rims and are checked for their ability to occlude with the opposing teeth. The denture, complete with anterior teeth, is constructed, sterilized, and readied for placement at surgery.

### Surgical Template

In addition to the denture, the laboratory prepares a surgical template. The surgical **template** resembles a clear plastic impression tray of the anterior area as this area should appear *after* the teeth have been extracted. The denture and the template must be sterilized before surgery. After the anterior teeth have been extracted, the oral surgeon uses the surgical template as a guide for properly contouring the remaining alveolar ridge.

### Placement

When the resulting alveolar ridge is satisfactory, the tissues are sutured into place. The sterilized denture is rinsed with saline solution and is positioned in the mouth. The patient is given postsurgical instructions and home care instructions.

The patient returns in 24 hours for a postoperative checkup. During this time, the denture should be worn continuously, except when it is removed for cleaning. Daily visits continue until initial healing has started and the sutures are removed, usually 48 to 72 hours after surgery. During each visit, the dentist irrigates the area with a mild antiseptic solution and checks the soft tissue for pressure points.

After the sutures have been removed and the dentist and the patient are satisfied with the prosthesis, the patient is scheduled for another appointment within a few months.

RECALL

**16** When is an immediate denture used?
**17** What is the normal length of time an immediate denture is worn?

## Overdentures

Patient satisfaction with a mandibular denture is enhanced when remaining teeth or *implants* improve retention and stability (see Chapter 53). An **overdenture** is a full denture that is supported by the bony ridge and oral mucosa plus two or more remaining natural teeth or implants. Most often, these remaining teeth are canines.

Preparation and placement of the denture for use with implants and for an overdenture are similar. To permit the denture to fit snugly over the teeth without excessive bulk, the natural teeth are prepared by removing much of their bulk. The remaining tooth structure is protected with a **coping**. In the *long coping technique,* only a minimal amount of tooth structure is removed, and the length of tooth remains almost the same. In the *short coping technique,* which is used only with endodontically treated teeth, tooth structure is greatly reduced and shortened.

The posts from an implant protrude through the gingiva much like teeth, and a casting is created to fit over the posts. In

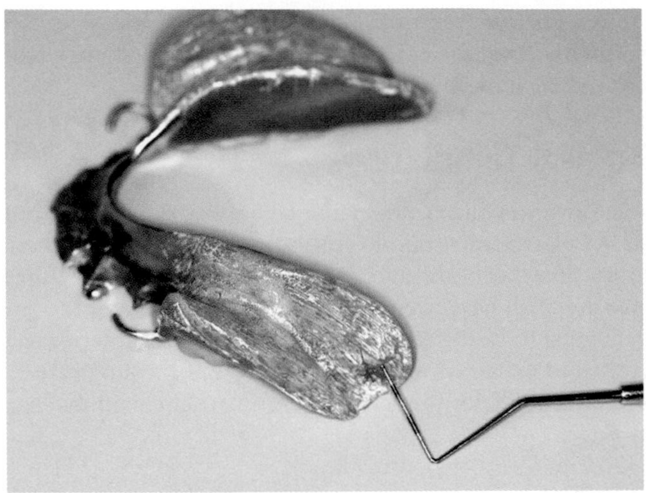

**FIG. 52.12** Example of denture with PID showing a sore spot. *(From Carr AB, Brown DT: McCracken's removable partial prosthodontics, ed 13, St Louis, 2016, Elsevier.)*

preparation for a mandibular denture, a *bar* to provide stability connects these castings; this forms the "male" portion of the appliance. The denture is prepared with a recessed *sleeve* in the anterior of the prosthesis, which serves as the receptor attachment; this is the "female" portion of the appliance. The denture is snapped over the bar and is stabilized in alignment with the opposing arch.

The in-office steps required for the fabrication of this special denture are similar to those for a normal denture.

# Denture Adjustment and Relining

If a denture puts too much pressure on a particular area in the mouth, the area will eventually become sore. A patient's input is helpful in identifying the general location of sore spots, but sometimes patients cannot precisely pinpoint the location of irritations. Pressure-indicating paste (PIP) is used for diagnosing problems with partials and dentures at insertion and adjustment appointments. PIP is a layer of white silicone paste that is placed over the entire tissue surface of the denture and seated back in the patient's mouth and allowed to set for approximately 2 minutes. The denture is removed from the patient's mouth, and the areas on the tissue surface of the denture where the paste has been displaced by heavy contact with the tissue will indicate a high area, causing it to rub (Fig. 52.12). That will require adjustment using an acrylic bur outside the patient's mouth.

Patients will assume that after they have received their denture, they are free from future dental visits. In reality, a patient should be scheduled once a year to evaluate the fit and to examine the oral tissues for subclinical irritation and dysplasia. The clinical indications for relining or rebasing are as follows:

- Dentures are loose or ill-fitting.
- A loss in vertical dimension occurs (angular cheilosis is an indication of this).
- Inflammatory hyperplasia is present.
- Traumatic ulcers appear after a long period of comfortable wear.

**Relining** is accomplished by placing a new layer of denture resin over the tissue surface of the appliance. **Rebasing** is a similar procedure that replaces the entire denture base material on an existing prosthesis without changing the occlusal relationship of the teeth. The difference is that a reline *resurfaces* the prosthesis, and a rebase *replaces* the denture base.

## Tissue Conditioners

The process of relining a denture must be done accurately to ensure a proper fit. The patient's supporting tissue must be healthy before impressions can be taken. One method used to rehabilitate unhealthy supporting tissues is to place a tissue-conditioning material for a short period, usually 3 or 4 days.

This material is a soft *elastomer* that is composed of a powder and a liquid. The mixed material is placed in the prosthesis and adapts to the supporting tissues and ridge, thereby providing a conditioning effect on unhealthy tissues.

## Impression

At the preliminary appointment, when it is agreed that relining is necessary, the patient is informed that the denture will be unavailable for at least 8 to 24 hours, while it is being processed in the laboratory. The impression is taken with the present (loose) denture used as the impression tray. The dentist flows a mix of zinc oxide–eugenol impression paste or an elastomeric impression material into the tissue side of the denture.

The denture is placed on the alveolar ridge, and the patient is instructed to close in normal occlusion and to hold the denture in place until the impression paste reaches a final set. The denture is removed from the mouth and disinfected. The denture and a written prescription are sent to the laboratory technician for relining.

## Delivery

When the relined denture is returned from the laboratory, it is disinfected and sealed in a precautionary bag. After removing the denture, make sure to rinse in cool water before returning it to the patient. The relined denture rarely needs adjustment because the only alteration to the original prosthesis is the addition of material within the tissue side of the denture.

If necessary, minor adjustments are made using an acrylic bur in a straight handpiece. Minor polishing may be done on the laboratory lathe with a sterile rag wheel with pumice paste; however, the tissue-bearing surfaces are *never* polished because this would alter the fit of the appliance.

The patient is dismissed and is advised to return within a period specified by the dentist for a checkup of the tissue and of the adaptation of the prosthesis.

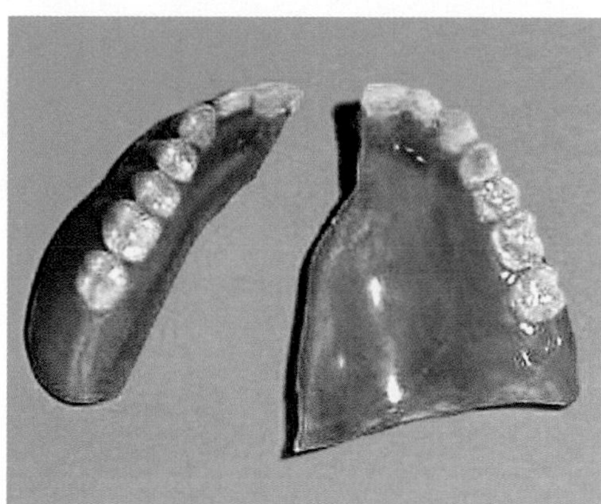

**FIG. 52.13** Broken denture.

18 How is an overdenture supported in the mouth?
19 What is the term for placing a new layer of resin over the tissue surface of a prosthesis?

## Denture Repairs

A patient may call the office upset because his or her denture or partial has fractured or has a missing or loose tooth (Fig. 52.13). The need for these repairs may be caused by changes in the oral tissues that place additional pressure on a certain area of the prosthesis, or just by careless handling. A broken acrylic denture can be repaired. Simple repairs are commonly handled in the dental office laboratory with the use of auto-cured or light-cured acrylics. More complicated repairs, particularly those involving replacement of teeth or a fracture in the framework, are sent to the dental laboratory technician for repair.

In most cases, the patient would be instructed to come to the office so the denture can be repaired. See Procedure 52.4: Repairing a Fractured Denture.

20 Who can repair a denture?

## Denture Duplication

Having a functional denture is important to the patient, and because dentures can break or may require time for relining, the patient can opt to have a duplicate denture. Although it involves an extra expense, many patients find that a duplicate is an excellent investment because they will not be without their denture if the original is damaged. To prevent warping while not in use, the spare denture should be stored in a moist, airtight container.

■ **Patient Education** Removable prosthodontics is an area of dentistry that can actually change a patient's self-perception. Some patients have never really "liked" the appearance of their teeth or have experienced a negative dental history regarding the care of their teeth. A removable prosthesis may make a "new person" out of these patients. By educating patients on the importance of taking care of their prosthesis and following a structured recall schedule, you will make them ever grateful for your assistance in meeting their dental needs. ■

■ **Legal and Ethical Implications** On the other hand, wearing a removable prosthesis can be one of the most aggravating and worst experiences of a patient's life. If patients expect a removable prosthesis to feel and function just as their natural teeth did, they will never be satisfied. You will find that patients who experience this negative reaction will not want to wear the prosthesis, because it fits poorly or the appearance is unappealing. If you have a patient who reacts in this manner, as part of the dental team, you have not provided the knowledge and service that this patient expected. ■

■ **Eye to the Future** With new advances in dental implants, patients who require a prosthetic appliance will be able to receive a prosthetic implant, partial or denture. Not only will this type of appliance be easier to maintain and be more natural looking for the patient than a denture, the cost will be greatly reduced, making it an option during the treatment planning stages. Increasingly, general dentists will receive training in implantology, thus making this option more readily available for a larger population. ■

■ **Critical Thinking**

1. Mr. Smith is scheduled for a lower partial denture. The partial will replace his molars on both sides. How many teeth will make up the partial denture? What teeth will become the abutment teeth for this prosthesis?
2. In reviewing the appointment stages for a partial and a full denture, what additional step is included for the making of a full denture that is not involved in the making of a partial?
3. Describe the different structures of the oral cavity that the dental laboratory technician requires from a final impression for a removable prosthodontic appliance, and compare these with requirements for a fixed-prosthesis case.
4. Discuss the importance of an immediate denture.
5. Why would a patient with a full set of dentures be placed on a recall system? What would be completed during this procedure? ■

PROCEDURE 52.1

# Assisting in the Delivery of a Partial Denture

## EQUIPMENT AND SUPPLIES

- Basic setup
- Articulating paper and holder
- Pressure indicator paste
- Low-speed and high-speed handpieces
- Pressure-indicating paste (PID)
- Acrylic burs
- Finishing burs
- Three-pronged pliers

## PROCEDURAL STEPS

1. Remove partial from laboratory packaging; disinfect and rinse to prepare for try-in.
2. Seat the patient.
3. The dentist places the new partial denture in the patient's mouth.
4. The patient is instructed to close his or her teeth together.
5. To check the *occlusion,* assist in placing articulating paper on the occlusal surface of the mandibular teeth, and ask the patient to simulate chewing motions. If the occlusion is too high, transfer handpiece with round carbide bur.
6. To detect *pressure points* (high spots) that could cause discomfort to the patient, apply pressure-indicator paste on the tissue surface of the prosthesis. The prosthesis is placed in the patient's mouth. As necessary, these high spots on the prosthesis are adjusted.
7. Retainers are examined for tension on the natural abutment teeth. Transfer pliers to the dentist to adjust the tension on the retainers.
8. After adjustments have been made, the partial denture is polished on the laboratory lathe with the appropriate pastes and sterile buffing wheels.
9. Scrub the partial denture with soap, water, and a brush; disinfect and rinse; return the partial denture to the treatment room for delivery to the patient.
10. Instruct the patient on placement, removal, and care of the partial denture.
11. Document the procedure.

| Date | Tooth | Surface | Charting Notes |
|---|---|---|---|
| 8/20/17 | — | | Delivered maxillary partial, minor adjustments made. Pt pleased with appearance and fit. Reschedule pt in 3 days for postdelivery check. T. Clark, CDA/L. Stewart, DDS |

PROCEDURE 52.2

# Assisting in a Wax Denture Try-in

## EQUIPMENT AND SUPPLIES

- Denture wax setup
- Basic setup
- Articulating paper and holder
- Wax spatula
- Heat source
- Low-speed handpiece with acrylic burs, discs, and stones

## PROCEDURAL STEPS

1. Remove wax setup from laboratory packaging; disinfect and rinse to prepare for try-in.
2. Seat the patient.
3. Assist in placing the wax setup of the denture for fit, comfort, and stability.
4. Assist with verifying the appearance of the denture teeth, which will include the shade selection, the size of the teeth, and alignment of the teeth.
5. Assist with the evaluation of the retention of the denture by asking the patient to articulate specific letters; *f, v, s,* and *th* sounds; swallows; and yawns.
6. Assist in checking the *occlusion,* assist in placing articulating paper on the occlusal surface of the mandibular teeth, and ask the patient to simulate chewing motions. If the occlusion is too high, transfer handpiece with round carbide bur.
7. Prepare the laboratory prescription for completion of the denture.
8. Disinfect the case, return it to the articulator, pack it, and return the case to the laboratory.
9. Document the procedure.

| Date | Tooth | Surface | Charting Notes |
|---|---|---|---|
| 8/20/17 | — | | Wax try-in of maxillary denture, base contoured and adjusted. Pt unhappy with canines. Noted on laboratory script for change in mold of #'s 6 and 11. Centric occlusion evaluated and adjusted. Pt rescheduled for delivery in 1 week. T. Clark, CDA/L. Stewart, DDS |

PROCEDURE 52.3

# Assisting in the Delivery of a Full Denture

## EQUIPMENT AND SUPPLIES

- Basic setup
- Dentures
- Hand mirror
- Articulating paper and holder
- High-speed and low-speed handpieces
- Pressure-indicating paste (PID)
- Finishing burs
- Acrylic burs

## PROCEDURAL STEPS

1 Remove denture from laboratory packaging; disinfect and rinse to prepare for try-in.

2 Seat the patient.

3 Assist the patient in inserting the new denture into the patient's mouth.

4 Hand the patient a mirror and evaluate the shade and mold of the artificial teeth for natural appearance.

5 Ask the patient to perform facial expressions and the actions of swallowing, chewing, and speaking, using *s* and *th* sounds.

**NOTE** These sounds also are appropriate for exercises to help the patient learn to speak normally with the new denture.

6 Assist in checking the *occlusion,* assist in placing articulating paper on the occlusal surface of the mandibular teeth, and ask the patient to simulate chewing motions.

**PURPOSE** Cusps that are too high in contact will be marked with the color of the articulating paper.

7 If the cusps are too high, the denture is removed from the mouth and is adjusted with a stone mounted on a straight handpiece.

8 The denture is replaced in the mouth, and the procedure is repeated until the cusps appear to be in occlusion with the opposing arch.

**NOTE** If the denture must be taken into the laboratory for adjustment, it must be disinfected again before it is returned to the patient.

9 When the patient is pleased with the appearance, function, and comfort of the denture, another appointment is made for the postdelivery checkup.

10 After adjustments have been made, the partial denture is polished on the laboratory lathe with the appropriate pastes and sterile buffing wheels.

11 Scrub the denture with soap, water, and a brush; disinfect and rinse; return the denture to the treatment room for delivery to the patient.

12 Instruct the patient on placement, removal, and care of the denture.

13 Before dismissal, the patient is informed that learning to wear a new denture will take several days or weeks.

14 Document the procedure.

| Date | Tooth | Surface | Charting Notes |
|---|---|---|---|
| 8/28/17 | | | Delivery of maxillary full denture. Pt pleased with change of canines. Teeth and shading good. Pt pleased with fit and appearance. Reschedule in 3 days for postdelivery check. |
| | | | T. Clark, CDA/L. Stewart, DDS |

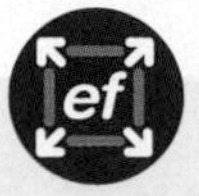

PROCEDURE 52.4

# Repairing a Fractured Denture (Expanded Function)

## EQUIPMENT AND SUPPLIES

- ✔ Fractured dentures
- ✔ Sticky wax
- ✔ Bunsen burner
- ✔ Plaster to pour a cast
- ✔ Low-speed handpiece
- ✔ Acrylic burs
- ✔ Auto-cured or light-cured acrylic

## PROCEDURAL STEPS

1. Disinfect the denture.
2. Align the fractured denture parts and apply sticky wax over the fracture line on the external surface of the denture.
3. Examine the denture and block out all undercuts on the internal surface that will be exposed to the plaster with a slurry mix or blockout wax.

   **PURPOSE** Blocking out the undercuts enables you to remove the plaster cast after it sets.

   **NOTE** Do not block out undercuts along the fracture line.
4. Prepare a plaster mix.
5. Slowly pour the plaster into the internal surface of the denture. The plaster should cover the fracture line, but not the entire denture.

   **NOTE** This is accomplished by holding the denture in your hand and gently resting it against the vibrator.
6. Place the denture in an upright position and allow the plaster to set.
7. Once the plaster is set, gently remove it from the cast.
8. Remove the sticky wax and pumice.
9. With an acrylic bur, widen the fracture lines on the denture and place retentive grooves along the fracture line.
10. Apply a thin coat of the acrylic monomer to the fracture lines, then place a small amount of the acrylic powder, alternating the liquid and powder until the fracture line is filled.
11. Once the material has cured, the area is smoothed and polished on the dental lathe.
12. The denture is cleaned and disinfected and tried in for fit.
13. Document the procedure.

| Date | Tooth | Surface | Charting Notes |
|---|---|---|---|
| 8/28/17 | | | Patient maxillary denture fractured at midline. Repaired with acrylic resin. Disinfected and polished. Pt pleased with fit and appearance.<br>T. Clark, CDA/L. Stewart, DDS |

53

# Dental Implants

## KEY TERMS

**Circumoral (sir-kum-OR-ul)** Surrounding the mouth.

**Endosteal (en-DOS-tee-ul)** Type of implant that is surgically embedded into the bone.

**Implant** A permanent replacement of one tooth or multiple teeth with a fixture and an abutment that are anchored into the bone or surrounding structure for the purpose of supporting a denture, bridge, or single tooth.

**Osseointegration (os-ee-oe-in-te-GRAY-shun)** The process of introducing certain metals, such as titanium, into living bone and forming a biocompatible bond with living bone.

**Stent** Clear acrylic template positioned over the alveolar ridge to guide in the proper angulation and axis for drilling into the bone and placing the implant.

**Subperiosteal (sub-per-ee-OS-tee-ul)** Type of implant that includes a metal frame, which is surgically placed under the periosteum.

**Titanium (tye-TAY-nee-um)** Type of metal used for implants.

**Transosteal (tranz-OS-tee-ul)** Type of implant in which the metal framework is surgically inserted through the inferior border of the mandible. This type of implant is used only on the mandible.

## LEARNING OUTCOMES

*On completion of this chapter, the student will be able to achieve the following objectives:*

1. Pronounce, define, and spell the key terms.
2. Discuss the indications for dental implants.
3. Discuss the contraindications to dental implants.
4. Describe the selection of patients to receive dental implants.
5. Explain the preparation for implants.
6. Identify the types of dental implants, and describe the surgical procedures for implantation.
7. Describe maintenance of dental implants, including home care procedures, routine office visits, and implant treatment failure.

## PERFORMANCE OUTCOME

*On completion of this chapter, the student will be able to achieve competency standards in the following skill:*

- Assist in endosteal implant surgery.

## ELECTRONIC RESOURCES

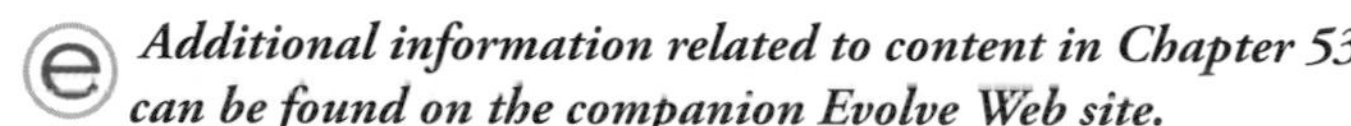
***Additional information related to content in Chapter 53 can be found on the companion Evolve Web site.***

- Practice Quiz

When natural teeth are lost, it is challenging to duplicate their function and appearance with a fixed bridge or removable partial or denture. Dental implants provide a natural-looking and functional replacement for missing teeth that incorporates principles from fixed and removable prosthodontics with the use of bone-anchored implants. Artificial teeth are attached to metal implants that are permanently secured in the jaw. These implants hold the artificial teeth in place as firmly as the root system holds natural teeth.

Dental **implants** are used to attach artificial teeth to anchors (similar to posts) that have been surgically embedded into the bone (Fig. 53.1). The implantation process involves several steps and can take anywhere from 3 to 9 months to complete. Depending on the type of implant, the steps will vary. Most dental implant procedures are performed in a dental office, but some could require an outpatient surgical setting, depending on the patient's general health and the type of implant.

The placement of dental implants involves both surgery and delivery of the prosthesis. Several specialists, which include the oral and maxillofacial surgeon, periodontist, prosthodontist, and *implantologist* (general dentist with specialized training) may perform these procedures. The dental laboratory technician will also be involved in this field of dentistry.

The type of specialist who performs the procedure is less important than the *ability, experience,* and *education* of the clinician involved. The clinician must have in-depth knowledge of both surgical and prosthodontic aspects of implants. A coordinated effort among specialists and general practitioners is necessary to obtain optimal results when implants are being considered.

## Indications for Implants

Dental implants are now considered as the standard of care. For example, the lower full denture yields a low rate

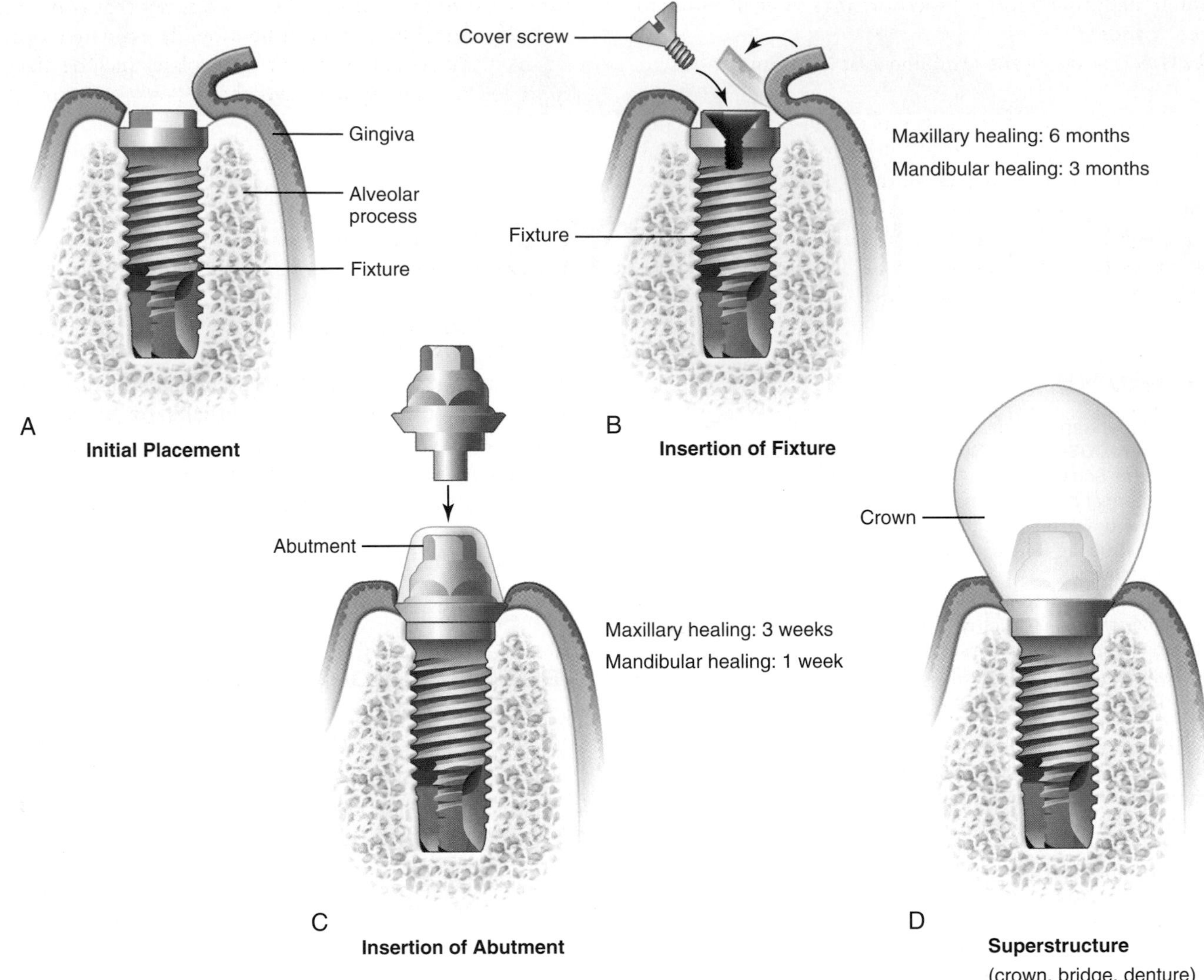


**FIG. 53.1** Dental implant. A, Initial placement. B, Insertion of cover screw. C, Insertion of the Abutment. D, Placement of final crown.

of patient satisfaction, where implant dentistry has a better chance of solving the problems associated with a mandibular denture.

A dental implant can have a success rate greater than 90 percent. Effective home care and regular dental visits are essential for the long-term success of dental implants; this should be conveyed to the patient during the treatment planning phase. Dental implants can last as long as 20 years and in some cases can last a lifetime. Indications for dental implants include the following:

- To replace one or more teeth as single units without affecting adjoining teeth
- To replace a bridge and eliminate the need for a removable partial denture
- To provide support for a denture, making it more secure and comfortable
- To prevent bone loss and gum recession that often accompany bridgework and dentures
- To enhance the patient's confidence in smiling and speaking
- To improve the patient's overall psychological health
- To improve the esthetic appearance of the patient's teeth and mouth

## Contraindications to Implants

As with any dental procedure, dental implants involve some risk. Because each patient is unique, any surgical success cannot be 100 percent guaranteed. The patient must be properly screened, and some patients may not be good candidates for an implant. The following contraindications should be considered when implant options are discussed:

- The financial investment is greater than that for a conventional bridge or denture.
- Treatment can take several months or longer to complete.
- As with any surgical procedure, implants convey a risk of infection and other complications.
- An implant may loosen, requiring replacement.

- Emotionally, the implant procedure may be challenging for some patients.
- *Bruxism* is a significant component of failed implants.

Patients with certain medical complications may not be good candidates for dental implants. Medical conditions that could contraindicate implants include diseases of the cardiovascular, respiratory, and gastrointestinal systems; a seriously compromised immune system; and other chronic conditions that impede healing. Lifestyle-related factors such as smoking and excessive alcohol can affect or impede periodontal health and healing factors.

RECALL

1 List the types of dental specialists who may receive training in dental implants.
2 What is the success rate for dental implants?
3 How long can dental implants last?
4 Is the financial investment for an implant greater or less than for a fixed bridge?
5 How long can an implant procedure take to complete?

# The Dental Implant Patient

A comprehensive evaluation is essential in the determination of whether the patient will benefit from dental implants. The ideal candidate to receive an implant should be in stable health and have adequate alveolar bone and is willing to commit to attentive oral hygiene and regular dental visits.

During treatment planning, the dentist and the patient should discuss the patient's needs, desires, and financial commitment. After these issues and existing problems have been evaluated, the treatment is decided on, and the prosthesis that satisfies these goals is started. Specific treatment options are available for the partially and completely edentulous patient, with the prosthesis being fixed or removable depending on existing oral conditions.

## Psychological Evaluation

The psychological evaluation takes place at the initial visit. The dentist assesses the patient's attitude, ability to cooperate during complex procedures, and overall outlook on dental treatment. The dentist also determines whether the patient has realistic expectations about dental implants and the end results.

## Dental Examination

During the examination, the dentist evaluates the condition of the teeth and soft tissues, areas of attached and unattached tissue, and the height and width of the edentulous alveolar bone ridge. This information is necessary for determining the best type of implant and for deciding the location in which to place the implants (Fig. 53.2).

## Medical History and Evaluation

The purpose of the medical history and evaluation is to assess any existing medical conditions that could worsen as a result of the stress of implant surgery. Any diseases that could interfere with normal healing must be carefully evaluated. Specific conditions that could interfere with implants include diabetes, suppressed immune system, and chemotherapy treatment for cancer.

## Specialized Radiographs and Imaging

The use of intraoral and extraoral radiographic images will be prescribed during the planning phase and throughout the treatment to evaluate and determine the height, width, and quality of bone in the area for the implant, as well as the exact positioning of the implant.

Types of images may include *periapical, panoramic, cephalometric,* and *tomographic* views (see Chapter 42). These radiographs are useful for locating the exact positions of anatomic structures such as the inferior alveolar nerve, mental foramen, maxillary sinus, and nasal floor, as well as any abnormalities (Fig. 53.3).

## Diagnostic Casts and Surgical Stents

A diagnostic cast is fabricated at the beginning of treatment to construct a surgical stent. A surgical **stent** is made from a clear acrylic resin and will be used as a guide or template that is positioned over the alveolar ridge to guide the proper angulation and axis for drilling into the bone and placing the implant screws in their proper position in bone (Fig. 53.4). The stent *must* be sterilized before use.

RECALL

6 What are the four types of extraoral radiographs that are used by the dentist in evaluating the dental implant patient?
7 Why would a dentist use a surgical stent during implant surgery?

# Preparation for Implants

## Informed Consent

Written informed patient consent is required before treatment begins. The consent form should advise and educate the patient about (1) background information on implants, (2) complications of implant surgery, (3) prognosis, (4) time frame, (5) home care, and (6) follow-up appointments.

## Surgical Preparation

Implant surgery must be completed under strict surgical sterile conditions with sterile instrumentation. The patient's mouth is rinsed with 0.1 percent chlorhexidine. The head is draped, and a sterile surgical drape is applied to the **circumoral** area, leaving only the mouth exposed.

It is recommended that the implant team consist of at least three persons: the clinician, the surgical dental assistant, and the nonsterile circulating assistant. The clinician and the

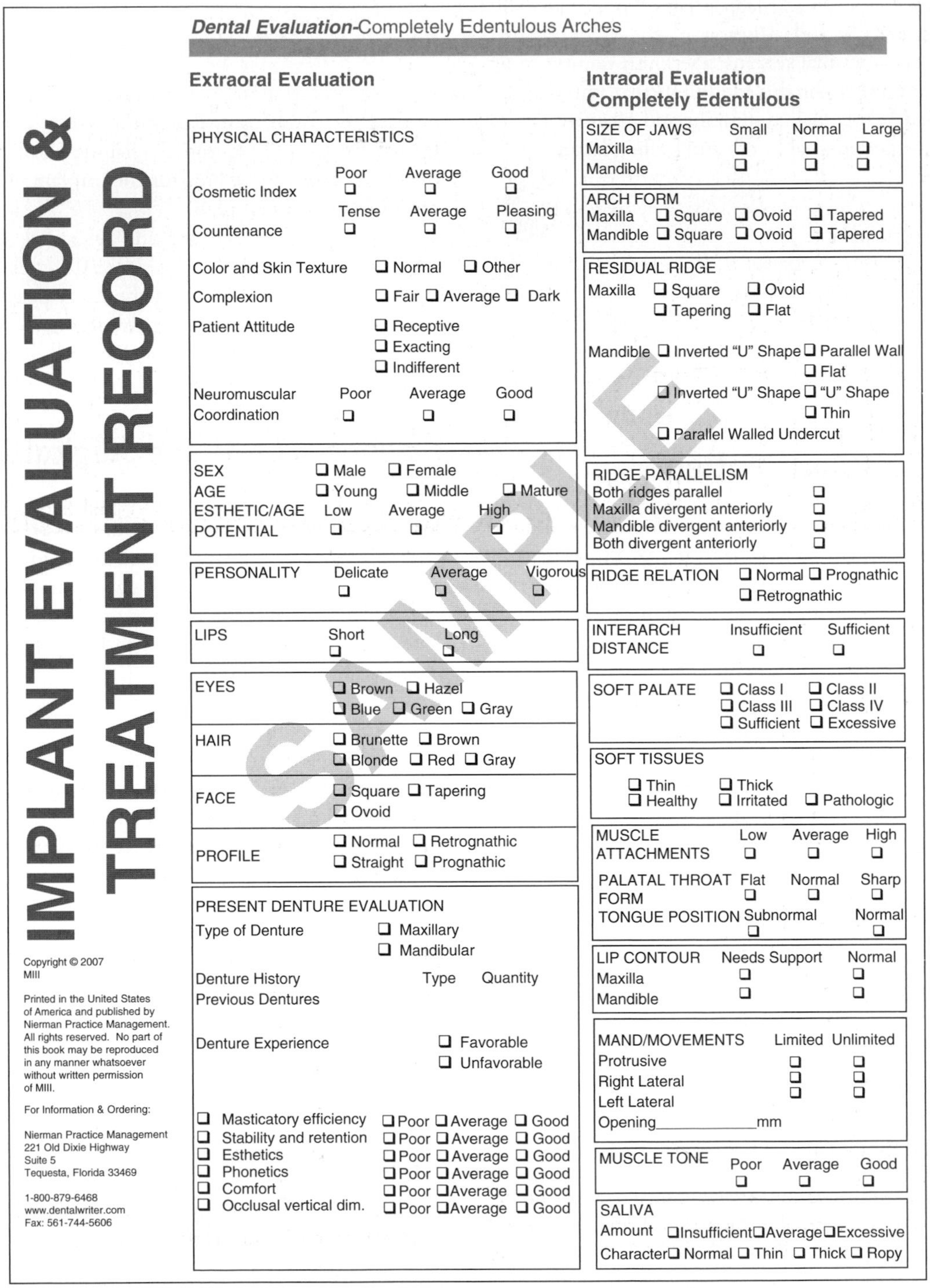

IMPLANT EVALUATION & TREATMENT RECORD

*Dental Evaluation*-Completely Edentulous Arches

**Extraoral Evaluation**

PHYSICAL CHARACTERISTICS

| | Poor | Average | Good |
|---|---|---|---|
| Cosmetic Index | ❑ | ❑ | ❑ |
| | Tense | Average | Pleasing |
| Countenance | ❑ | ❑ | ❑ |

Color and Skin Texture ❑ Normal ❑ Other

Complexion ❑ Fair ❑ Average ❑ Dark

Patient Attitude ❑ Receptive ❑ Exacting ❑ Indifferent

| | Poor | Average | Good |
|---|---|---|---|
| Neuromuscular Coordination | ❑ | ❑ | ❑ |

SEX ❑ Male ❑ Female

AGE ❑ Young ❑ Middle ❑ Mature

ESTHETIC/AGE POTENTIAL Low ❑ Average ❑ High ❑

PERSONALITY Delicate ❑ Average ❑ Vigorous ❑

LIPS Short ❑ Long ❑

EYES ❑ Brown ❑ Hazel ❑ Blue ❑ Green ❑ Gray

HAIR ❑ Brunette ❑ Brown ❑ Blonde ❑ Red ❑ Gray

FACE ❑ Square ❑ Tapering ❑ Ovoid

PROFILE ❑ Normal ❑ Retrognathic ❑ Straight ❑ Prognathic

PRESENT DENTURE EVALUATION

Type of Denture ❑ Maxillary ❑ Mandibular

Denture History Type Quantity

Previous Dentures

Denture Experience ❑ Favorable ❑ Unfavorable

| | | | |
|---|---|---|---|
| ❑ Masticatory efficiency | ❑ Poor | ❑ Average | ❑ Good |
| ❑ Stability and retention | ❑ Poor | ❑ Average | ❑ Good |
| ❑ Esthetics | ❑ Poor | ❑ Average | ❑ Good |
| ❑ Phonetics | ❑ Poor | ❑ Average | ❑ Good |
| ❑ Comfort | ❑ Poor | ❑ Average | ❑ Good |
| ❑ Occlusal vertical dim. | ❑ Poor | ❑ Average | ❑ Good |

**Intraoral Evaluation Completely Edentulous**

| SIZE OF JAWS | Small | Normal | Large |
|---|---|---|---|
| Maxilla | ❑ | ❑ | ❑ |
| Mandible | ❑ | ❑ | ❑ |

ARCH FORM

Maxilla ❑ Square ❑ Ovoid ❑ Tapered

Mandible ❑ Square ❑ Ovoid ❑ Tapered

RESIDUAL RIDGE

Maxilla ❑ Square ❑ Ovoid ❑ Tapering ❑ Flat

Mandible ❑ Inverted "U" Shape ❑ Parallel Wal ❑ Flat ❑ Inverted "U" Shape ❑ "U" Shape ❑ Thin ❑ Parallel Walled Undercut

| RIDGE PARALLELISM | |
|---|---|
| Both ridges parallel | ❑ |
| Maxilla divergent anteriorly | ❑ |
| Mandible divergent anteriorly | ❑ |
| Both divergent anteriorly | ❑ |

RIDGE RELATION ❑ Normal ❑ Prognathic ❑ Retrognathic

INTERARCH DISTANCE Insufficient ❑ Sufficient ❑

SOFT PALATE ❑ Class I ❑ Class II ❑ Class III ❑ Class IV ❑ Sufficient ❑ Excessive

SOFT TISSUES ❑ Thin ❑ Thick ❑ Healthy ❑ Irritated ❑ Pathologic

| | Low | Average | High |
|---|---|---|---|
| MUSCLE ATTACHMENTS | ❑ | ❑ | ❑ |
| | Flat | Normal | Sharp |
| PALATAL THROAT FORM | ❑ | ❑ | ❑ |
| | Subnormal | | Normal |
| TONGUE POSITION | ❑ | | ❑ |

| LIP CONTOUR | Needs Support | Normal |
|---|---|---|
| Maxilla | ❑ | ❑ |
| Mandible | ❑ | ❑ |

| MAND/MOVEMENTS | Limited | Unlimited |
|---|---|---|
| Protrusive | ❑ | ❑ |
| Right Lateral | ❑ | ❑ |
| Left Lateral | ❑ | ❑ |

Opening___________mm

MUSCLE TONE Poor ❑ Average ❑ Good ❑

SALIVA

Amount ❑Insufficient❑Average❑Excessive

Character❑ Normal ❑ Thin ❑ Thick ❑ Ropy



For Information & Ordering:

Nierman Practice Management
221 Old Dixie Highway
Suite 5
Tequesta, Florida 33469

1-800-879-6468
www.dentalwriter.com
Fax: 561-744-5606

**FIG. 53.2** Implant evaluation and treatment record. *(From Misch CE: Contemporary implant dentistry, ed 3, St Louis, 2008, Mosby.)*

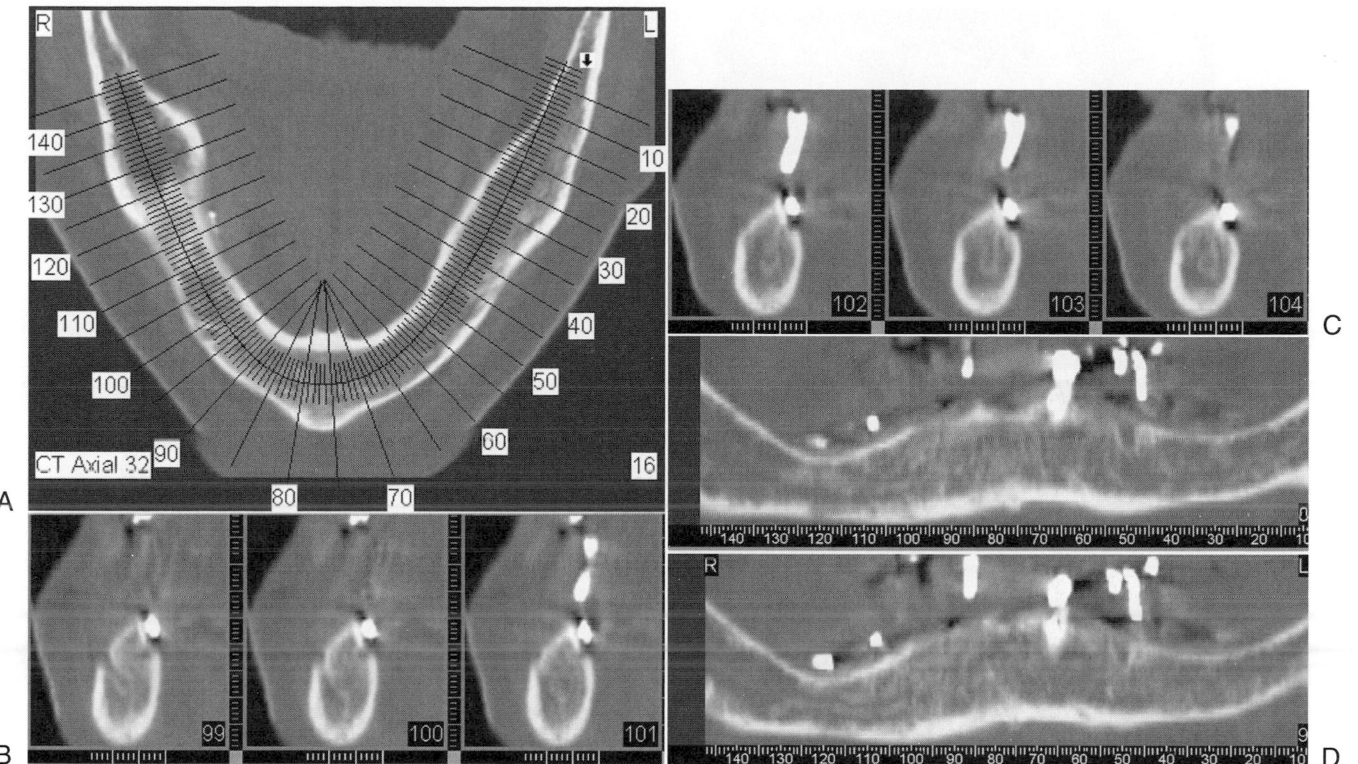


**FIG. 53.3** Programmed dental computed tomography. *(From Misch CE: Contemporary implant dentistry, ed 3, St Louis, 2008, Mosby.)*

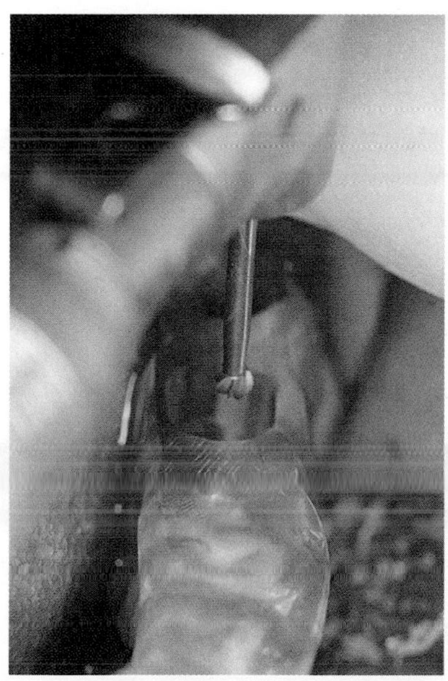

**FIG. 53.4** Custom stent used to aid the dentist in placing an implant. *(From Newman M, Takei T, Klokkevold P et al, editors: Carranza's clinical periodontology, ed 12, St Louis, 2015, Saunders.)*

surgical dental assistant should be gowned and masked and should wear talcum powder–free *sterile* gloves.

The implants are delivered in double-aseptic packaging. They must remain in this packaging until the actual time of placement. Just before placement, the inner vial is opened, and the implant is allowed to slide (untouched) onto a sterile surface. Depending on the type of implant to be placed, the surgical technique may vary slightly.

## Lack of Bone Density

Bone density is an important component of an implant's success or failure. Bone density can vary considerably on the location of the implant. For example, the density of bone in the mandibular anterior area is greater than that of the maxillary anterior. In a case where there is extensive alveolar bone loss, it may be necessary to provide bone augmentation before implant placement. Bone grafts are classified on the basis of how they produce new bone: osteoconduction, osteoinduction, and/or osteogenesis.

- Osteoconductive materials are synthetic biocompatible materials that allow bone growth from the existing bone.
- Osteoinductive materials are processed cadaver bone and come in three forms: frozen, freeze-dried, and demineralized freeze-dried material.
- Osteogenesis is an autogenous bone, which is a bone graft taken from other areas of the patient, for example, the iliac crest.

# Types of Dental Implants

## Endosteal Implant

**Endosteal** implants, also known as *osseointegrated implants,* are the most common type of implant placed. The implant is surgically placed into the jawbone (Fig. 53.5). Each implant holds one or more prosthetic teeth. This type of implant generally is

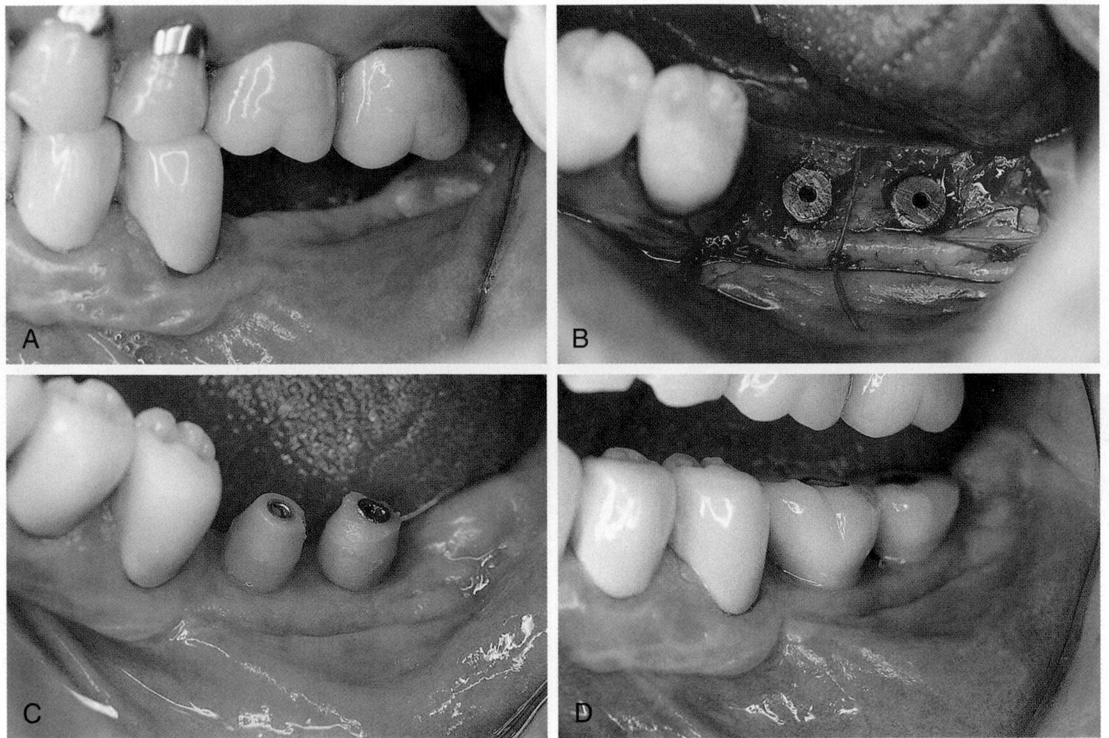


**FIG. 53.5** Second-stage surgery whereby two single endosseous units were placed for tooth #18 and tooth #19. A, Site for receiving implants. B, Initial placement of screws. C, Insertion of fixture. D, Final implant. *(From Newman M, Takei T, Klokkevold P et al, editors: Carranza's clinical periodontology, ed 12, St Louis, 2015, Saunders.)*

used as an alternative for patients requiring a crown, bridge or partial and full denture.

Implants and abutment screws are commonly made from the metal **titanium** because of its compatibility with bone and oral tissues. Titanium implants can be coated with *hydroxyapatite,* a ceramic substance that rapidly osseointegrates the implant to the bone. Endosteal implants have three components:

1. The *titanium implant* is surgically embedded into the bone during stage I surgery. This consists of a blade form, a cylinder form, or a screw form (Fig. 53.6).
2. The *titanium abutment screw* is screwed into the implant after osseointegration of the implant and during stage II surgery.
3. The *abutment post* or *cylinder* is attached to the artificial tooth or denture.

**Osseointegration** is the process by which the living cells of the jawbone naturally grow around the implanted dental supports (*osseo-* means bone). It refers to a bond that is developed between living bone and the surface of an implant fixture. Osseointegrated implants are used to support, stabilize, and retain removable dentures, fixed bridges, and single-tooth implants.

For this type of implant, three appointments are required to complete the procedure. At the *first surgery,* implant fixtures are placed within receptor sites in the jawbone at predetermined locations. The mucosa is sutured over the fixtures. After a 1- to 2-week healing period, the existing prosthesis (when applicable) may be removed and relined to adapt to the healed ridge.

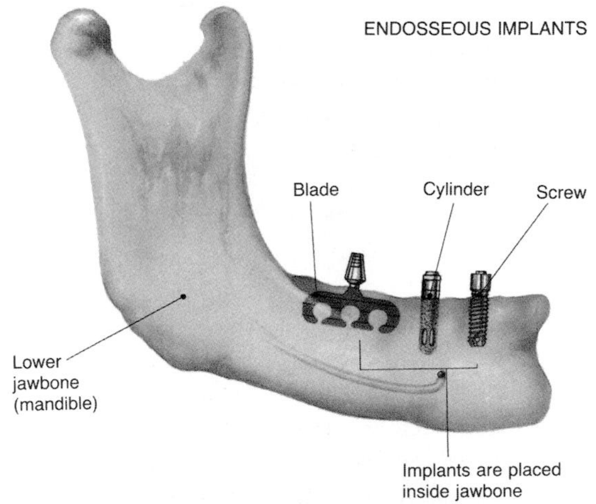


**FIG. 53.6** Diagram showing the types of endosteal implants. *(From Sakaguchi RL, Powers JM: Craig's restorative dental materials, ed 13, Philadelphia, 2012, Mosby.)*

A period of 3 to 6 months, the *osseointegration period,* is required to permit the fixture to osseointegrate or bond to the bone. Care must be taken during this healing period to avoid trauma to the mucosa overlying the implant sites.

At the *second surgery,* the endosteal implant fixture is exposed, and the abutment screw is connected to the anchor. This portion protrudes through the mucosa and will connect the fixture to the prosthesis. Because this is exposed in the mouth a provisional is placed until the final prosthetic is prepared.

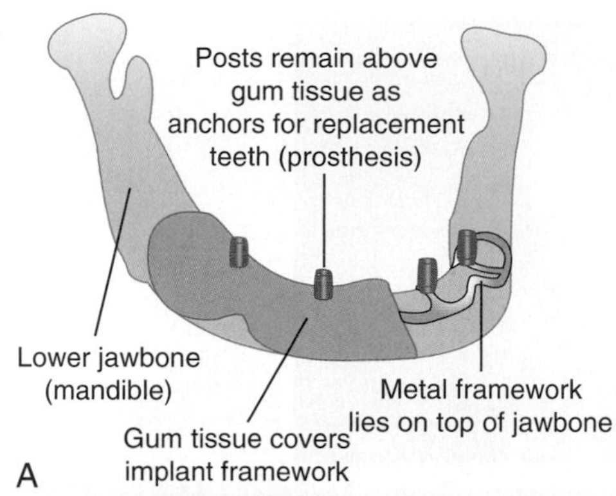


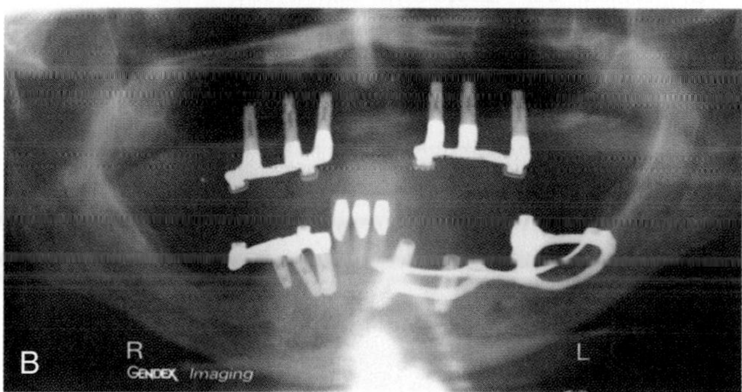


**FIG. 53.7** Diagram showing the position of the subperiosteal implant. A, Image to show framework of a mandibular implant. B, Radiographic image of the implant. *(From Darby ML, Walsh MM: Dental hygiene: theory and practice, ed 4, St Louis, 2015, Saunders.)*

After both surgeries have been completed and tissues have healed, the patient begins the *restorative phase,* during which the final crown, bridge, partial denture, or full denture is fabricated. The entire implant process can require 3 to 9 months to reach completion.

## Maxillary Implants

The maxillary sinus is a consideration when placing dental implants in the maxillary jaw. The floor of the maxillary sinus is close to the roots of maxillary molar and premolar teeth. Because of this, when these teeth are extracted there may not be adequate bone height to support dental implants in the posterior maxilla. A sinus lift or bone graft to the floor of the maxillary sinus may be indicated.

Procedure 53.1: Assisting in an Endosteal Implant Surgery describes the surgical components of a *two-stage* standard osseointegrated implant system for a single tooth.

## Subperiosteal Implant

A **subperiosteal** implant is a metal frame that is placed under the periosteum and *on top* of the bone. In contrast to an endosteal implant, a subperiosteal implant is *not* placed into the bone (Fig. 53.7).

Subperiosteal implants are indicated for patients who do not have sufficient alveolar ridge remaining to support the endosteal-type implant. This type of implant is used most frequently to support a mandibular complete denture (Fig. 53.8).

Two surgical procedures are required for this type of implant. During the *first surgery,* the alveolar ridge is exposed and impressions are taken of the alveolar ridge. After impressions are taken, the tissue is repositioned over the ridge and is sutured back into place. The impression is sent to a dental laboratory, where a metal frame with posts is fabricated.

After the frame has been fabricated, the *second surgery* is performed. The alveolar ridge again is surgically exposed, and the metal frame is placed over the ridge. When the frame is in place, the tissues are repositioned and sutured into place.

## Transosteal Implant

The **transosteal** implant is inserted through the inferior border of the mandible and into the edentulous area (Fig. 53.9). The most common type is the *transmandibular staple implant,* or fixed mandibular implant. These implants are used primarily in patients with severely resorbed ridges, and only when no other options exist.

RECALL

8 What material is commonly used to make an implant?
9 What does *osseo-* mean?
10 What component of the endosteal implant attaches to the artificial tooth or teeth?
11 When would a subperiosteal implant be recommended to a patient?

# Maintenance of Dental Implants

Long-term maintenance is an integral part of treatment for dental implant patients. This maintenance includes home care by the patient and periodic maintenance visits to the dental office.

The health of the peri-implant tissue is a critical factor in the success of dental implants. It is similar to the gingival sulcus that surrounds a natural tooth. Peri-implant tissue responds to bacterial plaque with inflammation and bleeding, similarly to gingival tissues around a normal tooth (Fig. 53.10).

Many implant patients have lost their natural teeth because of chronic periodontal disease, caused in part by poor oral hygiene. The task of educating and motivating these patients to practice proper home care is difficult but critical to the long-term success of the implants.

Dental *plaque* and *calculus* form on implants just as on natural teeth. Because the surface of implants is smooth, plaque is less adherent and is more easily removed than it is from natural teeth. Calculus is relatively easy to remove from implants because it cannot become embedded in the titanium surface. However, it is critical to remove plaque and calculus

**FIG. 53.8** Subperiosteal implant with full-arch denture prosthesis. *(From Newman M, Takei T, Klokkevold P, Carranza F, editors: Carranza's clinical periodontology, ed 11, St Louis, 2012, Saunders.)*

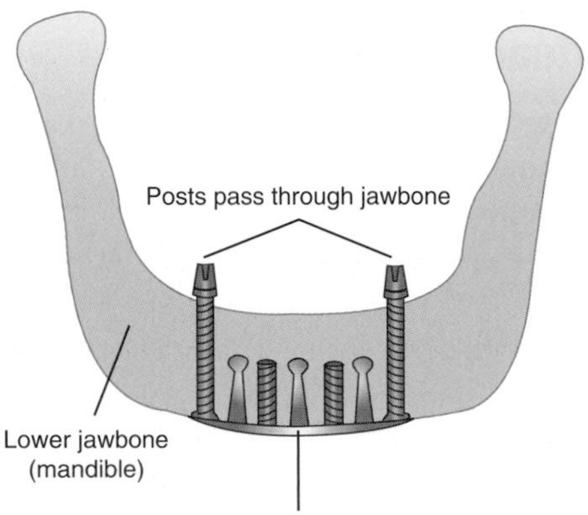


**FIG. 53.9** Diagram showing the position of the transosteal implant. *(From Darby ML, Walsh MM: Dental hygiene: theory and practice, ed 4, St Louis, 2015, Saunders.)*

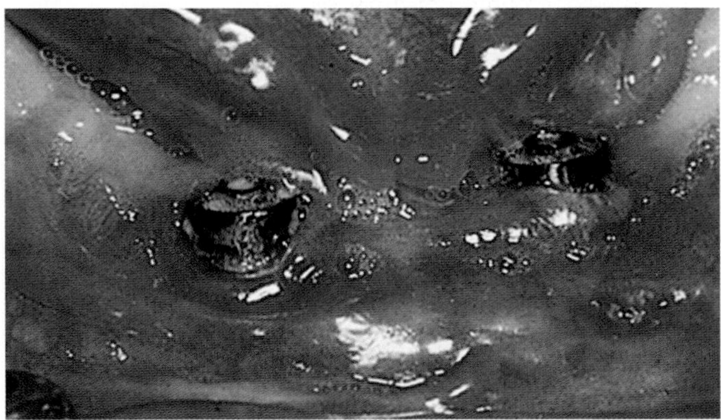

**FIG. 53.10** Peri-implantitis, showing redness and inflammation of tissue around the implant caused by plaque. *(Courtesy A. K. Lakha.)*

from the implant in such a way that the implant surfaces are not scratched (Fig. 53.11).

## Home Care

As with all home care, the goal is to remove all plaque and debris at least once daily. Patients are instructed in the use of home care aids, and their progress is monitored regularly. As discussed in Chapter 15, the following devices are essential in plaque removal for implant patients:

- Toothbrushes, manual or electric
- Single-tufted toothbrushes
- Partial denture clasp brushes
- Interproximal brushes
- Floss (thick, thin, or fuzzy)
- Dental implant floss, with a stiff, curved end

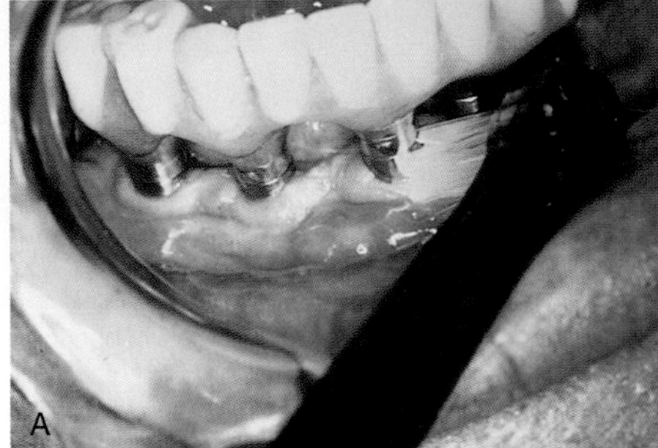


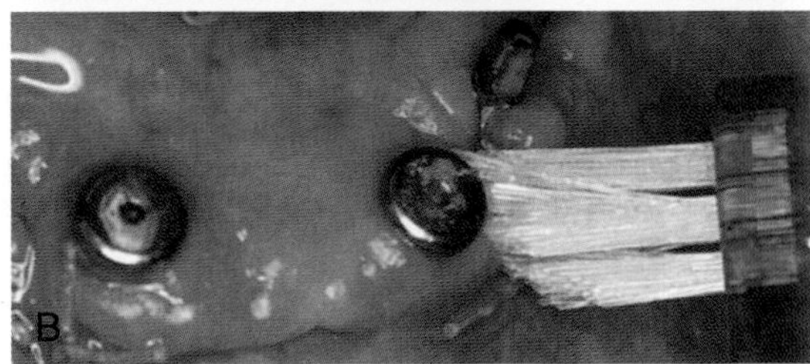


**FIG. 53.11** Implant sites should be cleaned daily. A, Using an implant toothbrush under a subperiosteal full arch denture. B, Technique for removing plaque and debris from around the implant. *(From Darby ML, Walsh MM: Dental hygiene: theory and practice, ed 4, St Louis, 2015, Saunders.)*

## Routine Office Visits

*Recall visits* are essential for the long-term success of implants. It is important that patients understand the need to maintain optimum plaque control through meticulous home care and frequent professional recalls. Patients are scheduled at regular intervals for examination, radiography, prophylaxis, removal of fixed components, replacement of components, and relines and remakes as recommended.

## Implant Treatment Failure

Implants can fail for a number of reasons. Implant failure can begin in the diagnostic stages, preparation of the site, placement of implant, and postsurgery. Listed are specific areas that affect the success of the implant:

- Patient health and lifestyle factors
- Comorbid periodontal disease
- Lack of osseointegration
- Fracture of bone during the osteotomy
- Graft failure
- Prosthetic design
- Postimplant soft tissue defects
- Miscalculation of bone density or tissue thickness
- Improper selection of type of implant
- Poor drilling technique
- Patient force factors

RECALL

12 Why are plaque and calculus easier to remove from an implant than from a natural tooth?
13 What cleaning accessories are used to clean implants?

**■ Patient Education** In American culture, people are often judged by their facial expressions. A smile can be a sign of competence, inner reflections, thoughts, and emotions. More people are becoming aware of dental implant procedures because of advertisements in the media. By providing this information to all of your patients through brochures, educational videos, and patient discussion, you are furthering their knowledge of dental care. ■

**■ Legal and Ethical Implications** Dental implants require a large investment of money and time for a patient, so it is important that the dental team present the complete plan for all stages of treatment. More dental insurance companies are handling dental implant procedures, but only for specific reasons. Dentists have a responsibility to their patients and should not deviate from providing this procedure for appropriate reasons. Negligence in providing proper care may cause undue harm to the patient. ■

**■ Eye to the Future** Modern advances in implant technology have made immediate implant placement possible. Once a tooth has been extracted, the bone underneath the space starts to shrink. If the implant is placed immediately after extraction and before any bone resorption has occurred, a maximum amount of bone is still available for support. Because the implant is placed at the same time the tooth is extracted, additional surgical procedures are not needed, and the implant can be placed while the patient is still anesthetized. ■

**■ Critical Thinking**

1. Describe your role as a clinical assistant in the procedure of implant surgery.
2. Discuss the reasoning behind the use of titanium metal over other metals for implants.
3. Your patient is considering implants. While updating the patient's medical and dental history, you find that the patient is taking fluoxetine (Prozac). For what condition is Prozac prescribed, and why would this information be important for the dentist to know before the implant process is begun?
4. Why is infection control so important during the preparation and procedure stages of implants?
5. Many types of specialists can actually provide implants; what does each specialist bring to this area of dentistry? ■

PROCEDURE 53.1

## Assisting in an Endosteal Implant Surgery

### EQUIPMENT AND SUPPLIES

- ✔ Basic setup
- ✔ Local anesthetic
- ✔ Sterile surgical gloves
- ✔ Sterile surgical drilling unit
- ✔ Surgical irrigation tip
- ✔ Scalpel
- ✔ Periosteal elevator
- ✔ Implant instrument kit
- ✔ Implant kit
- ✔ Sterile saline solution
- ✔ Low-speed handpiece with contra-angle attachment
- ✔ Inserting mallet
- ✔ Suture setup
- ✔ Electrosurgical unit and tips (or tissue punch)
- ✔ 3 percent hydrogen peroxide with syringe
- ✔ Sterile cotton pellets
- ✔ Sterile 2 × 2–inch gauze sponges

(Continued)

# PROCEDURE 53.1 Assisting in an Endosteal Implant Surgery—cont'd

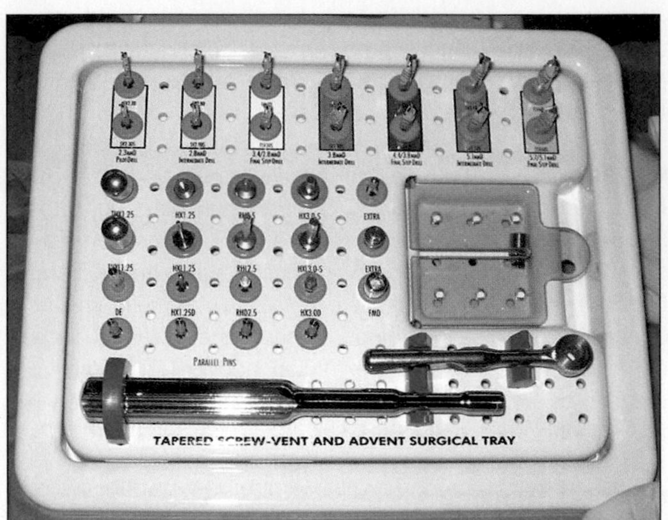


## PROCEDURAL STEPS

### Stage I Surgery: Implant Placement

1. The surgical stent (template) is placed in position in the patient's mouth.
2. After achieving adequate anesthesia, the surgeon uses a "pilot drill" (similar to a pesso bur) to drill through the stent and into the soft tissue on the ridge. This creates a target point on the bone for the implant site.

   **NOTE** All drilling of the bone is accomplished with generous amounts of sterile saline irrigation.
3. The surgeon removes the surgical stent and makes the incision at the implant site.

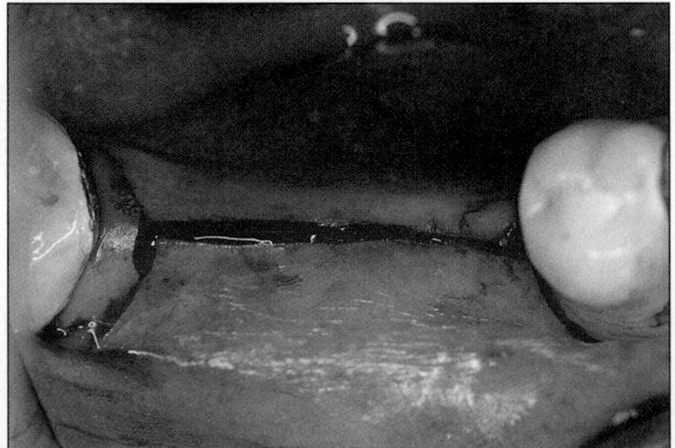

*From Newman M, Takei T, Klokkevold P et al, editors: Carranza's clinical periodontology, ed 12, St Louis, 2015, Saunders.*

4. The mucoperiosteal tissues are reflected.

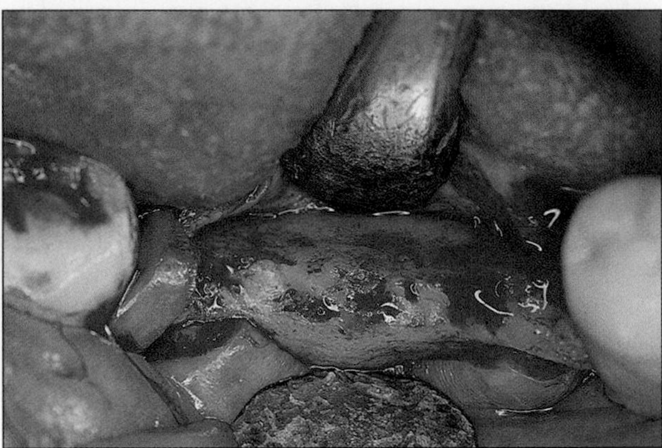

*From Newman M, Takei T, Klokkevold P et al, editors: Carranza's clinical periodontology, ed 12, St Louis, 2015, Saunders.*

5. The surgeon smooths any sharp edges on the crest of the ridge. The crest should be at least 2 mm wider than the implant that is being used.
6. A variety of drill tips (similar to burs) are used to prepare the osseous receptor site.
7. The implant cylinder (with a plastic cap over the top of it) is partially inserted into the osseous receptor site.
8. The plastic cap is removed, and the implant is tapped into its final position with the inserting mallet.
9. The sterile sealing screw (also called a *healing collar*) is placed into the implant cylinder with the contra-angle screwdriver. Final tightening of the sealing screw is accomplished with the handheld screwdriver.

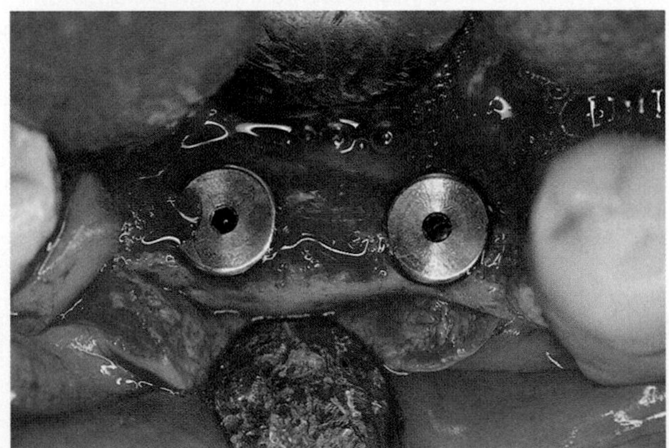

*From Newman M, Takei T, Klokkevold P et al, editors: Carranza's clinical periodontology, ed 12, St Louis, 2015, Saunders.*

10. The retraction suture is removed, and the mucoperiosteal flaps are repositioned and sutured in place. The implant receptor now is covered by the tissue and is not visible in the mouth.

## PROCEDURE 53.1 Assisting in an Endosteal Implant Surgery–cont'd

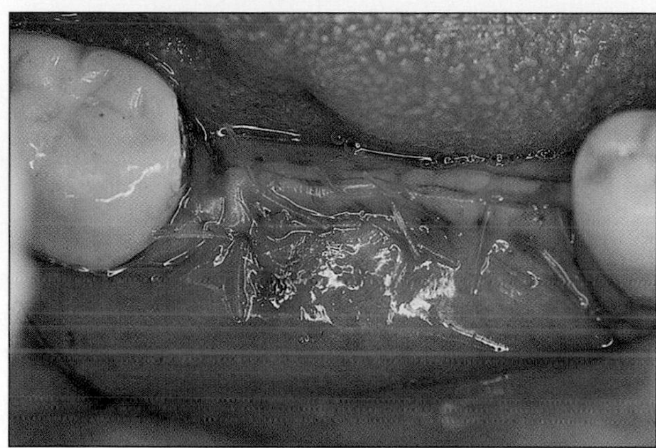

*From Newman M, Takei T, Klokkevold P et al, editors: Carranza's clinical periodontology, ed 12, St Louis, 2015, Saunders.*

### Osseointegration Period

**11** A period of 3 to 6 months is required to permit the fixture or fixtures to osseointegrate or bond to the bone. During this period, the existing denture or provisional coverage can be adapted to the healed alveolar ridge for temporary use—a procedure usually performed by the *restorative dentist.* The goal of the restorative dentist is to provide patients with beautiful teeth and a beautiful smile, so they can continue their normal activities without delay.

### Stage II Surgery: Implant Exposure

**12** After local anesthesia is administered, the surgical stent (template) is repositioned.

**13** A sharp instrument such as a periodontal probe is lowered through the opening in the stent to make bleeding points.

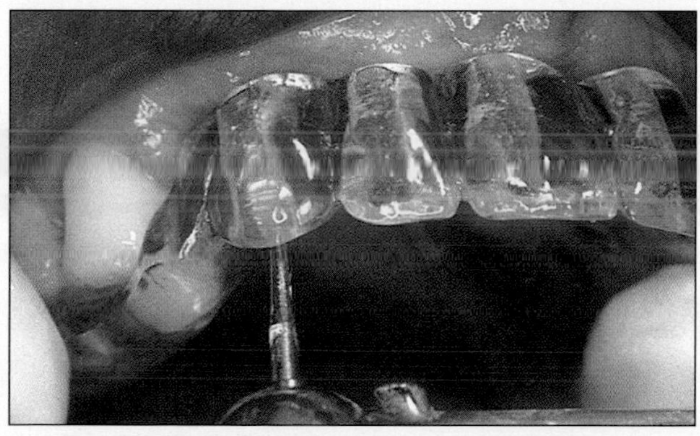

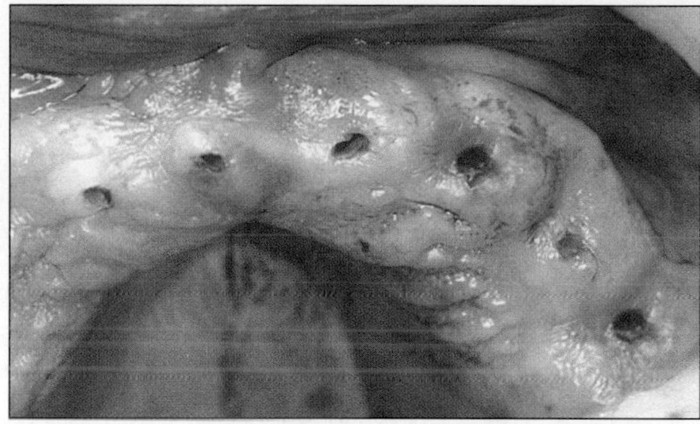

**14** The stent is removed, and the mark on the soft tissue shows the position of the previously placed implant.

**15** An electrosurgical loop is used to remove the soft tissue over the implant site by peeling it back one layer at a time until the titanium sealing screw is located. A special tissue punch can be used to remove the tissue from over the implant.

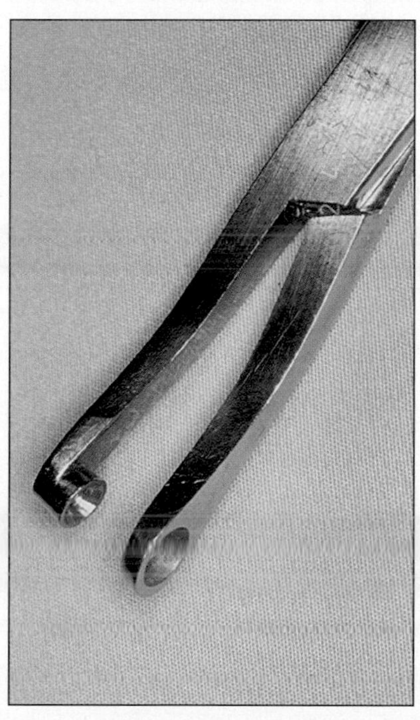

(Continued)

## PROCEDURE 53.1 Assisting in an Endosteal Implant Surgery—cont'd

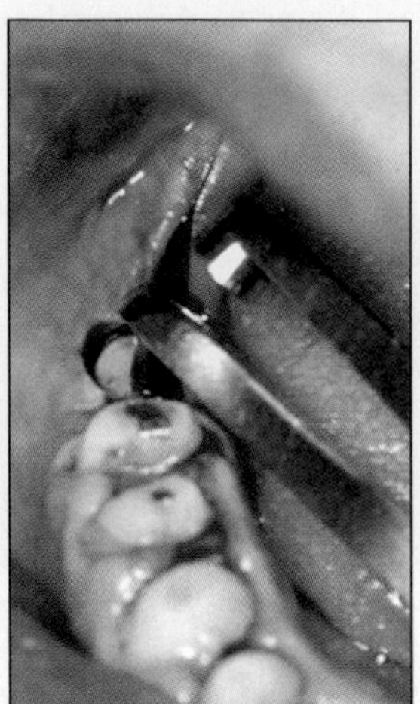

16 The implant is uncovered, and the sealing screw is removed.
17 The inside of the implant cylinder is cleaned with sterile cotton soaked in hydrogen peroxide.
18 A healing collar is screwed into the implant. This attachment now will extend above the mucosa.

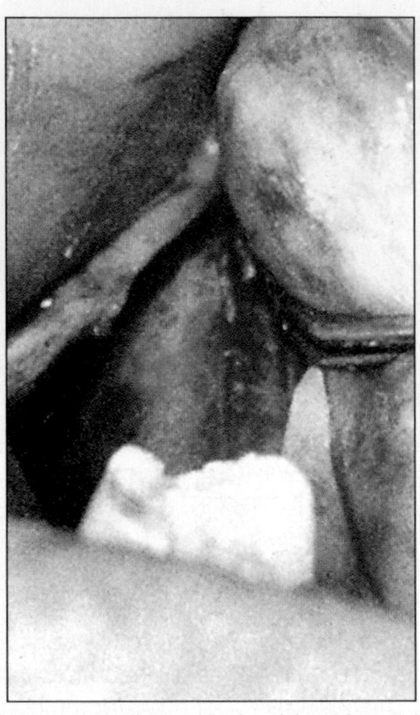

19 The soft tissues are allowed to heal for 10 to 14 days before a permanent crown is fabricated.

54

# Endodontics

## KEY TERMS

**Abscess (AB-ses)** Localized area of pus originating from an infection.

**Acute (uh-KYOOT)** Pertaining to a traumatic, pathologic, or physiologic occurrence or process that has a short and relatively severe course.

**Apical curettage (AP-i-kul kyoor-uh-TAHZH)** Surgical removal of infectious material surrounding the apex of a root.

**Apicoectomy (ap-i-ko-EK-tuh-mee)** Surgical removal of the apical portion of the tooth through a surgical opening made in the overlying bone and gingival tissues.

**Chronic** Pertaining to disease symptoms that persist over a long time.

**Control tooth** Healthy tooth used as a standard to compare questionable teeth of similar size and structure during pulp vitality testing.

**Debridement (day-breed-MAW, di-BREED-munt)** To remove or clean out the pulpal canal.

**Direct pulp cap** Application of dental material with an exposed or nearly exposed dental pulp.

**Endodontist** A dentist who specializes in the prevention, diagnosis, and treatment of diseases of the dental pulp and the periradicular tissues.

**Gutta-percha (guh-tuh-PUR-chuh)** Plastic type of filling material used in endodontics.

**Hemisection (hem-ee-SEK-shun)** Surgical separation of a multirooted tooth through the furcation area.

**Indirect pulp cap** Placement of a medicament over a partially exposed pulp.

**Irreversible pulpitis (pul-PYE-tis)** Infectious condition in which the pulp is incapable of healing, which would then require root canal therapy.

**Nonvital** Not living, as in oral tissue and tooth structure.

**Obturation (ob-tuh-RAY-shun)** Process of filling a root canal.

**Palpation (pal-PAY-shun)** Touching or feeling for abnormalities within soft tissue.

**Percussion (pur-KUH-shun)** Examination technique that involves tapping on the incisal or occlusal surface of a tooth to assess vitality.

**Perforation (pur-fuh-RAY-shun)** Making a hole, as in breaking through and extending beyond the apex of the root.

**Periodontal abscess** An inflammatory reaction to bacteria trapped in the periodontal sulcus.

**Periradicular (per-ee-ruh-DIK-yoo-lur)** Referring to the area of nerves, blood vessels, and tissues that surrounds the root of a tooth.

**Periradicular abscess** An inflammatory reaction to pulpal infection.

**Periradicular cyst** A cyst that develops at or near the root of a necrotic tooth.

**Pulpectomy (pul-PEK-tuh-mee)** Complete removal of vital pulp from a tooth.

**Pulpitis (pul-PYE-tis)** Inflammation of the dental pulp.

**Pulpotomy (pul-POT-uh-mee)** Removal of the coronal portion of a vital pulp from a tooth.

**Retrograde restoration (RET-roe-grayd res-tuh-RAY-shun)** Small restoration placed at the apex of a root.

**Reversible pulpitis** Form of pulpal inflammation in which the pulp may be salvageable.

**Root amputation (am-pyoo-TAY-shun)** Removal of one or more roots without removal of the crown of the tooth.

**Root canal therapy** Removal of the dental pulp and filling of the canal with material.

## LEARNING OUTCOMES

*On completion of this chapter, the student will be able to achieve the following objectives:*

1. Pronounce, define, and spell the key terms.
2. List the causes and symptoms of pulpal damage.
3. Describe the diagnostic testing performed for endodontic diagnosis.
4. Describe diagnostic conclusions for endodontic therapy.
5. List the types of endodontic procedures.
6. Identify the instruments and accessories used in endodontics.
7. Discuss microscopic endodontics.
8. Discuss the medicaments and dental materials used in endodontics.
9. Provide an overview of root canal therapy.
10. Describe surgical endodontics and how it affects treatment.

## PERFORMANCE OUTCOMES

*On completion of this chapter, the student will be able to achieve competency standards in the following skills.*

- Assist in electric pulp vitality test.
- Assist in root canal therapy.

## ELECTRONIC RESOURCES

e ***Additional information related to content in Chapter 54 can be found on the companion Evolve Web site.***

- Practice Quiz
- Tray Setup Drag-and-Drop Exercises: Opening/Sealing a Tooth for Endodontic Therapy
- Tray Setup Questions
- Canadian Content Corner

Endodontics was recognized as a specialty area in dentistry in 1963 by the American Dental Association. This specialty manages the prevention, diagnosis, and treatment of the dental pulp and the **periradicular** tissues that surround the root of the tooth. **Endodontic treatment,** often referred to as **root canal therapy**, provides an effective means of saving a tooth that might otherwise have to be extracted.

The general dentist is skilled and qualified to perform endodontic treatment; however, dentists will often refer patients in need of this treatment to an **endodontist**, a dentist who specializes in this area. An endodontist is a general dentist who has continued training for a minimum of 3 years in the clinical skill and research of pulp therapy.

# Pulpal Damage

## Causes

The two main sources of pulpal nerve damage are physical irritation and trauma.

**Physical irritation** can range from mild tooth sensitivity to complete nerve death of the tooth or even infection of the surrounding tissues. When bacteria reach the nerves and blood vessels, infection can result in an **abscess**, which is a localized area of pus (Fig. 54.1).

*Trauma,* such as a blow to a tooth or the jaw, can cause damage to surrounding tissues. Over time, this damage can affect the nerve tissue and blood vessels of the pulp (Fig. 54.2).

## Symptoms

Sensitivity, discomfort, and pain may be symptoms of **pulpal nerve damage.** Even though patients experience symptoms differently, the most common signs and symptoms of pulpal damage include the following:

- Pain when occluding
- Pain during mastication
- Sensitivity to hot or cold beverages
- Noticeable facial swelling
- Fever
- Tenderness of the surrounding gums
- Cracked or discolored teeth

RECALL

1 What are periradicular tissues?
2 Which specialist performs root canal therapy?
3 What can result if bacteria reach the nerves and blood vessels of a tooth?

# Endodontic Diagnosis

Diagnosis of a tooth that requires endodontic treatment is based on an examination that consists of subjective and objective components.

The **subjective examination** includes an evaluation of symptoms or problems *described by the patient,* which include the following:

- Chief complaint
- Character and duration of pain
- Painful stimuli
- Sensitivity to biting and pressure

The **objective examination** is conducted by the endodontist, who evaluates the status of the tooth and surrounding tissues with regard to the following:

- Extent of decay
- Periodontal conditions surrounding the tooth in question
- Presence of an extensive restoration

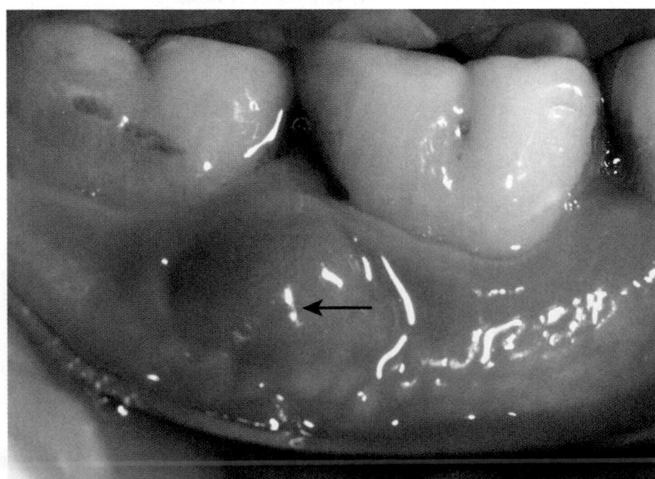

**FIG. 54.1** Abscess *(arrow)* associated with mandibular first molar resulting from extensive decay into the pulp. *(Courtesy Margaret J. Fehrenbach, RDH, MS.)*

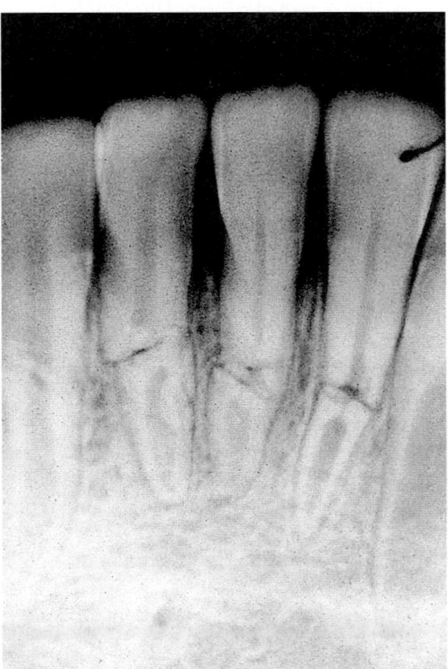

**FIG. 54.2** Radiograph of a necrotic tooth resulting from trauma. *(From Johnson W: Color atlas of endodontics, St Louis, 2002, Saunders.)*

- Tooth mobility
- Swelling or discoloration
- Pulp exposure

There are several clinical techniques used to test pulp vitality in determining whether endodontic therapy is required, or if the pulp is vital and is able to repair itself. When a questionable tooth is tested for vitality, a **control tooth** is selected to use for comparison. A healthy tooth, usually of the same type, in the opposite quadrant is selected as a control tooth. For example, if the maxillary right first premolar is the *suspect tooth,* the control tooth would be the maxillary left first premolar. The use of a control tooth shows that the stimulus is capable of achieving a response.

## Percussion and Palpation

Percussion and palpation tests are used to determine whether the inflammatory process has extended into the periapical tissues. A positive response to these tests indicates that inflammation is present in the periodontal ligament and that endodontic treatment is most likely required.

The dentist performs the **percussion** test by tapping on the incisal or occlusal surface of the tooth in question with the end of the mouth mirror handle, which is held parallel to the long axis of the tooth (Fig. 54.3).

The dentist completes the **palpation** test by applying firm pressure to the mucosa above the apex of the root (Fig. 54.4) and noting any sensitivity or swelling.

## Thermal Sensitivity

Tests using temperature can provide another method of determining the status of the pulp. A thermal stimulus is *never* used on a metallic restoration or on gingival tissue. Application of an altered temperature in this situation will result in an abnormal response and possible damage to the tissues.

In the *cold test,* the dentist uses ice, dry ice, or carbon dioxide to evaluate the response of a tooth to cold. First, the control tooth and the suspect tooth are isolated and dried. Next, the source of cold is applied first to the cervical area of the control tooth, then to the cervical area of the suspect tooth (Fig. 54.5).

A necrotic pulp will *not* respond to cold. Irreversible pulpitis is suspected when the cold relieves the pain; however, cold in teeth with irreversible pulpitis also can initiate severe, lingering pain.

The *heat test* is generally the least useful of the vitality tests because a painful response to heat could indicate *either* reversible pulpitis *or* irreversible pulpitis. A necrotic pulp will not respond to heat. A small (pea-sized) piece of **gutta-percha** is heated in a flame and then is applied to the facial surface of the tooth. Another method is to heat the end of an instrument and place it on the tooth. Petroleum jelly should be applied to the tooth surface before testing to prevent the material from sticking to the tooth surface.

## Electric Pulp Testing

Electric pulp testing is used in endodontic diagnosis to determine whether a pulp is vital or **nonvital**. Similar to other testing devices discussed, the pulp tester can produce a *false-positive* or a *false-negative* response (test results that show a positive or

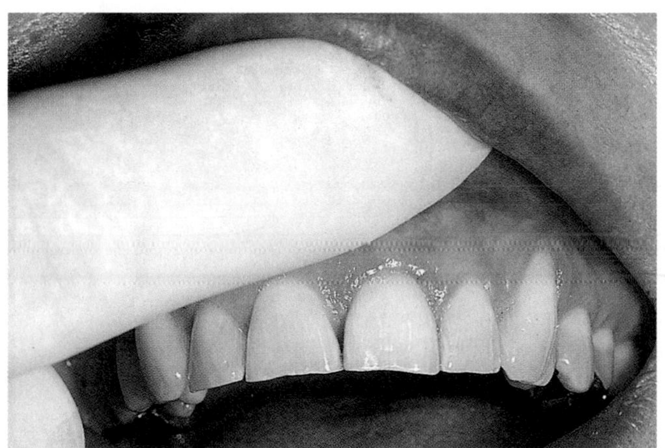

**FIG. 54.4** Palpation test. *(From Johnson W: Color atlas of endodontics, St Louis, 2002, Saunders.)*

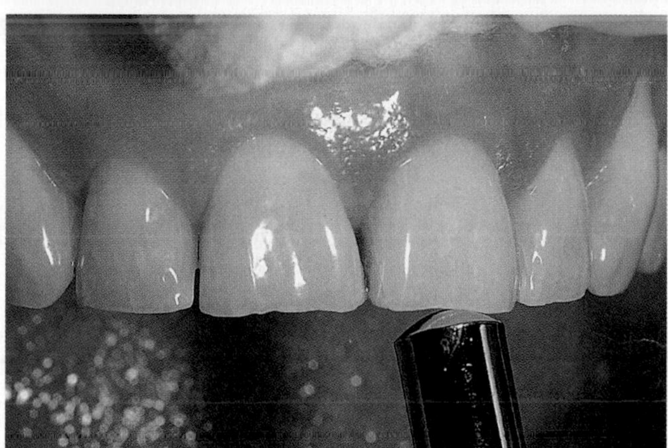

**FIG. 54.3** Percussion test. *(From Johnson W: Color atlas of endodontics, St Louis, 2002, Saunders.)*

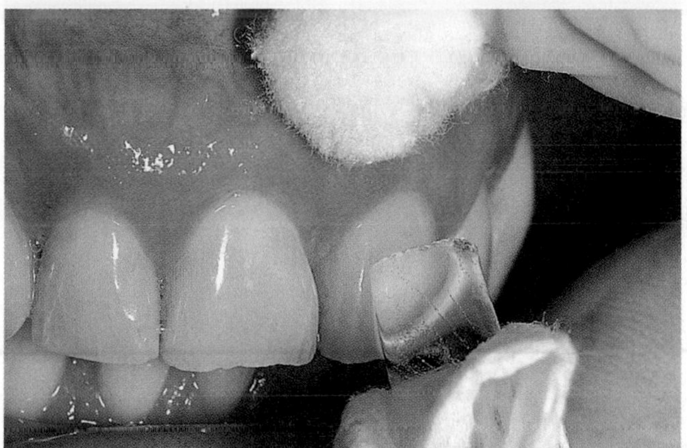

**FIG. 54.5** Ice used for testing thermal sensitivity. *(From Johnson W: Color atlas of endodontics, St Louis, 2002, Saunders.)*

a negative response incorrectly). Therefore test results must be supported by other diagnostic findings.

Electric pulp testers deliver a small electrical stimulus to the pulp (Fig. 54.6). Factors that influence the reliability of the pulp tester include the following:

- Teeth with extensive restorations can vary in response.
- Teeth with more than one canal can have one vital canal and other nonvital canals.
- A failing pulp can produce a variety of responses.
- Control teeth may not respond as anticipated.
- Moisture on the tooth during testing may produce an inaccurate reading.
- The batteries in the tester may weaken over time.

See Procedure 54.1: Assisting in Electric Pulp Vitality Test.

## Radiographic Imaging

Radiographic imaging is a necessity for diagnostic testing, as well as for root canal therapy. Good-quality images are required for attaining optimal information (Fig. 54.7) (see Chapter 41).

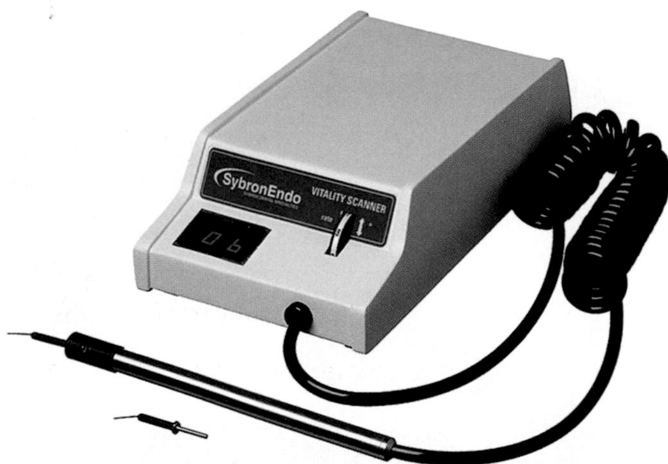


**FIG. 54.6** Pulp tester. *(Courtesy Kerr Endodontics.)*

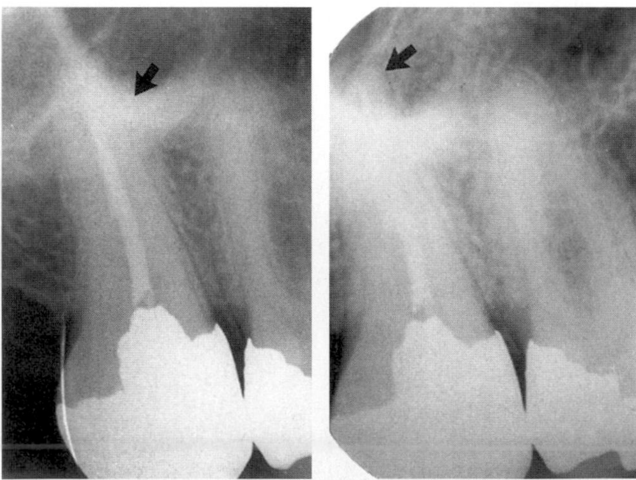

**FIG. 54.7** Good-quality radiographs are necessary for endodontic evaluation. *Left,* Showing good contrast around the apex; *right,* showing poor contrast around the apex.

The following images are required for the diagnosis and completion of endodontic treatment:

- **Initial radiograph:** This periapical radiograph is taken during the diagnostic stages before treatment.
- **Working length image:** This periapical radiograph is taken once the pulp has been opened. This image is used to determine the length of the canal. It is easier to detect canal length with the file remaining in the tooth.
- **Final instrumentation image:** This periapical radiograph is taken with the final size files in all canals receiving treatment.
- **Root canal completion image:** This final periapical radiograph is taken of the completed canal filled after the tooth has been temporized and the dental dam removed.
- **Recall image:** This radiographic image is taken at posttreatment evaluations.

### Requirements of Radiographic Images

- Show 4 to 5 mm beyond the apex of the tooth and the surrounding bone or pathologic condition
- Present an accurate image of the tooth without elongation or foreshortening
- Exhibit good contrast so that all pertinent structures are readily identifiable

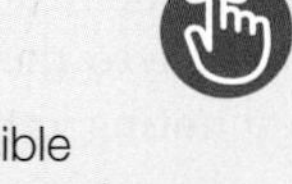


4 Would "pain" be a subjective or an objective component of a diagnosis?
5 Tooth #21 is the questionable tooth for possible endodontic treatment. What tooth would be used as a control tooth?
6 When the dentist taps on a tooth, what diagnostic test is being performed?
7 How many radiographic images may be taken through the course of root canal therapy?

## Diagnostic Conclusions

Once subjective and objective tests have been completed, a diagnosis of the pulp is presented to the patient.

A normal pulp will indicate no subjective symptoms or objective signs. The tooth responds normally to sensory stimuli, and a healthy layer of dentin surrounds the pulp.

**Pulpitis** indicates that pulpal tissues have become inflamed. Pulpitis can be described clinically as follows:

- **Reversible pulpitis** occurs when the pulp is irritated and the patient is experiencing pain to thermal stimuli. With reversible pulpitis, eliminating the irritant and placing a sedative material may save the pulp.
- **Irreversible pulpitis** displays symptoms of lingering pain. Clinical diagnostic findings will show that the pulp is incapable of healing, indicating root canal therapy or extraction as the only treatment options.

**Periradicular abscess** is an inflammatory reaction to pulpal infection. **Chronic** periradicular abscess is characterized by the presence of a draining sinus tract. The lesion is asymptomatic, with little or no discomfort, and an intermittent discharge of pus may be noticed. **Acute** periradicular abscess is an inflammatory response with pain, tenderness of the tooth to pressure, pus formation, and swelling of the tissue resulting from necrosis.

**Periodontal abscess** is an inflammatory reaction that is frequently caused by bacteria entrapped in the periodontal sulcus. Most often, a patient will experience rapid onset, pain, tenderness of the tooth to pressure, pus formation, and swelling.

**Periradicular cyst** develops at or near the root of a necrotic tooth. These types of cysts develop as an inflammatory response to pulpal infection and necrosis of the pulp.

**Pulp fibrosis** is the decrease of living cells within the pulp, causing fibrous tissue to take over the pulpal canal. Fibrosis is seen in older patients, as well as in patients with traumatic injury to a tooth.

**Necrosis**, also referred to as necrotic or nonvital, is used to describe a tooth that does not respond to a sensory stimulus. These terms can be confusing and inaccurate because even though the tooth may be considered "nonvital," the tooth continues to be attached to the alveolus by way of the cementum and periodontal ligaments, which are still vital tissues.

8 What diagnosis is given when pulpal tissues are inflamed?
9 Give another term used for necrotic or necrosis.

## Endodontic Procedures

The choice of endodontic treatment will depend on the diagnosis. The first line of treatment is **pulpal therapy,** which is an attempt to stimulate pulpal regeneration and save the pulp. When pulpal therapy is not effective, the endodontist will move to more extreme measures, which can include root canal therapy or surgery.

### Pulp Capping

In an attempt to save the pulp, a covering of calcium hydroxide is placed over an exposed or nearly exposed pulp to encourage the formation of new dentin at the site of injury.

**Indirect pulp cap** is a temporary procedure where most of the carious dentin in a deep cavity is not removed. A liner and a temporary restoration are placed, and the cavity is reopened after a period of time; the remaining carious dentin is then excavated. The goal for this treatment is to give the pulp a chance to form more dentin beneath the carious dentin, so that pulp exposure can be avoided. The aims of treatment are (1) to promote pulpal healing by removing most of the decay, and (2) to stimulate the production of reparative dentin through placement of calcium hydroxide.

**Direct pulp cap** is a procedure that is indicated when the pulp has been partially exposed. With a direct pulp cap, the tooth is still vital. Calcium hydroxide or an adhesive resin that is naturally compatible with pulpal tissue is placed to allow healing. When a direct pulp cap is performed, it is necessary to inform the patient that problems may develop later and that periodic monitoring is necessary.

### Pulpotomy

A **pulpotomy** involves removal of the coronal portion of an exposed vital pulp. This procedure is completed to preserve the vitality of the remaining portion of the pulp within the root of the tooth. Pulpotomy often is indicated for vital primary teeth, teeth with deep carious lesions, and emergency situations (see Chapter 57).

### Pulpectomy

A **pulpectomy**, also referred to as *root canal therapy,* involves complete removal of the dental pulp (see later in the chapter for complete discussion).

RECALL

10 What dental material is commonly selected for pulp capping?
11 What portion of the pulp is removed in a pulpotomy?

## Instruments and Accessories

Endodontic instruments and accessories are designed to be flexible and to fit into the pulpal canal.

### Hand Instruments

#### *Explorer*

The endodontic explorer is a double-ended instrument that is long and straight. The working ends are positioned at an angle to the handle that is unique to this instrument, which helps in locating canal openings (Fig. 54.8).

**FIG. 54.8** Endodontic explorer. *(From Boyd LRB: Dental instruments: a pocket guide, ed 6, St Louis, 2018, Elsevier.)*

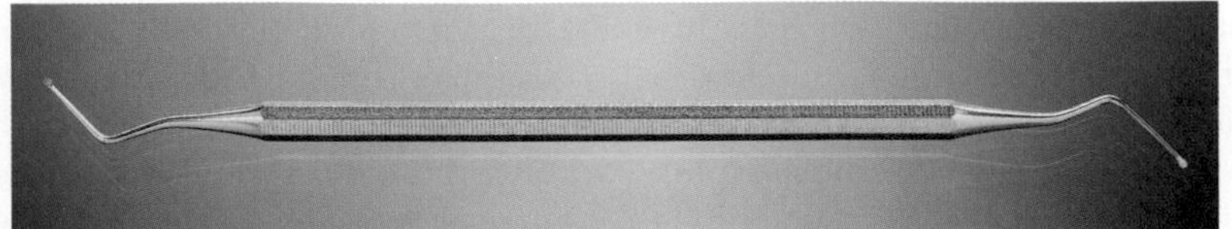

**FIG. 54.9** Endodontic spoon excavator. *(From Boyd LRB: Dental instruments: a pocket guide, ed 6, St Louis, 2018, Elsevier.)*

### Endodontic Spoon Excavator

The double-ended endodontic spoon excavator is similar to other spoon excavators. However, the endodontic spoon has a very long shank, which allows it to reach deep into the canal to remove coronal pulp tissue, decay, and temporary cements (Fig. 54.9).

### Spreaders and Pluggers

These instruments are used in the **obturation** of the canal. They condense and adapt the gutta-percha points into the canal. Pluggers and spreaders look similar but differ at the tip (Fig. 54.10). *Pluggers* have a flat tip like that of a condenser, but *spreaders* have a pointed tip, similar to that of an explorer.

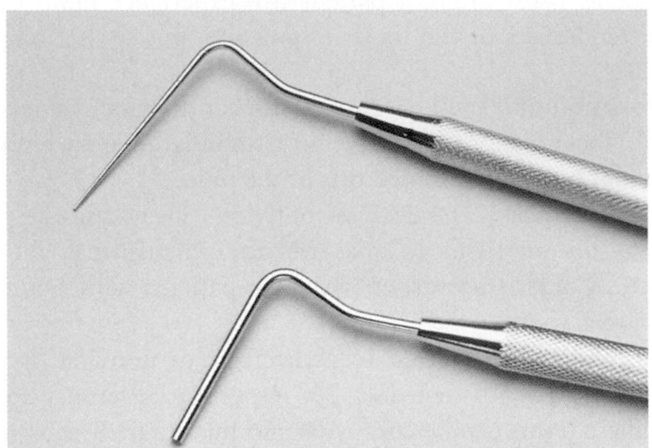

**FIG. 54.10** Spreader *(top)* and plugger *(bottom)* used to obturate the canal.

### Glick Number 1

The paddle-shaped end of the Glick Number 1 dental instrument is designed for placement of temporary restorations, and the rod-shaped plugger at the opposite end is ideal for removal of excess gutta-percha (Fig. 54.11). The plugger end is graduated at 5-mm increments and can be heated for placement or removal of gutta-percha.

## Hand-Operated Files

A series of hand files are used for cleaning and shaping the pulpal canal. Each file listed below is designed for a specific function once placed in the canal. The files are color-coded according to size (Table 54.1). The following files are available in stainless steel or nickel-titanium (Ni-Ti) alloy. Although they are more costly than stainless steel files, Ni-Ti files provide the advantages of (1) *extreme flexibility,* which enables them to better follow the contour of the canal; (2) *good strength,* which is an important safety factor in keeping the instrument from breaking while in the canal; and (3) a *longer working life.*

### K-type File

The **K-type file** has a twisted design and is used in the initial debridement (cleaning) of the canal and during later stages of shaping and contouring the canal. The *conventional* K-type file has a "stiff" feel that is very effective for straight canals (Fig. 54.12). For narrow canals and curved canals, some dentists prefer the *flexible K-type file.*

### Hedstrom File

The *Hedstrom file* provides greater cutting efficiency because of its design (Fig. 54.13). The Hedstrom file can be used for final enlargement of the canal after a Gates-Glidden bur or a Pesso reamer has been used (see later discussion). The H-type file has its spiral edges arranged so that cutting occurs only on the pulling stroke, making the dentinal walls smooth and easier to fill.

### Reamer File

The *reamer file* is similar in design to the K-type file, but its cutting edges are farther apart. Its functions are to remove dentin structure and to smooth and increase the size of the canal (Fig. 54.14).

### Broaches

A broach is a thin, flexible, tapered metal hand instrument. Broaches have tiny fishhook-like projections along the shaft that are used to remove vital, inflamed hemorrhagic pulp tissue from the canal (Fig. 54.15). Although broaches are not used as frequently as other files, they may be used to remove objects such as cotton pellets and paper points. Broaches should be discarded after a single use because of their fragile makeup.

## Rotary-Operated Files and Burs

Rotary files are similar to hand files but are latch-type files placed in a high-torque, low-rpm handpiece designed for Ni-Ti rotary instruments (Fig. 54.16). These groups of instruments are becoming more popular than traditional hand instruments because of their makeup, ease in use, and efficiency.

Besides the traditional files used to prepare the pulpal canal as mentioned earlier, a series of burs are used to open and enlarge the pulpal canal.

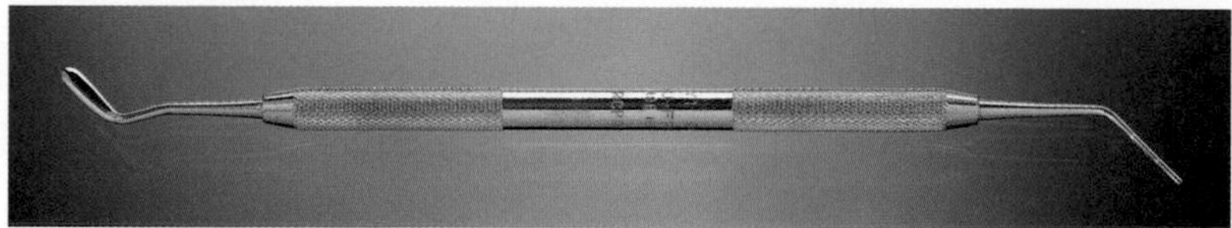

FIG. 54.11 Glick Number 1. *(From Boyd LRB: Dental instruments: a pocket guide, ed 6, St Louis, 2018, Elsevier.)*

**TABLE 54.1** Color Coding and Sizing of Hand-Operated Files

| Handle Color | Diameter |
|---|---|
| Gray | 08 |
| Purple | 10 |
| White | 15–45–90 |
| Yellow | 20–50–100 |
| Red | 25–55–110 |
| Blue | 30–60–120 |
| Green | 35–70–130 |
| Black | 40–80–140 |

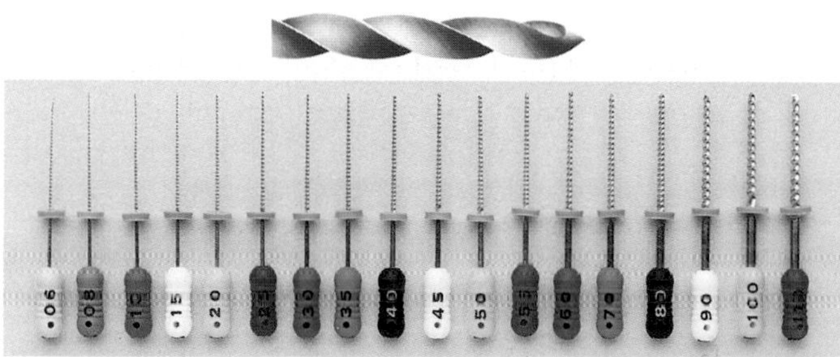

FIG. 54.12 K-type files. *(Courtesy Premier Dental, Plymouth Meeting, PA.)*

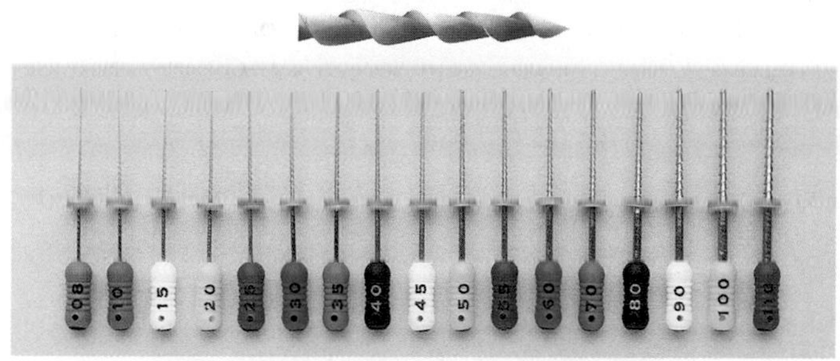

FIG. 54.13 Hedstrom files. *(Courtesy Premier Dental, Plymouth Meeting, PA.)*

*Gates-Glidden burs,* also known as *Gates-Glidden drills,* have a football-shaped working end with a very long shank (Fig. 54.17). These burs are designed to have the cutting edge on the sides, not on the end, to enlarge the walls of the pulp chamber. They are used in a handpiece with a latch-type attachment, and are operated in a clockwise direction.

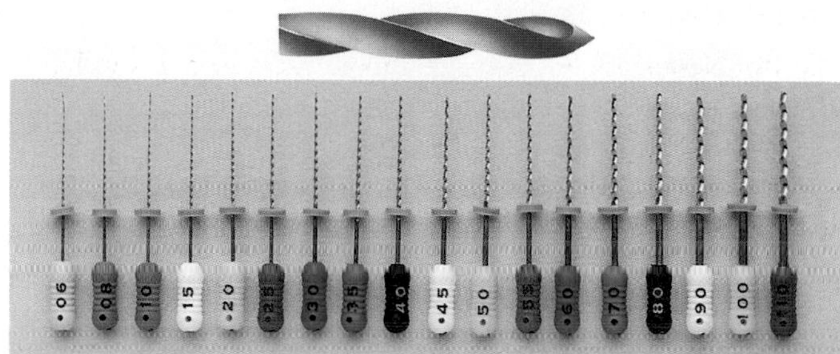

FIG. 54.14 Reamer files. *(Courtesy Premier Dental, Plymouth Meeting, PA.)*

*Pesso files,* also known as *Pesso reamers,* work in the same manner as Gates-Glidden burs, but are shaped slightly different to have their blades long and parallel with the noncutting ends (Fig. 54.18). These files are used primarily when the tooth requires a post preparation for placement of the final restoration.

## Ancillary Instruments

### Rubber Stops

A *stop* is a small, color-coded, round piece of rubber, silicone, or plastic that is slid onto hand-operated files to prevent **perforation** of the apex of the tooth during instrumentation (Fig. 54.19). The lengths of the files are carefully measured on a radiograph, and the stop is placed precisely at the predetermined working length of the canal (Fig. 54.20).

### Paper Points

Paper points are sterile absorbent pieces of paper rolled into long, narrow points (Fig. 54.21). A paper point is held with locking pliers and is inserted into the canal to absorb the irrigating solution and to dry the canal. This procedure is repeated with a fresh point until a paper point is completely dry when removed from the canal. Sterile paper points are available in a variety of sizes ranging from fine to coarse.

# Microscopic Endodontics

The development of the operating microscope in the field of endodontics has essentially changed the practice of endodontics, resulting in a more efficient, effective, and patient-friendly endodontic procedure. Operating microscopes are beneficial from diagnosis, to the location of canals or missed

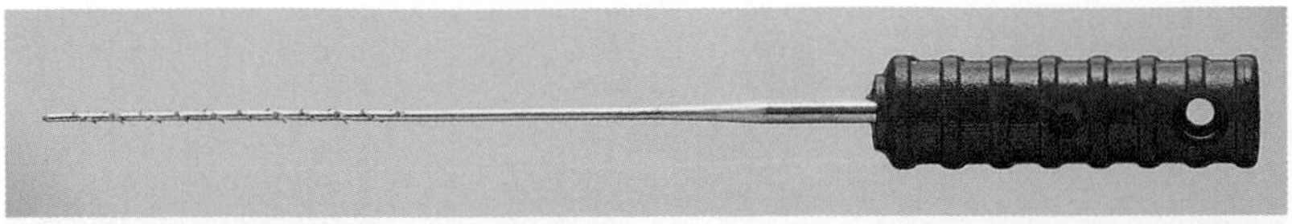

**FIG. 54.15** Dental broach. *(From Boyd LRB: Dental instruments: a pocket guide, ed 6, St Louis, 2018, Elsevier.)*

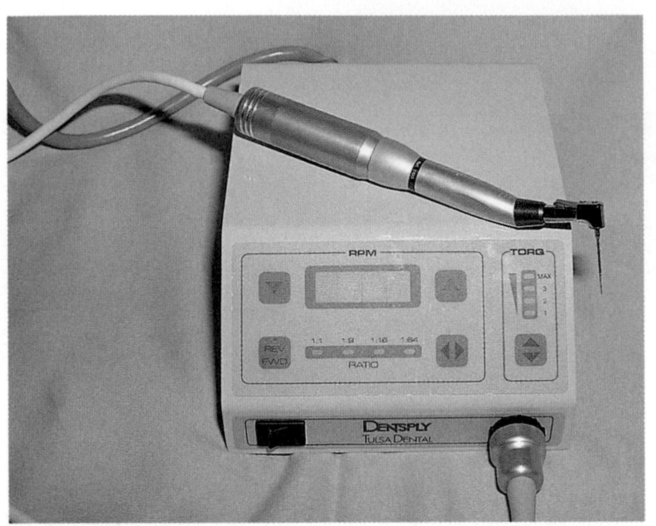


**FIG. 54.16** Rotary handpiece used for endodontics. *(From Johnson W: Color atlas of endodontics, St Louis, 2002, Saunders.)*

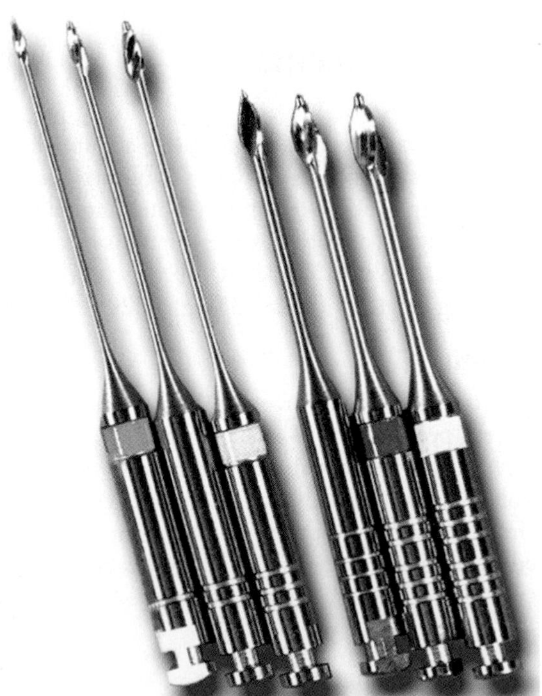

**FIG. 54.17** Gates-Glidden burs.

canals, for cleaning and shaping the canal, and to the filling of the canal. Endodontic procedures can be completed in less time because of the greater visibility of the root canal anatomy with the final product having reduced procedural errors (Fig. 54.22).

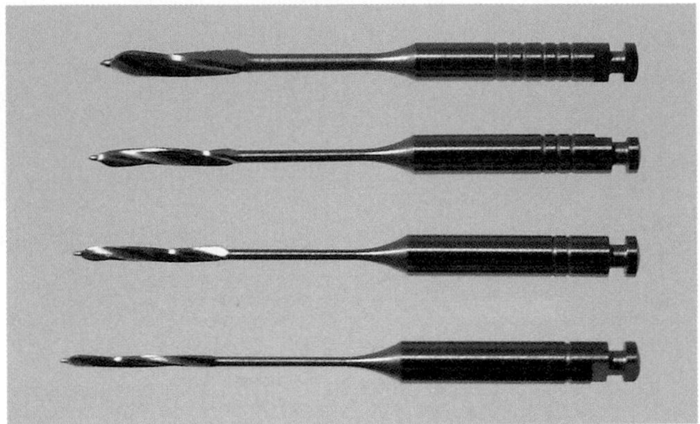

**FIG. 54.18** Peso files. *(From Boyd LRB: Dental instruments: a pocket guide, ed 6, St Louis, 2018, Elsevier.)*

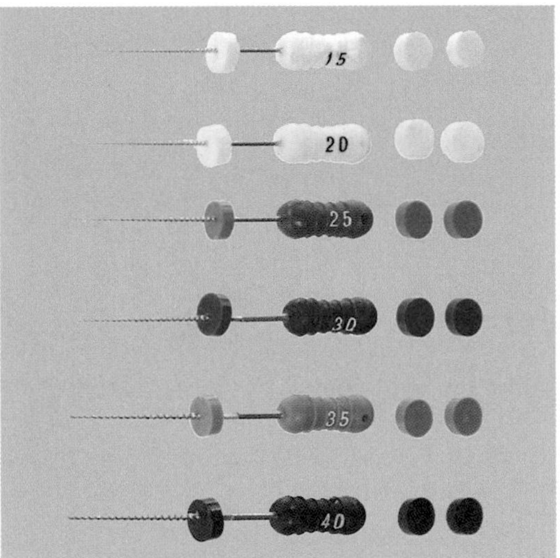


**FIG. 54.19** Rubber stops. *(From Boyd LRB: Dental instruments: a pocket guide, ed 6, St Louis, 2018, Elsevier.)*

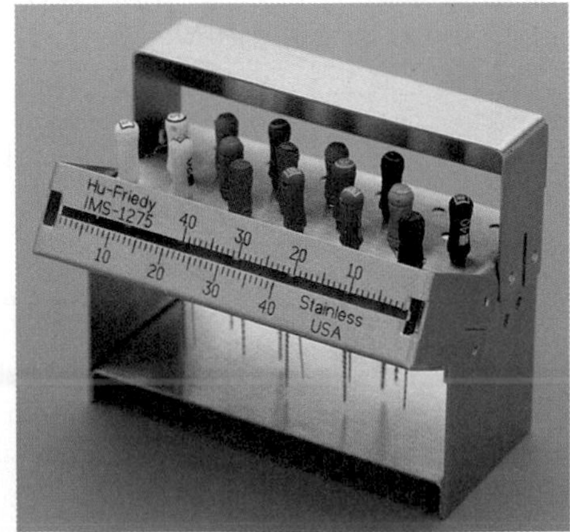


**FIG. 54.20** File stand for measuring files. *(Courtesy Hu-Friedy, Chicago, IL.)*

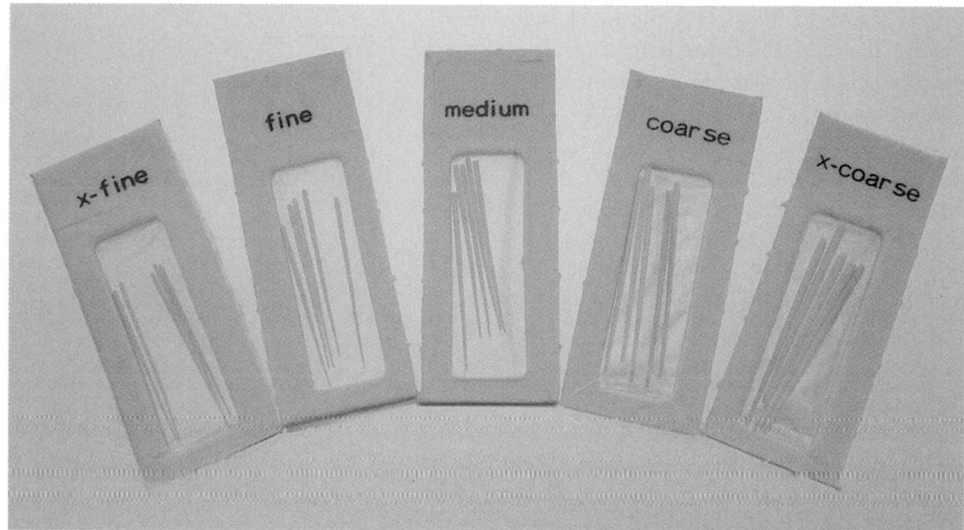


**FIG. 54.21** Paper points. *(From Boyd LRB: Dental instruments: a pocket guide, ed 6, St Louis, 2018, Elsevier.)*

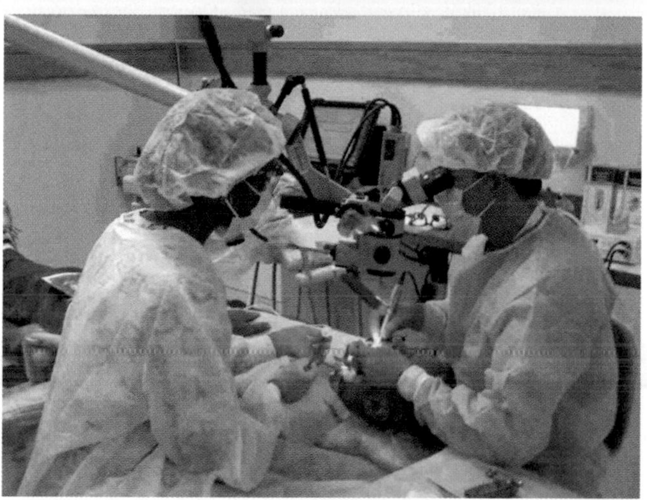

**FIG. 54.22** Operating an endodontic microscope. *(From Hargreaves KM, Berman LH, Rotstein I: Cohen's pathways of the pulp, ed 11, St Louis, 2016, Elsevier.)*

The operating microscope accomplishes three objectives:

- Magnification—acts like binoculars, allowing the endodontist to view the pulpal canal in a magnification mode.
- Illumination—the light from a 100-watt halogen bulb illuminates the canal, with the light intensity controlled by a rheostat and cooled by a fan.
- Addition of accessories—LCD monitor and a video camera for visualization and documentation.

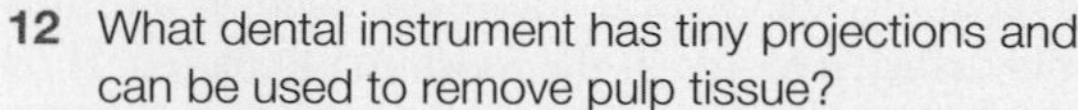

RECALL

12 What dental instrument has tiny projections and can be used to remove pulp tissue?
13 Can endodontic files be placed in a handpiece for use?
14 What type of file is best suited to shape and contour the pulpal canal?
15 Why is a rubber stop used on a file?
16 What does the term *obturate* mean?

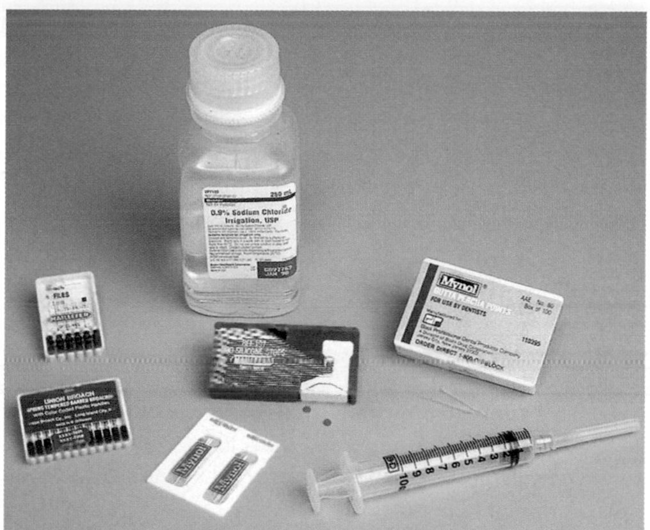


**FIG. 54.23** Materials needed for preparation and obturation of the pulpal canal. *Top,* Sterile irrigating solution. *Bottom,* Sterile paper points and syringe used with irrigating solution. *Left,* Files. *Right,* Gutta-percha.

## Medicaments and Dental Materials in Endodontics

Medicaments and dental materials used in endodontics include irrigation solutions, root canal filling materials, and root canal sealers (Fig. 54.23).

### Irrigation Solutions

In endodontics, irrigating the canal facilitates the removal of materials from the canal and provides tissue dissolution, bleaching, deodorizing, and hemorrhage control. The following solutions are used in this process:

- *Sodium hypochlorite,* commonly known as household bleach, is diluted with equal parts of sterile water for use as an irrigation solution. A 5- to 6-ml disposable plastic syringe with a special 27-gauge needle is used for irrigation. This solution is an antimicrobial agent that has a solvent action on necrotic pulp tissue and organic debris. It must be used with caution because a bleach solution causes skin irritation, and drips or splashes can ruin the patient's clothing.

- *Hydrogen peroxide* is a clear, colorless liquid with disinfectant and bleaching properties for endodontics.
- *Parachlorophenol (PCP)* is a colorless, crystalline toxic phenol compound that is used as an antimicrobial agent for disinfection of the pulp canal.

## Root Canal Filling Materials

*Gutta-percha points* are made from a rubber material taken from the *Palaquium gutta* tree. Gutta-percha is an organic substance that is solid at room temperature and becomes soft and pliable when heated. Gutta-percha points are used to obturate the pulpal canal after treatment has been completed. This *radiopaque* material is supplied in various sizes and is used with a sealer (Fig. 54.24, *A*). It is important to note that gutta-percha points are color coded to coincide with the file size.

Gutta-percha can be made to flow in the pulpal canal with the use of heat or solvents. The material that melts when heated above 140° F can be condensed with the use of an electronic heated spreader (Fig. 54.24, *B*).

## Root Canal Sealers

A *root canal sealer* is a cement-type material that seals out the unfilled voids during the obturation process. Several cements can be used as a sealer for root canal therapy, including calcium hydroxide, zinc oxide–eugenol, and glass ionomers. These materials undergo very little shrinkage. They also must be easy to place, radiopaque for detection on a radiograph, nonstaining to the teeth, bacteriostatic, gentle on the periapical tissues that surround them, and able to resist moisture.

### Types of Root Canal Sealers

**Calcium Hydroxide Sealers**

- Sealapex
- CRCS
- Apexit

**Resin Composite Sealer**

- Epipheny
- EndoRez

**Glass Ionomer Cement**

- Ketac Endo

*Formocresol* is a mixture of formaldehyde and cresol in a water-glycerin base. This type of solution was used as an intracanal medicament for the pulpotomy of primary teeth. Because of concerns about its toxic effects, it is not recommended for use.

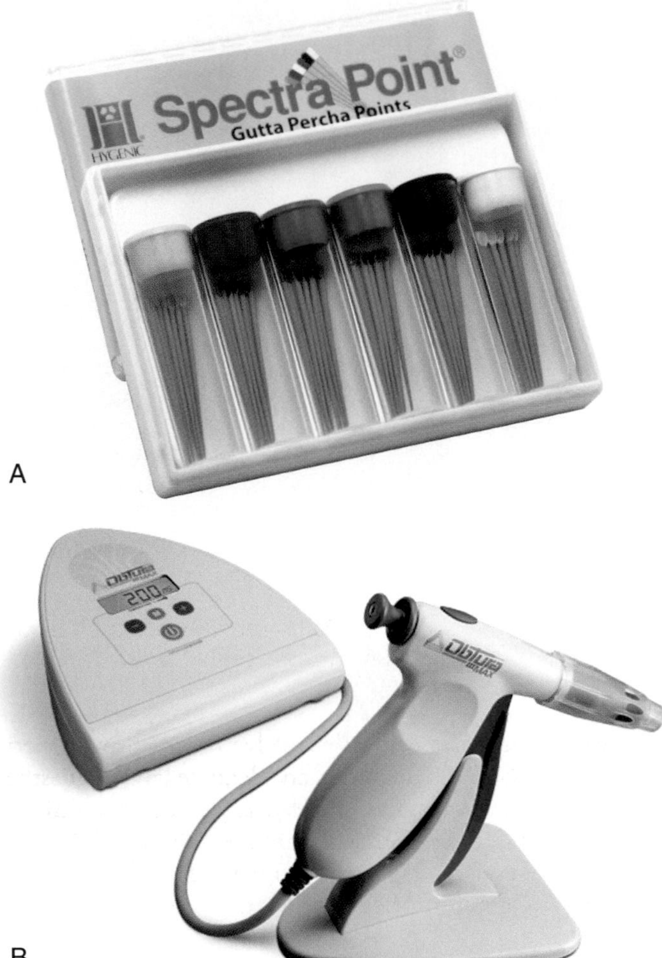


**FIG. 54.24** A, Gutta-percha in varying sizes. B, The Obtura Max is a heated gutta-percha delivery system used to deliver warm gutta-percha to the root canal system for obturation. *(A, Courtesy Coltène/Whaledent, Cuyahoga Falls, OH. B, Courtesy Obtura Spartan Endodontics, Algonquin, IL.)*

RECALL

**17** What type of irrigation solution(s) is available for root canal therapy?

**18** What material is used for the obturation of a canal?

# Overview of Root Canal Therapy

Root canal therapy involves specific treatment steps.

## Anesthesia and Pain Control

The anesthetic techniques of choice for endodontic treatment are *infiltration* for maxillary teeth and *nerve block* for mandibular teeth (see Chapter 37). A local anesthetic agent is administered any time vitality remains in the tooth to be treated. If the tooth is nonvital, the endodontist may advise the patient that a local anesthetic agent is not necessary.

After the pulp has been removed, a local anesthetic agent may or may not be administered during subsequent visits, depending on the patient's preference. Inflamed and infected tissues are difficult to anesthetize. Because endodontic

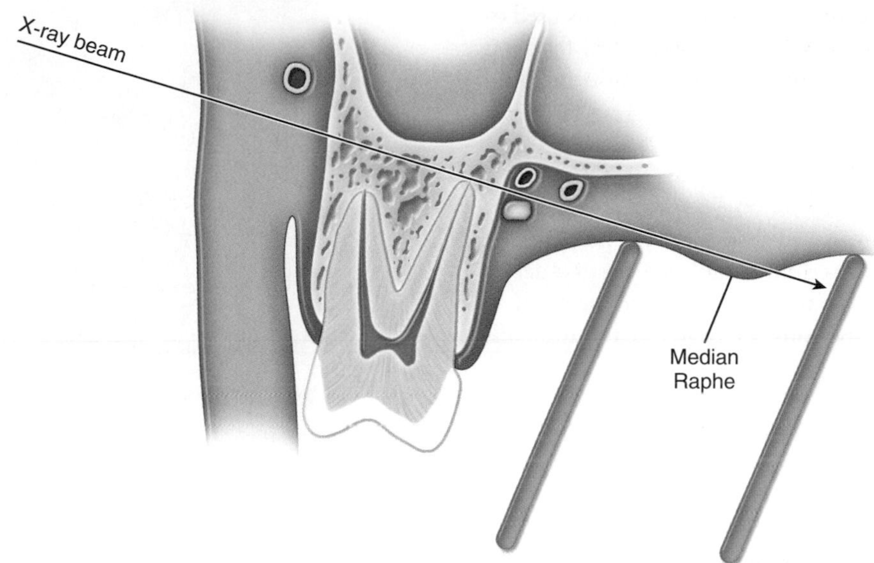


**FIG. 54.25** Position of XCP when taking a working length radiographic image. *(From Torabinejad M, Fouad A, Walton RE: Endodontics: principles and practice, ed 5, St Louis, 2015, Saunders.)*

treatment procedures generally involve inflamed pulp, periapical tissues, or both, obtaining an adequate level of anesthesia can be a problem. It may be necessary to inject additional local anesthetic solution directly into the pulp. In addition to local anesthesia, inhalation sedation may be used for patients who are extremely apprehensive.

## Isolation and Disinfection of the Operating Field

The standard of care established by the American Dental Association (ADA) for endodontic treatment requires the use of a *dental dam.* Once the dam is placed, it is necessary to disinfect the tooth, dental dam clamp, and surrounding dental dam material with the use of an iodine solution or a sodium hypochlorite solution.

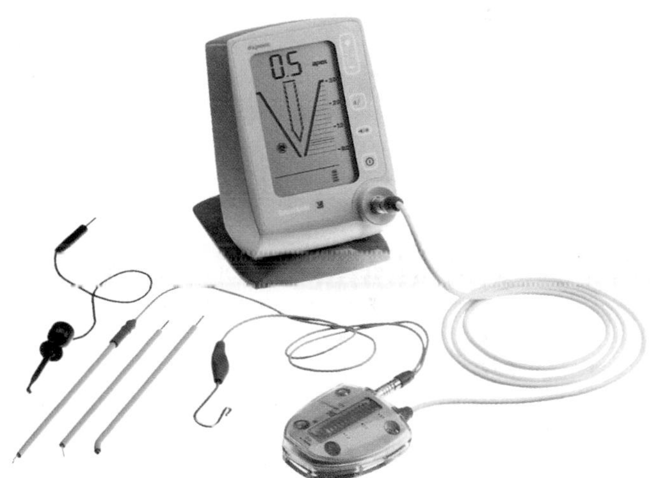

**FIG. 54.26** Electronic apex locator. *(Courtesy Kerr Endodontics.)*

## Access Preparation

During access preparation, the dentist will use the high-speed handpiece and a round bur to create an opening in the coronal portion of the tooth so that instrumentation can be used to reach the root canals. Access is gained through the occlusal surfaces of posterior teeth and the lingual surfaces of anterior teeth.

### *Estimated Working Length*

The dentist must know the length of the completed canal preparation and root canal filling. Problems that result from inaccurate measurement of length include (1) perforation of the apex, (2) overinstrumentation or underinstrumentation of canal length, (3) overfilling or underfilling of the canal, and (4) postoperative pain.

Because exact apex locations vary, and because these variations are not always visible on radiographs, the working length is assessed and is referred to as the *estimated working length.* The estimated working length is determined by selecting a reference point on the tooth, usually the highest point on the incisal or occlusal surface. On a periapical radiograph, a millimeter endodontic ruler is used to measure the distance from the reference point to the apex of the tooth. It is extremely important that the tooth length as represented on the radiograph be accurate and not distorted (Fig. 54.25).

## Electronic Apex Locator

An electronic apex locator is a supplemental technique that can be used to facilitate identification in the apex of the root canal (Fig. 54.26). Use of an electronic apex locator as an aid to endodontic therapy can reduce the number of diagnostic radiographs required for working length determination. It has been shown through numerous studies that when the combination of an electronic apex locator and a radiograph is used to determine working length, the location of the apical foramen is identified more accurately than when radiographs are used alone.

## Debridement and Shaping of the Canal

The purposes of **debridement** and shaping of the pulpal canal are (1) to remove bacteria, necrotic tissue, and organic debris from the root canal and (2) to smooth and shape the canal so that the filling material can be completely adapted to the walls of the canal.

## Obturation

The canal is now ready for obturation or to be filled by the endodontist. The objective is to place a fluid-tight seal in the canal from apical tip to the coronal surface, to prevent the reentry of microorganisms. If the tooth has more than one canal, each canal is filled individually, with each canal requiring a properly fitted and sealed gutta-percha point.

See Procedure 54.2: Assisting in Root Canal Therapy.

RECALL

**19** What type of moisture control is recommended for root canal therapy?
**20** What surface of an anterior tooth will the dentist enter when performing root canal therapy?

# Surgical Endodontics

Root canal therapy is successful approximately 90 to 95 percent of the time. In exceptional situations, however, surgical endodontic techniques must be used to save a tooth from extraction. Indications for surgical intervention include the following:

- **Endodontic failure:** Failure of nonsurgical endodontics may be caused by persistent infection, severely curved roots, perforation of the canal, fractured roots, extensive root resorption, pulp stones, or accessory canals that cannot be treated.
- **Exploratory surgery:** Surgery may be necessary to determine why healing has not occurred after root canal therapy. Canal medications that extend beyond the apex and into the periapical tissues may be the cause.
- **Biopsy:** A tissue sample for a biopsy may be required (see Chapter 56).

## Apicoectomy and Apical Curettage

**Apicoectomy** involves the surgical removal of the apical portion of the root with the use of a tapered fissure bur in a high-speed handpiece (Fig. 54.27). The dentist then can examine the apex for signs of (1) inadequate sealing of the canal, (2) accessory (additional) canals, or (3) fractures of the root.

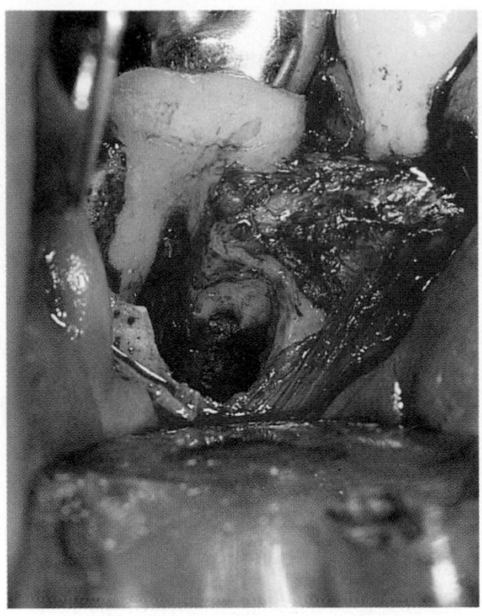

**FIG. 54.27** The apex of this mesiofacial root has been surgically removed. *(From Johnson W: Color atlas of endodontics, St Louis, 2002, Saunders.)*

Once the endodontist has entered the apical area of a tooth, **apical curettage** may be required to remove the pathologic soft tissue around the root apex. *Curettage* means the removal of diseased tissue by scraping with a curette.

## Retrograde Restoration

**Retrograde restoration**, also referred to as **root end filling,** is completed when the apical seal is not adequate. A small preparation is made at the apex and is sealed with filling materials such as gutta-percha, amalgam, or composite (Fig. 54.28).

## Root Amputation and Hemisection

**Root amputation** is a surgical procedure that is used to remove one or more roots of a multirooted tooth without removing the crown (Fig. 54.29, *A* and *B*). Amputation occurs at the point at which the root joins the crown. Root amputation most often is performed on maxillary molars.

**Hemisection** is a procedure in which the root and the crown are cut lengthwise and removed (Fig. 54.29, *C*). Hemisections most often are performed on mandibular molars.

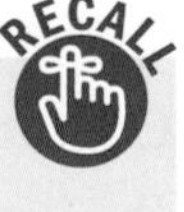


**21** What is the success rate of root canal therapy?
**22** What surgical procedure involves removal of the apex of a root?

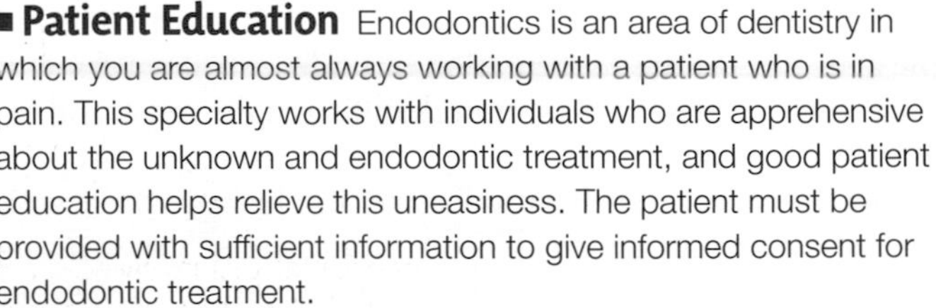

■ **Patient Education** Endodontics is an area of dentistry in which you are almost always working with a patient who is in pain. This specialty works with individuals who are apprehensive about the unknown and endodontic treatment, and good patient education helps relieve this uneasiness. The patient must be provided with sufficient information to give informed consent for endodontic treatment.

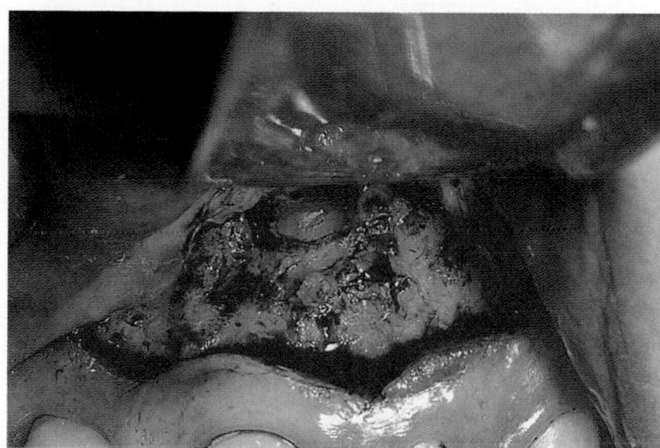

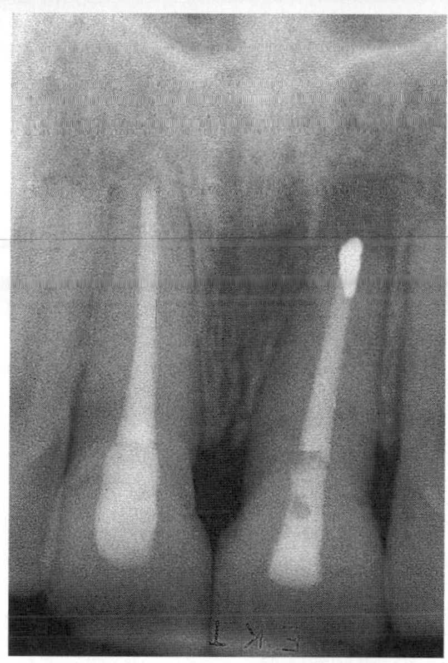

**FIG. 54.28** Root end filling is completed on a central incisor. *(From Johnson W: Color atlas of endodontics, St Louis, 2002, Saunders.)*

Always provide positive communication when discussing pulp therapy with a patient. *Do not say the following:*

- "All root canals are successful."
- "There is no pain in having a root canal."
- "Once the root canal is completed, the tooth will last forever."
- "There may be extreme pain and swelling from root canal treatment." ■

**■ Legal and Ethical Implications** For root canal therapy to be completed properly, it is imperative to remember that *accuracy* is the number one criterion when diagnostic and working radiographs are exposed, as well as when rubber stops are measured and placed on endodontic files.

Endodontics is deemed the "emergency room" of dentistry, and your patient may not always understand all that is being presented and discussed. Make sure you review diagnostic findings with the patient, and review the patient consent form. If the patient seems to be hesitant, stop and review again. ■

**■ Eye to the Future** New technology such as the apex finder, vitality scanner, and microscopic surgery is providing endodontists with the ability to diagnose and treat patients more efficiently and accurately. Because the dental laser is becoming a standard instrument in the field of dentistry, the next ideal area for its application will be endodontics. The dental laser will be introduced in endodontics as a quick, pain-free method by which to remove diseased pulpal tissue. ■

## ■ Critical Thinking

1. You have a new patient who has been treatment planned for root canal therapy. When discussing the procedure, she

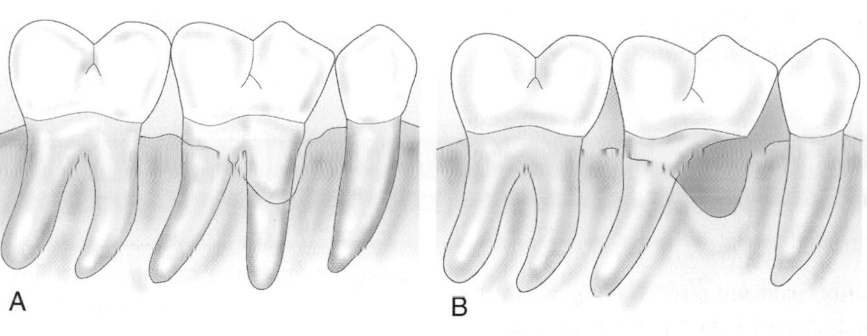


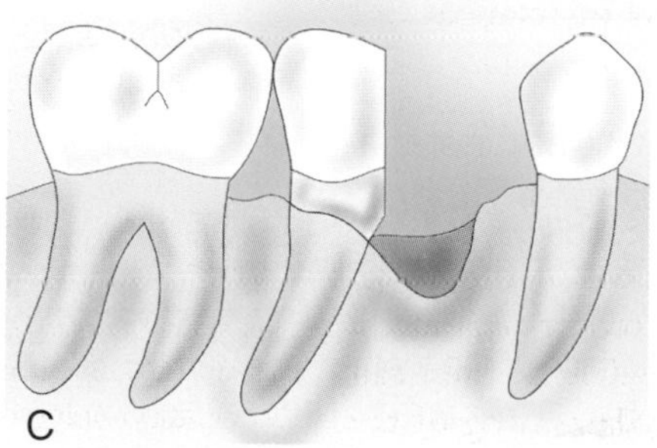


**FIG. 54.29** A, Periodontal loss involving the mesial root. B, Root amputation. C, Hemisection. *(From Johnson W: Color atlas of endodontics, St Louis, 2002, Saunders.)*

immediately says she will not allow radiographs to be taken because "they are harmful and of no use." How would you explain the necessity of x-rays to her, knowing the importance of radiographs during root canal therapy?
2. In root canal therapy, it is discussed that anesthesia may or may not be used during a procedure. Discuss why a dentist would *not* anesthetize the tooth and area before root canal therapy.
3. Why is it so important to use a dental dam in root canal therapy? Why is it imperative to keep saliva and other moisture away from a pulp exposure?
4. You are assisting the dentist in an endodontic diagnosis. The dentist has placed ice on the suspected tooth. The patient says that "the pain goes away" when the ice is on the tooth. What diagnostic conclusion would the dentist most likely reach?
5. You are assisting the endodontist in the therapy of a mandibular second molar. The patient record indicates that all roots will require treatment. How many roots are in a mandibular second molar? How would these roots appear on a periapical radiograph? ■

PROCEDURE 54.1

## Assisting in Electric Pulp Vitality Test

### EQUIPMENT AND SUPPLIES

- ✓ Electric pulp tester
- ✓ Toothpaste
- ✓ Electric pulp testing kit

### PROCEDURAL STEPS

1 Describe the procedure to the patient, and explain that the patient may feel a tingling or a warm sensation.

2 Identify the teeth to be tested (suspect tooth and control tooth), then isolate these teeth and thoroughly dry.

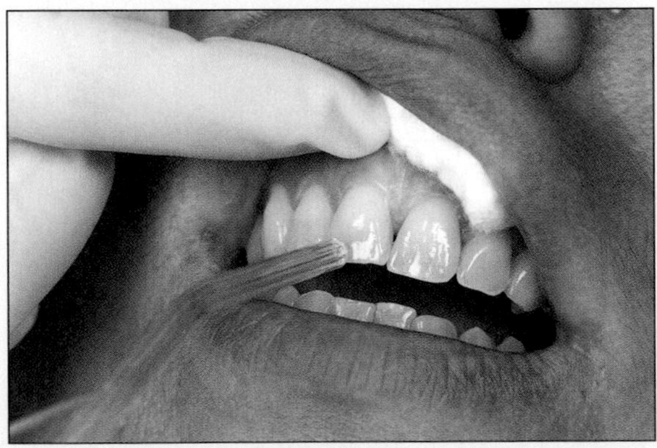

3 Set the dial (current level) at zero.

4 Place a thin layer of toothpaste on the tip of the pulp tester electrode.

**PURPOSE** To provide adequate contact to conduct a current from the pulp tester to the tooth.

5 Test the control tooth first.

6 Place the tip of the electrode on the facial surface of the tooth at the *cervical third*.

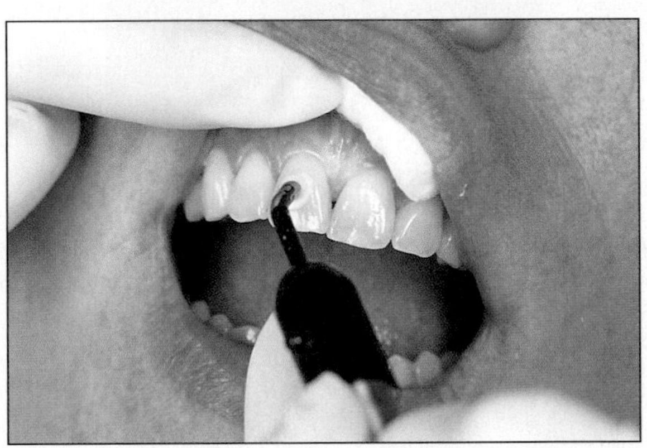

7 Gradually increase the level of the current until the patient feels a sensation. Document on the patient's record the level at which the response occurred.

8 Repeat the procedure on the suspect tooth.

9 Document the procedure.

| Date | Tooth | Surface | Charting Notes |
|---|---|---|---|
| 8/12/17 | 8 | — | Pt complained of pain, with sensitivity to hot beverages and also when chewing. Tooth #9 used as control tooth. Vitality tester showed tooth still responding to sensation. Periapical radiograph shows decay extending into pulp. T. Clark, CDA/L. Stewart, DDS |

All photos in this procedure from Boyd LRB: Dental instruments: a pocket guide, ed 6, St Louis, 2018, Elsevier.

PROCEDURE 54.2

# Assisting in Root Canal Therapy

## EQUIPMENT AND SUPPLIES

- Basic setup
- Local anesthetic agent setup *(optional)*
- Dental dam setup
- High-speed handpiece with burs (dentist's choice)
- Low-speed handpiece with latch attachment
- 5- to 6-ml syringe with 27-gauge needle
- Broaches and Hedstrom/K-type files (assorted sizes and lengths)
- Rubber instrument stops
- Paper points
- Gutta-percha points
- Endodontic sealer supplies
- Endodontic spoon excavator
- Endodontic explorer
- Glick Number 1
- Lentulo spiral
- Millimeter ruler
- Locking cotton pliers
- Sodium hypochlorite solution
- Hemostat
- High-volume oral evacuator (HVE) tip

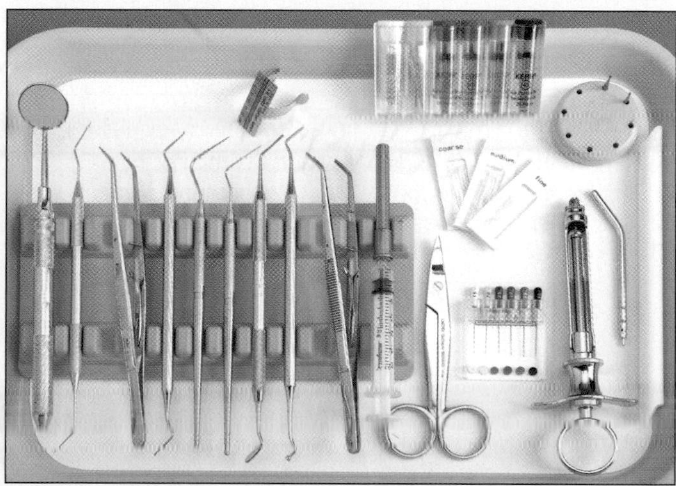

From Boyd LRB: *Dental instruments: a pocket guide, ed 6,* St Louis, 2018, Elsevier.

## PROCEDURAL STEPS

### Preparing the Field of Operation

1 Assist in administration of the local anesthetic agent (if applicable).

2 Assist with preparation and placement of the dental dam (expose only the tooth being treated).

3 Swab the antiseptic solution over the exposed tooth, the clamp, and the surrounding dental dam.

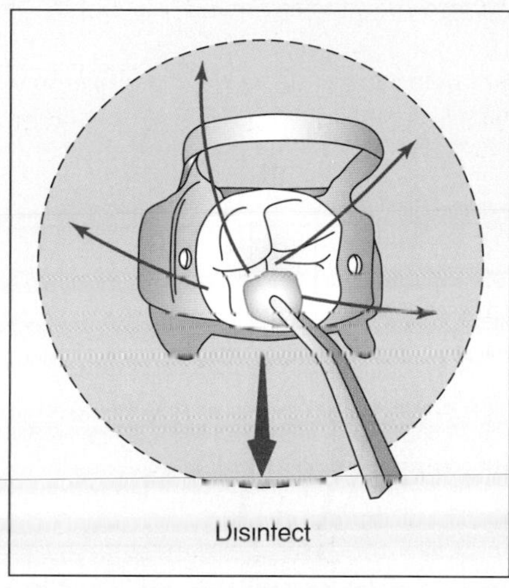


### Removing the Pulp

4 The dentist enters the coronal portion of the tooth with a carbide round bur, removing decay and infected tooth structure.

5 Once the canals are located and opened, the dentist will use the endodontic explorer and intracanal instruments to remove pulp tissue.

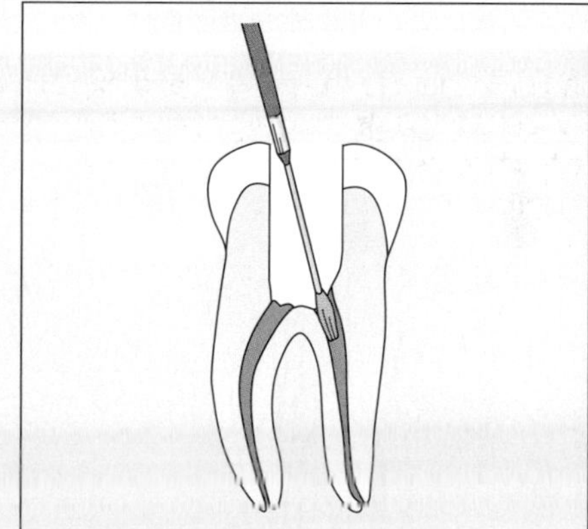

6 The canals are irrigated gently with an irrigation solution. Excess solution is removed with the HVE tip.

7 The dentist uses a small endodontic file to rub the irrigation solution against the walls of the canal and pulp chamber.

**PURPOSE** The solution acts as a disinfectant to destroy bacteria in the canal and to wash away debris. This step is called *biochemical cleaning.*

### Cleaning and Shaping the Canal

8 The dentist will use a series of files, beginning with the smallest and working to the largest as needed. The files are placed into the canal and are moved up and down with short strokes.

**PURPOSE** During this motion, the cutting edges of the files will remove dentin and debris from the walls of the canal.

**(Continued)**

## PROCEDURE 54.2 Assisting in Root Canal Therapy—cont'd

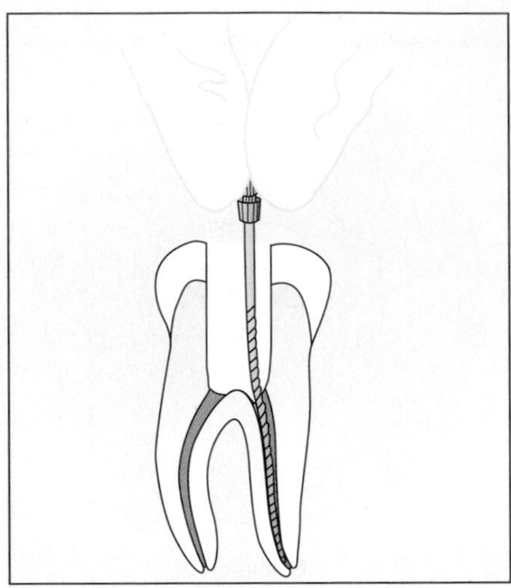

9 Transfer larger files to the dentist to clean and shape the canals.
**PURPOSE** The increase in size is intended to enlarge the diameter of the canal.

10 The rubber stop must be placed on the file at the desired working length for each canal.

11 Irrigate the canals thoroughly at frequent intervals during this shaping and cleaning process.
**PURPOSE** To prevent dentin shavings from clogging the cutting edges of the instruments.

12 Transfer paper points for insertion into the canals until the points come out dry.

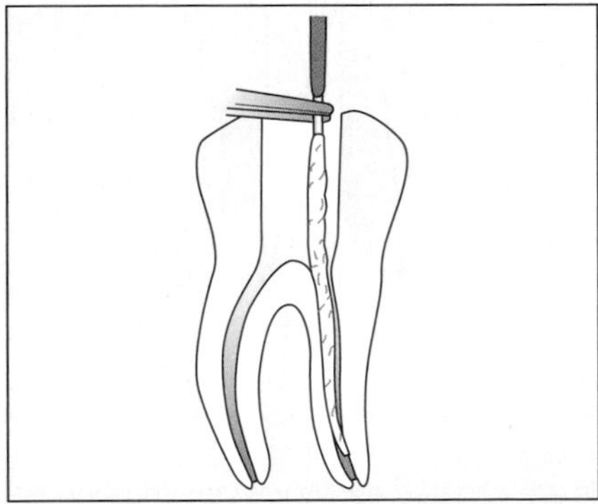

### Preparing to Fill the Canal

13 Select the appropriately sized gutta-percha point, and cut it to the predetermined length. This is called the *trial point.*

14 Take a periapical radiograph of the tooth with the trial point in the canal. This is the *working length radiograph.*

15 If the radiograph does not show the tip of the trial point within 1 mm of the apex of the root, the point is repositioned and another radiograph is taken.

16 At the signal from the dentist, prepare a thin mix of sealer on a sterile glass slab.
**PURPOSE** The sealer is used to ensure a perfect seal at the apical foramen.

### Filling the Canal

17 The master cone is removed from the canal, coated with sealer, and reinserted by the dentist.

18 The dentist inserts the finger spreader into the canal within 1 mm of the working length. The spreader is rotated counterclockwise to spread the sealer around the canal and to create space for the other cones.

19 Continue transferring gutta-percha points to fill the canal.

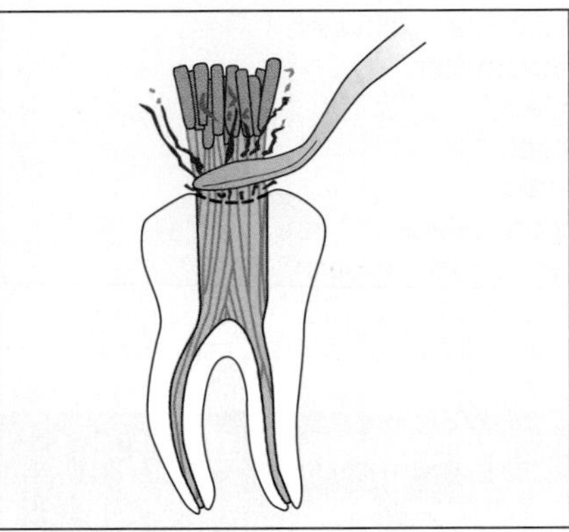

20 Transfer the Glick Number 1, heated at the working end, to remove the excess ends of the gutta-percha points.

21 Transfer the plugger for the dentist to compact vertically.

22 This routine continues until the canal is completely filled.

23 The dentist places a temporary restoration.

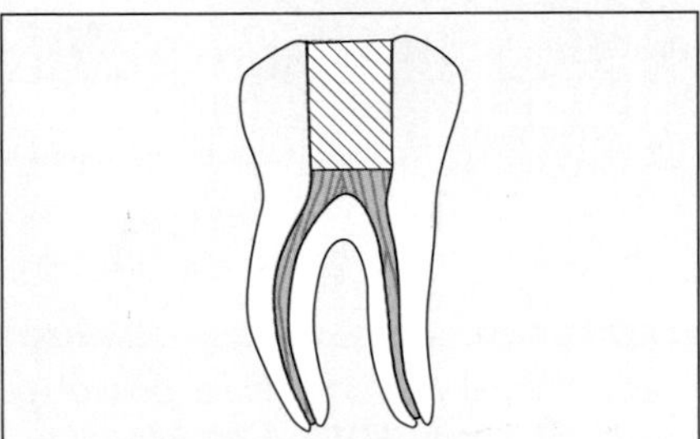

24 Expose a posttreatment radiograph.

25 The dentist checks the occlusion and adjusts as needed.

### Posttreatment Instructions and Follow-up

26 Instruct the patient to call the practice immediately if a problem, such as swelling or pain, is observed.

## PROCEDURE 54.2 Assisting in Root Canal Therapy—cont'd

27 Remind the patient that a return to his or her regular dentist is necessary to have a final restoration placed.

28 Request that the patient return to the endodontist for follow-up at intervals ranging from 3 to 6 months.

**PURPOSE** To enable the endodontist to determine that treatment was successful and that no complications developed.

29 Document the procedure.

| Date | Tooth | Surface | Charting Notes |
|---|---|---|---|
| 8/14/17 | 30 | | Root canal therapy, 2 carp. Xylocaine w/epi, dam isolation, tooth opened, maximum file used #70, working length 24 mm, irrigation solution, gutta-percha fill, closed with Cavit, initial, working/post-treatment radiographs. Pt tolerated procedure well. Return for postop check in 1 week. |
| | | | T. Clark, CDA/ L. Stewart, DDS |

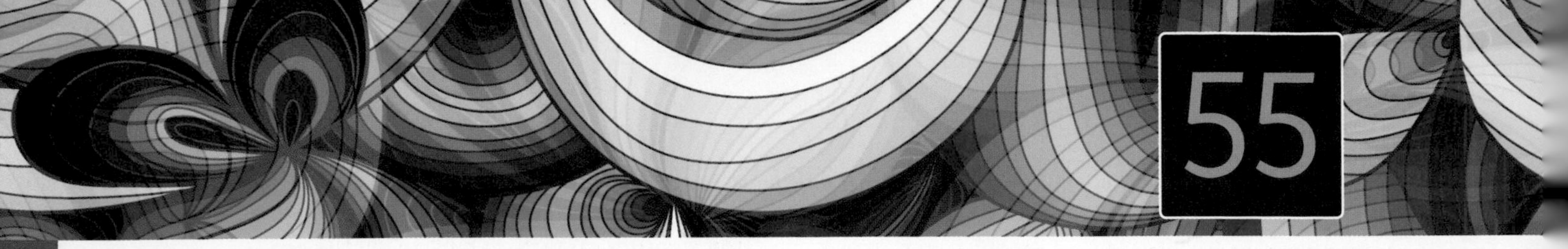

55

# Periodontics

## KEY TERMS

**Bleeding index** Method of scoring the amount of bleeding present.
**Bone augmentation** Addition of natural or synthetic bone to a surgical site.
**Chisel scaler** Instrument used to remove *supragingival* calculus in the contact area of anterior teeth. The blade on the chisel scaler is curved slightly to adapt to the tooth surfaces.
**Crown lengthening** Surgical procedure to expose more tooth surface.
**Curette (kyoo-RET)** Surgical instrument used to remove tissue from the tooth socket; also *curet.*
**File** A metal instrument of varying size and form with numerous ridges or teeth on its cutting surfaces.
**Furcation probe** Used to measure horizontal and vertical pocket depths of multirooted teeth in furcation areas.
**Gingivectomy (jin-ji-VEK-tuh-mee)** Surgical removal of diseased gingival tissues.
**Gingivoplasty (JIN-ji-vuh-plas-tee)** Surgical reshaping and contouring of gingival tissues.
**Gracey curette** Curette with one cutting edge, "area specific"; it is designed to adapt to specific tooth surfaces (mesial or distal).
**Hoe scaler** Type of scaler used to remove heavy supragingival calculus; it is most effective when used on buccal and lingual surfaces of the posterior teeth.
**Kirkland knife** Double-ended knife with kidney-shaped blades; commonly used in periodontal surgery.
**Laser (LAY-zur)** Highly concentrated beam of light; acronym for light amplification by stimulated emission of radiation.
**Mobility** To have movement.
**Occlusal trauma** Abnormal occlusal relationships of the teeth, causing injury to the periodontium.
**Orban knife** Knife with a spearlike shape and cutting edges on both sides of the blade; it is used to remove tissue from the *interdental* areas.
**Osseous (OS-ee-us) surgery** Surgical specialty of removing defects in bone.
**Ostectomy (os-TEK-tuh-mee)** Surgery involving the removal of bone.
**Osteoplasty (OS-tee-oe-plas-tee)** Surgery in which bone is added, contoured, and reshaped.
**Periodontal (per-ee-oe-DON-tul) charting** Commonly accepted notations that are made to the patient's chart to indicate the condition, position, and restorative history of individual teeth.
**Periodontal dressing (periopack)** Dressing applied to a surgical site for protection, similar to a bandage.
**Periodontal explorer** Fine, thin instrument that is easily adapted around root surfaces used to locate deposits of calculus.
**Periodontal flap surgery (flap surgery)** Incisional surgery performed when excisional surgery is not indicated. In flap surgery, the tissues *are not removed* but are pushed away from the underlying tooth roots and alveolar bone, similar to the flap of an envelope.
**Periodontal plastic surgery** Surgical procedures of mucogingival tissues.
**Periodontal pocket** Deepening of the gingival sulcus beyond normal; results from periodontal disease.
**Periodontal probe** Probe used to locate and measure the depth of periodontal pockets; tapered to fit into the gingival sulcus with a blunt or rounded tip.
**Periodontics (per-ee-oe-DON-tiks)** Dental specialty involved with the diagnosis and treatment of diseases of the supporting tissues.
**Periodontist (per-ee-oe-DON-tist)** Dentist with advanced education in the specialty of periodontics.
**Periotome** Instrument used to cut periodontal ligaments for atraumatic tooth extraction.
**Root planning** Procedure that smooths the surface of a root by removing abnormal toxic cementum or dentin that is rough, contaminated, or permeated with calculus.
**Scaling** Removal of calculus deposits from the teeth with the use of suitable instruments.
**Sickle scaler** A hook-shaped instrument that is available in various sizes and shapes and is used for the removal of tenacious supragingival deposits of calculus.
**Ultrasonic scaler** Device used for rapid calculus removal; it operates on high-frequency sound waves.
**Universal curette** Hand instrument used to treat subgingival surfaces; it has a blade with an unbroken cutting edge that curves around the toe and a flat face set at a 90-degree angle to the lower shank.

## LEARNING OUTCOMES

*On completion of this chapter, the student will be able to achieve the following objectives:*

1. Pronounce, define, and spell the key terms.
2. Describe the role of the dental assistant in a periodontal practice.
3. Explain the procedures necessary for a comprehensive periodontal examination, including the following:
   - Describe the early signs of periodontal disease.
   - Describe the role of radiographs in periodontal treatment.
4. Identify and describe the instruments used in periodontal therapy.
5. Discuss hand scaling and ultrasonic scaling, including the following:
   - Describe the advantages of hand scaling and ultrasonic scaling.
   - Describe the indications for and contraindications to use of the ultrasonic scaler.
6. Describe the types of nonsurgical periodontal treatment.
7. Discuss the types of surgical periodontal treatment, including the following:
   - Explain the purpose of crown lengthening.
   - Describe the purpose of soft tissue grafts.
   - Describe the postsurgical patient instructions.

- Identify the indications for placement of periodontal surgical dressings.
- Describe the technique for proper placement and removal of periodontal surgical dressings.
- Name the types of periodontal plastic surgery.

8 Discuss the use of lasers in periodontics.

## PERFORMANCE OUTCOMES

*On completion of this chapter, the student will be able to meet competency standards in the following skills:*

- Assist with a dental prophylaxis procedure.
- Assist with gingivectomy and gingivoplasty procedures.
- Prepare and place noneugenol periodontal dressings (expanded function).
- Remove a periodontal surgical dressing (expanded function).

## ELECTRONIC RESOURCES

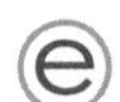
***Additional information related to content in Chapter 55 can be found on the companion Evolve Web site.***

- Practice Quiz
- Tray Setup Drag-and-Drop Exercise: Periodontal Surgical
- Tray Setup Questions
- Videos: Noneugenol Periodontal Dressings; Removing a Periodontal Dressing

**Periodontics** is the dental specialty involved in the diagnosis and treatment of diseases of the supporting tissues. The dental assistant in a periodontal specialty office must have a thorough understanding of periodontal diseases and the types of periodontal instruments and procedures. In a periodontal practice, the dental assistant assists with periodontal charting and periodontal surgeries and provides home care instructions to the patient. Depending on the particular state's dental practice act, the dental assistant also may place and remove periodontal dressings, remove sutures, perform coronal polishes, take impressions for study models, and administer topical fluoride applications.

Patients are usually referred to a periodontist's office by a general dentist or a dental hygienist for treatment of a periodontal condition that requires the skill and knowledge of a specialist. After periodontal treatment, the patient will return to the general dentist for routine dental care.

Frequently, a periodontal patient will alternate periodontal maintenance (cleaning and follow-up) appointments between the periodontist's office and the general dentist's office. The staff in both offices must coordinate periodontal maintenance therapy between the two practices to provide the most comprehensive care for the patient.

This chapter focuses on the *treatment* of patients with periodontal disease and includes a discussion of the instruments used and procedures commonly performed in a periodontal specialty office. It is recommended that you refer to Chapter 14 to review the types of periodontal disease, the associated risk factors, and the systemic factors that influence the progression of periodontal disease.

# The Periodontal Examination

In addition to a thorough dental examination (see Chapter 28), specialized periodontal examinations are necessary to diagnose periodontal disease and to determine the proper treatment. A periodontal examination includes the patient's medical and dental history, radiographic evaluation, examination of the teeth, examination of the oral tissues and supporting structures, and periodontal charting.

**Periodontal charting** includes pocket readings, furcations, tooth mobility, exudate (pus), and gingival recession. Clinical findings of the periodontal examination are recorded on the periodontal chart (Fig. 55.1). Software programs are available that provide computerized printouts of periodontal charting data (Fig. 55.2).

## Medical and Dental History

The **periodontist** reviews the medical history to detect any systemic conditions that may influence periodontal treatment. Systemic diseases, such as acquired immunodeficiency syndrome (AIDS), human immunodeficiency virus (HIV) infection, or diabetes, can lower resistance of the tissue to infection. Lowered resistance makes periodontal disease more severe and more difficult to treat.

The dental history is used to gather information about conditions that could indicate periodontal disease. For example, patients with periodontal disease often complain of bleeding gums, loose teeth, or a bad taste. They may describe a dull pain after eating or a burning sensation in the gingival tissue.

## Dental Examination

The dental examination focuses on the teeth for indications of periodontal disease or factors that could contribute to periodontal disease (Table 55.1).

### *Mobility*

Teeth normally have a slight amount of **mobility** (tooth movement) because of the cushioning effect of the periodontal membranes. However, excessive mobility can be an important sign of periodontal disease (Fig. 55.3).

### *Oral Tissues and Supporting Structures*

The periodontal examination includes an assessment of amounts of plaque and calculus, changes in gingival health and bleeding, and level of bone, as well as detection of periodontal pockets (Table 55.2).

### *Periodontal Probing*

A **periodontal pocket** occurs when disease causes the gingival sulcus to become deeper than normal. A normal sulcus measures

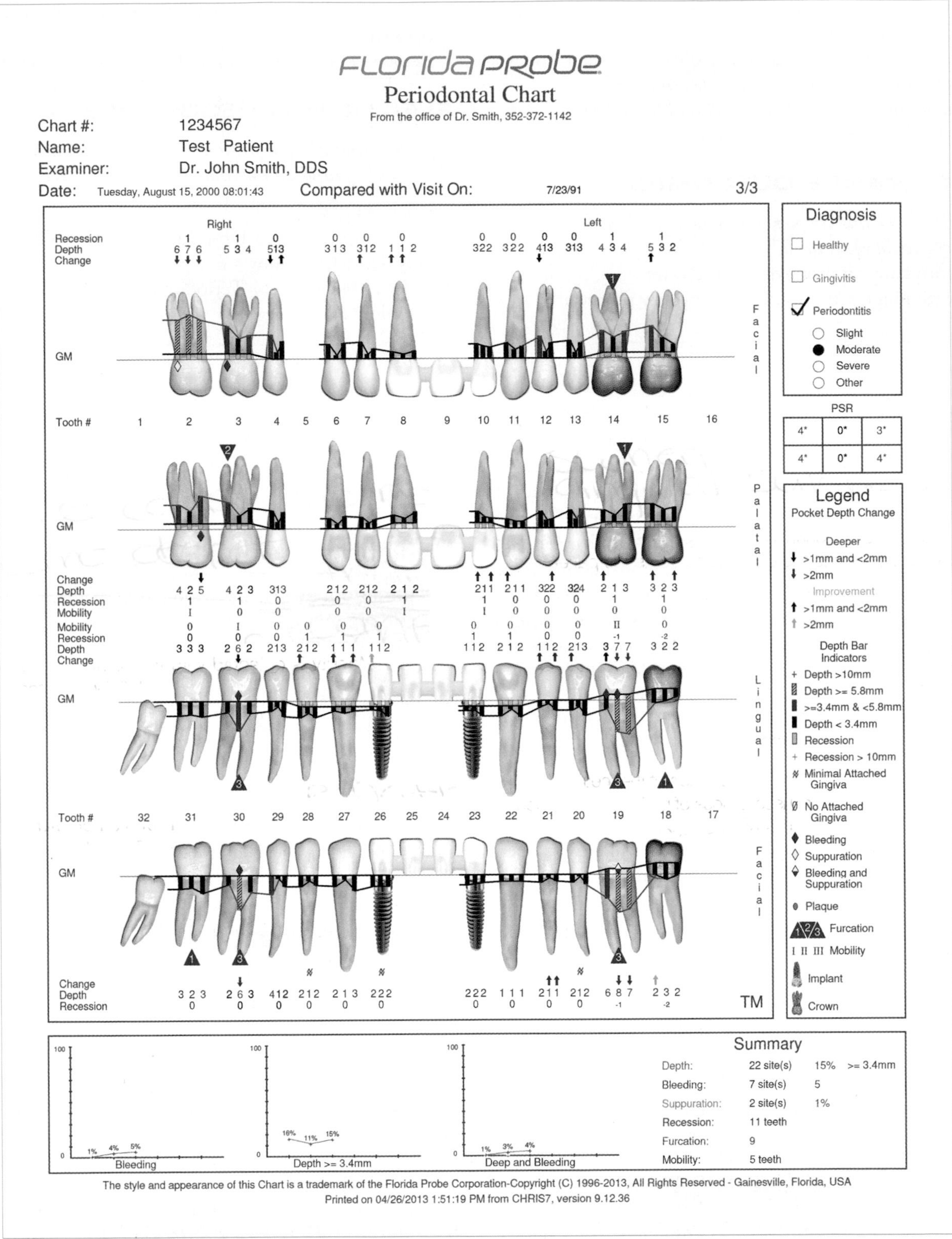


**FIG. 55.1** Computer generated periodontal chart. *(Courtesy Florida Probe Corporation, Gainesville, FL.)*

3 mm or less (Fig. 55.4). The purpose of periodontal probing is to measure how much epithelial attachment has been lost to disease. The greater the depth of the periodontal pocket, the greater is the loss of epithelial attachment and bone, and therefore the more severe is the periodontal disease (Fig. 55.5).

When periodontal pockets are present, it is very difficult and may be impossible for the patient to keep the pockets clean and free from bacteria and debris. The bacteria in the periodontal pockets will multiply, and, if left untreated, the disease will progress until the tooth is ultimately lost to periodontal disease.

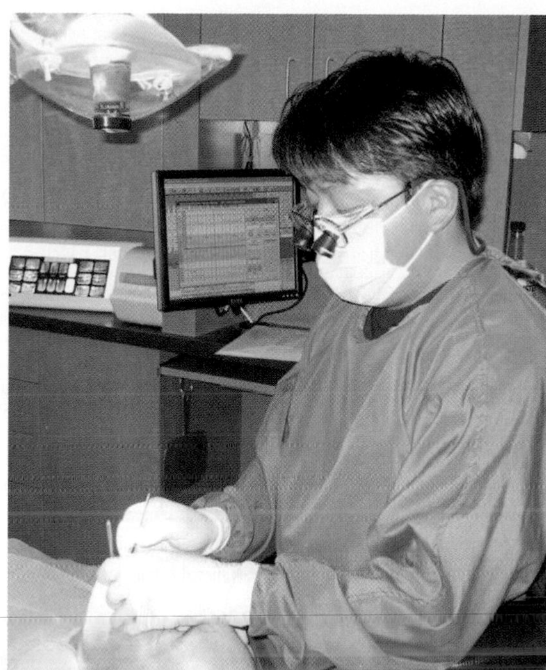

FIG. 55.2 A periodontal chart on a computer screen. This periodontist can easily refer to the chart as he treats the patient.

**TABLE 55.1 Dental Conditions That Contribute to Periodontal Disease**

| Condition | Description |
|---|---|
| Pathologic migration | A shift in the position of the teeth is caused by loss of periodontal support. |
| Clenching or grinding *(bruxism)* | Bruxism places excessive biting forces on the teeth and may accelerate bone loss. |
| Defective restorations or bridgework | Dental prostheses may retain plaque and increase the risk of periodontal disease. |
| Mobility | All teeth have some mobility (see Fig. 55.3). Mobility is recorded with the following scale: *0,* normal; *1,* slight mobility; *2,* moderate mobility; *3,* extreme mobility. |
| Occlusal interferences | Certain tooth areas can prevent the teeth from occluding properly. These interferences do not directly cause periodontal disease but can contribute to mobility, migration, and temporomandibular joint pain. |

### Early Signs of Periodontal Disease

- Changes in the gingiva (color, size, shape, texture)
- Gingival inflammation
- Gingival bleeding
- Evidence of exudates
- Development of periodontal pockets

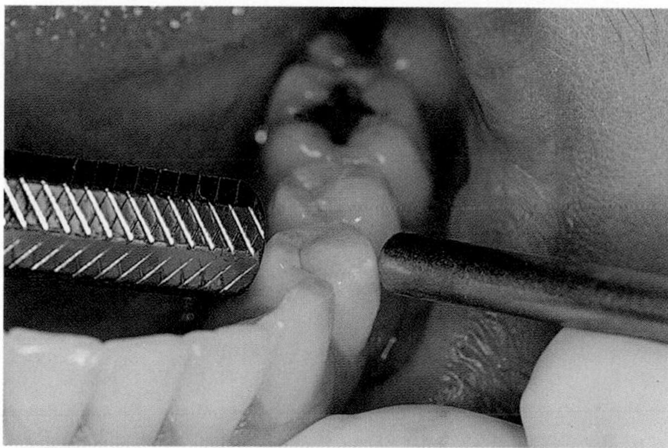

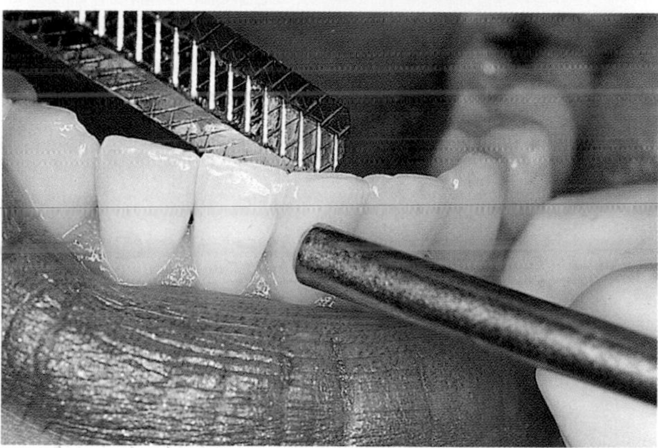

FIG. 55.3 Mobility is detected with the blunt ends of two instruments. *(From Daniel SJ, Harfst SA, Wilder R: Mosby's dental hygiene: concepts, cases, and competencies, ed 2, St Louis, 2008, Mosby.)*

## Bleeding Index

The severity of gingival inflammation can be measured by the **bleeding index**, or the amount of bleeding observed during probing (Fig. 55.6). Several different systems of recording bleeding scores are used. Each system is based on the principle that healthy gingiva does not bleed.

## Occlusal Adjustment

The patient's bite is evaluated for areas of unequal pressure. If excessive biting pressure is noted in a specific area, **occlusal trauma** can result. Occlusal adjustment, or *occlusal equilibration,* is a procedure that adjusts the patient's bite so that occlusal forces are equally distributed over all the teeth. Articulating paper, occlusal wax, stones, and burs are used to adjust the occlusion. Several appointments may be necessary to adjust the occlusion properly.

Occlusal trauma does *not cause* periodontal pocket formation, but it can cause tooth mobility, destruction of bone, migration of teeth, and temporomandibular joint pain.

## Radiographic Analysis

Radiographs are a valuable aid for evaluating periodontal disease. The accuracy of radiographs is critical in the diagnosis of periodontal disease because distortion of the image can result in an incorrect diagnosis (Fig. 55.7).

The *bitewing radiograph* is particularly valuable because it can accurately depict bone height along the root surface.

**TABLE 55.2** Periodontal Examination of Gingiva and Supporting Tissues

| Assessment | Description |
|---|---|
| Plaque | Plaque is the primary cause of gingival inflammation and most other forms of periodontal disease. |
| Calculus | Calculus is hard mineralized plaque. Calculus may be *supragingival* (above the gingivae) or *subgingival* (below the gingivae). Calculus adheres to the surfaces of natural teeth, crowns, bridges, and dentures. It is a contributing factor in periodontal disease because it is always covered with plaque. |
| Gingival recession | As disease progresses, the gingiva may recede, leaving portions of the roots of the teeth exposed below the cementoenamel junction. Gingival recession levels can be visualized on the chart by drawing a dotted or colored line to indicate the gingival margin (see Fig. 55.1). |
| Bleeding index | Severity of gingival inflammation is measured by the amount of bleeding observed during probing. Several different indices are used to measure bleeding. Each system is based on the principle that healthy gingivae do not bleed. |
| Measurement of periodontal pockets | A periodontal pocket occurs when disease causes the normal gingival sulcus to become deeper than normal. (A normal sulcus is 3 mm or less.) |
| Assessment of bone level | Radiographs are used to assess the patient's bone level. These also may be visualized on the computerized chart, or the paper chart by drawing a colored line to indicate the bone level (see Fig. 55.1). |
| Radiographs | Detect interproximal bone loss. Show changes in the bone as periodontitis progresses. Locate furcation involvements. Measure the crown-to-root ratio (the length of the clinical crown compared with the length of the root of the tooth). Show signs of traumatic occlusion. |

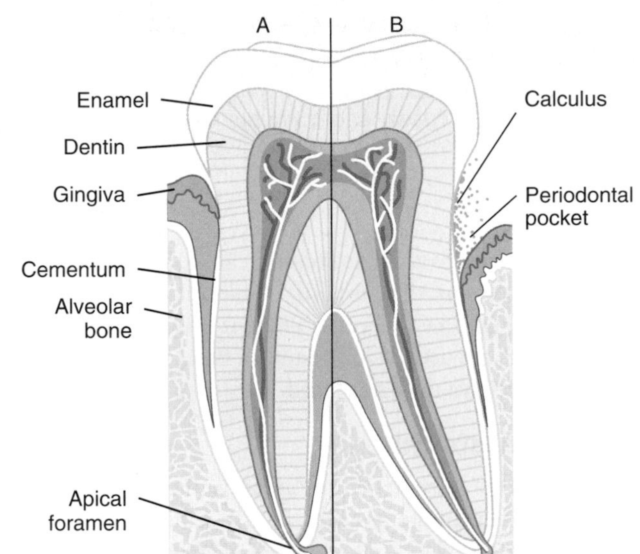


**FIG. 55.4** Cross section of a tooth, gingiva, and bone. The *A* side shows normal sulcus depth. The *B* side shows a periodontal pocket.

Vertical bitewing radiographs are excellent for determining the extent of crestal bone loss (Fig. 55.8).

RECALL

1 How do patients most often seek periodontal care?
2 What information is included in the periodontal charting?
3 Should teeth have any mobility?
4 What is the depth of a normal sulcus?
5 What units of measurement are used on the periodontal probe?
6 What type of radiograph is especially useful in periodontics?

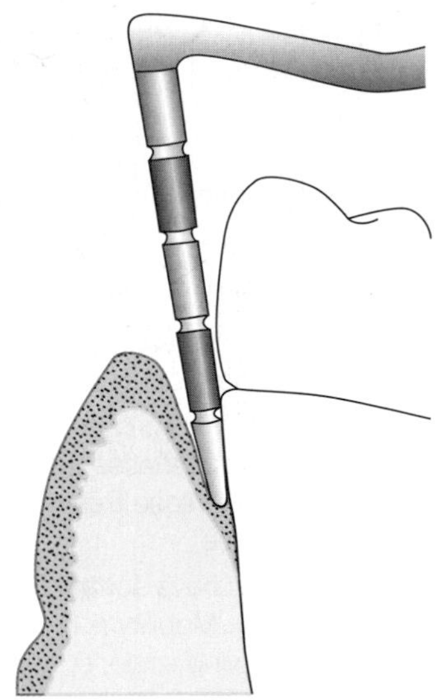

**FIG. 55.5** Diagram shows probing of the periodontal pocket depth. The millimeter measurement indicates the distance from the gingival margin to the base of the pocket. *(Modified from Perry DA, Beemsterboer PL: Periodontology for the dental hygienist, ed 4, St Louis, 2014, Saunders.)*

## Periodontal Instruments

Periodontal therapy requires the use of specialized instruments to remove calculus, smooth root surfaces, measure periodontal pockets, and perform periodontal surgery. These instruments must be sharp to perform periodontal procedures such as *scaling, root planing,* and *periodontal surgery.* In general, the dentist or registered dental hygienist who uses these instruments takes responsibility for maintaining their sharpness.

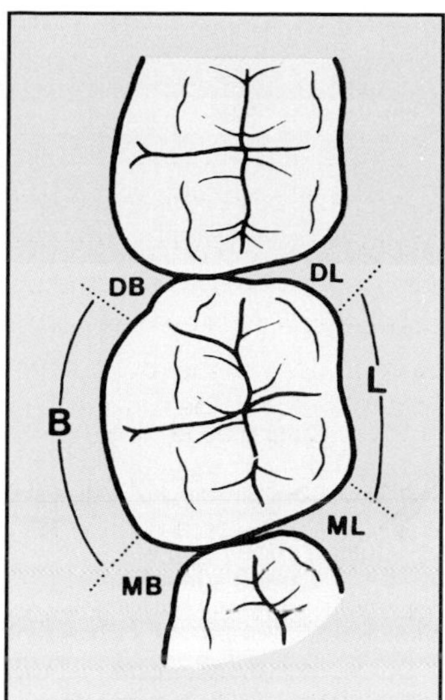


**FIG. 55.6** Six probing depths are taken for each tooth: *B,* buccal; *DB,* distobuccal; *DL,* distolingual; *L,* lingual; *MB,* mesiobuccal; *ML,* mesiolingual. *(From Perry DA, Beemsterboer PL, Carranza FA: Techniques and theory of periodontal instrumentation, Philadelphia, 1990, Saunders.)*

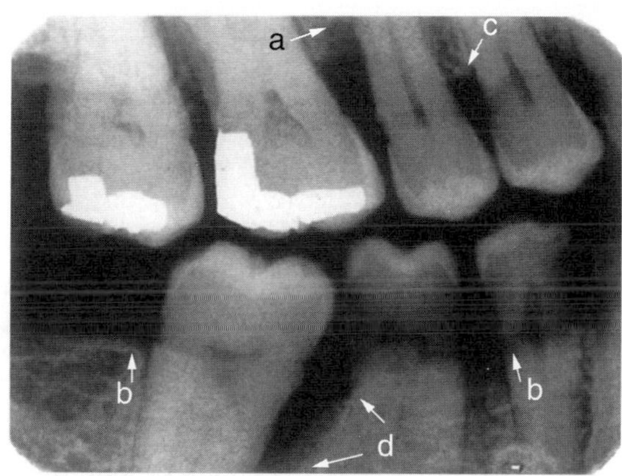


**FIG. 55.7** Bone loss in periodontal disease: *a,* Vertical bone defect. *b,* Crestal ridge at near-normal height. *c,* Alveolar crest. *d,* Severe vertical defect. *(From Miles DA, Van Dis ML, Williamson GF et al: Radiographic imaging for the dental team, ed 4, St Louis, 2009, Saunders.)*

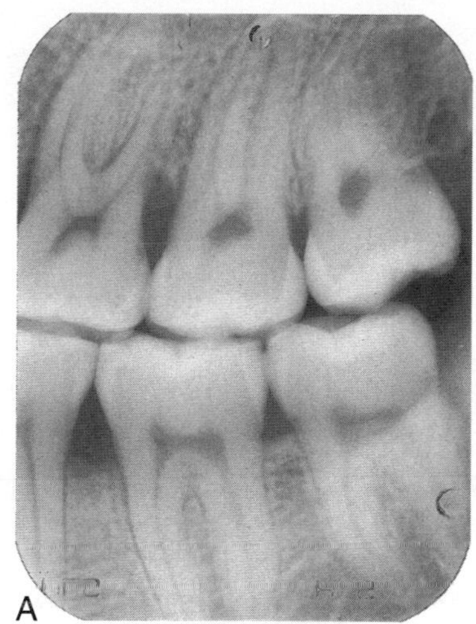


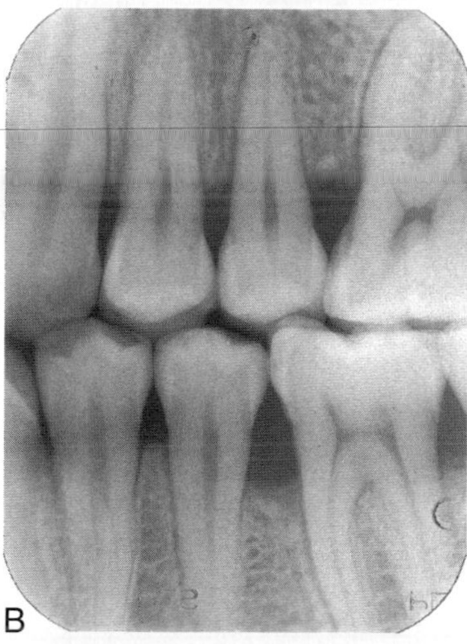


**FIG. 55.8** A, Molar vertical bitewing. B, Premolar vertical bitewing.

## Periodontal Probes

**Periodontal probes**, which are calibrated in millimeters, are used to locate and measure the depth of periodontal pockets. On some types of probes, the tip is color coded to make the measurements easier to read. The periodontal probe is tapered to fit into the gingival sulcus and has a blunt or rounded tip. Six measurements are taken and recorded for each tooth (Fig. 55.9). Periodontal probes are available in many designs; selection depends on the operator's personal preference.

**Furcation probes** are used to measure horizontal and vertical pocket depths of multirooted teeth in furcation areas. They have flat or rounded ends, and may be single or double ended (Fig. 55.10).

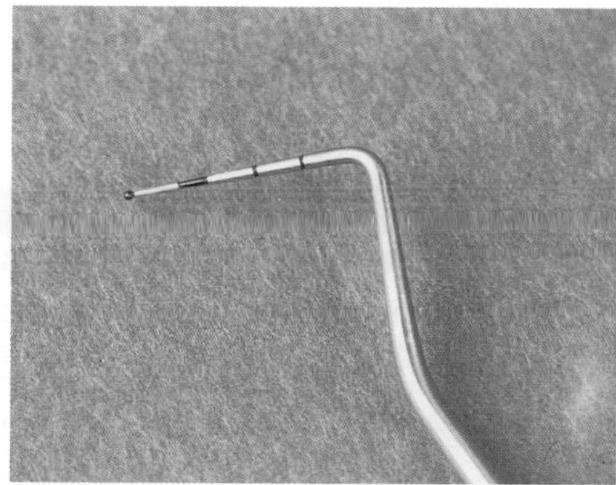

**FIG. 55.9** Working end of a periodontal probe.

## Explorers

**Periodontal explorers** are used in periodontics to locate deposits of calculus that may be *supragingival* or *subgingival.* Explorers also provide tactile information to the operator about the roughness or smoothness of root surfaces (Fig. 55.11).

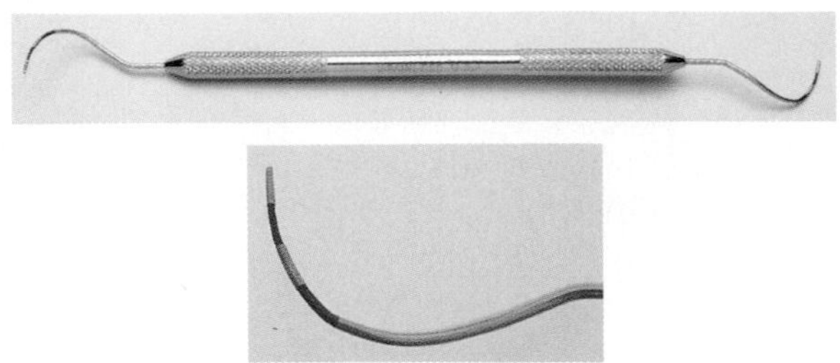

**FIG. 55.10** Furcation probe. *(From Boyd LRB: Dental instruments: a pocket guide, ed 6, St Louis, 2018, Elsevier.)*

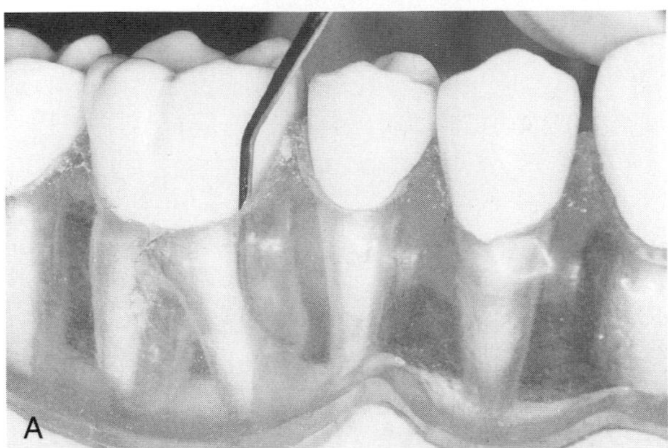


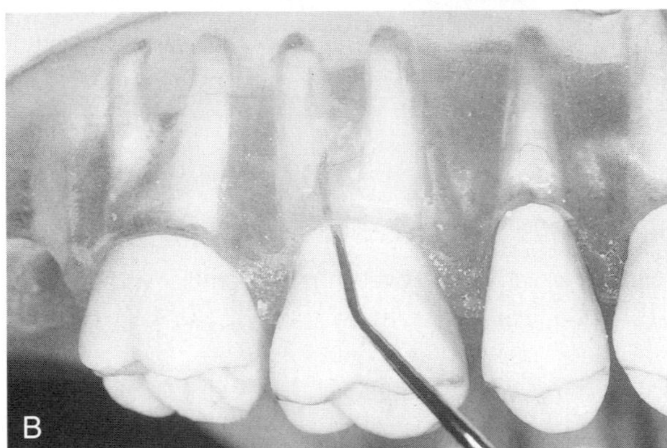


**FIG. 55.11** Various styles of periodontal explorers. A, EXC 11/12 AF explorer allows access to pockets deeper than 5 mm for evaluating root surfaces. B, Elongated design is useful for exploring the furcation area. *(Courtesy Hu-Friedy Manufacturing, Chicago, IL.)*

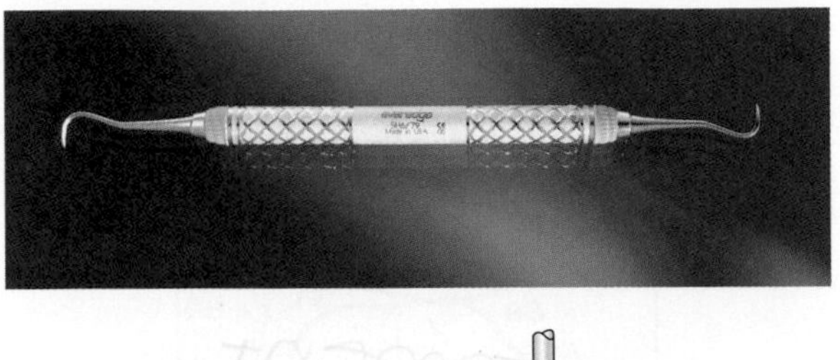

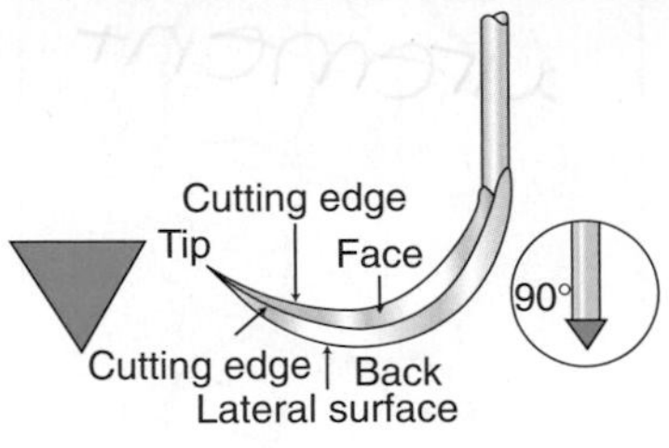


**FIG. 55.12** Curved sickle scaler. *(From Boyd LRB: Dental instruments: a pocket guide, ed 6, St Louis, 2018, Elsevier.)*

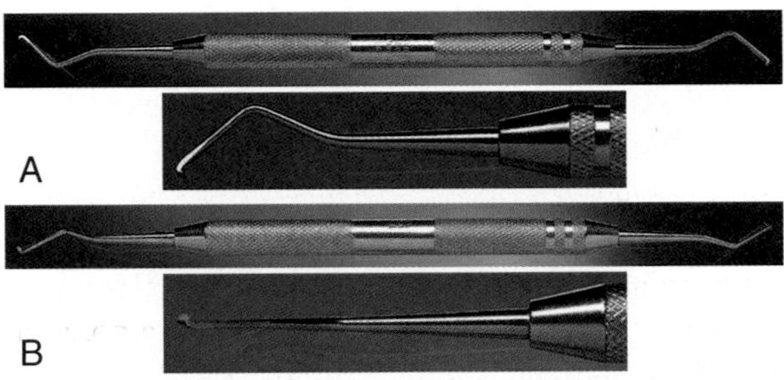


**FIG. 55.13** Hoes. A, Mesial/distal hoe. B, Buccal/lingual hoe. *(From Boyd LRB: Dental instruments: a pocket guide, ed 6, St Louis, 2018, Elsevier.)*

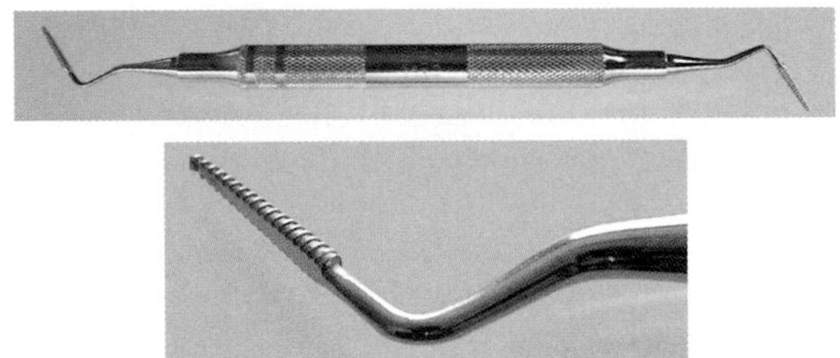

**FIG. 55.14** Interdental file. *(From Boyd LRB: Dental instruments: a pocket guide, ed 6, St Louis, 2018, Elsevier.)*

Many styles of explorers are used in periodontal treatment. Periodontal explorers are longer and more curved than explorers used for caries detection. (See Chapter 34 for other types of explorers.)

The working ends of periodontal explorers are thin, fine, and easily adapted around root surfaces. They also are long enough to be capable of reaching to the base of deep pockets and furcations. A *furcation* is the point at which the roots of a multirooted tooth diverge.

## Scalers and Files

- **Sickle scalers** are used primarily to remove large deposits of *supragingival* calculus. A sickle scaler with a long, straight shank is used to remove calculus from the anterior areas of the oral cavity. A *contra-angle* sickle scaler, which is angled at the shank, is designed to remove calculus from the posterior teeth (Fig. 55.12).
- **Chisel scalers** are used to remove *supragingival* calculus in the contact area of anterior teeth. The blade on the chisel scaler is curved slightly to adapt to tooth surfaces.
- **Hoe scalers** are used to remove *heavy supragingival* calculus. Hoes are most effective when used on buccal and lingual surfaces of posterior teeth (Fig. 55.13).
- **Files** are used to crush or fracture *extremely heavy* calculus. The fractured calculus is then removed from the tooth surface with curettes (Fig. 55.14).

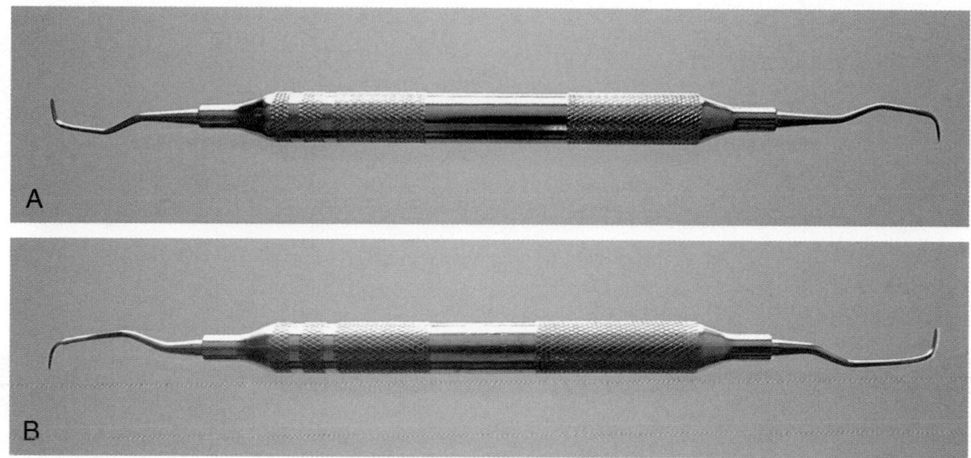


**FIG. 55.15** A, Anterior curette. B, Posterior curette. *(From Boyd LRB: Dental instruments: a pocket guide, ed 6, St Louis, 2018, Elsevier.)*

*Note:* The chisel, hoe, and files are used less frequently than scalers or curettes in periodontal procedures.

## Curettes

**Curettes** are used to remove *subgingival* calculus, to smooth rough root surfaces *(root planing),* and to remove the diseased soft tissue lining of the periodontal pocket *(soft tissue curettage)* (Fig. 55.15). In contrast to a scaler, which has a pointed end, curettes have a rounded end (Fig. 55.16). Curettes are available in two basic designs:

**Universal curettes** are designed so that one instrument is able to adapt to all tooth surfaces. These curettes have *two cutting edges,* one on each side of the blade. Universal curettes resemble the spoon excavators used in restorative dentistry (Fig. 55.17).

**Gracey curettes**, which have only *one cutting edge,* are *area specific;* that is, they are designed to adapt to specific tooth surfaces (mesial or distal). Treatment of the entire dentition requires the use of several Gracey curettes (Fig. 55.18).

## Surgical Knives

**Kirkland knives** are one of the most common types of surgical knives used in periodontal surgery. These instruments are usually double ended with kidney-shaped blades. **Orban knives** are used to remove tissue from *interdental* areas. These knives have a spearlike shape and cutting edges on both sides of the blade (Fig. 55.19).

**Periotomes** are used to cut periodontal ligaments for atraumatic tooth extraction. They are used when dental implant placement is indicated. They have thin, sharp blades that cause minimal damage to periodontal ligaments and surrounding alveolar bone (Fig. 55.20).

## Pocket Markers

Pocket markers are similar in appearance to cotton pliers; however, one tip is smooth and straight, and the other tip is sharp and is bent at a right angle. The smooth tip of the pocket marker is inserted at the base of the pocket. When pressure is applied to the instrument, the sharp tip makes small perforations in the gingiva. These perforations make *bleeding points* that are used to mark the area for an incision on the gingiva (Fig. 55.21).

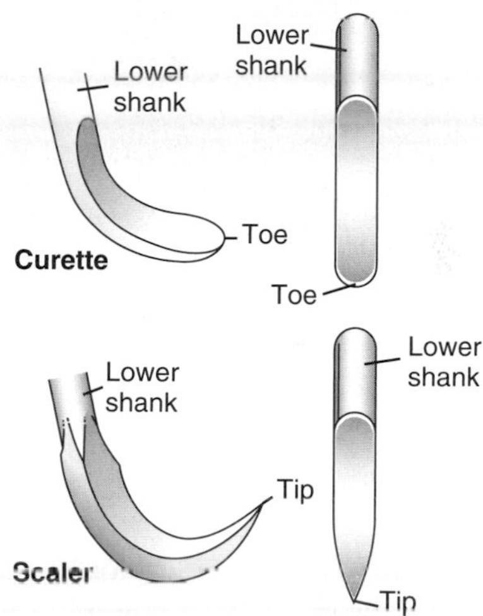


**FIG. 55.16** Comparison of the end of a scaler *(pointed)* and the end of a curette *(rounded).*

RECALL

7 What instruments are used to remove calculus from supragingival surfaces?
8 What instruments are used to remove calculus from subgingival surfaces?
9 What is the purpose of explorers in periodontal treatment?
10 What is the difference between a universal curette and a Gracey curette?
11 What is the purpose of a periodontal pocket marker?

# Hand Scaling and Ultrasonic Scaling

Ultrasonic and manual scaling techniques produce equally good results in calculus and dental plaque removal. A combination of both techniques is now preferred, and the patient benefits from treatment that incorporates the two approaches.

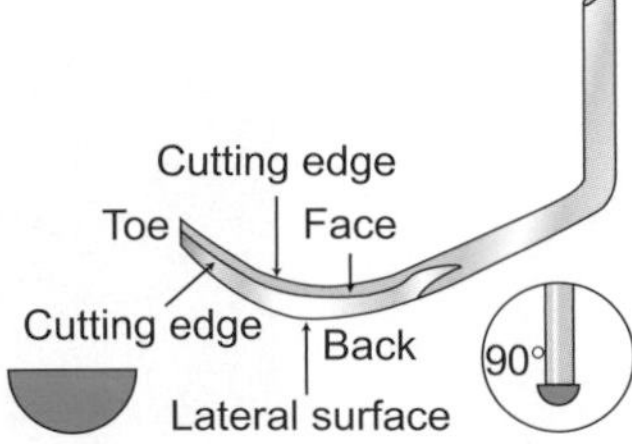


FIG. 55.17 Universal curette. Note the cutting edge on each side of the blade. *(From Boyd LRB: Dental instruments: a pocket guide, ed 6, St Louis, 2018, Elsevier.)*

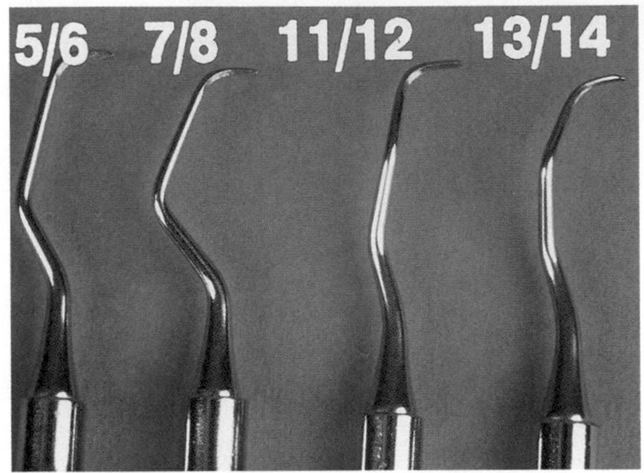


FIG. 55.18 Assorted Gracey curettes. *(Courtesy Hu-Friedy Manufacturing, Chicago, IL.)*

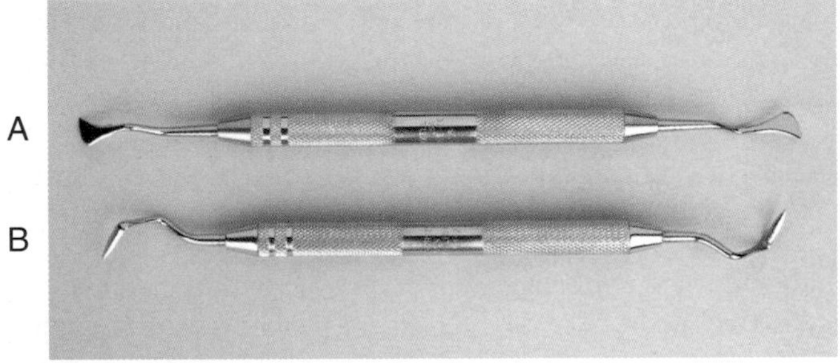


FIG. 55.19 Gingivectomy knives. A, Kirkland knife. B, Orban interdental knives. *(From Newman M, Takei T, Klokkevold P et al, editors: Carranza's clinical periodontology, ed 12, St Louis, 2015, Saunders.)*

### Advantages of Hand Scaling and Ultrasonic Scaling

**Advantages of Hand Scaling**

- Excellent tactile sensitivity
- Greater control
- Area-specific designs to enhance access

**Advantages of Ultrasonic Scaling**

- Improved healing time from lavage effect
- Operating field kept clean by water delivery
- Repetitive motions minimized with proper use
- Less tissue distention

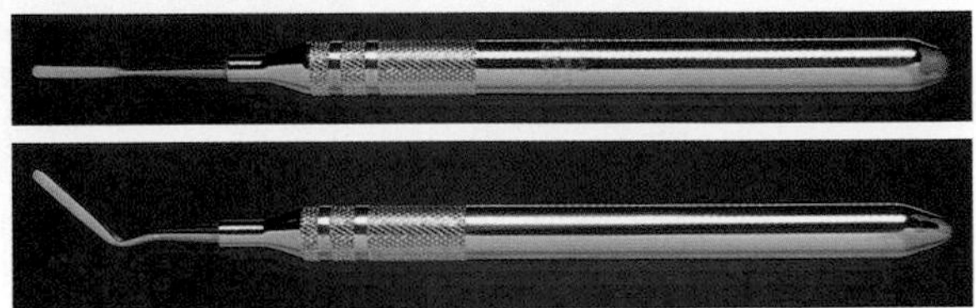

FIG. 55.20 Peritomes. *(From Boyd LRB: Dental instruments: a pocket guide, ed 6, St Louis, 2018, Elsevier.)*

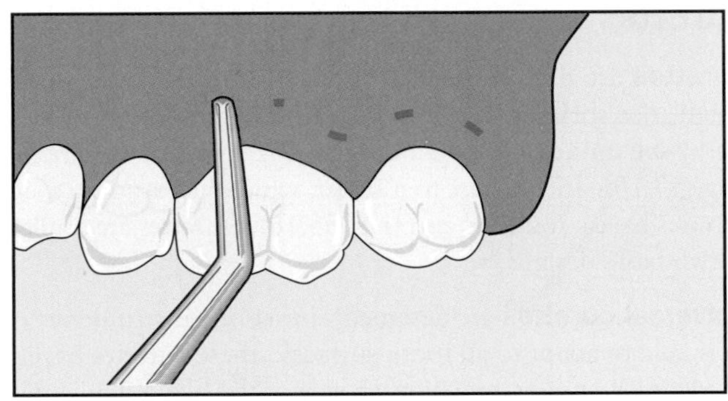

FIG. 55.21 Periodontal pocket marker makes pinpoint perforations that indicate the line for a surgical incision.

## Ultrasonic Scaler

The **ultrasonic scaler** provides rapid calculus removal and reduces hand fatigue for the operator. Newer styles and slimmer instrument tips have been designed to provide easier access to subgingival pockets. Use of these devices is rapidly increasing in periodontics (Fig. 55.22).

The ultrasonic scaler works by converting very-high-frequency sound waves into mechanical energy in the form of extremely rapid vibrations (20,000–40,000 cycles per second) at the tip of the instrument. A spray of water at the tip prevents the buildup of heat and continuously flushes debris and bacteria from the base of the pocket (Fig. 55.23).

Because of this spray of water at the tip, however, a large amount of potentially contaminated aerosol spray is released into the dental office environment. The operator of an ultrasonic scaler should have the dental assistant use the high-volume evacuator (HVE) to minimize aerosol contamination.

### *Indications*

Indications for use of an ultrasonic scaler include the following:

- Removal of supragingival calculus and difficult stains

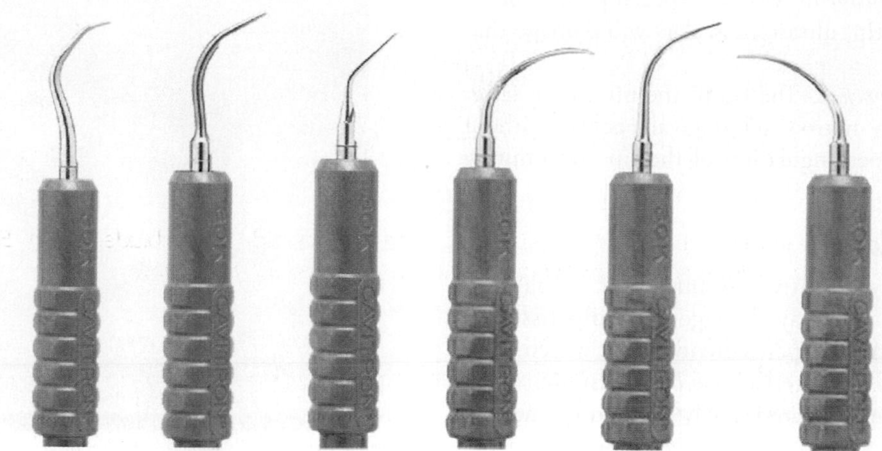

**FIG. 55.22** A series of ultrasonic tips designed to reach every area of the mouth. *(From Daniel SJ, Harfst SA, Wilder R: Mosby's dental hygiene: concepts, cases, and competencies, ed 2, St Louis, 2008, Mosby.)*

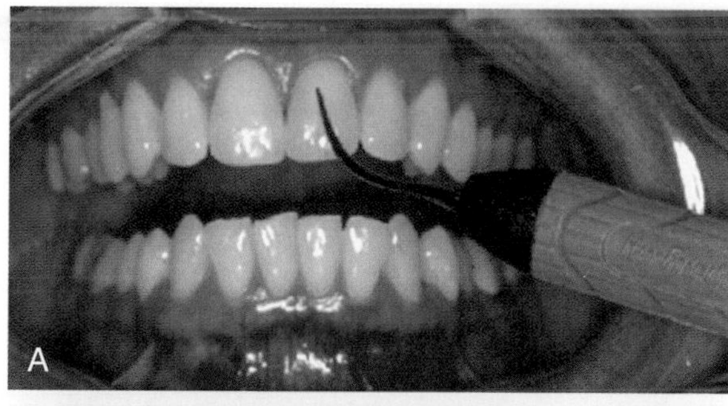

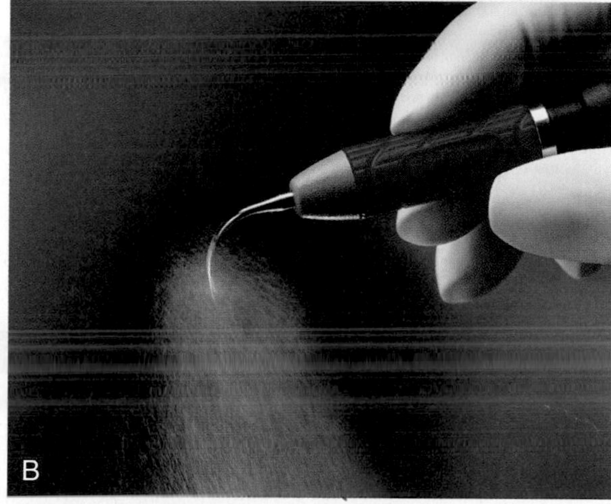

**FIG. 55.23** A, Positioning of the ultrasonic scaler. B, Ultrasonic scaler with water source turned on. *(Courtesy Hu-Friedy Manufacturing, Chicago, IL.)*

- Removal of subgingival calculus, attached plaque, and endotoxins from the root surface
- Cleaning of furcation areas
- Removal of deposits before periodontal surgery
- Removal of orthodontic cements, or *debonding*
- Removal of overhanging margins of restorations

## *Contraindications*

Contraindications to use of the ultrasonic scaler include the following *general health considerations:*

- *Communicable disease.* Patients with a known communicable disease, such as tuberculosis, can transmit contaminated aerosols. It is important to use an HVE to remove these aerosols.
- *Patients susceptible to infection.* Medically compromised patients, such as those receiving chemotherapy or with HIV infection, uncontrolled diabetes, debilitation, or organ transplants, are more susceptible to infection.
- *Respiratory problems.* Materials can be aspirated into the lungs of patients with chronic pulmonary disease, including asthma or other breathing problems, emphysema, and cystic fibrosis.
- *Swallowing difficulty.* Patients with muscular dystrophy, multiple sclerosis, paralysis, or amyotrophic lateral sclerosis may have swallowing problems or may have a severe gag reflex. The water flow and spray can be very uncomfortable for some patients.
- *Cardiac pacemaker.* Consultation with the patient's cardiologist is necessary because theoretically an ultrasonic scaler can disrupt a pacemaker, although no actual cases have been reported. The newer models of ultrasonic scalers have protective coatings to prevent this.

Oral conditions also may be contraindications to the use of ultrasonic scalers:

- *Demineralized areas.* The vibrations of the ultrasonic scaler may remove the areas of remineralization that begin to cover the demineralization.
- *Exposed dentinal surfaces.* Tooth structure may be removed, and this may cause tooth sensitivity.
- *Restorative materials.* Some restorative materials, including esthetic restorations such as porcelains, composite resins, and laminate veneers, may be damaged by ultrasonic scalers.

- *Titanium implant abutments.* Unless a special plastic sheath is used to cover the tip, ultrasonic scalers will damage titanium surfaces.
- *Narrow periodontal pockets.* The tip of the ultrasonic scaler will not fit into very narrow subgingival pockets without interfering with proper angulation of the tip and limiting visibility.

### Precautions for Children

Young tissues are very sensitive to ultrasonic vibrations. These vibrations and heat may damage the pulp tissue of primary and newly erupted permanent teeth, which have large pulp chambers. Therefore the use of ultrasonic scalers is contraindicated on primary and newly erupted permanent teeth.

RECALL

12 How do ultrasonic scalers work?
13 What oral conditions would contraindicate the use of an ultrasonic scaler?
14 Why should an ultrasonic scaler not be used on a patient with a communicable disease?

# Nonsurgical Periodontal Treatment

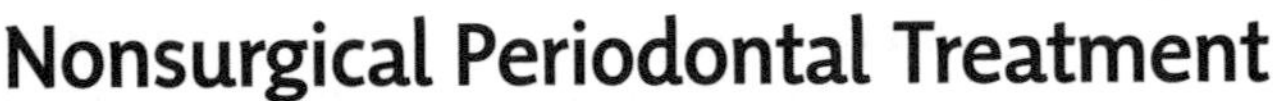

## Dental Prophylaxis

A dental prophylaxis procedure, commonly referred to as *prophy* or *cleaning,* is the complete removal of calculus, soft deposits, plaque, and stain from all supragingival and unattached subgingival tooth surfaces. The dentist and the dental hygienist are the *only* dental health team members licensed to perform a prophylaxis. See Procedure 55.1: Assisting with a Dental Prophylaxis.

A prophylaxis is indicated for patients with healthy gingiva as a preventive measure and is most often performed during recall appointments. A dental prophylaxis also is the primary treatment for gingivitis.

## Scaling and Root Planing

Scaling and root planing are done as part of a periodontal debridement. The goal of debridement is to remove deposits on the tooth and reduce the bioburden within the pocket. This procedure will help return the tissues to a healthy state. A local anesthetic is usually administered before this procedure is performed.

**Scaling** is done to remove *supragingival* calculus from the tooth surface with periodontal scalers. Curettes are used to remove *supragingival* and *subgingival* calculus. Areas on the root surface may remain rough after calculus removal because the cementum has become necrotic (dead), or because scaling has produced grooves and scratches in the cementum (Fig. 55.24).

**Root planing** follows scaling procedures to remove any remaining particles of calculus and necrotic cementum embedded in the root surface. After root planing, the surfaces are smoother and are free from endotoxins. Smooth root surfaces are easier for the patient to keep clean.

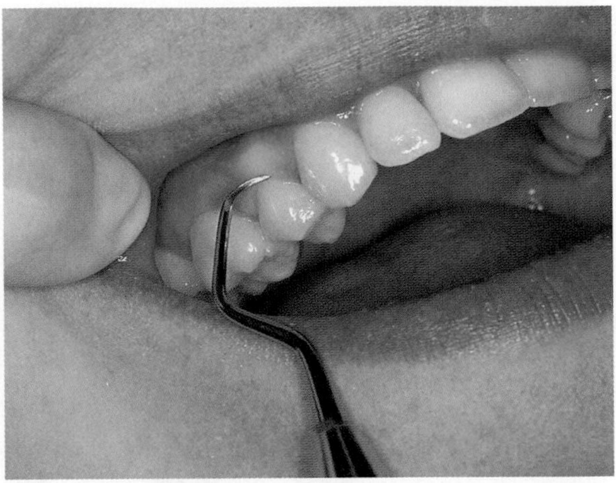

**FIG. 55.24** A Gracey currette is used during scaling and root planing. *(From Newman M, Takei T, Klokkevold P et al, editors: Carranza's clinical periodontology, ed 12, St Louis, 2015, Saunders.)*

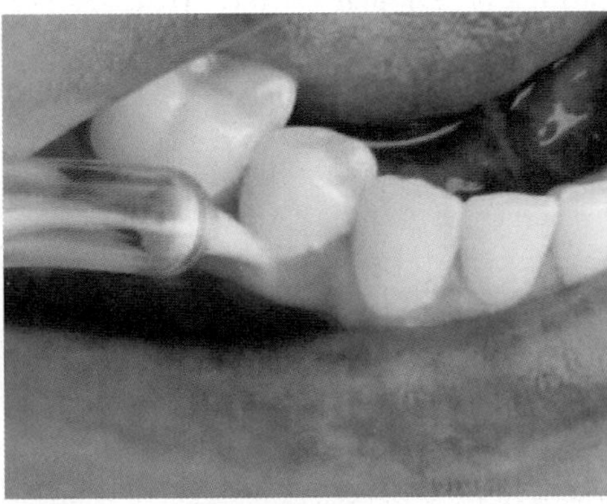

**FIG. 55.25** This irrigation tip is designed for low-pressure delivery of antimicrobial agents. The soft rubber tip is placed below the gingival margin and is ideal for cleaning periodontal pockets and furcations. It can be incorporated easily into a patient's self-care routine. *(Courtesy Water Pik, Inc., Fort Collins, CO.)*

## Gingival Curettage

In addition to scaling and root planing, which involve treating the surfaces of the tooth, some patients require gingival curettage. *Gingival curettage* involves scraping or cleaning the gingival lining of the pocket with a sharp curette to remove necrotic tissue from the pocket wall. Gingival curettage is also referred to as *subgingival curettage.*

## Antimicrobial and Antibiotic Agents

The periodontist may prescribe antimicrobial agents and antibiotics for use with periodontal treatment (Fig. 55.25). Several antibiotics have been used for the reduction of periodontal diseases, including metronidazole and amoxicillin, either alone or in combination.

*Tetracycline* is a particularly useful antibiotic for the treatment of early-onset periodontitis, as well as for rapidly destructive periodontitis. An important adverse effect of tetracycline is that it interferes with the effectiveness of birth control pills (i.e., oral contraceptives).

*Penicillin* is less effective against periodontal disease infection because many periodontal pathogens are resistant to it.

*Fluoride* mouth rinses have been shown to reduce bleeding by delaying bacterial growth within the periodontal pockets.

*Chlorhexidine* rinse (twice daily) is a highly effective antimicrobial therapy available to reduce plaque and gingivitis. Chlorhexidine can cause temporary brown staining of the teeth, tongue, and resin restorations. This stain can be removed by polishing.

## Locally Delivered Antibiotics

There are methods that now can be used to apply antibiotics directly into the periodontal pockets. These methods include using a syringe to insert *dissolvable materials* such as a gel (that contains an antibiotic similar to tetracycline) into the pocket. As the gel heats to body temperature, it becomes a semisolid. This material releases the antibiotic as it dissolves and does not have to be removed. With another technique, a dissolvable chip that releases chlorhexidine is inserted into deep pockets (Fig. 55.26).

Advantages of these methods include easy insertion and no need for removal. This local delivery of medications is particularly useful for patients with isolated areas of recurrent periodontitis, and for the treatment of medically compromised patients who cannot tolerate systemic medications.

RECALL

**15** What are the more common terms for dental prophylaxis?
**16** Who can legally perform a dental prophylaxis procedure?
**17** What are three nonsurgical periodontal treatments?
**18** How is tetracycline used in periodontal treatment?

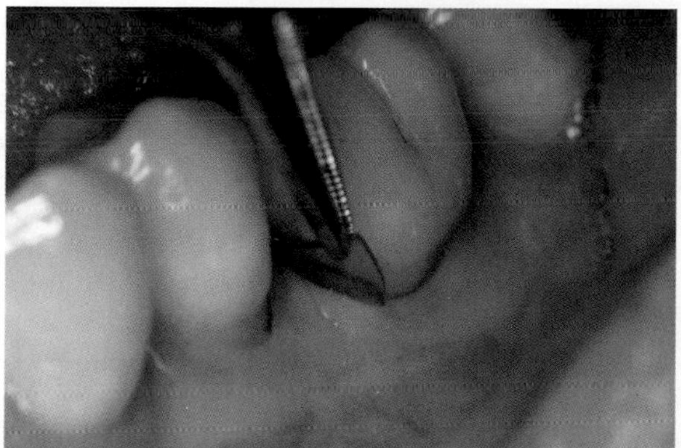

**FIG. 55.26** Chlorhexidine chip. *(From Rose LF, et al: Periodontics: medicine, surgery and implants, St Louis, 2004, Mosby.)*

# Surgical Periodontal Treatment

When nonsurgical treatment is ineffective in stopping the disease process, periodontal surgery is indicated to control the progress of periodontal destruction and loss of attachment.

## Advantages and Disadvantages

The primary advantage of periodontal surgery is that it allows one to *gain access* to the root surface by removing or lifting the gingival tissues. When root surfaces are exposed, they can be scaled and root-planed more easily and thoroughly. Surgery also improves access for the patient in cleaning areas that are difficult to reach.

Disadvantages of and contraindications to periodontal surgery include the patient's health status and age, as well as limitations of the procedures. From the patient's point of view, the disadvantages of surgery usually include time, cost, esthetics, and discomfort. The dental assistant usually has developed a good rapport with the patient and is in a unique position to discuss these concerns.

## Remaining Bone

The amount of bone remaining around a tooth is an important consideration in the decision to perform periodontal surgery. When large amounts of bone are present around a tooth, the dentist may take a "wait-and-see" approach to postpone or avoid periodontal surgery. When this approach is taken, it is important for the patient to maintain excellent home care techniques and to seek routine dental care. If the amount of bone is already reduced, delaying surgery may drastically reduce the chance of saving the tooth (Fig. 55.27).

## Excisional Surgery

Excisional periodontal surgery is a type of surgery that *removes* the excess tissue. It is the most rapid method for reduction of periodontal pockets. Gingivectomy and gingivoplasty are common types of excisional surgery.

### *Gingivectomy*

**Gingivectomy** is the surgical removal of diseased gingival tissue. This procedure is performed when it is necessary to reduce the depth of the periodontal pocket and when fibrous gingival tissue must be removed. The procedure involves making bleeding points with pocket markers and removing gingival tissue with periodontal knives and scissors. Recently, dental laser equipment has become popular for gingivectomy (see later discussion). After healing, the pockets are reduced, and it is easier for the patient to clean the area (Fig. 55.28).

### *Gingivoplasty*

**Gingivoplasty** involves the surgical reshaping and contouring of gingival tissues. The presence of *deep periodontal pockets* with

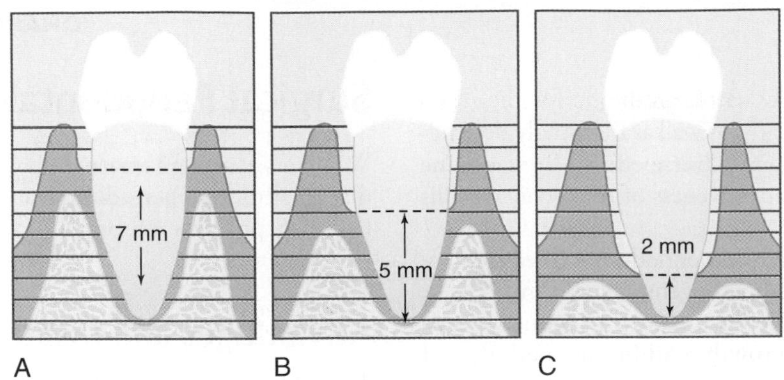


**FIG. 55.27** Prognosis based on amount of bone loss. A, When some bone is present, it may be safe to postpone surgery and take a wait-and-see approach. An additional bone loss of 2 mm may not alter the prognosis of the tooth. B, When half the bone has been lost, an additional 2 mm loss can seriously jeopardize the tooth; therefore surgery is highly recommended. C, With advanced bone loss, surgery may be performed in an effort to save the tooth, but the prognosis is poor. *(From Perry DA, Beemsterboer PL: Periodontology for the dental hygienist, ed 4, St Louis, 2014, Saunders.)*

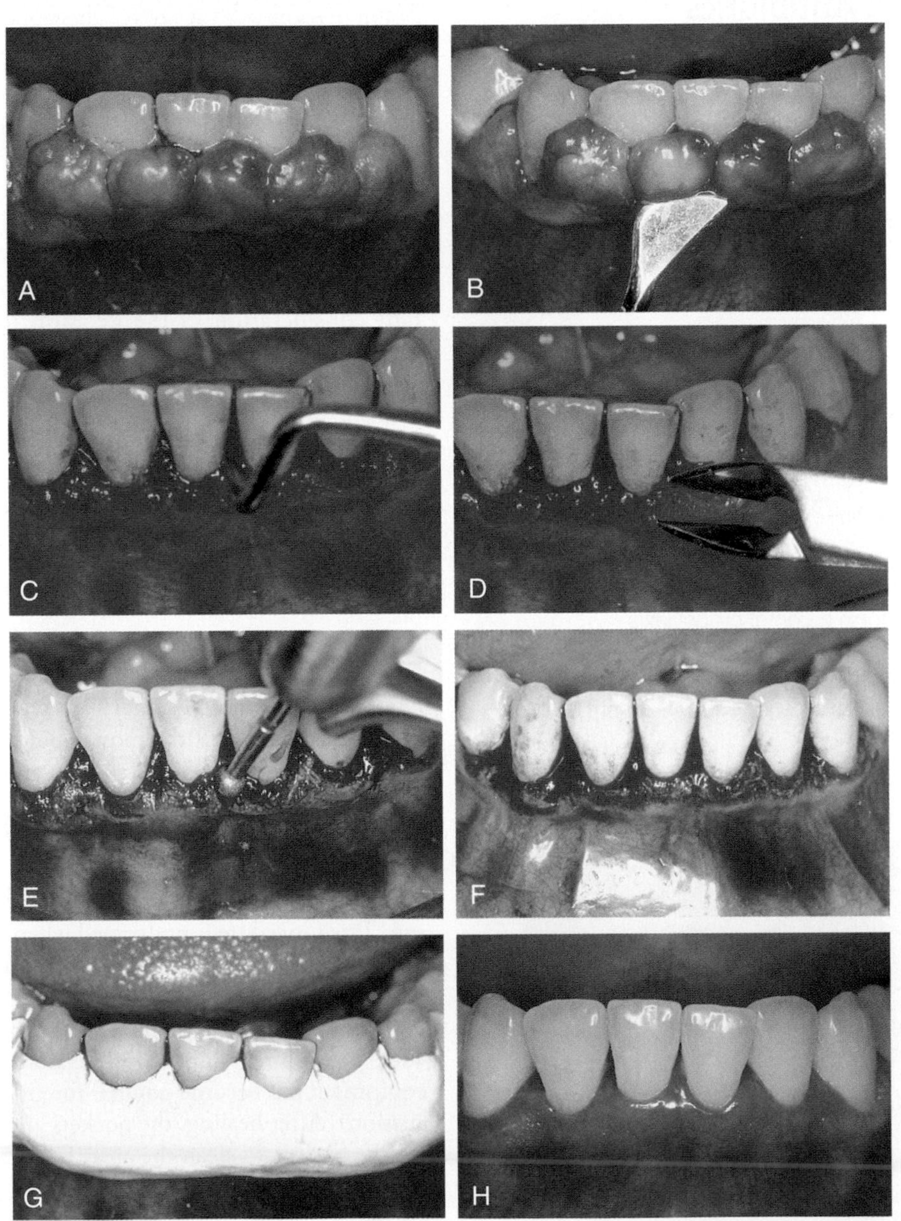


**FIG. 55.28** Gingivectomy surgery to treat gingival enlargement. A, Enlarged gingivae. B, Initial incision with a Kirkland knife. C, Interproximal tissue removed with an Orban knife. D and E, Gingivoplasty performed with tissue nippers and a round diamond bur. F, Surgery completed. G, Periodontal pack placed. H, Surgical area 3 months after surgery. *(From Newman M, Takei T, Klokkevold P et al, editors: Carranza's clinical periodontology, ed 12, St Louis, 2015, Saunders.)*

fibrous tissue is the main indication for both gingivectomy and gingivoplasty. Often, the two procedures are performed simultaneously. See Procedure 55.2: Assisting with Gingivectomy and Gingivoplasty.

During gingivoplasty, the gingivae are recontoured with the use of periodontal knives, rotary diamond burs, curettes, and surgical scissors. Gingival margins are thinned and are given a scalloped edge.

## Incisional Surgery

Incisional surgery, also known as **periodontal flap surgery** or simply **flap surgery**, is performed when excisional surgery is not indicated. In flap surgery, the tissues *are not removed* but are pushed away from underlying tooth roots and alveolar bone, similar to the flap of an envelope.

When the flap is elevated (lifted up), the dentist may perform one or more of the following procedures:

- Thorough scaling and root planing of exposed root surfaces
- Moving of the flap laterally (to the side) to cover the root surfaces of an adjacent tooth that does not have adequate tissue coverage (laterally sliding flap)
- Recontouring (reshaping) of underlying bone

After the procedure has been completed, the flap is closed and is sutured into place. A periodontal dressing usually is placed after flap surgery.

## Osseous Surgery

Periodontitis is a disease that involves the loss of connective tissue and alveolar bone. **Osseous surgery** is periodontal surgery that involves modification of the supporting bone. It is performed to eliminate pockets, remove defects, and restore normal contours in the bone. Types of periodontal surgeries that involve bone include *osteoplasty* and *ostectomy.* Each requires surgical exposure of the bone, along with recontouring or removal of bone with a rotary diamond bur or a bone chisel (Fig. 55.29).

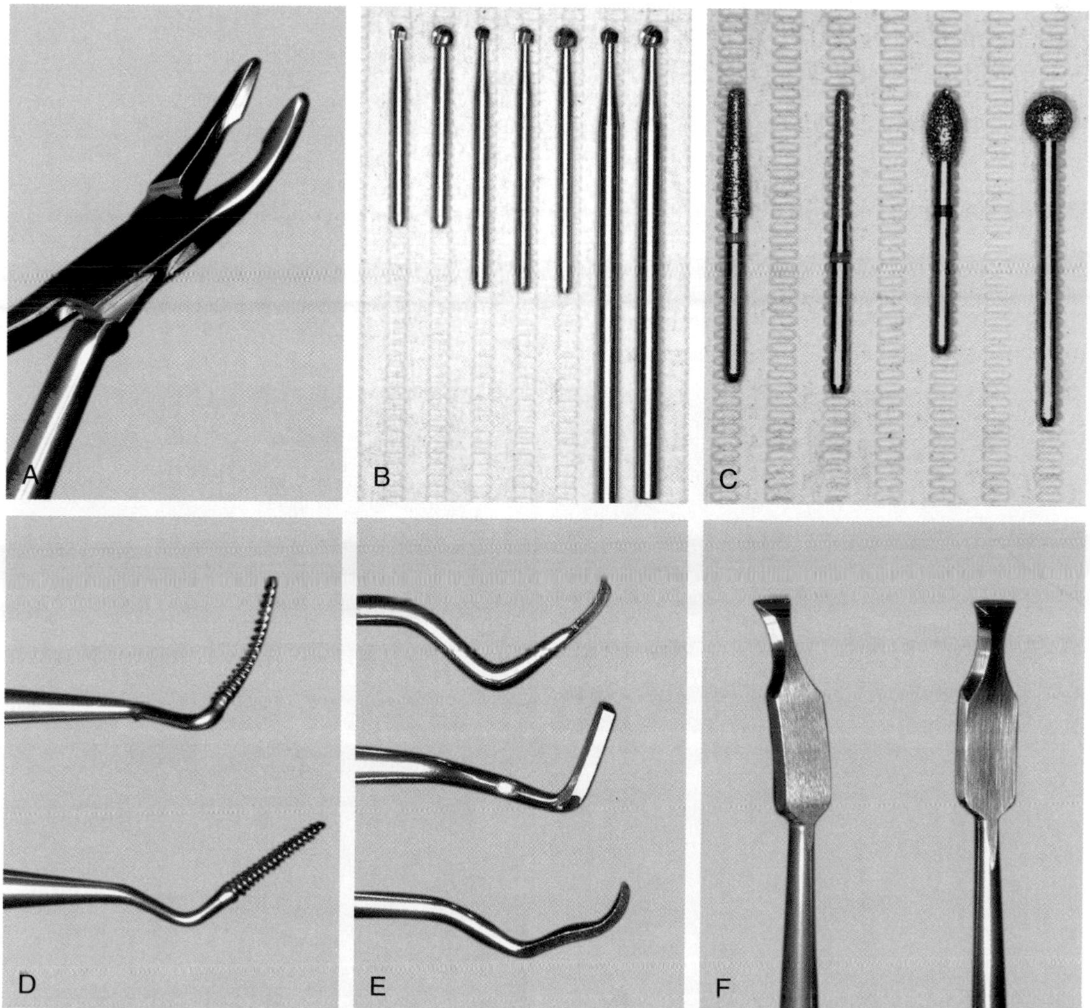


**FIG. 55.29** Instruments often used in osseous surgery. A, Rongeurs. B, Carbide round burs. *Left to right:* Friction grip, surgical-length friction grip, and slow-speed handpiece. C, Diamond burs. D, Interproximal files: Schluger and Sugarman. E, Back-action chisels. F, Ochsenbein chisels. *(From Newman M, Takei T, Klokkevold P et al, editors: Carranza's clinical periodontology, ed 12, St Louis, 2015, Saunders.)*

### Osteoplasty

In **osteoplasty**, or *additive bone surgery*, bone is contoured and reshaped. In addition, bone may be added through *bone grafting* (taking bone from one area and placing it in another) or *placement of artificial bone-substitute materials* through a procedure called **bone augmentation**. This procedure is useful for patients with bone defects caused by periodontal disease or during preparation for implants in patients without adequate bony support.

### Ostectomy

In **ostectomy**, or *subtractive bone surgery*, bone is removed. This procedure is necessary when the patient has large *exostoses* (bony growths). For example, an ostectomy is performed if a patient needs a full denture and the bony growth would interfere with the comfort and fit of the denture. Some patients require both an osteoplasty and an ostectomy (Fig. 55.30).

## Crown Lengthening

**Crown lengthening** is a surgical procedure that is designed to expose more tooth structure for the placement of a restoration such as a crown. Crown lengthening is becoming a very common procedure for esthetic anterior restorations. Surgical crown lengthening may involve the removal of soft tissue or of soft tissue and alveolar bone. In addition to esthetics, indications for crown lengthening include (1) a tooth that is fractured close to the gingival margin or alveolar crest, and (2) subgingival caries (Fig. 55.31).

## Soft Tissue Grafts

### Pedicle Graft

The pedicle graft is used to move gingivae from an adjacent tooth or edentulous area to a recipient site on another tooth. The pedicle graft is "freed" on three sides but remains attached on one side and thus retains its blood supply. The pedicle graft is best used for single-site recession for root coverage and for increasing the amount of attached gingivae.

### Free Gingival Soft Tissue Graft

In contrast to the pedicle graft, a free gingival graft has a donor site that is located away from the grafted site. Thus the blood supply is not attached to the graft and depends on the recipient site. The most common site for donor tissue is the patient's palate; however, edentulous areas also can be used (Fig. 55.32).

## Postsurgical Patient Instructions

After periodontal surgery, the periodontist most likely will prescribe an analgesic (pain medication) and possibly an antibiotic. Many periodontists recommend the use of an antibacterial rinse twice daily to help with plaque control. A chlorhexidine mouthwash may be used during the first week to freshen the mouth and inhibit plaque formation during the early stages of healing.

Postoperative instructions should be given to the patient to ease discomfort and promote healing.

### Patient Instructions After Periodontal Surgery

**Activity:** Limit your activities for the next few days to those requiring minimal exertion.

**Rinsing:** Do not rinse your mouth for 24 hours.

**Bleeding:** Some slight bleeding may occur during the first 4 or 5 hours after the operation. This bleeding is not unusual. If bleeding continues, apply firm pressure for 20 minutes with a piece of gauze. Repeat as necessary. Do not remove the gauze during this period. Do not rinse with water to stop the bleeding. If bleeding persists, call the office.

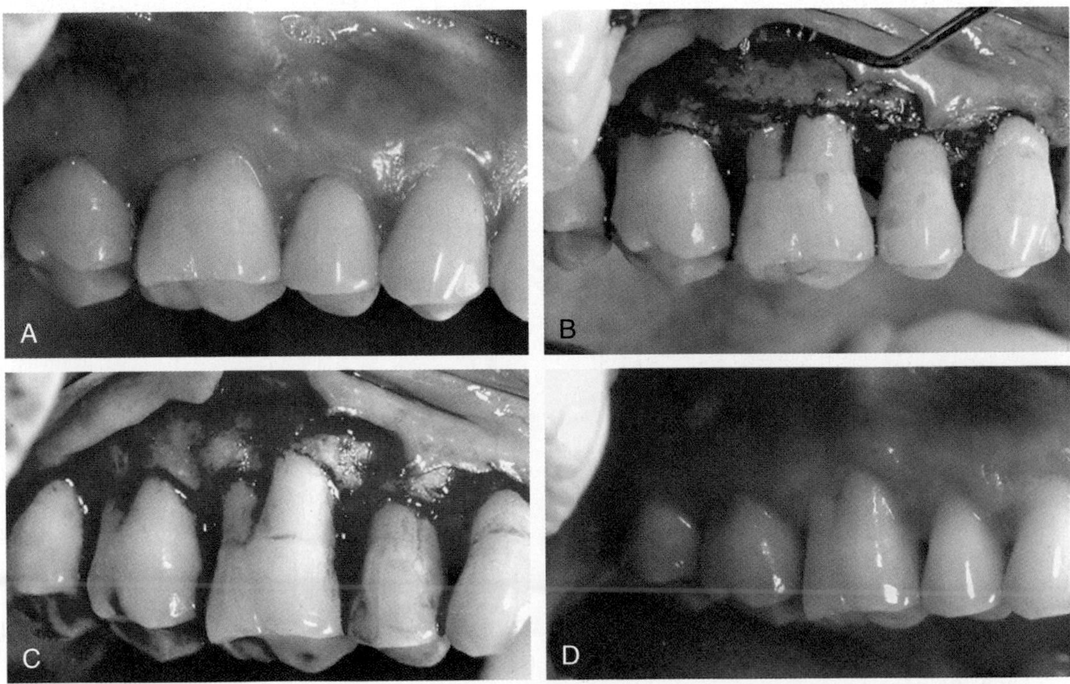


**FIG. 55.30** Reduction of bony ledges by osteoplasty. A, Buccal preoperative photograph showing two crowns and exostoses. B, Flap retracted to show a facial exostosis. C, After osseous surgery; the bulk of the bony removal was performed by osteoplasty, with minor ostectomy between the two molars. D, Postoperative photograph at 6 weeks. *(Courtesy Dr. Joseph Schwartz, Portland, OR.)*

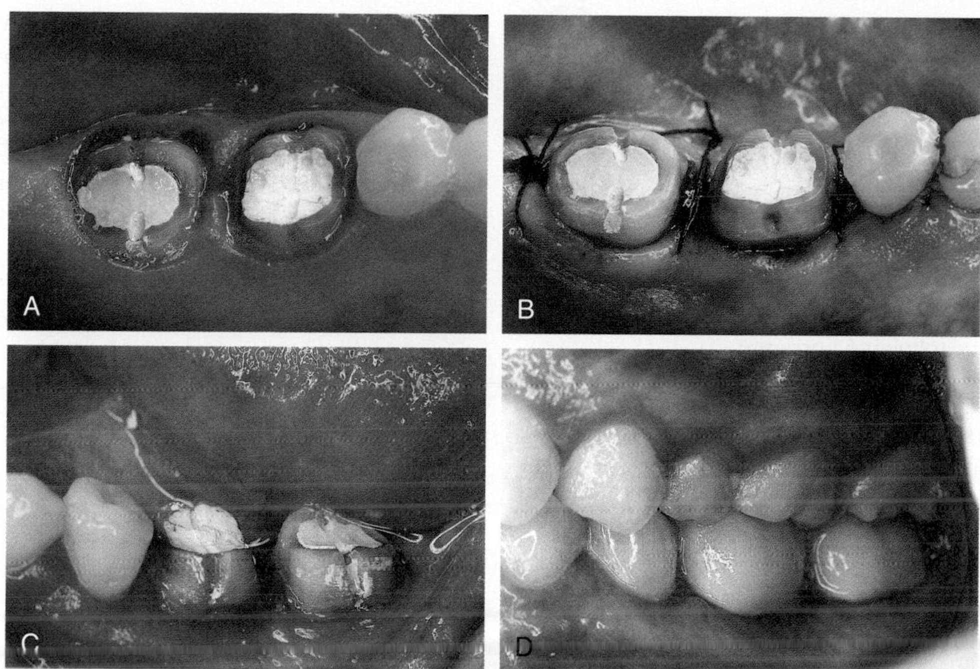

**FIG. 55.31** Surgical crown lengthening has provided these otherwise unrestorable mandibular molars with improved retention and restorative access for successful restorations. A, Before crown lengthening. B, Crown lengthening surgery completed. C, Buccal view after surgery. D, Final restoration. *(From Newman M, Takei T, Klokkevold P et al, editors: Carranza's clinical periodontology, ed 12, St Louis, 2015, Saunders.)*

## Patient Instructions After Periodontal Surgery—cont'd

**Discomfort:** Some discomfort is to be expected when the anesthesia wears off. If you have been given a prescription, fill it and take the medication as directed. If discomfort persists, call the office.

**Eating:** Limit yourself to a soft diet immediately after surgery. Avoid chewing in the area of surgery. Do not drink very hot beverages the first day. You may return to your regular diet as soon as you feel comfortable. Highly seasoned or spicy foods may irritate the area of surgery.

**Dressing:** A dressing material may have been placed around your teeth. It will become hard within about 2 hours and should not be disturbed. Although the dressing may remain in place until your next appointment, small parts may chip off. If a large portion of the dressing comes off, call the office for instructions.

**Swelling:** Swelling is expected after some procedures. You may use an ice pack on the outside of your face, 15 minutes on and 15 minutes off, for the next 4 hours. If excessive swelling develops in your neck or under your chin, call the office.

**Smoking:** Do not smoke. Smoking may interfere with the healing process and produce poor results.

**Home care:** If a surgical dressing is present, brush the top of the dressing lightly with a soft toothbrush. If no dressing is present, gently use a soft toothbrush to clean the area of surgery for the first few days. You may rinse gently with a medicated mouthwash if it was prescribed, or with warm salt water, starting the day after surgery.

IF YOU HAVE ANY QUESTIONS OR CONCERNS, CALL THE OFFICE. Telephone number: ___________.

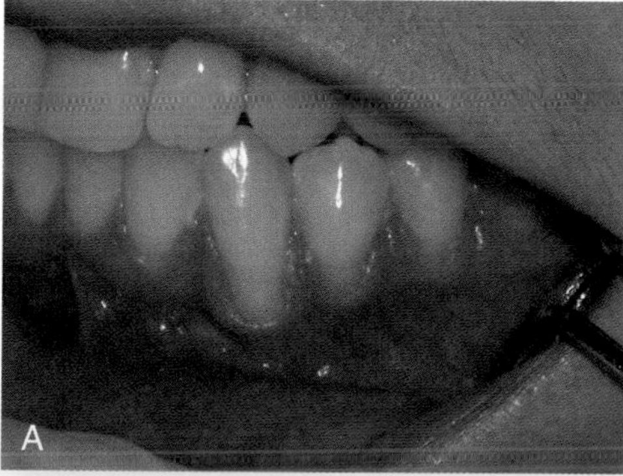

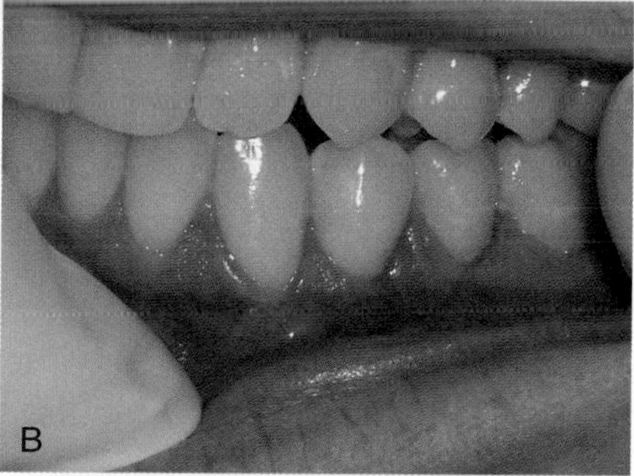

**FIG. 55.32** A, Gingival recession around #22 before soft tissue graft. B, After soft tissue graft. *(Courtesy Dr. Christine Ford, Santa Rosa, CA.)*

19 What is the primary goal of periodontal surgery?
20 From a patient's point of view, what are the primary disadvantages of periodontal surgery?
21 What is a gingivectomy?
22 What is the purpose of osseous surgery?

## Periodontal Surgical Dressings

A **periodontal dressing (periopack)** serves as a bandage over the surgical site. Periodontal dressings, also known as *periopacks,* are used for the following purposes:

- To hold the flaps in place
- To protect newly forming tissues
- To minimize postoperative pain, infection, and hemorrhage
- To protect the surgical site from trauma during eating and drinking
- To support mobile teeth during the healing process

A variety of materials are available on the market for periodontal dressings. The dressings most often used are those made with zinc oxide–eugenol (ZOE) and those made without eugenol.

### Zinc Oxide–Eugenol Dressing

The ZOE dressing is supplied as a powder and a liquid that are mixed before use. The material can be mixed beforehand, wrapped in waxed paper, and frozen for future use (Fig. 55.33).

ZOE has a slow set, which allows for a longer working time. It sets to a firm and heavy consistency and provides good support and protection for tissues and flaps. Some patients are allergic to the eugenol and will experience redness and burning pain in the area of the dressing.

### Noneugenol Dressing

The noneugenol dressing is the most widely used type of periodontal dressing. This material is supplied in two tubes—one for the base material and the other for the accelerator.

Noneugenol material is easy to mix and place and has a smooth surface for patient comfort. This material has a rapid setting time if exposed to warm temperatures, and it *cannot be mixed* and *stored in advance* (Fig. 55.34). See Procedure 55.3: Preparing and Placing a Noneugenol Periodontal Dressing and Procedure 55.4: Removing a Periodontal Dressing.

23 What is the function of a periodontal surgical dressing?
24 What materials are most commonly used in periodontal dressings?

## Esthetic and Plastic Periodontal Surgery

Today, more and more general dentists are increasing the scope of their practice by providing new esthetic and cosmetic procedures, including resin restorations, porcelain veneers and crowns, and dental implants. To enhance the patient's esthetic appearance, the teeth and tissues must appear natural and healthy. The relationship between periodontal health and the restoration of teeth is critical. For restorations to be functional and esthetic, the periodontium must be healthy. For the periodontium to remain healthy, restorations must be properly designed and placed. Together, general dentists and periodontists are working to provide optimum periodontal health and a focus on the esthetics and function of restorations. **Periodontal plastic surgery** procedures are used to correct defects in the shape, position, or amount of gingival tissue (Fig. 55.35).

### Types of Periodontal Plastic Surgery

- Crown lengthening
- Ridge augmentation
- Esthetic surgical correction
- Coverage of denuded root surfaces
- Reconstruction of papilla
- Esthetic correction around implants
- Surgical exposure of unerupted teeth for orthodontics
- Periodontal-prosthodontic correction

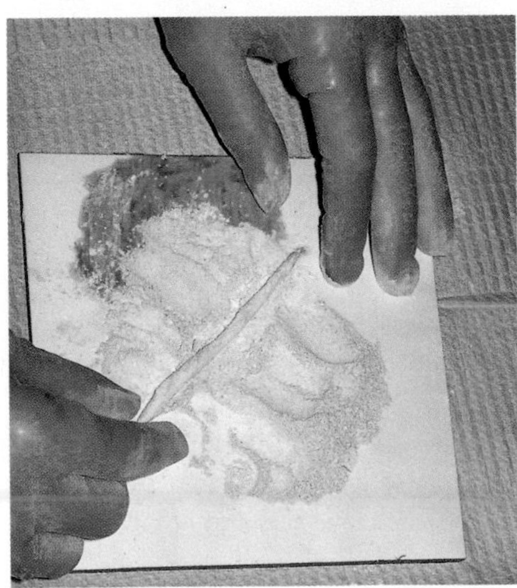

**FIG. 55.33** Zinc oxide powder and liquid eugenol are mixed in advance.

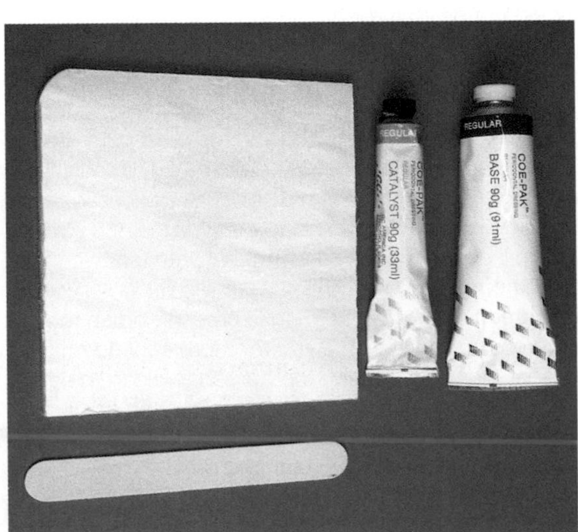


**FIG. 55.34** Paste for noneugenol dressing is ready to be mixed.

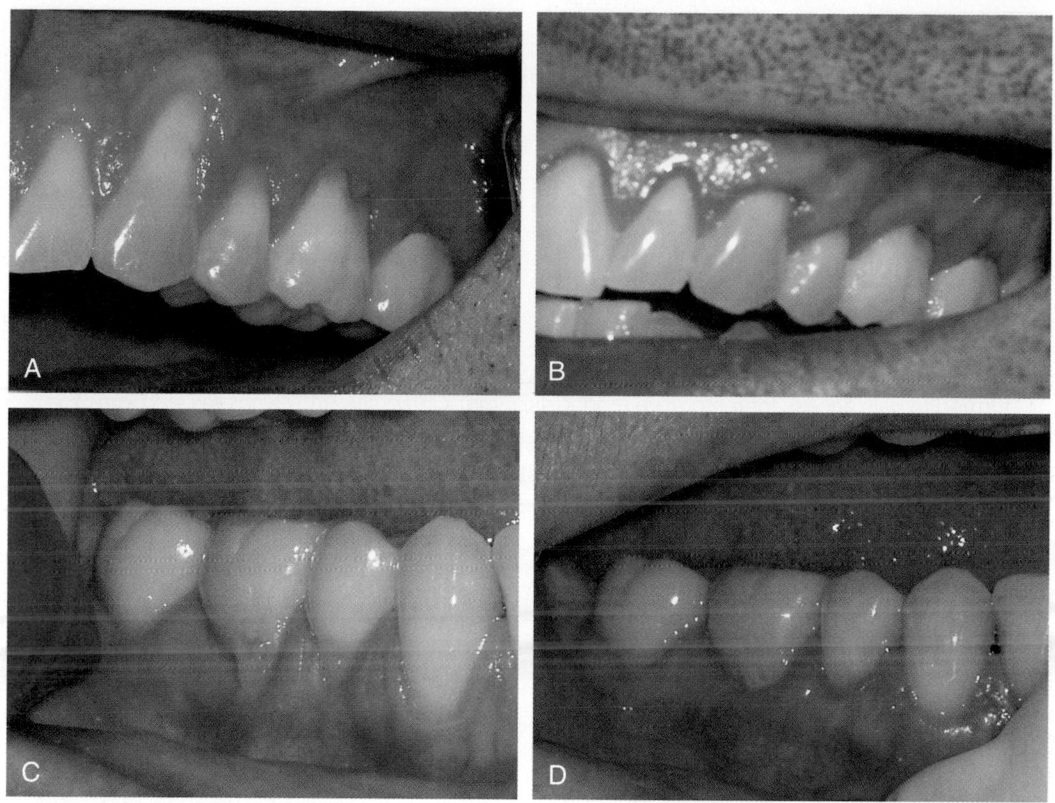


**FIG. 55.35** A and C, Presurgical recession of gingival tissues. B and D, Healed tissues after gingival graft surgery. *(Courtesy Dr. Christine Ford, Santa Rosa, CA.)*

## Lasers in Periodontics

The term **laser** is an acronym for *light amplification by stimulated emission of radiation.* A laser beam is a highly concentrated beam of light. The power of this beam can be adjusted to enable it to cut, vaporize, or cauterize tissue (Fig. 55.36).

The use of lasers offers a promising new technology for dentistry. Research is continuing that may lead to more widespread uses of lasers in clinical dentistry. Periodontal applications of lasers on soft tissue include the following:

- Removal of tumors and lesions
- Vaporization of excess tissues, as in gingivoplasty (Fig. 55.37), gingivectomy, and *frenectomy* (Fig. 55.38)
- Removal of or reduction in hyperplastic tissues (Fig. 55.39)
- Control of bleeding in vascular lesions (Fig. 55.40)

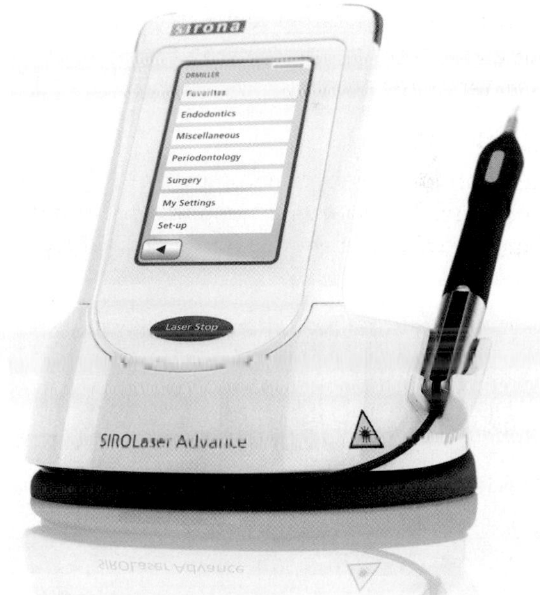


**FIG. 55.36** Laser unit. *(Courtesy Sirona Dental Inc., Charlotte, NC.)*

### Advantages of Laser Surgery

Lasers offer the following advantages over conventional surgical techniques:

- Laser incisions heal faster than incisions made with electrosurgery. (However, incisions made with scalpels heal faster than those made with lasers.)
- Hemostasis (control of bleeding) is rapid.
- The surgical field is relatively dry.
- The risk of blood-borne contamination is reduced.
- Less trauma occurs to adjacent tissues.
- Postsurgical swelling, scarring, and pain are reduced.
- Some procedures can be performed more quickly.
- Patients who are afraid of "surgery" may accept laser therapy.

### Laser Safety

Precautions must be taken to protect both the patient and the dental staff during laser procedures. Any person who operates

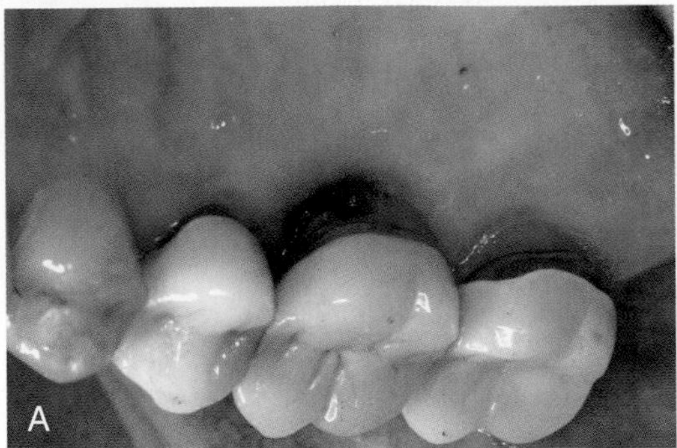


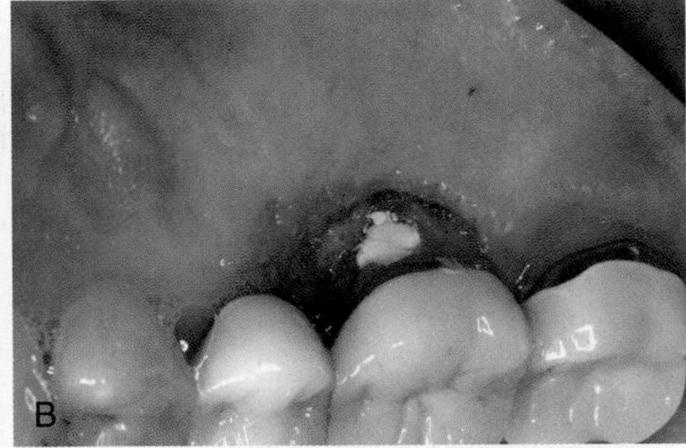


**FIG. 55.37** Preoperative (A) and immediate postoperative (B) views of a gingivectomy performed to gain access for restorative prognosis. *(From Convissar RA: Principles and practice of laser dentistry, St Louis, 2011, Mosby.)*

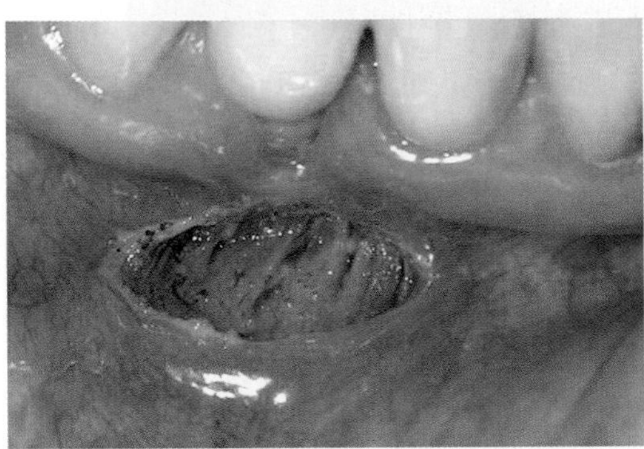

**FIG. 55.38** Immediate postoperative view of a frenectomy. Note the lack of bleeding. *(From Convissar RA: Principles and practice of laser dentistry, St Louis, 2011, Mosby.)*

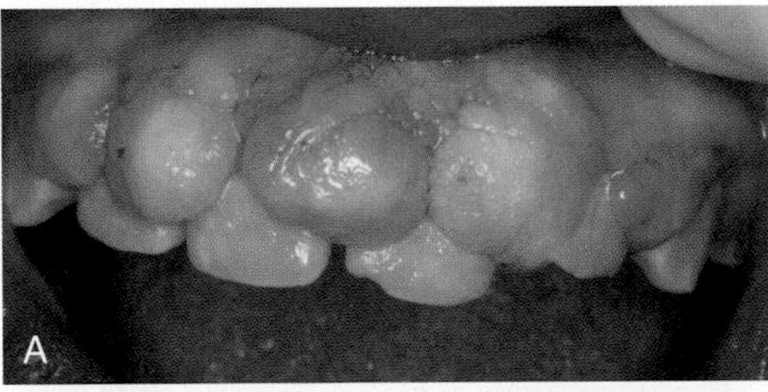


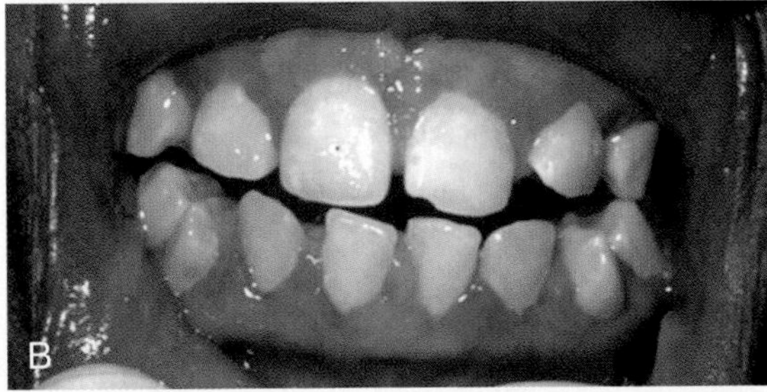


**FIG. 55.39** Laser removal of excess tissue caused by cyclosporine-induced gingival hyperplasia. A, Preoperative photo of excess tissue caused by cyclosporine-induced gingival hyperplasia. B, Postoperative photo following laser removal of excess tissue. *(From Convissar RA: Principles and practice of laser dentistry, St Louis, 2011, Mosby.)*

a laser or assists during a laser operation must be thoroughly trained in the use of this powerful instrument.

Guidelines for laser safety include the following protective devices and measures:

- *Shielded eyeglasses.* The dental staff and the patient must wear special shielded eyeglasses to protect the eyes (Fig. 55.41).
- *Matte-finished instruments.* Reflective surfaces such as instruments, mirrors, and even polished restorations can reflect laser energy. Matte-finished (nonshiny) instruments are recommended to avoid this reflection (Fig. 55.42).
- *Protection of nontarget tissues.* Nontarget oral tissue (tissues not being treated with the laser) should be shielded with wet gauze packs.
- *High-volume evacuation.* HVE should be used to draw off the *plume* (cloud) created when tissue vaporizes. This plume could be infectious.

**25** Are there any training requirements for persons who work with lasers?

■ **Patient Education** The dental assistant can play an important role in a periodontal office. Patients must be educated about the cause of their disease and about how to incorporate new oral hygiene techniques that will help them achieve good periodontal health (see Chapters 14 and 15).

Periodontal patients usually require more complex home care procedures than simple toothbrushing and flossing. These patients often have areas of attachment loss caused by the disease process or resulting from periodontal surgery. It can be very challenging for the patient to clean furcations, periodontal pockets, and areas of root exposure.

Patients with periodontal disease usually have had poor oral hygiene most of their lives that has contributed to their disease process. The dental assistant can help motivate the periodontal patient to begin and continue a lifelong process of improved daily oral hygiene. Thorough home care may require an additional 15 to 30 minutes a day. It is not easy for patients to change lifetime habits, and the dental assistant must be patient, understanding, and encouraging with each patient. ■

■ **Legal and Ethical Implications** Two of the most common types of malpractice suits result from failure to diagnose periodontal disease and failure to refer patients to a periodontist when necessary.

Accurate diagnosis of periodontal disease requires a comprehensive clinical examination. This examination should include

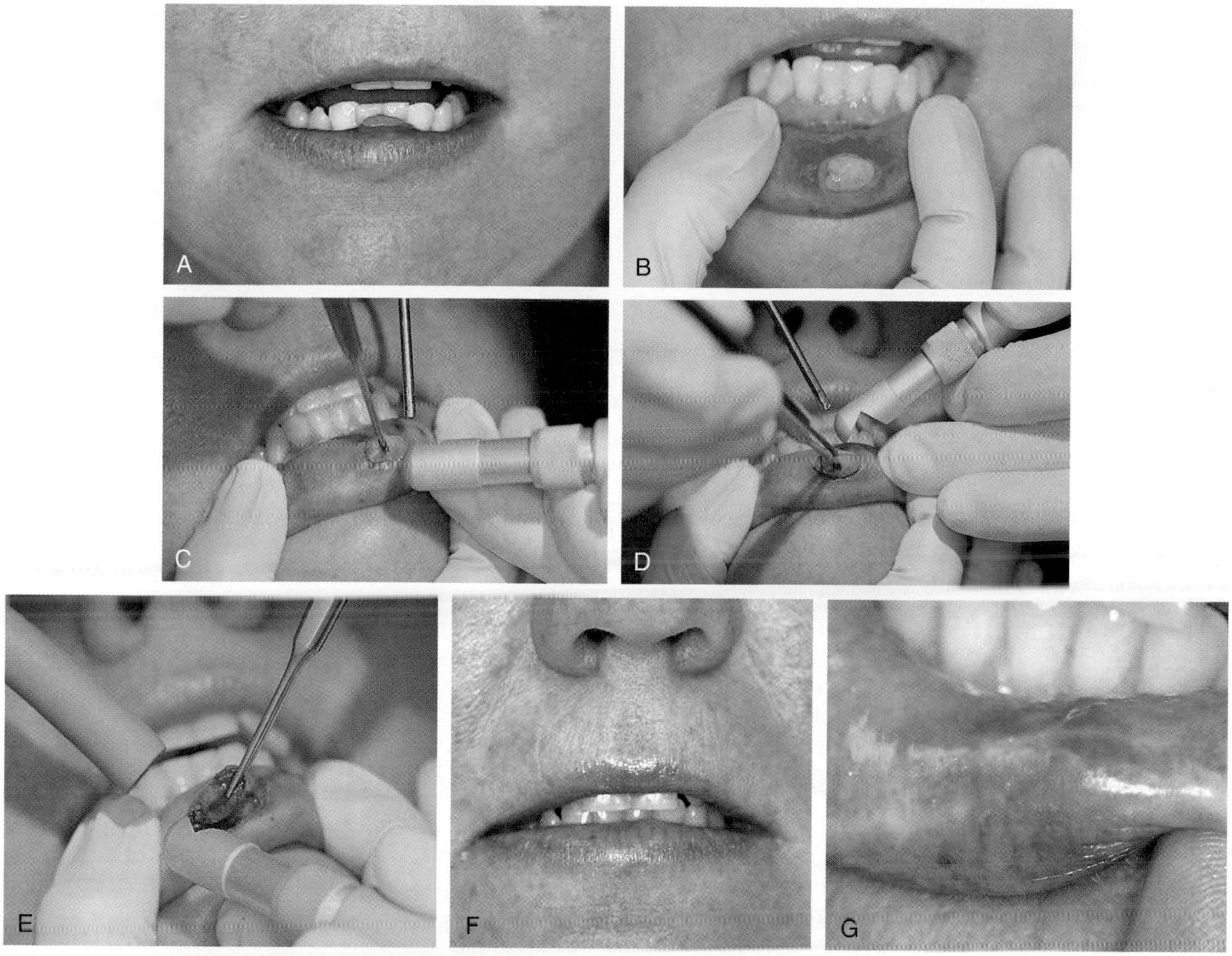

**FIG. 55.40** A and B, A lesion of the lower lip. C and D, Incision is performed using a laser. E, Complete removal of the lesion. F and G, At 10 days, sutures have been removed; note the favorable esthetic result. *(From Convissar RA: Principles and practice of laser dentistry, St Louis, 2011, Mosby.)*

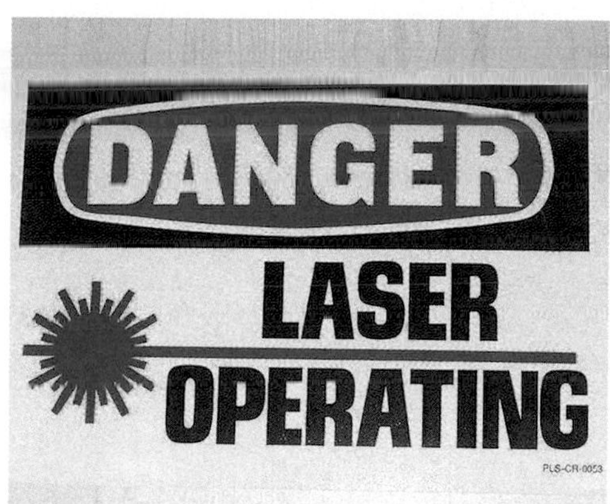


**FIG. 55.41** To prevent injury to the eyes of persons who are not wearing special light filter glasses, warning signs must be placed in areas where lasers are used.

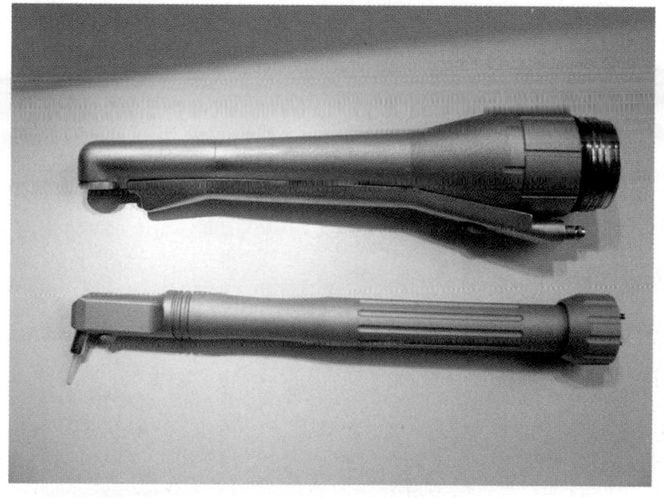

**FIG. 55.42** Matte-finished laser instruments. *(From Convissar RA: Principles and practice of laser dentistry, St Louis, 2011, Mosby.)*

extraoral, intraoral, oral mucosal, oral hygiene, and comprehensive periodontal and dentition assessments. Each of these assessments must be documented. It is unacceptable to assess the patient's oral health without documenting that information in the patient's record. Documentation serves many purposes in providing a historical record, a patient education tool, and a guide to treatment planning. It may also serve as an important part of a legal defense. ■

**■ Eye to the Future** New evidence suggests that periodontal disease is a risk factor in the development and management of serious systemic disease. In particular, periodontal infections have been implicated in cardiovascular disease, conditions affecting preterm low-birth-weight infants, and bacterial pneumonia. In addition, it appears to be more difficult to control non–insulin-dependent diabetes in patients with severe periodontitis.

Studies conducted by the National Institutes of Health suggest that in people older than 40 years of age, a relationship exists between periodontal conditions and the history of heart attacks. The inflammatory response in periodontal disease may influence buildup in the arterial walls. Research regarding the relationship between heart disease and periodontal disease will continue. It is obvious, however, that a healthy mouth is necessary for a healthy body. ■

## ■ Critical Thinking

1. Mrs. Camp has been a patient in your general dental office for longer than 20 years. She has a history of missing her regular appointments for dental cleanings, and her home care is not ideal. At her most recent visit, the dentist told Mrs. Camp that she is developing periodontal pockets of 4 to 6 mm and should be referred to a periodontist. Mrs. Camp does not want to seek periodontal care and promised that she will faithfully brush and floss her teeth. What do you think the dentist will say to her? Why?
2. Why do you think the dental hygienist in your office may ask you to assist with suction when she uses the ultrasonic scaler?
3. What would you say to a very nervous patient who has just been referred to a periodontist for a gingivectomy? ■

PROCEDURE 55.1

# Assisting with a Dental Prophylaxis

### GOAL

To assist competently with a dental prophylaxis procedure.

### EQUIPMENT AND SUPPLIES

- Mouth mirror
- Explorer
- Anterior scaler
- Universal curette
- Disposable prophy angle with rubber cup
- Disposable prophy angle with bristle brush
- Prophy paste
- Saliva ejector and/or high-volume evacuator (HVE)
- 2 × 2 gauze
- Dental floss or tape

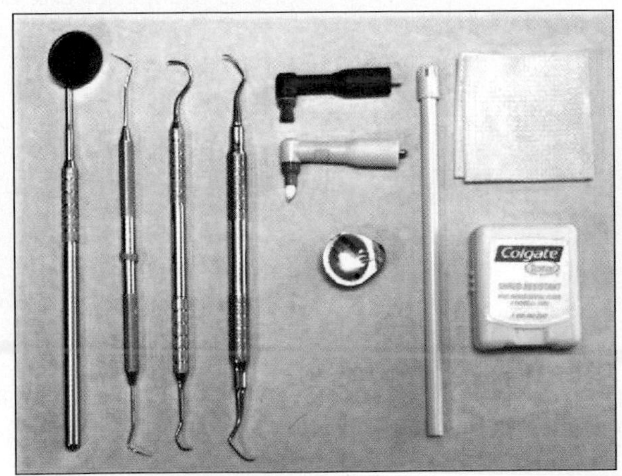


### PROCEDURAL STEPS

1. Assist with transfers as the operator uses an explorer to locate interproximal and subgingival calculus.
   **NOTE** The operator must have good access and visibility during this procedure.
2. Use the HVE as necessary and retract the lips, tongue, and cheeks to improve visibility and access as the operator uses scalers and curettes to remove all calculus and plaque.
3. The operator checks for and removes any remaining calculus.
4. The operator polishes the teeth using polishing paste, a rubber cup, and bristle brushes.
5. The operator removes any remaining interproximal debris with dental floss or tape.
6. Provide oral hygiene instructions appropriate to the individual needs of the patient.
7. Document the procedure.

PROCEDURE 55.2

# Assisting with Gingivectomy and Gingivoplasty

## GOAL

To assist the dentist competently in performing gingivectomy and gingivoplasty periodontal procedures.

## EQUIPMENT AND SUPPLIES

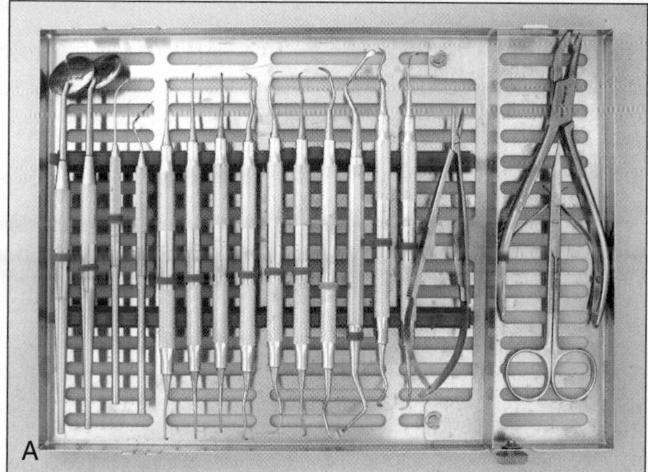


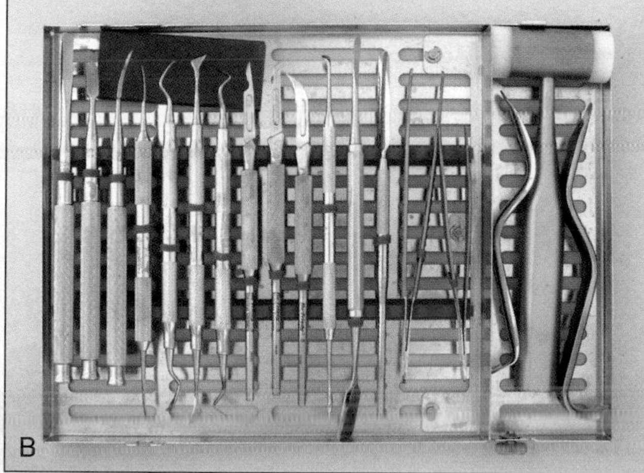


Typical series of periodontal surgical instruments, divided into two cassettes. A, *From left,* Mirrors, explorer, probe, series of curettes, needle holder, rongeurs, and scissors. B, *From left,* Series of chisels, Kirkland knife, Orban knife, scalpel handles with surgical blades (#15C, #15, #12D), periosteal elevators, spatula, tissue forceps, cheek retractors, mallet, and sharpening stone. *(A, Courtesy Hu-Friedy, Chicago, IL.* B, *Courtesy G. Hartzell & Son, Concord, CA.)*

## PROCEDURAL STEPS

### Role of the Dental Assistant

1 Set out the patient's health history, radiographs, and periodontal chart.
**PURPOSE** The dentist must review the case before surgery.

2 Assist in the administration of local anesthetic.

3 Anticipate the dentist's needs, and be prepared to transfer and retrieve surgical instruments when needed.
**PURPOSE** To save time and make the procedure less stressful.

4 Have gauze ready to remove tissue from the instruments as necessary.
**PURPOSE** Periodontal surgery can generate heavy bleeding.

5 Provide oral evacuation and retraction.
**PURPOSE** Good access and visibility are critical for the dentist, and the patient will be more comfortable.

6 Irrigate with sterile saline.
**PURPOSE** To keep the surgical site clean and free of debris.

7 If sutures are used, prepare the suture needle and suture material, and position them in a hemostat or needle holder. Transfer them to the dentist when requested.
**PURPOSE** To simplify the procedure for the dentist, and to aid in patient comfort.

8 Place, or assist with placement of, the periodontal dressing.
**PURPOSE** The dressing acts as a bandage to protect the surgical site.
**NOTE** Check your state's dental practice act before placing a periodontal dressing without assistance.

9 Wipe any blood or debris from the patient's face. Provide postoperative instructions to the patient.
**PURPOSE** To ensure that the patient clearly understands the postoperative instructions as necessary for personal well-being, and to address legal considerations.

10 Document the procedure.

### Role of the Dentist

1 The dentist administers the local anesthetic.
**PURPOSE** In addition to pain control, local anesthetic aids visibility by constricting blood vessels so there is less blood at the surgical site.

2 The dentist marks the pockets on the facial and lingual gingivae by using the periodontal pocket marker.
**PURPOSE** Bleeding points indicate the pocket depth and thus the point for the initial incision.

3 The dentist uses a scalpel or periodontal knife to incise the gingiva at a 45-degree angle, while following along the bleeding points. The incision is beveled to create a normally contoured, free gingival margin.

4 The dentist removes the gingival tissue along the incision line using surgical knives.

5 The dentist tapers the gingival margins and creates a scalloped marginal outline.
**PURPOSE** To create an attractive and healthy appearance.

6 The dentist shapes the interdental papillae using interdental knives.
**PURPOSE** To contour the interdental grooves.

7 The dentist performs scaling and root planing of the root surfaces.
**PURPOSE** To remove any residual calculus that was inaccessible before surgery.

8 The dentist places sutures if needed.

9 The dentist irrigates the surgical site and then covers it with a periodontal dressing.
**PURPOSE** To protect the surgical site.
**NOTE** In some states, placement and removal of the periodontal dressing are delegated to the dental assistant (expanded function).

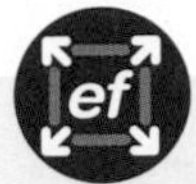

PROCEDURE 55.3 

# Preparing and Placing a Noneugenol Periodontal Dressing (Expanded Function*)

## GOAL

To prepare and assist the dentist in placing a noneugenol periodontal dressing.

## EQUIPMENT AND SUPPLIES

- ✔ Paper mixing pad (supplied by manufacturer)
- ✔ Wooden tongue depressor
- ✔ Noneugenol dressing (base and accelerator)
- ✔ Paper cup filled with room-temperature water
- ✔ Saline solution
- ✔ Plastic-type filling instrument

## PROCEDURAL STEPS

### Mixing the Material

1 Extrude equal lengths of the two pastes on the paper pad.

2 Mix the pastes with a wooden tongue depressor until a uniform color has been obtained (2 to 3 minutes).

3 When the paste loses its tackiness, place it in the paper cup filled with room-temperature water.

4 Lubricate gloved fingers with saline solution.

**PURPOSE** To prevent the material from sticking to the gloves.

5 Roll the paste into strips approximately the length of the surgical site.

### Placing the Dressing

6 Press small triangle-shaped pieces of dressing into the interproximal spaces.

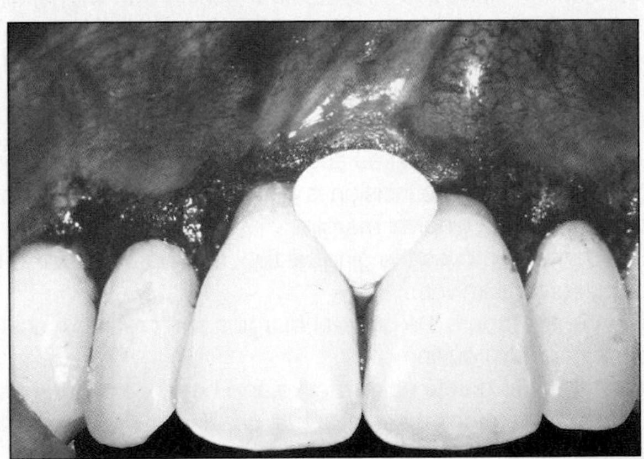

7 Adapt one end of the strip around the distal surface of the last tooth in the surgical site.

8 Bring the remainder of the strip forward along the facial surface, and gently press the strip along the incised gingival margin.

9 Gently press the strip into the interproximal areas.

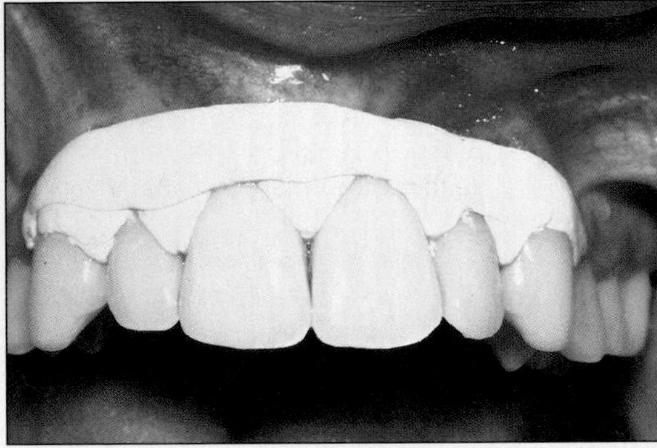

10 Apply the second strip in the same manner from the lingual side.

11 Join the facial and lingual strips at the distal surface of the last tooth at both ends of the surgical site.

12 Apply gentle pressure on the facial and lingual surfaces.

13 Check the dressing for overextension and interference with occlusion.

**PURPOSE** Excess packing irritates the mucobuccal fold and the floor of the mouth.

14 Remove any excess dressing, and adjust the new margins to remove any roughness.

**PURPOSE** If the pack is not adapted properly, it can break off.

### Documentation

15 Document the procedure.

*This procedure may not be considered an expanded function in your area. Check your local regulations.

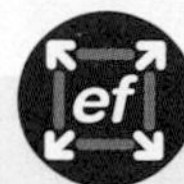

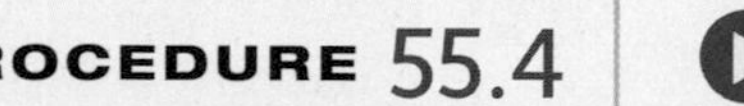
PROCEDURE 55.4

# Removing a Periodontal Dressing (Expanded Function*)

## GOAL

To remove a periodontal dressing.

## EQUIPMENT AND SUPPLIES

- ✔ Spoon excavator
- ✔ Suture scissors (for sutures if present)
- ✔ Dental floss
- ✔ Warm saline solution
- ✔ Irrigating solution
- ✔ High-volume evacuator (HVE) tip or saliva ejector

## PROCEDURAL STEPS

1 Gently insert the spoon excavator under the margin.

2 Use lateral pressure to pry the dressing gently away from the tissue.

**PURPOSE** The area may still be sensitive, and the newly healed tissue is delicate and easily injured.

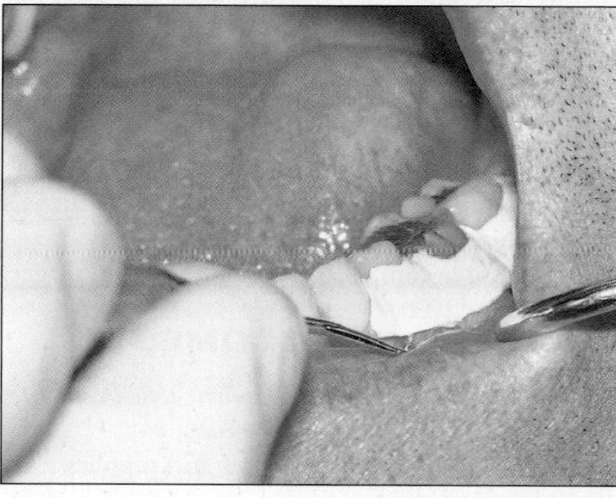

3 If sutures are embedded in the dressing material, cut the suture material free. Remove the sutures gently from the tissue.

**PURPOSE** Accidentally pulling the sutures could be painful for the patient and might open the wound.

4 Gently use dental floss to remove all fragments of dressing material from the interproximal surfaces.

**PURPOSE** Remaining fragments could cause discomfort for the patient and result in tissue irritation.

5 Irrigate the entire area gently with warm saline solution to remove superficial debris.

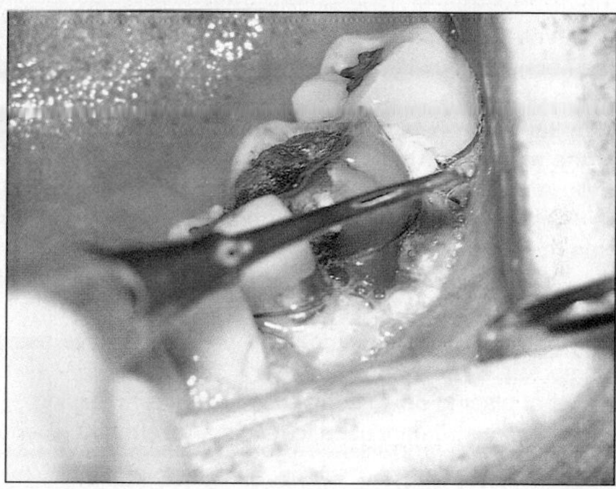

6 Use the HVE tip or saliva ejector to remove the fluid from the patient's mouth.

7 Document the procedure.

*This procedure may not be considered an expanded function in your area. Check your local regulations.

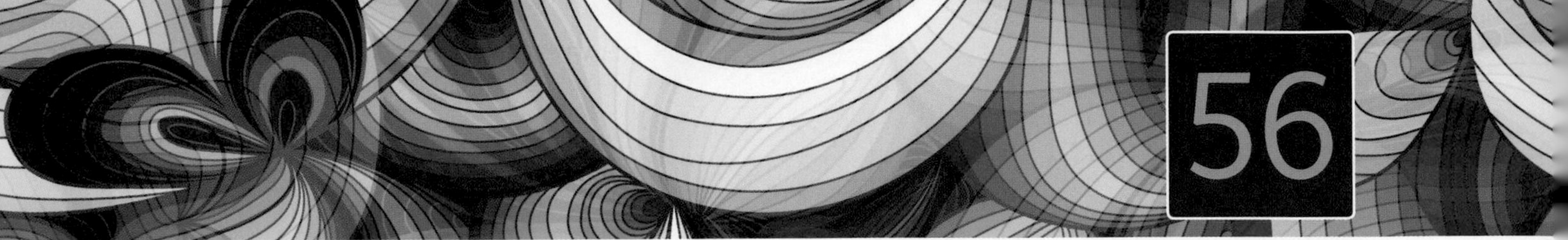

56

# Oral and Maxillofacial Surgery

## KEY TERMS

**Alveolar (al-vee-oh-lr) osteitis** Pain and inflammation resulting from exposed bone associated with the disturbance of a blood clot after extraction of a tooth.

**Alveoplasty (al-VEE-oh-plas-tee)** The surgical shaping and smoothing of the margins of the tooth socket after extraction of a tooth, generally in preparation for placement of a prosthesis.

**Bone file** Surgical instrument used to smooth rough edges of bone structure.

**Chisel** Surgical instrument used for cutting or severing a tooth and bone structure.

**Curette (kyoo-RET)** Surgical instrument used to remove tissue from a tooth socket.

**Donning** Act of placing on an item, such as gloves; dressing.

**Elevator** Surgical instrument used to reflect and retract the periodontal ligament and periosteum.

**Excisional biopsy (ek-SIZH-uh-nul BYE-op-see)** Surgical procedure in which tissue is cut from a suspected oral lesion.

**Exfoliative (eks-FOE-lee-uh-tiv) biopsy** Diagnostic procedure in which cells are scraped from a suspected oral lesion for analysis.

**Forceps (FOR-seps)** Surgical instrument used to grasp and hold onto teeth for their removal.

**Hard tissue impaction (im-PAK-shun)** Oral condition in which a tooth is partially to fully covered by bone and gingival tissue.

**Hemostat (HEE-moe-stat)** Surgical instrument used to hold or grasp items.

**Impacted tooth** Tooth that has not erupted.

**Incisional (in-SIZH-uh-nul) biopsy** Section of suspect oral lesion that is removed for evaluation.

**Luxate (LUK-sayt)** To dislocate, as a tooth from its socket.

**Mallet** Hammer-like instrument used with a chisel to section teeth or bone.

**Needle holder** Surgical instrument used to hold the suture needle.

**Oral and maxillofacial (MAK-sil-oe-fay-shul) surgeon (OMFS)** Dentist who has specialized in surgeries of the head and neck region.

**Oral and maxillofacial (MAK-sil-oe-fay-shul) surgery** Dental surgical specialty that diagnoses and treats conditions of the mouth, face, jaws, and associated areas.

**Outpatient** Patient seen and treated by a physician, then sent home for recovery.

**Retractor (ree-TRAK-tur)** Surgical instrument used to hold soft tissue away from the surgical site.

**Rongeur (raw-ZHUR, RON-gore)** Surgical instrument used to cut and trim the alveolar bone.

**Root tip picks** Surgical instrument used for the removal of root tips or fragments from the surgical site.

**Scalpel (SKAL-pul)** Surgical knife.

**Soft tissue impaction** Oral condition in which a tooth is partially to fully covered by gingival tissue.

## LEARNING OUTCOMES

*On completion of this chapter, the student will be able to achieve the following objectives:*

1. Pronounce, define, and spell the key terms.
2. Describe the specialty of oral and maxillofacial surgery and the roles of the oral surgeon and surgical assistant.
3. Describe surgical settings utilized in oral surgery.
4. Identify specialized instruments used for basic surgical procedures.
5. Explain the importance of the chain of asepsis during a surgical procedure.
6. Describe surgical procedures performed in a general practice.
7. Discuss sutures and suture removal.
8. Describe postoperative care given to a patient after a surgical procedure.
9. Discuss possible complications resulting from surgery.

## PERFORMANCE OUTCOMES

*On completion of this chapter, the student will be able to meet competency standards in the following skills:*

- Prepare a sterile field for instruments and supplies.
- Perform a surgical scrub.
- Perform sterile gloving.
- Assist in a forceps extraction.
- Assist in a multiple extraction procedure with alveoplasty.
- Assist in removal of an impacted tooth.
- Assist in suture placement.
- Perform suture removal.
- Assist in the treatment of alveolitis (dry socket).

## ELECTRONIC RESOURCES

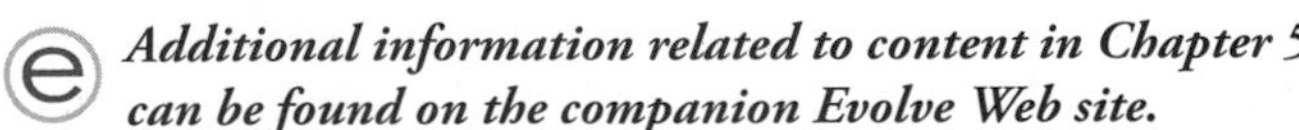

***Additional information related to content in Chapter 56 can be found on the companion Evolve Web site.***

- Practice Quiz
- Tray Setup Drag-and-Drop Exercises: Universal Surgical; Extraction of Maxillary Right First Molar/Impacted Mandibular Molar; Suture Removal
- Tray Setup Questions
- Video: Suture Removal

The specialty of **oral and maxillofacial surgery** is involved in the diagnosis and surgical treatment of diseases, injuries, and defects affecting the hard and soft tissues of the head and neck region.

### Indications for Oral and Maxillofacial Surgery

- Extraction of decayed teeth that cannot be restored
- Surgical removal of impacted teeth
- Extraction of nonvital teeth
- Preprosthesis surgery to smooth and contour the alveolar ridge
- Removal of teeth for orthodontic treatment
- Removal of root fragments
- Removal of cysts and tumors
- Biopsy
- Treatment of fractures of the mandible or maxilla
- Surgery to alter the size or shape of the facial bones
- Surgery of the temporomandibular joint
- Reconstructive surgery
- Cleft lip and cleft palate repairs
- Salivary gland surgery
- Surgical implant procedures

# Members of the Oral and Maxillofacial Surgical Team

## The Oral Surgeon

The **oral and maxillofacial surgeon (OMFS)**, also referred to as an oral surgeon, is a dentist who has received 4 to 6 years of postgraduate training in a hospital-based residency. The oral surgeon finishes a core surgical-medical year before program completion, with an emphasis on surgical techniques, anesthesiology, and oral medicine. The surgeon takes a national standardized examination of the American Board of Oral and Maxillofacial Surgery as a requirement to practice. It is common for oral surgeons to obtained their medical license as well.

The general dentist receives training in basic oral surgery procedures and can perform these in the private practice setting. For specific areas of the mouth and more complicated procedures, however, many dentists will refer their patients to an oral and maxillofacial surgeon.

## The Surgical Assistant

The surgical assistant is one of the most important members of the surgical team (Box 56.1). Surgical procedures are invasive and in-depth, requiring the surgical assistant to have advanced knowledge and skill in (1) patient assessment and monitoring, (2) use of specialized instruments, (3) surgical asepsis, (4) surgical procedures, and (5) pain control techniques.

After completion of a general dental-assisting program, dental assistants can further their education and training in a specialized program for surgical dental assistants, or through additional on-the-job training. Surgical dental assistants are often required to obtain certification in advanced cardiac life support and the use of additional monitoring procedures (see Chapter 27).

# The Surgical Setting

Surgical procedures are accomplished in two types of settings: the private dental office and the hospital or **outpatient** surgical suite.

## Surgical Preparation

Whether surgical procedures are performed in a private practice or in the operating room, an understanding of aseptic protocol, knowledge of needed supplies, and familiarity with the instruments used for a procedure are critical to the surgical assistant's role. The surgical team will follow a routine each time a patient is seen, and this routine should not be altered.

When you are preparing for a surgery, specific criteria must be met for smooth, efficient performance of procedural steps. Every surgical procedure requires preparation and advance planning by the dental team.

## Private Practice

An oral surgeon's private practice medicodental-surgical office consists of treatment areas similar to those in a general practice. In addition to treatment areas, the office will have a **surgical suite** that resembles an operating room, but on a much smaller scale. Specific items used only for surgical procedures, such as monitoring equipment, pain control units, and mobile trays, replace items seen in a general practice.

The patient who is receiving surgical care from an OMFS in an office setting is considered as having *minor surgery* and is being seen as an outpatient. The patient will be advised to arrive before the scheduled surgery, have a recovery period at the office, and then be escorted home to complete the recovery phase.

## Operating Room

The operating room of a hospital or ambulatory setting is quite different from a private practice (Fig. 56.1). To acquire permission from a hospital to use its clinical facility, the oral surgeon must submit an application for privileges to practice at a particular institution. The hospital will then grant privileges to the oral surgeon on the basis of his or her training, competency, and experience.

The environment is spacious enough to accommodate the (1) operating table; (2) anesthesiology equipment; (3) mobile surgical trays, holding instruments, and supplies; (4) overhead lighting; (5) monitoring equipment; and (6) standing room for the surgeon, surgical assistant, roving assistant, and anesthesiologist.

**BOX 56.1** Surgical Assistant's Role in Oral Surgery

**Advanced Preparation**

- Check that the patient record and radiographs are in order.
- Have necessary consent forms signed and available for review.
- Verify that any information requested from the patient's physician has been received.
- If a prosthesis will be delivered to the patient, determine whether the dental laboratory has returned it.
- Verify that the appropriate surgical setups have been prepared and sterilized.
- Contact the patient and provide preoperative instructions for taking any needed premedication and for eating or drinking after midnight.
- Instruct patient to have someone drive him or her and stay during the procedure.

**Treatment Room Preparation**

- Prepare the treatment room by placing protective barriers on anything that may be touched during the procedure.
- Keep surgical instruments in their sterile wraps until ready for use. If a surgical tray has been set out, open it and place a sterile towel over the instruments.
- Have the appropriate pain control medications ready for administration (local anesthesia, nitrous oxide/oxygen inhalation, intravenous sedation).
- Have the necessary postoperative instructions ready to provide to the patient.

**Patient Preparation**

- Update the patient's medical history and all laboratory reports.
- Check that the patient has taken prescribed premedication. If not, the surgeon should be alerted immediately.
- Have radiographic images on screen.
- Take vital signs to determine a baseline.
- Prepare any additional monitoring equipment to be applied.
- Seat and drape the patient. (To protect the patient's clothing, a large drape is often used, in addition to a patient towel.)
- Adjust the chair into a comfortable reclining position. If general anesthesia is to be administered, place the patient in a supine position.

**During Surgery**

- Maintain the chain of asepsis.
- Assist in the administration of local anesthetics.
- Monitor the administration of nitrous oxide and intravenous sedation (refer to Chapter 37 for a description of these procedures).
- Transfer and receive instruments.
- Aspirate and retract as needed.
- Maintain a clear operating field with adequate light.
- Monitor the patient's vital signs, oximetry, and electrocardiogram (ECG) (refer to Chapter 27 for a description of these procedures).
- Steady the patient's head and mandible if necessary during use of a mallet and chisel.
- Observe the patient's condition, and anticipate the surgeon's needs.

**Postoperative Surgery**

- Stay with the patient until he or she has recovered sufficiently to leave the office.
- Give verbal and written postoperative instructions to the patient and the responsible person who is accompanying the patient.
- Confirm a postoperative visit as directed by the dentist.
- Update the patient's treatment records, including a copy of any new prescription given to the patient.
- Return the patient's records to the business assistant.
- Break down and disinfect the treatment area.
- Transport all contaminated items to the sterilization center.

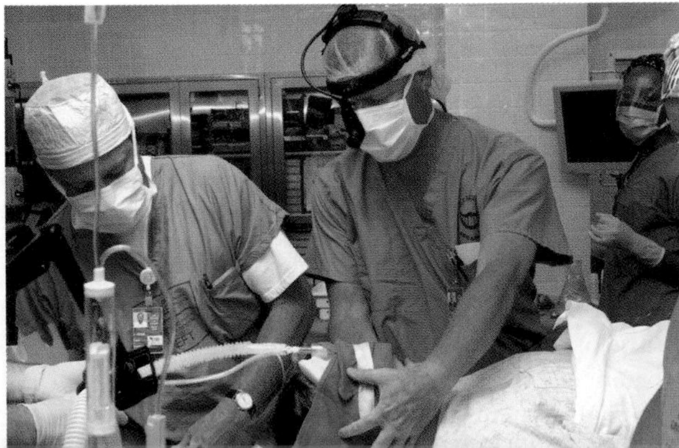

**FIG. 56.1** The operating room. *(From Hupp JR, Tucker MR, Ellis E: Contemporary oral and maxillofacial surgery, ed 6, St Louis, 2014, Mosby.)*

**RECALL**

1 Can a general dentist perform an extraction?
2 How can surgical assistants further their profession?
3 In which two settings could a patient receive oral surgery?
4 Are outpatient oral and maxillofacial surgical procedures considered major or minor surgeries?

## Specialized Instruments and Accessories

It is critical for the surgical assistant to have a working knowledge and understanding of surgical instruments. Such knowledge prepares the surgical staff for the sterilization and preparation of a surgical setup and ordering of the instruments and enables staff to be ready to assist.

Surgical instruments are designed to separate the tooth from the socket, retract surrounding tissue, loosen and elevate the tooth within the socket, or extract the tooth from the socket.

The instruments discussed in this chapter are the oral surgical instruments that are most commonly used. All surgical instruments are classified as **critical instruments** and must be sterilized after each use.

## Elevators

Periosteal **elevators** are available in many designs but are used to perform the same basic function (Fig. 56.2): to reflect *(separate)* and retract the *periosteum* from the surface of the bone. Before a surgical forcep is placed around the tooth, the dentist uses a periosteal elevator to detach the gingival tissues from around the cervix *(neck)* of the tooth.

Straight elevators are used to apply leverage against the tooth to loosen it from the periodontal ligament and ease the extraction (Fig. 56.3). Additional uses include removal of residual root fragments and removal of teeth that have been sectioned with a surgical handpiece and bur.

**Root tip picks** are instruments used for the removal of root tips or fragments that may break away from the tooth during the extraction procedure (Fig. 56.4).

## Forceps

Extraction **forceps** are available in many different shapes and designs and are able to accommodate the oral surgeon's needs in grasping teeth with different crown shapes, root configurations, and locations in the mouth. The goal is to remove the tooth in one piece with the crown and root intact.

The beaks of forceps are designed to grasp the crown of the tooth firmly at or below the cervical line. The inner surface of the beaks may be *plain* (smooth finished) or *serrated* (rough finished) to provide additional grasping power of the tooth being extracted. The handles can be *horizontal* (side by side) or *vertical.*

Forceps are used to remove teeth from the alveolus after they have been slightly loosened in the sockets by the application of elevators. The handles, which are held firmly in a palm grasp, provide the dentist with the leverage necessary to **luxate** and remove the tooth.

**Universal forceps** are designed to allow the surgeon to use the same instrument for the left and right sides of the same arch, as well as for a specific tooth. Fig. 56.5 illustrates forceps commonly used for specific areas of the mouth.

## Surgical Curette

The surgical **curette** resembles a large spoon excavator. It is a double-ended, scoop-shaped instrument with sharp edges that allow for a scraping motion. Curettes are used following the extraction to scrape the interior of the socket to remove diseased tissue or abscesses. Curettes come in varying sizes, and the shanks may be straight or angled to reach different areas of the mouth (Fig. 56.6).

## Rongeur

The **rongeur** is similar in its size to forceps, and its function resembles that of fingernail clippers. The rongeur has a spring between the handles and the blades have sharp cutting edges. The blades of the rongeur may be end cutting or side cutting, depending on the design (Fig. 56.7).

The rongeur is used to trim alveolar bone. It is widely used after multiple extractions to eliminate sharp projections and to shape the edentulous ridge. The beaks of the rongeur must be kept clean during the procedure. As necessary, the dentist holds the instrument toward the assistant with the beaks open. The assistant then carefully removes the debris by wiping the beaks with a sterile gauze sponge.

## Bone File

The **bone file** is used with a push-pull motion to smooth the surface of the bone after the rongeur has removed most of the undesirable bone. Bone files also can be used to smooth rough margins of the alveolus after an extraction. The working ends of bone files are rough and are available in a variety of shapes and sizes (Fig. 56.8).

## Scalpel

The **scalpel** is a surgical knife used to make a precise incision into soft tissue with the least amount of trauma to the tissue. The scalpel consists of a reusable handle with a disposable sterile blade (Fig. 56.9). The size and shape of the blade selected depends on the procedure that is being performed. The most commonly used scalpel blade for oral surgery is a #15 blade. A hemostat or needle holder is used to slide the blade cautiously onto the handle until is clicks into position. Care must be taken to avoid injury while the blades are attached and removed.

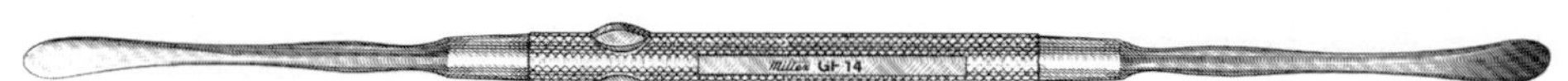


**FIG. 56.2** Periosteal elevators. *(Permission granted by Integra LifeSciences Corporation, Plainsboro, NJ.)*

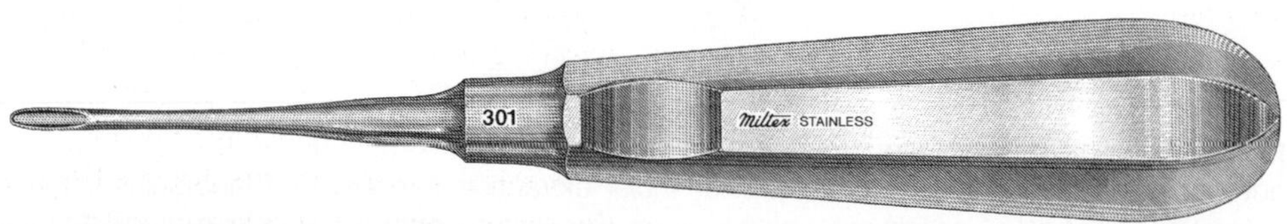


**FIG. 56.3** Straight elevator. *(Permission granted by Integra LifeSciences Corporation, Plainsboro, NJ.)*

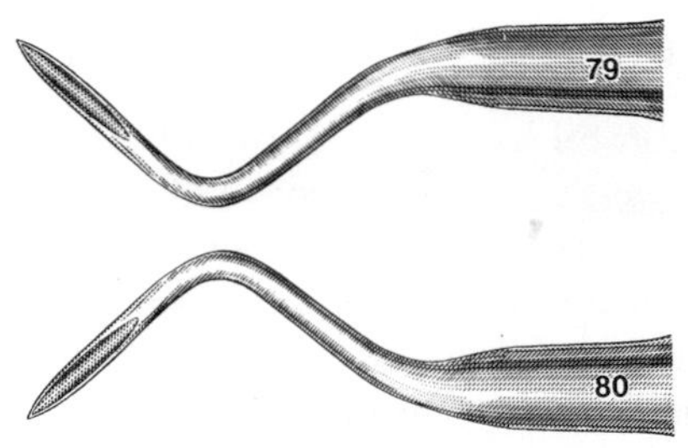


**FIG. 56.4** Root tip picks. *(Permission granted by Integra LifeSciences Corporation, Plainsboro, NJ.)*

Scalpels are also available as a single-use scalpel with a fixed blade attached. Disposable scalpels have plastic handles with metal blades and are supplied in sterile sealed packages. Individual blades and complete scalpel are designed to be used once and then discarded into the "sharps" container.

## Hemostat

Hemostats are multipurpose instruments that are used to grasp and hold things. During oral surgery, a hemostat is used to grasp a vessel, soft tissue, bone, and tooth fragments that have been removed during the procedure. A **hemostat** has grooves

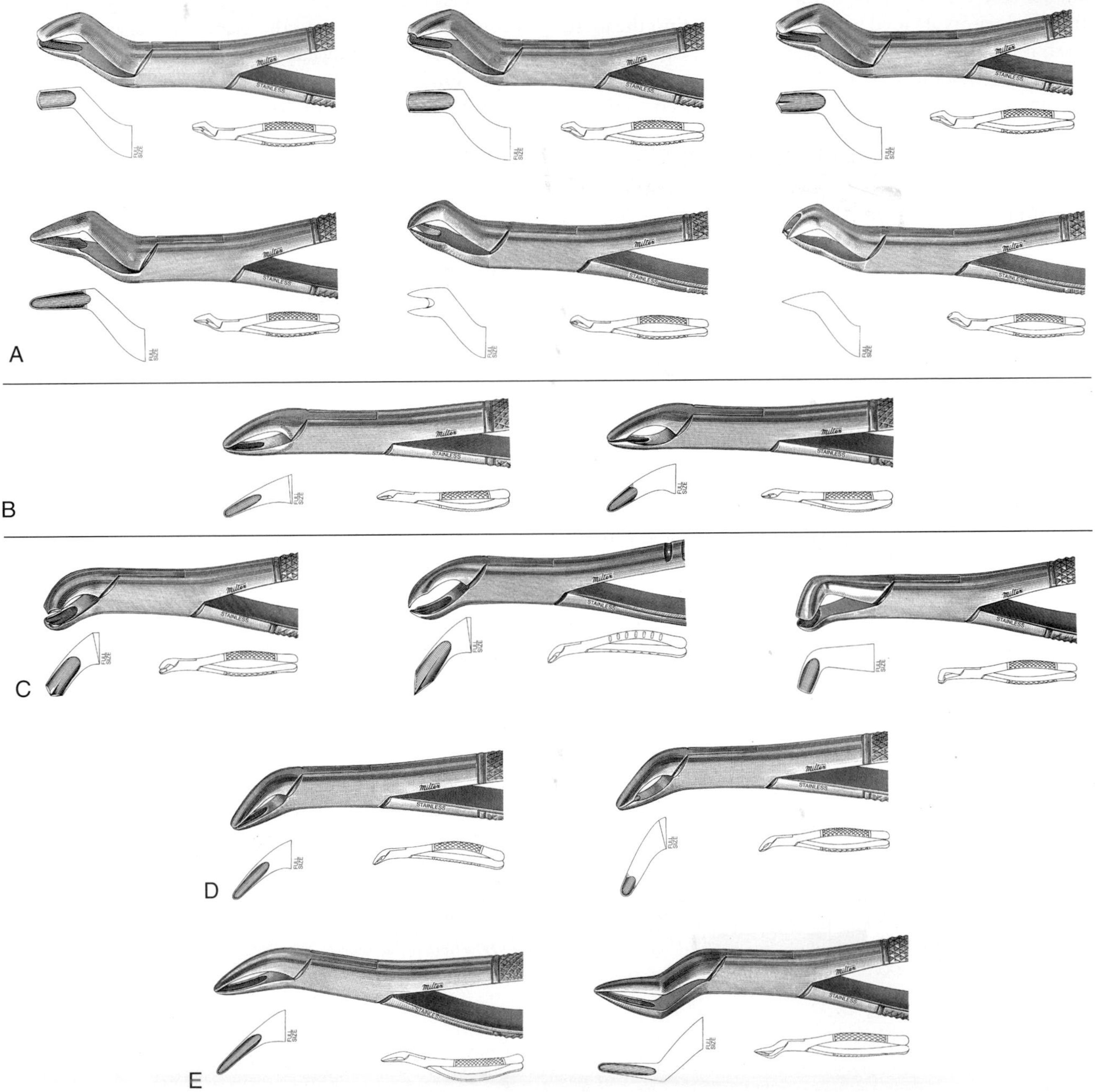

**FIG. 56.5** Types of extraction forceps. A, Maxillary molar extraction forceps. B, Maxillary anterior extraction forceps. C, Mandibular molar extraction forceps. D, Mandibular anterior extraction forceps. E, Root tip extraction forceps. *(Permission granted by Integra LifeSciences Corporation, Plainsboro, NJ.)*

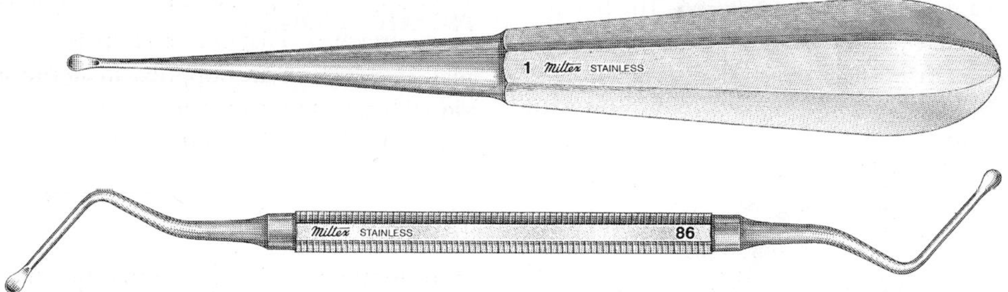


**FIG. 56.6** Surgical curettes. *(Permission granted by Integra LifeSciences Corporation, Plainsboro, NJ.)*

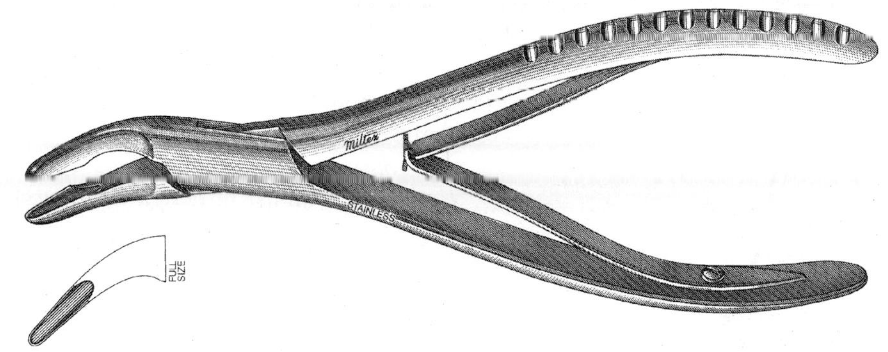


**FIG. 56.7** Rongeurs. *(Permission granted by Integra LifeSciences Corporation, Plainsboro, NJ.)*

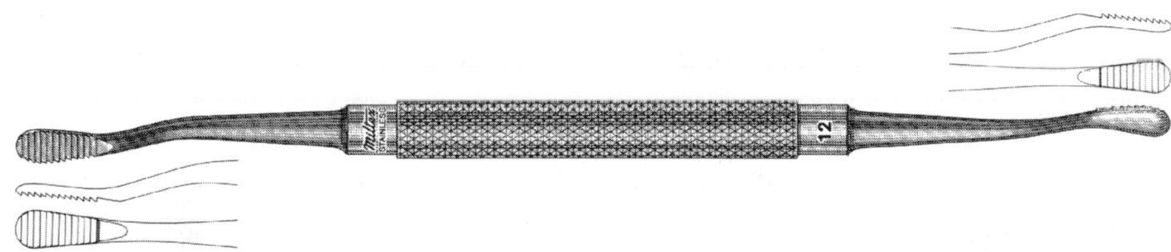


**FIG. 56.8** Bone files. *(Permission granted by Integra LifeSciences Corporation, Plainsboro, NJ.)*

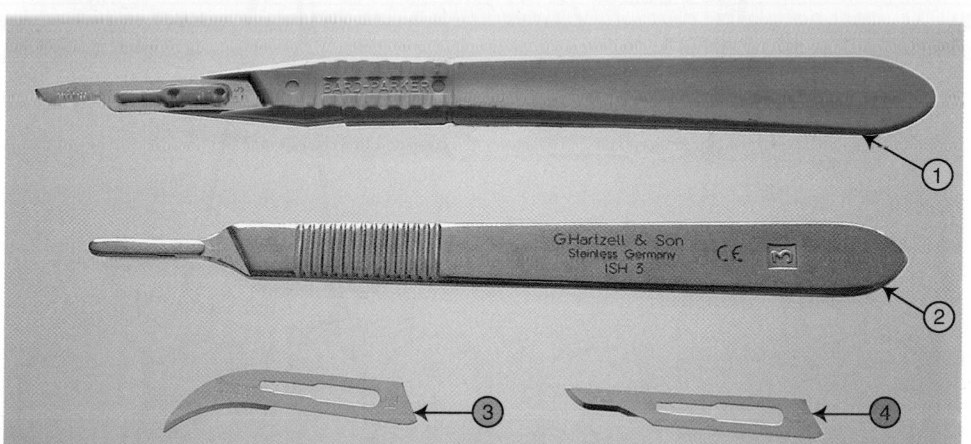


**FIG. 56.9** Scalpel handles and blades. *1,* Disposable handle. *2,* Bard Parker handle. *3,* #12 blade. *4,* #15 blade. *(From Boyd LRB: Dental instruments: a pocket guide, ed 6, St Louis, 2018, Elsevier.)*

in its beak that are used for grasping and holding. The handles have a mechanical lock that holds an object or tissue securely within the beaks (Fig. 56.10). These instruments are available in a variety of sizes, with straight and curved beaks and with handles of different lengths.

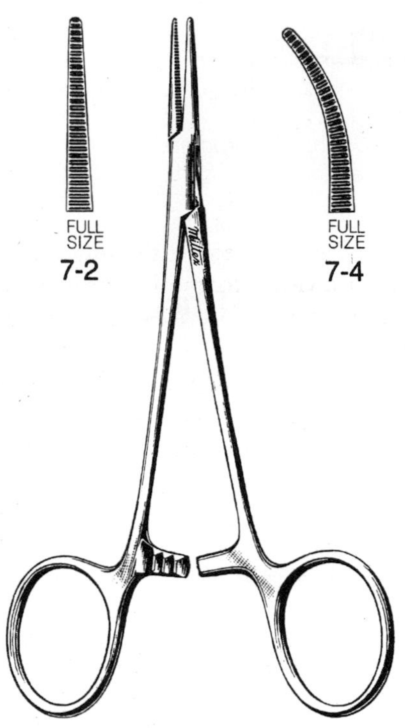


**FIG. 56.10** Hemostats. *(Permission granted by Integra LifeSciences Corporation, Plainsboro, NJ.)*

## Needle Holder

The **needle holder** looks and operates similarly to a hemostat. The difference is that the beaks have a cross-pattern serration on the surface, allowing the surgeon to grasp a suture needle firmly (Fig. 56.11). The handles are secured in place by a ratchet action that holds an object until the dentist releases it. This handle design allows the dentist to tie the suture material by using the needle holder without snagging it in the joint of the instrument.

## Surgical and Suture Scissors

**Surgical scissors** are available with straight or curved blades that have smooth or serrated cutting edges (Fig. 56.12). The handles range in length from approximately 3½ to 6¼ inches. These fragile scissors are used to trim soft tissue. Surgical scissors should never be used for nonsurgical tasks that would dull the cutting surfaces.

*Suture scissors* are designed to cut only suture material. Although similar in design to surgical scissors, suture scissors are sturdier and have a shorter cutting edge to slide under the suture to cut.

## Retractors

Tissue **retractors** are used during surgical procedures to handle soft tissue as carefully as possible to prevent trauma that may delay healing. These instruments resemble cotton pliers that have notched tips (Fig. 56.13).

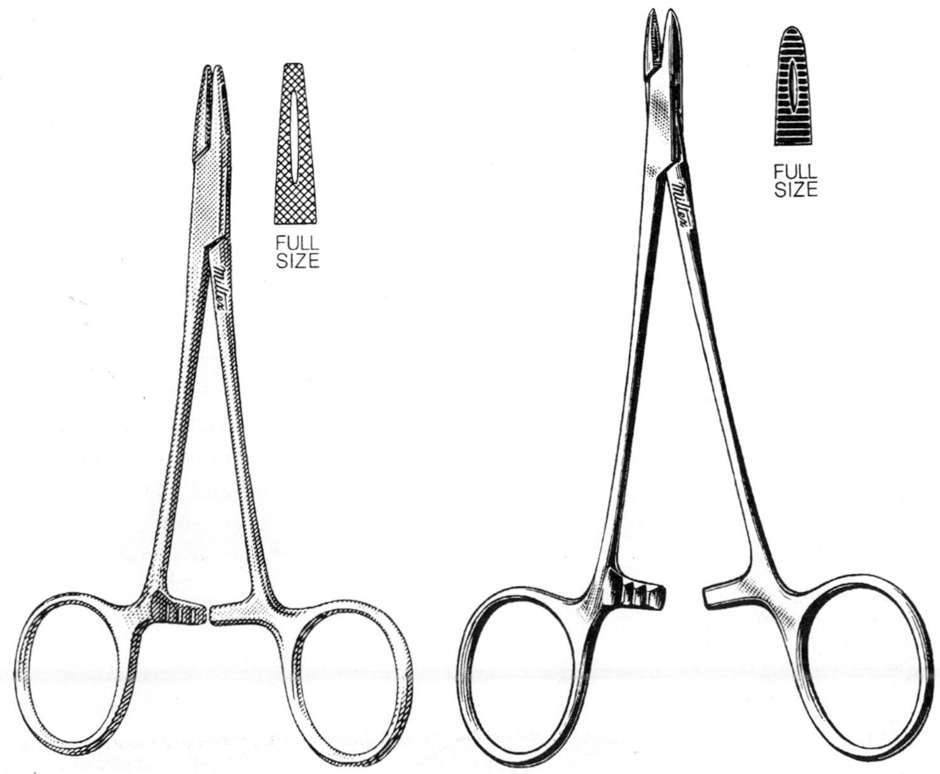


**FIG. 56.11** Needle holders. *(Permission granted by Integra LifeSciences Corporation, Plainsboro, NJ.)*

*Cheek and tongue retractors* are designed to hold and retract the cheeks and tongue during surgical procedures. They are large, curved, angled instruments made of metal or plastic. If plastic retractors are used during surgery, they must be able to withstand heat sterilization (Fig. 56.14).

## Mouth Props

During a surgical procedure, a rubber mouth prop, also known as a *bite-block,* allows the patient to rest and relax the jaw muscles (Fig. 56.15). The mouth prop is placed on the opposite side of the mouth being treated. A patient who is receiving nitrous oxide/oxygen, intravenous sedation, or general anesthesia should use a mouth prop to prevent involuntary closure of the mouth.

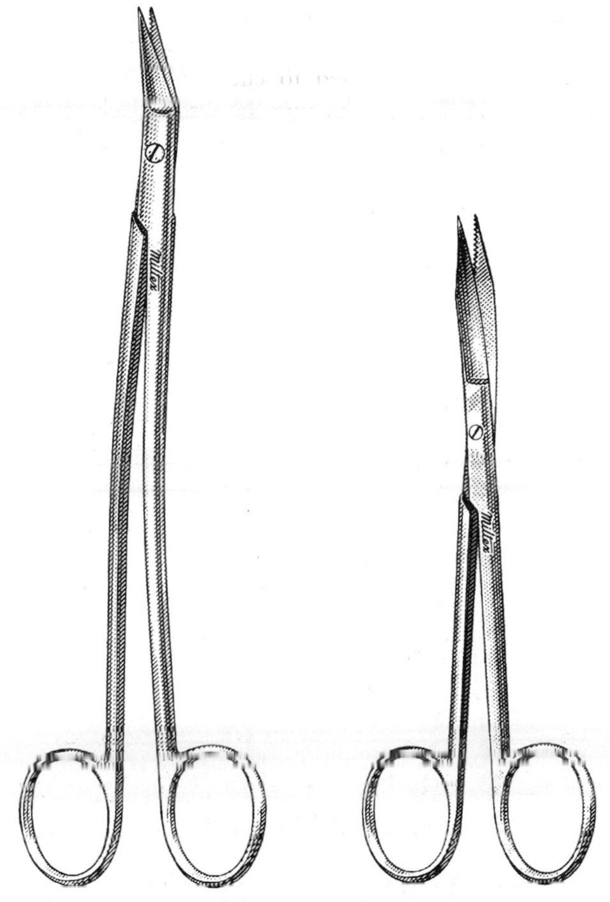

**FIG. 56.12** Surgical scissors. *(Permission granted by Integra LifeSciences Corporation, Plainsboro, NJ.)*

## Chisel and Mallet

When there is a need to remove or reshape bone, a surgical chisel and mallet can be used (Fig. 56.16). Surgical **chisels** are available in a single-bevel or bibevel design. The single-bevel type (bevel on one side of the edge) is used for removing bone. The bibevel type (bevel on both sides of the edge) is used for splitting teeth. Some chisels are designed for use with a hand **mallet**. Another type is driven by a surgical handpiece operated by an electrical system.

## Rotary Instruments

A surgical procedure may require the surgeon to use a handpiece and bur to divide a tooth or remove bone. A specially designed handpiece is used for this because of a sterile environment. Sterile saline water is required for cooling, and air must not be introduced into the surgical site. Surgical burs are also designed with extra long shanks to reach the surgical site. These burs are designed to fit into a surgical handpiece equipped for a sterile environment (Fig. 56.17).

RECALL

5 What does the periosteal elevator reflect and retract?
6 Why is the term "universal" used for forceps?
7 What surgical instrument resembles a spoon excavator?
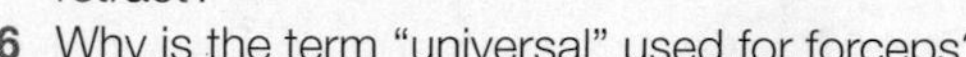
8 What surgical instrument is used to trim and shape bone?
9 What is the difference between a hemostat and a needle holder?
10 When the chisel is used, what additional surgical instrument must be used?

# Surgical Asepsis

You have become skilled in infection control practices in the general dentistry environment, but when a surgical procedure is performed, the surgical team must take these preventive measures a step further.

Establishing and maintaining the **chain of asepsis** for a procedure requires that the instruments, surgical drapes, and gloved hands of the surgical team must be sterile. Contact with nonsterile objects or surfaces breaks the chain of asepsis and contaminates the surgical area. Once established, the chain of asepsis must not be broken. Because surgical procedures invade open tissue, the surgical team *must* follow a sterile technique.

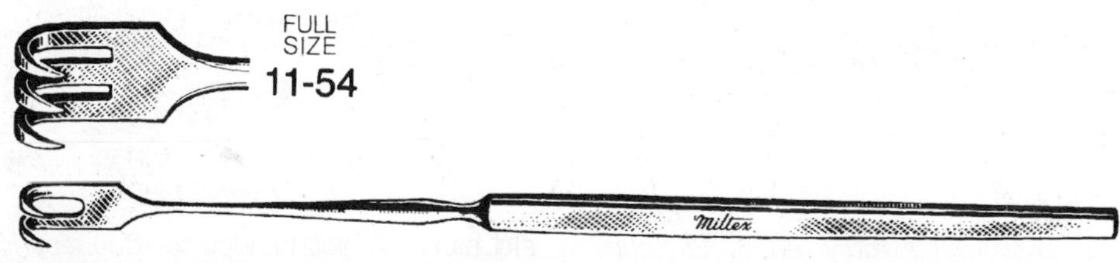


**FIG. 56.13** Tissue retractors. *(Permission granted by Integra LifeSciences Corporation, Plainsboro, NJ.)*

The purpose of this method of asepsis is to minimize the number of organisms that can enter an open wound.

## Sterile Field

A sterile field is prepared to hold surgical instruments and accessories that will be used during a surgery. Sterile setups are prepared just before assistants prepare themselves and begin a procedure. If a surgical setup has been open for longer than an hour because of delays or changes, the setup is considered unsterile at that point and should not be used.

See Procedure 56.1: Preparing a Sterile Field for Instruments and Supplies.

## Surgical Scrub

A surgical scrub is used to lessen the chance of infection. Even though sterile gloves are used for a surgical procedure, the number of organisms on a person's hands must be reduced in case of a tear or a break in the gloves.

See Procedure 56.2: Performing a Surgical Scrub.

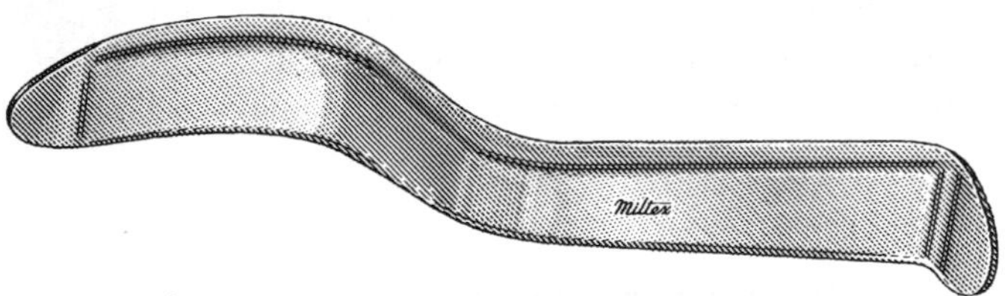


**FIG. 56.14** Cheek and tongue retractor. *(Permission granted by Integra LifeSciences Corporation, Plainsboro, NJ.)*

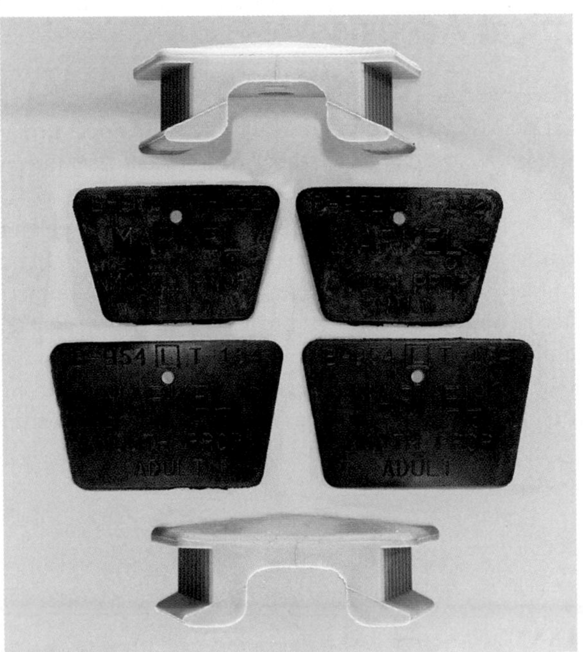

**FIG. 56.15** Mouth props. *(From Hupp JR, Tucker MR, Ellis E: Contemporary oral and maxillofacial surgery, ed 6, St Louis, 2014, Mosby.)*

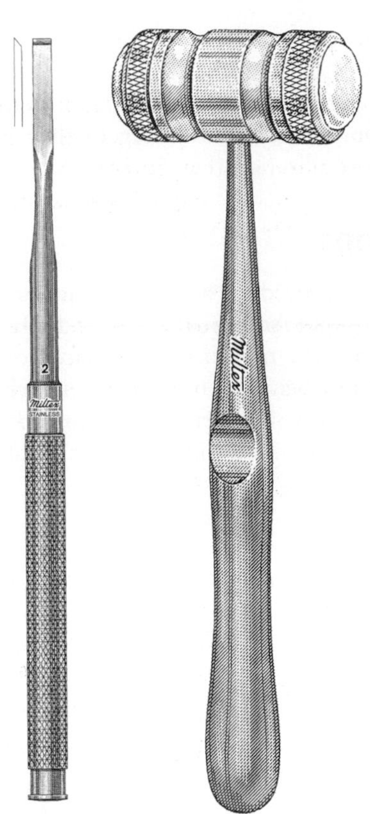


**FIG. 56.16** Chisel and mallet. *(Permission granted by Integra LifeSciences Corporation, Plainsboro, NJ.)*

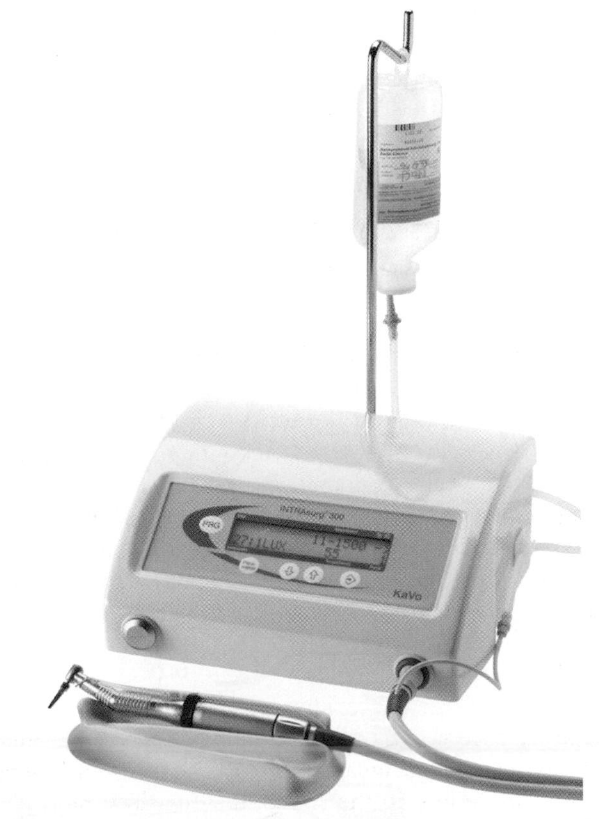


**FIG. 56.17** Surgical handpiece. *(Courtesy KaVo Dental, Charlotte, NC.)*

## Proper Gloving

Sterile gloves are prepackaged gloves that come in different sizes. When you are assisting in an invasive procedure, you must wear sterile gloves. The process of **donning** sterile gloves is important in the noncontamination process. See Procedure 56.3: Performing Sterile Gloving.

**11** What equipment is used when a surgical scrub is performed?
**12** What does the term *donning* mean?

# Surgical Procedures

## Forceps Extraction

Forceps extractions are often described as "routine" or "simple" extractions. These terms are misleading because all extractions are *surgical* procedures. Use of these terms implies that the extraction can be completed without extensive instrumentation. A forceps extraction is performed on a tooth that is fully erupted and has a solid, intact crown which is grasped firmly with forceps. Most "routine" forceps extractions do not require placement of sutures.

See Procedure 56.4: Assisting in Forceps Extraction.

## Multiple Extractions and Alveoplasty

A multiple extraction procedure is indicated when a patient will be receiving a partial denture, a full denture, or implants. Even though the teeth are fully erupted and the procedure is a routine forceps extraction procedure, the end result required for the patient's alveolar ridge changes the procedure. When several teeth have been extracted within the same quadrant, the alveolar crest remains intact, and the surgeon must perform an **alveoplasty** to contour and smooth the affected area. See Procedure 56.5: Assisting in Multiple Extractions and Alveoplasty.

## Removal of Impacted Teeth

The term *complex extraction* is used when conditions require additional skill, knowledge, and instrumentation to remove a tooth. The extraction of an impacted tooth is an example of a complex extraction. An **impacted tooth** is a tooth that has not erupted. A **soft tissue impaction** indicates that the tooth is located under the gingival tissue. A **hard tissue impaction** indicates that the tooth is partially or totally covered by tissue and bone.

See Procedure 56.6: Assisting in Removal of an Impacted Tooth.

## Biopsy

A **biopsy** is a process by which tissue is removed and examined to distinguish malignant *(cancerous)* from nonmalignant *(noncancerous)* lesions in the oral cavity. The three most common biopsy procedures used in dentistry are incisional biopsy, excisional biopsy, and exfoliative biopsy.

### Incisional Biopsy

When a lesion is located in an area that would be cosmetically or functionally impaired by surgery, an **incisional biopsy** is often indicated. An incisional biopsy is indicated when the lesion is larger than 1 cm in all dimensions. The surgeon will remove a wedge of tissue from the lesion, along with some normal tissue to be used for comparison. Complete surgical removal of the lesion is not performed until a final diagnosis of the type of lesion is made.

### Excisional Biopsy

An **excisional biopsy** involves removal of the entire lesion plus some adjacent normal tissue. This procedure is ideal for small lesions when complete removal will not create an esthetic or functional problem. For example, a small, nonhealing sore on the labial mucosa may be removed completely during the biopsy.

### Oral Brush Biopsy

The **exfoliative biopsy** was introduced as a noninvasive technique to recognize oral cancer. With new technology and design, the oral brush biopsy is able to penetrate and remove tissue from all three epithelial layers of the oral mucosa (Fig. 56.18). The oral brush does not require anesthesia and produces minimal to no bleeding or discomfort to the patient. The brush is pressed against the lesion in question and rotated; the cells gathered on the brush are then rotated onto the enclosed glass slide, fixed, and sent to a laboratory for analysis.

### Biopsy Results

The pathology report indicates whether the lesion is malignant or benign. Nonmalignant tumors and cysts are removed if their size and location interfere with appearance and normal function. If they do not interfere and do not pose a threat to the patient, removal may be postponed. However, the situation must be reviewed regularly to determine whether the tumor has changed in size or shape.

Informing the patient of a malignant tumor requires kindness, empathy, and a tactful explanation from the dentist. In general, this is not done by phone; ideally, the dentist informs the patient in person with a close family member present. A malignant tumor dictates immediate treatment by a qualified specialist.

RECALL

**13** What procedure is commonly completed after multiple teeth have been removed from the same quadrant or arch?
**14** Which type of impaction is it when a tooth is located directly under the gingival tissue?
**15** Which type of biopsy is completed when a surface lesion is scraped to attain cells?

# Sutures

The term *suture* refers to the act of stitching. As a rule, if a scalpel has been used, sutures are placed to control bleeding and promote healing. Therefore when a scalpel is on the setup tray, suture equipment will be added.

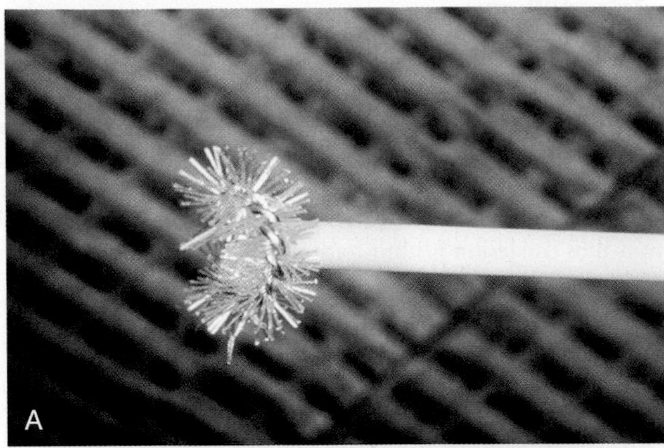


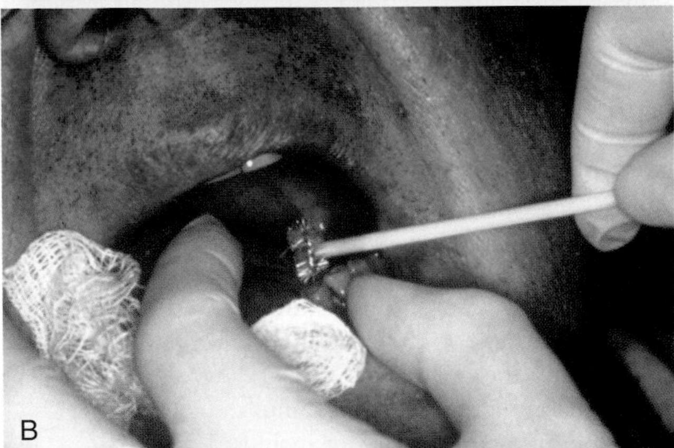


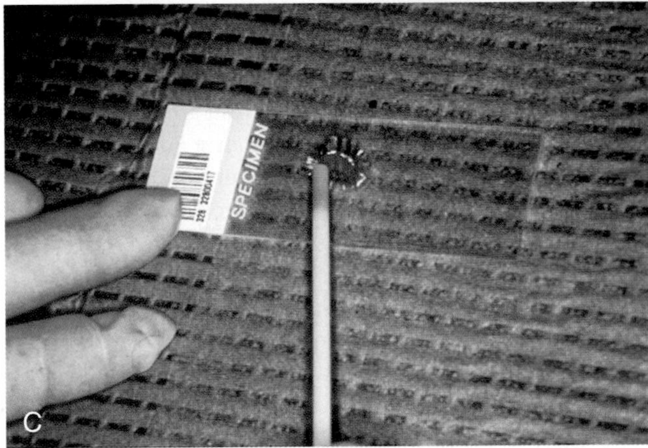


**FIG. 56.18** Brush used to gather surface cells. *(From Hupp JR, Tucker MR, Ellis E: Contemporary oral and maxillofacial surgery, ed 6, St Louis, 2014, Mosby.)*

## Suture Placement

Suture needles are supplied already threaded and in a sterile pack (Fig. 56.19). Suture material is available in absorbable and nonabsorbable varieties.

*Absorbable* suture materials dissolve and become absorbed by the body's enzymes during the healing process. The most common types of absorbable suture materials are (1) **plain catgut,** which provides the fastest healing for mucous membrane and subcutaneous tissues; (2) **chromic catgut,** which provides a slower healing process, allowing the internal tissues to heal first; and (3) **polyglactin 910 (Vicryl),** a synthetic absorbable material.

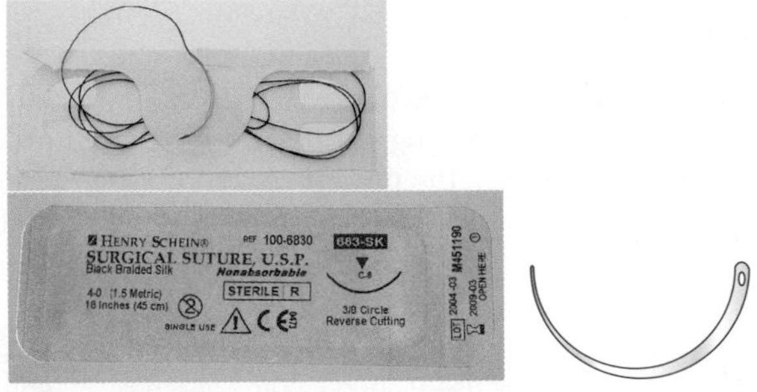


**FIG. 56.19** An example of suture material labeled according to size, type, length, and type of needle. *(From Boyd LRB: Dental instruments: a pocket guide, ed 6, St Louis, 2018, Elsevier.)*

**Nonabsorbable** suture materials include (1) **silk,** for its strength and easy application; (2) **polyester fiber,** which is one of the strongest sutures; and (3) **nylon,** for its strength and elasticity. Nonabsorbable sutures require the patient to return to the office for removal. This type of suture is usually removed 5 to 7 days after surgery.

The type of extraction performed will determine the suture technique used by the surgeon. *Interrupted* and *horizontal mattress sutures* are the most commonly placed sutures for a single tooth socket. The *mattress suture* and the *figure-eight suture* are used for suturing two or more papillae together (Fig. 56.20). See Procedure 56.7: Assisting in Suture Placement.

## Suture Removal

If nonabsorbable sutures were placed, the patient will be scheduled to return to the office and have the sutures removed in approximately 5 to 7 days. The surgeon will discuss the healing process with the patient and examination the area for proper healing.

An important step when removing sutures is to prepare the area of the suture placement by preparing the surface site with a sterile cotton-tip applicator and antiseptic solution.

Suture removal may be an *expanded function* in the state, province, or territory in which you practice. If so, specific steps must be followed in the suture removal process.

See Procedure 56.8: Performing Suture Removal (Expanded Function).

RECALL

16 What does the term *suture* mean?

17 What are the three types of nonabsorbable suture materials?

18 What is the approximate time frame for removing nonabsorbable sutures?

## Postoperative Care

When surgery has been completed, the patient will be moved to the recovery area to rest and to allow the sedation to wear

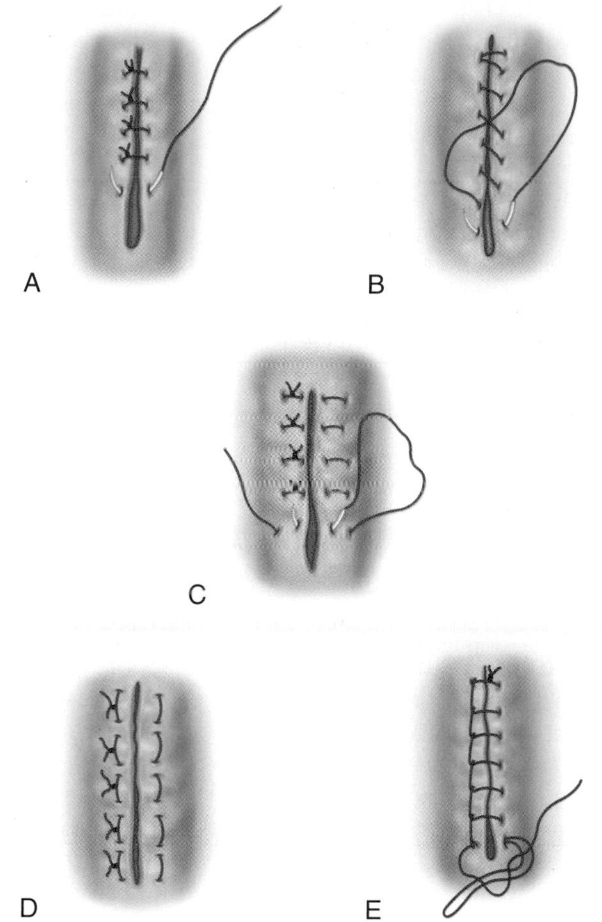


**FIG. 56.20** Types of suture techniques A, Interrupted suture. B, Continuous suture. C, Vertical/mattress suture. D, Horizontal/mattress suture. E, Continuous box suture. *(From Singh PP, Cranin AN: Atlas of oral implantology, ed 3, St Louis, 2010, Mosby.)*

off. Postoperative care and instructions are provided for the *total* recovery period, before the patient leaves the office. Verbal and written postoperative instructions, along with a package of sterile gauze, are provided to the patient and the individual accompanying him or her.

## Control of Bleeding

Immediately after an extraction is performed, sterile 2 × 2–inch gauze is folded and placed over the socket to control bleeding and to promote clot formation and healing. The patient should receive the following instructions:

- After leaving the office, keep the pack in place for 30 to 45 minutes. Removing the pack too soon could disturb clot formation and may increase bleeding.
- Do not disturb the clot with your tongue or by rinsing your mouth vigorously.
- If bleeding continues and does not stop, call the dental office.
- Restrict strenuous work or physical activity for that day.

## Control of Swelling

After extensive surgery, expected swelling can be controlled with cold packs. The patient receives the following instructions regarding the control of swelling:

- During the first 24 hours, place a cold pack on a cycle of 20 minutes on and 20 minutes off.
- After the first 24 hours, apply external heat to the area of the face to enhance circulation in the tissues and to promote healing.
- After the first 24 hours, begin gently rinsing the oral cavity with warm saline solution (1 tsp salt to 8 oz warm water) every 2 hours to promote healing.

### *Control of Pain*

The patient should be provided instructions on pain control. The procedure and extent of the surgery will determine what type of pain control is provided. It can be an over-the-counter type of analgesic, or it may require a prescription. Whichever type of pain medication is prescribed, the first dose should be taken before the effects of the local anesthetic wears off.

#### Common Analgesics for Postextraction Pain

**Mild Pain**
- Ibuprofen
- Acetaminophen

**Moderate Pain Situations (by Prescription)**
- Acetaminophen with Codeine
- Hydrocodone

**Severe Pain Situations (by Prescription)**
- Oxycodone (Percocet)

### *Postoperative Diet*

On the day of surgery, instruct the patient that he or she can drink liquids and eat soft foods (such as Jell-O, pudding, and broth), trying to eat on the other side of the mouth. Make sure not to eat anything too hot or too cold, and especially not to drink anything through a straw.

After 24 hours, or as soon as the patient can chew comfortably, the patient can begin to eat solid foods. Try to chew on the opposite side of the surgical site. It is important to avoid alcoholic beverages. If troubled by nausea and vomiting, the patient should call the office for further instructions.

RECALL

**19** How long should a pressure pack remain on a surgical site to control bleeding?
**20** What over-the-counter analgesics may be prescribed by the surgeon for pain?
**21** Would you instruct a patient to use a hot compress or a cold compress for swelling?

# Postsurgical Complications

## Alveolar Osteitis

When a tooth has been extracted, healing begins immediately, with blood filling the socket and forming a clot. The clot is important because it protects the wound and is later replaced by granulation tissue and ultimately bone.

Failure of the healing process can result in **alveolar osteitis**, also known as a **dry socket.** When the blood clot at the site of the tooth extraction has been dislodged or has dissolved before the wound has healed. The underlying bone and nerves are exposed resulting in pain, not only in the socket but also radiating to the side of the face. This painful condition can occur 2 to 4 days after removal of the tooth. Specific factors that can initiate this condition can occur for the following reasons:

- Not caring for the extraction site as instructed
- Not following home care instructions
- Smoking, sneezing, coughing, spitting, or drinking from a straw within the first 24 hours
- Women who take oral contraceptives (may be more susceptible)

Treatment of dry socket focuses on reducing symptoms, particularly pain. Dry socket treatment may include the following:

- **Flushing out the socket.** The surgeon will use a sterile saline solution and flush the socket to remove any food particles or other debris that may contribute to pain or infection.
- **Medicated dressings.** A surgical dressing either as a paste or saturated gauze strips with a medicated dressing that includes an antibacterial and topical anesthetic is packed into the socket for up to 5 days providing immediate relief for the patient. The patient may need to have the dressings changed several times over a 2-week period.
- **Pain medication.** The surgeon may prescribe a pain medication.
- **Self-care.** A sterile disposable syringe will be provided with instructions on how to flush the socket with warm saline solution at home to promote healing and eliminate debris.

See Procedure 56.9: Assisting in the Treatment of Alveolar Osteitis.

**■ Patient Education** When preparing for surgery, patients have many fears and apprehensions. Some have heard "stories" from friends or family who have undergone the same surgery with a negative outcome. As the surgical assistant, one of your many important roles is to talk with the patient, answer questions, and help eliminate fears. Be sure that you are confident and explicit when providing preoperative and postoperative instructions to a patient. ■

**■ Legal and Ethical Implications** When a surgical procedure moves from the treatment room to the hospital operating room, legal awareness and responsibilities become more consequential for the oral surgeon and the surgical team. Before beginning any surgery, confirm the following with the patient:

- The surgeon has explained the procedure and answered all questions.
- The patient has signed all consent forms with a witness, and the surgeon's signature and date are on the form.
- Another person is present to escort the patient home.
- All postsurgical instructions have been given verbally and in writing. ■

**■ Eye to the Future** The oral and maxillofacial surgeon will become the medicodental expert in head and neck diseases and treatment. No longer will a patient seek care from a medical surgeon regarding head and neck diseases.

Because of advances in surgical dentistry, surgical assistants will have to expand their knowledge and skill to maintain their level of competence. Because more time will be spent in the operating room than in the office setting, it is advantageous for the surgical assistant to acquire additional credentialing. ■

**■ Critical Thinking**

1. You are assisting in a surgical procedure, and an instrument has dropped on the floor. No duplicate is available on the tray. What do you do?
2. A patient is scheduled to have multiple extractions and an alveoplasty for the preparation of a denture. What may be the patient's concerns about the procedure? How can you alleviate these concerns?
3. You are assisting in a forceps extraction. List what you would place on the tray setup for this procedure.
4. Which personality traits are required for a surgical assistant? Do you think you have the necessary traits to make a good surgical assistant?
5. Contrast the operating room in a hospital with the treatment area of a private practice. ■

PROCEDURE 56.1

# Preparing a Sterile Field for Instruments and Supplies

## PROCEDURAL STEPS

1 Wash and dry hands.
2 Position the mobile cart behind the patient chair, and place a sterile pack on the tray.
3 Turn the outside wrapping so the first section of the packaging will be opened away from you.

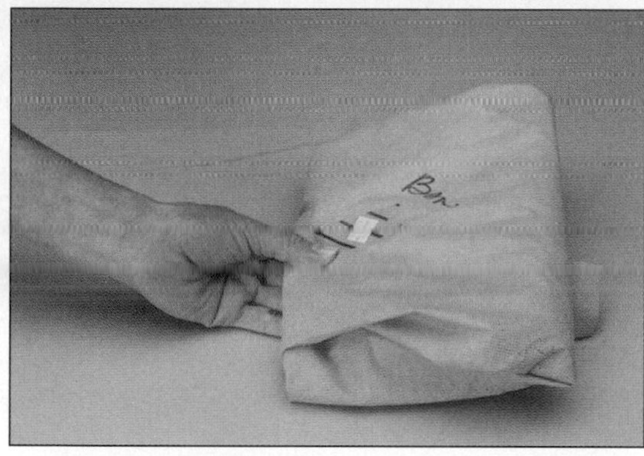

4 Allow the paper to open completely so the sterile field is facing up.
5 Holding the outside flaps of the internal wrapping, allow the sterile contents to fall onto the tray.

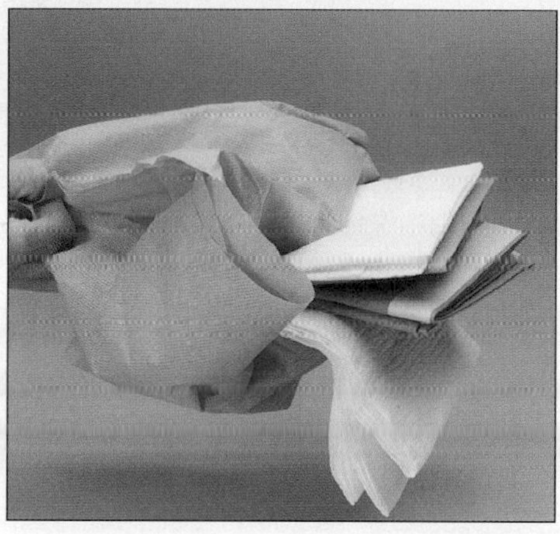

6 You can now begin adding items, such as additional surgical instruments and suture material, to the sterile field.

Photos from Proctor DB, et al: Kinn's the medical assistant: an applied learning approach, ed 13, St Louis, 2017, Elsevier.

PROCEDURE 56.2

# Performing a Surgical Scrub

## EQUIPMENT AND SUPPLIES

- ✓ Orange stick
- ✓ Antimicrobial soap (such as chlorhexidine gluconate)
- ✓ Sterile surgical scrub brush
- ✓ Sterile disposable towels

## PROCEDURAL STEPS

1 Cover your hair and don protective eyewear and mask before performing a surgical scrub.
**PURPOSE** Once your hands are scrubbed, they should not touch anything.
2 Remove all jewelry.
3 With water running, use the orange stick to clean under your nails. Discard the stick and rinse your hands without touching the faucet or the inside of the sink.

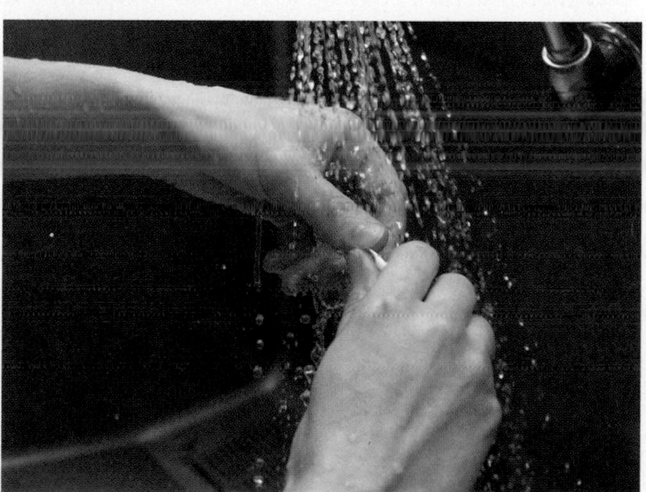

4 Wet hands and forearms up to the elbows with warm water, then dispense about 5 ml of antimicrobial soap into cupped hands.

(Continued)

## PROCEDURE 56.2 Performing a Surgical Scrub–cont'd

5 Use the surgical scrub brush to scrub hands and forearms for 7 minutes.

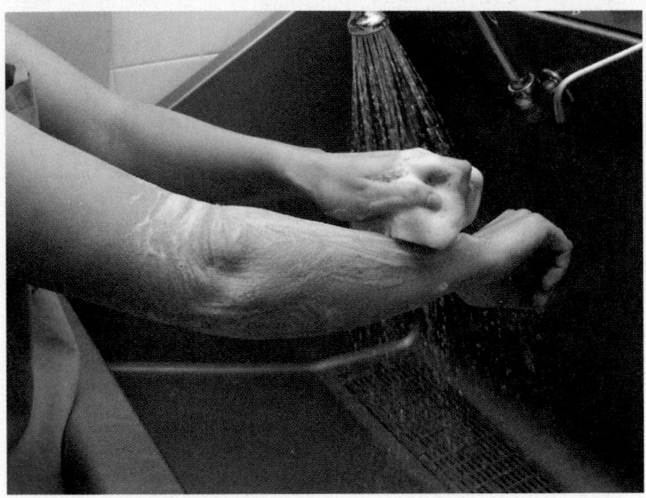

6 Rinse thoroughly with warm water. Keep your hands up and above waist level.

**PURPOSE** This allows the water to run toward the elbows, keeping the hands clean.

7 Dispense another 5 ml of antimicrobial soap, and repeat the scrub.

8 Wash for an additional 7 minutes without using a brush. Rinse so the contaminated water runs down the arms and off the elbows.

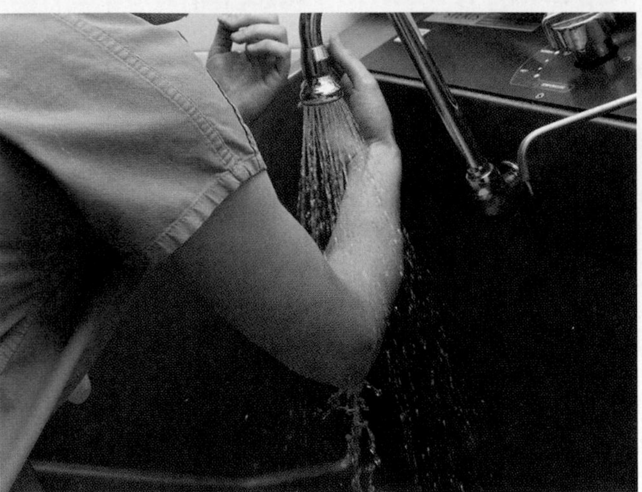

9 Dry hands and arms with a sterile towel. Use a patting motion, and continue up the forearms.

10 Keep your hands above your waist before donning your sterile gown.

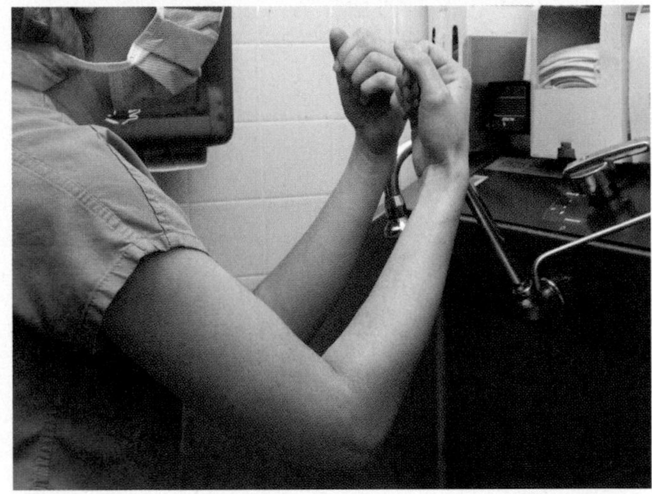

All photos from Hupp JR, Ellis E III, Tucker M: Contemporary oral and maxillofacial surgery, ed 6, St Louis, 2014, Mosby.

# PROCEDURE 56.3

## Performing Sterile Gloving

### PROCEDURAL STEPS

1 The glove package should already be opened before the surgical scrub is completed. Be sure to touch *only* the inside of the package at this point.
**PURPOSE** The open glove pack is a sterile field.

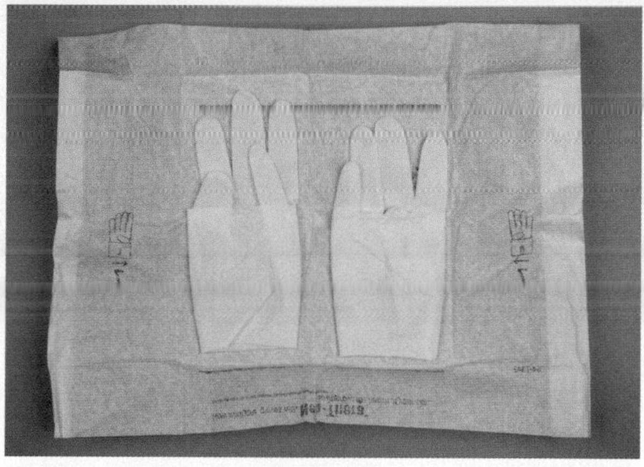

2 Glove your *dominant* hand first.
**PURPOSE** Applying the second glove is more difficult, in that you have greater dexterity with your dominant hand.

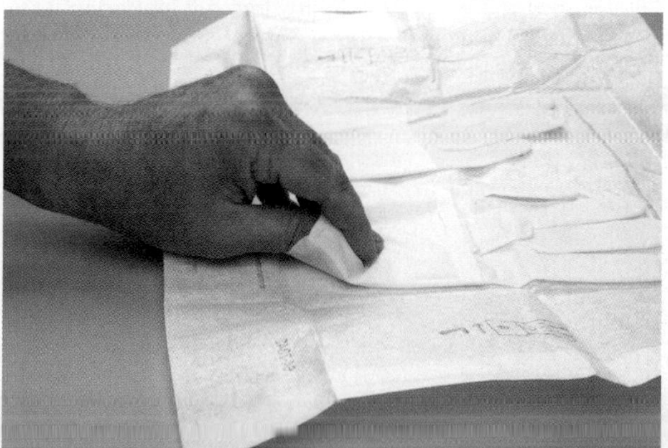

3 Pull the glove over the hand, touching only the folded cuff.
**PURPOSE** Remember that you want to touch only the *inside* of the glove.

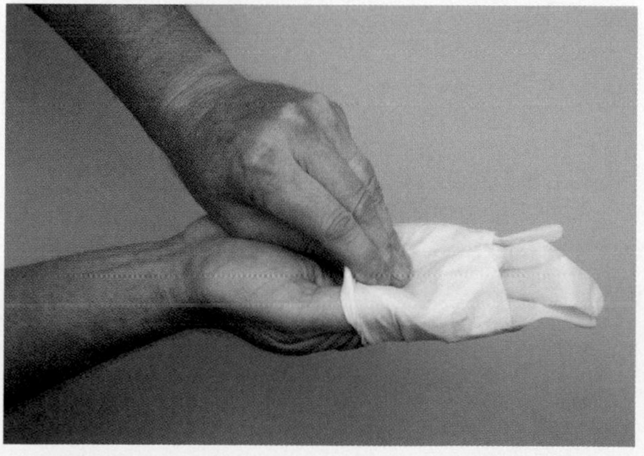

4 With your dominant hand gloved, slide your forefingers under the cuff of the other glove.
**PURPOSE** You can touch only the sterile portion of the glove with your dominant hand.

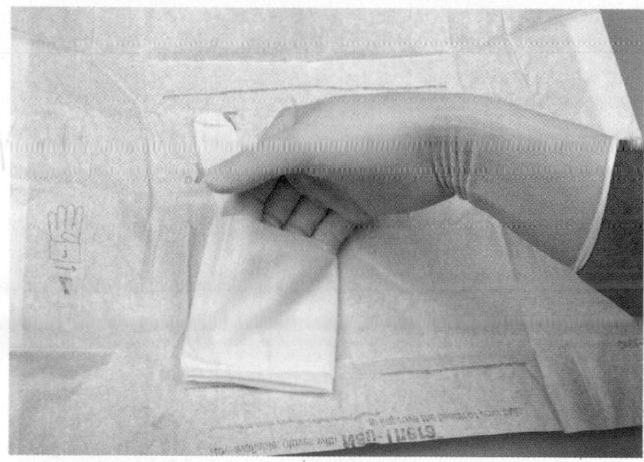

5 Pull the glove up over your other hand.

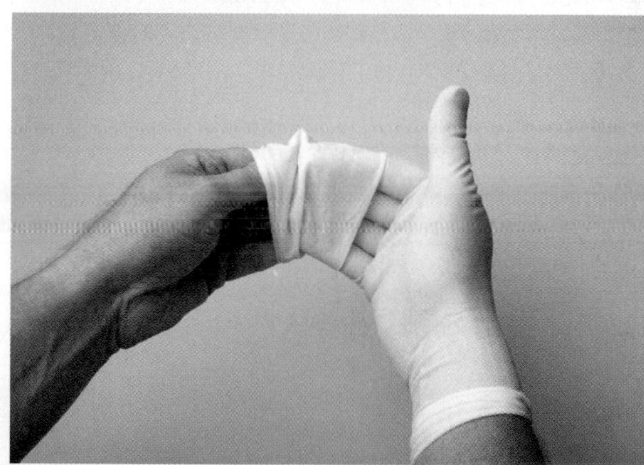

6 Unroll the cuff from your gloves.

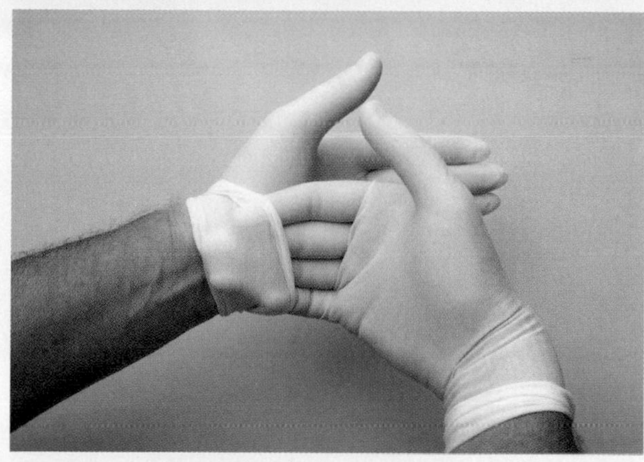

All photos from Hupp JR, Ellis E III, Tucker M: Contemporary oral and maxillofacial surgery, ed 6, St Louis, 2014, Mosby.

  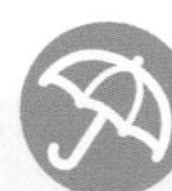 

PROCEDURE 56.4

# Assisting in Forceps Extraction

## EQUIPMENT AND SUPPLIES

- ✔ Local anesthetic agent setup
- ✔ Basic setup
- ✔ Periosteal elevator
- ✔ Elevator (dentist's choice)
- ✔ Forceps (dentist's choice)
- ✔ Surgical curette
- ✔ Sterile gauze sponge
- ✔ Surgical aspirator tip

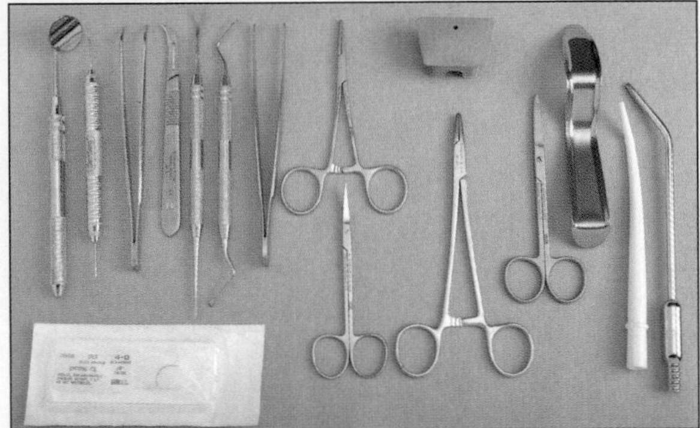

*From Boyd LRB: Dental instruments: a pocket guide, ed 6, St Louis, 2018, Elsevier.*

## PROCEDURAL STEPS

1. The local anesthetic agent is administered.
2. Transfer the explorer for the dentist to probe the area to determine the level of anesthesia.
3. Transfer the periosteal elevator for the dentist to loosen the gingival tissue gently and to compress the alveolar bone surrounding the neck of the tooth.

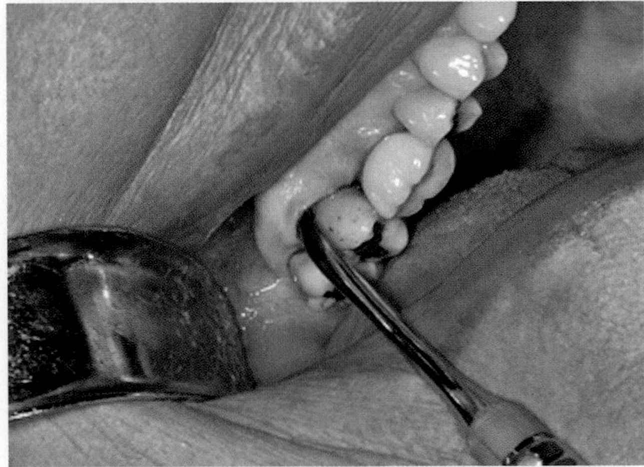

*Courtesy Dr. Edward Ellis III.*

4. Transfer an elevator (most often straight) as requested by the dentist to loosen the tooth.
5. The dentist places the beaks of the forceps on the tooth and firmly grasps the tooth around and below the cementoenamel junction.

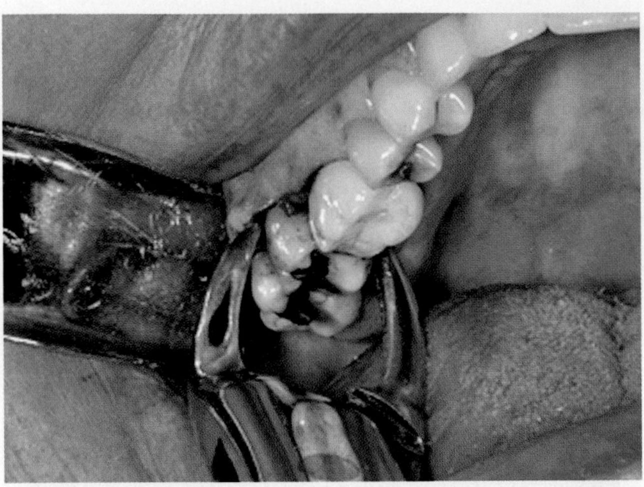

*Courtesy Dr. Edward Ellis III.*

6. The tooth is luxated in the socket to compress the bone and enlarge the socket. When this has been done, the tooth can be freely lifted from the socket.
7. The dentist examines the tooth to ensure that the root is intact.
8. When the tooth has been removed, use the aspirating tip to debride the surgical site.
9. Fold several sterile gauze squares into a tight pad to form a pressure pack. Retract the cheek, and place the folded gauze over the extraction site.

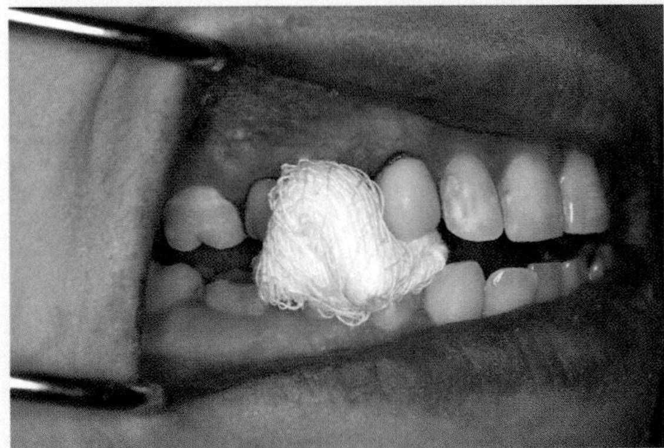

*From Hupp JR, Tucker MR, Ellis E: Contemporary oral and maxillofacial surgery, ed 6, St Louis, 2014, Mosby.*

10. Instruct the patient to bite firmly on the pack for at least 30 minutes.

    **PURPOSE** This pressure aids in control of bleeding and in blood clotting.
11. Slowly move the dental chair to an upright position.
12. Provide the patient with postoperative instructions.
13. Document the procedure.

| Date | Tooth | Surface | Charting Notes |
|---|---|---|---|
| 8/26/17 | 4 | — | Extraction, 2 cartridges Xylocaine 1/50,000. Pt tolerated procedure well. Postop instructions given. Pt instructed to return in 1 wk. |
| | | | T. Clark, CDA/L. Stewart, DDS |

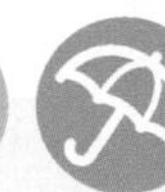

PROCEDURE 56.5

# Assisting in Multiple Extractions and Alveoplasty

## EQUIPMENT AND SUPPLIES

- ✓ Forceps extraction setup
- ✓ Additional elevators and forceps (dentist's choice)
- ✓ Rongeur
- ✓ Curettes
- ✓ Bone file
- ✓ Scalpel
- ✓ Suture material and needle
- ✓ Needle holder or hemostat
- ✓ Suture scissors
- ✓ Sterile saline solution

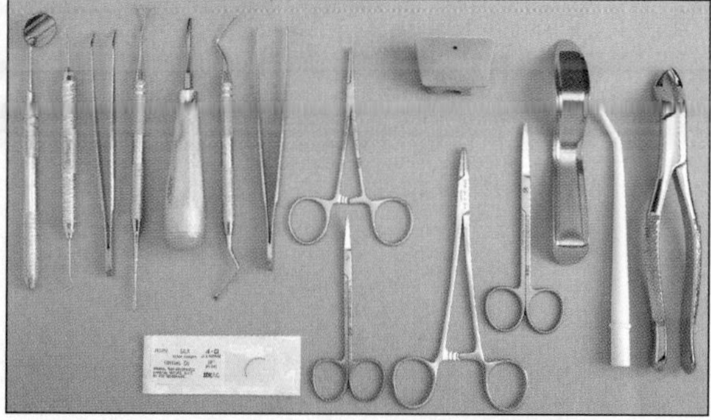

*From Boyd LRB: Dental instruments: a pocket guide, ed 6, St Louis, 2018, Elsevier.*

## PROCEDURAL STEPS

1. Follow steps 1 through 9 in Assisting in Forceps Extraction (see Procedure 56.4) until all teeth have been extracted.
2. After the teeth have been extracted, the dentist will use the rongeur to trim the alveolus. After each cut with the rongeur, have sterile gauze available to carefully remove debris from the cutting ends.

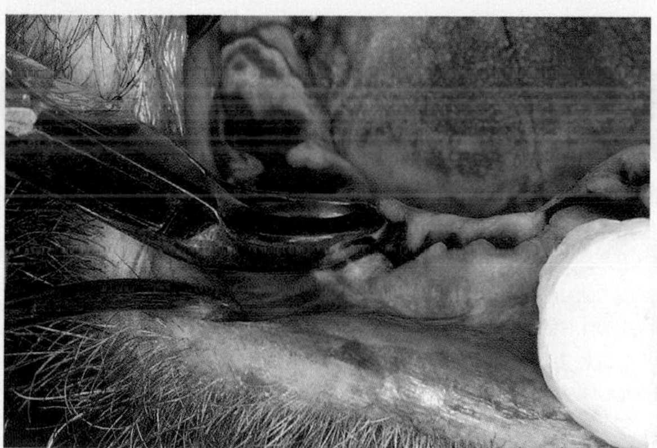

*From Hupp JR, Tucker MR, Ellis E: Contemporary oral and maxillofacial surgery, ed 6, St Louis, 2014, Mosby.*

3. Following use of the rongeur, transfer the bone file for the dentist to finish smoothing rough margins. After each stroke with the file, use a clean sterile gauze square to remove debris from the grooves.
4. Irrigate and aspirate the surgical site with sterile saline solution to remove bone fragments.
5. The dentist repositions the mucosa over the ridge and sutures it into place.

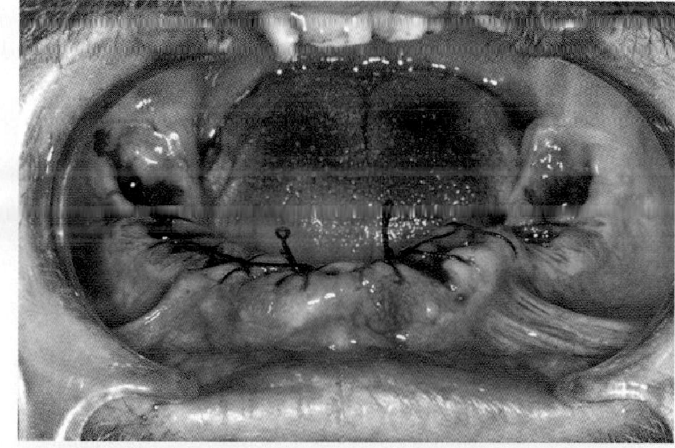

*From Hupp JR, Tucker MR, Ellis E: Contemporary oral and maxillofacial surgery, ed 6, St Louis, 2014, Mosby.*

6. Place pressure packs made of sterile gauze sponges as needed. Provide the patient with postoperative instructions, verbal and written, and complete the patient's dismissal process.
7. Document the procedure.

| Date | Tooth | Surface | Charting Notes |
|---|---|---|---|
| 8/26/17 | 22–27 | — | Vitals: P 90, BP 140/90. Multiple extractions, 6 teeth, 2 cartridges Xylocaine 1:20,000, alveoplasty, 8 nylon sutures placed. Pt tolerated procedure well. Postop instructions given. Pt to return in 1 wk for suture removal and check. |
| | | | T. Clark, CDA/L. Stewart, DDS |

PROCEDURE 56.6

# Assisting in Removal of an Impacted Tooth

## EQUIPMENT AND SUPPLIES

- ✓ Forceps extraction setup
- ✓ Scalpel, #15 blade and handle
- ✓ Additional elevators and forceps (surgeon's choice)
- ✓ Rongeur
- ✓ Bone file
- ✓ Curettes
- ✓ Root tip picks
- ✓ Surgical scissors
- ✓ Surgical high-speed handpiece with surgical bur or mallet and chisel
- ✓ Irrigating syringe
- ✓ Sterile saline solution
- ✓ Sterile suture material and needle
- ✓ Needle holder or hemostat
- ✓ Suture scissors
- ✓ Sterile gauze sponges

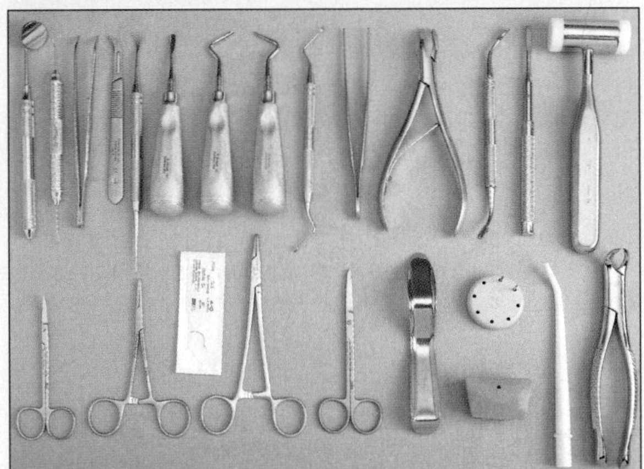

*From Boyd LRB: Dental instruments: a pocket guide, ed 6, St Louis, 2018, Elsevier.*

## PROCEDURAL STEPS

### Surgical Preparation

1. The surgeon determines that adequate anesthesia has been achieved.
2. Transfer the scalpel for the surgeon to make the initial incision along the ridge through the gingival mucosa and the periosteum.
3. The periosteal elevator is used to retract the tissues away from the bone.
4. Once the incision has been made continuously, evacuate blood, debris, and saliva from the surgical site.
5. A surgical mallet and chisel or a surgical handpiece with surgical burs will be used to remove the bony covering from the impacted tooth.

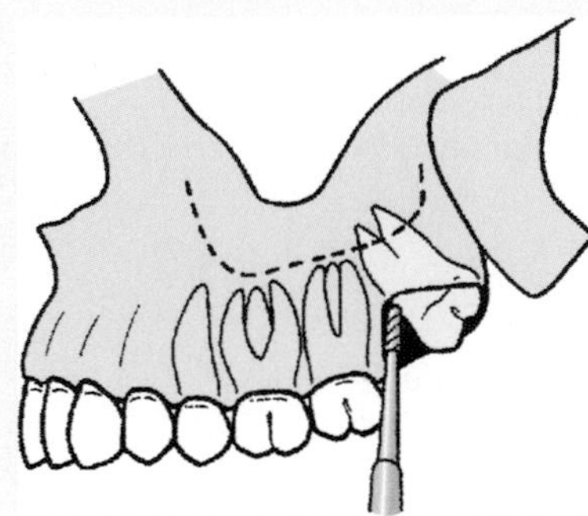

*From Hupp JR, Tucker MR, Ellis E III: Contemporary oral and maxillofacial surgery, ed 6, St Louis, 2014, Mosby.*

### Removing the Impacted Tooth

6. When the surgeon has uncovered the impacted tooth, it can be luxated and lifted from the alveolus with the use of an elevator or extraction forceps.

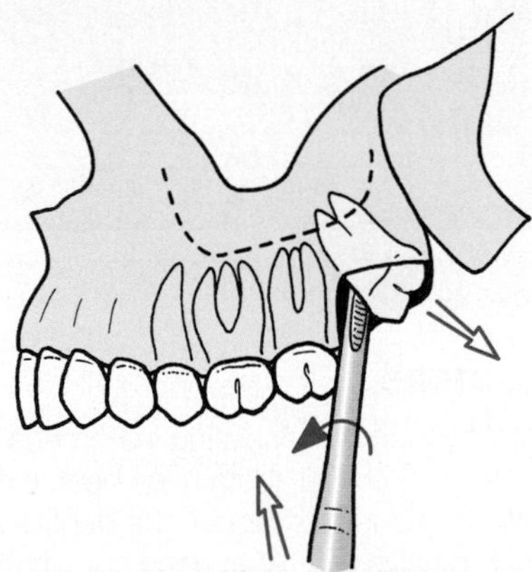

*From Hupp JR, Tucker MR, and Ellis E III: Contemporary oral and maxillofacial surgery, ed 6, St Louis, 2014, Mosby.*

7. If the tooth is lodged between bone and another tooth, this may require the surgeon to section the crown of the impacted tooth with the mallet and chisel or a surgical bur.
8. After the tooth has been removed, the surgical site is curetted, irrigated, and evacuated to remove all debris and infectious material.
9. After a thorough debridement, the surgeon returns the mucoperiosteal flap to its normal position over the wound and sutures it into place.
10. Return the patient slowly to an upright position.
11. Provide the patient with postoperative instructions.
12. Document the procedure.

| Date | Tooth | Surface | Charting Notes |
|---|---|---|---|
| 8/26/17 | 16, 17 | — | Vitals: P 80, BP 130/82. Extraction, $N_2O$ sedation, 4 cartridges Xylocaine 1:20,000; incision using #12 blade, teeth removed in sections; 2 gut sutures placed per site. Pt tolerated procedure well. Pt to return in 1 wk. Postop instructions given. |

T. Clark, CDA/L. Stewart, DDS

PROCEDURE 56.7

# Assisting in Suture Placement

## EQUIPMENT AND SUPPLIES

- ✓ Suture material
- ✓ Hemostats
- ✓ Needle holder
- ✓ Suture scissors
- ✓ Sterile gauze sponges

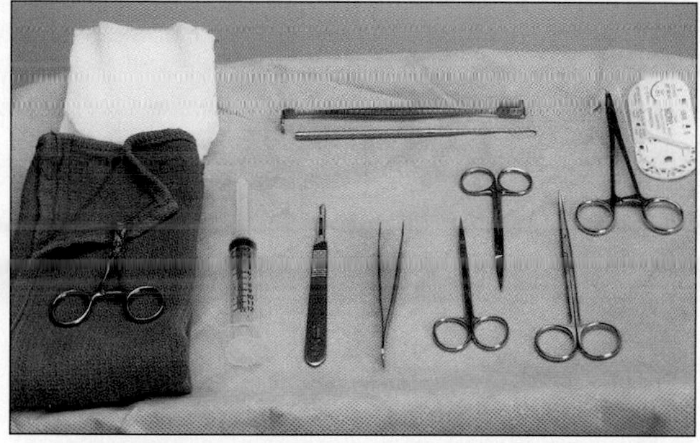

## PROCEDURAL STEPS

1 Remove the suture material from its sterile package.

2 Using the needle holder, clamp the suture needle at the upper third.

**PURPOSE** If you clamp too close to the thread, you may cause the suture to detach from the needle; if you clamp too close to the needle end, you may damage the needle point.

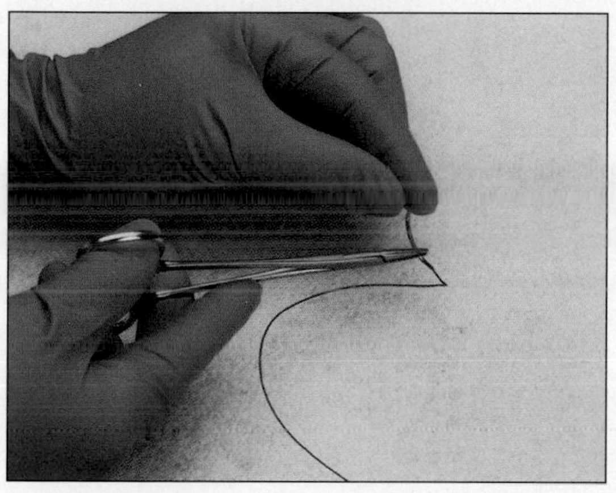

3 Transfer the needle holder to the surgeon; while you are grasping the hinge, allow the surgeon to grasp the handle of the instrument.

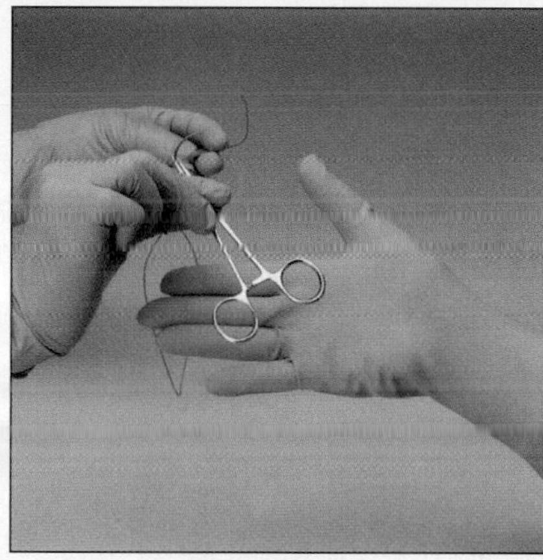

4 Retract the tongue or the cheek to provide a clear line of vision for the surgeon as the sutures are placed.

5 After the tying of each suture, if directed by the surgeon, use the suture scissors to cut the sutures, leaving approximately 2 to 3 mm of suture material beyond the knot.

6 Retrieve the suturing supplies from the surgeon, and replace them on the surgical tray.

7 Record in the patient's record the numbers and types of sutures placed.

Photos from Proctor DB, et al: Kinn's the medical assistant: an applied learning approach, ed 13, St Louis, 2017, Elsevier.

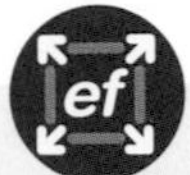  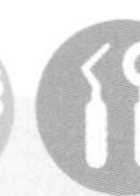 

PROCEDURE 56.8 

# Performing Suture Removal (Expanded Function)

## PREREQUISITES FOR PERFORMING THIS PROCEDURE

- ✔ Operator positioning
- ✔ Knowledge of technique
- ✔ Intraoral instrumentation
- ✔ Mirror skills
- ✔ Fulcrum placement

## EQUIPMENT AND SUPPLIES (Suture tray setup)

- ✔ Basic setup
- ✔ Suture scissors
- ✔ Sterile cotton gauze
- ✔ Cotton-tip applicator
- ✔ Antiseptic solution

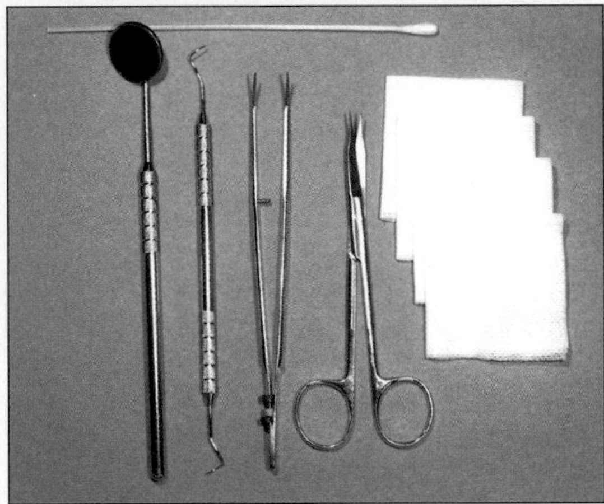

## PROCEDURAL STEPS

1. The surgeon will examine the surgical site to evaluate healing. If healing is satisfactory, the sutures may be removed.
2. Swab the site with an antiseptic agent to remove any debris.
3. Use cotton pliers to hold the suture gently away from the tissue to expose the attachment of the knot.

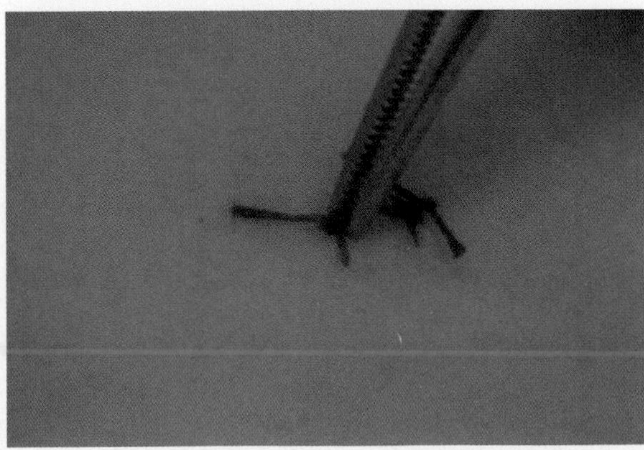

4. Slip one blade of the suture scissors gently under the suture. Cut near the tissue.

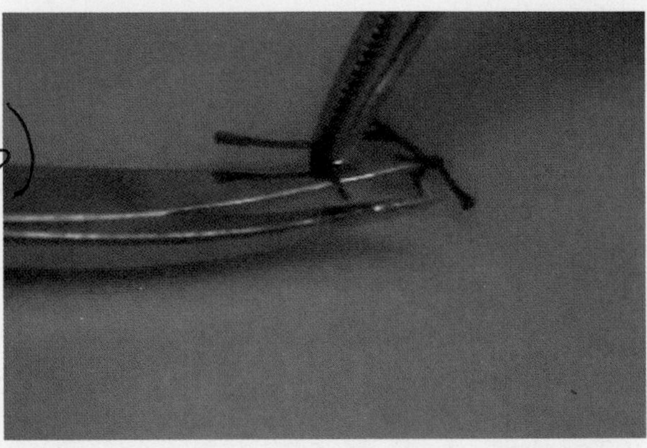

5. Use the cotton pliers to grasp the knot, and gently tug it so the suture slides through the tissue.
   **NOTE** Never pull ("yank") the knot through the tissue.

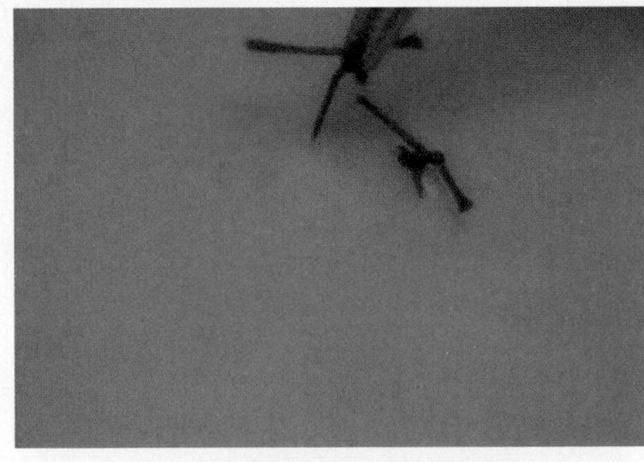

6. If bleeding occurs, irrigate the surgical site with an antiseptic solution or warm saline solution. Apply a compress briefly to the surgical site to promote clotting.
7. Count the sutures that have been removed, and compare this number with the number documented in the patient's record.

| Date | Tooth | Surface | Charting Notes |
|---|---|---|---|
| 9/3/17 | — | — | Suture removal, 4 nylon sutures removed. Pt healing well, with no complications. |
| | | | T. Clark, CDA/L. Stewart, DDS |

PROCEDURE 56.9

# Assisting in the Treatment of Alveolar Osteitis

## EQUIPMENT AND SUPPLIES

- ✓ Basic setup
- ✓ Scissors
- ✓ Irrigation syringe
- ✓ Warm saline solution
- ✓ Iodoform gauze
- ✓ Medicated dressing
- ✓ High-volume oral evacuator (HVE) tip

## PROCEDURAL STEPS

1 The socket is gently irrigated with warm saline solution.
**PURPOSE** To remove accumulated debris from the alveolus.

2 A narrow strip of iodoform gauze is cut to a length that fills the socket.
**PURPOSE** Iodoform gauze contains a topical antiseptic that soothes the nerve endings and prevents infection.

3 The gauze is dipped in the medication and is gently packed in the socket.
**PURPOSE** The medication soothes the exposed bone. Packing the gauze in the socket prevents food from becoming lodged in the wound.

4 The dentist may prescribe analgesics to relieve the pain, antibiotics to treat the infection, or both.

5 The patient is instructed to return so this procedure can be repeated and healing can be evaluated.

6 Document the procedure.

| Date | Tooth | Surface | Charting Notes |
|---|---|---|---|
| 9/4/17 | — | — | Pt having discomfort from surgery. Diagnosed with alveolitis. Surgical site irrigated with warm saline solution, iodoform gauze packed in socket, prescription for Tylenol with codeine. Reschedule for evaluation and change of dressing. |
| | | | T. Clark, CDA/L. Stewart, DDS |

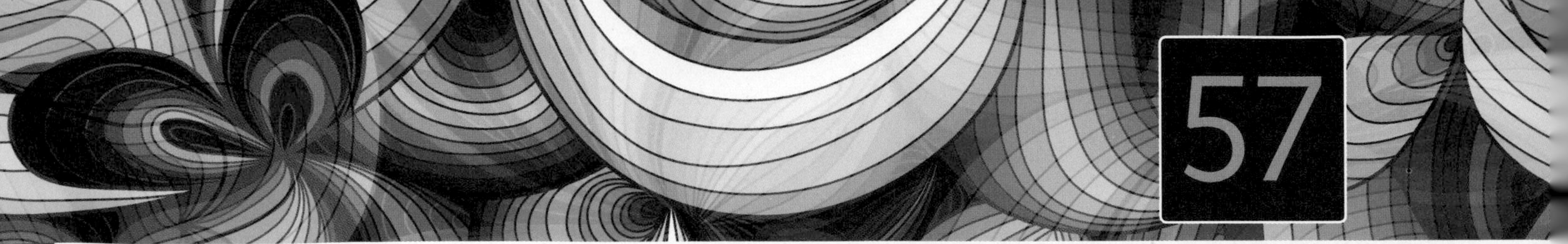

57

# Pediatric Dentistry

## KEY TERMS

**Analogy (uh-NAL-uh-jee)** Comparison of similarities between things that are otherwise not alike.

**Athetosis (ATH-e-toe-sis)** Type of involuntary movement of the body, face, and extremities.

**Autonomy (aw-TON-uh-mee)** Childhood process of becoming independent.

**Avulsed (uh-VULST)** Torn away or dislodged by force.

**Cerebral palsy (suh-REE-brul PAWL-zee)** Neural disorder of motor function caused by brain damage.

**Chronologic (KRON-uh-loj-ik) age** Actual age (months, years) of pediatric patients.

**Contour (KON-toor)** To shape or conform an object.

**Down syndrome** Chromosomal defect that results in abnormal physical characteristics and mental impairment; also called *trisomy 21.*

**Emotional age** Measure of the level of emotional maturity of pediatric patients.

**Extrusion (ek-STROO-zhun)** Displacement of a tooth from its socket as a result of injury.

**Frankl (FRANG-kul) scale** Scale designed to evaluate patient behavior.

**Intellectual disability** Disorder in which an individual's intelligence is underdeveloped.

**Intrusion (in-TROO-zhun)** Displacement of a tooth into its socket as a result of injury.

**Luxation (luk-SAY-shun)** Dislocation.

**Mental age** Measure of the level of intellectual capacity and development of pediatric patients.

**Neural (NUR-uhl)** Referring to the brain, nervous system, and nerve pathways.

**Open bay** Concept of open design used in pediatric dental practices.

**Papoose (pa-POOS) board** Type of protective stabilization device that holds the pediatric patient's hands, arms, and legs still.

**Pediatric (pee-dee-AT-rik) dentistry** Dental specialty concerned with neonatal through adolescent patients, as well as patients with special needs in these age groups.

**Postnatal (post-NAY-tul)** After birth.

**Prenatal** Before birth.

**Pulpotomy (pul-POT-uh-mee)** Removal of the coronal portion of a vital pulp from a tooth.

**Spasticity (spas-TIS-i-tee)** Exaggerated movement of the arms and legs.

**T-band** Type of matrix band used for primary teeth.

## LEARNING OUTCOMES

*On completion of this chapter, the student will be able to achieve the following objectives:*

1. Pronounce, define, and spell the key terms.
2. Discuss the pediatric dental team and the appearance and setting of a pediatric dental office.
3. Discuss the pediatric patient, including the following:
   - List the stages of childhood from birth through adolescence.
   - Discuss specific behavior techniques that work as positive reinforcement when treating children.
4. Explain why children and adults with special needs are treated in a pediatric practice.
5. Describe what is involved in the diagnosis and treatment planning of a pediatric patient.
6. Discuss the importance of preventive dentistry in pediatrics.
7. List the types of procedures that are performed for the pediatric patient compared with those performed to treat patients with permanent teeth.
8. Discuss types of pediatric dental trauma and their treatments.
9. Discuss how to handle suspected child abuse and neglect.

## PERFORMANCE OUTCOMES

*On completion of this chapter, the student will be able to meet competency standards in the following skills:*

- Assist in a pulpotomy of a primary tooth.
- Assist in the placement of a stainless steel crown.

## ELECTRONIC RESOURCES

***Additional information related to content in Chapter 57 can be found on the companion Evolve Web site.***

- Practice Quiz
- Canadian Content Corner

**Pediatric dentistry** is the specialized area of dentistry that focuses on providing oral healthcare according to the needs of infants, children, adolescents, and individuals with special needs. Emphasis of the pediatric dental practice is placed on prevention, early detection, diagnosis, and treatment. Although many of the procedures completed for children are similar to those for adult patients, pediatric patients require special adaptations and techniques in the way dentistry is provided (Fig. 57.1).

# The Pediatric Dental Team and Office

## The Pediatric Dentist

A pediatric dentist will continue his or her education for an additional 2 to 3 years after dental school in an accredited pediatric program based in a dental school setting. The program of study and hands-on experience prepares the specialist to meet the needs of infants, children, adolescents, and persons with special needs.

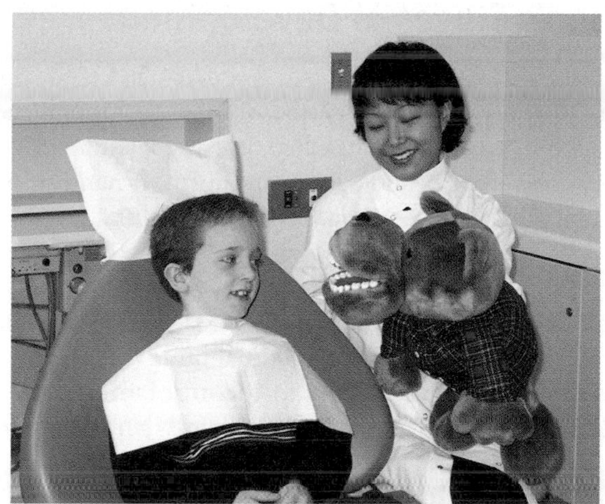

**FIG. 57.1** Patient at a pediatric dental office.

## The Pediatric Dental Assistant

As a dental assistant in a pediatric setting, you must have the compassion and patience to enjoy working with children, adolescents, and patients with special needs. Pediatric dentistry provides a clinical practice ("hands-on") environment where you will have an active role in the patient's dental care. Many pediatric dental offices employ a certified dental assistant to perform preventive procedures that are legal to perform in that state, province, or territory. If coronal polishing, application of sealants, and taking of preliminary impressions are legal functions, these *expanded functions* would be completed in a pediatric setting.

## The Pediatric Dental Office

The pediatric dental office will display a cheerfulness and pleasant environment with a nonthreatening decor. Many offices will have a "theme" in the overall decor, such as a rain forest, outer space, or even a popular movie character (Fig. 57.2).

When entering a pediatric dental practice, you will notice that the treatment areas are not confining or structured. Many practices are designed with the **open bay** concept, in which several dental chairs are arranged in one large area. The advantage of this design is that it provides reassurance by allowing pediatric patients to see other children who are receiving care. This can be psychologically effective because children are often hesitant to express fear or to misbehave in the presence of other children.

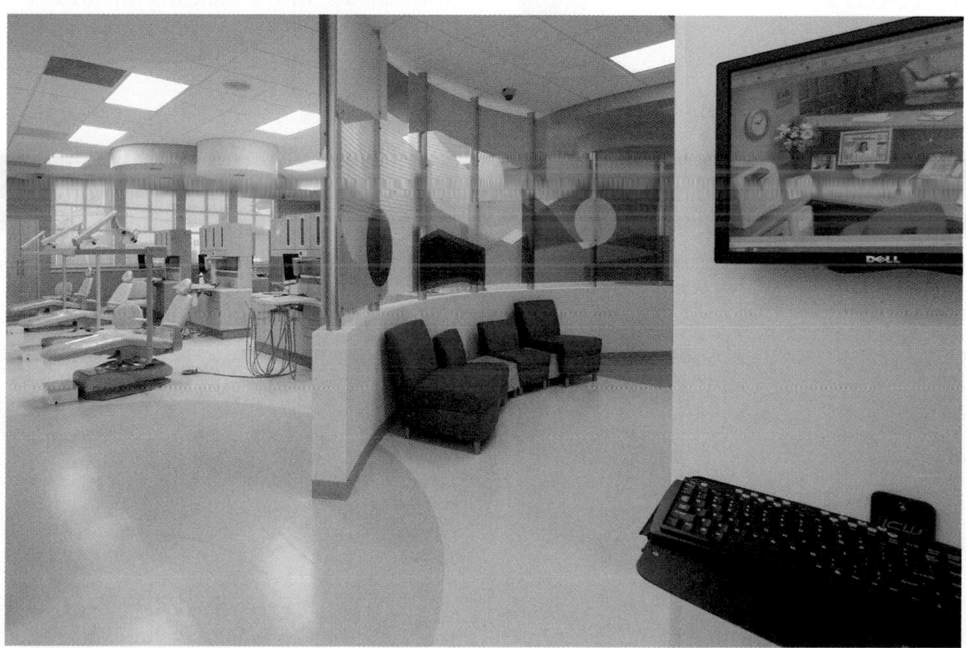

**FIG. 57.2** Example of pleasing, patient-friendly reception area of a pediatric dental office. *(Courtesy Patterson Dental, St Paul, MN.)*

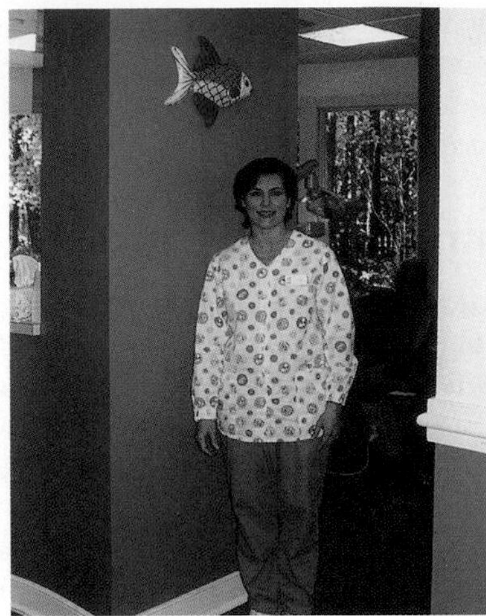

**FIG. 57.3** Clinical assistants should dress professionally but in a nonthreatening manner for the pediatric dental patient.

If an isolated area is required for patient care, most practices will use a "quiet room." This room is separate from the open area and can be used for children whose behavior may upset other children.

A variety of reading materials, such as magazines and educational brochures, should be available for both the pediatric patient and the parent. Some offices install computer and video equipment with programs intended for patient education and entertainment.

Many pediatric offices are less "medical looking" with regard to how dental personnel dress. It is common for "scrubs" to be worn in bright coordinating colors or designs (Fig. 57.3). Name tags worn by the staff may even resemble a tooth, with the assistant's name inscribed.

RECALL

1 Would it be possible to see a 21-year-old patient in a pediatric office?
2 What is unique about the treatment setting of a pediatric practice?
3 What types of patients are seen in a pediatric practice?

## The Pediatric Patient

Children constitute an important and special portion of the dental population. As with adults, children have individual likes and dislikes, as well as fears and complex personalities. The pediatric patient is treated with the same respect of dignity and individuality as is provided to an adult. The child must be understood in terms of his or her chronologic, mental, and emotional ages:

- **Chronologic age** is the child's actual age in terms of years and months.
- **Mental age** refers to the child's level of intellectual capacity and development.
- **Emotional age** describes the child's level of emotional maturity.

These ages are not necessarily the same for each child. For instance, a child at the chronologic age of 6 may have a mental age of 8 (i.e., *mentally,* the child is comprehending information at the level of the average 8-year-old) and an emotional age of 4 (i.e., *emotionally,* he or she is reacting at the level of the average 4-year-old).

According to well-known psychiatrist Erik Erikson, the socialization process consists of stages. These stages were formulated to understand the social and emotional development of children and teenagers. A guideline *(norm)* for the average child's development can be used as a simple index to the child's anticipated behavior level at a certain age. A child who differs widely from these norms may be physically or emotionally challenged. It is important to remember that some children may be under the stress of a dental appointment and could temporarily regress to a more immature level of behavior.

### Erikson's Stages of Development

#### Learning Basic Trust

Chronologically, this is the period of infancy through the first year of life. The child, well handled, nurtured, and loved, develops trust and security and a basic optimism. If handled poorly, the infant will become insecure and mistrustful.

#### Learning Autonomy

During this period, children learn to sit, stand, walk, and run. Vocally, they progress from babbling to using simple sentences. Socially, they learn to identify familiar faces and alternate through periods of being friendly and being fearful of strangers.

Around the age of 2 years old, children begin to have basic fears associated with separation from the parent and a related fear of strangers. These "toddlers" are too young to be expected to cooperate with dental treatment. It is easier for the parent to be with the child during the initial examination. If further treatment is required, the child may require premedication.

#### Play Age

A child 3 to 5 years of age has two primary and somewhat conflicting needs (Fig. 57.4). First, the child has gone through a process of developing **autonomy** and initiative. Second, the child requires control and structure in his or her environment. Children are able to follow simple instructions, and they welcome having an active role in the treatment experience. The child's role is to help by following directions and "sitting still," "keeping your hands by your side," and "opening your mouth wide." By allowing the child to have choices, the dental team shows regard for the child's need for autonomy and initiative.

#### School Age

The child ages 6 to 11 is in a period of **socialization,** which involves learning to "get along" with people, learning the rules and regulations of society, and learning to accept these social requirements. Through their experiences with others, children at this age have learned to overcome fears of objects

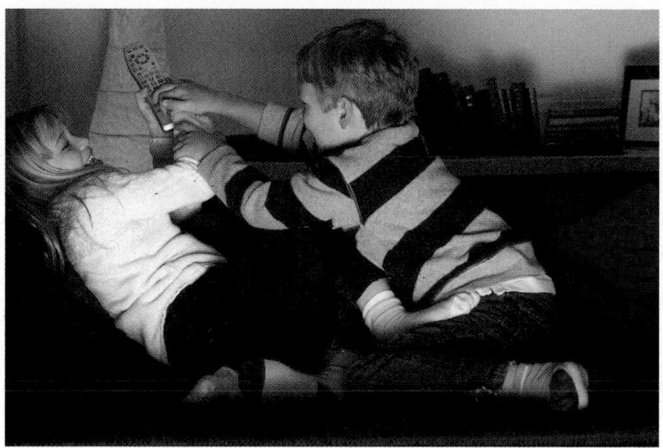

**FIG. 57.4** During the period in which children are developing autonomy, conflicts with siblings, peers, and parents can seem never-ending. *(Copyright © Monkey Business Images/Monkey Business/Getty Images.)*

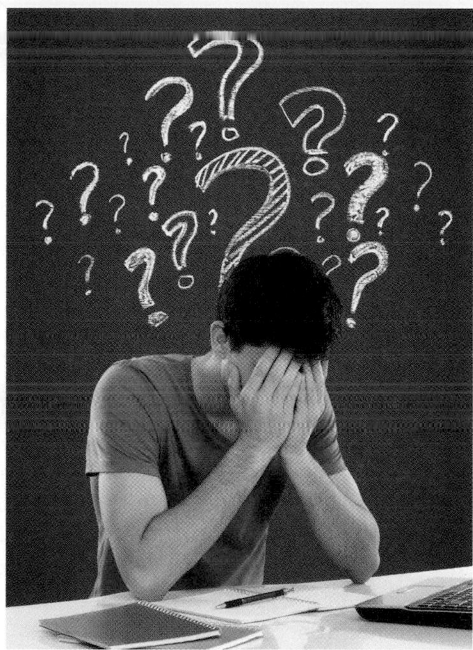

**FIG. 57.5** Adolescence is an extremely complex stage of development because of the many new opportunities and challenges thrust on the teenager. *(Copyright © ferlistockphoto/iStock/Getty Images.)*

and situations that were once quite frightening to them. They have learned that situations usually are less threatening than they had imagined, and that generally they need not be afraid.

### Adolescence

This is a transitional stage of physical and psychological human development generally occurring during the period from puberty to young adulthood. The period of adolescence is most closely associated with the teenage years, although its physical, psychological, and cultural expressions can begin earlier and end later. From ages 12 to 20, young people acquire self-certainty (Fig. 57.5). They experiment with different roles. Clear sexual identity is established. The adolescent will seek leadership (someone to inspire them) and will gradually develop a set of ideals.

## Behavior Management

The initial examination is important for both the child and the dental team. Remember that this often is the first dental experience for the child. The rapport developed during the initial examination can establish an attitude toward dental health that will last for a child's lifetime.

Many dentists will follow a **behavior scale** early in the treatment of a pediatric patient. The child's behavior then can be evaluated and followed through the child's experience in the practice. Dr. Spencer Frankl developed one of the most widely used systems, the **Frankl scale**, to measure a pediatric patient's behavior (Table 57.1).

### Guidelines for Child Behavior

The development of trust between the parent/child and the dentist serves as the basis for a productive, effective means of providing dental healthcare. Dental procedures can be accomplished for patients of all ages if the dental team practices the following procedural guidelines:

- **Be honest with the child.** Make sure that what is said to the child is true from the child's point of view.
- **Consider the child's point of view.** Words that unnecessarily evoke fear in the child should be avoided. Also, the child must understand the words that are used. For example, it is

**TABLE 57.1** Frankl Scale for Pediatric Dental Patient Behavior

| Rating | Definition | Patient Behavior |
|---|---|---|
| 1 | Definitely negative | Refusal of treatment; crying forcefully; fearful; other evidence of extreme negativism |
| 2 | Negative | Reluctance to accept treatment; uncooperative; some evidence of negative attitude but not pronounced, that is, no sudden withdrawal |
| 3 | Positive | Acceptance of treatment; cautious at times; willingness to comply, at times with reservation, but follows directions |
| 4 | Definitely positive | Good rapport with dentist; interested in dental procedures; laughing and enjoying the situation |

Courtesy Dr. Spencer Frankl.

better to use a word such as "pinch" rather than "mosquito bite," especially if the child does not clearly understand that a "mosquito bite" hurts.

- **Always "tell, show, and do." Tell** the child what is to be done, **show** the child what is to be done, and then proceed to **do** exactly what the child has been led to expect. The dental team should not assume that a procedure or instrument is so harmless that it will not concern a child. The team should include this "tell, show, and do" process in any new procedure.
- **Give positive reinforcement.** Reinforce and reward appropriate behaviors; avoid rewarding undesirable behavior.

### Examples of Ways to Include a Young Child in a Procedure

- Have the child select the type of safety eyewear that he or she would like to wear today.
- Say to the child, "Point to the tooth you would like me to start with."
- Have the child point to the tooth that was "smiling for the camera" (radiograph).
- Allow the child to choose the flavor of fluoride.
- Ask the child to hold the saliva ejector during the procedure.

### *The Challenging Patient*

Treating an anxious, fearful, or uncooperative child can be challenging for the dentist, assistant, parents, and especially for the child. In some situations, a child will remain uncooperative despite the fact that the dental team has used every possible approach to provide a positive dental experience. Occasionally, a child's behavior during treatment requires a firmer management style to be used to protect him or her from possible injury. Voice control (speaking calmly but firmly) will usually prevent the need for additional steps.

In certain cases, a form of restraint may be required for a patient's protection. The use of **restraint** can be either pharmacologic or physical to help lessen a patient's movement or activity to a minimum. If the dentist knows that restraint will be needed, premedication can be prescribed to calm and ease the patient before treatment. Mild sedation, such as nitrous oxide/oxygen or a sedative, may benefit an anxious child. If a child is especially fearful and/or requires extensive dental treatment, other sedative techniques or intravenous (IV) sedation may be recommended (see Chapter 37).

Physical restraint can be as simple as the dentist or assistant holding a child's hands during treatment. By holding the child's hands, you can prevent possible injury to the child, the dentist, and yourself, if, for instance, the child were to quickly reach for the syringe during an injection or for the dentist's arm while using the handpiece.

For young toddlers and preschool-age children, a parent may be asked to help keep the child calm and under control. A problem with this scenario is that if a parent is anxious or nervous about the child's care, bringing him or her back into the clinical setting may actually impair the situation and create an even more nervous environment.

Additional steps for restraining a child can be taken with the use of protective stabilization. Protective stabilization is any manual method, physical or mechanical device, material, or equipment that immobilizes or reduces the ability of a patient to move his or her arms, legs, body, or head freely. The **papoose board** is a device that gently "hugs" or wraps around the child's arms, legs, and middle section during a procedure. The papoose board uses Velcro straps that fasten over the child and restrains the movement of the child's hands, arms, and legs (Fig. 57.6). This device can be adapted for the younger child who has been sedated or for the patient with special needs who may have limited control of his or her movement.

When the dentist takes steps in using pharmacologic or protective stabilization with a child, the parents must be made aware and must provide consent. An immediate and documented explanation should be given to parents as to why such actions are to be taken. The child should also be informed appropriately.

RECALL

4 Is it possible for a child to be 10 years old but to act like a 7-year-old? If so, what are you describing about this patient?
5 At what developmental stage do children first want control and structure of their environment?
6 How would Dr. Frankl describe a "positive" child?
7 When would a papoose board be used?

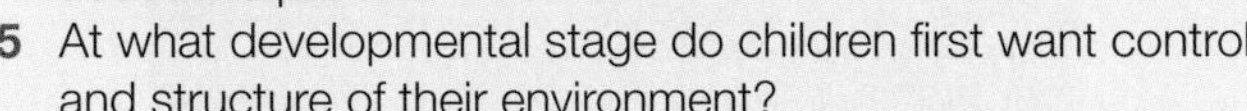

## Patients with Special Needs

Certain physical and mental disorders can slow or challenge a child's psychological and social growth. When a child has been diagnosed with a condition such as intellectual disability, Down syndrome, autism, or cerebral palsy, parents and families become responsible for assisting with more of the child's daily physical and oral health needs.

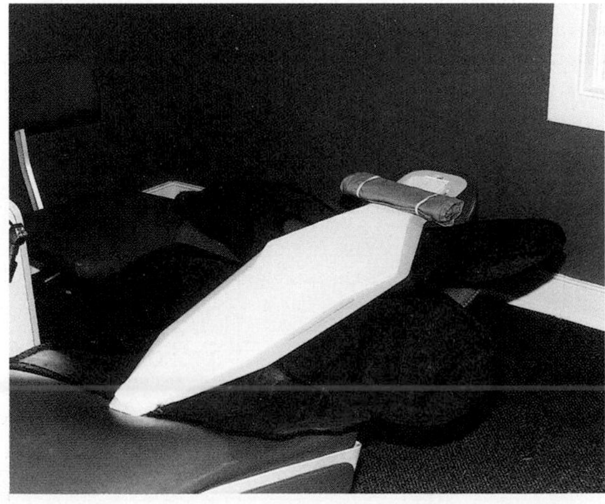

**FIG. 57.6** The papoose board provides a way of holding the arms and legs still to prevent patients from injuring themselves or others.

The environment of a pediatric dental office better suits a patient who has been diagnosed with special needs. The severity of each patient's disorder dictates whether treatment is provided in the pediatric dental office or in the hospital setting. Evaluation of a patient's medical and social history helps reveal whether modifications to the treatment plan are needed.

## Intellectual Disability

**Intellectual disability** is a particular state of functioning that begins in childhood and is characterized by limitations in intelligence and in adaptive skills. For descriptive purposes, *intellectual disabled* individuals are classified into four groups that reflect their degree of intellectual impairment: mild, moderate, severe, and profound.

*Mild intellectual disability* describes individuals with intelligence quotients (IQs) ranging from 50 up to 70. These individuals typically develop social and communication skills during the preschool years and have minimal impairment in sensorimotor areas; they often are indistinguishable from normal children until a later age. They are capable of receiving dental care in the usual manner. Because comprehension is slow, a patient may require extra patience, understanding, and reassurance. With help from the dental team, a person with mild intellectual disability can become a good dental patient.

When communicating with the patient who has mild intellectual disability, do the following:

- Minimize distractions
- Use short explanations
- Use simple language
- Take more time to present information
- Avoid explanation of causes
- Focus on effects of lack of oral hygiene
- Teach activities rather than concepts
- Encourage consistency
- Use "tell-show-do"
- Use positive reinforcement
- Use verbal praise

*Moderate intellectual disability* describes individuals with IQs ranging from 35 up to 55. These individuals talk or learn to communicate during the preschool years. They may profit from vocational training and, with moderate supervision, can take care of themselves; however, they are unlikely to progress beyond the second-grade level in academic subjects. They adapt well to life in the community, but they need supervision and guidance when under stress and usually live in supervised group homes. A patient with moderate intellectual disability probably will require special care in receiving dental treatment, including premedication, restraints, or care while under general anesthesia.

*Severe intellectual disability* describes individuals with IQs ranging from 20 up to 40. During the preschool period, these individuals display poor motor development and acquire little or no communicative speech. In their adult years, they may be able to perform simple tasks under close supervision. Specialized dental treatment involving general anesthesia is frequently necessary for patients with severe intellectual disabilities.

*Profound intellectual disability* describes individuals with IQs below 20 to 25. During the early years, these children display minimal capacity for sensorimotor functioning. A highly structured environment with constant aid and supervision is necessary throughout life. These individuals require specialized dental care, which usually is provided in an institutional setting.

## Down Syndrome

Patients with **Down syndrome**, also known as *trisomy 21,* have a chromosomal deficit that commonly results in certain abnormal physical characteristics and mental impairment. The intellectual disability may range from mild to moderate. The common physical characteristics unique to a Down patient are: the back of the head is flattened, the eyes are slanted and almond shaped, and the bridge of the nose is slightly depressed. Muscle strength and muscle tone usually are reduced, and one third of these children are diagnosed with heart problems.

Frequently, patients with Down syndrome have anomalies in dental development. Eruption of teeth may be delayed, with the primary incisors not erupting until after 1 year of age. Teeth may be small and peg-shaped, often with malocclusion. Periodontal problems are common because of malaligned teeth, mouth breathing, or poor dental care at home. The forward position of the mandible and underdeveloped nasal and maxillary bones do not provide sufficient space for the tongue. The resulting open-mouth, forward-tongue position gives the appearance of an enlarged tongue.

Dental treatment for patients with Down syndrome depends on the person's psychological development and physical problems. The patient should be approached in terms of *mental* age and abilities, not in terms of chronologic age.

## Autism

Autism is a developmental disorder that affects how information is processed in the brain by altering how nerve cells and their synapses connect and organize. Signs of this disorder are evident before a child reaches 3 years of age, and the disorder can be characterized by difficulty in social interaction, difficulty in verbal and nonverbal communication, and repetitive behaviors.

This patient may exhibit behavioral problems with management difficulties. Behavior management techniques may include behavior modification, positive reinforcement, and desensitization; however, sedation, restraint, and general anesthesia may be necessary when oral disease is extensive.

Patients who have autism have a known desire for sweet foods and generally have poor oral hygiene. Therefore these patients are at risk for increased dental caries and periodontal disease. Patients with autism are often receiving psychotropic medications, which can cause xerostomia.

## Cerebral Palsy

**Cerebral palsy** is a broad term that is used to describe a group of nonprogressive **neural** disorders caused by **prenatal** or

**postnatal** brain damage before the central nervous system has reached maturity. The resultant brain damage *manifests* (presents) as a malfunction of motor centers and is characterized by paralysis, muscle weakness, lack of coordination, and other disorders of motor function.

In addition to motor disabilities, many individuals with cerebral palsy have other symptoms of brain damage, such as seizure disorders, intellectual disability, and sensory and learning disorders. These conditions may be complicated further by behavioral and emotional disorders.

Cerebral palsy most often is classified according to the type of *motor disturbance.* The two most common types are spasticity and athetosis. **Spasticity** is characterized by a state of increased muscle tension that manifests as an exaggerated stretch reflex. **Athetosis** is marked by uncontrollable, involuntary, purposeless, and poorly coordinated movements of the body, face, and extremities; grimacing, drooling, and speech defects are present.

Premedication frequently is used to help control and relax the patient with cerebral palsy. Along with patience, understanding, and flexibility of the dental team, premedication makes routine dental care possible. For some patients, however, general anesthesia may be necessary.

Oral hygiene in most patients with cerebral palsy is poor, in part because of the nature of their disease and the resultant physical limitations. The patient and the caregiver should receive a thorough orientation to a home care program, with modifications as necessary to meet the patient's special needs. Frequently, an electric toothbrush can be used effectively. Special adaptations of toothbrush handles and other aids to hygiene also may be helpful.

RECALL

8 What types of skills are limited in an intellectual disabled child?
9 What is another term for Down syndrome?
10 Would it be common for you to treat a cerebral palsy patient in a wheelchair? If so, why?

# Diagnosis and Treatment Planning

According to the American Academy of Pediatric Dentistry (AAPD), the first dental appointment for a child should take place around his or her first birthday or when their first tooth erupts. This appointment is scheduled to collect information, introduce the child to the dentist and staff, and help the child feel comfortable in the office surroundings. It also gives the dental team an opportunity to educate the parents on preventive techniques and pediatric care. It is then recommended that the child begin regular examinations at age 2. Once dental care has begun, the patient will be instructed to return for recall appointments.

The child's parent or legal guardian must give consent before any dental care is provided for a child younger than 18 years of age. Introduce yourself to the child and the parent and welcome them to the office. While interacting with the parent and the child, establish a friendly but professional rapport to aid in the development of confidence among dental team members.

## Medical and Dental History

The medical and dental history should include information about the child's general medical and dental health background; these details are reviewed with the parent and the child.

### Specific Information Noted in the Pediatric Medical and Dental History

**Medical History**

- Past hospitalizations and procedures while under general anesthesia
- Date of last visit to the physician and current treatment
- Medications taken in the past
- Daily medications
- Unfavorable reaction to any medicine
- Allergies, including to any prescribed or over-the-counter medications taken
- Weight at birth and any problems that occurred at birth
- Parental report on level of learning

**Dental History**

- Primary concern about the child's dental health
- Satisfaction with appearance of teeth
- Bleeding gums with brushing
- Finger, thumb, or pacifier habits
- Fluoride and toothbrush habits
- Inherited family dental characteristics

## Initial Clinical Examination

Depending on the child's age, the dentist will take radiographic images and will complete an extraoral examination, an intraoral soft tissue examination, and a clinical examination, which includes charting of the teeth (Fig. 57.7).

### *Radiographic Imaging*

In general, children often require radiographs on a more routine basis than adults. Because their mouths grow and change rapidly, children can be more susceptible to tooth decay. The AAPD recommends radiographs every 6 months for children with a high risk for tooth decay (less frequently in children at low risk).

A radiographic examination is necessary if a complete diagnosis is to be made. Young children often have difficulty cooperating with the radiographic procedure, which may have to be postponed until the child is better able to withstand the size of the film in the mouth and to refrain from any movement. When radiographs are possible, the following steps are helpful in introducing the child to the procedure:

- Use words such as "camera" and "taking a picture" as an **analogy** to help explain the equipment and the process.
- Use the "tell, show, do" concept. By positioning the film and the x-ray unit, you can determine whether the child will sit for the exposure, without actually exposing the child to unnecessary radiation.

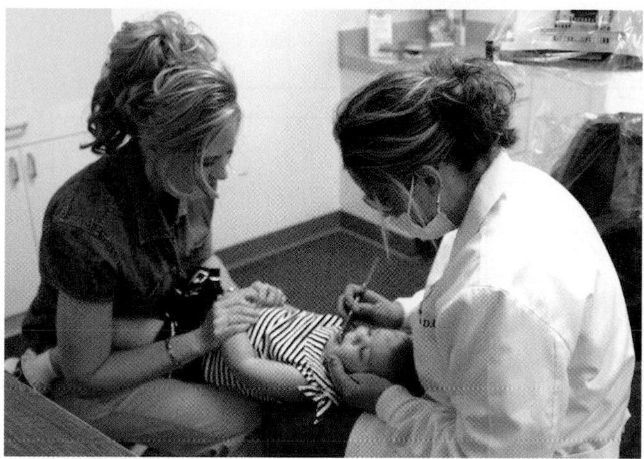

**FIG. 57.7** Positioning the child so the child can see his or her mother while being examined. *(From Dean JA, Avery DR, McDonald RE: McDonald and Avery dentistry for the child and adolescent, ed 10, St Louis, 2016, Elsevier.)*

- Match the size of the film to the child's level of comfort. In some cases, bending the anterior corners facilitates bitewing placement.
- Expose the easiest films first. Usually, occlusal projections are most comfortable for the child (Fig. 57.8).

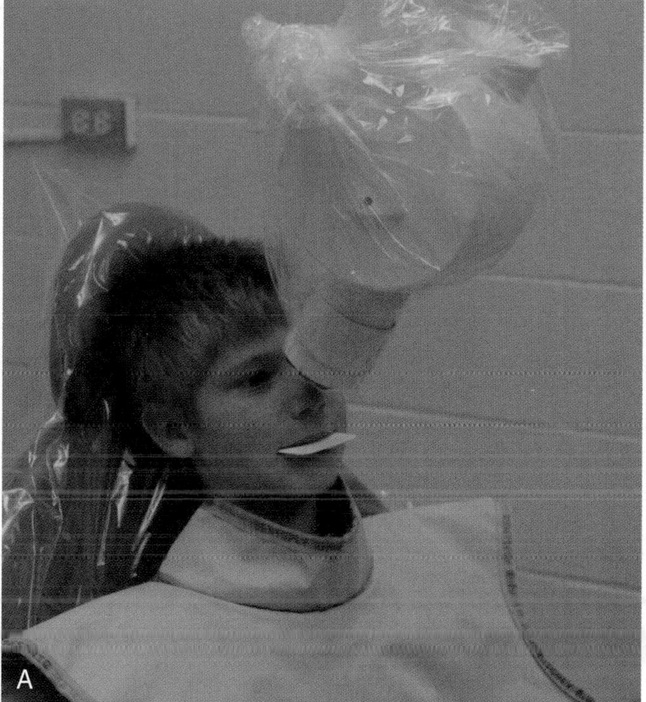


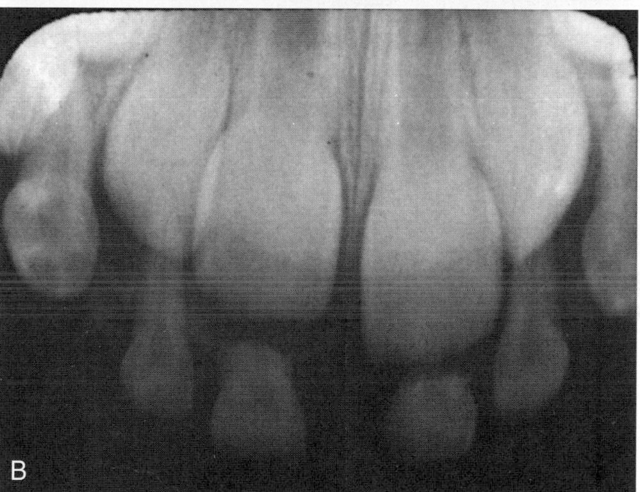


**FIG. 57.8** Maxillary occlusal projection. A, Technique. B, Radiographic image. *(From Dean JA, Avery DR, McDonald RE: McDonald and Avery dentistry for the child and adolescent, ed 9, St Louis, 2011, Elsevier.)*

### Extraoral Examination

The extraoral examination is used to evaluate the patient's profile to determine skeletal characteristics. Any facial deviation or asymmetry of the eyes, ears, or nose may be a symptom of an undiagnosed syndrome, and the child should be referred to an appropriate professional for complete evaluation.

### Intraoral Soft Tissue Examination

It is important for the dentist or the hygienist to evaluate the child's gingiva and periodontium through the use of a gingival score and/or a periodontal plaque score (see Chapter 55).

### Examination and Charting of Teeth

The initial clinical examination requires the use of a mouth mirror and an explorer. Very young children may be hesitant in allowing the dentist or hygienist to place an instrument and instead may allow "only fingers" in their mouth.

The primary or mixed dentition is examined with the occlusion to determine spacing and crowding of teeth. Chapter 28 describes the type of charting system used with the primary dentition.

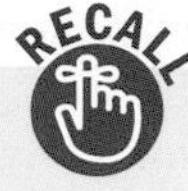


**11** When should a child first see the dentist?
**12** If a patient is at high risk for decay, how often should radiographs be taken?

## Preventive Dentistry for Children

Prevention is one of the most encompassing areas for a pediatric dental practice. It not only involves the complete dental team in educating the patient and parents, it also reaches to the community and to local school systems. The role of the pediatric dentist is to communicate the importance of preventive dental health in such areas as oral hygiene, fluoride use, diet, and preventive procedures.

## Oral Hygiene

Oral hygiene instructions are geared toward improving a child's brushing and flossing techniques. This teaching eventually will lead to cleaner teeth and healthier gums, thus preventing decay. By learning the habit of brushing effectively twice a day with fluoride toothpaste and flossing once a day, children will maintain proper oral habits throughout their lives (see Chapter 15).

The AAPD recommends a dental checkup twice a year for most children (Fig. 57.9). Some children need more frequent

DENTAL REPORT CARD

For: ______________________ Date: ____________

TREATMENT PERFORMED

PLAQUE SCORE

Upper

Right

Left

Lower

Scoring
2 = No plaque
1 = Detectable plaque
0 = Visible plaque

Today's Score _____
9-10 Excellent
7 - 8 Good
5 - 6 Fair

☐ Clinical Evaluation
- Evaluate tooth and jaw development
- Cavity detection examination
- Orthodontic screening
- Pathology screening
- Monitoring restorative treatment

☐ Dental prophylaxis (cleaning)

☐ Topical fluoride treatment
- Foam–wait 30 minutes to eat, drink, or rinse.
- Varnish–wait 10 minutes to eat, drink, or rinse. Do not brush for 12 hours. A yellowish tint is normal.

Necessary X-rays (radiographs) taken:
☐ Bitewings to evaluate for "tooth decay"
☐ Panorex to evaluate "jaw development and tooth development" and "pathology"
☐ Periapicals to evaluate "tooth development" and/or "pathology"

TREATMENT RECOMMENDATIONS AND FINDINGS

CURRENT STATUS

Patient's Oral Hygiene Evaluation:
☐ Needs Improvement ☐ Satisfactory ☐ Good
Cavities ☐ Yes ☐ No

Gums and Supporting Tissues:
☐ Normal and Healthy
☐ Inflamed/gingivitis
☐ Thin gum tissues ____
☐ Prominent frenum ____
☐ Other ____

Tooth Development:
☐ Normal and Healthy ☐ Hypoplastic enamel
☐ Mottling ☐ Missing teeth ☐ Extra teeth
☐ Abnormal shape ☐ Other ____

Tooth Eruptions:
☐ Normal ☐ Ankylosed teeth ____
☐ Ectopic eruption ____
☐ Abnormal ____

ORTHODONTIC EVALUATION

☐ Problems noted at this time
☐ Crowding ☐ Jaw Relation (bite off)
☐ Notes ____

RECOMMENDATIONS
☐ Observation
☐ Preventive/interceptive treatment
☐ Full treatment
Records fee ____
Treatment fee ____
Approximate treatment time ____
Other ____

Treatment fee and treatment time are estimates.

RECOMMENDATIONS FOR PROFESSIONAL CARE

___ Sealants
___ Fillings
___ Stainless steel crowns
___ Pulp therapy
___ Extractions
___ Space maintainers
Fee ____
# of appts. ____

Home Care Improvement Recommendations

___ Brush 2x a day (once in morning and once at bedtime)
___ Brush 3 minutes
___ Brush gumlines
___ Brush incisors
___ Brush molars
___ Floss nightly
___ Parents assist in brushing and flossing
___ Fluoride mouth rinse (ACT or Fluoriguard) (Use at bedtime after brushing and flossing)

**FIG. 57.9** Example of dental report card used for recall appointments. *(Courtesy Dr. John Christensen.)*

dental visits because of increased risk for tooth decay, unusual growth patterns, or poor oral hygiene.

## Fluorides

As discussed in Chapter 15, fluoride is safe and necessary, but only at appropriate levels. Children between the ages of 6 months and 16 years should have a daily intake of fluoride. Discuss with the parent how much fluoride is in their drinking water. If they drink well water or bottled water, assist them in getting an analysis of its fluoride content. After knowing how much fluoride the child receives, the pediatric dentist can decide whether the child needs a fluoride supplement.

Instruct the parent to watch the child's use of fluoridated toothpaste as the second step. A pea-sized amount on the brush is plenty for fluoride protection. Teach the child to spit out the toothpaste and not to swallow after brushing.

### *Fluoride Varnish*

Some patients are more susceptible to decay, and for them, fluoride rinses may not be as beneficial. Fluoride varnish is being used on a routine basis for caries prevention. The varnish is a gel-like substance designed to release fluoride on enamel and root structure (see Chapters 15 and 44 for additional information).

## Diet

A healthy diet is one that is balanced and that naturally supplies all the nutrients a child needs for growth. Chapter 16 describes the types of foods that children should eat for normal growth and identifies foods that may increase caries activity. An important role for the pediatric dental team is to do the following.

- Help assess the child's diet.
- Instruct parents to "shop smart" and not to routinely stock their pantry with sugary or starchy snacks. It is okay to buy "fun foods," but just for special times.
- Discuss limiting the number of snack times and choosing nutritious snacks.
- Review a balanced diet, and talk about saving foods with sugar or starch for mealtimes.
- Encourage parents to not put a young child to bed with a bottle of milk, formula, or juice.
- Discuss whether the child chews gum or drinks soda, and talk about choosing other options without added sugar.

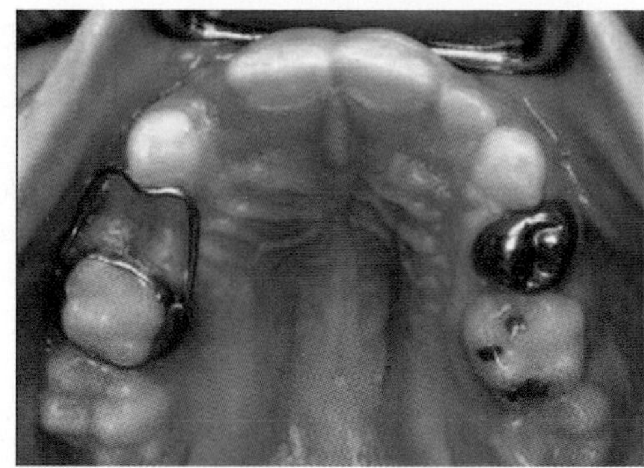

**FIG. 57.10** Space maintainer used to "reserve" the space until the permanent tooth erupts. *(From Dean JA, Avery DR, McDonald RE: McDonald and Avery dentistry for the child and adolescent, ed 10, St Louis, 2016, Elsevier.)*

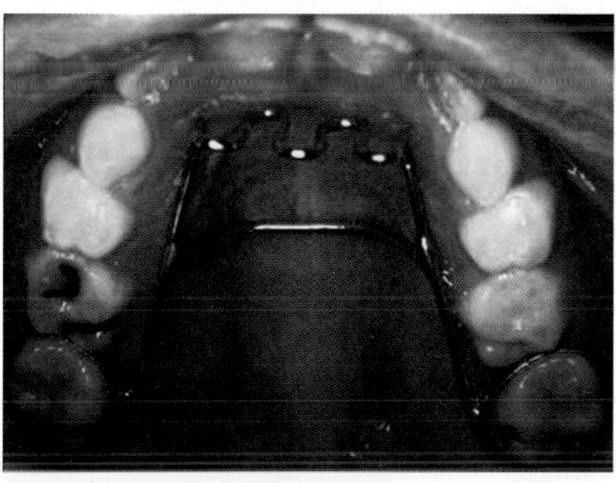

**FIG. 57.11** An appliance is placed to interfere with the finger position during thumb sucking. *(From Dean JA, Avery DR, McDonald RE: McDonald and Avery dentistry for the child and adolescent, ed 10, St Louis, 2016, Elsevier.)*

## Sealants

Sealants protect the grooved and pitted surfaces of teeth, especially the chewing surfaces of back teeth, where most cavities in children are found. Made of clear or shaded plastic, sealants are applied to the teeth to help keep them cavity-free (see Chapter 59).

## Orofacial Development

It is never too early for the pediatric dentist to start to evaluate a child's oral and facial *(orofacial)* development. The pediatric dentist will be the first to identify malocclusion, crowded or crooked teeth, and habits that can affect the dentition later on. The pediatric dentist can actively intervene or can refer the patient to an orthodontist to guide the teeth as they emerge in the mouth. Early preventive and interceptive orthodontic treatment can prevent the need for more extensive treatment later.

**Preventive** treatment allows the dentist to prevent or eliminate irregularities and malpositions in the developing dentofacial region. Preventive orthodontics includes the following:

- Control of decay to prevent the premature loss of primary teeth, which may result in loss of space for the eruption of permanent teeth.
- Use of a space maintainer to save space for the eruption of permanent teeth (Fig. 57.10). Space maintainers most often are cemented into place and are retained until the permanent tooth erupts.
- Use of appliances to correct oral habits such as thumb sucking that may be damaging to the permanent dentition (Fig. 57.11).
- Early detection of genetic and congenital anomalies that may influence dental development.
- Supervision of the natural exfoliation (shedding) of the primary teeth. If retained for too long, primary teeth may cause permanent teeth to erupt out of alignment or to become impacted (Fig. 57.12).

**Interceptive** treatment allows the dentist to intercede or correct problems as they develop. Examples of problems include the following:

- Extraction of primary teeth that may be contributing to malalignment or crowding of the permanent dentition
- Correction of a cross-bite through the use of a removable or fixed appliance (Fig. 57.13)

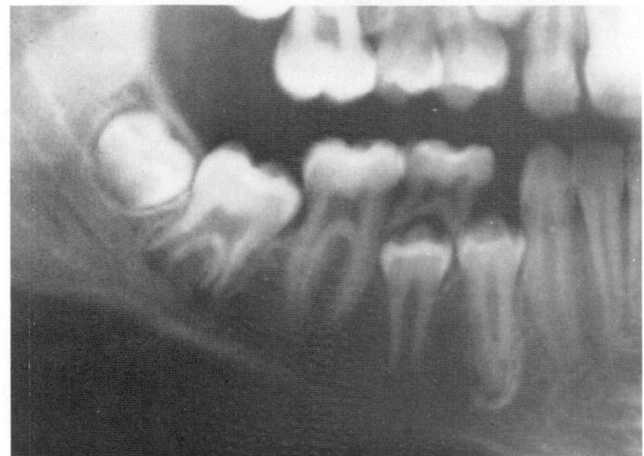

**FIG. 57.12** The lower permanent premolars erupted lingual to the primary teeth. *(From Proffit WR, Fields HW, Sarver DM: Contemporary orthodontics, ed 5, St Louis, 2013, Mosby.)*

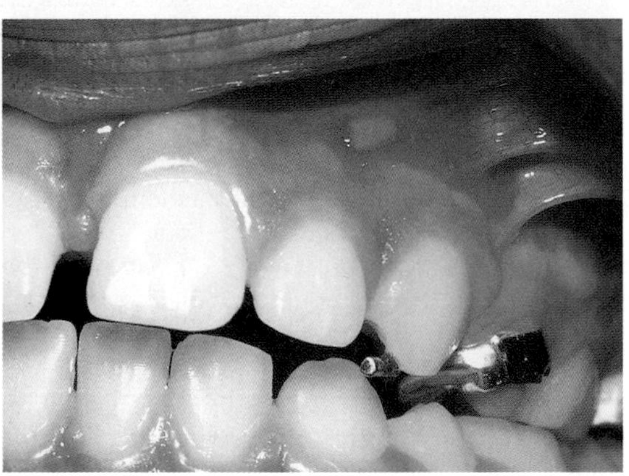

**FIG. 57.13** Example of fixed appliance used to correct cross-bite. (Courtesy Dr. Frank Hodges, Santa Rosa, CA.)

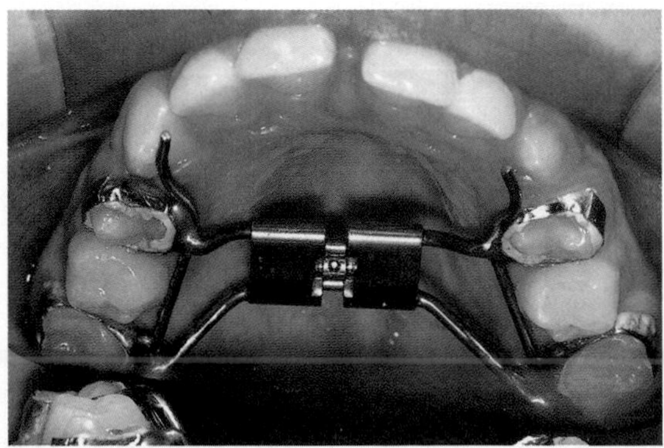

**FIG. 57.14** Palatal expansion appliance used to widen the maxillary arch. *(Courtesy Dr. Frank Hodges, Santa Rosa, CA.)*

- Correction of a jaw size discrepancy through the use of a removable or fixed appliance (Fig. 57.14)

## Sports Safety

The fields of sports medicine and dentistry have documented the benefits of wearing protective face equipment during recreational sports that might injure the mouth area. Mouth protectors are an important piece of protective face gear. Many states have regulations that require student athletes in contact sports to wear protective mouth guards to help prevent traumatic injuries to the teeth. Professional athletes in sports that expose them to potential oral injury are required to wear mouth guards.

Three types of mouth guards are used: commercial mouth guards, mouth-formed protectors, and custom-fitted vacuum-formed guards. Custom mouth guards can be fabricated easily in the dental office (Fig. 57.15).

RECALL

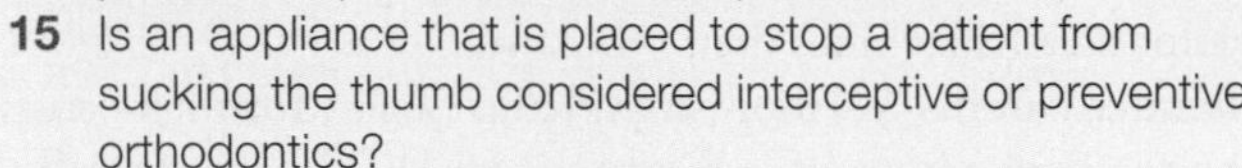

**13** Would fluoride varnish be used on a child?
**14** What procedure is recommended for children to protect the pits and fissures of posterior teeth?
**15** Is an appliance that is placed to stop a patient from sucking the thumb considered interceptive or preventive orthodontics?
**16** As a swimmer, should you wear a mouth guard?

# Pediatric Procedures

The basic principles of operative or restorative treatment of primary teeth are generally the same as those for permanent teeth. Primary teeth are charted with the same classifications as permanent teeth, and amalgam and composite resin materials are used for restorative purposes. The only difference is that the pediatric dentist adapts to a smaller dentition and mouth size by using special instruments, accessories, and techniques.

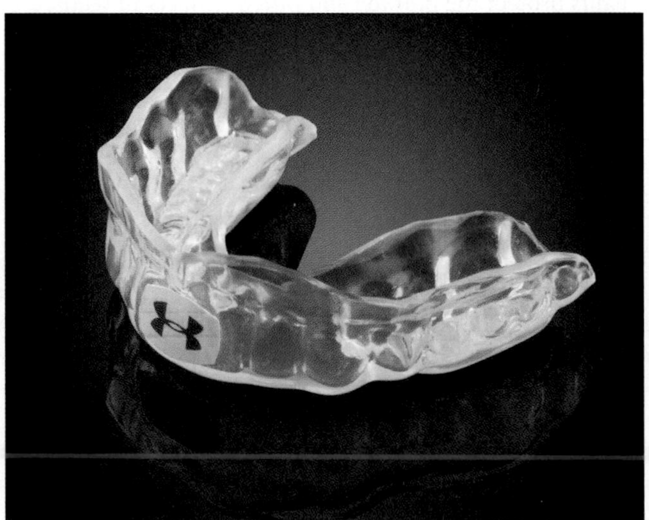

**FIG. 57.15** Under Armour mouth guard. *(Courtesy Bite Tech Inc., Exclusive Licensee, Under Armour Performance Mouthwear™.)*

## Restorative Procedures

### Anesthesia and Pain Control

It is important to create a positive, painless experience early on in a child's dental visit. Using simple distraction techniques can help divert the patient to lessen the experience. Depending on the age, some of the following techniques provide a positive experience:

- Refer to the procedure as placing "sleepy juice" on the tooth.
- Have the topical and syringe prepared and covered with a patient napkin when seating the patient.
- Position the patient with the chin up. Provide a poster or mobile on the ceiling for the patient to look at.
- Transfer the syringe behind the patient's head to prevent the patient looking to see what you are doing.
- Continue talking to the patient to keep the child preoccupied.
- During the application of anesthesia, place your arm closest to the patient across the patient to provide security and support.

At the conclusion of a procedure, it is important to instruct the parent and the patient that the patient's lip may be numb and will feel funny. Instruct the patient not to chew or bite the lip at this time.

### Use of the Dental Dam

The placement of the dental dam in pediatric dentistry offers many advantages for the pediatric patient:

- Refer to the procedure as a "raincoat" for the tooth; the child can understand the need for the tooth to stay dry.
- The dam can decrease the time of a procedure.
- It can help keep the child from talking throughout the procedure.
- It provides protection from saliva and debris during the procedure.
- It protects the patient from aspirating dental materials or items used in the procedure.

### Instrument Size

Dental instruments, handpieces, and rotary instruments are scaled down in size for use with the pediatric patient. Smaller sizes provide the dentist easier access to areas within the mouth and do not require the child to open the mouth as wide.

### Matrix System

Two types of matrices are used when primary teeth are restored: the **T-band** and the spot-welded band (see Chapter 49). Both of these custom bands are designed to better fit the width and height of the primary tooth.

## Endodontic Procedures

### Pulp Therapy

Pulp therapy is an attempt to stimulate and preserve pulpal regeneration in primary teeth. The two factors that most commonly affect the pulpal health of teeth are deep caries and traumatic injury. Deep caries is much more likely to affect the posterior teeth, and trauma is much more likely to affect the anterior teeth.

Indirect and direct **pulp capping** can also be indicated for a newly erupted permanent tooth to promote pulpal healing and stimulate the production of reparative dentin (see Chapter 54).

### Pulpotomy

**Pulpotomy** is the complete removal of the coronal portion of the dental pulp. The goal of this procedure is to remove the portion of the pulp that is inflamed while maintaining the healthy vital pulp tissue within the canals of the primary tooth. A pulpotomy can be accomplished with two different types of medicaments:

- Mineral trioxide aggregate (MTA) is replacing the popular use of a formocresol pulpotomy, which was most often used for primary teeth. Because of the material's toxicity, it is not recommended. MTA is an endodontic cement that is biocompatible and is capable of stimulating healing and osteogenesis.
- The *calcium hydroxide pulpotomy* is used primarily for young permanent teeth with open apices (Fig. 57.16). A common indication on the fractured tooth is significant exposure of the pulp. This type of treatment allows continued apical development so that endodontic treatment can be performed later.

See Procedure 57.1: Assisting in Pulpotomy of a Primary Tooth.

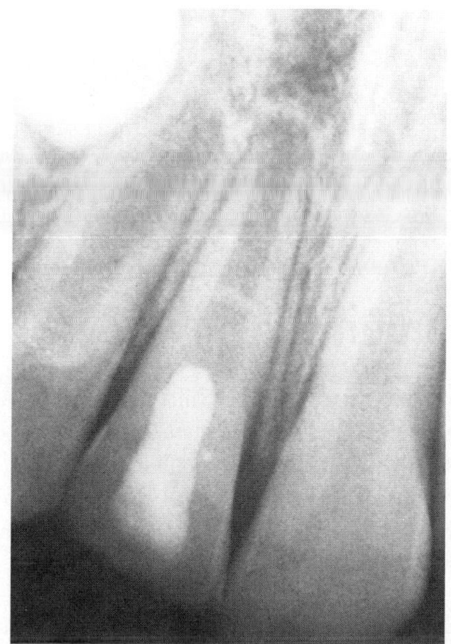

**FIG. 57.16** A deep calcium hydroxide pulpotomy completed on the central incisor. *(From Hargreaves KM, Cohen S: Cohen's pathways of the pulp, ed 10, St Louis, 2011, Mosby.)*

# Prosthodontic Procedures

### Stainless Steel Crown

Because of the importance of maintaining primary teeth throughout adolescent years, the dentist may use a crown system to cover severely decayed and endodontically treated teeth without the cost and time investment of a fixed prosthesis. A stainless steel crown is the restoration of choice for the following reasons:

- Stainless steel crowns can be prepared and placed at a single appointment, which is especially important in young children, patients with behavioral problems, and patients with special needs.
- Crowns are sufficiently durable to last until the primary teeth are replaced by the permanent teeth.
- Crowns are almost always well tolerated by the gingiva of young patients.
- Stainless steel crowns are much less expensive than cast restorations.

### Types of Crowns

Stainless steel crowns are available in a variety of sizes for the various primary and permanent teeth. The two types typically used in pediatric dentistry are pretrimmed and precontoured stainless steel crowns.

- *Pretrimmed crowns* have straight sides but undergo festooning to follow a line parallel to the gingival crest. These must be trimmed and contoured to fit the tooth.
- *Precontoured crowns* are already festooned and **contoured**. Some additional trimming and contouring may be necessary, but this need is usually minimal.

See Procedure 57.2: Assisting in Placement of a Stainless Steel Crown.

RECALL

17 What types of matrices are commonly used on primary teeth?
18 What endodontic procedure would most likely be performed on a primary tooth?
19 Would a child be referred to a prosthodontist for placement of a stainless steel crown?

# Dental Trauma

An injury to the tooth of a young child can have serious and long-term consequences, including discoloration and possible loss. Many injuries to primary teeth occur around 1 to 2 1/2 years of age—the "toddler" stage. The teeth that are injured most frequently in the primary dentition are the maxillary central incisors (Fig. 57.17).

The concern with this type of injury to a primary tooth is that the permanent tooth is developing directly under the injured tooth and may also become damaged. Causes of dental injury to children include bicycle accidents, sports injuries, automobile accidents, and child abuse. It is important to educate parents and school nurses on proper actions to take when a dental emergency occurs (Fig. 57.18).

## Fractured Anterior Teeth

Fractures of the anterior teeth are common emergencies in a pediatric dental practice (Fig. 57.19). The dentist should see children with fractured teeth as soon as possible. Complete documentation of the accident, clinical examination, vitality testing, and radiographic examination are completed at the emergency visit.

The dentist often prefers to delay restorative treatment for 3 to 6 weeks to avoid any further trauma to the pulp of an injured tooth. This time gives the delicate pulp an opportunity to recover without additional injury. During this recovery period, the dentist (1) provides temporary relief by covering all exposed dentin with calcium hydroxide to prevent thermal sensitivity, and (2) places an interim covering of resin material. Radiographs and vitality tests are provided at subsequent appointments to determine the status of the injured tooth. If the pulp is still vital, more definitive restorative procedures can be performed.

## Traumatic Intrusion

Traumatic **intrusion** is the result of an injury where the tooth is forcibly driven into the alveolus so that only a portion of the crown is visible. Traumatic intrusion can occur to primary and permanent dentition. Teeth that are intruded should be allowed to re-erupt naturally; these teeth often require endodontic treatment later. Damage to the developing permanent tooth can occur when a primary tooth is intruded. The extent of damage to the permanent tooth cannot be determined until it erupts.

## Extrusion and Lateral Luxation Injuries

**Extrusion** and lateral **luxation** injuries occur when the teeth are displaced from their position. Severe damage to the

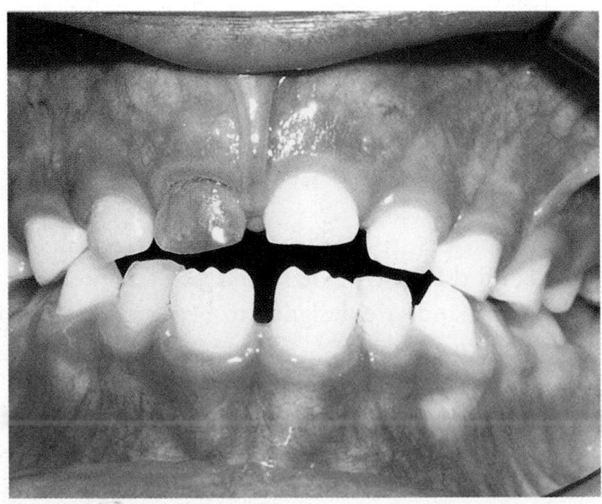

**FIG. 57.17** Traumatized maxillary incisor. *(Courtesy Dr. Frank Hodges, Santa Rosa, CA.)*

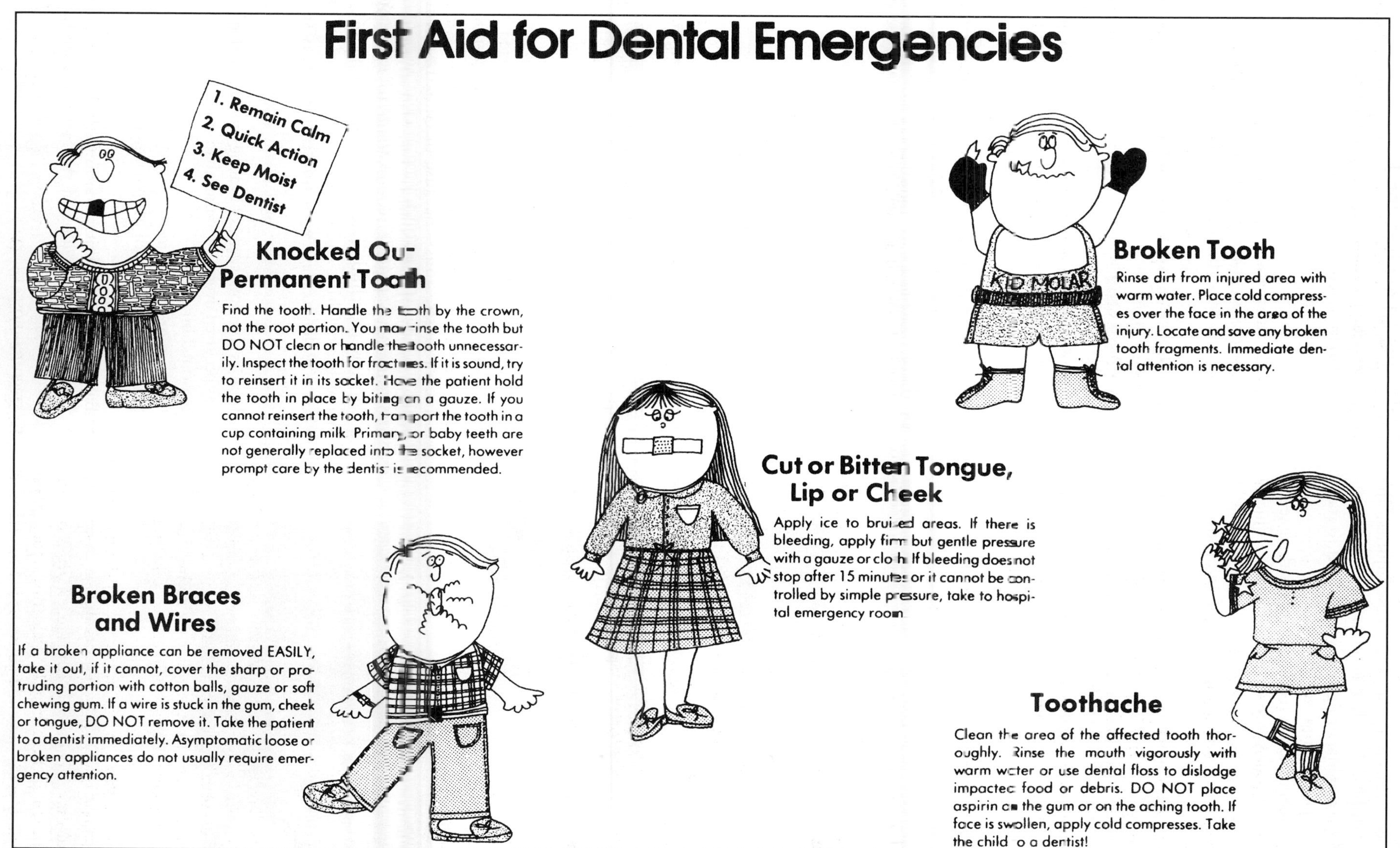


**FIG. 57.18** Flyer describing actions to take in a dental emergency as distributed to school personnel. *(Courtesy Dr. John Christensen.)*

periodontal ligaments usually occurs with these injuries. The dentist repositions displaced teeth as soon as possible. A temporary splint of resin material or ligature wire is used to stabilize the repositioned permanent teeth.

Endodontic treatment is often required later for these teeth. Primary teeth tend to undergo root resorption more quickly after injuries of this type, and they tend to become mobile. These teeth should be observed for signs of infection and removed if indicated.

## Avulsed Teeth

Permanent teeth that have been **avulsed** can be replanted with varying degrees of success (Fig. 57.20). Primary teeth usually will not be replanted. The more quickly a tooth can be replanted, the greater is the chance for success. Therefore when an injury of this type occurs, the adult who is present should be instructed to do the following:

- Recover the tooth immediately.
- Wrap the tooth in moistened gauze.
- Go immediately to the dentist's office.

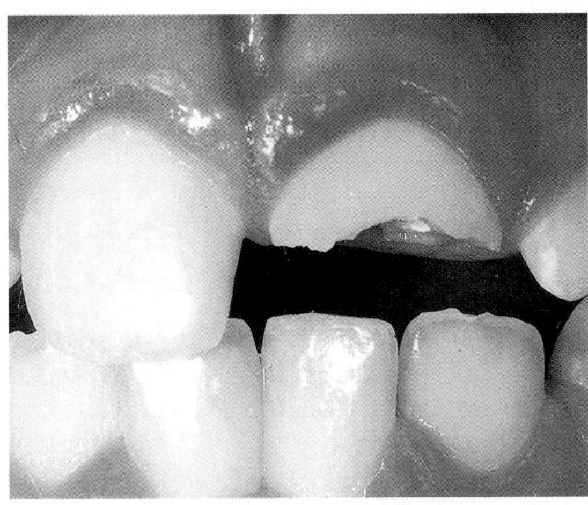

**FIG. 57.19** Fracture of an anterior tooth. *(Courtesy Dr. Frank Hodges, Santa Rosa, CA.)*

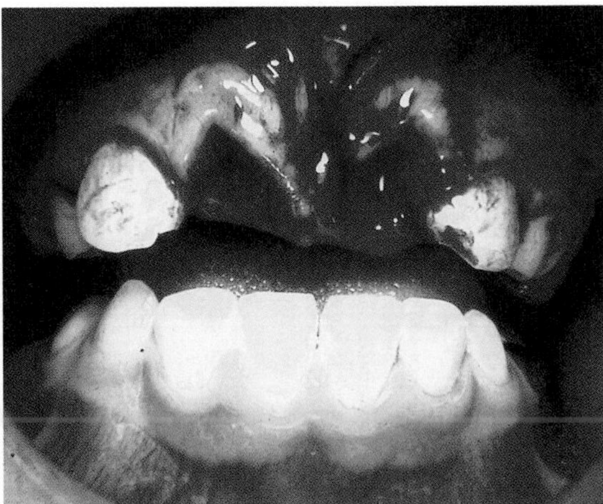

**FIG. 57.20** Avulsion of maxillary central incisors. *(Courtesy Dr. Frank Hodges, Santa Rosa, CA.)*

### Replanting an Avulsed Tooth

The success rate for replantation of permanent teeth is highest when the tooth is replanted within 30 minutes of the accident. The procedure for replantation is as follows:

- The local anesthetic agent is administered.
- Radiographs are taken. Often, both periapical and occlusal radiographs are indicated to reveal any fragments of tooth or bone.
- Clotted blood is removed from the alveolus (socket) with a surgical curette.
- The avulsed tooth is washed in saline solution and is inserted into the alveolus.
- The tooth is splinted into place with wire, acrylic, or orthodontic splints.
- Postoperative radiographs are taken.
- Endodontic treatment is performed 6 to 8 weeks after replantation.

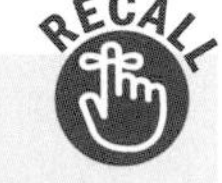


**20** Which teeth are injured most frequently?
**21** What happens when a tooth is avulsed?
**22** How would a dentist stabilize a tooth after an injury?

## Child Abuse and Neglect

By law, in all 50 states, healthcare professionals (physicians, dentists, nurses, and social workers) are required to report any case in which they suspect that a child is being neglected or abused. The state or county child protective services agency is the government body that should be contacted.

The name of the person who makes the report will not be revealed. Although dental assistants and clerical staff are not legally required to report abuse, each member of the dental team has a moral responsibility to report known or suspected abuse cases to the dentist. Reporting of suspected child abuse may be done by telephone, in person, or in writing. Specific information is required to file a report.

For various reasons—because of embarrassment, fear of losing custody of the child, or the wish to avoid a fine or imprisonment—abusive parents tend to make up stories about how the child "fell" or sustained some other injury to the head. Child abuse must be suspected as the cause when a child presents with unexplained signs such as the following:

- Injuries at various stages of healing (indicating that the trauma has occurred over time rather than as a single incident)
- Repeated injuries
- Chipped or injured teeth
- Scars inside the lips or on the tongue
- Tears of labial frena
- Battering or other injuries around the head and neck
- Facial bruising, swelling of the facial structures, or blackened eye(s)
- Fractured nose

- Bite marks
- Injuries not consistent with the explanation presented by the parent

### What to Include When Reporting Child Abuse

- Name, address, gender, age, height, and weight of the child
- Name and address of the adult who has custody of the child
- Description of the current physical and emotional abuse or neglect of the child
- Evidence of previous injuries or negligence
- Information that may assist in establishing the causes of injuries
- Sketches or photographs documenting the nature and location of injuries

RECALL

**23** Are you legally required to report child abuse?
**24** Could a fractured or broken nose be a result of child abuse?
**25** Who in the dental office should report child abuse?

**■ Patient Education** Children are sponge-like in that they absorb and remember everything you say and do. Always be mindful of their presence when they are in the dental chair. Allow children to feel comfortable about asking questions. When you answer their questions, think about their age, how they grasp concepts, and how you can make them more interested in taking better care of their oral health. ■

**■ Legal and Ethical Implications** Because the clinical assistant takes on such an important role in the clinical component of the pediatric patient, it is easy to acquire responsibilities that may not be legal for an assistant to practice. Review your state, province, or territory laws and discuss with your dentist what role you want to take in the practice. Come up with a plan for how you can be legally involved to your maximum potential. ■

**■ Eye to the Future** For many years, the rate of tooth decay has declined, primarily because of water fluoridation and the use of products with fluoride. However, pediatric and general dentists now are seeing an increase in problems of rampant decay in children and adolescents. The problem is the result of candy, sodas, fruit juices, and sports drinks. Preteens and teenagers are taking in large quantities of sugar-containing products; therefore interproximal and cervical decay rates are rising. Caries has become such an epidemic that the American Dental Society and the American Academy of Pediatric Dentistry are emphasizing that dental professionals must educate their patients about their nutrition and diet. ■

## ■ Critical Thinking

1. You are assisting today with a new patient named Katie. After reviewing the patient registration form, you see that she is 3 years old. When you go out to call Katie, she runs to her mother and clings to her leg. What techniques could you use to encourage her to come with you for her appointment?
2. You are applying sealants to the primary molars of a 6-year-old boy. You are using cotton rolls for moisture control. When you place the cotton roll on the lower lingual side, the boy pushes it up with his tongue. How can you maintain a dry area and still complete the procedure?
3. An emergency patient has just arrived. The patient, 1-year-old Lori, has fallen and hit primary tooth E. You have been asked to take a periapical radiograph of the area. How will you take a periapical view of this very young girl?
4. Your next oral hygiene patient is Luke, a 10-year-old boy with Down syndrome. Describe how you will prepare for this patient, and identify what techniques can be used to make Luke feel more comfortable and have a positive experience.
5. Explain why a different type of matrix system is used with primary teeth. Which additional supplies would you require to set up this system? ■

PROCEDURE 57.1

## Assisting in Pulpotomy of a Primary Tooth

### EQUIPMENT AND SUPPLIES

- ✓ Local anesthetic agent setup
- ✓ Basic setup
- ✓ Dental dam setup
- ✓ Low-speed handpiece
- ✓ Round burs
- ✓ Spoon excavators (various sizes)
- ✓ Sterile cotton pellets
- ✓ MTA pulpal material
- ✓ Zinc oxide–eugenol (ZOE) base
- ✓ Final restorative material and instruments for placement

(Continued)

## PROCEDURE 57.1 Assisting in Pulpotomy of a Primary Tooth—cont'd

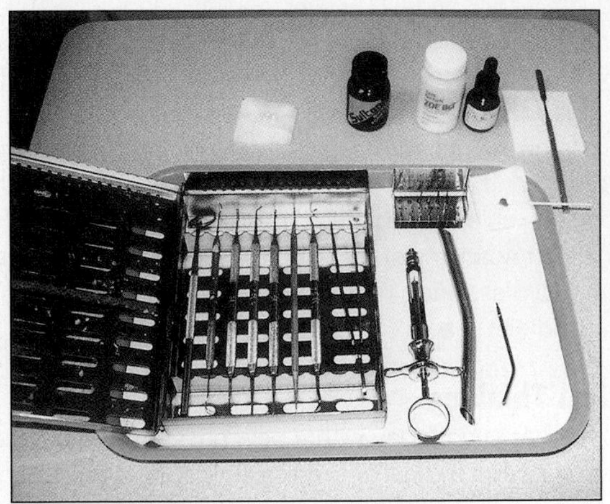

### PROCEDURAL STEPS

1 The local anesthetic agent is administered.
2 The dental dam is placed.
3 The dentist will use a round bur in the low-speed handpiece to remove the dental caries and expose the pulp chamber.
4 Transfer a spoon excavator for the dentist to remove all pulp tissue inside the coronal chamber.
5 Prepare MTA pulpal material (1:1 ratio).
6 Prepare a sterile cotton pellet with chlorhexidine solution and transfer to dentist to wipe the cavity preparation.
7 Transfer applicator for the material to be placed over the floor of the cavity preparation.
8 The pulp chamber is filled with the ZOE base.
9 The final restoration is placed.
10 Document the procedure.

| Date | Tooth | Surface | Charting Notes |
|---|---|---|---|
| 9/4/17 | C | — | Pulpotomy, 1 cartridge Xylocaine, 1:100,000 w/o epi. Dam isolation, tooth opened, MTA placed. ZOE base, amalgam. Pt tolerated procedure well. |
| | | | T. Clark, CDA/L. Stewart, DDS |

  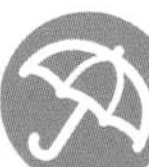 

## PROCEDURE 57.2

# Assisting in Placement of a Stainless Steel Crown

### EQUIPMENT AND SUPPLIES

- Basic setup
- Local anesthetic agent setup
- Dental dam setup
- Low-speed and high-speed handpieces
- High-volume oral evacuator (HVE) tip
- Friction grip burs (dentist's choice of diamond or carbide)
- Spoon excavator
- Selection of stainless steel crowns
- Crown and bridge scissors
- Contouring and crimping pliers
- Mandrel
- Finishing and polishing discs
- Mounted green stones
- Cotton rolls
- Cementation setup
- Dental floss
- Articulating paper and holder

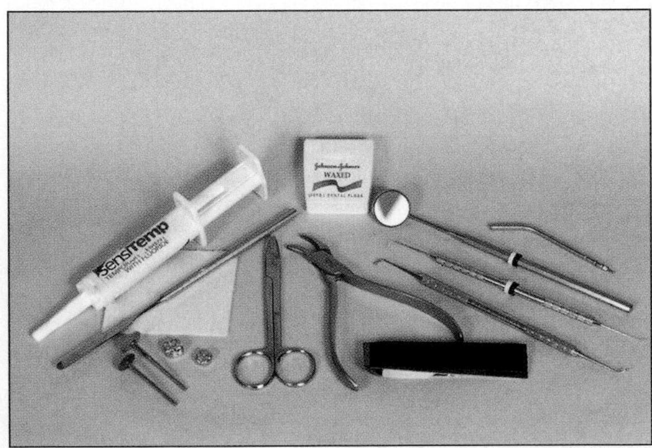


### PROCEDURAL STEPS

#### Preparing the Tooth

1 After the local anesthetic agent has been administered and has taken effect, cotton rolls or the dental dam is placed.

## PROCEDURE 57.2 Assisting in Placement of a Stainless Steel Crown—cont'd

2 The dentist will use the high-speed handpiece and a tapered diamond or carbide bur to prepare the tooth in a method similar to that used for a cast crown.
3 The dentist reduces the entire circumference of the tooth, as well as the height of the tooth.
4 All dental caries are removed with hand instruments and burs.

### Selecting and Sizing the Stainless Steel Crown

5 The crown is selected and is tried on the prepared tooth for fit.
6 The stainless steel crown is properly sized when it fits snugly on the prepared tooth and has *both* mesial and distal contact.
7 Clean and sterilize any crowns that were tried in the mouth but not used; then return them to storage.

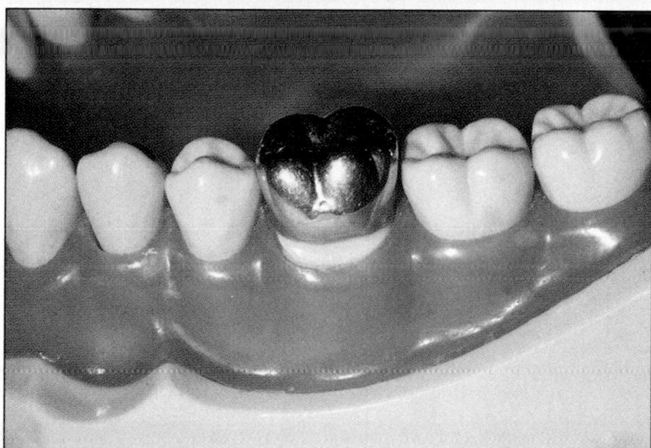

### Trimming and Contouring the Crown

8 The dentist will use crown and bridge scissors to reduce the height of the crown until it is approximately the same as that of adjacent teeth.

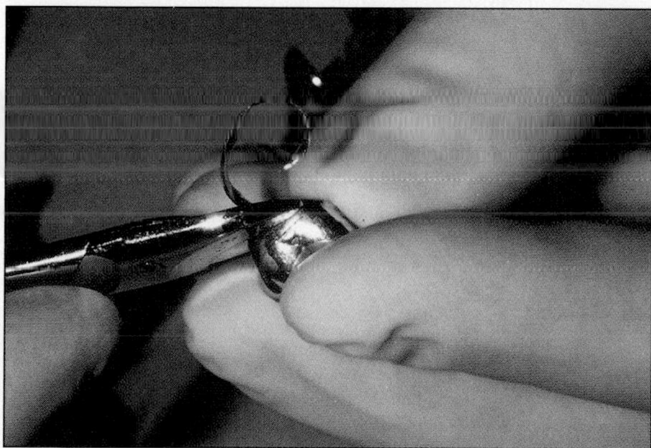

9 The dentist may use a green stone to smooth the rough edges of the crown along the cervical margin.
10 The cervical margin of the crown may be polished with a rubber abrasive wheel.
11 The occlusion is checked and adjusted as needed.
12 The dentist uses the contouring pliers to crimp the cervical margins of the crown toward the tooth to obtain a tight fit and a proper cervical contour.

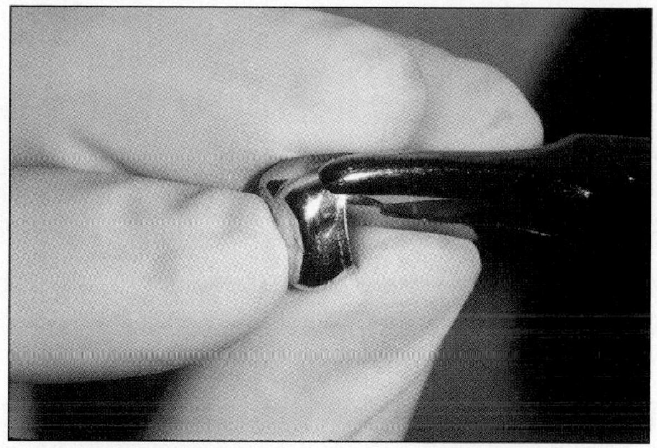

### Cementation

13 Rinse and dry the tooth thoroughly. Place cotton rolls to maintain dry conditions.
14 Mix the permanent cement (polycarboxylate is often selected).
15 Line the crown with the cement and transfer to the dentist for placement.

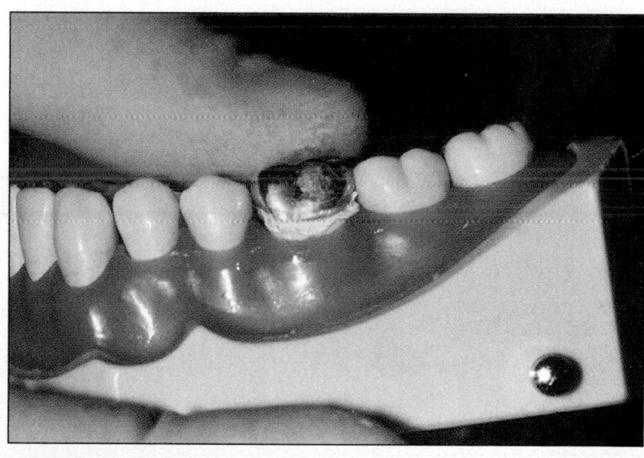

16 Transfer an explorer to the dentist to remove the excess cement from around the tooth.
17 Use dental floss to remove any remaining cement from the interproximal areas.

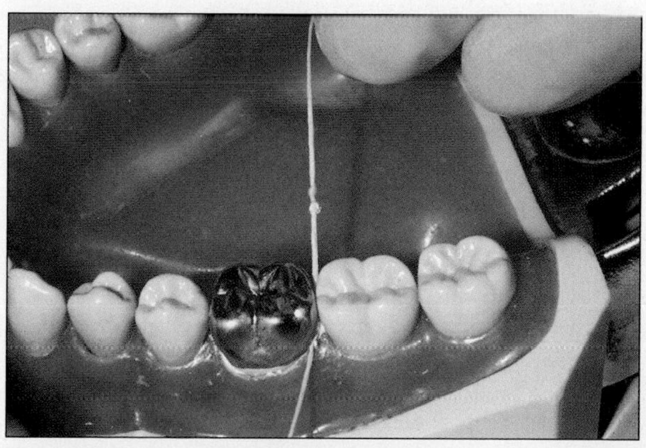

(Continued)

## PROCEDURE 57.2 Assisting in Placement of a Stainless Steel Crown—cont'd

**18** Use the air-water syringe and the HVE tip to rinse the patient's mouth before dismissal.

**19** Document the procedure.

| Date | Tooth | Surface | Charting Notes |
|---|---|---|---|
| 9/5/17 | B | | Stainless steel crown, 1 cartridge Xylocaine 1:100,000 w/o epi. Cotton roll isolation, crown cemented w/Duralon. Pt tolerated procedure well. |
| | | | T. Clark, CDA/L. Stewart, DDS |

All photos in this procedure from Hatrick CD, Eakle WS: Dental materials: clinical applications for dental assistants and dental hygienists, ed 3, St Louis, 2016, Elsevier.

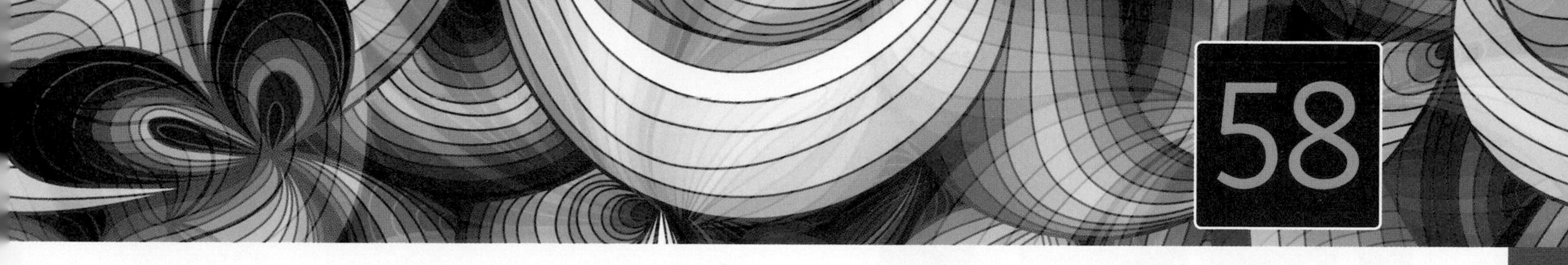


# Coronal Polishing

## KEY TERMS

**Calculus (KAL-kyoo-lus)** Calcium and phosphate salts in saliva that become mineralized and adhere to tooth surfaces.

**Clinical crown** That portion of the tooth that is visible in the oral cavity.

**Coronal (kuh-ROE-nuhl) polishing** A technique used to remove plaque and stains from the coronal surfaces of the teeth.

**Endogenous (en-DOJ-en-us) stains** Stains developed from within the structure of the tooth.

**Exogenous (ek-SOJ-uh-nus) stains** Stains developed from external sources.

**Extrinsic (ek-STRIN-zik) stains** Stains that occur on the *external* surfaces of the teeth that may be removed by polishing.

**Fulcrum (FUL-krum)** Finger rest used when an instrument or handpiece is held for a specified time.

**Intrinsic (in-TRIN-zik) stains** Stains that occur within the tooth structure that may not be removed by polishing.

**Nasmyth's (NAS-miths) membrane** Residue from epithelial tissue on the crowns of newly erupted teeth that may become extrinsically stained.

**Oral prophylaxis (proe-fi-LAK-sis)** The complete removal of calculus, debris, stain, and plaque from the teeth.

**Prophy paste** Commercial premixed abrasive paste used for polishing teeth and restorations.

**Rubber cup polishing** A technique that is used to remove plaque and stains from the coronal surfaces of the teeth.

## LEARNING OUTCOMES

*On completion of this chapter, the student will be able to achieve the following objectives:*

1. Pronounce, define, and spell the key terms.
2. Discuss coronal polishing, including the following:
   - Explain the difference between a prophylaxis and coronal polishing.
   - Explain the indications for and contraindications to a coronal polish.
   - Explain the principal of selective polishing.
3. Name and describe the types of extrinsic stains, the two categories of intrinsic stains, and the methods used to remove plaque and stains.
4. Name the handpieces and attachments used for coronal polishing.
5. Explain the importance of selecting an appropriate polishing agent.
6. Discuss polishing esthetic restorations, including the following:
   - Name materials to be avoided when one is polishing esthetic restorations.
   - Describe the technique used for polishing esthetic restorations.
7. Discuss the steps of coronal polishing, including safety precautions, correct sequence, flossing after polishing, and evaluation of polishing.

## PERFORMANCE OUTCOMES

*On completion of this chapter, the student will be able to meet competency standards in the following skills:*

- Demonstrate the handpiece grasp and positioning for the prophy angle.
- Demonstrate the fulcrum or finger rest used in each quadrant during a coronal polish procedure.
- Demonstrate the proper seating positions for the operator and the assistant during a coronal polish procedure.
- Be able to determine that the teeth are free from stains and plaque.
- Complete coronal polishing without causing tissue trauma.

## ELECTRONIC RESOURCES

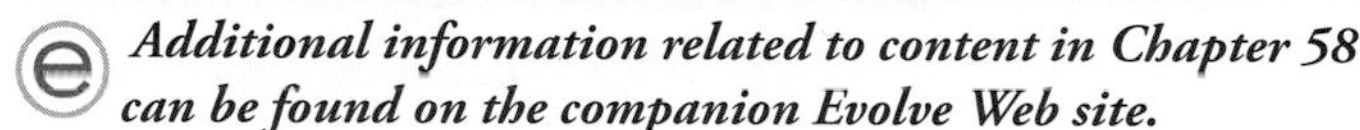
***Additional information related to content in Chapter 58 can be found on the companion Evolve Web site.***

- Practice Quiz
- Video: Coronal Polishing

## Coronal Polishing

**Coronal polishing** is a technique that is used to remove plaque and stains from the coronal surfaces of the teeth. (Refer to Chapter 15 for a discussion of dental plaque.) Polishing the crowns of teeth is considered to be primarily a cosmetic procedure. However, a smooth tooth surface is less likely to retain plaque, calculus, and stain.

In addition, patients like the feel of smooth, polished teeth. Coronal polishing is most commonly done with the use of a

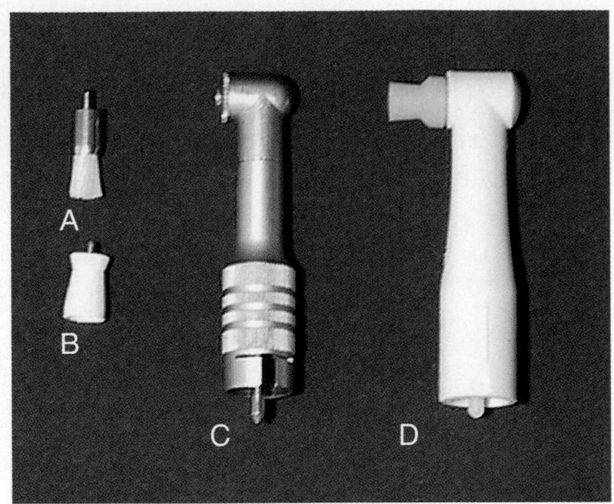


**FIG. 58.1** A, Bristle brush. B, Rubber polishing cup. C, Reusable prophy angle. D, Disposable prophy angle.

dental handpiece with a prophy angle (Fig. 58.1), a rubber cup, and a polishing material (abrasive agent). Specific indications for and contraindications to a coronal polish are listed in Box 58.1.

Coronal polishing is strictly limited to the clinical crowns of the teeth. (The **clinical crown** is that portion of the tooth that is visible within the oral cavity.) In some states, coronal polishing is delegated to registered or expanded-functions dental assistants (EFDAs) who have had special training in this procedure.

It is very important to understand the difference between a prophylaxis and a coronal polishing. A coronal polish is *not* a substitute for an oral prophylaxis. An **oral prophylaxis**, commonly known as a *prophy* or a *cleaning,* is the complete removal of calculus, debris, stain, and plaque from the teeth. (**Calculus** is a hard mineralized deposit that is attached to the teeth.) In almost every state, the dentist and the registered dental hygienist are the only members of the dental team who are licensed to perform an oral prophylaxis.

### Benefits of Coronal Polishing

- Polishing prepares the teeth for placement of dental sealants.
- Smooth tooth surfaces are easier for the patient to keep clean.
- Formation of new deposits is slowed.
- Patients appreciate the smooth feeling and clean appearance.
- Polishing prepares the teeth for placement of orthodontic brackets and/or bands.

## Selective Polishing

Selective polishing is a procedure in which *only* those teeth or surfaces with stain are polished. Studies have shown that the abrasive agent used during coronal polishing actually removes a small amount of the fluoride-rich outer enamel layer. The purpose of selective polishing is to avoid unnecessary removal of even small amounts of surface enamel. Therefore when the stain is very light and is not of esthetic concern to the patient, selective polishing should be considered. The basic principle of selective polishing is that teeth should not be polished unless it is necessary. For some individuals, stain removal may cause dentinal hypersensitivity during and after the appointment. The needs of the patient must always be reviewed before stain removal. If you encounter a patient who does not have visible stain but is accustomed to polishing and chooses to have it done, you should use a very fine abrasive such as a commercial toothpaste.

### BOX 58.1 Indications for and Contraindications to Coronal Polishing

**Indications**

- Before placement of dental sealants
- Before placement of the dental dam
- Before cementation of orthodontic bands
- Before application of acid etching solution on enamel (if indicated by the manufacturer's instructions)
- Before cementation of crowns and bridges

**Contraindications**

- When no stain is present
- Patients who are at high risk for dental caries, such as nursing bottle caries, root caries, or areas of thin demineralized enamel (because small amounts of enamel are removed during the polishing procedure)
- Sensitive teeth (because abrasive agents can increase the areas of sensitivity)
- Newly erupted teeth (because mineralization of the surfaces may be incomplete)

Historically, teeth were polished to remove all soft deposits and stains before fluoride was applied because it was believed that uptake of the fluoride into the enamel would be increased. As scientific knowledge has evolved, it has been shown that polishing does *not* improve the uptake of professionally applied fluoride. Therefore polishing is no longer necessary before fluoride is applied.

In addition to cosmetic value, coronal polishing can have therapeutic value. *Therapeutic polishing* refers to polishing of the root surfaces that have been exposed during periodontal surgery. (Refer to Chapter 55 for a review of periodontal surgery.) Polishing reduces the endotoxins and the bacteria on the cementum. Whether polishing for cosmetic or therapeutic purposes, it is important to understand the polishing process and its effects on the tooth surface (Box 58.2).

## Dental Stains

Stains are primarily an esthetic problem. Some types of stain can be removed, whereas others cannot. It is important for the dental assistant to be able to correctly identify stains, to provide the patient with accurate information about the

**BOX 58.2 Possible Damaging Effects of Coronal Polishing**

**Tooth Surfaces**

- Newly erupted teeth are incompletely mineralized, and excessive polishing with an abrasive could remove a small amount of surface enamel.
- Avoid polishing exposed cementum in areas of recession because cementum is softer than enamel and is removed more easily.
- Avoid polishing areas of demineralization because of the possibility of loss of surface enamel.

**Gingival Tissues**

- Gingival tissue may be damaged if the cup is run at a high speed and/or is applied too long.
- Fast rotation may force particles of the polishing agent into the sulcus, thereby creating a source of irritation.

**Restorations**

- Abrasive pastes can leave scratches or rough surfaces on gold, composite restorations, acrylic veneers, and porcelain surfaces.

From Robinson D, Bird D: Essentials of dental assisting, ed 6, St Louis, 2017, Saunders.

cause of the stains and possible options for removing them. For stains that cannot be removed, other treatment options are available. These include professional and at-home bleaching procedures, enamel microabrasion, and cosmetic restorative procedures such as laminate veneers and composite restorations.

## Types of Stains

Dental stains are categorized as endogenous or exogenous in nature.

**Endogenous stains** originate within the tooth through developmental and systemic disturbances. Types of endogenous stains include those caused by an excessive amount of fluoride during formation of the tooth. Another example of an endogenous stain would be that resulting from medications taken by the mother or the child during tooth development. Tetracycline is an example of a medication that is known to cause developmental staining. Endogenous stains may be seen in both deciduous and permanent dentitions and cannot be removed by polishing (Figs. 58.2 through 58.7).

**Exogenous stains** are those that originate outside the tooth and are caused by environmental agents. These can be subdivided even further into extrinsic and intrinsic stains, depending on whether or not the stain can be removed.

**Extrinsic stains** are those stains that appear on the exterior of the tooth and *can* be removed. Examples include staining from food, drink, and tobacco.

There is another type of extrinsic stain that can occur during the eruption process. **Nasmyth's membrane** is

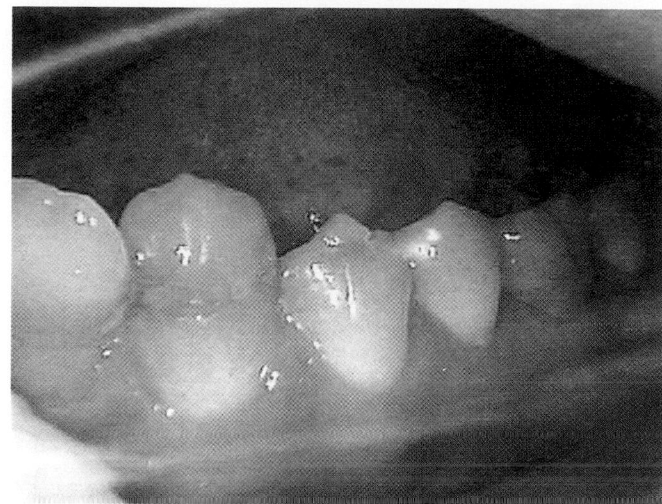

**FIG. 58.2** Endogenous developmental stain: tetracycline. Note how the stained area corresponds to the period of tooth development and the time the drug was taken. *(Courtesy Santa Rosa Junior College, Santa Rosa, CA.)*

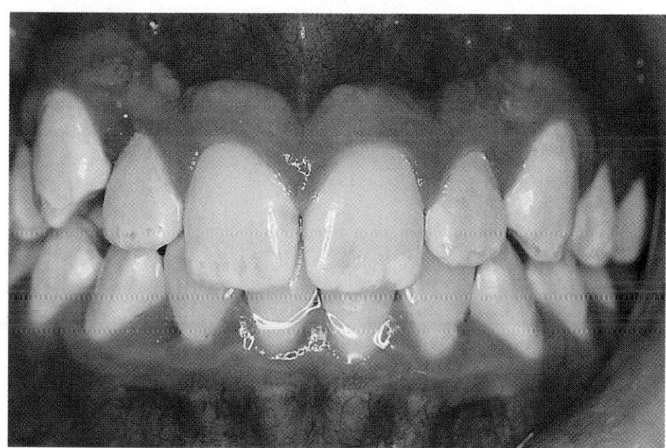

**FIG. 58.3** Endogenous developmental stain: enamel hypoplasia. *(Courtesy Dr. George Taybos, Jackson, MS.)*

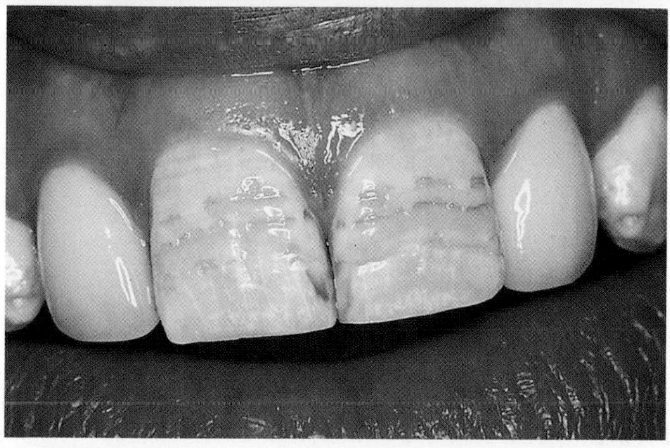

**FIG. 58.4** Endogenous developmental stain: dental fluorosis. *(Courtesy Dr. George Taybos, Jackson, MS.)*

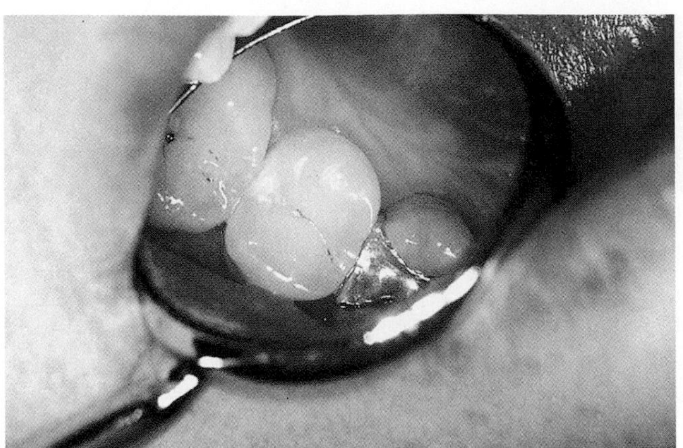

**FIG. 58.5** Endogenous developmental stain: secondary caries. *(Courtesy Dr. George Taybos, Jackson, MS.)*

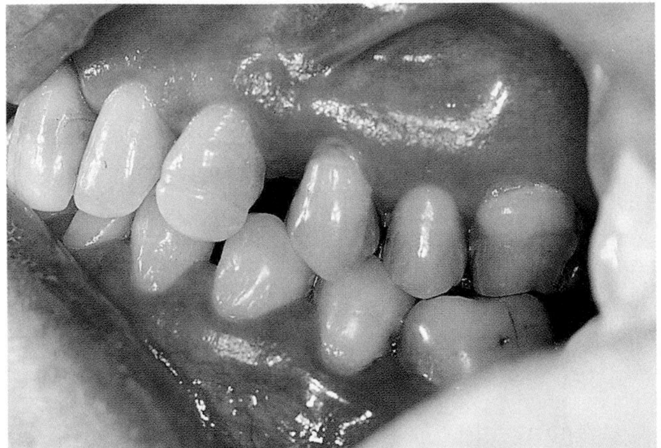

**FIG. 58.6** Exogenous stain: amalgam restoration. *(Courtesy Dr. George Taybos, Jackson, MS.)*

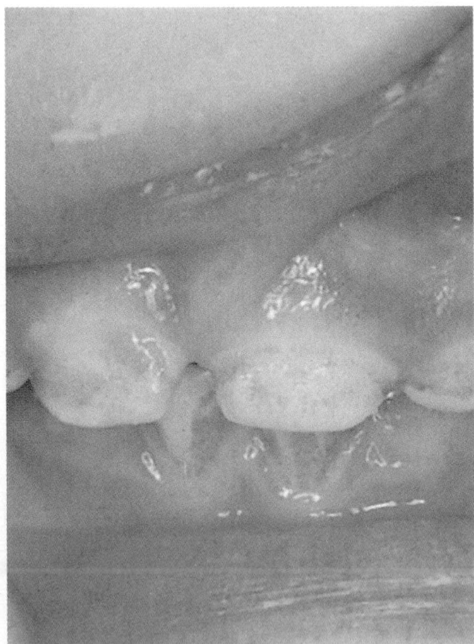

**FIG. 58.7** Staining of Nasmyth's membrane after eruption of the teeth. The entire crown area of the primary dentition is affected. *(Courtesy of Margaret J. Fehrenbach, RDH, MS.)*

a residue from the oral epithelium on the newly erupted enamel. This residue is easily stained from food and drink, and can be difficult to remove with toothbrushing. However, it can be removed by selective polishing of those teeth (see Fig. 58.7).

In these cases, the source of the stain is external, and the stain may be removed (Table 58.1).

**Intrinsic stains** are those that are caused by an environmental source but *cannot* be removed because the stain has become incorporated into the structure of the tooth. Examples include tobacco stains from smoking, chewing, or dipping and stains from dental amalgam that have become incorporated into the tooth structure. The dental assistant must be able to recognize these conditions because these stains cannot be removed by polishing or scaling (Table 58.2).

### Tooth Stains

Stains of the teeth occur in three basic ways:

1. The stain adheres directly to the surface of the tooth.
2. The stain is embedded in calculus and plaque deposits.
3. The stain is incorporated within the tooth structure.

1 What is a coronal polish?
2 What is the difference between a coronal polish and an oral prophylaxis?
3 What is the purpose of selective polishing?
4 What is an extrinsic stain?
5 What is an intrinsic stain?

## Methods of Removing Plaque and Stains

Two methods of stain removal are air-powder polishing and **rubber cup polishing**.

With any type of stain and plaque removal procedure, you must be careful (1) not to remove the surface enamel of the tooth, and (2) to avoid trauma to the gingiva.

Remember, you must check the regulations in your state regarding whether coronal polishing is delegated to qualified dental assistants and, if so, which technique is permitted.

### *Air Polishing*

Air polishing is an alternative to traditional rubber cup polishing (Box 58.3). The air-powder polishing technique uses a specially designed handpiece with a nozzle that delivers a slurry of warm water and sodium bicarbonate (Fig. 58.8). This slurry will remove surface stains, plaque, and other soft deposits such as food particles trapped in between teeth. Under pressure, the slurry of water and sodium bicarbonate removes stains rapidly and efficiently. The flow rate of the sodium bicarbonate powder is adjusted to control the rate of abrasion. Air polishing is also recommended for cleaning and removing extrinsic stain from pits and fissures before placement of sealants. The manufacturer's instructions caution against the use of air polishing for patients with respiratory diseases because of the potential for aspiration.

**TABLE 58.1 Extrinsic Stains**

| Type of Stain | Appearance | Cause |
|---|---|---|
| Black stain | Thin black line on the teeth near the gingival margin. More common in girls. Frequently found in clean mouths. Difficult to remove. | Caused by natural tendencies. |
| Tobacco stain | A very tenacious dark brown or black stain. | Caused by the products of coal tar in tobacco and by the penetration of tobacco juices into pits and fissures, enamel, and dentin of the teeth. Use of any tobacco-containing products causes tobacco stains on the teeth and restorations. |
| Brown or yellow stain | Most commonly found on the buccal surfaces of the maxillary molars and the lingual surfaces of the lower anterior incisors. | Caused by poor oral hygiene or by the use of a toothpaste with inadequate cleansing action. |
| Green stain | Appears as a green or green-yellow stain, usually on the facial surfaces of the maxillary anterior teeth. Most common stain in children. | Caused by poor oral hygiene when bacteria or fungi are retained in bacterial plaque. |
| Dental plaque agents | Reddish-brown stain appears on the interproximal and cervical areas of the teeth. Also can appear on restorations, in plaque, and on the surface of the tongue. | Caused by the use of prescription mouth rinses that contain chlorhexidine. (Chlorhexidine is a disinfectant with broad antibacterial action.) |
| Food and drink | Light brownish stain. Stain is lessened with good oral hygiene. | Caused by tea, coffee, colas, soy sauce, berries, and other foodstuffs. |
| Nasmyth's membrane | Light green or brownish stain that is removed with gentle polishing. | Caused by food stains in the residue of epithelium during tooth eruption. |

Modified from Robinson D, Bird D: Essentials of dental assisting, ed 6, St Louis, 2017, Saunders.

**TABLE 58.2 Intrinsic Stains**

| Type of Stain | Appearance | Cause |
|---|---|---|
| Pulpless teeth | Not all pulpless teeth discolor. A wide range of colors exists: light yellow, gray, reddish brown, dark brown, or black; sometimes an orange or greenish color is seen. | Blood and pulpal tissues break down as a result of bleeding in the pulp chamber or death of pulp tissue. Pigments from the blood and tissue penetrate the dentin and show through the enamel. |
| Tetracycline antibiotics | Light green to dark yellow or a gray brown. Discoloration depends on the dosage, the length of time the drug was used, and the type of tetracycline given. | Can occur in the child when the mother is given tetracycline during the third trimester of pregnancy, or when this agent is given in infancy or early childhood. |
| Dental fluorosis | Also referred to as *mottled enamel;* results from ingestion of excessive fluoride during the mineralization period of tooth development. | Varying degrees of discoloration ranging from a few white spots to extensive white areas or distinct brown stains. |
| Imperfect tooth development | Teeth are yellowish brown or gray brown. Teeth appear translucent or opalescent and vary in color. | May result from genetic abnormality or environmental influences during development. |
| Silver amalgam | Appears as a gray or black discoloration around a restoration. | Metallic ions from the amalgam penetrate into the dentin and enamel. |
| Other systemic causes | Appear as a yellowish or greenish discoloration of the teeth. | Conditions of prolonged jaundice early in life and erythroblastosis fetalis (Rh incompatibility). |

From Robinson D, Bird D: Essentials of dental assisting, ed 6, St Louis, 2017, Saunders.

### *Rubber Cup Polishing*

The most common technique for removing stains and plaque and for polishing the teeth is the use of an abrasive polishing agent in a *rubber polishing cup* that is rotated slowly and carefully by a prophy angle attached to the slow-speed handpiece. This is the form of coronal polishing that is described in detail in this chapter.

## Handpieces and Attachments for Coronal Polishing

### Polishing Cups

Soft, webbed polishing cups are used to clean and polish the smooth surfaces of the teeth. The polishing cup attaches to the reusable prophy angle with a snap-on or screw-on attachment.

**BOX 58.3 Indications for and Contraindications to Air Polishing Use**

**Indications**

- Cleaning of pits and fissures before sealant placement
- Removal of temporary cement residues
- Cleaning of bands and brackets inside the mouth
- Surface cleaning (for exact tooth color selection before selection from the shade guide)
- Removal of difficult stain

**Contraindications**

- Patients with restricted sodium diets
- Patients with respiratory, renal, or metabolic disease
- Children
- Areas of exposed cementum or dentin
- Prolonged polishing of root surfaces

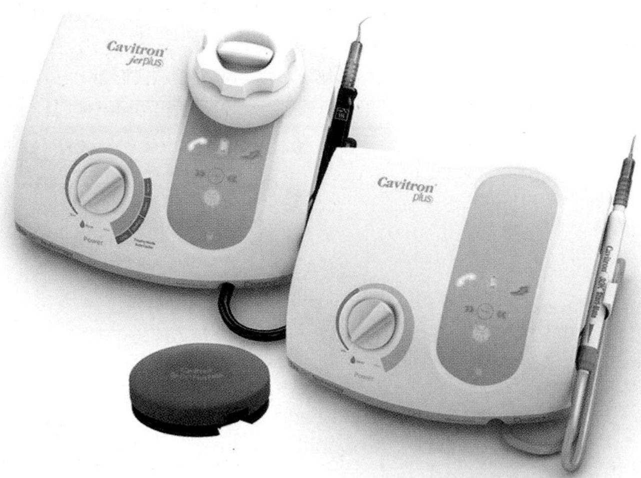


**FIG. 58.8** Air polisher unit *(left)* and magnetostive scaler *(right)*. *(Courtesy Dentsply Professional Division, York, PA.)*

Polishing cups are made from natural or synthetic rubber. Natural rubber polishing cups are more resilient and do not stain the teeth. Synthetic polishing cups are stiffer than natural polishing cups. Synthetic polishing cups should be used for patients with latex allergies.

## Bristle Brushes

Bristle brushes are made from natural or synthetic materials and may be used to remove stains from the deep pits and fissures of enamel surfaces. Bristle brushes can cause cuts on the gingivae and must be used with special care. Brushes are *not* recommended for use on exposed cementum or dentin because these surfaces are soft and are easily grooved.

### Bristle-Brush Polishing Stroke

- If necessary, soak stiff brushes in hot water to soften them.

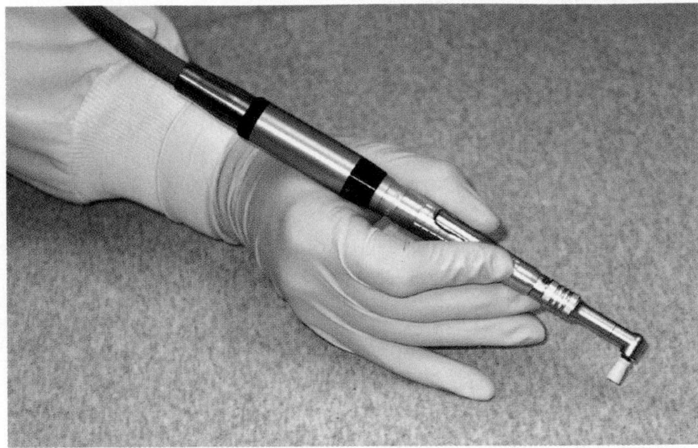

**FIG. 58.9** Close-up of hand with handpiece and proper grasp.

- Apply a mild abrasive polishing agent to the brush and, using a light wiping stroke, spread the polishing agent over the occlusal surfaces to be polished.
- Use the free hand and fingers to retract and protect the cheek and tongue from the revolving brush.
- Establish a firm finger rest and bring the brush almost into contact with the tooth surface before activating the brush.
- Using the slowest speed, apply the revolving brush lightly to the occlusal surfaces. Take care to avoid contacting the gingiva.
- Use a short-stroke brushing motion, moving from the inclined planes to the cusps of the tooth.
- Move frequently from tooth to tooth to avoid generating frictional heat.
- Frequently replenish the supply of polishing agent to minimize frictional heat.

## Prophylaxis Angle and Handpiece

The prophylaxis angle, commonly called a *prophy angle,* attaches to the low-speed handpiece (see Chapter 35).

The two basic types of prophy angles are *reusable* and *disposable.* The reusable type of prophy angle must be properly cleaned and sterilized after each use. (Handpiece maintenance is discussed in Chapter 35.) The disposable angle is simply discarded after a single use. The disposable angle is manufactured with a polishing cup or a brush already attached.

When attaching the polishing cup or the brush to the reusable type of prophy angle, you must ensure that the polishing cup or brush is securely fastened. If a polishing cup or brush falls off during the procedure, the patient could swallow or aspirate it.

### Grasping the Handpiece

The handpiece and the prophylaxis angle are held in a pen grasp with the handle resting in the U-shaped area of the hand between the thumb and the index finger (Fig. 58.9).

Proper grasp is important; if the grasp is not secure and comfortable, the weight and balance of the handpiece can cause loss of control, possibly resulting in hand and wrist fatigue.

### Handpiece Operation

- A low-speed handpiece that operates at a maximum of 20,000 revolutions per minute (rpm) is recommended. The low speed minimizes frictional heat and gingival trauma caused by the polishing cup.
- The rheostat (foot pedal) is used to control the speed (rpm) of the handpiece.
- The toe of the foot is used to activate the rheostat. The sole of the foot remains flat on the floor, similar to its position when one is operating a gas pedal on a car.
- Apply steady pressure with the toe on the rheostat to produce a slow, even speed. Release the rheostat immediately when the handpiece is removed from the tooth for longer than a moment. This prevents splattering of prophy paste and saliva.
- Use intermittent pressure on the tooth to allow the heat that is generated to dissipate between strokes. Constant pressure of the rubber cup or the brush on the tooth builds up frictional heat that may cause discomfort and possible pulpal damage.
- The speed of the cup is important in minimizing frictional heat and in polishing effectively. Operating the cup at high speeds may be harmful and ineffective.

### The Fulcrum and Finger Rest

The terms **fulcrum** and *finger rest* are used interchangeably to describe the placement of the third, or ring, finger of the hand, which holds the instrument or handpiece.

The fulcrum provides stability for the operator and must be placed in such a way as to allow movement of the wrist and forearm. The fulcrum is repositioned throughout the procedure as necessary and usually is maintained as close as possible to the working area. The fulcrum may be intraoral or extraoral, depending on a variety of circumstances:

- The presence or absence of teeth
- The area of the mouth that is being treated
- The patient's ability to widen the mouth when open

When possible, an intraoral fulcrum is preferable. Improper positioning of the hand and fingers greatly increases operator fatigue and can cause painful inflammation of the ligaments and nerves of the wrist over time.

## Polishing Agents

Selecting an appropriate polishing agent is important. The recommended polishing pastes are those with high polish and low abrasion levels. All polishing materials are abrasives, and it is through a process of abrasion that they reduce scratches, remove stains, and smooth surfaces.

Polishing agents (abrasives) are available in various grits. (*Grit* refers to the degree of coarseness of an agent.) These agents are available in extra coarse, coarse, medium, fine, and extra fine. The coarser the agent, the greater is the abrasion to the surface.

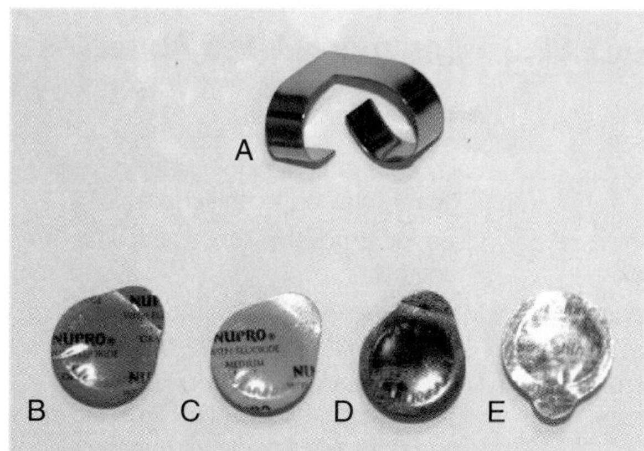


**FIG. 58.10** Prophy pastes and equipment. A, Finger ring that holds the individual container of prophy paste. B, Mild grit. C, Medium grit. D, Coarse grit. E, Soft polishing paste for esthetic restorations.

Even a fine-grit agent removes small amounts of enamel surface. Therefore the goal is to always use the abrasive agent that will produce the *least* amount of abrasion to the tooth surface.

Polishing agents are available as commercial premixed pastes (**prophy paste**) or as powders mixed with water or mouthwash to form slurry used on the polishing cup. Powder abrasives should be as wet as possible (i.e., the texture should be similar to moist cake mix) to minimize frictional heat. If the mixture is too wet, spatter will occur, and it will be difficult to keep the material inside the cup. The commercial type of premixed paste is available in ready-to-use packages (Fig. 58.10 and Table 58.3).

## Polishing Esthetic Restorations

Esthetic dentistry has become an important part of today's dental practice, and this trend will continue to grow. Many patients have crown and bridge restorations, and many are choosing to have cosmetic resin, composite, bonding, and veneers placed to enhance their smile. Identifying esthetic restorations can be challenging because tooth-colored restorations are not easy to recognize. Before polishing, the dental assistant must be able to differentiate between tooth structure and the restorative material by carefully examining the margins and the outline of the tooth surface with an explorer and relying on tactile sensitivity. Radiographs and reflection of light with the mouth mirror also can help in identifying the location of a restoration (Fig. 58.11). A review of the patient's dental record can reveal the locations of esthetic restorations.

Improper oral care can quickly damage many of these types of restorations. Dental assistants who perform rubber cup coronal polishing must understand the maintenance requirements associated with esthetic dentistry.

Regular prophy paste generally is not recommended for polishing most esthetic restorations. Low-abrasive pastes such as micron-fine sapphire or diamond paste or aluminum oxide paste should be used for these restorations. The polishing agent should be applied directly to the

TABLE 58.3 Commonly Used Abrasives

| Agent | Action |
|---|---|
| Silex | Fairly abrasive; used for cleaning more heavily stained tooth surfaces. |
| Superfine Silex | Used for removal of light stains on tooth enamel. |
| Fine pumice | Mildly abrasive; used for more persistent stains, such as tobacco stains. |
| Zirconium silicate | Used for cleaning and polishing tooth surfaces (this material is highly effective and does not abrade tooth enamel). |
| Chalk | Also known as *whiting;* chalk is precipitated calcium carbonate (frequently incorporated into toothpaste and polishing pastes to whiten the teeth). |
| Commercial premixed preparations | Contain an abrasive, water, a humectant (to keep the preparation moist), a binder (to prevent separation of the ingredients), flavoring agents, and color. Commercial preparations are available in small plastic containers or individual packets. These are available in a variety of grits; some are made especially for esthetic restorations. |
| Fluoride prophylaxis pastes | Replace some of the fluoride that is lost from the surface layer during the polishing process. These pastes are not a substitute for topical application of fluoride. Use of fluoride paste is contraindicated before acid etching of the enamel when followed by bonding of sealants or other bonded materials. |

restoration and then polished thoroughly with the use of a rubber cup for 30 seconds. Sapphire or diamond polishing paste is suggested when only porcelain is being polished. Aluminum oxide paste is recommended for use on filled hybrid composites and resin restorations. Always follow the manufacturer's suggestions regarding polishing of esthetic restorations.

Esthetic and porcelain restorations should be polished first. Then, the remaining teeth may be polished with the use of appropriate methods for any stain present. This is done to reduce the possibility that a coarse abrasive may remain in the rubber cup when one is polishing esthetic restorations.

### Factors That Influence the Rate of Abrasion

- The amount of abrasive agent used (the more agent used, the greater the degree of abrasion)
- The amount of pressure applied to the polishing cup (the lighter the pressure, the less abrasion)
- The rotation speed of the polishing cup (the slower the rotation of the cup, the less abrasion)

### Polishing Tips

- Use approximately one cupful of polishing agent for one or two teeth. An empty cup generates more heat.
- Use moderate intermittent pressure to permit heat dissipation. Heavy pressure creates more heat and greater abrasion to the tooth.
- Use the lowest possible handpiece speed that will move the cup or brush against the tooth without stalling. A whine or whistle in the handpiece indicates excessive speed.
- Usually 20 pounds per square inch (psi) of air pressure is sufficient for stain removal.
- Polish each tooth for approximately 3 to 5 seconds. The more time spent polishing a tooth, the greater will be the abrasive effect.

RECALL

6 Which is the most common technique for stain removal?
7 Which type of grasp is used to hold the handpiece?
8 What is the purpose of a fulcrum?
9 What precaution should be taken when esthetic-type restorations are polished?

# Coronal Polishing Steps

## Polishing Stroke

- Begin with the distal surface of the most posterior tooth in the quadrant, and work forward toward the anterior.
- The stroke should occur from the gingival third toward the incisal third of the tooth (Fig. 58.12).
- Fill the polishing cup with the polishing agent, and spread it over several teeth in the areas to be polished.
- Establish a finger rest, and place the cup almost in contact with the tooth.
- Using the slowest speed, apply intermittent strokes with the revolving cup lightly to the tooth surface for approximately 1 to 2 seconds between strokes. *Purpose:* Higher speeds produce frictional heat that can damage the tooth and burn the gingiva. Intermittent strokes allow the heat to dissipate.
- Use intermittent pressure that is sufficient to cause the edges of the polishing cup to flare slightly. Each tooth should be completed in approximately 3 to 5 seconds (Fig. 58.13).
- Move the cup to another area on the tooth, using a patting, wiping motion and an overlapping stroke. *Purpose:* This motion avoids creating heat that could harm the tooth.
- Reapply polishing agent frequently as needed.
- Turn the handpiece to adapt the polishing cup to fit every area of the tooth. *Purpose:* Doing so ensures that the cup covers all areas of the tooth.

If you are using two polishing agents with different degrees of coarseness, always use a separate polishing cup for each. Use the most abrasive agent first; finish with the finest (least abrasive). Always rinse between polishing agents. *Purpose:* The finer abrasive removes tiny scratches left by the more coarse abrasive.

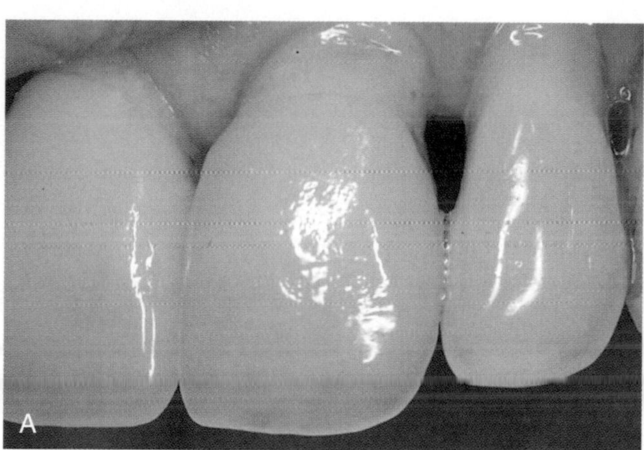


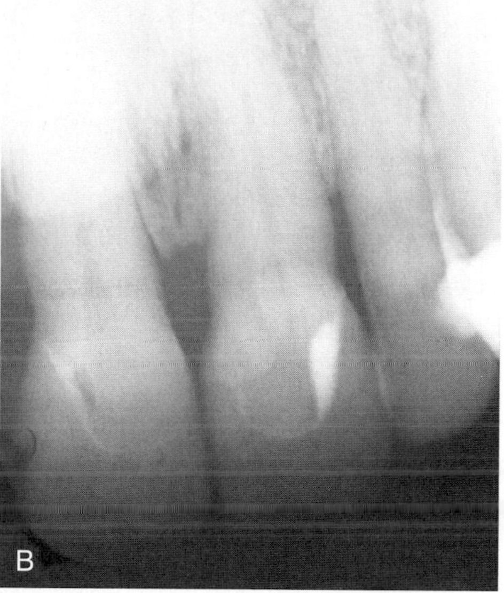


**FIG. 58.11** A, It can be difficult to detect esthetic restorations. Two of these teeth have crowns. B, Note the opaque white line of cement on teeth #8 and #9, which shows that these teeth have porcelain crowns. *(Courtesy Dr. Peter Pang, Sonoma, CA.)*

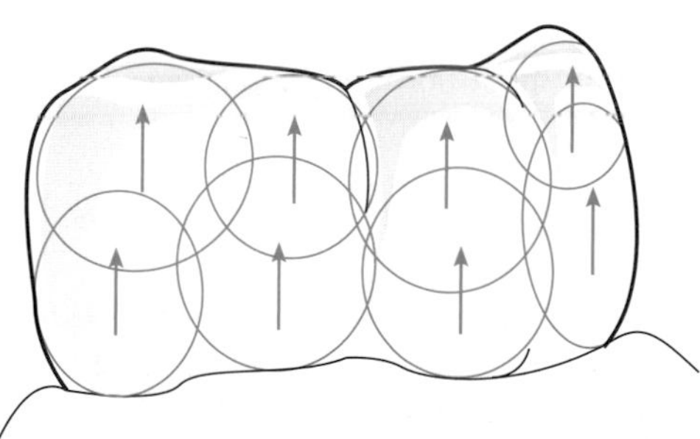

**FIG. 58.12** Use overlapping strokes to ensure complete coverage of the tooth.

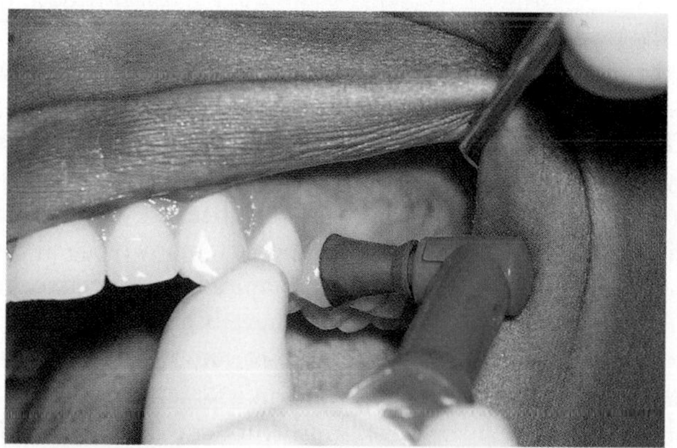

**FIG. 58.13** Stroke from the gingival third with just enough pressure to cause the cup to flare.

## Positioning the Patient and Operator

Proper positioning of both the operator and the patient during coronal polishing procedures is necessary for maximum comfort and efficiency.

### *Positioning the Patient*

- The dental chair is adjusted so the patient is approximately parallel to the floor with the back of the chair raised slightly.
- The movable headrest is adjusted for patient comfort and operator visibility.
- For access to the *mandibular arch,* position the patient's head with the chin down. When the mouth is open, the lower jaw is parallel to the floor (Fig. 58.14).
- For access to the *maxillary arch,* position the patient's head with the chin up (Fig. 58.15).

### *Positioning the Operator*

- The operator positions described in this chapter refer to the face of a clock. (This concept is discussed in Chapter 33.)
- The operator should be seated comfortably at the patient's side and must be able to move around the patient to gain access to all areas of the oral cavity.
- The seated operator's feet should be flat on the floor with the thighs parallel to the floor.
- The operator's arms should be at waist level and even with the patient's mouth.

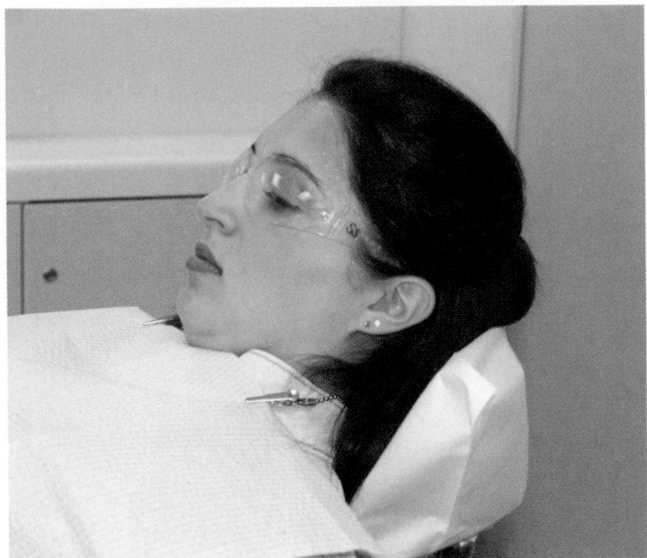

**FIG. 58.14** For the mandibular arch, the patient's head is positioned so the lower jaw is parallel to the floor when the mouth is open.

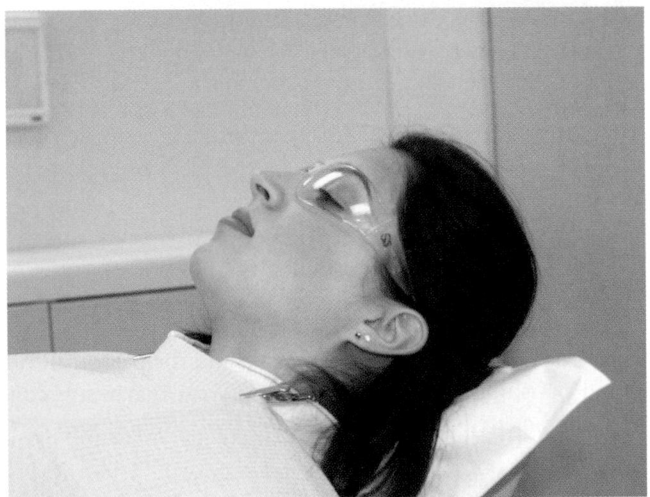

**FIG. 58.15** For access to the maxillary arch, position the patient's head with the chin up.

- When performing a coronal polish procedure, the right-handed operator generally begins by being seated at the eight o'clock or nine o'clock position (Fig. 58.16).
- When performing a coronal polish procedure, the left-handed operator generally begins by being seated at the three o'clock or four o'clock position.

*Tip:* For maximum support and safety, keep the fulcrum as close to the area you are polishing as possible, preferably on the same dental arch.

## Sequence of Polishing

If full-mouth coronal polishing is indicated, it must be done in a predetermined sequence to be certain that no area is missed. The best sequence is based on the operator's preference and the individual needs of the patient.

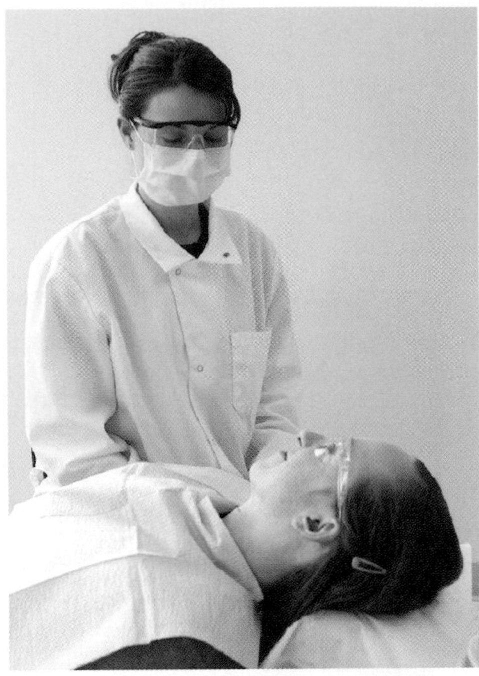

**FIG. 58.16** The right-handed operator is seated at the nine o'clock position.

One very effective sequence is described in Procedure 58.1: Rubber Cup Coronal Polishing (Expanded Function). Positions and fulcrums described are for a right-handed operator. The concepts of direct and indirect vision are discussed in Chapter 33.

The patient's mouth is rinsed with water from the air-water syringe as necessary to maintain patient comfort throughout the procedure. The high-volume evacuator (HVE) tip is used to remove excess water and debris.

**10** In which direction should the polishing stroke move?
**11** What damage can result from use of the prophy cup at high speed?
**12** How should the patient's head be positioned for access to the maxillary mandibular arch?

## Flossing After Polishing

Dental floss or tape can be used after coronal polishing to polish the interproximal tooth surfaces and to remove any abrasive agent or debris that may be lodged in the contact area.

To polish these areas, abrasive is placed on the contact area between the teeth, and floss or tape is worked through the contact area with a back-and-forth motion. Because operators' and patients' preferences for floss and tape vary, many types are available. When used properly, floss and tape are equally effective.

After the interproximal surfaces have been polished, a fresh piece of dental floss or tape is used to remove any remaining abrasive particles between the teeth.

If necessary, a floss threader can be used to pass the floss under fixed bridgework to gain access to the abutment teeth. Flossing techniques are further discussed in Chapter 15.

## Evaluation of Polishing

When you have completed polishing and flossing, evaluate the effectiveness of your technique by reapplying the disclosing agent and checking for the following criteria:

- After the tooth surfaces have been dried with air, no disclosing agent remains.
- The teeth are glossy and reflect light from the mirror uniformly.
- No evidence of trauma to the gingival margins or to any other soft tissues in the mouth is apparent.

**■ Patient Education** Most patients are self-conscious about stains on their teeth and appreciate any tips you can give them about how they can keep their teeth as white as possible.

You can explain to the patient that the causes of extrinsic stains are often controllable sources, such as coffee, tea, and tobacco. Patients may then choose to eliminate the causes of these stains, or they may have you show them how to improve their oral hygiene procedures. It is important that patients understand the causes of stains on their teeth. When stains are intrinsic, the dentist may want you to mention possible cosmetic dental care options to satisfy the patient's desire for attractive and stain-free teeth. ■

**■ Legal and Ethical Implications** Laws regarding coronal polishing performed by dental assistants vary widely among states. In some states, the dental assistant may have to be certified or registered to perform this function. It is your responsibility to understand and comply with the regulations of your state.

It is also important to remember that a coronal polish is not the same as a prophylaxis. Dental assistants are not allowed to perform a prophylaxis. A dentist or a dental hygienist must complete this procedure ■

**■ Eye to the Future** Every day, patients see and hear advertisements in the media for products that will clean, polish, whiten, and remove stains from their teeth. Some of these products are effective; many are not. This trend of consumer interest will continue to grow, and patients will look to the dental professionals who provide their care to help them make wise choices. The role of the dental healthcare professional is to help patients realize that good oral health means more than just white teeth. ■

### ■ Critical Thinking

1. Before performing a coronal polish on Michelle, a 16-year-old girl, the certified dental assistant (CDA) notices in the health history that Michelle was given the drug tetracycline as a very young child. Michelle states that she took the drug repeatedly over several months. What, if any, conditions might the CDA expect to see on Michelle's teeth?
2. The dentist asks the CDA to perform a coronal polish on a patient who will have some orthodontic brackets placed. The CDA notices some formation of light calculus on the facial surfaces of the anterior teeth. What should the CDA do?
3. You are getting ready to perform a coronal polish procedure by beginning on the facial surfaces of the maxillary right quadrant. How would you position yourself and your patient? ■

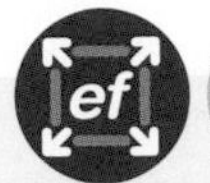

PROCEDURE 58.1 

# Rubber Cup Coronal Polishing (Expanded Function)

## PREREQUISITES FOR PERFORMING THIS PROCEDURE

- Mirror positioning
- Operator positioning
- Dental anatomy
- Fulcrum positioning
- Instrumentation

## EQUIPMENT AND SUPPLIES

- Prophy angle, sterile or disposable
- Polishing cup accessory, snap-on or screw-on
- Bristle brush, snap-on or screw-on
- Prophy paste or other abrasive in slurry
- High-volume evacuator (HVE) tip or saliva ejector
- Disclosing agent (tablets, gel, or solution)
- Cotton-tip applicator (if disclosing solution is used)
- Dental tape
- Dental floss
- Bridge threader
- Air-water syringe and sterile tip

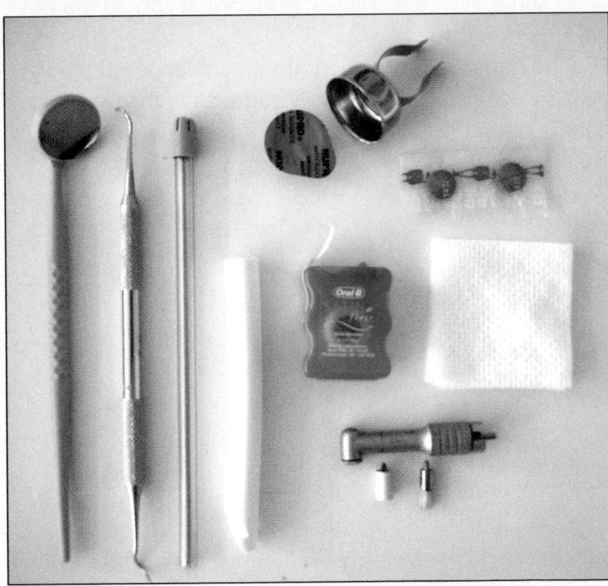

## PROCEDURAL STEPS

1. Check the patient's medical history for any contraindications to the coronal polish procedure.
2. Seat and drape the patient with a waterproof napkin. Ask the patient to remove any dental prosthetic appliance that he or she may be wearing. Provide the patient with protective eyewear.
3. Explain the procedure to the patient and answer any questions.
4. Inspect oral cavity for lesions, missing teeth, tori, and so forth.
5. Apply a disclosing agent to identify areas of plaque.

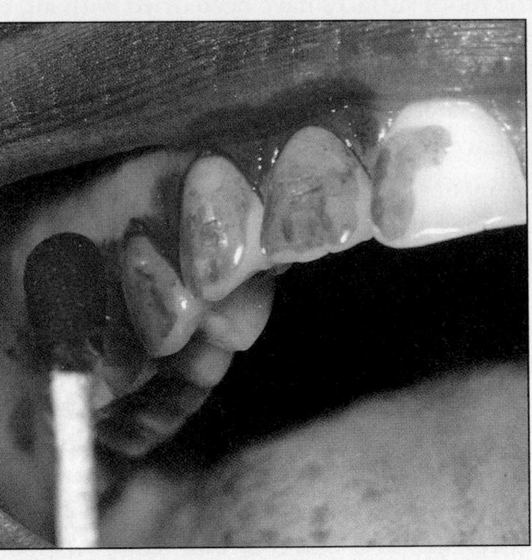

### Maxillary Right Posterior Quadrant, Buccal Aspect (Eleven O'clock or Twelve O'clock Position May Be Used)

6. Sit in the eight o'clock to nine o'clock position.
7. Ask the patient to tilt the head up and turn slightly away from you.
8. Hold the dental mirror in your left hand. Use it to retract the cheek or for indirect vision of the more posterior teeth.

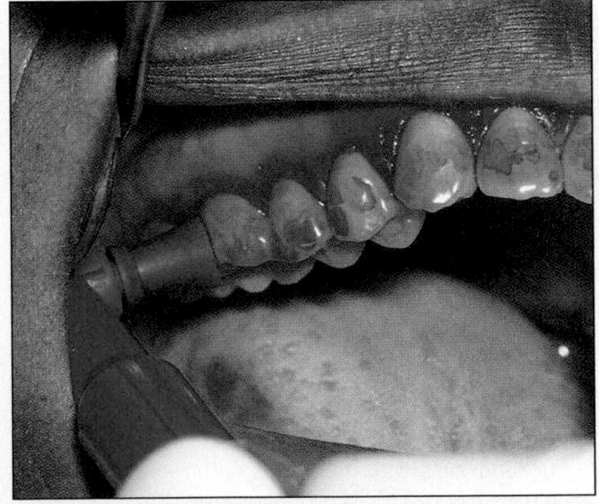

9. Establish a fulcrum on the maxillary right incisors.

### Maxillary Right Posterior Quadrant, Lingual Aspect (Eleven O'clock or Twelve O'clock Position May Be Used)

10. Remain seated in the eight o'clock to nine o'clock position.
11. Ask the patient to turn the head up and toward you.
12. Hold the dental mirror in your left hand. Direct vision in this position with use of the mirror provides a clear view of the distal surfaces.
13. Establish a fulcrum on the lower incisors, and reach up to polish the lingual surfaces.

# PROCEDURE 58.1 Rubber Cup Coronal Polishing (Expanded Function)–cont'd

### Maxillary Anterior Teeth, Facial Aspect

**14** Remain in the eight o'clock to nine o'clock position.
**15** Position the patient's head tipped up slightly and facing straight ahead. Make necessary adjustments by turning the patient's head slightly toward or away from you.
**16** Use direct vision in this area.
**17** Establish a fulcrum on the incisal edge of the teeth adjacent to the ones being polished.

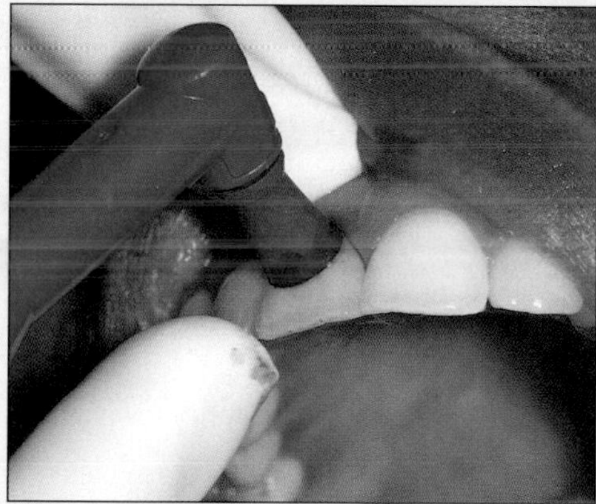

### Maxillary Anterior Teeth, Lingual Aspect

**18** Remain in the eight o'clock to nine o'clock position, or move to the eleven o'clock to twelve o'clock position.
**19** Position the patient's head so it is tipped slightly upward.
**20** Use the mouth mirror for indirect vision and to reflect light on the area.
**21** Establish a fulcrum on the incisal edge of the teeth adjacent to the ones being polished.

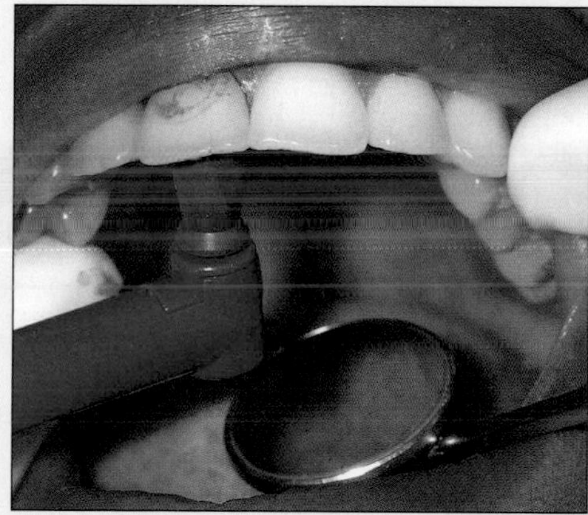

### Maxillary Left Posterior Quadrant, Buccal Aspect

**22** Sit in the nine o'clock position.
**23** Position the patient's head tipped upward and turned slightly toward you to improve visibility.
**24** Use the mirror to retract the cheek and for indirect vision.
**25** Rest your fulcrum finger on the buccal occlusal surface of the teeth toward the front of the sextant.

**ALTERNATIVE** Rest your fulcrum finger on the lower premolars, and reach up to the maxillary posterior teeth.

### Maxillary Left Posterior Quadrant, Lingual Aspect

**26** Remain in the eight o'clock to nine o'clock position.
**27** Ask the patient to turn the head away from you.
**28** Use direct vision in this position. Hold the mirror in your left hand for a combination of retraction and reflecting light.
**29** Establish a fulcrum on the buccal surfaces of the maxillary left posterior teeth or on the occlusal surfaces of the mandibular left teeth.

### Mandibular Left Posterior Quadrant, Buccal Aspect (Eleven O'clock or Twelve O'clock Position May Be Used)

**30** Sit in the eight o'clock to nine o'clock position.
**31** Ask the patient to turn the head slightly toward you.
**32** Use the mirror to retract the cheek and for indirect vision of distal and buccal surfaces.
**33** Establish a fulcrum on the incisal surfaces of the mandibular left anterior teeth, and reach back to the posterior teeth.

### Mandibular Left Posterior Quadrant, Lingual Aspect

**34** Remain in the nine o'clock position.
**35** Ask the patient to turn the head slightly away from you.
**36** For direct vision, use the mirror to retract the tongue and reflect more light to the working area.
**37** Establish a fulcrum on the mandibular anterior teeth, and reach back to the posterior teeth.

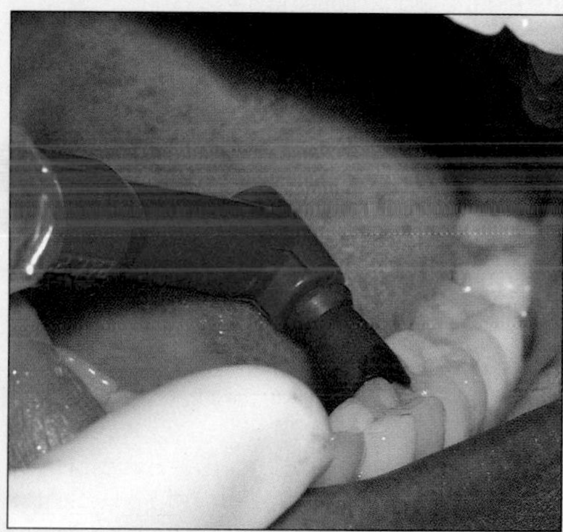

### Mandibular Anterior Teeth, Facial Aspect

**38** Sit in the eight o'clock to nine o'clock position, or in the eleven o'clock to twelve o'clock position.
**39** As necessary, instruct the patient to make adjustments to head position by turning toward or away from you or by tilting the head up or down.

**(Continued)**

## PROCEDURE 58.1 Rubber Cup Coronal Polishing (Expanded Function)–cont'd

**40** Use your left index finger to retract the lower lip. Direct and indirect vision can be used in this area.

**41** Establish a fulcrum on the incisal edges of the teeth adjacent to the ones being polished.

### Mandibular Anterior Teeth, Lingual Aspect

**42** Sit in the eight o'clock to nine o'clock position, or in the eleven o'clock to twelve o'clock position.

**43** As necessary, instruct the patient to make adjustments to the head position by turning toward or away from you or by tilting the head up or down.

**44** Use the mirror for indirect vision, to retract the tongue, and to reflect light onto the teeth. Direct vision often is used in this area when the operator is seated in the twelve o'clock position, but indirect vision also can be helpful.

**45** Establish a fulcrum on the mandibular cuspid incisal area.

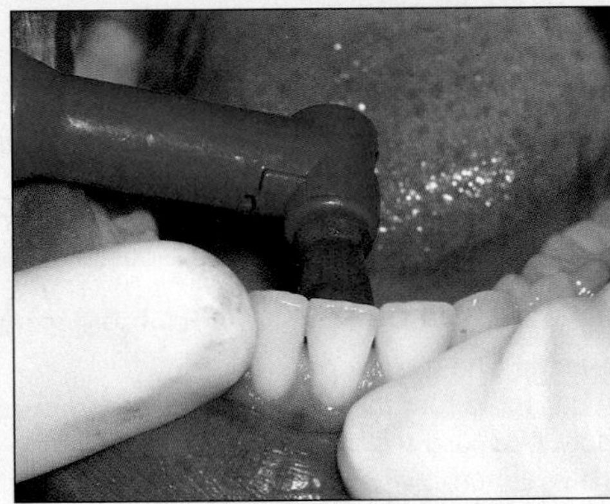

### Mandibular Right Quadrant, Buccal Aspect

**46** Sit in the eight o'clock position.

**47** Ask the patient to turn the head slightly away from you.

**48** Use the mirror to retract tissue and reflect light. The mirror also may be used to view the distal surfaces in this area.

**49** Establish a fulcrum on the lower incisors.

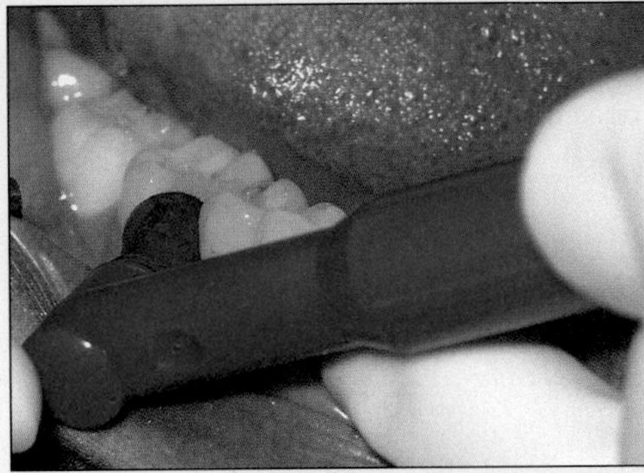

### Mandibular Right Quadrant, Lingual Aspect

**50** Remain in the eight o'clock position.

**51** Ask the patient to turn the head slightly toward you.

**52** Retract the tongue with the mirror.

**53** Establish a fulcrum on the lower incisors.

### Mandibular Right Quadrant, Lingual Aspect (Eleven O'clock or Twelve O'clock Position May Be Used)

**54** Sit in the eight o'clock to nine o'clock position.

**55** Ask the patient to turn the head slightly toward you.

**56** Retract the tongue with the mirror.

**57** Establish a fulcrum on the lower incisors.

### Documentation

**58** Document the procedure.

59

# Dental Sealants

## KEY TERMS

**Acrylate (AK-ri-layt)** A salt or ester of acrylic acid.
**Dental sealant** Coating that covers the occlusal pits and fissures of teeth.
**Filled resin (REZ-in)** Sealant material that contains filler particles.
**Light-cured** Type of material that is polymerized by a curing light.
**Microabrasion (air abrasion)** Technique used to open fissures before sealant placement.
**Microleakage (mye-kroe-LEE-kuj)** Microscopic leakage at the interface of the tooth structure and the sealant or restoration.
**Polymerization (puh-LIM-ur-i-zay-shun)** Process of changing a simple chemical into another substance that contains the same elements.
**Sealant retention** Sealant firmly adhering to the tooth surface.
**Self-cured** Type of material that is polymerized by chemical reactions.
**Unfilled resin (REZ-in)** Sealant material that does not contain filler particles.

## LEARNING OUTCOMES

*On completion of this chapter, the student will be able to achieve the following objectives:*

1. Pronounce, define, and spell the key terms.
2. Explain the ways that dental sealants prevent caries development.
3. Describe indications and contraindications for dental sealants.
4. Discuss the types of sealant materials, including the following:
   - Describe the two methods of polymerization of sealant materials and their advantages and disadvantages.
   - Discuss the rationale for filled and unfilled sealant materials.
   - Describe the technique and criteria for placement of dental sealants.
5. Discuss preventing problems with sealants.
6. Describe the precautions for dental personnel and patients with the use of sealants.
7. Explain the most important factor in sealant retention.

## PERFORMANCE OUTCOME

*On completion of this chapter, the student will be able to meet competency standards in the following skill:*

- Describe and demonstrate the steps and safety precautions necessary for the patient and the operator during sealant placement (expanded function).

## ELECTRONIC RESOURCES

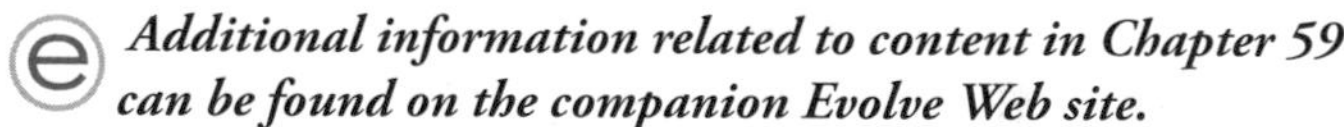

***Additional information related to content in Chapter 59 can be found on the companion Evolve Web site.***

- Practice Quiz
- Tray Setup Drag-and-Drop Exercise: Sealant
- Tray Setup Questions
- Video: Applying Dental Sealants

**Dental sealants** represent one of the greatest advances in modern dentistry. Unfortunately, too many children, particularly low-income children, do not receive the protective benefits of dental sealants. The purpose of a dental sealant is to prevent dental caries in the pits and fissures. Dental sealants are clear protective coatings that are easily applied; they cover the tooth surface, preventing bacteria and food particles from settling into the pits and fissures (grooves) of the teeth (see Chapter 8).

Although fluoride has caused the overall rate of dental caries to drop, the greatest benefits from fluoride occur on the smooth surface of the enamel. The pits and fissures of the teeth do not benefit from the effects of fluoride as much as smooth enamel surfaces do. Scientific studies have proved that properly placed dental sealants are 100 percent effective in preventing development of cavities in sealed tooth surfaces.

## How Sealants Work

The narrow width and uneven depth of pits and fissures make them ideal places for the accumulation of food and acid-producing bacteria. Saliva, which helps remove food particles from other areas of the mouth, cannot clean deep pits and fissures. Pits and fissures are often deep, narrow channels in the enamel surface that can extend close to the dentinoenamel junction (Fig. 59.1). The enamel that lies at the base of the fissures is thinner than the enamel around the rest of the tooth. This means that deep, narrow fissures can make it more likely that tooth decay will occur, and any decay that does form will penetrate through the thin enamel and progress more quickly into the pulp.

Pits and fissures on the teeth are so tiny that even a single toothbrush bristle is too large to enter for cleaning purposes (Fig. 59.2).

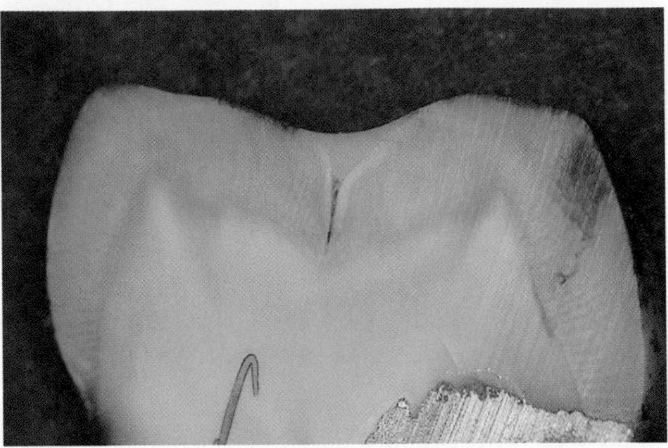

**FIG. 59.1** Section of tooth showing long, narrow fissure containing debris. A sealant is present and covers the opening of the fissure. *(Courtesy Steve Eakle, University of California, San Francisco, CA.)*

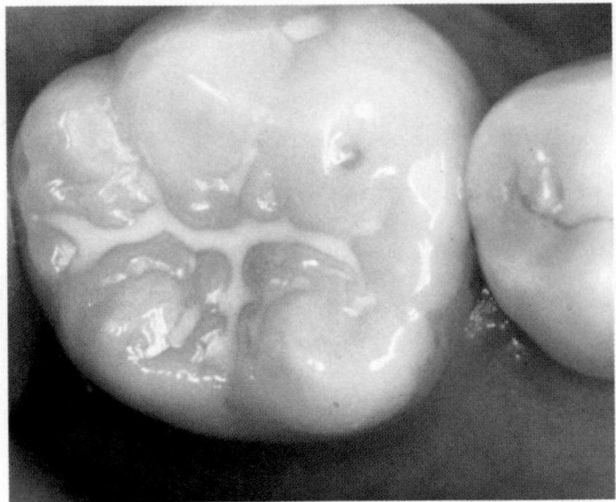

**FIG. 59.3** Molar with a properly placed sealant.

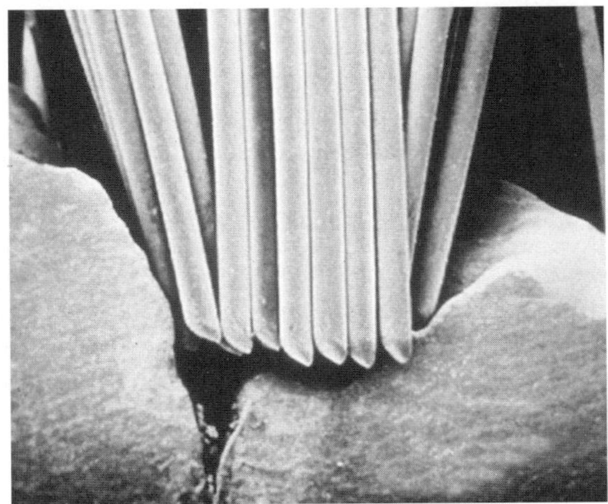

**FIG. 59.2** Micrograph showing toothbrush bristle in a groove.

The sealant acts as a physical barrier that prevents decay (Fig. 59.3). Small food particles and plaque (bacteria) cannot penetrate through or around a sealant. As long as the sealant remains intact, the tooth is protected. However, if part of the sealant or bond is broken, the sealant protection is lost.

Sealants are not as widely used as they should be among low-income children (utilization of sealants is only about 30 percent); this is the high-risk group that could benefit the most from sealants.

In many states, application of dental sealants is a duty that may be delegated to the educationally qualified dental assistant (see Procedure 59.1: Application of Dental Sealants [Expanded Function] later in this chapter).

RECALL

1 What is the purpose of dental sealants?
2 Why are pits and fissures susceptible to caries?

## Dental Caries and Sealants

On occasion, teeth with very small initial carious lesions may be inadvertently sealed, or some bacteria may remain beneath the sealant. It was once believed that if this were to occur, decay would develop under the sealant. However, numerous studies have shown that this does not occur. Bacteria cannot survive beneath a *properly placed sealant* because the carbohydrates that they need to survive cannot reach them. Studies have shown that the number of bacteria in small, existing carious lesions that had been properly sealed actually *decreased* dramatically over time. The most important factor is that the sealant must be properly placed.

Pit and fissure sealants are especially useful through the caries-active period (i.e., ages 6 to 15 years) and may delay the need for an occlusal restoration unless a proximal lesion develops. Surfaces on teeth that have large, overt dental caries should *not* be sealed. Scientific research on the use of pit and fissure sealants has proved that sealants are an effective way of preventing the development of dental caries.

# Indications for Sealants

Sealants are used primarily on children, but in certain circumstances, adults can benefit from their use. Some maxillary central and lateral incisors may have deep pits that could be protected by sealants. The dental professional must exercise proper patient selection. Sealants are indicated for teeth with deep pits and fissures, preferably in recently erupted teeth (i.e., within previous 4 years). Teeth that are well coalesced (fused together) are less likely candidates for sealants (Fig. 59.4). Premolars are not generally high-risk teeth. Although sealant therapy is aimed at permanent teeth, primary molars may also be sealed to reduce the caries rate and premature tooth loss. Even though the occlusal surface of the primary molars is flatter than that of the permanent molars, sealants are still indicated if deep or stained fissures are found (see Chapter 12). Sealants should be used as part of a preventive program that includes the use of fluorides, dietary considerations, plaque control, and regular dental examinations (see Chapter 15).

### Indications for Sealant Placement

- The tooth on the opposite side of the mouth has similar pits and fissures. This indicates that the tooth on the other side has a similar risk for decay. If the tooth on the opposite side has decay or a filling, the tooth in question may decay and may also need a filling.
- Adjacent molars have or need occlusal restorations. When the teeth beside the tooth in question have fillings or need fillings, that tooth also may develop decay.
- The tooth is newly erupted. The highest risk period for decay occurs within the first 3 years of eruption.
- The tooth is fully erupted. If a sealant is to be placed, the entire occlusal surface must be exposed. If it is not, the sealant cannot be placed.
- No proximal decay (decay between the teeth) is noted. If a filling must be placed to restore the proximal surface after the sealant has been placed, the sealant will break off.
- Sealants are used in conjunction with a fluoride program. This is an indication because fluoride helps reduce the risk of decay and will complement the role of the sealant in preventing decay.

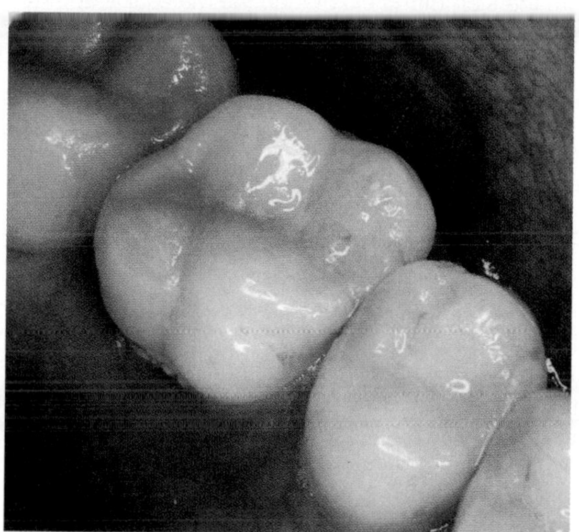

**FIG. 59.4** Enamel without significant fissures (well coalesced). *(Courtesy Steve Eakle, University of California, San Francisco, CA.)*

## Contraindications to Sealants

The cooperation of the patient during sealant placement is very important because proper placement requires a well-isolated, dry field. Patients and their parents should be advised that dental sealants are not a substitute for other caries control measures. Dental sealants are an *additional* part of the patient's overall preventive care.

### Contraindications to Sealant Placement

- Lack of deep pits and fissures
- Obvious dental decay
- Any proximal surface decay
- Insufficiently erupted teeth
- Primary teeth expected to be lost soon
- Poor patient cooperation in the dental chair

## Types of Sealant Materials

A wide variety of sealant materials are available (Table 59.1). The dental assistant should have a thorough understanding of the types and characteristics of the various sealant products (Fig. 59.5).

### Method of Polymerization

One major difference among materials is the method of **polymerization** (setting or curing) used (Box 59.1). Some brands are self-cured (also called chemical cured or auto-polymerizing), whereas others are light-cured. These types are comparable in terms of bond strength and rate of retention.

**TABLE 59.1** Troubleshooting Problems with Sealants

| Problem | Cause | Solution |
|---|---|---|
| Sealant comes off when retention is checked at placement visit. | Moisture contamination (saliva) | Maintain good isolation, and re-etch and apply the sealant. |
| Sealant blocks the contact area. | Applying too much sealant; lack of finger rest to control placement | Use just enough sealant to cover fissure and 1 mm beyond. Use good finger rest. Remove excess material before curing it. Remove hardened sealant in contact area with a scaler. |
| Sealant has holes in surface. | Air bubbles in wet sealant; vigorous scrubbing with application brush | Carefully dispense material to avoid bubbles. Gently work sealant into fissures with brush or explorer. Repair by working fresh sealant into holes with explorer tip (re-etch first if isolation was lost). |
| Sealant is high in the bite. | Too much sealant was applied | Do not puddle the sealant. Use just enough to cover the fissure and 1 mm beyond. |

From Hatrick CD, Eakle WS: Dental materials: clinical applications for dental assistants and dental hygienists, ed 3, St Louis, 2016, Elsevier.

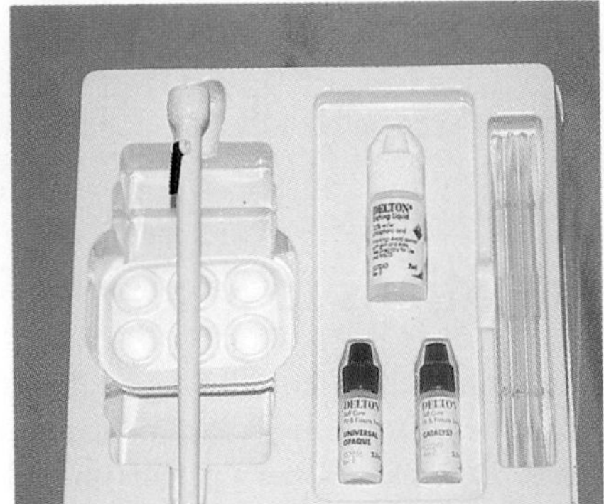

**FIG. 59.5** Universal liquid and catalyst vials shown with mixing wells and a mixing stick. *(From Darby ML, Walsh MM: Dental hygiene theory and practice, ed 4, St Louis, 2015, Saunders.)*

**Self-cured** materials are supplied as a two-part system (base and catalyst). When these pastes are mixed together, they quickly *polymerize* (harden). This usually occurs within 1 minute, and the material must be in place before the initial setting occurs.

**Light-cured** sealants do not require mixing. Visible light–cured sealants are polymerized by photo initiators in the resin that are sensitive to the visible blue light spectrum. Currently, a one-step delivery system is available in which the material is provided in a light-protected preloaded syringe and is ready for direct application to the tooth. After the material has been applied to the tooth, the curing light activates the setting of the material. A vast majority of sealants in use today are light-cured.

## Color

Sealants may be clear, tinted, or opaque (white). Tinted or opaque sealants are more popular because they are easier to see during application and during checks for sealant retention on subsequent office visits. Some brands have a tint that is visible during application but that turns clear after polymerization.

## Fillers

Sealant materials are available as **filled resins** or **unfilled resins**. The purpose of filler material in the sealant is to make it more wear resistant. Some filler particles may be radiopaque (white) and can be seen on radiographs. However, filled and unfilled sealants penetrate the fissures equally well, with no difference in **microleakage** (leakage between the tooth surface and the sealant material) and similar rates of retention.

Some dentists believe that a filled sealant is better because of a lower wear rate on occlusal surfaces. Other dentists believe that the occlusal wear is insignificant because sealants flow deep into the pits and fissures to form a barrier.

An important clinical consideration in deciding between the two types is that the unfilled sealant material does *not* require occlusal adjustment after placement because the natural wear is sufficient to establish occlusion, whereas a filled resin sealant *does* require checking of the occlusion and possible adjustment with a stone or bur.

### BOX 59.1 Advantages and Disadvantages of Chemical-Cured and Light-Cured Sealants

**Chemical-Cured (Self-Cured or Auto-Polymerizing) Sealants**

Advantages

- No need for the curing light.
- No risk of damage to the retina from the curing light.
- Sealants can be applied to several teeth without the need to go back and individually cure each one with a light.

Disadvantages

- Setting time can vary greatly with variations in room temperature; the warmer the material, the faster the set.
- Setting time of 2 minutes may be too long if you are having trouble maintaining a dry field or controlling an active child.
- Mixing two liquids together introduces bubbles into the material that could produce voids in the completed sealant.
- Viscosity (thickness) of the material increases continuously from the start of the mix. When the material is applied to several teeth, the ability of the material to flow well into tight fissures diminishes with time, and a new mix may be needed.

**Light-Cured Sealants**

Advantages

- Material sets in a short period of time (typically 20 seconds). These are particularly useful when working on an active child or trying to control a heavy salivary flow.
- Time for application is not limited as with chemical-cured sealants.
- Mixing is not required, so fewer bubbles are introduced into the material.
- Viscosity remains low throughout the application period until light is applied.

Disadvantages

- The curing light can cause damage to the retina if protection is not used.
- The curing light and filter are added expenses.
- Only the material directly under the light tip is completely cured, so when several teeth are done, the total curing time may be significantly increased. It may be difficult to manipulate the light tip to reach the distal pits of the maxillary second molars in small mouths.

From Hatrick CD, Eakle WS: Dental materials: clinical applications for dental assistants and dental hygienists, ed 3, St Louis, 2016, Elsevier.

## Working Time

Self-cured sealants polymerize to final set within approximately 2 minutes from the start of mixing the two components. An experienced operator can apply the material to one or two quadrants of posterior teeth with a single mix of material, so it has the advantage of being faster than the light-cured material when used on a comparable number of teeth.

Light-cured material has the following advantages: (1) It does not require mixing (thus bubbles are already incorporated into the material), and (2) it allows the operator to place and cure the material when the operator is ready.

## Placement Technique

Placement of dental sealants requires attention to detail (see Procedure 59.1). The surface to be sealed must first be cleaned with a rubber cup and pumice, or by air polishing to remove any surface debris that would interfere with acid etching (see Chapter 58 for a discussion of polishing techniques). Retention of the sealant is attained by etching the enamel with 37 percent phosphoric acid to roughen it and open the pores in the enamel for penetration of the resin sealant. After etching, rinsing, and drying of the enamel, isolation of the field is very important. The sealant is applied to the pits and fissures and the surrounding enamel and is cured. Any moisture on the tooth could result in failure of the sealant to adhere. Moisture could come from saliva, from an air-water syringe that leaks water into the air, or even from the patient's breath. If moisture contamination occurs, the sealant could be lost immediately or partially lost at a later date, or leakage could occur around the partially retained sealant, resulting in decay beneath the sealant. Maxillary and mandibular second molars are the teeth that most frequently lose sealants, probably because they are the most difficult teeth for which to maintain isolation when a rubber dam is not used. It is very important to carefully check the sealants at recall visits. Some manufacturers have added an agent to the sealant kit that enhances the sealant bond and evaporates moisture from fissures. This procedural step follows drying of the etched enamel.

# Preventing Problems with Sealants

## Etching

Use care in placement of the etchant, so that it does not contact adjacent teeth or soft tissue. Mylar matrix strips or metal matrix bands can be placed in the interproximal spaces to prevent this from happening.

### Remineralization of Etched Unsealed Enamel

What happens to the portions of the tooth that are etched and not covered with sealant material? Studies have shown that the etched enamel begins remineralization after 24-hour exposure to calcium phosphate salts in the saliva.

## Bite Interference by Sealant

If the sealant is too high, it might interfere with the patient's bite. Unfilled sealants that are too high will wear down in a few days or weeks. Sealants with filler particles are much more wear resistant. Ideally, all high sealants should be adjusted so that they are compatible with the patient's bite. Sealants that are too high can cause sore teeth or jaws. Articulating paper should be used to identify the high spots, and an appropriate stone or bur can be used to adjust them.

## Failures

Most sealant failures will occur within the first 3 to 6 months, and all or part of the sealant comes off. The most serious failure is the one that leaks but does not come off. The leak can go undetected and decay can occur significantly underneath the sealant before it is detected.

## Blocked Contacts

Placing too much sealant material can result in the flow of excess material into the contact area between adjacent teeth, where the patient could not floss (Fig. 59.6 and see Table 59.1).

RECALL

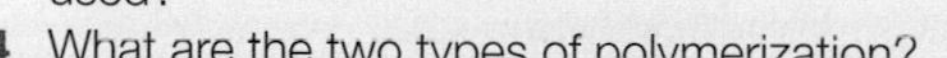

3 Should sealants be the only preventive measure used?
4 What are the two types of polymerization?
5 Why is clear sealant material less desirable?
6 Is there a difference in retention rates between filled and unfilled sealants?

## Fluoride Release

Some brands of sealant materials contain fluoride that is released after polymerization. The theory is that fluoride released from the sealant may create a fluoride-rich layer at the base of the sealed groove, helping to remineralize incipient enamel caries. This fluoride-rich layer is also thought to make the pit or fissure more resistant to decay if the sealant is lost. Clinical studies are under way to compare the effectiveness of these two types of sealants.

Some manufacturers recommend that fluoride-containing polishing paste should not be applied to the enamel surface immediately before a sealant procedure is performed. Other manufacturers do not consider fluoride polishing pastes to be contraindicated. Always follow the sealant manufacturer's instructions for each product you use.

## Microabrasion

**Microabrasion (air abrasion)** units are sometimes used by the dentist before dental sealants are applied to open the fissures, to remove any slight decay, and/or to prepare the site for placement of a sealant. The cutting ability can be controlled to remove minimal amounts of tooth structure. High-pressure alpha-alumina particles are delivered through a small handpiece-like device (Fig. 59.7).

# Precautions for Dental Personnel and Patients

## Etchant Precautions

Because etching agents contain phosphoric acid, patients and dental personnel should always wear protective eyewear when etching agents are used. Avoid contact with oral soft tissue, eyes, and skin. In case of accidental contact, immediately flush

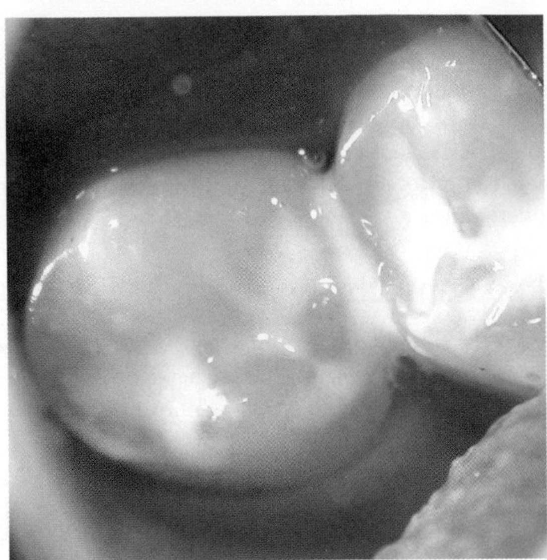

FIG. 59.6 Excess sealant blocking the contact area. *(Courtesy Steve Eakle, University of California, San Francisco, CA.)*

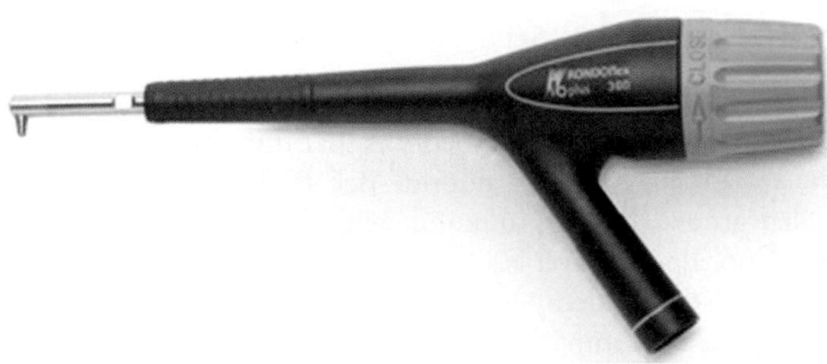

FIG. 59.7 Air abrasion tip. *(Courtesy KaVo Kerr, Orange, CA.)*

the area with large amounts of water. If eye contact is involved, immediately rinse with plenty of water and seek medical attention.

## Sealant Precautions

Sealant material contains **acrylate** resins. Do *not* use sealants on patients with known acrylate allergies. To reduce the risk for an allergic response, minimize exposure to these materials. In particular, avoid exposure to uncured resin. Use of protective gloves and a *no-touch technique* are recommended. If skin contact occurs, wash the skin with soap and water. Acrylates may penetrate gloves. If the sealant contacts the gloves, remove and discard the gloves, wash hands immediately with soap and water, and then put on new gloves. If accidental eye contact or prolonged contact with oral soft tissue should occur, flush with large amounts of water. If irritation persists, contact a physician.

*Protective glasses* should be used by operators when light-cured resins are applied. Protective eyewear also should be provided for the patient during sealant procedures.

## Storage and Use

Because products and recommendations differ among manufacturers, it is very important that you read the instructions specific to the brand that is being used. Following are some general tips regarding sealant materials:

- Replace caps on syringes and bottles immediately after use.
- Do not expose materials to air or light.
- Do not store materials in proximity to eugenol-containing products.
- Most etchant and sealant materials are designed to be used at room temperature. Check the manufacturer's recommendations.
- The shelf life of most sealant products at room temperature ranges from 18 to 36 months.
- Some brands of sealants must be stored in a refrigerator.

### Manufacturer's Instructions

**Always read and carefully follow the manufacturer's instructions when applying dental sealants.** The application technique and etching times may vary among manufacturers. For example, some manufacturers recommend against using a polishing paste that contains fluoride. Other manufacturers do not consider fluoride polishing pastes to be contraindicated.

## Factors in Sealant Retention

The effectiveness of dental sealants depends on how well and how long the sealant remains on the tooth. This is referred to as **sealant retention**. Dental caries will not occur if the sealant remains in place and completely covers the pits and fissures.

Moisture contamination is the *primary cause* of failure of sealant retention. Inadequate etching is also a factor in loss of sealant retention. Dental sealants should be examined at each recall visit to make certain that the sealant material is not partially or totally lost. When dental sealants are *properly placed,* it is not uncommon for them to last from 5 to 10 years.

7 What is the reason for putting fluoride in dental sealant material?
8 What is the range of shelf-life of sealant materials?
9 What are two patient safety precautions to keep in mind when one is using sealants?
10 What determines the effectiveness of dental sealants?

**■ Legal and Ethical Implications** Dental sealants are nontoxic, are extremely effective, and have been recommended by the American Dental Association for 20 years. Although dental sealants significantly reduce caries, very few children are protected by dental sealants. Many dentists say this is because of a lack of public awareness, and the fact that parents simply do not know that this is an effective method of protecting their children's teeth.

Application of dental sealants is considered to be an expanded function for dental assistants in many states. In other states, however, dental assistants are allowed only to assist with the placement of dental sealants. It is your professional responsibility to check the regulations in your state and to practice accordingly.

Whether or not you are legally allowed to place dental sealants, you can certainly educate your patients about the importance of sealants, explain the application process, and answer their questions. ■

**■ Eye to the Future** Dental sealants also protect the margins of dental restorations. Microleakage can occur around the margins of composite restorations because the material shrinks slightly during the visible light–curing process. These tiny gaps can lead to recurrent decay and marginal staining. Clinical researchers have shown that sealing the margins of amalgam and composite restorations with unfilled resins will (1) reduce microleakage, (2) arrest the progression of caries, (3) preserve existing restorations, and (4) preserve tooth structure.

This type of treatment may increase the longevity of the restoration, especially if the sealant is reapplied at 1-year intervals. ■

## ■ Critical Thinking

1. Carol Tyler is a single mom with limited financial means. Her young son, Phillip, has deep grooves and pits on his newly erupted first molars, and the dentist has recommended dental sealants. After the dentist leaves the room, Carol explains that she is on a very tight budget and asks you why it is necessary to add sealants when the teeth have just erupted and there is no decay. What will you tell her?
2. Emily Schmidt is a very lively 8-year-old child who does not sit still in the dental chair. About 6 months ago, when two dental sealants were placed, Emily was very uncooperative and difficult to manage. Now, on her 6-month recall, the dentist notes that one of the two sealants is gone. What do you think might have happened to make the sealant fail in such a short period?
3. Lorraine Yee and her friend Margaret Printz are talking about their children's first dental visit to Dr. McBride's office. Both children are 5 years old, and both of them saw Dr. McBride. Lorraine was advised to have dental sealants placed on her child's teeth; however, Dr. McBride did not tell Margaret that her child needed sealants. Why would Dr. McBride recommend sealants for one child, but not for another? ■

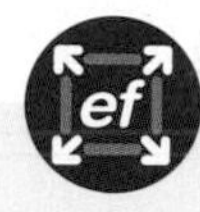

PROCEDURE 59.1 

# Application of Dental Sealants (Expanded Function)

### PREREQUISITES FOR PERFORMING THIS PROCEDURE

- ✔ Mirror positioning
- ✔ Operator positioning
- ✔ Dental anatomy
- ✔ Fulcrum positioning
- ✔ Instrumentation

### EQUIPMENT AND SUPPLIES

- ✔ Protective eyewear for patient and operator
- ✔ Basic setup
- ✔ Cotton rolls or rubber dam setup
- ✔ Etching agent (liquid or gel)
- ✔ Sealant material
- ✔ Applicator syringe or device
- ✔ Prophy brush
- ✔ Pumice and water
- ✔ High-volume oral evacuator (HVE)
- ✔ Curing light and appropriate shield
- ✔ Low-speed dental handpiece with contra-angle attachment
- ✔ Articulating paper and holder
- ✔ Round white stone (latch type)
- ✔ Dental floss
- ✔ Materials for occlusal adjustments (when a filled resin product is used)

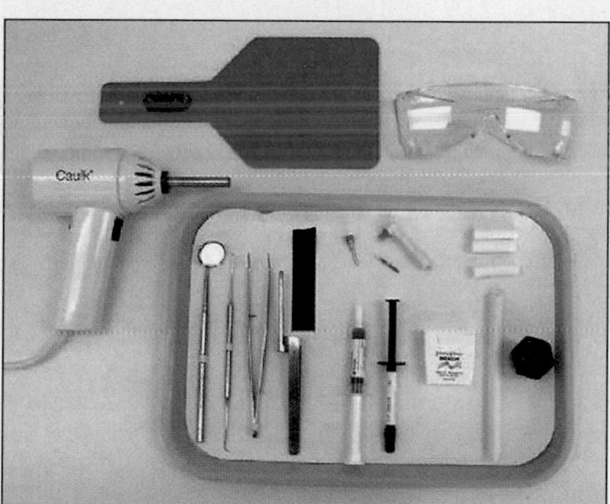


(Continued)

## PROCEDURE 59.1 Application of Dental Sealants (Expanded Function)–cont'd

### PROCEDURAL STEPS

1 Place dental dam or cotton rolls and saliva ejector to isolate teeth to be sealed.

**NOTE** Moisture contamination with saliva or water can cause a lost or leaking sealant.

2 Clean the surfaces of the teeth to be sealed with pumice or oil/fluoride-free paste.

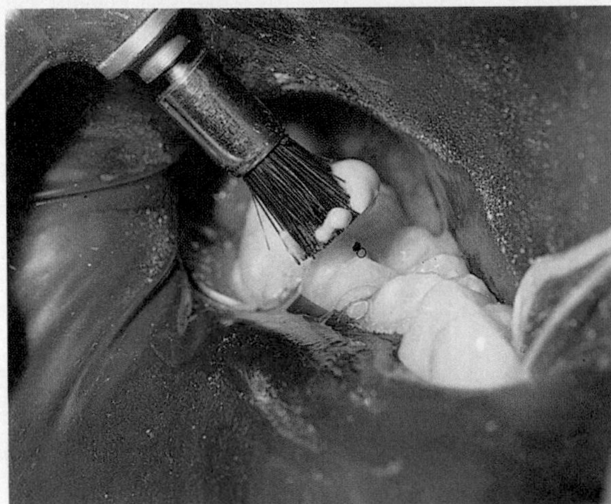

3 Use three-way syringe and HVE to rinse and dry teeth thoroughly. Remove any retained polishing paste.

**NOTE** Some dentists prefer to clean out the fissures with a small round or needle-shaped bur or diamond rotary instrument. This allows them to inspect the fissures for the presence of caries.

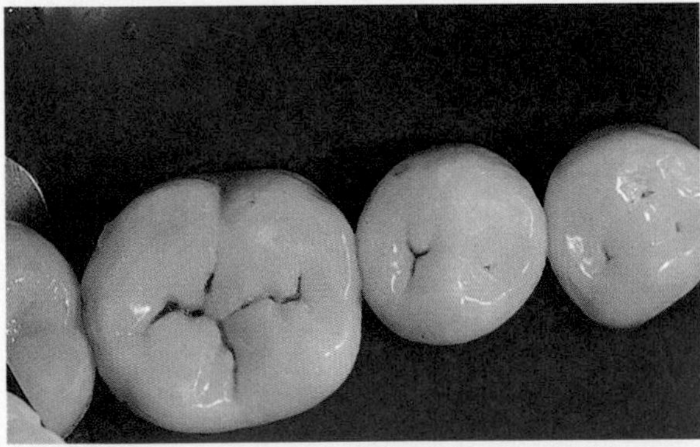

4 Place etchant on enamel to be sealed for 20 to 30 seconds.

**NOTE** Some teeth need longer etching times, such as primary teeth and teeth with fluorosis.

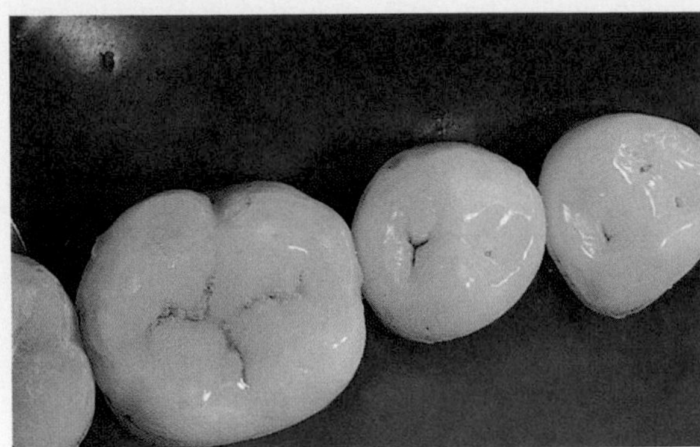

5 Rinse with water for 10 to 15 seconds.

6 If using cotton rolls, carefully replace them or dry them out with the HVE.

**NOTE** Be certain that saliva does not contaminate the freshly etched surfaces or the enamel will need to be re-etched for 15 seconds.

7 Dry the teeth thoroughly.

**NOTE** Properly etched enamel should appear frosty. If not adequately etched, re-etch for an additional 30 seconds. The fissures in this photo were opened minimally with a small bur before etching.

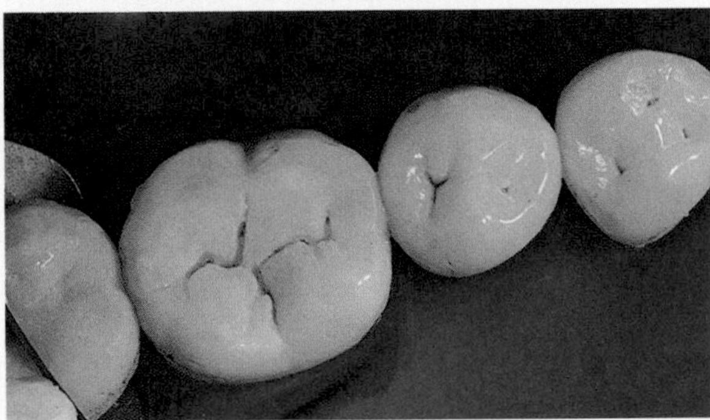

8 Apply sealant according to the manufacturer's instructions.

**NOTE** Sealant should be gently worked into the pits and fissures to displace trapped air. It should cover the entire fissure but should not overfill the groove pattern because that will probably interfere with the occlusion.

9 Cure appropriately for the required length of time (self-cure or light-cure).

**NOTE** If light-curing, each area under the light probe should be cured for at least 20 seconds. High-powered curing lights may require less time. Follow manufacturer's recommendations.

# PROCEDURE 59.1 Application of Dental Sealants (Expanded Function)–cont'd

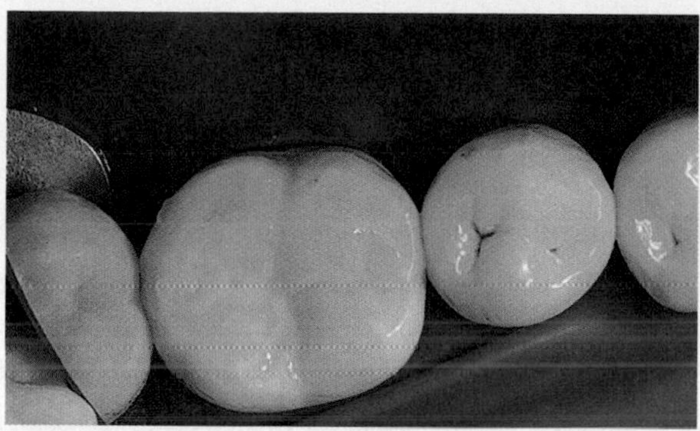

10 Check with explorer to ensure that all fissures and pits are covered, no holes in the material exist, and sealant is well retained. Apply more material, if needed.
11 Remove dental dam or cotton rolls and thoroughly rinse.
12 Check occlusion with articulating paper and adjust sealant where needed.

**NOTE** Follow state laws as to which healthcare practitioners are allowed to do adjustment.

13 Check contact areas with floss.

**NOTE** Excess material may have blocked these areas.

14 Check retention at each subsequent visit.

**NOTE** Sealants should be checked for partial or complete loss. Make sure fissures are still covered. With retained sealants, check periphery for staining that may indicate leakage. Extensive decay can occur under leaking sealants if not detected early. Replace lost or leaking sealants.

15 Document the procedure.

| Date | Charting Notes | Signature |
|---|---|---|
| 8/15/17 | Sealant applied to # 30 | PJL |

All photos in this procedure from Hatrick CD, Eakle WS, Bird WF: Dental materials: clinical applications for dental assistants and dental hygienists, ed 3, St Louis, 2016, Saunders.

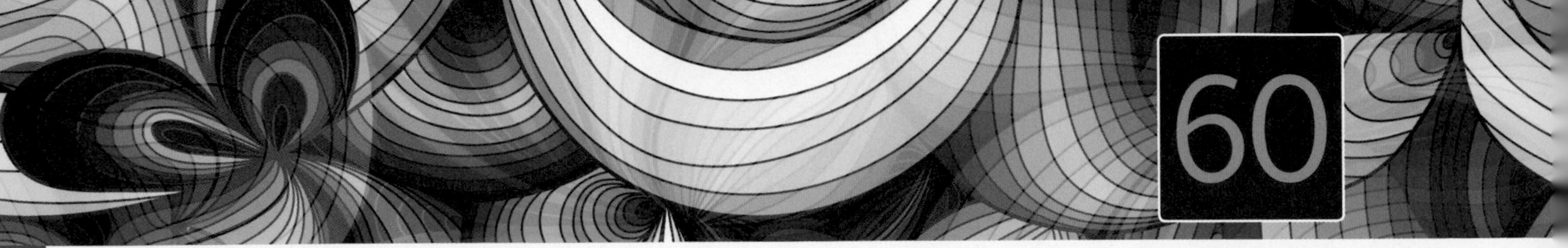


# Orthodontics

## KEY TERMS

**Arch wire** A contoured metal wire that provides force when teeth are guided in movement for orthodontics.
**Auxiliary (awg-ZIL-yuh-ree)** Attachments located on brackets and bands that hold arch wires and elastics in place.
**Band** Stainless steel ring attached to molars to hold the arch wire and auxiliaries for orthodontics.
**Braces** Another term for fixed orthodontic appliances.
**Bracket** A small device bonded to teeth to hold the arch wire in place.
**Cephalometric (seph-uh-loe-MET-rik) projection** An extraoral radiograph of the bones and tissues of the head.
**Cross-bite** Condition that occurs when a tooth is not properly aligned with its opposing tooth.
**Crowding** Condition that occurs when teeth are not properly aligned within the arch.
**Dentofacial** Structures that include the teeth, jaws, and surrounding facial bones.
**Distoclusion (dis-toe-KLOO-shun)** A class II malocclusion in which the mesiobuccal cusp of the maxillary first molar occludes mesial to the mesiobuccal groove of the mandibular first molar.
**Ectopic** An abnormal direction of tooth eruption.
**Fetal molding** Pressure applied to the jaw, causing a distortion.
**Headgear** An external orthodontic appliance that is used to control growth and tooth movement.
**Ligature (LIG-uh-chur) tie** Light wire used to hold the arch wire in its bracket.
**Mesioclusion (mee-zee-oe-KLOO-zhun)** Term used for class III malocclusion.
**Open bite** A lack of vertical overlap of the maxillary incisors, creating an opening of the anterior teeth.
**Orthodontics (or-thoe-DON-tiks)** Specialty of dentistry designed to prevent, intercept, and correct skeletal and dental problems.
**Overbite** Increased vertical overlap of the maxillary incisors.
**Overjet** Excessive protrusion of the maxillary incisors.
**Positioner** An appliance used to retain teeth in their desired position.
**Retainer** An appliance used for maintaining the positions of the teeth and jaws after orthodontic treatment.
**Separator** A device made from wire or elastic used to separate molars before fitting and placement of orthodontic bands.

## LEARNING OUTCOMES

*On completion of this chapter, the student will be able to achieve the following objectives:*

1. Pronounce, define, and spell the key terms.
2. List the benefits of orthodontic treatment.
3. Explain the roles of the orthodontist and orthodontic assistant, and describe the environment of an orthodontic practice.
4. List the causes and habits that can affect occlusion.
5. Describe the types of malocclusion.
6. Discuss corrective orthodontics, and describe what type of treatment is involved.
7. List the types of records that are used to assess orthodontic problems and put together treatment plans.
8. Discuss case presentation and financial arrangements for orthodontic treatment.
9. Name the specialized instruments and accessories used in orthodontics.
10. Describe the components of each type of appliance used in orthodontic treatment.
11. Discuss the clear aligner treatment and its effects on orthodontic alignment.
12. Explain the importance of an adjustment visit.
13. Describe ways to convey the importance of good dietary and oral hygiene habits in the practice of orthodontics.
14. Describe the use and function of headgear.
15. Discuss the completion of treatment and how retention is achieved.

## PERFORMANCE OUTCOMES

*On completion of this chapter, the student will be able to meet competency standards in the following skills:*

- Place and remove steel separating springs.
- Place and remove elastomeric ring separators.
- Assist in the fitting and cementation of orthodontic bands.
- Assist in the direct bonding of orthodontic brackets.
- Place an arch wire.
- Place and remove ligature ties.
- Place and remove elastomeric ties.

## ELECTRONIC RESOURCES

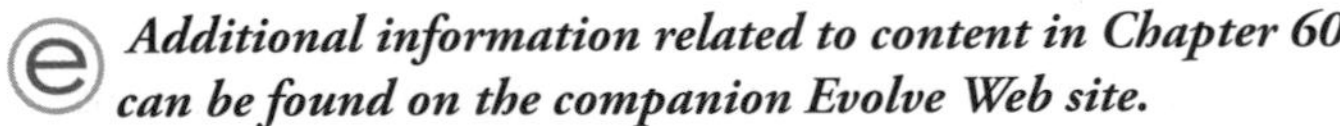

***Additional information related to content in Chapter 60 can be found on the companion Evolve Web site.***

- Practice Quiz
- Tray Setup Drag-and-Drop Exercises: Orthodontic Tooth Separating; Orthodontic Cementing and Bonding Brackets; Orthodontic Tying-in Arch Wire; Orthodontic Removing Bands and Brackets
- Tray Setup Questions
- Videos: Placing and Removing Ligature Ties; Placing and Removing Elastomeric Ties

**Orthodontics** is the specialized branch of dentistry that diagnoses, prevents, and treats dental and oral facial irregularities. Orthodontics includes **dentofacial** orthopedics, which is a term used when a fixed or removable appliance is positioned inside or outside the mouth to correct problems that involve movement of teeth or growth of the jaws.

Orthodontic treatment includes the following types of treatment:

- Straightens teeth that are rotated, tilted, or otherwise improperly aligned
- Corrects crowded or unevenly spaced teeth
- Corrects bite problems
- Aligns the upper and lower jaws

As insurance companies increase their benefits for continued orthodontic care, more people are choosing orthodontic treatment throughout their lifetime, at any age.

# Benefits of Orthodontic Treatment

Orthodontic treatment can eliminate or reduce adversity for the patient in three areas: psychosocial problems, oral malfunction, and dental disease.

## Psychosocial Problems

Severe malocclusion and dental facial deformities can be a social handicap. The impact of these types of problems may have a strong influence on patients' self-esteem and their positive feelings about themselves.

## Oral Malfunction

Malocclusion can compromise all aspects of oral function:

- Chewing can be difficult if teeth do not occlude properly.
- Jaw discrepancies can force changes in the manner of swallowing.
- Malocclusion can make it more difficult for particular speech sounds to be made.
- Temporomandibular joint (TMJ) pain can arise from minor imperfections in occlusion that trigger clenching and grinding activities.

## Dental Disease

Malocclusion can contribute to dental decay and periodontal disease. When the teeth and tissues do not receive the benefits of normal occlusion and natural cleansing, proper plaque removal becomes difficult.

# The Orthodontic Team and Office

## The Orthodontist

The orthodontist works closely with the pediatric and general dentist in providing an opportunity to change a person's "smile." As a specialist, the orthodontist will continue his or her education after dental school. Most accredited orthodontic programs are 3 years in length. The emphasis of study for the orthodontist is with orofacial growth and development, new techniques, biomechanics, and research. After receiving a certificate or a master's degree, the orthodontist will go into private practice or remain in academia.

## The Orthodontic Assistant

If you are looking for an area of dentistry with greater autonomy, orthodontics is the specialty of choice. The orthodontic assistant has the ability to participate in many "hands-on" skills. Depending on the expanded functions that are legally permitted in the state, province, or territory in which you practice, the clinical assistant is able to participate in various procedures, which involve diagnostic records, preliminary appointments, and adjustment visits.

If advancing in the profession of orthodontics is your goal, you have opportunities to (1) continue specialized training within a program and (2) take the Dental Assisting National Boards specialty examination in Orthodontic Assisting to obtain an additional credential of certified orthodontic assistant (COA).

## The Orthodontic Office

The orthodontic office is designed to accommodate many patients at a time. Because very little equipment is required for orthodontic procedures, the orthodontic office follows the "open bay" concept, along with pediatric dentistry. The patient care area of the office can be sectioned off to serve three functions: (1) to obtain records and create a more private setting, (2) to take radiographs, and (3) to provide clinical care at all stages of treatment. In larger practices, it is common to see up to 30 patients a day. Longer appointments, such as obtaining records or the bonding of brackets, are scheduled in the morning and early afternoon; shorter appointments, such as adjustments and emergencies, are kept for the early morning and late afternoon.

One area of the practice that is more expansive in the orthodontic setting is the dental laboratory. Some orthodontic practices fabricate their own diagnostic casts and fixed and removable appliances to keep overhead costs down. A laboratory technician may be hired to complete all laboratory prescriptions in house.

# Understanding Occlusion

Most malocclusions are caused by hereditary factors that affect the contours of the face and the size of the teeth and jaw. The most common cause of malocclusion is a disproportion in size between the jaw and the teeth or between the upper and lower jaws. Orthodontic problems result from the interaction of developmental, genetic, and environmental influences.

## Developmental Causes

Disturbances in dental development can accompany major congenital defects; however, they occur more frequently as isolated findings. The most common developmental disturbances include the following:

- Congenitally missing teeth
- Malformed teeth
- Supernumerary teeth
- Interference with eruption (e.g., an impaction in which eruption is blocked or the tooth is forced to erupt into an abnormal position)
- **Ectopic** eruption

## Genetic Causes

Genetic causes are responsible for malocclusion when discrepancies in the size of the jaw and/or the size of the teeth are evident. A child who inherits a mother's small jaw and a father's large teeth may have teeth that are too big for the jaw, causing overcrowding. If you have a missing tooth, it is likely that one of your parents or grandparents has the same missing tooth.

## Environmental Causes

### *Birth Injuries*

Injuries can occur at birth in two major categories: fetal molding and trauma during birth.

1. **Fetal molding** occurs when an arm or leg of the fetus is pressed against another part of the body, such as when an arm is abnormally pressed against the mandible. This pressure can lead to distortion of rapidly growing areas.
2. Trauma during birth, such as an injury to the jaw, may occur during the actual birth, particularly with the use of forceps in delivery.

### *Injury Throughout Life*

Trauma to the teeth can occur throughout life. Dental trauma can lead to the development of malocclusion in three ways:

1. Damage to permanent tooth buds when an injury to primary teeth has occurred
2. Movement of a tooth or teeth as the result of premature loss of a primary tooth
3. Direct injury to permanent teeth

## Habits

Habits that contribute to malalignment must be corrected if orthodontic treatment is to be successful. As a general rule, sucking habits that involve the thumb, tongue, lip, or finger during the primary dentition years are considered normal. These habits have few, if any, long-term effects beyond the mixed dentition; however, if they persist beyond this stage, it may be necessary to seek guidance in eliminating the habit. Table 60.1 describes habits that affect the dentition.

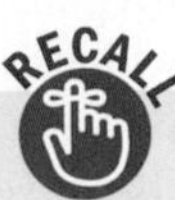


1 What age groups seek orthodontic care?
2 Give a type of genetic cause for malocclusion.

## Malocclusion

As described in Chapter 11, the maxillary and mandibular teeth, when closed correctly, are referred to as being **occluded** or as having **normal occlusion** (Fig. 60.1, *A*).

Orthodontists are concerned with teeth that do not occlude properly because of the size of the patient's jaws or because of crowding or displacement of teeth. Malocclusion refers to the abnormal or malpositioned relationship of the maxillary teeth to the mandibular teeth when occluded.

According to Angle's classification, any deviation from normal occlusion is regarded as malocclusion.

## Class I Malocclusion

Class I malocclusion consists of a normal relationship with the molars, but the anterior teeth will be out of alignment with malpositioned or rotated teeth (Fig. 60.1, *B*).

**TABLE 60.1 Habits That Affect the Dentition**

| | |
|---|---|
| **Tongue thrusting** | *Anterior tongue thrust:* The tongue rests on the lingual surfaces of the maxillary teeth. Pressure causes the teeth to move forward.<br>*Lateral tongue thrust:* The pressure of the tongue causes the bite to close down, preventing the permanent teeth from erupting.<br>*Fan tongue thrust:* The tongue thrusts out at the occlusal surfaces. |
| **Tongue thrust swallowing** | The tongue presses forward against the anterior teeth with each swallow, placing a forward pressure against the teeth. |
| **Thumb and finger sucking** | Beyond age 5, the facial structure will be affected, particularly the maxillary arch, the palate, and the anterior teeth. |
| **Bruxism** | Involuntary grinding or clenching of the teeth in movements other than chewing. This occurs most frequently during sleep. The grinding of teeth causes unnatural wear of the enamel and pressure on the periodontium. |
| **Mouth breathing** | May be a result of narrowing of the maxilla, which can cause a pinched facial appearance. Mouth breathing prolonged over a number of years can cause a change in the dentofacial structure of the child. |

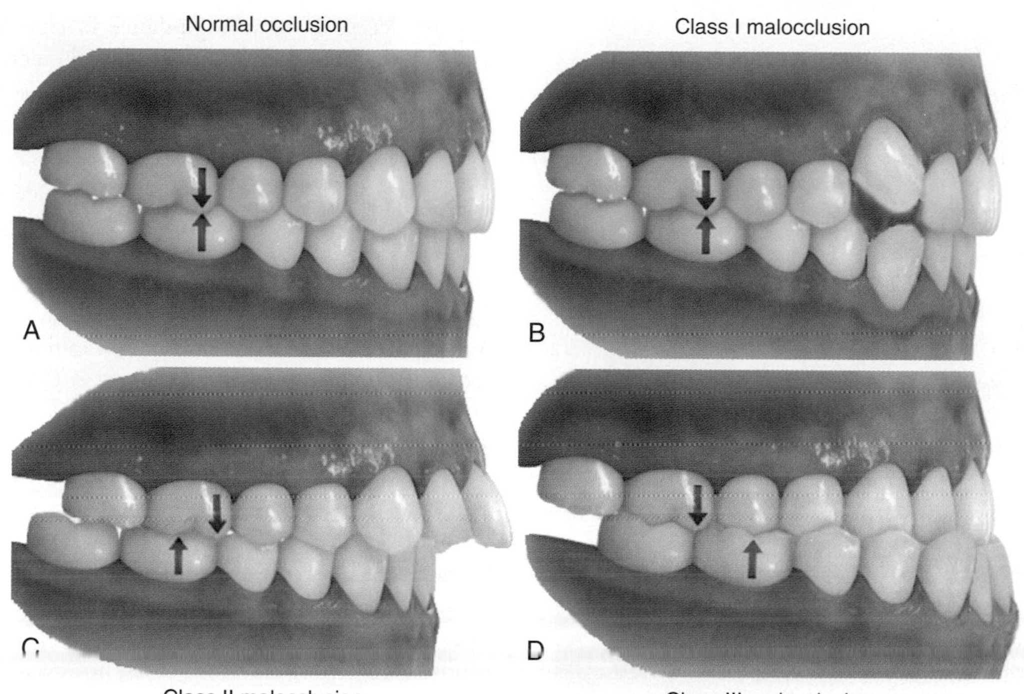


**FIG. 60.1** A, Angle's classification of normal occlusion. B, Class I malocclusion. C, Class II malocclusion. D, Class III malocclusion. *(From Graber LW, Vanarsdall RL, Vig KWL: Orthodontics: current principles and techniques, ed 5, Philadelphia, 2012, Mosby.)*

## Class II Malocclusion

In class II malocclusion, also known as **distoclusion**, the mandible is in an abnormal distal relationship to the maxilla. The mesiobuccal cusp of the maxillary first molar occludes in the interdental space between the mandibular second premolar and the mesial cusp of the mandibular first molar. This gives the appearance of the maxillary anterior teeth protruding over the mandibular anterior teeth (Fig. 60.1, *C*).

## Class III Malocclusion

In class III malocclusion, also known as **mesioclusion**, the body of the mandible is in an abnormal mesial relationship to the maxilla. The mesiobuccal cusp of the maxillary first molar occludes in the interdental space between the distal cusp of the mandibular first permanent molar and the mesial cusp of the mandibular second permanent molar. This frequently gives the appearance of the mandibular anterior teeth protruding in front of the maxillary anterior teeth, also referred to as an **underbite** (Fig. 60.1, *D*).

## Malaligned Teeth

In addition to evaluating a patient's occlusion, the orthodontist examines specific alignment of the teeth and arches. The most common malalignment problems are as follows:

- **Crowding** is the most common contributor to malocclusion. One or many teeth can be involved in misplacement (Fig. 60.2).
- **Overjet** is excessive protrusion of the maxillary incisors, causing space or distance between the facial surface of the mandibular incisors and the lingual surface of the maxillary incisors (Fig. 60.3).
- **Overbite** is an increased vertical overlap of the maxillary incisors. With an extreme overbite, the mandibular incisors may not be visible (Fig. 60.4).
- **Open bite** is a lack of vertical overlap of the maxillary incisors, creating an opening of the anterior teeth when the posterior teeth are closed (Fig. 60.5).
- **Cross-bite** indicates that a tooth is not properly aligned with its opposing tooth. An example of this occurs when a person closes the teeth; the maxillary arch should be slightly wider and longer so that it properly occludes the mandibular arch. If a maxillary tooth is inward or touches end to end with another tooth, a cross-bite exists (Fig. 60.6).

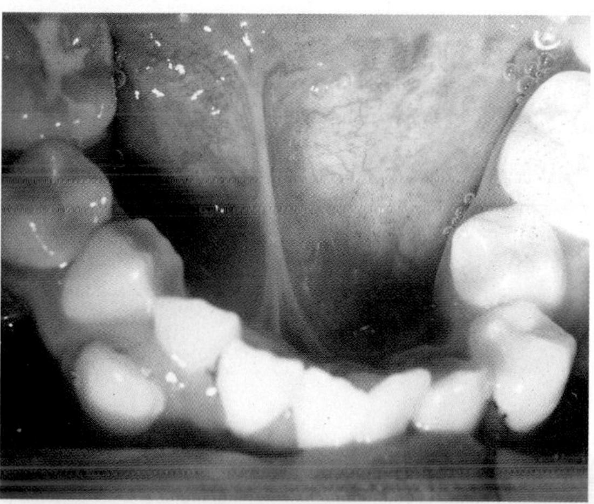

**FIG. 60.2** Crowding of teeth in the mandibular arch.

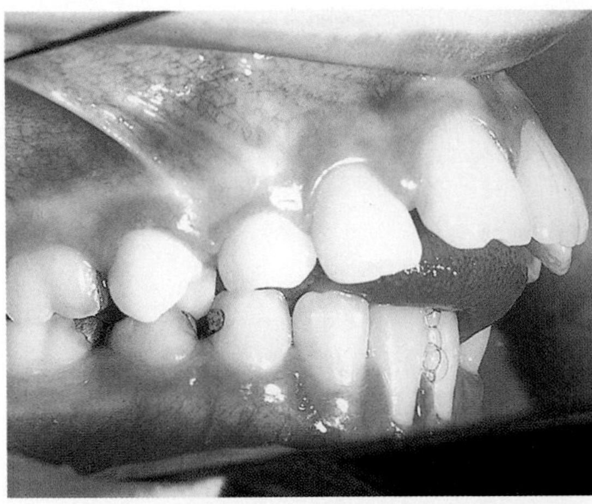

**FIG. 60.3** Excessive protrusion of the maxillary incisors creates an overjet.

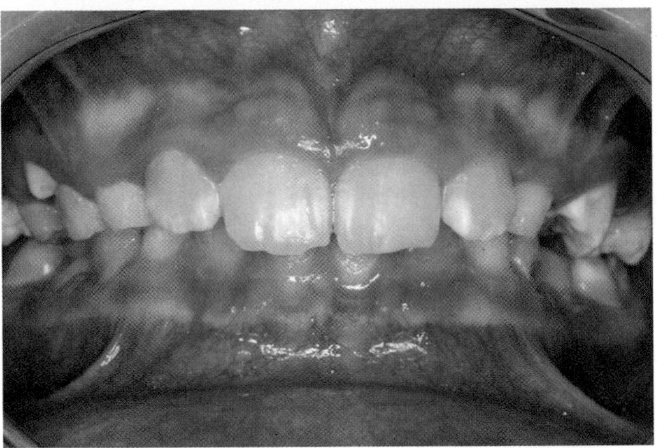

**FIG. 60.4** Complete coverage of the lower anterior teeth is caused by an overbite. *(From Freedman G: Contemporary esthetic dentistry, St Louis, 2012, Mosby.)*

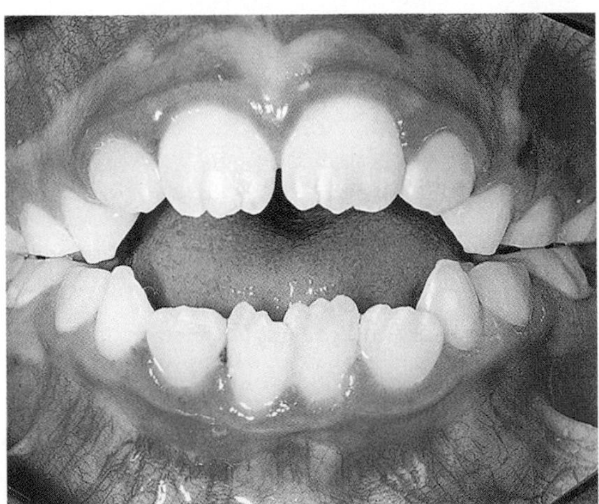

**FIG. 60.5** An open bite is created when the patient's anterior teeth make an opening.

RECALL

3 What term is used for abnormal occlusion?
4 What tooth is used to determine a person's occlusion?
5 If a tooth is not properly lined up with its opposing tooth, it is said to be in ________.
6 If a person occludes and you cannot see the mandibular anterior teeth, what is the patient's malalignment?

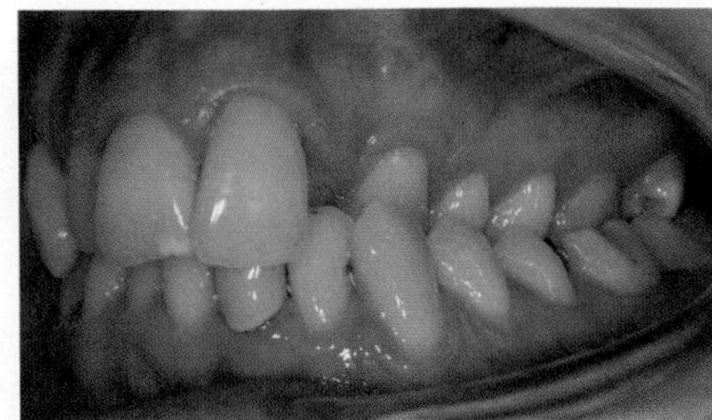

**FIG. 60.6** An example of a cross-bite showing improper alignment of the maxillary and mandibular teeth. *(From Cobourne MT, DiBiase AT: Handbook of orthodontics, ed 2, Oxford, 2016, Elsevier.)*

# Management of Orthodontic Problems

Pediatric and general practitioners are trained in the recognition and treatment of preventive and interceptive orthodontic cases (see Chapter 57 for information on preventive and interceptive care). More extensive cases, however, are referred to the orthodontist for diagnosis and treatment.

## Corrective Orthodontics

The scope of corrective orthodontics includes conditions that require the movement of teeth and the correction of malrelationships and malformations. Adjustments between and among teeth and facial bones are made through the application of fixed appliances with force and sometimes through stimulation and redirection of functional forces within the dentofacial structure. Responsibilities of personnel in the orthodontic practice include treatment of all forms of malocclusion of the teeth and surrounding structures.

Corrective orthodontics includes the following:

- Fixed appliances (e.g., cemented or bonded in place; cannot be removed by the patient)
- Removable appliances for the correction or maintenance of orthodontic treatment
- Orthognathic surgery when the orthodontic problem is too severe to be corrected by other means

# Orthodontic Records and Treatment Planning

The first step in determining a treatment plan is for the orthodontist to learn as much about the orthodontic condition as possible. The patient's first orthodontic appointment is devoted to obtaining records. These records are needed for the orthodontist to make a diagnosis and develop a treatment plan.

## Medical and Dental History

Careful medical and dental histories are necessary to obtain a comprehensive understanding of the physical condition and to evaluate specific orthodontic concerns.

Patient Name: Date:

**Are you interested in: (Please indicate all that apply)**
[ ] Information
[ ] Treatment at this time
[ ] Clarification of previously received or conflicting information

**If your child's teeth were to be changed, how would you like them changed?**
[ ] Upper teeth Forward/Backward
[ ] Lower teeth Forward/Backward
[ ] Upper teeth up because gums show too much
[ ] Close spaces Upper/Lower
[ ] Straighten crowded teeth Upper/Lower
[ ] Improve the appearance of chipped/cracked/stained/dark/pointed teeth

**Do you realize that growth has a strong influence on the success of orthodontic treatment?**
Yes _____ No _____

**Is it likely that your son or daughter will be an early maturer or late maturer?**
Early _____ Late _____

**How tall do you think this child will be when growth is completed?** ___ ft ___ inches

**Are you aware that orthodontic treatment can to some extent alter facial appearance?**
Yes _____ No _____

**If any features of the face could be changed, what would you like to see:**
[ ] Upper lip Forward/Backward
[ ] Lower lip Forward/Backward
[ ] Upper jaw Forward/Backward
[ ] Lower jaw Forward/Backward
[ ] Chin Larger/Smaller
[ ] Nose Larger/Smaller/Different Shape

**Would you prefer that facial appearance NOT be discussed in front of your child?**
Yes _____ No _____

**Is there any significant family history of jaw or teeth problems?**

**Are you interested in improving the appearance of the teeth at this time even if more treatment will be needed later?** Yes _____ No _____

Signature Relationship to Patient

**FIG. 60.7** An example of a form used to acquire information about the perception of a person's teeth. *(From Proffit WR, Fields HW, Sarver DM: Contemporary orthodontics, ed 5, St Louis, 2013, Mosby.)*

## Physical Growth Evaluation

Because orthodontic treatment in children is closely related to growth stages, it is necessary to evaluate the child's physical growth status. Questions are asked about how rapidly the child has grown recently and about signs of sexual maturation.

## Social and Behavioral Evaluation

Motivation for seeking treatment is very important. What does the patient expect as a result of treatment? How cooperative or uncooperative is the patient likely to be? A major motivation for orthodontic treatment of children is the parent's desire for treatment; however, it is essential that the child is willing and cooperative. Normally, children accept orthodontic treatment in a positive way (Fig. 60.7).

Adults tend to seek orthodontic treatment for themselves for other reasons, including the need to improve personal appearance or function of the teeth. It is important to explore the reasons an adult patient seeks treatment.

## Clinical Examination

The purpose of the orthodontic clinical examination is to document, measure, and evaluate the facial aspects, the occlusal relationship, and the functional characteristics of the jaws. At the initial (records) visit, the orthodontist decides which diagnostic evaluations are required for the patient.

### Evaluation of Oral Health

A thorough hard and soft tissue examination, oral hygiene assessment, and prophylaxis must be completed before orthodontic treatment can begin. Charting of periodontal pockets must be noted. If necessary, the patient is to be referred for treatment and follow-up procedures before orthodontic treatment is started.

### Evaluation of Jaw and Occlusal Function

The orthodontist will examine the patient's occlusion and the TMJ to evaluate its function. Lateral or anterior shifts of the mandible on closure are of special interest for orthodontic purposes.

## Diagnostic Records

Before the clinical evaluation can be completed, diagnostic records are required in the form of photographs, radiographs, and diagnostic casts. When possible, it is best to have these available at the time of the intraoral examination. Diagnostic records document features such as tooth angulation, dental crowding, and the presence of unerupted teeth.

### Photographs

Photographs capture the color, shape, texture, and characteristics of intraoral and extraoral structures. Photography is also useful as an aid in patient identification, treatment planning, case presentation, case documentation, and patient education.

Two standard extraoral photographs are taken as follows (Fig. 60.8):

- The frontal view, with the lips in a relaxed position
- A profile view of the patient's right side, with the lips in a relaxed position

Three standard intraoral photographs are also routinely taken (Fig. 60.9):

- The full direct view, which includes all teeth in occlusion
- The maxillary occlusal view, which includes the palate and all maxillary occlusal surfaces
- The right buccal view, which includes the distal of the canine to the distal of the last molar view

When intraoral photographs are taken, it is important that the cheeks and lips are retracted sufficiently to show all structures.

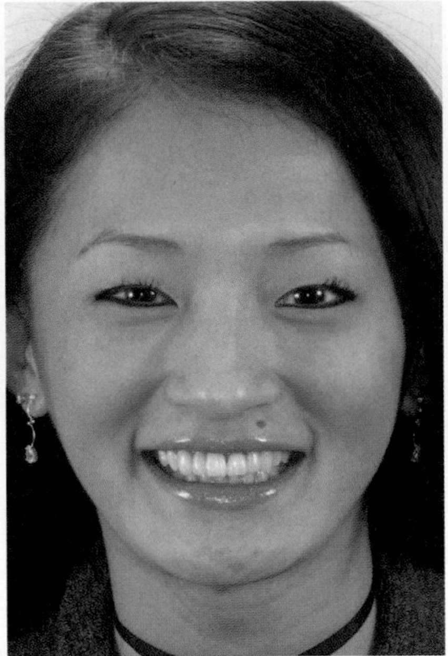

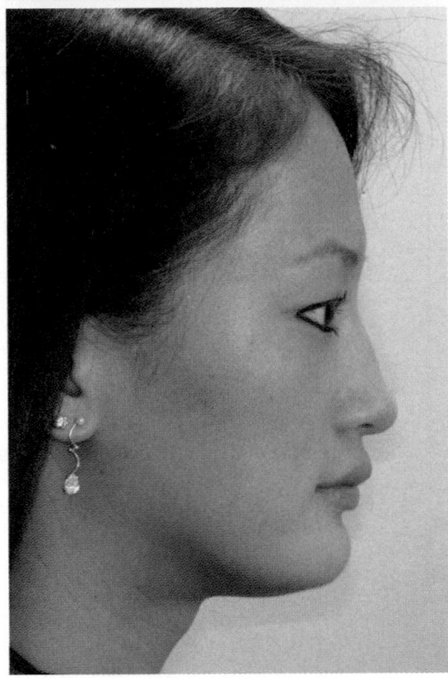

**FIG. 60.8** Standard extraoral photographs. *(From Graber LW, Vanarsdall RL, Vig KWL: Orthodontics: current principles and techniques, ed 5, Philadelphia, 2012, Mosby.)*

### Analysis of Facial Proportions

A reasonable goal for orthodontic treatment is to recognize and improve facial symmetry by correcting disproportion (Fig. 60.10).

In **frontal analysis,** the face is examined for the following:

- Bilateral symmetry
- Size proportion of midline to lateral structures
- Vertical proportionality

In **profile analysis,** the profile relationship is examined for the following reasons:

- To determine whether the jaws are proportionately positioned
- To evaluate lip protrusion (excessive lip protrusion most often is caused by protrusion of the incisors)
- To evaluate the vertical facial proportions and the mandibular plane angle

### Craniofacial Images

The types of radiographic images commonly taken in the orthodontic setting are as follows:

- The panoramic projection is used to view the eruption process of primary and permanent teeth, as well as to

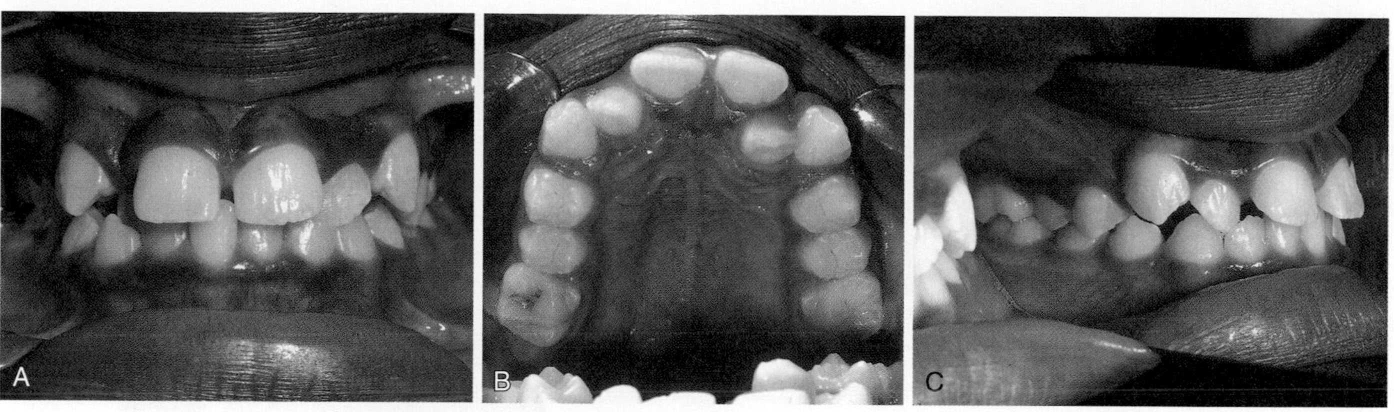


**FIG. 60.9** Intraoral photographs showing a patient's front view in occlusion (A), the maxillary occlusal view (B), and the right buccal view (C).

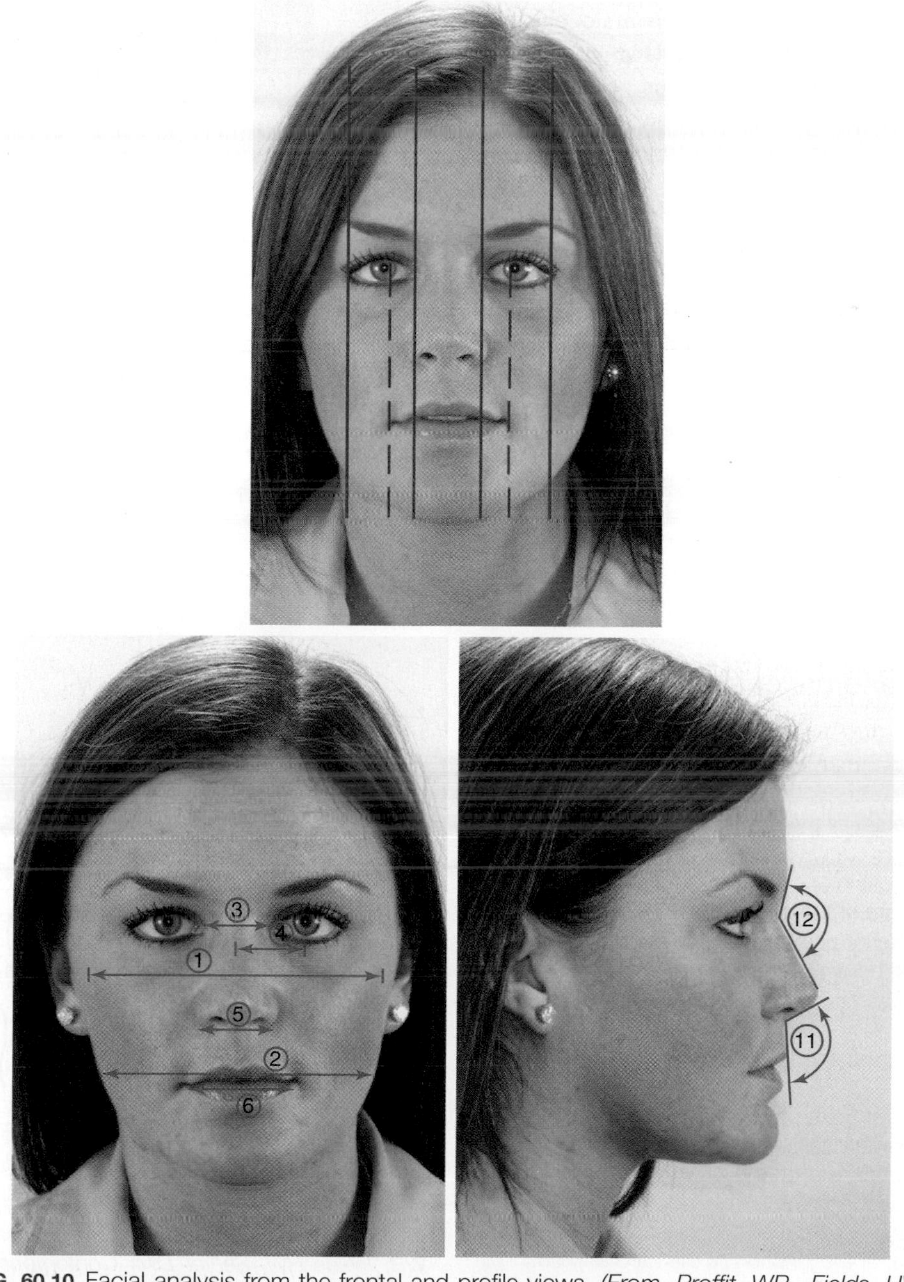


**FIG. 60.10** Facial analysis from the frontal and profile views. *(From Proffit WR, Fields HW, Sarver DM: Contemporary orthodontics, ed 5, St Louis, 2013, Mosby.)*

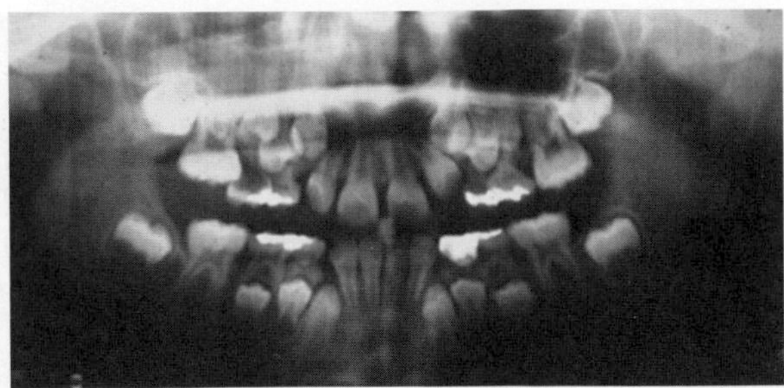

**FIG. 60.11** A panoramic radiograph showing the eruption process. *(From Proffit WR, Fields HW, Sarver DM: Contemporary orthodontics, ed 5, St Louis, 2013, Mosby.)*

evaluate the amount of space available for the eruption process (Fig. 60.11).

- The **cephalometric projection** is an extraoral radiograph to evaluate the anatomical bases for malocclusion, as well as skull, bones, and soft tissue (Fig. 60.12, *A*). Serial cephalometric radiographs taken at intervals before, during, and after treatment can be superimposed for study of changes in jaw and tooth positions. (See Chapter 42 for techniques for exposing panoramic and cephalometric radiographs.)

## Cephalometric Analysis

Cephalometric analysis is not completed on the radiograph but instead is performed as a tracing or a computerized drawing that emphasizes relationships among selected points. Specific landmarks are represented as a series of points, making it possible for the orthodontist to compute mathematical descriptions and measurements of the status of the skull (Fig. 60.12, *B* and *C*). From these measurements, the orthodontist can analyze growth patterns in the planning of the type of treatment to be provided for the patient.

### Cephalometric Landmarks and Points

- **Anterior nasal spine (ANS):** the median bony process of the maxilla at the lower margin of the anterior nasal opening
- **Gnathion (Gn):** the center of the inferior contour of the chin
- **Gonion (Go):** the center of the inferior contour of the mandibular angle
- **Menton (Me):** the most inferior point on the mandibular symphysis (the bottom of the chin)
- **Nasion (Na):** the anterior point of the intersection between the nasal and frontal bones
- **Orbitale (Or):** the lowest point on the inferior margin of the orbit
- **Pogonion (Pog):** the most anterior point on the contour of the chin
- **Point A:** the innermost point on the contour of the premaxilla between the anterior nasal spine and the incisor
- **Point B:** the innermost point on the contour of the mandible between the incisor and the bony chin
- **Posterior nasal spine (PNS):** the tip of the posterior spine of the palatine bone, at the junction of the hard and soft palates

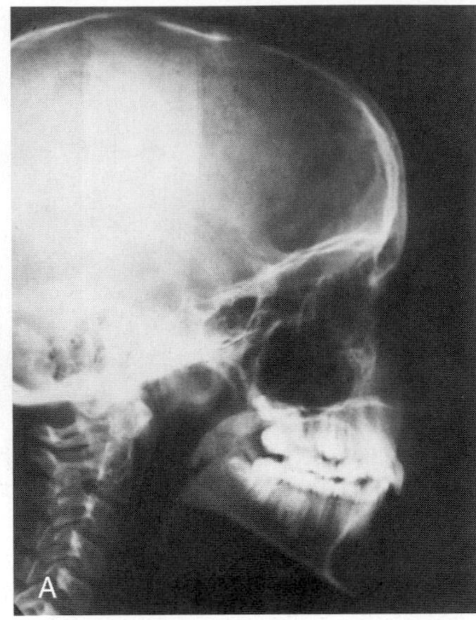


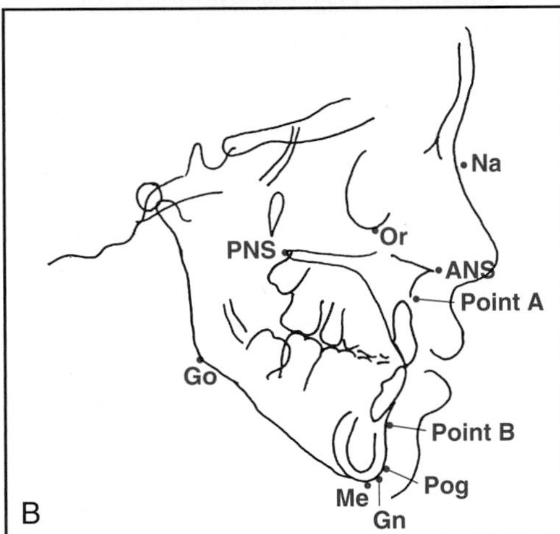


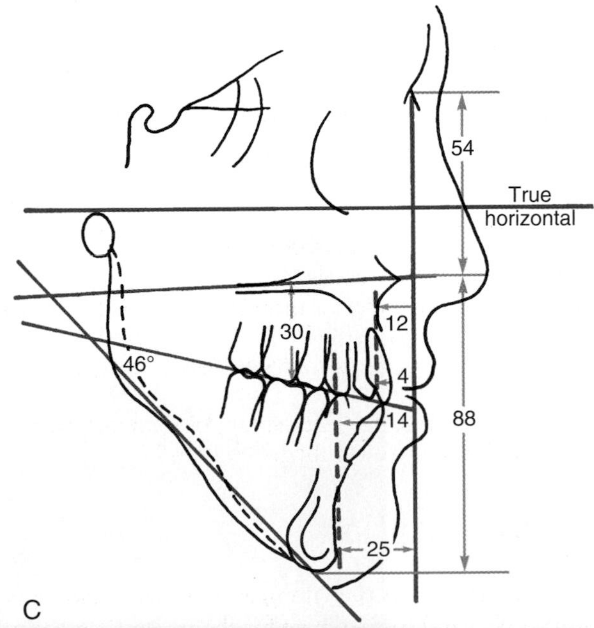


**FIG. 60.12** A, Cephalometric radiograph. B, Cephalometric landmarks and points. C, Cephalometric analysis. *(C, From Proffit WR, Fields HW, Sarver DM: Contemporary orthodontics, ed 5, St Louis, 2013, Mosby.)*

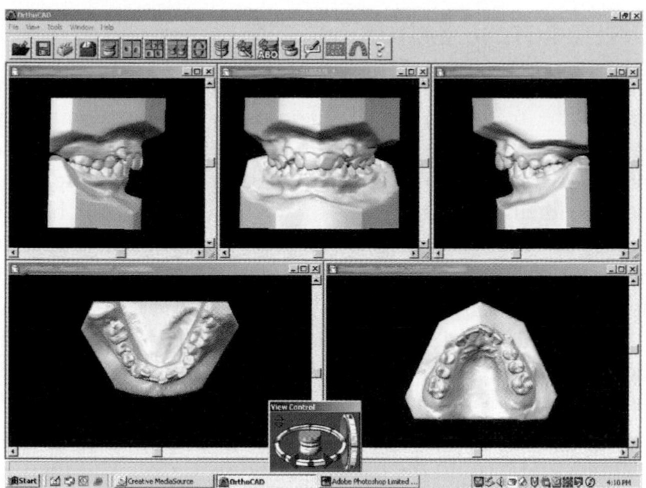

**FIG. 60.13** Diagnostic cast that has been digitally produced from a laser scan of the cast and displayed for space analysis. *(From Proffit WR, Fields HW, Sarver DM: Contemporary orthodontics, ed 5, St Louis, 2013, Mosby.)*

### Computed Tomography

Computed tomography can provide state-of-the-art images for comprehensive orthodontic treatment with minimal increase in radiation dose. Specific information the orthodontist can gain from this technology includes accurate measurements, localization of impacted teeth, asymmetry, periodontal structures, placement sites for anchorage devices, and views of the condylar joint and TMJ. See Chapter 42 for complete description.

### Diagnostic Casts

Diagnostic casts are used for the diagnosis and case presentation of the orthodontic patient, as well as for space analysis of the dentition (Fig. 60.13). The orthodontic diagnostic cast is commonly made from plaster and is constructed in a precise and finished manner. Chapter 47 provides detailed instructions regarding the taking of preliminary impressions and the fabrication of diagnostic casts.

RECALL

7 What two positions does the orthodontist evaluate for facial symmetry?
8 What type of radiograph is used to review the anatomical base for malocclusion?
9 How many photographs are taken during the records appointment?
10 What gypsum material is commonly used for fabricating diagnostic casts in the orthodontic office?

## Case Presentation

The orthodontist reviews the information gathered and develops a treatment plan and cost estimate for the patient in preparation for the case presentation. Approximately 1 hour is reserved for the case presentation visit. If the patient is younger than 18 years of age, the parent or guardian should also be present. At this visit, the orthodontist will use the photographs, radiographs, cephalometric tracing, diagnostic models, and other aids to present the diagnosis and treatment plan. This presentation includes the approximate length of treatment and a clear statement of the responsibility of the patient in helping to ensure successful completion.

Once treatment has been accepted, the adult or the legal guardian signs a consent form. This consent form clearly states the information delineated during the case presentation.

## Financial Arrangements

In addition to the case presentation and the consent form, a formal contract for payment of the treatment fee is presented and is discussed with the individual responsible for the finances. The most frequently used payment plan involves divided payments. Once the patient and responsible persons agree that treatment should proceed, the person who is legally responsible for the account signs the contract.

Some dental insurance plans cover the cost of orthodontic treatment. When insurance coverage is in place, it is usually the responsibility of the subscriber, not the orthodontic practice, to submit periodic progress claims for reimbursement.

## Specialized Instruments and Accessories

Orthodontics requires the use of highly specialized instruments. The most commonly used types of instruments and pliers are shown in Tables 60.2 and 60.3.

RECALL

11 What instrument is used to seat a molar band?
12 Is the orthodontic scaler used for removing calculus from around the fixed appliance?
13 What is another name for 110 pliers?

## Orthodontic Treatment

**Orthodontic treatment** refers to the use of fixed or removable appliances or a combination of the two types to mechanically move the teeth or jaw.

### Fixed Appliances

Fixed appliances, also referred to as **braces**, are a combination of bands, brackets, arch wires, and auxiliaries that can move a tooth in six directions: mesially, distally, lingually, facially, apically, and occlusally (Fig. 60.14).

#### Sequence of Appointments and Procedures for the Orthodontic Patient

1. Placement of separators
2. Cementation of molar bands
3. Bonding of brackets
4. Insertion of arch wire and tying in with ligature ties or elastomeric ties

### Sequence of Appointments and Procedures for the Orthodontic Patient—cont'd

5. Adjustment checks
6. Removal of appliance
7. Retention of teeth

## Separators

Tight interproximal contacts can make it impossible to properly seat a band; therefore the teeth must be separated before fitting bands. A **separator** is used for this purpose. Although separators are available in many varieties, the principle is the same in each case: A device is placed to force or wedge the teeth apart long enough for initial tooth movement to occur. The separator slightly separates the teeth *before* the time of the appointment during which bands are to be fitted. It is important to instruct the patient to call the office promptly if a separator falls out and to schedule an appointment to have it replaced.

The two main methods of separation used for posterior teeth are steel separating springs and elastomeric separators.

See Procedure 60.1: Placing and Removing Steel Separating Springs (Expanded Function) and Procedure 60.2: Placing and Removing Elastomeric Ring Separators (Expanded Function).

## Orthodontic Bands

Orthodontic **bands** are preformed stainless steel bands fitted around the teeth and cemented into place. Most commonly, bands are placed on the first and second molars. Bands are divided into maxillary and mandibular, and right and left, to compensate for individual tooth anatomy. The occlusal edge of the band is slightly rolled or contoured, whereas the gingival edge is straight and smooth. Buttons, tubes, and cleats also may be attached for the arch wire and for power products (Fig. 60.15).

Bands to be fitted are selected from the manufacturer's tray with sterile cotton pliers. At the chairside, bands can be selected through visual inspection and estimation of the size of the tooth and then they are fitted; or bands may be selected, adapted, and fit onto the patient's diagnostic cast. This method eliminates the lengthy process at chairside, and minor alterations can be accomplished at chairside as necessary.

### Fitting Molar Bands

The maxillary molar band is seated on the tooth by finger pressure from the mesial and distal surfaces. This brings the band down close to the height of the marginal ridges. The band pusher is used on the mesiobuccal and distolingual edges to seat the band into place (Fig. 60.16). Mandibular molar bands are designed to be

**TABLE 60.2 Intraoral Instruments**

**Orthodontic scaler**

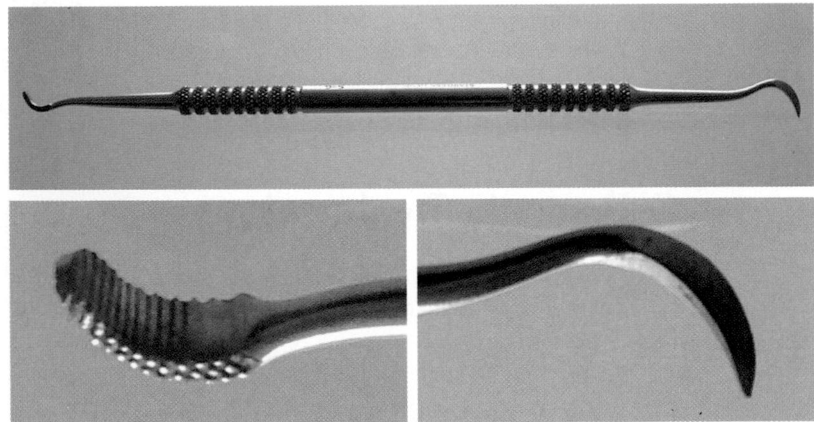

Aids in bracket placement, removal of elastomeric rings, and removal of excess cement or bonding material.

**Ligature director**

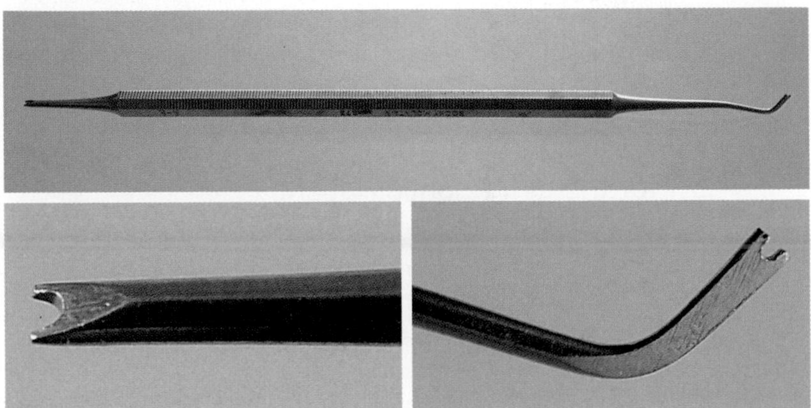

Guides the elastic or wire ligature tie around the bracket. Additionally, the operator can tuck the twisted and cut ligature tie under the arch wire.

**TABLE 60.2** Intraoral Instruments—cont'd

| Instrument | Description |
|---|---|
| **Band plugger**<br>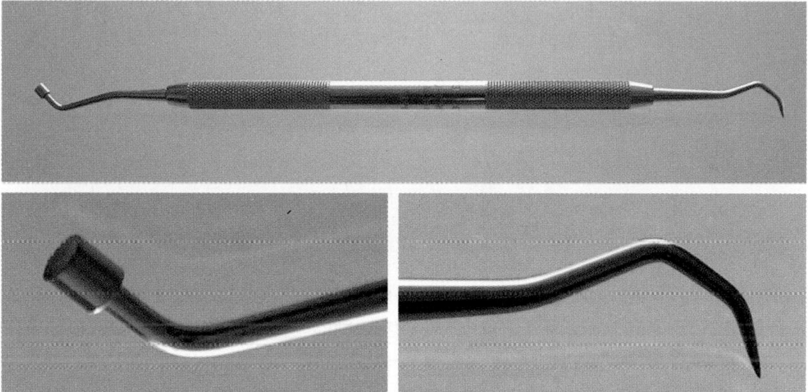 | Round serrated end helps seat a molar band for a fixed appliance. |
| **Bite stick**<br>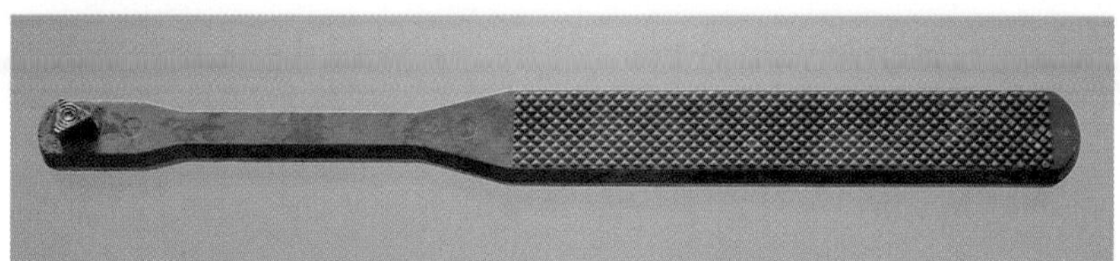<br>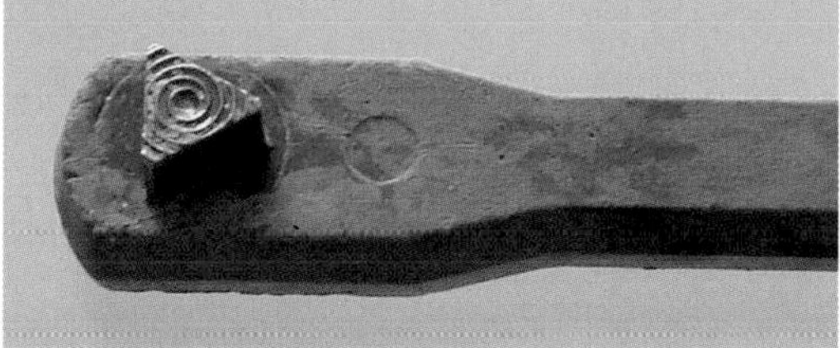 | Consists of a molded plastic handle with a triangular stainless steel serrated working area. This is used to aid in seating a molar band for a fixed appliance. |
| **Bracket placement tweezers**<br>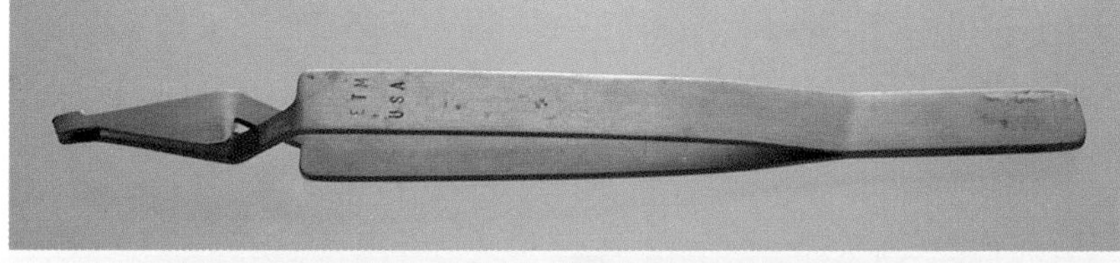 | Long-tip, reverse-action tweezers with fine serrated beaks. They are used to carry and place the bonded bracket onto the tooth. |

Photos from Boyd LRB: Dental instruments: a pocket guide, ed 6, St Louis, 2018, Elsevier.

**TABLE 60.3** Pliers

| Instrument | Description | Instrument | Description |
|---|---|---|---|
| **Bird-beak pliers**<br>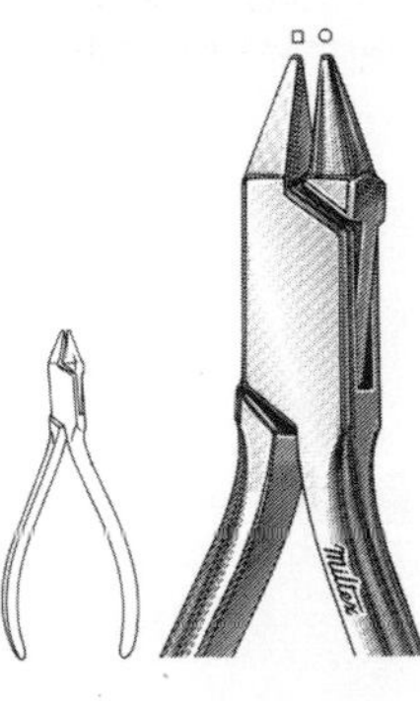 | Useful in forming and bending wires for fixed or removable appliances. | **Contouring pliers**<br>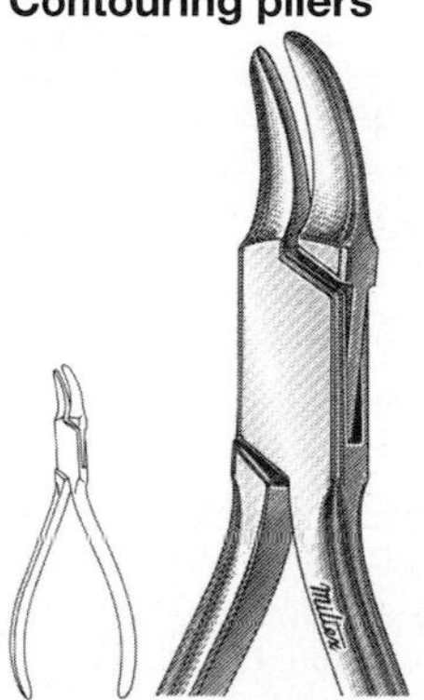 | Aid in fitting bands for fixed or removable appliances. |

*Continued*

**TABLE 60.3** Pliers—cont'd

**Weingart utility pliers**

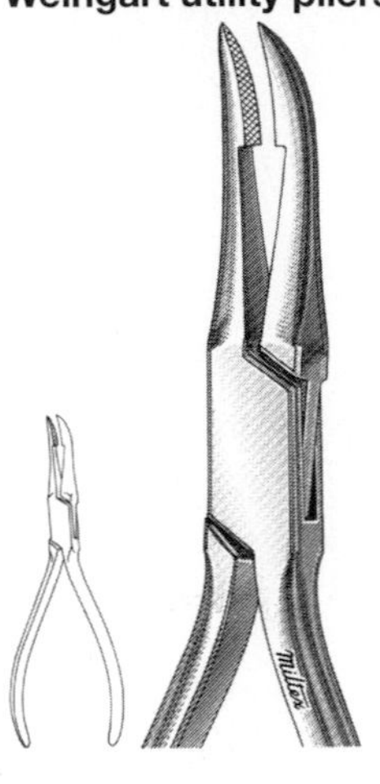
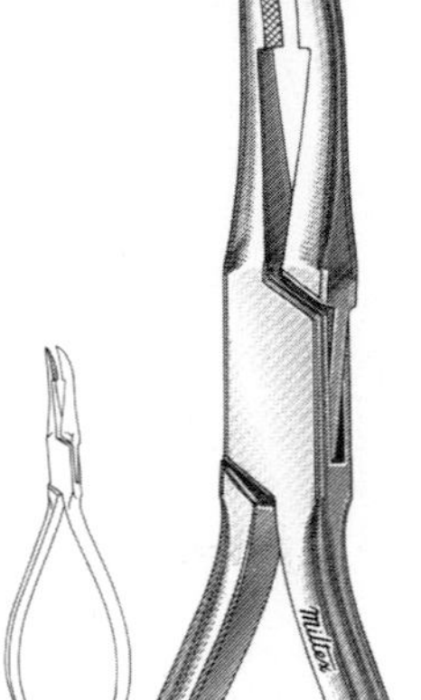

Finely serrated narrow beaks allow accessibility to all areas. They are used in the placement of arch wires.

**Three-pronged pliers**

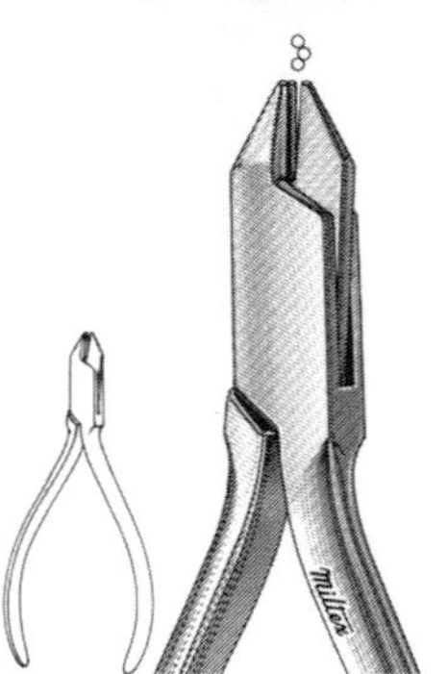

Used primarily in closing and adjusting clasps.

**Posterior band remover pliers**

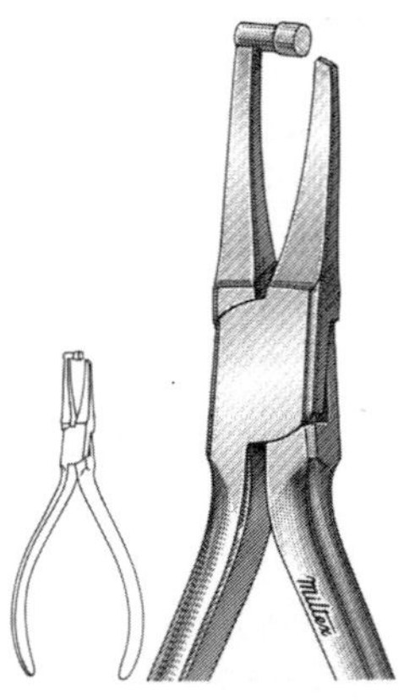

Remove bands without placing stress on the tooth or providing discomfort to the patient.

**Pin-and-ligature cutter**

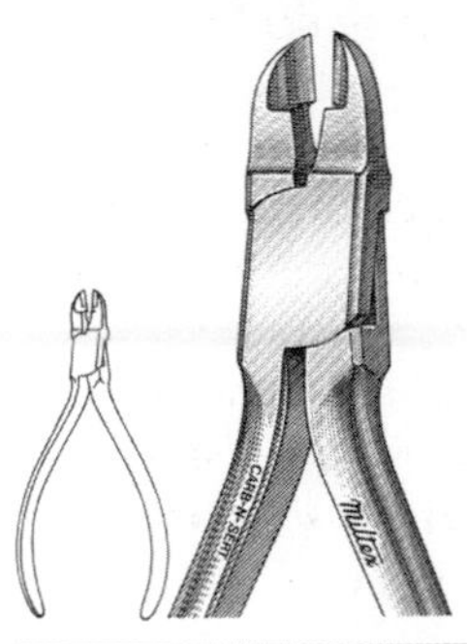

Cuts the ligature wire once it has been ligated around the bracket.

**Howe (110) pliers**

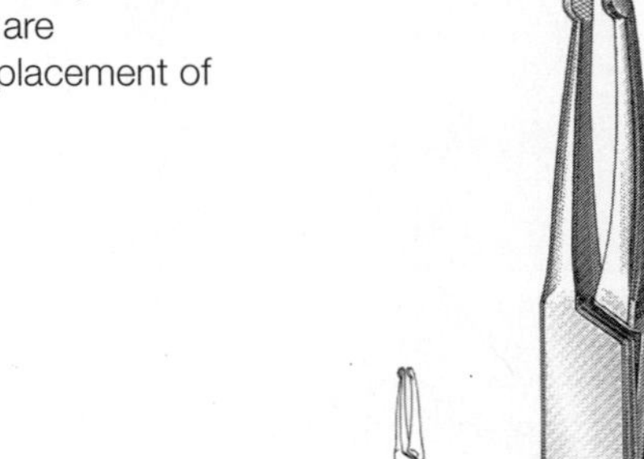

Flat, rounded serrated tip allows placement and removal or creation of adjustment bends in the arch wire.

**Wire-bending pliers**

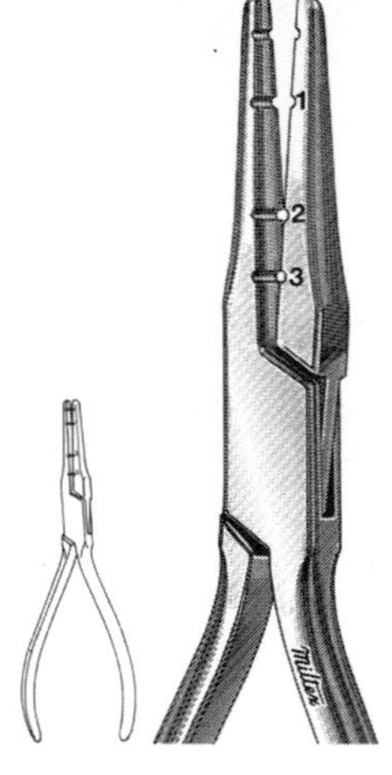


Used for holding and bending and adjusting arch wires to create movement.

**Ligature-tying pliers**

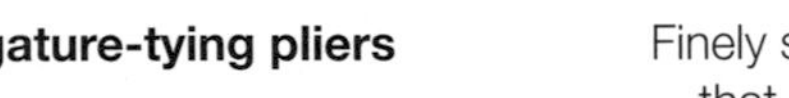
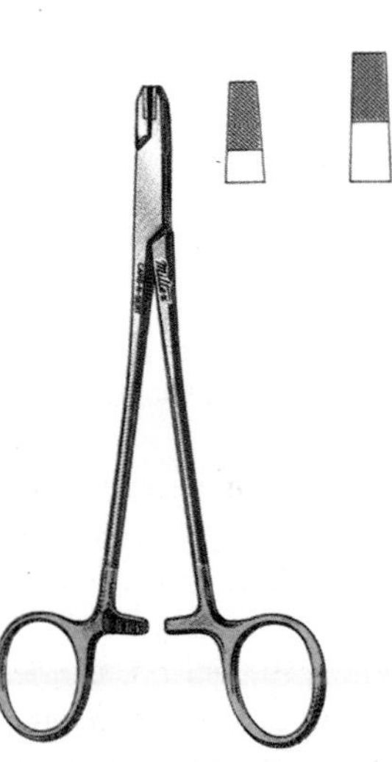

Finely serrated narrow beaks that allow ease in ligature tying.

Permission for illustrations granted by Integra LifeSciences Corporation, Plainsboro, NJ.

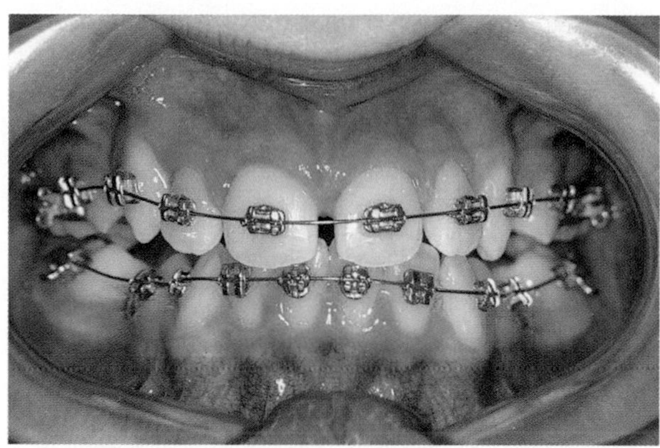

**FIG. 60.14** Full braces. *(From Graber LW, Vanarsdall RL, Vig KWL: Orthodontics: current principles and techniques, ed 5, St Louis, 2011, Mosby.)*

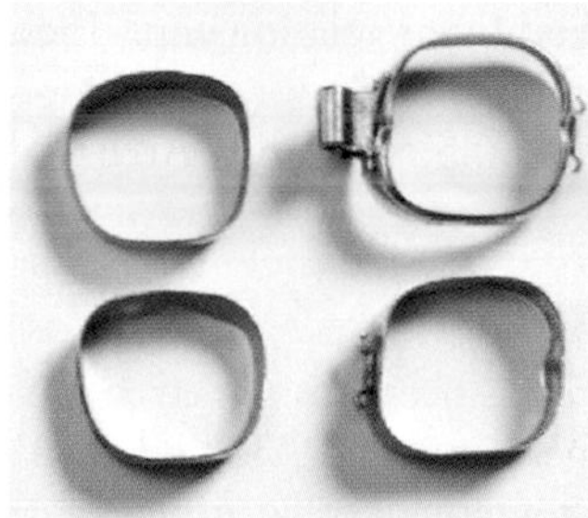

**FIG. 60.15** Molar bands showing the attachments of tubes and cleats to hold the arch wire and head gear. *(From Miller M, Scully C: Mosby's textbook of dental nursing, ed 2, Oxford, 2015, Mosby.)*

seated initially with finger pressure on the proximal surfaces. A band seater is placed along the buccal margins, and the patient's heavy biting force is used to drive the band into place.

### Cementation of Orthodontic Bands

Cementation of orthodontic bands is similar to cementation of a cast restoration; the difference is that the cement adheres exclusively to enamel. Glass ionomer cement is commonly selected because of its strength to aid in retention with enamel, and its timed-release fluoride properties to aid in preventing decay under the band. The cement to be used is determined by the orthodontist. The type selected must be mixed in accordance with the manufacturer's directions.

See Procedure 60.3: Assisting in the Fitting and Cementation of Orthodontic Bands (Expanded Function).

## Bonded Brackets

The bonded **bracket** is the most resourceful component of the fixed appliance (Fig. 60.17). Brackets can be constructed from stainless steel, titanium, ceramic, or a combination of these. Most commonly, brackets are bonded onto the anterior teeth and premolars. The bracket is attached to a backing pad, which is bonded to the enamel of the tooth. The bracket is designed differently depending on the type and use. The edgewise bracket, which consists of four tie wings, allows the arch wire to be placed horizontally through the wings of the bracket and then is **ligated** into place.

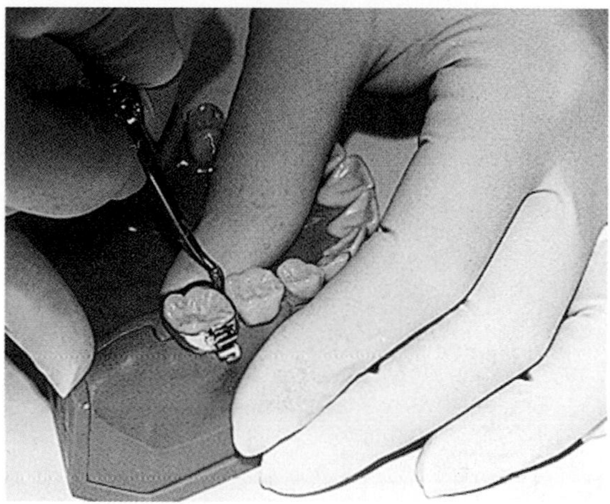

**FIG. 60.16** The band pusher is used to seat the band interproximally.

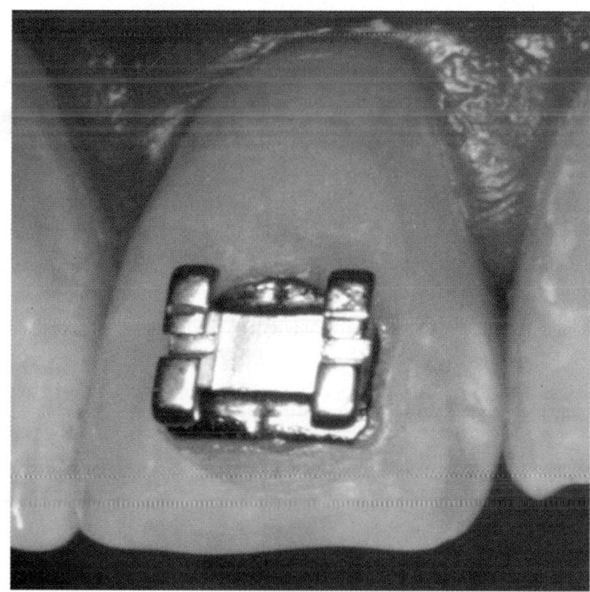

**FIG. 60.17** Example of bonding on tooth #9. *(From Proffit WR, Fields HW, Sarver DM: Contemporary orthodontics, ed 5, St Louis, 2013, Mosby.)*

This stabilization of the arch wire initiates tooth movement by allowing forces from the arch wire to be transmitted to the tooth.

See Procedure 60.4: Assisting in the Direct Bonding of Orthodontic Brackets.

## Auxiliary Attachments

**Auxiliary** attachments are an integral part of the contemporary edgewise appliance. These can be attached to molar bands or to single brackets (Fig. 60.18).

- *Headgear tubes* are round tubes that are placed routinely on maxillary first molar bands. They are used for insertion of the inner bow of a face-bow appliance.
- Edgewise tubes are rectangular tubes that are placed gingival to the plane of the main arch wire. These tubes should be present on the facial surfaces of the upper and lower first molars to receive the arch wire.

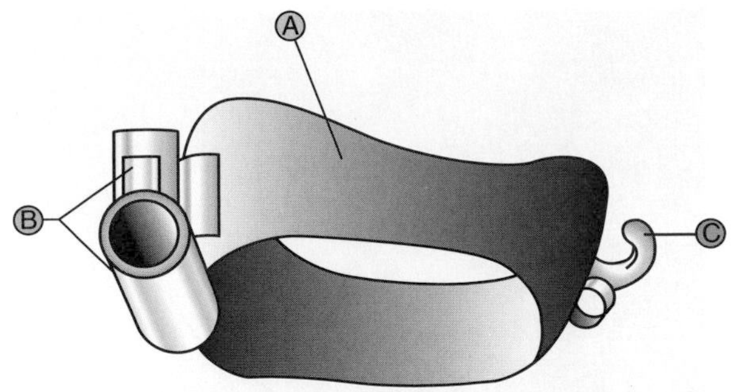


**FIG. 60.18** Auxiliary attachment on a molar band. A, Band. B, Tubing. C, Brackets. *(From Boyd LRB: Dental instruments: a pocket guide, ed 6, St Louis, 2018, Elsevier.)*

- Labial hooks are located on the facial surfaces of the first and second molar bands and brackets for both arches. These hooks hold the interarch elastics.
- A lingual arch attachment is a button or bracket that is located on the lingual portion of the bands to stabilize the arch and to reinforce anchorage and tooth movement.

## Arch Wire

The **arch wire** is an essential component of fixed orthodontics. It serves as the pattern from which the dental arch will take its shape. When the arch wire is placed into the slots of each bracket and then is held in position by a ligature or an elastomeric tie, a force is created that guides the teeth in movement.

Several shapes and materials are used in the design of arch wires. Each type has properties that are unique to a particular application (Fig. 60.19).

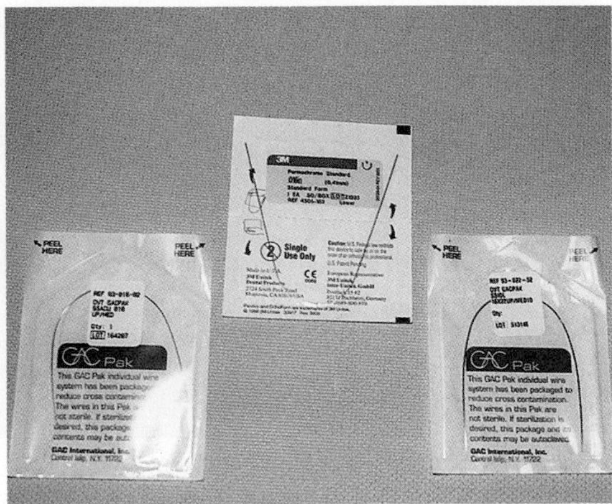


**FIG. 60.19** Type of arch wires packaged.

### Types of Arch Wires

**Nickel titanium,** also referred to as **NiTi,** is very useful for movement because of its flexibility. This type of arch wire is used during the initial stages of tooth movement for malaligned and/or crowded teeth.

**Stainless steel wire** is stiffer and stronger than other types of wire and is used to apply greater force and give better stability to control the teeth. It can withstand greater force and is called the *working arch wire.*

**Beta titanium (TMA)** provides a combination of strength, flexibility, and memory. The orthodontist may choose this type of arch wire when many bands have to be placed.

**Optiflex** is a newer type of arch wire that is made from a composite material with a top coating of optical glass fibers, making it esthetically pleasing. This type of wire is used for light force in the initial stages of alignment.

### Shapes of Arch Wires

**Round wires** are used during initial and intermediate stages of treatment. Their main functions are to correct crowded and crooked teeth and to level the arch. They also can be used for opening a bite and for sliding teeth along to close spaces.

**Square** or **rectangular wires** are used during the final stages of treatment to position the crown and the root in the correct maxillary and mandibular relationship. These wires also give the tooth better stability and apply greater force.

See Procedure 60.5: Placing Arch Wires (Expanded Function).

### Ligating the Arch Wire

Once the arch wire has been positioned in each bracket, it must be ligated to be held in place. Methods used for this include ligature ties or elastomeric ties (Fig. 60.20). Ligature ties are thin wires that are twisted around the bracket to hold the arch wire in place. Elastomeric ties are made from a rubber-like material that is stretched around the bracket to hold the arch wire in place.

**Ligature ties** are 0.01-gauge stainless steel wires that are used to "tie" arch wires in two unique ways. The dentist can indicate each bracket to be tied with a ligature tie or can designate a quadrant or a group of teeth to be tied with one ligature tie, creating a figure-eight to form a chain. With either application, the operator begins from the most posterior tooth and works toward the midline. This makes for a much easier application process and greater uniformity in technique.

**Kobayashi hooks** are ligature ties that have been spot-welded at the tip to form a hook for the attachment of elastics. These hooks are ligated on a bracket as necessary to attach elastics. See Procedure 60.6: Placing and Removing Ligature Ties (Expanded Function) and Procedure 60.7: Placing and Removing Elastomeric Ties (Expanded Function).

## Power Products

Power products are accessory items made of elastic materials that help in tooth movement (Fig. 60.21).

**Elastic chain ties** are continuous "O's" that form a chain. They are used to close space between teeth or to correct rotated teeth.

**Elastics,** commonly referred to as *rubber bands,* are placed from one tooth to another in the same arch, or from one tooth to another in the opposing arch. Elastics help in closing space between teeth and in correcting occlusal relationships. Placement is determined by the orthodontist to create a specific direction of movement.

**Elastic thread** is a type of tubing that is used to close space or aid in the eruption of impacted teeth.

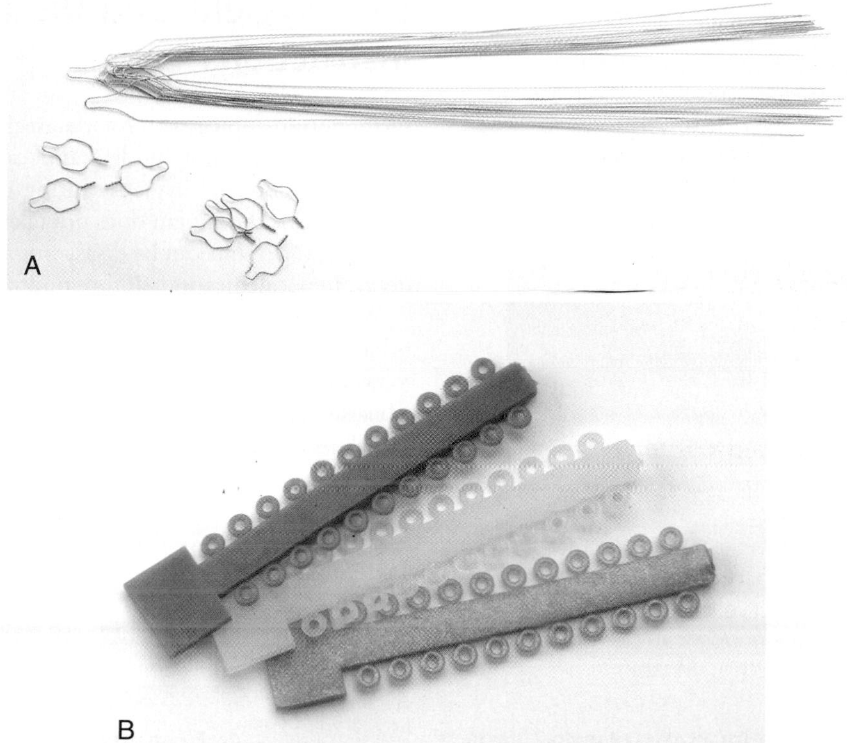


FIG. 60.20 Examples of types of ligature ties. A, Wire ligature tie. B, Elastic ligature tie. *(Courtesy DynaFlex, St Louis, MO.)*

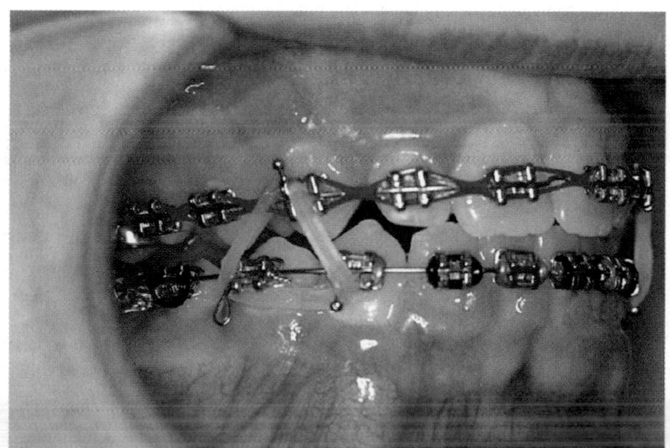

FIG. 60.21 An example of different power products used for movement *(From Proffit WR, Fields HW, Sarver DM: Contemporary orthodontics, ed 5, St Louis, 2013, Mosby.)*

**Comfort tubing** enhances patient comfort by covering an arch wire that may be causing discomfort.

# Clear Aligner Treatment

Recent technology has devised a new way to straighten teeth without the use of fixed appliances.

An orthodontic alignment technique highly profiled today for simple alignment of teeth is the vacuum-formed clear aligner (similar in design and fit to the thermoplastic vacuum–formed tray). The positive aspect of this type of treatment is that it is less visible, and the aligner can be removed during eating and oral hygiene. The Invisalign is a brand of this technology. A series of clear "aligners" is computer generated to gradually guide the teeth into alignment (Fig. 60.22).

## Steps in Preparing the Aligner

- Records, which include the following:
  - Impression taken with a polyvinyl siloxane impression putty material
  - Bite registration
  - Radiographic images
  - Intraoral and extraoral radiographic images
- Records downloaded into the software.
- A digital scan of the impressions using a computed tomography (CT) scanner.
  - From this information a three-dimensional model is created of the upper and lower teeth.
- A technician creates an on-screen animation showing a sequence of tooth movements as proposed in the treatment plan.
- Once approved, a series of upper and lower dental casts are fabricated.
  - Depending on the complexity of the case, there can be from 10 to 30 pairs of casts, representing each stage of treatment.
  - Individual aligners are then prepared for each cast.
- A series of aligners are shipped for the entire course of treatment.
- The customized aligners are worn at 2-week intervals.

### Steps in Preparing the Aligner—cont'd

- The patient's teeth gradually move as a result of the pressure that the aligner creates, until the desired result is achieved. When movement of a tooth or teeth has reached the maximum stage of movement, the next aligner in the series is used to create new movement.

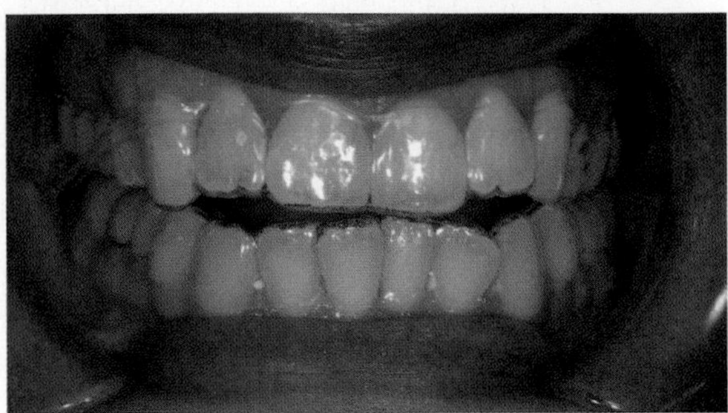

**FIG. 60.22** Invisalign trays for corrective treatment. *(From Graber LW, Vanarsdall RL, Vig KWL: Orthodontics: current principles and techniques, ed 5, St Louis, 2011, Mosby.)*

This type of system is not suitable for all cases of malocclusion, but advancement in this technique includes the use of power products as well as the insertion of mini screws for stabilization.

RECALL

**14** To prepare for the placement of orthodontic bands, what procedure is completed to wedge teeth apart?
**15** When bands are cemented, what can be used to prevent cement from getting into the buccal tubes or attachments?
**16** Are brackets cemented or bonded to a tooth?
**17** Where would most auxiliary attachments be found on braces?
**18** What shape of wire is commonly used for the initial stage of treatment?
**19** In what two ways can you measure an arch wire without placing it in the patient's mouth?
**20** Besides the use of ligature ties, what technique can be used to hold an arch wire in place?

## Adjustment Visits

Throughout active orthodontic treatment, the patient must return regularly for adjustments. At these appointments, the orthodontist reviews the patient's progress and makes adjustments as necessary.

### Checking the Appliance

At each adjustment appointment, it is the responsibility of the chairside assistant to check the patient's appliance to determine whether any of the following exist:

- Broken or missing arch wires
- Loose brackets and bands
- Loose, broken, or missing ligatures
- Loose, broken, or missing elastics

## Oral Hygiene and Dietary Instructions

Orthodontic appliances provide areas for food and plaque to become trapped and hidden and can make brushing more difficult. Good oral hygiene during orthodontic treatment is imperative. If the patient does not take care of his or her mouth properly, the results can be disastrous and may involve rampant decay, hypocalcification, and periodontal disease.

A concern with patients in orthodontic treatment is poor eating habits. The patient should be urged to use good sense in selecting foods and to avoid eating anything that could loosen a band, pop off a bracket, or bend an arch wire. Table 60.4 provides simple dietary guidelines that should be followed during orthodontic treatment.

### Toothbrushing Instructions

- Floss your teeth using a floss threader for easy application.
- Brush your teeth after meals.
- After brushing, rinse and swish water around your mouth to remove any debris.
- Inspect your teeth and braces carefully to make sure they are spotless.

## Headgear

Another aspect of the treatment phase in fixed appliances is the **headgear**. This is an orthopedic device used to control growth and tooth movement. Headgear is composed of two parts: the face bow and the traction device.

### Face Bow

The face bow is used to stabilize or move the maxillary first molar distally and to create more room in the arch. The intraoral part of the face bow fits into the buccal tubes of the maxillary first molars. The outer part of the bow attaches to the traction device.

### Traction Devices

Traction devices apply the extraoral force needed to achieve desired treatment results. Fig. 60.23 illustrates the four types of traction.

RECALL

**21** What additional appliance might the orthodontist use to control growth and tooth movement?
**22** How can hard foods possibly harm braces?
**23** How can a patient make flossing easier with braces?

## Completed Treatment

Once the patient has completed the treatment phase of orthodontics, the bands and bonded attachments are removed. Band removal is accomplished by breaking the seal of cement and lifting the bands off the tooth with the band remover.

**TABLE 60.4 Dietary Habits and Orthodontics**

| Types of Foods to Avoid | Reasons | Examples |
|---|---|---|
| Sugar-containing foods | Weaken cement beneath the bands, causing bands to loosen. Adhere to tooth enamel, causing cavities. | Candy, cookies, cakes, pies, ice cream, soda, sugar-coated cereals, candy apples |
| Sticky foods | Loosen bands, pull out ligature ties, may bend arch wires. | Caramel, caramel corn, taffy, licorice, Gummy Bears, Starbursts, Sugar Daddies, chewy fruit snacks |
| Hard foods | Loosen bands and bend and occasionally break arch wires. | Ice, hard breads, hard-shell tacos, jawbreakers, peanut brittle, chips, frozen candy bars |
| Husk foods | May lodge between bands and beneath arch wires, causing irritation to gum tissues. | Peanuts, popcorn, corn on the cob, meat on the bone |
| Chewing gum | Loosens bands, pulls out the wires, and bends arch wires. | Large pieces of gum |

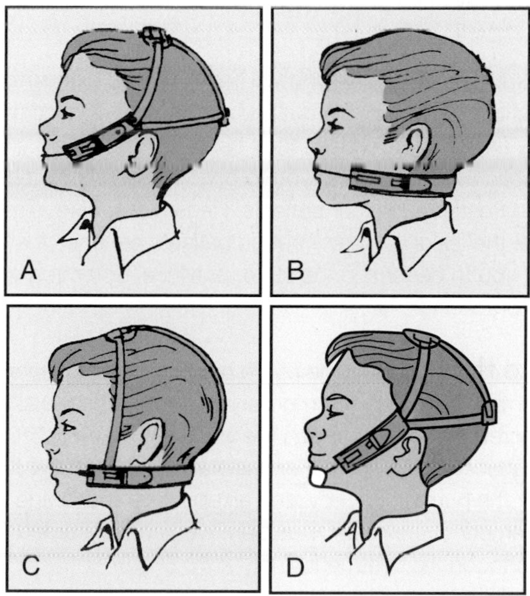


**FIG. 60.23** A, High-pull headgear. The high-pull traction device is a caplike device that fits around the top of the patient's head and hooks perpendicular to the occlusal plane. It can be used in controlling the growth of the maxilla or in retraction of the anterior teeth. B, Cervical traction. The cervical traction device fits around the patient's neck. The exerted force is parallel to the occlusal plane of the patient's teeth. This type of traction is used when the maxillary first molars are stabilized or moved distally. C, Combination headgear. A combination traction device combines the features of high-pull and cervical traction devices. It exerts a force along the occlusal plane and upward. D, Chin cap. The chin cap traction device is a combination of a high-pull strap and a chin cup that fits on the mandible. This helps control growth of the mandible in patients with class III malocclusion.

Bonded brackets are removed by creating a fracture within the resin bonding material. This is done carefully so as not to damage the enamel surface. Any cement or resin material can be removed with a scaling instrument or an ultrasonic scaler.

## Retention

A patient may think that treatment is complete when the fixed appliances are removed, but at that point, an important stage in orthodontic treatment still lies ahead. Orthodontic control of tooth position and occlusal relationships must be withdrawn gradually, not abruptly, if excellent long-term results are to be achieved. Retention is necessary for the following reasons:

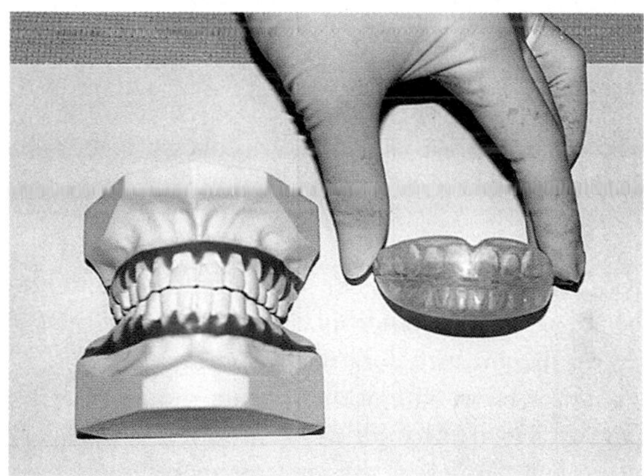

**FIG. 60.24** An orthodontic positioner.

- To allow gingival and periodontal tissues the required time for reorganization
- To support the teeth that are in an unstable position, so pressure of the cheeks and tongue does not cause a relapse
- To control changes caused by growth

### Orthodontic Positioner

The **positioner** is a custom appliance that is made of rubber or pliable acrylic and fits over the patient's dentition after orthodontic treatment (Fig. 60.24). The positioner is designed to accomplish the following:

- Retain the teeth in their desired position
- Permit the alveolus to rebuild support around the teeth before the patient wears a **retainer**
- Massage the gingiva

### Hawley Retainer

The Hawley retainer is a removable retainer worn to passively retain the teeth in their new position after fixed appliances have been removed. The retainer allows some tooth movement to close band spaces and provides control of the incisors (Fig. 60.25). A Hawley retainer is constructed of clear, self-polymerizing acrylic designed to hold wire clasps on molar

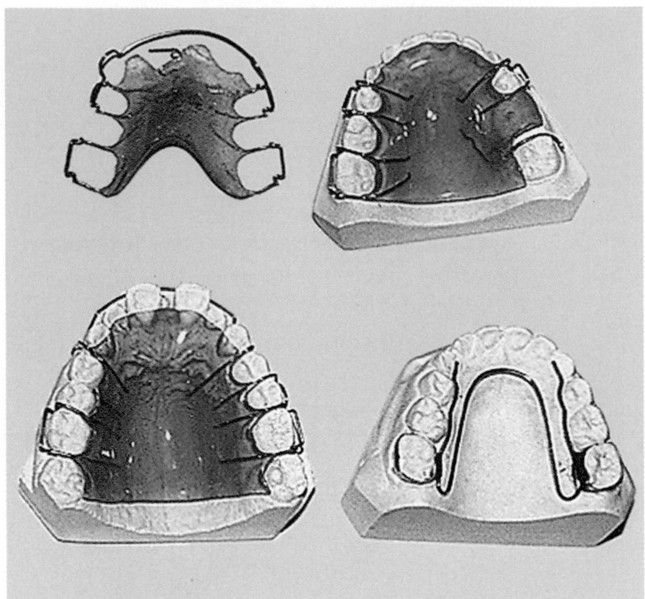

FIG. 60.25 Examples of Hawley retainers.

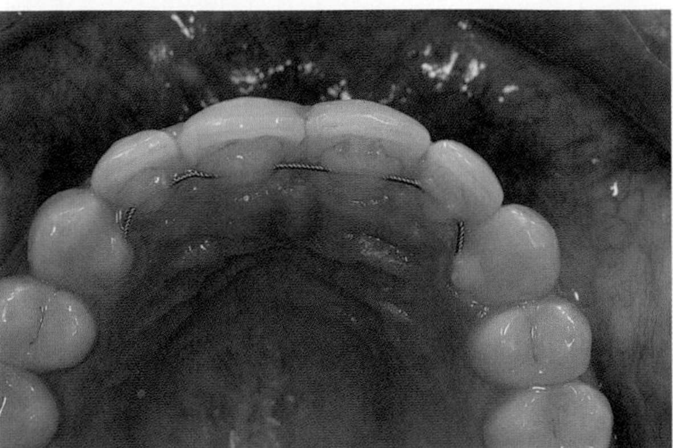

FIG. 60.26 The lingual retainer is bonded into place. *(From Graber LW, Vanarsdall RL, Vig KW: Orthodontics: Current principles and techniques, ed 5, Philadelphia, Mosby, 2012.)*

teeth. On a maxillary retainer, the acrylic portion is placed over the palate. On a mandibular retainer, the acrylic portion is placed on the anterior floor of the mouth.

The anterior facial wire of the retainer should rest lightly on the facial surfaces at the midline of the anterior maxillary teeth and the lingual surface of the anterior mandibular teeth. The wire should fit lightly between the contact areas of the canines and the first premolars.

### *Lingual Retainer*

A fixed lingual canine-to-canine retainer is designed to be bonded to the lingual surfaces (Fig. 60.26). This provides lower incisor position during late growth. The fabrication consists of light steel wiring that is bent so it rests against the flat portion of the lingual surface of the incisors with a long loop over the cingulum of the canines.

RECALL

**24** When a patient's braces come off, does this mean that treatment is over?
**25** Give an example of a retention appliance.

**■ Patient Education** Most individuals who have worn "braces" believe that their orthodontist was the "greatest." Patients seek orthodontic treatment because they want to—not because they are in pain. Because of this attitude, in most cases, you will find that patients are willing participants in their treatment. A problem occurs when a patient is receiving orthodontic treatment as a result of the decision of someone else, such as a parent. When this takes place, your patient probably will not be as compliant in oral hygiene care and diet, and the dental team will have to take on a more enforcing role through the process of treatment. ■

**■ Legal and Ethical Implications** Patients who are receiving orthodontic care may be seen in the office every month for several years. Because you will have such an extensive relationship with your patients, they will become very comfortable with you and with your role in their treatment. Being an orthodontic assistant allows you to become more involved in the care and treatment of your patients. Regardless, *always* make sure that the tasks you carry out on patients are ones that are legal for you to perform in the state, province, or territory in which you are practicing. ■

**■ Eye to the Future** One of the newest developments in orthodontics is the use of temporary anchorage devices ("TADs"). These screws, which are much like implants, measure 3 to 4 mm and are placed in the cortical or skeletal bone. TADs are fixed to bone for the purpose of providing an absolute anchorage point for movement of teeth. TADs are removed and discarded at the end of orthodontic treatment. ■

### ■ Critical Thinking

1. As a certified orthodontic assistant, what expanded functions might you be responsible for during the records appointment?
2. A patient is scheduled to have separators placed. The patient record notes that bands are to be placed on the permanent first and second molars. How many separators will be placed, and where?
3. When you sit down to examine a patient at an adjustment appointment, you note that the patient's buccal mucosa adjacent to tooth #18 is inflamed and irritated. What could be the cause of this? How could this be corrected?
4. Amy is 12 years old and soon will be getting braces. She is very concerned about her appearance once she gets them. How can you help her through this adjustment period? How can braces become more personalized?
5. Sheila is 35 years old and has always been displeased with her appearance because of her crowded teeth. Because of financial reasons, she was unable to get braces as a child, but now she has dental insurance through her job. Because Sheila is an adult patient, what issue(s) would not be a concern in her case (as opposed to the case of a child patient)? ■

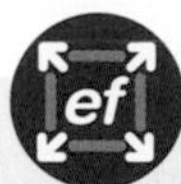

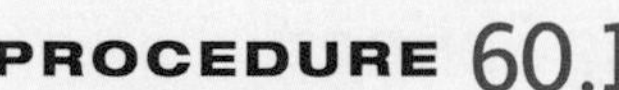


# Placing and Removing Steel Separating Springs (Expanded Function)

## PREREQUISITES FOR PERFORMING THIS PROCEDURE

- ✔ Mirror skills
- ✔ Operator positioning
- ✔ Dental anatomy
- ✔ Instrumentation
- ✔ Fulcrum

## EQUIPMENT AND SUPPLIES

- ✔ Separating springs
- ✔ Bird-beak pliers
- ✔ Orthodontic scaler

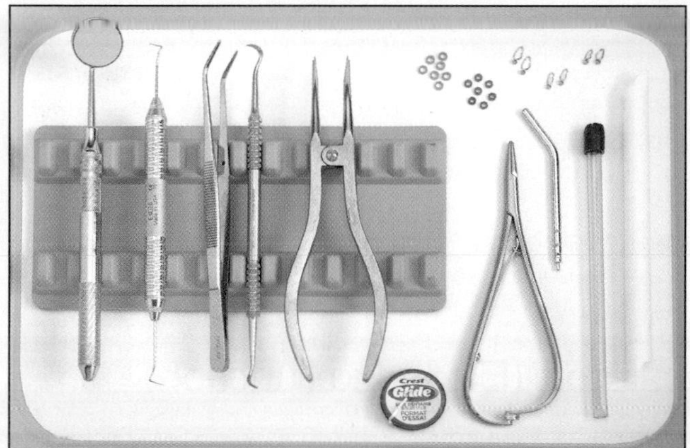


*From Boyd LRB: Dental instruments: a pocket guide, ed 6, St Louis, 2018, Elsevier.*

## PROCEDURAL STEPS

### Placing Steel Separating Springs

1 Grasp the spring with bird-beak pliers at the base of its shorter leg.

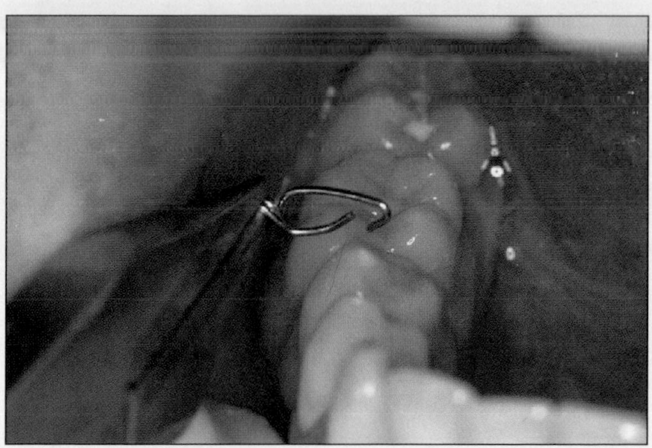

2 Place the bent-over end of the longer leg into the lingual embrasure. Pull the spring open so the shorter leg can slip beneath the contact from lingual to facial.

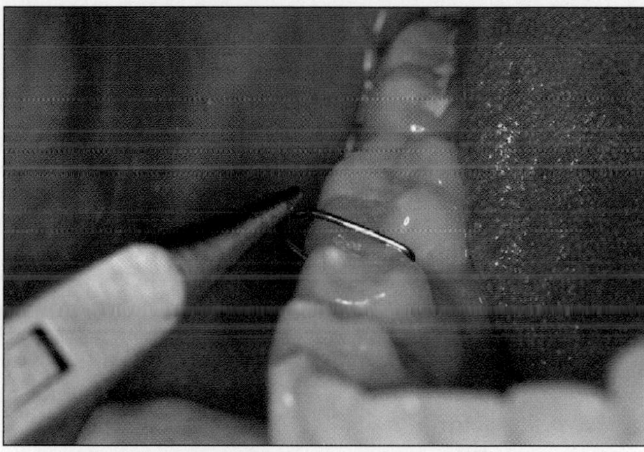

3 Slip the spring into place with the helix to the facial side.

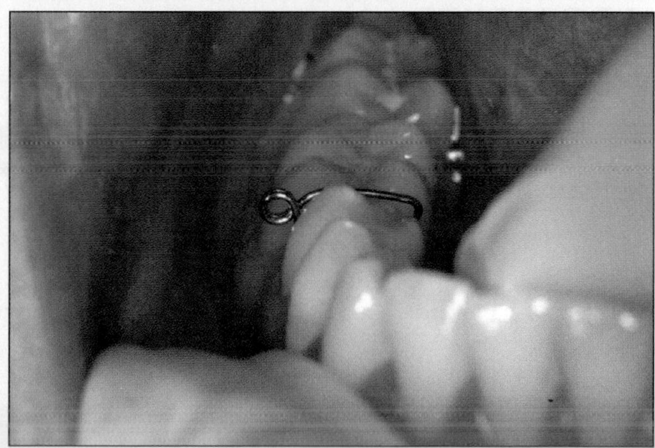

4 This type of separator is normally left in place for 3 to 5 days.

**(Continued)**

## PROCEDURE 60.1 Placing and Removing Steel Separating Springs (Expanded Function)–cont'd

### Removing Steel Separating Springs

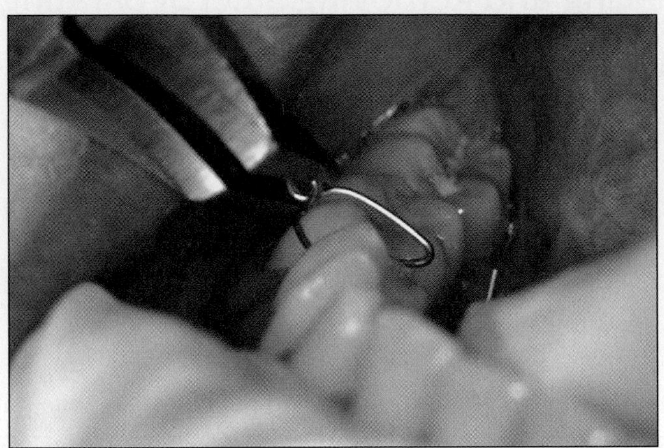

1. During this procedure, keep the fingers of the other hand over the separator to prevent it from coming off the tooth unexpectedly.
2. Use an orthodontic scaler to engage the helix of the separator. Lift upward until space is apparent between the upper arm and the occlusal aspect of the marginal ridge.
3. Support the separator on the helix with the index finger. Disengage the upper arm from the lingual embrasure, and pull the separator toward the facial surface.

## PROCEDURE 60.2

## Placing and Removing Elastomeric Ring Separators (Expanded Function)

### PREREQUISITES FOR PERFORMING THIS PROCEDURE

- ✔ Mirror skills
- ✔ Operator positioning
- ✔ Dental anatomy
- ✔ Instrumentation
- ✔ Fulcrum

### EQUIPMENT AND SUPPLIES

- ✔ Elastomeric separators
- ✔ Separating pliers
- ✔ Floss
- ✔ Orthodontic scaler

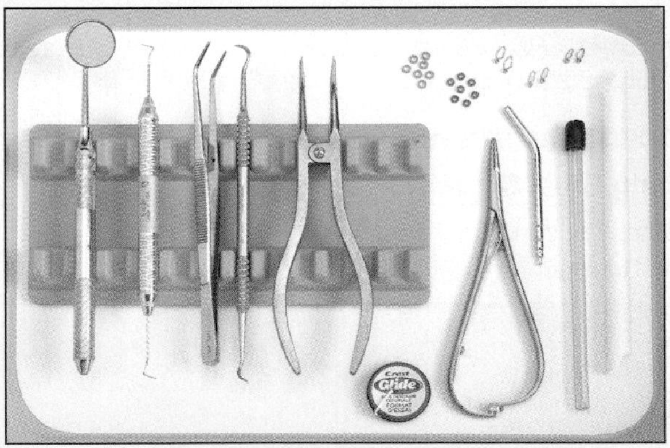

*From Boyd LRB: Dental instruments: a pocket guide, ed 6, St Louis, 2018, Elsevier.*

## PROCEDURE 60.2 Placing and Removing Elastomeric Ring Separators (Expanded Function)—cont'd

### PROCEDURAL STEPS

#### Placing Elastomeric Ring Separators

1 Place the separator over the beaks of the separating pliers.
2 Stretch the ring; then use a see-saw motion to gently force it through the contact.

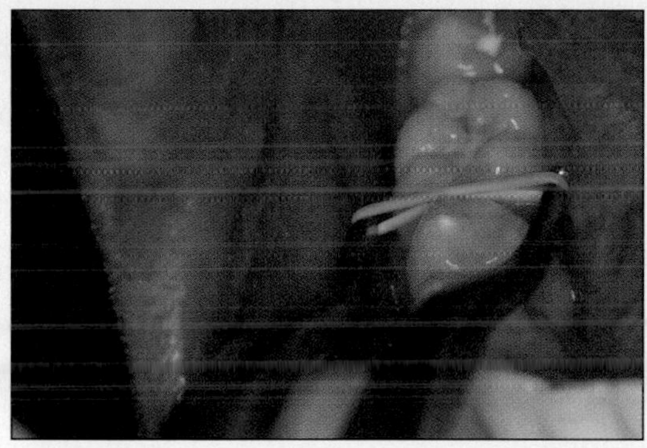

3 An alternative method is to use two loops of dental floss to stretch the ring and guide it into place.

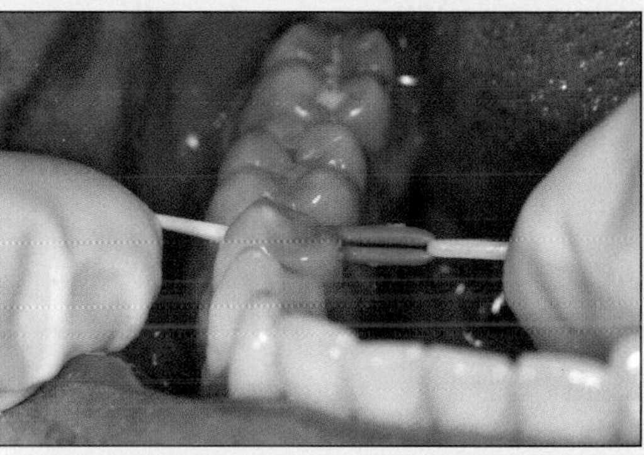

4 This type of separator can be left in place for up to 2 weeks.

#### Removing Elastomeric Ring Separators

1 Slide an orthodontic scaler into the doughnut-shaped separator.
2 Use slight pressure to remove the ring from under the contact.

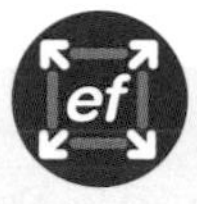

## PROCEDURE 60.3

## Assisting in the Fitting and Cementation of Orthodontic Bands (Expanded Function)

### EQUIPMENT AND SUPPLIES

- ✔ Basic setup
- ✔ Preselected orthodontic bands
- ✔ Chilled glass slab or paper pad
- ✔ Spatula (stainless steel)
- ✔ Gauze sponges
- ✔ Band pusher
- ✔ Band seater
- ✔ Scaler
- ✔ Band remover
- ✔ Contouring pliers
- ✔ Isopropyl alcohol
- ✔ Masking tape
- ✔ Chapstick or utility wax
- ✔ Selected cement

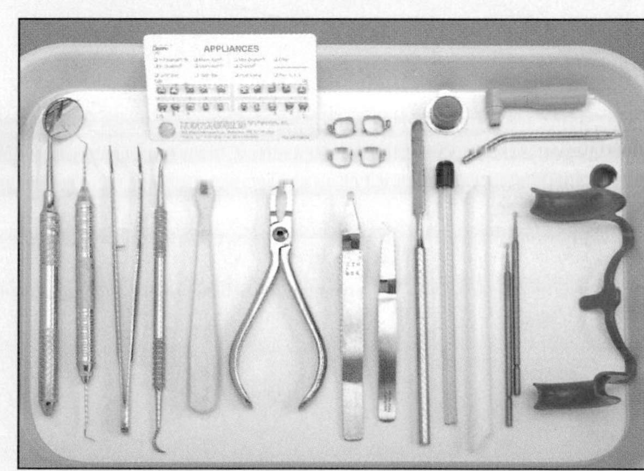


*From Boyd LRB: Dental instruments: a pocket guide, ed 6, St Louis, 2018, Elsevier.*

(Continued)

# PROCEDURE 60.3 Assisting in the Fitting and Cementation of Orthodontic Bands (Expanded Function)–cont'd

## PROCEDURAL STEPS

### Preparation

1 Place each preselected orthodontic band on a small square of masking tape with the occlusal surface on the tape and the gingival margin of the band upright.

**PURPOSE** This keeps the bands in order and prevents the cement from flowing out the other side.

2 Wipe any buccal tubes or attachments with ChapStick or utility wax.

**PURPOSE** This prevents cement from getting into or around these areas.

### Mixing and Placing the Cement

3 The teeth are isolated and dried.

4 At a signal from the orthodontist, dispense the cement according to the manufacturer's directions; then quickly mix the cement until it is homogeneous.

5 Hold the band by the margin of the masking tape. The gingival surface is upright, and the cement spatula is placed on the margin of the band.

6 Wipe the spatula over the margin, allowing the cement to flow into the circumference of the band.

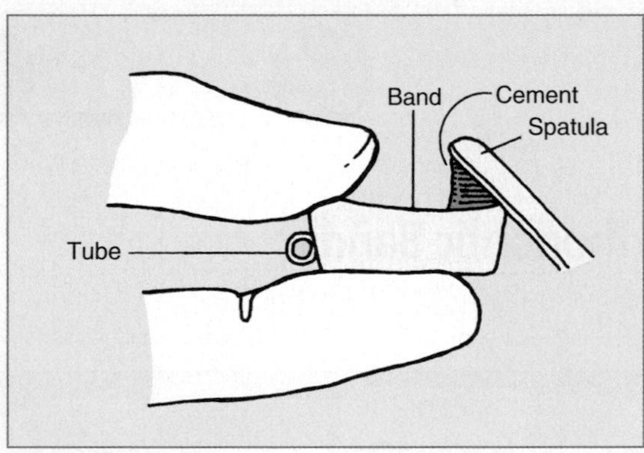


7 Transfer the cement-filled band to the orthodontist, who inverts the band over the tooth.

8 Transfer the band seater. The orthodontist places it on the buccal margin of the band.

9 The patient is instructed to bite gently on the band. This action forces the band down onto approximately the middle third of the tooth crown.

10 Excess cement is forced out from under the gingival and occlusal margins of the bands and is allowed to harden.

11 This process is repeated until all bands have been seated.

### Removing Excess Cement

12 After the cement has reached its final stage of setting, a scaler or explorer is used to remove the excess cement from the enamel surfaces.

13 The patient's mouth is rinsed, flossed, and checked to ensure that all excess cement has been removed.

### Documentation

14 Document the procedure.

| Date | Tooth | Surface | Charting notes |
|---|---|---|---|
| 9/6/17 | | | Upper and lower bands cemented w/glass ionomer on first molars, UR-22, UL-24, LL-21, LR-22. Schedule for bonding. |
| | | | T. Clark, CDA/L. Stewart, DDS |

PROCEDURE 60.4

# Assisting in the Direct Bonding of Orthodontic Brackets

## EQUIPMENT AND SUPPLIES

- ✔ Brackets (type specified by the orthodontist)
- ✔ Cotton rolls or lip retractors
- ✔ Prophy cup
- ✔ Pumice
- ✔ Bonding setup
- ✔ Bracket placement tweezers
- ✔ Orthodontic scaler

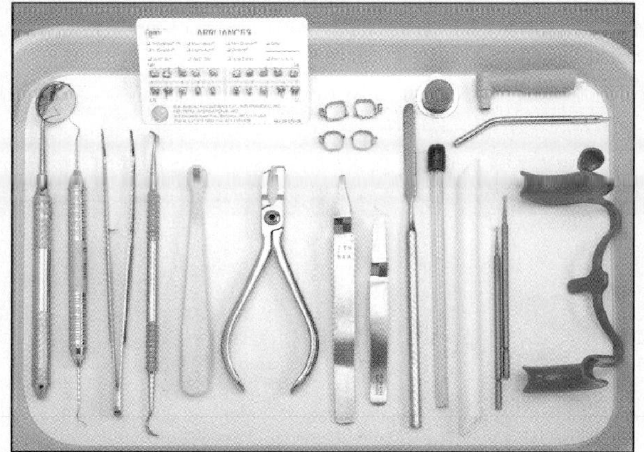

*From Boyd LRB: Dental instruments: a pocket guide, ed 6, St Louis, 2018, Elsevier.*

## PROCEDURAL STEPS

### Preparing the Teeth

1 The tooth surface must be cleaned with prophy cup and pumice slurry and then rinsed and dried.

2 Use cotton rolls or retractors to isolate the teeth.

3 An etchant gel is placed on the facial area of the tooth that is to receive the bonding. This remains on the tooth for the manufacturer's specified time; the tooth then is rinsed and dried thoroughly.

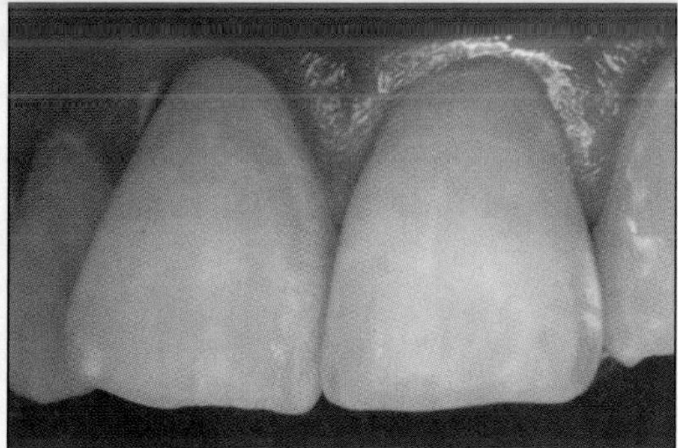

*From Proffit WR, Fields HW, Sarver DM: Contemporary orthodontics, ed 5, St Louis, 2013, Mosby.*

### Bonding the Brackets

4 The orthodontist applies a liquid sealant, usually the monomer of the bonding agent, to the prepared tooth surface.

5 Express a small quantity of bonding material and place it on the back of the bracket. Bracket placement tweezers are used to transfer the bracket to the orthodontist.

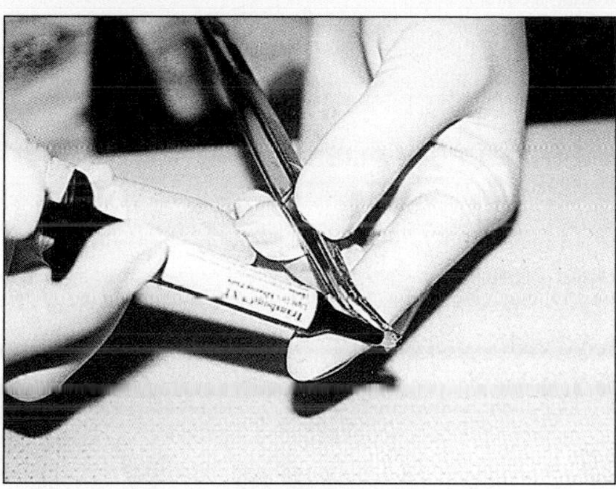

*From Proffit WR, Fields HW, Sarver DM: Contemporary orthodontics, ed 5, St Louis, 2013, Mosby.*

6 Transfer the orthodontic scaler. The orthodontist places the bracket and moves it into final position with a scaler.

7 The orthodontist uses the scaler to immediately remove the excess bonding material before light-curing the material.

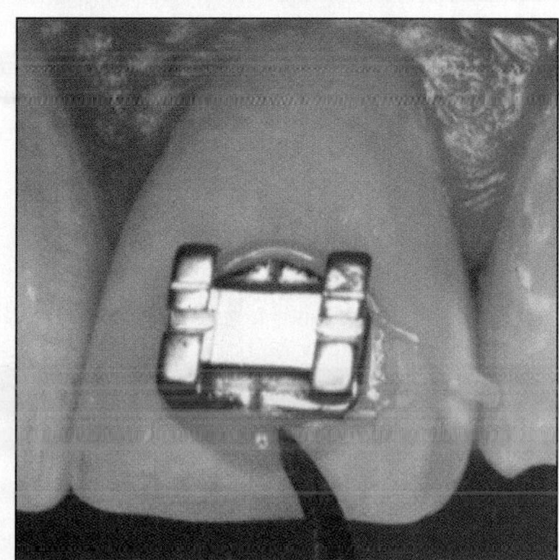

*From Proffit WR, Fields HW, Sarver DM: Contemporary orthodontics, ed 5, St Louis, 2013, Mosby.*

### Documentation

8 Document the procedure.

| Date | Tooth | Surface | Charting notes |
|---|---|---|---|
| 9/7/17 | | | Edgewise brackets bonded on Max. 5–1/1–5 and Mand. 4–1/1–4. Light arch wire placed. |
| | | | T. Clark, CDA/L. Stewart, DDS |

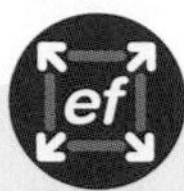

PROCEDURE 60.5

# Placing Arch Wires (Expanded Function)

## PREREQUISITES FOR PERFORMING THIS PROCEDURE

- ✔ Mirror skills
- ✔ Operator positioning
- ✔ Dental anatomy
- ✔ Instrumentation
- ✔ Fulcrum

## EQUIPMENT AND SUPPLIES

- ✔ Preformed arch wires
- ✔ Patient's diagnostic casts (or previously used arch wire)
- ✔ Weingart pliers
- ✔ Bird-beak pliers
- ✔ Torquing pliers
- ✔ Distal end cutter

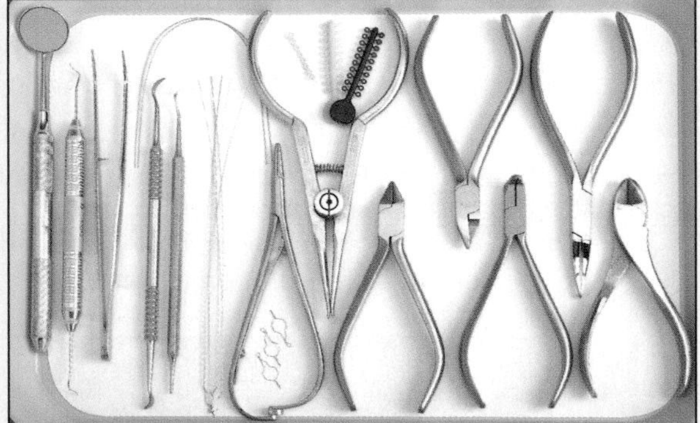

*From Boyd LRB: Dental instruments: a pocket guide, ed 6, St Louis, 2018, Elsevier.*

## PROCEDURAL STEPS

### Measuring the Arch Wire

**1** Preformed wires are measured before they are placed into the mouth. The wire should be long enough to extend past the end of the buccal tube on the molar band but not so long that it injures the patient's tissues.

**2** Measure the wire by trying it on the patient's diagnostic model or by holding it against the arch wire that is being replaced.

**3** If the orthodontist will need to place bends in the wire, additional wire must be allowed for the length.

### Positioning the Arch Wire

**4** Locate the mark at the center of the arch wire.

**PURPOSE** This indicates the midline or the center of the arch form.

**5** Position the wire in the mouth with the mark between the central incisors.

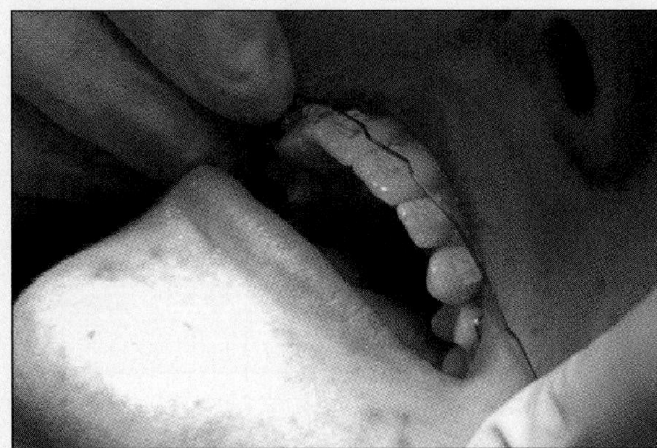

*From Proffit WR, Fields HW, Sarver DM: Contemporary orthodontics, ed 5, St Louis, 2013, Mosby.*

**6** Place the arch wire in the main arch wire slot of the buccal tube.

**7** Use the Weingart pliers to slide the wire in on either side of the arch and to position the wire within the bracket slots.

**8** Check the distal ends to determine whether they are securely positioned or are too long or too short.

**PURPOSE** You need to retrieve the distal end cutters to cut the wire if it is impinging the mucosa.

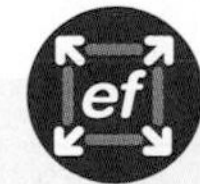

PROCEDURE 60.6 

# Placing and Removing Ligature Ties (Expanded Function)

## PREREQUISITES FOR PERFORMING THIS PROCEDURE

- ✔ Mirror skills
- ✔ Operator positioning
- ✔ Dental anatomy
- ✔ Instrumentation
- ✔ Fulcrum

## EQUIPMENT AND SUPPLIES

- ✔ Ligature ties
- ✔ Ligature director
- ✔ Hemostat
- ✔ Ligature cutter

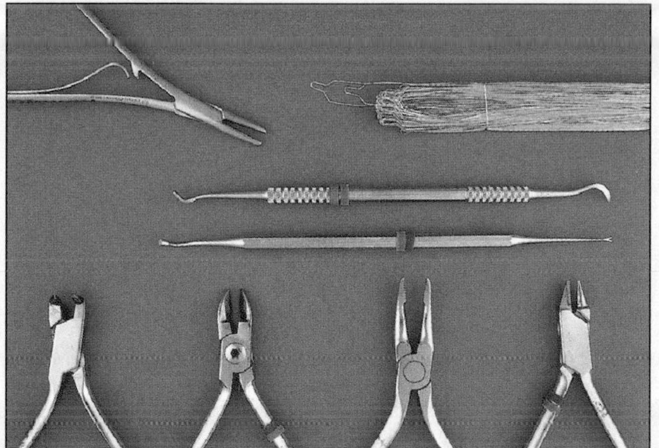

## PROCEDURAL STEPS

### Placing Wire Ligatures

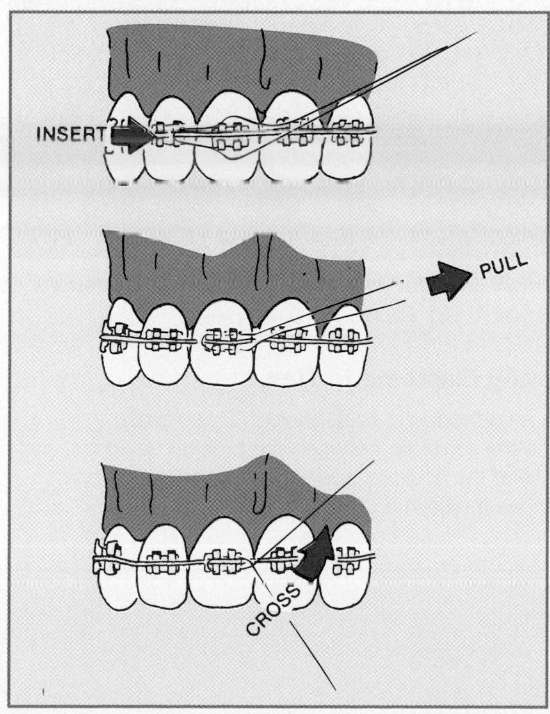


1 While holding the ligature between the thumb and index finger, slide the wire between these fingers so only the section that wraps around the bracket is exposed. Make sure to work toward the midline.

2 Slide the ligature around the bracket, using the ligature director to push the wire against the tie wing.

3 Twist together the ends of the ligature. Place the hemostat about 3 to 5 mm from the bracket, and twist the wire snugly against the bracket.

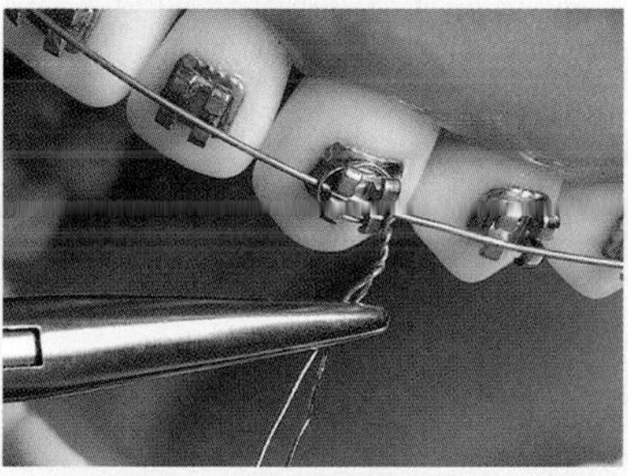

*From Boyd LRB: Dental instruments: a pocket guide, ed 6, St Louis, 2018, Elsevier.*

4 After all teeth have been ligated, use a ligature cutter to remove the excess wire, leaving a 4- to 5-mm pigtail.

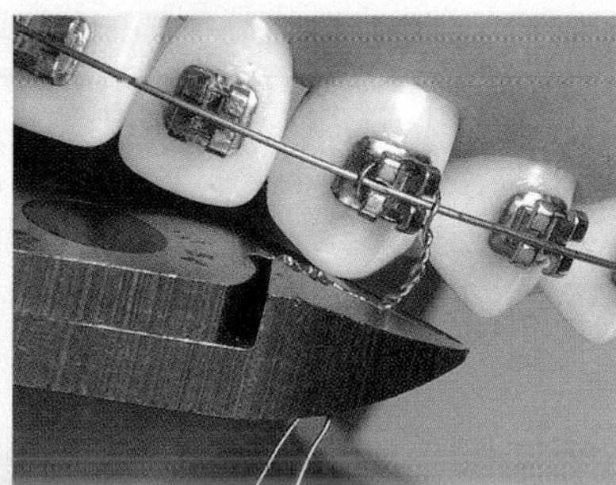

*From Boyd LRB: Dental instruments: a pocket guide, ed 6, St Louis, 2018, Elsevier.*

(Continued)

## PROCEDURE 60.6 Placing and Removing Ligature Ties (Expanded Function)–cont'd

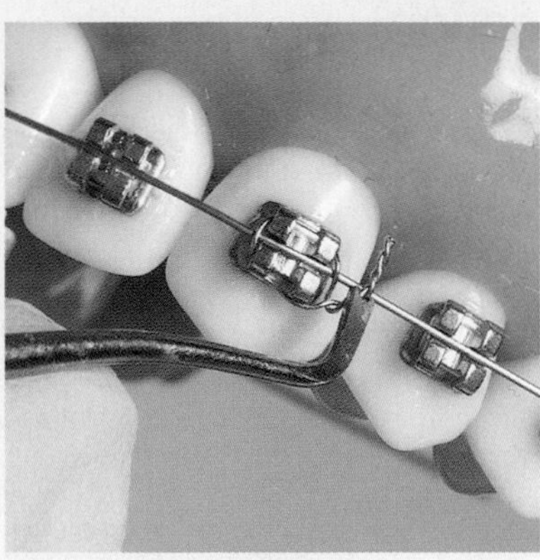

*From Boyd LRB: Dental instruments: a pocket guide, ed 6, St Louis, 2018, Elsevier.*

5 Use the ligature director to tuck the pigtails under the arch wire toward the gingiva at the interproximal space.
6 Repeat this procedure until all ligatures have been cut and tucked away.
7 Run a finger along the arch to make sure that no protruding wires could injure the patient.

### Removing Ligature Ties

1 Using the ligature cutter, place the beaks of the pliers at the end of the twisted wire and snip it off, making sure to hold on to the cut portion.
2 Carefully remove this portion of the wire.
3 Do not twist or pull as you cut and remove the ligatures.

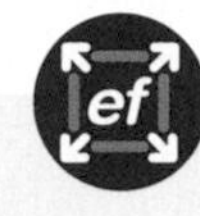

## PROCEDURE 60.7 

# Placing and Removing Elastomeric Ties (Expanded Function)

### PREREQUISITES FOR PERFORMING THIS PROCEDURE

- Mirror skills
- Operator positioning
- Dental anatomy
- Instrumentation
- Fulcrum

### EQUIPMENT AND SUPPLIES

- Elastomeric tie for each bracket
- Hemostat
- Orthodontic scaler

### PROCEDURAL STEPS

### Placing Elastomeric Ties

1 Use a hemostat to place the pliers' beak on a tie; lock the pliers.
2 Do not place the beaks too close to the center of the "O," or it will become impossible to stretch the tie around the bracket.
3 Place the tie on the occlusal portion of one tie wing; then slide the tie under the edge of the bracket.
4 To get the tie started, support it with your finger.
5 Pull the tie up and over the tie wing and then over and down the other tie wing.
6 Release the pliers.

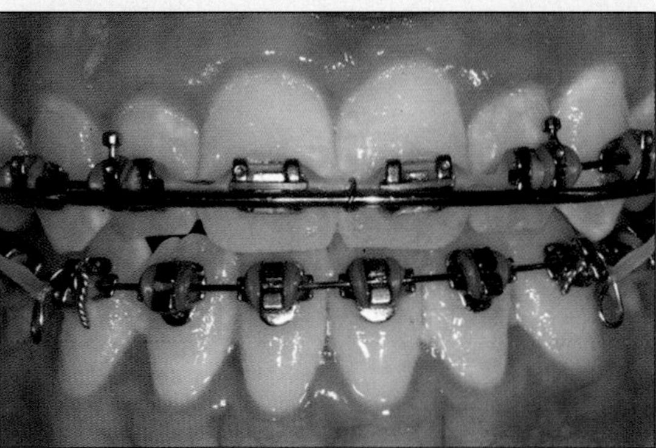

*From Proffit WR, Fields HW, Sarver DM: Contemporary orthodontics, ed 5, St Louis, 2013, Mosby.*

### Removing Elastomeric Ties

1 Use an orthodontic scaler held in a pen grasp.
2 Place the scaler tip between the bracket tie wings, and pull the tie at the occlusal position with a rolling motion.
3 Remove the tie in a gingival direction.

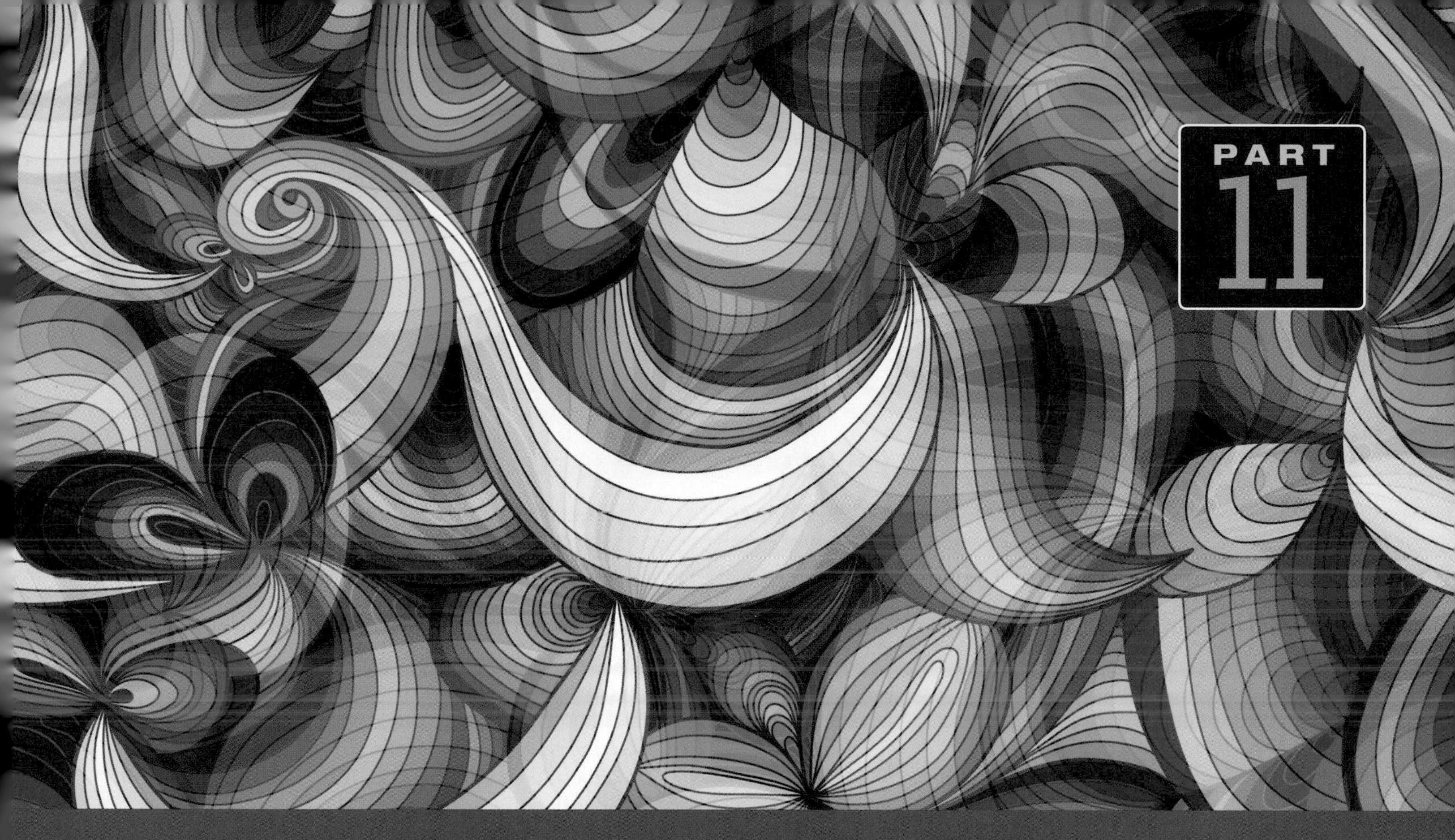


# Dental Administration and Communication Skills

The business aspect of a dental practice must be managed and operated efficiently to make a practice run successfully. A career as a dental business assistant can provide you with an opportunity to practice your business skills while working in the dental field.

The chapters in this section provide an overview of how human relations play an important role when working and communicating with colleagues and patients. By understanding the communication methods used in the dental setting, learning the technology of the dental practice, managing the financial aspects of a practice, and marketing your personal skills for lifelong learning, you will become an advocate for the profession of dentistry and the patients you care for.

61

# Communication in the Dental Office

## KEY TERMS

**Copier** A business machine that can make duplicates (copies) from an original.

**Fax machine** A business machine attached to a phone line that transmits hard copy written messages (handwritten or typed); "fax" is short for "facsimile."

**Human behavior** The collection of behaviors exhibited by human beings who have been influenced by a person's culture, attitudes, emotions, values, ethics, and authority.

**Letterhead** The part of a letter (or printed stationery) that contains the name and address of the person sending the letter.

**Marketing** A way of advertising or recruiting people to a business.

**Nonverbal communication** Type of communication in which body language is used as a form of expression.

**Salutation (sal-yoo-TAY-shun)** The part of the letter that contains the introductory greeting.

**Socialization** The process through which society influences individuals.

**Verbal communication** Type of communication in which words are used as a form of expression.

**Word processing software** A computer program designed to create most types of business documents.

## LEARNING OUTCOMES

*On completion of this chapter, the student will be able to achieve the following objectives:*

1. Pronounce, define, and spell the key terms.
2. Explain why it is important to understand human behavior.
3. Describe cultural diversity.
4. Discuss communication pathways and identify the differences between verbal and nonverbal communication.
5. Describe the importance of communicating effectively with colleagues.
6. Discuss communicating with patients, including identifying and meeting patient needs.
7. Discuss phone skills, including the following:
    - Describe good phone courtesy.
    - Describe and compare the handling of different types of phone calls.
    - Describe the types of available phone message systems.
    - Describe phone equipment.
8. Discuss written communication, including the following:
    - Describe different formats of business letters.
    - Describe the parts of a business letter.
9. Discuss marketing your dental practice, including external and internal marketing.

## PERFORMANCE OUTCOMES

*On completion of this chapter, the student will be able to meet competency standards in the following skills:*

- Use correct phone techniques when talking with a patient.
- Compose a business letter that includes the appropriate parts of a letter.

## ELECTRONIC RESOURCES

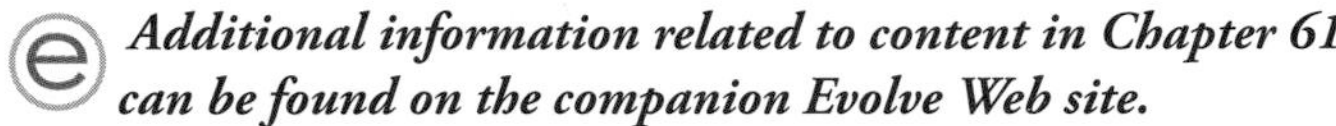

***Additional information related to content in Chapter 61 can be found on the companion Evolve Web site.***

- Practice Quiz

Appropriate communication, in all forms, is the backbone of a well-run organization. By having effective interpersonal skills, you are able to improve the quality of relationships, establish connections, solve problems, and create possibilities. Interpersonal communication teaches you how to communicate and interpret what others say and do; this trait is important not only to everyday social relationships, but also to business and professional relationships.

This chapter describes the importance of understanding human behavior, especially when it pertains to oral and written communication skills in the dental practice.

## Understanding Human Behavior

**Human behavior** is the collection of actions performed by human beings that have been influenced by a person's culture, attitudes, emotions, values, ethics, and authority. The behavior of people can be viewed as "normal," common, acceptable, or even unusual or unacceptable.

## Significant People in Psychology

Several psychologists have been instrumental in researching the way we understand how individuals behave in their personal and professional life.

- According to **Sigmund Freud** (1856–1939), people have conscious and unconscious thoughts, and our purpose in life is to control our instincts and the power of these thoughts.
- **Erik Erikson** (1902–1994) believed that a person's identity is individual and that it comes from the past and from one's heritage. This would include culture, religion, and status.
- **Carl Rogers** (1902–1987) believed that human beings are intrinsically good and friendly. A person is born with these qualities; it is society and their surroundings that impact these behaviors.
- **B. F. Skinner** (1904–1990) assumed that behavior is learned. Any behavior that is a threat can be changed by learning to solve problems; positive behavior is acknowledged by positive reinforcement.
- **Abraham Maslow** (1908–1970) is the founder of social learning psychology. He believed that humans cannot live without needs. He categorized these needs in groups with different rankings and titled them "Maslow's Hierarchy of Needs" (Fig. 61.1).

### Social Attitudes

As a person grows and develops in life, social attitudes begin to influence behavior and a cultural way of thinking. We tend to internalize the attitudes of others around us by making their attitudes our own. The process through which society influences individuals is called **socialization**.

### Peer Pressure

We often have the tendency to adapt our behavior to fit in with a particular group. Peer pressure is seen when a person conforms to the general behavior of a group of peers in an attempt to feel more acceptable within that group. Peer pressure can have a negative or a positive effect.

RECALL

1. Which psychologist believed that human beings are intrinsically good and friendly?
2. What is the first basic need a person has according to Maslow's Hierarchy of Needs?
3. What psychological term is used to describe the process by which society influences individuals?

## Cultural Diversity

Another aspect of effective understanding and communication is our respect for a highly diverse society. Social diversity is an important factor for a professional to consider. Differences in gender, race, cultural heritage, age, physical abilities, and spiritual beliefs are differences that must be appreciated and understood when working with patients, staff members, and other professionals in dentistry.

Verbal and nonverbal language varies among cultures. When working with such a diverse population as that of the United States, it is an advantage to have someone in the practice who is bilingual. If no one in the office speaks another language, it is good to have a multiple-language dictionary on hand. Encourage all members of the team to learn various cultural traditions and to always show respect for these traditions when providing patient care.

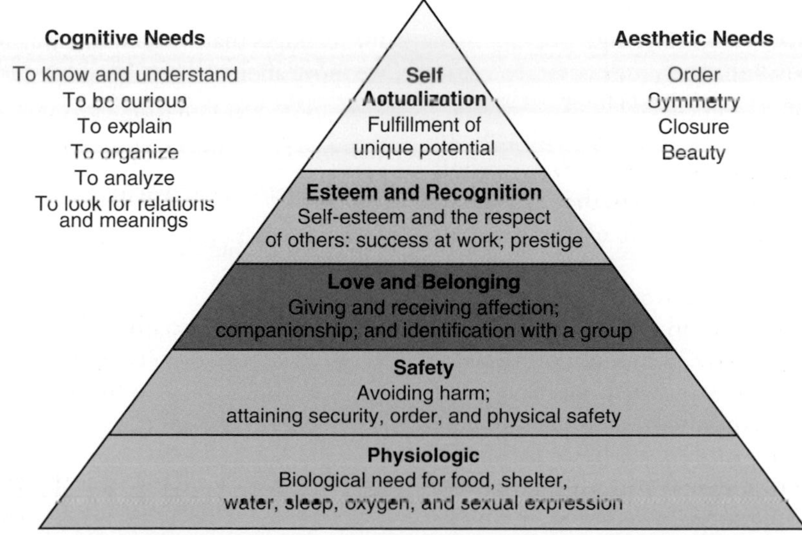


**FIG. 61.1** Maslow's Hierarchy of Needs. *(From Gaylor LJ: The administrative dental assistant, ed 4, St Louis, 2016, Elsevier.)*

**Basic Dental Terms in Other Languages**

| English | Spanish |
|---|---|
| Mouth | la boca |
| Tooth | el diente |
| Pain | el dolor |
| Open | abierto/a |
| Bite | la mordedura |
| Decay | la descomposición |
| Filling | la empastadura |
| X-ray | la radiografía |

# Communication Pathways

Effective communication can be one of the most important aspects of a dental assistant's job. We spend most of our working day communicating with others.

Communication is the sending of a message by one individual and the receiving of the same message by another individual. Every message we send has two parts that must coincide in time:

- The **statement proper,** or the "This is what I have told you" portion, consists of the words that are being used.
- The **explanation** is the part of the message that conveys, "Now, this is how I expect you to understand it." This part of the message is sent nonverbally.

We communicate with words, facial expressions, appearance, gestures, mannerisms, listening, voice inflection, attitudes, and actions. The two parts of the message identified above are grouped into the two general categories of verbal and nonverbal communication.

## Verbal Communication

**Verbal communication** is made up of the words we use. Most verbal communication is perceived by "hearing."

### *Words Are Important*

Words are verbal symbols that are used to represent an object or a meaning. Unfortunately, these verbal symbols usually are not checked against the things they represent; often, the result is confusion, distortion of meaning, or misunderstanding.

It is important to remember that words mean different things to different people—and they can mean different things in different situations. Good verbal communication depends on the basis of a common language, in which the sender and the receiver are using words that they both understand to have the same meaning.

When communicating with a dental patient, take care to select words that he or she understands, rather than confusing the person with the technical language and specialized terminology of dentistry. Be careful to select words that will not frighten, intimidate, or upset the patient. Box 61.1 lists effective words for patient interaction.

### *Voice Quality*

Voice quality accounts for more than one third of the impact of the total message and reveals a lot about the individual. Try to develop a pleasant voice (tone) quality, and speak slowly, distinctly, and loudly enough to be heard easily without being harsh or too loud.

In the event of a true emergency in the dental office, it is particularly important that you be extremely careful to keep your voice calm, because it is not *what* is said but *how* it is said that may alarm the patient or the person accompanying the patient.

### *Asking Questions*

Questions are used to gather information. Often, the way you phrase a question determines the type of answer you will get. By being aware of this, you can be more effective in gathering information and in helping patients to feel more at ease.

**Closed-ended questions** are questions that can be answered with "Yes" or "No." These questions are best used to confirm information, to limit a conversation, or to close a conversation. Closed-ended questions often begin with the words *is, do, has, have, can,* or *will.* For example, "Is next Monday at 9 AM convenient for you, Mr. Thomas?" is a closed-ended question that can be answered simply with "Yes" or "No."

**Open-ended questions** are those that require more than a "Yes" or "No" for an answer. These questions are best used to obtain information, maintain control of the conversation, or build rapport. Open-ended questions usually begin with words such as *what, when, how, who, where,* or *which.* For example, "Mrs. Jackson, what time of day is best to schedule your next appointment?" is an open-ended question.

## Nonverbal Communication

**Nonverbal communication** is perceived at an almost subconscious level through all the senses. Nonverbal communication is conveyed by our body language. Body language consists of the messages that we send, the way we carry ourselves, and how we move about.

**BOX 61.1 Effective Words**

| Instead of this ... | Try this ... |
|---|---|
| Pain | Discomfort |
| Shot | Anesthetic |
| Pull | Remove |
| Drill | Prepare tooth |
| Filling | Restoration |
| False teeth | Denture |
| Operatory | Treatment area |
| Waiting room | Reception area |

**TABLE 61.1** Nonverbal Communication

| Message | Low-Level Behavior | High-Level Behavior |
|---|---|---|
| **Empathy** | Frown resulting from lack of understanding | Positive head nods; facial expressions that reflect the content of the conversation |
| **Respect** | Mumbling; patronizing tone of voice | Devoting full attention |
| **Warmth** | Apathy; fidgeting; signs indicating a desire to leave | Smiling; physical contact |
| **Genuineness** | Avoidance of eye contact | Congruence between verbal and nonverbal behaviors |
| **Self-disclosure** | Bragging gestures; pointing to oneself | Gestures that minimize references to oneself |
| **Confrontation** | Pointing a finger or shaking a fist; speaking in a loud tone of voice | Speaking in a natural tone of voice |

From Proctor DB et al: Kinn's the medical assistant, ed 13, St Louis, 2017, Elsevier.

Posture, movements, and attitudes transmit major messages. For example, the person who is depressed often moves slowly with a restrained gait that reflects his or her mental attitude. The happy, healthy individual with a bright outlook on life tends to demonstrate this attitude with a free-moving walk that mirrors a sense of well-being. Hands grasping chair arms and restless shifting of body position are reliable indicators of inner tension and uneasiness in a patient. Rapid, shallow breathing also is a sign of tension and stress; you can help the patient relax by encouraging him or her to breathe slowly and deeply in a more normal pattern. Table 61.1 describes specific behaviors that may be observed in nonverbal communication.

Facial expressions indicate a wide variety of emotional states at which words can only hint. The eyes are particularly expressive of emotion and the patient's mental state of well-being.

Although many patients become capable of hiding their true emotions, the assistant should be aware of the signs of tension, stress, pain, boredom, lack of interest, or anxiety. At chairside, be careful not to convey a feeling of alarm on your face as a reaction to operative or surgical procedures, because this response could unnecessarily alarm the patient.

## Listening Skills

It has been estimated that 90 percent of all spoken words are never heard; listening is one of the greatest arts of communication and one of the most difficult to master. Good listening requires that you concentrate entirely on the patient. To be a good listener, focus on the following:

- **Do not let your mind wander.** Put aside personal concerns while the patient is talking.
- **Do not concentrate on formulating a reply.** Instead, concentrate on what the patient is actually saying. This shows the patient that you care.
- **Look as well as listen.** In this way, you will pick up both the verbal and the nonverbal information that the patient is transmitting.
- **Do not stereotype.** A person's appearance, cultural background, race, or religion should not influence your response to what he or she is saying.
- **Be careful of selective hearing.** Sometimes we hear only parts of what someone is saying.
- **Do not get impatient.** When you are in a hurry or are trying to obtain a specific answer, it is easier to become annoyed with a patient, especially if the patient is a child or an older adult.

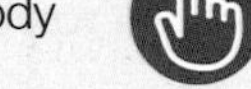


4 What type of communication describes our body language?
5 What percentage of spoken words do we never hear?
6 Can anxiety be communicated through facial expression?
7 Give a more effective word for "pulling" a tooth.

# Communicating with Colleagues

Americans spend more time with their coworkers than with their own families. Working in a positive, challenging, and stress-free environment is what everyone wants from their place of employment. How you communicate and get along with your coworkers will be evident to your patients and will influence their perception of the practice (Fig. 61.2). A patient can tell right away what level of harmony exists in a particular dental setting.

The one key to a successful work environment is teamwork. Teamwork results when everyone feels needed and respected and is given an opportunity to fulfill his or her role along with the others in a specific setting.

## Being a Team Member

- Be flexible and receptive to altering the way responsibilities are performed.
- Be self-confident and use self-initiative when it is time to get things done. Do not wait to be told what to do.
- Show appreciation to coworkers; do not take advantage of them.
- Think before speaking.
- Do not let your emotions get overly involved.
- Remember that the first impression is not always the right one.

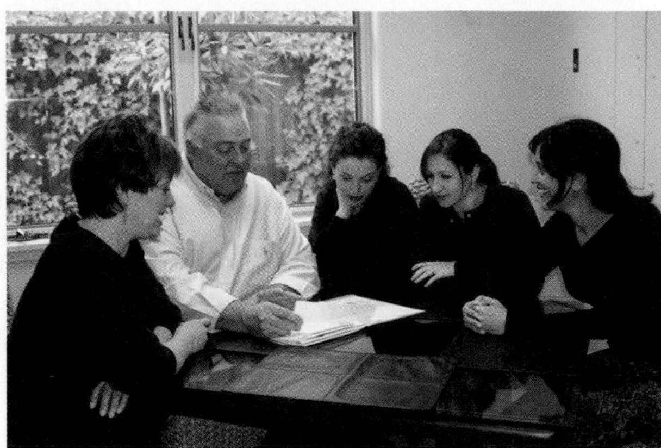

FIG. 61.2 Team meeting.

- Share the ups and downs of the day.
- Remember that "your way" may not always be the right way.

## Stress in the Dental Office

An important aspect of good communication is how you handle stress in your personal life and at work. The dental atmosphere can be a stressful environment, and this can affect the way you respond to your patients and coworkers.

### *Causes*

Stress is common in the workplace. Many dental team members feel stressed at times and need to find an outlet for their emotions. Causes of stress in the dental office include, but are not limited to, the following:

- Lack of sufficient staff
- Appointment overbooking
- Multiple tasks required simultaneously
- Lack of good communication
- Perceived lack of job advancement

### *Methods of Stress Reduction*

You can reduce stress by maintaining a lifestyle that includes regular exercise, taking time for yourself, leaving the office behind at the end of the day, eating properly, and setting realistic expectations. Learning to control stress will enable you to make intelligent decisions regarding patient management, patient care, and patient relationships.

## Conflict among Coworkers

If differences or **conflicts** among colleagues are creating stress, learn how to work through those differences by engaging in team-building dialogue. Conflict is necessary for effective problem solving and for effective interpersonal relationships. Unfortunately, unresolved conflict tends to escalate. Learning to control stress will enable you to make intelligent decisions regarding patient management, patient care, and patient relationships. Box 61.2 lists conflict resolution tips to make your work environment a less stressful, more productive environment.

**BOX 61.2 Conflict Resolution**

- **Be specific about your conflict.** "I'm never included when the sales rep comes in" is not as effective as "I feel I could contribute to the dental materials being used in the office."
- **Resist the temptation to involve yourself** in conflicts that do not directly involve you. Even if someone has clearly been wronged, allow the person to resolve the situation as he or she chooses.
- **Try to depersonalize conflicts.** Instead of a "me versus you" scenario, visualize an "us versus the problem" scenario. Not only is this a more professional attitude, but it will also improve productivity and reflects the best interests of the office.
- **Be open and listen** to another's point of view, and think about how the person responded to the conflict. This important clarification skill leads to less misunderstanding with the other person.
- **Don't always involve the dentist or office manager** in conflict resolution. You'll quickly give the impression that you are unable to resolve the smallest difficulties.
- **Take it outside and away from the group** of curious coworkers if they are not involved in the problem.
- **Limit your complaints** to those directly involved in the conflict. You need to protect a working relationship rather than a personal one, which means that your opinion of a coworker's character is generally irrelevant.
- **Know when conflict is more than conflict.** If conflict arises as the result of sexual, racial, or ethnic issues, or if someone behaves inappropriately, that's not conflict—it's harassment.
- **Consider a mediator** if the problem gets out of control, or if the issue is too emotional to resolve in a mutual discussion. At this step, the office manager or dentist should be involved.
- **It's not all about you.** You may think it's a personal attack, but maybe your coworker is just having a bad day.

RECALL

8 What is the key to a successful work environment?
9 Describe stressors in a dental office.

# Communicating with Patients

A solid foundation of excellence in dental care and communication skills is necessary for a dental practice to achieve its goals and for the needs of patients to be fulfilled at all levels. Effective communication is important in achieving patient satisfaction. Patients who have good relationships with their dentist and the dental staff are likely to stay with the practice, accept the treatment presented to them, pay for the treatment on time, and refer other patients to the practice (Fig. 61.3).

## Patient Needs

Patients build a relationship with their dentist and dental staff through confidence and trust. Patients base their perceptions about a practice on the following factors:

- How they are treated on the phone
- How they are greeted

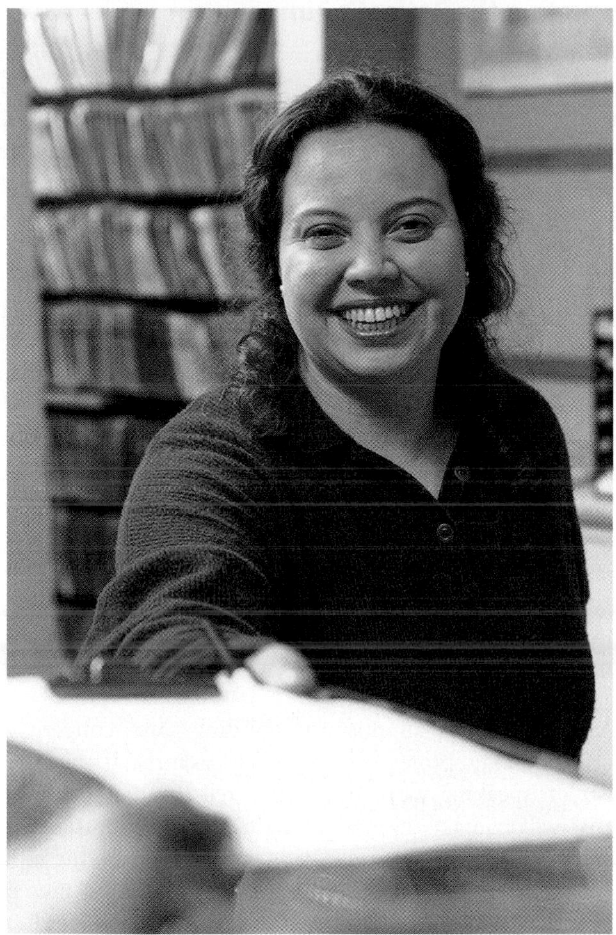

**FIG. 61.3** Communication is the most important tool in a practice. *(From Proctor DB et al: Kinn's the medical assistant: an applied learning approach, ed 13, St Louis, 2017, Elsevier.)*

- How they are made to feel in the office
- How efficiently the staff manages business aspects, such as billing and insurance

Establishing a positive professional/patient relationship is part of understanding the needs of the patient. As a dental professional, you must recognize that patients are different and have different needs.

## Psychological Needs

Psychological reactions are more obvious when a patient appears tense, suspicious, apprehensive, and resistant to suggested treatment. All individuals have emotional needs, and these needs must be considered even when a patient seems confident, comfortable, and agreeable. One factor of major importance is the patient's current life situation; this includes the many stresses, tensions, conflicts, and anxieties that may be present in any part of the patient's life.

Other important factors that can influence the patient's reactions to the current situation are his or her *previous dental experiences* and the patient's *attitudes and beliefs* about the importance of his or her teeth. These attitudes and beliefs are strongly influenced by the patient's socioeconomic and cultural background, as well as by the attitudes of peers or relatives. For example, if a patient grew up in a family in which going to the dentist was a dreaded experience, he or she may have difficulty overcoming this attitude.

## Anxiety and Fear of Pain

The fear of pain is a frequently stated cause of anxiety regarding dental treatment. For many patients, however, it is the *expectation* of pain, not *actual* pain, that causes the greatest distress. Unfortunately, the more fearful and anxious the patient becomes, the more sensitive he or she may be to pain.

**Subjective fears,** also known as **acquired fears,** are based on feelings, attitudes, and concerns that have developed at the suggestion of peers, siblings, parents, or other individuals. These fears are based on anecdotal evidence (hearing stories or seeing dental care depicted in movies or television shows). Subjective fears, imaginative as they are, can cause irreparable damage to a patient's composure and conduct during a routine dental visit. Small children especially have an intense fear of the unknown. Whether the patient is a child or an adult, he or she should be informed in a general and positive way about the dental procedure, the use of equipment, and the sequence of events that can be expected.

**Objective fears,** also known as **learned fears,** are those related to the patient's experiences and his or her own memories of those experiences. If the experience was traumatic, the patient dreads subsequent treatment. If the experience was a positive one, the patient is not fearful. The best way to address objective fear is to be honest when communicating with the patient. Never lie to a patient. For example, it is always better to say, "This will pinch for just a moment," than to say, "This won't hurt at all."

Despite their concerns and feelings of uneasiness, most patients are able to seek and receive treatment. The dental team can help these patients by seeking to understand patient behavior and by actively working to enable the patient to cope with the experience in a positive manner.

## Dental-Phobic Patients

For some patients, the mere suggestion of a routine dental visit can bring an overwhelming sensation of panic and terror. These patients are described as **dental-phobic.** Patients with the most severe cases of dental phobia avoid routine treatment completely and will seek urgent or emergency treatment only with the most aggressive dental symptoms.

## Patient's Responses

The patient's responses to dental treatment and to the dental team are not limited to what is being said and done at the moment; rather, responses are influenced by the patient's total personality and by his or her background of experiences. When working with patients, it is particularly important to remember the following:

- The patient's response to the situation results primarily from causes that are not part of the present situation.
- These causes are probably not fully understood by the patient and most likely will remain unknown to the dental team.

- The patient's anxieties concerning treatment may result in hostile, irrational, and inappropriate behavior.
- This hostility is an expression of the patient's anxieties and is not caused by, or directed at, dental personnel.

### Physical and Mental Needs

Maintenance of high standards of care requires sensitivity to the patient's physical and mental needs. The patient registration form and the medical-dental history form should include questions about the patient's dental and medical health. With this information, it is easier to determine whether a patient requires extra attention because of specific physical needs. Patients with physical or mental impairment have complicated and special needs that must be considered before and during provision of dental treatment.

### Financial Needs

Often, a major obstacle to patient acceptance is the cost of treatment. Patients may believe that the fees are too high, that they are unable to afford the treatment, or that they do not need the treatment. Employment, payment, and insurance information are relevant to patient care. Many people do not equate dental care with basic human needs such as shelter and food. Getting patients to understand the benefits and advantages of appropriate treatment requires good communication skills.

## Meeting Patient Needs

The following sections describe ways that you can help the dental team to meet patient needs.

### Positive Atmosphere

The physical appearance of the office speaks very clearly to patients. To ensure that patients feel welcome, create an environment and a decor that reflect a warm, hospitable atmosphere. Worn or shabby floor covering should be replaced or cleaned when necessary. Plants and fresh floral arrangements reflect a healthy and inviting practice atmosphere. Plants, magazines, and other reception area amenities must be well maintained to keep this area as comfortable and pleasant as a living room in a private home.

### Sincerity

Each action and word that takes place in the dental office is a reflection of the dental practice's level of sincerity. Patients are especially sensitive to tone of voice and remarks that could be misinterpreted (e.g., a humorous remark could be mistaken for a serious comment). Every member of the dental team must make a conscious effort to think before speaking or acting.

### Showing Respect

Patients prefer to be treated as "friends of the practice." Every effort should be made to help patients feel welcome and important. It is advisable to address adults as "Mr.," "Mrs.," "Miss," or "Ms." at the initial greeting. If, after that time, the patient expresses a desire to be called by a first name or a nickname, then do so. (Make a note of this on the patient's chart for future reference.)

### Respecting the Patient's Time

Patients expect the value of their time to be respected and not wasted by unnecessary waiting. Scheduling of appointments and staying on time are two essential components of helping patients feel welcome. By keeping a patient "waiting," the dental office is sending the message that the patient's time is not important.

### Resolving Complaints and Misunderstandings

It has been studied and shown that 95 percent of patients who are unhappy or dissatisfied never say so; they simply leave the practice. Thus it makes good sense to listen carefully to those few patients who do attempt to express dissatisfaction. One of the best ways to calm an irate patient is to listen silently, use good eye contact, and occasionally nod your head. Do not interrupt. Let the patient finish. Often, this helps the patient calm down slowly. It then is appropriate to say to the patient, for example, "If I hear correctly what you are saying, Mr. Harris, you feel upset about the charge that appeared on last month's statement. Is that right?" This will give the patient a sense of control over the situation.

Make sure that all misunderstandings and concerns are resolved quickly, professionally, and pleasantly. If the patient insists on speaking with the dentist, tell the patient that the dentist will contact the patient by a specific time (later that same day, ideally); then take steps to ensure that this indeed takes place. (Dentists should be interrupted only to take calls that meet specific predetermined criteria. See further discussion later.)

### Remaining Approachable

Many patients are afraid of approaching professionals or of asking questions that they fear may seem "dumb." One of the best communication techniques the dental office can practice is to display a sense of approachability at all times. Patients' questions should be encouraged. The dental team should respond to the patient with a sense of genuine care and concern. If the dentist has a "call-in" or "call-back" time each day for handling phone calls, this time should be used to reach patients. Most patients want to feel reassured that the dental team cares about them.

### Respecting Patient Confidentiality

In a time of increasing litigation, it is more important than ever to keep conversations and patient records confidential. If patients believe that their concerns are not taken seriously, or if they detect or sense a lack of confidentiality, the practice/patient relationship may experience irreparable damage (see Chapters 4 and 40).

**10** How can a patient be psychologically influenced by others' attitudes?
**11** Are objective fears acquired or learned?
**12** Describe a few techniques that can be used to calm an irate patient.

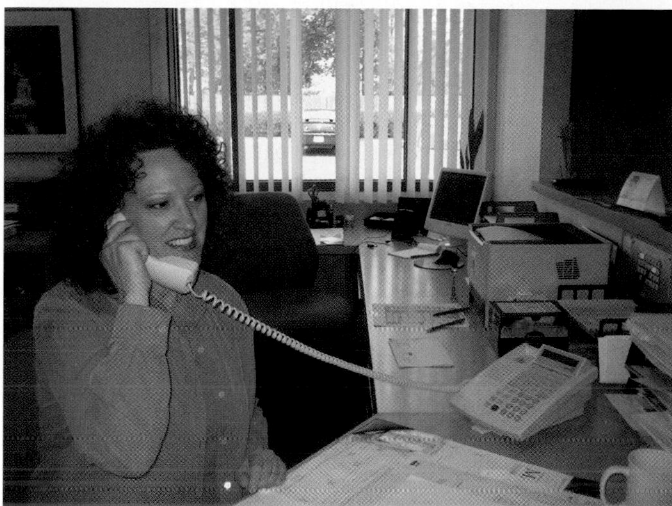

FIG. 61.4 The business assistant answers the phone.

## Phone Skills

The phone is your most important device used in public relations. Most patients make their first contact with the dental office by phone. On the basis of this first contact, the patient forms an opinion of the practice. This opinion reflects on the dentist and the dental team and even on the quality of care provided—although no actual care has yet been provided.

The business assistant is responsible for answering the phone and ensuring that all patient contacts have a positive experience (Fig. 61.4).

### Etiquette

Phone calls should be governed by the same rules of courtesy that apply to face-to-face meetings. This courtesy should begin with a prompt and pleasant response to the ring of the phone and should continue until the receiver is gently replaced at the end of the call. When answering the phone, your voice should convey the equivalent of a warm smile, and the perceived message should be, "I'm glad you called!" You never want to send the message that the call is an unwanted interruption, or that you are tired, angry, preoccupied, or in a hurry. Remember the following:

- Smile; it shows in your voice.
- Never chew gum, eat, drink, or have a pen or pencil in your mouth while talking on the phone.
- Speak directly into the receiver (mouthpiece), keeping your mouth 1 to 2 inches away.
- Ask the name of the person who is calling, and talk to him or her, not to the phone.
- Speak clearly and slowly; guard against slurring your words.
- Do not speak too quietly or too loudly.
- Do not talk with others in the office while on the phone.
- Do not have background noise.
- Do not speak too quickly.
- Use the caller's name in the conversation and give him or her complete attention.
- When completing a call, always allow the person who originated the call to hang up first.

### Incoming Calls

- The phone should be answered promptly, preferably after the first ring.
- Greet the patient pleasantly.
- Identify the practice and yourself. (Properly identifying yourself at the beginning of the conversation will prompt the caller to identify himself or herself as well.)
- Ask how you may help the caller.

### Working with Difficult Callers

Sometimes a caller will come across on the phone as difficult. This is most common if they are in pain, or there is a billing question. First, remember that this caller is a patient, so your handling of the call could result either in the patient continuing his or her relationship with the office or going elsewhere. Do the following:

- Listen without interrupting.
- Gather the facts and take notes.
- Organize your notes, so they can be relayed to the appropriate person.
- Sympathize with the caller and offer to act as quickly as you can.
- Stay calm even though the caller may be angry and possibly abusive.

### Placing a Caller on Hold

Before placing a caller on hold, ask for his or her permission: "May I put you on hold for just a moment, Mr. Johnson?" Then wait for the caller's response before pressing the "hold" or "mute" button.

Always be courteous, and do not expect the caller to remain on hold for longer than a few minutes. If necessary, ask whether you can return the call, and give a specific time when you will do so.

#### *On-Hold Message Systems*

On-hold message systems consist of recorded messages or music used by the practice to make "on-hold" time educational and more pleasant for callers than a waiting signal. These messages may explain a variety of treatments and services available at the practice. The messages or musical interludes are broken occasionally by recordings by professional announcers who apologize for any delay and thank the caller for waiting.

### Callers Wanting to Speak to the Dentist

The dentist should not be interrupted at chairside to come to the phone. Phone interruptions (1) reduce productivity and cause treatment delays, (2) are inconsiderate to the seated

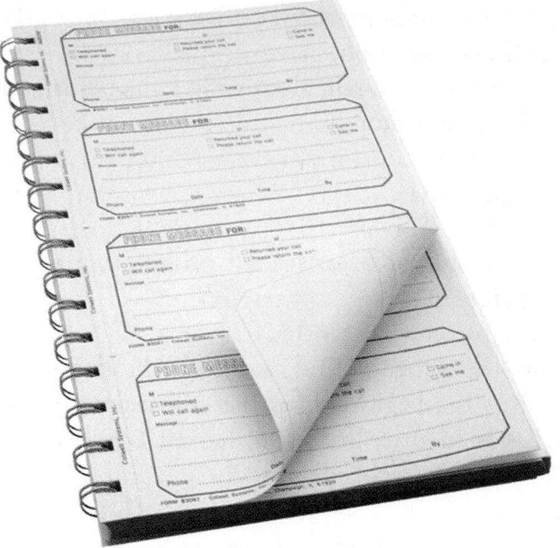

**FIG. 61.5** An example of a printed form for taking messages. *(Courtesy Patterson Dental, St Paul, MN.)*

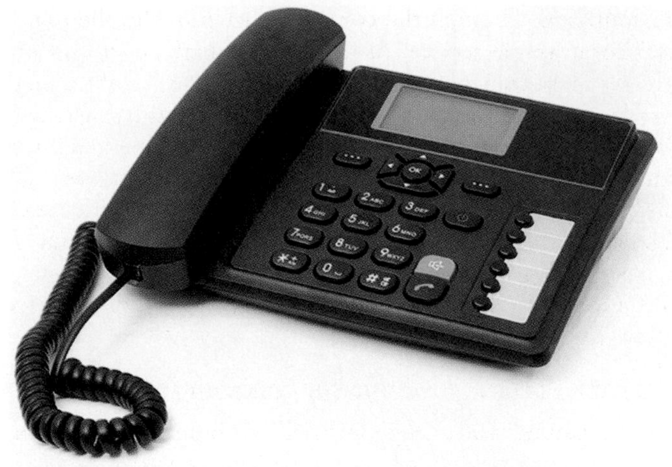

**FIG. 61.6** A multipurpose phone system with multiple lines and answering machine. *(From BigStockPhoto.com.)*

patient, and (3) make it difficult for the dental team to maintain infection control protocols.

The most common exceptions for which a dentist should come to the phone are to talk to another dentist, the dental laboratory technician, or an immediate family member. It is the business assistant's responsibility to know the dentist's policy on this and to handle all other calls tactfully.

Select your words and phrases with care. If the request of a caller to speak with the dentist does not meet the dentist's specified criteria for interruption, be polite. A statement such as, "Dr. Garcia is with a patient. How may I help you?" is appropriate.

## Taking Messages

Make a written notation of all incoming calls, particularly those that require further action. Many practices use a printed form or a phone log to organize this information (Fig. 61.5). Many of these types of form systems create a duplicate copy of the message as you write, so that the original message can be torn off and delivered. At the beginning of the conversation, note the caller's name, and then ask the appropriate questions. Be sure to record the information completely and accurately. After you take a message, deliver it promptly and accurately.

If you promise to follow through on a call, be sure to do just that! Do not promise that the dentist will call back at a certain time unless you are positive that this is possible, and that the dentist will be willing to follow through. When the dentist is expected to return a call to a patient, have the appropriate patient records ready for the dentist when you deliver the message.

See Procedure 61.1: Answering the Phone.

## Phone Message Systems

### Answering Service

When the dental office is closed, some form of phone coverage must be provided. If an answering service is used, learn how to use these services properly. In general, it is necessary to call the service and notify service staff when the office is closing. Relay the following information to the service:

- When the office will reopen
- Whom to contact in case of an emergency (and how to contact that person)

When the office reopens, call the service immediately to notify service staff that you are back and will be taking incoming calls again. At this time, service staff will give you the messages they have taken during your absence. As messages are dictated, record them accurately and return calls promptly as appropriate.

### Answering Machine

The phone answering machine is a recording device that is located in the dental office (Fig. 61.6). When the office is closing, the business assistant dictates an appropriate message into the machine, providing the following information:

- The identification of the office
- Why the phone is being answered by a recording (e.g., the office is closed)
- The time at which the office will reopen
- Whom to contact in case of an emergency (and how to contact that person)
- Basic instructions on how to leave a message (e.g., "After the tone, please leave your name, a brief message, and the number where you can be reached.")

After you have dictated the message, play it back to check for accuracy and clarity. Remember that even during a recording, you want to create a good impression. Then turn on the machine so that it will answer and record all incoming calls. When you return to the office, listen to the messages that have been left, log them, and promptly take any necessary follow-through action.

### Voice Mail

Many dental practices prefer to use a voice mail service to allow the caller to select a variety of options. These services are contracted through the company that provides the practice's local phone service. As a rule, calls may be forwarded directly to various parties to answer questions, or the caller may leave a message for the dentist or one of the assistants. Voice mail services allow you to leave a recorded greeting, similar to that used with an answering machine; however, no physical machine is kept in the dental office. Instead, messages are retrieved by calling an access number and entering a security code number. As with other message systems, listen to the messages, log them, and promptly take any necessary follow-through action.

### Patients' Preferred Method of Communication

Do not assume that a single method of communication will meet everyone's needs. Collect your patients' preferred method of communication. Some will prefer a voice message or email. Some will want the traditional postcard. Many of your patients will want a text message. Your capability to respect this preference will not only demonstrate good customer service but also exhibit your practice's technological sophistication.

### Emailing

Email communication has grown to be an essential tool in this age of technology. The use of email can increase productivity, decrease costs, and be included in new marketing ways for a dental practice.

There is an increasing awareness of privacy issues when sharing patient records between specialists, dentists, and laboratories through email. A violation occurs when transmitting protected health information by email. Regulations, such as HIPAA, and the Canadian equivalent PIPEDA, have established very specific guidelines for the handling of patient information. Electronic transmission of patient information creates multiple opportunities for the potential loss of data. An office should look into a HIPAA-compliant system that requires a secure login when using email.

**EMAIL ETIQUETTE.** Because your correspondence says a lot about you and the dental practice, you should be aware of some basic email etiquette:

- *Mind Your Manners:* Think of the basic rules you learned growing up, such as saying please and thank you. Address people you don't know as Mr., Mrs., or Dr.; address someone by first name only if they imply that it is okay to do so.
- *Watch Your Tone:* The dictionary defines *tone* as an "accent or inflection expressive of a mood or emotion." It is very difficult to express tone in writing. You want to come across as respectful, friendly, and approachable. You don't want to sound curt or demanding.
- *Be Concise:* Get to the point of your email as quickly as possible, but don't leave out important details that will help your recipient answer your query.
- *Be Professional:* This means stay away from abbreviations and don't use emoticons (those little smiley faces). Don't use a cute or suggestive email address for business communications.
- *Use Correct Spelling and Proper Grammar:* Use a dictionary or a spell checker—whichever works better for you. While you can write in a conversational tone (contractions are okay), pay attention to basic rules of grammar.
- *Ask Before You Send an Attachment:* Because of computer viruses, many people won't open attachments unless they know the sender. Even that can be a mistake because many viruses come disguised in email messages from someone you know. Before sending an attachment, ask the recipient if you may do so.
- *Wait to Fill in the "TO" Email Address:* Never fill in the "TO" email address until you are completely through proofing the email and positive that it is exactly the way you want it. This will keep you from accidentally sending an email prematurely.

### Automatic Dialing Services

An automated appointment reminder service can help a practice by reducing missed appointments, thus increasing revenue. With a patient appointment phone reminder service, patients can be contacted in a professional manner reminding them of their upcoming appointment. Prerecorded messages can be played to either answering machines or to individuals informing them of upcoming appointments. Simple to complex scripts can be developed for touch phone response.

If a patient finds it necessary to cancel an appointment, the patient can be directed back to a staff member or transferred to outside third parties such as an office answering service.

### Text Messaging

Whether we like it or not, text messaging or texting is all around us. Everyone has to admit that for quick messages such as "I'm running late" or "Does anyone need anything at the store?" it is a great tool. So, when we look at its application in the *dental practice,* we should focus on its use for *quick reminders, alerts, and appointment confirmations.* This can also be used to notify a patient that the office is running late for an *upcoming appointment.*

## Phone Equipment

### Headsets

For a business assistant who may be handling more than one task at a time, a headset may be very useful. A headset is a lightweight combination of an earphone and a microphone that rests on the assistant's head and allows a person to move about the office and talk on the phone (Fig. 61.7). The advantage of a headset is that the business assistant's hands are free to do other things. For many users, a headset also creates less neck and elbow strain than a traditional handpiece/receiver.

### Pager

Many dentists need to be "on call" during weekends or while away from the practice. A pager is a mobile system that contacts the dentist through an answering service or by calling a special number that is left on the answering machine.

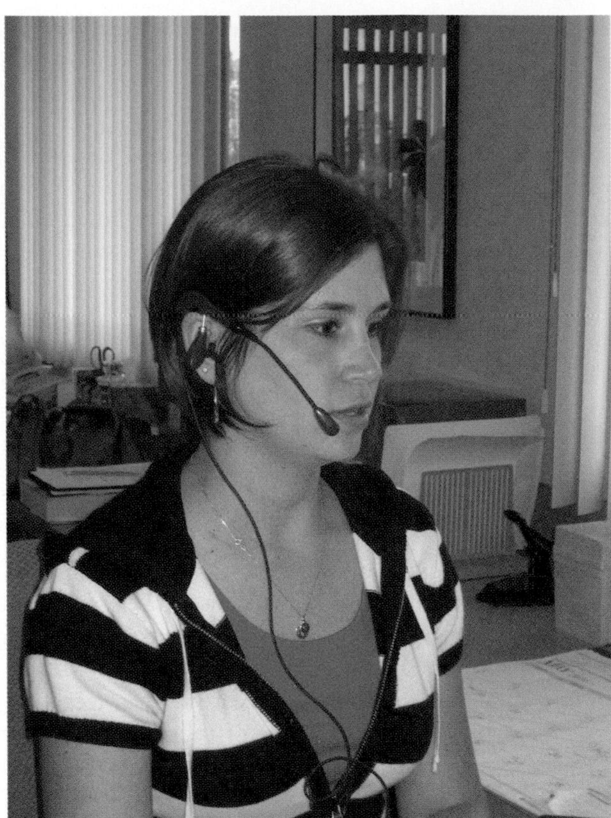

**FIG. 61.7** The office assistant using a headset system.

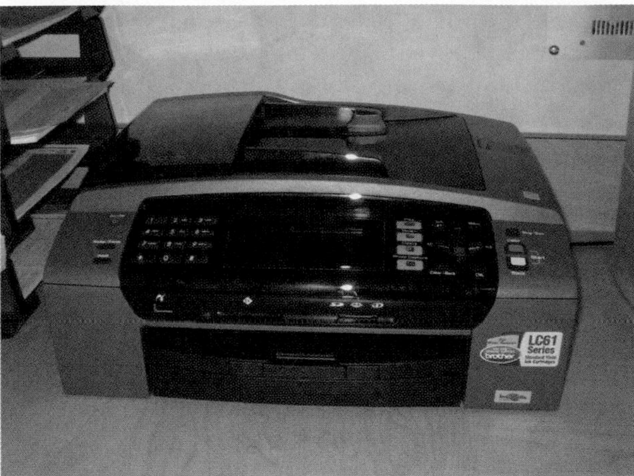

**FIG. 61.8** A facsimile (fax) machine.

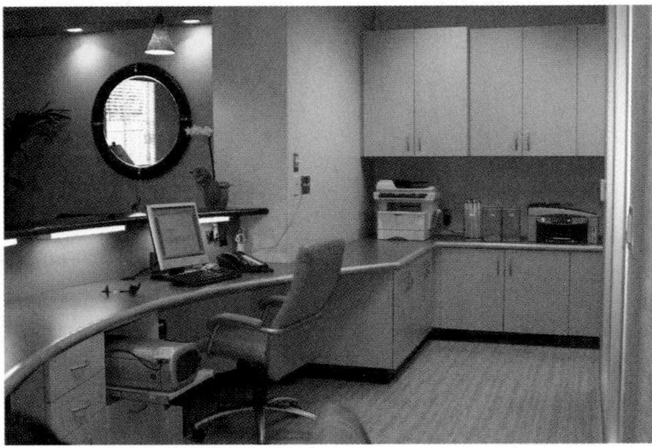

**FIG. 61.9** Business equipment is set up within the office management area.

### *Facsimile ("Fax") Machine*

A **fax machine** can be a great asset for enhancing communication in your office (Fig. 61.8). Many dental practices work closely with other specialty offices and must convey patient information to other dentists or healthcare professionals. Sending this information by fax can save time and labor. The fax unit is joined to the phone system and is used to electronically send and receive hard copy messages (handwritten or typed).

Uses of the fax machine in the dental office include placing orders with suppliers, relaying and receiving patient information, and sending information to insurance companies. When sending a fax, remember that it should be neat and professional in appearance (similar to other forms of written communication).

RECALL

13 What is the most important piece of office equipment that can be used for public relations?
14 On which ring should you answer the phone?
15 When the dental office is closed, how are messages obtained?
16 What piece of equipment allows you to transmit hard copy written messages?

## Written Communications

Many types of written communication originate from the dental practice. It is important to realize that, other than speaking with someone on the phone, written communication is the most important public relations tool of a practice. Thus the practice's image or the perception it creates is based to a great degree on the type and quality of printed communications that it generates.

## Equipment

If one of your responsibilities in the dental office is to correspond through written communication, you will be required to learn how to use the necessary business equipment within the office (Fig. 61.9).

The **computer** is the operating system used for all forms of written communication (Fig. 61.10). This useful and most versatile piece of equipment allows the business assistant to handle all types of written communication. There are multiple dental software companies that can set up a customized program for the dental office. Learning basic keyboarding is useful for typing effectively with the computer.

A **copier** allows you to make duplicates (copies) of documents that must be sent to a patient, another dentist, a dental laboratory, or a supply company (Fig. 61.11). Maintenance of copy machines can be time-consuming and costly. Make sure

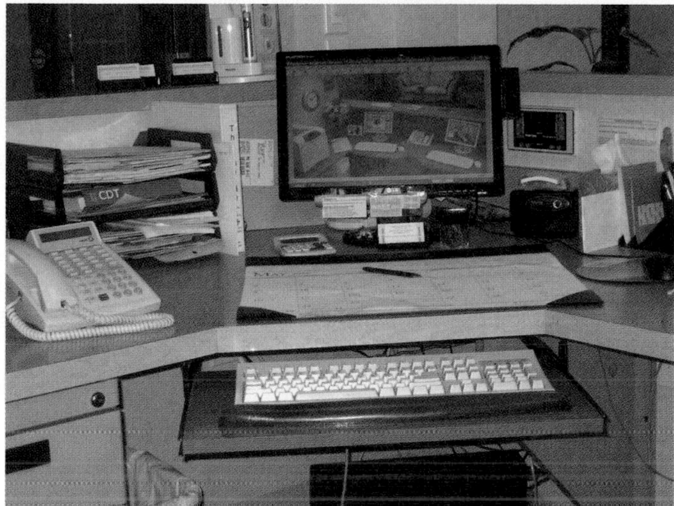

FIG. 61.10 A desktop computer system used in the dental office.

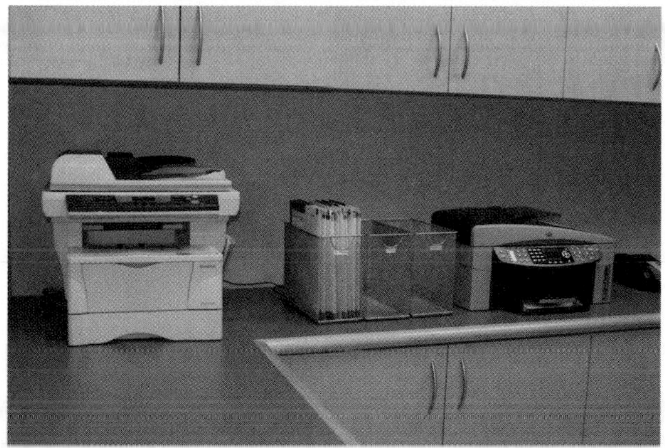

FIG. 61.11 Copier, printer, scanner, and fax machine all in one.

the office invests in a copier that will withstand the amount of work generated by that practice.

## Business Letters

An appropriate business letter is essential when conveying a professional image. Every letter or correspondence mailed from your dental office must be produced on high-quality, professionally designed stationery. Letters must be concise, accurate, and neat, and should be proofread for spelling and grammatical errors. Misspelled words and poor grammar convey the image of an office that does not care about quality. Patients and referring dentists may see this as unprofessional and even as a reflection on the quality of dental care provided.

### Types of Business Letters

Many practices send letters to their patients for a variety of reasons:

- Welcome to the practice
- Congratulations
- Acknowledgment of a referral
- Completion of an extensive case
- Continuing care (recall)
- Missed appointment
- Proposed treatment
- Collection of payment (see Chapter 63)

To save time when composing letters, many practices keep sample letters on file under specific headings. Other commercially prepared sample letters (often called *templates*) are available in books ("hard copy" format) or in electronic format (discs, CDs, or downloadable files) for use with a **word processing software** program. The word processing program enables users to quickly create form letters and to personalize them automatically by merging appropriate information from patient data files.

A blank paper is bare and an important document printed on it lacks the seriousness of the correspondence. A **letterhead** shows an importance and urgency to whatever is written on the paper. A simple design and arrangement of the dental practice name, the logo, and other important information is placed at the top of the page.

### Letters to Colleagues

Dentists frequently communicate with other professionals in writing. It is the job of the alert dental assistant to ensure that these communications take place in an expedient and professional manner. Letters to the dentist's colleagues may include examination findings or referral to specialists. It is important to double-check for spelling accuracy and consistency when sending written communications to other professional practices.

### Letters to Insurance Carriers

When completing written correspondence to insurance carriers, make sure that the following items are included:

- Patient identification information: patient's name, address, date of birth, and contract number or identification number (*Note:* Be careful not to include a patient's social security number when submitting information.)
- Case information: nature and extent of the case, any unusual circumstances or conditions, and an estimate of the fees to be incurred
- Radiographs: included only if required

### Format of a Business Letter

Using the proper business letter format is one step in making your business more professional. You can simplify the entire process of creating a properly formatted business letter by using your word processing program. By going to the letter wizard under the "Tools" function, select "Letters & Mailings" and click on the Letter Wizard. The wizard will prompt you through each field and allow you to choose a format.

- *Block Letter Format:* The common block letter format places all of your text flush with the left margin. Paragraphs are double spaced, and all line text is single spaced. The margins use a standard word processor setting of 1 inch (Fig. 61.12).

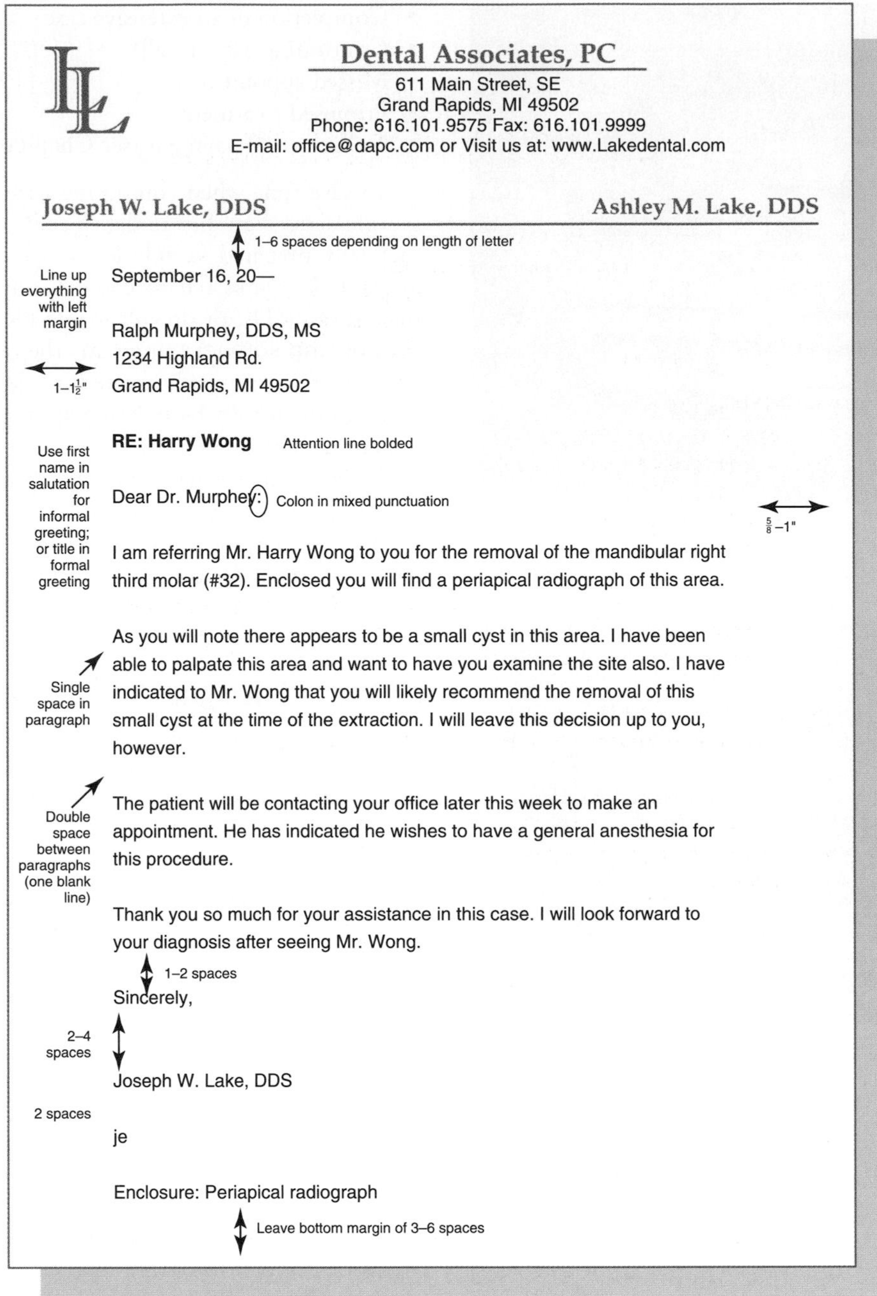
Dental Associates, PC
611 Main Street, SE
Grand Rapids, MI 49502
Phone: 616.101.9575 Fax: 616.101.9999
E-mail: office@dapc.com or Visit us at: www.Lakedental.com

Joseph W. Lake, DDS Ashley M. Lake, DDS

September 16, 20—

Ralph Murphey, DDS, MS
1234 Highland Rd.
Grand Rapids, MI 49502

**RE: Harry Wong**

Dear Dr. Murphey:

I am referring Mr. Harry Wong to you for the removal of the mandibular right third molar (#32). Enclosed you will find a periapical radiograph of this area.

As you will note there appears to be a small cyst in this area. I have been able to palpate this area and want to have you examine the site also. I have indicated to Mr. Wong that you will likely recommend the removal of this small cyst at the time of the extraction. I will leave this decision up to you, however.

The patient will be contacting your office later this week to make an appointment. He has indicated he wishes to have a general anesthesia for this procedure.

Thank you so much for your assistance in this case. I will look forward to your diagnosis after seeing Mr. Wong.

Sincerely,

Joseph W. Lake, DDS

je

Enclosure: Periapical radiograph



**FIG. 61.12** A full-blocked business letter. *(From Finkbeiner BL, Finkbeiner CA: Practice management for the dental team, ed 8, St Louis, 2016, Mosby.)*

- *Semi–Block Letter Format:* The only difference between the semi–block letter and the alternative block letter format is that instead of placing the body text justified left, the first line of each paragraph is indented (Fig. 61.13).
- *Alternative Block Letter Format:* The alternative block letter format moves the return address, date, closing, name, title, and signature to the left side of the page.
- *Simplified Letter Format:* This format has the same properties as the block letter with one exception: The greeting or **salutation** is eliminated. This is a helpful format when you don't know the recipient's gender or marriage status.

### Anatomy of a Business Letter

A business letter contains many crucial parts. Fig. 61.14 provides a visual presentation of a letter along with descriptions for each section.

See Procedure 61.2: Composing a Business Letter.

## Preparing Envelopes for Mailing

With the automation equipment that the United States Postal Service uses to sort letters, there are some right and wrong ways to send an envelope so that it will safely and quickly travel through the U.S. mail.

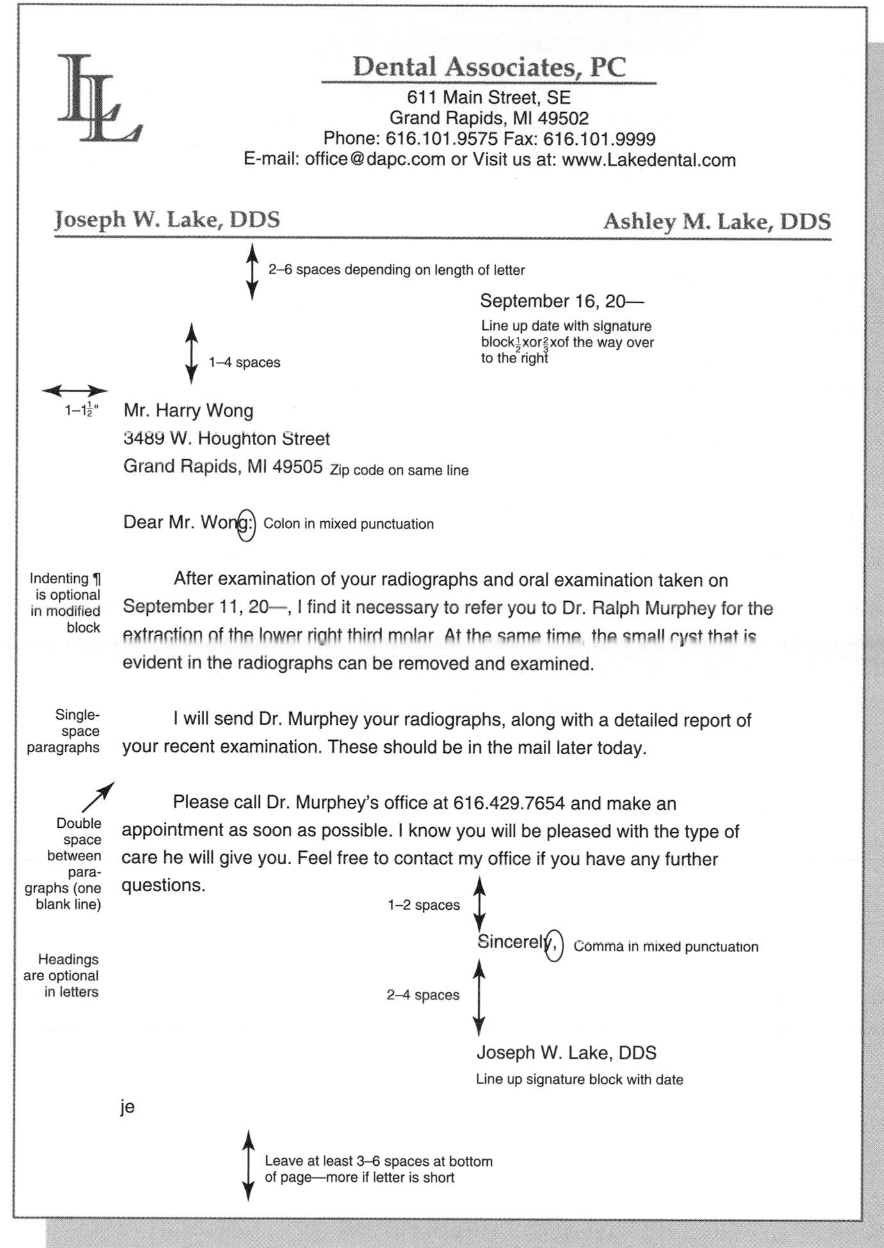

Dental Associates, PC
611 Main Street, SE
Grand Rapids, MI 49502
Phone: 616.101.9575 Fax: 616.101.9999
E-mail: office@dapc.com or Visit us at: www.Lakedental.com

Joseph W. Lake, DDS    Ashley M. Lake, DDS

2–6 spaces depending on length of letter

September 16, 20—
Line up date with signature block $\frac{1}{2}$xor$\frac{2}{3}$xof the way over to the right

1–4 spaces

1–$1\frac{1}{2}$"

Mr. Harry Wong
3489 W. Houghton Street
Grand Rapids, MI 49505 Zip code on same line

Dear Mr. Wong: Colon in mixed punctuation

Indenting ¶ is optional in modified block

After examination of your radiographs and oral examination taken on September 11, 20—, I find it necessary to refer you to Dr. Ralph Murphey for the extraction of the lower right third molar. At the same time, the small cyst that is evident in the radiographs can be removed and examined.

Single-space paragraphs

I will send Dr. Murphey your radiographs, along with a detailed report of your recent examination. These should be in the mail later today.

Double space between paragraphs (one blank line)

Please call Dr. Murphey's office at 616.429.7654 and make an appointment as soon as possible. I know you will be pleased with the type of care he will give you. Feel free to contact my office if you have any further questions.

1–2 spaces

Sincerely, Comma in mixed punctuation

Headings are optional in letters

2–4 spaces

Joseph W. Lake, DDS
Line up signature block with date

je

Leave at least 3–6 spaces at bottom of page—more if letter is short

**FIG. 61.13** A semi-blocked business letter. *(From Finkbeiner BL, Finkbeiner CA: Practice management for the dental team, ed 8, St Louis, 2016, Mosby.)*

Place the correct name and address on the front, placing it roughly in the middle of the envelope. Include the zip code; if you don't know what it is, you can look it up online at USPS.com. Handwriting and nonstandard fonts are harder for automated machinery to read and could cause delay. Also, do not use periods or commas. For example, instead of writing,

john doe
2015 N. 3rd St.
St. Louis, MO. 63110

You should write,

Mr. John Doe
2015 North 3rd Street
St. Louis MO 63110

Be sure your return address is on the envelope in the extreme upper left-hand corner on the front. Apply the correct postage using stamps, a postage meter, or PC postage. The postage should be placed in the upper right-hand corner of the envelope. If you are not sure what the proper postage is, you can check current rates on the USPS.com Web site, or take it to your local post office to have them weigh it and apply the correct postage.

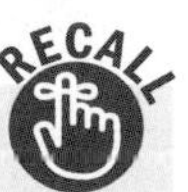


**17** What would be an example of a salutation on a letter?

**18** In addition to the patient, to what other individual might you send a business letter?

## ANATOMY OF A BUSINESS LETTER

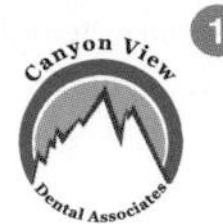

1 Canyon View Dental Associates
4546 North Avery Way
Canyon View, California
Telephone (987) 654-3210

2 April 28, 2016

3 Canyon View Medical Group
2908 Circle Drive
Canyon View, CA 91783
4 Lynn Saunders, M.D.
Director of Pediatric Medicine

5 Dear Dr. Saunders:

6 Subject: NURSING BOTTLE SYNDROME

7 BODY OF THE LETTER

7a Keeping smiles is our business and recently we have treated several young children with rampant decay. We are treating cavities caused by nursing bottle syndrome.

7b As you know, this is caused by giving a baby a bottle with milk, formula, or juice at bedtime. The sugars in these liquids feed the mouth bacteria-producing acids that dissolve tooth enamel in a relatively short period of time.

Babies and young children should be given only water at bedtime or before a nap. If a child falls asleep with a bottle containing anything else, the potential for nursing bottle syndrome increases.

7c Thanks for passing this information to the parents of your young patients. If you need more information or pamphlets, please call us at 987-654-3210.

8 Sincerely,

9 Canyon View Dental Associates

10 Mary A. Edwards, D.D.S.

11 MAE/lg
Enclosure 12

13 CC:

**1 LETTERHEAD**

Identifies the company or dental practice sending the letter. The letterhead style will vary in color, font style, and size. The name and address of the dental practice (company) are included, but telephone number, fax number, email address, web address, or company logo are optional. Traditionally the letterhead is placed at the top of the paper, but this may vary. Letterheads are used only on the first page.

**2 DATELINE**

The date the letter was written is placed a few lines below the letterhead (if the letterhead is at the top of the page). Rules for spacing the dateline are flexible, to allow for a well-balanced, appealing letter.

**3 INSIDE ADDRESS**

The same as the address on the outside of the envelope. When addressing the letter to an individual, several different methods can be used:

1) The name of the intended reader is listed, followed by the company name and address.
2) The company name and address is listed, followed by an attention line to identify the intended reader.

These styles vary and may be determined by the type of computer software being used. Most software packages can print envelopes with information from the inside address.

**4 ATTENTION LINES**

Used to draw attention to the person you wish to read the letter. The full name should be typed and underlined, or typed in all capital letters. Do not include redundant titles such as Dr. Mary A. Edwards, DDS. A person's company title can be placed on a second line, for example:

Lynn Saunders, M.D.
Director of Pediatric Medicine
2908 Circle Drive
Canyon View, CA 91783

**5 SALUTATION**

Greets the reader. When the reader's name is known, it is best to use the name: Dear Ms. Jones, Dear Tom Smith. If the reader is familiar with you and this is a less formal letter, Dear Tom is appropriate. If the reader is unknown, general titles may be used: Dear Sir, Dear Madam, Dear Sir or Madam, Dear Ladies and Gentlemen, Gentleman, To Whom It May Concern.

**6 SUBJECT LINE**

Draws attention to the subject of the letter. Its use is optional. It can be underlined or typed in all capital letters.

**7 BODY OF THE LETTER**

Within the body of the letter there are three sections, the introduction, the main body, and the closing. The introduction is the first paragraph and states the reason you are writing. This section is one paragraph long and should contain a brief list of the important points you will cover in the main body of the letter. The main body gives details of the points that you stated in the introduction. This section is one or two paragraphs long, depending on the number of points that you cover. This section should be concise and to the point.

7a **The introduction** is the first paragraph and states the reason you are writing. This section is one paragraph long and should contain a brief list of the important points you will cover in the main body of the letter.

7b **The main body** gives details of the points that you stated in the introduction. This section is one or two paragraphs long, depending on the number of points that you cover. This section should be concise and to the point.

7c **The closing paragraph** describes the next step or expected outcome. Clearly state what action will be taken. For example, if you are sending a letter of referral to a specialist introducing a patient, inform the dentist what the patient will do next (call for an appointment, wait for the dental office to call and set up an appointment, or explore options and then decide what to do). The closing paragraph should enable the reader to determine what to do next.

**8 COMPLIMENTARY CLOSING**

Closes the letter courteously. Typical complimentary closings are Yours truly, Truly yours, Sincerely yours, and so on. The type of complimentary closing should follow the overall intent of the correspondence. For example, you would not close a collection letter with Best wishes.

**9 COMPANY SIGNATURE**

Identifies the company of the person who is sending the letter and is optional. It is used when the sender of the letter represents the company.

**10 SIGNER'S IDENTIFICATION**

Occurs four lines below the previous item (complimentary close or company signature) to allow room for a signature. Type the signer's name and appropriate title (if needed).

**11 REFERENCE INITIALS**

Identify the sender and the typist of the letter. Type the sender's initials in capital letters, followed by a slash (/) or a colon (:) and the typist's initials in lower case. The purpose is to identify the preparer.

**12 ENCLOSURE REMINDER**

Alerts the reader that there is more to the letter. Use a reminder line when attachments or enclosures are included with the letter.

**13 COPY NOTATION**

Notifies the reader that a copy of the document is being forwarded to another party. CC is the notation used. It stands for "carbon copy" or "computer copy" and states that a copy of the letter has been forwarded to the recipient whose name follows the CC notation.

**FIG. 61.14** Anatomy of a business letter. *(From Gaylor LJ: The administrative dental assistant, ed 4, St Louis, 2017, Elsevier.)*

## Marketing Your Dental Practice

The term **marketing** usually brings to mind large advertising campaigns; however, that is not how this term applies to dentistry. In dentistry, marketing encompasses all activities involved in attracting new patients to the practice and retaining satisfied ones. Communication skills are an essential part of the marketing of a dental practice.

Initiation and development of a marketing plan are the responsibilities of the dentist; however, for a marketing plan to be successful, all members of the dental team must be actively and enthusiastically involved in planning, implementing, and monitoring that plan.

Although this is a team effort, one person (usually the office manager or the business assistant) may be given responsibility for ensuring the overall smooth functioning of the marketing program.

## Goals of Practice Marketing

A primary goal of any marketing plan is to create a positive image of the practice as a place where patients receive quality treatment in a caring atmosphere. The positive and cooperative attitudes of all staff members are vital in successfully creating this image; however, the business assistant is a key person because he or she usually has the all-important first contact with the patient.

A secondary goal is to enroll new patients at the practice. An important part of achieving this goal is determining the perceived needs of potential patients and seeking out ways to meet these needs.

## Logistics of Marketing

Most practices with successful marketing programs attribute this success to good organization, attention to detail, determination of a budget, and tracking of the results.

### The Plan

For a marketing plan to succeed, written goals and dates must be established. Attention to detail is essential.

### Marketing Budget

The average amount of investment budgeted by dentists for a practice marketing plan ranges between 3 and 5 percent of the previous year's gross revenues.

### Tracking Responses

Tracking determines the success of the marketing plan and provides a response to each marketing activity. This may be accomplished by counting the number of new patient referrals that result from a marketing promotion; for example, "Thirty new patients entered the practice after [a specific] marketing event" is a measurable response regarding success.

## Types of Practice Marketing

**External marketing** activities are those that take place outside of the office that are directed to reach people who are not patients. It can include any of the following tools:

- Advertising
- Web site
- Blog
- Social media marketing
- Marketing material such as business cards, letterhead, and logo
- Health fairs
- Presentations to schoolchildren or senior citizen groups

**Internal marketing** strategies are those activities and promotions that are targeted toward current patients of the practice. These also may require staff participation. Such activities may include, but are not limited to, the following (Fig. 61.15):

- Publishing a practice newsletter
- Developing promotional materials for insertion into monthly statements
- Sending flowers or other appropriate "thank you" gifts to those who refer new patients to the practice
- Sending birthday or other special occasion cards to patients
- Sponsoring giveaways, office open houses, and other promotional events

### Dental Office Newsletter

A newsletter represents a valuable communication tool for the practice. Patients enjoy reading about newly available techniques and learning about the "human" side of the practice. The purposes of a practice newsletter include the following:

- Keeping patients aware of new technology and treatment advances
- Keeping in touch with the dentist and members of the dental team
- Listing patients' names as referral sources or contest winners (*Note:* Names are used *only* with patients' permission.)
- Announcing other changes that have taken place within the practice

Most practices will publish a newsletter for their patients on a quarterly basis. A number of professional newsletter preparation organizations are available to produce a newsletter that incorporates the dentist's masthead and practice information.

### Patient Education Materials

Printed pamphlets, brochures, and statement "stuffers" are printed communication tools that have been used successfully by many dental practices. The American Dental Association provides a series of educational brochures that can be purchased and have available for your patients. These can be personalized with your office information, in a different language, and cover all aspects of the type of dentistry that is practiced in the office.

## Services

**Preventive Services**
- Comprehensive oral examination with cancer screening
- Routine dental cleaning
- Periodontal maintenance
- Sealants

**Restorative Cosmetic Services**
- Bleaching
- Bonding
- Porcelain Crowns
- Implants
- Bridges
- Partial Dentures
- Full Dentures

**Other Services**
- Fresh Breath Evaluation and Treatment
- Periodontal Services
- Endodontics
- Extractions

## Prescriptions

Please remember that all prescriptions and authorizations for renewals should be requested during normal office hours.

## Financial & Insurance Policies

We make every effort to keep the costs down while maintaining a high level of professional care. If your treatment program requires several visits, you will be given an estimate. We accept all major credit cards and also offer financing options.

Please bring your insurance plan information with you on your first visit. We will be happy to submit your insurance forms for you. All co-pays or deductibles will be due at the time services are rendered and it will be your responsibility to pay any remaining balance after insurance benefits have been credited.

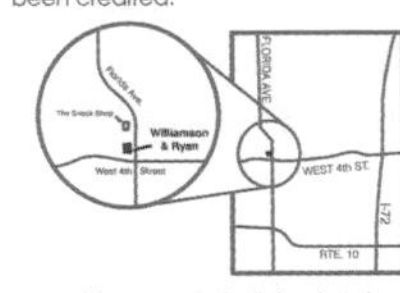

*We are conveniently located at* ***1234 West 4th Street*** *in Champaign. We are on the west side of Florida Ave. and next to "The Snack Shop."*

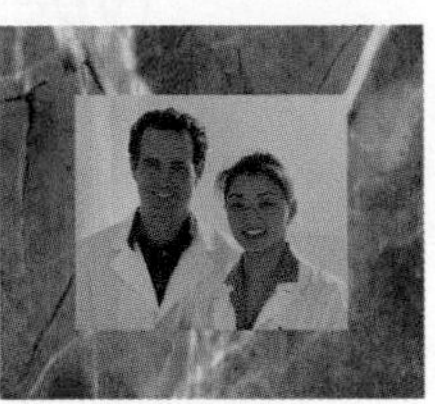

*Williamson & Ryan*

*Dentistry for all Ages*

*Dr. Derek R. Williamson*

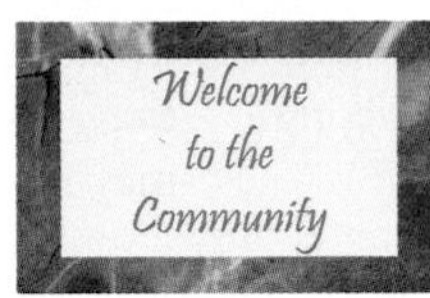


We are committed to providing optimum care for all our patients in a compassionate manner. Your health and comfort are foremost in our minds. We will thoroughly evaluate your dental needs and make recommendations to provide you with a complete care program to achieve your goals.

Together we know how important your smile can be to project confidence, optimism, and openness. We're here to provide comfortable dental care for the whole family and have been serving the Champaign-Urbana area for over 10 years. Modern technology and education provide many options to improve your smile and dental health.

Our office has made professional and financial commitments to provide to you safe and effective dental care. We will continue to update our techniques and procedures as necessary.

## Technology

We take great pride in our professionalism through continuing education. We strive to stay current with the latest dental techniques and services available.

Air abrasion, no drill/no needle cavity preparation, is one of the newest technological advancements. It allows for removal of decay without the discomfort associated with injections or the use of a drill. Patients who have experienced this new cavity preparation agree that it is much more pleasant than the traditional form of treatment.

Digital radiographs use 95% less radiation than traditional x-rays and allow us to see, in sharp vivid detail, the radiograph on the computer monitor within seconds. We also use our intra-oral camera, and our laser fluorescence system for cavity detection, which has helped us to diagnose hidden decay without x-rays.

Not only do we take pride in our technology in the office, but, we also take pride in how we attempt to educate our patients. We have many different patient brochures to help address questions which you might have and to help you make informed decisions about your dental care.

## Appointments

We see all patients on an appointment basis, and ask that you call and schedule an appointment in advance. We also ask that if you must cancel your appointment that you give us 24 hours notice so that your previously reserved time might be made available for another patient. If an emergency should arise; please call our office, even if it is not our normal working hours. Our answering service will notify us and we will contact you as soon as possible.

On your first visit we will have you fill out a questionnaire which includes your medical and dental history. We will then do a complete exam of your teeth, gums, and supporting bones. After your exam, we will ask you a few questions about what your goal is in dental care - whether it is to simply maintain your teeth and smile, or to

## Office Hours

| | |
|---|---|
| 8:00 - 5:00 | Monday, Wednesday & Friday |
| 10:00 - 7:00 | Tuesday & Thursday |
| 9:00 - 1:00 | Saturday |

**FIG. 61.15** An example of a dental practice brochure for marketing. *(Courtesy Patterson Dental, St Paul, MN.)*

RECALL

**19** Which members of the dental office team should be involved in marketing of the practice?
**20** What percentage of the office's gross revenue should be invested in marketing?
**21** Give an example of an external marketing activity.

**■ Patient Education** The dental team serves as the front door to a practice. As a member of the team, everything you say and do represents the dentist and the practice. The entire staff should work as a team to create an atmosphere of patient confidence and trust. Offer information about appointment schedules, billing, insurance services, phone hours, office hours, and emergency coverage. Information about fees and office policies should be readily available to patients. The more information you can offer to your patients, the more they will feel confident about care received at the dental practice. ■

**■ Eye to the Future** Technology today allows us to communicate with people very easily. For example, a dental practice can maintain its own Web site that introduces the staff, presents philosophies of practice, and describes the specialty or focus of the practice. Through use of the Internet, most information will be conveyed via email in the future. As patients update their patient registration forms, they will be required to include their email address. The business assistant then can email appointment reminders, recall notifications, insurance information, and billing questions. ■

**■ Legal and Ethical Implications** Remember that all types of communication with patients are confidential, whether it is conveyed by phone, through written letters, or via the documentation in a patient's record. The Health Insurance Portability and Accountability Act (HIPAA) of 1996 has increased our awareness of privacy in speaking with a patient. Make sure that you are discreet in discussing specific treatment or financial information. Every means of communication should project a professional image. ■

**■ Critical Thinking**

1. Go through your personal "junk mail"; select examples that show a powerful marketing technique that gets your attention.

2. Write down a specific dialogue that you would use when answering the phone in a dental office.
3. Think back to your last visit to the dentist or doctor, and discuss how the business tasks of the office were handled. Describe how the reception area was maintained and how staff members treated one another.
4. List possible reasons why a patient might feel apprehensive about his or her visit to the dentist, and describe how you could make the visit less stressful.
5. Have you ever observed a situation in which someone was being discriminated against by another person? If so, describe the situation and your feelings, and suggest ways that this problem could have been prevented. ■

## PROCEDURE 61.1

## Answering the Phone

### EQUIPMENT AND SUPPLIES

- ✓ Phone
- ✓ Message pad
- ✓ Pen or pencil
- ✓ Appointment book

### PROCEDURAL STEPS

1 Answer the phone on the first ring.

**PURPOSE** This shows the patient that your office is prompt and ready to please.

2 Speak directly into the receiver with your mouth approximately 1 inch from the mouthpiece.

3 Identify the office and yourself.

**PURPOSE** This lets the caller know whether he or she has reached the correct number.

4 Acknowledge the caller by name.

**PURPOSE** This shows interest in the caller and initiates the first relationship.

5 Follow through on the caller's request by answering specific questions about new patient information, appointments, or financial information.

6 Take a message if appropriate.

7 Complete the call in a professional manner, and replace the receiver after you hear that the caller has done so.

## PROCEDURE 61.2

## Composing a Business Letter

### EQUIPMENT AND SUPPLIES

- ✓ Computer
- ✓ Letterhead paper
- ✓ Pen

### PROCEDURAL STEPS

1 Using your word processing document set your margins, font, spacing, and order of the letter (if this is a function of your particular software).

2 Prepare a draft of the letter on the computer; then have a peer review it and make comments.

**PURPOSE** This provides practice in writing skills and helps you to develop your verbal and nonverbal skills with the help of another person.

3 Check the draft for correct information, grammar, spelling, and punctuation.

4 Create the final letter from the corrected draft.

5 Type your name and sign by hand (or, if you are writing the letter for someone else, type the sender's name at the closing, and have that person sign by hand).

62

# Business Operating Systems

## KEY TERMS

**Active files** Files of patients who have been seen within the past 2 to 3 years.
**Buffer time** Time reserved on the daily schedule for emergency patients.
**Call list** List of patients who can come in for an appointment on short notice.
**Chronologic file** Filing system that divides materials into months (and possibly days of the month).
**Cross-reference file** A file in which each item is listed in alphabetic order by name and its document number is provided.
**Daily schedule** Printed schedule that is copied and placed throughout the office for viewing by staff only.
**Downtime** Waiting period between patient procedures.
**File guides** An insert placed between files that displays the letters or numbers of the patient records that follow it.
**Filing** The act of classifying and arranging records to be easily retrieved when needed.
**Inactive files** Files of patients who have not been seen over the past 3 years.
**Lead time** A time estimate that allows for delays in ordering or shipping of materials.
**Ledger** A financial statement that documents all account transactions.
**Outguide** Device used for a filing system; similar to a bookmark.
**Patient of record** Individual who has been examined and diagnosed by the dentist and for whom treatment has been planned.
**Purchase order** A form that authorizes the purchase of products from a supplier.
**Rate of use** The quantity of a product that is used within a given time.
**Reorder tags** A notation system that is used when the supply of a particular item is getting low and the item must be reordered.
**Requisition (re-kwi-ZI-shun)** A formal request for supplies.
**Shelf life** How long a product may be stored before use.
**Units of time** Time increments used in planning appointments.
**Want list** A list of supplies to be ordered and questions to be asked of the representative.
**Warranty** A written statement that explains the manufacturer's responsibility for replacing and repairing a particular product.

## LEARNING OUTCOMES

*On completion of this chapter, the student will be able to achieve the following objectives:*

1. Pronounce, define, and spell the key terms.
2. Discuss the elements of the operating procedure manual.
3. Discuss computer applications in the dental office.
4. Discuss record keeping, including types of practice records and files.
5. Discuss guidelines to efficient filing and describe how to use these filing systems: alphabetic, color-coded, numeric (cross-reference), chronologic, and electronic.
6. Describe the process of scheduling appointments for maximum productivity.
7. Identify the types of preventive recall systems and state the benefits of each.
8. Discuss the management of inventory systems.
9. Explain the components of the dental supply budget.
10. Discuss the record keeping necessary for repairing and maintaining dental equipment.

## ELECTRONIC RESOURCES

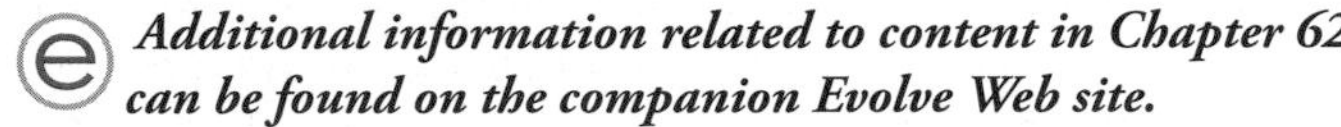

***Additional information related to content in Chapter 62 can be found on the companion Evolve Web site.***

- Dentrix Exercise
- Practice Quiz

The business office, also referred to as the "front office," is the core of the business side of the dental practice. For a dental practice to be successful, effective management is necessary to achieve organizational goals, team-oriented employee satisfaction, and financial profits. This chapter introduces business operating systems that are vital to the day-to-day operations of a dental practice. Efficient and effective business systems can enhance productivity, decrease stress, and maximize patient confidence.

The person responsible for the business of the office is titled the *administrative assistant* or *business assistant.* Responsibilities are divided differently, depending on the size of the practice; a smaller practice would commonly have one individual who would handle all of the functions, and in some larger practices, responsibilities would be divided among the receptionist, bookkeeper, appointment clerk, file clerk, and insurance clerk. These responsibilities can include, but are not limited to, the following:

- Greeting patients and answering the telephone
- Scheduling patients
- Managing patient records
- Managing accounts receivable and accounts payable
- Managing the recall and inventory control systems
- Overseeing and monitoring practice marketing activities
- Managing payroll
- Presenting fees and making financial arrangements to patients
- Overseeing insurance submissions

## Operating Procedure Manual

For a dental practice to run smoothly, it is essential to have an office procedure manual on hand. This manual will include policies and procedures that the dentist has defined in writing for the staff to follow within the practice. The manual should outline individual job descriptions for business and clinical personnel. Information included in this office manual may include, but is not limited to, the following:

- Objective or purpose of the manual
- Office communications
- Staff policies
- Employment policies
- Office records
- Health Insurance Portability and Accountability Act (HIPAA) procedures
- Occupational Safety and Health Administration (OSHA) and infection control policy
- Clinical procedures
- Professional organizations

The American Dental Association (ADA) offers a *Practical Guide to Creating an Employee Office Manual.* This program assists dental practices in creating customized employee office manuals. Written and reviewed by a team of ADA professionals, *Creating an Employee Office Manual* addresses many common employment issues and contains sample forms, checklists, policies, and procedures. These documents can be acquired in a Microsoft Word format with an accompanying CD-ROM for quick and easy customization for each dental practice's unique needs. Specific features include updated sample job descriptions and interview questions; policies on using cell phones, electronic communications, and social media—both on and off the clock; patient management; sections on HIPAA and OSHA policies; employee performance evaluation forms; and a section on natural disaster preparation.

### HIPAA Compliance

The Health Insurance Portability and Accountability Act of 1996 (commonly known as HIPAA) was adopted to enhance and protect the rights of patients. Knowing state and federal law requirements eases implementation of this act into the dental practice.

The ADA has played an integral part in the implementation of HIPAA. Through involvement of the ADA, dental practices have acquired the flexibility to create their own privacy procedures tailored to fit the size and needs of the practice on an individual basis.

The dentist must follow a specific format when putting HIPAA policies into practice. The dental staff must be informed of specific security and confidentiality issues. HIPAA-related training of existing dental staff must be reinforced continuously. New staff is trained as soon as possible.

#### *HIPAA Privacy Compliance List*

Specific areas included in the procedure manual include the following:

- **Know the law.** Become familiar with HIPAA regulations. Know the requirements of your state privacy laws.
- **Adopt or create the required forms** to put into action the privacy policies and procedures of the practice.
- **Train dental staff** regarding privacy policies and procedures, and designate a privacy officer and a contact person to receive complaints. Make sure to document the training provided.
- **Notify patients of the new policies** by posting and distributing a Notice of Privacy Practice, and obtain written permission to enforce this through the signed patient's Acknowledgment of Receipt of Notice of Privacy Practice.
- **Make sure that policies and procedures are fully implemented and up to date .** If changes have to be made, make sure modifications are documented.

### Personnel Manual

Personnel issues may be discussed in the employment section of the office procedure manual or in a separate personnel manual. Personnel topics include a job description for each employee, details regarding pay periods and working hours, and information concerning employee benefits such as paid holidays, vacation, and sick leave. Also included should be policies on provisional employment, maternity leave, disciplinary measures, sexual harassment, and termination.

Some practices use a commercially prepared manual, whereas others customize their own personnel manual. Whichever type is preferred, it is helpful to use a ring binder, which allows pages to be added or deleted as office policy is updated or information becomes obsolete. To prevent miscommunication among staff, make sure that each new employee reviews the office manual during the first week of employment, and that all employees continue to review any new information that is added. Any areas that are not clear should be addressed during that time.

## Computer Applications in the Dental Office

Computers continue to be used in the dental practice to replace many of the manual tasks that were completed by the business assistant for so many years. The computer, which can receive, store, process, and send information, can handle nearly all the business aspects of the practice (Fig. 62.1). Specific applications that the computer can handle in a dental practice include the following:

- Appointment scheduling
- Electronic patient records
- Word processing
- Networking and marketing
- Bookkeeping tasks
- Database management
- Billing and collection
- Patient ledger
- Processing of insurance claims

## Characteristics of the Computer

A computer is a programmable machine that consists of two main components: (1) the **hardware** that houses the wires, transistors, and circuits and responds to a specific set of instructions, and (2) the **software,** which introduces data to the hardware to execute a list of instructions.

A general purpose computer requires the following hardware components:

- **Memory,** which enables a computer to store temporary data and programs.
- **Central processing unit (CPU),** also referred to as the heart of the computer. This is the component that actually executes instructions.
- **Mass storage device,** which allows the computer to permanently retain large quantities of data. An example of this is a disc drive.
- **Input device,** which includes the keyboard and the mouse. The input device is a channel through which data and instructions enter a computer.
- **Output device,** which is a display screen and printer that allow you to see what the computer has accomplished.

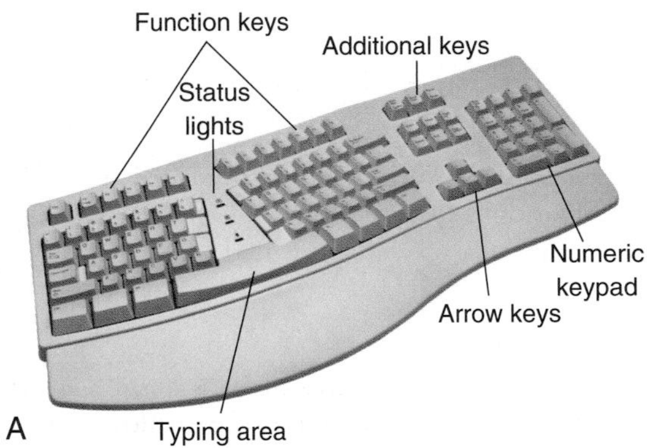


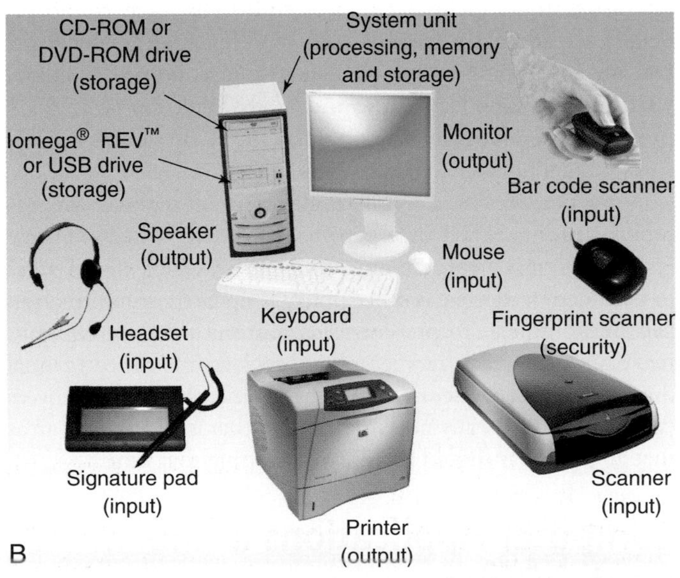


**FIG. 62.1** A, Computer keyboard. B, Computer system. *(A, From Finkbeiner BL, Finkbeiner CA: Practice management for the dental team, ed 7, St Louis, 2011, Mosby. B, Courtesy Patterson Dental, St Paul, MN.)*

RECALL

1. Is overseeing financial activities the responsibility of the clinical assistant or the business assistant?
2. What is the best way for a new employee to learn about office protocol?
3. What continues to replace "handwritten" operating procedures in the handling of business?

# Record Keeping

Maintenance of adequate records is one of the business assistant's most important responsibilities. Because so much information is maintained in a hard copy or electronic file, the office must decide which types of records and filing system best suit the needs of the practice. Maintenance of accurate and complete records is a sign of quality care.

## Types of Records and Files

### *Patient Dental Records*

The patient record includes multiple forms. Each form is sequenced and includes the patient registration form, the medical and dental history form, examination findings, diagnosis and treatment plans, a record of treatment provided, correspondence, consent forms, and radiographs. (Chapter 26 provides a detailed explanation of the forms within a patient record.)

### *Patient Financial Records*

Financial information regarding a patient's account is maintained separately as part of the practice business records. This information should never be filed with patient clinical records.

A patient statement, or **ledger**, contains the financial information for each patient or family (Fig. 62.2). The electronic ledger works just like a paper ledger (Fig. 62.3). You can enter payments, file claims, and print statements and reminder letters all from one location. Insurance benefits are automatically updated as you enter payments, and the system will accurately calculate the carrier

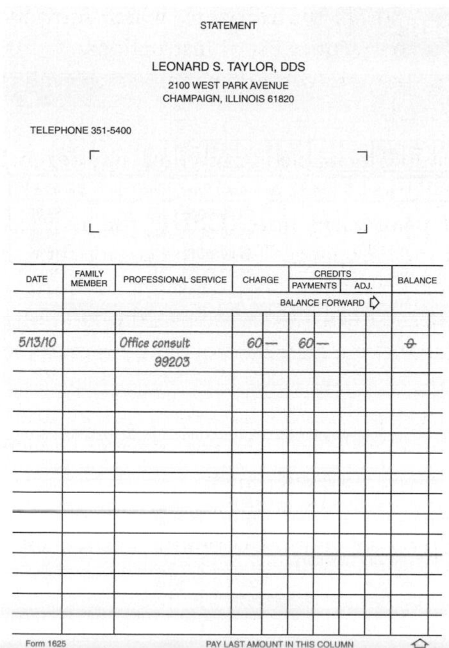

STATEMENT

LEONARD S. TAYLOR, DDS
2100 WEST PARK AVENUE
CHAMPAIGN, ILLINOIS 61820

TELEPHONE 351-5400

| DATE | FAMILY MEMBER | PROFESSIONAL SERVICE | CHARGE | CREDITS PAYMENTS | CREDITS ADJ. | BALANCE |
|---|---|---|---|---|---|---|
| | | | | BALANCE FORWARD | | |
| 5/13/10 | | Office consult 99203 | 60— | 60— | | -0- |

Form 1625 PAY LAST AMOUNT IN THIS COLUMN

**FIG. 62.2** Patient ledger. *(Courtesy Patterson Dental, St Paul, MN.)*

portion of the fee each time a treatment plan is entered. An automatic alert will even appear if secondary insurance coverage exists.

### Practice Business Records

Accurate business and financial records enable the business assistant to operate the practice in a well-organized and business-like manner. These records are either stored through the use of a subject file system, under specific categories such as "accounts receivable" and "business office supplies," or they are stored electronically. Business records include, but are not limited to, the following (Fig. 62.4):

- Accounts receivable records
- Practice expenses awaiting payment
- Expense records (receipts and paid bills)
- Payroll records
- Business correspondence
- Canceled checks and bank statements
- Records of income and expenses
- Financial statements, tax records, and possibly corporate records
- Computer printouts of practice reports
- Personnel records

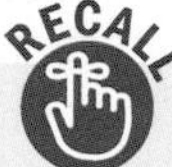


4 What is another term that is used for a patient statement?

## Filing Systems

Even if a dental office has transitioned to an electronic system, there may be specific records for which a dental office will continue to use a traditional filing system. **Filing** is the method of classifying and arranging records so that they are preserved safely and can be quickly retrieved when needed.

## Basic Filing Methods

The basic methods of filing used in dental offices are alphabetic by last name, color coding, numeric, and chronologic.

### Alphabetic

The alphabetic filing system is by far the easiest and most commonly used system for filing patient records and ledger cards. In alphabetic filing, all items are filed in straight alphabetic (A-B-C) order in accordance with the basic rules of indexing. Standard rules must be followed for this system (Fig. 62.5). Table 62.1 provides the rules for alphabetic filing.

### Color Coding

Color coding is used to make filing and retrieval of patient records easier and faster (Fig. 62.6). With color coding, the tabs combine colors and letters, which are used to indicate the first two letters of the patient's last name. In addition to speeding up filing and finding of records, color coding makes it easier to spot a misfiled record. Color coding may be used with numeric filing; in this case, the color tabs are labeled with the last two digits of the chart number.

### Numeric

In numeric filing, each patient record or document is assigned a number. In straight numeric filing, all items are filed in strict 1-2-3 order. Numeric filing is used most often for patient records in a large group practice. Through this system, to locate items you must maintain a **cross-reference file**, in which each item is listed in alphabetic order by name along with its document number.

### Chronologic

A **chronologic file** can be divided into months, quarters, and years. This type of file may be used for the recall system or as a "reminder" system for miscellaneous tasks, such as routine maintenance, which must be performed at specific times during the year. Other special files such as cross-reference files, inventory control files, and short-notice appointment lists may be maintained for various purposes (Fig. 62.7).

### Electronic

You most likely will use at least one type of electronic filing or storage system. Electronic files are stored on the computer's hard drive (at least temporarily); they should be stored additionally on a zip drive or CD. To keep track of these files, label each unit with a subject name or number (Fig. 62.8).

## Guidelines for Efficient Filing

- **Keep the filing system simple.** The simpler the system, the easier it is to work with.
- **Label folders clearly.** Each file folder should have a neatly typed label that shows the patient's full name or subject. This saves time and avoids having to go through the chart to make certain that you have the right one. Use an adequate number of **file guides**. Approximately 1 file guide should be used for every 5 to 10 folders, depending on the size of the folders.

**ANATOMY OF AN ELECTRONIC LEDGER**

Dentrix Ledger + History - Crosby, Brent L [CR001]

File Options View Transaction Insurance Print Month End Help

| Date | Name | Tooth | Surface | Check # | Code | * | Description | N | R | D | M | Amount | Prov | Ins | Balance |
|---|---|---|---|---|---|---|---|---|---|---|---|---|---|---|---|
| 08/02/2010 | Brent L Crosby | | | | D0274 | | Bitewing Four Image | ♪ | | | | 59.00 | DDS1 | No | 59.00 |
| 08/02/2010 | Brent L Crosby | | | | D1110 | | Prophylaxis-adult | ♪ | | | | 85.00 | DDS1 | No | 144.00 |
| 08/04/2014 | Brent L Crosby | | | | D0120 | | Periodic oral evaluation | ♪ | | | △ | 46.00 | DDS1 | No | 190.00 |
| 02/02/2015 | Brent L Crosby | | | | D0120 | | Periodic oral evaluation | ♪ | | | △ | 46.00 | DDS1 | No | 236.00 |
| 04/17/2015 | Brent L Crosby | 18 | | | D2792 | | Crown-full cast noble metal | ♪ | | | | 950.00 | DDS1 | No | 1186.00 |
| 08/02/2015 | Brent L Crosby | | | | D0120 | | Periodic oral evaluation | ♪ | | D | △ | 46.00 | DDS1 | No | 1232.00 |

1

2A

| 0-->30 | 31-->60 | 61-->90 | 91--> | Family Balance |
|---|---|---|---|---|
| 1232.00 | 0.00 | 0.00 | 0.00 | 1232.00 |

3

| | |
|---|---|
| Today's Charges | 950.00 |
| Est. Dental Ins. Portion | 160.00 |
| Est. Patient Portion | 790.00 |

2

Billing Type (1) Standard Billing - finance charges
Last Payment 0.00 Date
Last Ins. Payment 0.00 Date
Last Statement Date
Outstanding Billed to Medical/Dental 0.00/950.00
Expected from Dental Insurance * 160.00
Family Portion of Balance * 1072.00
* Based on Pending Claims and Today's Charges

4

Payment Agreement Summary
Monthly Pmt 50.00 Pmt Due 100.00
Amt Past Due 0.00 Due Date 10/01/2004

5

Future Due Payment Plans Summary
Original Bal. 500.00 Payment 100.00
Remain Bal. 500.00 Due Date Fri, 10th

1 The Transaction Log lists all transactions posted to the patient/family's account. For each transaction, the Ledger lists the date, patient or guarantor name, tooth number (when applicable), procedure code or type, a description, amount of the transaction, and the transaction provider. It also indicates whether or not insurance has been billed. Several symbols can appear in the Description column to provide additional information about the transaction.

2 Account Information includes the Billing Type, the amount and date of the last guarantor payment, and the amount and date of the last insurance payment. The Last Statement Date is the last time a Billing Statement was printed for the account. Outstanding Billed to Insurance is the estimated amount that insurance will pay on all outstanding dental claims. Family Portion of Balance is the estimated amount the patient will owe after insurance has paid.

2A The account balance is shown in the appropriate aging bracket(s). The total account balance is shown under Family Balance.

3 Today's Charges is the total of all transactions with today's date. Est. Dental Ins. Portion is the estimated amount that dental insurance will pay according to the coverage setup in the Family File. Est. Patient Portion is the estimated amount the patient owes according to the coverage setup in the Family File.

4 If a Payment Agreement exists for the account, the current status of the agreement is shown here.

5 If a Future Due Payment Plan exists for the account, the current status of the payment plan is shown here.

**FIG. 62.3** Anatomy of an electronic ledger. *(From Gaylor LJ: The administrative dental assistant, ed 4, St Louis, 2016, Elsevier. Dentrix screen capture courtesy Henry Schein Practice Solutions, American Fork, UT.)*

- **Leave adequate working space within each file.** If too little space is allowed for each file, papers become tightly wedged, which slows the process of filing, makes records more difficult to find, and may damage filed materials. Leave at least 4 inches of working space on each shelf or in each drawer.
- **Label shelves or drawers.** All files should be clearly, neatly, and accurately labeled as to the contents or other appropriate designation.
- **Use outguides.** An **outguide** is like a bookmark for the filing system. When a folder is removed from the file, place an outguide to mark its place. This makes it faster to return records to the file and easy to spot where records are missing (Fig. 62.9).
- **Presort.** Presorting folders into approximate order before you start to file will speed the filing process.

## Active and Inactive Files

Patient records are **permanent records** of the dental practice, which means they should never be discarded or destroyed without the dentist's specific instruction. To reduce the number of charts that must be sorted through daily, many practices will subdivide patient records into active and inactive files.

**Active files** are files of patients who have been seen recently (usually within the past 2 to 3 years). These are maintained in the areas of easiest accessibility.

**Inactive files** are records of patients who have not been seen in the last 3 years. These files are maintained in a less convenient area but can be accessed if needed.

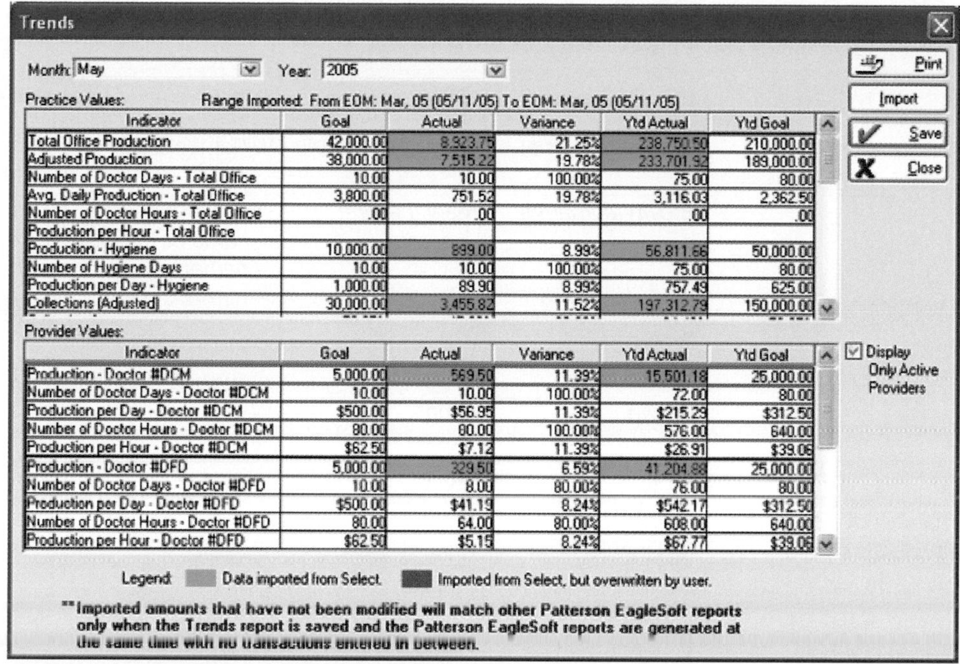


| Indicator | Goal | Actual | Variance | Ytd Actual | Ytd Goal |
|---|---|---|---|---|---|
| Total Office Production | 42,000.00 | 8,923.75 | 21.25% | 238,750.50 | 210,000.00 |
| Adjusted Production | 38,000.00 | 7,515.22 | 19.78% | 233,701.92 | 189,000.00 |
| Number of Doctor Days - Total Office | 10.00 | 10.00 | 100.00% | 75.00 | 80.00 |
| Avg. Daily Production - Total Office | 3,800.00 | 751.52 | 19.78% | 3,116.03 | 2,362.50 |
| Number of Doctor Hours - Total Office | .00 | .00 | | .00 | .00 |
| Production per Hour - Total Office | | | | | |
| Production - Hygiene | 10,000.00 | 899.00 | 8.99% | 56,811.66 | 50,000.00 |
| Number of Hygiene Days | 10.00 | 10.00 | 100.00% | 75.00 | 80.00 |
| Production per Day - Hygiene | 1,000.00 | 89.90 | 8.99% | 757.49 | 625.00 |
| Collections (Adjusted) | 30,000.00 | 3,455.82 | 11.52% | 197,312.79 | 150,000.00 |

| Indicator | Goal | Actual | Variance | Ytd Actual | Ytd Goal |
|---|---|---|---|---|---|
| Production - Doctor #DCM | 5,000.00 | 569.50 | 11.39% | 15,501.18 | 25,000.00 |
| Number of Doctor Days - Doctor #DCM | 10.00 | 10.00 | 100.00% | 72.00 | 80.00 |
| Production per Day - Doctor #DCM | $500.00 | $56.95 | 11.39% | $215.29 | $312.50 |
| Number of Doctor Hours - Doctor #DCM | 80.00 | 80.00 | 100.00% | 576.00 | 640.00 |
| Production per Hour - Doctor #DCM | $62.50 | $7.12 | 11.39% | $26.91 | $39.06 |
| Production - Doctor #DFD | 5,000.00 | 329.50 | 6.59% | 41,204.88 | 25,000.00 |
| Number of Doctor Days - Doctor #DFD | 10.00 | 8.00 | 80.00% | 76.00 | 80.00 |
| Production per Day - Doctor #DFD | $500.00 | $41.19 | 8.24% | $542.17 | $312.50 |
| Number of Doctor Hours - Doctor #DFD | 80.00 | 64.00 | 80.00% | 608.00 | 640.00 |
| Production per Hour - Doctor #DFD | $62.50 | $5.15 | 8.24% | $67.77 | $39.06 |

**FIG. 62.4** An example of a software program to show the business side of a practice. *(Courtesy Patterson Dental, St Paul, MN.)*

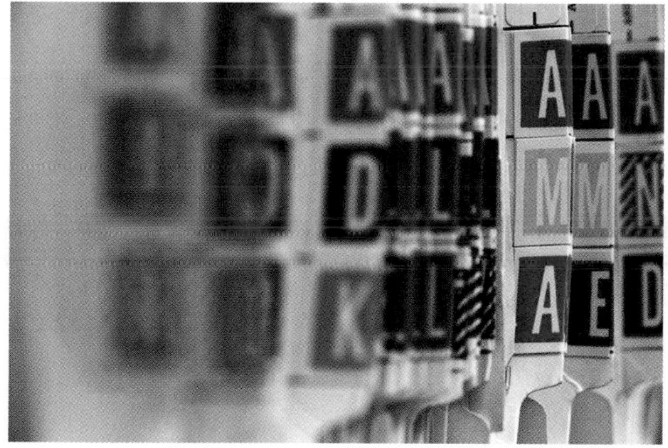

**FIG. 62.5** Keep filing systems simple. *(From Proctor DB et al: Kinn's the medical assistant: an applied learning approach, ed 13, St Louis, 2017, Elsevier.)*

## Purge Tabs

Color-coded purge tabs, also known as **aging tabs,** make it easier to sort records into active and inactive categories. For example, at a patient's first visit in 2016, a red 2016 tag is placed on the folder. At the first visit in 2017, a green 2017 tag is placed over the previous one. When it is time to sort out the charts for all patients not seen since 2016, it is easy to go through the file and quickly identify those folders still labeled with only a red 2016 tag.

## Record Protection and Confidentiality

The destruction of records through loss, fire, or other catastrophe could seriously handicap a dental practice. For this reason, it is vital that all records be protected at all times. Patient records and all other practice information are confidential and should be treated with appropriate care.

### HIPAA Electronic Safeguards

Safeguards must be put in place to ensure the confidentiality and protection of electronic files. The specific protocol of HIPAA compliance states that the dental office must have physical and technical safeguards to ensure the safety and confidentiality of the patient's personal information. Passwords are put into practice and changed often. It is important to maintain up-to-date antivirus protection software on your computer system. Firewalls should be constructed if you are working from a network. Also, computer screens in the business area must not be in plain sight of patients. Even if you are certain that your computer screen is out of public sight, never leave patient files open on your screen unless you are currently using them. Once you have finished using a file, close it.

### Protecting Electronic Files

If the practice system is computerized, it is advisable to back up all files at the end of each business day. To *back up* means to make a copy of the computer files. The backup file is then available if there is a problem with the system. Many practices keep two sets of backup files: one set in the office and a second set in a safe place outside of the office. Thus in the event of fire or other catastrophe, a remaining set of files is available.

### Protecting Paper Files

Never leave paper records outside their appropriate file space. As you finish using a record, return it to its proper place. When leaving for the day, make certain that all records are protected in file cabinets and that the cabinets are properly closed. Precautions also

**TABLE 62.1** Indexing* Rules for Alphabetic† Filing

| Indexing Rules | Unit 1‡ (Caption)§ | Unit 2 | Unit 3 | Unit 4 |
|---|---|---|---|---|
| Names | Brown *(surname)* | John *(first name)* | William *(middle name)* | Senior *(term denoting seniority)* |
| Married woman | Brown *(surname)* | Mary *(her first name)* | Harris *(her middle name or maiden name)* | Mrs. John W. *(for information only, not an indexing unit)* |
| Nothing comes before something | Brown | | | |
| | Brown | J. | | |
| | Brown | John | | |
| | Brown | John | W. | |
| | Brown | John | William | |
| | Brown | John | William | Senior |
| The prefix is part of surname, not a separate unit *(maintain strict alphabetic order!)* | Macdonald<br>McDonald | Peter<br>Paul | | |
| Abbreviated prefix *(index as if spelled out)* | St. Andrew *(Saint Andrew)* | Francis | Lee | |
| Hyphenated names (treat as one unit) | Vaughan-Eames | Henry | David | |
| Titles are not indexing units | Douglass | James | Richard | Ph.D. *(for information only, not for indexing)* |

*Indexing is the process of selecting a caption under which a paper will be filed. It is also the process of determining the order in which the units of that name are to be considered.

†Alphabetizing is the arrangement of captions and indexing units in strict alphabetic order: A-B-C.

‡A unit is a single important element in a name or subject. Material to be indexed is handled in units. A name can be arranged out of normal order for indexing; however, once it is assigned a unit number, the units are then handled in their normal numeric order.

§The caption is the name or phrase under which a paper is filed. This constitutes the first indexing unit.

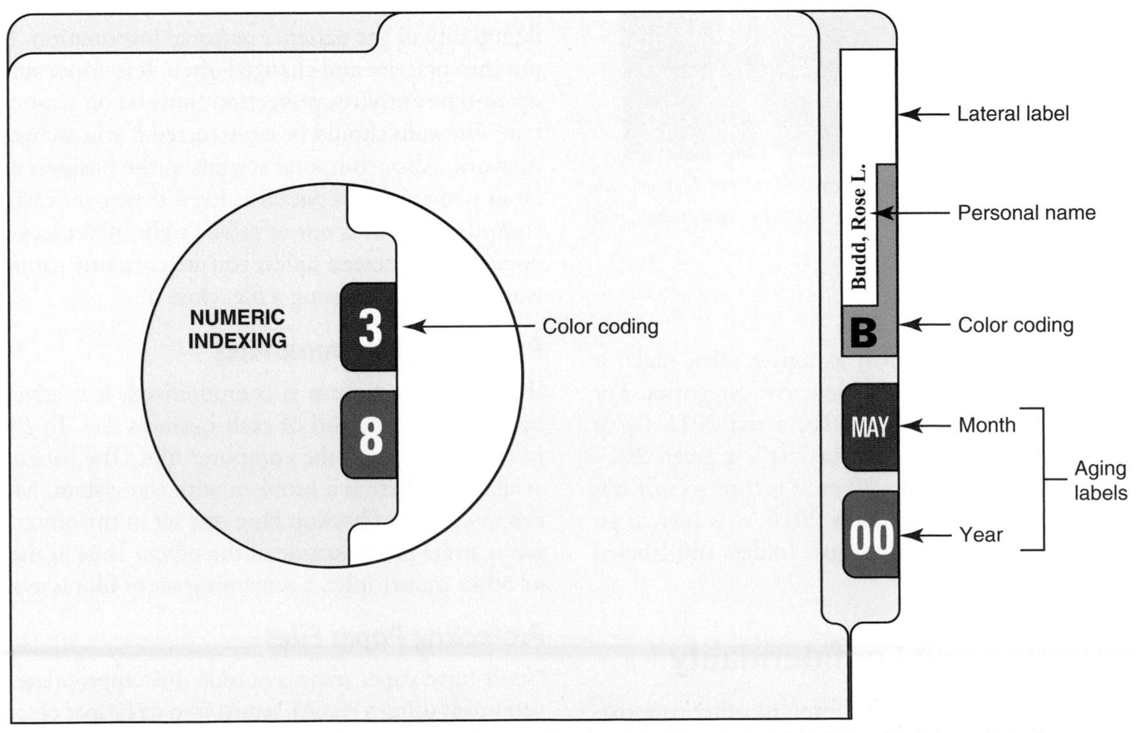


**FIG. 62.6** File showing color coding. *(From Gaylor LJ: The administrative dental assistant, ed 4, St Louis, 2016, Elsevier.)*

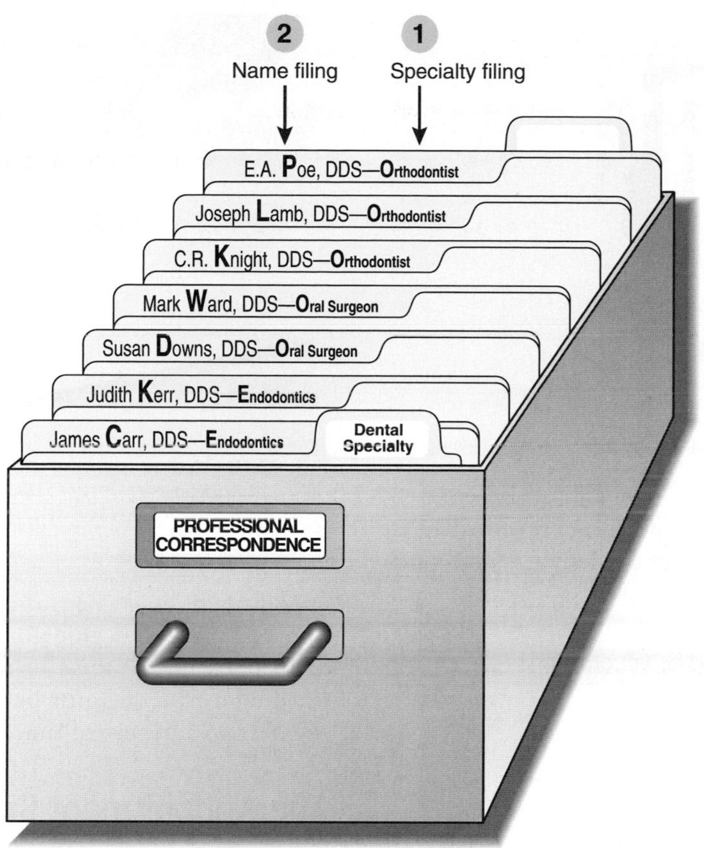


**FIG. 62.7** Chronologic filing. *(From Gaylor LJ: The administrative dental assistant, ed 4, St Louis, 2016, Elsevier.)*

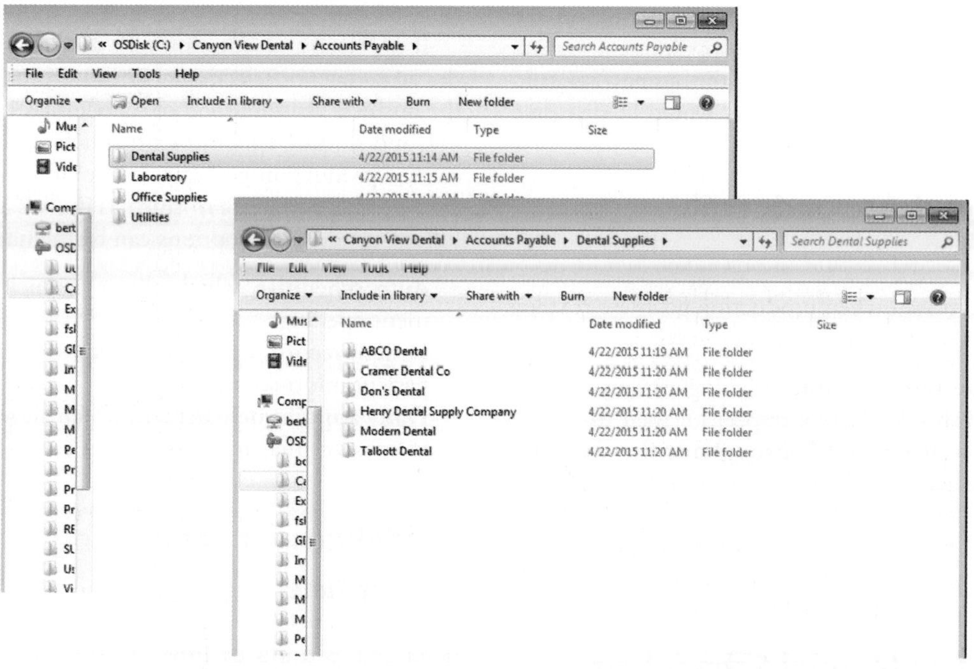


**FIG. 62.8** Computerized filing. *(From Gaylor LJ: The administrative dental assistant, ed 4, St Louis, 2016, Elsevier.)*

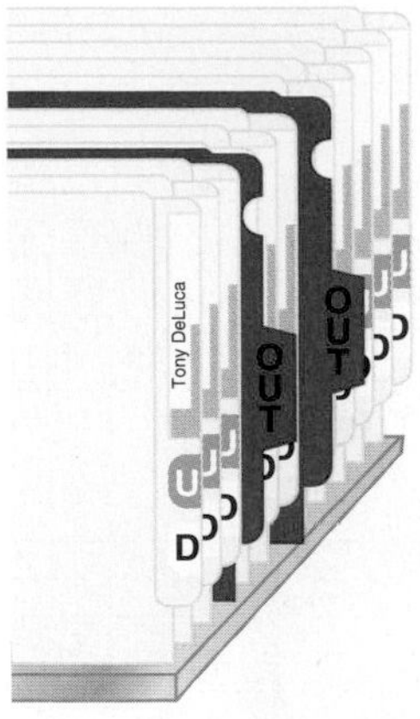

FIG. 62.9 Use an outguide.

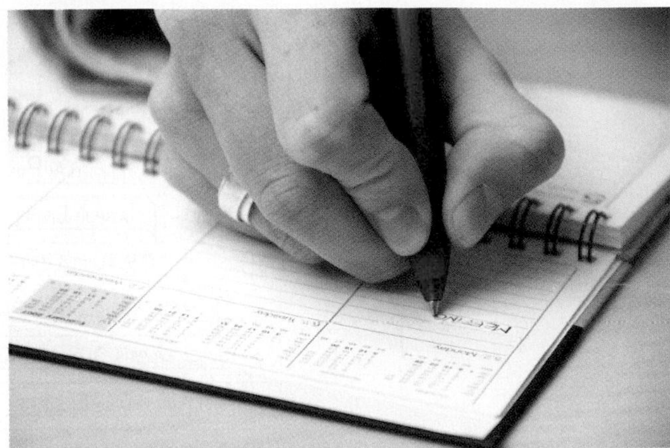

FIG. 62.10 An example of a manual appointment book for scheduling. *(Copyright © 2007 SilviaJansen, iStock.com. All rights reserved.)*

should be taken to prevent cross-contamination when files are moved from the treatment area and returned to the business area.

RECALL

5 How much free space should be left on each shelf of a filing cabinet?
6 What is used to mark a space from which a record has been taken?
7 Which filing system is easiest to use?
8 If a patient was seen in 2013, would that patient be considered active or inactive?

# Appointment Scheduling

Effective appointment scheduling is vital to the smooth functioning and success of the entire dental practice. If the appointment schedule is not productive the office will eventually lose money.

Scheduling is most effective when one person oversees the appointment planning and entries in the appointment system. This responsibility is commonly assumed by the business assistant, or in larger practices, an appointment clerk would be delegated for this task.

## Goals of Efficient Appointment Scheduling

The stress level is decreased when production goals are reached and patients are happy with good customer service.

- **Patients must be seen on time.** Making patients wait is discourteous and shows a lack of respect for their time.
- **Patient load is well balanced throughout the day.** This provides an even pace, and the day is completed without undue tension or hurry.
- **The dentist and the staff are able to make good use of their time.** This enables the clinical team to maximize their productivity while providing quality care for patients.

## Computerized or Manual Scheduling

Appointment control can be managed with a computerized scheduling system or manually with a traditional appointment book. Regardless of the system used, the basic understanding and guidelines are the same: The appointment book format must be selected, the days must be outlined, and patients must be scheduled efficiently to ensure the best possible use of time.

## The Appointment Book

If a manual appointment book is used, it must be selected to ensure sufficient space for all necessary entries and to facilitate efficient scheduling of patients for the dental practice. The most efficient format is the so-called week-at-a-glance design. This allows the business assistant to view all days of the week at once. Ideally, the book should have ring binders or be spiral bound to allow it to lie flat when fully open (Fig. 62.10).

If an electronic appointment system is selected, you have the advantage of selecting a software program that will make the business assistant's job of scheduling, canceling, rescheduling, and shifting appointments much easier. Additionally, you can set production goals by controlling when and where specific procedures are performed (Figs. 62.11 and 62.12). The following additional options can be included:

- **Auto scheduler,** which allows a quick search of appointment openings
- **Patient record,** which allows you to view demographic and patient information
- **Daily appointment screen,** which allows you to color-code columns as they relate to patient care

## Guidelines for Scheduling

### *Units of Time*

The basic time increments used in planning appointments are described as **units of time**. A unit of time may be 10, 15, or 30 minutes, depending on the dentist's preference. With 10-minute increments, the hour consists of six units. With 15-minute increments, the hour consists of four units, and

## ANATOMY OF AN APPOINTMENT BOOK PAGE

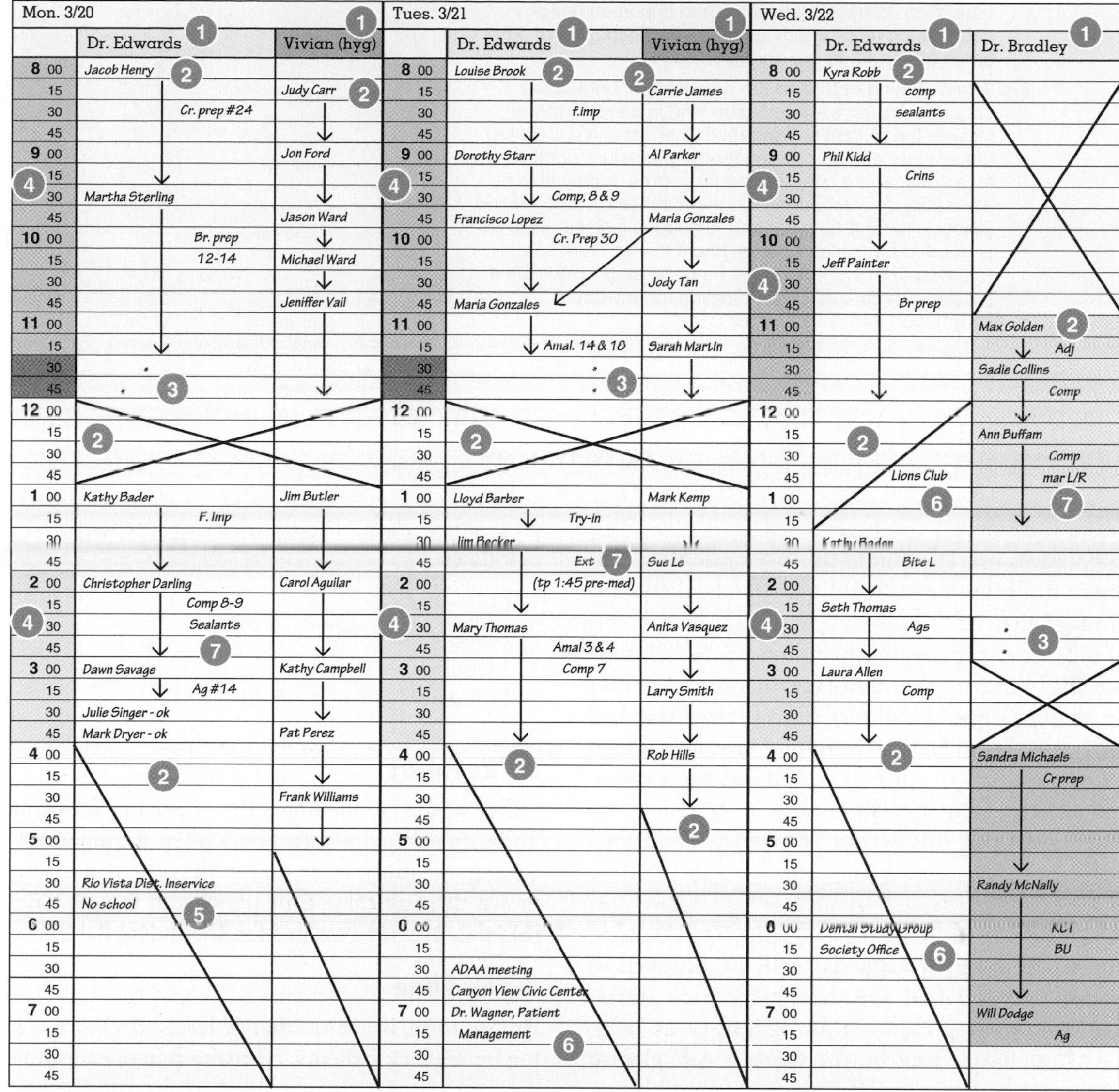


**Appointment Book Matrix**

Once the style of the appointment book is selected, the next step in the organization of the appointment book is to custom configure the pages. This is referred to as the **appointment book matrix.** The purpose of the matrix is to configure or outline the pages. Electronic schedulers are matrixed during the initial computer setup function. The program will customize the appointment book following the specifications of the dental practice.

**Steps in matrixing an appointment book**

1. Assign each practitioner a column for the day and clearly identify. If you are scheduling by treatment room, identify the treatment room assigned to each column.
2. Mark the columns so it can be easily determined by anyone looking at the appointment book what time the first procedure begins, when lunch or dinner will be scheduled, and when the last procedure ends.
3. During the course of the day it may be necessary to schedule emergency patients. The appointment book can be matrixed to identify a specific block of time each day in anticipation of an emergency. Dovetailing is another method used for short appointments and emergencies. For example, the dentist will need to wait 10 to 20 minutes after giving anesthetic before proceeding with the procedure, allowing time to check another patient.
4. With careful planning and attention to detail, the appointment book can be matrixed to identify when and where specific procedures should be scheduled. Colored highlighters, small colored sticky notes or colored book tabs (sticky notes and book tabs can be reused) will help identify blocks of time and procedures to be scheduled. When using a computerized scheduler, this type of function can be programmed into the system.
5. Identify when the local schools are on break or have days off. This is useful because teachers and children will be available for appointments without missing school.
6. Information other than patient appointments can be placed in the appointment book, which will help organize the function of the office. Items included are: professional meetings for the dentist and auxiliary, such as dental society meetings, dental assistant and dental hygienist society meetings; study clubs and continuing

**FIG. 62.11** Anatomy of an appointment book page. *(From Gaylor LJ: The administrative dental assistant, ed 4, St Louis, 2016, Elsevier.)*

ANATOMY OF AN APPOINTMENT BOOK PAGE (cont'd)

education courses; vacations; and important deadline dates, such as quarterly taxes, payroll deposits, or other dates important to the dental office.

7 When making entries in the appointment book, care should be taken to write legibly and in pencil. Entries include the patient's name (both the first and last name), the amount of time needed for the procedure (indicated by an arrow), and a code for the procedure. It may also be advisable to include a telephone number for confirmation (especially for a new patient), a code to indicate if lab work is needed for the procedure, and if the lab work has returned from the lab. It may be necessary to indicate if the patient requires premedication, or any other information that is vital to the case.

Some common codes are:

C – appointment needs confirmation
Ȼ – confirmed
cr – crown
ag – amalgam
comp – composite
ext – extraction
prophy – prophylaxis
RP – root planing
rc – root canal (rct)
fl – fluoride treatment
p.o. – post operative appointment
br – bridge
prep – preparation (crown, bridge, inlay, or onlay)
ins – insertion (placement of crown, bridge, inlay, or onlay)
tp – told patient
L – lab work
Ⓛ – lab work returned from the lab

**FIG. 62.11, cont'd**

with 30-minute increments, the hour consists of two units. Most dental practices use 15-minute units because they provide maximum flexibility in scheduling, which allows for enhanced productivity.

The key to efficient patient scheduling is to schedule patients according to the time necessary for their complete procedure rather than trying to fit all procedures into a standard 30-minute or 1-hour formula. If a 15-minute time unit is used in the practice and a patient must be scheduled for a procedure that will take approximately 40 minutes to complete, the dentist should request that this patient be given a "three-unit" appointment.

### Columns per Day

Appointment scheduling for each day will be assigned to a separate column designated specifically for each operator, with each column representing an operatory or treatment area. An "operator" may be the dentist, a hygienist, or an assistant with expanded-function responsibilities. For example, in a typical solo practice, one column per day is scheduled for the dentist, and one is scheduled for the dental hygienist. If an expanded-functions assistant is also employed in the practice, a separate column may be designated for that person.

To make the most efficient use of everyone's time, many dentists prefer to use several treatment areas simultaneously. This preference is reflected in the appointment book when one column represents each operatory. In larger practices with many providers, it is necessary to use a computerized system or multiple appointment books.

## Outlining the Appointment Schedule

The business assistant should go through the appointment schedule several months in advance and outline basic information. Computer scheduling allows the business assistant to block out operatories and times for specific procedures; this helps the practice to customize the schedule to meet specific production goals. The four basic elements to be outlined are as follows:

- Office hours
- Buffer time
- Meetings
- Holidays

### Office Hours

**Office hours** are the hours that a practice is open for business. These do not include the hours when the practice is opening or closing, the lunch hour, and routine days off. A diagonal line is drawn through these time periods on the schedule to indicate that they are not available for scheduling patients.

### Buffer Time

**Buffer time** is a time that is reserved each day for scheduling emergency patients. In many practices, a buffer period of one or two units is scheduled in the late morning or in the early afternoon. These times are bracketed or highlighted in the appointment book. Buffer time not needed for emergencies may be used at the last minute for short appointments, such as denture adjustments or suture removal. This time should *not* be filled more than 24 hours in advance.

An experienced business assistant may not need to have specific buffer times actually marked in the appointment book. This assistant can determine the best time to schedule a patient just by looking at the existing appointment sequence.

### Meetings

Regular meetings that occur during the workday and those that require the dentist to leave the office early should be marked. Time needed for staff meetings also should be blocked out well in advance.

### Holidays

Major holidays on which the office is closed should be crossed out. Other holidays and school vacations, when school is closed

## ANATOMY OF AN ELECTRONIC APPOINTMENT BOOK

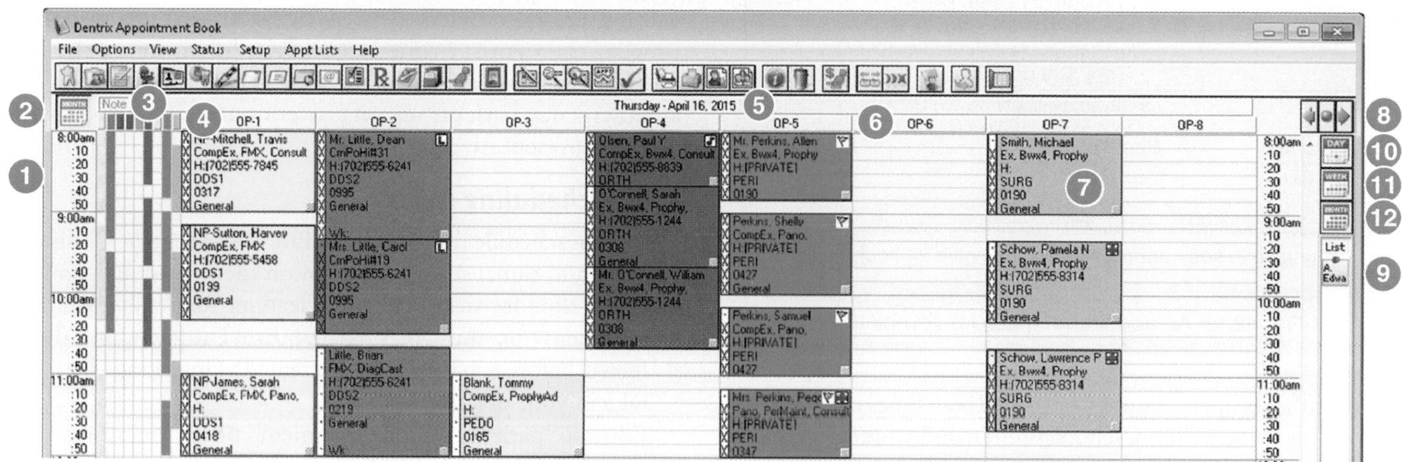


1. The Time Bars on the left and right sides of the Appointment Book separate hour intervals into selected time block size.
2. Click the Calendar button to open a monthly Calendar. From the Calendar dialog, you can view production goals, scheduled production, and actual production, making it easy to quickly evaluate your progress in meeting production objectives. In addition, you can click a date square to quickly move to the selected date in the Appointment Book.
3. Click the Note button to enter a note applicable for that day. The Note button turns yellow when a note is entered, indicating to staff members that a note has been entered for that day. There is also an option to print the Appointment Book Day Note when printing the Appointment Book View.
4. A unique color can be used for each treatment provider in your office. These colors will be used to flag each appointment, so you can tell which provider the patient is seeing. Similarly, on the left side of the Appointment Book is a color column for each provider. A colored block in that column indicates that the provider is scheduled to be working on a patient during the blocked time.
5. The Date Bar displays the date being viewed.
6. A column is displayed for each operatory added to the system. Operatories are displayed in numerical, then alphabetical, order by Operatory ID.
7. Each time an appointment is scheduled, a colored block appears in the appropriate operatory column for the amount of time scheduled. This new appointment will be the color assigned to the provider in the Provider Setup. Depending on the length of the appointment, up to nine lines of customizable information may be displayed, including Name, Appointment Reason, Home Phone, Work Phone, Provider, Production Amount, Appointment Type, Staff, Chart Number, Preferred Name, Name/Preferred Name, Referred By, and Social Security Number. In addition, a red cross on the appointment block indicates that the patient has a Medical Alert. Similarly, a blue musical note indicates that the patient has a note attached to the displayed appointment.
8. The Navigation buttons are used to move from day to day in the Appointment Book. Click the left arrow button to move back one day. Click the right arrow to move forward one day. Click the circle button to return to the current day.
9. The Appointment Book pin board can be used to temporarily store appointment information until a new appointment time can be found. An appointment can be quickly moved to a different day by dragging the appointment to the pin board, switching to another date, and then dragging the appointment to a new time. A scheduled appointment can be moved to any place on the schedule by clicking and dragging the appointment to a new time, a new operatory, or a new day (using the pin board).
10. Opening the Appointment Book in the day view allows you to see detailed information pertaining to an individual day and its scheduled appointments. Appointments can be scheduled by double clicking an available time.
11. The week view option allows you to see a week's worth of appointments. In the week view, the Appointment Book window displays large columns for each day of your work week. Each day column is further divided into operatory columns that show provider color blocks, indicating already scheduled appointments, making it easy to see free scheduling opportunities. To schedule an appointment, double click an available time.
12. Click the Month button to display an entire month's worth of appointment times for each provider. On the left side of the Appointment Book, each provider is listed by ID for each workday in the month. On the top of the Appointment Book, the time of day is shown. To view the appointments on a particular day, click the desired date to move to that date in the day view.

**FIG. 62.12** Anatomy of an electronic appointment book. *(From Gaylor LJ: The administrative dental assistant, ed 4, St Louis, 2016, Elsevier. Dentrix screen capture and associated text courtesy Henry Schein Practice Solutions, American Fork, UT.)*

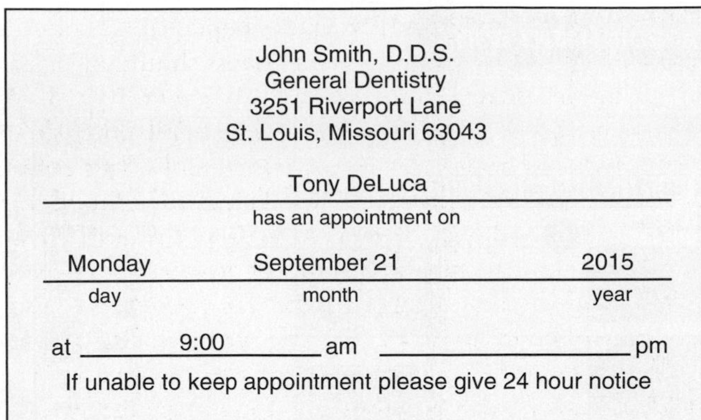
John Smith, D.D.S.
General Dentistry
3251 Riverport Lane
St. Louis, Missouri 63043

Tony DeLuca
has an appointment on

Monday September 21 2015
day month year

at 9:00 am pm
If unable to keep appointment please give 24 hour notice

**FIG. 62.13** An appointment card is completed.

but the office is open, should be noted. These times may be more convenient for scheduling schoolchildren and working people.

## Making Appointment Book and Appointment Card Entries

- All appointment book entries must be accurate, legible, complete, and made in pencil.
- Entries must be clearly written so they are easy to read.
- Manual entries must be made in pencil that is sufficiently legible to read, yet erasable if necessary.
- Entries must be complete and accurate so it is clear who is scheduled and for what treatment.

Entries should be complete but should be limited to information that is directly applicable to the scheduled appointment. Generally, the appointment book entry includes (1) the patient's name, (2) the patient's business and telephone numbers, (3) an abbreviated code for the treatment to be provided, (4) the length of the appointment, and (5) special notations such as whether the patient is new or requires premedication.

The proper sequence for recording entries is as follows:

1. Make the complete entry in the appointment book.
2. Write the appointment card for the patient.
3. Double check to ensure that the information is the same in both places.

When the appointment book entry is complete, the patient is handed an appointment card that states the day, date, and time of the appointment (Fig. 62.13). As the business assistant hands this to the patient, he or she orally confirms that the patient understands the information.

## Special Considerations for Scheduling

Difficult procedures, such as extensive crown and bridge preparation, implants, or surgeries, require careful scheduling, especially if the patient has been premedicated. These types of procedures often are scheduled in the morning, when the dentist and staff are at their highest energy levels.

Scheduling must also be engineered to allow efficient use of "idle" time for greater productivity. For example, during a restorative procedure, the dentist will inject the patient with a local anesthetic agent and then will wait 3 to 5 minutes for the anesthetic agent to take effect. This waiting period is referred to as **downtime**. During downtime, if the dentist's time is well scheduled, he or she can check a hygiene patient, make a prosthetic adjustment, see an emergency patient, return a telephone call, or meet with a sales representative.

### *Daily Scheduling Rules*

- Do not schedule difficult procedures close together. This can place additional stress and strain on the dentist and staff.
- Allow time for treatment area cleanup. Remember that the treatment area must be prepared, broken down, and disinfected before a patient can be seated. How long does this take in your practice?
- Educate patients about treatment times; reinforce this teaching regularly.
- Protect the appointment book from the eyes of others; this is private information.

### *New Patients*

New patients should be scheduled as soon as possible after they call for an appointment, even if it is not an emergency. Some practices accomplish this by reserving a "new patient time" each day. New patients should be asked to come to the dental office at least 15 minutes before the beginning of their appointment time so they can complete the necessary patient registration forms. Some practices also send an introductory packet of information to new patients before the first appointment. This packet may contain information such as the following:

- A letter welcoming the patient to the practice
- Practice information such as the dentist's educational and licensure credentials
- Office policies such as payment plans and management of insurance claims
- A map or printed directions to the office (including information about parking facilities if applicable)
- Patient registration forms (so the patient can fill them out before the time of the appointment)

### *Scheduling for the Dental Hygienist*

Effective appointment scheduling for the dental hygienist is important. The business assistant must pay close attention to the time needed for these appointments. It is recommended that the hygienist and the business assistant work out a list of average times required for certain types of hygiene visits. Hygiene patients may be scheduled as follows:

- New adult patient
- New child patient
- Adult prophylaxis
- Child prophylaxis
- Fluoride treatment
- Pit-and-fissure sealants

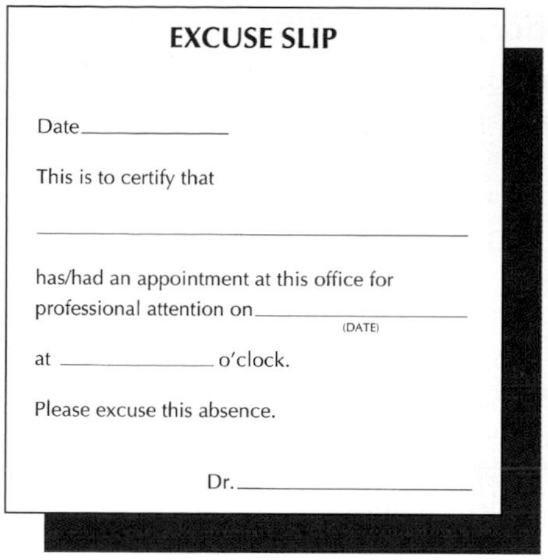

EXCUSE SLIP

Date____________

This is to certify that

____________________________

has/had an appointment at this office for professional attention on____________ (DATE)

at ____________ o'clock.

Please excuse this absence.

Dr.________________

**FIG. 62.14** Excuse slip for student. *(Courtesy Patterson Dental, St Paul, MN.)*

The scheduling list should cover all types of procedures commonly performed by the hygienist and should include the time required for the dentist to check the hygiene patient. On the basis of this information, the business assistant can schedule a hygiene patient for the correct amount of time so the hygienist is neither rushed nor wasting time waiting for the next patient.

### Recall Patients

Recall patients customarily are scheduled with the hygienist for prophylaxis, review of home care, and routine radiographs. However, it is also necessary to include time in this appointment for the dentist to see the patient. A recall patient always must be asked whether any changes in his or her health history have occurred, whether address or insurance coverage information has changed, and whether the patient is taking any new or different medications.

### Children

Young children are usually at their best in the morning, so most dentists prefer to schedule them early in the day. Whenever possible, parents prefer to schedule older schoolchildren after school or at times when school is closed. Having a copy of the school calendar is helpful in planning such appointments. Sometimes it is necessary to have a child dismissed from school for dental treatment. To minimize disruption of the school day, it is best to schedule the child at the beginning of the day (before he or she goes to school) or near the end of the school day. If a child misses a portion of the school day, provide a printed excuse slip for the child as a reference for missing school (Fig. 62.14).

### Emergency Patients

Emergency patients must be seen as quickly as possible. Buffer time is reserved in the appointment book for this purpose. Regardless of buffer time, a patient with an acute emergency must be seen immediately. An emergency obviously can delay the treatment of regularly scheduled patients. If this happens, the situation should be explained to the scheduled patients, and their cooperation should be requested. If necessary, scheduled patients should be offered the option of rescheduling.

The patient in pain who has been seen before in the practice should be scheduled as soon as possible. This caller is known as a **patient of record**, and failure to accommodate him or her could leave the dentist open to charges of abandonment. An emergency caller who is not a patient of record could actually become a regular patient of the practice if specific procedures are followed. For this reason, many practices make every effort to accommodate any patient in pain. If the dentist is out of town or is not able to see a patient with an urgent problem, another dentist should be on call.

When you receive a telephone call from a patient in pain, gather as much information as possible that will help the dentist diagnose the patient's problem. Ask the following questions:

- Where is the pain?
- How long has it continued?
- Is there fever or swelling?
- Is the pain constant or "on and off"?
- Does the pain occur in response to heat? Cold? Sweets? Chewing? Pressure?
- Has recent treatment or injury occurred in the area of pain?

A patient with a true emergency generally will come at the first available time. If a patient tries to negotiate a time that is more convenient, it may not be a true emergency. The business assistant must use good judgment in identifying a true emergency case.

### Scheduling an Appointment Series

Certain procedures, such as the fabrication of a prosthetic device or the restoration of multiple teeth, may require a series of appointments. It is more efficient to plan the entire series at the beginning of treatment. To do this, the business assistant must become knowledgeable about the following:

- How many appointments will be required?
- How long (the number of units) will each appointment take?
- How many laboratory working days must be allowed between appointments?

When scheduling a series of appointments, try to give the patient the same day of the week and the same time of day for each appointment. This makes it easier for the patient to remember the appointments. With the exception of prosthodontics, it generally is not recommended to schedule more than two appointments in advance. Otherwise, the dentist's schedule becomes overbooked and appointment time is not available for new patients and emergencies. In addition, the chance that a patient may miss an appointment is greater if it is scheduled too far in advance.

### Scheduling for the Expanded-Functions Dental Assistant

When scheduling for an expanded-functions dental assistant, entries in the appointment book are made "by the chair." To do this, a separate appointment book column is designated for each operatory. Appointments must be planned so that only one patient is scheduled per chair and per expanded-functions assistant. Before scheduling an appointment, the business assistant must determine the following:

- What treatment is planned?
- How much time must be reserved for the entire appointment?
- Which units of the visit will be spent with the dentist?
- Which units will be solo time for the expanded-functions assistant before the dentist enters or after the dentist leaves the treatment room?

For example, a patient who is having teeth prepared for the placement of a bridge first must have an alginate impression taken to create a diagnostic cast that can be used in fabricating provisional coverage. The first 10 minutes of the appointment may be scheduled with the assistant who can legally perform this function.

## Confirmation of Appointments

One of the greatest obstacles to good appointment control is failure of the patient to keep the appointment. Sometimes, missed appointments are unavoidable; however, confirming all appointments by telephone, email, or texting the day before the appointment catches many cancellations far enough in advance to allow the time to be used effectively. Noting the patient's telephone number and/or email address next to his or her name in the appointment book facilitates the task of placing these confirmation calls.

## Patient Circumstances

### *Late Patients*

An office that consistently runs late is disrespectful of its patients' time. In turn, the dentist will soon find that patients begin to come in late for their appointments rather than having to wait. If the dentist is able to see patients on time, the same courtesy should be expected of the patients. Patients who are chronically late should be tactfully reminded that their tardiness is depriving them, as well as others, of treatment.

### *Canceled Appointments*

If a patient has not appeared within 10 minutes of the appointed time, the patient should be contacted immediately in the hope that he or she will still be able to be seen for the remainder of the scheduled time. If not, the patient usually is offered another appointment, and every effort is made to schedule another patient into the remainder of the reserved time.

When a patient fails to keep an appointment, this information should be recorded on the patient record as "BA" (broken appointment) along with the date, as well as specific reasons noted why. These are important clinical data because in case of a malpractice suit, repeated breaking of appointments can be considered contributory negligence on the part of the patient.

### *Short-Notice Appointments*

Although scheduling patients on short notice is not as efficient as careful prior planning, it is to the office's advantage to maintain a list of patients who are available to take an appointment on short notice. Information on such available patients may be placed on file cards or kept on a **call list**. This listing should include the patient's name, work and home telephone numbers, notes of the treatment to be provided, and times when the patient is available.

The list should be kept up to date at all times, and the patient's name should be removed when he or she no longer needs an appointment. A patient who comes in on short notice should be thanked for changing his or her plans for the convenience of the dental office.

## Daily Treatment Area Schedule

Appointment book information for the next day is transferred to the **daily schedule** form (Fig. 62.15). A sufficient number of copies are printed or posted electronically so that it can be posted in each treatment area, the laboratory, and the dentist's private office. On this form, the patient's name and an abbreviated code for treatment should be provided next to the appointment time. However, remember the HIPAA privacy rules, and do not indicate specific types of appointments for other patients to see. This list is updated throughout the day as changes in the schedule are made. A checkmark is placed to the left of the patient's name when the appointment has been confirmed. A circle around the time indicates that the appointment has not been confirmed.

### *Appointment Preparations*

At the end of the day, the business assistant must make certain preparations for patients who are scheduled for the next day.

### *Daily Meeting*

Many practices make a point of starting each workday with a team meeting. This is usually a brief meeting of 5 to 10 minutes during which the dentist and staff review the daily schedule and any specific treatment procedures to be completed and patient concerns to be addressed.

RECALL

9 What are the most common time lengths used for scheduling units of time in a dental practice?
10 What four elements should be outlined in an appointment book?
11 If a patient does not keep an appointment, where should this information be recorded?

# Preventive Recall Programs

Regularly scheduled preventive care is important for a patient's dental health. The recall system, which is also referred to as the *continuing care program,* is designed to help patients return in a timely manner for treatment. It is the responsibility of the business assistant to ensure that patients are placed on recall, and that those who are due to return are notified promptly.

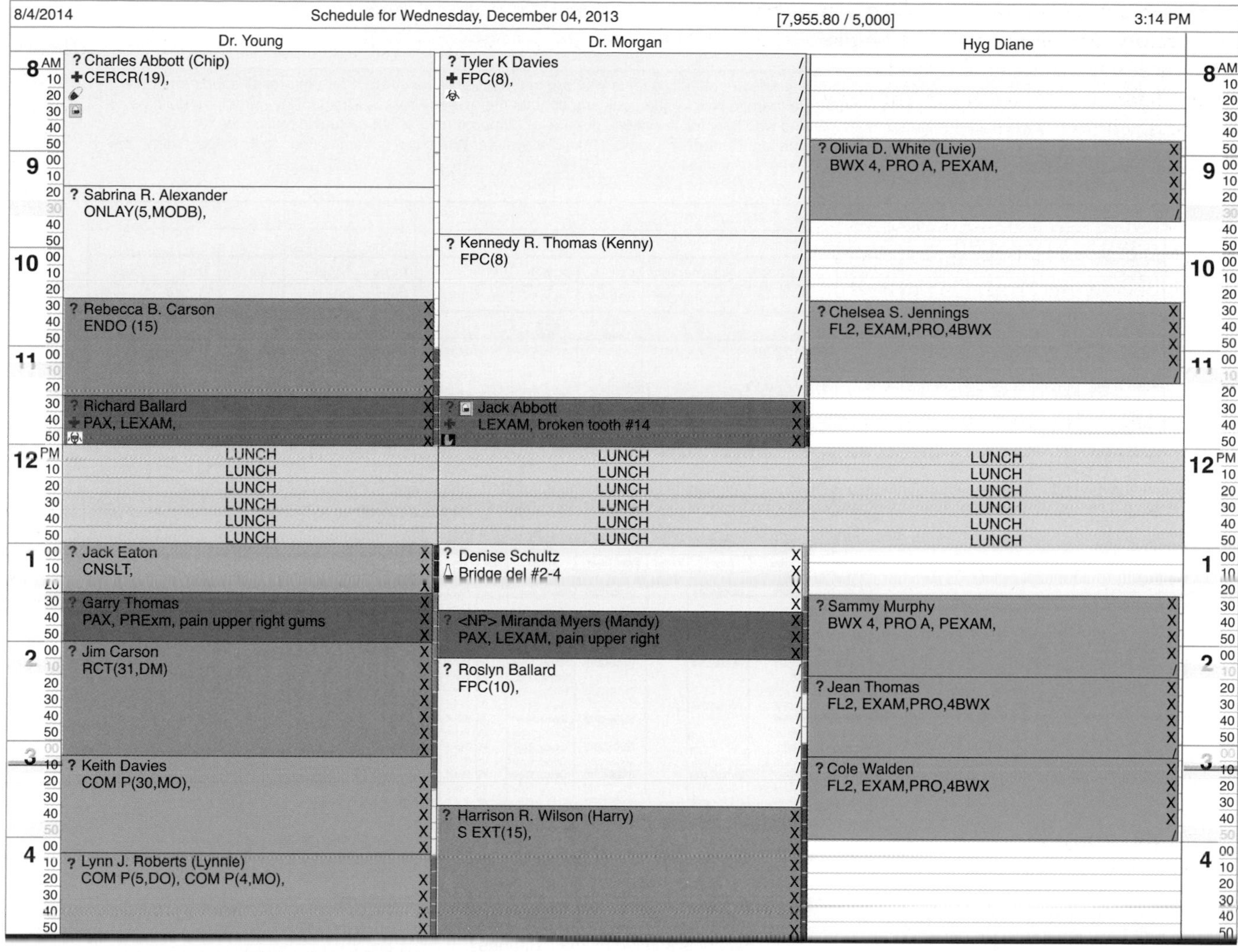


**FIG. 62.15** A computer-generated daily schedule. *(Courtesy Patterson Dental, St Paul, MN.)*

**BOX 62.1** Calculating 6-Month Recall Time

| January | February | March | April | May | June |
|---|---|---|---|---|---|
| (1) | (2) | (3) | (4) | (5) | (6) |
| July | August | September | October | November | December |
| (7) | (8) | (9) | (10) | (11) | (12) |

From the first half of the year, add 6 to the number of the month.
From the second half of the year, subtract 6 from the number of the month.

The patient should be placed on recall when current dental treatment is completed or on instruction from the dentist. Box 62.1 can be used to calculate when a patient is due to return. The most common period of recall is 6 months; however, patients who require more periodic visits may be placed on a 3- or 4-month recall. All steps necessary to place the patient on recall should be completed before the patient's treatment is filed for insurance. Doing this helps ensure that the patient's information is indeed placed into the recall system.

# Types of Recall Systems

## *Continuing Appointment System*

This method is also known as the **advance** or **preappointment recall** appointment system (Fig. 62.16). At the time of the last visit in the current series, the patient is given a specific appointment time and date for the recall visit. This is noted in the appointment book, and the patient is provided an appointment card. These appointments are coded either in the appointment book or completed in the electronic appointment system. The patient is then sent a reminder 2 weeks before the appointment. These appointments also should be confirmed by telephone.

## *Written Recall Notification*

Many practices send a recall card or a postcard to remind the patient to return for continuing care (Figs. 62.17 and 62.18). With a computerized recall system, the cards for each month can be quickly prepared by the system. With a manual system, at the time of the last visit in the current series, the patient may be asked to self-address a recall card. This card is then filed behind the month of recall. At the beginning of each month,

## ANATOMY OF A RECALL TRACKING SYSTEM

The ultimate purpose of the tracking system is to ensure that all patients who are in the recall system return for their recall appointments. It is easy for any member of the dental healthcare team to pick up the book and contact the overdue recall patients. Any member should be able to identify who has completed the recall and who has not. A system, manual or computerized, is set up that identifies the type of second notice, third notice, and so on until the patient is seen or removed from the system. When the system is used to its fullest extent, the status of the patient is always known and the patient is not lost.

(1) Monthly Recall Tracking Form

RECALLS FOR THE MONTH OF APRIL, 20XX

| Patient | type of recall | unit time | x-rays | telephone # | prescheduled appointment | call patient | pt will call | recall completed | other work | appt Dr./Hyg. | 1st notice | 2nd notice | 3rd notice |
|---|---|---|---|---|---|---|---|---|---|---|---|---|---|
| (2) | (3) | (4) | (5) | (6) | (7) | (8) | (9) | (10) | (11) | (12) | (13) | (14) | (14) |
| Rose Budd | prophy | 3 | no | 555-1233(H) | 4/4/99 | | | 4/4/XX | bridge | hyg | #### | | |
| Bill Frank | endo | 1 | yes | 555-4987(W) | | x | | 4/22/XX | crown | doctor | #### | | |
| Jose Gomez | prophy | 3 | bw/2 | 555-6794(VM) | | | x | 4/18/XX | | hyg | #### | | |
| Sam Jones | prophy | 3 | FMX | 555-0908(W) | | | x | | | hyg | #### | | |

Dentrix Continuing Care

File Edit View Status Office Journal

(1) > ALL (3) (7) (2) (12) (6)

| Date (1) | Type (3) | Appt? (7) | Status | Prior Treat. | Name (2) | Age | Prov. (12) | Phone (6) |
|---|---|---|---|---|---|---|---|---|
| 04/01/2014 | BITEWINGS | 04/08/2014 | | 01/03/2010 | *Abbott, Ken S | 40 | Prov1 | (02)555-1586 |
| 04/01/2014 | PROPHY | 04/08/2014 | | 01/03/2010 | *Abbott, Ken S | 40 | Prov1 | (02)555-1586 |
| 04/01/2014 | BITEWINGS | | | 01/03/2010 | Abbott, Patricia | 37 | Prov1 | (02)555-1586 |
| 04/01/2014 | BITEWINGS | 04/08/2014 | | 01/03/2010 | Abbott, Timoth | 16 | Prov1 | (02)555-1586 |
| 04/01/2014 | PANOREX | 04/08/2014 | | | Abbott, Patricia | 37 | Prov1 | (02)555-1586 |
| 04/01/2014 | PROPHY | | | 01/03/2010 | Abbott, Patricia | 37 | Prov1 | (02)555-1586 |
| 04/01/2014 | PROPHY | 04/08/2014 | | 01/03/2010 | Abbott, Timoth | 16 | Prov1 | (02)555-1586 |
| 10/29/2013 | FMX | | | | *Brown, Mary | 30 | Prov1 | (02)555-4509 |
| 04/02/2014 | BITEWINGS | | | 01/04/2010 | *Brown, Mary | 30 | Prov1 | (02)555-4509 |
| 04/02/2014 | PANOREX | 04/08/2014 | | | *Brown, Mary | 30 | Prov1 | (02)555-4509 |
| 04/02/2014 | PROPHY | | | 01/04/2010 | *Brown, Mary | 30 | Prov1 | (02)555-4509 |
| 11/10/2013 | PANOREX | + | | | *Crosby, Brent | 45 | Prov1 | (02)555-5969 |
| 02/28/2014 | PERIO | + | | 08/02/2010 | *Crosby, Brent | 45 | Prov1 | (02)555-5969 |
| 04/04/2014 | BITEWINGS | 04/08/2014+ | | 01/06/2010 | *Crosby, Brent | 45 | Prov1 | (02)555-5969 |
| 04/04/2014 | PROPHY | 04/08/2014+ | | 01/06/2010 | *Crosby, Brent | 45 | Prov1 | (02)555-5969 |
| 04/04/2014 | BITEWINGS | 04/09/2014 | | | Crosby, Shirley | 42 | Prov1 | (02)555-5969 |

**(1) MONTH**

Identify the month and year the patient is due for recall.

**(2) PATIENTS' NAMES**

Patients' names are listed in alphabetical order. Adding an account number will help to locate the patient in the computer file, or the numerical number of the patient if the dental practice utilizes a numerical filing system.

**(3) TYPE OF RECALL**

Identifies the category of recall needed.

**(4) UNIT TIME**

States the amount of time that will be needed to complete the appointment.

**(5) X-RAYS (radiographs)**

Indication of whether x-rays are needed and what type.

**(6) TELEPHONE NUMBER**

The telephone number of the patient. Indicate if the telephone is home, work, voice mail, or message center.

**(7) PRESCHEDULED**

Type of recall method. The appointment was made at the patient's last recall appointment. In a modified version of this system, the patient selects a general day of the week and time for the next appointment. When the recall cards are processed for a given month the assistant schedules the appointment. The patient is notified by mail and has the opportunity to keep the selected time or call the office to reschedule.

**(8) CALL PATIENT**

Type of recall method. The patient has indicated that he or she wants to be called a few weeks prior to the recall to schedule an appointment.

**(9) PATIENT WILL CALL**

Type of recall method. The patient has stated that he or she will call for an appointment after receiving a reminder in the mail.

**(10) RECALL COMPLETED**

The date the patient is seen in the office for the recall. This is the most important element of the system. If this portion is not completed it will be impossible to determine if the patient has returned as scheduled. Time must then be taken to check the clinical record or the computer system.

**(11) OTHER WORK**

Identify if there is any other treatment that needs to be scheduled at the time of the recall. It is also a good tracking tool for clinical treatment. Patients may delay treatment for a variety of reasons.

**(12) APPOINTMENT WITH**

Identify which dental professional needs to see the patient.

**(13) 1ST NOTICE**

Record the date that the first recall card was sent or telephone call was made.

**(14) 2ND NOTICE, 3RD NOTICE**

The dates that follow-up contacts were made with the patient regarding the recall appointment. A system is designed by the dental practice to notify patients (via postcard, letter, or personal telephone call) that they need to schedule an appointment. For example, a 2nd notice is mailed if they have not returned to the dental practice within 3 months of their original recall month. At 6 months, a third attempt is made. This can be a combination of a reminder card or letter followed by a telephone call. At this point, patients on a 6-month recall have not had their teeth cleaned or examined for 1 year.

**FIG. 62.16** Anatomy of an electronic recall tracking system. *(From Gaylor LJ: The administrative dental assistant, ed 4, St Louis, 2016, Elsevier. Dentrix screen capture and associated text courtesy Henry Schein Practice Solutions, American Fork, UT.)*

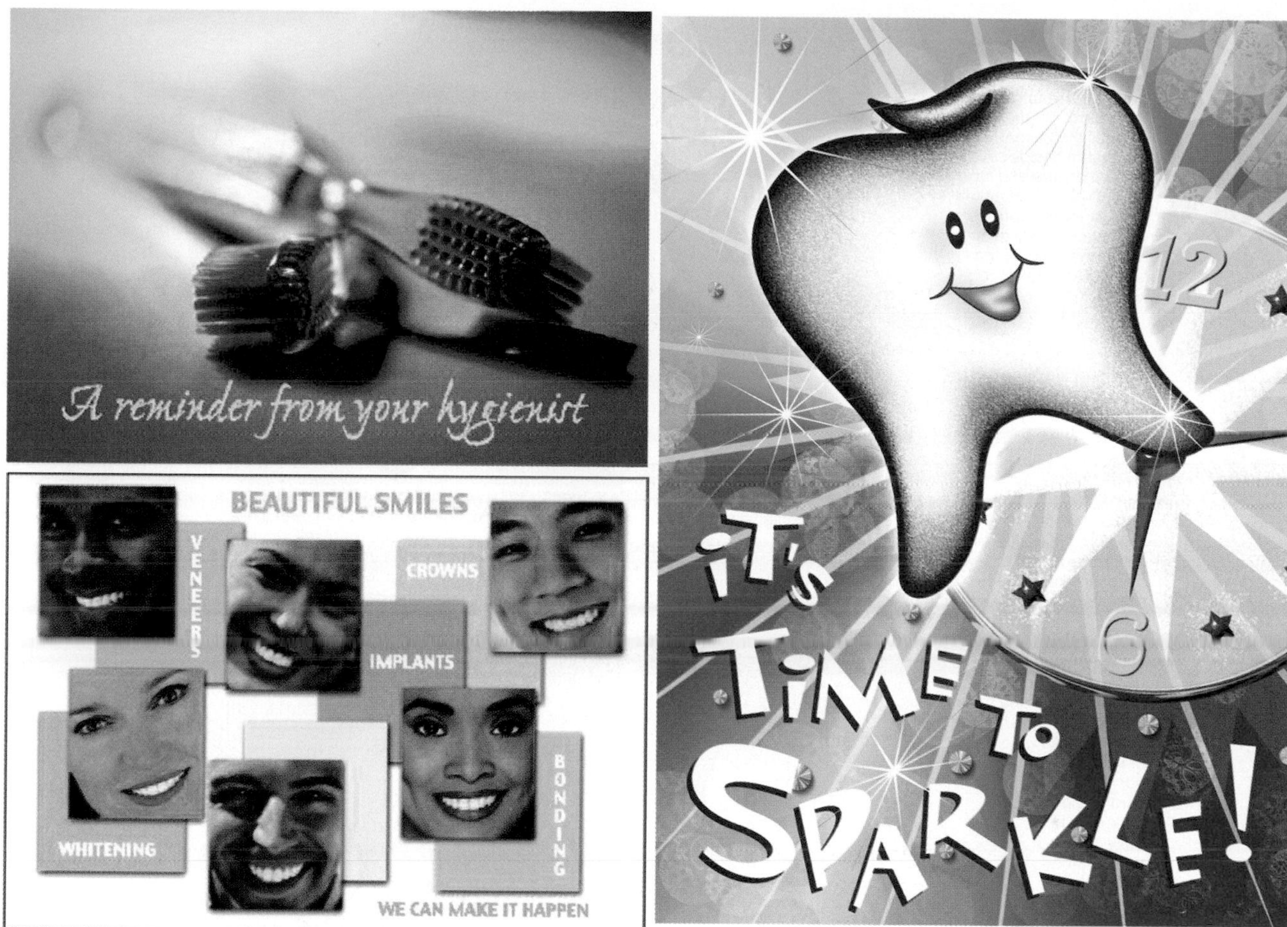


**FIG. 62.17** Styles of recall cards. *(Courtesy Patterson Dental, St Paul, MN.)*

the business assistant removes the cards from the file for that month and mails them out.

### Recall by Telephone

Another option is to maintain a list of the names and telephone numbers of all patients due to be recalled each month. As time permits, the business assistant calls each patient and tries to schedule the recall appointment. A note is made next to the patient's name regarding the results of the call, and the patient's name is crossed out when he or she has been contacted. Although recall by telephone is time-consuming, it is usually more effective than repeatedly sending written reminders.

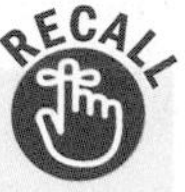


**12** What is the most common time period for recall?
**13** If a patient was last seen in March, what recall time would be used?

## Inventory Management

Running out of supplies can create embarrassing situations and unnecessary crises in the dental office. An adequate quantity of all necessary dental supplies is essential for the smooth functioning of the practice.

An inventory system should be simple, readily workable, and kept up to date at all times; it is advisable that one person should be responsible for maintaining the inventory control and ordering supplies. However, the cooperation of the entire staff is necessary if the system is to work. Frequently, the coordinating assistant or clinical assistant is assigned to handle the inventory of clinical area supplies, and the business assistant is assigned to manage the inventory of business office supplies.

Of major concern in organizing the inventory system are the expendable and disposable items that are used up in a relatively short time and that must be reordered regularly; these include restorative and impression materials, disposable needles, local anesthetic solutions, radiograph film, laboratory supplies, paper products, and business office supplies. A simple system should be developed that maintains the following information for ordering a product:

- Full brand name of the product
- All applicable descriptive information, such as name of the manufacturer, size, gauge, color, grit, length, shank type, fast or regular set, and container size
- Reorder point for that product
- Purchase source, including the name, telephone number, and, if necessary, the address of the supplier of that product (it also is helpful to note the name of the contact person who usually handles the order)

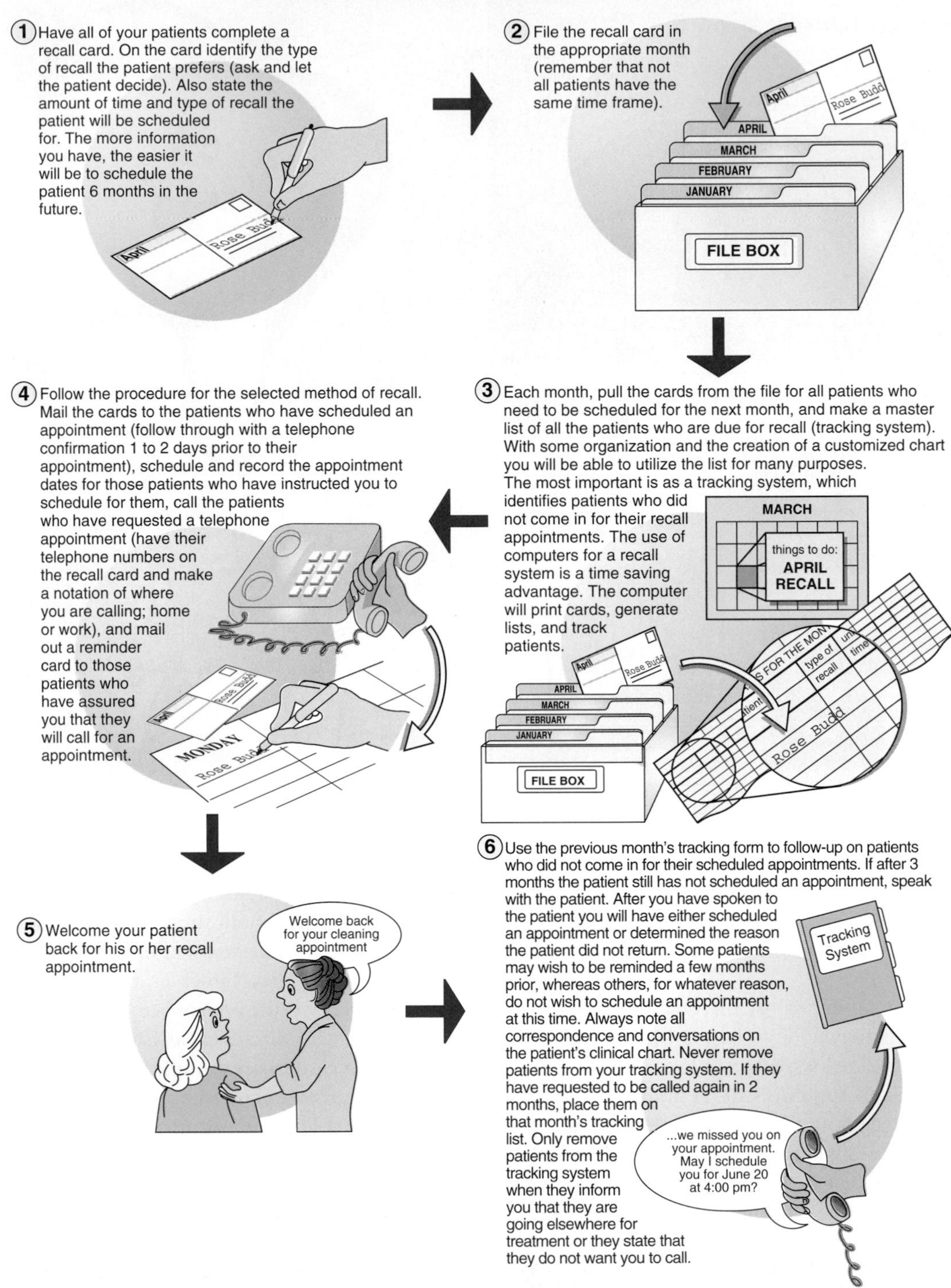


**FIG. 62.18** Anatomy of a manual recall system. *(From Gaylor LJ: The administrative dental assistant, ed 4, St Louis, 2016, Elsevier.)*

- Any necessary catalog numbers for that product
- Quantity purchase rates and reorder quantity

## Computerized Inventory System

A computerized inventory system is a computer software program that tracks inventory and then creates an automated replenishment order (Fig. 62.19). This type of program allows the staff to enter all expendable supplies used in the office and to maintain an inventory report on a monthly basis.

When an item is removed from inventory, the staff person scans the item using the bar code technology for dental supply items. The assistant uses a bar code wand to "read" the product and reorder information, which then is transmitted electronically to the supplier.

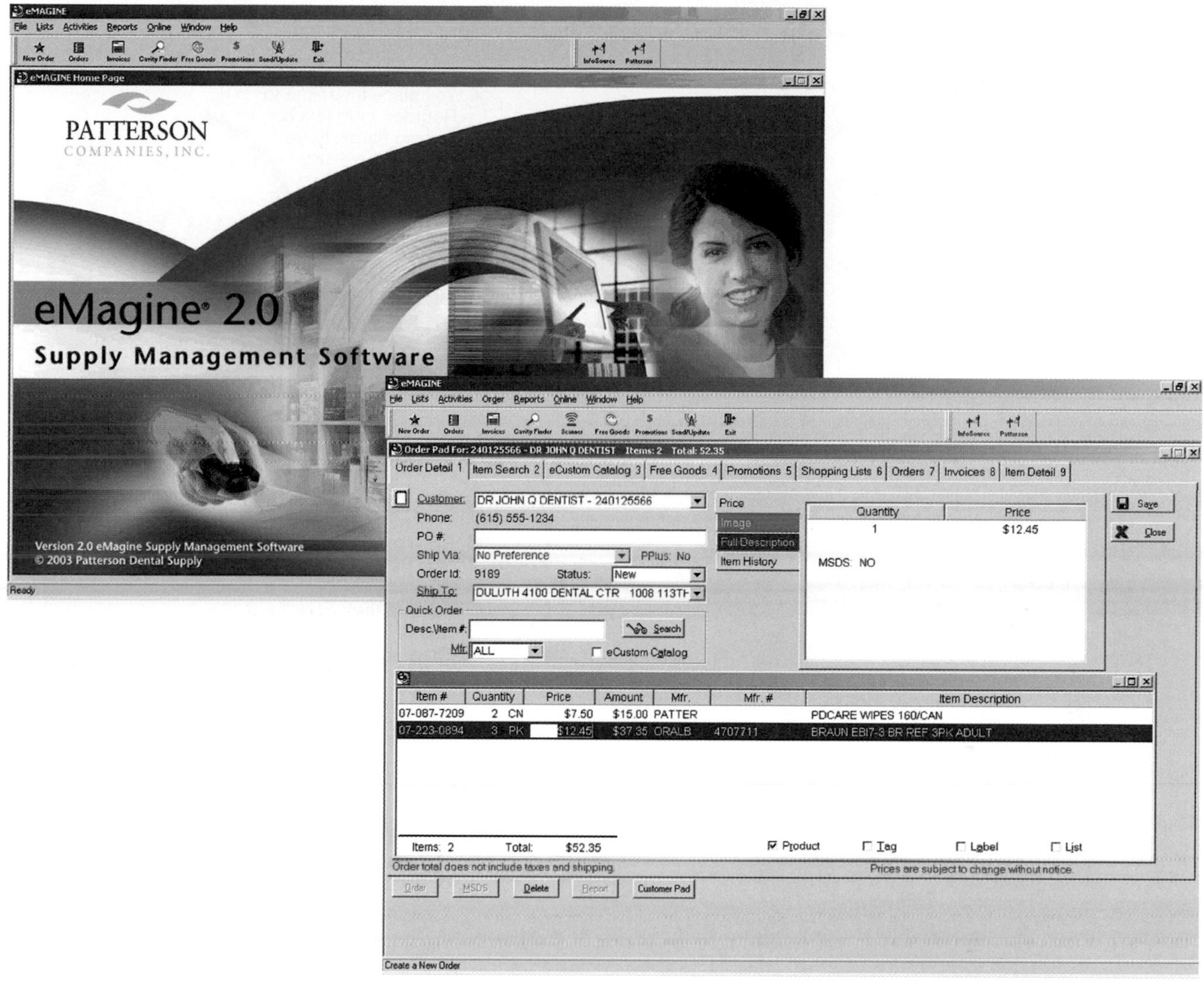


**FIG. 62.19** An example of a computerized inventory management system. *(Courtesy Patterson Dental, St Paul, MN.)*

## Guidelines for Ordering Dental Supplies

Supplies may be ordered (1) through a dental supply sales representative; (2) from a catalog by telephone, fax, mail order, or bar code scanning; and (3) online (Internet). When you are ordering and managing dental supplies in the office, it is important to keep all items in one central storage place. This eliminates the need to look through several places in the office to locate a needed product. It also makes treatment room restocking and tray setups more efficient. Many offices make use of alphabetically labeled and arranged plastic storage bins to keep supplies neat and organized. The dentist should specify his or her preference as to the purchase source, quantity, and brand information.

Journals and catalogs should be reviewed for ideas that can be adapted to the needs of the practice. The assistant should check regularly with the sales representative and make a point of reviewing the exhibits at dental meetings for new products and ideas.

### When Ordering Supplies

- *Be prepared.* Have a **want list** ready and check with the dentist before the sales representative is due to call.
- *Be specific.* Know what you need and how much is needed. Be sure to supply all the necessary information, including the correct catalog or item number, descriptive information, and the quantity desired.
- *Be alert.* Be on the lookout for "specials" and authentic savings (a special on something that is not needed or is not used is no bargain). The assistant should plan ahead to take advantage of seasonal savings and convention specials.
- *Be informed.* Just as the dentist will want to keep abreast of new product information, the assistant should be alert for new products and ideas that can make business office responsibilities easier to manage.

### Reorder Point

The reorder point for any given item is the minimum amount that represents an adequate reserve for that product. Thus a reorder point, or minimum quantity, should be established for each expendable item used in the practice. This point, which ensures an adequate supply while the new order is being processed, is based on two factors:

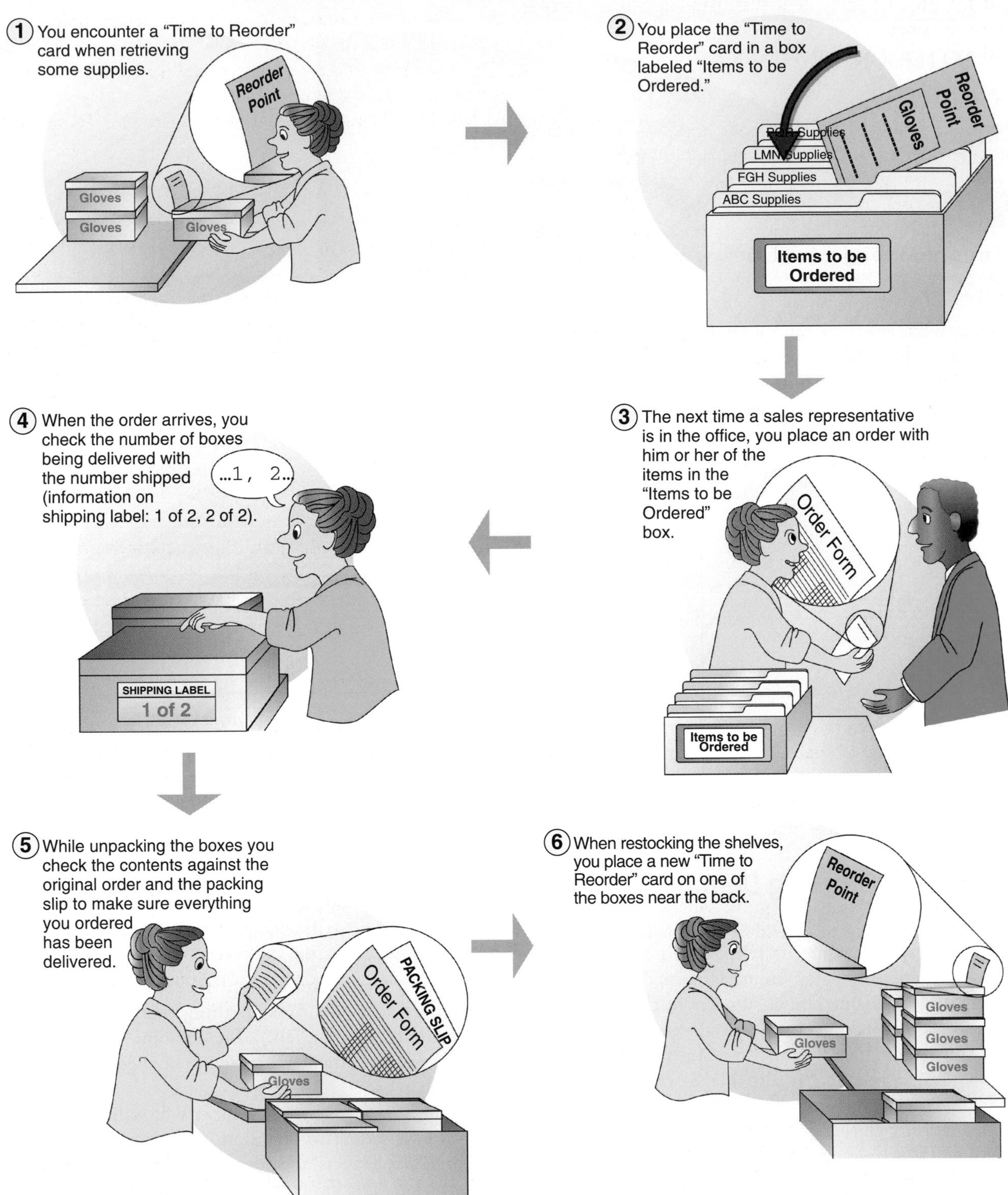


**FIG. 62.20** Steps for an inventory management system. *(From Gaylor LJ: The administrative dental assistant, ed 4, St Louis, 2016, Elsevier.)*

1. The **rate of use** of the product on a daily, weekly, or monthly basis
2. The **lead time** necessary to order and receive a new supply of that product; this time estimate should include a generous allowance for delays in ordering or shipping or the possibility of backordering

## Marking the Reorder Point

The reorder point for each item should be clearly marked on the supply of that item. This task can be accomplished with **reorder tags** (Fig. 62.20). These tags, also known as *red flag reorder tags* or *tie tags,* are usually bright red. The reorder tag is attached to the minimum quantity of the item with a rubber band or tape, or is placed into a stack of a flat product (such as a supply of ledger cards). This tag may be marked with the name of the product only, or it may contain full reordering information. When the reorder point is reached, this tag is removed and is processed immediately for reordering.

### Automatic Shipments

Many suppliers offer dentists the advantage of bulk quantity pricing with automatic shipments of a portion of the total order. This ensures the practice a constant supply of the amount of a product necessary to meet the practice's need. It also eliminates bulk storage problems and spreads the billing over a sequence of monthly or quarterly payments.

### Quantity Purchase Rate

The quantity purchase rate is the savings that can be attained by purchasing a product in larger quantities. The price break is the point at which the greater savings becomes effective. Although it is often wise for the office manager to take advantage of the best price per unit on supplies, it also is necessary to take into consideration the available storage space in the office and the rate at which the product is used.

### Reorder Quantity

Reorder quantity is the maximum quantity of a product to be ordered at one time. This should be reviewed periodically and increased or decreased as needed, depending on changes in these determining factors. The reorder quantity is determined by the following:

- Rate of use
- **Shelf life** and any storage problems for that product
- Availability of storage space (a consideration with bulky items that take up a lot of space [e.g., patient bibs])
- Availability of proper storage conditions (a concern with items that are particularly sensitive to heat and light [e.g., radiograph film])
- Best quantity purchase rate
- Investment involved (e.g., the purchase of a large quantity of a supply may tie up too much of the practice's cash flow to make it a "good buy")

### Backorders

When an item is not available for delivery with the rest of an order, it is placed on **backorder** and will be delivered as soon as it becomes available. A backorder notice usually is sent to the dentist to advise him or her of this situation. If sufficient lead time has been allowed, a backorder does not create a major problem. However, if the item is in critically short supply, it may be necessary to purchase it elsewhere. In this case, to avoid duplication, the backorder must be canceled.

### Order Exchange, Return, or Replacement

Sometimes it is necessary to exchange, return, or replace an ordered product. This can occur as the result of a variety of factors, including the following:

- The wrong item was ordered.
- The right item was ordered, but the wrong item was shipped.
- The size, color, or quantity was wrong.
- The product was broken or damaged in shipment.

When it is necessary to correct the supply order, the office manager must contact the supplier regarding the order and the reason for the exchange, replacement, or request for a credit on account. Until the supplier has made good on the request, a record should be maintained to trace and, if necessary, follow up on the transaction.

### Requisitions and Purchase Orders

In a large group practice, institution, or clinic with a central supply source, dental supplies are obtained by **requisition**. The requisition form usually is completed in duplicate. One copy is submitted to procure the supplies, and the person who requests the supplies retains the other copy. In institutions with central purchasing, a requisition may be submitted to the purchasing agent, who in turn issues a **purchase order**. These forms are numbered, and when an order is placed, the supplier may refer to the purchase order number.

# Dental Supply Budget

Institutions and well-organized practices operate on a budget. The budget request for dental supplies is based on how much money was spent in the previous year and an estimate of the increased rate of use, plus consideration for inflation.

## Consumables and Disposables

Consumable supplies are those that are literally "used up" as part of their function, such as restorative and impression materials. Disposables are items that are used once and then are discarded, such as local anesthetic agents, needles, a saliva ejector, and cotton rolls.

## Expendables

Expendable items are materials of relatively low cost that are used up in a short time. Minor dental instruments, such as mouth mirrors and burs, are examples of expendable items. For budget purposes, expendable items may be classified as those items that cost less than a certain amount, such as $50, and are ordered regularly. In some institutions, consumable, disposable, and expendable items are classified together under the single heading of "Expendables."

## Nonexpendables

Nonexpendable items are smaller pieces of equipment or instruments that eventually will be replaced as the items wear out or are broken, such as a calculator or a curing light.

## Major Equipment

This category includes larger pieces of equipment that are costly to purchase and will depreciate over a 5- to 10-year period. In the treatment area, this includes items such as dental chairs, radiograph units, and the air compressor. In the business office, this might include the computer and the printer.

RECALL

14 What two factors must be determined when a product must be reordered?
15 How is an item marked for reorder?
16 Identify three ways that supplies can be ordered.
17 If an item you ordered is not currently available from a supply company, the item is placed on ________.
18 Is a handpiece considered an expendable item? Why or why not?

## Equipment Repairs

The breakdown of dental equipment can result in major expense, loss of income, and inconvenience for the dental staff and patients. The best way to control this situation is through a sound preventive maintenance program.

## Equipment Records

When a new piece of equipment is purchased, the following information regarding that equipment should be entered on a service record:

- Date of purchase
- Name of supplier
- Expiration date of manufacturer's warranty
- Model and serial numbers

A **warranty** is a written statement that explains the manufacturer's responsibility for replacement and/or repair of a piece of equipment over a limited time. A warranty card, which registers this warranty with the manufacturer, usually is enclosed with the instruction manual. This should be completed and mailed promptly. Instructions for use, care, and cleaning of the equipment should be filed systematically so they are available for ready reference. Persons responsible for preventive maintenance of a piece of equipment should read the instructions and care manual thoroughly and add this item to the preventive maintenance schedule.

### Service Contracts

Some dental equipment is protected by a service contract. Under the terms of this contract, emergency repairs and possibly some routine maintenance are provided on a fixed-fee basis. An example would be a service contract for a computer system that guarantees emergency service within a specified period.

### Service Call

The expense of service calls is high because the cost is based on mileage, time, the expertise of the technician, and the materials and parts involved. Naturally, service calls should be avoided if possible. If a piece of equipment does not work, check the following points *before* calling for repair service:

- Is the equipment properly plugged in and turned on?
- Is there a *reset* button that must be pushed?
- Did you check the equipment for a blown fuse?
- Did someone check the fuse box or circuit breaker to ensure that the electrical circuit is functioning properly?

If you still must call for service after checking these points, be prepared to give complete information so the service technician can ensure the best use of his or her time without the need for a second trip. Necessary information includes the following:

- The brand name of the piece of equipment
- The model number and approximate age of the equipment or year of installation
- A brief description of the problem

■ **Legal and Ethical Implications** When discussing dental information or financial information concerning a specific patient, it is important to understand the ownership of the documents. Patient records and financial statements belong to the dentist; the information that is included in these documents belongs to the patient. Always make certain that every paper placed in a file provides the date, the name of the patient, and the name of the person who entered the information. ■

■ **Eye to the Future** More and more, the business aspects of dentistry and the smooth day-to-day operation of a dental practice are accomplished by a computer. In the future, these functions will become completely computerized. Because of these challenges, the role of the business assistant will require new levels of skill and knowledge. It has always been advantageous for the business assistant to first be a dental assistant or a dental hygienist. Having this background allows the business assistant to be knowledgeable when answering questions about patients' dental needs. However, in the future, the business assistant also will be required to have a background in information technology so he or she is competent in operating new equipment. ■

### ■ Critical Thinking

1. Describe how color coding can speed up the filing and retrieval of patient records.
2. When preparing the daily schedule for the treatment areas, what two items will you include, in addition to the patient's name?
3. Describe three reasons why patients commonly fail to keep appointments, and discuss how the business assistant should deal with each of these situations.
4. Discuss the importance of buffer time. Where in the daily schedule is this time best placed?
5. Discuss why the number of patients seen in a dental practice may best determine the filing method used. ■

63

# Financial Management in the Dental Office

## KEY TERMS

**Accounting** A system designed to maintain the financial records of a business.
**Accounts payable** Expenses and disbursements paid out from a business.
**Audit trail** Method of tracking the accuracy and completeness of bookkeeping records.
**Bonding** Form of insurance that reimburses an employer for loss resulting from theft by an employee.
**Bookkeeping** The process of managing the financial accounts of a business.
**Carrier** The insurance company that pays the claims and collects premiums.
**Change fund** Fixed amount of cash.
**Check** A draft or an order drawn on a bank account for payment of a specified amount of money.
**Check register** Record of all checks issued on and deposits made to a specific account.
**Coordination of benefits (COB)** Coordinating insurance coverage between two insurance carriers.
**Current Dental Terminology (CDT)** Publication that lists the procedure codes assigned to dental services for the processing of dental insurance.
**Customary fee** A fee that is within the range of the usual fee charged for the service.
**Deposit slip** An itemized memorandum of funds to be deposited into the bank.
**Disbursements** Payments on any outstanding accounts payable.
**Expenses** The overhead costs of a business that must be paid to keep operating.
**Fixed overhead** Business expenses that are ongoing.
**Gross income** The total of all professional income received.
**Invoice** An itemized list of goods that specifies the prices and terms of sale.
**Ledger** A financial statement that maintains all account transactions.
**Net income** Gross income minus expenses.
**Packing slip** An itemized listing of shipped goods.
**Payee** The person (or business) named on the check as the recipient of the amount shown.
**Pegboard system** A manual bookkeeping system.
**Petty cash fund** A limited amount of cash that is kept on hand for small daily expenses.
**Posted** Describes the documentation of money transactions within a business.
**Provider** The dentist who provides treatment to the patient.
**Reasonable fee** A fee that is considered justified for an extensive or complex treatment.
**Responsible party** Person who has agreed to pay for services or for an account.
**Statement** A summary of all charges, payments, credits, and debits for the month.
**Transaction** Any charge, payment, or adjustment made to a financial account.
**Usual fee** A fee that the dentist charges for a specific service.
**Variable overhead** Business expenses that change depending on the types of services needed.
**Walkout statement** A written indication of any balance due on an account, given to a patient as he or she leaves the practice at the end of an appointment.

## LEARNING OUTCOMES

*On completion of this chapter, the student will be able to achieve the following objectives:*

1. Pronounce, define, and spell the key terms.
2. Discuss account management, including the gathering of financial information.
3. Discuss accounts receivable, including types of systems and recording of payments.
4. Describe the importance and management of collections in the dental office, and demonstrate ways to make financial arrangements with a patient.
5. Discuss accounts payable management, including overhead, disbursements, and expenditure records.
6. Discuss the writing of checks in the dental office, including the purpose of business summaries.
7. Discuss payroll, including the following:
   - Discuss the financial responsibility of the employer.
   - Identify common payroll withholding taxes.
8. Discuss dental insurance, including the following:
   - Explain the purpose of dental insurance.
   - Identify the parties involved with dental insurance.
   - Identify the types of available prepaid dental programs.
   - Define managed care.
   - Discuss and define basic dental insurance terminology.

- Explain dual coverage.
- Identify dental procedures and coding.
- Detail claim forms processing.
- Describe the procedure and purpose of claim forms follow up.
- Identify insurance fraud.

## ELECTRONIC RESOURCES

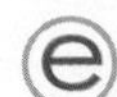

***Additional information related to content in Chapter 63 can be found on the companion Evolve Web site.***

- Dentrix Exercise
- Practice Quiz

The financial management of a dental practice is the foundation in how a dental office increases its profitability in relation to production. The business staff assumes the responsibility of maintaining complete, accurate, and up-to-date financial records in the following areas:

- Billing and collection procedures
- Financial planning
- Declaring money earned to federal and state agencies

# Account Management

Account management begins with a clearly defined financial strategy established by the dentist. Once these guidelines have been determined, it is the responsibility of the business assistant to follow through with specific objectives. Basic practice financial policies should include the following: statements on gathering financial information; presenting the fee; making financial arrangements with patients; and collecting overdue accounts.

## Gathering Financial Information

When a new patient calls to schedule an appointment, this is the time to provide the financial services offered. Inquire about dental insurance and inform the patient to bring their identification card to the appointment. This material should be reviewed to determine eligibility and available benefits for coverage. The registration form gathers all the basic financial information needed to manage the account history and complete the patient identification portion of an insurance claim form.

Information on the form includes the following:

- The name, address, telephone number(s), and place of employment of the person responsible for the account
- Information specifying the patient's coverage under a dental insurance plan
- Identification information for all individuals included on the account

### Credit Reports

Dentistry today is costly, especially in the area of specialty procedures such as implants, surgical procedures, and orthodontics. A credit report of the responsible party may be requested. If this is the dentist's policy, the responsible party should be informed before the credit report is applied for. Consumer credit reporting agencies, commonly referred to as **credit bureaus** or **agencies,** will provide a financial profile of the patient. The report provides information on the consumer's paying habits and accounts placed for collection, plus other pertinent information such as lawsuits, judgments, and bankruptcies.

### Fee Presentation

Before a case is presented to the patient, an estimate is developed as part of the treatment plan. This estimate is prepared in duplicate: One copy is provided to the patient, and the other is retained with the office records.

The fee for service represents a fair return to the dentist for professional treatment provided. After the dentist has completed the case presentation to the patient, the business assistant will discuss the fees involved and make financial arrangements with the patient to the satisfaction of both the dentist and the patient.

### Making Financial Arrangements

Financial arrangements are made with each patient when professional services are performed. These arrangements are made before treatment is initiated, except in such instances as emergency treatment. Realistic financial arrangements are made in an unhurried manner with the person responsible for the account. This information remains confidential and should take place in a private setting where others cannot overhear the discussion.

When making financial arrangements, it is necessary to take into consideration the dentist's stated payment plans, along with the sound business principles used in the management of the practice. It is also necessary to consider the patient's ability to pay. The resulting arrangements should be reasonable to both parties. The patient must realize that once these arrangements have been made, he or she is responsible for following through as agreed. All financial agreements should be recorded on the account **ledger**. (See Chapter 62 for more information on the ledger.) The patient will sign a contract for the agreed amount. A copy is provided to the patient, and the original is retained with the office records.

# Accounting

**Accounting** is the means or process of recording, classifying, and summarizing financial transactions. **Bookkeeping** is the recording of the accounting process. The business assistant conducts bookkeeping procedures on a daily basis to maintain dental practice accounts. The two types of bookkeeping systems used in a dental practice are the accounts receivable and accounts payable systems.

RECALL

1 What two types of bookkeeping systems are used in dental practices?
2 What form in the patient record is used to gather financial information from a patient?
3 Where in the dental practice is it best for the business assistant to discuss financial arrangements with a patient?

## Accounts Receivable

The accounts receivable system manages all money owed to the practice. Accounts receivable management, which is frequently referred to as **bookkeeping,** involves maintaining financial records regarding all **transactions** related to collecting fees for professional services provided to a patient. This information must be arranged systematically so it is accurate at all times and provides the data needed for effective management of these financial matters. The business assistant assumes the responsibility of handling other people's money. In this way, he or she is responsible for making every effort to keep this money safe, to record it accurately, and to respect the confidence in which all of this information must be held.

The dentist may choose to obtain **bonding** insurance on staff members who handle practice funds by receiving and banking patient payments or writing **checks**. This insurance will cover a loss, and the employee can be prosecuted under the law for any such theft.

## Types of Accounts Receivable Systems

The most frequently used type of accounts receivable bookkeeping system in a dental practice is the computerized system or a manual **pegboard system**. Increasingly, offices are using an electronic practice management system because of the capability of integrating technology with accounting.

### *Pegboard Accounts Receivable Management*

Pegboard accounting, also known as a **one-write system,** is a manual bookkeeping system in which all records are completed with a single entry. Through positioning of the daily journal page, ledger card, and a carbonized receipt, all financial records for each patient visit are completed by writing the information just one time (Fig. 63.1). Entries for additional records, such as daily totals and monthly summaries, must be completed manually. The totals then must be calculated and verified for accuracy.

### *Computerized Accounts Receivable Management*

With a computerized accounts receivable system, data entered into the system is used to maintain account histories and practice records (Fig. 63.2). It is essential that the information be entered into the system accurately because it is used to generate account totals and daily and monthly summaries. These and other management reports are automatically calculated and produced by the system. It is also important that the data stored on the hard drive of the computer are protected by being backed up (copied for safekeeping) daily. An additional set of backup files (zip drives or flash drives) should be stored in a safe place outside the office. These backup records are vital in the event of theft, fire, or other disaster that makes it necessary to reconstruct information that may have been lost from the system.

## Accounts Receivable Management Basics

Whether you are using a manual or a computerized system, the same information requirements and organizational format are necessary. Learning to use either system begins with an understanding of the basics of accounts receivable bookkeeping. The accounting process begins when the patient leaves the treatment area.

### *Charge Slips*

A charge slip, also referred to as a **routing slip** or **superbill,** is used to transmit financial information from the treatment area to the business office. The form contains information about the patient, such as name, account number and previous balance, current charges, and payment. The form can be designed to include all of the procedures completed in the office along with the insurance CDT code. The form provides space for the dentist or assistant to note the treatment provided at the visit. The form consists of three color-coded pages (white for the patient's permanent record, yellow for the office or patient to submit to the insurance company, and pink for the patient's copy) (Fig. 63.3).

The completed charge slip is returned to the business office, and the information is **posted** to the accounts receivable system. Charge slips are a part of the **audit trail**. A charge slip is generated for each patient. At the end of the day, a number must account for each charge slip. In this way, the dentist knows that all patient visits have been entered into the system.

### *Daily Journal Page*

The daily journal page is the practice record of all patient transactions each day; this record includes the name of each patient seen and any charges, payments, and adjustments made to that account. Throughout the day, all transactions are posted to the bookkeeping system. In addition to maintaining the patient account record, this posting generates the daily journal page entry. A computerized system automatically totals this form and uses the information to generate other practice reports.

### *Receipts and Walkout Statements*

A **walkout statement** is similar to a receipt, except that it shows the current account balance. It is provided to patients who do not provide payment in full (Fig. 63.4). A walkout statement should be provided with a postage-paid reply envelope, allowing the patient to mail the outstanding payment within a specified time period. The use of walkout statements improves cash flow because it speeds payments. It also reduces the number of statements that must be prepared and mailed at the end of the month.

## Recording Payments

All payments are entered promptly into the bookkeeping system so they are documented in the account history and on

## ANATOMY OF A PEGBOARD ACCOUNTS RECEIVABLE SYSTEM

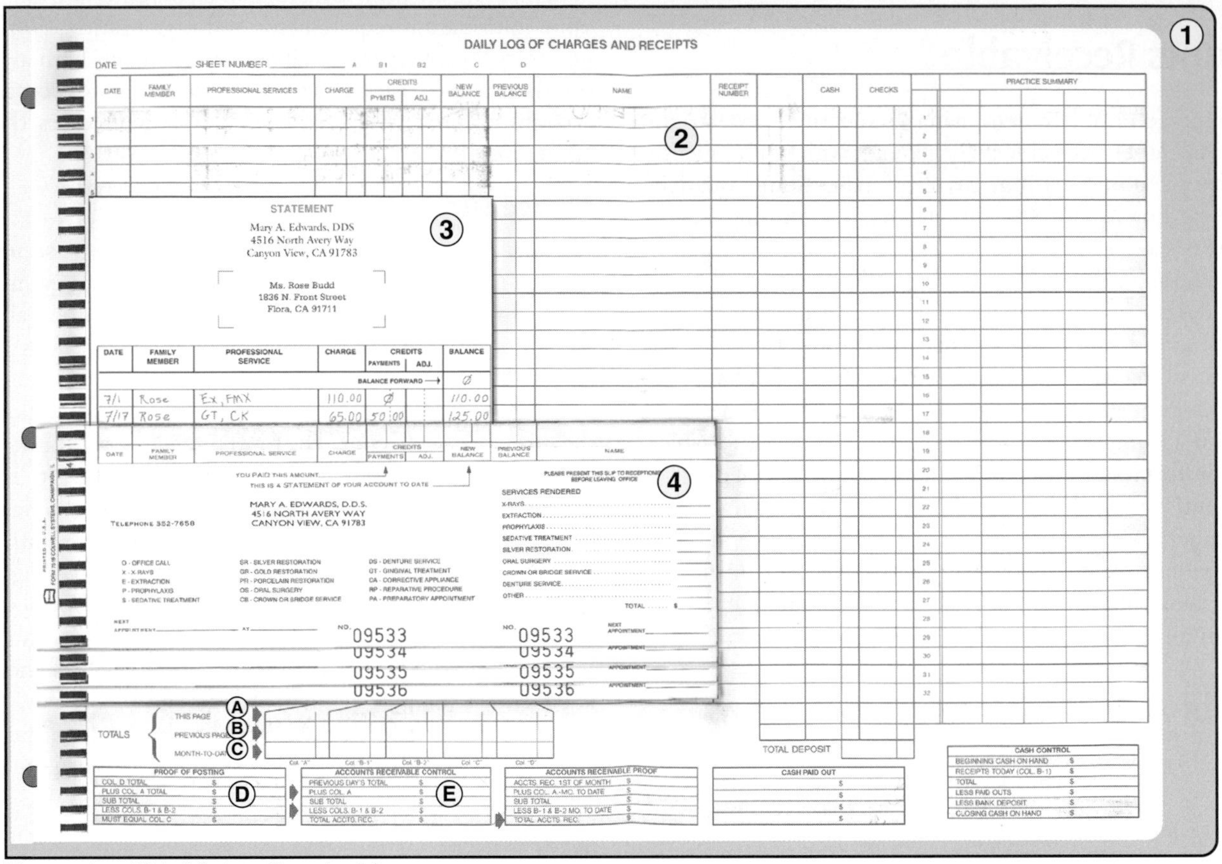

(Forms courtesy of Colwell Systems, Champaign, IL.)

### ① PEGBOARD

The pegboard is a flat board with a series of pegs on the left-hand side of the board. The pegs align and hold the forms in place. The alignment facilitates the "one write" concept.

### ② DAILY JOURNAL

The daily journal (day sheet, daily log of charges and receipts) is a large sheet that is placed over the pegs. The daily journal contains information that identifies all financial transactions that have taken place during the day (or other identified period of time). At the end of the recording period (day), columns are totaled, balanced, and placed in a journal for storage. Information stated in the journal becomes an important document and must be safeguarded against loss or damage.

### ③ ACCOUNT RECORD

Ledger cards contain individual account information. Information listed on the ledger card identifies the patient, treatment, payment information, and account balance.

Ledger cards are placed alphabetically in trays (Fig. 14-4). The information on the ledger card is considered confidential and is important documentation. The cards are stored in metal boxes which can be tightly closed at the end of the day to protect them from fire and damage.

### ④ RECEIPT AND CHARGE SLIPS

This portion of the system is used as a communication and audit tool. The clinical assistant or administrative assistant enters transaction information onto the charge slip (communicating with the front office). The information is used to post transactions. The receipt portion of the slip is used to communicate transactions with the patient. Control numbers are printed on each slip, providing a tracking system to ensure that all transactions are posted.

Superbills are used in the same way as receipts. With the addition of insurance coding (CDT Procedure Codes), they can also be used for insurance billing. The completed superbill is given to the patient and it becomes the responsibility of the patient to submit the form to the insurance carrier.

### ANATOMY OF DAILY JOURNAL CALCULATIONS

Ⓐ Add each column vertically and place the totals in the corresponding boxes.

Ⓑ Bring previous page totals forward (found in the corresponding box on the previous day's journal).

Ⓒ Add the columns, enter the total in the corresponding box.

Ⓓ Complete "Proof of Posting."

Ⓔ Complete "Accounts Receivable Control."

**FIG. 63.1** Anatomy of pegboard accounts receivable system. *(Modified from Gaylor LJ: The administrative dental assistant, ed 4, St Louis, 2016, Elsevier.)*

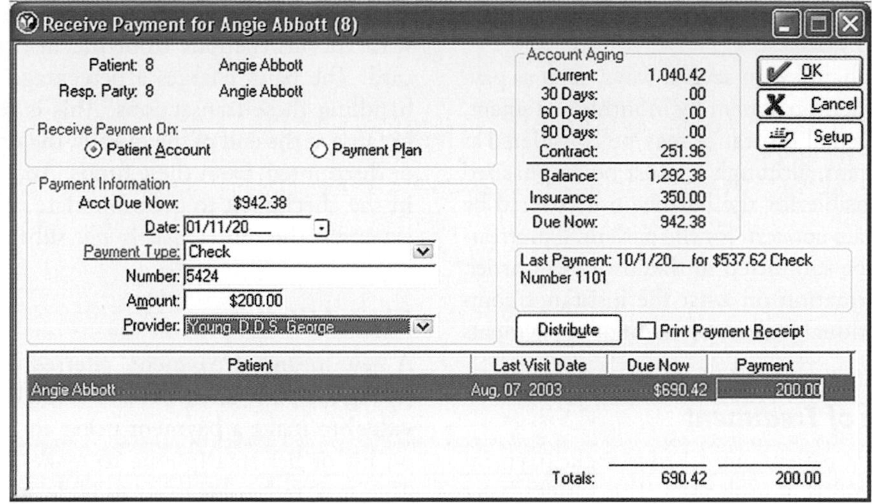


FIG. 63.2 Computerized accounts receivable management system. *(Courtesy Patterson Dental, St Paul, MN.)*

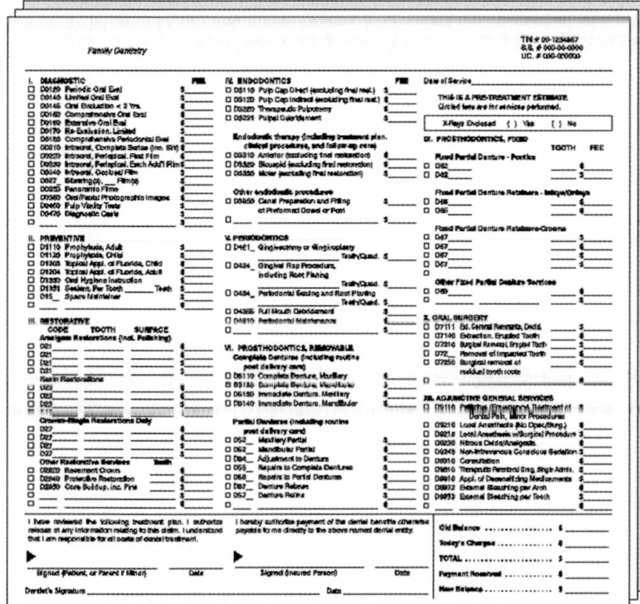

FIG. 63.3 A sample superbill form is used to transmit financial information from the treatment area to the business office. *(Courtesy Patterson Dental, St. Paul, MN.)*

the daily journal page. Payments received by mail are entered in the same manner as those made in person. As a safeguard, checks should be stamped immediately with a **restrictive endorsement,** which prevents anyone from cashing a check if stolen.

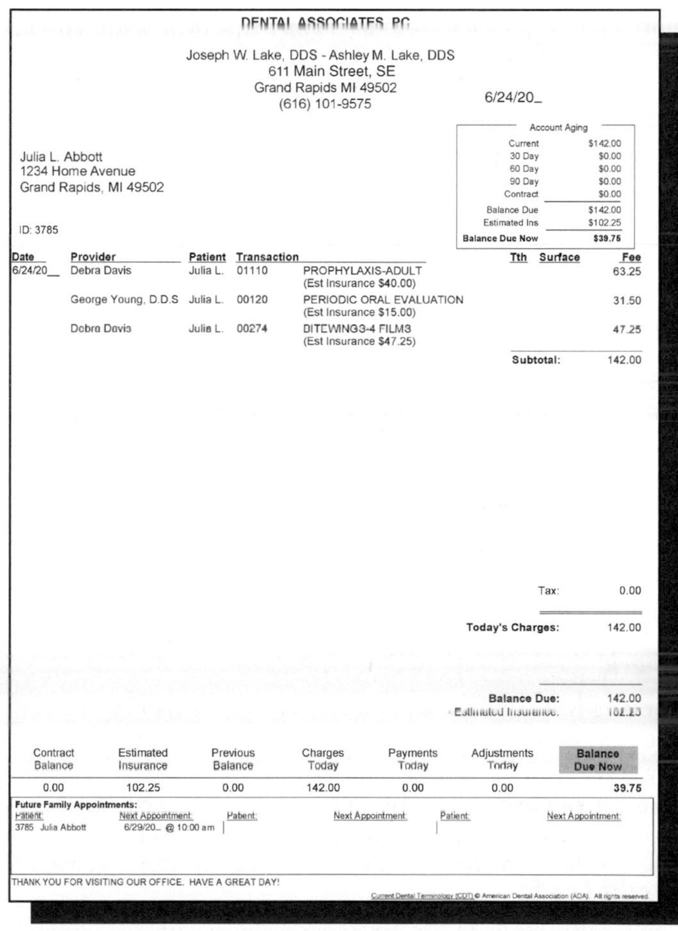

DENTAL ASSOCIATES PC

Joseph W. Lake, DDS - Ashley M. Lake, DDS
611 Main Street, SE
Grand Rapids MI 49502
(616) 101-9575

6/24/20_

Julia L. Abbott
1234 Home Avenue
Grand Rapids, MI 49502

ID: 3785

| Account Aging | |
|---|---|
| Current | $142.00 |
| 30 Day | $0.00 |
| 60 Day | $0.00 |
| 90 Day | $0.00 |
| Contract | $0.00 |
| Balance Due | $142.00 |
| Estimated Ins | $102.25 |
| **Balance Due Now** | **$39.75** |

| Date | Provider | Patient | Transaction | | Tth | Surface | Fee |
|---|---|---|---|---|---|---|---|
| 6/24/20__ | Debra Davis | Julia L. | 01110 | PROPHYLAXIS-ADULT (Est Insurance $40.00) | | | 63.25 |
| | George Young, D.D.S | Julia L. | 00120 | PERIODIC ORAL EVALUATION (Est Insurance $15.00) | | | 31.50 |
| | Debra Davis | Julia L. | 00274 | BITEWINGS-4 FILMS (Est Insurance $47.25) | | | 47.25 |

Subtotal: 142.00

Tax: 0.00

Today's Charges: 142.00

Balance Due: 142.00
Estimated Insurance: 102.25

| Contract Balance | Estimated Insurance | Previous Balance | Charges Today | Payments Today | Adjustments Today | Balance Due Now |
|---|---|---|---|---|---|---|
| 0.00 | 102.25 | 0.00 | 142.00 | 0.00 | 0.00 | 39.75 |

Future Family Appointments:

| Patient: | Next Appointment: | Patient: | Next Appointment: | Patient: | Next Appointment: |
|---|---|---|---|---|---|
| 3785 Julia Abbott | 6/29/20_ @ 10:00 am | | | | |

THANK YOU FOR VISITING OUR OFFICE. HAVE A GREAT DAY!

Current Dental Terminology (CDT) © American Dental Association (ADA). All rights reserved

FIG. 63.4 A walkout statement is presented to the patient for his or her records. *(Courtesy Patterson Dental, St Paul, MN.)*

## Patient Account Records

Patient account records are organized on the basis of information regarding the responsible party. The **responsible party,** also known as the **guarantor,** is the person who has agreed to be responsible for payment of the account. This is not always the patient. The patient account record is used to track all account transactions. A current account balance is maintained at all times, and this information is used to generate statements, insurance claims, and other collection efforts. In a manual system, patient account records are maintained on account ledger cards. In a computerized system, these are organized as account histories or ledgers.

## Payment

Patients' accounts can be handled in several ways, such as payment at the time of treatment, payment by monthly statement, and divided payments. Dental insurance may be considered as another method of payment, although it must be emphasized that the patient is responsible for the balance not covered by the insurer. To help alleviate concern for the patient, a pretreatment estimate form can be submitted to the insurance carrier. This would provide information on what the insurance company covers and any additional patient payment or copayments that will be required.

### Payment at the Time of Treatment

Under this payment policy, patients are asked to make payment in full for treatment provided at each visit. This system helps control practice costs by improving cash flow and reducing the cost of sending statements or using other collection methods. Patients must be notified of this type of payment plan before the first visit. In many practices, this is completed during the initial telephone conversation. Under this plan, cash, checks, and credit cards are accepted for payment.

### Cash

Although few patients pay for dental treatment in cash, it is necessary to be alert to the needs of cash-paying patients. When you are accepting payment in cash for services, it is essential to ensure that the office has correct change available for the patient. The patient who is paying cash must be provided a written (or computer-generated) receipt.

A **change fund** or **petty cash fund** is a fixed amount of cash (usually $50 or less) that is maintained in small bills so that money will be available when a patient pays in cash. Each morning, the change fund is placed in the cash drawer, and it is used as needed during the day. At the end of the day, the change fund is removed and placed in safekeeping. Money from the change fund does *not* become part of the daily deposit, and the amount in the change fund at the end of the day must be the same as it was at the beginning of the day.

### Check

Patients will pay for dental services with a personal check to the dentist or to the name of the professional practice. In some practices, it is office policy to review the payer's driver's license number and one other form of identification. The patient paying by check is provided a receipt for the payment.

### Credit Cards

Another option is to pay for dental services with a credit card. Credit card transactions are listed as payments, but the posting code is different from that used for cash or a check. The credit card system is now electronically able to verify immediately if the card is valid and that the credit limit has not been exceeded. When a dentist agrees to be a bankcard merchant, the participating bank will explain the procedure of verification and submittal.

The credit card charge form is completed, and a copy is handed to the patient. Credit card charges are not part of the regular bank deposit. Instead, they are managed in accordance with the instructions from the institution issuing the credit card. The bank charges a percentage rate as a service fee for handling these transactions. This is referred to as *discounting* because at the end of the month, the service charge is deducted, or discounted, from these funds. An adjustment entry is made in the checkbook to accommodate this discount as a practice expense. This difference is *not* subtracted from the patient's account.

### Digital Wallet

A new means of payment, referred to as the *digital wallet,* is taking the place of checks and credit cards. This allows an individual to make a payment using an "app" that is downloaded on his or her smartphone to make an electronic transaction. This new technology can provide security and encryption of personal information making it a safer means of financial transactions. The individual's bank account is linked to the digital wallet allowing the money to move directly from one account to another.

### Professional Courtesy and Discounts

Occasionally, the dentist will extend a professional courtesy in the form of a discount to professional colleagues or members of their families. The dentist makes this determination and places a notation on the chart after completing the treatment for the day. For example, if the usual fee for a procedure is $50 and the dentist wishes to give a **professional courtesy** of $10, the amount owed is $40.

A practice may offer a discount if payment is made in full before the beginning of planned treatment. For example, if a patient is having a complete upper and lower denture fabricated at a cost of $1400, the dentist might extend a 5 percent discount ($70) for payment in full. In this case the patient would pay $1330 in advance, for a savings of 5 percent off the total charge.

To enter this discount into the bookkeeping system, the total fee of $1400 is posted. Then an adjustment representing the discount is entered for $70. This adjustment acts as a credit and leaves an account balance of $1330 to be paid.

## Daily Proof of Posting

At the end of each workday, the entries on the daily journal page are compared with the appointment book to ensure that all patient visits have been entered. Computerized systems total all figures automatically and can print various reports as needed. The total for receipts must match the amount in the cash drawer minus the change fund. If these two numbers do not match, or "balance," it is necessary to go back and find the error.

## Bank Deposits

All receipts should be deposited daily. When the amount of receipts exactly matches the amount of deposits, the account has met the auditor's critical test to verify bookkeeping accuracy. A **deposit slip** is an itemized memorandum of the currency and checks taken to the bank to be credited to the practice's account (Fig. 63.5). This slip is generated from the computer after all checks have been posted. After the deposit has been made, the date and amount of the deposit should be entered in the practice check register as follows:

- The deposit slip must be imprinted with the practice name, address, and account number.
- The information on the deposit slip must be legible.
- All cash (bills and coins) is listed together under "Currency."
- Checks are listed separately, usually by the last name and first initial of the person writing the check. Computer systems do this automatically when checks are posted.
- In many practices, the deposit slip is completed in duplicate so a copy can be retained with the practice records.

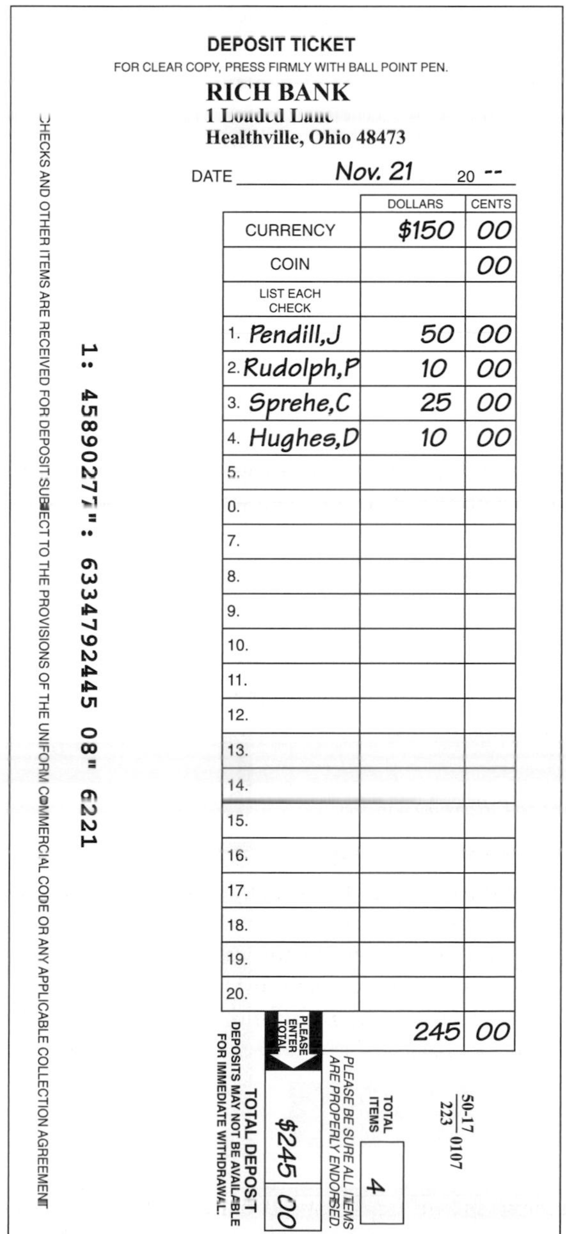

DEPOSIT TICKET

FOR CLEAR COPY, PRESS FIRMLY WITH BALL POINT PEN.

RICH BANK
1 Loaded Lane
Healthville, Ohio 48473

DATE Nov. 21 20 --

| | DOLLARS | CENTS |
|---|---|---|
| CURRENCY | $150 | 00 |
| COIN | | 00 |
| LIST EACH CHECK | | |
| 1. Pendill,J | 50 | 00 |
| 2. Rudolph,P | 10 | 00 |
| 3. Sprehe,C | 25 | 00 |
| 4. Hughes,D | 10 | 00 |
| 5. | | |
| 6. | | |
| 7. | | |
| 8. | | |
| 9. | | |
| 10. | | |
| 11. | | |
| 12. | | |
| 13. | | |
| 14. | | |
| 15. | | |
| 16. | | |
| 17. | | |
| 18. | | |
| 19. | | |
| 20. | | |
| PLEASE ENTER TOTAL | 245 | 00 |

TOTAL DEPOSIT $245 00

DEPOSITS MAY NOT BE AVAILABLE FOR IMMEDIATE WITHDRAWAL.

PLEASE BE SURE ALL ITEMS ARE PROPERLY ENDORSED.

TOTAL ITEMS 4

50-17/223 0107

CHECKS AND OTHER ITEMS ARE RECEIVED FOR DEPOSIT SUBJECT TO THE PROVISIONS OF THE UNIFORM COMMERCIAL CODE OR ANY APPLICABLE COLLECTION AGREEMENT

1: 458902771": 6334792445 08" 6221

**FIG. 63.5** Deposit slip.

## Monthly Statement

The monthly statement represents a request for payment of the balance due on the accounts receivable. Under this plan, the patient is expected to pay the balance in full on receipt of the statement. A computer-generated statement shows this data, plus an age analysis of the account balance. Financial arrangements can also be printed on a computer-generated statement. Some practices add a finance charge (usually 1 percent) to accounts that are not paid within 30 days of receipt of the first statement.

When a charge such as this is incorporated on an account, or when more than four payment installments are set up, the patient will receive a **Truth in Lending** statement (Fig. 63.6).

### *Divided Payment Plans*

Divided payment plans are arrangements by which the patient pays a fixed amount on a regular basis. For example, orthodontic treatment is commonly divided into a monthly payment plan. These arrangements are made at the time of the case presentation. After the patient has accepted the proposed treatment plan, the business assistant will work with the patient to develop a divided payment plan. When a divided payment plan is set up, the primary information to be determined is as follows:

- Total fee for services to be rendered
- Balance after deduction of the down payment; the resulting amount is to be financed
- Annual percentage rate of the finance charge (if there is one)
- Number of payments to be made
- Amount of each payment
- Date on which each payment is due

Once this information has been gathered, the payment plan agreement is completed, and both the patient and the dentist must provide a signature to confirm the agreement. A copy is provided to the patient, with the original kept in the patient's record.

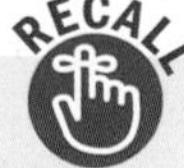


4 Is money that is owed to the practice considered part of accounts payable?
5 If a dental office does not have a computerized accounts receivable system, what type of system would be used?
6 What form is used to transmit a patient's fee from the treatment area to the business office?
7 What methods of payment can a patient use to pay on an account?
8 How often should bank deposits be made?

## Collections

It is essential for the business assistant to have the skills to manage the money owed to the practice and to collect it in a timely and organized manner.

## Accounts Receivable Report

The accounts receivable report is a valuable management report that shows the total balance due on each patient account plus an analysis of the "age of the account." This shows how much of the balance is current (recent charges not yet billed), 30 days old, 31 to 60 days old, 61 to 90 days old, and older. This information is helpful in tracking and taking action on overdue accounts.

A computer can generate this report automatically with a breakdown of account age. Although creation of the report is not automatic with a pegboard system, it is possible to generate one manually.

### *Management of Collection Efforts*

All collection efforts must be handled tactfully and in keeping with the dentist's wishes and policies, because the dentist is ultimately responsible for the actions of his or her employees. The dentist does not want to lose a patient's goodwill because of poor collection tactics. Under the federal **Fair Debt Collection Practice Act,** it is illegal for anyone to carry out the following:

- Telephone the debtor at inconvenient hours (before 8:00 PM is considered an acceptable time).
- Threaten violence or use obscene language.
- Use false pretenses to get information.
- Contact the debtor's employer, except to verify employment or residence.

**FINANCIAL AGREEMENT**

DATE ________

PATIENT NAME ________

RESPONSIBLE PARTY ________

ADDRESS ________

________

HOME PHONE ________ WORK PHONE ________

CELL PHONE ________ E-MAIL ________

| | |
|---|---|
| COST OF TOTAL TREATMENT | $________ |
| INITIAL PAYMENT | –________ |
| APPROXIMATE INSURANCE PAYMENTS | –________ |
| BALANCE DUE | =________ |
| INTEREST RATE PERCENTAGE | ________ |
| TOTAL AMOUNT OF FINANCE CHARGE | +________ |
| AMOUNT REMAINING TO BE PAID BY PATIENT | =________ |

AMOUNT DUE TO BE PAID IN________ MONTHLY PAYMENTS OF $ ________ STARTING________. BALANCE TO BE PAID IN FULL BY ________.

I understand the financial arrangements above and agree to comply with them. I agree that parents are responsible for all fees and services rendered for treatment of a child. I understand that I am responsible for ALL fees regardless of insurance coverage. I also understand that as treatment progresses the above fees may have to be adjusted, but that I will be informed of these adjustments and how they will affect my payment plan. In the event that my payments are not received within 30 days of their due date, I agree to pay all costs of collections, including, but not limited to, reasonable attorney's fees.

________ Responsible Party Signature ________ Date

**FINANCIAL AGREEMENT**

ITEM 07-0513739/9054

**FIG. 63.6** Example of a truth-in-lending form. *(Adapted from a form provided courtesy Patterson Dental, St. Paul, MN. From Finkbeiner BL, Finkbeiner CA: Practice management for the dental team, ed 8, St Louis, 2016, Mosby.)*

### Collection Telephone Calls

Telephone calls can be more effective than letters when collecting money because they provide direct contact with the debtor and therefore are not as easily ignored. When you are placing a collection call, be certain to speak only to the person responsible for the account. Never leave a message that could be misunderstood, could reveal confidential information, or could be considered damaging.

Before you pick up the phone, it is critical that you have all the specifics of the debt you are calling about. Having the facts in front of you keeps you in control. You do not want the conversation to get disrupted by a question you cannot answer. Many debtors know how to use this to their advantage. Suddenly they cannot discuss payment on their account without details you do not have and they do not "have in front of them" either. So the call is over.

If you hear yourself saying, "I'll have to get back to you on that," you have just given the debtor an extension without a commitment to pay—and you will have to start from the beginning with that person when you call back. At minimum, be sure to have the following information in front of you before you make the call:

- Exact amount owed
- Payment due date
- Notes from previous conversations

Once the appropriate person has been reached, the business assistant should identify himself or herself and wait. The person who is being called knows what is wanted, and it is best to let that person make the first statement. The debtor may react with anger or hostility. It is important to remember that this is part of a defense mechanism and not a personal attack. Regardless of what the debtor says or does, do not become argumentative or defensive. Try to be understanding but firm and never permit yourself to be insulting, no matter what the provocation. Note any agreement made over the telephone on the patient's account ledger. Promises should be followed up carefully, and if they are not kept, the account should be taken to the next step in the collection process (Box 63.1).

### Collection Letters

All collection letters should be phrased in a firm, positive, business-like manner that makes every effort to persuade the patient to pay the debt and allows the patient to avoid embarrassment (Fig. 63.7 and Box 63.2).

#### BOX 63.1 Specific Responses to Say When Calling to Collect Money

Patient: The check is in the mail.
Collector: Great! May I have the check number, amount, and date it was mailed so I can ensure it is posted correctly?
Patient: I have a cash flow problem right now.
Collector: I understand that times are difficult. Can I set you up on a payment plan, or can you make at least a partial payment today?
Patient: I don't have a copy of the invoice.
Collector: I'll fax/mail the invoice right now. Will you be mailing the check today?

### Final Collection Options

The final decision regarding turning accounts over for collection must be made by the dentist, and an account is never turned over without the dentist's specific approval.

### Collection Agency

A collection agency makes additional efforts to collect the balance on an overdue account. The agency's charge is a percentage of the amount collected, and this is deducted before the balance is remitted to the dental office. Some attorneys also attempt to collect overdue accounts in exchange for a percentage of the amount collected.

### Small Claims Court

Another option is to take the debtor to small claims court. Sometimes, arrangements are made so that the business assistant, not the dentist, appears for the hearing. One drawback to the option of seeking a small claims court judgment is that even if the court rules that the debtor must pay, it is still up to the practice to collect the amount of the judgment.

#### Collection Follow-through

Here is a collection follow-through timetable that can be used to collect money:

- 30 days: The regular statement, which is sent at the end of the month, within 30 days, or on completion of treatment with financial arrangements printed on the statement.
- 60 days: A second statement, with a kindly printed collection message or a telephone call.
- 75 days: Another telephone call and an amiable collection letter mailed.
- 90 days: A third statement with a stronger note or a collection letter; often, this letter states that unless payment is made within 10 days, the account will be turned over to a collection agency for action.
- 105 days: Another telephone call; in this call, the message should be, "Unless the account is paid by the specified date, it will be necessary to turn the account over to a collection agency for action."
- 120 days: If no payment has been made and promises have not been kept, the account is turned over to a collection agency for action.

9 What is the time frame for an office to begin collection efforts?
10 Give four ways that a business can follow through on the collection of fees.

## Accounts Payable Management

**Accounts payable** systems manage all of the money that is owed by the practice. **Expenses** and **disbursements** determine the cost of doing business in the dental practice.

Expenses are called **overhead,** which is the actual cost of doing business. As these expenses are incurred, they become accounts payable. Disbursements are the payments made for these accounts payable. It is the responsibility of the office manager or the business assistant to ensure accuracy in all accounts payable transactions within the practice and in the management of day-to-day expenses and disbursements.

## Dental Office Overhead

Dental office overhead consists of all expenses incurred in running a dental practice; these expenses are categorized as *fixed overhead* and *variable overhead.* Fee schedules must reflect both of these overhead factors, plus a fair return to the dentist.

### Fixed Overhead

**Fixed overhead** includes business expenses that continue at all times; these are costs (such as the rent or mortgage, utilities, insurance, and salaries) that are incurred regardless of whether the dentist is in the office or whether professional services are actually being provided. *Note:* Not all salaries are part of fixed overhead. Salaries that are not fixed are those of professionals who work as independent contractors, on a commission basis, or as part-time workers, who are employed on an hourly rate "as needed."

### Variable Overhead

**Variable overhead** expenses are those that change according to the types of services procured or obtained, for example, dental and stationery supplies, independent contractor fees, dental laboratory fees, and equipment repair fees.

### Gross versus Net Income

The money the dentist receives for professional services is calculated as **gross income** (the total of *all* professional income received). Gross income minus the payment of all practice-related expenses yields the dentist's **net income**

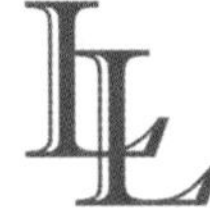

Dental Associates, PC
611 Main Street, SE
Grand Rapids, MI 49502
Phone: 616.101.9575 Fax: 616.101.9999
E-mail: office@dapc.com or Visit us at: www.Lakedental.com

Joseph W. Lake, DDS    Ashley M. Lake, DDS

November 5, 20__

Mr. Marvin Beattie
1407 Colorado Street N.W.
Grand Rapids, MI 49505

Dear Mr. Beattie:

Your account of $565.00 is over 90 days past due. If you are unable to pay this account in full, perhaps we can help you in making arrangements to take care of this account.

Please contact us before November 15, 20__ at 5:00 p.m.

Sincerely,

Jennifer Ellis, RDA
Administrative Assistant

**FIG. 63.7** Two examples of collection letters showing the intensity of the wording. *(From Finkbeiner BL, Finkbeiner CA: Practice management for the dental team, ed 8, St Louis, 2016, Mosby.)*

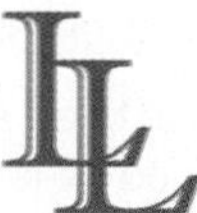

Dental Associates, PC
611 Main Street, SE
Grand Rapids, MI 49502
Phone: 616.101.9575 Fax: 616.101.9999
E-mail: office@dapc.com or Visit us at: www.Lakedental.com

Joseph W. Lake, DDS    Ashley M. Lake, DDS

November 26, 20__

**REGISTERED**

Mr. Marvin Beattie
1407 Colorado Street N.W.
Grand Rapids, MI 49505

Dear Mr. Beattie:

Since we have not heard from you regarding your account of $565.00 from June 1, 20__, please be informed that it will be necessary to transfer this account to a collection agency.

This account must be paid in full by Friday, December 1, 20__ to avoid such legal action.

Sincerely,

Jennifer Ellis, RDA
Administrative Assistant

**FIG. 63.7, cont'd**

from the practice. Unless the dentist earns an adequate net income, he or she will not be able to afford to maintain a practice.

A **certified public accountant (CPA)** is often employed on a retainer basis. It will be the CPA's responsibility to handle the major financial records, such as annual profit and loss statements, tax returns, and other government reports. These reports are based on financial information supplied by the dental practice. This information must be accurate, up-to-date, complete, and presented in a usable format. The business assistant can help the accountant by having the required information and records in good order and ready on time.

## Disbursements

Effective management of a dental practice requires organized handling and prompt payment of all bills for practice-related expenses. Payment of major expenses should be made by check, with records kept up to date and balanced at all times. Minor expenses are handled through the use of petty cash. All expenses should be documented as completely as possible with bills and receipts or canceled checks.

### *Packing Slips, Invoices, and Statements*

A **packing slip** is a form used in a warehouse operation that lists the items to be shipped and the recipient of the shipment. The packing slip may also include the amount due for a credit order and any shipping and handling charges, as well as a shipment control number. The packing slip travels with the shipment and, at the destination, is used to confirm that the shipment is complete. It is matched with the invoice before payment is made. When materials are received, they should be carefully checked against the packing slip to ensure that everything has been received as ordered and that everything is in good condition. Discrepancies or damage should be reported immediately to the supplier.

An **invoice** may be included with the shipment, or it may be mailed separately, but it is a detailed list of goods shipped or services rendered, with an account of all costs on an itemized bill. Once an invoice has been verified, it should be paid promptly unless other arrangements have been made (Fig. 63.8).

## BOX 63.2 Suggestions for Composing Collection Letters

- Your account has always been paid promptly in the past, so this must be an oversight. Please accept this note as a friendly reminder of your account due in the amount of $_____.
- Since your care in this office in March, we have had no word from you in regard to how you are feeling or your account payment. If it is impossible for you to pay the full amount of $______ at this time, please call this office before June 15 so that satisfactory arrangements can be worked out.
- Medical bills are payable at the time of service unless special credit arrangements are made. Please send your check in full or call this office before June 30, 20__.
- If you have some question about your statement, we will be happy to discuss it with you. If not, may we have a payment before the end of this month?
- Unless some definite arrangement is made to reduce your balance of $_____, we can no longer carry your account on our books. Delinquent accounts are turned over to our collection agency on the 25th of the month.
- When a payment plan has been established, it can be reinforced by recognizing the first remittance with a letter of acknowledgment: Thank you for the recent payment of $_____ on your account. We are glad to cooperate with you in this arrangement for clearing your account. We will look for your next check at about the same time next month, and your final payment the following month.
- When a payment schedule has been arranged by a telephone call, it can be confirmed by letter: As agreed upon in our telephone conversation today, we will expect you to mail a payment of $50 on February 10; $50 on March 10; and the balance on April 10. If some emergency should prevent your making one of these payments on time, please notify us immediately by telephone.

### Do's and Don'ts

**Do**

- Individualize letters to suit the situation.
- Design your early letters as mere reminders of debt.
- Always imply that the patient has good intentions to pay, until lack of response over a period of time proves otherwise.
- Send letters with a firmer tone only after you have sent one or two friendly reminders.

**Don't**

- Use the same collection letter for a patient with good paying habits as for one who is known to neglect financial obligations.
- Place an overdue notice of any kind on a postcard or on the outside of an envelope. This is an invasion of privacy.

From Adams AP, Proctor DB: Kinn's the medical assistant: an applied learning approach, ed 11, St Louis, 2011, Saunders.

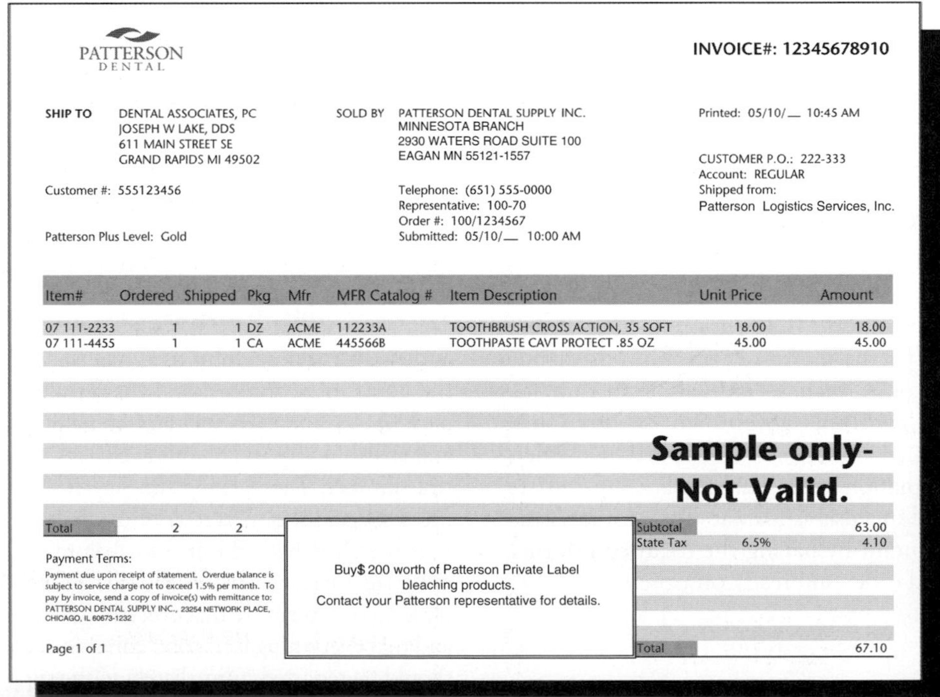

PATTERSON DENTAL

**INVOICE#: 12345678910**

**SHIP TO** DENTAL ASSOCIATES, PC
JOSEPH W LAKE, DDS
611 MAIN STREET SE
GRAND RAPIDS MI 49502

Customer #: 555123456

Patterson Plus Level: Gold

SOLD BY PATTERSON DENTAL SUPPLY INC.
MINNESOTA BRANCH
2930 WATERS ROAD SUITE 100
EAGAN MN 55121-1557

Telephone: (651) 555-0000
Representative: 100-70
Order #: 100/1234567
Submitted: 05/10/__ 10:00 AM

Printed: 05/10/__ 10:45 AM

CUSTOMER P.O.: 222-333
Account: REGULAR
Shipped from:
Patterson Logistics Services, Inc.

| Item# | Ordered | Shipped | Pkg | Mfr | MFR Catalog # | Item Description | Unit Price | Amount |
|---|---|---|---|---|---|---|---|---|
| 07 111-2233 | 1 | 1 | DZ | ACME | 112233A | TOOTHBRUSH CROSS ACTION, 35 SOFT | 18.00 | 18.00 |
| 07 111-4455 | 1 | 1 | CA | ACME | 445566B | TOOTHPASTE CAVT PROTECT .85 OZ | 45.00 | 45.00 |
| Total | 2 | 2 | | | | | | |

**Sample only-**
**Not Valid.**

| | | |
|---|---|---|
| Subtotal | | 63.00 |
| State Tax | 6.5% | 4.10 |
| Total | | 67.10 |

Payment Terms:
Payment due upon receipt of statement. Overdue balance is subject to service charge not to exceed 1.5% per month. To pay by invoice, send a copy of invoice(s) with remittance to: PATTERSON DENTAL SUPPLY INC., 23254 NETWORK PLACE, CHICAGO, IL 60673-1232

Buy$ 200 worth of Patterson Private Label bleaching products.
Contact your Patterson representative for details.

Page 1 of 1

**FIG. 63.8** Example of an invoice statement. *(Courtesy Patterson Dental, St Paul, MN.)*

A **statement** is a summary of all invoices (charges), payments, credits, and debits for the month (Fig. 63.9).

## Organizing Expenditure Records

Statements and invoices that have not yet been paid are placed in the **accounts payable folder.** As part of the organization of expenditure records, expenses are classified into categories; these usually include groups such as professional supplies, laboratory fees, salaries, rent and maintenance, utilities, and business office supplies. Category headings, which are determined by the dentist, are placed on file folders to store expense records in an organized manner. At the end of the year, this expense documentation is removed and filed, in the same categories, with other business records for that year.

The same categories are used to organize disbursements in the check register and for budget purposes. If the practice has a computer system that handles disbursements, this information is entered by category and is used when disbursements are made and records for financial management of the practice are maintained.

### Payment of Accounts

In the dental office, the accounts payable is routinely paid once or twice a month. Before writing checks to pay these accounts, the business assistant removes all invoices and statements from the accounts payable folder. These statements and invoices are verified by checking the numbers and amounts of the invoices received from each supplier during that period against the monthly statement. It also is necessary to verify that all payments, credits, and returns have been properly entered. To facilitate the handling and storage of records, the invoices are stapled to the statement that covers them.

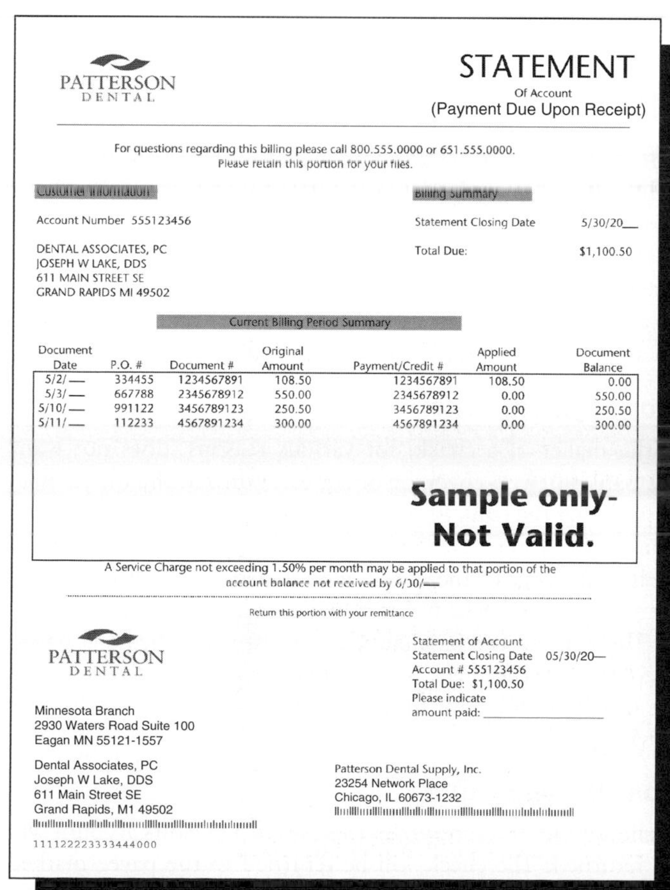

PATTERSON DENTAL

STATEMENT
Of Account
(Payment Due Upon Receipt)

For questions regarding this billing please call 800.555.0000 or 651.555.0000.
Please retain this portion for your files.

Customer Information

Account Number 555123456

DENTAL ASSOCIATES, PC
JOSEPH W LAKE, DDS
611 MAIN STREET SE
GRAND RAPIDS MI 49502

Billing Summary

Statement Closing Date 5/30/20__

Total Due: $1,100.50

Current Billing Period Summary

| Document Date | P.O. # | Document # | Original Amount | Payment/Credit # | Applied Amount | Document Balance |
|---|---|---|---|---|---|---|
| 5/2/— | 334455 | 1234567891 | 108.50 | 1234567891 | 108.50 | 0.00 |
| 5/3/— | 667788 | 2345678912 | 550.00 | 2345678912 | 0.00 | 550.00 |
| 5/10/— | 991122 | 3456789123 | 250.50 | 3456789123 | 0.00 | 250.50 |
| 5/11/— | 112233 | 4567891234 | 300.00 | 4567891234 | 0.00 | 300.00 |

**Sample only- Not Valid.**

A Service Charge not exceeding 1.50% per month may be applied to that portion of the account balance not received by 6/30/—

Return this portion with your remittance

PATTERSON DENTAL

Statement of Account
Statement Closing Date 05/30/20—
Account # 555123456
Total Due: $1,100.50
Please indicate amount paid: ______

Minnesota Branch
2930 Waters Road Suite 100
Eagan MN 55121-1557

Dental Associates, PC
Joseph W Lake, DDS
611 Main Street SE
Grand Rapids, M1 49502

Patterson Dental Supply, Inc.
23254 Network Place
Chicago, IL 60673-1232

111122223333444000

**FIG. 63.9** Example of a statement from a dental supply company. *(Courtesy Patterson Dental, St Paul, MN.)*

The dentist should review and approve all bills before payment is made. Once these accounts have been approved for payment, the business assistant writes the necessary checks. As each statement is paid, the number of the check and the date the payment was made are noted on the statement. Customarily, the business assistant writes the checks but does not sign them; the prepared checks are given to the dentist for his or her signature. The office manager who has been given limited power of attorney by the dentist and has proper authorization on file with the bank may sign checks.

### Cash on Delivery

Sometimes goods are shipped cash on delivery (COD), which means that at the time of delivery, the person who receives the goods must pay the cost of the merchandise plus a COD handling fee. Some delivery services that handle COD merchandise will accept a check for the exact amount; others insist on cash. If a check is acceptable, it should be made out to the supplier and not to the delivery service.

The business assistant should never accept a COD package unless it is something that has been ordered and is expected. When paying for a COD, the business assistant should receive a signed receipt of payment.

### Petty Cash

As stated earlier in the chapter, **petty cash** is a limited supply of cash that is kept on hand to reimburse patients with change. It is also available to meet frequent small expenses for which immediate cash is needed (e.g., postage due). The amount in the fund should be large enough to last weekly but not large enough to invite theft. In most offices, this amount is no more than $50. If more than this is needed within 1 week, it is likely that the concept of petty cash is misunderstood or that the cash is being misused.

A petty cash voucher must be submitted for all payments made from the fund. Each voucher must include the date, the amount spent, to whom it was paid, for what it was spent, and who spent it. A receipt should be attached to each voucher (Fig. 63.10).

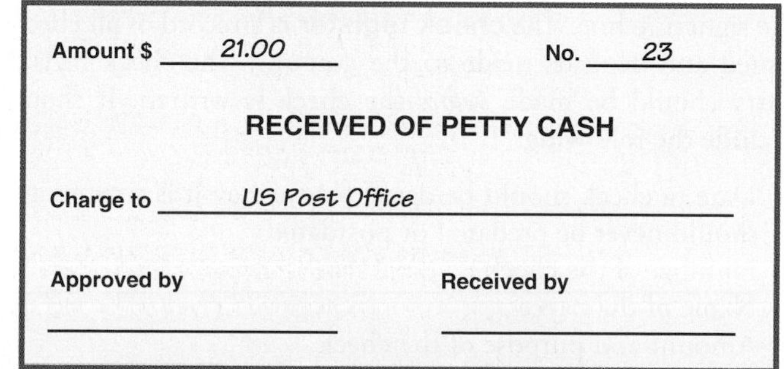

Amount $ 21.00 No. 23

RECEIVED OF PETTY CASH

Charge to US Post Office

Approved by ______ Received by ______

**FIG. 63.10** Petty cash voucher.

**REPLENISHING PETTY CASH FUNDS.** Petty cash should be balanced and replenished on a regular basis. Because a voucher is completed for each petty cash payment, the sum of all the vouchers plus the cash on hand should always equal the total amount of the petty cash fund. When these have been balanced, a check is written to refill the fund. If the fund is balanced, the check (which will return the fund to its original amount) should be written for a sum equal to that of the vouchers for that month. The vouchers and attached receipts are stapled together, and the date and total are noted. These are filed under the "Business Office" expense category.

RECALL

11 Give an example of fixed overhead.
12 After a dental practice pays all practice-related expenses, what type of income is rendered?
13 What type of itemized listing of goods may be included in a shipment of supplies?
14 What does C.O.D. mean?

# Writing Checks

Some practices have computerized check-writing capabilities. Advantages of computerized check writing include savings in time, reduced possibility of error, and ease of storage and retrieval of specific information. Other practices use a manual pegboard check-writing system or a business checkbook.

## Check Terminology

A **check** is a draft, or an order, drawn on a specific bank account for payment of a specified sum of money to the payee or to the bearer. Payment is made on demand, that is, when the check is presented to the bank, that amount of money must be paid provided the account includes sufficient funds to cover the amount of the check.

The **payee** is the person named on the check as the intended recipient of the amount shown. The payee's name is written after the words "Pay to the order of." The name of the payee should be written out in full; however, titles such as Mr., Mrs., and Ms. are best omitted. It is preferable to make a check out to "Mary Jones" rather than to "Mrs. John Jones."

The *maker* of the check is the one from whose account the amount of the check will be withdrawn. The maker of the check, or his or her authorized agent, must sign the check on the signature line. The **check register** is a record of all checks issued and deposits made to the account. The check register entry should be made *before* the check is written. It should include the following:

- Date (a check should be dated for the day it is written and should never be predated or postdated)
- Number of the check
- Name of the payee
- Amount and purpose of the check

Whether a manual or computerized system is used to process check writing, the utmost care should be taken in stating the amount of the check in both figures and words and in making certain that the amount stated agrees in the following three places (Fig. 63.11):

- On the check register
- In numbers on the right side of the check next to the dollar sign
- Written out in words on the line before the word "dollars"

Note that the number of cents usually is written as a fraction so that no mistake can be made about the placement of the decimal point.

Checks that are written carelessly or with conflicting numbers can be "raised" or otherwise altered. A **raised check** is one on which extra numbers have been added, for example, changing the check's value from $100 to $1000. Specifying the amount accurately in both words and numbers is one way of safeguarding against this.

## Check Endorsement

Before the payee can receive cash for the check, he or she must *endorse* (sign) it. Endorsement is made on the back left side of the check and must match the name shown on the face of the check. A check signed in this manner has a **blanket endorsement,** and anyone holding that check may cash it (including someone who may have stolen it).

With a **restrictive endorsement,** which may read "For deposit only to the account of [*the name of the payee*]," the check can be deposited only to the account of the named individual. This type of endorsement makes the check nonnegotiable, that is, it can be deposited only to that account, and if it is stolen, it cannot be cashed.

A rubber stamp with the appropriate restrictive phrase and the payee's name may be used in place of the payee's signature. As a safeguard, such a restrictive endorsement should be placed on all checks as soon as they are received.

### Stop Payment Order

If the maker of a check, for various reasons, does not want the bank to pay a check he or she has written, the maker may request that the bank issue a stop payment order for that check. The stop payment order must give all necessary information, such as number of the check, date issued, name of the payee, amount of the check, and reason for stopping payment.

The written stop payment order must reach the bank bookkeeper before the check is presented for payment. These orders are usually in force for 90 days, and the bank charges for this service.

### Nonsufficient Funds

A check written for more than what is in a person's account will be returned. The check will be returned to the payee marked NSF **(nonsufficient funds).** This means that not enough money is in the account to cover the check, and the payee cannot collect any of the amount due. A check that has been returned for this reason is known as a *returned item;* however, it is commonly referred to as having "bounced" (come back). The bank will add a charge against the account of the person (or company) who wrote the N.S.F. check; however, no charge is usually applied to the person who received the check.

For accounting purposes, when a check from a patient is returned, the amount of that check must be "charged back" against the patient's account. Do this by making an entry in the ledger, noting the date on which the check was returned. Then make an adjustment, which acts as a charge and increases the account balance by the amount of the returned check. It also is necessary to make a check register entry; here, the amount of the returned check is subtracted from the checking account balance.

Often a telephone call to the maker will resolve the problem, and the check may be redeposited. A check that is to be redeposited should be listed on a separate deposit slip and clearly marked so that it is not credited twice to income. When the check is redeposited, this should be noted on the account history, and the amount of the check again should be subtracted from the balance.

If a returned check cannot be redeposited, the outstanding balance on that account requires immediate attention.

### Business Summaries

All checks must be accounted for in a specific expense category. With a computerized system, posting to the appropriate category is part of the check-writing process. With the pegboard system, check-writing expenses are posted into categories at the time the check is written. Totals from monthly summaries are carried forward to an annual summary. By keeping these records, the dentist and the accountant at any time can quickly tell what the practice expenses have been to date. This is important information for management, budgeting, and tax purposes.

RECALL

**15** Where in the checkbook do you record the checks written and deposits made on an account?

**16** What term is used to indicate that an account does not have enough money in it to cover a check?

## Payroll

Payroll is the sum of all financial records of salaries, wages, bonuses, and deductions. From the accounting perspective,

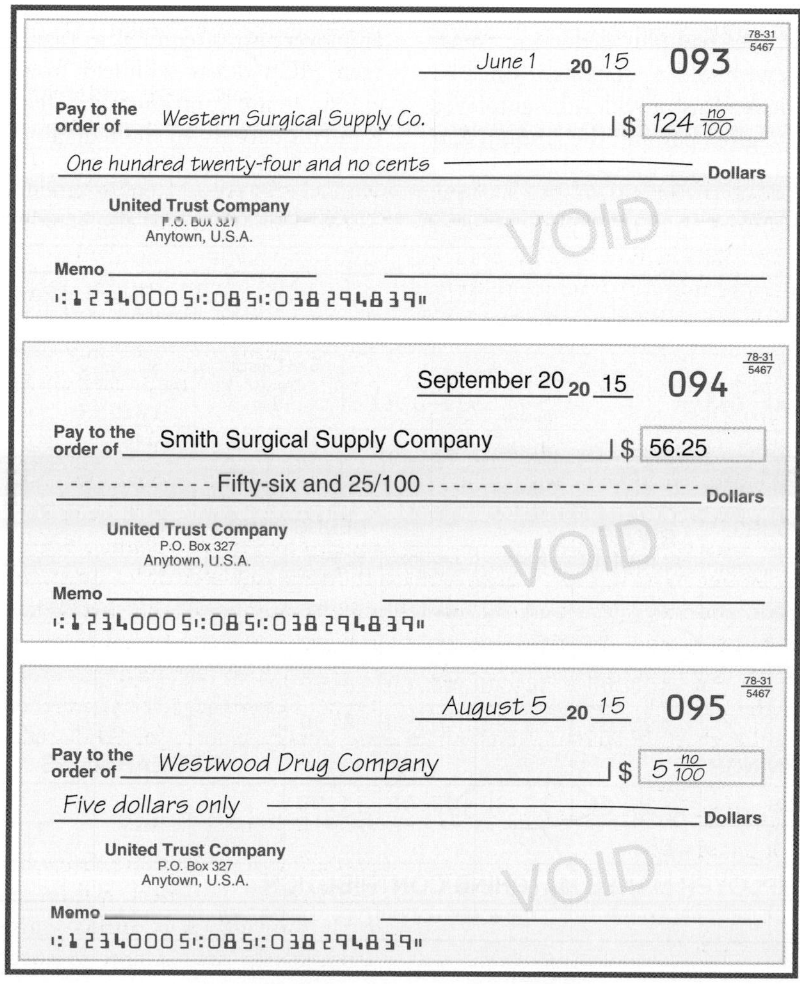


**FIG. 63.11** Correct way to write a check.

payroll refers to the amount paid to employees for services provided during a specified period of time. From an accounting point of view, payroll is crucial because payroll and payroll taxes considerably affect the net income of a dental practice, plus they are subject to laws and regulations.

Federal regulations require that an employer must make certain deductions from an employee's pay, and that the employer also must pay certain payroll taxes. These federal requirements are explained in the *Circular E* booklet issued by the Internal Revenue Service (IRS). Most states publish similar booklets that explain the requirements for state income tax.

The business assistant who is responsible for handling payroll should study these booklets carefully and ask questions about any point that is not clear. It is better to ask questions first than to make an expensive mistake that can be corrected only with great difficulty later. The government requires that each employer keep records of the hours worked, the amounts paid, and the amounts deducted for tax purposes. Complete and accurate employee records must be kept at all times, and back records should be stored with other important financial papers. A separate payroll sheet is maintained for each employee (Fig. 63.12). The headings on this form show the employee's full name (spelled correctly), social security number, address, and the number of exemptions claimed.

The gross *(total pretax)* pay for each pay period is entered on this form, as are each of the deductions and the net *(gross pay minus all deductions)* pay. Net pay plus deductions must equal the earned gross pay. A withholding statement must be included with each payroll check. This provides the employee with information regarding the gross pay and the amount and reason for each deduction.

## Payroll Deductions

### *Income Tax Withholding*

All employees must file a federal income tax return before April 15 of each year. A portion of the estimated tax is withheld directly from each paycheck during the year. By the end of the year, the amount withheld should approximate the annual tax that the employee will actually owe. Amounts withheld are determined from a schedule in *Circular E.* These amounts are based on earnings and the number of exemptions claimed. It is the responsibility of the employer to withhold this tax and to remit it to an authorized bank or directly to the IRS.

Each employee must complete an *employee's withholding exemption certificate (W-4 form)* at the following times: (1) at the beginning of employment, (2) within 10 days of any change of status (such as marriage), and (3) before December 1 of the following year. This form authorizes the employer to deduct the tax and indicates the number of exemptions that the employee is claiming. These completed forms must be kept with other payroll records.

### *Federal Insurance Contributions Act*

Under the **Federal Insurance Contributions Act (FICA),** commonly known as **Social Security,** the employer is required to deduct a certain percentage of the employee's gross pay. This is a fixed amount regardless of the number of exemptions. The employer also is required to match the contribution. Thus for each FICA dollar withheld from the employee's wages, the employer also contributes a dollar. Both contributions are forwarded quarterly to the federal government to be credited to the employee's account.

| NAME Patricia Andrews, CDA | Social Sec. Number 123-45-6789 | | | Record of Pay Rate Changes | |
|---|---|---|---|---|---|
| | | | | DATE | RATE |
| STREET 305 Oak Drive | Phone Number 933-0111 | No. of Exempt 1 | | 7/1/9X | 9.00 |
| | | | | 1/1/9X | 10.00 |
| CITY Centerville, NJ 08511 | Date Started 7/1/9X<br>Date Left | M | F<br>X | | |

| DATE | HOURS reg | HOURS over | GROSS AMOUNT | DEDUCTIONS Social Sec. | Fed. Inc. Tax | State Inc. Tax | | | | NET AMOUNT |
|---|---|---|---|---|---|---|---|---|---|---|
| 1/8/9X | 40 | | 400.00 | 33.20 | 40.00 | 8.50 | | | | 318.30 |
| 1/15/9X | 40 | | 400.00 | 33.20 | 40.00 | 8.50 | | | | 318.30 |
| 1/22/9X | 40 | | 400.00 | 33.20 | 40.00 | 8.50 | | | | 318.30 |
| 1/29/9X | 40 | | 400.00 | 33.20 | 40.00 | 8.50 | | | | 318.30 |
| JANUARY TOTALS | | | 1600.00 | 132.80 | 160.00 | 34.00 | | | | 1273.20 |
| | | | | | | | | | | |
| | | | | | | | | | | |
| | | | | | | | | | | |

GROSS EARNINGS

NET EARNINGS

EMPLOYER MAKES MATCHING CONTRIBUTION

**FIG. 63.12** Sample payroll report.

For FICA earnings to be properly credited, it is important to keep the Social Security Administration informed of any change of name. The employee will receive a **Statement of Earnings** from the Social Security Administration annually. This is a written record of the amount "credited" to the employee's account. Should an error be found here, it must be reported and corrected through the Social Security Administration.

### Other Deductions

Additional federal, state, and local taxes may be withheld from the employee's pay. The person in charge of payroll computations is responsible for having current information about the regulations that govern these deductions. Personal deductions, such as the employee's contribution to health or life insurance coverage, an automatic personal savings plan, or pretax retirement contributions, may be taken directly from the employee's earnings.

The employer must pay additional payroll taxes such as **workers' compensation, federal unemployment taxes (FUTA),** and **state unemployment insurance (SUI).** These amounts are not deducted from the employee's earnings, except in states in which a portion of the SUI tax is paid by the employee.

### Government Remittance

All government reports must be completed accurately and neatly (preferably typewritten or computer generated) and filed *on time.* Stiff penalties are issued for late reports. All employers are required to file an "Employer's Quarterly Federal Tax Return." This is a report of all taxable wages paid during the quarter. Withheld taxes and FICA contributions must be deposited regularly; the frequency of these deposits depends on the total amount owed.

Within 30 days of the end of the calendar year or on termination of employment, the employee must be furnished with a statement of total earnings and taxes withheld for that year (W-2 form). Many computer systems have the capabilities to process payroll and taxes, creating computer-generated reports and business summaries that fit the individual practice.

# Dental Insurance

Dental insurance is an assistance program that supports the patient or family with the cost of dental care. There are different forms of dental insurance policies available for individuals in the United States, with each one designed to help offset the costs associated with necessary dental care. They are the traditional dental insurance dental plan, managed care dental insurance plan, and government programs.

## Traditional Insurance Plan

The traditional insurance plan, also referred to as the *indemnity* plan, provides benefits for dental treatment that the covered individual has received from his or her own dentist. These plans are considered fee-for-service and come with limitations and copayment options. This means that the patient pays a flat fee for the dental visit, but has an annual limit on coverage for dental spending, and specific coverage limits that may apply to individual dental procedures. The total dollar amount of coverage one of these policies provides is typically limited by its deductible and maximum benefit.

## Managed Care Dental Insurance Plan

With escalating medical and dental premiums affecting the healthcare system, managed care is a method of providing low- to medium-cost healthcare coverage to everyone. Under these plans, the type, level, and frequency of treatment can be limited, and disease prevention is encouraged. The plans also try to control the level of reimbursement for services.

### Capitation Plans (Dental HMOs)

**Capitation plans (dental HMOs)** involve an arrangement in which a dentist (dental office, several dental offices, a network of dentists) has contracted to provide dental services for the plan's members. The dentist is paid (usually monthly) a fixed amount per dental plan participant who has selected the dentist as their treatment provider. In return, it is the dentist's obligation to provide any and all needed dental treatment for these individuals (as specified by the conditions of the plan) during the negotiated time frame.

### Preferred Provider Organizations (Dental PPOs)

**Preferred provider organizations (dental PPOs)** are technically a "closed panel" type of plan. This is a variation of a fee-for-service practice. A dentist may join a PPO in hopes of attracting new patients or in an effort to retain his or her current patients who are covered by the PPO plan. These patients are seen in the dentist's office. The dentist also may continue to see other fee-for-service patients who are not part of the PPO contract. These fee-for-service patients are charged the dentist's usual fees.

### Exclusive Provider Organizations (EPOs)

**Exclusive provider organizations (EPOs)** are another form of "closed panel" dental insurance. They are similar in nature to dental PPOs with the exception that the patients are offered no option other than receiving their treatment from a dentist who is a member of the plan's network of providers.

### Direct Reimbursement Plan

A **direct reimbursement plan** is a self-funded program in which the individual is reimbursed by his or her employer on the basis of a percentage of dollars spent for dental care provided. This type of plan allows beneficiaries to seek treatment from the dentist of their choice. Under a direct reimbursement plan, no insurance carrier is involved. Instead, the employee pays the dentist, and the employer reimburses a portion of this expense. The amount of reimbursement depends on the benefit design established by the employer.

### Individual Practice Associations

An **individual practice association (IPA)** is an organization that is formed by groups of dentists or, in some cases, dental societies for the primary purpose of collectively entering into contracts to provide dental services to enrolled populations. Frequently, services are provided on a capitation basis. These dentists may practice in their own offices. In addition to treating patients enrolled in the IPA, they may provide care to patients who are not covered by the contract. Treatment of patients who are not covered is provided on a traditional fee-for-service basis.

### Affordable Care Act

On March 23, 2010, President Barack Obama signed a comprehensive health reform, Patient Protection and Affordable Care Act, into law. This law is intended to expand coverage, control healthcare costs, and improve the healthcare delivery system. The American Dental Association states that "a number of provisions will directly impact dentistry and it is very likely that changes in the larger delivery and payment systems will have ripple effects on dentistry in the future."

Continue to view http://www.ada.org/ to see what changes will affect dental care in the private sector.

### Government Programs

Millions of individuals lack access to dental care due to lack of health insurance, or because their income is too low to pay for any type of medical or dental bills.

**Medicare** is funded by the federal government, but the terms of the program and what is or is not covered is established by each state government. It is a health insurance program that is available for people who are 65 years and older or for those patients who have specific disabilities or a special need.

**Medicaid Dental Coverage** serves low-income children, pregnant women, the disabled, and the impoverished elderly. Medicaid is a voluntary partnership program between the federal government and individual states.

Medicaid calls for each state's medical assistance program to cover at least 50 percent of associated payments. However, due to funding crises, critical health programs have been reduced or eliminated, with dental benefits often the first to go. As of 2013 Medicaid has declined in reimbursements in 37 or the 50 states. Medicaid dental care for children is required by law and offers comprehensive coverage (involving early screening, diagnosis, and treatment).

## Parties Involved in Dental Insurance

A working knowledge of the parties involved in dental insurance is necessary for an understanding of basic insurance concepts. In most instances, the following parties are involved: The person who receives the dental treatment is the **subscriber** who carries the dental insurance plan or the **dependent** of the subscriber, such as a spouse or a child. The **group** is the union or employment organization that has negotiated the dental insurance as part of its benefits package. The **carrier** is the party (usually an insurance company) who pays the claims and collects the premiums. The **provider** is the dentist who provides the treatment to the patient. Table 63.1 provides a list of the terms most commonly used for dental insurance.

## How Benefits Are Calculated

The three most commonly used methods of calculating fee-for-service benefits are (1) usual, customary, and reasonable (UCR) fees; (2) schedule of benefits; and (3) fixed fee schedules.

### Usual, Customary, and Reasonable Fees

The term **usual fee** refers to the fee that the dentist charges private patients for a given service. These fees are determined by the individual dentist and are the fees that are routinely charged by the practice. The dentist files a confidential list of these fees with the carrier. The carrier uses this information, called **prefiled fees,** to determine the customary fee for the area.

A **customary fee** is one that is within the range of the usual fees charged for the same service by dentists with similar training and experience within the same geographic area (such as a city or county). Using information from the prefiled fees, the carrier determines what is customary on the basis of a percentile of the fees charged by dentists within that area.

A **reasonable fee** is one that is considered justified by special circumstances necessitating extensive or complex treatment. These apply to unusual cases for which the dentist would charge more than the usual fee, even to a private patient, because of the extent of treatment involved. For instance, a particularly difficult extraction might justify an unusual fee. In these instances, the dentist is able to charge whatever is *reasonable* for the situation; however, the carrier may request written documentation to explain why the unusual fee was necessary.

In a UCR system, the payment can still be low, and the patient is responsible for the difference between the insurance payment and the dentist's fee. The **limitations** of the policy also influence the amount that the dentist receives from the carrier and how much the patient must pay.

### Schedule of Benefits

This also is known as a **table of allowances** or a **schedule of allowances.** A schedule of benefits is a list of fixed specified amounts that the carrier will pay toward the cost of *covered services.* A schedule of benefits is not related in any way to the dentist's actual fee schedule. Under most schedule of benefit plans, the patient is responsible for the difference between what the carrier will pay and what the dentist actually charges.

### Fixed Fee Schedule

A fixed fee schedule is an established fee for any treatment received by the patient. Under government programs, such as Medicaid, the dentist must accept the amount paid by the carrier as payment in full and may not bill the patient for the difference.

## Determining Eligibility

When a subscriber starts a new job, a 30- to 60-day waiting period is commonly required before coverage becomes effective. If a subscriber changes jobs, is laid off, or retires, his or

## TABLE 63.1 Insurance Terms

| Term | Definition |
|---|---|
| **Accepted fee** | The dollar amount that the contracting dentist has agreed to accept as payment in full from the insurance and the patient. This amount is shown on the notice that accompanies payment of a claim. |
| **Annual maximum** | The total dollar amount that an insurance plan will pay for dental care incurred by an individual patient or family (under a family plan) in a specified benefit period, typically a calendar year. |
| **Balance billing** | When a dentist bills the patient for an amount above fee and the enrollee's coinsurance, the dentist is balance billing and violating his or her contract with the insurance company |
| **Basic services/ basic benefits** | A category of dental services in an open network dental benefits contract that usually includes restorations (fillings), oral surgery (extractions), endodontics (root canals), periodontal treatment (root planing), and sealants. (This may vary by contract.) Typically, the same coinsurance percentage applies to all services grouped as basic services. |
| **Benefits** | The amounts that the insurance pays for dental services covered under a patient's contract. |
| **Capitation** | Compensation paid to general dentists in a closed network dental benefit plan (such as a DHMO) for providing covered services to enrollees assigned to their office. |
| **Claim/claim form** | A standard form that provides an itemized statement submitted by an enrollee or a dentist requesting payment of benefits for dental services provided. |
| **Closed network plan** | A type of dental plan where enrollees must visit a preselected or assigned network dentist in order to receive benefits. |
| **Coinsurance** | The enrollee's share, expressed as a fixed percentage, of the contract allowance. For example, a benefit that is paid at 80% by the plan creates a 20% coinsurance obligation for the enrollee. Coinsurance applies after the enrollee meets a required deductible. |
| **Contract benefit level** | The percentage of the maximum contract allowance that the insurance company pays after the deductible has been satisfied. |
| **Contracted dentist** | A dentist who has a contract with the insurance company to participate in a network. |
| **Contracted fee** | The fee for each single procedure that a contracted dentist has agreed to accept as payment in full for covered services provided to an enrollee. |
| **Coordination of benefits (COB)** | A process that carriers use to determine the order of payment and amount each carrier will pay when a person receives dental services that are covered by more than one benefit plan (dual coverage). COB ensures that no more than 100% of the charges for services are paid when an enrollee has coverage under two or more benefits plans—for example, a child who is covered by both parents' plans. |
| **Copayment** | A fixed dollar amount that an enrollee under certain dental plans (such as a DHMO-type plan) is required to pay at the time the service is rendered. |
| **Deductible** | A dollar amount that each enrollee (or, cumulatively, a family for family coverage) must pay for certain covered services before insurance begins paying benefits. |
| **Diagnostic and preventive services** | A category of dental services in an open network dental benefits contract that usually includes oral evaluations, routine cleanings, x-rays, and fluoride treatments. |
| **Dual choice** | A program that allows enrollees to select one of two or more dental plans. (Also may be referred to as "dual option.") |
| **Dual coverage** | When dental treatment for an enrollee is covered by more than one dental benefits plan, such as when dental services are provided to a child who is covered by both parents' benefit plans. |
| **Effective date** | The date a dental benefits contract begins; may also be the date that benefits begin for a plan enrollee. |
| **Eligibility** | The circumstances or conditions that define who and when a person may qualify to enroll in a plan and/or a specific category of covered services. These circumstances or conditions may include length of employment, job status, length of time an enrollee has been covered under the plan, dependency, child and student age limits, etc. |
| **Eligible enrollee** | An enrollee who has met the eligibility requirements under the insurance plan. |
| **Fee-for-service** | Compensation paid to dentists based on an amount per service. A fee-for-service plan generally permits enrollees to freely select a network or noncontracted dentist to provide the service. |
| **Health maintenance organization (HMO)** | An entity that is authorized to issue a benefit plan in which enrollees receive all or most treatment through a preselected or preassigned dental office. The dentist receives a monthly capitation payment for each patient who selects or is assigned to that office, no matter how many services that patient receives. |
| **In-network/out-of-network** | Services provided in a plan either by a contracted or noncontracted dentist. In-network dentists have agreed to participate in a plan and to provide treatment according to certain administrative guidelines and to accept their contracted fees as payment in full. |
| **Lifetime maximum** | The cumulative dollar amount that a plan will pay for dental care incurred by an individual enrollee or family (under a family plan) for the life of the enrollee or the plan. Lifetime maximums usually apply to specific services such as orthodontic treatment. |

*Continued*

TABLE 63.1 Insurance Terms—cont'd

| Term | Definition |
|---|---|
| **Limitations and exclusions** | Dental plans typically do not cover every dental procedure. Each plan contains a list of conditions or circumstances that limit or exclude services from coverage. Limitations may be related to time or frequency (the number of procedures permitted during a stated period)—for example, no more than two cleanings in 12 months or one cleaning every 6 months. |
| **Network** | A panel of dentists that contractually agree to provide treatment according to administrative guidelines for a certain plan, including limits to the fees they will accept as payment in full. |
| **Open access** | A plan feature that allows enrollees to visit the dentists of their choice (freedom of choice). Also sometimes used to describe an enrollee's ability to seek treatment from a specialist without first obtaining a referral from his/her primary care dentist. |
| **Open enrollment** | A period (usually a 2-week or 1-month period during the year) when qualified individuals (eligible employees) can enroll in or change their choice of coverage in group benefits plans. |
| **Open network plan** | A type of dental plan where enrollees can visit any licensed dentist and can change dentists at any time without contacting the benefits carrier. |
| **Out-of-pocket costs** | Any amount the enrollee is responsible for paying, such as coinsurance or copayments, deductibles, and costs above the annual maximum. |
| **Patient's share** | The portion of a dentist's fee that an enrollee must pay for covered services, including coinsurance or copayment, any remaining deductible, any amount over plan maximums and/or any services the plan does not cover. |
| **Preauthorization** | A requirement that recommended treatment must first be approved by the plan before the treatment is rendered in order for the plan to pay benefits for those services. |
| **Preferred provider organization (PPO) plan** | A reduced fee-for-service plan that allows enrollees to visit any dentist, but encourages them to visit PPO network dentists to minimize out-of-pocket expenses. Enrollees usually pay less when visiting a PPO dentist. |
| **Prepaid plan** | A term used to describe a benefits plan in which a carrier prepays network dentists a capitated amount for each patient enrolled in (assigned to) his or her office. |
| **Pretreatment estimate** | The insurance company's written estimate of benefits available as of a specific date, given to an enrollee or treating dentist in advance of proposed treatment. |
| **Primary enrollee** | An individual (commonly, an employee or member of an association) who meets the eligibility requirements for enrollment in a dental plan. Family members of a primary enrollee are called dependents. |
| **Provider** | Any licensed dentist who performs dental health services for an enrollee. This includes general dentists and dental specialists. |
| **Submitted fee** | The amount that the dentist bills and is entered on a claim as the charge for a specific procedure. |
| **Table program** | A dental plan where benefits are based on a specific table or schedule of allowances or fees. |
| **Usual fee** | The amount commonly charged for a particular service by a dentist. |
| **Waiting period** | A stated period of time that a person must be enrolled in a plan before being eligible for benefits or for a specific category of benefits. |

her coverage is customarily terminated within 30 days of the change. However, the subscriber has the option to continue coverage under the Consolidated Omnibus Budget Reconciliation Act (COBRA) of 1985. This entitles the subscriber to continue the same coverage, but he or she is responsible for paying the premiums. If any question regarding eligibility arises, the carrier should be contacted *before* routine dental care is started.

The rules for eligibility under other government programs, such as Medicaid and the Civilian Health and Medical Program of the Uniformed Services (CHAMPUS), vary greatly. Medicare does *not* include dental coverage.

When working with clients enrolled in government programs, you must be familiar with the specific form of identification that should be requested to determine eligibility. This usually is an identification card or a proof-of-eligibility sticker. Because the individual's eligibility may change from month to month, it is essential that this identification be verified at each visit.

## Determining Benefits

The employer who purchases coverage as a benefit for employees negotiates the limitations and benefits of the plan. The carrier is responsible for covering *only* the level of treatment that is included in that plan. Information that explains the coverage under a specific plan is found in the *benefits booklet* supplied to the subscriber. The patient is asked to bring this booklet to the first dental visit so that coverage can be reviewed and discussed before the start of treatment.

The two major factors that determine how much the carrier will pay and how much the patient must pay are the **method of payment** and the **limitations** within the plan.

### *Limitations*

In addition to different methods of payment, other factors influence the level of benefits that the beneficiary is entitled to receive under the plan, and how much he or she must pay as a share of these costs.

**LEAST EXPENSIVE ALTERNATIVE TREATMENT.** The least expensive alternative treatment (LEAT), also known as an **alternative benefit policy,** is a limitation in a dental plan that allows benefits only for the least expensive treatment. For example, a patient needs a replacement for a missing tooth. Treatment alternatives include a fixed bridge costing $3000 or a removable partial for $1200. Under LEAT, the carrier will pay benefits only for the partial denture. The patient may choose to have the bridge, but the carrier will pay only $1200 (as if the patient had a partial denture made), and the patient is responsible for the difference in the fee.

**DUAL COVERAGE.** If a patient has dental insurance coverage under more than one plan, this is known as **dual coverage.** In this case it is necessary to take steps to be certain that the appropriate benefits are paid.

***Determining Primary and Secondary Carriers.*** With situations involving dual coverage, it is necessary to determine which carrier is **primary** (and should pay first) and which carrier is **secondary** (and should pay at least a portion of the balance). Specific questions on a claim form ask for this information. When the *patient* is the insured, his or her carrier is always primary and the spouse's carrier is secondary. When spousal coverage is in place for patients with insurance of their own, their insurance must be billed first. After payment from the primary insurance company is received, a claim is sent to the other insurance company if any balance is still due.

***Birthday Rule.*** The birthday rule was established to explain which insurance carrier is the primary carrier when both parents have insurance to cover a child. The rule stipulates that when a child is covered under both parents' plans, the plan of the parent whose birthday (month and day, not year) falls earlier in the calendar year is billed first. This rule applies to parents who are *not* divorced. Other factors are considered when parents are divorced or separated and when step-parents are involved. It is important to work with parents to determine the appropriate sequencing of insurance form filing by clearly defining office billing policies for the parent accompanying the child.

***Coordination of Benefits.*** Under **coordination of benefits (COB)**, the patient will receive payment from both carriers, but the total received may *not* be more than 100 percent of the actual dental expenses. For example, the fee is $250. Benefits from the primary carrier are $175 for this service. No matter what benefits the secondary carrier usually pays for this service, under coordination of benefits, the second carrier will pay no more than the difference between the fee and the amount paid by the primary carrier. This comes to $75, after which the patient has been reimbursed for 100 percent of the fee.

### *Nonduplication of Benefits*

Under plans that call for nonduplication of benefits, also known as **benefit-less benefit,** a provision relieves the carrier from responsibility for paying for services that are covered under another program. Under these plans, reimbursement is limited to the higher level allowed by the two plans rather than to a total of 100 percent of the charges. For example, the fee is $250. The primary carrier allows $175 for this service. The secondary carrier allows $190 for this service. In this situation, the primary carrier pays $175. The secondary carrier pays only $15, which is the total amount of the allowed benefit minus the amount that has already been paid. If the primary carrier allowed the higher of the two benefits, the secondary carrier would not pay anything. The result is that the patient is reimbursed for the higher of the two allowed amounts but not for 100 percent of the fee.

Many patients are not aware of the nonduplication of benefits clause, which can cause confusion regarding their benefits. It is important to explain this clause to patients after their predetermination results are returned.

## Dental Procedure Codes

The **Code on Dental Procedures and Nomenclature** was developed by the American Dental Association (ADA) to speed and simplify the reporting of dental procedures. These codes are provided in **Current Dental Terminology (CDT)**, which is published and periodically updated by the ADA. These codes are *very* specific. The CDT should be reviewed carefully before specific dental treatment is coded. Each procedure has a designated code number. The codes are divided into categories of service and are listed in Table 63.2.

In many practices, encounter forms (also known as *charge slips* or *routing slips*) are preprinted with the codes used in the practice. One of these forms is clipped to the outside of the patient's file folder before the dentist sees the patient. After the visit, the dentist simply checks the boxes for services and charges and makes notations. This reduces the possibility that coding errors will be made by the clinical assistant or front office personnel.

## Claim Forms

### *Claim Form Preparation*

Claims for dental treatment are filed in one of two ways: by submission on a claim form that is mailed to the carrier (paper claim) or by electronic transmission, in which information is submitted electronically to the carrier (electronic claim). Both types of transmission require the same three primary areas of information: patient and subscriber identification, dentist identification, and details concerning the treatment provided.

### *Paper Claim*

If completed manually, a dental insurance claim form is used to submit a predetermination of benefits for planned treatment

**TABLE 63.2 Dental Procedure Codes**

| Code | Procedure(s) |
|---|---|
| **Diagnostic**<br>D0100–D0999 | • Clinical oral evaluations<br>• Radiographs/diagnostic imaging (including interpretation)<br>• Tests and examinations<br>• Oral pathology laboratory |
| **Preventive**<br>D1000–D1999 | • Dental prophylaxis<br>• Topical fluoride treatment (office procedure)<br>• Other preventive services |
| **Restorative**<br>D2000–D2999 | • Amalgam restorations (including polishing)<br>• Resin-based composite restorations—direct<br>• Gold foil restorations<br>• Inlay/onlay restorations<br>• Crowns—single restorations only<br>• Other restorative services |
| **Endodontics**<br>D3000–D3999 | • Pulp capping<br>• Pulpotomy<br>• Endodontic therapy on primary teeth<br>• Endodontic therapy (including treatment plan, clinical procedures, and follow-up care)<br>• Endodontic retreatment<br>• Apexification/recalcification procedures<br>• Apicoectomy/periradicular services<br>• Other endodontic procedures |
| **Periodontics**<br>D4000–D4999 | • Surgical services (including usual postoperative care)<br>• Nonsurgical periodontal service<br>• Other periodontal services |
| **Removable Prosthodontics**<br>D5000–D5899 | • Complete dentures<br>• Partial dentures (including routine postdelivery care)<br>• Adjustments to dentures<br>• Repairs to complete dentures<br>• Repairs to partial dentures<br>• Denture rebase procedures<br>• Denture reline procedures<br>• Interim prosthesis<br>• Other removable prosthetic services |
| **Maxillofacial Prosthetics**<br>D5900–D5999 | • Prosthetic replacements<br>• Radiation<br>• Surgical splinting |
| **Implant Services**<br>D6000–D6199 | • Presurgical services<br>• Surgical services<br>• Implant supported prosthetics supporting structures<br>• Implant/abutment supported removable dentures<br>• Implant/abutment supported fixed dentures (hybrid prosthesis)<br>• Single crowns, abutment supported<br>• Single crowns, implant supported<br>• Fixed partial denture, abutment supported<br>• Fixed partial denture, implant supported<br>• Other implant services |
| **Fixed Prosthodontics**<br>D6200–D6999 | • Fixed partial denture pontics<br>• Fixed partial denture retainers—inlays/onlays<br>• Fixed partial denture retainers—crowns<br>• Other fixed partial denture services |

**TABLE 63.2** Dental Procedure Codes—cont'd

| Code | Procedure(s) |
|---|---|
| **Oral Surgery** D7000–D7999 | • Extractions (includes local anesthesia, suturing, if needed, and routine postoperative care)<br>• Surgical extractions (includes local anesthesia, suturing, if needed, and routine postoperative care)<br>• Other surgical procedures<br>• Alveoloplasty—surgical preparation of ridge for dentures<br>• Vestibuloplasty<br>• Surgical excision of soft tissue lesions<br>• Surgical excision of intraosseous lesions<br>• Excision of bone tissue<br>• Surgical incision<br>• Treatment of fractures—simple<br>• Treatment of fractures—compound<br>• Reduction of dislocation and management of other temporomandibular joint dysfunctions<br>• Repair of traumatic wounds<br>• Complicated suturing (reconstruction requiring delicate handling of tissues and wide undermining for meticulous closure)<br>• Other repair procedures |
| **Orthodontics** D8000–D8999 | • Limited orthodontic treatment<br>• Interceptive orthodontic treatment<br>• Comprehensive orthodontic<br>• Minor treatment to control harmful habits<br>• Other orthodontic services |
| **Adjunctive General Services** D9000–D9999 | • Unclassified treatment<br>• Anesthesia<br>• Professional consultation<br>• Professional visits<br>• Drugs<br>• Miscellaneous services (bleaching, desensitizing, occlusal analysis) |

or to request payment of claims for services that have been rendered. The ADA provides a standardized claim form that is accepted by most carriers (Fig. 63.13).

The completed claim form is generated in duplicate; one copy is submitted to the carrier, and the other copy is retained with the practice records. The claim form includes two boxes for patient signatures. These relate to the release of information and the assignment of benefits.

**Release of information** regarding the patient's treatment is confidential and may be done only with the patient's written consent. The patient's signature in the "release of information" box gives the dentist permission to reveal to the insurance carrier information regarding the patient's dental treatment.

**Assignment of benefits** is a procedure by which the subscriber authorizes the carrier to make payment of allowable benefits directly to the dentist. If no assignment of benefits occurs, the check goes directly to the patient. To assign benefits, the subscriber signs the appropriate box on the insurance claim form. If no assignment of benefits occurs, financial arrangements are made for the total amount of the fee, just as if the patient did not have dental insurance.

**SIGNATURE ON FILE.** The patient registration form has signature boxes similar to those on the claim form; specific signature authorization forms can also be used. The patient should sign these when completing the form. These signatures are kept on file, and when the claim form is prepared, "Signature on File" can be used. When claims are submitted electronically, there is no place for a patient signature. The "Signature on File" option covers the need to have the patient's permission for the release of this information.

### Electronic Claim

With electronic claims processing, data stored in the practice's computer are used to generate and submit claims from the practice's computer to the carrier's computer (Fig. 63.14). This provides the advantages of speeding claim submission and payment and reducing paperwork and the possibility of errors. As part of claims preparation on the computer, the system checks each claim for missing information before electronic submission. When claims have been verified as complete, they are transmitted by modem. This transmission may occur directly to the carrier's computer; however, because a practice contracts with many carriers, claims are transmitted through a clearinghouse that is set up through the individual practice software. Your software vendor will assist you with this process.

Dental practices that see a large number of patients transmit their claims on a daily basis. Dentists who see a small number of patients per day may decide to transmit their claims once a

## ADA. Dental Claim Form

**HEADER INFORMATION**

1. Type of Transaction (Mark all applicable boxes)

☐ Statement of Actual Services ☐ Request for Predetermination/Preauthorization

☐ EPSDT/Title XIX

2. Predetermination/Preauthorization Number

**INSURANCE COMPANY/DENTAL BENEFIT PLAN INFORMATION**

3. Company/Plan Name, Address, City, State, Zip Code

**OTHER COVERAGE**

4. Other Dental or Medical Coverage? ☐ No (Skip 5-11) ☐ Yes (Complete 5-11)

5. Name of Policyholder/Subscriber in #4 (Last, First, Middle Initial, Suffix)

6. Date of Birth (MM/DD/CCYY) | 7. Gender ☐ M ☐ F | 8. Policyholder/Subscriber ID (SSN or ID#)

9. Plan/Group Number | 10. Patient's Relationship to Person Named in #5 ☐ Self ☐ Spouse ☐ Dependent ☐ Other

11. Other Insurance Company/Dental Benefit Plan Name, Address, City, State, Zip Code

**POLICYHOLDER/SUBSCRIBER INFORMATION** (For Insurance Company Named in #3)

12. Policyholder/Subscriber Name (Last, First, Middle Initial, Suffix), Address, City, State, Zip Code

13. Date of Birth (MM/DD/CCYY) | 14. Gender ☐ M ☐ F | 15. Policyholder/Subscriber ID (SSN or ID#)

16. Plan/Group Number | 17. Employer Name

**PATIENT INFORMATION**

18. Relationship to Policyholder/Subscriber in #12 Above ☐ Self ☐ Spouse ☐ Dependent Child ☐ Other | 19. Student Status ☐ FTS ☐ PTS

20. Name (Last, First, Middle Initial, Suffix), Address, City, State, Zip Code

21. Date of Birth (MM/DD/CCYY) | 22. Gender ☐ M ☐ F | 23. Patient ID/Account # (Assigned by Dentist)

**RECORD OF SERVICES PROVIDED**

| | 24. Procedure Date (MM/DD/CCYY) | 25. Area of Oral Cavity | 26. Tooth System | 27. Tooth Number(s) or Letter(s) | 28. Tooth Surface | 29. Procedure Code | 30. Description | 31. Fee |
|---|---|---|---|---|---|---|---|---|
| 1 | | | | | | | | |
| 2 | | | | | | | | |
| 3 | | | | | | | | |
| 4 | | | | | | | | |
| 5 | | | | | | | | |
| 6 | | | | | | | | |
| 7 | | | | | | | | |
| 8 | | | | | | | | |
| 9 | | | | | | | | |
| 10 | | | | | | | | |

**MISSING TEETH INFORMATION**

| | Permanent | | | | | | | | | | | | | | | | Primary | | | | | | | | | | |
|---|---|---|---|---|---|---|---|---|---|---|---|---|---|---|---|---|---|---|---|---|---|---|---|---|---|---|---|
| 34. (Place an 'X' on each missing tooth) | 1 | 2 | 3 | 4 | 5 | 6 | 7 | 8 | 9 | 10 | 11 | 12 | 13 | 14 | 15 | 16 | A | B | C | D | E | F | G | H | I | J | 32. Other Fee(s) |
| | 32 | 31 | 30 | 29 | 28 | 27 | 26 | 25 | 24 | 23 | 22 | 21 | 20 | 19 | 18 | 17 | T | S | R | Q | P | O | N | M | L | K | 33. Total Fee |

35. Remarks

**AUTHORIZATIONS**

36. I have been informed of the treatment plan and associated fees. I agree to be responsible for all charges for dental services and materials not paid by my dental benefit plan, unless prohibited by law, or the treating dentist or dental practice has a contractual agreement with my plan prohibiting all or a portion of such charges. To the extent permitted by law, I consent to your use and disclosure of my protected health information to carry out payment activities in connection with this claim.

X ______________________________

Patient/Guardian signature Date

37. I hereby authorize and direct payment of the dental benefits otherwise payable to me, directly to the below named dentist or dental entity.

X ______________________________

Subscriber signature Date

**ANCILLARY CLAIM/TREATMENT INFORMATION**

38. Place of Treatment ☐ Provider's Office ☐ Hospital ☐ ECF ☐ Other | 39. Number of Enclosures (00 to 99) Radiograph(s) ☐ Oral Image(s) ☐ Model(s) ☐

40. Is Treatment for Orthodontics? ☐ No (Skip 41-42) ☐ Yes (Complete 41-42) | 41. Date Appliance Placed (MM/DD/CCYY)

42. Months of Treatment Remaining | 43. Replacement of Prosthesis? ☐ No ☐ Yes (Complete 44) | 44. Date Prior Placement (MM/DD/CCYY)

45. Treatment Resulting from ☐ Occupational illness/injury ☐ Auto accident ☐ Other accident

46. Date of Accident (MM/DD/CCYY) | 47. Auto Accident State

**BILLING DENTIST OR DENTAL ENTITY** (Leave blank if dentist or dental entity is not submitting claim on behalf of the patient or insured/subscriber)

48. Name, Address, City, State, Zip Code

49. NPI | 50. License Number | 51. SSN or TIN

52. Phone Number ( ) – | 52A. Additional Provider ID

**TREATING DENTIST AND TREATMENT LOCATION INFORMATION**

53. I hereby certify that the procedures as indicated by date are in progress (for procedures that require multiple visits) or have been completed.

X ______________________________

Signed (Treating Dentist) Date

54. NPI | 55. License Number

56. Address, City, State, Zip Code | 56A. Provider Specialty Code

57. Phone Number ( ) – | 58. Additional Provider ID



A J400 (Same as ADA Dental Claim Form – J401, J402, J403, J404)

To Reorder, call 1-800-947-4746 or go online at www.adacatalog.org

**FIG. 63.13** American Dental Association (ADA) standard claim form. *(Copyright © 2012 American Dental Association, Chicago, IL.)*

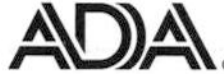

American Dental Association
www.ada.org

Comprehensive completion instructions for the ADA Dental Claim Form are found in Section 4 of the ADA Publication titled *CDT-2007/2008*. Five relevant extracts from that section follow:

**General Instructions**

A. The form is designed so that the name and address (Item 3) of the third-party payer receiving the claim (insurance company/dental benefit plan) is visible in a standard #10 window envelope. Please fold the form using the 'tick-marks' printed in the margin.

B. In the upper-right of the form, a blank space is provided for the convenience of the payer or insurance company, to allow the assignment of a claim or control number.

C. All Items in the form must be completed unless it is noted on the form or in the following instructions that completion is not required.

D. When a name and address field is required, the full name of an individual or a full business name, address and zip code must be entered.

E. All dates must include the four-digit year.

F. If the number of procedures reported exceeds the number of lines available on one claim form, the remaining procedures must be listed on a separate, fully completed claim form.

**Coordination of Benefits (COB)**

When a claim is being submitted to the secondary payer, complete the form in its entirety and attach the primary payer's Explanation of Benefits (EOB) showing the amount paid by the primary payer. You may indicate the amount the primary carrier paid in the "Remarks" field (Item # 35)

**National Provider Identifier (NPI)**

49 and 54 NPI (National Provider Indentifier): This is an identifier assigned by the Federal government to all providers considered to be HIPAA covered entities. Dentists who are not covered entities may elect to obtain an NPI at their discretion, or may be enumerated if required by a participating provider agreement with a third-party payer or applicable state law/regulation. An NPI is unique to an individual dentist (Type 1 NPI) or dental entity (Type 2 NPI), and has no intrinsic meaning. Additional information on NPI and enumeration can be obtained from the ADA's Internet Web Site: **www.ada.org/goto/npi**

**Additional Provider Identifier**

52A and 58 Additional Provider ID: This is an identifier assigned to the billing dentist or dental entity other than a Social Security Number (SSN) or Tax Identification Number (TIN). It is not the provider's NPI. The additional identifier is sometimes referred to as a Legacy Identifier (LID). LIDs may not be unique as they are assigned by different entities (e.g., third-party payer; Federal government). Some Legacy IDs have an intrinsic meaning.

**Provider Specialty Codes**

56A Provider Specialty Code: Enter the code that indicates the type of dental professional who delivered the treatment. Available codes describing treating dentists are listed below. The general code listed as 'Dentist' may be used instead of any other dental practitioner code.

| Category / Description Code | Code |
|---|---|
| **Dentist**<br>A dentist is a person qualified by a doctorate in dental surgery (D.D.S.) or dental medicine (D.M.D.) licensed by the state to practice dentistry, and practicing within the scope of that license. | 122300000X |
| **General Practice** | 1223G0001X |
| **Dental Specialty** (see following list) | Various |
| Dental Public Health | 1223D0001X |
| Endodontics | 1223E0200X |
| Orthodontics | 1223X0400X |
| Pediatric Dentistry | 1223P0221X |
| Periodontics | 1223P0300X |
| Prosthodontics | 1223P0700X |
| Oral & Maxillofacial Pathology | 1223P0106X |
| Oral & Maxillofacial Radiology | 1223D0008X |
| Oral & Maxillofacial Surgery | 1223S0112X |

Dental provider taxonomy codes listed above are a subset of the full code set that is posted at: **www.wpc-edi.com/codes/taxonomy**

Should there be any updates to ADA Dental Claim Form completion instructions, the updates will be posted on the ADA's web site at: **www.ada.org/goto/dentalcode**

B

**FIG. 63.13, cont'd**

## ADA Dental Claim Form

**HEADER INFORMATION**

1. Type of Transaction (Check all applicable boxes)
[X] Statement of Actual Sevices [ ] Request for Predetermination/Preauthorization
[ ] EPSDT/Title XIX

2. Predetermination/Preauthorization Number

**PRIMARY PAYER INFORMATION**

3. Name, Address, City, State, Zip Code
Dental Support
P.O. Box 313
Denver, CO 39720

**OTHER COVERAGE**

4. Other Dental or Medical Coverage? [X] No (Skip 5-11) [ ] Yes (Complete 5-11)

5. Other Insured's Name (Last, First, Middle Initial, Suffix)

6. Date of Birth (MM/DD/CCYY) 04/25/1960
7. Gender [X] M [ ] F
8. Subscriber Identifier (SSN or ID#) 543-20-9765
9. Plan/Group Number FBOC
10. Patient's Relationship to Other Insured (Check applicable box) [X] Self [ ] Spouse [ ] Dependent [ ] Other
11. Other Carrier Name, Address, City, State, Zip Code

**PRIMARY INSURED INFORMATION**

12. Name (Last, First, Middle Initial, Suffix), Address, City, State, Zip Code
Ralph Henderson
287 Oak Drive
Centerville, IL 61822

13. Date of Birth (MM/DD/CCYY) 04/25/1960
14. Gender [X] M [ ] F
15. Subscriber Identifier (SSN or ID#) 543-20-9765
16. Plan/Group Number FBOC
17. Employer Name First Bank of Centerville

**PATIENT INFORMATION**

18. Relationship to Primary Insured (Check applicable box) [X] Self [ ] Spouse [ ] Dependent Child [ ] Other
19. Student Status [ ] FTS [ ] PTS
20. Name (Last, First, Middle Initial, Suffix), Address, City, State, Zip Code
Ralph Henderson
287 Oak Drive
Centerville, IL 61822

21. Date of Birth (MM/DD/CCYY) 04/25/1960
22. Gender [X] M [ ] F
23. Patient ID/Account # (Assigned by Dentist) 543-20-9765

**RECORD OF SERVICES PROVIDED**

| | 24. Procedure Date (MM/DD/CCYY) | 25. Area of Oral Cavity | 26. Tooth System | 27. Tooth Number(s) or Letter(s) | 28. Tooth Surface | 29. Procedure Code | 30. Description | 31. Fee |
|---|---|---|---|---|---|---|---|---|
| 1 | 01/10/20xx | | | | | D0150 | Comprehensive oral evaluation | 70 00 |
| 2 | 01/10/20xx | | | | | D0210 | Intraoral FMS - Complete Series | 80 00 |
| 3 | 01/10/20xx | | | | | D1330 | Oral Hygiene Instructions | 35 00 |
| 4 | 01/10/20xx | | | | | D1110 | Prophylaxis - adult | 80 00 |
| 5 | 01/10/20xx | | | | | D0470 | Diagnostic Casts | 75 00 |
| 6 | | | | | | | | |
| 7 | | | | | | | | |
| 8 | | | | | | | | |
| 9 | | | | | | | | |
| 10 | | | | | | | | |

**MISSING TEETH INFORMATION**

34. (Place an 'X' on each missing tooth)

Permanent: 1 2 3 4 5 6 7 8 9 10 11 12 13 14 15 16 / 32 31 30 29 28 27 26 25 24 23 22 21 20 19 18 17

Primary: A B C D E F G H I J / T S R Q P O N M L K

32. Other Fee(s)
33. Total Fee 340 00

35. Remarks

**AUTHORIZATIONS**

36. I have been informed of the treatment plan and associated fees. I agree to be responsible for all charges for dental services and materials not paid by my dental benefit plan, unless prohibited by law, or the treating dentist or dental practice has a contractual agreement with my plan prohibiting all or a portion of such charges. To the extent permitted by law, I consent to your use and disclosure of my protected health information to carry out payment activities in connection with this claim.

X Signature on File 2/1/XX
Patient/Guardian signature Date

37. I hereby authorize and direct payment of the dental benefits otherwise payable to me, directly to the below named dentist or dental entity.

X Signature on File 2/1/XX
Subscriber signature Date

**ANCILLARY CLAIM/TREATMENT INFORMATION**

38. Place of Treatment (Check applicable box) [ ] Provider's Office [ ] Hospital [ ] ECF [ ] Other
39. Number of Enclosures (00 to 99) Radiograph(s) Oral Image(s) Model(s)
40. Is Treatment for Orthodontics? [ ] No (Skip 41-42) [ ] Yes (Complete 41-42)
41. Date Appliance Placed (MM/DD/CCYY)
42. Months of Treatment Remaining
43. Replacement Prosthesis? [ ] No [ ] Yes (Complete 44)
44. Date Prior Placement (MM/DD/CCYY)
45. Treatment Resulting from (Check applicable box) [ ] Occupational illness/injury [ ] Auto accident [ ] Other accident
46. Date of Accident (MM/DD/CCYY)
47. Auto Accident State

**BILLING DENTIST OR DENTAL ENTITY** (Leave blank if dentist or dental entity is not submitting claim on behalf of the patient or insured/subscriber)

48. Name, Address, City, State, Zip Code
Leonard S Taylor
2100 W. Park Avenue
Champaign, IL 61820

49. Provider ID
50. License Number IL-3456
51. SSN or TIN 203-55-9278
52. Phone Number (217)351-5400

**TREATING DENTIST AND TREATMENT LOCATION INFORMATION**

53. I hereby certify that the procedures as indicated by date are in progress (for procedures that require multiple visits) or have been completed and that the fees submitted are the actual fees I have charged and intend to collect for those procedures.

X
Signed (Treating Dentist) Date

54. Provider ID
55. Liscense Number
56. Address, City, State, Zip Code
57. Phone Number ( )
58. Treating Provider Specialty



To Reorder, call 1-800-947-4746 or go online at www.adacatalog.org

**FIG. 63.14** Computerized claim form submitted for payment. *(Copyright © 2012 American Dental Association, Chicago, IL.)*

week. Although no paper claim is generated, the practice must have a record of each claim that was submitted. Transmission problems can arise periodically when electronic claims are submitted. Therefore this record is essential in the event that a claim is lost or disputed and must be submitted again. It also is important in tracking claims for payment. A daily or weekly status report of claims is sent electronically from the clearinghouse to be checked against your record.

## HIPAA and Electronic Transactions

Under the Health Insurance Portability and Accountability Act of 1996 (HIPAA), the U.S. Department of Health and Human Services (HHS) has implemented transaction standards to protect the integrity and promote the standardization of electronic claims submissions. The goal of this program is to allow one standardized format for each specific transaction, along with a standard set of procedure codes. When this is done, electronic data transmissions are more efficient, which results in a cost savings for healthcare providers. For dentistry, the CDT codes are used to simplify transaction processing.

Dental offices that are not filing electronically are not affected by this particular section of the law but must still comply with the privacy rule and with the other aspects of administrative simplification that address security standards. Medicaid accepts only electronic claims, so any office that accepts Medicaid will have to submit all insurance claims electronically.

### HIPAA Electronic Transfers

Under the Health Insurance Portability and Accountability Act (HIPAA), electronic claim submissions must be standardized. For dentistry, Current Dental Terminology (CDT) codes are used to standardize submission processing.

## Claim Form Processing

At the end of the patient's visit, all charges are entered into the patient's account history or ledger (with or without insurance). A claim for payment then is submitted to the insurance company. If this is the patient's first visit, it also may be necessary to file a predetermination for planned additional treatment. If so, the predetermination is submitted on a separate claim. Make definite financial arrangements with the patient for payment of his or her portion of the fee.

### *Tracking Claims in Process*

Insurance claims are another form of accounts receivable—that is, money that has been earned and must now be collected. It is important that these claims be handled in a business-like manner. Most computerized programs generate the reports needed to track these claims, including the following:

- Claims that have been submitted for predetermination but have not yet been returned
- Claims that have been submitted for payment but have not yet been paid
- Charges for claims that have been generated but have not yet been submitted
- Claims that have been returned for any reason and have not yet been resubmitted

These reports should be printed and reviewed on a regular basis. It is important that you follow up promptly on any claims process that has not been completed in a reasonable length of time.

## Payments from Insurance Carriers

Checks received from insurance carriers should be accompanied by an explanation of benefits that tells which benefits have been paid and which have been denied. The explanation of benefits breaks down how payment was determined and contains the following information:

- Patient's name and policy number
- Provider of services
- Dates of services
- Procedures
- Amount billed by the provider
- Amount allowed by the insurance carrier
- Amount disallowed or not eligible for payment
- Deductible amount deducted
- Copayment or coinsurance amount due from the patient
- Total amount paid by the insurance carrier
- Comments explaining why payment was denied, asking for more information, or specifying coordination of benefits

This report should be reviewed carefully to determine whether further action is necessary. Each check is entered into the bookkeeping system by patient account with a notation that shows the source of the payment. If, after making this payment, the patient owes a balance, he or she should be notified that the insurance carrier has paid its portion, and that the patient is now responsible for the unpaid balance.

Occasionally, it is necessary to make adjustments in the bookkeeping system to write off *(deduct)* amounts that cannot be collected. The balance of the patient's account is reduced by the amount of the adjustment.

## Handling Overpayments

If the patient has paid his or her account and a check also arrives from the insurance carrier, this procedure must be followed to handle the resulting overpayment:

1. Credit the check from the carrier to the patient's account, and deposit it as any other payment on account. Crediting the check to the patient's account will create a credit; insurance carriers report to the IRS how much they paid to each dentist, and it is important that the practice records show receipt of these funds.
2. Write a check from the practice to the patient to refund the amount of the overpayment. This check is taken from

the accounts payable system and shows up as a practice expense.
3. Make an entry on the account ledger to show that the check was sent. This will eliminate the credit balance on the account.

Because the funds received are equal to the amount of the refund check, the total amount of taxable income for the practice is not increased.

## Insurance Fraud

The business assistant is responsible for accurate and honest claims submission. It is important for the assistant to understand the consequences of submitting fraudulent claims even if it is the dentist's idea. An assistant cannot escape liability by pleading ignorance; therefore it is necessary for the assistant to understand what constitutes fraud. To commit fraud is to lie to or deceive someone for unlawful gain. Some examples of dental insurance fraud are as follows:

- Billing for services not provided
- Changing fees on a claim form to obtain a higher payment
- Disregarding a copayment or deductible, accepting only the insurance payment, and writing off the difference

RECALL

17 What three methods are most commonly used to calculate fee-for-service insurance benefits?
18 _____ is a specified amount of money that an insured person must pay before the insurance goes into effect.
19 A child or spouse of an insurance subscriber is considered to be a _____.
20 Is it possible to be covered under two insurance policies?
21 How is insurance submitted?
22 What CDT section of service would include radiographs?
23 What CDT section of service would include an amalgam restoration?
24 What CDT section of service would include a full denture?
25 What CDT section of service would include root planing and curettage?

**■ Patient Education** The office manager or business assistant has the important task of discussing financial obligations with the patient. Discussion of money can be one of the most time-consuming and stressful parts of a job. Because discussing finances involves the personal realm of a patient, it is important to remember that patients must be respected for who they are, not for what they have. Try to present as much information as possible before treatment is provided; for example, ask about insurance coverage, explain what the patient is responsible for, and discuss how payments can be handled. ■

**■ Legal and Ethical Implications** The responsibility placed on the business assistant in keeping financial records current and up to date shows great trust in that person. It is in turn important to keep accurate and completed daily procedures for all accounts receivable and accounts payable systems. Keep an open communication network with the dentist and accountant regarding all transactions in the day-to-day business of a dental practice. ■

**■ Eye to the Future** In the area of financial matters, you will never see an automatic self-checkout in the medical and dental setting as you see in some grocery and department stores. Dental and medical services are personal and require a more respectful and individual way of handling finances. Even so, with increasing use of electronic payment, the traditional paper check will one day be a thing of the past, and deductions will be made directly from a patient's personal account. ■

### ■ Critical Thinking

1. A patient is checking out and wishes to pay today's fees ($76), as well as an outstanding account balance ($320). The patient writes a check for $400.How do you enter this payment in the management system?
2. It takes a certain type of person to collect money from a patient. Examine your thoughts and feelings regarding collections, and describe your style when asking a patient of the practice who has recently lost his job for payment of $700 that is 6 months past due.
3. Discuss your thoughts on searching a patient's credit background. When do you think it would not be necessary, and when would it be necessary in a dental practice?
4. As the business assistant, one of your responsibilities is to prepare the staff payroll. Do you think that this should be a job of the business assistant? Why or why not? If so, how important is it for you to maintain confidentiality regarding each staff member's salary?
5. A woman who is not a patient of the practice came in today for an emergency. When checking out, she hands you her dental insurance card. Your dental office does not accept this type of insurance, and she does not have any other means of payment. How could this have been prevented, and what should you do now? ■

64

# Marketing Your Skills

## KEY TERMS

**Career** A profession or occupation that requires specific education or training.
**Employment** An activity or job performed, usually for payment.
**Interview** A formal meeting in person to assess the qualifications of an applicant.
**Professional** Person who meets the standards of a profession.
**Résumé** A brief description of one's professional or work experience and qualifications.
**Termination** The end of an employee/employer relationship, which can be initiated by the employee or employer.

## LEARNING OUTCOMES

*On completion of this chapter, the student will be able to achieve the following objectives:*

1. Pronounce, define, and spell the key terms.
2. Discuss aspects of a professional career, including the following:
   - Determine career goals and develop a personal philosophy.
   - List the eight steps to follow when seeking employment.
   - Identify potential career opportunities.
3. Name possible sources of employment opportunities.
4. Discuss strategies for seeking employment and résumé preparation, including the following:
   - Describe the preparation and demeanor needed for a job interview.
   - Prepare a follow-up letter.
5. Discuss factors that should be considered in salary negotiations.
6. Discuss the elements of an employment agreement.
7. Explain the importance of the Americans with Disabilities Act.
8. Describe the steps of job termination.
9. Describe the attributes necessary for achieving career objectives.

## PERFORMANCE OUTCOME

*On completion of this chapter, the student will be able to meet competency in the following skill:*

- Prepare a professional résumé.

## ELECTRONIC RESOURCES

***Additional information related to content in Chapter 64 can be found on the companion Evolve Web site.***

- Practice Quiz

As you complete your education, you will begin to identify and consider the type of employment you will be seeking. Your knowledge and skills will allow you to select a job in which your needs and capabilities are met and a setting in which you will be recognized as a valuable employee.

## Your Professional Career

You have many resources to offer to a potential employer. It is important to analyze your qualifications and career direction. By doing this, you can determine what type of employment you are looking for and what type of environment is compatible with your needs.

### Goals and Philosophy

Ultimately, you are responsible for your personal and professional development. This means that you need to ask yourself what you want to accomplish in your work and personal life. You can establish concrete professional goals that focus on your talents and accomplishments. Your personal philosophy should reflect your commitments, values, and concerns as they relate to future employment.

### Marketing Yourself

You've graduated and the **résumé** is ready. What more do you need? You need to stand out. Be different—the type of employee that your prospective employer can't do without. Learn what your perspective employer is looking for, then market yourself appropriately. The trick is to stay true to your capabilities and skills, but rise above everyone else. It is your responsibility to identify what capability you can offer to your "patient."

The process of marketing yourself can be similar to the kind of marketing plan developed for a product or service. There are eight steps to follow when seeking employment:

1. **Define your mission and the benefits you offer:** Start with self-knowledge: aptitudes, interests, personality, values, and

specific skills within dental assisting. Consider what type of job fits you best: generalist or specialist or a combination; clinical or the business side of dentistry. Ask yourself, "What do I have to offer?"

2. **Set your marketing objective:** What exactly do you want to achieve? Be specific, make it measurable, make it realistic, and build in a timeline with deadlines.
3. **Design performance measures:** What will be the observable, objective indicators that show that you are accomplishing or have accomplished your goal?
4. **Gather, analyze, and interpret information about your situation:** Identify your personal strengths and weaknesses: How do you stack up against your competition? Identify external opportunities and threats: What trends may affect you and your career positively or negatively?
5. **Identify your target markets:** Who needs to know you, your capabilities, and your professional goals? This may mean that you focus your efforts on key managers, mentors, or human resources staff solely, or that you broaden your outreach through membership in professional organizations, depending on your goal.
6. **Develop your marketing strategy and activities aimed at your target market:** Volunteer, take on leadership or committee roles in professional organizations, and attend conferences and continuing education events, even if you have to pay for them.
7. **Define implementation strategies:** What will you do, when, what resources will you need, and what might be obstacles to overcome?
8. **Evaluate your efforts and modify them if needed:** What's working? What do you need to do differently? Do you need to do more, or scale back your efforts?

Once you have committed to your personal marketing plan, discuss it with at least three people you respect, such as an instructor, mentor, or family member. Incorporate their feedback and suggestions, and then begin to implement your plan. As you make progress, evaluate your results and revise your plan accordingly.

## Career Opportunities

Given your education and the many opportunities available within dental assisting, you have a wide range of employment options from which to choose. This range of choices will open doors to new and exciting **career** choices.

### Factors to Remember When You Are Seeking Employment

You want to feel physically, psychologically, and socially comfortable in your work environment.
You want to select an employer whom you respect and whose philosophy of practice parallels your beliefs.
You want to find the type of employment situation that will be the most stimulating, interesting, and rewarding for you—one that will provide professional and personal growth.
You want to be able to work well with other members of the dental health team to achieve mutual respect and shared values.

### Private Practice

Traditionally, independent private practitioners have delivered dental care in the United States. These practitioners provide a wide range of professional services for their patients. A private practice can take the form of a solo practice or a group practice; a group practice can involve additional dentists as associates, or a partnership. The American Dental Association definition states that a nonsolo dentist works "in a practice with at least one other dentist. Some of these dentists may be employed by the owner dentist in the practice."

A group practice may be composed of almost any number and variety of general practitioners and specialists working in a shared facility. The benefits of being employed in a larger group setting include the following:

- Opportunities to develop more specialized skills
- Professional stimulation and sociability of working with many other auxiliaries
- Greater opportunity for advancement
- Potential for a more extensive program of employee benefits than can be offered by a solo practitioner

### Insurance

Dental insurance companies are continually looking for skilled dental assistants to contribute to their organizations. Depending on your expertise and interests, you could consider a challenging career in business and administrative procedures that incorporates your knowledge of dentistry, processing of claims, and customer service.

### Sales

Many dental manufacturing companies seek out individuals with a background in dentistry. If you are outgoing, find it easy to approach new people, have experience in dental assisting, and like to travel, you may find sales to be a rewarding career.

### Research

Dental schools and hospitals with dental clinics hire dental assistants to work in their dental clinics or within research settings. These positions generally require you to be in charge of coordinating patients within a research study, report writing, and entering a wide range of data.

### Management Consulting

Experienced dental assistants with managerial and clinical backgrounds bring their expertise to dental practices through consulting firms. Many assistants join an existing consulting firm or obtain the resources and support to start their own. Their purpose is to develop customized practice management concepts for individual dental practices that are interested in enhancing employee satisfaction, achieving economic success, and improving communication and management skills.

### Teaching

Employment as an instructor in a dental-assisting program is a challenging and rewarding career option for the motivated dental assistant. Each school and state has requirements for teacher certification. These vary and may include prescribed college courses in educational methods, at least a bachelor's degree, and certification or registration as a dental assistant.

An assistant who would enjoy teaching should consider taking college courses in related sciences and education on a part-time basis while simultaneously gaining valuable work experience in the dental office.

### Dental Schools

Educationally qualified and experienced dental assistants are employed by dental schools to work in clinical settings to provide dental students with experience in four-handed dentistry. **Employment** at a dental school provides the assistant with the stimulation of working in an educational setting with faculty, students, and patients.

### Hospitals

A hospital setting that has a dental clinic will hire qualified assistants to work with special patients who may be in the hospital for another health-related illness or with patients who require a specialized setting to be treated, such as those with human immunodeficiency virus (HIV) or another type of immune disorder.

### Public Health and Government Programs

Public health and other government-supported dental facilities function at the federal, state, and local levels. Dental public health programs promote dental health through organized community efforts. Dental assistants may be employed by programs in which dental services are provided at no cost or minimal cost to patients who are eligible to receive care. Public health practices almost always involve a team effort with other professionals such as physicians, nurses, social workers, and nutritionists.

Professionals in these settings generally also collect data and report statistics on specific public health issues and services such as fluoridation, incidence of acquired immunodeficiency syndrome (AIDS), and care for older adults or specific population groups, which could include Native Americans and immigrants.

1 List the types of employment choices from which a dental assistant may choose.

## Locating Employment Opportunities

Once you have determined potential areas of employment, it is important to be knowledgeable about employment sources. This type of assistance will help you find the position and the employer that you seek.

### Newspaper Advertisements

Newspaper advertisements are an excellent employment source. Frequently, dentists place classified advertisements describing the available position and the requirements. The employer will include a telephone number if he or she wishes to speak to you directly or will ask that you send your letter of application and résumé to a box address or email address. This is known as a *blind box* advertisement; it gives the employer an opportunity to screen prospective employees before scheduling an **interview**.

### Campus Placement

If you are attending a dental-assisting program, the school will commonly offer a placement service or will provide a list of employment opportunities with practicing dentists in the area. Dentists frequently contact dental-assisting schools for new employees. It is common for a clinical rotation that is taking place in the curriculum to result in employment.

### Employment Agencies

Employment agencies are located in all regions of the United States, and most states offer employment services and employment opportunity information free of charge. Private employment agencies charge a fee to help you find a position, but over the past decade, employment agencies have changed their fee policy from applicant-paid to employer-paid. These agencies are paid on a contingency-fee basis, and placement fees are calculated on the basis of a percentage of the projected monthly or annual starting salary of the applicant.

### Temporary Agencies

Temporary employment can be an ideal route to finding permanent employment. It is not always possible to be certain on the basis of a résumé and one interview whether the dental practice and the prospective employee are a good match for each other. By working temporarily in a variety of settings, you have a chance to evaluate firsthand the responsibilities and challenges involved in a given position.

Many assistants prefer temporary work because it is usually short-term or part-time and ideal for employees with the responsibility of caring for young children. However, temporary services can offer a temporary-to-permanent transition if desired.

### Dental Supply Companies

The sales representatives who call on dental offices in the area frequently know when a dentist is looking for a qualified assistant. When you are seeking employment, inform the salesperson about the type of employment you prefer.

### Professional Organizations

Local dental societies and dental assistant organizations frequently serve as informal employment information centers. Many local dental societies publish monthly newsletters in which it may be possible to place a classified advertisement or be placed on a hiring list. **Professional** journals also have a classified section with possible job opportunities.

## Social Media

Social media broadly refers to a form of communication and networking. Social media is an extremely powerful tool when looking for employment opportunities and has become a fast and inexpensive background check. Employers search social media to verify facts on resumes, to check out knowledge and attitudes publicly expressed, and to evaluate communication skills. It helps employers gain a clearer idea of who you are and what you have done before talking with you. They can also pick up clues about your personality and how you might fit into their dental practice.

In general, the three major social media associated with job searches are LinkedIn, Facebook, and Twitter.

### LinkedIn

LinkedIn is the largest professional network site in the world. Members connect with each other and directly with employers. Most employers prefer LinkedIn, and it is widely viewed as the most businesslike and professional of the social networks. Most importantly, your profile must be professional and up to date. Remove any photos or items that are politically divisive or could be considered offensive (https://www.linkedin.com).

### Facebook

Facebook is the largest social networking Web site. Your Facebook wall must be either suitable for viewing by potential employers or sufficiently protected by your privacy settings (https://www.job-hunt.org/social-networking/facebook-job-search/facebook-job-search.shtml).

### Twitter

Twitter is a free social networking service that enables its users to send and read messages known as tweets (https://www.job-hunt.org/social-networking/twitter-job-search.shtml).

RECALL

**2** Where might a dentist advertise for a job position?

## Seeking Employment

The following sections describe specific methods that will assist you in your job search.

## Telephone Contact

Your first contact with a prospective employer will probably be made by telephone. When you call, identify yourself and explain your reasons for calling. The first impression over the telephone is very important because if you do not make a good impression here, you may not get a second chance to prove yourself in an interview. You may be asked to submit a completed application or a résumé before the interview.

## Résumé

The résumé is an important marketing tool designed to gain interest from prospective employers (Fig. 64.1). It should present a summary of your skills and qualifications in a positive and professional manner. The primary purpose of the résumé is to convince a potential employer that you are a qualified candidate for employment, and that it would be well worth his or her time to interview you in person. Different résumé styles may be considered, but the style you choose should fit the type of job you want, your qualifications, and the actual job opening. The appearance of the résumé is extremely important because it may represent the first physical contact you have with a prospective employer; therefore a well-organized, concise, neat résumé is vital. Include the following information:

- *Heading:* This consists of three items: your full name (with credentials if appropriate), complete address, and appropriate telephone number or numbers. This information most often is centered at the top of the page.
- *Professional Objective:* This is a clear statement of the type of job you are seeking; however, it should not be so narrowly stated that it limits your job opportunities.
- *Education:* List your most recent educational level obtained. You may list all degree programs you have completed, but if you have a college degree, do not list your high school graduation. If you took special courses or received honors that may be of interest to your potential employer, you may wish to make note of them here.
- *Professional Experience:* List your work experiences in order, beginning with the most recent. For each job, provide the dates (months and years only) of your employment, your position or title, the employer's name and location, and your responsibilities and accomplishments.
- *Skills:* To stand out or capture the reader, you need to provide specific areas that make you more employable than the next person. List the specific areas that you excel in, such as advanced functions, business skills, or people skills.
- *Certifications:* List your certification, registration, cardiopulmonary resuscitation (CPR) certification, and any other appropriate certification information. Emphasize career-related affiliations. It is not recommended that personal data be included on your résumé. Under Federal Equal Employment Opportunity regulations, employers may not ask questions regarding race, color, religion, gender, national origin, marital status, and child care arrangements unless they relate to bona fide occupational qualifications. However, you may be required to submit verification of citizenship or appropriate alien status.
- *Volunteer Experience:* If you have completed any volunteer work, list it even if it does not pertain to dentistry. This will show your future employer that you are a caring and concerned individual. Do not list this as a category if it does not apply.
- *Awards/Scholarships:* List any scholarships or awards that you received in high school or college. Do not list this as a category if it does not apply to you.
- *References:* It is not required that references be included on the résumé, but you may wish to have a list of references available should the prospective employer request them.

See Procedure 64.1: Preparing a Professional Résumé.

## ANATOMY OF A RESUME

1234 Valley Boulevard
Canyon View, CA 12345 (1)
Cell phone (123) 555-7890
imagraduate@comcast.com

**Ima Graduate** (1)

**Objective** (2) Interested in obtaining a position as an administrative dental assistant. Offering excellent skills in patient communication, appointment scheduling, and computer applications. Enjoy working as a member of a professional healthcare team.

**Education** (3)
2014–2015 Canyon View Junior College, Canyon View, CA
Administrative Dental Assistant
Certification of Completion

2010-2014 Canyon View High School, Canyon View, CA
Diploma

**Work Experience** (4) January–September 2015, Canyon View Dentistry, Canyon View, CA
Administrative Dental Assistant
- Patient scheduling
- Computer data entry and management
- Patient relations

**Skills and Abilities** (5)
- Computer skills
- Telephone procedures
- Patient communications
- Enthusiastic team member
- Organized
- Able to work unsupervised

**Professional Affiliations and Certification** (6)
- ADAA, American Dental Assistants Association
- CDPMA, Certified Dental Practice Management Assistant
- American Heart Association, CPR–Healthcare Provider
- Radiology Certification

**References**  Available upon request

A resume is a summary of your skills, abilities, education, and work experience. The completed resume serves as an introduction; depending on your resume, you may or may not obtain an interview.

### 1 HEADING

The heading will include full name, address, cell phone number, and e-mail address. For security reasons if the resume is posted online, omit your address.

### 2 JOB OBJECTIVE

A job objective focuses on the type of job you are seeking and what you can offer the prospective employer. The statements made should be specific and concise. Information listed in the objective will be supported in the body of the resume. **The objective** is considered one of the most important sections of the resume.

### 3 EDUCATION

Information included in your education statement: dates attended, diplomas, degrees, awards and certificates earned. Workshops and seminars that contribute to your qualifications should also be included in this section. List the information in chronological order (start with the most recent date and work back in time).

### 4 WORK HISTORY

This section can also come under the heading **Work Experience, Employment History, Professional Experience,** or **Experience.** In this section you will list the name and location of each company or organization, starting and ending dates, and a brief description of your duties. You can also list volunteer work experience, especially if it demonstrates skills and abilities that will enhance your job qualifications (non-paid training can also be listed). List the experience in chronological order.

### 5 SKILLS AND ABILITIES

Use this section to highlight skills, abilities, and strengths that are pertinent to the job you are applying for. Statements should be action-oriented, begin with verbs, and be concise.

### 6 MISCELLANEOUS

Headings and information include such items as extracurricular activities, clubs, memberships in professional organizations, certification, volunteer activities, awards, and achievements.

### 7 REFERENCES

You can include two professional references or state: References furnished upon request. The use of references is optional. When listing references state the name, title or occupation, address, and telephone number.

**ORDER OF INFORMATION**
Prime space is the top one-third of the page, so list the most important sections first.

**MECHANICS**
Typed on one page, easy to read, with correct spelling, grammar, and punctuation. Eliminate unessential words or phrases.

**MARGINS**
The finished resume should appear balanced, centered from top to bottom and left to right.

**PAPER**
Use heavy stock standard size (8.5" x 11") resume paper of good quality (white, cream, or light gray). Print on high-quality setting or have professionally printed. Pages should be free of streaks, fading, or correction fluid.

**FIG. 64.1** An example of a professional résumé. *(From Gaylor LJ: The administrative dental assistant, ed 4, St Louis, 2017, Elsevier.)*

1 **Your Contact Information**
Name
Address
City, State, Zip code
Phone number
Email address

2 **Date**

3 **Employer Contact Information**
Name
Address
City, State, Zip code

4 **Salutation**
Dear Dr. last name

5 **First Paragraph**
The first paragraph of your letter should include information on why you are writing. Mention the position you are applying for and where you found the job listing. Include the name of a mutual contact, if you have one.

6 **Middle Paragraph(s)**
The next section of your cover letter should describe what you have to offer the employer. Mention specifically how your qualifications match the job you are applying for. Remember, you are interpreting your resume, not repeating it.

7 **Final Paragraph**
Conclude your cover letter by thanking the employer for considering you for the position. Include information on how you will follow up.

8 **Complimentary Close**
Respectfully yours,

9 **Signature**
Handwritten signature (for a mailed letter)
Typed signature

1 **Alicia Moore, CDA**
121 Pleasant Drive
Any City, US 27740
(000) 555-1212
almoore@internet.com

2 Date, 20XX

3 Dr. Name
123 Cherry Lane
Any City, US 27740

Re: Clinical Assistant Position

4 Dear Dr. Name:

5 I am applying for the Clinical Assistant position advertised in the Any City newspaper.

6 I am a Certified Dental Assistant and a graduate of the Area Accredited School of Dental Assisting. My enclosed resume provides additional information about my experience and background in the dental field.

I would appreciate the opportunity to schedule an interview with you and your staff at your earliest convenience. I can also be reached on my cell phone at (000) 965-1255.

7 Thank you in advance for your consideration, and I look forward to hearing from you.

8 Sincerely,

9 *Alicia Moore*

Alicia Moore, CDA

**FIG. 64.2** Sample of a cover letter.

### *Electronic Résumé*

Many companies process incoming résumés by using electronic scanners and computers. Knowing how to post your résumé electronically will be beneficial because an increasing number of dental offices are going online to look for potential employment candidates.

## Cover Letter

A well-written cover letter serves to introduce you to your prospective employer and markets your skills and qualifications at the same time. It also serves to create interest on the part of the reader to look at your résumé. A variety of approaches and styles are available (Fig. 64.2).

## Completing a Job Application Form

Before your interview, you may be asked to complete an application form. This will serve as the initial basis of your conversation with the interviewer. In completing this form, be sure that you *follow directions exactly,* and that the information you provide is accurate, neat, and complete.

## The Interview

Even the smartest and most qualified person needs to prepare for a job interview. Interviewing is a learned skill, and there are no second chances when making a first impression. The employment interview is an all-important exchange of information and impressions. This is the time when you gather information to help you determine whether you would be happy working for this dentist, with his or her staff, and in this practice. At the same time, the dentist is trying to determine whether you are the right employee for this position.

If you have not already sent a résumé, take a cover letter and résumé along when you go to the interview, and leave it with the interviewer. The strategies listed will better prepare you and enhance your interview skills.

### Promptness

Plan to arrive 10 to 15 minutes before the scheduled time of the interview. If the interview is scheduled in a geographic area with which you are unfamiliar, it is advisable to take a "dry run" to find the office before the scheduled interview.

### Appearance

It is important to know what to wear to an interview and to look professional. What you wear depends on the office environment and the position you are seeking. When selecting your clothing, you want your appearance to reflect the fact that you are a neat, well-organized, and competent professional. Do not wear scrubs to an interview. It is best to wear conservative business attire. Keep jewelry and makeup to a minimum.

### Interviewing Professionally

The first 10 minutes of your interview is the most critical time because during this time, both you and the interviewer will form a first impression. You may be nervous, but try to relax and be natural. You can create a positive and professional impression by smiling, maintaining direct eye contact, offering a firm yet gentle handshake, and using words such as, "Hi, I'm [*first name, last name*]; it's a pleasure to meet you."

During the interview, many questions will be asked and answered on both sides. Try to answer all questions courteously, completely, and honestly. Be prepared for a variety of questions, and feel free to ask questions yourself if it seems to be an appropriate time. Remember that your attitude and motivation during the interview are important determining factors. You want to convey a positive attitude without overselling yourself.

### Listen

From the very beginning of the interview, your interviewer is giving you information, either directly or indirectly. If you are not hearing it, you are missing a major opportunity. Good communication skills include listening and letting the person know you heard what was said.

### Don't Talk Too Much

Telling the interviewer more than he or she needs to know could be a fatal mistake. When you have not prepared ahead of time, you may ramble when answering interview questions, sometimes talking yourself right out of the job. Prepare for the interview by reading through the job posting, matching your skills with the position's requirements, and relating only that information.

### Don't Be Too Familiar

The interview is a professional meeting to talk business. This is not about making a new friend. Your level of familiarity should mimic the interviewer's demeanor. It is important to bring energy and enthusiasm to the interview and to ask questions, but do not overstep your place as a candidate looking for a job.

### Use Appropriate Language

You should use professional language during the interview. Be aware of any inappropriate slang words or references to age, race, religion, politics, or sexual orientation—these topics could send you out the door very quickly.

### Don't Be Arrogant

Attitude plays a key role in your interview success. There is a fine balance between confidence, professionalism, and modesty. Even if you are putting on a performance to demonstrate your ability, overconfidence is as bad as, if not worse than, being too reserved.

### Take Care to Answer the Questions

When interviewers ask for an example of a time when you did something, they are asking behavioral interview questions, which are designed to elicit a sample of your past behavior. If you fail to relate a specific example, you not only don't answer the question, but you also miss an opportunity to prove your ability and talk about your skills.

### Ask Questions

If you are asked if you have any questions, "No" would be the wrong answer. Part of knowing how to interview is being ready to inquire about what goes on in the practice. Asking questions also gives you the opportunity to find out if this is the right place for you. The best questions come from listening to what you are asked during the interview and asking for additional information.

### Don't Appear Desperate

When you interview with the "please, please hire me" approach, you will come across as desperate and less confident. You know you can do the job; make sure the interviewer believes you can, too.

### Concluding the Interview

Let the prospective employer (or office manager) conclude the interview. If you believe the interview has concluded, you could say, "Do you have any additional questions you would like to ask at this time?" Usually, the interviewer stands up to signal the conclusion of the interview. Make sure to extend your hand for a final handshake, and again use direct eye contact as you say, "I look forward to hearing from you." Within

**Alicia Moore, CDA**
121 Pleasant Drive
Any City, US 27740
(000) 555-1212
almoore@internet.com

Date, 20XX

Dr. Name and Staff
123 Cherry Lane
Any City, US 27740

Dear Dr. Name and Staff:

Thank you for taking time out of your busy schedule to interview me last Tuesday, October 25th. I enjoyed our conversation and am very enthusiastic about the possibility of working with you and your staff.

I know that my clinical and communication skills would be an asset to your practice. Please do not hesitate to call me should you have any other questions.

Again, thank you for your consideration. I look forward to hearing from you in hopes that you have reached a decision favorable to both of us.

Sincerely,

Alicia Moore

Alicia Moore, CDA

**FIG. 64.3** An example of a follow-up letter.

the first week after the interview, you will have developed some intuition regarding how the interview went, as well as whether the office is one in which you would like to pursue employment.

### Follow-up Letter

A thank you letter is an excellent way to follow up with an employer after an interview. It serves to remind the employer of your interview, to accentuate your qualifications, to reaffirm your interest in the position, and to help you stand out in the interviewer's mind. The letter should be mailed within 48 hours, and it should be addressed to the person with whom you interviewed and should reaffirm your interest in the position in the practice. Make sure the letter is thoughtful and sincere (Fig. 64.3).

3 What is the most common means of communication for your first contact with a future employer?
4 What does a cover letter do?
5 Should a résumé list your gender, race, religion, and marital status?
6 How many pages should a résumé be?
7 What is the most critical part of the interview?

## Salary Negotiations

Although salary and benefits are not the only factors to be considered when you are accepting a job, they are very important issues that must be clarified. The interviewer may ask, "What do you expect in terms of salary?" If you have a definite and realistic idea, by all means state it. Keep in mind that education, experience, and skills are important factors that should be considered in a fair and equitable salary and benefits package.

As you negotiate your compensation package with the dentist, you should realize the importance of the total dollar value when benefits are added to salary, the number of hours you will be working, and the working conditions that you will encounter. This is also the time to ask about the frequency of reviews and salary increases and opportunities to advance with the practice. Specific benefits to inquire about include the following:

- Health insurance
- Dental care for self and family
- Retirement plan
- Uniform allowance
- Dues toward professional organizations
- Travel expenses for professional meetings
- Bonuses

## Employment Agreement

Before you accept a position, you need to explore several topics with the dentist or office manager. Reaching a clear understanding of these topics at the time when you are offered the position is important because it can prevent later misunderstandings.

This process is best managed through the completion of an employment agreement. An employment agreement is prepared in duplicate and is signed by both the employer and employee (Fig. 64.4). One copy is retained in the personnel file and the other is given to the employee for his or her records. The agreement should cover the following topics:

- *Job Description:* Your job description states specifically what your employment duties and responsibilities will be.
- *Work Schedule:* This is a list of the hours and days you will routinely be expected to work. If this schedule varies, it is important to know how far in advance these changes will be announced.
- *Compensation:* This section covers agreements regarding salary and benefits plus provisions for performance reviews and salary increases. It also may cover items such as payment of required registration fees, association dues, and continuing education costs.
- *Professional Attire:* Required personal protective equipment must be provided and maintained by the employer. If other uniform requirements apply, you need to know who is responsible for supplying and maintaining them.
- *Interim Employment:* Most employers routinely consider the first several weeks to 90 days as interim employment, during which either party may terminate the relationship without notice. At the end of this period, the new employee should undergo a performance review.
- *Summary Dismissal:* Summary dismissal is termination without notice or severance pay. Causes for summary dismissal include stealing, use of illegal drugs, and any other form of unprofessional behavior.
- *Giving Notice:* The agreement should clarify how much notice you are expected to give should you decide to terminate your employment. The agreement also should cover what happens if the dentist decides to terminate your employment. One common agreement is that you will receive 2 weeks' notice or severance pay.

8 What time frame is usually considered interim employment?
9 What is the term for termination without notice or severance pay?

## Americans with Disabilities Act

The 1992 American with Disabilities Act (ADA) is commonly believed to pertain only to disabled people who seek access to public accommodations and healthcare, but the act also applies to job applicants and current employees.

*Title I* of the act specifically makes it illegal for an employer to discriminate against prospective job applicants on the basis of disability. An employer is required to make an accommodation to the known disability of a qualified applicant or employee if it would not impose an "undue hardship" on the operation of the employer's business. Undue hardship is defined as an action that requires significant difficulty or expense when factors such as an employer's size, financial resources, and the nature and structure of the operation are considered. An employer is not required to lower quality or production standards to make an accommodation, nor is an employer obligated to provide personal use items such as eyeglasses or hearing aids.

Title I also make it illegal for the employer to discriminate against employees of the practice who may become disabled. If a dental staff member becomes disabled while employed, the law requires that the employer must make reasonable accommodations (i.e., take action within reason) to continue employment of that person at the same rate of pay. The dentist may not discharge an employee on the basis of disability without the employee's consent.

This law applies to companies that employ at least 15 people and thus may not apply to the practice for which you work. However, legal and economic realities are pushing small businesses into realizing the value of skilled workers with disabilities.

## Job Termination

If **termination** of your employment becomes necessary, this should be done in keeping with the terms of the employment agreement. The most common time frame is 2 weeks' notice. If you are leaving under friendly conditions, give adequate notice, and, if asked, help select and train your replacement. It also is appropriate to request a letter of recommendation

**EMPLOYMENT AGREEMENT**
**(Complete form in duplicate: one copy for the employer; one copy for the employee.)**

**EMPLOYEE'S NAME** Debbie Quigley, CDA

**Date** 11/08/xx **Full time/Part time** full time

**JOB TITLE** Chairside assistant to Dr. Hernandey
**See attached list for details of duties and responsibilities:**

**PRACTICE WORK SCHEDULE**
**(Your hours will be scheduled within these times.)**

**Usual days per week:** S ____ M √ T √ W 1/2 Th √ F √ S 1/2

**Usual working hours:** 8:30 to 5:30; lunch 1 hr; breaks ________.

**Work schedules are posted:** two weeks in advance; assigned hours may vary

**SALARY AND BENEFITS**

**Pay days:** every other Friday **Starting rate:** $ XX. per hour

**Basis for increases:** review at 6 months, then annually

**Vacation days:** 5; **Sick days:** 5; **Personal time:** 2.

**Additional benefits:** group insurance is available

retirement plan after 3 years

**TERMINATION**

For each new employee, the first 6 weeks are a provisional period of employment.
During this time, the new employee may leave or be dismissed without notice.

After this period, the employee is expected to give 2 weeks notice.

If dismissed, the employee will receive 2 weeks notice or the equivalent in severance pay.

In the event of fraud, theft, illegal drug use, or unprofessional conduct, the employee may be dismissed without notice or severance pay.

Debbie Quigley, CDA — Employee's signature

J. Hernandey, DDS — Employer's signature

**FIG. 64.4** An example of an employment agreement.

that may be helpful in finding other employment. If you are leaving under other circumstances, it is best to leave quickly and quietly.

If your employer terminates your employment, your departure should be handled in accordance with the terms of your employment agreement. Severance pay, which is the equivalent of salary for the notice period, is paid if you are asked to leave immediately on being notified of your dismissal. This is usually paid with the final paycheck. Your benefits termination also should be outlined in the employment agreement.

## Achieving Career Objectives

Achieving and maintaining career objectives and employment represents a two-sided situation. Team members have responsibilities as employees, and the dentist (or other group) has responsibilities as the employer. Before accepting employment, try to determine, through observation and by talking to other employees, whether the dentist does indeed carry out the responsibilities of a good employer. If it is apparent that the dentist does not, perhaps you should consider employment elsewhere.

## Positive Attitude

A positive attitude is important in all aspects of our lives, including work. No single factor is more important in determining your professional success and achieving your career objectives than your own attitude. As a team player, a positive attitude goes a long way. It can reduce stress for the dental team and enhance your communication skills with patients.

## Professional Responsibilities

The dental assistant has many responsibilities as an employee of a dental practice. Following is a list of the responsibilities of a truly professional employee:

- To comply with local, state, and federal laws and regulations governing the practice of dentistry in the region in which the practice is located
- To acquire and maintain all required professional credentials, such as in cardiopulmonary resuscitation, and appropriate state registration
- To maintain high personal and professional ethical standards that result in pleasant, respectful, and professional interactions with *all* patients and staff members
- To be honest, cooperative, and responsible
- To be punctual and on duty at all assigned times (If an absence is unavoidable, the employee should make advance arrangements to ensure that his or her position is covered.)
- To carefully follow the instructions given and work to the best of his or her ability
- To realize that supervision, feedback, and criticism are occasionally necessary, and to be able to respond to these in a constructive manner
- To give proper due notice to the employer should it become necessary to seek other employment

The dentist also has responsibilities as the employer of the practice. Following are some of the duties of a truly professional employer:

- The employer must comply with local, state, and federal laws and regulations governing the practice of dentistry and the hiring of employees.
- The employer must treat all employees with professional and personal dignity and respect in an atmosphere that will motivate and encourage employees to do their best.
- The employer must establish and maintain fair employment policies and practices to provide safe and pleasant working conditions for all.
- The employer or office manager should conduct a performance review for each employee at least once a year. This review, which is conducted in private, is a discussion of the employee's job skills, attitudes, contributions to the practice, and areas of strength and weakness. A written copy of this report is given to the employee, and another copy is maintained in the personnel file.

## Physical Well-Being

Physical well-being is reflected in all aspects of your life. Maintaining a healthy lifestyle is an important part of successful employment. As a dental professional, you need to focus on areas of your life that will lead to a lifelong commitment to sound physical and mental health. In day-to-day terms, the attainment and maintenance of health include exercising regularly, making wise food choices, getting sufficient sleep, maintaining friendships, and indulging in a diversity of interests.

Your professional image is very important. You should always look professional by having healthy skin, a neat and clean hairstyle that does not fall in your face or that of the patient, and appropriate clothing. Clinical personnel should follow Occupational Safety and Health Administration (OSHA) regulations, and business personnel should dress in professional, business-like clothes. As a healthcare professional, you should be a reflection of the quality of care provided in your practice.

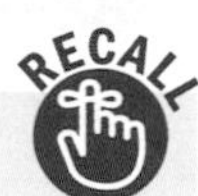


**10** What is the most important factor in determining your professional success?

**■ Patient Education** As a professional healthcare provider, it will be up to you to educate your patients about your profession. Your patients are unaware of your educational background, your qualifications, and your role in a dental practice. Begin by displaying your credentials and by describing your role in their care when they first come to the practice, and by introducing new technologies as you use them. The more patients are aware of their surroundings, the more they feel confident in the care that is provided for them. ■

**■ Legal and Ethical Implications** As an employee, plan to observe all office protocols, such as presenting yourself professionally, working the scheduled hours, practicing business or clinical functions, and representing the dentist and his or her practice. If the state in which you will practice has regulations and guidelines, know those boundaries, so that you perform only what is legal for you to practice. ■

**■ Eye to the Future** Developments in technology, procedures, new materials, and research will continue to challenge the practice of dentistry. The role of the dental assistant will become more complex and efficient. Research has shown that the productivity and income of dentists can be greatly improved through the use of qualified assistants and hygienists. This should encourage states to permit a wider range of expanded functions and challenging job opportunities for assistants. ■

### ■ Critical Thinking

1. Review the Wednesday or Sunday classified section of your local newspaper. Select the dental-assisting job opportunities that interest you. Discuss why those ads appeal to you.

2. List the strengths and weaknesses of your extern sites. On the basis of these, try to develop criteria for your ideal working environment.
3. Your instructor has told you that a local dentist has a clinical position available. What is your plan of action in pursuing this position?
4. You have been on the job now for 2 weeks, and you are just not happy with your position. What should you do?
5. At the end of the day, your dentist calls you in to his or her office and asks you to have a seat. The dentist indicates that you are not working out as well as hoped and that your last day will be this Friday. You are completely shocked by this comment and are not sure why this has happened. How should you handle the situation? ■

**PROCEDURE 64.1**

## Preparing a Professional Résumé

### GOAL

To prepare a résumé to be used for seeking employment.

### PROCEDURAL STEPS

**1** Keep the résumé to one page.
**2** Use standard 8½ × 11–inch white or ivory rag paper.
**3** Use common typefaces.
**4** Use 1-inch margins on all sides.
**5** Use a 12-point font size.
**6** Ensure that the résumé is neat and error free.
**7** Make the résumé concise and easy to read.

# BIBLIOGRAPHY


Abrahams PH, Boon JM, Spratt JD. *McMinn's color atlas of human anatomy*. 6th ed. St Louis: Mosby; 2008.

American Dental Association. Meth mouth: overview. Chicago: ADA. From http://www.ada.org/2386.aspx.

American Heart Association. 2010 American Heart Association guidelines for cardiopulmonary resuscitation and emergency cardiovascular care. *Circulation*. 2010;18(suppl 3):S640.

Bloodborne infectious diseases—universal. From www.cdc.gov/niosh/topics/bbp/universal.html.

Boyd LRB. *Dental instruments: a pocket guide*. ed 6. St Louis: Elsevier; 2018.

Budenz A. Local anesthetics and medically complex patients. *J Calif Dent Assoc*. 2000.

California Dental Association. *Waste management guide for dental offices*. Sacramento, CA: CDA; 2004.

Carr AB, Brown DT. *McCracken's removable partial prosthodontics*. 13th ed. St Louis: Elsevier; 2016.

Centers for Disease Control and Prevention. Dental sealants. From www.cdc.gov/OralHealth/publications/faqs/sealants.htm.

Centers for Disease Control and Prevention. National Center for Emerging and Zoonotic Infectious Diseases (NCEZID), Division of Vector-Borne Diseases (DVBD). Zika virus. From https://educatorgoldarchives.wordpress.com/2016/09/05/medical.

Centers for Disease Control and Prevention. Retention of natural teeth among older adults. *MMWR Morb Mortal Wkly Rep*. 2003;52(50):1226.

Chobanian AV, Bakris GL, Black HR, et al. The seventh report of the Joint National Committee on Prevention, Detection, Evaluation, and Treatment of High Blood Pressure: the JNC 7 report. *JAMA*. 2003;289:2560.

Dahm TS. Skip the sugary drinks. *Dimens Dent Hyg*. 2015;13(3).

Daniel SJ, Harfst SA, Wilder R. *Mosby's dental hygiene: concepts, cases, and competencies*. 2nd ed. St Louis: Mosby; 2008.

Darby M, Walsh M. *Dental hygiene: theory and practice*. 4th ed. St Louis: Saunders; 2015.

Dean JA. *McDonald and Avery's dentistry for the child and adolescent*. 10th ed. St Louis: Elsevier; 2016.

Featherstone JBD. The caries balance: contributing factors and early detection. *J Calif Dent Assoc*. 2003;31:129.

Fehrenbach MJ, Herring SW. *Illustrated anatomy of the head and neck*. 5th ed. St Louis: Saunders; 2017.

Fehrenbach MJ, Popowics T. *Illustrated dental embryology, histology, and anatomy*. 4th ed. St Louis: Elsevier; 2016.

Finkbeiner BL. Four handed dentistry revisited. *J Contemp Dent Pract*. 2000;1(4).

Finkbeiner BL, Finkbeiner CA. *Practice management for the dental team*. 7th ed. St Louis: Mosby; 2011.

Gaylor LJ. *The administrative dental assistant*. 4th ed. St Louis: Saunders; 2017.

Globally Harmonized System (GHS). OSHA hazard communication, safety and health fact sheet. From www.dir.ca.gov/dosh/dosh_publications/ghs_fs.pdf.

Guidelines for infection control in dental health-care settings. 2003. *MMWR Morb Mortal Wkly Rep 52(RR-17)*. December 19, 2003.

Hatrick CD, Eakle WS. *Dental materials: clinical applications for dental assistants and dental hygienists*. 3rd ed. St Louis: Saunders; 2016.

Heyman HO, Swift EJ, et al. *Sturdevant's art and science of operative dentistry*. 6th ed. St Louis: Mosby; 2013.

Iannucci JM, Jansen HL. *Dental radiography: principles and techniques*. 5th ed. St Louis: Saunders; 2017.

Ibsen O, Phelan J. *Oral pathology for the dental hygienist*. 6th ed. St Louis: Saunders; 2014.

Johnson WT. *Color atlas of endodontics*. St Louis: Saunders; 2002.

Lynch H, Milgrom P. Xylitol and dental caries: an overview for clinicians. *J Calif Dent Assoc*. 2003;31(3):205–209.

Malamed SF. *Handbook of local anesthesia*. 6th ed. St Louis: Mosby; 2013.

Malamed SF. *Sedation: a guide to patient management*. 5th ed. St Louis: Mosby; 2010.

Miller C, Palenik C. *Infection control and management of hazardous materials for the dental team*. 5th ed. St Louis: Mosby; 2014.

Misch CE. *Contemporary implant dentistry*. 3rd ed. St Louis: Mosby; 2008.

Mosby. *Spanish terminology for the dental team*. 2nd ed. St Louis: Mosby; 2011.

National Institute for Occupational Safety and Health (NIOSH): Workplace safety. DHHS (NIOSH) Publication Number 2015-236.

National Institutes of Health Consensus Statement. Diagnosis and management of dental caries throughout life. *NIH Consens Statement*. 2001;18(1):24.

Neville B, Damm DD, Allen CM, et al. *Oral and maxillofacial pathology*. 3rd ed. St Louis: Saunders; 2009.

Organization for Safety, Asepsis and Prevention (OSAP): *From policy to practice: OSAP's guide to the guidelines*. Annapolis, MD: OSAP; 2003.

Perry D, Beemsterboer P, Essex G. *Periodontology for the dental hygienist*. 4th ed. St Louis: Elsevier; 2014.

Proffit W, Fields HW, Sarver DM. *Contemporary orthodontics*. 5th ed. St Louis: Mosby; 2013.

Ring ME. *Dentistry: an illustrated history*. St Louis: Abradale Press, Mosby; 1985.

Rosenstiel SF, Land MF, Fujimoto J. *Contemporary fixed prosthodontics*. 5th ed. St Louis: Elsevier; 2016.

Samaranayake LP. *Essential microbiology for dentistry*. 4th ed. St Louis: Churchill Livingstone; 2012.

Wallace S, Cyr W. Green practice. *Dimens Dent Hyg*. 2014;12(3).

White SC, Pharoah MJ. *Principals and interpretation*. 7th ed. ; 2014.

Wilson W, Taubert KA, Gewitz M, et al. Prevention of infective endocarditis: guidelines from the American Heart Association. A guideline from the American Heart Association. *Circulation*. 2007;10:1161. From globalwebsupport@heart.org.

# GLOSSARY

**Abandonment** Withdrawing a patient from treatment without giving reasonable notice or providing a competent replacement. (5)

**Abdominal cavity** Contains the stomach, liver, gallbladder, spleen, and most of the intestines. (6)

**Abdominopelvic cavity** Part of the ventral cavity that contains the abdominal and pelvic cavities. (6)

**Abscess (AB-ses)** Localized area of pus originating from an infection. (17, 54)

**Absorption** Process by which the body takes in or receives (absorbs) a drug. (30)

**Abutment (uh-BUT-munt)** A tooth, root, or implant used for support and retention of a fixed or removable prosthesis. (50)

**Accounting** A system designed to maintain the financial records of a business. (63)

**Accounts payable** Expenses and disbursements paid out from a business. (63)

**Acquired immunity** Immunity that is developed during a person's lifetime. (19)

**Acrylate (AK-ri-layt)** A salt or ester of acrylic acid. (59)

**Active files** Files of patients who have been seen within the past 2 to 3 years. (62)

**Acute (uh-KYOOT)** Referring to a condition with a rapid onset. (31) Pertaining to a traumatic, pathologic, or physiologic phenomenon or process that has a short and relatively severe course. (54)

**Acute exposure** High levels of exposure over a short period. (23)

**Acute infection** An infection of short duration that is often severe. (19)

**Acute inflammation** Minimal and short-lasting injury to tissue. (17)

**Adhere** To stick or glue two items together. (43)

**Administrative law** Category of law that involves regulations established by government agencies. (5)

**Aerobes (AYR-oebz)** Bacteria that require oxygen to grow. (18)

**Agar (AG-ahr)** Gelatin-type material derived from seaweed. (46)

**Ala (AY-lah) (plural, *alae*)** Winglike tip of the outer side of each nostril. (10)

**ALARA concept** Concept of radiation protection that states that all exposures should be kept "*as low as reasonably achievable*." (38)

**Alert** To bring attention to a specific medical or clinical condition. (26)

**Alginate (AL-ji-nayt)** Irreversible hydrocolloid material used for taking preliminary impressions. (46)

**Allergen (AL-ur-jen)** A substance, such as pollen, that causes an allergy. (31)

**Allergy (AL-ur-jee)** High sensitivity to a certain substance. (31)

**Alloy** A solution composed of two metals that are dissolved in each other when in the liquid state. (43)

**Alveolar crest** Highest point of the alveolar ridge. (8)

**Alveolar process** Portion of the maxillary bones that form the support for teeth of the maxillary arch. (9)

**Alveolar socket** Cavity within the alveolar process that surrounds the root of a tooth. (8)

**Alveolitis (al-vee-ah-LI-tis) osteitis** Pain and inflammation resulting from exposed bone associated with disturbance of a blood clot after extraction of a tooth. (56)

**Alveoplasty (al-VEE-uh-plas-tee)** The surgical shaping and smoothing of the margins of the tooth socket after extraction of the tooth, generally in preparation for the placement of a prosthesis. (52, 56)

**Alzheimer's (AHLTS-hie-merz) disease** Form of progressive mental deterioration that occurs in middle to older age. (29)

**Amalgam (uh-MAL-gum)** An alloy, one of the constituents of which is mercury. (43)

**Ameloblasts (uh-MEL-oe-blasts)** Cells that form enamel. (8)

**American Dental Assistants Association (ADAA)** Professional organization that represents the profession of dental assisting on a national level. (2, 22)

**American Dental Association (ADA)** Professional organization for dentists. (22)

**American Dental Hygienists Association (ADHA)** Professional organization for dental hygienists. (22)

**Amino (uh-MEE-noe) acids** Compounds in proteins used by the body to build and repair tissue. (16)

**Anaerobes (AN-uh-roebz)** Bacteria that grow in the absence of oxygen and are destroyed by oxygen. (18)

**Analgesia (an-ul-JEE-zee-uh)** Stage of anesthesia in which the patient is relaxed and conscious. (37)

**Analogy (uh-NAL-uh-jee)** Comparison of similarities between things that otherwise are not alike. (57)

**Anaphylaxis (an-uh-fi-LAK-sis)** Extreme hypersensitivity to a substance that can lead to shock and life-threatening respiratory collapse. (19, 31)

**Anatomic (an-uh-TOM-ik)** Pertaining to the anatomy of a structure.

**Anatomic (an-uh-TOM-ik) portion** A structural portion of a dental model created from the alginate impression. (47)

**Anatomical crown** Portion of the tooth that is covered with enamel. (8)

**Anatomical (anatomic) (an-uh-TOM-i-kul) position** The body standing erect with face forward, feet together, arms hanging at the sides, and palms forward. (6)

**Anatomy (uh-NAT-uh-mee)** Study of the shape and structure of the human body. (6)

**Anemia (uh-NEE-mee-uh)** Shortage of red blood cells or hemoglobin in the blood, resulting in paleness and weakness. (29)

**Anesthesia (an-es-THE-zhuh)** Temporary loss of feeling or sensation. (37)

**Anesthetic** Medication that produces a temporary loss of feeling or sensation. (37)

**Angina (an-JYE-nah)** Severe chest pain associated with an insufficient supply of blood to the heart. (29, 31)

**Angle of the mandible** The lower posterior of the ramus. (10)

**Angle's classification** System developed by Dr. Edward H. Angle to describe and classify occlusion and malocclusion. (11)

**Angular cheilosis** Inflammation at the corners of the mouth that may be caused by nutritional deficiency of the B-complex vitamins but most commonly is a fungal condition. (10)

**Angulation** Alignment of central ray of x-ray beam in horizontal and vertical planes. (41)

**Anode (AN-oed)** Positive electrode in the x-ray tube. (38)

**Anorexia nervosa (an-uh-REK-see-uh nur-VOE-suh)** Eating disorder caused by an altered self-image. (16)

**Antecubital (an-tee-KYOO-bi-tul) space** Small groove or fold in the inner arm, at or "in front of" *(ante)* the elbow *(cubitus).* (27)

**Anterior** Toward the front surface. (6, 11)

**Anterior faucial pillar** Anterior arch of the soft palate. (10)

**Anterior naris (NAY-ris) (*plural,* nares)** The nostril. (10)

**Antibodies** Immunoglobulins produced by lymphoid tissue in response to a foreign substance. (31)

**Antigen (AN-ti-jen)** Substance introduced into the body to stimulate the production of an antibody. (31)

**Antiretraction device** Mechanism that prevents entry of fluids and microorganisms into waterlines as a result of negative water pressure; also called "suck back." (24)

**Antiseptic** Substance used for killing microorganisms on the skin. (20)

**Apex** Tapered end of each root tip. (8)

**Apical curettage (AP-i-kul kyoor-uh-TAHZH)** Surgical removal of infectious material surrounding the apex of a root. (54)

**Apical foramen** Natural opening in the root. (8)

**Apical third** Division of the root nearest the tip of the root. (11)

**Apicoectomy (ap-i-ko-EK-tuh-mee)** Surgical removal of the apical portion of the tooth through a surgical opening made in the overlying bone and gingival tissues. (54)

**Apocrine sweat glands** Large sweat glands that are found under the arms, around the nipples, and in the genital region. (7)

**Appendicular (ap-en-DIK-yoo-ler)** Pertaining to the body region that consists of the arms and legs. (6)

**Appendicular (ap-en-DIK-yoo-ler) skeleton** Portion of the skeleton that consists of the upper extremities and shoulder girdle plus the lower extremities and pelvic girdle. (7)

**Arch wire** Contoured metal wire that provides force when teeth are guided in movement for orthodontics. (60)

**Arrhythmia (uh-RITH-mee-uh)** Irregularity in the force or rhythm of the heartbeat. (27)

**Arteries** Large blood vessels that carry blood away from the heart. (7)

**Arthritis (ahr-THRYE-tis)** Inflammation of a joint or many joints, resulting in pain and swelling. (29)

**Articular (ahr-TIK-yoo-ler) disc** Cushion of dense, specialized connective tissue that divides the articular space into upper and lower compartments; also known as the *meniscus.* (9)

**Articular eminence** Raised portion of the temporal bone just anterior to the glenoid fossa. (9)

**Articular space** Space between the capsular ligament and the surfaces of the glenoid fossa and condyle. (9)

**Articulation (ahr-tik-yoo-LAY-shun)** Another term for *joint.* (7)

**Articulator (ar-TIK-yoo-lay-tur)** Dental laboratory device that simulates mandibular and temporomandibular joint movement when models of the dental arches are attached to it. (47, 50)

**Artifact** A blemish or unintended radiographic image that is not present in the actual structure. (40)

**Artificially acquired immunity** Immunity that results from a vaccination. (19)

**Aspirate (AS-pi-rayt)** To draw back or to draw within. (36, 37)

**Aspiration (as-pi-RAY-shun)** The act of inhaling or ingesting, as of a foreign object. (31)

**Assessment** Process of making an official evaluation of someone or a particular situation. (26)

**Asthma (AZ-muh)** Respiratory disease often associated with allergies and characterized by sudden recurring attacks of labored breathing, chest constriction, and coughing. (29, 31)

**Athetosis (ATH-e-toe-sis)** Type of involuntary movement of the body, face, and extremities. (57)

**Atom** Basic unit of matter. (38)

**Atrophy (AT-ruh-fee)** Wasting away or deterioration. (29)

**Audit trail** Method of tracking the accuracy and completeness of bookkeeping records. (63)

**Autoclave (AW-toe-klayv)** Instrument used for sterilization by means of moist heat under pressure. (21)

**Auto-cured** Hardened or set by a chemical reaction of two materials. (43)

**Automatic processor** Device that automates all film processing steps. (39)

**AutoMatrix (aw-toe-MAY-triks)** Matrix system designed to establish a temporary wall for tooth restoration without use of a retainer. (49)

**Autonomy (aw-TON-uh-mee)** Self-determination. (4) Childhood process of becoming independent. (57)

**Auxiliary (awg-ZIL-yuh-ree)** Attachments located on brackets and bands that hold arch wires and elastics in place. (60)

**Avulsed (uh-VULST)** Torn away or dislodged by force. (57)

**Axial (AK-see-ul)** Referring to the body region that comprises the head, neck, and trunk. (6)

**Axial skeleton** Portion of the skeleton that consists of the skull, spinal column, ribs, and sternum. (7)

**Axial wall** Internal surface of a cavity preparation positioned in the same vertical direction as the pulp within the tooth. (48)

**Bacilli (singular, *bacillus*)** Rod-shaped bacteria that cause tuberculosis and other diseases. (18)

**Bacteremia (bak-tur-EE-mee-uh)** Presence of bacteria in the blood. (29)

**Band** Stainless steel ring attached to molars to hold the arch wire and auxiliaries for orthodontics. (60)

**Base** Foundation or basic ingredient of a material. (46)

**Baseplate** A temporary resin form representing the base of a denture used to help establish jaw relationships and the arrangement of teeth. (52)

**Beam alignment device** Assists in positioning of the position indicator device (PID). (39)

**Beneficence** Of benefit to the patient. (4)

**Bevel (BEV-ul)** Enamel margin of a tooth preparation. (50)

**Beveled (BEV-uld)** Characterized by an angle of a surface that meets another angle. (34)

**Bicanineate** Two-cusp type of mandibular second premolar. (12)

**Bifurcated** Divided into two. (12)

**Bifurcation** Area in which two roots divide. (12)

**Bioburden** Blood, saliva, and other body fluids. (20)

**Biofilm (BYE-oe-film)** Slime-producing bacterial communities that may also harbor fungi, algae, and protozoa. (24)

**Biologic indicators** Vials or strips, also known as *spore tests,* that contain harmless bacterial spores; used to determine whether sterilization has occurred. (21)

**Biologic monitoring** Verifies sterilization by confirming that all spore-forming microorganisms have been destroyed. (21)

**Biopsy (BYE-op-see)** Removal of tissue from living patients for diagnostic examination. (17)

**Bisecting (bisection of the angle) technique** Intraoral technique of exposing periapical films. (41)

**Bitewing** Image view that shows the crowns of both arches on one film. (39) Type of image used for interproximal examination. (41)

**Blade** Flat edge of instrument sharp enough to cut. (34)

**Bleeding index** Method of scoring the amount of bleeding present. (55)

**Blood-borne disease** Disease such as HBV, HCV, or HIV infection that is caused by microorganisms such as viruses or bacteria that are carried in blood. (19)

**Blood-borne pathogens** Disease-causing organisms transferred through contact with blood or other body fluids. (19)

**Blood pressure (BP)** Pressure exerted by the blood against the walls of the blood vessels. (27)

**Board of dentistry** State agency that adopts rules and regulations and implements the specific state's Dental Practice Act. (5)

**Bonding** Form of insurance that reimburses an employer for loss resulting from theft by an employee. (63)

**Bone augmentation** Addition of natural or synthetic bone to a surgical site. (55)

**Bone file** Surgical instrument used to smooth rough edges of bone structure. (56)

**Bone marrow** Gelatinous material that produces white blood cells, red blood cells, or platelets. (7)

**Bookkeeping** Process of managing the financial accounts of a business. (63)

**Border molding** Process of using fingers to contour a closer adaptation of the margins of an impression while still in the mouth. (46, 52)

**Bow** Rounded part of clamp that extends through the dental dam. (36)

**Braces** Another term for fixed orthodontic appliances. (60)

**Brachial (BRAY-kee-uhl)** Relating to the arm (brachium), as in brachial artery. (27)

**Bracket** Small device bonded to teeth to hold the arch wire to the teeth. (60)

**Bremsstrahlung radiation** *Braking radiation.* Sudden deceleration of electrons as they interact with highly positively charged nuclei. (38)

**Broad-spectrum activity** Capable of killing a wide range of microbes. (20)

**Bronchitis (bron-KYE-tis)** Inflammation of the mucous membranes of the bronchial tubes. (29)

**Buccal (BUK-ul)** Region of the head that refers to structures closest to the inner cheek. (9)

**Buccal surface** Tooth surface closest to the inner cheek. (11)

**Buccal vestibule** Area between the cheeks and the teeth or alveolar ridge. (10)

**Buccolingual division** Lengthwise division of the crown in a labial or buccal-lingual direction, consisting of the *facial* or *buccal/labial* third, *middle* third, and *lingual* third. (11)

**Buffer time** Time reserved on the schedule for emergency patients. (62)

**Bulimia (buh-LEE-mee-uh)** Eating disorder characterized by binge eating and self-induced vomiting. (16)

**Bur** Rotary instrument used in all aspects of dentistry. (35)

**Calcium tungstate** Common type of phosphor. (39)

**Calculus (KAL-kyoo-lus)** Calcium and phosphate salts in saliva that become mineralized and adhere to tooth surfaces. (14, 58)

**Call list** List of patients who can come in for an appointment on short notice. (62)

**CAMBRA** Caries management by risk assessment. (13)

**Canadian Dental Assistants Association (CDAA)** Professional organization for dental assistants in Canada. (22)

**Cancellous (KAN-sil-us) bone** Lightweight bone found in the interior of bones; also known as *spongy bone.* (7)

***Candida*** Yeast commonly found in the oral cavity, gastrointestinal tract, and female genital tract, and sometimes in the skin. (18)

**Candidiasis (kan-di-DYE-i-sis)** Superficial infection caused by a yeastlike fungus. (17)

**Canine eminence (EM-i-nens)** External vertical bony ridge on the labial surface of canines. (12)

**Canthus (KAN-thus)** Fold of tissue at the corner of the eyelids. (10)

**Capillaries** System of microscopic vessels that connects the arterial and venous systems. (7)

**Carcinoma (kahr-si-NOE-muh)** Malignant tumor in epithelial tissue. (17)

**Cardiopulmonary resuscitation (CPR) (kahr-dee-oe-PUL-muh-nar-ee ree-suh-si-TAY-shun)** Planned action for restoring consciousness or life. (31)

**Career** Profession or occupation that usually requires a specific educational background. (64)

**Caries (KAR-eez)** Tooth decay. (13)

**Caries risk test (CRT)** Test for cariogenic bacteria. (13)

**Cariogenic** Producing or promoting tooth decay. (16)

**Cariology (KAR-ee-all-o-gee)** The science and study of dental caries. (13)

**Carious (KAR-ee-us) lesion** White spots, brown spots, decay on tooth surfaces. (13)

**Carotid (kuh-ROT-id)** Relating to either of the two major arteries on each side of the neck that carry blood to the head. (27)

**Carpal tunnel syndrome (CTS)** Pain associated with continued flexion and extension of the wrist. (25)

**Carrier** Insurance company that pays the claims and collects premiums. (63)

**Cartilage** Tough, connective, nonvascular elastic tissue. (7)

**Cassette** Holder for extraoral films during exposure. (39)

**Cast post** Metal post placed into the root canal of an endodontically treated tooth to improve the retention of a cast restoration. (50)

**Catalyst (KAT-uh-list)** Substance that modifies or increases the rate of a chemical reaction. (46)

**Cathode (KATH-oed)** Negative electrode in the x-ray tube. (38)

**Cavitation (ka-vi-TAY-shun)** Formation of a cavity or hole. (13)

**Cavity** Pitted area in a tooth caused by decay. (48)

**Cavity preparation** Process of decay removal and tooth design in preparation for restoring a tooth. (48)

**Cavity wall** Internal surface of a cavity preparation. (48)

**CDT (Current Dental Terminology)** Publication that lists the procedure codes assigned to dental services for the processing of dental insurance. (63)

**Cellulitis (sel-yoo-LYE-tis)** Inflammation of cellular or connective tissue. (17)

**Celluloid (SEL-yoo-loid) strip** Clear plastic strip used to provide a temporary wall for the restoration of an anterior tooth. (49)

**Cementoblasts (se-MEN-toe-blasts)** Cells that form cementum. (8)

**Cementoclasts (se-MEN-toe-klasts)** Cells that resorb cementum. (8)

**Cementum** Specialized, calcified connective tissue that covers the anatomic root of a tooth. (8)

**Centers for Disease Control and Prevention (CDC)** Federal agency that is nonregulatory and issues recommendations on health and safety. (22)

**Central groove** Most prominent developmental groove on the posterior teeth. (12)

**Central nervous system (CNS)** Brain and spinal cord. (7)

**Central ray** X-ray at center of beam. (38, 41)

**Centric (SEN-trik)** Having an object centered, such as maxillary teeth centered over mandibular teeth in correct relation. (46)

**Centric occlusion** Maximum contact between the occluding surfaces of the maxillary and mandibular teeth. (11)

**Centric (SEN-trik) relation** Having the jaws in a position that produces a centrally related occlusion. (52)

**Cephalometric (seph-uh-loe-MET-rik) film** Shows the bony and soft tissue areas of the facial profile. (39)

**Cephalometric projection** Extraoral radiograph of the bones and tissues of the head. (60)

**Cephalostat** Special device that allows the operator to easily position both film and patient. (42)

**Ceramic** Hard, brittle, heat- and corrosive-resistant material such as clay. (43)

**Cerebral palsy (suh-REE-brul PAWL-zee)** Neural disorder of motor function caused by brain damage. (57)

**Certified dental assistant (CDA)** Nationally recognized credential of the dental assistant who has passed the DANB certification examination and keeps current on practice through continuing education. (2)

**Certified dental technician** Dental laboratory technician who has passed a written national examination and who performs dental laboratory services such as fabricating crowns, bridges, and dentures, as specified by the dentist's written prescription. (3)

**Cervical third** Division of the root nearest the neck of the tooth. (11)

**Chain of infection** Conditions that all must be present for infection to occur. (19)

**Chamfer (CHAM-fur)** Tapered finish line of the margin at the cervical area of a tooth preparation. (50)

**Chancre** Painless ulcerating sore. (18)

**Change fund** Fixed amount of cash. (63)

**Charge-coupled device (CCD)** Solid-state image sensor used in intraoral digital imaging. (39)

**Check** Draft or order drawn on a bank account for payment of a specified amount of money. (63)

**Check register** Record of all checks issued on and deposits made to a specific account. (63)

**Chemical** Any substance or mixture of substances. (23)

**Chemical inventory** Comprehensive list of every product used in the office that contains chemicals. (23)

**Chemical vapor sterilization (ster-i-li-ZAY-shun)** Sterilization by means of hot formaldehyde vapors under pressure. (21)

**Child abuse** Any act that endangers or impairs a child's physical or emotional health or development. (5)

**Chisel** Surgical instrument used for cutting or severing a tooth and bone structure. (56)

**Chisel scaler** Instrument used to remove *supragingival* calculus in the contact area of anterior teeth. The blade on the chisel scaler is curved slightly to adapt to the tooth surfaces. (55)

**Chlorine dioxide** Effective, rapid acting environmental surface disinfectant or chemical sterilant. (20)

**Chronic** Persisting over a long time. (26) Pertaining to disease symptoms that persist over a long time. (54)

**Chronic exposure** Repeated exposures, generally to lower levels, over a long time. (23)

**Chronic infection** Infection of long duration. (19)

**Chronic inflammation** Continuous injury or irritation to tissue. (17)

**Chronologic (KRON-uh-loj-ik)** Arranged according to time of occurrence; earliest to most recent. (26)

**Chronologic age** Actual age (months, years) of pediatric patients. (57)

**Chronologic file** Filing system that divides materials into months (and possibly days of the month). (62)

**Cingulum (SING-gyoo-lum)** Raised, rounded area on the cervical third of the lingual surface. (12)

**Circumoral (sir-kum-OR-ul)** Surrounding the mouth. (53)

**Circumvallate lingual papillae (sir-kum-VAL-ayt LING-gwul puh-PIL-ee)** Large tissue projections on the tongue. (9)

**Civil law** Category of law that deals with relations of individuals, corporations, or other organizations. (5)

**Classification** To identify the properties of a chemical to determine the degree of hazard.

**Clean area** Place where sterilized instruments, fresh disposable supplies, and prepared trays are stored. (21)

**Clinical contact surface** Surface touched by contaminated hands, instruments, or spatter during dental treatment. (20)

**Clinical crown** That portion of the tooth that is visible in the oral cavity. (8, 58)

**Cocci (singular, *coccus*)** Spherical bacterial cells that reproduce by dividing into two. (18)

**Code of ethics** Voluntary standards of behavior established by a profession. (4)

**Colloid (KOL-oid)** A suspension of particles in a dispersion medium such as water. Its two phases are sol and gel. (46)

**Colony-forming units (CFUs)** A number of separable cells on the surface of a semisolid agar medium that create a visible colony. (24)

**Commission on Dental Accreditation of the American Dental Association** Commission that accredits dental, dental assisting, dental hygiene, and dental laboratory educational programs. (1)

**Communicable disease** Condition caused by an infection that can be spread from person to person or through contact with body fluids. (19)

**Compact bone** Outer layer of bones, where needed for strength; also known as *cortical bone.* (7)

**Computed tomography (CT)** Radiographic technique that allows imaging of one layer or section of the body while blurring images from structures in other planes. (42)

**Concave** Curved inward. (11)

**Conception** Union of the male sperm and the female ovum. (8)

**Condensation (kon-dun-SAY-shun)** Process by which liquid is removed from vapor. (32)

**Condyloid process** The posterior process of each ramus; articulates with a fossa in the temporal bones to form the temporomandibular joint; also known as the *mandibular condyle.* (9)

**Cone beam computed tomography (CBCT)** Three-dimensional digital imaging method that uses a cone-shaped beam of radiation that rotates around the patient. (42)

**Confidentiality** Never revealing any personal information about the patient. (4, 40)

**Congenital (kun-JEN-i-tul) disorders** Disorders that are present at birth. (17)

**Connective tissue** Major support material of the body. (6)

**Connector** Piece of metal that joins the various parts of a partial denture; also called a *bar.* (52)

**Console (KON-sole)** Freestanding cabinet that holds contents or control devices, such as the laser handpiece. (35)

**Consultation (kon-sul-TAY-shun) room** Meeting room or specified area where diagnostic and treatment information is discussed with the patient. (32)

**Contact area** Area of the mesial or distal surface of a tooth that touches the adjacent tooth in the same arch. (11, 41)

**Contaminated area** Place where contaminated items are brought for precleaning. (21)

**Contaminated waste** Items such as gloves and patient napkins that may contain potentially infectious body fluids of patients. (19, 23)

**Contour (KON-toor)** To shape or conform an object. (57)
**Contract law** Category of law that involves an agreement for services in exchange for a payment (contract). (5)
**Contrast** Differences in degrees of blackness on a radiograph. (38)
**Control panel** Portion of the x-ray unit that contains the master switch, the indicator light, the selector buttons, and the exposure button. (38)
**Control tooth** Healthy tooth used as a standard to compare questionable teeth of similar size and structure during pulp vitality testing. (54)
**Convenience form** Cavity preparation step that allows the dentist easier access when restoring a tooth. (48)
**Convex** Curved outward. (11)
**Convulsion (kun-VUL-shun)** Involuntary muscular contraction. (31)
**Coordination of benefits (COB)** Coordinating insurance coverage between two insurance carriers. (63)
**Copier** Business machine that can make duplicates (copies) from an original. (61)
**Coping (KOPE-ing)** Thin metal covering or cap placed over a prepared tooth. (52)
**Core** Portion of a post that extends above the tooth structure. (50)
**Coronal (kuh-ROE-nuhl) polishing** Technique used to remove plaque and stains from the coronal surfaces of the teeth. (58)
**Coronal pulp** Part that lies within the crown portion of the tooth. (8)
**Coronal suture** Line of articulation between the frontal bone and the parietal bones. (9)
**Coronavirus (kuh-ROE-nuh-vye-rus)** Type of virus that causes respiratory infection.
**Cortical plate** Dense outer covering of spongy bone that makes up the central part of the alveolar process. (8)
**Cosmetic dentistry** Type of dentistry limited to improving patients' appearance.
**Coupling agent** Agent that strengthens resin by bonding filler to the resin matrix. (43)
**Cranial (KRAY-nee-ul) cavity** Space that houses the brain. (6)
**Cranium (KRAY-nee-um)** Eight bones that cover and protect the brain. (9)
**Crestal bone** Coronal portion of alveolar bone found between the teeth. (41)
**Creutzfeldt-Jakob (KROITS-felt YAH-koeb) disease** Rare chronic brain disease with onset in middle to late life (40 to 60 years). (18)
**Criminal law** Category of law that involves violations against the state or government. (5)
**Critical instrument** Item used to penetrate soft tissue or bone. (21)
**Cross-bite** Condition that occurs when a tooth is not properly aligned with its opposing tooth. (60)
**Cross-reference file** File in which each item is listed in alphabetic order by name and its document number is provided. (62)
**Crowding** Condition that occurs when teeth are not aligned properly within the arch. (60)
**Crown lengthening** Surgical procedure to expose more tooth surface. (55)
**Crystallization (kris-tul-i-ZAY-shun)** Chemical process in which crystals form a structure. (47)
**Cumulative (KYU-myeh-luh-tiv) trauma disorders (CTDs)** Painful conditions that result from ongoing stresses to muscles, tendons, nerves, and joints. (25)
**Cupping** Condition created by a concave tooth surface that has not been contoured properly. (49)
**Cured** Preserved or finished by a chemical or physical process. (43)
**Curette (kyoo-RET)** Surgical instrument used to remove tissue from the tooth socket; also *curet.* (55, 56)
**Current Dental Terminology (CDT)** Publication that lists the procedure codes assigned to dental services for the processing of dental insurance. (63)
**Curve of Spee** Curvature formed by the maxillary and mandibular arches in occlusion. (11)
**Curve of Wilson** Cross-arch curvature of the occlusal plane. (11)
**Cusp** Major elevation on the masticatory surfaces of canine and posterior teeth. (12)
**Cusp of Carabelli** The fifth supplemental cusp found lingual to the mesiolingual cusp. (12)
**Custom provisional** Pertaining to coverage designed from a preliminary impression or thermoplastic tray resembling the tooth that is being prepared. (51)
**Customary fee** Fee that is within the range of the usual fee charged for the service. (63)
**Cyst (sist)** Closed cell or pouch with a definite wall. (17)
**Cytoplasm (SI-toe-plaz-em)** Gel-like fluid inside the cell. (6)
**Daily schedule** Printed schedule that is copied and placed throughout the office for viewing by staff only. (62)
**Debridement (day-breed-MAW, di-BREED-munt)** To remove or clean out the pulpal canal. (54)
**Deciduous (duh-SID-yoo-us)** Pertaining to first dentition of 20 teeth; often called "baby teeth" or primary teeth. (11)
**Delegate** To authorize or entrust another person to perform a specific skill or procedure. (33)
**Dementia (duh-MEN-shuh)** Mental disorder characterized by loss of memory, concentration, and judgment. (29)
**Demineralization (dee-min-ur-ul-i-ZAY-shun)** Loss of minerals from the tooth. (13)
**Demographics** Personal information about patients that includes address, phone, and work information; also, statistical characteristics of populations. (26)
**Density** Overall darkness or blackness of a radiograph. (38)
**Dental assistant** Oral healthcare professional trained to provide supportive procedures to the dentist and to patients. (3)
**Dental Assisting National Board (DANB)** National agency responsible for administering the certification examination and issuing the credential of certified dental assistant. (2)
**Dental auxiliary (awg-ZIL-yuh-ree)** Dental assistant, dental hygienist, or dental laboratory technicians. (5)
**Dental equipment technician** Specialist who installs and maintains dental equipment. (3)
**Dental handpiece** Electrical device that rotates a selection of rotary equipment for dental procedures. (35)
**Dental hygienist (hy-JEN-ist)** Licensed oral healthcare professional who provides preventive, therapeutic, and educational services. (3)
**Dental laboratory technician** Professional who performs dental laboratory services such as fabricating crowns, bridges, and dentures, as specified by the dentist's written prescription. Most frequently trained on the job as an apprentice. (3)
**Dental lamina** Thickened band of oral epithelium that follows the curve of each developing arch. (8)
**Dental operatory (OP-ur-uh-tor-ee)** Dental treatment room and control center of the clinical area. (32)
**Dental papilla** Gingivae between the teeth. (8)
**Dental public health** Specialty that promotes oral health through organized community efforts. (3)
**Dental radiography (ray-dee-OG-ruh-fee)** Process of making radiographs of the teeth and adjacent structures by exposure to radiographs. (38)

**Dental sac** Connective tissue that envelops the developing tooth. (8)

**Dental sealant** Coating that covers the occlusal pits and fissures of teeth. (15, 59)

**Dental spa** New trend in dentistry that treats patients to a variety of amenities, including massages and herbal masks, in a spalike atmosphere. (3)

**Dental supply person** Representative of a dental supply company who provides dental supplies, product information, services, and repairs. (3)

**Dental treatise (TREE-tis)** Formal article or book based on dental evidence and facts. (1)

**Dental unit waterline (DUWL)** Small-bore tubing, usually made of plastic, used to deliver dental treatment water through a dental unit. (24)

**Dentin** Hard portion of the root that surrounds the pulp and is covered by enamel on the crown and by cementum on the root. (8)

**Dentinal fibers** Fibers found in dentinal tubules. (8)

**Dentinal tubules** Microscopic canals found in dentin. (8)

**Dentist** Oral healthcare provider licensed to practice dentistry. (3)

**Dentition (den-TI-shun)** Natural teeth in the dental arch. (11)

**Dentofacial** Structures that include the teeth, jaws, and surrounding facial bones. (60)

**Deposit slip** Itemized memorandum of funds to be deposited into the bank. (63)

**Deposition** Process by which the body adds new bone. (8)

**Depth** In respiration, amount of air in a breath. (27)

**Desiccate (DES-i-kayt)** To remove all moisture from an item, or to dry out. (44)

**Detail person** Representative of a specific company who provides information concerning the company's product. (3)

**Detection** Act or process of discovering tooth imperfections or decay. (28)

**Developmental disability** Impairment of mental or physical functioning that usually occurs before adulthood and lasts indefinitely. (41)

**Diabetes mellitus (dye-uh-BEE-teez MEL-e-tus, me-LYE-tus)** Metabolic disorder characterized by high blood glucose and insufficient insulin. (29)

**Diagnosis** Identification or determination of the nature and cause of a disease or injury through evaluation of a patient's history and examination findings. (26)

**Diagnostic quality** Referring to radiographs with the proper images and necessary density, contrast, definition, and detail for diagnostic purposes. (41)

**Diastema (dye-uh-STEE-muh)** A space between two teeth. (12, 48)

**Diastolic (dye-uh-STOL-ik, dye-uh-STAHL-ik)** Normal rhythmic relaxation and dilation of the heart chambers. (27)

**Die** Accurate replica of the prepared portion of a tooth used in the laboratory during the fabrication of a cast restoration. (47, 50)

**Differentiation** Term for the specialization function of cells. (6)

**Diffuse (di-FYOOZ)** To spread from an area of high concentration to one of low concentration. (37)

**Digital image** Electronic signals captured by sensors and displayed on computer monitors. (39)

**Digital imaging** Filmless method of capturing an image and displaying it by using an image sensor, an electronic signal, and a computer to process and store the image. (38)

**Digital panoramic units** Filmless method of recording a panoramic image and displaying it by using an electronic sensor and a computer to process and store the image. (42)

**Digitized (DIJ-i-tized)** Scanning of traditional film-based radiographs into a digital image. (39)

**Dihydrate (dye-HYE-drayt)** Related to gypsum products and indicating two parts of water to one part of calcium sulfate. (47)

**Dimensionally (di-MEN-shun-uh-lee) stable** Resistant to changes in width, height, and length. (47)

**Direct contact** Touching or contact with a patient's blood or saliva. (19)

**Direct digital imaging** Technique in which the image is captured on an intraoral sensor and then is viewed on a computer monitor.

**Direct pulp cap** Application of dental material with an exposed or nearly exposed dental pulp. (54)

**Direct supervision** Level of supervision in which the dentist is physically present when the dental auxiliary performs delegated functions. (5, 33)

**Disbursements** Payments on any outstanding accounts payable. (63)

**Disclosing agent** Coloring agent that makes plaque visible when applied to teeth. (15)

**Disclosure** Process of informing the patient about a procedure, for example, the procedure for taking x-rays. (40)

**Disinfectant** Chemical used to reduce or lower the number of microorganisms on inanimate objects. (20)

**Dissipate (DI-suh-payt)** To cause something to scatter or become dispersed, and gradually disappear. (45)

**Distal** Farther away from the trunk of the body; opposite of *proximal.* (6)

**Distal surface** Surface of tooth distant from the midline. (11)

**Distoclusion (DIS-toe-kloo-shun)** Class II malocclusion in which the mesiobuccal cusp of the maxillary first molar occludes (by more than the width of a premolar) mesial to the mesiobuccal groove of the mandibular first molar. (11, 60)

**Distortion** Change in the size of an image on a radiograph caused by incorrect vertical angulation. (38)

**Distribution** Action by which a drug is released throughout the body. (30)

**Donning** Act of placing on an item, such as gloves; dressing. (56)

**Dorsal cavity** Cavity located in the back of the body. (6)

**Dosage** Amount of drug to be administered within a specific time, often according to body weight. (30)

**Dose** Specified quantity of a drug or medicine. (30)

**Dose (of radiation)** Amount of energy absorbed by tissues. (38)

**Dosimeter** Device used to detect and measure an accumulated dosage of radiation. (38)

**Down syndrome** Chromosomal defect that results in abnormal physical characteristics and mental impairment; also called *trisomy 21.* (57)

**Downtime** Waiting period between patient procedures. (62)

**Droplet infection** Infection that occurs through mucosal surfaces of the eyes, nose, or mouth. (19)

**Drug** Substance used in the diagnosis, treatment, or prevention of a disease. (30)

**Dry heat sterilizer** Instrument for sterilization by means of heated air. (21)

**Dual-cured** A composite resin material that has both light-cure and auto-cure properties.

**Due care** Just, proper, and sufficient care, or the absence of negligence. (5)

**Duplicating film** Film designed for use in film duplicating machines. (39)

**Duration (duh-RAY-shun)** Time from induction to complete reversal of anesthesia. (37)

**Early childhood caries (ECC)** Decay in any primary teeth. (13)

**Ebola** A rare but deadly virus that causes bleeding inside and outside the body. (18)

**Ecchymosis (ek-i-MOE-sis)** Technical term for bruising. (17)

**Ectopic** An abnormal direction of tooth eruption. (60)

**Edentulous (ee-DEN-tyoo-lus)** To be without teeth. (52)

**Elastomeric (ee-las-tuh-MER-ik)** Material having elastic properties from rubber. (46)

**Elder abuse** Includes physical or sexual abuse, financial exploitation, emotional confinement, passive neglect, or willful deprivation of an elderly person. (5)

**Electrocardiogram (ee-lek-tro-KAHR-dee-oe-gram)** Instrument used in the detection and diagnosis of heart abnormalities. It generates a record of the electrical currents associated with heart muscle activity. (27)

**Electron** Negatively charged particle in the atom. (38)

**Elevator** Surgical instrument used to reflect and retract the periodontal ligament and periosteum. (56)

**Embrasure (em-BRAY-zhur)** Triangular space in a gingival direction between the proximal surfaces of two adjoining teeth in contact. (11)

**Embryo** Organism in the earliest stages of development. (8)

**Embryology (em-bree-OL-uh-jee)** The study of prenatal development. (8)

**Embryonic (em-bree-ON-ik) period** Stage of human development that occurs from the beginning of the second week to the end of the eighth week. (8)

**Emotional age** Measure of the level of emotional maturity of pediatric patients. (57)

**Emphysema (em-fi-ZEE-muh)** Abnormal increase in the size of the air spaces in the lungs, resulting in labored breathing and increased susceptibility to infection. (29)

**Employment** Activity or job performed, usually for payment. (64)

**Emulsion (ee-MUL-shun)** Coating on the x-ray film that contains energy-sensitive crystals. (39)

**Enamel lamellae** Thin, leaflike structures that extend from the enamel surface toward the dentinoenamel junction and consist of organic material with little mineral content. (8)

**Enamel organ** Part of a developing tooth destined to produce enamel. (8)

**Enamel spindles** The ends of odontoblasts (dentin-forming cells) that extend across the dentinoenamel junction a short distance into the enamel. (8)

**Enamel tufts** The hypocalcified or uncalcified ends of groups of enamel prisms that start at the dentinoenamel junction and may extend to the inner third of the enamel. (8)

**Endocarditis (en-doe-kahr-DYE-tus)** Inflammation of the endocardium. (29)

**Endodontics (en-do-DON-tiks)** Dental specialty that diagnoses and treats diseases of the pulp. (3)

**Endodontist** A dentist who specializes in the prevention, diagnosis, and treatment of diseases of the dental pulp and periradicular tissues. (54)

**Endogenous (en-DOJ-en-us) stains** Stains developed from within the structure of the tooth. (58)

**Endospores** Resistant, dormant structures formed inside of some bacteria that can withstand adverse conditions. (18, 21)

**Endosteal (en-DOS-tee-ul)** Type of implant that is surgically embedded into the bone. (53)

**Energy** The ability to do work. (38)

**Environmental Protection Agency (EPA)** Federal regulatory agency whose responsibility it is to protect and restore the environment and public health through environmental laws. (22)

**Environmental surface** Surface within a healthcare facility that is not directly involved in patient care, but that may become contaminated during the course of treatment (e.g., countertops, floors, walls, instrument control panels). (20)

**Epidemiologic (ep-i-dee-mee-oe-LOJ-ic) studies** Studies of the patterns and causes of diseases. (19)

**Epilepsy (E-pi-lep-see)** Neurologic disorder with sudden recurring seizures of motor, sensory, or psychic malfunction. (29, 31)

**Epithelial (ep-i-THEE-lee-ul) tissue** Type of tissue that forms the covering of all body surfaces. (6)

**Ergonomics (er-guh-NAH-miks)** Adaptation of work environment and tasks to the human body. (25)

**Erosion** Wearing away of tissue. (17)

**Erythema (er-i-THEE-muh)** Skin redness, often caused by inflammation or infection. (31)

**Esthetic (aesthetic) (es-THET-ik)** Artistically pleasing and beautiful appearance. (43)

**Esthetic dentistry** Type of dentistry that improves the appearance of teeth by camouflaging defects and whitening teeth. (48)

**Etchant (ECH-unt)** Chemical agent used in etching. (44)

**Etching (ECH-ing)** Process of cutting into a surface with the use of an acid product. (44)

**Ethical drug** Drug that requires a prescription. (30)

**Ethics** Moral standards of conduct; rules or principles that govern proper conduct. (4)

**Eugenol (YOO-je-nol)** Colorless liquid made from clove oil and used for its soothing qualities. (44)

**Event-related packaging** Instruments in packages should remain sterile indefinitely unless an event causes them to become contaminated (e.g., torn or wet packaging). (21)

**Evidence based** Information based on documented evidence from critically reviewed research. (13)

**Excisional biopsy (ek-SIZH-uh-nul BYE-op-see)** Surgical procedure in which tissue is cut from a suspect oral lesion. (56)

**Excretion (ek-SKREE-shun)** Action by which a drug leaves the body. (30)

**Exfoliation (eks-foe-lee-AY-shun)** Normal process of shedding the primary teeth. (8)

**Exfoliative (eks-FOE-lee-uh-tiv) biopsy** Diagnostic procedure in which cells are scraped from a suspect oral lesion for analysis. (56)

**Exogenous (ek-SOJ-uh-nus) stains** Stains developed from external sources. (58)

**Exothermic (ek-so-THUR-mik)** Characterized by the release of heat from a chemical reaction. (45)

**Expanded functions** Specific intraoral functions delegated to an auxiliary that require increased skill and training. (5, 33)

**Expenses** Overhead costs of a business that must be paid to keep operating. (63)

**Exposed** Pertaining to selected teeth visible through the dam; *isolated.* (36)

**Exposure controls** Feature that allows the operator to adjust the milliamperage and kilovoltage settings. (42)

**Expressed contract** Contract that is established through verbal or written words. (5)

**Extension arm** Flexible arm that is attached to the x-ray tubehead. (38)

**External auditory meatus** Bony passage of the outer ear. (9)

**Extraoral** Outside the oral cavity. (28)

**Extraoral film** Film designed for use in cassettes. (39)

**Extraoral images** Images taken when large areas of the skull or jaw must be examined. (42)

**Extraoral imaging** Image of the teeth and bones made by placing the film or cassette against the face or the head and projecting the x-rays from the opposite side. (42)

**Extrinsic (ek-STRIN-zik) stains** Stains that occur on the *external* surfaces of the teeth that may be removed by polishing. (58)

**Extrusion (ek-STROO-zhun)** Displacement of a tooth from its socket as a result of injury. (57)

**Face bow** Portion of articulator used to measure the upper teeth as compared with the temporomandibular joint. (47)

**Facial surface** Tooth surface closest to the face. Facial surfaces closest to the lips are called *labial surfaces,* and facial surfaces closest to the inner cheek are called *buccal surfaces;* therefore, the term *facial* can be substituted for *labial* and *buccal,* and vice versa. (11)

**Facultative anaerobes** Organisms that can grow with or without oxygen. (18)

**Fats** Lipids. (16)

**Fax machine** Business machine that is attached to a phone line and that transmits hard copy written messages (handwritten or typed); "fax" is short for "facsimile." (61)

**Felony** A major crime, such as fraud or drug abuse. Conviction can result in imprisonment of 1 year or longer. (5)

**Fermentable (fur-MEN-tuh-bul) carbohydrates** Simple carbohydrates, such as sucrose, fructose, lactose, and glucose. (13)

**Festooning (fes-TOO-ning)** The process of carving the base material of a denture or denture pattern to simulate the contours of the natural tissues. (52)

**Fetal molding** Pressure applied to the jaw, causing a distortion. (60)

**Fetal period** Stage of human development that starts at the beginning of the ninth week and ends at birth. (8)

**Fibroblast** Type of cell in connective tissue responsible for the formation of the intercellular substance of pulp. (8)

**Field of view** The area that can be shown when performing imaging procedures. (42)

**File** A metal instrument of varying size and form with numerous ridges or teeth on its cutting surfaces. (55)

**File guides** Insert placed between files that displays the letters or numbers of the patient records that follow it. (62)

**Filiform papillae** Threadlike elevations that cover most of the tongue. (10)

**Filing** The act of classifying and arranging records to be easily retrieved when needed. (62)

**Filled resin (REZ-in)** Sealant material that contains filler particles. (59)

**Filler** Inorganic material that adds strength and other characteristics to composite resins. (43)

**Film holder** Device used to position and hold dental x-ray films.

**Film speed** The sensitivity of the emulsion on the film to radiation. (39)

**Fixed bridge** Dental prosthesis with artificial teeth fixed in place and supported by attachment to natural teeth. (50)

**Fixed overhead** Business expenses that are ongoing. (63)

**Flammables** Readily capable of catching fire. (23)

**Flange (flanj)** Parts of a full or partial denture that extend from the teeth to the border of the denture. (52)

**Fluoride (FLOOR-ide)** Mineral used in dental products to make teeth more resistant to decay. (13)

**Fluoride varnish** Method of administration of topical fluoride. (15)

**Flutes** Blades on the working end of a finishing rotary instrument that resemble pleats. (35)

**Focal trough (trof)** Imaginary three-dimensional horseshoe-shaped zone used to focus panoramic radiographs. (42)

**Food and Drug Administration (FDA)** Federal regulatory agency that regulates food, drugs, medical devices, animal feed and drugs, cosmetics, and radiation-emitting products (e.g., cell phones, lasers, microwaves). (22)

**Foramen (plural, *foramina*)** Small round opening in a bone through which blood vessels, nerves, and ligaments pass. (9)

**Foramen magnum** Large opening in the occipital bone that connects the vertical canal and the cranial cavity. (9)

**Force** Any push or pull on an object. (43)

**Forceps (FOR-seps)** Surgical instrument used to grasp and hold onto teeth for their removal. (56)

**Fordyce's (FOR-dise-ez) spots** Normal variations that may appear on the buccal mucosa. (10)

**Forensic (fuh-REN-zik)** Pertaining to establishment of the identity of an individual on the basis of scientific methods. (26)

**Forensic dentistry** Area of dentistry that establishes the identity of an individual on the basis of dental evidence such as dental records, impressions, bite marks, and so forth. (1)

**Fossa (FOS-ah, FAW-suh)** Hollow, grooved, or depressed area in a bone. (9, 12)

**Four-handed dentistry** Process by which the operator and the assistant work together to perform clinical procedures in an ergonomically structured environment. (33)

**Framework** Metal skeleton of a removable partial denture. (52)

**Frankfort plane** Imaginary plane that passes through the top of the ear canal and the bottom of the eye socket. (42)

**Frankl (FRANG-kul) scale** Scale designed to evaluate patient behavior. (57)

**Frenum (FRE-num) (plural, *frenula*)** Band of tissue that passes from the facial oral mucosa at the midline of the arch to the midline of the inner surface of the lip; also called *frenulum.* (10)

**Frontal** Region of the head pertaining to the forehead. (9)

**Frontal plane** Vertical plane that divides the body into anterior (front) and posterior (back) portions. (6)

**Frontal process** Process of the zygomatic bone that extends upward to articulate with the frontal bone at the outer edge of the orbit. (9)

**Fulcrum (FUL-krum)** Finger rest used when an instrument or handpiece is held for a specified time. (33, 58)

**Full crown** Cast restoration that covers the entire anatomic crown of the tooth. (50)

**Full denture (DEN-chur)** Prosthesis that replaces all of the teeth in one arch. (52)

**Functional occlusion** Contact of the teeth during biting and chewing movements. (11)

**Fungi (singular, *fungus*)** Plants, such as mushrooms, yeasts, and molds, that lack chlorophyll. (18)

**Fungicidal (fun-ja-SI-dal)** Product that is capable of killing fungi. (20)

**Fungiform papillae** Knoblike projections on the tongue. (10)

**Furcation (fur-KAY-shun)** Area between two or more root branches. (12, 28)

**Furcation probe** Used to measure horizontal and vertical pocket depths of multirooted teeth in furcation areas. (55)

**Gait** A particular way of walking, or *ambulating.* (31)

**Galvanic (gal-VA-nik)** An electrical current that takes place when two different or dissimilar metals come together. (43)

**Gauge** Standard dimension or measurement of the thickness of an injection needle. (37)

**General supervision** Level of supervision in which the dental auxiliary performs delegated functions according to the instructions of the dentist, who is not necessarily physically present. (5)

**Generic (jeh-NAIR-ik)** Drug sold without a brand name or trademark. (30)

**Genetic (juh-NE-tik) effects** Effects of radiation that are passed on to future generations through genetic cells. (38)

**Gestation (jes-TAY-shun)** Stage of human development that starts at fertilization and ends at birth. (8)

**Gingiva (JIN-ji-vuh) (*plural,* gingivae)** Masticatory mucosa that covers the alveolar processes of the jaws and surrounds the necks of the teeth. (10)

**Gingival retraction (jin-JI-vul ree-TRAK-shun)** Means of displacing gingival tissue away from the tooth. (50)

**Gingivectomy (jin-ji-VEK-tuh-mee)** Surgical removal of diseased gingival tissues. (55)

**Gingivitis (jin-ji-VYE-tis)** Inflammation of the gingival tissue. (14)

**Gingivoplasty (JIN-ji-voh-plas-tee)** Surgical reshaping and contouring of gingival tissues. (55)

**Glabella (glah-BEL-uh)** Smooth surface of the frontal bone; also, the anatomic part directly above the root of the nose. (10)

**Glenoid fossa** Area of the temporal bone where condyles of the mandible articulate with the skull. (9)

**Globally Harmonized System of Classification and Labeling of Chemicals (GHS)** An international approach to hazard communication. (23)

**Glossitis (glos-EYE-tis)** Inflammation of the tongue. (17)

**Glutaraldehyde (gloo-tuh-RAL-duh-hide)** Environmental Protection Agency (EPA)–registered high-level disinfectant. (20)

**Gold** Soft, yellow, corrosive-resistant metal that is used in the making of indirect restorations. (43)

**Gomphosis** Type of fibrous joint such as a tooth into the alveolus. (7)

**Gracey curette** Curette with one cutting edge, "area specific"; it is designed to adapt to specific tooth surfaces (mesial or distal). (55)

**Gram negative** Classification of bacteria that do not hold a dye stain under a microscope. (18)

**Gram positive** Classification of bacteria that hold a dye stain and appear dark purple under a microscope. (18)

**Gram stain** Four-step staining process developed by Hans Christian Gram and used to separate bacteria into groups. (18)

**Gram variable** Classification of bacteria that are not consistently stained. (18)

**Granuloma (gran-yoo-LOE-muh)** Granular tumor or growth. (17)

**Grasp** The correct way for an instrument or handpiece to be held. (33)

**Greater palatine (PA-luh-tine) nerve** Nerve that serves the posterior hard palate and the posterior lingual gingiva. (9)

**Greener infection control** Minimizing the environmental impact of infection control products and procedures. (20)

**Gross income** The total of all professional income received. (63)

**Gurney (GUR-nee)** Mobile table to transport patients.

**Gutta-percha (guh-tuh-PUR-chuh)** Plastic type of filling material used in endodontics. (54)

**Gypsum (JIP-sum)** Mineral used in the formation of plaster of Paris and stone. (47)

**H1N1** A form of swine influenza virus. (18)

**Hamulus** A hook-shaped process. (9)

**Handle** Part of a dental instrument that the operator grasps. (34)

**Hard tissue impaction (im-PAK-shun)** Oral condition in which a tooth is partially to fully covered by bone and gingival tissue. (56)

**Hazard class** The nature of the physical or health hazards, e.g., flammable solid, carcinogen, oral acute toxicity. (23)

**Hazard classification** To identify the properties of a chemical to determine the degree of hazard. (23)

**Hazard Communication Standard (HCS)** Recently revised Occupational Safety and Health Administration (OSHA) standard regarding employees' "right to know" about hazardous chemicals in the workplace. (23)

**Hazard statement** A statement assigned to a hazard class and category that describes the nature of the hazard(s) of a chemical, including, where appropriate, the degree of hazard. (23)

**Hazardous waste** Waste that poses a danger or risk to humans or to the environment. (19, 23)

**Headgear** External orthodontic appliance that is used to control growth and tooth movement. (60)

**Health hazard** A chemical for which acute or chronic health effects may occur in an exposed employee. (23)

**Hematoma (hee-muh-TOE-muh)** Swelling or mass of blood collected in one area or organ. (17)

**Hemihydrate (hem-ee-HYE-drayt)** Removal of one-half part water to one part of calcium sulfate, forming the powder product of gypsum. (47)

**Hemisection (hem-ee-SEK-shun)** Surgical separation of a multirooted tooth through the furcation area. (54)

**Hemophilia (hee-moe-FIL-ee-uh)** Blood coagulation disorder in which the blood fails to clot normally. (29)

**Hemostat (HEE-moe-stat)** Surgical instrument used to hold or grasp items. (56)

**Herpesvirus** Virus that causes infection in humans, such as herpes, cytomegalovirus, chickenpox, shingles, mononucleosis, measles, and Kaposi's sarcoma. (18)

**Heterotrophic (het-ur-oe-TRO-fik) bacteria** Bacteria that use organic carbon as a source of nutrients. Protozoa, fungi, and most bacteria fall into this category. (24)

**High-level disinfectant** Hospital disinfectant with tuberculocidal activity. (20)

**HIPAA** The Health Insurance Portability and Accountability Act of 1996 specifies federal regulations that ensure privacy regarding a patient's healthcare information. (2, 4, 5, 26, 61, 62, 63)

**Histology (his-TOL-uh-jee)** Study of the structure and function of body tissues on a microscopic level. (8)

**Hoe scaler** Type of scaler used to remove heavy supragingival calculus; it is most effective when used on buccal and lingual surfaces of the posterior teeth. (55)

**Homogenous (hoe-MOJ-uh-nus), homogeneous (hoe-moe-JEE-nee-us)** Having a uniform quality and consistency throughout. (47)

**Horizontal plane** Plane that divides the body into superior (upper) and inferior (lower) portions. (6)

**Hospital disinfectant** Disinfectant with the ability to kill *Staphylococcus aureus, Salmonella choleraesuis,* and *Pseudomonas aeruginosa.* (20)

**Housekeeping surface** Surface that is not contaminated during dental treatment (e.g., floors, walls). (20)

**Human behavior** Collection of behaviors exhibited by human beings who have been influenced by a person's culture, attitudes, emotions, values, ethics, and authority. (61)

**Hunter-Schreger bands** Alternating light and dark bands in the enamel that are produced when enamel prisms intertwine or change direction. (8)

**Hybrid (HYE-brid)** Material that produces a similar outcome to its natural counterpart. (44)

**Hydro-** Prefix meaning "water." (46)

**Hydroxyapatite** Mineral compound that is the principal inorganic component of bone and teeth. (8)

**Hyoid arch** The second branchial arch, which forms the styloid process, stapes of the ear, stylohyoid ligament, and part of the hyoid bone. (8)

**Hyperglycemia (hye-pur-glye-SEE-mee-uh)** Abnormally high blood glucose level. (31)

**Hyperplasia (hye-pur-PLAY-zh[ee-]uh)** Abnormal increase in the number of cells in an organ or a tissue.

**Hypersensitivity** State of being excessively sensitive to a substance, often with allergic reactions. (31)

**Hyperthyroidism (hye-pur-THYE-roid-iz-em, hye-pur-THYE-roi-di-zem)** Condition that results from excessive activity of the thyroid gland. (29)

**Hypertrophied (hye-PUR-troe-feed)** Referring to overgrown oral tissues. (50)

**Hyperventilation** Abnormally fast or deep breathing. (31)

**Hypoglycemia (hye-poe-glye-SEE-mee-uh)** Abnormally low blood glucose level. (31)

**Hypotension (hye-poe-TEN-shun)** Abnormally low blood pressure. (31)

**Hypothyroidism (hye-poe-THYE-roid-iz-em, hi-poe-THYE-roi-di-zem)** Condition that results from severe thyroid hormone insufficiency. (29)

**Hysteresis** Change in temperature that causes reversible hydrocolloid material to transform from one physical state to another. (46)

**Image** Film-based or digitally produced recordings of anatomic images. (38)

**Image receptor** Recording medium for an image—a digital sensor, a phosphor storage plate (PSP), or conventional dental x-ray film. (38, 39, 40)

**Imbibition (im-bi-BI-shun)** Absorption of water, causing an object to swell. (46)

**Imbrication (im-bri-KAY-shun) lines** Slight ridges that run mesiodistally in the cervical third of the teeth. (12)

**Immediate denture** Temporary denture placed after extraction of anterior teeth. (52)

**Immersion disinfectant** Disinfectant used for immersion (soaking) of heat-sensitive instruments. (20)

**Immunity (i-MYOO-ni-tee)** Ability of the body to resist disease. (19)

**Immunocompromised** Having an immune system that is weakened. (24)

**Impacted tooth** Tooth that has not erupted. (56)

**Implant** A permanent replacement of one tooth or multiple teeth with a fixture and an abutment that are anchored into the bone or surrounding structure for the purpose of supporting a denture, bridge, or single tooth. (53)

**Implied consent** Type of consent in which the patient's action indicates consent for treatment. (5)

**Implied contract** Contract that is established by actions, not words. (5)

**Inactive files** Files of patients who have not been seen over the past 3 years. (62)

**Incipient (in-SIP-ee-ent) caries** Tooth decay that is beginning to form or become apparent. (13)

**Incisal edge** Ridge on permanent incisors that appears flattened on labial, lingual, or incisal view after tooth eruption. (12)

**Incisal surface** Chewing surface of anterior teeth. (11)

**Incisional (in-SIZH-uh-nul) biopsy** Section of suspect oral lesion that is removed for evaluation. (56)

**Incisive papilla** Pear-shaped pad of tissue that covers the incisive foramen. (10)

**Inclined cuspal planes** Sloping areas between cusp ridges. (12)

**Indirect contact** Touching or contact with a contaminated surface or instrument. (19)

**Indirect digital imaging** An existing radiograph is scanned and converted into a digital form with the use of a charge-coupled device (CCD) camera.

**Indirect pulp cap** Placement of a medicament over a partially exposed pulp. (54)

**Indirect supervision** Overseeing an assistant's work by working in the immediate area. (33)

**Indirect vision** Viewing an object with the use of a mirror. (33)

**Induction (in-DUK-shun)** Time from injection to effective anesthesia. (37)

**Infection control** Policies and practices designed to prevent the spread of infectious agents. (19)

**Infection prevention** Ultimate goal of all infection control procedures and policies. (19)

**Infectious disease** Disease that is communicable. (19)

**Infectious waste** Waste that is capable of transmitting an infectious disease. (19, 23)

**Inflammation** Protective response of the tissues to irritation or injury. (17)

**Informed consent** Permission granted by a patient after he or she is informed about the risks, benefits, and alternatives of a procedure. (5, 40)

**Infraction** Minor offense that usually results in only a fine. (5)

**Infraorbital (in-fruh-OR-bi-tul)** Region of the head below the orbital region. (9)

**Infuser (in-FYOO-zur)** Syringe that applies hemostatic solution on the gingival retraction cord. (50)

**Inherited immunity** Immunity that is present at birth. (19)

**Inlay (IN-lay)** Cast restoration designed to replace a conservative class II cavity. (50)

**Innervation (in-ur-VAY-shun)** Supply or distribution of nerves to a specific body part. (37)

**Inscription** The name and quantity of a drug listed on the prescription. (30)

**Insulating** Preventing the passage of heat or electricity. (44)

**Integumentary (in-teg-yoo-MEN-tuh-ree) system** The skin system. (7)

**Intellectual disability** Disorder in which an individual's intelligence is underdeveloped. (57)

**Intensifying screen** Device used to convert x-ray energy into visible light, which in turn exposes screen film. (39)

**Intensity** The total energy of the x-ray beam. (38)

**Intermediate-level disinfectant** Liquid disinfectant with EPA registration as a hospital disinfectant with tuberculocidal activity. It is used for disinfecting operatory surfaces. (20)

**Interproximal (in-tur-PROK-si-mul)** Between two adjacent surfaces. (41)

**Interproximal space** Area between adjacent tooth surfaces. (11)

**Intersecting** Cutting across or through. (41)

**Interview** Formal meeting in person to assess the qualifications of an applicant. (64)

**Intraoral** Within the oral cavity. (28)

**Intraoral film** Film designed for placement in the patient's mouth. (39)

**Intrinsic (in-TRIN-zik) stains** Stains that occur within the tooth structure that may not be removed by polishing. (58)

**Intrusion (in-TROO-zhun)** Displacement of a tooth into its socket as a result of injury. (57)
**Invert (in-VURT)** To reverse position, order, or condition. To turn inside out or upside down. (36)
**Investment material** Special gypsum product able to withstand extreme heat. (50)
**Invoice** Itemized list of goods that specifies the prices and terms of sale. (63)
**Involuntary muscles** Muscles that function automatically without conscious control. (7)
**Iodophor (eye-oe-doe-FOR)** EPA-registered, intermediate-level hospital disinfectant. (20)
**Ion (EYE-on)** An electrically charged particle. (38)
**Ionization (eye-uh-ni-ZAY-shun)** Process by which electrons are removed from atoms, causing the harmful effects of radiation in humans. (38)
**Ionizing (EYE-uh-nye-zing) radiation** Radiation that produces ionization, resulting in harmful effects. (38)
**Irregular** Not straight, uniform, or symmetric. (43)
**Irreversible pulpitis (pul-PYE-tis)** Infectious condition in which the pulp is incapable of healing and a root canal is required. (54)
**Isolated** Pertaining to selected teeth visible through the dam; *exposed.* (36)
**Isthmus of fauces** The opening between the two arches of the soft palate. (10)
**Jaws** Part of a clamp that is shaped into four prongs to help stabilize the clamp on the tooth. (36)
**Joints** Structural areas where two or more bones come together. (7)
**Justice** Fair treatment of the patient. (4)
**Kilovoltage (KIL-uh-vole-tuj) peak (kVp)** Highest voltage of radiograph tube used during a radiograph exposure. (38)
**Kirkland knife** Double-ended knife with kidney-shaped blades; commonly used in periodontal surgery. (55)
**Korotkoff (kuh-ROT-kof) sounds** Specific sounds heard when one is taking a blood pressure. (27)
**Label elements** The pictogram, hazard statement, signal word, and precautionary statement for each hazard class and category. (23)
**Label side** Colored side of the film that faces the tongue. (39)
**Labia** Gateway to the oral cavity; commonly known as "lips." (10)
**Labial commissure (LAY-bee-ul kom-i-shur)** Angle at the corner of the mouth where the upper and lower lips join. (10)
**Labial frenum (plural, *frenula*)** Band of tissue that passes from the facial oral mucosa at the midline of the arch to the midline of the inner surface of the lip; also called *frenulum.* (10)
**Labial surface** Facial surface closest to the lips. (11)
**Labioversion** Inclination of the teeth to extend facially beyond the normal overlap of the incisal edge of the maxillary incisors over the mandibular incisors. (11)
**Lacrimal (LAK-ri-mul) bones** Paired facial bones that help form the medial wall of the orbit. (9)
**Lactobacilli (lak-toe-buh-SIL-eye)** Bacteria that produce lactic acid from carbohydrates. (13)
**Lambdoid suture** Line of junction between the occipital and parietal bones. (9)
**Lamina dura** Thin, compact bone that lines the alveolar socket; also known as the *cribriform plate.* (8)
**Laser (LAY-zur)** Highly concentrated beam of light; acronym for light amplification by stimulated emission of radiation. (35, 55)
**Latent (LAY-tent)** Dormant. (18)
**Latent image** Invisible image on the x-ray film after exposure but before processing. (39)
**Latent infection** Persistent infection with recurrent symptoms that "come and go." (19)
**Latent period** Time between exposure to ionizing radiation and appearance of symptoms. (38)
**Lateral excursion (ek-SKUR-zhun)** Sliding position of the mandible to the left or right of the centric position. (52)
**Lateral pterygoid plate** Point of origin for internal and external pterygoid muscles. (9)
**Lathe (layth)** Machine used for cutting or polishing dental appliances. (47)
**Laws** Minimum standards of behavior established by statutes for a population or profession. (4)
**Lead apron** Device used to protect the reproductive and blood-forming tissues from scatter radiation. (38)
**Lead time** Time estimate that allows for delays in ordering or shipping of materials. (62)
**Ledger** Financial statement that documents all account transactions. (62, 63)
***Legionella* (lee-juh-NEL-uh)** Genus of bacteria responsible for the disease legionellosis. (24)
**Lesion (LEE-zhun)** An area of pathology. (17)
**Letterhead** The part of a letter (or printed stationery) that contains the name and address of the person sending the letter. (61)
**Leukemia (loo-KEE-mee-uh)** Progressive disease in which the bone marrow produces an increased number of immature or abnormal white cells. (17, 29)
**Leukoplakia (loo-koe-PLAY-kee-ah)** Formation of white spots or patches on the oral mucosa. (17)
**Liability** Accountable or legally responsible. (40)
**Licensure** License to practice in a specific state. (5)
**Lichen (LI-kun) planus** Benign, chronic disease that affects the skin and oral mucosa. (17)
**Ligature (LIG-uh-chur) tie** Light wire used to hold the arch wire in its bracket. (60)
**Light-cured** Type of material that is polymerized by a curing light. (59)
**Line angle** Junction of two walls in a cavity preparation. (11, 48)
**Linea alba** Normal variation noted on the buccal mucosa. (10)
**Lingual frenum** Thin fold of mucous membrane that extends from the floor of the mouth to the underside of the tongue. (10)
**Lingual surface** Surface of mandibular and maxillary teeth closest to the tongue; also called *palatal surface.* (11)
**Linguoversion** Position in which the maxillary incisors are behind the mandibular incisors. (11)
**Lining mucosa** Mucous membrane that covers the inside of the cheeks, vestibule, lips, soft palate, and underside of the tongue and acts as a cushion for underlying structures. (8)
**Liquid sterilant (STER-i-lunt)** Chemical used at room temperature used for items that are damaged by heat sterilization. (20)
**Litigation (li-ti-GAY-shun)** Act of initiating legal proceedings, as in a lawsuit. (26)
**Long axis of the tooth** Imaginary line dividing the tooth longitudinally (vertically) into two equal halves. (41)
**Low-level disinfectant** Disinfectant that destroys certain viruses and fungi; used for general housecleaning (e.g., walls, floors). (20)
**Lumen (LOO-men)** The hollow center of the injection needle. (37)
**Luting (LOO-ting) agent** Cement-type substance used to seal a surface. (45)
**Luxate (LUK-sayt)** To dislocate, as a tooth from its socket. (56)
**Luxation (luk-SAY-shun)** Dislocation. (57)
**Lymphadenopathy (lim-fad-uh-NOP-uh-thee)** Disease or swelling of the lymph nodes. (9, 17)

**Lymphoma (lim-FOE-muh)** Malignant disorder of the lymphoid tissue. (17)

**Magnification** Proportional enlargement of a radiographic image. (38)

**Malaligned (mal-uh-LINED)** Displaced out of line, especially teeth displaced from normal relation to the line of the dental arch; also called *malposed.* (36)

**Malleability (mal-ee-uh-BIL-uh-tee)** The ability of a material to withstand permanent deformation under compressive stress without sustaining permanent damage. (43)

**Mallet** Hammer-like instrument used with a chisel to section teeth or bone. (56)

**Malocclusion (MAL-o-kloo-zhun)** Occlusion that is deviated from a class I normal occlusion. (11)

**Malpractice** Professional negligence. (5, 40)

**Mamelon (MAM-uh-lon)** Rounded enamel extension on the incisal ridges of incisors. (12)

**Mandated reporters** Designated professionals who are required by law to report known or suspected child abuse. (5)

**Mandibular (man-DIB-yoo-lur) arch** The lower jaw. (8, 11)

**Mandrel (MAN-drul)** Metal shaft on which a sandpaper disc or other abrasive materials are mounted. (35)

**Marginal groove** Developmental groove that crosses a marginal ridge and serves as a spillway, allowing food to escape during mastication. (12)

**Marginal ridge** Rounded, raised border on the mesial and distal portions of the lingual surfaces of anterior teeth and the occlusal table of posterior teeth. (12)

**Marketing** A way of advertising or recruiting people to a business. (61)

**Masseter (muh-SEE-tur)** The strongest and most obvious muscle of mastication. (9)

**Master cast** Cast created from a final impression used to construct baseplate, bite rims, wax setups, and finished prostheses. (50)

**Master switch, indicator light, selector buttons, exposure button** Components of control panel. (38)

**Mastication (mas-ti-KAY-shun)** Chewing. (52)

**Masticatory (MAS-ti-kuh-tor-ee) mucosa** Oral mucosa that covers the hard palate, dorsum of the tongue, and gingiva. (8)

**Masticatory (MAS-ti-kuh-tor-ee) surface** Chewing surface of the teeth. (11)

**Mastoid process** Projection on the temporal bone located behind the ear. (9)

**Matrix (MAY-triks)** Foundation that binds a substance together; continuous phases (organic polymer) in which particles of filler are dispersed in composite resin. (43)

**Matter** Anything that occupies space and has form or shape. (38)

**Maxillary (MAK-si-lar-ee) arch** The upper jaw. (11)

**Maxillary tuberosity** Large, rounded area on the outer surface of the maxillary bones in the area of the posterior teeth. (9)

**Maximum horizontal reach** Reach created when the upper arm is fully extended. (25)

**Maximum vertical reach** Reach created by a vertical sweep of the forearm while the elbow is kept at midtorso level. (25)

**Meatus** External opening of a canal. (9)

**Medial** Toward or nearer to the midline of the body. (6)

**Medial pterygoid plate** Plate that ends in the hook-shaped hamulus. (9)

**Meiosis (mye-OE-sis)** Reproductive cell production that ensures the correct number of chromosomes. (8)

**Mental** Region of the head pertaining to or located near the chin. (9)

**Mental age** Measure of the level of intellectual capacity and development of pediatric patients. (57)

**Mental protuberance** Part of the mandible that forms the chin. (9, 10)

**Mesial surface** Surface of the tooth toward the midline. (11)

**Mesioclusion (MEE-zee-oe-kloo-zhun)** Term used for class III malocclusion. (11, 60)

**Mesiodistal division** Lengthwise division of the crown in a mesial-distal (front-to-back) direction, consisting of the *mesial* third, *middle* third, and *distal* third. (11)

**Metabolism (muh-TAB-uh-liz-um)** Physical and chemical processes that occur within a living cell or organism and are necessary for the maintenance of life. (27, 30)

**Metastasize (muh-TAS-tuh-size)** To spread (disease) from one part of the body to another. (17)

**Methamphetamine** Potent central nervous system stimulant. (17)

**Methicillin-resistant *Staphylococcus aureus*** Type of staph infection that is resistant to several common antibiotics. (18)

**Meth mouth** Informal name for the rampant tooth decay caused by heavy methamphetamine use. (17)

**Microabrasion (air abrasion)** Technique used to open fissures before sealant placement. (59)

**Microbiology** Study of microorganisms. (18)

**Microcephaly** Abnormal smallness of the head, a congenital condition associated with incomplete brain development. (18)

**Microfiltration** Use of membrane filters to trap microorganisms suspended in water. (24)

**Microleakage (mye-kroe-LEE-kuj)** Microscopic leakage at the interface of the tooth structure and the sealant or restoration. (43, 59)

**Micromechanical (mye-kroe-me-KAN-i-kul)** Means by which a material and a structure lock onto one another through minute cuttings. (44)

**Middle third** Division of the root in the middle. (11)

**Midsagittal plane** Imaginary line that divides the patient's face into equal right and left sides. (6, 42)

**Milliampere (mil-ee-AM-peer) (mA)** One one-thousandth (1/1000) of an ampere, a unit of measurement used to describe the intensity of an electrical current. (38)

**Misdemeanor** Offense that may result in imprisonment of 6 months to 1 year. (5)

**Mixed dentition** Mixture of permanent teeth and primary teeth that occurs until all primary teeth have been lost, usually between the ages of 6 and 12. (11)

**Mobility** To have movement. (28, 55)

**Model** Replica of the maxillary and mandibular arches made from an impression. (47)

**Modeling** Bone changes that involve deposition and resorption of bone and occur along articulations as they increase in size and shape to keep up with the growth of the surrounding tissues; also known as *displacement.* (8)

**Molars** Teeth located in the posterior aspect of the upper and lower jaws. (12)

**Monomer (MON-oe-mur)** Molecule that, when combined with other molecules, forms a polymer. (47)

**Morphologically (mor-fuh-LOJ-i-kul-lee), morphologic (mor-fuh-LOJ-ik), morphology (mor-FOL-uh-jee)** Branch of biology that deals with form and structure. (12, 28)

**Mucobuccal fold** Base of the vestibule where the buccal mucosa meets the alveolar mucosa. (10)

**Mucogingival junction** Distinct line of color change in the tissue where the alveolar membrane meets with attached gingivae. (10)

**Multiparameter indicators** Strips placed in packages that change color when exposed to a combination of heat, temperature, and time. Also known as *process integrators.* (21)

**Muscle insertion** Location where the muscle ends; the portion away from the body's midline. (7)

**Muscle origin** Location where the muscle begins; the portion toward the body's midline. (7)

**Muscle tissue** Tissue with the ability to lengthen or shorten to provide movement to body parts. (6)

**Musculoskeletal (mus-kyu-loh-SKEH-leh-tul) disorders (MSDs)** Painful conditions that affect both muscles and bones, such as neck or back pain and carpal tunnel syndrome. (25)

**Mutagenicity** Ability to cause a random change in a gene or chromosome resulting in a new trait or characteristic that can be inherited.

***Mutans streptococci* (strep-toe-KOK-sye)** Type of bacteria primarily responsible for caries. (13)

**Mylar (MYE-lahr)** Brand name for clear plastic strip used to provide a temporary wall for restoration of an anterior tooth. (49)

**Myocardial infarction (mye-oe-KAHR-dee-ul in-FAHRK-shun)** Condition in which damage occurs to the muscular tissue of the heart, commonly caused by obstructed circulation; also referred to as a *heart attack.* (29, 31)

**MyPlate** The U.S. government's primary food group symbol. (16)

**Nasal** Region of the head that pertains to or is located near the nose. (9)

**Nasal conchae (singular, *concha*)** Projecting structures found in each lateral wall of the nasal cavity and extending inward from the maxilla. (9)

**Nasion (NAY-ze-on)** Midpoint between the eyes just below the eyebrows. (10)

**Nasmyth's (NAS-miths) membrane** Residue from epithelial tissue on the crowns of newly erupted teeth that may become extrinsically stained. (11, 58)

**Nasolabial sulcus** Groove extending upward between the labial commissure and the nasal ala. (10)

**National Institute for Occupational Safety and Health (NIOSH)** Federal agency that is nonregulatory and provides national and worldwide leadership to prevent work-related illnesses and injuries. (22)

**National Institute of Dental and Craniofacial Research (NIDCR)** Federal agency whose mission is to improve oral, dental, and craniofacial health through research, research training, and dissemination of health information. (6, 22)

**National Institutes of Health (NIH)** One of the world's foremost research centers. (22)

**Naturally acquired immunity** Immunity that occurs when a person has contracted and is recovering from a disease. (19)

**Needle holder** Surgical instrument used to hold the suture needle. (56)

**Negligence** The failure to provide a proper or reasonable level of care. (40)

**Nerve tissue** Responsible for coordinating and controlling body activities. (6)

**Net income** Gross income minus expenses. (63)

**Neural (NUR-uhl)** Referring to the brain, nervous system, and nerve pathways. (57)

**Neurons** Direct nerve impulses. (7)

**Neutral position** Position in which the body is properly aligned and the distribution of weight throughout the spine is equal. (25)

**Neutroclusion** An ideal mesiodistal relationship between the jaws and the dental arches. (11)

**Nib** Blunt point or tip. (34)

**Noncritical instrument** Item that comes into contact with intact skin only. (21)

**Nonmaleficence** To do no harm to the patient. (4)

**Nonpathogenic (non-path-oe-JEN-ik)** Pertaining to microorganisms that do *not* produce disease. (18)

**Nonsuccedaneous (non-suk-se-DAY-nee-us)** Pertaining to a permanent tooth that does not replace a primary tooth. (12)

**Nonverbal communication** Type of communication in which body language is used as a form of expression. (61)

**Nonvital** Not living, as in oral tissue and tooth structure. (54)

**Normal horizontal reach** Reach created by a sweep of the forearm with the upper arm held at the side. (25)

**Nucleus (NOO-klee-us)** "Control center" of the cell. (6)

**Nutrients (NOO-tree-ents)** Organic and inorganic chemicals in food that supply energy. (16)

**Obliterating (oe-BLIT-uh-rayt-ing)** Removing something completely. (44)

**Obturation (ob-tuh-RAY-shun)** Process of filling a root canal. (54)

**Occipital (ok-SIP-i-tul)** Region of the head overlying the occipital bone and covered by the scalp. (9)

**Occlusal (o-KLOO-sul; o-KLOO-zul)** Radiographic view that shows large areas of the maxilla or mandible. (39)

**Occlusal registration** Reproduction of a patient's bite with the use of wax or elastomeric material. (46)

**Occlusal rim** Rim built on the baseplate to register vertical dimension and occlusal relationships of the mandibular and maxillary arches. (52)

**Occlusal surface** Chewing surface of posterior teeth. (11)

**Occlusal technique** Used to examine large areas of the upper or lower jaw. (41)

**Occlusal trauma** Abnormal occlusal relationships of the teeth, causing injury to the periodontium. (55)

**Occlusion (o-KLOO-zhun)** Natural contact of the maxillary and mandibular teeth in all positions. (11)

**Occlusocervical division** Crosswise division of the crown that is parallel to the occlusal or incisal surface, consisting of the *occlusal* third, *middle* third, and *cervical* third. (11)

**Occupational exposure** Any reasonably anticipated skin, eye, or mucous membrane contact or percutaneous injury involving blood or any other potentially infectious materials. (19)

**Occupational Safety and Health Administration (OSHA)** Federal regulatory agency whose mission is to ensure the safety and health of America's workers by setting and enforcing standards. (22)

**Odontoblasts (o-DON-to-blasts)** Cells that form dentin. (8)

**Odontogenesis (o-don-to-JEN-eh-sis)** Formation of new teeth. (8)

**Onlay (ON-lay)** Cast restoration designed to replace a class II cavity that includes the occlusal, one or more cusp, and proximal surfaces of posterior teeth. (50)

**Opaquer (oe-PAY-kur)** Resin material placed under a porcelain restoration to mask tooth discoloration. (50)

**Open bay** Concept of open design used in pediatric dental practices. (57)

**Open bite** Lack of vertical overlap of the maxillary incisors, creating an opening of the anterior teeth. (60)

**Operating zones** Concept by which the face of a clock is used to position the dental team, equipment, and supplies. (33)

**Operative dentistry** Term commonly used to describe restorative and esthetic dentistry. (48)

**Oral** Region of the head pertaining to or located near the mouth. (9)

**Oral and maxillofacial (MAK-sil-oe-fay-shul) radiology (ray-dee-OL-o-jee)** Dental specialty that deals with the diagnosis of disease through various forms of imaging, including x-ray films (radiographs). (3)

**Oral and maxillofacial surgeon (OMFS)** Dentist who has specialized in surgeries of the head and neck region. (56)

**Oral and maxillofacial surgery** Dental surgical specialty that diagnoses and treats conditions of the mouth, face, upper jaw (maxilla), and associated areas. (3, 56)

**Oral Biofilm** Also called plaque, a highly organized complex of microorganisms that adheres to surfaces where moisture and nutrients are available. (13, 14)

**Oral candidiasis (kan-di-DYE-uh-sis)** *Candida* yeast infection of the oral mucosa. (18)

**Oral cavity proper** Space on the tongue side within the upper and lower dental arches. (10)

**Oral pathology (puh-THOL-uh-jee)** Dental specialty that diagnoses and treats diseases of the oral structures. (3)

**Oral prophylaxis (proe-fi-LAK-sis)** Complete removal of calculus, debris, stain, and plaque from the teeth. (58)

**Orban knife** Knife with a spearlike shape and cutting edges on both sides of the blade; it is used to remove tissue from the *interdental* areas. (55)

**Orbital** Region of the head pertaining to or located around the eye. (9)

**Organelle (or-guh-NEL)** Specialized part of a cell that performs a specific function. (6)

**Organic (or-GAN-ik)** Describes food products that have been grown without the use of chemical pesticides, herbicides, or fertilizers. (16)

**Organization for Safety and Asepsis Procedures (OSAP)** The premier infection control educational organization in dentistry. (22)

**Orthodontics (or-thoe-DON-tiks)** Specialty within dentistry that focuses on preventing, intercepting, and correcting skeletal and dental problems. (3, 60)

**OSHA Blood-Borne Pathogens Standard** Guidelines designed to protect employees against occupational exposure to blood-borne pathogens. (19)

**Osseointegration (os-ee-oe-in-te-GRAY-shun)** The process of introducing certain metals, such as titanium, into living bone and forming a biocompatible bond with living bone. (53)

**Osseous (OS-ee-us) surgery** Surgical specialty of removing defects in bone. (55)

**Ossicles** Bones of the middle ear. (9)

**Ostectomy (os-TEK-tuh-mee)** Surgery involving the removal of bone. (55)

**Osteoblasts (OS-tee-oe-blasts)** Cells that form bone. (7, 8)

**Osteoclasts (OS-tee-oe-klasts)** Cells that resorb bone. (8)

**Osteoplasty (OS-tee-oe-plas-tee)** Surgery in which bone is added, contoured, and reshaped. (55)

**Outguide** Device used for a filing system; similar to a bookmark. (62)

**Outline form** Design and initial depth of sound tooth structure used by the dentist when restoring a tooth. (48)

**Outpatient** Patient seen and treated by a physician, then sent home for recovery. (56)

**Overbite** Increased vertical overlap of the maxillary incisors. (60)

**Overdenture** Full denture supported by two or more remaining natural teeth. (52)

**Overhang** Excess restorative material that extends beyond the cavity margin. (49)

**Overjet** Excessive protrusion of the maxillary incisors. (60)

**Oxidizers** To react or cause a chemical to react with oxygen. (23)

**Oximetry (ok-SIM-uh-tree)** Measurement of oxygen concentration in the blood. (27, 37)

**Packing slip** Itemized listing of shipped goods. (63)

**Palatal surface** Lingual surface of maxillary teeth. (11)

**Palladium (puh-LAY-dee-um)** Soft, steel-white, tarnish-resistant metal that occurs naturally with platinum. (43)

**Palodent (PAL-uh-dent)** Small, oval-shaped matrix made of stainless steel used interproximally during tooth restoration. (49)

**Palpate (PAL-payt)** To examine or explore by touching. (27)

**Palpation (pal-PAY-shun)** Touching or feeling for abnormalities within soft tissue. (28, 54)

**Pandemic (pan-DEM-ik)** Condition that occurs throughout the people of a country or the world. (18)

**Panoramic film** Provides a wide view of the upper and lower jaws. (39)

**Papoose (pa-POOS) board** Type of restraining device that holds a pediatric patient's hands, arms, and legs still. (57)

**Parallel** Moving or lying in the same plane, always separated by the same distance. (41)

**Paralleling technique** Intraoral technique of exposing periapical and bitewing radiographs. (41)

**Parietal (puh-RYE-e-tul)** Pertaining to the walls of a body cavity. (6, 9)

**Parotid (puh-ROT-id) duct** Duct associated with the parotid salivary gland, which opens into the oral cavity at the parotid papilla. (9)

**Parotid papilla** Small elevation of tissue located on the inner surface of the cheek. (10)

**Partial denture** Removable prosthesis that replaces teeth within the same arch. (52)

**Patent medicine** Drug that can be obtained without a prescription; also called *over-the-counter drug.* (30)

**Pathogens (PATH-uh-jens)** Disease-producing microorganisms. (18, 19)

**Pathology (pa-THOL-uh-jee)** Study of disease. (17)

**Patient of record** Individual who has been examined and diagnosed by the dentist and has had treatment planned. (5, 62)

**Payee** Person (or business) named on the check as the recipient of the amount shown. (63)

**Pediatric (pee-dee-AT-rik) dentistry** Dental specialty concerned with neonatal through adolescent patients, as well as patients with special needs in these age groups. (3, 57)

**Pegboard system** Manual bookkeeping system. (63)

**Pegged laterals** Incisors with a pointed or tapered shape. (12)

**Pellicle (PEL-i-kul)** Thin film coating of salivary materials deposited on tooth surfaces. (13)

**Pelvic cavity** Contains portions of the large and small intestines, the rectum, the urinary bladder, and reproductive organs. (6)

**Penumbra (puh-NUM-bruh)** Blurred or indistinct area that surrounds an image. (38)

**Percolation (PER-ko-LAY-shun)** The process of a liquid substance passing through a porous substance. (43)

**Percussion (pur-KUH-shun)** Examination technique that involves tapping on the incisal or occlusal surface of a tooth to assess vitality. (54)

**Percutaneous (pur-kyoo-TAY-nee-us)** Through the skin, such as a needle stick, a cut, or a human bite. (18, 19)

**Perforation (pur-fuh-RAY-shun)** Making a hole, as in breaking through and extending beyond the apex of the root. (54)

**Periapical (per-ee-AP-i-kul)** Radiographic view that shows the crown, root tip, and surrounding structures. (39)

**Pericardium (per-ee-KAHR-dee-um)** Double-walled sac that encloses the heart. (7)

**Peri-implant tissue** Gingival sulcus surrounding the implant.

**Periodontal (per-ee-oe-DON-tul)** Referring to the periodontium. (14)

**Periodontal abscess** An inflammatory reaction to bacteria trapped in the periodontal sulcus. (54)

**Periodontal charting** Commonly accepted notations that are made to the patient's chart to indicate the condition, position, and restorative history of individual teeth. (55)

**Periodontal disease** Infections and other conditions of structures that support the teeth (gums and bone). (1)

**Periodontal dressing (periopack)** Surgical dressing applied to a surgical site for protection, similar to a bandage. (55)

**Periodontal explorer** Fine, thin instrument that is easily adapted around root surfaces and is used to locate deposits of calculus. (55)

**Periodontal flap surgery (flap surgery)** Incisional surgery performed when excisional surgery is not indicated. In flap surgery, the tissues *are not removed* but are pushed away from the underlying tooth roots and alveolar bone, similar to the flap of an envelope. (55)

**Periodontal plastic surgery** Surgical procedures of mucogingival tissues. (55)

**Periodontal pocket** Deepening of the gingival sulcus beyond normal; results from periodontal disease. (55)

**Periodontal probe** Probe used to locate and measure the depth of periodontal pockets; tapered to fit into the gingival sulcus with a blunt or rounded tip. (55)

**Periodontics (per-ee-oe-DON-tiks)** Dental specialty involved with the diagnosis and treatment of diseases of the supporting tissues. (3, 55)

**Periodontist (per-ee-oe-DON-tist)** Dentist with advanced education in the specialty of periodontics. (55)

**Periodontitis (per-ee-oe-don-TYE-tis)** Inflammatory disease of the supporting tissues of the teeth. (14)

**Periodontium (per-ee-oe-DON-shee-um)** Structures that surround, support, and are attached to the teeth. (8, 14)

**Perioscopy (per-ee-OS-kuh-pee)** Procedure in which a dental endoscope is used subgingivally. (14)

**Periosteum (per-ee-OS-tee-um)** Specialized connective tissue that covers all bones of the body. (7)

**Periotome** Instrument used to cut periodontal ligaments for atraumatic tooth extraction. (55)

**Peripheral nervous system (PNS)** Cranial nerves and spinal nerves. (7)

**Periradicular (per-ee-ruh-DIK-yoo-lur)** Referring to the area of nerves, blood vessels, and tissues that surround the root of a tooth. (54)

**Periradicular abscess** Inflammatory reaction to pulpal infection. (54)

**Periradicular (per-ee-ruh-DIK-yoo-lur) cyst** A cyst that develops at or near the root of a necrotic tooth. (54)

**Peristalsis (per-i-STAHL-sis)** Rhythmic action that moves food through the digestive tract. (7)

**Permanent dentition** The set of 32 secondary teeth. (11)

**Permeate (PUR-mee-ayt)** To spread or flow throughout. (37)

**Permucosal (per-myoo-KOE-sul)** Contact with mucous membranes, such as the eyes or mouth. (19)

**Perpendicular** Intersecting at or forming a right angle. (41)

**Personal protective equipment (PPE)** Items such as protective clothing, masks, gloves, and eyewear used to protect employees. (19)

**Personal radiation monitoring badge** A device that measures exposure of personnel to ionizing radiation by measuring the intensity of visible light emitted from a crystal in the detector when heated. The intensity of light emitted is dependent upon the radiation exposure. (38)

**Pestle (PES-ul, PES-tul)** Object that is moved vertically to pound or pulverize a material. (43)

**Petechiae (pe-TEE-kee-uh)** Small, pinpoint red spot on the skin or mucous membrane. (17)

**Petri plate** Small, flat dish made of thin glass or plastic that contains sterile solid medium for the culture of microorganisms; also called *petri dish.* (18)

**Petty cash fund** Limited amount of cash that is kept on hand for small daily expenses. (63)

**Pharmacology** Branch of medicine concerned with the uses, effects, and actions of drugs. (30)

**Philtrum (FIL-trum)** Rectangular area from under the nose to the midline of the upper lip. (10)

**Phosphor storage plates (PSP)** Reusable film-sized plates coated with phosphor as the image receptor. (39, 40)

**Photon (FOE-ton)** A minute (tiny) bundle of pure energy that has no weight or mass. (38)

**Physical disability** Impairment in certain function(s) of the body, such as vision, hearing, or mobility. (41)

**Physical hazard** A chemical that is a combustible liquid, a compressed gas, or an explosive material or is flammable-reactive or water-reactive. (23)

**Physiology (fiz-ee-OL-uh-jee)** Study of the functions of the human body. (6)

**Pictograms** Graphic elements used on a hazard label, used to identify the specific hazard class and category. (23)

**Plane** Flat or level surface of the working end of an instrument. (34)

**Planes** Three imaginary lines used to divide the body into sections. (6)

**Planktonic (plank-TON-ik)** Describes bacteria that are freely floating in water. (24)

**Plaque (plak)** Soft deposit on teeth that consists of bacteria and bacterial by-products. (13, 14)

**Plasma** Straw-colored fluid that transports nutrients, hormones, and waste products. (7)

**Platinum (PLAT-i-num)** Silver-white noble metal that does not corrode in air. (43)

**Point** Sharp or tapered end. (34)

**Point angle** Angle formed by the junction of three surfaces. (11)

**Polycarbonate (pol-ee-KAHR-buh-nayt) crown** Provisional crown made from a hard plastic tooth-colored material used for anterior teeth. (51)

**Polymer (POL-i-mur)** Compound of many molecules. (47)

**Polymer crown** Provisional coverage designed in a shell-like form. (51)

**Polymerization (pah-LIM-ur-i-zay-shun)** Process of changing a simple chemical into another substance that contains the same elements. (59)

**Polymerize (pah-LIM-uh-rize)** To subject a material to the bonding process of two or more monomers. (44)

**Pontic (PON-tik)** Artificial tooth that replaces a missing natural tooth. (15, 50)

**Porcelain (POR-se-lun)** Hard, white, translucent ceramic material fabricated by firing and then glazing to match the tooth color. (43)

**Porcelain-fused-to-metal (PFM) crown** Indirect restoration in which a thin porcelain material is fused to the facial portion of a gold crown. (50)

**Porous (POR-us)** An object with minute openings that allow the passage of gas or fluid. (37)

**Positioner** Appliance used to retain teeth in their desired position. (60)

**Positioning device/positioning instrument** Intraoral device used to position and hold the film, sensor, or PSP. (39, 40, 41)

**Post dam** Seal in back of a full denture that holds it in place; also called *posterior palatal seal.* (52)

**Posted** Describes the documentation of money transactions within a business. (63)
**Posterior** Toward the back. (6, 11)
**Posterior faucial pillar** Posterior arch of the soft palate. (10)
**Postnatal (post-NAY-tul)** After birth. (57)
**Precautionary statement** A phrase that describes recommended measures to be taken to minimize or prevent adverse effects resulting from exposure to a hazardous chemical, or improper storage or handling of a hazardous chemical. (23)
**Preceptorship (PREE-sep-tor-ship)** Study under the guidance of a dentist or other professional. (1)
**Precleaning** Removal of bioburden before disinfection. (20)
**Preformed** Referring to provisional coverage that is already shaped as needed. (51)
**Preimplantation period** Stage of development that occurs during the first week after fertilization. (8)
**Prenatal (pree-NAY-tul)** Before birth. (57)
**Prenatal development** Stage of human development that starts at pregnancy and ends at birth. (8)
**Prescription** Written order for a specific drug. (30)
**Pressure points** Specific areas in the mouth where a removable prosthesis may rub or apply more pressure. (52)
**Preventive dentistry** Program of patient education, use of fluorides, application of dental sealants, proper nutrition, and plaque control. (15)
**Primary beam** The most penetrating beam produced at the target of the anode. (38)
**Primary cementum** Cementum that covers the root of the tooth and is formed outward from the cementodentinal junction for the full length of the root. (8)
**Primary dentin** Dentin that forms before eruption and that makes up the bulk of the tooth. (8)
**Primary dentition** The first set of 20 primary teeth. (11)
**Primary palate** Shelf that separates the oral and nasal cavities. (8)
**Primary radiation** Same as *primary beam.* (38)
**Prions (PRYE-ons)** Infectious particles of proteins that lack nucleic acids. (18)
**Prism** Calcified column or rod. (8)
**Probing** Use of a slender, flexible instrument to explore and measure the periodontal pocket. (28)
**Process** Prominence or projection on a bone. (9)
**Process indicators** Tapes, strips, or tabs with heat-sensitive chemicals that change color when exposed to a certain temperature. (21)
**Process integrators** Strips placed in packages that change color when exposed to a combination of heat, temperature, and time. (21)
**Processing** Series of steps that change exposed film into a radiograph. The steps include developing, rinsing, fixing, washing, and drying. (39)
**Product identifier** The name or number used for a hazardous chemical on a label or in the SDS. (23)
**Professional** Person who meets the standards of a profession. (2, 64)
**Prophy paste** Commercial premixed abrasive paste used for polishing teeth and restorations. (58)
**Prophylaxis (pro-fah-LAK-sus)** Administration of drugs to prevent disease or protect a patient. (30)
**Prosthesis (pros-THEE-sis)** Fabricated replacement for a missing tooth. (50)
**Prosthodontics (pros-thoe-DON-tiks)** Dental specialty that provides restoration and replacement of natural teeth. (3)
**Protozoa (proe-toe-ZOE-uh)** Single-celled microscopic animals without a rigid cell wall. (18)
**Protrusion (proe-TROO-zhun)** Position of the mandible placed forward as related to the maxilla. (52)
**Provider** The dentist who provides treatment to the patient. (63)
**Provirus** Virus that is hidden during the latency period. (18)
**Provisional** Referring to temporary coverage made for crown or bridge preparations and worn during cast preparation. (45, 51)
**Proximal** Closer to the trunk of the body; opposite of *distal.* (6)
**Proximal surfaces** The surfaces next to each other when teeth are adjacent in the arch. (11)
**Pterygoid process** Process of the sphenoid bone, consisting of two plates. (9)
**Public Health Agency of Canada** The main federal agency responsible for public health in Canada. (22)
**Pulp chamber** The space occupied by pulp. (8)
**Pulpal (PUL-pul) wall** Surface of the cavity preparation perpendicular to the pulp of a tooth. (48)
**Pulpectomy (pul-PEK-tuh-mee)** Complete removal of vital pulp from a tooth. (54)
**Pulpitis (pul-PYE-tis)** Inflammation of the dental pulp. (54)
**Pulpotomy (pul-POT-uh-mee)** Removal of the coronal portion of a vital pulp from a tooth. (54, 57)
**Pulse** Rhythmic throbbing of the arteries produced by regular contractions of the heart. (27)
**Purchase order** Form that authorizes the purchase of products from a supplier. (62)
**Quadrant** One quarter of the dentition. (11)
**Quality (of x-ray beam)** The mean energy or penetrating ability of the x-ray beam. (38)
**Quality assurance** Program in place for monitoring and evaluating a project, service, or facility to ensure that standards of quality are being met. (26) A plan to ensure that the dental office produces consistent, high-quality images with a minimum of exposure to patients and personnel. (40)
**Quality control tests** Specific tests used to ensure quality in dental x-ray equipment, supplies, and film processing. (40)
**Quantity (of x-ray beam)** The number of x-rays produced in the dental unit; the quantity of x-rays produced is controlled by milliamperage. (38)
**Radial** Related to the radius *(bone)* or forearm *(antebrachium),* as in *radial artery.* (27)
**Radiation** Forms of waves of energy emission through space or material. (38)
**Radicular pulp** The other portion of pulp known as *root pulp.* (8)
**Radiograph (RAY-dee-oe-graf)** Image produced on photosensitive film by exposing the film to radiation and then processing it. (38, 39)
**Radiology (ray-dee-OL-uh-jee)** The science or study of radiation as used in medicine. (38)
**Rampant (RAM-punt) caries** Decay that develops rapidly and is widespread throughout the mouth. (13)
**Rate** A quantity measured, as in breaths and heartbeats. (27)
**Rate of use** The quantity of a product that is used within a given time. (62)
**Reasonable fee** Fee that is considered justified for an extensive or complex treatment. (63)
**Rebasing (ree-BAY-sing)** Procedure to replace the entire denture base material on an existing prosthesis. (52)
**Recession** Process of withdrawal or wearing away from its normal location.
**Reciprocity (re-si-PROS-i-tee)** System that allows individuals in one state to obtain a license in another state without retesting. (5)
**Red blood cells** Cells that contain the blood protein *hemoglobin,* which plays an essential role in oxygen transport; also known as *erythrocytes.* (7)

**Regenerative medicine** Process of creating living, functional tissues to repair or replace tissue or organ function through the use of stem cells. (6)

**Registration** Act of completing forms by providing personal information. (26)

**Regulated waste** Infectious waste that requires special handling, neutralization, and disposal. (23)

**Relining (ree-LYE-ning)** Procedure to resurface the tissue side of a partial or full denture so that it fits more accurately. (52)

**Remineralization** Replacement of minerals in the tooth. (13)

**Remodeling** Growth and change in shape of existing bone that involves deposition and resorption of bone. (8)

**Reorder tags** Notation system that is used when the supply of a particular item is getting low and the item must be reordered. (62)

**Requisition (re-kwi-ZI-shun)** Formal request for supplies. (62)

***Res gestae*** Latin for "things done." Statements made by a person present at the time of an alleged negligent act that are admissible as evidence in a court of law. (5)

***Res ipsa loquitur*** Latin phrase for "the thing speaks for itself." (5)

**Residual activity** Action that continues long after initial application, as with disinfectants. (20)

**Resin-bonded bridge** Fixed dental prosthesis with wings that are bonded to the lingual surfaces of adjacent teeth; also known as *Maryland bridge.* (50)

**Resistance (ree-ZIS-tuns) form** Shape and placement of cavity walls in the preparation of tooth restoration. (48)

**Resorption (ree-SORP-shun)** The body's processes of eliminating existing bone or hard tissue structure. (8, 52)

**Respiration** Act or process of inhaling and exhaling; breathing. (27)

***Respondeat superior*** Latin for "Let the master answer." Legal doctrine that holds an employer liable for acts of the employee. (5)

**Responsible party** Person who has agreed to pay for services or for an account. (63)

**Rest** Metal projection on or near the retainer of a partial denture. (52)

**Restoration** The use of dental material to restore a tooth or teeth to a functional permanent unit. (28, 48)

**Restorative (re-STOR-uh-tiv)** To restore or bring back to its natural appearance. (43)

**Restorative dentistry** Type of dentistry that restores teeth by removing decay and restoring defects. (48)

**Résumé** A brief description of one's professional or work experience and qualifications. (64)

**Retainer (ree-TAY-nur)** Device used to hold attachments and abutments of a removable prosthesis in place. (52) An appliance used for maintaining the positions of the teeth and jaws after orthodontic treatment (60).

**Retard (ree-TAHRD)** To slow down a process. (45)

**Retention (ree-TEN-shun)** The act of holding something by means of an adhesive, or mechanical locking, or both. (43)

**Retention form** Shaping of the cavity walls to aid in retaining the restoration. (48)

**Retention (retentive) pin** Basis of a stronger system used to retain and support a tooth restoration. (48)

**Retractor (ree-TRAK-tur)** Surgical instrument used to hold soft tissue away from the surgical site. (56)

**Retrograde restoration (RET-roe-grayd res-tuh-RAY-shun)** Small restoration placed at the apex of a root. (54)

**Retrusion (ree-TROO-zhun)** Position of the mandible posterior from the centric position as related to the maxilla. (52)

**Reuse life** Time period that a disinfectant should remain effective during use and reuse. (20)

**Reversible pulpitis** Form of pulpal inflammation in which the pulp may be salvageable. (54)

**Rheostat (REE-uh-stat)** Foot-controlled device used to operate dental handpieces. (32)

**Rheumatoid arthritis** A disease that causes pain, stiffness, swelling, and loss of function in the joints. (29)

**Rhythm** A sequence or pattern, such as the heartbeat or breathing. (27)

**Right angle** Angle of 90 degrees formed by two lines perpendicular to each other. (41)

**Risk management** Policies and procedures that will reduce the chance that a malpractice lawsuit will be brought against the dentist. Key areas of risk management include *patient informed consent, patient records, confidentiality, liability issues*, and *patient education.* (40)

**Rongeur (raw-ZHUR, RON-gore)** Surgical instrument used to cut and trim the alveolar bone. (56)

**Root** Facial landmark commonly called the "bridge" of the nose. (10)

**Root amputation (am-pyoo-TAY-shun)** Removal of one or more roots without removal of the crown of the tooth. (54)

**Root canal therapy** Removal of the dental pulp and filling of the canal with material. (54)

**Root caries** Decay on the root surface of teeth that have gingival recession. (13)

**Root planning** Procedure that smooths the surface of a root by removing abnormal toxic cementum or dentin that is rough, contaminated, or permeated with calculus. (55)

**Root tip picks** Surgical instrument used for the removal of root tips or fragments from the surgical site. (56)

**Rotary (ROE-tuh-ree)** Part or device that rotates around an axis. (35)

**Rubber cup polishing** Technique that is used to remove plaque and stains from the coronal surfaces of the teeth. (58)

**Safety Data Sheet (formerly known as Material Safety Data Sheet)** Form that provides printed information regarding the hazards of materials that contain chemicals. (23)

**Sagittal (SADJ-ih-tal) plane** Any vertical plane parallel to the midline that divides the body into unequal left and right portions. (6)

**Sagittal suture** Suture that is located at the midline of the skull, where the two parietal bones are joined. (9)

**Saint Apollonia** Recognized as the Patroness of Dentistry. (1)

**Saliva flow rate test** Determines flow rate of saliva in milliliters per minute. (13)

**Salutation (sal-yoo-TAY-shun)** Part of the letter that contains the introductory greeting. (61)

**Sarcoma (sahr-KOE-muh)** Malignant tumor in connective tissue such as muscle or bone. (17)

**Scaling** Removal of calcareous deposits from the teeth with the use of suitable instruments. (55)

**Scalpel (SKAL-pul)** Surgical knife. (56)

**Scatter radiation** Form of secondary radiation that occurs when an x-ray beam has been deflected from its path by interaction with matter. (38)

**Sealant retention** Sealant firmly adhering to the tooth surface. (59)

**Sebaceous glands** Oil glands that keep the hair and skin soft and are associated with sex hormones. (7)

**Secondary cementum** Cementum that is formed on the apical half of the root; also known as *cellular cementum.* (8)

**Secondary dentin** Dentin that forms after eruption and continues at a very slow rate throughout the life of the tooth. (8)

**Secondary palate** The final palate formed during embryonic development. (8)

**Secondary radiation** X-radiation that is created when the primary beam interacts with matter. (38)
**Sedative (SED-uh-tiv)** Having a soothing effect. (44)
**Seizure** Sudden attack, spasm, or convulsion that occurs in specific disorders. (29)
**Self-contained water reservoir** Container attached to a dental unit that is used to hold and supply water or other solutions to handpieces and air-water syringes. (24)
**Self-cured** Type of material that is polymerized by chemical reactions. (59)
**Semicritical instrument** Item that comes in contact with oral tissues but does not penetrate soft tissue or bone. (21)
**Sensor** Solid-state image receptor that contains a silicon chip with an electric circuit. (38)
**Separator** Device made from wire or elastic and used to separate molars before fitting and placement of orthodontic bands. (60)
**Septum (SEP-tum)** Dental dam material located between the holes of the punched dam. (36) Tissue that divides the nasal cavity into two nasal fossae. (10)
**Serrated (suh-RAY-ted)** Having notchlike projections that extend from a flat surface. (34)
**Sextant** One sixth of the dentition. (11)
**Shade guide** Accessory dental item that contains different shades of teeth and is used to match the color of a patient's teeth for the laboratory technician. (50)
**Shank** Part of an instrument where the handle attaches to the working end. (34, 35)
**Sharpey's fibers** Tissues that anchor the periosteum to the bone. (7)
**Sharpness** A measure of how well the radiograph reproduces the fine details or outlines of an object. (38)
**Sharps** Pointed or cutting instruments, including needles, scalpel blades, orthodontic wires, and endodontic instruments. (19)
**Shelf life** How long a product may be stored before use. (20, 62)
**Shoulder** Margins of a tooth preparation for a cast restoration. (50)
**Sickle scaler** Hook-shaped instrument that is available in various sizes and shapes and is used for the removal of tenacious supragingival deposits of calculus. (55)
**Signal word** Two words used on the Safety Data Sheet: "Warning" for less severe hazard categories, and "Danger" for more severe hazard categories. (23)
**Signature** Instructions on a prescription explaining how to take a specific medicine. (30)
**Silver amalgam (uh-MAL-gum) paste** Mixture of mercury, silver, and tin. (1)
**Single-parameter indicators** Tapes, strips, or tabs with heat-sensitive chemicals that change color when exposed to a particular temperature. Also known as *process indicator.* (21)
**Single-use items** Items that are used on only one patient and then are thrown away. (20)
**Slurry (SLUR-ee)** Mixture of gypsum and water used in the finishing of models. (47)
**Smear layer** Very thin layer of debris on newly prepared dentin. (44)
**Socialization** Process through which society influences individuals. (61)
**Sodium hypochlorite (hye-poe-KLOR-ite)** Surface disinfectant commonly known as *household bleach.* (20)
**Soft tissue impaction** Oral condition in which a tooth is partially to fully covered by gingival tissue. (56)
**Somatic (soe-MAT-ik) effects** Effects of radiation that cause illness and are responsible for poor health (such as cancer, leukemia, and cataracts) but are not passed on to offspring. (38)
**Spasticity (spas-TIS-i-tee)** Exaggerated movement of the arms and legs. (57)
**Spatulate (SPACH-uh-layt)** To mix using a spatula-type instrument. (45)
**Specialized mucosa** Mucous membrane on the tongue in the form of lingual papillae, which are structures associated with sensations of taste. (8)
**Sphenoid sinuses** Sinuses that are located in the sphenoid bone. (9)
**Spherical (SFER-i-kul)** Round. (43)
**Sphygmomanometer (sfig-moe-muh-NOM-e-tur)** Instrument for measuring blood pressure in the arteries. (27)
**Spinal cavity** Space in the body that contains the spinal cord. (6)
**Spirochetes** Spiral-shaped bacteria. (18)
**Splash, spatter, and droplet surface** Surface that does not contact members of the dental team or contaminated instruments or supplies. (20)
**Sporicidal** Capable of killing bacterial spores. (20)
**Spousal abuse** Domestic violence intentionally inflicted by a family member or members. (5)
**Sprains** Injuries caused by sudden twisting or wrenching of a joint with stretching or tearing of ligaments. (25)
**Stainless steel crown** Thin crown made from a medium-hard material for good durability. (51)
**Standard of care** Level of knowledge, skill, and care comparable with that of other dentists who are treating similar patients under similar conditions. (5, 40)
**Standard Precautions** Standard of care designed to protect healthcare providers from pathogens that can be spread by blood or any other body fluid via excretion or secretion; expands on the concept of Universal Precautions. (19)
**Staphylococci** Cocci that form irregular groups or clusters. (18)
**State Dental Practice Act** Document of law that specifies legal requirements for practicing dentistry in a particular state. (5)
**Statement** A summary of all charges, payments, credits, and debits for the month. (63)
**Statutory law** Law enacted by legislation through U.S. Congress, state legislature, or local legislative bodies. (5)
**Stem cell** Immature, unspecialized cells capable of replication and differentiation into other types of cells or tissues. (6)
**Stent** Clear acrylic template positioned over the alveolar ridge to guide in the proper angulation and axis for drilling into the bone and placing the implant. (53)
**Stepwedge** Device constructed of layered aluminum steps to demonstrate film densities and contrasts. (40)
**Sterilant (STER-i-lunt)** Agent that kills all microorganisms. (20)
**Sterilization (ster-i-li-ZAY-shun)** Process that kills all microorganisms. (20)
**Sternocleidomastoid (stur-noe-klye-doe-MAS-toid)** Major cervical muscle. (9)
**Stethoscope** Instrument used for listening to sounds produced within the body. (27)
**Stomodeum** The primitive mouth. (8)
**Storage phosphor imaging** Technique in which a digital image is captured on phosphor-coated plates and then is placed into an electronic processor, where a laser scans the plate and produces an image on a computer screen.
**Strain** Distortion or change produced as a result of stress. (43)

**Strains** Injuries caused by extreme stretching of muscles of ligaments. (25)
**Stratified squamous (SKWA-mus) epithelium** Layers of flat formed epithelium. (8)
**Streptococci** Cocci that form chains as they divide. (18)
**Stress** Internal reaction or resistance to an externally applied force. (43)
**Striae of Retzius** Incremental rings that represent variations in deposition of the enamel matrix during tooth formation. (8)
**Stroke** Sudden loss of brain function caused by blockage or rupture of a blood vessel to the brain; also called *cerebrovascular accident.* (29)
**Styloid process** Process that extends from the undersurface of the temporal bone. (9)
**Stylus (STYE-lus)** Sharp, pointed tool used for cutting. (36)
**Subgingival (sub-JIN-ji-vul)** Referring to the area below the gingiva. (14)
**Subperiosteal (sub-per-ee-OS-tee-ul)** Type of implant that includes a metal frame, which is surgically placed under the periosteum. (53)
**Subscription** Directions to the pharmacist for mixing the medication; this is seldom done by the pharmacist anymore. (30)
**Subsupine (sub-SOO-pine) position** Lying-down position in which the patient's head is lower than the feet (below the heart); used in emergency situations. (32)
**Succedaneous (suk-se-DAY-ne-us) teeth** Permanent teeth that replace primary teeth. (8, 11, 12)
**Sudoriferous (soo-doe-RIF-ur-us) glands** Sweat glands that are widely distributed over the body and provide heat regulation. (7)
**Superficial** On or near the surface.
**Superior** Above another portion, or closer to the head. (6)
**Superscription** The patient's name, address, date, and Rx symbol on a prescription. (30)
**Supine (SOO-pine) position** Lying-down position in which the patient's head, chest, and knees are at the same level. (32)
**Supragingival (soo-pruh-JIN-ji-vul)** Referring to the area above the gingiva. (14)
**Surface barrier** Fluid-resistant material used to cover surfaces likely to become contaminated. (20)
**Symmetric (si-MET-rik)** Balanced or even on both sides. (28)
**Symphysis menti (SIM-fi-sis MEN-tee)** Separation of the mandible at the chin that occurs at birth. (9)
**Syncope (SING-kuh-pee)** Loss of consciousness caused by insufficient blood to the brain. (31)
**Syneresis (si-ner-E-sus)** Loss of water, causing something to shrink. (46)
**Synthetic phenol (sin-THEH-tik FEE-nol) compound** EPA-registered intermediate-level hospital disinfectant with broad-spectrum disinfecting action. (20)
**Systemic (sis-TEM-ik)** Referring to a drug that affects a specific system (or multiple systems) of the body. (30)
**Systemic fluoride** Fluoride that is ingested and then circulated throughout the body. (15)
**Systemic toxicity (sis-TEM-ik tok-SIS-i-tee)** A harmful reaction to a drug that affects one or more of the body systems. (37)
**Systolic (sis-TOL-ik)** Rhythmic contraction of the heart, especially of the ventricles. (27)
**Tactile (TAK-til)** Having a sense of touch or feeling. (34)
**Tarnish (TAR-nish)** A discoloration. (43)
**T-band** Type of matrix band used for primary teeth. (57)
**Teledentistry** Process of using electronic transfer of images and other information for consultation and/or insurance purposes in dentistry. (1, 39)
**Temperature** Degree of hotness or coldness of a body or an environment. (27)
**Tempering (TEM-pur-ing)** Bringing a material to a desired consistency. (46)
**Template (TEM-plut)** Clear plastic tray that represents the alveolus as it should appear after teeth have been extracted. (52)
**Temporal** Region of the head superior to the zygomatic arch (9)
**Temporal process** Process that articulates with the zygomatic process of the temporal bone to form the zygomatic arch, which creates the prominence of the cheek. (9)
**Temporomandibular (tem-puh-roe-man-DIB-yoo-lur) joint (TMJ)** Joint on each side of the head that allows for movement of the mandible. (9, 42)
**Termination** The end of an employee/employer relationship, which can be initiated by the employee or the employer. (64)
**Tertiary dentin** Dentin that forms in response to irritation and appears as a localized deposit on the wall of the pulp chamber; also known as *reparative dentin.* (8)
**Thenar eminence (THEE-nar EH-meh-nents)** Fleshy mound on the palm at the base of the thumb. (25)
**Thermal (THUR-mul)** Related to heat. (44)
**Thermometer** Instrument used for measuring temperature. (27)
**Thoracic cavity** Contains the heart, lungs, esophagus, and trachea. (6)
**Three-dimensional digital imaging** An image that demonstrates the anatomy in three dimensions. (42)
**Three-quarter crown** Cast restoration that covers the anatomic crown of a tooth except for the facial or buccal portion. (50)
**Thyroid collar** Flexible lead shield that is placed securely around the neck. (38)
**Tidal volume** Amount of air inhaled and exhaled with each breath. (37)
**Titanium (tye-TAY-nee-um)** Type of metal used for implants. (53)
**Titrate (TYE-trayt)** To determine the effective dosage of analgesic by increasing the dosage until the desired effect is achieved. (37)
**Tomography (toe-MOG-ruh-fee)** Radiographic technique that allows imaging of one layer or section of the body while blurring images from structures in other planes.
**Tooth buds** Enlargements produced by the formation of dental lamina. (8)
**Topical fluoride** Fluoride that is applied directly to the tooth. (15)
**Tori (TOR-eye, TOR-ee)** Abnormal growths of bone in a specific area. (17)
**Torque (tork)** Twisting or turning force. (35)
**Tort law** Involving an act that brings harm to a person or damages to property. (5)
**Touch surface** Surface directly touched and contaminated during procedures. (20)
**Toxic chemicals** Chemicals that can have a fatal or toxic effect to humans. (23)
**Toxic waste** Waste that can have a poisonous effect. (23)
**Tragus (TRAY-gus)** Cartilaginous projection anterior to the external opening of the ear. (10)
**Transaction** Any charge, payment, or adjustment made to a financial account. (63)
**Transfer surface** Surface not directly touched but often contacted by contaminated instruments. (20)
**Transosteal (tranz-OS-tee-ul)** Type of implant in which the metal framework is surgically inserted through the inferior border of the mandible. (53)
**Trapezius (truh-PEE-zee-us)** Major cervical muscle. (9)
**Triangular groove** Developmental groove that separates a marginal ridge from the triangular ridge of a cusp. (12)
**Tricanineate** A three-cusp type of mandibular second premolar. (12)

**Trifurcated** Divided into three. (12)
**Trifurcation** Area in which three roots divide. (12)
**Trigeminal nerve** Nerve that is the primary source of innervation for the oral cavity. (9)
**Triglycerides** Neutral fats. (16)
**Triturate (TRICH-ur-ayte, TRI-chuh-rayt)** Process of mechanically mixing a material, as when an amalgamator is used to mix an alloy and mercury to create dental amalgam. (32)
**Trituration (trich-uh-RAY-shun)** To mix together, as in the process of mixing an alloy with mercury to form an amalgam.
**Tube side** Solid white side of the film that faces the x-ray tube. (39)
**Tubehead** Part of the x-ray unit that contains the x-ray tube, high-voltage and low-voltage transformers, and insulating oil. (38)
**Tuberculocidal (too-bur-kyoo-loe-SYE-dul)** Capable of inactivating tuberculosis-causing microorganisms. (20)
**Tuberosity (too-buh-ROS-i-tee)** Rounded bony protrusion behind the last molar in the maxilla. (52)
**Tungsten target** A focal spot in the anode. (38)
**Tympanic (tim-PAN-ik)** Related to or resembling a drum, as in the *tympanic membrane,* or eardrum. (27)
**Tyndallization (tin-duhl-i-ZAY-shun)** Intermittent, or fractional, sterilization. (18)
**Ultrasonic (ul-truh-SON-ik)** Referring to mechanical radiant energy of water and sound vibrations used to break down material or tissue. (35)
**Ultrasonic cleaner** Instrument that loosens and removes debris by sound waves traveling through a liquid. (21)
**Ultrasonic scaler** Device used for rapid calculus removal; it operates on high-frequency sound waves. (55)
**Unfilled resin (REZ-in)** Sealant material that does not contain filler particles. (59)
**Unit** Each component of the fixed bridge. (50)
**Units of time** Time increments used in planning appointments. (62)
**Universal** Pertaining to the same clamp that can be placed on the same type of tooth in the opposite quadrant. (36)
**Universal curette** Hand instrument used to treat subgingival surfaces; it has a blade with an unbroken cutting edge that curves around the toe and a flat face set at a 90-degree angle to the lower shank. (55)
**Universal Precautions** Guidelines based on treating all human blood and body fluids (including saliva) as potentially infectious. (19)
**Universal retainer** Dental device used to hold a matrix band in place during restoration of a class II cavity. (49)
**Upright position** Vertical, seated position in which the back of the dental chair is upright at a 90-degree angle. (32)
**Use-life** Period of time during which a germicidal solution is effective after it has been prepared for use. (21)
**Usual fee** Fee that the dentist charges for a specific service. (63)
**Uvula** Pear-shaped projection at the end of the soft palate. (10)
**Vallate papillae** Largest papillae on the tongue, arranged in the form of a V. (10)
**Variable overhead** Business expenses that change depending on the types of services needed. (63)
**Vasoconstrictor (vay-zoe-kun-STRIK-tor)** Type of drug that constricts (narrows) blood vessels; used to prolong anesthetic action. (37)
**Veins** Blood vessels that carry blood to the heart. (7)
**Veneer (vuh-NEER)** Thin layer of composite resin or porcelain bonded or cemented to a prepared facial surface. (48, 50)
**Ventral cavity** Cavity located at the front of the body. (6)
**Ventricular fibrillation (ven-TRIK-yoo-lur fib-ri-LAY-shun)** Abnormal cardiac rhythm that prevents the heart from pumping blood. (31)
**Veracity** Truthfulness; not lying to the patient. (4)
**Verbal communication** Type of communication in which words are used as a form of expression. (61)
**Vermilion (vur-MIL-yun) border** Darker-colored border around the lips. (10)
**Vestibule** Space between the teeth and the inner mucosal lining of the lips and cheeks. (10)
**View box** An illuminated boxlike device used to view radiographs. (40)
**Virucidal** Capable of killing some viruses. (20)
**Virulence (VIR-yoo-lens)** Strength of a pathogen's ability to cause disease; also known as *pathogenicity.* (19)
**Virulent (VIR-yoo-lent)** Capable of causing serious disease. (18)
**Viruses** Ultramicroscopic infectious agents that contain DNA or RNA. (18)
**Visceral (VIS-er-ul)** Pertaining to internal organs or the covering of these organs. (6)
**Viscous, viscosity (vis-KOS-i-tee)** Physical property of fluids responsible for resistance to flow. (43, 46)
**Volatile (VOL-uh-til)** Substance that can evaporate easily and is very explosive. (47)
**Volume** Quantity or amount, as in force of a heartbeat. (27)
**Walkout statement** A written indication of any balance due on an account, given to a patient as he or she leaves the practice at the end of an appointment. (63)
**Want list** A list of those supplies to be ordered and questions to be asked of the representative. (62)
**Warranty** Written statement that explains the manufacturer's responsibility for replacing and repairing a particular product. (62)
**Wedge** Wooden or plastic triangular device placed in the embrasure to provide the contour needed when a class II lesion is restored. (49)
**Wetting** Covering or soaking something with a liquid. (43)
**White blood cells** Cells that have the primary function of fighting disease in the body; also known as *leukocytes.* (7)
**Wicking** Process of microorganisms being drawn through wet or damp paper packaging contaminating the instruments inside. (21)
**Winged clamp** Type of dental dam clamp that has extensions to help retain the dental dam. (36)
**Word processing software** A computer program designed to create most types of business documents. (61)
**Working end** Part of a dental instrument that is used on the tooth or when dental materials are mixed. (34)
**Written consent** Consent that involves a written explanation of the diagnostic findings, prescribed treatment, and reasonable expectations about treatment results. (5)
**Xerostomia (zeer-oe-STOE-mee-uh)** Dryness of the mouth caused by reduction of saliva. (13, 17, 29)
**X-radiation** High-energy ionizing electromagnetic radiation. (38)
**Xylitol (ZY-li-tol)** Ingredient in chewing gum that has an antibacterial effect against decay-causing bacteria. (13)
**Zika** A virus that is spread to people primarily through the bite of an infected *Aedes* species mosquito. (18)
**Zygomatic** Region of the head pertaining to or located near the zygomatic bone (cheekbone). (9)
**Zygomatic arch** Arch formed when the temporal process of the zygomatic bone articulates with the zygomatic process of the temporal bone. (9, 10)
**Zygomatic process** Process of the maxillary bones that extends upward to articulate with the zygomatic bone. (9)
**Zygote** Fertilized egg. (8)

# INDEX



*Note:* Page numbers followed by *f* indicate figures, *t* indicate tables, and *b* indicate boxes.

**J**



**K**



**L**

## Q



## R

# Tooth Numbering for the Primary Dentition

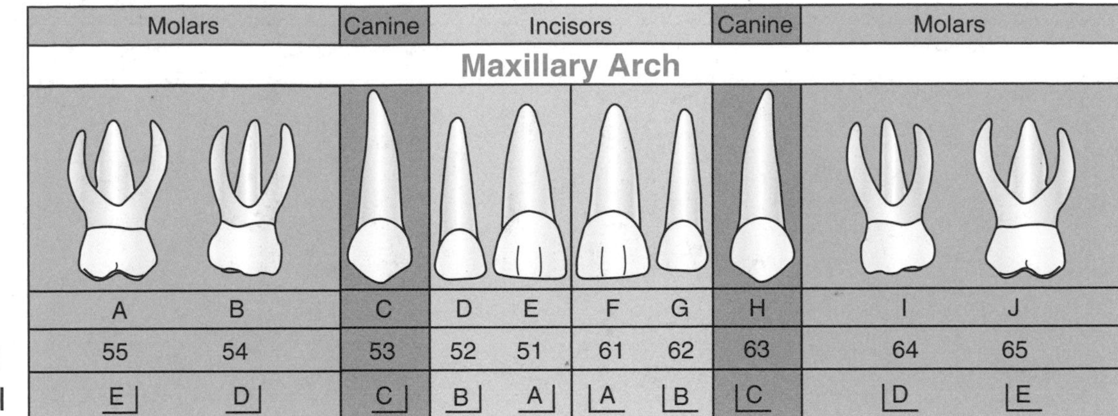


| | Molars | | Canine | Incisors | | | | Canine | Molars | |
|---|---|---|---|---|---|---|---|---|---|---|
| III | E⌉ | D⌉ | C⌉ | B⌉ | A⌉ | ⌈A | ⌈B | ⌈C | ⌈D | ⌈E |
| II | 85 | 84 | 83 | 82 | 81 | 71 | 72 | 73 | 74 | 75 |
| I | T | S | R | Q | P | O | N | M | L | K |

Mandibular Arch

| Right | Left |
|---|---|

I Universal tooth numbering system

II International Standards Organization

III Palmer Method

From Fehrenbach MJ, Popowics T: *Illustrated dental embryology, histology, and anatomy,* ed 4, St Louis, 2016, Saunders.